Textbook of

Medical Laboratory Technology

Ramnik Sood MD
Formerly
Sr Pathologist
Maulana Azad Medical College
New Delhi

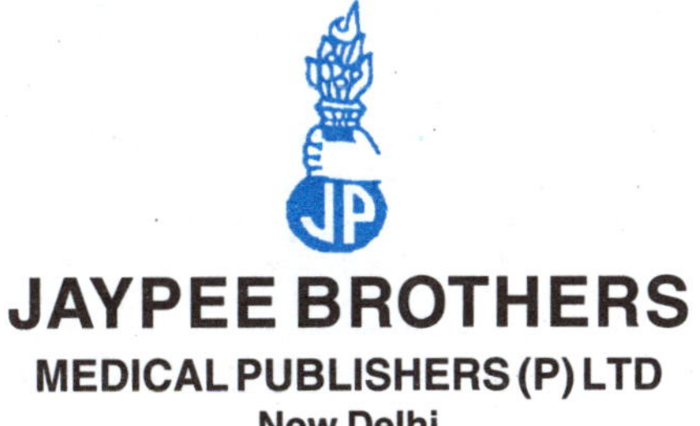

JAYPEE BROTHERS
MEDICAL PUBLISHERS (P) LTD
New Delhi

Published by

Jitendar P Vij
Jaypee Brothers Medical Publishers (P) Ltd
EMCA House, 23/23B Ansari Road, Daryaganj
New Delhi 110 002, India Phones: +91-11-23272143,
+91-11-23272703, +91-11-23282021, +91-11-23245672
Fax: +91-11-23276490, +91-11-23245683
e-mail: jaypee@jaypeebrothers.com
Visit our website: www.jaypeebrothers.com

Branches

- 202 Batavia Chambers, 8 Kumara Krupa Road, Kumara Park East, **Bangalore** 560 001, Phones: +91-80-22285971, +91-80-22382956, +91-80-30614073 Tele Fax: +91-80-22281761 e-mail: jaypeebc@bgl.vsnl.net.in
- 282 IIIrd Floor, Khaleel Shirazi Estate, Fountain Plaza Pantheon Road, **Chennai** 600 008, Phones: +91-44-28262665, +91-44-28269897 Fax: +91-44-28262331 e-mail: jpmedpub@md3.vsnl.net.in
- 4-2-1067/1-3, Ist Floor, Balaji Building, Ramkote Cross Road, **Hyderabad** 500 095, Phones: +91-40-55610020, +91-40-24758498 Fax: +91-40-24758499 e-mail: jpmedpub@rediffmail.com
- 1A Indian Mirror Street, Wellington Square **Kolkata** 700 013, Phones: +91-33-22456075 , +91-33-22451926 Fax: +91-33-22456075 e-mail: jpbcal@cal.vsnl.net.in
- 106 Amit Industrial Estate, 61 Dr SS Rao Road, Near MGM Hospital Parel, **Mumbai** 400 012, Phones: +91-22-24124863, +91-22-24104532, +91-22-30926896 Fax: +91-22-24160828 e-mail: jpmedpub@bom7.vsnl.net.in

Textbook of Medical Laboratory Technology

© 2006, Ramnik Sood

All rights reserved. No part of this publication should be reproduced, stored in a retrieval system, or transmitted in any form or by any means: electronic, mechanical, photocopying, recording, or otherwise, without the prior written permission of the author and the publisher.

This book has been published in good faith that the material provided by author is original. Every effort is made to ensure accuracy of material, but the publisher, printer and author will not be held responsible for any inadvertent error(s). In case of any dispute, all legal matters are to be settled under Delhi jurisdiction only.

First Edition : **2006**

ISBN 81-8061-591-X

Typeset at JPBMP typesetting unit
Printed at Gopsons Papers Ltd., Noida.

to
My Father and my friend
Deepak G Tripathi

Preface

The current medical laboratory practice has significantly changed from what it was say a decade ago. Now most of the inputs that come for lab technicians are ready-made. They do not have to prepare anything at all, dipsticks estimate simple things like urine albumin and sugar and for complicated procedures like estimation of tumour markers—ready to use kits are available. To run these kits, automated instruments are also available. I was lucky to have a partner in Tulip Diagnostics Pvt. Ltd—a pioneering company related to medical laboratory diagnostic technology. They have very kindly permitted me to use their products and their associated technical literatures for use in this textbook as technology demonstrator. Fortunately, Tulip Diagnostics makes products from A to Z of medical laboratory technology, one of their sister concerns—Lilac Medicare—provides imported high end technological products to the Indian consumers. My very special thanks are due to my very special friend and director of the Tulip Group Mr Deepak G Tripathi who very kindly offered me the products and papers from his repertoire. The completeness of the book is due to the presence of in-use products as on date from the range of Tulip Diagnostics. Gone are the days when we used to import important products, we now export to the very same countries from where we used to source finished products earlier. Gradually the diagnosis making is shifting to the bedside. With the availability of RDTs a confirmed diagnosis can now be established at the bedside or even at the primary health center level without the use of expensive instruments. Diagnosis of malaria, leptospirosis, dengue fever or acute myocardial infarction at the patient's residence, etc. is possible these days.

While methodologies are important, more important is their interpretation. One must also understand the problems that can creep while working and should be in a position to troubleshooting them. The book discusses the relevance of tests, gives various methods available, talks about interpretation of the reports generated and tells ways of troubleshooting the accompanying problems.

Wish to start a laboratory, you shall know everything as to what hardware, consumables and other materials are needed from within the covers of this book. The book also tells as to what to source from where. Medico-legal aspects are also considered.

Normal reference ranges have been provided considering the latest acceptable values. They are given according to the age and sex of individuals for all parameters as applicable. SI units are mentioned, as are the conversion factors. Wherever important panic level values are given.

Laboratory technologists, medical undergraduates, postgraduates and practitioners alike shall find the book useful. Few may want the methods while others may want to go through the interpretations. All routine and most sophisticated investigations have been covered under relevant chapters. The monotony of reading through a single colour has been avoided by presenting the entire book in two colours. Parasitology segment provides indepth understanding by way of pictorial representation of their lifecycles and the pathologies caused. AIDS/HIV has been dealt with in ample detail—the disease, diagnosis and precautionary measures have been discussed in detail. Clinical chemistry goes as far as trace elements. Endocrinology delves deep till thyroid antibodies and C-peptide. Sero-immunology aptly details third generation tests for HIV/AIDS. Diagnostic immunology mentions all about turbidimetry. Need one ask for more!

While going to press, the author and the publisher have made all efforts to weed out all typographic and other textual errors, however, in a volume of this size, inadvertently an error may creep in. The same should kindly be overlooked. The author and the publisher disclaim any or all responsibility for the same. It would be ideal for the end-user to judge the quality of various products mentioned personally.

Enjoy the most up-to-date and comprehensive book the *Textbook of Medical Laboratory Technology*.

Ramnik Sood

Contents

1. Laboratory ... *1*
2. Sterilisation ... *29*
3. SI Units ... *35*
4. Fundamental Chemistry ... *49*
5. Urine Analysis ... *50*
6. Renal Function and its Evaluation ... *85*
7. Stool Examination ... *90*
8. Medical Parasitology ... *100*
9. Clinical Haematology ... *196*
10. Clinical Haematology: Bleeding Disorders ... *264*
11. Blood Banking (Immunohaematology) ... *322*
12. Cerebrospinal and other Body Fluids ... *397*
13. Semen Analysis ... *408*
14. Sputum Examination ... *411*
15. Pregnancy Tests ... *418*
16. Examination of Gastrointestinal Contents ... *442*
17. The Endocrine System ... *452*
18. Diabetes Mellitus Laboratory Diagnosis ... *598*
19. Liver Function Tests ... *609*
20. Clinical Chemistry ... *617*
21. Enzymology ... *673*
22. Blood Gases and Electrolytes ... *717*
23. Serology/Immunology ... *731*
24. Histopathology ... *1030*
25. Cytology ... *1048*
26. Microbiology and Bacteriology ... *1061*
27. Mycology ... *1119*
28. Diagnostic Skin Tests ... *1123*
29. Diagnostic Immunology (Immunodiffusion, Electrophoresis and Turbidimetry) ... *1129*
30. Cytogenetics ... *1192*

Appendices ... *1199*

Index ... *1275*

CHAPTER 1

Laboratory

INTRODUCTION

The definition of health includes a state of complete and perfect physical, mental, social and spiritual well-being and not just the absence of disease or infirmity and good health is a fundamental right of every living human being on earth. However, modern world, though, has to an extent eliminated infectious diseases. But the focus has now shifted to lifestyle diseases. Pollution of every nature too has taken its toll. About half a century back, the predominant diseases used to be infective ones but now you may find individuals in midtwenties waiting for their turn for open heart surgeries. Also, modern medicine has increased the longevity of life accompanied by attendent geriatric diseases like Alzheimer's disease and malignancies. The polluted and toxic world has not spread the fetuses *in utero* and neonates. A new face of disease has emerged, diseases like HIV-AIDS and SARS are new entrants in the long list of infective diseases. We may have eradicated smallpox but tuberculosis and malaria have raised their heads with a vengeance. So, do what you might. Some form of disease, mild or severe will strike every human being living. On getting sick, the patient first comes in contact with a clinician—medical or surgical. The clinician gives a patient hearing (if the patient is conscious) to his problems and symptoms and also takes note of various signs which he sees or elicits. Sometimes, he may immediately arrive at a diagnosis and may under emergency circumstances institute treatment at first instances. In most cases, however, he will have a differential diagnosis in mind and to arrive at a specific diagnosis he usually orders for a battery of tests.

Various means of diagnosis are available.

1. Most important: Clinical laboratory tests which include any tissue or fluid obtained from the body
2. Imaging sciences: X-rays, ultrasound, colour Doppler, CAT scan, MRI scan and the latest PET scan
3. Electrical signal processing techniques ECG, EMG, EEG and nerve transmission techniques, etc.

4. Direct visualisation techniques: With the availability of fibreoptic-based technologies, the clinician is now capable of passing small tubes (called scopes) through natural passage ways of the human body (without actually surgically opening up the part), e.g. gastroscopy, cystoscopy, etc. These techniques, eventually culminate in taking small tissue samples (biopsies) which are sent to histopathology laboratories.

So, whenever, any sample from a human body is taken (either voided naturally or obtained by the clinician or the laboratarian), it is referred to the clinical laboratory for investigation. On receipt of a report from the laboratarian, the clinician, then, makes up his mind and starts a unidirectional or specific treatment against the disease thus diagnosed. It would not be wrong to designate medical laboratory personnel as the backbone of the clinicians. But for these technologists, the clinicians would forever grope in the dark. Gone are the days when diabetes mellitus was presented with the classsical triad of symptoms—increased thirst, hunger and urination; likewise, typhoid seldom presents with a step-ladder pattern fever. Blood testing is absolutely mandatory, to know that they exist, their severity and eventually, after treatment to know that they are under control or cured. Investigations are diagnostic as well as prognostic tools.

Clinical laboratory investigations now-a-days are being utilised as future predictors. On getting warning signals, one can take necessary corrective measures (lifestyle and/or dietary) and can prevent diseases from striking or at least deferring or postponing their arrival.

HELP! AND YOU DID. AND YOU ALWAYS WILL. When a clinician is lost, you shall show him the way in the best possible way, you lead him to a diagnosis and let him do his job thereafter. He may come back to you later to determine that his efforts have been fruitful.

The following pages within the covers of this book will show you the right path on how to be an excellent laboratarian. Do your best in serving mankind. As you yourself may be a patient tomorrow. This book shall also serve you well by providing interpretation of the results obtained by you. This book shall be true to its title "Medical Laboratory Technology—Methods and Interpretations".

While *physiology* is the study of essentially normal structures and functions of a body, *pathology* deals with the study of a diseased organ or system of the body, its abnormal functions, their mode of origin, their progress to recovery or otherwise. All these studies come under the ambit of a *clinical pathology laboratory*. A clinical laboratory has further sub-branches such as: haematology, biochemistry, seroimmunology, microbiology, cytogenetics, histopathology, cytopathology, blood banking and last but not the least—clinical microscopy.

A clinical laboratory can be manned by a qualified doctor specialising in clinical pathology, biochemistry, immunology, blood banking, histopathology, cytopathology, haematology, microbiology or cytogenetics. The pathologist is usually assisted by laboratory technicians or technologists (they are also qualified for the job) and lastly the cleaning and documentation staff. Only by collective efforts of the individuals mentioned above, a proper report can be generated. Be grateful to the clinician for having faith in you and give back nothing except an accurate and correct report.

The cycle of health disease with all intermediaries is given below. Just as there are primary, secondary and tertiary health centres, there are also the primary, secondary and tertiary laboratories too. In India, there are no specific guidelines as to what or how

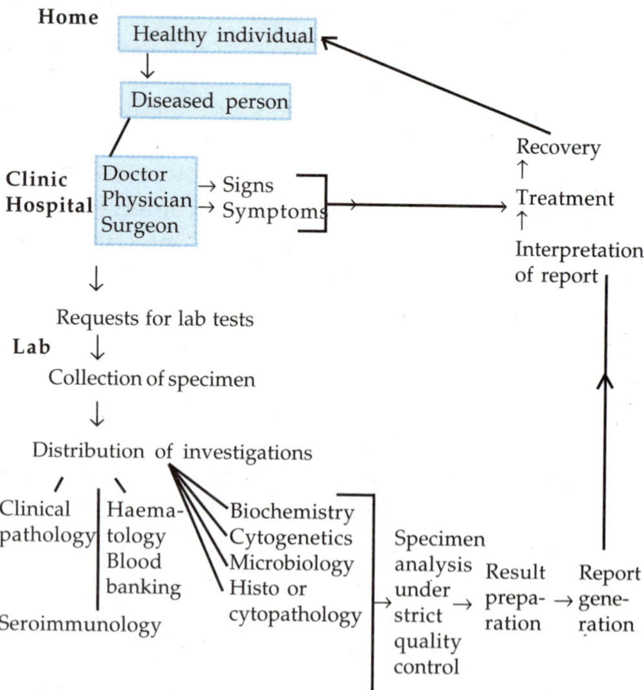

much they can do and overlaping can occur. A superior laboratory may perform all functions of an inferior laboratory too.

Primary Laboratory

In rural setups, for instance, a primary laboratory may provide only the basic investigations. These investigations are simple to perform and do not involve expensive machinery usage. Such laboratories are also attached to physician chambers now-a-days, so that clinicians may obtain basic inputs right in their own premises. These primary laboratories may provide the following simple investigations:

- Haemograms (haemoglobin estimation, total and differential counts, erythrocyte sedimentation rate and packed cell volume with basic peripheral smear study including the reporting of haemoparasites)
- Routine and microscopic studies of urine and stool. Routine examination also entails chemical examination either by laborious and time-consuming old chemical methods or by new generation dipstick tests. These may include tests for glucose, bilirubin, ketones, haemoglobin, leukocytes, pH, nitrites, protein, urobilinogen and specific gravity in case of urine. For stool samples, reducing substances, pH and occult blood may be performed. Basic spot/latex/device tests (e.g. pregnancy test) may be conducted.

Secondary Laboratory

These are laboratories that assist a clinician to confirm a clinical suspicion or establish a diagnosis. Therapy and prognosis monitoring can also be provided from these laboratories. Such laboratories are staffed by qualified personnel who are trained and experienced to perform the tests. They also have a perfect knowledge of the equipment and machines they use. They should be aware of quality control essentials and be well versed with interpretational aspects of the reports generated by their laboratories.

In addition to what has been mentioned under primary laboratories, secondary laboratories also perform:

- routine immunohaematological tests
- routine examination of all body fluids, e.g. semen, CSF, sputum, etc.
- routine bacteriologic studies including stains, cultures and antibiograms. Routine mycological investigations would include—primary cultures, isolation and identification techniques along with microscopic evaluation.
- routine immunoserological tests. These can include tests like Widal, STS, ELISA or strip or device tests HIV I and II, Hepatitis B and Hepatitis C, etc.
- routine biochemistry investigation and organ profile tests, e.g. lipid, cardiac, liver and renal profiles
- under haematology, these laboratories may also provide RBC indices, platelet, retic and absolute eosinophil counts. They can also classify anemias and generally speaking should be able to indicate haematologic malignancies. When headed by a pathologist, they should be in a position to report bone marrow smears/preparation too.

Tertiary Laboratory

These kinds of laboratories should be able to and do perform all kinds of sophisticated and delicate/precise investigations. The tertiary laboratories can branch out in very special fields and not cater to all aspects of specialised tests. Besides doing all investigations that are conducted in secondary laboratories, they also carry out the following:

- Specialised haematological (e.g. leukemia typings), coagulation profiles and immunohaematological investigations. They are equipped with 18 parameter cell counters with differentials and flow cytometry
- Complete biochemical assays, commonly referred to as SMA-12, SMA 27, etc. Also included are elemental assays, e.g. zinc, magnesium, iron, TIBC, lithium, etc. special enzymes like HBDH, lipase and isoenzymes, etc.
- Complete immunology based assays for hormones, cancer markers, hepatitis markers, rheumatic/autoimmunity etiology-based profiles, TORCH profiles, rare infectious diseases (e.g. brucellosis leptospirosis, cysticercosis, ecchinococosis, etc.)
- All microbiological processes, e.g. cultures—aerobic, anaerobic, fungal, tubercular, etc. with antibiograms.

The techniques for these investigations may vary. They may be ELISA, chemiluminescence, turbidimetry, PCR, etc. These laboratories are totally automated and have sizable workload. Furthermore, they also undertake all histopathology (simple H and E, special staining techniques, immunohistochemistry methods) and cytopathology processing and reportings. They may also undertake cytogenetic investigations, e.g. chromosomal analysis.

The dissemination of reports from these laboratories is in keeping with recent trends in telecommunications, e.g. fax, e-mail, etc.

In the United States of America, these laboratories though classified differently (with a few differences) are covered under the Clinical Laboratory Improvement Act (CLIA) of 1988.

LABORATORY SET-UP

Unless the laboratory is hygienic and provides necessary physical and operative comfort, it would be wrong to expect perfect results. To get perfect results, one has to provide a perfect set-up for people to work in.

Laboratory Building and Space

Ample working space is absolutely essential. For smaller laboratories up to 25 square meters, the working platforms can be arranged along the walls while the central area is kept free for movement.

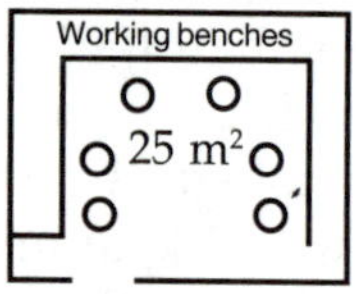

Working benches

25 m^2

A typical small laboratory

For larger areas, partitions can be made which would create separate spaces for different sections. The chief pathologist must have free and easy access to all sub-units of the laboratory. If possible, he should be able to directly see into the cabins either through glass windows or through closed circuit cameras. In the cabins again, the central region should be kept free and benches be placed against the walls and away from the doors.

Sero-immunology ELISA's, PCRs, drugs Cancer markers	Biochemistry	Microbiology
Pathologist's chamber	Collection of specimens and report delivery	Haematology + Clinical pathology
Histopathology Cytopathology		Toilet

A typical large/complete laboratory plan

- Hygiene is of utmost importance. The whole facility should be absolutely clean, uncrowded and devoid of any hindrances to movement of men and materials. Never, should a chance arise where two people would clash or contaminated material would be spilt all over
- Scratch proof matt finish vitrified floor (slip resistant) should be provided. The walls should preferably have white ceramic tiles. Such provisions are resistant to chemicals and disinfectants
- All benches should be preferably 2½ feet high and those to be used while standing should be at least 3 feet high. The bench surfaces should be solvent and acidproof
- Every laboratory and/or its section must have at least one sink and one hand wash basin. The hand wash basin should not be used for any other purpose, the sink can be utilised for laboratory purposes like washing off stains from slides or washing glassware or dischanging non-contaminated laboratory refuse.

Physical Aspects of a Laboratory

- The ambient temperature should be within the comfort zone of a human body. It should between 21 and 27 degrees Celsius. If the laboratory is in a cold zone, it must have heating provision, and conversely, if it is in a hot zone, it must have cooling or air conditioning. The environment control appliances like air conditioners or heaters must not directly discharge air at the working bench zone.
- A good exhaust system is a must for all laboratories. This removes dirty air (aerosols) which may at times be foul smelling. The sample collection zone too, must have excellent exhaust provision.
- Adequate ventilation is also essential but without strong currents of air.
- Lighting should be more than adequate and places where very delicate or fine processes are being conducted should have additional lighting provision. As far as possible, do not use excessive heat producing bulbs and lamps. The new CFLs are ideal.
- Windows that are exposed to bright sunlight can be internally fitted with reflective films or blinds.

- There should be sufficient running water for the laboratory and all must have sufficient number of sinks and hand wash basins.
- As most machines consume a lot of electricity, sufficient power load (a little is excess) must be available to the laboratory.

Provisions and Precautions

Every working room or cabin should have adequately spaced provision of water, electricity, gas, sinks lighting and exhausts. All aspects, whether plumbing, electrical systems or gas connection must pass through regular inspections and a log book should be maintained of such preventive exercises. Preventive maintenance should be carried out by knowledgeable and qualified persons.

Fire Prevention

- Install appropriate fire extinguishing system and timely testing of such a system be conducted at regular intervals.
- Colour code and place fire fighting equipment at an easily visible and reachable location. Check the working capability of all such systems at regular intervals.
- Provide adequate ventilation in zones where flammable chemicals are used. Before these substances reach combustible or explosive concentration, they should be removed by mechanical exhausts.
- Post "No-smoking" signs in zones where smoking can be hazardous.
- Lastly, mark clearly the emergency exit points. Keep the emergency exit route free from obstructions.

Electrical Installations

- Hire a proper, qualified electrical engineer and explain to him the pupose of the premises being taken. As far as possible, all points where sparks can be generated should be kept out of room/cabins where explosive chemicals are likely to be used.
- Use earthing everywhere and install fire-resistant cables in the laboratory.
- Employ only certified products.
- Use one electrical socket for a single device or machine. Overloading is usually the cause of accidents.

Liquefied and Compressed Gases

- Colour code and identify each gas container. Check their values regularly.
- Keep all such cylinders away from sources of heat and electrical sparks.
- When not in use, replace protection/safety caps back on the cylinder mouths.

Chemicals and Radioactive Substances

- Label all bottles with proper names of contents and affix warning signs and symbols as applicable to them.
- Clearly display the warning charts (both chemical and radioactive) next to such containers. All staff members working in such areas should be well trained to handle accidents of any kind that can happen.
- A stringent record of stocks should be maintained of all persons and radioactive substances being used in the laboratory. A bottle lost or stolen is invitation to problem.

Stores

- Every bottle/container should be labeled. Affix the hazard intensity on the bottle or the container.
- Ensure in every possible way that the containers cannot under any circumstances fall or spill. This can be done by placing the most dangerous chemical at the bottom or at the floor level.
- Proper ventilation should be ensured in storage zones that house flammable chemicals. Keep fire extinguishing equipment handy. Post "No smoking" signs that are clearly visible. Make sure that the place remains free from pests.

Staff Safety and Facilities

The most important asset of any institution is the manpower that works for it. It holds true for laboratories too. Absence of staff due to morbidity or mortality can stiffle your working capacity, capability and reputation. Provide adequate facilities to your team. (Designate a room or space meant exclusively for retiring or resting and consuming foodstuffs).

- Hot and cold running water with soap and desinfectants should always be provided.

Clean hand towels should be replaced daily.

- A clean toilet for use by staff members is mandatory as are the changing rooms. If possible, separate units for male and female members should be provided.
- Biomedical wastes and nonbiomedical wastes should be discarded properly and safely. Chemical treatment of liquid wastes and incineration of solid wastes should not be overlooked. Wastes handled properly ensures good health of your working team
- Designate a room or space meant exclusively for retiring or resting and consuming foodstuffs. Under no circumstances laboratorians should eat or drink on their workbenches. Provide safe drinking water to all.
- Each room/cabin must have a first-aid box kept at an identified place that is easily accessible. Every person working in the laboratory must be aware of all hazards that exist and must also know about the remedial measures that should be taken if something happens. What can be managed in house should be managed, when required, assistance of other specialists must be taken. Contact numbers of such institutions/specialists must be displayed prominently.
- All members of your team must be immunised as relevant to the laboratory work. Make sure no single person works alone in a room or cabin. Two compatible persons should work together always.

Basic Laboratory Safety

- Use only certified safe equipment in the laboratory.
- Decontaminate all equipment regularly and before their servicing or maintenance, use appropriate disinfectants correctly.
- As far as possible, use disposable plasticware to avoid contamination (chemical, biological, etc.) and breakages with ensuing dangers.
- Regularly test and service biological safety cabinets and fume cupboards.

APPROPRIATE SAFETY MEASURES TAKEN BY YOU WILL GO A LONG WAY IN ENHANCING PRODUCTIVITY.

As a rule, the place for receiving or withdrawing the specimens should be separate from the working compartment. TO AVOID specimen mixing (hazardous), each sample should be carefully labeled. The label should clearly mention the alloted specimen number, the date and time of receipt of specimen, the investigations to be done and most important the name of the patient.

Both, the clinical and the paraclinical workers are equally at risk of acquiring transmissible diseases through the patient or through the test samples. The risk of these can be lessened by taking appropriate *vaccinations*. In addition, one should attend to one's general hygiene and prevent fomite transmission of any infectious disease. Disinfect the working benches and as far as possible autoclave (or chemically disinfect) various glassware used in the laboratory. Use a rubber teet for sucking/filling the pipettes. To avoid strain on the eyes, keep both eyes open while doing microscopic work. Before leaving the laboratory, one should thoroughly wash one's hands with soap and water, then rinse them well in a disinfectant lotion.

CODE OF CONDUCT FOR MEDICAL LABORATORY PERSONNEL

1. Place the well-being and service of the sick above your own interests.
2. Be loyal to your medical laboratory profession by maintaining high standards of work and strive to improve your professional knowledge.
3. Work scientifically and with complete honesty.
4. Do not misuse your professional skills or knowledge for personal gain.
5. Never take anything from your place of work that does not belong to you.
6. Do not disclose to a patient or any unauthorised person the result of your investigations.
7. Treat with utmost confidentiality and personal information that you may learn about a patient.
8. Respect and work in harmony with the other members of your hospital staff or health center team.
9. Be at all times courteous, patient, and considerate to the sick and their relations.
10. Promote health care and the prevention and control of disease.
11. Follow safety procedures and know how to apply first aid.

12. Do not drink alcohol during laboratory working hours or when on emergency stand-by.
13. Use equipment and laboratory-ware correctly and with care.
14. Do not waste reagents or other laboratory supplies.
15. Fulfil reliably and completely the terms and conditions of your employment.

ALWAYS REMEMBER THAT YOU CAN BE A PATIENT TOMORROW. TREAT OTHERS AS YOU WOULD WANT THEM TO TREAT YOU.

ACCIDENTS

SAFETY MEASURES IN THE LABORATORY

You must remain alert and cautious while working in the laboratory. You must know that careless handling of reagents, glassware or specimens to be tested in the laboratory can cause serious injury and is dangerous to life.

HAZARDS IN THE CLINICAL LABORATORY

Clinical laboratory workers may encounter three types of hazards:

1. Physical
2. Chemical and
3. Biological.

Physical Hazards

Physical hazards are present in ordinary equipment or surroundings. Electrical equipment, open flames, laboratory instruments and glassware can all be hazardous if improperly used.

Electricity

- All electrical equipment must be properly grounded following the manufacturer's instructions
- Even minor repairs, such as replacement of the microscope bulbs, require that instrument be disconnected from the power supply before the work is begun
- All electrical cords and plugs be kept in good shape and order with no frayed cords or exposed wires
- Avoid overloaded circuits
- Extension cords present several safety hazards and should not be used except in emergency.

Fire

Fire is a potential danger in the workplace.

- Though rare, they can occur when open flames are used in the vicinity of flammable liquids
- Make sure that loose clothing and long hair do not catch fire
- Instead of open flames, use hot plates, microwave ovens, electric incinerators and slide warmers
- Store flammable chemicals in a flameproof cabinet, away from heat sources and well-ventilated area. A falmeproof cabinet can protect flammable chemical from flames until firefighters arrive and also allow workers more time to escape
- All laboratory workers must know about the escape route and procedure to follow if that exit is blocked
- All workers must know the location of fire extinguishers and how to use them
- Inspect all fire extinguishers periodically and log the date of inspection.

Usual Causes of Fire in the Laboratory

- Naked flames (do not work with loose clothing and long hair near naked flames). Naked flames can also ignite flammable liquids and gases
- Electrical overloading. Use one socket for one equipment only. Do not operate a 15 amp equipment from a 5 amp socket
- Poor electrical maintenance. No frayed or open/exposed wires be ever used
- Leaving equipment switched when not in use. Out of mind is out of sight
- Deteriorated gas tubing. Leakage of gas is an open invitation to fire hazard. If you suspect gas leakage, do not operate any electrical equipment (do not ever switch on a light or a fan)
- Smoking in the laboratory.
- Misusing matches. Use carbonised matches as far as possible
- Storing flammable and explosive chemicals is an ordinary refrigerator.

Fire Fighting Equipment

Fire fighting material	*Used for*	*Contraindicated for*
Fire blanket	Clothing fire, a small blaze	Electrical fires, flammable liquids, burning metals, alkali metal
Water	Paper, wood, fabric	Electrical fires, flammable liquids, burning metal, alkali metal
CO_2 fire extinguisher	Flammable liquids and gases, electrical fire	—
Dry powder	As above	—
Foam	Flammable liquids	—
Halon spray	All kinds of fires	—

Should a Fire Occur

- For tiny blazes; water, sand and a fire blanket can be employed to put out the fire. For larger blaze, a fire extinguisher can be used
- Never use water on an electrical fire or one caused by organic solvents (ether, alcohol, petrol, etc). For electrical fires, use carbon dioxide fire extinguisher. For organic solvents, use sand or Halon
- Escape via the fire exit route. Stay close to the floor, cover your mouth and nose with a damp cloth to filter out some of the harmful fumes
- Inform fire fighting department of your area if you feel the fire can go out of hand. Medium to large fires should be reported irrespective of your preparedness to handle them.

Laboratory Equipment

- Use all laboratory equipment as per manufacturer's recommendation
- Any instrument with moving parts, such as a centrifuge, must be operated with a special regard for safety. Latch, the lid before turning it on. On turning it off, do not open the lid before it has come to a complete stop.
- Autoclaves present special hazards. Strictly adhere to manufacturer's instruction to present explosions and burns. Use insulated gloves while removing hot items from the autoclave.

Glassware

- Use glassware that is free of chips and cracks. Damaged glassware is weakened and may break, resulting in injury
- Broken glass should be cleaned with a brush and dustpan and not with bare hands
- Glass should not be discarded into regular trashcans, but into rigid cardboard or plastic containers
- Wherever possible, replace glassware with plasticware.

Equipment-Related Hazards

- Hypodermic needles: Accidental inoculation, aerosol or spillage
- Centrifuges: Aerosols, splashing and tube bridge
- Culture stirrers, shakers, agitators: Aerosols, splashing and spillage
- Refrigeration: If flammable Chemicals are stored within them; the light switches, thermostats, etc. can provide sparks to ignite them.
- Water baths: Provide ground for microorganismal growth.
  (The risk of acquiring hepatitis B from a needlestick is 30%, hepatitis C is 2-10% and HIV is 0.3%)

Equipment/Materials Employed to Eliminate/ Reduce Hazards

- Laboratory apron: Assists in diminishing skin contacts to a certain extent
- Biological safety cabinets: Prevent dangers arising out of aerosols and splatters
- Splatter shields: Provide protection from splatter of specimen and chemicals
- Pipetting aids (teet or electromechanical devices). Prevent from hazards arising out of mouth pipetting
- Goggles: Protect eyes from impacts and splashes
- Face shields: Protect the face from impacts and splashes.

SAFETY WITH CHEMICALS/REAGENTS

Excepting just a couple of reagents, almost all chemicals/reagents used even in the most basic laboratory are lethal poisons if consumed by anyone. Even if they are splashed on the skin/eye, they can cause irreversible damage. There is an appropriate way of handling and storage of hazardous chemicals to avoid injury and damage to self and others. In our country (and other tropical nations) excessive heat

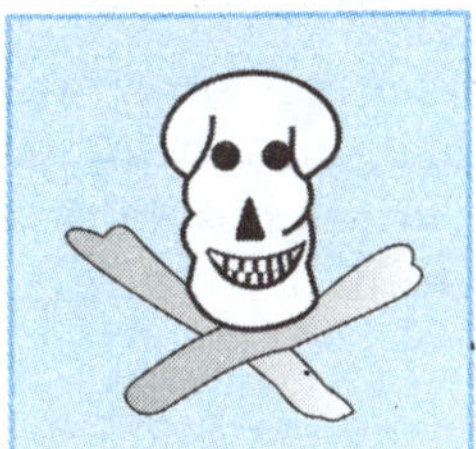
Toxic

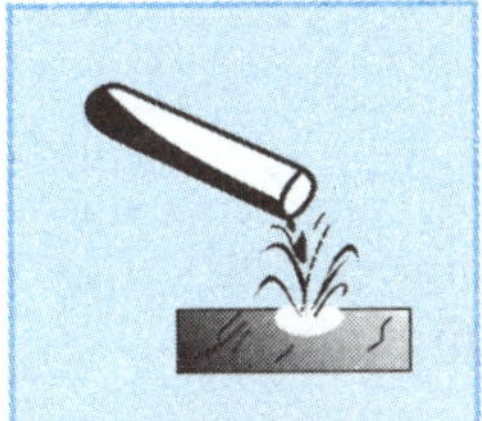
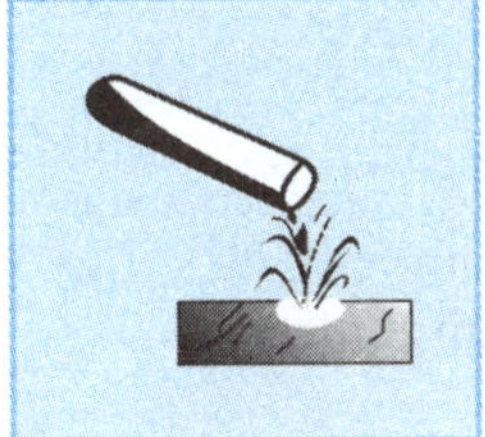
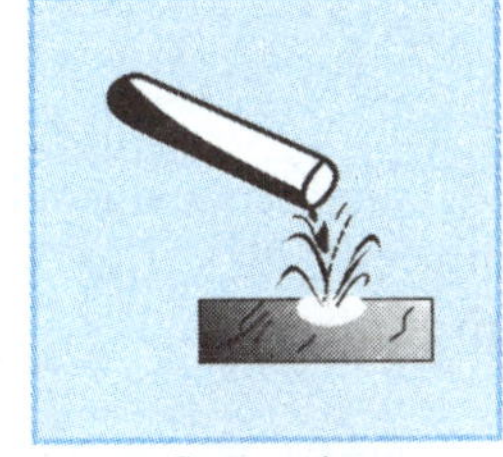
Corrosive

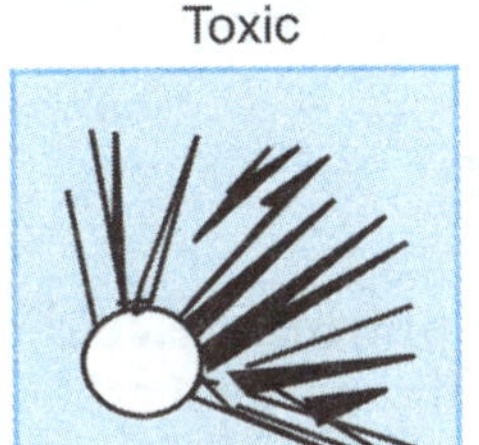
Explosive

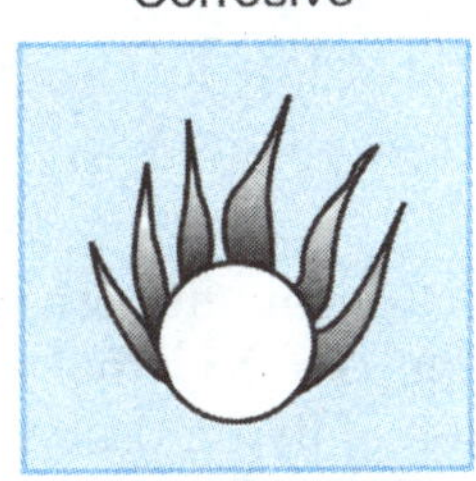
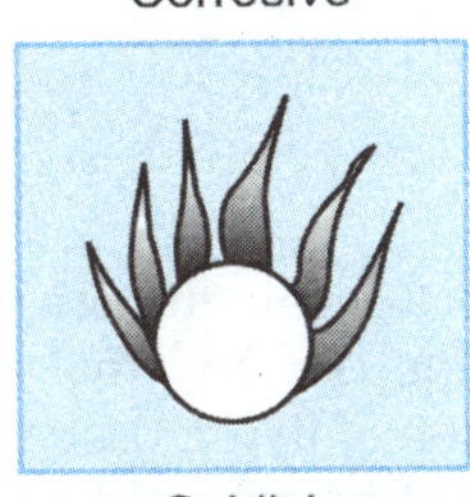
Oxidising

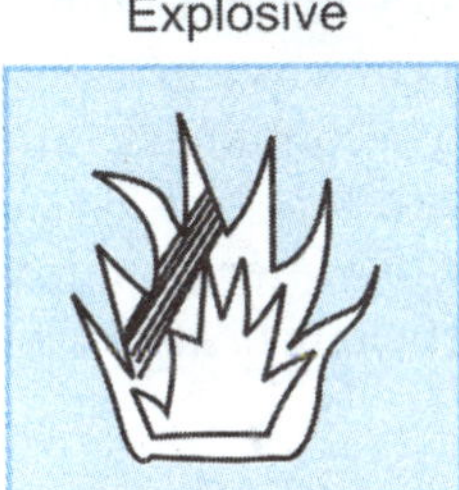
Highly inflammable

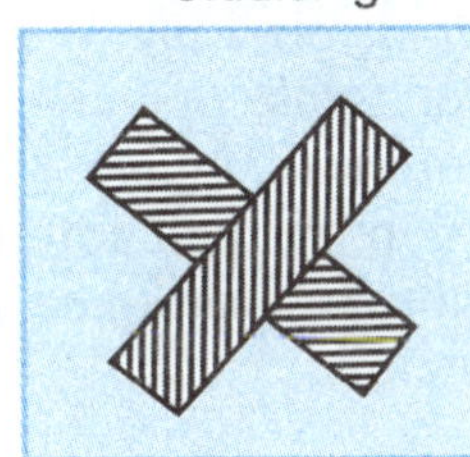
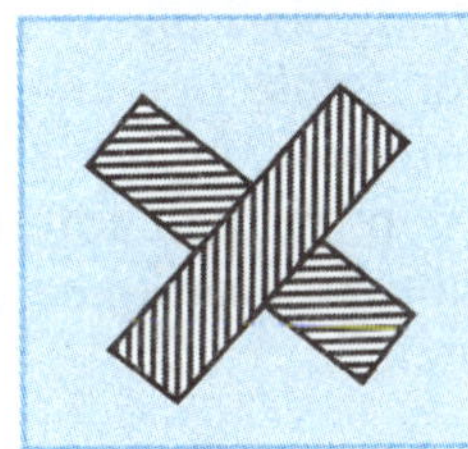
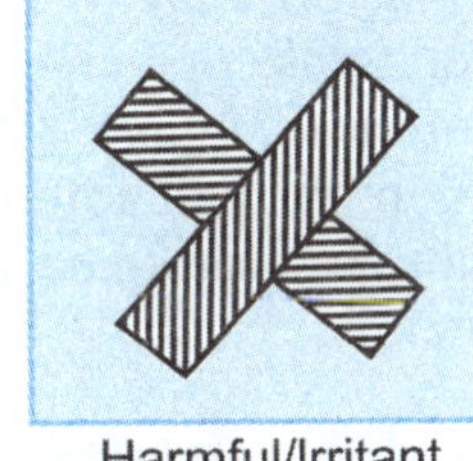
Harmful/Irritant

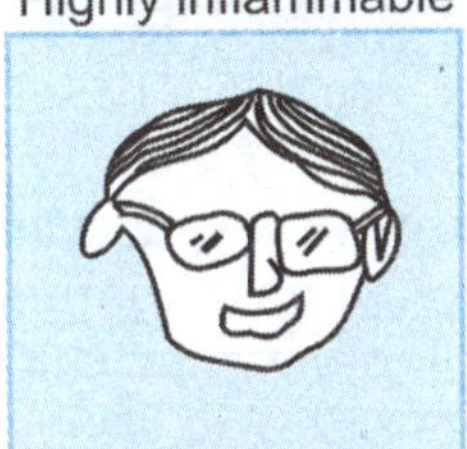
Eye protection mandatory

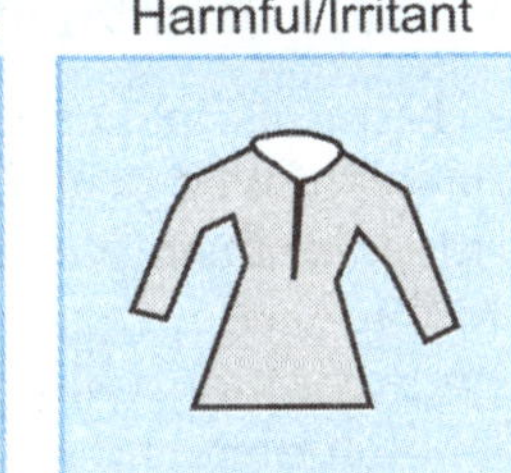
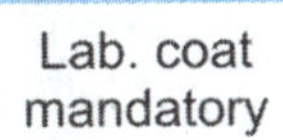
Lab. coat mandatory

Risk of danger

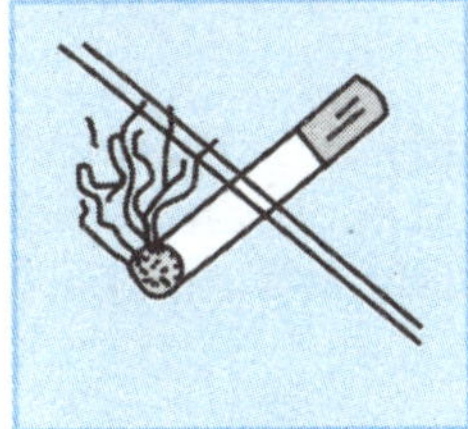
No smoking

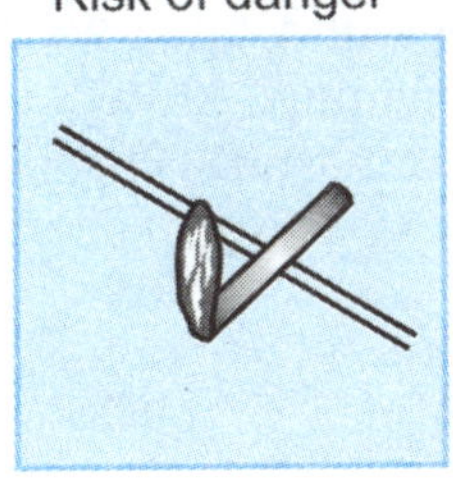
Naked flames prohibited

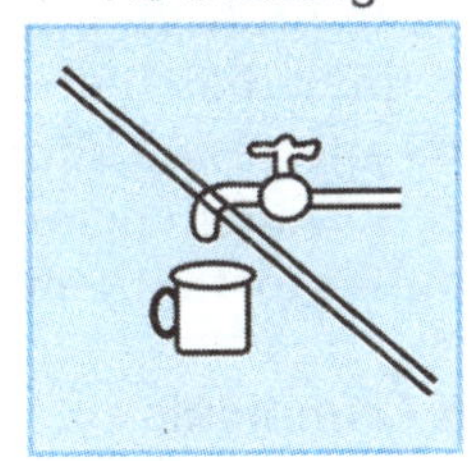
Not drinking water

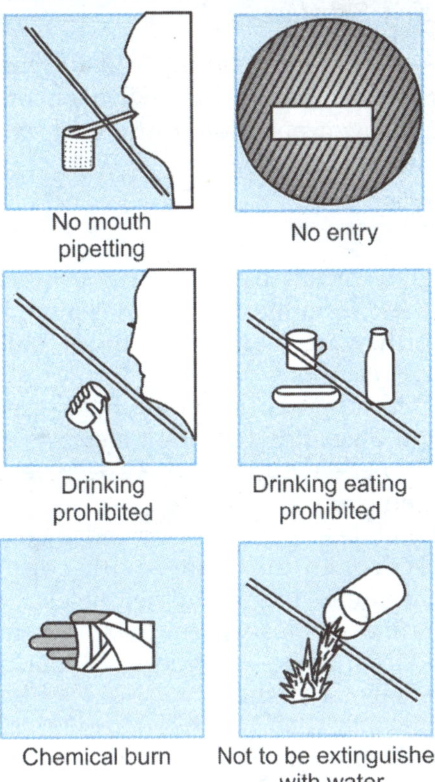
No mouth pipetting

No entry

Drinking prohibited

Drinking eating prohibited

Chemical burn

Not to be extinguished with water

can decompose many chemicals, cause explosions, or lead to the formation of toxic fumes.

LABELING OF HAZARDOUS REAGENTS/CHEMICALS

At appropriate places, display the prohibition signs; and on all dangerous reagents or chemicals, stick *Hazard* warning symbols.

Incompatible Chemicals

Fair number of common laboratory chemicals react dangerously if they come in contact with specific chemical. Ensure that you keep such chemicals away from each other.

A few examples are listed below.

Acids

- Acetic acid-with chromic acid, nitric acid, hydroxyl compounds, ethylene glycol, peroxides and permanganates.
- Chromic acid—with acetic acid, alcohol, glycerol and other flammable liquids
- Sulfuric acid—with chlorates, perchlorates, permanganates and water.

Vapourizing Substances

- Acetone—with sulfuric acid and nitric acid.
- Flammable liquids—with chromic acid, hydrogen peroxide, nitric acid, ammonium nitrate and halogens

Others

- Alkali metals, e.g. calcium, potassium, sodium (these form hydroxides on coming in contact with water) and with other chlorinated hydrocarbons
- Chlorine—with ammonia, hydrogen, benzene and other finely divided metals
- Copper—with azides, hydrogen peroxide and acetylene
- Cyanides—with all acids and alkalies
- Hydrogen peroxide—with copper, iron, chromium and most other metals
- Iodine—with acetylene and ammonia
- Sodium azide—with lead, copper and other metals

Flammable Chemicals

These include ether, xylene, toluene, methanol, ethanol, glacial acetic acid, acetic acid, acetone, acetic anhydride, alcoholic Romanowsky stains and acid alcohol, etc.

Storage

These should be stored in a fireproof metal box at ground level, preferrably in a cool store. A container well lined with tin foil can also be used. Store only small quantities of such solvents on the shelves.

Safe Use

Ensure that there is no open flame nearby while opening a bottle containing flammable solvent. Nearest flame should be at least 10 feet away. Never heat a flammable liquid over any flame. Use a water bath or electric hot plate.

Control of Fire Caused by Flammable Chemicals

Best controlled by smothering them. Use sand, thick blanket or the now available multipurpose fire extinguishers. Pouring water on such fires will spread them. Every laboratory should be equipped with the commercially available fire extinguishers. If these are not available, there should be sand buckets in accessible places.

Corrosive Chemicals

These include strong acids, e.g. concentrated sulphuric acid, hydrochloric acid, nitric acid, glacial acetic acid, trichloroacetic acid, orthophosphoric acid, and strong alkalies like sodium hydroxide and potassium hydroxide.

Storage

Store these at low levels.

Safe Use

Never attempt mouth pipetting. Accidental swallowing can be lethal as these Chemicals cause destruction of living tissue. Always pour a corrosive chemical at below eye level, slowly, and with great care to avoid splashing. Wear protective eye glasses/ eye shields while opening such containers. *Always add the corrosive substance to water and that too slowly.* The addition of small amount of water to sulphuric acid is enough to produce sufficient heat to break a glass container.

Toxic, Harmful, and Irritating Chemicals

These are chemicals that can cause death or serious ill-health if swallowed or inhaled or if they come in contact with skin. Examples are potassium cyanide, mercuric nitrate, sodium azide, sodium nitroprusside, formaldehyde solution, chloroform, barium chloride and methanol. Iodine and sulphanic acid also fall in this category. Skin and mucous membrane irritants are xylene, formaldehyde and ammonia vapors.

Storage

Store highly toxic chemicals, e.g. potassium cyanide in a locked cupboard. Stock solutions should also be stored safely in a cupboard, not on an open shelf.

Safe Use

Always wear protective gloves and after working with them immediately lock them up. Always wash your hands after using a toxic or harmful chaemical. Keep fume forming chemicals in a fume cupboard. Never mouth pipette them.

Oxidising Chemicals

These include chlorates, perchlorates, strong peroxides, potassium dichromate, and chromic acid.

Storage

Keep these away from organic materials and reducing agents. They can produce much heat when in contact with other chemicals, especially flammable chemicals.

Safe Use

Handle them with utmost care. Most of them are dangerous to skin and eyes and when in contact with reducing agents.

Explosive Chemicals

These chemicals can explode on being heated or on getting exposed to flame or friction. A good example is picric acid, which must be stored under water. If picric acid is allowed to dry, it can explode.

Carcinogens

These chemicals can cause cancer by ingestion, inhalation, or by skin contact.

Such chemicals include benzidine, O-toluidine, O-dianisidine, α and β naphthylamine, nitrosamines, nitrosophenols, nitronaphthalenes, and selenite. The carcinogenic risk is directly proportional to the length and frequency of exposure and the concentration of the chemical.

Storage

Label their containers "CARCINOGENIC" and handle with special precautions.

Safe Use

Must wear protective plastic or rubber gloves, a face mask and eyeshields when handling carcinogenic chemicals. Do not let them come in contact with skin. After handling a carcinogen, wash well in cold water all the apparatus, bench, bottles and protective gloves (before removing them) and change your overall. Rinse your hands in cold running water before using soap. Should a carcinogen come in contact with skin, wash the affected part in cold running water for 5 minutes.

ACCIDENTS IN THE LABORATORY

They may be caused by:

1. Acids or 2. Alkalis }
   - splashes on the skin
   - splashes in the eye
   - swallowing
3. Toxic substances
4. Heat
   - open flames
   - hot liquids
   - inflammable liquids
   - explosions
5. Broken glass
6. Contamination by infected material
7. Electric shock

A suggested list of first aid equipment is given later in the chapter. The items should be readily available in the laboratory. They must not be kept in a locked cupboard.

FIRST AID IN LABORATORY ACCIDENTS

Acid Burns

Nitric, sulphuric, hydrochloric and trichloroacetic acids)

In all cases: Wash immediately with large quantities of water.

Acid Splashes on the Skin

a. Wash thoroughly and repeatedly with water.
b. Bathe the affected skin with cotton wool soaked in 5% aqueous sodium carbonate.

Acid Splashes in the Eye

a. Wash the eye immediately with large quantities of water sprayed from a wash bottle or rubber bulb. Squirt the water into the corner of the eye near the nose.
b. After washing, put 4 drops of 2% aqueous sodium bicarbonate into the eye.
c. Refer the patient to a physician. Continue to apply bicarbonate solution to the eye while waiting for the doctor.

Alternatively, hold the eye under the running tap.

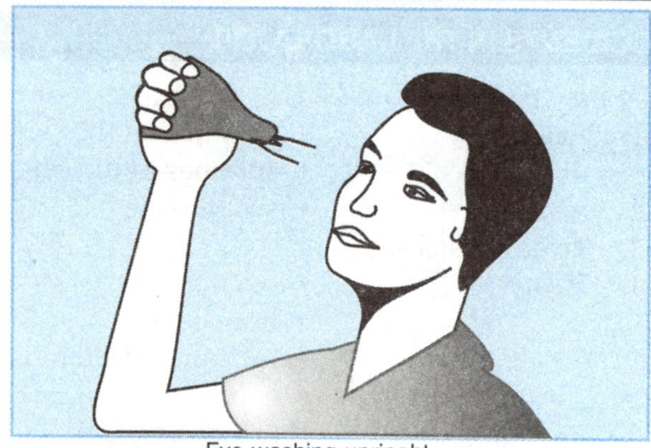

Eye washing upringht

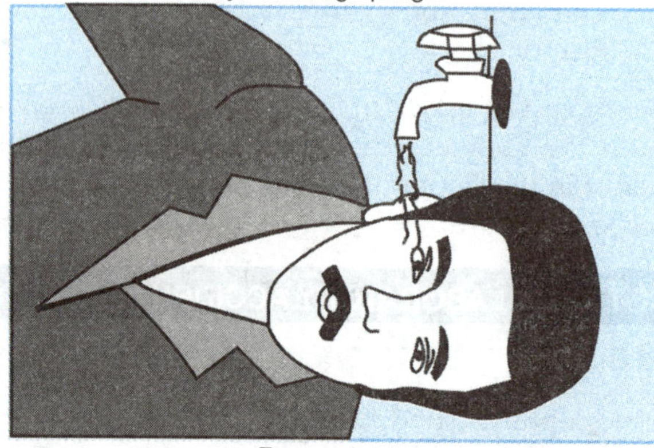

Eye wash-lying

Swallowing Acids

Accidental swallowing while using a pipette:

a. Call a physician.
b. Make the patient drink some 5% soap solution immediately. Alternatively, give him two whites of egg mixed with 500 ml of water or milk. If neither of these is available, he should drink ordinary water.
c. Make him gargle with the soap solution.
d. Give him 3 or 4 glasses of ordinary water.
e. If the lips and tongue are burned by the acid:
   - rinse thoroughly with water
   - bathe with 2% aqueous sodium bicarbonate.

Alkali Burns

Sodium, potassium and ammonium hydroxide.

In all cases: Wash immediately with large quantities of water.

Important: Alkali burns are as serious as, and often more serious than, acid burns.

Alkali Splashes on the Skin

a. Wash thoroughly and repeatedly with water.
b. Bathe the affected skin with cotton soaked in 5% acetic acid (or undiluted vinegar).

Alkali Splashes in the Eye

a. Wash immediately with large quantities of water sprayed from a wash bottle or rubber bulb. Squirt the water into the corner of the eye near the nose.
b. After washing with water, wash the eye with a saturated solution of boric acid (apply drops repeatedly).
c. Refer the patient to a physician at once.

Swallowing Alkalis

Accidental swallowing while using a pipette:

a. Send for a physician.
b. Make the patient drink at once:
   - a 5% solution of acetic acid or lemon juice or dilute vinegar (1 part vinegar to 3 parts water).
c. Make him gargle with the same acid solution.
d. Give him 3 or 4 glasses of ordinary water.
e. If the lips and tongue are burned by the alkali:
   - rinse thoroughly with water
   - bathe with 5% acetic acid.

Poisoning

This can be caused by:

- inhaling toxic vapours or gases (e.g. chloroform)
- accidental swallowing while pipetting a poisonous solution.

In all cases:

a. Send for a physician or qualified nurse, specifying the toxic substance involved.
b. Place the victim in the open air while waiting for the physician.

Burns Caused by Heat

They fall into two categories:

- Severe burns—affecting large areas of skin, e.g. burns caused when burning ether or boiling water is spilled over the victim.
- Minor burns—affecting a small area of skin, e.g. burns caused by hot glassware or a Bunsen flame.

Severe Burns

a. If the victim is on fire, e.g. if splashed with burning ether or other inflammable solvent, roll him in a blanket or overall to smother the flames.
b. Inform the physician on duty immediately.
c. Lay the victim on the ground. Do not remove his clothing. Cover him if he is cold.
d. Do not apply any treatment to the burns. This must be left to the physician.

Minor Burns

a. Plunge the affected part into cold water or ice-water to soothe the pain.
b. Apply mercurochrome or acriflavine ointment to the burn.
c. Apply a dry gauze dressing loosely.
d. If the burn becomes infected or does not heal, refer the patient to a physician.

Note: Never tear off the blisters that form over the burns.

Injuries Caused by Broken Glass

These are caused by broken test tubes, syringes or other glassware.

a. Wash the wound immediately to remove any glass pieces.
b. Apply mercurochrome or acriflavine ointment to the wound.
c. Cover with gauze and adhesive tape.
d. If the cut bleeds profusely, stop the bleeding by pressing down on it with a compress. Refer the patient to a physician.
e. If the cut bleeds heavily with the blood spurting out at intervals, try to stop the bleeding with a compress and call a physician or qualified nurse.
f. Continue to press on the wound while awaiting the physician's or nurse's arrival. He or she will decide whether a tourniquet should be applied.

Contamination by Infected Material

Wounds caused by broken glassware containing stools, pus, etc.:

a. Wash the wound immediately.
b. Check whether the cut is bleeding. If not, squeeze hard to make it bleed for several minutes.
c. Bathe the whole area, i.e. the edges of the cut and inside the cut, with antiseptic lotion.
d. Wash thoroughly with soapy water.
e. Bathe again with antiseptic lotion.
f. Refer the patient to a physician if the material involved is known to be very infective, e.g. pus.

If infected material is accidentally sucked into the mouth:

a. Spit it out immediately.
b. Wash out the mouth with diluted antiseptic lotion.
c. Wash out the mouth thoroughly with large amounts of clean water.

Bodily Damage by Electric Shock

A low-voltage alternating electric current (220 V) is usually used in the laboratory and electric shocks are rare. They may occur when faulty equipment is being handled, particularly with wet hands. The symptoms are fainting and asphyxia.

a. Before doing anything else, put off the main switch.
b. Send for a physician.
c. Begin giving mouth-to-mouth respiration immediately (as given below).

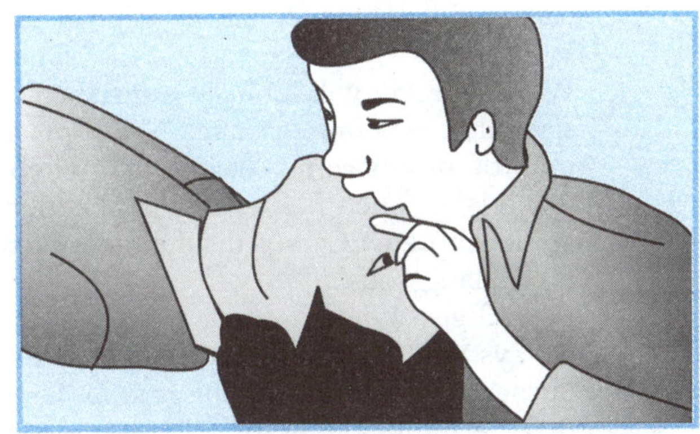

Precautions for the Avoidance of Accidents

1. Handling acids and alkalis
   a. Diluting sulphuric acid with water: Always add the sulphuric acid to the water drop by drop, stirring the mixture after each drop. Do this preferably in a sink. *Never pour water into sulphuric acid* (because of the danger of splashing).

b. Bottles of acids and alkalis: Keep them on the lower shelves of the cupboards. When you take one out, hold it firmly upright with a dry hand. Do not keep acids and alkalis in bottles with ground glass stoppers as they may get stuck.

c. Pipetting: Where possible, use small measuring cylinders for measuring acids and alkalis. If more accurate measurement is required, use a pipette plugged with non-absorbent cotton wool or with a rubber tube attached. Pipette slowly, watching the level of the liquid.

2. Heating glassware and liquids
   a. Test tubes: Never heat the bottom of a test tube. The liquid inside might sputter. Heat the middle of the tube, shaking gently. The mouth of the tube should be facing away from the worker and any other person, towards an empty space or a sink.
   b. Ordinary glass and Pyrex: Only Pyrex glassware and porcelain receptacles can be heated over a Bunsen flame. Ordinary glass will break.
   c. Inflammable liquids: Only small quantities of inflammable liquids such as ether, ethanol, acetone, benzene, toluene and carbon disulphide should be kept in the laboratory.
   Warning: Ether will ignite at a distance of several meters from a flame. Never place a bottle of ether on a workbench where there is an open flame (Bunsen burner, spirit lamp, etc.). Carbon disulphide is even more dangerous.
   d. Butane gas: When lighting a gas burner, always light the match and hold it to the burner before turning on the gas tap. Turn off the main valves of all butane gas cylinders every evening. Replace the rubber connecting pipes once a year.
3. Do not use broken, cracked or chipped laboratory glassware.
4. Put clear labels on poisons. Keep them in a locked cupboard.
5. Do not use nylon clothes while working as these are easily inflammable. Always use a laboratory apron.
6. Always ensure that electrical wiring and electrical appliances are in good condition.

Suggested List of First Aid Equipment for Laboratory

1. 5% aqueous sodium carbonate
2. 2% aqueous sodium bicarbonate in an eyedrop bottle
3. 5% acetic acid
4. Saturated solution of boric acid in an eyedrop bottle
5. Soap powder solution (5 gm per litre of water)
6. Acriflavine ointment
7. Mercurochrome 2%
8. Antiseptic lotion
9. Cotton wool
10. Gauze
11. Roller bandage
12. Adhesive tape
13. Scissors

CONTAMINATION FROM INFECTIVE MATERIAL

If contamination has occurred, then:

1. *Disinfect* the part with the disinfectant available in the lab. Thoroughly clean the affected area with a stream of running water.
2. *Sucking the contaminated material:* Spit out all that has been sucked. Use a disinfectant liquid (*e.g.* diluted dettol) for mouth washing. If the infected material has been swallowed accidentally, forced vomiting to be done, ascertain the kind of infection and take advise from a medical person.
3. *If skin is infected* by highly virulent organisms, touch the involved part with pure carbolic acid.

PRECAUTIONARY MEASURES

1. A fire extinguisher should always be handy.
2. Keep sand bucket in the laboratory.
3. Take measures to prevent electrical short circuiting.
4. No smoking in the working zone of the laboratory.
5. Breakable items should be kept in proper racks and never at the edge of the working table.
6. Do not suck anything with the mouth, use rubber teets and bulbs for sucking.
7. Do not place eatables on the working bench.
8. Keep fingernails short.
9. At the end of the day, clean all working benches with a disinfectant. See that nothing except the required electrical appliance is on.

10. Dispose all infected material properly. Can put such material in hypochlorite solution or in an acidic solution, e.g. diluted sulphuric acid (25%). Burn off all dried contaminated articles, e.g. filter papers.
11. The glassware should be disinfected with a suitable disinfectant and be cleaned thoroughly with running water.
12. Use rubber gloves and a nose mask while working with infective samples, e.g. serum of viral hepatitis patient.

UNIVERSAL WORK PRECUATIONS (UWP) FOR LAB PERSONNEL (ESPECIALLY IN RELATION TO HIV TRANSMISSION)

Introduction

Health care personnel (HCP) can acquire certain illnesses beyond those acquired by all others who live and work in our society, by virtue of their profession. HCPs are at risk of acquiring any of the whole gamut of infections from patients/specimens which may be viral, bacterial, parasitic or fungal. However, this risk due to occupational exposure can be minimized if not obliterated altogether, if we follow universal work precautions (UWP).

Today, with the WHO estimates of above 4 million HIV positive persons in India, there is an urgent need to review UWP. Besides HIV, there is the very real danger of acquiring Hepatitis B and Hepatitis C in exactly the same way as HIV and could also be fatal. Hepatitis B is 100 times more infectious than HIV. Besides, Hepatitis B is also far more prevalent in India in comparison to HIV with estimated carriers being between 30 and 40 million, a considerable number being infectious. However, fortunately, effective vaccination is available for Hepatitis B; therefore, it is strongly recommended for all levels of health care workers.

Much of the contamination in the laboratory occurs as a result of penetrating injuries caused by sharp objects and the spilling and splashing of specimen materials.

Components of UWP

1. Handwashing.
2. Barrier precautions (mask, cap, plastic apron and protection of feet).
3. Careful handling of all kinds of sharps and needles.
4. Effective infection.
5. Sterilization.
6. Correct disposal of different kinds of wastes generated in a health care facility.

Guidelines of Basic Practices and Procedures

- Prevention of puncture wounds, cuts and abrasions and protection of existing wounds, skin lesions, conjunctiva and mucosal surfaces.
- Application of simple protective measures designed to prevent contamination of the person and his/her clothing.
- Good basic hygiene practises, including regular handwashing.
- Control of surface contamination by containment and disinfection procedures.
- Safe disposal of contaminated waste.

Biosafety Regulations for Laboratory Procedures

- Wear gloves when handling infectious materials or where there is a possibility of exposure to blood and other body fluids. All laboratories that work with material that is potentially infected with HIV require a generous supply of good quality gloves.
- Discard gloves whenever they are thought to have become contaminated or perforated, wash your hands and put on new gloves. Alternatively, where there are economic constraints, wash gloved hands whenever they get contaminated with blood/body fluids before collecting further samples.
- Do not touch your eye, nose, or other exposed membranes or skin with your gloved hands.

Sterilization (For Nondisposable Items)

- For sharps, reusable blades, cystoscopy instruments, endoscopy instruments, use CIDEX (2% glutaraldehyde) or 5% Korsolex. Disinfection in 30 minutes.
- Use autoclaving for other reusable items (e.g. needle holders, gowns, etc.).
- Wherever autoclaving is not possible, boiling must be for 30 minutes at the least.

Waste Disposal

Divide waste into three parts at source.

i. Household type noninfectious waste:
   - Not to be decontaminated.
   - To be disposed off as such.

ii. Infected sharp waste disposables (needles/surgical instruments)
   - Place in puncture proof container containing disinfectant (1% bleach prepared every morning). Needles should ideally be burnt (machines are available that operate on electricity).
   - Final disposal

iii. Infected nonsharp waste:
   - Is to be decontaminated.
   - Placed in disinfectant 5-10% bleach as the case may be (left over blood, tissues, etc).

Final Disposal

- Purchase of needle destroyer if resources permit.
- Incineration of all infected waste.
- Deep burial in controlled land fill sites (protected from all sides)
- Shredding of disposable plasticware waste.

Post-Exposure Care

- Minor bleed with percutaneous inoculation, open skin wound, breached skin, exposed mucous membranes.

First Aid

- Allow to bleed by squeezing.
- Wash with water
- Antiseptic

Report

- Employee identification, date, time with place of accident.
- Circumstances around accident.
- Action taken.

Initial Consultation

- Easy access to medical advise with counselling. Consult, physician for AZT prophylaxis regime if medication available.

Laboratory Testing

- After consent with counselling within 2 weeks, 5 weeks, 12 weeks, or 24 weeks

Clinical Follow-up

- For fever, pharyngitis, rash, malaise, lymphadenopathy, myalgia and arthralgia within 6 months.
- Do not leave the workplace or walk around the laboratory while wearing gloves.
- Wash hands with soap and water immediately after any contamination and after work is finished. If gloves are worn, wash your hands with soap and water after removing the gloves. This is a vital and simple precaution that is often overlooked.
- Wear a laboratory gown or uniform when in the laboratory. Wrap-around gowns are preferable. Remove this protective clothing before leaving the laboratory.
- When work with material that is potentially infected with HIV is in progress, close the laboratory door and restrict access to the laboratory. The door should have a sign BIOHAZARD: NO ADMITTANCE.
- Keep the lab clean, neat and free from extraneous materials and equipment.
- Disinfect work surfaces when procedures are completed at the end of each working day. An effective all purpose disinfectant is a hypochlorite solution with a concentration of at least 0.1% available chlorine (1 g/litre, 1000 ppm)
- Whenever possible, avoid using needles and other sharp instruments. Place used needles, syringes and other sharp instruments and objects in a puncture resistant container. Do not recap used needles and do not reuse needles from syringes for disposal.
- Never pipette by mouth.
- Perform all technical procedures in a way that minimizes the risk of creating aerosols, droplets, splashes or spills.
- Use a biosafety cabinet while working on aerosolizing specimen.
- Do not eat, drink, smoke, apply cosmetics or store food or personal items in the laboratory.
- Make sure that there is an effective insect and rodent control programme.
- If a laboratory personnel has lesions on hand and feet, then:
  a. If superficial, he or she should wear protective dressing and wear gloves over it.

b. If wound is deep or raw then the the concerned person should not handle samples till the wound heals.

- If there is a pregnant health care worker then in view of the occupational risk to the woman and the developing fetus, on compassionate grounds, where possible she should be involved in clerical tasks or stay away from work for the duration of her pregnancy.

Containing Spills

- Cover the spill immediately with absorbent material to avoid aerosolization.
- Soak the material by pouring disinfectant on it.
- Leave the area for 30 minutes.
- Mop with more adsorbent material after wearing gown, mask and gloves.
- Place material in appropriate bin for disposal (autoclaving or incineration).

Collection of Specimen

- Always keep labeled bottle ready on the bedside.
- Wear disposable gloves
- Keep adequate cotton with spirit at collection site.
- Keep a bucket full of disinfectant [CIDEX (glutaraldehyde)], one for at the most 5 beds.

Transport of Specimen

- Specimens should be collected in plastic; screw-capped containers prelabeled with patient identification data, should be packaged and transported in puncture, resistant containers in upright position with the sign of biohazard on the container.

MEDICO-LEGAL ASPECTS OF CLINICAL PRACTICE

Under the Consumer Protection Act (CPA), India, 1986; any patient, registered consumer organisation, state or central government or patient's legal heirs can sue the undermentioned persons for shortcomings in "service" provided by them.

- A technician, microbiologist, biochemist or pathologist running a laboratory.
- Any private polyclinic, nursing home or hospital, registered or otherwise
- As government hospitals provide service without consideration (free of cost), they cannot be held responsible under CPA 1986.
- Doctors appointed by the government, however, can be held accountable under other civil and criminal laws for proven negligence
- Medical practitioners delivering new service without any consideration in a charitable hospital or medical camps are exempted from the provisions under CPA
- As per clause 2(d) (ii) of the CPA 1986, a consumer implies any person who hires or avails of any service for a consideration which has been paid or promised, or partly paid and partly promised, or under any system of deferred payment, and includes any beneficiary of such services other than the person who hires or avails of the service for consideration paid or promised or partly paid and partly promised or under any system of deferred payment, when such services are availed of with the approval of the first mentioned person.
- The time limit stipulated for filing a complaint is two years from the date of alleged negligence.
- Patients can be dealt with severely if they file frivolous and false complaints just to harass the medical practitioner
- Free services provided are exempted under CPA
- A laboratarian is also a consumer as he buys various instruments, equipment, diagnostic kits/reagents/devices. He too can file a complaint under CPA for any defect or deficiency in service related to that purpose.
- Ignorance is not held as an excuse as an established legal principle. Concurrently, law does not expect a very high degree of knowledge but expects only average knowledge from a medical practitioner.
- Medical negligence is a civil wrongdoing classified as 'tort', where a medical practitioner fails to take proper care in respect of examination, diagnosis, investigation, treatment, etc., resulting in injury or mortality.
- Laboratarians are expected to keep all reports confidential (legally and ethically). The reports can be divulged to the refering clinician or to the patient or the relatives of

the patient (with patient's consent). Reports pertaining to sexually transmitted diseases or HIV / AIDS should be handed over only to the patient.

- Legally, only authorised or registered blood banks can supply units of blood. All mandatory information must be clearly mentioned on the bottle label legibly.
- These days doctors have 'Malpractice Insurance Covers'. In case a legal notice is received by such a doctor, he should immediately notify the insurance company. The insurance company must take all necessary actions in such a case. The company should appoint a lawyer to give reply or to take legal steps and inform the doctor about it. The doctor, by permission of the company, can appoint a lawyer of his choice
- What constitutes a legal notice? Any letter received by a medical practitioner from a patient or a voluntary registered organisation or an advocate, demanding explanation about treatment given or demanding some explanation about treatment for alleged injury or death constitutes a legal notice
- Section 27 of the civil procedure code provides that when a suit has been duly instituted, a summon may be issued to be defendent to answer the claim, and such summon is to be served in the prescribed manner. When a complaint is lodged before the commission or the forum, the defendent practitioner is informed by a registered letter by the office, which is called a summon in legal parlance. In this summon, time for the reply and date of hearing is mentioned. Usually, the time given for filing the reply is 30 days.

LABORATORY INSTRUMENTS

Microscope

Micro = Small, Scope = to view.
It magnifies the image of the object to be visualized through it. Normally, the laboratory microscopes provide a magnification of × 40 (scanner), × 100 (low power), × 400 (high power) and × 1000 (oil immersion). The total magnification is obtained by multiplying the magnification of the objective with that of the eyepiece.

Parts of the Microscope

It has three sets of parts. They are the:
1. Stand
2. Mechanical adjustments and
3. Optics or the lenses

Stand

It consists of:
1. The tube—supports objectives and eyepiece.
2. The body—gives support to the tube.
3. The arm—gives correct height and angulation to the body and the tube.
4. The stage with a pair of spring clips or a mechanical stage.
5. The substage holds the condenser lens with its iris diaphragm and a holder for light filters and stops.
6. The foot on which other parts rest, can be in tripod or horseshoe shape.

Mechanical Adjustments

Focusing adjustments: These are coarse and fine adjustments.

Coarse adjustment: Controlled by a pair of large knobs, one on each side of the body. On rotating this, the tube moves with its lenses. Some microscopes have this attached to the stage; so that instead of the tube, the stage moves up and down. Coarse adjustment is enough for low power lenses.

Fine adjustment: Necessary for high power and oil immersion lenses. This is usually controlled by two smaller knobs on each side of the body. They may be graduated to indicate the movement in microns.

Draw tube: It is used to adjust the distance between the objective lens and the eyepiece lens.

Inclination: The arm can be tilted upon the foot by a hinge.

Condenser adjustments: Focusing of condenser is done by rotating a knob present on one side below the stage.

Aperture adjustment: It is done by the iris diaphragm (made up of leaves).

Centring of condenser: It is done to bring the light beam accurately through the instrument. In some microscopes it is permanently fixed.

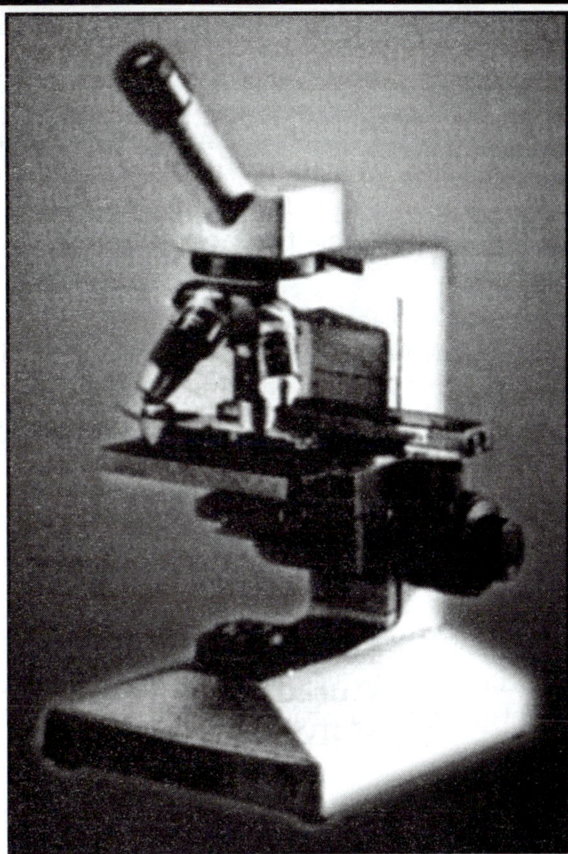

Fig. 1.1: Monocular microscope with substage lamp

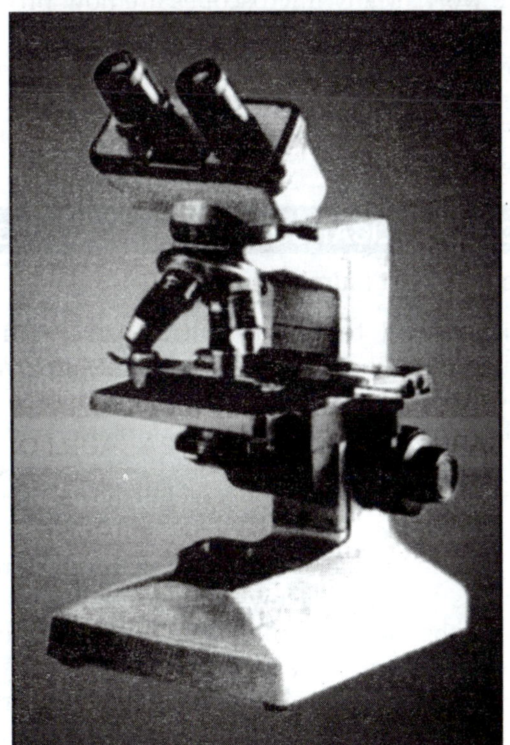

Fig. 1.2: Binocular microscope with substage lamp

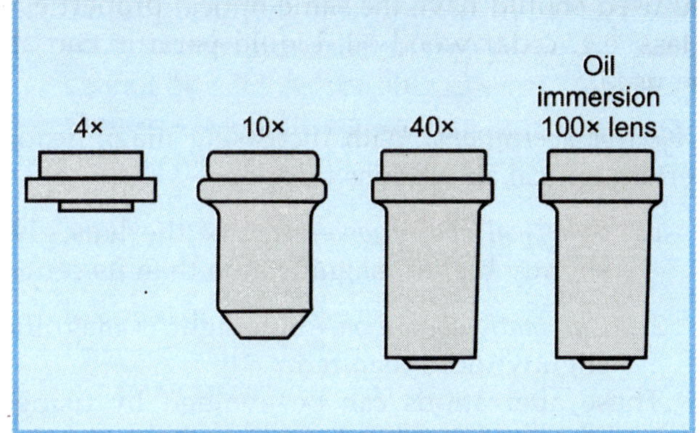

Fig. 1.3: Microscope objectives

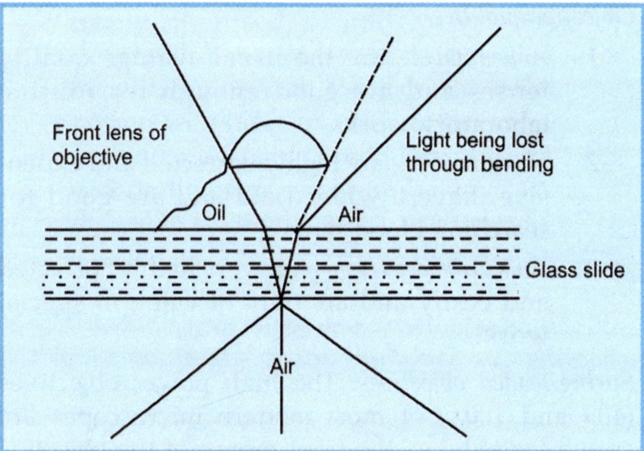

Fig. 1.4: Working of an oil immersion objective

Mechanical stage: It has knobs for moving the slide across or along the stage.

Monocular and binocular microscopes
Monocular—has only one eyepiece (Fig. 1.1).
Binocular—has 2 eyepieces, the only advantage it offers is that it causes less strain on the eyes (Fig. 1.2).

Microscope Optics

Objective: On objective quality, depends, the quality of the image. These are usually made up of more than one lens. On each objective is engraved the magnification power.

Numerical aperture: (NA) of the objective is important, for on this, depends, among other things, the amount of light which the lens passes and the detail which it can make visible, on which it is said to resolve.

Oil immersion objectives: They are used to avoid bending of light beam (with higher magnification). The oil used should have the same optical properties as glass, e.g. cedar wood oil. Liquid paraffin can also be used.

Objective aberrations: With increasing magnification certain optical aberrations creep in:

1. *Spherical aberration*—edge of the lens gives slightly higher magnification than its center.
2. *Chromatic aberration*—blue light is magnified slightly more than red.

These aberrations can be avoided by using a series of lenses made of special glass, carefully calculated and designed.

Objective qualities

1. *Achromatic*—are the usual average quality lenses and are good enough for routine laboratory work.
2. *Fluorite (Fi)*—are highly corrected and expensive, have a wider field and are good for searching blood films.
3. *Apochromatic (Apo)*—are very highly corrected and costly and are only of value in special work.

Spring-loaded objectives: The high power objectives (40× and 100×) of most modern microscopes are spring loaded, i.e., the front mount of the objective will be pushed in rather than pushed through a specimen if such an objective is accidentally pressed against a specimen when focusing (Fig. 1.3).

Working of oil immersion objectives: A beam of light passing from air into glass is bent; and while passing from glass to air, it is bent back again. The bending effect and its limitations can be avoided by replacing the air between the specimen and lens with an oil which has optical properties similar to that of glass, i.e., immersion oil. When an appropriate oil is used, the light passes in a straight line from glass through the oil and back to glass as though it were passing through glass all the way. Whenever possible, the immersion oil recommended by the manufacturer of a microscope should be used (Fig. 1.4).

Eyepiece: The most commonly used eyepiece is known as Huyghens eyepiece which has 2 lenses mounted at a correct distance apart, with a circular diaphragm between, which give a sharp edge to the image. These are available in different magnifications. Lesser the magnification, brighter and sharper is the image. For routine work, a 10x Huyghens is good enough. The 15x eyepieces are also available, as are wide field ones.

Condenser and iris: Condenser is a large lens mounted below the stage, with an iris and diaphragm. There may be 2 or more lenses. Its function is to deliver the light beam to the objective at a sufficiently wide angle.

The mirror: It is placed below the condenser and iris, it can be turned in any direction. It reflects the light beam from the source to the iris and condenser. It usually has two mirrors mounted back to back, one flat and the other concave. Flat mirror is used in the presence of condenser and the concave without the condenser.

Light Source

Daylight: Use of direct sunlight is bad for the microscope and the eye. It is best to use reflected sunlight of a dull white background. It is not sufficient for oil immersion lens and it is not available during evening or night.

Electric light: A 60 watt frosted electric lamp placed 18" away from the microscope is sufficient for most routine work. Many microscopes are now provided with built-in sources of illuminations. In the absence of electricity, a battery lamp or an oil lamp can be utilized. The light from these artificial sources is rather yellow but may be used. Best, however, are halogen lamps.

SPECIAL APPLICATIONS OF THE MICROSCOPE

Phase Contrast Illumination

This is needed to visualize transparent microorganisms suspended in a fluid. Ray of light travels in a wave form in a straight line. Two such rays travelling together are said to be in phase, and they produce a brighter illumination. If, however, these rays are out of step with each other, they are said to be out of phase. They interfere and produce less bright illumination. Phase contrast microscopy makes use of this property of rays to help or hinder each other and thereby resulting increased contrast in the microscopic image.

The desired effect is brought about by placing an annulus in the condenser and a phase plate in the objective. A circle is engraved in the phase plate which matches the ring of beam coming through the condenser and annulus. This circle makes the wave take a longer or a shorter step, so becoming out of phase with those waves which pass through the rest of the plate.

Supposing that the specimen is suspension-free fluid, the only light that reaches the eye is that which goes from the annulus through the phase plate. Whereas presence of organisms would diffract and scatter the light. The light passing through the fluid gets out of phase with the light that has the organisms stand out in contrast to their background.

Equipment Needed

An annulus, a phase plate and a telescope that is needed for adjusting the rings of both annulus and the phase plate.

Method

1. Focus the specimen with the right objective after illuminating the microscope.
2. Place the matching annulus at its position.
3. Remove the eyepiece and put the telescope in its place, adjust it till the two rings, one bright and one dark are in focus.
4. Adjust condenser screws till the bright annulus ring fits exactly into the darker ring of the phase plate.
5. Remove the telescope, replace the eye piece, focus and examine the specimen.

Importance

This method is made use of for examining live organisms, e.g.

a. Cholera vibrios
b. Amoebae
c. Trypanosomes
d. Trichomonas and
e. Other flagellates

It can also be used for platelet counting and for examining routine urine specimens.

Demerits

a. A halo is seen around each particle, it gives a false appearance of its structure.
b. In addition, some resolution power is lost but this is more than compensated for by the increased contrast that is produced.

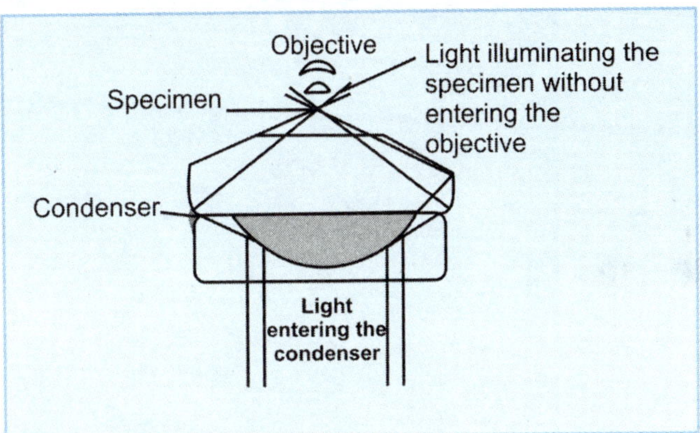

Fig. 1.5: The principle of dark ground illumination

Dark Ground Illumination

This method too, is used for visualising organisms suspended in fluid, both the structure and the motility of the organisms can be seen. In this method the light enters the special condenser which has a central blacked-out area so that light cannot pass directly through it to enter the objective. Instead the light is reflected to pass through the outer rim of the condenser at a wide angle which illuminates the microorganisms by a ring of light surrounding them (Fig. 1.5).

In this method the light that is seen comes only from the microorganisms themselves and not from the light source. Hence, the organisms are brightly illuminated against a dark background. Though useful, this method is rather cumbersome.

Equipment Needed

1. An oil immersion dark ground condenser with the centring screws.
2. A funnel stop for insertion in 100x objective to reduce its NA and exclude light coming directly from the source.
3. A brightly illuminated microscope lamp.
4. Scratchless slides not more than 1 mm thick.

Method

1. Fit the dark ground condenser, raise it to stage level.
2. Place the coverslipped specimen on the thin polished glass slide. Both, the coverslip and the slide should be absolutely clean.

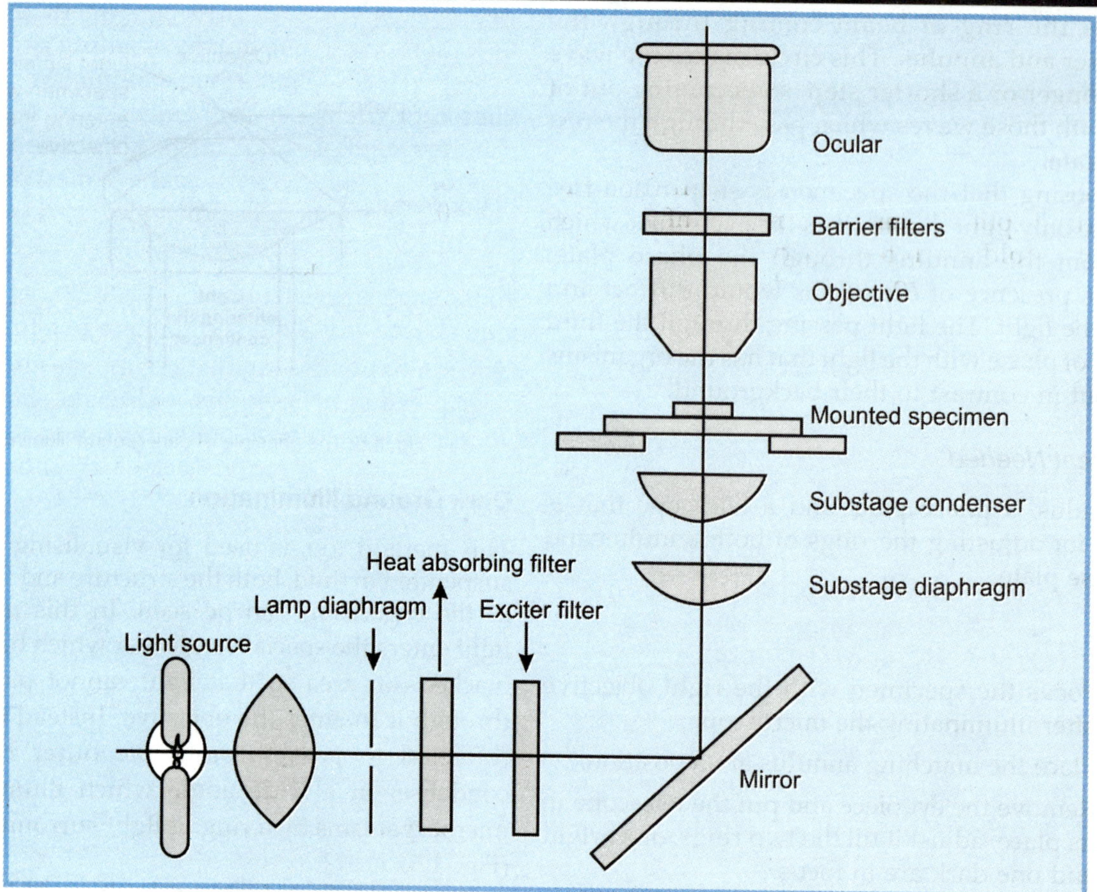

Fig. 1.6: Components of fluorescence system

3. Place a drop of immersion oil between the condenser and the slide.
4. Adjust light source and the mirror properly.
5. Focus 10x objective and observe.
6. Focus condenser up or low so that the ring ultimately becomes just a spot of light. Focus this spot right in the centre.
7. Use 40x objective; if needed, use the 100x oil immersion by inserting the funnel stop into it.

Demerits

1. Focusing and/or centring of condenser is difficult as is the alignment of the lamp.
2. Difficulties may arise under the following circumstances:
   - Smear traces on the slide or coverslip.
   - If the specimen is dense.
   - A bubble is present in the immersion oil.
   - Insufficient oil contact below or above the slide.

Importance

1. This method is of particular importance for the examination of *Treponema* group of organisms.
2. It can also be of use for microfilariae, for the sheath of the pathogenic forms can be clearly seen which otherwise needs to be stained.
3. For examining the rapid movement of *Vibrio cholerae*
4. In addition, this method can be used for:
   - *Leptospira*
   - *Borrelia* and
   - *Spirillum* species.

   (The ideal objective for dark ground illumination is the 50x fluorite as this lens gives a clear, sharp and a well-illuminated image)

Fluorescence Microscopy

This method entails the illumination of particles/microorganisms (previously stained with a fluorescent dye) with ultraviolet (UV) light into visible light (yellow or orange), by lengthening their wavelength. This procedure is made use of for visualizing mycobacteria glowing against a black background.

All other wavelengths emitted by the lamp except the ultraviolet (UV) are to be filtered off (by using appropriate optical filters) and no harmful rays of UV light should reach the observer's eye (by using an immersion dark ground condenser as described for previous method). Again, another filter is used to remove all unwanted fluorescent light by placing a secondary or a barrier filter above the eyepiece (Fig. 1.6).

Equipment Needed

1. A fluorescent lamp (mercury vapour or quartz iodine, the latter is better, being cheaper, lighter and easier to use).
2. A blue (primary or exciting) filter, generally a BG 12.
3. A yellow (secondary or barrier) filter.
4. An immersion dark ground condenser.
5. A nonfluorescent immersion oil, e.g. liquid paraffin.

Importance

1. For identifying mycobacteria.
2. It is used extensively in fluorescent antibody techniques used in parasitology and bacteriology.
3. It is also used widely in histopathology of kidney, skin, etc., where immune/autoimmune basis of disease is expected. In fact, anything can be confirmed with high degree of sensitivity and specificity, if antibodies against it (later tagged with a fluorescent dye) can be produced.
4. Used widely in cytogenetics.

ELECTRON MICROSCOPE

Basic Principle

The resolution of the light microscope has been shown to be limited by the NA and the wavelength of light employed. As the degree of correction in glass lenses is very high, the main limitation is imposed by the light (e.g., half wavelength of light), giving a normal resolution of approximately 250 nm; and when UV light is used, a resolution of about 100 nm. By the substitution of an electron beam for light rays, a much greater degree of resolution can be obtained; since at an acceleration of 50,000 volts, electrons have a wavelength of only 0.001 nm; therefore, a theoretical resolving power of .0005 nm could be attained, which would enable molecules to be seen. Unfortunately, the degree of correction that is currently feasible with transmission electron microscope (TEM) lenses will permit a resolution of only 0.25 nm, but this is still a thousand times greater than that possible with the light microscope. A further difficulty with the TEM is that, since electrons have poor penetrating power, the sections to be examined must be very thin, less than 50 nm thick. This necessitates the use of special hard embedding media (plastics) and special ultra microtomes to cut such thin sections. Steel knives cannot be used to cut these sections; either glass or diamond knives are used.

WEIGHING SCALES OR ANALYTICAL BALANCE

Weighing scales: For weighing large quantities.

Analytical balance: For accurate weighing of smaller quantities.

Use and Care

1. The weighing equipment must be placed on a firm bench, away from vibration, draughts, direct sunlight and dust.
2. It should be kept perfectly horizontal by altering the screws on which the equipment stands.
3. Chemicals, etc. should never be placed directly on the pans. Weigh them in a container.
4. Never touch the weights with hands, handle them with forceps.
5. The balance should be at rest before adding or removing the weights or Chemicals.
6. Before taking the reading, the glass window of the instrument should be closed.

   Electronic analytical balances are also available. Made by various companies, these are very accurate.

CENTRIFUGE

Centrifuge is used to sediment or deposit rapidly particles such as cells which may be suspended in a fluid. The speed is expressed as rpm, i.e. revolutions per minute.

Relative Centrifugal Force (RCF)

More important than rpm is relative centrifugal force (RCF). RCF is expressed as the acceleration due to gravity or G (dynes per cm). The formula is:

$G = 0.00001118 \times (r) \times (n)^2$
where r = radius in centimeters
and n = revolutions per minute

The time of centrifugation is equally important. The tubes should be spun for a definite period to obtain the desired effect.

TYPES OF CENTRIFUGE

1. *Hand centrifuge*—fixed to the bench, the handle is rotated manually. It gives low speeds only.
2. *Motor-driven centrifuge*—operated through mains electricity supply. The tubes may be kept in a fixed angle head or in a swing out head (Figs 1.7 and 1.8).

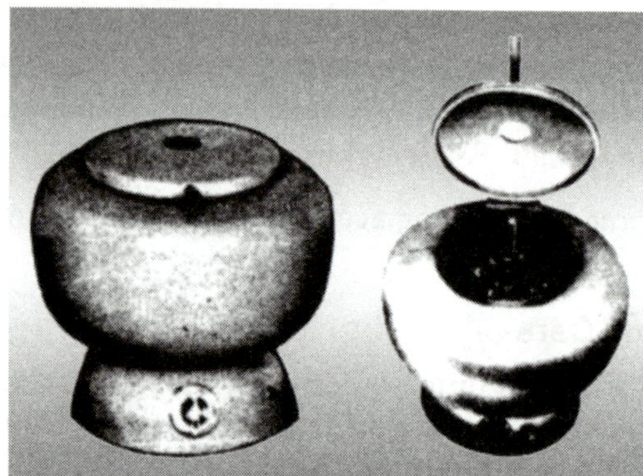

Fig. 1.7: Motor-driven ordinary centrifuge

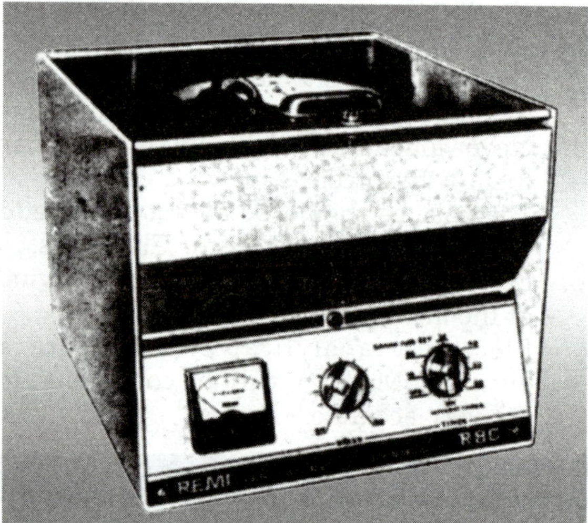

Fig. 1.8: Motor driven centrifuge with rpm. indicator and auto (timed) shut off

3. *Microhematocrit centrifuge*—also motor driven for finding out packed cell volume (PCV) of red blood cells (RBCs). In this, blood-filled capillary tubes are spun and later the percentage of RBC-filled column is estimated (Figs 1.9 and 1.10).

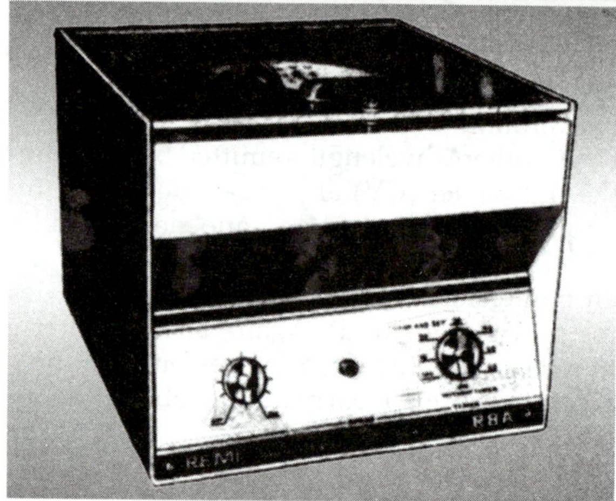

Fig. 1.9: Microhematocrit centrifuge

Use and Care

1. Use centrifuge tubes made of strong glass and they should not be too long.
2. The opposite tubes should be balanced properly.
3. The centrifuge speed should be increased gradually.
4. The instrument should be kept clean. If something spills over inside, it should be cleaned and the instrument disinfected if necessary.

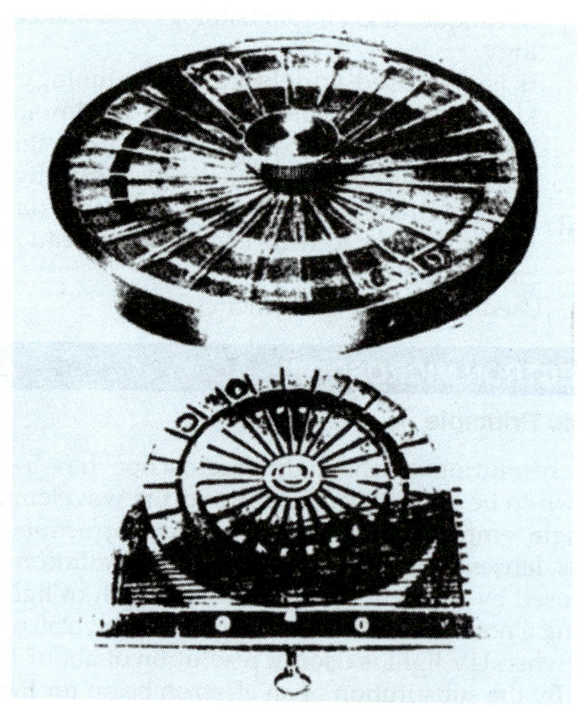

Fig. 1.10: Microhematocrit centrifuge parts

GLASSWARE (MANY ITEMS ARE NOW MADE OF PLASTIC)

1. *Flasks*—are of different sizes and shapes.
   a. Erlenmeyer or conical flasks—for heating and boiling liquids (Fig. 1.11).

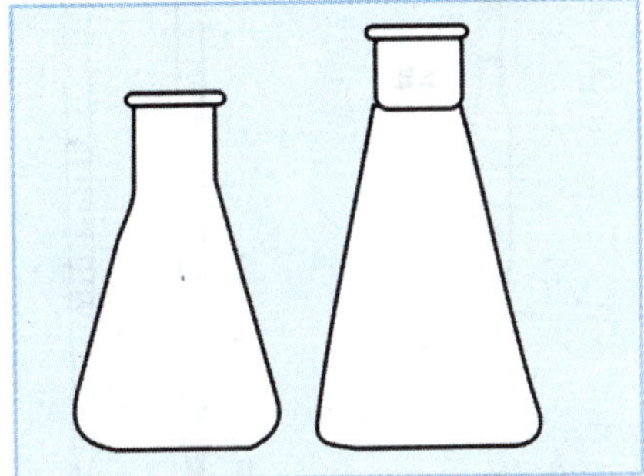

Fig. 1.11: Conical flasks

   b. Volumetric flasks—are graduated for getting exact volume of liquids (Fig. 1.12).

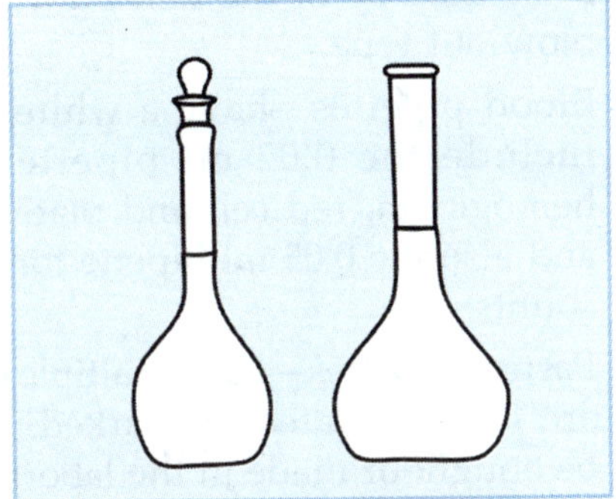

Fig. 1.12: Volumetric flasks

   c. Round and flat-bottomed flasks for preparing solutions (Figs 1.13A and B).

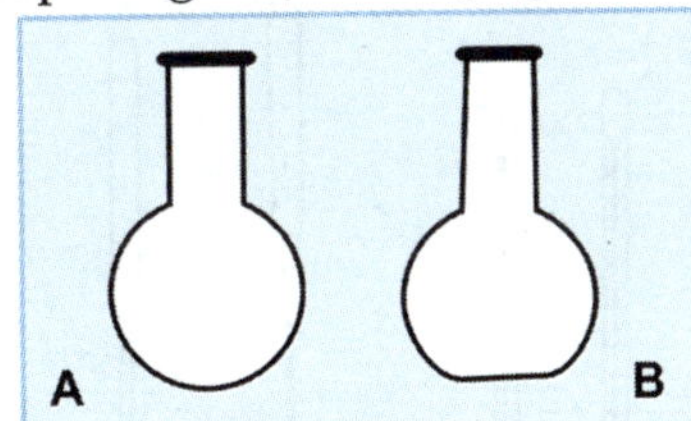

Fig. 1.13: (A) Round bottomed flask and (B) Flat bottomed flask

2. *Beakers*—available in different sizes (Fig. 1.14).
3. *Bottles*
   a. Specimen bottles—with top screws, e.g. the universal type containers.
   b. Reagent bottles—have ground glass or plastic stoppers, available in different sizes and may be made of amber colored glass (Figs 1.15A and B).

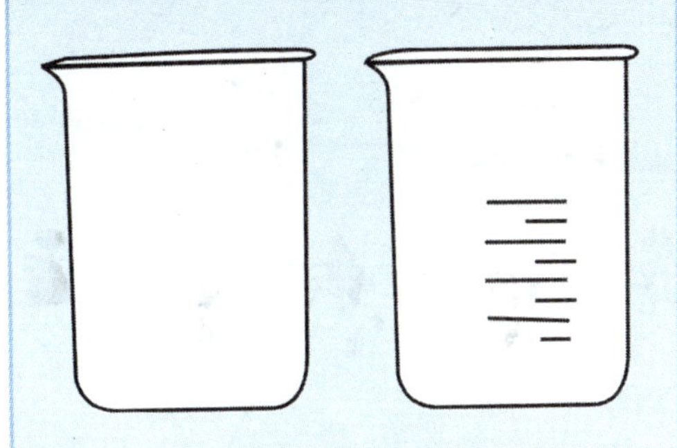

Fig. 1.14: Beakers

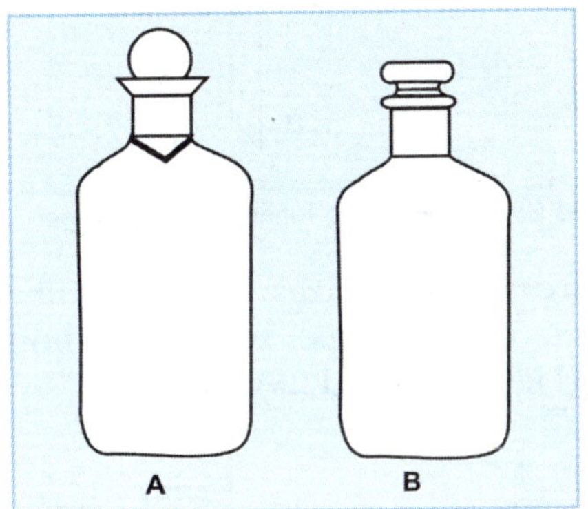

Fig. 1.15: (A) Specimen bottles and (B)Reagent bottles

   c. Drop bottles—fitted with special tops through which drops can be delivered (Fig. 1.16).

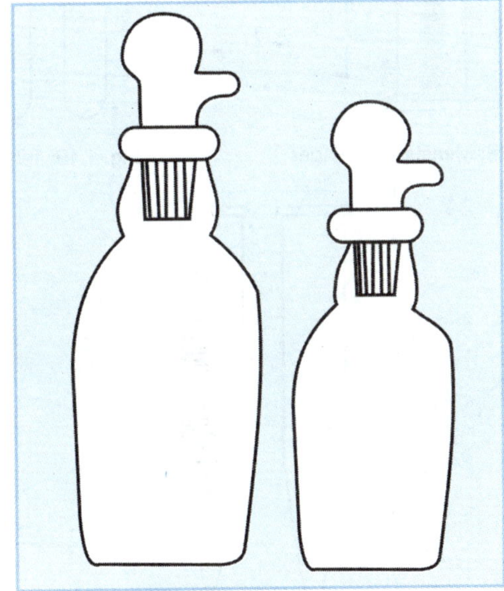

Fig. 1.16: Drop bottles

4. *Funnels*—used to hold filter papers when filtering fluids or for pouring liquids into narrow neck containers (Figs 1.17A and B).
5. *Cylinders*—used for measuring liquids, they have a pouring spot (Fig. 1.18).

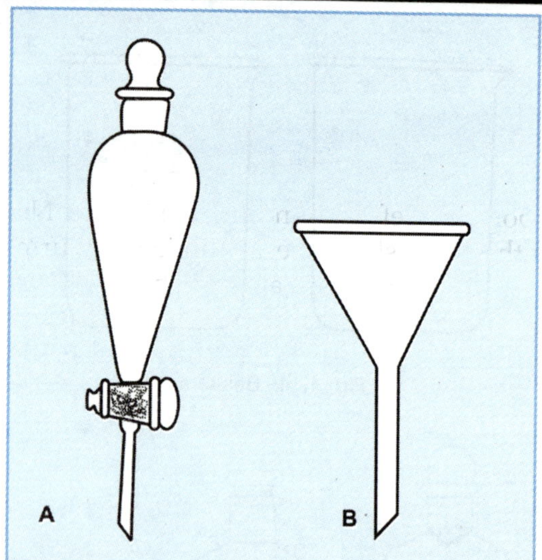

Figs 1.17A and B: (A) Separating funnel and (B) Funnel

6. *Tubes*—are of various sizes; of the test tube or centrifuge (conical) type, with or without a top rim (Figs 1.19 and 1.20).

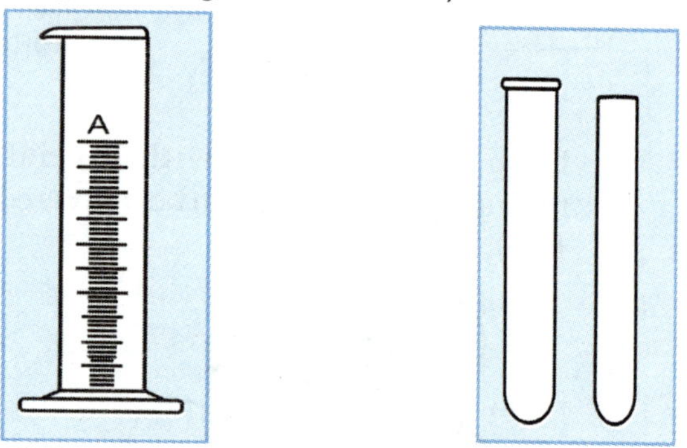

Fig.1.18: Measuring cylinder

Fig. 1.19: Test tubes

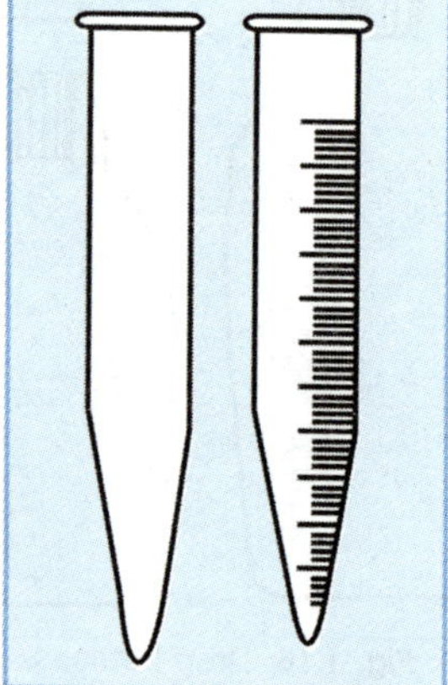

Fig. 1.20: Centrifuge tubes

7. *Pipettes*—are used to measure and deliver a given volume of fluid.
   a. Volumetric pipettes—have a bulb shape in the stem. Each pipette is marked to show the given volume of fluid it contains or delivers (Figs 1.21A and B).

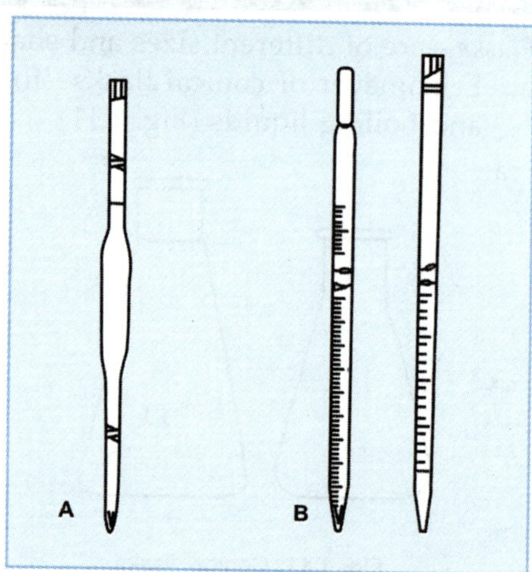

Figs 1.21: (A) Volumetric pipette and (B) Measuring pipette

   b. Graduated pipettes—are of various sizes. They may be of the non blow out or the blow out type.
   c. Blood pipettes—have a white back and include the 0.02 ml pipette used for hemoglobin, red cell and platelet counts, and also the 0.05 ml pipette for white cell counts.
   d. Pasteur pipettes—have multiple uses. They are not graduated or marked. These can be bought or made in the laboratory (Figs 1.22 A and B).

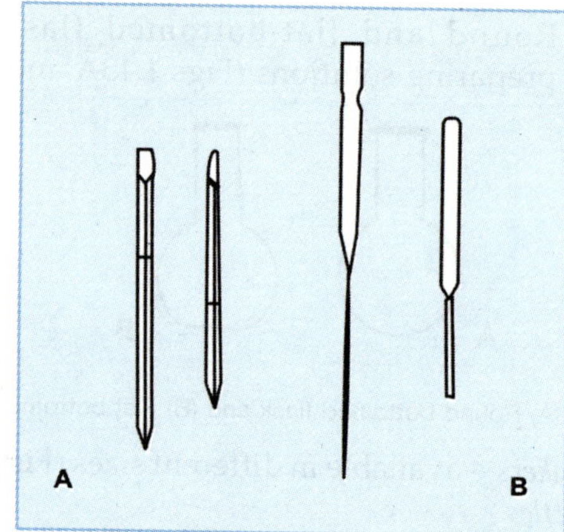

Figs 1.22 A and B: (A) Blood pipettes and (B) Pasteur pipttes

OTHER NECESSARY EQUIPMENT

1. **Serological water bath:** It is electrically heated and has a thermostatic temperature regulator.

It can provide temperature ranging from room temperature to 100°C. Various sizes to suit various workloads are available (Fig. 1.23).

2. **Incubator:** Works on electricity and regulates temperature thermostatically. Necessary for various investigations where body temperature 37°C (or otherwise) incubation is required (Fig. 1.24).

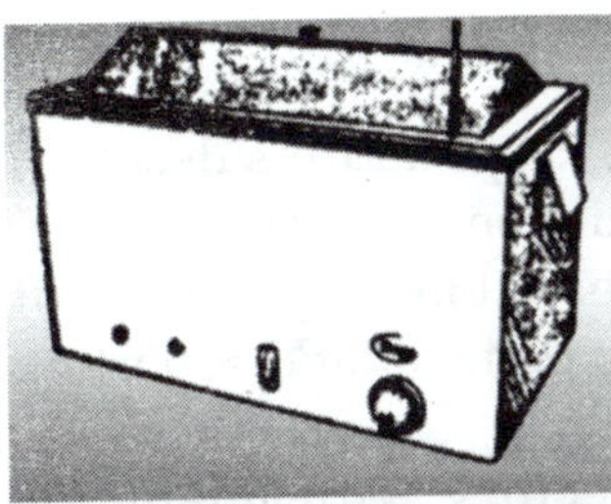

Fig. 1.23: Serological water bath

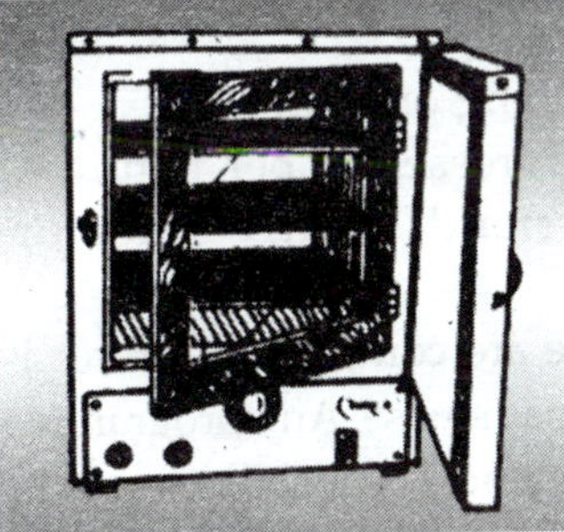

Fig. 1.24: Incubator

3. **Hot air oven:** This is used for drying and sterilizing glassware. This too is thermostatically controlled and electrically heated.

REPORTING LABORATORY TESTS AND KEEPING RECORDS

Standardisation

Standardisation in the reporting of laboratory tests contributes to the efficiency of the laboratory service and is of great value when patients are referred from one place to another.

Whenever possible, request forms and other laboratory printed stationery should be prepared and issued by a central stationery office.

Use of Rubber Stamps

When stationery is not supplied from a central source, standardization in presenting and reporting results can be achieved by the use of rubber stamps. Adequate ink must be used and the stamp must be positioned carefully.

Format

The top part of the report card must prominetly give the name, address and telephone number's of the laboratory. It should then have place for printing the patient's name, age, sex, name of the referring doctor, the laboratory reference number and date. Next, the title of the report should be mentioned, e.g., urinalysis, stool examination, haematology, biochemistry, etc. After this, print the investigation name, leave space for patient's values, print normal values followed by the units. The report must end with the signatures of the person in-charge of the laboratory.

Keeping Records in the Laboratory

A record of all test results must be kept by the laboratory as carbon copies, work sheets, or in simple exercise books. A day book is ideal as it has the necessary ruled lines. In your record put the date, reference number, patient's name, name of the referring doctor, investigations asked for, reports given and payment status (if privately owned lab).

Lab Reporter

An ideal laboratory computer programme helps in reporting and recording diagnostic centre, pathology lab and other diagnostic imaging fields. The programme should also keep history records of the patients. It must have facilities of making and reporting profiles, e.g. lipid, renal, cardiac, hepatic and diabetic profile. A programme can be called ideal if:

It Reduces Overload

- Avoids manual operations by printing booking slips, receipts, bills, envelopes, etc.
- Prints daily register of patients
- Prints rate lists
- Reports only the tests required and not the whole group of tests
- A comprehensive reporting option for day end operations including daily collection report and doctorwise daily collection.

It Helps Referencing Doctor

- Provides clear reports with normal values
- Abnormal values are underlined or highlighted automatically
- Prints history reports of the patients.

It Makes Working Easy

- Reports as per your own method of grouping of tests, profiles, etc.
- Automatic calculation of charges
- Keeps list of referencing doctors
- Maintains daily collection on referencing doctor/institution
- Provides workload report.

The Computerised System is Easy to Operate

- Simple menu based operations and does not require any detailed knowledge of computers
- Help facility at every stage of working for beginners
- Can find a patient detail on the basis of reference number, name, date and referencing doctor.

Features and Provisions

- Keeps the results for as long as you want
- Keeps normal values for male/female and adult/child for all tests
- Can change any normal value as per your equipment, techniques and methods
- Provision for reporting by different doctors
- Reports can be printed on simple paper or on preprinted letter heads (computer stationery).

Graphs

- Prints graphs, e.g. GTT for to the point reporting
- Can make/design your own graphs
- Can see the graph on screen as well as print

Accounts

- Maintains your bank, cash accounts
- Provides all ledgers
- Makes trial balance for final accounts.

Address Manager

- A mail list program, keeps address details
- Provides easy working on the basis of name
- Keeps addresses for labmate program of referencing doctors, patients and reporting doctors
- Prints address directory with telephone numbers, etc.
- Prints labels for sticking on your mail
- Can group your addresses as per nature of address such as friend, relative, doctor, patient, etc.

The features given above are complete. All records can be retrieved datewise or namewise. Any programme that provides the above-mentioned capabilities can be considered as an ideal laboratory reporter.

Caution: All medical electronic diagnostic devices need a stable constant voltage, therefore, proper protective cover must be provided. CVT (constant voltage transformer), servo stabilizers, and UPS (uninterrupted power supply) should be installed in the mainline or with specific instruments.

CHAPTER 2

Sterilisation

The terms *sterilisation* and *disinfection* are used to indicate the treatment of material so as to destroy or otherwise eliminate any living organisms present. However, the term sterilisation is used where physical methods are used and disinfection is used where chemical agents are made use of.

METHODS COMMONLY USED FOR STERILISATION

The methods used commonly in practice are:

1. *Killing organisms by heat:* Heat may be dry or moist
2. *Destroying organisms by employing chemical antiseptics,* e.g. lysol, phenol, perchloride of mercury, etc.
3. *Removing organisms mechanically by filtration:* e.g. Seitz, unglazed porcelain.

Sterilisation by Heat

Adequate heat is the most certain and rapid method for sterilisation. The time needed for sterilisation is inversely related to the temperature of exposure—the higher the temperature, the shorter the time needed. High temperature kills bacteria by coagulating their proteins. Different types of bacteria show considerable differences in heat susceptibility. In general, vegetative forms are destroyed at lower temperatures, whereas high temperatures are needed for sporing organisms.

Dry Heat

This is the preferred method for sterilising glassware, e.g. of glass syringes and of materials such as oils, jellies and powders which are impervious to steam. Dry heat requires a much higher temperature or a much longer time at the same temperature than does moist heat. Dry heat can be used in the following ways:

1. *Flaming:* The articles are passed through the Bunsen flame, without letting them become red hot. It is used for scalpels, needles, mouths of culture tubes, glass slides, coverslips and points of forceps. Only the surfaces actually touched by the flame are sterilised.

2. *Red heat:* Platinum loops, inoculating wires and needles are heated in the bunsen flame until red hot.
3. *Hot air oven:* These are electrically heated and thermostatically controlled. The oven itself is a double-walled steel chamber with a stout door. The top or side contains a ventilator which is left open during sterilisation to disperse any moisture or volatile matter. Air circulates within the oven by convection currents. Suitable sterilising times in the hot air oven are 3 hours at 140°C, 1 hour at 160°C and 30 minutes at 180°C. All dry glassware, such as test tubes, petri-dishes, flasks, pipettes and throat swabs, etc. are made sterile by using hot air oven.

This method is not suitable for sterilizing culture media, liquids, rubber connections, glass to metal fitting and fabrics, e.g., masks, towels or gowns.

Moist Heat

a. *A temperature of 60-65°C* kills most vegetative bacteria (made use of in pasteurisation of milk and preparation of vaccines).
b. *Boiling* is frequently used for sterilizing syringes etc. but is not adequate as many spores withstand this temperature.
c. *Steam* is the most effective technique of moist heat sterilisation. Steam may be employed in three ways.
   1. *Steam at 100°C:* The apparatus used commonly is called Koch's steamer. It has a vertical metal cylinder with a conical lid. It is fitted with a thermometer and has a small opening for escape of steam.
      Sterilisation by free steam can be done in two ways.
      - *Prolonged exposure* for 1½ hours, used for broth or nutrient agar.
      - *Intermittent heat or tyndallisation:* It involves exposure for 20 minutes on three successive days and is used to sterilize sugars and gelatin which decompose on higher temperatures.
      - *Principle:* Spores would germinate after first steaming and destroyed on the next, three steamings would eliminate all spores and their vegetative forms.
   2. *Low temperature steam:* This method is employed for sterilizing materials (blankets, polyethene tubing, etc.) which would be damaged at higher temperatures.
   3. *Steam at temperatures above 100°C (Autoclaving):* Autoclaves are made of strong metal jackets; strong enough to withstand high pressures required (Fig. 2.1). The autoclave door is hermetically sealed. It has a safety valve set to blow off at a predetermined pressure. The principle is that water boils when its vapour pressure is equal to the pressure of the surrounding atmosphere. If the pressure is raised inside a closed vessel, the temperature at which water boils will rise above 100°C. At 15 lbs. pressure water boils at 120°C.
      Following are the measures that must be taken care of during autoclaving:
      a. The steam must be saturated.
      b. There must be complete discharge of air from the sterilizing chamber.
      c. The autoclave must be loaded in such a way that all the materials to be sterilized can be adequately penetrated by steam.
      d. The duration of autoclaving would depend on the pressure inside and hence on the steam temperature.

Method

1. Fill boiler with water to a point just below the basket bottom.
2. Place articles within the basket, bottles should not be more than 3/4 full and should have loosely screwed on caps.
3. Close the lid and tighten the screws.
4. Open outlet valve and adjust safety valve to the required pressure.

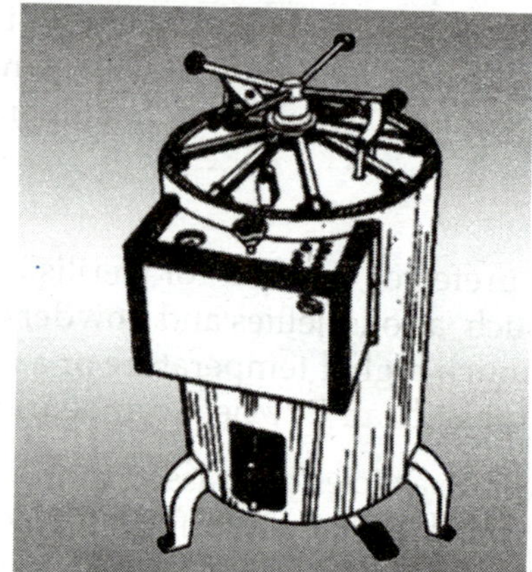

Fig. 2.1: Vertical autoclave

5. Turn on the heat source and when steam flows smoothly, close the ventcock and let the internal pressure rise. See that all air has been expelled from the cylinder.
6. Let pressure rise to the required level and maintain at that level for the required period of time.
7. Switch off the heat source and let the pressure meter register zero. Open the ventcock and the lid slowly.

(If the autoclave pressure is taken down very quickly—the fluid-filled bottles may burst).

Timings
10 lbs. Pressure for 10 minutes—culture media.
15 lbs. Pressure for 20 minutes—infected material.
20 lbs. Pressure for 30 minutes—rubber gloves

4. *Inspisation:* Used to sterilize serum containing media e.g., Loeffler's for diphtheria and Dorset's, or Lowenstein's media for TB. The inspissator consists of a double-walled copper box, with water flowing between the 2 walls; the temperature is controlled between 75-80°C thermostatically. Sterilisation is done for 2-3 hours on each of 3 successive days. A higher temperature may cause bubbling of the surface of the media.

Cold

Not used clinically
Cold shock: A sudden drop of temperature (e.g. 45-15°C) without actual freezing causes irregular contraction of cytoplasmic organelles leading to disorganization of cellular structures (95% drop in *E. coli* viable number is reported by using this method).

Freezing: This helps by (1) formation of ice crystals outside the cell by the withdrawal of water from the cell interior, increases the intracellular salt concentration—protein denaturation and (2) formation of ice within the cell.

Ultraviolet Radiation

Ultraviolet (UV) rays of wavelength 2400 to 2800 Angstrom units are most effective. Low pressure mercury vapour type lamps can be used to produce UV rays. Take care that the UV rays do not directly enter the eyes. Gram-negative bacteria are destroyed more rapidly than gram-positive bacteria, spores are highly resistant and susceptibility of viruses is variable.

Ionising Radiations

Cathode rays and gamma rays are the most effective and are being increasingly used to sterilise disposable items. These radiations have considerable disinfectant action.

Filtration

It may be used for the preparation from cultures of cell-free bacterial products, e.g. toxins and enzymes, to free virus containing fluids from bacteria and for the sterilisation of media or media ingredients which would be damaged by heating. For this purpose, filters with pores sufficiently small to hold back bacteria must be employed. Filtration is usually carried out under negative pressure, the fluid being sucked through the filter into a receiving flask, which is connected to an exhaust pump. During filtration, the filter surface may adsorb material carrying an opposite charge—the material adsorbed may be the one desired in the filtrate.

Seitz filter: This employs filter that consists of a flat disc or asbestos material of special composition and is inserted into metal holders which ensure a tight joint (Fig. 2.2). The disc is used only once. The discs are available in three grades, viz., (1) clarifying (2) normal and (3) special. This method is good for obtaining bacteria-free filtrates. The large pore filters are good for filtration of serum for making media.

Fig. 2.2: Seitz filter

Colloidion or Gradocol membranes: These are virtually free of any adsorptive effects and have replaced Seitz filters considerably. These, too, are replaced after a single use.

Berkefeld and Mandler filters: These are made from diatomaceous earth. Grades available are V—coarse, N—medium and W—fine.

Chamberland and Doulton filters— These are made of unglazed porcelain. Available in various grades:

L/a—coarse clarifying.
L/a L2 and L3—medium.
L5 to L15—very fine.

Sintered glass: It is made of a pad of finely ground glass fused into a glass cup.

Sand and paper pulp filter: They used for removing large particles and clearing emulsions, etc.

Chemical Sterilisation

Chemical agents can exert bactericidal or bacteriostatic effect. The bactericidal agents in lower concentrations exert bacteriostatic effect. The bactericidal effect is probably because of enzyme inactivation either by protein denaturation, oxidation or by a combination of the antibacterial agent with specific groups of enzyme proteins.

Chemicals Used

Various chemicals used are:

1. *Chloroform (volatile antiseptic):* Used in preservation of serum for culture media at 0.25% concentration. Can be removed by heating to 56°C).
2. *Phenol group:* Cresol, lysol (strong antiseptics) are mainly employed for surgical instruments, discarded routine cultures, and pipettes, slides, etc., and disinfecting hands. Phenol 0.5% is used for preserving sera and vaccines.
3. *Metallic salts:* Perchloride of mercury in 1:1000 strength solution.
4. *Glycerol:* A 50% solution is used for preservation of certain viruses. Glycerol also kills contaminating organisms.
5. *Formalin:* It is the only method for sterilising perspex or polythene and for killing cultures on plates. Can also be used for fumigation purposes.
6. *Sulphur:* Burning in air form sulphur dioxide (SO_2) for fumigation.
7. *Halogens:* Chlorine and iodine. Chlorine for water disinfection and iodine for skin.
8. *Acids and alkalies:* Most bacteria grow in pH range of 5 to 9 and many grow at pH 7. Strong acids and alkalies can be used to disinfect contaminated materials.
9. *Alcohols:* These are used for disinfecting skin before injecting and before operations. Alcohols act by protein denaturation.
10. Two groups of dyes (a) the aniline dyes and (b) the acridines have been widely used as skin and wound disinfectants.
11. Quaternary ammonium compounds are active against both gram-positive and gram-negative species but are not effective against spores and *Mycobacteria*. They are used for sterilising food utensils in restaurants and hotels and for disinfecting blankets in hospitals.
12. Glutaraldehyde (Cidex) affects even spores and *Mycobacteria*. It is employed as 2% solution and is recommended for sterilising cystoscopes, etc.
13. Ethylene oxide gas is being widely used to sterilise disposable plastic syringes, petridishes, etc.

GLASSWARE PREPARATION FOR USE

1. *Selection:* Grade A glassware needs no testing. Grade B is satisfactory for most routine work. Others should be heat resistant, have a low coefficient of expansion and be free from soluble metals and free alkali; in addition, they should be mechanically strong.
2. *Cleaning Glassware*

   New: Look for cracks if any. Soak in 2% HCl for overnight to neutralize any alkali present. Wash in running water. Boil in synthetic detergent for 30 minutes, rinse in tap water and finally in distilled water.

   Used glassware should be rinsed immediately after use. Boil in a detergent for 30 minutes and clean thoroughly with a brush, rinse in tap water and finally in distilled water. Dry them in the oven with temperature not exceeding 80°C.

Dichromate Cleaning Solution

Dissolve 25 gm potassium dichromate in 25 ml of water. Add 50 ml conc. sulphuric acid (slowly, always add acid to water and not (*vice-versa*), cool, store it in a stoppered bottle; discard when it starts turning green.

Petridishes

- Autoclave to remove infected material
- Wash in soapy water
- Rinse in running water, let dry
- Rinse in methylated spirit, let dry
- Sterilize in hot air oven.

Pipettes

- Soak in chromic acid solution overnight
- Wash in running water
- Rinse in distilled water
- Dry on suction pump using methylated spirit, or ether, or methylated acetone
- To sterilize—plug mouth piece with nonabsorbent cotton wool, wrap in kraft paper and hot air sterilize (160ºC for 1 hour).

Test tubes

- Autoclave to remove infected material
- Boil in detergent solution for 30 minutes
- Clean with a brush
- Rinse in running water, rinse in distilled water and place them in a wire basket upside down and dry in an oven
- Cotton plug them and sterilize in the hot air oven.

Pasteur pipettes

- Soak in 3% lysol for 1 hour
- Wash as before (as for test tubes).

Screw-capped bottles

- Wash the liners separately
- Dry quickly to avoid corrosion
- Sterilize metal caps and their bottles in hot air oven
- Rubber liners—autoclaved.

Glass slides

New

- Boil in a detergent for 30 minutes
- Place in dichromate for overnight
- Wash in running water
- Keep in methylated spirit
- For using, take them out with a forceps and hold them only by the edges.

Used

- As for used glassware.

Infected slides

- Should be autoclaved and then cleaned as mentioned earlier (never use slides used for examining acid-fast bacilli for the same purpose).

Infected Glassware

Contaminated material—may be disposed in paper or cardboard wrappers and incinerated.

Autoclave the glassware that has been contaminated. Having autoclaved, wash and prepare in the usual way.

Syringes

Complete bacterial sterility can be achieved either by sterilising them in the hot air oven or in an autoclave. Keep injection syringes separate from blood withdrawing syringes. Fresh syringes (sterilised) should be used for withdrawing blood for each patient. Before re-using them, clean them properly and then sterilise them. Needles used should be sharp and not with blunted ends.

Choice of Syringes and Needles

All glass syringes are preferred over glass and metal ones. Preferrably keep size 5 ml or more syringes for withdrawing blood. Needles should be of size less than 21 (SWG). A needle with a smaller diameter would cause lysis of blood when used for blood withdrawing. Withdrawing needles should be at least an inch long.

New syringes These are washed in the usual way. Dried with acetone. Wrap the plunger and the barrel in a paper and sterilise in hot air oven.

Used syringes Immediately after use, wash them thoroughly with cold water (hot water will coagulate proteins and will make the syringes difficult to clean). Clean them thoroughly in a detergent, brush the barrel properly, rinse in tap water and then in distilled water. Rinse in acetone and let dry. Sterilise in hot air oven as mentioned above.

Infected syringes These should be washed at first with cold 2% lysol solution and then clean as above. Syringes infected with highly virulent material should at first be autoclaved. The syringes should be placed in the cold oven and be heated at 160ºC for 90 minutes. Syringes not used for 3 months should be resterilised before use.

Glass barrel and metal plunger syringes The only precaution to be taken here is that metal corrosion should be avoided and the barrel and the plunger should be sterilised separately (kept in a wrapper) by autoclaving them.

Needles

- Should first be rinsed in cold water.
- Clean the mounts with a cotton-wool swab.
- Wash again, rinse in acetone.
- Pass a styllete through the hole to remove any plugs if present.
  (It is important to discard all needles with blunted tips, a hand lens can be used to examine needle tips).
- Serum hepatitis and HIV can be transmitted through using imperfecty cleaned and sterilised needles.
- The needle should be sterilised in hot air oven.

Disinfection of syringes by boiling In an emergency, syringes can be fairly effectively sterilised by boiling them in distilled water for at least 5 minutes after having cleaned them in the usual way.

Disposable Sterile Syringes

This is the world and time of disposables. In the interest of the patient every laboratory should ideally use disposable syringes only.

As far as possible use disposable, sterilised plasticware instead of glassware.

Chapter 3

SI Units

The SI units (Système International d'Unités) have replaced the old system of reporting and measurements. This is in accordance with a World Health Organization resolution which recommends the adoption of the International System of Units by the medical community throughout the world. Consequently, reports and measurements from any corner of the world can be safely understood anywhere else.

The SI system is based on metre-kilogram-second system and replaces both the foot-pound-second system and the centimetre-gram-second system. There are seven SI base units, i.e. meter, kilogram, second, mole, ampere, Kelvin and Candela. The symbols for these units and what they measure are listed in Table 3.1.

LITRE

The SI unit of volume is cubic metre (m^3). This is a very large unit, hence, the litre (L) although not an SI unit, has been recommended for use in the laboratory.

The litre is equal to a cubic decimetre (1 dm^3). Volume measurements are made in litres or multiples and submultiples of the litre, e.g. dl (10^{-1}l), ml (10^{-3}l), μl (10^{-6}l).

One litre is, therefore, equivalent to 10 dl, 1000 ml or 1000 000 μl. One dl is equivalent to 100 ml, and 1 ml to 1000 μl.

SI unit	*Old unit*
dl	100 ml
ml or cm^3	cc
μl	lambda
nl	—
pl	$\mu\mu$l

GRAM

The kilogram (kg) is the SI unit for mass and the gram (gm) is the working unit.

Formerly, the gram (gm) was written as gramme, or gm.

Table 3.1: The symbols of units and what they measure

SI base units		
	Symbol	*Quantity measured*
metre	m	length
kilogram	kg	mass
second	s	time
mole	mol	amount of substance
ampere	A	electric current
Kelvin	K	temperature
Candela	cd	luminous intensity
SI derived units		
square metre	m^2	area
cubic metre	m^3	volume
metre per second	m/s	speed
Named SI derived units		
Hertz	Hz	frequency
Joule	J	energy, quantity of heat
Newton	N	force
Pascal	Pa	pressure
Watt	W	power
Volt	V	electric potential difference
degree Celsius	°C	Celsius temperature

SI unit prefixes			
Prefix	*Symbol*	*Function*	*Divide by*
deci	d	10^{-1}	10
centi	c	10^{-2}	100
milli	m	10^{-3}	1000
micro	μ	10^{-6}	1000 000
nano	n	10^{-9}	1000 000 000
pico	p	10^{-12}	1000 000 000 000
femto	f	10^{-15}	1000 000 000 000 000
			Multiply by
deca	da	10^{1}	10
hecto	h	10^{2}	100
kilo	k	10^{3}	1000
mega	M	10^{6}	1000 000
giga	G	10^{9}	1000 000 000
tera	T	10^{12}	1000 000 000 000
peta	P	10^{15}	1000 000 000 000 000

Mass measurements are made in grams or in multiples and submultiples of the gram, e.g. mg (10^{-3}gm), μg (10^{-6}gm), ng (10^{-9}gm), pg (10^{-12}gm).

One g is, therefore, equivalent to 1000 mg, 1000 000 μg, or 1000 000 000 ng. One mg is equivalent to 1000 μg.

SI unit	*Old unit*
nm	m μ
μm	μ (micron)

MOLE (MOL)

The mole (mol) is the SI unit for amount of substance and measurements of the amounts of substances are made in moles, or in mmol (10^{-3} mol), μmol (10^{-6} mol), or nmol (10^{-9} mol).

One mol is, therefore, equivalent to 1000 mmol, 1000 000 μmol, or 1000 000 000 nmol. One mmol/L is equivalent to 1000 μmol/L.

Earlier, the results of tests expressed in mmol/L or μmol/L were expressed in mg/100 ml or μg/100 ml. The formula used to convert mg/100 ml to mmol/L is as follows:

$$\text{mmol/L} = \frac{\text{mg/100 ml} \times 10}{\text{molecular weight of substance}}$$

where the molecular weight of a substance cannot be accurately determined (e.g. albumin), results are expressed in gm/L.

SI unit	*Old unit*
mol	M
mmol	m Eq
μmol	μM
nmol	nM

INTERNATIONAL UNIT (U)

This unit is used to express enzyme activity. An International Unit of enzyme activity is that amount of enzyme which under defined assay conditions will catalyze the conversion of 1 µmol of substrate per minute. Results are expressed in International Units per litre (U/L).

CONVERSION FACTORS BETWEEN CONVENTIONAL AND SYSTÈME INTERNATIONAL UNITS (SIU)

This list is included to assist the reader to convert values between conventional units and the newer SI units that have been mandated by many journals. Only common analytes are included.

Hematology

Analyte	Conventional units	SI units	Conversion factors: Conventional to SI units	Conversion factors: SI to Conventional units
WBC count (leucocytes) (B)	μl or / cu mm or / mm³	cells 10⁹L	0.001	1000
(CSF)	/ cu mm or	10⁶ / L	1	1
	→cu μl	10⁶ / L	10⁶	10⁻⁶
(SF)	# / μ1	# / L	10⁶	10⁻⁶
Platelet count	10³ / cu mm	10⁹ / L	1	1
Reticulocytes	/ cu mm	10⁹ / L	0.001	1000
RBC count (erythrocytes) (B)	10⁶ / μl or / cu mm	10¹² / L	1	1
(CSF)	or / mm³ / cu mm	10⁶ / L	1	1
Haematocrit [packed cell volume (PCV)]	%	Volume fraction	0.01	100
Mean corpuscular volume (MCV) (volume index)	μ³ (cubic microns)	fl	1	1
Mean corpuscular haemoglobin (MCH)	pg (or μg)	pg	1	1
(colour index)	pg	fmol	0.06206	16.11
Mean corpuscular haemoglobin	gm / dl	gm / L	10	0.1
concentration (MCHC) (saturation index)	gm / dl	mmol / L	0.6206	1.611
Haemoglobin	gm / dl	gm / L	10	0.1
(whole blood)	gm / dl	mmol / L	0.155	6.45
(plasma)	mg / dl	μmol / L	0.155	6.45
Foetal haemoglobin	%	mol / mol (may omit symbol)	0.01	100
Haptoglobin	mg / dl	mg / L	10	0.1
Fibrinogen	mg / dl	gm / L	0.01	100

Chemistry

Analyte	Conventional units	SI units	Conversion factors: Conventional to SI units	Conversion factors: SI to Conventional units
Adrenocorticotropic hormone (ACTH)	pg / ml	ng / L	1	1
	pg / ml	pmol / L	0.2202	4.541
Aldosterone				
(S)	ng / dl	nmol / L	0.0277	36.1
(U)	mEq / 24 hr	mmol / d	1	1
(U)	μg / 24 hr	nmol / d	2.77	0.36
Angiotensin	ng / dl	ng / L	10	0.1
	pg / ml	ng / L	1	1
Angiotensin-converting enzyme (ACE)	nmol / min / ml	U / L	1	1
Antidiuretic hormone (ADH) (vasopressin)	pg / ml	ng / L	1	1
Albumin				
(S)	gm / dl	gm / L	10	0.1
(CSF, AF)	mg / dl	mg / L	10	0.1
Alpha antitrypsin	mg / dl	gm / L	0.01	100
Alpha-fetoprotein (AFP)	ng / ml	μg / L	1	1
(S)	ng / dl	ng / L	10	0.1
	mg / dl	gm / L	0.01	100

Contd...

Contd...

	mg/dl	mg/L	10	0.1
	μg/dl	μg/L	10	0.1
Ammonia	μg/dl	μmol/L	0.714	1.4
(P)	μg/dl	μmol/L	0.5872	1.703
Anion gap	mEq/L	mmol/L	1	1
Base excess	mEq/L	mmol/L	1	1
Bicarbonate	mEq/L	mmol/L	1	1
Bilirubin	mg/dl	μmol/L	17.1	0.0584
Calcitonin	pg/ml	ng/L	1	1
Catecholamines (U)	μg/24 hr	nmol/d	5.91	0.169
Norepinephrine	μg/mg creatinine	μmol/mol creatinine	669	0.00149
	pg/ml	pmol/L	5.91	0.169
	ng/ml	nmol/L	5.91	0.169
Epinephrine	μg/24 hr	nmol/d	5.46	0.183
	μg/mg creatinine	μmol/mol creatinine	617	0.00162
	pg/ml	pmol/L	5.46	0.183
	ng/ml	nmol/L	5.46	0.183
Normetanephrine	ng/ml	nmoj/L	5.46	0.183
Dopamine	μg 24 hr	nmol/d	6.53	0.153
	μg/mg creatinine	μmol/mol creatinine	783	0.00136
	pg/ml	pmol/L	6.53	0.153
	ng/ml	nmol/L	6.53	0.153
Chorionic gonadotrophin (HCG), beta, subunit	mU/ml	IU/L	1	1
	U/24 hr	IU/d	1	1
Calcium				
(S)	mg/dl	mmol/L	0.25	4.0
	mEq/L	mmol/L	0.5	2.0
(U)	mg/24 hr	mmol/d	0.025	40
Carbon dioxide total (content; CO_2 + bicarbonate)	mEq/L	mmol/L	1	1
CO_2 partial pressure, tension (PCO_2)	mmHg	kPa	0.133	7.52
Standard bicarbonate (hydrogen carbonate)	mEq/L	mmol/L	1	1
Chloride	mEq/L or mg/dl	mmol/L	1	1
CEA	ng/ml	μg/L	1	1
	μg/ml	mg/L	1	1
Ceruloplasmin	mg/dl	mg/L	10	0.1
Cholesterol	mg/dl	mmol/L	0.0259	38.61
HDL-cholesterol	mg/dl	mmol/L	0.0259	38.61
LDL-cholesterol	mg/dl	mmol/L	0.0259	38.61
Copper				
(S)	μg/dl	μmol/L	0.157	6.37
(U)	μg/24 hr	μmol/d	0.0157	63.69
Coproporphyrins (I and III)	μg/dl	nmol/L	15	0.067
(U)	μg/24 hr	nmol/d	1.5	0.67
(F)	μg/gm	nmol/gm	1.5	0.67
Porphobilinogen (PBG)				
(U)	mg/24 hr	μmol/d	4.42	0.226
Cortisol				
(S)	μg/dl	μmol/L	0.028	35.7
	ng/ml	nmol/L	2.76	0.362

Contd...

Contd...

17-OHKS (cortisol)	mg/24 hr	μmol/d	2.759	0.3625
(U)	μg/24 hr	nmol/d	2.759	0.3625
Creatine	mg/dl	μmol/L	76.3	0.0131
(S)				
Creatinine				
(S, AF)	mg/dl	μmol/L	88.4	0.0113
(U)	gm/24 hr	mmol/d	8.84	0.1131
(U)	mg/24 hr	mmol/d	0.00884	113.1
(U)	mg/kg/24 hr	μmol/kg/d	8.84	0.113
(C)	ml/min/1.73 m^2	ml/sec/m^2	0.00963	104
cAMP (cyclic adenosine monophosphate)				
(S)	μg/L	nmol/L	3.04	0.329
(B)	ng/ml	nmol/L	3.04	0.329
(U)	mg/24 hr	μmol/d	3.04	0.329
(U)	mg/gm creatinine	μmol/mol creatinine	344	0.00291
Dehydroepiandrosterone sulfate (DHEA-S)				
(S)	μg/ml	μmol/L	2.6	0.38
(AF)	ng/ml	nmol/L	2.6	0.38
17-Ketosteroids (as DHEA)				
(U)	mg/24 hr	μmol/d	3.467	0.2904
17-Ketogenic steroids (as DHEA)				
(U)	mg/24 hr	μmol/d	3.467	0.2904
17-Hydroxycorticosteroids (17-OHCS)				
(U)	mg/d of creatinine	mg/mol of creatinine	113.1	0.00884
11-Deoxy corticosterone (DOC)				
(S)	pg/ml	pmol/L	3.03	0.33
Glucose	mg/dl	mmol/L	0.0555	18.02
Ferritin	ng/ml	μg/L	1	1
Gastrin	pg/ml	ng/L	1	1
Growth hormone	ng/ml	μg/L	1	1
Homovanillic acid (HVA)				
(U)	mg/24 hr	μmol/d	5.49	0.182
	μg/24 hr	μmol/d	0.00549	182
	μg/mg of creatinine	mmol/mol of creatinine	0.621	1.61
5-Hydroxyindoleacetic acid (5-HIAA)				
(U)	mg/24 hr	μmol/d	5.2	0.19
Hormone receptors (T)				
Progesterone receptor assay (PRA)	fmol/mg of protein	nmol/kg of protein	1	1
Estrogen receptor assay (ERA)	fmol/mg of protein	nmol/kg of protein	1	1
Iron	μg/dl	μmol/L	0.179	5.587
Iron-binding capacity	μg/dl	μmol/L	0.179	5.587
Iron saturation	%	fraction saturation	0.01	100
Lactate	mg/dl	mmol/L	0.111	9.01
Lead				
(S)	μg/dl	μmol/L	0.0483	20.72
(S)	mg/dl	μmol/L	48.26	
(U)	μg/24 hr	μmol/d	0.00483	
Lipids (total)	mg/dl	gm/L	0.01	100
Magnesium	mEq/L	mmol/L	0.5	2
	mg/dl	mmol/L	0.411	2.433

Contd...

Contd...

Osmolality	mOsml/kg	same		
O_2 partial pressure (PaO_2)	mm Hg	kPa	0.133	7.5
Parathyroid hormone	pg/ml	ng/L	1	1
	µlEq/ml	mlEq/L	1	1
Phosphate (inorganic phosphorus)				
(S)	mg/dl	mmol/L	0.323	3.10
(U)	gm/24 hr	mmol/d	32.3	0.031
pH	nEq/L	nmol/L	1	1
Porphobilinogen	µg/d	µmol/d	4.42	0.226
Potassium				
(S)	mEq/L	mmol/L	1	1
(U)	mEq/24 hr	mmol/L	1	1
(U)	mg/24 hr	nmol/d	0.02558	39.1
Protein, total				
(S)	gm/dl	gm/L	10	0.1
(U)	mg/24 hr	gm/d	0.001	1000
CSF	mg/dl	mg/L	10	0.1
Renin [plasma-renin activity (PRA)]	ng/ml/hr	µg/L/hr	1	1
Sodium				
(S)	mEq/L	mmol/L	1	1
(U)	mEq/24hr	mmol/L	1	1
(U)	mg/24 hr	mmol/d	0.0435	22.99
Serotonin				
(S)	ng/ml	µmol/L	0.00568	176
Testosterone (total)				
(S)	ng/dl	nmol/L	0.0347	28.8
Thyroid-binding globulin (TBG)	mg/dl	mg/L	10	0.1
	µg/dl	µg/L	10	0.1
Thyroglobulin	ng/ml	µg/L	1	1
TSH (thyroid-stimulating hormone)	µU/ml	mIU/L	1	1
Thyrotropin-releasing hormone (TRH)	pg/ml	ng/L	1	1
Triiodothyronine, total (T-3)	ng/dl	nmol/L	0.0154	65.1
Reverse T-3 (rT-3)	ng/dl	nmol/L	0.0154	65.1
Thyroxine, total (T-4)	µg/dl	nmol/L	12.9	0.0775
Transferrin (TIBC)	mg/dl	gm/L	0.01	100
Triglycerides	mg/dl	mmol/L	0.0113	88.5
Urea nitrogen				
(S)	mg/dl	mmol/L	0.357	2.8
(U)	gm/24 hr	mol/d	0.0357	28
Uric acid				
(S)	mg/dl	mmol/L	0.05948	16.9
(U)	mg/24 hr	mmol/d	0.0059	169
Vanillylmandelic acid (VMA)				
(U)	mg/24 hr	µmol/d	5.05	0.198
	µg/mg of creatinine	mmol/mol of creatinine	0.571	1.75
Viscosity (S)	centipoise	same		
Vitamin B_{12} (cyanocobalamin)	pg/ml	pmol/L	0.738	1.355
Unsaturated B_{12} binding capacity				
(S)	pg/ml	pmol/L	0.738	1.355
Vitamin C (ascorbic acid)	mg/dl	µmol/L	56.78	0.176
Vitamin A	µg/dl	µmol/L	0.0349	28.65

Contd...

Contd...

Vitamin D (calcitriol; 1,25-dihydroxy)	pg/ml	pmol/L	2.4	0.417
Xylose (U)	mg/dl	mmol/L	0.0666	15.01
	gm/5 hr	mmol/5 hr	6.66	0.15

(μ = microns; μmol = micromoles; mmol = millimoles; nmol = nanomoles; fmol = fentamoles; mg = milligrams; gm = grams; pg = picograms; ng = nanograms; L = liter; ml = milliliter; mEq = milliequivalent; ml/sec = milliliter/second; ml/min = milliliter/minute; U = units; mU = milliunits; IU = international units; d = day; 24 hr = 24 hours; S = serum; U = urine; B = blood; C = clearance; F = feces; AF = amniotic fluid; SF = synovial fluid; T = tissue. All references are to serum unless otherwise indicated.

Enzyme

Conventional unit	*IU/L Equivalent*	
Acid phosphatase (prostatic)		
Bodansky	5.37	
Shinowara-Jones-Reinhart	5.37	
King-Armstrong	1.77	
Bessey-Lowry-Brock	16.67	
Alkaline phosphatase		
Bodansky	5.37	
Shinowara-Jones-Reinhart	5.37	
King-Armstrong	7.1	
Bessey-Lowry-Brock	16.67	0.14
Babson	1.0	
Aldolase		
Sibley-Lehninger	0.74	
Amylase		
Somogyi (saccharogenic)	1.85	
Somogyi	20.6	0.541
Creatine kinase (CK)	1.0	
Hydroxybutyric dehydrogenase (d-HBD)		
Rosalki-Wilkinson	0.482	
Isocitrate dehydrogenase (ICD)		
Wolfson-Williams-Ashman	0.0167	
Taylor-Friedman	0.0167	
Lactate dehydrogenase (LDH)		
Wroblewski	0.482	
Lipase		
Cherry-Crandal	278	
Malic dehydrogenase (MD)		
Wacker-Ulmer-Valee	0.482	
Transaminases		
Reitman-Frankel	0.482	
Karmen	0.482	

Therapeutic and Toxic Drugs

			Conversion factors	
Analyte	*Conventional units*	*SI units*	*Conventional to SI units*	*SI to conventional units*
Acetaminophen	μg/ml	μmol/L	6.62	0.151
Amikacin	μg/ml	μmol/L	1.71	0.585
Amitriptyline	ng/ml	nmol/L	3.61	0.277
Amobarbital	μg/ml	μmol/L	4.42	0.226
Amphetamine	ng/ml	nmol/L	7.4	0.135
	μg/ml	μmol/L	7.4	0.135
Bromide	μg/ml	mmol/L	0.0125	79.9
Caffeine	μg/ml	μmol/L	5.15	0.194
Carbamazepine (Tegretol)	μg/ml	μmol/L	4.23	0.236
Carbenicillin	μg/ml	μmol/L	2.64	0.378
Chloral hydrate	μg/ml	μmol/L	6.69	0.149
Chloramphenicol	μg/ml	μmol/L	3.09	0.323
Chlordiazepoxide (Librium)	ng/ml	μmol/L	0.00334	300
Chlorpromazine (Thorazine)	ng/ml	nmol/L	3.14	0.319
Chlorpropamide (Diabinese)	μg/ml	μmol/L	3.61	0.227
Cimetidine (Tagamet)	μg/ml	μmol/L	3.96	0.252
Clonazepam (Clonopin)	ng/ml	nmol/L	3.17	0.316
Clonidine (Catapres)	ng/ml	nmol/L	4.35	0.230
Cocaine	ng/ml	nmol/L	3.3	0.303
Codeine	ng/ml	nmol/L	3.34	0.299
Demerol (Meperidine)	ng/ml	nmol/L	4.04	0.247
Desipramine (Norpramin)	ng/ml	nmol/L	3.75	0.267
Diazepam (Valium)	ng/ml	μmol/L	0.0035	285
Digitoxin	ng/ml	nmol/L	1.31	0.765
Digoxin	ng/ml	nmol/L	1.28	0.781
Dilaudid	ng/ml	nmol/L	4.85	0.206
Disulfiram	μg/ml	μmol/L	12.12	0.0761
Doxepin (Sinequan)	ng/ml	nmol/L	3.58	0.279
Ethanol	mg/dl	mmol/L	0.217	4.61
Ethchlorvynol (Placidyl)	μg/ml	μmol/L	6.92	0.145
Ethosuximide (Zarontin)	μg/ml	μmol/L	7.08	0.141
Gentamicin	μg/ml	μmol/L	2.09	0.478
Glutethimide (Doriden)	μg/ml	μmol/L	4.60	0.217
Haloperidol (Haldol)	ng/ml	nmol/L	2.66	0.376
Ibuprofen	μg/ml	μmol/L	4.85	0.206
Imipramine (Tofranil)	ng/ml	nmol/L	3.57	0 28
Isoniazid	μg/ml	μmol/L	7.29	0.137
Kanamycin (Kantrex)	μg/ml	μmol/L	2.06	0.485
Lidocaine (Xylocaine)	μg/ml	μmol/L	4.27	0.234
Lithium	mEq/L	mmol/L	1	1
Lorazepam	ng/ml	nmol/L	3.11	0.321
LSD (lysergic acid diethylamide)	μg/ml	μmol/L	3.09	0.323
Meprobamate	mg/L	μmol/L	4.58	0.218
Methadone	ng/ml	μmol/L	0.00323	309
Methaqualone (Quaalude)	μg/ml	μmol/L	4.0	0.250
Methotrexate	ng/ml	nmol/L	2.2	0.454
Methsuximide	μg/ml	μmol/L	5.29	0.189
Methyldopa (Aldomet)	μg/ml	μmol/L	4.73	0.211

Contd...

Contd...

Morphine	ng/ml	nmol/L	3.5	0.285
	ng/ml	μmol/L	0.0035	285
Nortriptyline	ng/ml	nmol/L	3.8	0.263
Oxazepam	μg/ml	μmol/L	3.49	0.287
Paraldehyde	μg/ml	μmol/L	7.57	0.132
Pentobarbital (Nembutal)	μg/ml	μmol/L	4.42	0.179
Percodan	ng/ml	nmol/L	3.17	0.315
Phenacetin	μg/ml	μmol/L	5.58	0.179
Phenobarbital (Luminal)	μg/ml	μmol/L	4.31	0.232
Phenylbutazone (Butazolidin)	μg/ml	μmol/L	3.08	0.324
Phenytoin (Dilantin)	μg/ml	μmol/L	3.96	0.253
Primidone	μg/ml	μmol/L	4.58	0.218
Procainamide (Pronestyl), procaine (Novacain)	μg/ml	μmol/L	4.23	0.236
Propoxyphene (Darvon)	μg/ml	μmol/L	3.07	0.326
Propranolol	ng/ml	nmol/L	3.86	0.259
Quinidine	μg/ml	μmol/L	3.08	0.324
Quinine	μg/ml	μmol/L	3.08	0.324
Salicylic acid	μg/ml	μmol/L	7.24	0.138
Secobarbital (Seconal)	μg/ml	μmol/L	4.2	0.238
Theophylline (Aminophylline)	μg/ml	μmol/L	5.55	0.180
Tobramycin	μg/ml	μmol/L	2.14	0.467
Valproic acid	μg/ml	μmol/L	6.93	0.144
Vancomycin	μg/ml	mg/L	1	1
Warfarin (Coumadin)	μg/ml	μmol/L	3.24	0.308

CHAPTER 4

Fundamental Chemistry

INDICATORS

These are usually acids of weak strength whose molecules in solution are of a different colour than their anions.
(pH. Neutral pH = 7.0, less than 7.0 is acidic, more than 7.0 is alkaline).

The colour of an indicator solution depends on the degree of dissociation of the indicator, and on the pH of the solution. Supposing the weak acid indicator is H Indic′, it would dissociate as:

H Indic′	H^+	+	+Indic⁻
(colour-X)	(hydrogen ion)		(Colour Y)

All acids contain hydrogen ions, so addition of an acid would make the reaction shift from right to left (change of colour from Y to X) and addition of an alkali (alkalies contain OH^- or hydroxyl ions) would lead to production of water ($H_2O \rightarrow H^+ + OH^-$) as the OH^- radicals will associate with and remove H^+ ions causing a shift to the right of the reaction (change of colour from X to Y). Indicators that just show whether a solution is an acid or alkali are called broad indicators while some indicators change colour at a precise pH.

Given in Table 4.1 is a list of commonly employed indicators.

Solutes, Solvents and Solutions

Solute—is any substance that dissolves in a liquid

Solvent—is any liquid in which a solute dissolves

Solution—a solvent becomes a solution after dissolving a solute.

Buffer solution: At any given temperature these solutions retain their definite pH and maintain it even after adding considerable amounts of acids or alkalies. These solutions generally consist of a weak acid mixed with its sodium or potassium salt.

Table 4.1: Commonly employed indicators

Indicator	Colour in acid solution	Colour in alkaline solution	pH ranges
Litmus	Red	Yellow	5.5-8.0
Phenophthalein	Colourless	Red	8.0-9.8
Methyl red	Red	Yellow	4.2-6.3
Methyl orange	Red	Orange	3.1-4.4
Phenol red	Yellow	Blue	6.8-8.4
Bromthymol blue	Yellow	Blue	6.0-7.6

STRENGTH OF A SOLUTION

Solution strength can be expressed in four ways: (1) Per cent solutions, (2) Part dilutions, (3) Molar solutions, and (4) Normal solutions.

Per cent Solutions

This is the most usual way of expressing solution strength. Per cent implies per hundred and a 30 per cent solution of anything should contain 30 parts of solute per hundred parts of the final solution.

Per cent solution can further be expressed in three ways.

1. *Weight per unit weight (w/w):* This implies that the weight of both, solute and solvent add up to 100, regardless of the final volume produced. A 25% solution would be 25 grams of solute dissolved in 75 grams of solvent. These solutions are made by weighing both the solute and the solvent and the resultant solution may not have a volume of 100 ml.
2. *Weight per unit volume (w/v):* This is a commoner method of preparing laboratory solutions. In this method a weight of the solute is dissolved in a final volume of 100 ml (it is wrong to dissolve the weight of solute in 100 ml of solvent as is often done).

   A volumetric flask is the most accurate and convenient container for preparing such solutions. Put the weighed solute in the flask, add the solvent (keeping volume less than the final volume required), dissolve the solvent completely and then make up the total volume by adding more of the solvent.

   Wherever necessary, deduct the molecular weight of water if the amount indicated is of anhydrous solute.
3. *Volume per unit volume (v/v):* This is used when the ultimate solution is to be prepared from liquids. A volume of the liquid solute is made up to 100 ml final volume with solvent. Here too, a volumetric flask/beaker should be used and the final volume be made up by adding the solvent. Care should be taken to work under temperature conditions as indicated on the glass equipment.

The type of per cent solution should be ascertained first, as a different type used instead of the required way would cause substantial error ultimately, for instance, a 50 per cent w/w solution of sodium hydroxide is 75 per cent w/v; similarly a 22½ per cent w/v solution of sodium sulphate is only 10 per cent w/w.

Part Dilutions

In this method, the dilution is expressed as that part of the whole volume into which one part (or more parts) of the solution is dissolved, e.g. WBC dilution is 1:20, implying that there is one volume or part of blood in 20 volumes or parts of final solution, though actually mixed with 19 volumes or parts of the diluting fluid.

Molar Solutions

A molar solution contains the molecular weight of the solute (dissolved substance) in grams per litre of solution. The molecular weight is found by adding the atomic weights of the different atoms present in the compound.

Example: The molecular weight of sodium chloride is 58.454. Hence, 1 molar solution of the salt contains 58.454 grams of NaCl in one litre.

Formula to convert a percentage solution into a mol/L solution:

$$\text{mol/L solution} = \frac{\text{gm\% (w/v) solution} \times 10}{\text{molecular weight of substance}}$$

To change a normal solution into a mol/L solution:

$$\text{mol/L solution} = \frac{\text{Normality of solution}}{\text{valence of substance}}$$

Normal Solutions

A normal solution is one which contains the gram equivalent weight (equivalent weight in grams) of a substance per litre of solution. The equivalent weight is the number of units of the substance which will combine with or replace a single unit of hydrogen, 35.5 units of chlorine, 8 units of oxygen, etc., or the number of units of that substance which will contain a single unit of hydrogen, 35.5 units of chlorine, 8 units of oxygen, etc.

1. The equivalent weight of an element is calculated by dividing the atomic weight by the valency (valency is the number of atoms of hydrogen one atom of the element will combine with or displace).

   Example: The atomic weight of sulphur is 32.006 and its valency is 2, the equivalent weight would be 32.006/2 = 16.003.

2. The equivalent weight of an acid is the weight of it in grams which contains 1.008 gm (one atomic weight) of replaceable hydrogen. It is calculated by dividing the molecular weight by the number of replaceable hydrogen atoms in the molecule.

   Example: The molecular weight of sulphuric acid (H_2SO_4) is 98.082 and the number of replaceable hydrogen atoms is 2, hence its equivalent weight would be 98.082/2 = 49.041.

3. Equivalent weight of an alkali is that weight of it which will neutralize the equivalent weight of an acid. It is calculated by dividing the molecular weight by the number of OH^-(hydroxyl) radicals in the molecule.

   Example: Calcium hydroxide; Ca $(OH)_2$, has a molecular weight of 91.014 and 2 hydroxyl groups, its equivalent weight would be 91.014/2 = 45.507.

4. Equivalent weight of a salt is calculated by dividing its molecular weight by the number of metal ions (cations) per molecule, multiplied by the valence of the ion (cation).

   Example: Sodium sulphate has a molecular weight of 142.060, has 2 cations and the valency of the cation is one, hence its equivalent weight would be:

   $$\frac{142.060 \times 1}{2} = 71.030$$

Saturated solution: In these the weight of the solute is not specified nor is the volume of the solvent. It states that it contains as much as will dissolve.

Standard solution: These are solutions, the exact strength of which is known and are used for comparing strengths of other similar solutions.

Period	1 1A 1A	2 IIA 2A	3 IIIB 3B	4 IVB 4B	5 VB 5B	6 VIB 6B	7 VIIB 7B	8 — —	9 VIII 8	10 — —	11 1B 1B	12 IIB 2B	13 IIIA 3A	14 IVA 4A	15 VA 5A	16 VIA 6A	17 VIIA 7A	18 vIIIA 8A
1	1 H 1.008										Atomic Number Atomic Symbol Atomic mass							2 He 4.003
2	3 Li 6.941	4 Be 9.012											5 B 10.81	6 C 12.01	7 N 14.01	8 O 16.00	9 F 19.00	10 Ne 20.18
3	11 Na 22.99	12 Mg 24.31											13 Al 26.98	14 Si 28.09	15 P 30.97	16 S 32.07	17 Cl 35.45	18 Ar 39.95
4	19 K 39.10	20 Ca 40.08	21 Sc 44.96	22 Ti 47.88	23 V 50.94	24 Cr 52.00	25 Mn 54.94	26 Fe 55.85	27 Co 58.93	28 Ni 58.69	29 Cu 63.55	30 Zn 65.39	31 Ga 69.72	32 Ge 72.59	33 As 74.92	34 Se 78.96	35 Br 79.90	36 Kr 83.80
5	37 Rb 85.47	38 Sr 87.62	39 Y 88.91	40 Zr 91.22	41 Nb 92.91	42 Mo 95.94	43 Tc (98)	44 Ru 101.1	45 Rh 102.9	46 Pd 106.4	47 Ag 107.9	48 Cd 112.4	49 In 114.8	50 Sn 118.7	51 Sb 121.8	52 Te 127.6	53 I 126.9	54 Xe 131.3
6	55 Cs 132.9	56 Ba 137.3	57 La *138.9	72 Hf 178.5	73 Ta 180.9	74 W 183.9	75 Re 186.2	76 Os 190.2	77 Ir 190.2	78 Pt 195.1	79 Au 197.0	80 Hg 200.5	81 Tl 204.4	82 Pb 207.2	83 Bi 209.0	84 Po (210)	85 At (210)	86 Rn (222)
7	87 Fr (223)	88 Ra (226)	89 Ac ~(227)	104 Rf (257)	105 Db (260)	106 Sg (263)	107 Bh (262)	108 Hs (265)	109 Mt (266)	110 Ds (271)	111 Uuu (272)	112 Uub (277)		114 Uuq (296)		116 Uuh (298)		118 Uuo (?)
Lanthanide Series*			58 Ce 140.1	59 Pr 140.9	60 Nd 144.2	61 Pm (147)	62 Sm 150.4	63 Eu 152.0	64 Gd 157.3	65 Tb 158.9	66 Dy 162.5	67 Ho 164.9	68 Er 167.3	69 Tm 168.9	70 Yb 173.0	71 Lu 175.0		
Actinide Series~Th			90 Pa 232.0	91 U (231)	92 Np (238)	93 Pu (237)	94 Am (242)	95 Cm (243)	96 Bk (247)	97 Cf (247)	98 Es (249)	99 Fm (254)	100 Md (253)	101 No (256)	102 Lr (254)	103 (257)		

List of Periodic Table Elements Sorted by Atomic Number

No.	Atomic Weight	Name	Symbol	MP (°C)	BP (°C)	Density* (g/cm^3)	Earth crust (%)*
1	1.0079	Hydrogen	H	–259	–253	0.09	0.14
2	4.0026	Helium	He	–272	–269	0.18	
3	6.941	Lithium	Li	180	1347	0.53	
4	9.0122	Beryllium	Be	1278	2970	1.85	
5	10.811	Boron	B	2300	2550	2.34	
6	12.0107	Carbon	C	3500	4827	2.26	0.094
7	14.0067	Nitrogen	N	–210	–196	1.25	
8	15.9994	Oxygen	O	–218	–183	1.43	46.71
9	18.9984	Fluorine	F	–220	–188	1.7	0.029
10	20.1797	Neon	Ne	–249	–246	0.9	
11	22.9897	Sodium	Na	98	883	0.97	2.75
12	24.305	Magnesium	Mg	639	1090	1.74	2.08
13	26.9815	Aluminium	Al	660	2467	2.7	8.07
14	28.0855	Silicon	Si	1410	2355	2.33	27.69
15	30.9738	Phosphorus	P	44	280	1.82	0.13
16	32.065	Sulfur	S	113	445	2.07	0.052
17	35.453	Chlorine	Cl	–101	–35	3.21	0.045
18	39.948	Argon	Ar	–189	–186	1.78	
19	39.0983	Potassium	K	64	774	0.86	2.58
20	40.078	Calcium	Ca	839	1484	1.55	3.65
21	44.9559	Scandium	Sc	1539	2832	2.99	
22	47.867	Titanium	Ti	1660	3287	4.54	0.62
23	50.9415	Vanadium	V	1890	3380	6.11	
24	51.9961	Chromium	Cr	1857	2672	7.19	0.035
25	54.938	Manganese	Mn	1245	1962	7.43	0.09
26	55.845	Iron	Fe	1535	2750	7.87	5.05
27	58.9332	Cobalt	Co	1495	2870	8.9	
28	58.6934	Nickel	Ni	1453	2732	8.9	0.019
29	63.546	Copper	Cu	1083	2567	8.96	
30	65.39	Zinc	Zn	420	907	7.13	
31	69.723	Gallium	Ga	30	2403	5.91	
32	72.64	Germanium	Ge	937	2830	5.32	
33	74.9216	Arsenic	As	81	613	5.72	
34	78.96	Selenium	Se	217	685	4.79	
35	79.904	Bromine	Br	–7	59	3.12	
36	83.8	Krypton	Kr	–157	–153	3.75	
37	85.4678	Rubidium	Rb	39	688	1.63	
38	87.62	Strontium	Sr	769	1384	2.54	
39	88.9059	Yttrium	Y	1523	3337	4.47	
40	91.224	Zirconium	Zr	1852	4377	6.51	0.025
41	92.9064	Niobium	Nb	2468	4927	8.57	
42	95.94	Molybdenum	Mo	2617	4612	10.22	
43	*98	Technetium	Tc	2200	4877	11.5	
44	101.07	Ruthenium	Ru	2250	3900	12.37	
45	102.9055	Rhodium	Rh	1966	3727	12.41	
46	106.42	Palladium	Pd	1552	2927	12.02	
47	107.8682	Silver	Ag	962	2212	10.5	
48	112.411	Cadmium	Cd	321	765	8.65	
49	114.818	Indium	In	157	2000	7.31	
50	118.71	Tin	Sn	232	2270	7.31	

Contd...

Contd...

51	121.76	Antimony	Sb	630	1750	6.68	
52	127.6	Tellurium	Te	449	990	6.24	
53	126.9045	Iodine	I	114	184	4.93	
54	131.293	Xenon	Xe	–112	–108	5.9	
55	132.9055	Cesium	Cs	29	678	1.87	
56	137.327	Barium	Ba	725	1140	3.59	0.05
57	138.9055	Lanthanum	La	920	3469	6.15	
58	140.116	Cerium	Ce	795	3257	6.77	
59	140.9077	Praseodymium	Pr	935	3127	6.77	
60	144.24	Neodymium	Nd	1010	3127	7.01	
61*	145	Promethium	Pm	1100	3000	7.3	
62	150.36	Samarium	Sm	1072	1900	7.52	
63	151.964	Europium	Eu	822	1597	5.24	
64	157.25	Gadolinium	Gd	1311	3233	7.9	
65	158.9253	Terbium	Tb	1360	3041	8.23	
66	162.5	Dysprosium	Dy	1412	2562	8.55	
67	164.9303	Holmium	Ho	1470	2720	8.8	
68	167.259	Erbium	Er	1522	2510	9.07	
69	168.9342	Thulium	Tm	1545	1727	9.32	
70	173.04	Ytterbium	Yb	824	1466	6.9	
71	174.967	Lutetium	Lu	1656	3315	9.84	
72	178.49	Hafnium	Hf	2150	5400	13.31	
73	180.9479	Tantalum	Ta	2996	5425	16.65	
74	183.84	Tungsten	W	3410	5660	19.35	
75	186.207	Rhenium	Re	3180	5627	21.04	
76	190.23	Osmium	Os	3045	5027	22.6	
77	192.217	Iridium	Ir	2410	4527	22.4	
78	195.078	Platinum	Pt	1772	3827	21.45	
79	196.9665	Gold	Au	1064	2807	19.32	
80	200.59	Mercury	Hg	–39	357	13.55	
81	204.3833	Thallium	Ti	303	1457	11.85	
82	207.2	Lead	Pb	327	1740	11.35	
83	208.9804	Bismuth	Bi	271	1560	9.75	
84	*209	Polonium	Po	254	962	9.3	
85	*210	Astatine	At	302	337		
86	*222	Radon	Rn	–71	–62	9.73	
87	*223	Francium	Fr	27	677		
88	*226	Radium	Ra	700	1737	5.5	
89	*227	Actinium	Ac	1050	3200	10.07	
90	232.0381	Thorium	Th	1750	4790	11.72	
91	231.0359	Protactinium	Pa	1568		15.4	
92	238.0289	Uranium	U	1132	3818	18.95	
93	*237	Neptunium	Np	640	3902	20.2	
94	*244	Plutonium	Pu	640	3235	19.84	
95	*243	Americium	Am	994	2607	13.67	
96	*247	Curium	Cm	1340		13.5	
97	*247	Berkelium	Bk	986		14.78	
98	*251	Californium	Cf	900		15.1	
99	*252	Einsteinium	Es	860			
100	*257	Fermium	Fm	1527			
101	*258	Medelevium	Md				
102	*259	Nobelium	No	827			
103	*262	Lawrencium	Lr	1627			
104	*261	Rutherfordium	Rf				
105	*262	Dubnium	Db				

Contd...

Contd...

106	*266	Seaborgium	Sg
107	*264	Bohrium	Bh
108	*277	Hassium	Hs
109	*268	Meitnerium	Mt

Abbreviations and Definition

No. – Atomic Number
M.P. – melting point
B.P. – boiling point

- Density of elements with boiling points below 0°C is given in g/1
- Earth crust composition average values are from a report by F.W. Clarke and HS Washington, 1924. Elemental composition of crustal rocks differ between different localities.
- Group: There are only 18 groups in the periodic table that constitute the columns of the table. Lanthanoids and Actinoids are numbered as 101 and 102 to separate them in sorting by group.

Atomic number: The number of protons in an atom each element is uniquely defined by its atomic number.

Atomic mass: The mass of an atom is primarily determined by the number of protons and neutrons in its nucleus. Atomic mass is measured in Atomic Mass Units (amu) which are scaled relative to carbon, 12C, that is taken as a standard element with an atomic mass of 12. This isotope of carbon has 6 protons and 6 neutrons. Thus, each proton and neutron has a mass of about 1 amu.

Isotope: Atoms of the same element with the same atomic number, but different number of neutrons. Isotope of an element is defined by the sum of the number of protons and neutrons in its nucleus. Elements have more than on isotope with varying numbers of neutrons. For example, there are two common isotopes of carbon, 12C and 13C which have 6 and 7 neutrons respectively. The abundances of different isotopes of elements vary in nature depending on the source of materials. For relative abundances of isotopes in nature see reference on Isotopic Composition of the Elements.

Atomic weight: Atomic weight values represent weighted average of the masses of all naturally occurring isotopes of an element. The values shown here are based on the IUPAC Commission determinations (Pure Appl. Chem. 73:667-683, 2001). The elements marked with an asterisk have no stable nuclides. For these elements the weight value shown represents the mass number of the longest-lived isotope of the element.

Electron configuration: The distribution of electrons according to the energy sublevels (subshells) in uncharged atoms. The noble gas shown in square brackets (e.g. [He]), marks that all the subshells associated with that element are fully occupied by electrons.

CHAPTER 5

Urine Analysis

COMPOSITION OF URINE

Urine composition is affected mainly by three factors:

1. Nutritional status
2. State of metabolic processes
3. Ability of the kidney to selectively handle the material presented to it.

Physicochemical Characteristics of Urine

Dry weight	55-70 gm/24 hr
Osmolality	38-1400 mOsm/kg water (Average = 500-800 mOsm/kg water)
pH	4.6-8.0 (mean = 6.1)
Specific gravity	
Neonates	1.012
Infants	1.002-1.006
Adults	1.003-1.030
Volume:	Per day
Neonates	30-60 ml
10-60 days	250-450 ml
60-365 days	400-500 ml
Children	
1-3 years	500-600 ml
3-5 years	600-700 ml
5-8 years	650-1000 ml
8-14 years	800-1400 ml

Adults	600-2500 ml (Avg: 1200 ml)

Inorganic Constituents per 24 Hours

Iron	0.06-0.1 mg
Chlorides	6 (4-10) gm on usual diet
Sodium	4 gm on usual diet
Phosphate	0.8-1.3 gm on usual diet
Sulphur	2 gm
Calcium	< 150 mg.

Organic Constituents per 24 Hours

Nitrogenous—total	25-35 gm
Urea	15-30 gm
Creatinine	1.4 (1-1.8) gm
Ammonia	0.7 (0.3-1) gm
Uric acid	0.45 (0.3-0.6) gm
Protein (albumin)	0-0.1 gm
Creatine, in children	10-50 mg (Excreted in urine in adults in hepatic or muscle disorders or thyrotoxicosis)
Glucose Fasting range	2-20 mg% (Diabetic may lose up to 100 gm/day)
Amylase (diastase)	40-260 units/hour.

Cells and Casts

	Range	*Mean*
RBC	up to 1 million /day (more in females)	130,000/day
Casts hyaline and occasionally granular	up to 5,000/day	2,000/day
Leucocytes	up to 5 million /hour (more in females)	108,000/hr, females; 28,000/hr, males
Epithelial cells	up to 2.5 lakh /hour (more in males)	68,000/hr, females;78,000/hr. males.
Squamous epithelial variable.		

Collection of Urine

The urine sample should be collected in a clean, dry container and should be examined fresh. For cultures sterile containers should be used. With time, RBC, and leucocytes tend to be destroyed due to hypotonicity of the urine. Casts too tend to get decomposed. Bacterial contamination of stale urine is frequent and causes alkalinization of the urine due to conversion of urea to ammonia and loss of glucose. This rise in pH accelerates loss of leucocytes and epithelial cells. For ordinary qualitative, tests a random sample is enough. For diabetes mellitus, a 2 hour postprandial sample is desirable; for nephritis, a morning specimen is best as it has higher specific gravity and lower pH desirable for preservation of formed elements.

Repeated samples are necessary sometimes, as for orthostatic proteinuria.

Whenever needed, a 24 hour urine should be collected in a large container. Have patient void and discard urine at any particular time, save all urine for the next 24 hours, and then void at the same hour to finish the collection.

Preservation of Specimen

Urinary decomposition occurs quickly in warm temperatures. Hence, fresh specimens should be examined, if not, then it should be refrigerated. As far as possible, the need for preservation should not arise. However, the following preservatives can be used:

1. *Toluol* best for preservation of chemical constituents. Add 2 ml toluol/100 ml urine.
2. *Thymol* a small floating lump of thymol can preserve the urine for several days in a bottle. Thymol may, however, cause a false-positive reaction for protein.
3. *Formalin* 1 drop/30 ml urine. Is good for preserving formed elements. It can precipitate proteins and can reduce Benedict's solution.
4. *Boric acid* 0.3 gm/120 ml of urine. However, yeasts can still grow and uric acid crystals get precipitated.

GROSS EXAMINATION OF URINE

Colour and Appearance

Normal urine is clear and pale yellow (straw) in colour.

1. *Colourless* Dilution; diabetes mellitus/insipidus, nervousness, diuretic or alcohol intake.
2. *Milky* Purulent genitourinary tract disease; chyluria.

3. *Orange* Urobilinogenuria, fever, excessive sweating, concentrated urine.
4. *Red* Beet root ingestion, haematuria, haemoglobinuria, phenophthalein, pyridium, sulfonal.
5. *Greenish* Jaundice, phenol poisoning.
6. *Dirty blue or green* Putrefying urine, in typhus or cholera, methylene blue.
7. *Dark brown, brown red, or yellow* Very concentrated urine. Acute febrile diseases. Bilirubinuria.
8. *Brown-yellow or brown red (if acidic) or bright red (if alkaline)* Due to rhubarb, cascara, aloes.
9. *Brown, brown black or black* Haemorrhage in urinary tract if urine is acidic (Acid-haematin); haemoglobinuria; porphyria, methaemoglobinuria; myoglobinuria, melanin, phenol poisoning, homogentisic acid (alkaptonuria). In porphyria, urine turns dark brown on exposure to sunlight or boiling.

Interfering Factors

- Normally, urine darkens on standing. This occurs because of oxidation of urobilinogen to urobilin. Decomposition of urine commences in half an hour.
- Some foods cause change in urine colour
  - Beets turn the urine red
  - Rhubarb changes colour of urine to brown
- Many drugs are also responsible for urinary colour change
  - Cascara and senna laxatives in acidic urine will turn the urine reddish-brown, in alkaline urine they will turn the urine red
  - Phenazopyridine (pyridium), amido-pyrine turn urine orange in colour
  - Pyridium, ethoxazene turn urine to orange/ orange red
  - Orange to purple red may occur due to chlorzoxazome
  - Salicylazosulfapyridine, anisindone, or phenindione turn urine colour to orange-yellow in alkaline urine
  - Sulphonamides and nitrofurantoins produce rust-yellow to brownish colour
  - Dilantin (dephenydantoin) dioctyl calcium sulphosuccinate, phenolphthalein and phenothiazine turn urine colour to pink to red or red-brown
  - Phenolphthalein may also produce magenta colour
  - Amidopyrine, pyridium, aniline dyes, BSP, PSP in alkaline urine or phenophthalein and pyridium in acid urine or deferoxamine can produce red urine.
  - Phenolphthalein in alkaline urine produces purple red colour
  - Phenylhydrazine and phenolic drugs produce dark brown urine
  - Cascara may produce brown-black urine
  - Riboflavin or pyridium in alkaline urine produce bright yellow colour
  - Methylene blue and amitriptyline produce blue or green coloured urine
  - Levodopa causes urine to darken on standing
  - Iron salt consumption produces dark coloured urine
  - Phenothiazine tranquilizers cause pink to brown colour
  - Triametrene causes pale blue coloured urine.

Reaction

Average range: 4.6-8, Average pH = 6.0

Litmus paper or other pH indicator papers broad range (pH 1-12 or narrow range pH papers) can be used. Another simple method is to add 2 drops of 0.4% alcoholic solution of methyl red to 5 ml of urine. Note the colour change—if red = acidic; orange = neutral; yellow = alkaline. Digital electronic pH meters for better accuracy can be used—here, the electrode is dipped in urine and pH read off directly from the digital display.

Amongst urinary tract infections, *Escherichia coli* produces acidic urine, while *Proteus* (urea splitting) produces alkaline urine. Meat protein diet causes urinary acidification, while consumption of citrus fruits makes the urine alkaline.

Urine pH

Finding and condition	Causes and comments.

Acidic Urine

Ketosis	Diabetes, starvation, febrile illness in children.
Systemic acidosis	Except with impaired renal tubular function, respiratory or metabolic

Acidification	acidosis provokes intense urine acidity and decreased NH_4^+ excretion. Use in treating urinary tract infections, and to prevent precipitation of calcium carbonate or phosphates or magnesium ammonium phosphate.

Alkaline Urine

Postprandial Alkaline tide	Normal finding in specimens voided shortly after meals.
Vegetarianism	Meats produce fixed acid residue, vegetarian diet does not.
Systemic	As may occur in severe vomiting, hyperventilation, excess alkali ingestion.
Urinary tract infection	*Proteus* or *Pseudomonas* infections, they split urea to HCO_3^- and ammonia.
Alkalinization	Used to prevent crystallization of uric acid, oxalate, cystine, sulphonamides, streptomycin.
Stale specimen	Bacterial overgrowth. If true infection exists, the sediment should show pus cells.
Renal tubular	Impaired tubular acidification causes inappropriately high urine pH with systemic acidosis and low serum HCO_3^-.

Interfering Factors

- On standing, urinary pH becomes alkaline because CO_2 will diffuse into the air
- Alkaline urine specimens tend to cause hemolysis of red cells and disappearance of casts
- High protein diets will cause excessively acidic urine
- Ammonium chloride and mandalic acid may produce acidic urines
- Alkaline urine after meals is a normal response to the secretions of HCl in gastric juices
- Sodium bicarbonate, potassium citrate, and acetazolamide may produce alkaline urines.

Be Careful

- Only a freshly voided sample is suitable for measuring pH. Refrigerate the sample if any delay is expected
- Alkaline urine occurs from vegetarian diets, citrus fruits, milk and other dairy products
- Highly concentrated urine such as that formed in hot, dry environments is strongly acidic and may be irritating
- While sleeping, decreased pulmonary ventilation causes respiratory acidosis and urine becomes highly acidic
- Chlorothiazide diuretic will cause acidic urine to be excreted
- Bacterial contamination and overgrowth will result in alkaline urine. Bacteria in urine will convert to ammonia.

Odour

Important in fresh specimens only and is aromatic because of volatile fatty acids. Bacterial action causes ammoniacal odour, while ketosis leads to a fruity odour in urine.

Specific Gravity

It depends upon the concentration of various solutes in the urine.

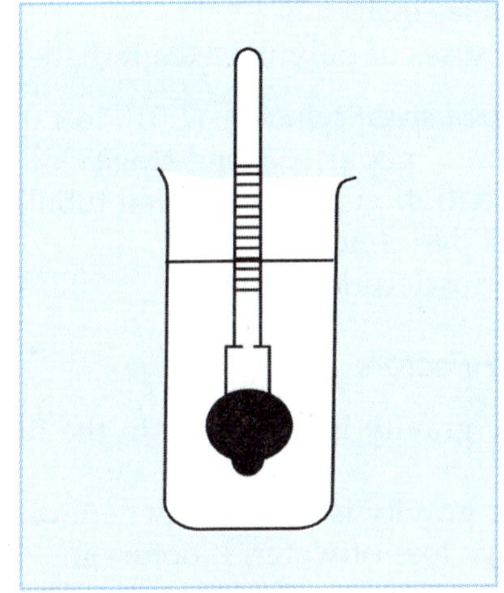

Fig. 5.1: Urinometer

1. *Urinometer:* Urine should be foamless. Transfer urine (about 70-80 ml) into the urinometer container and let the urinometer float freely without touching the sides or the bottom of the container (Fig. 5.1). Read graduations at the lowest level of urinary meniscus. If the urine amount is less, dilute the urine to raise the volume till 70-80 ml, take the reading and multiply the last two digits by the dilution factor.
2. *Refractometer:* Only small amount of urine is needed. It measures the concentration of solutes

(related to refractive index). In Goldberg refractometer the specific gravity of urine can be read directly from the calibration.
3. Can be tested with *Dipsticks* also.
4. *Osmometry:* Give the most accurate assessment.

Correction factor for temperature: While using urinometer, add or subtract 0.001 for each 3°C above or below the standardization temperature of the instrument.

Urines of low specific gravity are called hyposthenuric (< 1.007) while urines of fixed specific gravity of about 1.010 are known as isothenuric.

High specific gravity
- Excessive sweating
- Glycosuria
- Acute nephritis
- Albuminuria
- All causes of oliguria

Low specific gravity: (less than 1.010)
- Excessive water intake
- Chronic nephritis
- Diabetes insipidus
- All causes of polyuria except diabetes mellitus

Low and fixed specific gravity: (1.010 to 1.012)
- Chronic nephritis (end-stage kidney) when concentration power of renal tubules is low
- ADH deficiency
- Arteriosclerotic kidney

Interfering Factors

- Specific gravity is maximum in the first morning sample
- Specific gravity is increased whenever there is an excessive loss of water. It occurs in:
  - sweating
  - fever
  - vomiting
  - diarrhoea
- Drugs leading to false positive:
  - Dextran
  - Radiopaque contrast media used in X-rays of the urinary tract.
- Temperature of urine specimens affects specific gravity when specific gravity is measured in urine removed from the refrigerator. Specific gravity will be falsely higher.
- Reagent strip testing of urine containing glucosed urea greater than 1% may cause a low specific gravity. Highly buffered alkaline urine may also cause a low reading.
- Elevated reading may occur in presence of moderate (100-750 mg/dl) amounts of proteinuria.

Urinary Volume

The average 24 hour urinary output in an adult is around 1200 to 1500 ml and the night urine should not be more than 400 ml.

A volume more than 2000 ml is termed *polyuria. Oliguria* implies excretion of urine less than 500 ml and *anuria* is complete cessation. *Nocturia* is excretion by an adult of urine more than 500 ml with a specific gravity of less than 1.018 at night (characteristic of chronic glomerulonephritis).

Polyuria

- Neurotic polydipsia.
- Diabetes mellitus/insipidus
- Diuretics
- Intravenous saline/glucose
- Chronic renal failure
- Addison's disease, decrease of adrenocortical hormones.

Oliguria

- Dehydration:
  - vomiting
  - diarrhoea
  - excessive sweating
- Renal ischaemia
- Acute renal tubular necrosis
- Acute glomerulonephritis
- Obstruction to urinary outflow

Turbidity

Normal value—fresh urine is clear

The appearance of cloudy urine provides a warning of possible abnormality such as the presence of pus, RBCs or bacteria. Sometimes, however, excretion of cloudy urine may not be abnormal since the change in urine pH may cause precipitation within the bladder of normal urinary constituents. Alkaline urine may appear cloudy because of presence of phosphates, and urine may appear cloudy because of urates.
- Pathologic urines are often turbid or cloudy, but so are many normal urines. Cloudy urine may appear from precipitation of crystals due to rapid cooling of the urine.

- Occasionally, urine turbidity may result from urinary tract infections.
- Abnormal urines may be cloudy on account of presence of RBCs, pus cells or bacteria.

Interfering Factors

- After ingestion of food, urates or phosphates may produce cloudiness in normal urine.
- Vaginal contamination in female patients is often a cause of turbidity
- Greasy cloudiness may be caused by lipiduria
- Many normal urines will develop haziness or turbidity after being refrigerated or on standing at room temperature.

CHEMICAL EXAMINATION OF URINE

Tests for Protein

Normal values—Negative (2-8 mg/dl)
If urine is not clear—filter or centrifuge the specimen.
Both bile and protein cause urine to froth.

Heat and Acetic acid Test

Take a test tube 2/3rd full with urine, boil upper portion of urine for 2 minutes (lower portion is not heated so that it can be used as a control for comparing). Now turbidity can arise because of phosphates, carbonates or protein. Add a few drops of 10% acetic acid, persistence or development of turbidity implies proteinuria.

False-positive tests may occur with X-ray contrast media and tolbutamide derivatives. Sensitivity = 5-10 mg%

Interpretation

- — No cloudiness.
- ± Cloudiness barely visible
- \+ Definite cloudiness, but no granularity and no flocculation.
- ++ Granular cloudiness, but no flocculation. Seen from above, the cloud is dense but not opaque. Protein content = about 0.1%.
- +++ Dense opaque cloud, clearly flocculated. About 0.2-0.3% protein.
- ++++ Very thick precipitation, almost a solid. Protein concentration > 0.5%.

Sulphosalicylic Acid Test

Urine should be clear and acid.

To 1 ml of urine, add 3 drops of 20% sulfosalicylic acid.

Absence of cloudiness means absence of protein. If the turbidity persists after boiling, it is due to protein. If the cloudiness vanishes on heating and reappears on cooling, it is due to Bence Jones (BJ) protein.

False-positive test may appear if the urine contains tolbutamide derivatives, high concentration of penicillin or X-ray contrast media.

Paper Strip Method

Paper strips impregnated with Bromphenol blue and salicylate buffer are dipped in urine. Presence of protein is indicated by change of colour from light yellow to blue. Tolbutamide, X-ray contrast media and preservatives do not react, hence no false-positive tests. However, highly alkaline urine may cause a false-positive test; (sensitivity—30 mgm% or more). Tablets of similar reagents producing the same colour are also available.

Quantitative Estimation of Protein in Urine

1. *Turbidimetric and chemical procedures:* Provide an accurate estimation. Colorimetric readings taken against blanks and calculations done accordingly give the result (example; sulphosalicylic acid turbidity method).
2. *Esbach's quantitative method*: Acidify the urine if necessary. Cover the bottom of the Esbach tube with pumice, fill urine till the 'U' mark and add Esbach's or Tsuchiya's regent till the 'R' mark. Stopper the tube and invert it about a dozen times slowly.

Set the tube vertically and read after 30 minutes (if pumice has not been used, read after 24 hours). The tube is graduated to read in per cent or in grams of protein per liter at the top of the sediment. Urine may be diluted for obtaining greater accuracy. After diluting, the Esbach tube reading may be multiplied by the dilution factor (Fig. 5.2). Dilutions can be made according to the specific gravity as follows:

1. 1.010 to 1.014—1:1 dilution.
2. 1.015 to 1.021—1:2: : urine : water.
3. 1.022 or more—1:3: : urine : water.
4. If the qualitative test reading is +++, dilute as 1:4::urine : water.

Bence Jones Protein Tests

Seen in multiple myeloma classically.

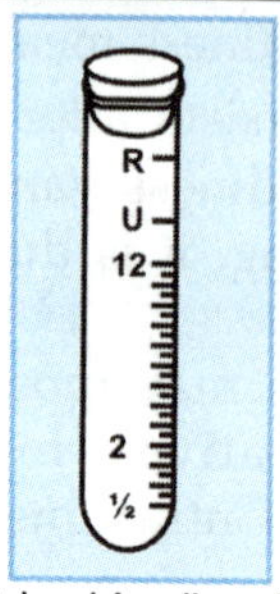

Fig. 5.2: Esbach's albuminometer

1. *Heat and sulphosalicylic acid:* As for albumin, the precipitate formed will contain both BJ proteins and albumin. Mix the specimen of urine with the precipitate and divide equally in two test tubes. Place both in a water bath and heat to boiling. Remove one from the bath, cool to below 40°C and compare the turbidity in the two tubes in good light against a dark background. Cool the other hot tube and heat the cold one and compare again. If the cold tube both the times shows persistently a more densely turbid flocculum of protein, BJ protein is most likely present. If albumin is present also, add 10% acetic acid to a fresh urine sample (pH to be less than 6.0) and bring to boil, keep shaking and break the floc the BJ protein goes into solution. Filter off albumin while it is still hot, BJ proteins will come in the filtrate. Repeat the sulphosalicylic acid test as described above.
2. *Toluenesulfonic acid:* Add 1 ml of TSA reagent to 2 ml of urine, let the reagent flow slowly by the side of the test tube. Mix. A precipitate appearing within 5 minutes indicates presence of BJ protein. A negative test excludes.

   Sensitivity > 500 mg%.
3. *Electrophoresis:* of concentrated urine for proteins would show the dense gammaglobulin band.

Bence Jones protein is often seen in multiple myeloma and rarely in chronic leukemia, osteomalacia, osteosarcoma, cancer metastases to bone, and hypertension.

Interpretation of Proteinuria

Minimal proteinuria (< 0.5 gm/day)

- Following exercise or in highly concentrated urine, in healthy persons
- Fever, severe emotional/thermal stress, in otherwise healthy persons
- Postural proteinuria; young adults may pass protein while ambulatory but not while lying
- Hypertension
- Renal tubular dysfunction, including genetic and drug-induced
- Polycystic kidneys
- Lower urinary tract infections
- Hemoglobinuria with severe haemolysis.

Moderate proteinuria (0.5-3 gm/day)

- Chronic glomerulonephritis, moderate.
- Congestive heart failure
- Diabetic nephropathy, mild.
- Pyelonephritis
- Multiple myeloma
- Pre-eclampsia

Marked proteinuria (> 3 gm/day)

- Acute glomerulonephritis.
- Chronic glomerulonephritis, severe
- Lipoid nephrosis } & other causes of nephrotic syndrome
- Severe diabetic nephropathy }
- Renal amyloidosis
- Lupus nephritis

Nonrenal causes of proteinuria

- Fever
- Trauma
- Severe anaemias and leukemia
- Toxaemia
- Abdominal tumours
- Convulsive disorders
- Hyperthyroidism
- Intestinal obstruction
- Cardiac disease
- Poisoning from turpentine, phosphorus, mercury, sulfosalicylic acid, lead, phenol, opiates and drug therapy.

Other Important Related Aspects

- Large numbers of leucocytes accompanying proteinuria usually imply infection at some level in the urinary tract. Large numbers of leucocytes and erythrocytes usually indicate a non-infectious inflammatory disease of glomerulus. Proteins with pyelonephritis may have as many RBCs as white blood cells.

- Proteinuria does not necessarily always accompany renal diseases. Pyelonephritis, obstructions, nephrolithiasis, tumours and congenital malformation can cause severe illness without causing protein leakage.
- Proteinuria is associated with the finding of casts on the sediment examination as protein is necessary for cast formation.
- Postural proteinuria is the excretion of protein by patients who are standing or moving during daytime. This proteinuria is intermittent and disappears when the patient lies down. Postural proteinuria has an incidence of 3% to 5% of all normal healthy subjects.

Collecting specimen for orthostatic proteinuria

1. Instruct the patient to void at bedtime and discard sample.
2. Next morning sample is collected immediately as the patient awakes and assumes a standing posture.
3. A second specimen is collected after the patient has been standing or walking for a considerable period of time.

Differentiation from other types of proteinuria is done by testing for protein in two urine specimens; one collected before and one after the person is erect. In postural proteinuria the first sample would be devoid of protein while second one would be positive.

Interfering Factors

a. Functional, mild and transitory protein in the urine, because of renal vasoconstriction, is associated with:
   - Violent exercise
   - Severe emotional stress
   - Cold baths
b. Increased protein in urine occurs:
   - After eating large amounts of protein
   - In pregnancy or immediately following delivery
   - In neonates
   - In premenstrual state
   - In orthostatic proteinuria
c. False or accidental proteinuria may occur because of a mixture of pus and RBCs in urinary tract infections and the menstrual flow.
d. False-positive results can occur from incorrect use and assessment of colour strip test.
   - Prolonged dipping or allowing the strip to be held too long in the urine stream.
   - Failing to accurately match the reactive area with the colour chart.
e. Alkaline urine can give a false-positive test on the colour strip test due to alkaline, highly buffered urine.
f. A very dilute urine may give a falsely low protein value.
g. Drugs that may cause false-positive tests for protein (acid turbidity methods only) include:
   - Gold
   - Arsenic
   - Sodium bicarbonate
   - Acetazolamide
   - Radiopaque contrast media for up to 3 days (no false positives with dipsticks, only with sulphosalicylic acid test)
   - Sulfisoxazole
   - Thymol
   - Chlorpromazine
   - This list includes many other drugs also.

MECHANISMS OF PROTEINURIA

a. *Glomerular proteinuria:* There may be increased filtration of plasma proteins when there is disruption of normal glomerular capillary permeability, as occurs with antigen-antibody, with infiltrative processes such as amyloid or with ischaemic glomerular injury.
b. *Tubular proteinuria:* There is increased renal excretion of plasma protein in the presence of normal glomerular permeability, increased filtered load of small proteins, light chain proteinurias, multiple myeloma.
   Normal filtered load of small proteins with a decreased capacity for tubular absorption of these proteins. Chronic cadmium poisoning, Fanconi's syndrome, cystinosis, and some patients with Wilson's disease.
c. *Postglomerular proteinuria:* There is secretion of protein by the structures of upper and lower urinary tract in response to infection or the presence of renal calculi.

MICROALBUMINURIA

Definition

Microalbuminuria is the earliest sign of nephropathy before it manifests overtly as proteinuria, a condition where significant kidney damage has already occurred.

Microalbuminuria is classified as:

- Albumin excretion rate: 20-200 μg/min or 30-300 mg/day
- Albumin/Creatinine ratio: 2.5-25 mg/mmol
- Albumin/ Creatinine ratio: 30-300 mg/g
- Albumin concentration (early morning urine): 30-300 mg/L

Microalbuminuria can only be detected by specific immunochemical assays for urinary albumin using antibodies to human albumin. The existing biochemical tests for detection of microprotein are nonspecific as they also detect other proteins apart from albumin.

Although dye binding and protein precipitation assays have been described, these are insensitive and nonspecific and should not be used.

Microalbuminuria: Diagnostic Relevance

Microalbuminuria indicates high probability of damage of the glomerular filtration capacity of the kidney and is of great diagnostic relevance;

- in diabetic patients for early diagnosis of nephropathy,
- in hypertensive patients as indicator of end organ damage associated with lower life expectancy, and
- is probably associated with cardiovascular diseases in general population.

MICROALBUMINURIA DETECTION

It is recommended in the following subjects.

Diabetic Subjects

- Insulin-dependent diabetes mellitus (IDDM): Annually in all patients suffering from diabetes for 5 years or more and over 12 years of age
- Noninsulin-dependent diabetes mellitus (NIDDM): As soon as diabetes is diagnosed, and at regular intervals (1-2 times) annually thereafter incase of negative test results.

Nondiabetic Subjects

- All patients with potential disease involvement of the kidneys for early diagnosis.
- Patients at risk of cardiovascular complications.

Indirect Latex Slide Test for Detection of Microalbuminuria Microtex® (Courtsey: Tulip Group of Companies)

Summary

Urinary albumin excretion between 30-300 mg/day (microalbuminuria), far below the levels found in clinical proteinuria (> 300 mg/day) is a strong predictor of development of diabetic nephropathy and vascular complications. These low levels of albumin excretion are detectable only by sensitive immunoassays for microalbuminuria.

Diabetic nephropathy leads to progressive loss of renal function or end-stage renal disease (ESRD) and may necessitate need for dialysis or transplantation in most cases. The progression of microalbuminuria is closely associated with progressive hypertension and loss of blood glucose control. The early presence of microalbuminuria can be reversed by strict metabolic control and timely intervention of drugs early in the course of disease can arrest the progression of diabetic renal disease. Annual screening of microalbuminuria is recommended by the **'WHO'** and **'International Diabetes Foundation'** in all patients with IDDM over the age of 12 years and who have had diabetes for five years or more.

Microalbuminuria is also a significant risk marker of cardiovascular diseases. Its presence can be regarded as an index of increased cardiovascular vulnerability and a signal for correction of known risk factors.

Microtex is a sensitive immunoassay useful for the detection of microalbuminuria.

Reagent

1. *Antihuman albumin reagent:* The concentration of antibodies to human albumin is adjusted to provide sensitivity of about 25 mg/L and above of microalbuminuria.
2. *Albumin latex reagent:* A uniform suspension of polystyrene latex particles to which human albumin has been chemically coupled. Each batch of reagent undergoes rigorous quality control at various stages of manufacture for its specificity, sensitivity and performance.

Reagent Storage and Stability

Store the reagents at 2-8°C. DO NOT FREEZE.

The shelf life of the reagents is as per the expiry date mentioned on the reagent vial labels.

Principle

Microtex slide test for the detection of microalbuminuria is based on the principle of agglutination inhibition. The urine specimen to be tested is first mixed with antibody reagent containing antibodies directed against human albumin. The latex coupled with human albumin is added to the mixture and is allowed to react. When the urine specimen does not contain albumin, antibodies to human albumin would be free to react with the latex coupled with human albumin causing agglutination. When the urine specimen contains at least 25 mg/L of albumin, the antibodies to human albumin will be neutralized and will not be available to react with latex couple with human albumin. Hence, no agglutination will be observed.

Note

1. *In vitro* diagnostic reagent for laboratory and professional use only. *Not for medicinal use.*
2. All the materials derived from human source have been tested for HBsAg and anti-HIV antibodies and found to be nonreactive.
3. The reagents contain 0.1% sodium azide as preservative. Avoid contact with skin or mucosa. On disposal, flush with large quantities of water.
4. The reagents can be damaged due to microbial contamination or on exposure to extreme temperatures. It is recommended that the performance of reagents should be verified with positive and negative controls provided with the kit.
5. Use reagents of same lot numbers. Do not interchange reagents of different lot numbers.
6. Do not interchange vial droppers.
7. Shake the albumin latex reagent vial well before use to disperse the latex particles uniformly and improve test readability.
8. Only a clean and dry glass slide must be used. Slide should be free from even traces of protein compounds.

Sample Collection and Preparation

For Qualitative Method

Though random urine specimens can be used, first morning urine specimen is preferable. Specimens should be collected in clean glass or plastic containers free of detergents. Specimens should be tested immediately preferably within 12 hours of collection. Should a delay in testing occur, add thimerosal (0.01%) or sodium azide (0.1%) to the specimen and store at 2-8°C up to 72 hours. Do not use grossly contaminated specimens. If specimen is cloudy or contains blood, centrifuge the specimen at 1000 rpm (revolutions per minute) for one minute and use clear supernatant for testing.

For Semiquantitative Method

Urine specimens collected over a 24 hour period should be pooled in a clean detergent free container and refrigerated at 2-8°C. Thimerosal (0.01%) or sodium azide (0.1%) are recommended as urine preservatives.

Materials Provided with the Kit

Reagents

Antihuman albumin reagent, albumin latex reagent, positive control reactive with antihuman albumin reagent, negative control non-reactive with antihuman albumin reagent.

Accessories

Glass slide with six reaction circles, pipettes for dispensing urine specimen, mixing sticks and rubber teats.

Additional Materials Required

A high intensity direct light source, and stop watch.

Test Procedure

Bring all reagents and samples to room temperature before use.

Qualitative Method

1. Place one drop of clear urine under test on the glass slide using disposable pipettes provided with the kit. Deliver the drop vertically.

2. Add one drop of antihuman albumin reagent to the drop of urine under test on the slide. Deliver the drop vertically.
3. Using a mixing stick, mix the antihuman albumin reagent and urine over the circle for 30 seconds.
4. Add one drop of well mixed albumin latex reagent to the mixture. Mix uniformly over the entire circle.
5. Immediately start the stopwatch, rock the slide gently back and forth observing for agglutination macroscopically at three minutes.

Semiquantitative Method

Measure and record the total volume of patient urine collected over a 24-hour period. Centrifuge an aliquot of the 24 hour urine specimen. Using isotonic saline, prepare progressive dilutions from the centrifuged urine specimen. Perform the qualitative test procedure using each dilution as specimen.

Interpretation of Results

Qualitative Method

Agglutination is a negative test result indicating the absence of detectable levels of albumin in urine signifying absence of microalbuminuria. No agglutination is a positive test result indicating the presence of albumin in concentrations above 25 mg/L in urine signifying microalbuminuria.

Semiquantitative Method

No agglutination in the highest urine dilution corresponds to the titre of microalbumin per litre of the specimen. To calculate the concentration of microalbumin in the specimen use the following formula:

Microalbumin (mg/L) = S × D
where S = Sensitivity of the test, i.e. 25 mg/L
D = Highest dilution of urine showing no agglutination.

Remarks

1. Microalbuminuria also occurs in response to acute inflammatory conditions such as ischaemia, trauma and thermal injury, surgery, pancreatitis and inflammatory bowel disease. In many of these conditions the albumin excretion increases within minutes or hours of the initiating stimulus and only lasts for 24-72 hours.
2. Use only urine as test specimen. Do not use serum.
3. Albumin excretion is increased after physical activity. It is, therefore, recommended to use urine sample that has been produced at rest whenever random urine specimen is used.
4. As albumin excretion is subject to physiological fluctuations, it is necessary to take two measurements in consecutive days; in case of contradictory results, three measurements on different days must be done preferably within a week.
5. Liquid intake of the patient must be in the normal range, i.e. 1.5-2 litres /day.
6. To diagnose incipient nephropathy microalbuminuria must be present in at least 2 out of 3 specimens over a 3-6 month period.
7. It is recommended that results of the tests should be correlated with clinical findings to arrive at the final diagnosis.
8. It is recommended that reagents should be tested with positive and negative controls periodically to validate their performance.
9. The agglutination pattern in negative urines will vary from sample to sample since it is affected by the salt concentration and pH of the urine under test.

TESTS FOR GLUCOSE

Normal values
Random : negative
24 hr specimen: 100 mg/24 hours.

Benedict's Qualitative (Semiquantitative) Glucose Test

In this method the cupric ion is reduced to Cu_2O (cuprous oxide). If only 0.1% or less of glucose is present, the precipitate may not appear until cooling. To 5 ml of Benedict's qualitative reagent, add 8 drops of urine (0.5 ml). Heat to boiling and set in a boiling water bath for 5 minutes or else boil it over a flame for 2 minutes.

Read as follows:
Blue to cloudy green colour = Negative, O
Yellow-green = + (< 0.5% glucose)

Greenish yellow = ++ (0.5-1% glucose)
Yellow = +++ (1-2% glucose)
Orange to brick red = ++++ (over 2% glucose)
Sensitivity of this test is 50 mg% or more.

Glucose oxidase methods: Glucose oxidase reacts with glucose to yield gluconic acid and hydrogen peroxide. Hydrogen peroxide and orthotolidine yield a blue colour. This is a specific test. The reagents may be impregnated on paper strips (as mentioned above) and dipping them in urine provide the result in lesser time as compared to Benedict's method (sensitivity = 0.1%).

Benedict's Quantitative Glucose Test

Place a small quantity of powdered pumice, 10 gm of anhydrous sodium carbonate and 25 ml of quantitative Benedict's reagent in a 250 ml container and heat. While the mixture is boiling, add urine rapidly from a buret until the blue colour begins to fade, then add urine drop by drop until all blue colour is gone and only a grey colour remains. At this point, all cupric ion originally in solution is reduced. The amount of urine used contains 0.05 gm of glucose. To calculate grams of glucose per 100 ml of urine, divide 5 by the number of ml of urine used.

Sugar Tests in Urine

Sugars detected	*Benedict's qualitative test*	*Glucose oxidase strips*
	Glucose Galactose Lactose Fructose Maltose Pentose	Glucose
False positive	Ascorbic acid Homogentisic acid Many antibiotics (Antitubercular drugs) Phenothiazines Salicylates Levodopa X-ray contrast media	Hydrogen peroxide or hypochlorite in container
False negative		Ascorbic acid Homogentisic acid, Large amounts of salicylates

Significance of Sugars in Urine

Glycosuria with Hyperglycaemia

Diabetes mellitus

Other endocrine disorders: Acromegaly, Cushing's syndrome, hyperthyroidism, pheochromocytoma.

Pancreatic disease: Cystic fibrosis—advanced stage, haemochromatosis, severe chronic pancreatitis, carcinoma.

CNS dysfunction: Asphyxia, tumors or haemorrhage, especially of hypothalamus.

Massive metabolic derangement: Severe burns, uraemia, advanced liver disease, sepsis, cardiogenic shock.

Drug induced: Corticosteroids and ACTH, thiazides, oral contraceptives.

Glycosuria without Hyperglycaemia

- Renal tubular dysfunction
- Pregnancy (differentiate from gestational diabetes).

Nonglucose Sugars in Urine

Galactose: Detecting galactosaemia in newborn period may prevent irreversible liver and CNS damage. Galactose spills into urine only if milk is being taken.

Fructose: Essential fructosuria (rare).

Pentose: Very high fruit intake may cause pentosuria in normal persons.

Interfering Factors

a. Pregnancy and lactation may cause a false positive in enzymatic tests. About 70% of women show a temporary glucosuria that appears to be of no clinical value.
b. Ascorbic acid, keflen, creatinine in concentrated urine, streptomycin and homogentisic acid may cause a false-positive reduction test (Benedict's), usually it will only be a trace reaction.
c. Stress excitement, testing after a heavy meal, and following the administration of IV glucose may cause false positives of all tests. Usually, it is a trace reaction.
d. Ascorbic acid in large amounts may cause a false negative in the enzyme tests.

e. False negatives may be obtained if deteriorated reagents strips have been used, or directions not followed exactly.

KETONE BODIES IN URINE

Normal values: Negative

The three ketone bodies that can be detected in urine are:

1. Acetone (2%)
2. Acetoacetic acid (20%)
3. β-Hydroxybutyric acid (78%)

$$\text{Acetoacetic acid} \xrightarrow{-CO_2} \text{acetone}$$

$$\text{Acetoacetic acid} = \underset{-2H}{\text{Hydroxybutyric acid}}$$

Ketone bodies are products of incomplete fat metabolism and their presence is indicative of acidosis.

Tests for Ketone Bodies

(Never heat urine specimen before performing the tests)

1. *Rothera's test:* Saturate 5 ml of urine with ammonium sulfate, add a few crystals of sodium nitroprusside, shake. Add liquor ammonia from the side of the test tube, formation of a purple ring at the junction indicates a positive test.
   Sensitivity > 1-5 mg% acetoacetic acid, or > 10-25 mg% of acetone.
2. *Legal's test:* Take 10 ml of urine in a test tube and add a few crystals of sodium nitroprusside. Acidify with glacial acetic acid, invert to mix. Overlay with strong liquor ammonia, let stand for 5 minutes. A violet ring indicates a positive test. The degree of positivity depends upon the speed of the reaction.
3. *Paper strip/tablet methods (Ketur test—Boehringer):* These contain sodium nitroprusside, amino-acetic acid and disodium phosphate. A positive test is indicated by development of a purple colour.
4. *Diacetic acid test (Gerhardt's test)*: Not a very sensitive test. Perform this test if the test for acetone was positive. Precipitate the phosphates in 5 ml of urine with 10% ferric chloride solution, drop-by-drop, filter and add more ferric chloride. If a purple-red colour appears, it indicates presence of 0.05% or more of diacetic acid. False-positive test may appear with salicylates, sodium bicarbonate, etc.

Causes of Ketonuria

1. *Diabetic:* Ketonuria indicates ketoacidosis and if unchecked may go on to coma. Juvenile diabetics are more susceptible to develop this. Whenever glycosuria is more than 2+, always test for ketone bodies also.
2. *Nondiabetic:* In infants and children in:
   - Acute febrile states
   - Toxic states with vomiting, diarrhoea, etc.
   - Hyperemesis gravidarum
   - Cachexia with vomiting
   - Post-anaesthesia vomiting
   - Conditions where there is limited availability of glucose, e.g. glycogen storage disease
   - Sometimes following exposure to cold or severe exercise.

Clinical Implications

a. Ketosis and ketonuria may occur whenever increased amounts of fat are metabolized, carbohydrate intake restricted, or the diet is fat rich.

b. Ketonuria occurs in association with:
   - Fever
   - Anorexia
   - Starvation
   - Prolonged vomiting
   - Gastrointestinal disturbances
   - Following anaesthesias
   - Fasting.

c. In nondiabetics, ketonuria will frequently occur in acute illness. Fifteen per cent of hospitalized cases will show ketone bodies in urine even though they are nondiabetics.

d. Children are particularly prone to developing ketonuria and ketosis.

e. Ketone bodies appear in urine before there is any significant increase of ketone bodies in the blood.

Interfering Factors

a. Carbohydrate-free diets as well as high protein and fat will cause ketonuria.

b. Drugs that may cause false-positive tests.
   - Levodopa
   - BSP or PSP
   - Isopropyl alcohol
   - Metformin
   - Paraldehyde
   - Ether
   - Pyridium

- Insulin
- Phenformin

Clinical Relevance

1. Presence of ketone bodies in the urine is helpful in differentiating between a diabetic coma and an insulin shock (hypoglycaemia).
2. Any stressful condition that distorts the normal regulation of a diabetic can be recognised at any early point by a positive urine ketone test.
3. Urine ketones indicate caution, not a crisis situation, in either a diabetic or a non-diabetic patient
   - Appearance of ketones in a diabetic imply that the patient is not adequately controlled, and that adjustments of either the medication or the diet should be made immediately.
   - In a nondiabetic, ketone bodies, indicate a small amount of CHO metabolism and excessive fat metabolism.

Bile Salts

Bile salts when present decrease the surface tension of urine. When sulphur powder is added on the surface of urine, sulphur particles sink to the bottom of the test tube. In normal urine sample sulphur particles float on the surface of the urine.

Method

1. Take about 10 ml urine in a test tube
2. Sprinkle a little dry sulphur powder on the surface of urine
3. Observe the sulphur particles.

Interpretation

1. Sulphur particles sink to the bottom: Bile salts present
2. Sulphur particles remain floating: Bile salts absent

   Dipstick tests are available.

Bile Pigments

Bile pigments (always use fresh specimen) Normal level of bile pigments is urine in < 0.02 mg%.

1. *Foam test*: Not very accurate as proteins can also form foam. Shake 5 ml of urine in a test tube, bile produces a yellowish foam which persists.
2. *Iodine ring test*: A sensitive cum reliable test. Layer a solution of 10% alcoholic iodine on urine in a test tube. A green ring indicates presence of bile.
3. *Harrison test:* A sensitive test. To 5 ml of urine, add 5 ml of 10% barium chloride in a test tube. Shake. Filter it off. Let the filter paper dry. When dry, add 1-2 drops of Fouchet's reagent to the dried precipitate. A green (disregard all other colours) colour indicates bilirubinuria.
4. *Diazo test:* p-nitrobenzene diazonium p-toluene sulphonate is the active reagent. Place 5 drops of the urine on the mat provided in the kit. Bilirubin, if present shall be absorbed onto the mat surface. Place a reagent tablet on it. Let 2 drops of water flow over the tablet. A positive test is indicated by the appearance of a blue to purple colour within 30 seconds. Pink/red colour is negative. Sensitivity > 0.1 to 0.05 mg% of bilirubin in urine.
5. *Paper strip method:* After dipping the strip in urine, match with the colour chart provided by the manufacturers.

	Diazo method	*Harrison/Fouchet's test*
False positive	Chlorpromazine	Aspirin metabolites, Urobilin or indican, urobilinogen
False negative	Ascorbic acid High levels of nitrites Oxidation of bilirubin, if examination is delayed by over 4 hours.	Oxidation of bilirubin if examination is delayed

Causes of Hyperbilirubinuria

1. Moderate to severe hepatocellular damage.
2. Obstruction of bile ducts, extrahepatic or intrahepatic.

In early hepatocellular damage and in haemolysis, urine bilirubin may be negative.

Urobilinogen and Urobilin

Urobilinogen is colourless, and on standing it gets oxidised to urobilin which has a brown colour. It is best to perform tests for urobilinogen on fresh specimens. If delay is inevitable, collect the sample in a dark bottle, provide a surface layer of petroleum ether and add sodium carbonate (5 gm for 24 hours volume) and refrigerate the sample.

Urobilinogen

Ehrlich's test: Nitrites and bilirubin interfere with this test. Sulphonamide and procaine cause yellowish colour reactions. Pyridium, indole, porphobilinogen and PAS yield pink-red colour not different from that produced by urobilinogen.

To 10 ml of fresh sample at room temperature add 1 ml of Ehrlich's reagent, invert several times and let stand for 5 minutes. A pink colour is normal, cherry or darker red colour indicate abnormal amounts of urobilinogen. Dilutions may be used. Colour reactions are normal in dilutions upto 1:20 (Sensitivity > 1.3 mgm%).

Urobilin (Schlesinger's Test)

Convert urobilinogen to urobilin by adding a few drops of Lugol's solution. Mix 10 ml of urine with an equal quantity of saturated alcoholic solution of zinc acetate filter into a dry test tube.

Abnormal amounts of urobilin give the filtrate a green fluorescence which is best seen against a dark background with a light source from the side, or in sunlight against a black background.

The filtrate obtained from Harrison's test for bilirubin can be used for urobilinogen or urobilin.

Paper strip method (Dipstick tests are available).

Estimated Urobilinogen

Normal values: 0.1-1 Ehrlich unit/dl

Urinary urobilinogen is an important tool in routine urinalysis since it serves as a guide in detecting and differentiating liver disease, haemolytic disease, and biliary obstruction. Sequential determination assists in evaluating progress of disease and response to treatment. Both urobilinogen and bilirubin in urine may be regarded as bile pigments, but the tests provide different information.

Increased values of urobilinogen occur in:

- Cirrhosis: Bilirubin in urine may or may not be present
- Haemolytic jaundice: Bilirubin does not appear in urine

A number of drugs produce false positives or negatives.

Urobilinogen (Quantitative)

Normal values
2 hour specimen: 0.1-1.0 Ehrlich units/2 hours
24 hour specimen: 1-4 mg/24 hours.

This is one of the most sensitive tests employed to determine impaired liver function. Bilirubin, formed from the metabolism of hemoglobin entering the intestine in the bile, is transformed through the action of bacteria into urobilinogen. Part of the urobilinogen formed in intestine is excreted with the faeces; another portion is absorbed into the portal blood stream and carried to the liver where it is metabolised and excreted in bile. Traces of urobilinogen that escape removal from the blood by the liver are carried to the kidneys and excreted in the urine.

Clinical Relevance

Increase in Urinary Urobilinogen

This occurs in any condition that causes an increase in the production of bilirubin and by any disease that prevents the liver from normally removing the reabsorbed urobilinogen from the portal circulation.

a. Increased urobilinogen is found whenever there is excessive destruction of RBCs as in
   - Haemolytic anaemias
   - Pernicious anaemia
   - Malaria
b. Values above normal also occur in:
   - Infectious and toxic hepatitis
   - Pulmonary infarction
   - Biliary disease
   - Cholangitis
   - Haemolytic jaundice and anaemia
   - Chemical injury to liver due to chloroform and carbon tetrachloride poisoning.
   - Cirrhosis
   - Congestive heart failure
   - Infectious mononucleosis
c. An increased urobilinogen level is one of the earliest signs of acute liver cell damage.

Decrease in Urinary Urobilinogen

This occurs when normal amounts of bilirubin are not excreted into the intestinal tract. It usually indicates partial or complete obstruction of the bile ducts. As occurs in:

- Cholelithiasis
- Severe inflammatory disease
- Cancer of head of pancreas
- During antibiotic therapy. Suppression of normal gut flora may prevent breakdown of bilirubin to urobilinogen, leading to its absence in urine
- Decreased values are also associated with:
  - Severe diarrhoea
  - Renal insufficiency

Interfering Factors

a. Drugs and foods that may cause urobilinogen to be increased include:
   - Para-aminosalicylic acid (PAS)
   - Antipyrine
   - BSP
   - Cascara
   - Phenothiazines
   - Sulphonamides
   - Drugs causing haemolysis of RBC
   - Bananas
   - Phenazopyridine

b. Drugs that may cause decreased urobilinogen include those that cause cholestasis and those that reduce bacterial flora in the GI tract (e.g. chloramphenicol and antibiotics).

c. Peak excretion is said to occur from noon to 16:00 hours. The urinary urobilinogen is subject to diurnal variation.

d. Strongly alkaline urine will show higher value and strongly acid urine will show a lower level.

PORPHYRINS

Perform Ehrlich's test for urobilinogen by mixing equal parts of urine and Ehrlich's reagent. Add 2 parts of saturated sodium acetate solution and mix. If turbid, filter. Shake with a small quantity of chloroform. Urobilinogen is soluble in chloroform, porphobilinogen is not. If after several extractions with chloroform the aqueous phase is still pink, the test is positive for porphobilinogen.

Causes

Conditions producing increased levels of any of the haeme precursors are called porphyrias. The two rare major categories of genetically determined porphyria and erythropoietic porphyrias, in which the major diagnostic abnormalities occur in red cell chemistry, and hepatic porphyrias, in which haeme precursors are found in urine or faeces. In acquired disorders, precursors accumulate more in urine and faeces than in red cells.

Normal Values

Porphobilinogens	: 2 mg/24 hr or negative
Porphyrins	: 50-300 mg/24 hr
DAL or ALA	: 1-710 mg/24 hr
Fluorescent	: Negative

Porphyrins are cyclic compounds formed from delta-aminolevulinic acid (DAL or ALA), which is important in the formation of haemoglobin and other haemoproteins that function as carriers of oxygen in the blood and tissues. In health, insignificant amounts of porphyrin are excreted in the urine. However, in conditions like porphyria (disturbance in metabolism of porphyrin), liver disease, lead poisoning, and pellagra, there is an increased level of prophyrins as well as DAL and ALA in the urine. Disorders of porphyrin metabolism also result in porphobilinogen. In acute attacks of porphyria, the patient may suffer skin lesions, abdominal pain, neuropathy, and mental disturbances. The urine of patients with this disease usually has a pinkish to reddish-black tinge and will become darker upon standing. In the laboratory the urine is tested for the presence of porphyrins, porphobilinogen, and DAL or ALA. It is also given the black light screening test (porphyrins fluorescence when exposed to black or ultraviolet light).

A random sample or 24 hours sample may be submitted to the laboratory. Porphobilinogens are always done with porphyrin test. Should a single, fresh-voided specimen be ordered, only a porphobilinogen will be done. Protect specimen from light. The test must be performed within 60 minutes. Random sample should be obtained between 10:00 and 14:00 hours. Observe and record the colour of urine. If porphyrins are present, the urine may have a grossly recognisable amber red or burgundy colour. It may vary from pale pink to almost black. Some patients will excrete a urine of normal colour that turns dark after standing in the light.

Clinical Relevance

Porphyria

1. In the porphyrias, the urine contains increased amounts of porphyrins and porphobilinogens and may not contain increased amounts of DAL or ALA.
2. ALA and DAL excretion is elevated in acute intermittent porphyria, a hepatic porphyria that is aggravated by alcohol, barbiturates, and other drugs affecting the liver.

Lead Poisoning

1. ALA or DAL will be present in the urine
2. Porphyrins may or may not be present in the urine.

Other Conditions with Increased Levels of Porphyrins

- Cirrhosis
- Infectious hepatitis
- Hodgkin's disease
- Some cancers
- CNS disorders
- Heavy metal poisoning
- Carbon tetrachloride or benzene poisoning.

Interfering Factors

1. During menstruation and pregnancy porphyrins may be normally increased
2. Drugs that can cause false-positive test are:
   - Acriflavine
   - Ethoxazene
   - Phenazopyridine
   - Sulphamethoxazole
   - Tetracyclines
   - Antipyretics
   - Barbiturates
   - Phenylhydrazine
   - Sulphonamides.

BLOOD IN URINE (HAEMATURIA)

Haematuria can be gross, urine appears reddish due to blood, it can also be microscopic, when it is not visible to the naked eye, here various tests are performed for confirmation.

1. *Guaic test:* In one test tube, mix 2 ml of 10% acetic acid, 5 ml of urine and 5 ml ether. In a second test tube place 5 ml of 95% alcohol, 2 ml fresh hydrogen peroxide and a pinch of powdered guaic. Now pour the guaic solution slowly down the side of the first tube. Blood in the urine causes blue colour to appear at the zone of contact between the guaic and ether.
2. *Benzidine test:* Saturate 2 ml of glacial acetic acid with benzidine and pour off the clear supernatant fluid. Add 1 ml of fresh hydrogen peroxide and 2 ml of urine (if the blue colour develops before the addition of urine, the glassware is contaminated).
3. *Paper strips*: (Sangur test-Boehringer). Blood reacts with the peroxide-orthotolidine reagent to produce a blue colour.

Causes

a. Bleeding diathesis.

b. Local disorders of kidney and genitourinary tract.
   1. Trauma
   2. Cystitis
   3. Renal calculi
   4. Genitourinary tumours
   5. Heritable disorders
      - Haemoglobinopathies
      - Osler-Weber-Rendu disease
      - Polycystic kidney.

Diffuse Renal Lesions

1. Acute and chronic glomerulonephritis
2. Systemic lupus erythematosus
3. Polyarteritis
4. Goodpasture's syndrome
5. Tuberculous pyelonephritis
6. Allergic nephropathies (Henoch-Schonlein's purpura)
7. Thrombotic thrombocytopenic purpura
8. Focal embolic glomerulitis
9. Malignant hypertension
10. Chemical/Drug induced
    - Carbon-tetrachloride
    - Sulphonamides
    - Dicoumarol, etc.

NITRITE/BACTERIA

Normal values: Negative for bacteria.

Explanation of test: There are two methods that are used to detect bacteria in the urine during routine urinalysis—microscopic examination and clinical testing. The sediment when examined microscopically can reveal bacteria when present. Chemical dipstick testing is also commonly done. The nitrite area in the multiple reagent strip is calibrated so that any shade of pink colour that develops within 30 seconds indicates an amount of nitrite produced by 10^5 or more organisms per ml in the urine specimen.

Procedure

1. A first morning specimen is preferred because urine that has been in the bladder for several hours is more likely to yield a positive result. A clean catch or a midstream urine is needed to avoid bacterial contamination.
2. Follow procedure as stated by the dipstick manufacturer.

Clinical Implications

1. The finding of 20 or more bacteria per high power field may indicate a urinary tract infection.
2. The presence of only a few bacteria should be interpreted with caution and suggests a urinary tract infection that cannot be confirmed or excluded until more definitive studies, such as cultures and sensitivity tests are performed.
3. A positive result from the nitrite test is a reliable indication of a significant bacteriuria and is an indication for urine culture.
4. A negative result should never be interpreted as indicating absence of bacteriuria because:
   a. If an overnight sample was not used, there may have been insufficient time for the conversion of nitrate to nitrite to have occurred.
   b. There may be a rare instance when nitrite does not appear in urine, and a person of this type could have significant bacteria without a positive test.
   c. Some strains of urinary pathogens do not produce enzymes necessary to change nitrate to nitrite and can cause a negative result.

RAPID DIAGNOSTICS

Rapidity of diagnosis is of utmost importance in today's context.

Many manufacturers now provide rapid strip test (qualitative and semiquantitative). Important amongst them are as follows.

Boehringer-Knoll Limited

	Product	*Determines*
a.	Combur 9 test	Leucocytes, nitrite, pH, protein, glucose, ketone bodies, urobilinogen, bilirubin, blood.
b.	Combur 8 test	All of A except leucocytes
c.	Combur 7 test	All of B except nitrite
d.	Combur 6 test	All of C except bilirubin
e.	Combur 4 test	Protein, glucose urobilinogen, blood
f.	Ecur test	Protein, glucose, blood
g.	Combur test	Glucose, protein, pH

Various other combinations or single test strips are also available, e.g. pertaining only to liver/kidney disorders.

Bayer India Limited

Now with improved pad order and efficacy

a.	Diastix	Glucose
b.	Hemastix	Blood
c.	Ictotest (tablets)	Bilirubin
d.	Keto-diastix	Glucose and ketones
e.	Multistix	pH, protein, glucose, ketones, bilirubin, blood, urobilinogen.
f.	Uristix	Glucose and protein
g.	Combistix SG	Glucose, protein, pH and specific gravity
h.	Multistix SG	All of (E) + Specific gravity
i.	Neostix 3	Blood, glucose and protein

SPECIAL URINE TESTS

Calcium in Urine (Sulkowitch Test)

Fasting or random samples may be tested. Before the test, the patient should be on neutral low-calcium diet for 3 days. Collect 24 hour urine specimen. Mix equal parts of urine and Sulkowitch reagent, let stand for 2-3 minutes and read as under.

0	=	No precipitate, no urine calcium; serum calcium level 5-7.5 mg%
1+	=	Fine white cloud, normal urine and blood calcium level.
2+ & 3+	=	Thicker, coarser precipitate, raised urinary calcium.
4+	=	Precipitate like milk, strongly positive.

Normal Values

24 hour levels

100-250 mg/24 hours on average diet

< 150 mg/24 hours on low calcium diet.

Most of the calcium discharged by the body is excreted via stool. However, there is a small quantity of calcium that is normally excreted in the urine, this varies with the variation in dietary calcium. The 24-hour test is most often required to determine the function of the parathyroid gland, which maintains a balance between calcium and phosphorus by means of parathormone.

Clinical Relevance

Increased Levels

1. Caused by:
   - Hyperparathyroidism (results in constant 3 + to 4 + Sulkowitch test).
   - Sarcoidosis
   - Primary cancers of breast and lung
   - Metastatic malignancies
   - Myeloma with bone metastasis
   - Wilson's disease
   - Renal tubular acidosis
   - Glucocorticoid excess
2. Increased urinary calcium almost always accompanies elevated blood calcium levels.
3. Calcium excretion greater than intake is always excessive, and excretion above 400-500 mg/24 hr is reliably abnormal.
4. Increased levels of calcium occur whenever calcium is mobilised from the bone, as in metastatic cancer and prolonged skeletal mobilisation.
5. When calcium is excreted in increasing amounts, a potential for nephrolithiasis or nephrocalcinosis is created.

Decreased Levels

Caused by:

1. Hypoparathyroidism (hypocalcaemia caused by hypoparathyroidism is usually associated with a negative reaction).
2. Vitamin D deficiency (Vitamin D is essential for absorption of calcium).
3. Malabsorption syndrome.

Interfering Factors

a. Falsely high values are seen in:
   - High sodium and magnesium intake
   - Very high milk intake
   - Levels are often high immediately after meals
   - Drugs:
     - Androgens
     - Cholestyramine
     - Vitamin D
     - Parathyroid injection
     - Nandrolone, in some cancer patients.

B. False negative (lowered) values are seen in
   - Increased dietary phosphate
   - Alkaline urine
   - Drugs:
     - Sodium phytate
     - Thiazides
     - Viomycin

Be Careful

1. Urine calcium test is not a substitute for serum calcium, it can, however, be done in an emergency. Hypercalcaemia can be life threatening.
2. Low urinary calcium patients should be observed for tetany.
3. The first sign of calcium imbalance may be the occurrence of pathological fractures that can be related to calcium excess.

SEROTONIN (5-HYDROXYTRYPTAMINE)

Carcinoids

Carcinoids: (argentaffinomas) may produce serotonin, which is metabolised to 5-hydroxy-indoleacetic acid (5-HIAA). Presence of this compound in urine in more than traces indicates *malignant carcinoid metastatic to the liver.*

Test

Acidify 2 ml of filtered urine with 2 drops of 10% HCl and extract twice with 20-25 ml of ether. Evaporate the dry residue in 1 ml of 0.1 N HCl. Add 1 ml Ehrlich's reagent. Boil for 2-3 minutes. A distinct blue colour indicates the presence of 5-HIAA in abnormal amounts in urine.

Normal Values
Qualitative— Negative
Quantitative—2-10 mg/24 hr.
60-100 mEq/24 hr.

For screening purposes, a random test may be enough. Serotonin is a vasoconstricting hormone produced normally by argentaffin cells of the GI tract. The principal function of the cells is to regulate smooth muscle contraction and peristalsis. In carcinoid tumour (tumour of the argentaffin cells), there is rise in levels of 5-hydroxy-indoleacetic acid (5-HIAA) which happens to be a denatured product of serotonin.

Method

1. No bananas, pineapples, tomatoes, eggplants, or avocados to be consumed during the 24-hour test because they contain serotonin.
2. A 24-hour urine container with preservative is labelled with the name of patient, test and date.
3. General instructions for 24-hour sample collection are observed.

Clinical Relevance

1. Levels in excess of 100 mg per 24 hours are indicative of large carcinoid tumour, especially when metastatic. However, this increase is found only in 5-7% cases of carcinoid tumour.
2. Levels between 10 mg and 100 mg per 24 hours may be seen in:
   - Haemorrhage
   - Thrombosis
   - Nontropical sprue
   - Severe pain of sciatica or skeletal and smooth muscle spasm.

Interfering Factors

False Positives
1. Bananas, pineapples, plums, walnut, and avocados may increase 5-HIAA levels, for all of them contain serotonin.
2. Drugs that may lead to false-positive result
   - Acetanilide
   - Acetophenetidin
   - Caffeine
   - Glyceryl guaicolate
   - Fluorouracil (5 FU)
   - Mephenesin
   - Melphelan
   - Methocarbamol
   - Methamphetamine
   - Reserpine
   - Phenacetin solution
   - Lugol's iodine
   - Phenmetrazine
   - Methysergide maleate

False Negatives
Drugs that may falsely decrease 5-HIAA levels:
- ACTH
- Chlorpromazine
- Heparin
- Imipramine
- Isoniazid
- MAO inhibitor
- Methanamine mandelate
- Methyldopa
- Phenothiazines
- Promethazine
- P-chlorophenylaniline

Ideally, the patient should take no drugs for 72 hours prior to test if possible.

CYSTINE

To 5 ml of urine, add 2 ml of 5% sodium cyanide solution and let them react for 10 minutes. Add 5 drops of 5% sodium nitroprusside solution and mix thoroughly. Cystine produces a magenta colour. If no cystine is present, a pale brown or pale pink colour results. All solutions should be freshly prepared. Also, examine the urinary sediment for cystine crystals. Urinary cystine is raised in cystinurias.

Normal values
Qualitative : Negative
Quantitative : Children under 8 years: 2-13 mg/24 hr.
Individuals above 8 years: 7-28 mg/hr.

These tests of urine are useful in the differential diagnosis of cystinuria, an inherited disease from cystinosis. Cystinuria is a hereditary disease, characterised by bladder calculi. In cystinosis, cytine is deposited in lung tissues.

Clinical Relevance

Values are increased in:
1. Cystinuria (up to 20 times normal) in which there is excessive urinary excretion of lysine, ornithine, arginine, and cystine.

2. Cystinosis (no excess of lysine, arginine or ornithine)

FAT IN URINE

Take equal parts of urine and ether, cloudiness due to fat disappears, decant ether onto a watch glass, evaporate, fat leaves a greasy deposit. Fat may be seen microscopically.

HEREDITARY METABOLIC DISORDERS

Errors of Carbohydrate Metabolism

1. *Galactosuria:* Positive test for reducing substance (Benedict's qualitative). Negative glucose-oxidase test. Positive phloroglucinol test.
2. *Pentosuria:* Positive Benedict's qualitative test. Negative glucose-oxidase test. Positive orcinyl-HCl test.
3. *Fructosuria:* Positive Benedict's test. Negative glucose-oxidase test. Positive resorcinol-HCl test (Seliwanoff).

Errors of Amino Acid Metabolism

1. *Cystinuria*: Positive cyanide-nitroprusside test. Cystine crystals in urine.
2. *Fanconi's syndrome:* Positive glucose-oxidase test. Paper chromatography for amino acids.
3. *Wilson's disease*: Positive glucose-oxidase test. Paper chromatography for amino acids.
4. *Phenylketonuria*: Positive ferric chloride test.
5. *Hartnup disease*: Paper chromatography
6. *Alkaptonuria (Homogentisic acid):* Positive Benedict's test. Urine darkens on standing. Negative glucose-oxidase test. Urine reduces silver on sensitised plate.
7. *Tyrosinosis*: Paper chromatography. Positive Millon test.
8. *Maple syrup disease*: Maple syrup odour of urine. Paper chromatography.

Abnormal Porphyrin Metabolism

1. Acute porphyria—urine darkens on exposure to sunlight. Positive porphobilinogen test. Spectroscopic and fluorimetric identification.
2. Cutaneous porphyria—red urine. Spectroscopic and fluorimetric tests.

FERRIC CHLORIDE TESTING

Many amino acids react with ferric chloride to give distinctive colours. Ferric chloride testing is a screening test not only for aminoacidurias but also for many abnormal metabolites and drug excretion products. Definitive diagnosis requires specific identification and measurement of the relevant materials in blood or urine.

Substance	*Colour alteration*
Amino acids	
α-Ketobutyric acid	Purple, fading to red brown
Homogentisic acid (alkaptonuria)	Rapidly fading blue or green
p-Hydroxyphenylpyruvic acid (tyrosinosis)	Rapidly fading green
Valine, leucine, and isoleucine (maple syrup disease)	Blue
Phenyl pyruvic acid (phenylketonuria)	Stable green or blue green
Other metabolites	
Acetoacetic acid	Red or red-brown
Melanin	Grey, changing to black
Indican (Hartnup disease, intestinal stasis, malabsorption)	Violet or blue
Drugs	
Aspirin, salicylates	Stable red-wine colour
Phenothiazine derivatives	Immediate purple pink
p-Aminosalicylic acid (PAS)	Red-brown
Phenol derivatives	Violet

URIC ACID

Normal values

0.4 — 1.0 gm/24 hr on normal diet

0.2 — 0.5 gm/24 hr on purine free diet

2.0 gm/24 hr on high purine diet

Uric acid formation occurs as a result of the metabolic breakdown of nucleic acids, purines are the main sources of this breakdown. The test is required in the investigation of metabolic disturbances to identify gout and diagnose kidney disease. It also reflects the effect of uricosuric agents when these drugs are used, by indicating the total amount of uric acid excreted. A 24-hour sample is needed.

Clinical Relevance

Increased Levels (uricosuria)

- Found in:
  - Gout
  - Chronic myeloid leukaemia
  - Polycythaemia vera
  - Liver disease
  - Febrile illness
  - Toxaemias of pregnancy
  - Fanconi's syndrome
- Cytotoxic drugs used to treat lymphoma and leukaemia often cause greatly increased urinary uric acid levels.
- High uric acid concentration plus low urine pH may lead to uric acid stones in the urinary tract.

Decreased Levels

Found in kidney disease (chronic glomerulonephritis) because hampered renal function diminishes uric acid excretion.

Interfering Factors

1. Drugs
   - Salicylates
   - Thiazide diuretics
   - Chronic alcohol consumption
2. X-ray contrast media can markedly increase uric acid levels
3. Many other drugs can also influence these results.

VANILLYLMANDELIC ACID (VMA)

(Catecholamines or 3-Methoxy-4-Hydroxymandelic acid)

Normal values
VMA up to 9 mg/24 hr

Catecholamines

Epinephrine	100-230 mg/24 hr
Norepinephrine	100-230 mg/24 hr
Metanephrine	24-96 mg/24 hr
Normetanephrine	12-288 mg/24 hr

These investigations for adrenal medullary function are usually needed for a person with hypertension suspected to be having phaeochromocytoma (a tumour of chromaffin cells of the adrenal medulla). Incidence is about 1% amongst hypertensives. The compounds mentioned above contain a catechol nucleus and an amine group and are, therefore, called catecholamines. The major portion of the hormones are changed into metabolites, mainly 3-methoxy-4-hydroxy-mandelic acid or VMA.

Method/Principle

Catecholamines are adsorbed from untreated urine on to a column of Amberlite IRC 50, eluted and condensed in alkaline solution with ethylenediamine and the resulting fluorescence read. However, spectrophotometric methods are less subject to drug interference than fluorimetry. Samples should be collected in 10 ml hydrochloric acid and refrigerated.

Clinical Relevance

Elevated VMA levels
1. High levels found in phaeochromocytoma
2. Mild to moderate elevations seen in:
   - Neuroblastomas
   - Ganglioneuromas
   - Ganglioblastomas

Elevated catecholamines
Found in:
- Phaeochromocytoma
- Neuroblastomas
- Ganglioneuromas
- Ganglioneuroblastomas
- Progressive muscular dystrophy
- Myasthenia gravis

Interfering Factors

Increased VMA levels are caused by
1. Starvation (patients on nil orally-therapy should not undergo this test).
2. Foods: Tea, coffee, cocoa, vanilla, gelatin foods, fruit juice, chocolate, fruit, especially bananas, cider vinegar, salad dresssing, carbonated drinks, jelly and jam, candy gum, artificially flavoured or coloured foods, foods containing liquorice.
3. *Drugs causing increased VMA levels*
   - Aspirin
   - BSP
   - Glyceryl guaicolate
   - Phenazopyridine

- PSP
- Sulphonamides
- Levodopa
- Lithium
- Nitroglycerin
- Mephenesin
- Chlorpromazine
- Para-aminosalicylic acid (PAS)
- Methocarbamol
- Methylene blue
- Nalidixic acid
- Oxytetracycline
- Penicillin

False decreased levels of VMA are caused by

- Alkaline urine
- Uraemia (impairs VMA excretion)
- Radiographic contrast agents
- Drugs:
  - Clofibrate
  - Guaneshidine drugs
  - Imipramine
  - Methyldopa
  - MAO inhibitors
  - Clonidine
  - Reserpine
  - Imipramine

Interfering Factors in Determining Catecholamine Levels

- Vigorous exercise may increase catecholamine levels
- Drugs:
  - Ampicillin
  - Ascorbic acid
  - Chloral hydrate
  - Epinephrine
  - Erythromycin
  - Hydralazine
  - Methenamine
  - Methyldopa
  - Nicotinic acid
  - Quinine
  - Tetracycline
  - Vitamin B complex

Be Careful

- Explain that it is a 24-hour collection test
- Explain diet and drug restrictions
- Exclude all restricted foods for at least 3 days before test date
- Exclude all drug intake for 3 to 7 days before the test date
- Rest and adequate food and fluids are encouraged, and stress is to be avoided during the test.
- Patients can resume all restricted foods, drugs, and activity as soon as test is completed.

17-ketosteroids (17-KS)
17-Ketogenic Steroids (17-KGS)
17-Hydroxycorticosteroids (17-OHCS)

Normal values

17-ketosteroids

Men	: 8-18 mg/24 hr
Women	: 5-15 mg/24 hr

17-ketogenic steroids

Men	: 5.5-23 mg/24 hr
Women	: 3-15 mg/24 hr

17-hydroxycorticosteroids: 10 mg/24 hr

The above-mentioned substances are urinary steroids and their estimation is indicated in investigation of endocrine disturbances of the adrenals and testes.

17-ketosteroids have 19 carbon atoms with a ketone group at C-17. These steroids are composed of adrenal hormones and metabolites of testicular androgens. In men the adrenals produce 2/3rd of these hormones, while the testes produce the remainder. In women the adrenals produce all of the hormones.

17-ketogenic steroids are composed of glucocorticoid derivatives and pregnanedriol, have 21 carbon atoms and a hydroxyl group at C-17. Their estimation gives a good reflection of adrenal cortex activity.

17-hydroxycorticosteroids have 21 carbons with hydroxy groups at C-17 and C-21 and a ketone at C-20. These are also known as Porter-Silber chromogens.

Method/Principle 17 KS

Their assessment is a colorimetric assay. Urine is subjected to acid hydrolysis and the steroids are extracted with ethylene dichloride. A solvent aliquot is evaporated to dryness under a nitrogen stream and the resultant residue is reacted with m-dinitrobenzene (Zimmerman reaction), which in the presence of alkali gives a red colour with compounds containing an active methylene group. This colour obtained has an absorption maximum at 520 μ.

Method/Principle 17-OHCS

Porter-Silber reaction: The glucuronide conjugates of urinary corticosteroids are hydrolysed with β-glucuronidase. The "freed" steroids and free steroids (i.e. tetra and dihydro derivatives) normally present in the urine are extracted in methylene chloride. This extract is washed with a dilute aqueous alkali to remove a considerable amount of blank material which consists of oestrogens, bile acids, and other interfering chromogens. A portion of methylene chloride is shaken with a phenylhydrazine hydrochloride—sulphuric acid—ethanol reagent. For correction of the residual blank material, another portion of the extract is shaken with just the ethanol sulphuric acid reagent. The upper layer of methylene chloride is removed, and the lower phase after colour development is measured spectrophotometrically at 410 mm. No need to add preservative for 24-hour urine collection for 17-OHCS, but stop all medication 2-3 days prior to test day.

Clinical Relevance

- There is decrease in 17-KGS and 17-KS excretion in Addison's disease, hypopituitarism, Simmond's diseases and cretinism.
- There is an increase in 17-KGS excretion in precocious puberty on account of adrenal hyperplasia, surgery, excessive burns and infection.
- Increased 17-OHCS and 17-KGS usually imply hyperplasia of the adrenal cortex, tumour, cancer, or some variation of the adrenogenital syndrome.
- Steroid levels are also enhanced in Cushing's syndrome, eclampsia, acute pancreatitis, and ACTH therapy. If the beta-alpha ratio is >0.4, it is indicative of adrenal carcinoma. Unless the 17-KS are increased, the beta-alpha ratio is not likely to be abnormal.

Interfering Factors

a. Severe stress will cause increased levels of KS and KGS
b. KS levels are often increased in third trimester of pregnancy.
c. Drugs:
   1. Increasing 17-KS levels:
      - Chloramphenicol
      - Meprobamate
      - Spironolactone
      - Chlorpromazine
      - Nalidixic acid
      - Phenaglycodol
      - Cloxacillin
      - Penicillin
      - Erythromycin
      - Quinidine
      - Ethinamate
      - Secobarbitol
      - Oleandomycin
      - Phenazopyridine
      - Spironolactone
   2. Decreasing 17-KS levels:
      - Chlordiazepoxide
      - Probenecid
      - Estrogen
      - Meprobamate
      - Promazine
      - Metyrapone
      - Reserpine
   3. Increasing 17-OHCS levels:
      - Acetazolamide
      - Ascorbic acid
      - Chloral hydrate
      - Chloramphenicol
      - Chlordiazepoxide
      - Chlormerodrin
      - Chlorpromazine
      - Chlorthalidone
      - Colchicine
      - Cloxacillin
      - Erythromycin
      - Spironolactone
      - Digitoxin
      - Digoxin
      - Cortisone
      - Ethinamate
      - Etryptamine
      - Glutethimide
      - Meprobamate
      - Hydralazine
      - Oleandomycin
      - Paraldehyde
      - Quinine
      - Quinidine
   4. Decreasing 17-OHCS levels:
      - Aminoglutethimide
      - Diphenhydantoin
      - Estrogen

- Dexamethasone
- Calcium gluconate
- Phenothiazines
- Oral contraceptives
- Reserpine
- Corticosteroids
- Mitotane

CHLORIDES

Normal values
—110-250 mEq/24 hours
—10-20 gm NaCl/24 hours

Vary widely with intake amount and perspiration. The test findings have meaning only in relation to salt intake and output.

Clinical Relevance

Results are meaningful only when considered in relation to other data such as state of health/illness, salt intake and urine volume.

1. Normal findings: Urinary excretion of chloride decreases to a very low level whenever the serum level is much below 100 mEq/litre.
2. Decreased levels:
   a. In some conditions, urinary excretion of chloride increases even when the serum level is as low as 85 mEq/litre or less. Occurs in Addison's disease when there is a deficiency of adrenal hormones that controls the excretion of sodium and chloride.
   b. Decreased levels are also associated with:
      - Malabsorption syndrome
      - Pyloric obstruction
      - Prolonged gastric suction
      - Diarrhoea
      - Diaphoresis
      - Congestive heart failure
      - Emphysema
3. Increased levels are associated with:
   - Dehydration
   - Starvation
   - Salicylate toxicity
   - Mercurial and chlorothiazide diuretics.

Interfering Factors

1. Urinary chloride concentration varies with dietary salt intake, perspiration and to some extent, with urine volume.
2. False elevations may occur if the patient has taken bromides.

SODIUM

Normal values
130-200 mEq/24 hr.

The test is indicated in the study of renal and adrenal disturbances and of water and acid-base imbalances.

Clinical Relevance

Results have significance only when considered in relation to other data, such as a state of health/illness, salt intake, and urine volume.

1. *Increased levels*
   Caused by:
   - Dehydration
   - Starvation
   - Salicylate toxicity
   - Adrenal cortical insufficiency
   - Mercurial and chlorothiazide diuretics
   - Chronic renal failure
   - Diabetic acidosis
2. *Decreased levels of sodium associated with:*
   - Malabsorption syndrome
   - Congestive heart failure
   - Pyloric obstruction
   - Diarrhoea
   - Diaphoresis
   - Acute renal failure
   - Pulmonary emphysema
   - Aldosteronism
   - Cushing's disease
3. *Decreased levels:*
   Often accompanied by an equivalent loss of chloride.

Interfering Factors

1. Dietary salt intake
2. Altered renal function.

POTASSIUM

Normal values
40-80 mEq/24 hour

Test is required to assess electrolyte balance of the body by measuring the amount of potassium excreted in 24 hours. This measurement is useful in the study of renal and adrenal disorders and of water and acid-base imbalances.

Clinical Relevance

1. Increased levels:
   - Chronic renal failure

- Diabetic and renal tubular acidosis
- Dehydration
- Starvation
- Primary aldosteronism
- Cushing's disease
- Salicylate toxicity
- Mercurial chlorthiazide, ammonium chloride, and Diamox diuretics

2. Decreased levels:
   - Malabsorption syndrome
   - Diarrhoea
   - Acute renal failure
   - Adrenal cortical insufficiency (in some cases)
   - Excessive mineralocorticoid activity (aldosterone)
   - In patients with potassium deficiency, regardless of the cause
3. Cautionary finding:
   - In excessive vomiting or stomach suctioning, the accompanying alkalosis maintains urinary potassium excretion at levels inappropriately high for the degree of actual potassium depletion
   - In diabetes insipidus, urinary potassium is normal

Interfering Factors

Varies with dietary intake.

FOLLICLE-STIMULATING HORMONE (FSH) LUTEINISING HORMONE (LH)

Normal values

FSH

Men	: 4-25 IU/ml
Women	: 4-30 IU/ml
Postmenopausal	: 40-250 mu/ml
Midcycle	: Two times baseline

LH

Men	: 7-24 IU/ml
Women	: 6-30 IU/ml
Postmenopausal	: Over 30 IU/ml
Midcycle	: Over three times baseline.

These investigations are required in determining whether a gonadal insufficiency is primary or due to deficient stimulation by the pituitary hormones. The production of these hormones is under control of pituitary gland. In women, FSH promotes maturation of the ovarian follicle, and the maturing follicle produces oestrogens. As the levels of oestrogen rise, luteinising hormones are produced. Together, FSH and LH induce ovulation. In men, FSH produces spermatogenesis, and LH induces the secretion of androgens.

FSH is an aid in studying various causes of hypothyroidism in women as well as endocrine dysfunction in men. In primary ovarian failure or testicular failure, FSH is increased.

Kits for hormone determination ELISA/RIA based are available from *Spectral Diagnostics* and *Ranbaxy diagnostics.*

Clinical Relevance

Blood and urine estimation are used.

Decreased FSH levels occur in

- Feminising and masculinising ovarian tumours when production is inhibited as a result of increased oestrogen
- Failure of pituitary or hypothalamus
- Anorexia nervosa
- Neoplasm of testes or adrenal glands that secrete oestrogens or androgens

Increased FSH levels occur in

- Turner's syndrome (ovarian dysgenesis). Approximately 50% of patients with primary amenorrhoea have Turner's syndrome.
- Hypogonadism and primary gonadal failure
- Complete testicular feminisation syndrome
- Precocious puberty, either idiopathic or secondary to a central nervous system lesion
- Klinefelter's syndrome.

PREGNANEDIOL

Normal values

Standardisation extremely difficult

Proliferative phase	: 0.5-1.5 mg/24 hr
Luteal phase	: 2-7 mg/24 hr
Post-menopausal	: 0.2-1.0 mg/24 hr
Pregnancy	: 5-63 mg/24 hr.

The test helps in assessing ovarian and placental function. It is indicated when a deficiency of progesterone is suspected. Combined deficiency of oestrogen and progesterone is hinted by menstrual irregularities and difficulty in conceiving and maintaining a pregnancy. To be specific, it measures the hormone progesterone and its principal excreted metabolite, pregnanediol. Progesterone has its main effect on the endometrium by causing the endometrium to enter the secretory phase and become ready for implantation of the blastocyte if fertilisation has taken place. Pregnanediol excretion is high in pregnancy and low in luteal deficiency or placental failure. A 24-hour urine sample collection is needed.

Clinical Relevance

Increased levels
Associated with:
- Luteal cysts of ovary
- Arrhenoblastomas of the ovary
- Hyperadrenocorticism

Decreased levels
Associated with:
- Amenorrhoea
- Threatened abortion (not always)
- Foetal death
- Toxaemia

PREGNANETRIOL

Normal values
Adult : Up to 2 mg/24 hr
Children : Up to 1.0 mg/24 hr
Infants : Up to 0.2 mg/24 hr.

Do not confuse this with pregnanediol. Pregnanetriol reflects one segment of adrenocortical activity. This is a precursor in adrenal corticoid synthesis and arises from 17-hydroxyprogesterone, not from progesterone. The 24-hour urine test is conducted to diagnose adrenogenital syndrome, a defect in 21-hydroxylation.

The diagnosis of adrenogenital syndrome is considered in:
- Adult women who show signs and symptoms of excessive androgen production with or without hypertension
- Craving for salt
- Sexual precocity in boys
- Infants who exhibit signs of failure to thrive
- External genitalia in women (pseudoher-maphroditism). In boys, differentiation must be made between a virilising tumour of the adrenal gland, neurogenic and constitutional types of sexual precocity, and interstitial cell tumour of the testes.

Clinical Relevance

Elevated pregnanetriol levels occur in:
- Congential adrenocortical hyperplasia
- Stein-Leventhal syndrome.

OESTROGEN FRACTIONS

Normal values
Women - Total: 4-60 mg/24 hr.
Estron (E): 2-25 mg/24 hr.
Estradiol (E2) : 0-10 mg/24 hr.
Pregnancy - Estriol (E3): 2-30 mg/24 hr.
Men: 4-24 mg/24 hr.

To evaluate ovarian function and gynaecologic problems, estradiol, estron, and estriol are routinely measured. Oestrogens will be normally increased in pregnancy and in some tumours of the ovary and adrenal cortex.

Oestrogens are decreased in the absence of deficiency of ovarian hormones. Estriol levels are used in the management of high-risk pregnancies as a method of assessing placental function. A fall in estriol should be judged by at least two different serial measurements. A falling estriol excretion signifies impending foetal death.

Clinical Relevance

1. *Decreased oestrogen values are seen with:*
   - Hypo or dysfunction of pituitary and adrenal glands
   - Primary ovarian malfunction
   - Agenesis of the ovaries
2. *Increased oestrogen levels are found in:*
   - Solid ovarian tumours, granulosa/theca cell
   - Tumour/hyperplasia of the adrenal cortex
3. *Decreasing estriol levels:* of more than 40% of previous values is associated with placental insufficiency. An abrupt drop of 40% or more is associated with foetal distress.
4. *Miscellaneous causes of estriol levels decline are:*
   - Anaemia
   - Malnutrition
   - Pyelonephritis
   - Intestinal disease
   - Haemoglobinopathies

Interfering Factors

Drugs interfering are:
- Ampicillin
- Hydrochlorothiazide
- Exogenous corticosteroids

- Meprobamate
- Meth. mandelate
- Cascara
- Phenazopyridine
- Diethylstilbestrol
- Prochlorperazine
- Hexamine
- Senna
- Tetracyclines

HEAVY METALS, BLOOD AND 24-HOURS URINE

Norm:

	Blood	*SI units*
Antimony	0.052 ± 0.019 μg/dl	4.35 ± 1.6 nmol/L
Arsenic	2-23 μg/L	0.03-0.31 μmol/L
Chronic poisoning	100-500 μg/L	1.33-6.65 μmol/L
Acute poisoning	600-9300 μg/L	7.98-124 μmol/L
Bismuth	0.1-3.5 μg/L	0.5-16.7 nmol/L
Cadmium		
Smokers	0.6-3.9 μg/L	5.3-34.7 nmol/L
Nonsmokers	0.3-1.2 μg/l	2.7-10.7 nmol/L
Toxic	100-3000 μg/L	0.9-26.7 μmol/L
Cobalt	0.11-0.45 μg/L	1.9-7.6 noml/L
Copper		
Infants	20-70 μg/dl	3.1-11 μmol/L
Child 6 years	90-190 μg/dl	14.1-29.8 μmol/L
Child 12 years	80-160 μg/dl	12.6-25.1 μmol/L
Adult male	70-140 μg/dl	11-22 μmol/L
Adult female	80-155 μg/dl	12.6-24.3 μmol/L
Pregnant	118-302 μg/dl	18.5-47.4 μmol/L
Lead		
Child	<25 μg/dl	<1.21 μmol/L
Adult	<40 μg/dl	<1.93 μmol/L
Industry exposure	<60 μg/dL	<2.90 μmol/L
Toxic concentration	>100 μg/dl	>4.83 μmol/L
Toxic concentration in children	>25 μg/dl	1.21 μmol/L
Mercury	0 6-59 μg/L	3-294 μmol/L
Non-fish eaters	<5 μg/L	<25 nmol/L
Selenium	58-234 μg/L	0.74-2.97 μmol/L
Thallium	<0.5 μg/dl	<24.5 nmol/L
Toxic concentration	10-800 μg/dl	0.5-39.1 μmol/L
Zinc	70-150 μg/dl	10.7-23 μmol/L
Antimony	<10 μg/L	<82.1 μmol/L
Toxic concentration	>10 μg/L	>82.1 μmol/L
Arsenic	5-50 μg/L	0.067-0.665 μmol/L
Chronic poison	50-5000 μg/L	0.67-66.5 μmol/L
Acute poison	1000-20,000 μg/L	13.3-266 mmol/L
Bismuth	0.3-4.6 μg/L	1.4-22 nmol/L
Cadmium	0.5-4.7 μg/L	4.4-41.8 nmol/L
Industrial exposure	10-580 μg/L	0.09-5.16 μmol/L
Cobalt	1-2 μg/L	17-34 nmol/L
Copper	2-80 μg/L	0.03-1.26 μmol/L
Lead	<80 μg/L	<0.39 μmol/L
Industrial exposure	<120 μg/L	<0.58 μmol/L
Mercury		
Adult	<20 μg/L	<0.10 μmol/L
Toxic concentration	>150 μg/L	>0.75 μmol/L
Lethal concentration	>800 μg/L	>4 μmol/L
Selenium	7-160 μg/L	0.09-2.03 μmol/L
Toxic concentration	>400 μg/L	5.08 μmol/L
Thallium	<2 μg/L	<9.8 nmol/L
Toxic concentration	1-20 mg/L	4.9-97.8 μmol/L
Zinc	150-1200 μg/L	2.3-18.4 μmol/L
Toxic concentration	>1200 μg/L	18.4 μmol/L

TOXIC/POISONING SYMPTOMS AND TREATMENT

Symptoms

Antimony: Vomiting.

Arsenic: Gastric pain, vomiting, diarrhoea, convulsions, coma, and death in acute poisoning; and diarrhoea, scaling and pigmentation of skin, hair loss, and peripheral neuropathy in chronic poisoning.

Bismuth: Weakness, decreased appetite, fever, halitosis, black gum line, rheumatic type pain, and renal damage.

Cadmium: Pneumonia, pulmonary oedema, and cardiovascular collapse from inhalation, violent gastrointestinal symptoms from acute ingestion, and osteomalacia and renal dysfunction from chronic ingestion.

Cobalt: Thyroid gland hyperplasia, cardiomyopathy, nerve damage, and myxoedema.

Copper: Nausea, vomiting, headache, diarrhoea, and abdominal pain.

Lead: Anorexia, abdominal pain, vomiting, irritability, and apathy.

Mercury: Fatigue, headache, loss of memory, apathy, emotional instability, paraesthesia, ataxia, deafness, dysarthria, visual deterioration, dysphagia, coma, and death.

Selenium: Garlic smell in breath and urine, metallic taste, headaches, nausea, vomiting, pneumonia, and pulmonary oedema.

Thallium: Ataxia, pulmonary oedema, vomiting, constipation, restlessness, delirium, and coma.

Zinc: Cough, chest discomfort, tachycardia, hypertension, gastrointestinal irritation, nausea, vomiting, diarrhoea, and metallic taste in mouth.

Treatment

Antidotes for heavy metal poisoning include BAL (British antilewisite), deferoxamine, dimercaprol, and EDTA. Heavy metals respond to haemodialysis and/or haemoperfusion in varying degrees (poor to well).

Usage

Screening for heavy-metal toxicity from over-exposure, ingestion, or occupational exposure. Disorders for individual metals found under test listings for individual metals. Drugs that may further increase some values include carbamazepine, oestrogens, oral contraceptives, penicillamine, phenobarbital, phenytoin, and sodium salts.

Description

Heavy metals include antimony, arsenic, bismuth, cadmium, cobalt, copper, lead, mercury, selenium, thallium, and zinc.

Antimony exposure occurs in miners, smelters, and ore refinery workers.

Arsenic is found naturally in food and the environment as well as in pesticides.

Bismuth exposure occurs in workers in cosmetic, disinfectant, and pigment industries. It may also occur as a result of treatment for syphilis.

Cadmium accumulates in the lungs, liver and kidneys via exposure to food, water, air, and cigarette smoke.

Cobalt, a component of vitamin B_{12}, is found in most foods. It is also used to treat some resistant anaemias and some radiosensitive malignancies.

Copper is a trace element found in normal diets. It is one of the few heavy metals that are potentially harmful at low levels as well as at toxic levels. Toxic levels may be caused by the use of copper IUDs, ingestion of contaminated substances, or fungicide exposure.

Lead is absorbed into the body through the ingestion of lead-containing paint or through industrial exposure.

Mercury is found in fungicides, industrial processes, and in fish (polluted water). It can also be ingested in the form of mercury salts. High mercury levels have been noted among dental workers.

Selenium is a metal used for the activity of human glutathione peroxidase. Exposure occurs as a result of the manufacture of glass, paints, dyes, electronic equipment, fungicides, rubber, and semiconductors.

Thallium is present in cosmetics, pesticides, and in some medications. It is absorbed through intact skin and mucous membranes.

Zinc is a trace metal important for cellular growth and metabolism. Toxicity can occur from industrial exposure and consumption of acidic food or beverages from galvanised containers.

MICROSCOPY OF THE URINARY SEDIMENT

Use a clean, fresh morning specimen. Obtain urinary sediment by centrifuging urine at 3000 rpm for 5 minutes. Draw off the clear supernatant fluid, place a drop of the sediment on a glass slide and cover it with a coverslip. Examine first under low power, then under high power, vary the light intensity for seeing casts. If protein is present, look for casts, RBCs, pus cells and epithelial cells.

In most instances an unstained sediment is sufficient. However, should a difficulty arise or the examiner is inexperienced, staining can be done with Sternheimer and Malbin stain.

A drop of methylene blue solution can be added to the sediment and would help in identifying cellular structure and bacteria. A crystal violet saffranine stain is used to identify cellular elements; a peroxidase stain will differentiate renal tubular cells that are peroxidase negative and neutrophils (pus cells) that are peroxidase positive. In most cases qualitative or semiquantitative examination of the urine is enough. For following the progress of active renal disease, Addis' count may be used. Cell counts can be expressed as occasional, 1+, 2+, 3+ or full field. Count in at least 10 high power fields for cells and express the average as the number of cells per high power field.

Red blood cells: Under high power they appear as pale discs. If the specimen is stale, because of dissolution of haemoglobin, these cells will appear as ghost cells. These red cells may show crenated margins.

RBCs may be confused with oil droplets or yeast cells. Oil droplets are variable in size and are refractile. Yeast cells usually show budding. Alkaline haematin stains dark purple in alkaline urine.

Neutrophilic leucocytes (Pus cells): Unstained neutrophilic leucocytes appear as round granular 12 μ spheres, larger than RBC. These may look like small epithelial cells—let a drop of glacial acetic acid flow under the coverslip—the segmented nucleus of a leucocyte becomes clearer.

Epithelial cells have a single, rounded nucleus. Glitter cells are larger neutrophils, cytoplasmic granules may show brownian movement.

Renal tubular epithelial cells: Unstained cells are almost the same size as that of a neutrophil but contain a large round nucleus. Oval fat bodies are those cells containing fat globules, the nucleus, then, is not visible.

Bladder epithelial cells: Unstained cells are larger than renal tubular cells, have a round nucleus and vary in size depending on depth of origin in transitional epithelium. Superficial cells are large and flat with small nucleus.

Squamous epithelial cells: Unstained, these are large, flattened cells with abundant cytoplasm and a small round nucleus. The cell may be folded or rolled.

Casts: These are cylindrical, diameter varies according to the size of the renal tubule or duct of their origin. The ends are usually rounded but may be flat, irregular or tapered.

Hyaline: Are colourless, homogeneous, transparent.

Finely granular casts: Contain fine granules in all or in part of the cast.

Coarse granular casts: Contain fat, degenerated cell or protein aggregates which appear as dark granules.

Fatty casts: Contain highly refractile globules of varying size. Fat droplets will stain bright orange with Sudan III.

Red cell casts: Yellow under LP objective. If many cells are present in each cast, the matrix will not be visible.

Blood casts: Contain haemoglobin from degenerated RBCs. Are yellow to orange in colour, best seen with LP objective.

Leucocyte casts: Contain small granular cells in a clear matrix. The leucocytes may be admixed with red cells or epithelial cells. Clumps of leucocytes may sometimes look like casts.

Tubular epithelial casts: Resemble leucocyte or mixed cell casts. They often appear as two rows of cells in a narrow cast.

Waxy casts: Are yellow and homogeneous, have sharper outlines than hyaline casts with irregular ends and cracks.

Structures commonly confused with casts are mucous threads and rolled, cigar-shaped squamous epithelial cells. Mucous threads are long, ribbon-like strands with poorly defined edges and have pointed or split ends. Often, they appear to have longitudinal striations.

Fat: Free globules are seen in grape-like clusters. They vary in size more than the yeast cells or red cells.

DETAILED STUDY OF IMPORTANT URINARY MICROSCOPY CONSTITUENTS

Red Cells and Red Cell Casts

Normal values of RBCs

1-2/LPF (low powered field)
0-1/HPF (high powered field)
Red cell casts Nil (zero)/LPF

In a healthy subject, red cells are only occasionally found in the urine, but persistent finding needs to be investigated. Examine sediment under low and high power. RBCs are studied under high power.

Clinical Relevance

Red cell casts

- Casts composed largely of RBCs are rarely found normally and indicate haemorrhage or desquamative conditions of the nephron.
- RBC casts imply acute inflammatory or vascular disorder in the glomerulus.
- They may be the only manifestation of:
  - Acute glemerulophritis
  - Renal infarction
  - Collagen disease
  - Kidney involvement in subacute bacterial endocarditis
- The usual finding in SLE is RBC casts and epithelial cell casts.

Red Blood Cells

The finding of more than one to two RBCs per HPF is an abnormal condition that can indicate:

- Renal or systemic disease
- Trauma to kidney

Increased red cells are found in:

- Pyelonephritis

- SLE
- Renal stones
- Cystitis
- Haemophilia
- Prostatitis
- Tuberculosis of urinary tract
- Malignancies of urinary tract

Red cells in excess of WBCs imply bleeding into the urinary tract as may occur in:

- Trauma
- Tumours
- Aspirin consumption
- Anticoagulant therapy
- Thrombocytopenia.

Interfering Factors

- Increased numbers of RBCs can be found following violent exercise, a traumatic catheterisation, passage of stones, or contamination by menstrual fluid
- Alkaline urine haemolyses RBCs and dissolves casts
- Many drugs can cause RBC appearance in urine
- Red cell casts may occur after strenuous physical activity and contact sports.

White Cells and White Cell Casts

Normal values
WBCs : 0-5/high powered field (HPF)
WBC casts : none (zero)/LPF

WBCs may come from anywhere in the genitourinary field. While white cell casts always come from renal tubules.

Clinical Relevance

Leucocytes

- Large numbers of WBCs indicate bacterial infection of urinary tract
- If infection is in the kidney, WBCs may be associated with cellular and granular casts, bacteria, epithelial cells and relatively few red cells
- Usually, presence of abnormal numbers of WBCs in urine necessitates urine culture.

WBC casts

- White cell casts indicate renal parenchymal infection
- May be found in:
  - Pyelonephritis most common cause
  - Acute glomerulonephritis
  - Interstitial inflammation of the kidney.
- It is difficult to differentiate between WBC and epithelial cell casts
- As pyelonephritis may remain completely asymptomatic even though renal tissue is being progressively destroyed, careful examination (using low power) of urinary sediment for leucocyte casts is mandatory.

Interfering Factors

Vaginal discharge can contaminate the sample. Either a "clean catch" (midstream sample) or a catheterised specimen should be taken to rule out contamination.

Epithelial Cells and Epithelial Cell Casts

Normal values
Occasional renal epithelial cell may be found

Renal epithelial cell casts are formed by cast-off tubular cells. Since tubular cells are being replaced, it is of little importance, therefore, to find an occasional epithelial cells or clumps.

Clinical Relevance

Large numbers of epithelial cells are abnormal.
May be seen in:

- Nephrosis
- Amyloidosis
- Poisoning from heavy metals and toxins.

Squamous epithelial cells (squames) are usually seen when urine is contaminated with vaginal discharge.

Hyaline Casts

Normal value
Occasional hyaline cast/LPF may be found

These are clear, colourless casts and are formed when protein (Tamm-Horsfall) within the tubules precipitates and gels. Their appearance in the urine depends on the rate of urine flow, urine pH, and the degree of proteinuria. Examine under low power.

Clinical Relevance

- Hyaline casts imply possible damage to the glomerular capillary membrane, which is permitting leakage of proteins through the glomerular filter.

- Hyaline casts may be temporarily seen in:
  - Fever
  - Postural strain
  - Emotional fatigue
  - Strenuous exercise
  - Palpation of kidney
- When large numbers of hyaline casts appear in the urine along with heavy proteinuria, fine granular casts, fatty casts, or oval fat bodies or fat droplets, nephrotic syndrome should be considered.
- Casts may not be found even if proteinuria is heavy because of dilute urine or because pH is alkaline.
- In cylindruria, large numbers of casts are seen, but there may not be any protein in the urine.

Granular Casts

Normal value
Occasional granular cast may be seen.

Granular casts result from the disintegration of the cellular material of WBCs and epithelial cells into coarse and fine particles.

Clinical Relevance

- Acute tubular necrosis
- Advanced glomerulonephritis
- Pyelonephritis
- Malignant nephrosclerosis
- Chronic lead poisoning.

Waxy Cysts

Never seen in healthy subjects. Seen in terminal diseases of kidney.

- Chronic renal disease
- Tubular inflammation and degeneration.

Oval Fat Bodies and Fatty Casts

Never seen in urines of healthy individuals. In nephrotic syndrome, fat accumulates in the tubular cells and eventually sloughs off, forming oval fat bodies. This fat is probably a cholesterol ester. Fatty casts usually composed of individual droplets. The presence of fat droplets, oval fat bodies, or fatty casts is the hallmark of the nephrotic syndrome.

Clinical Relevance

Fatty casts are found in chronic renal disease and indicate tubular inflammation and degeneration.

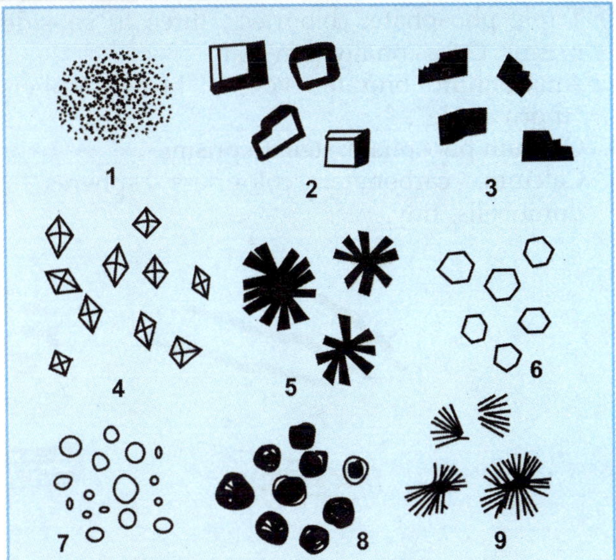

Fig. 5.3: Crystals etc., Usually found in acidic urine: (1) Amorphous urates, (2) Uric acid, (3) Cholesterol, (4) Calcium oxalate (5) Sodium urate, (6) Cystine (7) Fat droplets, (8) Leucin spheres, and (9) Tyrosine needles

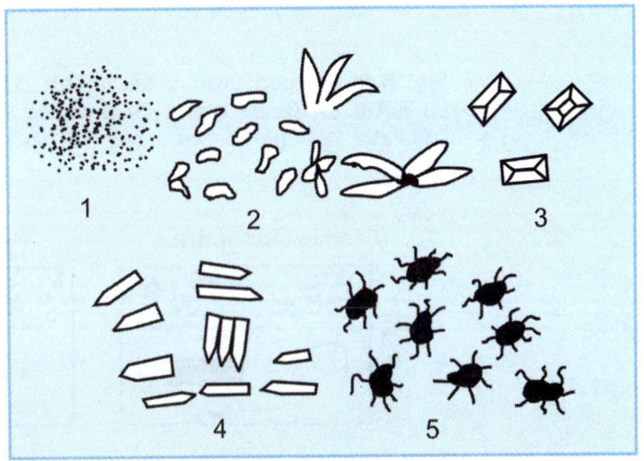

Fig. 5.4: Crystals usually found in alkaline urine: (1) Amorphous phosphate, (2) Calcium carbonate, (3) Triple phosphate, (4) Calcium phosphate, and (5) Ammonium urate

CRYSTALS

Crystals seen in normal acid urine (Fig. 5.3):

1. Amorphous urates: yellow-red granules.
2. Uric acid: yellow or red-brown irregular but usually whetstone crystals or rhomboids.
3. Calcium oxalate: refractile, octahedral "envelopes".

Crystals seen in Normal Alkaline Urine (Figs 5.4 to 5.6)

1. Amorphous phosphates: fine precipitate.

2. Triple phosphate: colourless, three to six-sided prisms. Occasionally fern leaf.
3. Ammonium biurate: yellow brown spheres "thorn apple".
4. Calcium phosphate: stellate prisms.
5. Calcium carbonate: colourless spheres or dumbbells, tiny.

Crystals seen in Abnormal Urine

1. Cystine: colourless, refractile, hexagonal plate.
2. Tyrosine: fine needles arranged in sheaves or clumps, usually yellow, silky.
3. Leucine: yellow, oily appearing spheres with radial and concentric striations.

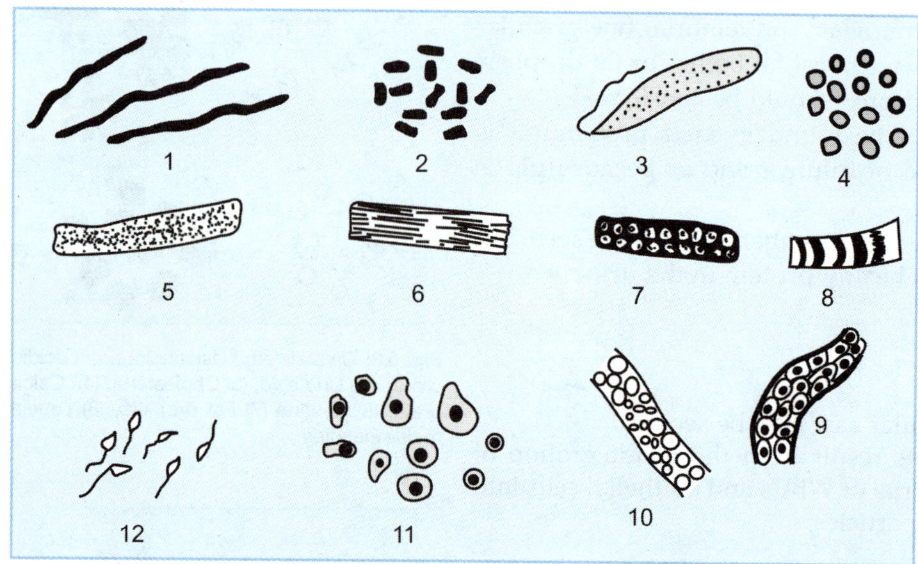

Fig. 5.5: Formed urinary sediment; (1) Mucous threads, (2) Bacteria, (3) Cylindroid, (4) RBCs. (5-10, are casts), (5) Granular, (6) Hyaline, *(7)* Pus cell, (8) Waxy, (9) Epithelial cell, (10) Fatty, (11) Epithelial cells, and (12) Spermatozoa

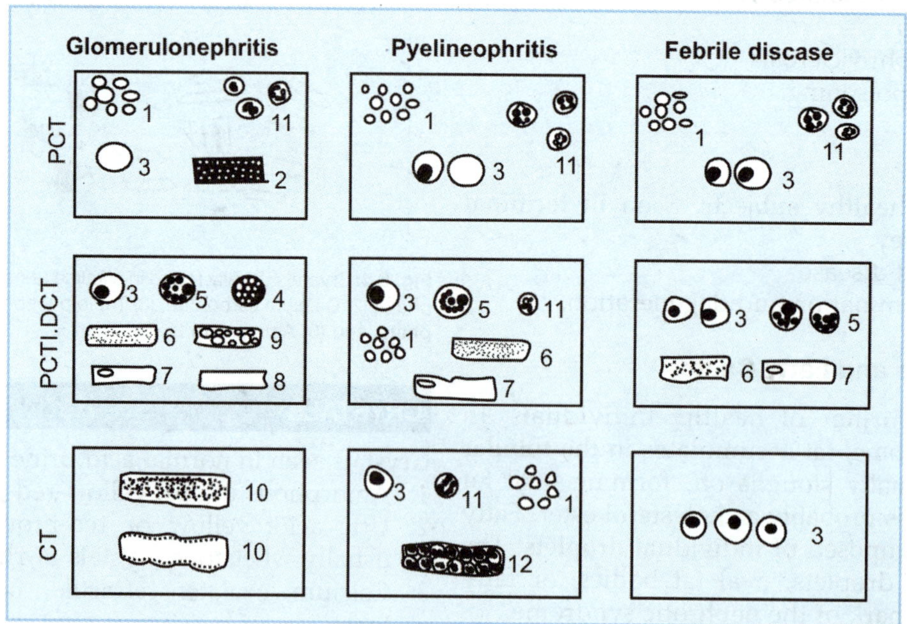

Fig. 5.6: Microscopic urinary sediment in Glomerulonephritis, Pyelonephritis and Febrile Disease: (1) Red blood cells, (2) RBC cast, (3) Tubule cell, (4) Oval fat body, (5) Tubule cell full of protein(6) Granular cast, (7) Hyaline case, (8) Waxy cast, (9) Fatty cast, (10) Broad cast, (11) WBC, (12) Pus cell cast. PCT Proximal convoluted tubule, L—Loop of Henle, DCT—Distal convoluted tubule, CT—Collecting tubule

COMMON PATTERNS OF ABNORMAL URINE COMPOSITION IN DISEASE

Disease	*Daily volume*	*Colour*	*Sp Gr*	*Protein*	*Red cell*	*Casts*	*Microscopic & other findings*
Normal	600-2500	Yellow amber	1.003 1.030	O-trace	O to Occ	O to Occ	Hyaline, casts, must be acid and fresh or preserved
Hyper-pyrexia	Decreased	Amber	Increased	Trace to+	O to +	None to few	Hyaline casts, tubular cells
Congestive heart failure	↓	Amber	↑-varies with renal function	1-2+	None to +	+	Hyaline and granular casts
Eclampsia	↓	Amber	↑	3-4+	None to +	3-4+	Hyaline casts
Diabetic coma	↓ or ↑	Light	↑	+	O	None to +	Hyaline casts, glucose, ketonuria
Acute glomeru-lonephritis (Ac. GN)	↓	Smoky red	↑	2-4+	1-4+	2-4+	Blood, cellular, granular, hyaline casts, renal, tubul epith
Degenerative phase (De. GN)	Normal or ↓	Light	Normal or ↑	4 +	1-2 +	4 +	Granular, waxy, fatty casts, broad casts
Lipoid nephrosis	↓	Light to dark	Very high	4 +	O to trace	4 +	Hyaline, granular, fatty, waxy casts, fatty tubule cells
Collagen disease	Normal, ↓ or ↑	Light to dark	Normal or ↓	1-4+	1-4+	1-4+	Blood, cellular, granular, hyaline, waxy, fatty, broad casts, fatty tubule cells
Pyelonephritis	Normal or ↑	Cloudy, dark	Normal or ↓	1-2+	None to+	None to+	Pus casts and hyaline casts. Many pus cells, bacteria
Benign hypertension	Normal or ↑	Normal or Light	Normal or ↓	None to+	O to trace	None to+	Hyaline and granular casts
Malignant hypertension	Normal ↓ or ↑	Light	Low, fixed	1-2+	Trace to+	1-2+	Hyaline and granular casts

Occ = Occasional. ↓ = Reduced or decreased. ↑ = Increased or raised O= Nil/Zero

4. Sulphonamide crystals (sulphadiazine): yellow-brown asymmetrical, striated sheaves and round forms with radial striations.

Cholesterol appears as flat notched plates in acid urine, calcium oxalate and calcium hydrogen phosphate crystals are found in neutral urine. Uric acid and urates redissolve on warming at 60°C. Ampicillin is occasionally seen as masses of long, tiny colourless crystals in acid urine when given parenterally.

Bacteria, Fungus and Parasites

Bacteria may or may not (contaminated, overgrown) be important. A dry film may be madeby spreading a drop or two of the urine sediment on a glass slide, fixed and stained with Gram's stain. If bacteria are identified in an uncentrifuged specimen under an oil immersion lens, it suggests that more than 100,000 organisms/ml are present, i.e. significant bacteriuria.

Acid-fast bacilli may be seen but urine should always be cultured as smegma also contains some acid-fast bacilli.

Yeast cells may be seen in UTI (e.g. in diabetes mellitus) but yeasts are also common contaminants.

Parasites and Parasitic Ova

May be seen as faecal or vaginal contaminants. In *Schistosoma haematobium*, typical ova may be seen in urine accompanied by RBCs from urinary bladder. *Trichomonas vaginalis* may come from vagina when urethral or bladder infection is suspected, the protozoa should be searched for immediately in a wet preparation. Spermatozoa are generally present in the urine of men after nocturnal emissions.

Casts in Urine

Hyaline

- Normal people after strenuous exercise.
- Congestive heart failure.
- Diabetic nephropathy.
- Chronic renal failure.
- Glomerulonephritis and pyelonephritis.

Red Cell

- Acute glomerulonephritis.
- Lupus nephritis.
- Goodpasture's syndrome.
- Subacute bacterial endocarditis.
- Renal infarction.

White Cell

- Acute pyelonephritis.
- Interstitial nephritis.
- Lupus nephritis.

Epithelial Cell

- Tubular necrosis.
- Cytomegalovirus infection.
- Toxicity from heavy metals, salicylates.
- Transplant rejection.

Granular

- Nephrotic syndrome.
- Pyelonephritis.
- Glomerulonephritis.
- Transplant rejection.
- Lead toxicity.

Waxy Casts

- Severe tubular atrophy.
- Renal failure.
- Transplant rejection.

CHAPTER 6

Renal Function and Its Evaluation

Assessment of renal function involves urine analysis; both routine and microscopic, blood chemistry, urography and special renal function tests.

Renal Physiology in Brief

Each kidney contains about 1 million nephrons. A nephron has a glomerulus and a long tubule that has three parts: (1) the proximal convoluted tubule (PCT), (2) the thin loop of Henle (LH), and (3) the distal convoluted tubule (DCT).

The glomeruli are the ultrafilter and the filtrate produced is like plasma except that it has almost no protein, 180 litres of this filtrate is produced in 24 hours, of which 178 litres of water and most of the organic and inorganic solutes are reabsorbed. Normally, some components of the filtered solutes are actively absorbed (completely or almost so)—glucose, phosphate and amino acids, sodium, etc. For some solutes, such as glucose, phosphate and amino acids, the maximum reabsorptive capacity of the tubule is limited and filtered material in excess of this limit is passed on in the urine. Normal renal threshold for glucose is 180 mg%, if excess is presented to the nephron, it would result in glycosuria. Other solutes are not reabsorbed, or are only passively and partially reabsorbed or are actively secreted by the tubule. Inulin (a carbohydrate) used for renal function studies is not at all reabsorbed by the tubules. Some urea is passively reabsorbed, but most of the filtered urea escapes reabsorption. Exogenous creatinine, H^+, K^+, phenol red (PSP), iodopyracet (Diodrast), para-aminohippurate and penicillin are actively secreted by the tubule cells, thus increasing excretion over the amount filtered.

Functions of the Kidney

1. Removal in solution of solid waste substances (e.g., end products of protein metabolism and foreign substances like dyes).

2. Regulation of water balance.
3. Regulation of acid-base equilibrium and electrolyte excretion. This includes secretion of H^+ and production of ammonia from amino acids, principally glutamine. The H^+ and NH_4^+ produced are exchanged for Na^+ in the DCT, thus providing for conservation of this essential cation.

Urinalysis

This has already been dealt in depth in previous chapter.

Impaired Renal Function and Blood Chemistry

1. Reduction in glomerular filtration rate or renal blood flow is accompanied by a rise in blood urea nitrogen (BUN), creatinine and non-protein nitrogen (NPN). Phosphate and sulphate retention is common.
2. Low serum protein concentrations occur commonly. Oedema may occur if serum albumin drops below 2.5 gm% or total serum proteins become less than 5.5 gm%.
3. Acid-base equilibrium is disturbed in nephritis. Renal acidosis is partly due to failure to conserve sodium during excretion of anions (e.g., chlorides and phosphates).
4. Anaemia accompanies chronic renal disease.

CONCENTRATION: DILUTION TESTS

If the patient's routine urine specimens contain no sugar or protein and have a specific gravity of 1.025 or higher, a concentration test is unnecessary.

Principle

Urine specific gravity is a measure of capacity of the tubules to reabsorb water from glomerular filtrate, thus concentrating the urine. Determination of osmolality is better but equipment needed for this is generally not available.

Concentration Test

It is contraindicated in uraemia and is unreliable in a case of heart failure with oedema.

1. No fluids for 24 hours after the morning meal (uraemic patients are not to be dehydrated, they may have a large obligatory renal water loss).
2. Collect urine specimens during the last 12 hours of the period and determine specific gravity of each.
3. Specific gravity should reach 1.025 or more. In some patients with oedema, nocturnal diuresis will invalidate the test.

Dilution Test (Water Test)

It is contraindicated in patients with renal/cardiac oedema. The test may be modified for use in the diagnosis of adrenal insufficiency.

1. Evening meal as desired. Nothing orally after 8.00 pm.
2. At 8.00 am empty bladder and drink 1500 ml water within 45 minutes.
3. Void every half an hour until noon (Save 8 specimens).
4. Specific gravity should be 1.003 in at least one of the specimens.
5. Total quantity of voided specimens should be over 80% of intake (i.e., over 1200 ml).

Mosenthal Modification of Concentration—Dilution Tests

1. The patient follows his usual eating and drinking habits.
2. Collect urine every 2 hours from 8.00 am to 8.00 pm. Collect night urine as one specimen (8.00 pm to 8.00 am).

Results:

3. Specific gravity in one specimen should exceed 1.020.
4. A difference of 0.009 or more should exist between lowest and highest specific gravities.
5. Volume of 12-hour night urine should not exceed 725 ml.

Vasopressin Concentration Test

This is contraindicated in pregnancy and coronary artery disease. It depends on the antidiuretic effect of posterior pituitary extract.

No preparation is needed other than abstinence from diuretics.

Empty the bladder. Inject subcutaneously 10 USP units of vasopressin. Collect urine after 60 and 120 minutes. The highest specific gravity should exceed 1.020.

Interpret as in concentration test above. This vasopressin test gives reliable results in the presence of cardiac oedema or ascites. A further application of the test is in diabetes insipidus, where urine concentration is normal after giving vasopressin but not after fluid restriction.

Conditions that Impair Concentrating Ability

Renal diseases:
- Pyelonephritis.
- Acute or chronic glomerular failure.
- Nephrogenic diabetes insipidus.
- Renal tubular acidosis.

Metabolic disturbances:
- Osmotic diuresis (especially diabetes mellitus).
- Hypokalaemia.
- Hypercalcaemia (especially hyperparathyroidism).
- Lithium use.
- Ethanol use.
- Prolonged overhydration.
- Severe hypoproteinaemia.

Systemic diseases affecting renal medulla:
- Multiple myeloma.
- Amyloidosis.
- Sickle cell anaemia or trait.

PHENOL RED TEST [Phenolsulphonphthalein (PSP)]

Principle

This is a measure of tubular excretion. PSP is removed from peritubular capillary blood by the renal tubules and excreted into the urine.

Intravenous Method

Make sure that no residual volume remains in the bladder and evacuation is complete. At the beginning of the test, the bladder should not be empty for it is necessary that the patient be able to void for the 15-minute collection.

1. The patient should drink 2 glasses of water and additional water during the test to ensure a urine volume sufficient to permit collection of urine specimen at the stated time. Larger urine volumes reduce error resulting from incomplete bladder emptying.
2. Inject 1 ml of dye (6 mg) intravenously. Collect the total volume of urine voided at 15, 30 and 60 minutes after injection of the dye. Determine the PSP content of each specimen.

Interpretation

	% PSP excretion			
	15 min.	30 min.	60 min.	Total
Normal	15-27+	12-20	13-20	55-60
Renal insufficiency	< 15	< 12	< 12	< 40

Ureteral Catheterisation Method (Cystoscopy)

The method can be used to study function of a single kidney at a time. Have the 2 ureteral catheters dripping into separate test tubes containing dilute NaOH and inject 1 ml of PSP I/V. Normally, the dye appears within 3 minutes, as indicated by pink colouration in the tubes.

Phenol Red Test for Residual Urine

(Modified PSP test to serve as a measure of residual urine).

Let the patient empty his bladder. Give I/V 1 ml of PSP (6 mg of dye). The water intake here is limited to 200 ml or less during each of the 2 subsequent half-hour periods; this is necessary because the rapid filling of the bladder in the presence of uretheral obstruction may result in a loss of bladder tone and a consequent increase in residual urine.

Collect all urine that the patient can pass half an hour and 1 hour after the injection of the dye.

Normally, the PSP excretion is 50-60% in the first half-hour, plus another 10-15% during the second half-hour.

Interpretation

		First specimen (½ hour)	*Second specimen (1 hour)*
Normal		50-60%	10-15%
Residual urine present	(a)	15%	25%
	(b)	35%	25%
	(c)	25%	25%

If the initial half-hour excretion is less than, equal to, or only slightly more than the second half-hour excretion, residual urine must be present. In case the excretion curve is flat and the morning specific gravity low, catheterisation should be done after collection of the second half-hour specimen to confirm the presence or absence of residual urine, since under these circumstances one cannot distinguish between severely depressed renal function and a large residual volume of urine. If the specific gravity of the morning urine is high, renal insufficiency is unlikely and a flat excretion curve is a reliable index of residual urine volume.

A rough estimate of residual urine volume can be calculated from the following formula:

$$\frac{Vol^{(½\,h.)}\ (60\text{-}PSP^{(½\,h.)})}{PSP^{(½\,h.)}} = \text{ml residual urine}$$

$Vol^{(1/2\,h.)}$ = Volume of first half-hour specimen.
$PSP^{(1/2\,h.)}$ = % of PSP recovered in first specimen.
60 = Expected normal PSP excretion in the first half-hour.

(values of the second half-hour are not used in this calculation).

CLEARANCE TESTS

By these tests, the capacity of the kidneys to clear waste products or foreign materials (inulin, etc.) from the blood into the urine is found. From the determination of blood concentration of the test material and the quantity eliminated in the urine "clearance" can be calculated in terms of millimetres of blood cleared per unit time.

Creatinine Clearance

Creatinine is filtered through the glomerulus. Under ordinary circumstances, the clearance of endogenous creatinine approximates the glomerular filtration rate. The clearance formula is:

$$\text{Clearance} = \frac{UV}{P}$$

where U= mg% creatinine in urine
P= mg% creatinine in plasma
V= ml of urine excreted per minute or per 24 hours.

Methods

1. Twenty four hour endogenous creatinine clearance. The entire volume of 24 hours period is collected. A blood sample is withdrawn during the forenoon of the day of the test. Creatinine concentrations in plasma/serum and urine are found and the volume of the urine is measured and the clearance estimated as per the formula given.
2. Two to 6-hour clearance periods may be used. Fasting state is preferred for the brief clearance period. A 2-to 6-hour urine collection is completed and a blood sample withdrawn at about the midpoint of the urine collection period. Creatinine concentrations are estimated in urine and plasma and the urine volume is found and clearance estimated.

Interpretation

Normal values for men and women corrected to 1.73 sq m body surface area range from 140-180 litres/24 hours (100-150 ml/minute). To correct clearance to standard 1.73 sq. m. body surface area.

$$\text{Clearance observed} \times \frac{1.73\ \text{sq m}}{\text{Estimated surface area}} = \text{Corrected clearance.}$$

(This test is superior to urea clearance).

Creatinine Clearance Test

Normal range: 110-150 ml/min (males)
105-132 ml/min (females)

Effect of age on normal function
Ages 50-75, subtract 5 ml for each 5-yr interval. Age 75 and above, subtract 8 ml for each 5-yr interval.

Artefacts that lower calculated figure:
- Incomplete urine collection.
- Bacterial multiplication in collecting vessel.
- Ketones, barbiturates, PSP in urine at higher levels than is plasma.

Causes for reduced creatinine clearance
Acute: Shock, hypovolaemia, nephrotoxic chemicals, acute glomerulonephritis, malignant hypertension, eclampsia.

Chronic: Glomerulonephritis, pyelonephritis, hypertensive nephrosclerosis, polycystic kidneys.

PRINCIPLES OF PRECISE TESTS OF RENAL FUNCTION

Clearance of inulin or endogenous creatinine and of iodopyracet (Diodrast) or PAH helps differentiate diseases of glomeruli and tubules.

Renal Function Tests

Determination		*Normal values*
Phenolsulphonphthalein (PSP, Phenol red)	1 ml I/V	15 min 35% (28-51) 30 min 17% (13-24) 60 min 12% (9-17) 120 min 6% (3-10) } 55-60%
Clearance tests Inulin clearance Iothalamate ^{131}I Endogenous creatinine clearance }	Glomerular filtration rate -do- -do-	Corrected to 1.73 sq m SA. Male: 110-150 ml/min Female: 105-132 ml/min
Iodohippurate^{131}I PAH clearance	Renal Plasma flow	Male: 560-830 ml/min Female: 490-700 ml/min
Filtration fraction	$FF = \frac{GFR}{PRF}$	Male: 17-21% Female: 17-23%
Urea clearance (Cu)		Standard: 40-65 ml/min Maximal: 60-100 ml/min
Maximal glucose reabsorptive capacity	TmG	Male: 300-450 mg/min Female: 250-350 mg/min
Maximal iodopyracet capacity	TmD	Male: 43-59 mg/min Female: 33-51 mg/min
Maximal PAH excretory capacity	Tm PAH	80-90 mg/min.

Glomerular Filtration Rate (GFR)

Inulin, a polysaccharide is eliminated exclusively through the glomeruli, is neither excreted nor absorbed by the tubules. Inulin clearance is therefore a measure of the glomerular filtration rate. Other radioactive labelled substances can be used. Normal in adults is 100-130 ml/minute per 1.73 sqm of body surface.

Renal Plasma Flow (RPF)

Para-aminohippurate (PAH), iodopyracet and ^{131}I or ^{125}I labelled sodium iodohippurate at low concentration in plasma are cleared almost completely by filtration and tubular secretion as the plasma flows through kidney.

If, for example, at a plasma PAH concentration of 1 mg%, 6-mg PAH appear, in urine per minute, 600 ml of plasma must be passing the kidneys per minute. The normal range is 500-800 ml of plasma per minute per 1.73 sq m of body surface. Varying with the haematocrit, this indicates a flow through the kidneys of 1000-1500 ml of whole blood per minute or almost one-third of the cardiac output at rest.

Filtration Fraction

Ratio of volume of glomerular filtration to the volume of plasma from which the filtrate was obtained is expressed as GFR/RPF. This ratio is called the filtration fraction. The normal filtration fraction is:

$$\frac{120 \text{ ml/min}}{600 \text{ ml/min}} = 0.2$$

Maximal Tubular Capacity (Tm)

At high concentrations of iodopyracet, iodo-hippurate, or PAH in plasma, the excretory capacity of the renal tubule is exceeded. By measuring the amount of test material excreted under these conditions and correcting for the amount of test material simultaneously filtered through the glomerulus, the maximal excretory capacity of the tubule is obtained. Tm for reabsorption of glucose, amino acids, etc. can be determined similarly, although in this instance the amount filtered minus the amount excreted per unit of time equals the maximal reabsorptive capacity.

Chapter 7

Stool Examination

Average healthy adults defecate from three times a day to three times a week. Common pattern is once a day. The stool tends to be soft and bulky on a diet high in vegetables and small and dry on a diet high in meat. Two thirds of the stool weight is attributable to its water content. The normal brown colour is of still undetermined origin. The odour results from indole and skatole, produced by bacteria from tryptophan.

Faeces are Composed of

1. Waste residue of indigestible material in food
2. Bile (pigments and salts)
3. Intestinal secretions, including mucus
4. Leucocytes that migrate from the bloodstream
5. Shed epithelial cells
6. Large numbers of bacteria that make up to one-third of total solids
7. Inorganic material (10-20%) that is chiefly calcium and phosphates
8. Digested food (present in very small quantities).

Specimen Collection

A wide mouthed jar with a screw cap is good enough, provided it is neat, clean, and without any extraneous material in it. It should, however, never be overfilled and should be opened slowly to release the gas that accumulates frequently in it (if not done so, the contents may be released explosively). Since rectal evacuation is not completely at will and faeces passed correlate very poorly with the food consumed; hence, collection should be done over a period of 3 days. The accuracy of this method can be enhanced somewhat by having the patient ingest carmine dye (0.3 gm) and charcoal (1 gm) at the beginning and the end of a collecting period, respectively, collecting the stools from the beginning of the appearance of the dye to the beginning of the appearance of the charcoal.

Be Careful

- Faeces should be urine free when collected. Collect the entire stool and transfer to another container by a tongue blade. Deliver to the laboratory immediately after collection.
- Warm stools are best for detecting ova and parasites. Do not refrigerate for ova and parasites
- Some coliform bacilli produce antibiotic substances that destroy enteric pathogens
- Refrigerate stool if it cannot be examined immediately. Never place a stool in an incubator.
- A diarrhoeal stool will usually give good results.
- A freshly passed stool is the specimen of choice.
- Preferably, stool specimens should be collected before antibiotic therapy is initiated and as early in the course of disease as possible.
- Only a small amount of stool is needed; the size of a walnut. If mucus and blood are present, they should be included in part of the specimen to be examined.
- Do not use a stool that has been passed into the toilet bowl or that has been contaminated with barium or other X-ray medium.
- Label all stool specimens with patient's name, date, and reason for examination/testing.

Interfering Factors

- Meat interferes with some tests and should usually be omitted from the diet for 3 days before a test for blood (not necessary for the guaiac method)
- Stool specimens from patients receiving barium, bismuth, oil, or antibiotics are not satisfactory
- Bismuth from paper towels and toilet tissues interferes with tests.

Normal Values in Stool Analysis

See Table 7.1.

Inspection of Faeces

A simple inspection of faeces may lead to a diagnosis of parasitic infection, obstructive jaundice, diarrhoea, malabsorption, rectosigmoidal obstruction, dysentery or ulcerative colitis or gastrointestinal tract bleeding.

Note the quantity, form, consistency and colour of the stool (Table 7.2).

Table 7.1: Normal values in stool analysis

Macroscopic examination	*Normal*
Colour	Brown
Odour	Varies with pH stool and depends upon bacterial fermentation and putrefaction
Consistency	Plastic; not unusual to see seeds and vegetable skins; soft and bulky in a high vegetable diet; small and dry in a high meat diet
Size and shape	Formed
Gross blood	Absent
Mucus	Absent
Pus	Absent
Parasites	Absent
Fat	Colourless, neutral fat (18%) and fatty acid crystals and soaps
Undigested	None to small amount food, meat fibres, starch, trypsin
Eggs and segments of parasites	Absent
Yeasts	Absent
Leucocytes	Absent
Chemical examination	*Normal*
pH	Neutral to weakly alkaline
Adult	7.0–7.5
Newborn	5.0–7.0
Bottle-fed infants	Neutral to slightly alkaline pH of 7.0–8.0
Breast-fed infants	Slightly acidic
Occult blood	Negative
Urobilinogen	50-300 mg/24 hr
Porphyrins	Coproporphyrins < 200 μg/24 hr. Protoporphyrins < 1500 μg/24 hr. Uroporphyrins < 100 μg/24 hr.
Nitrogen	1-2 gm/24 hr
Bile	Negative in adults, positive in children
Trypsin	Positive in small amounts in adults, in greater amounts in normal children.

Interfering Factors

1. Stool darkens on standing
2. Colour is influenced by diet, food dyes, certain foods, and drugs.
   a. Yellow to yellow green colour occurs in the stool of breast-fed infants who lack normal intestinal flora. It also occurs in sterilisation of bowel by antibiotic
   b. Green colour occurs in diets high in chlorophyll-rich vegetables and with use of the drug calomel

Table 7.2: Inspection of faeces

Type of stool	*Likely reason*
Watery stool	Diarrhoea
Large amount of mushy, foul smelling, grey stool that floats on water	Steatorrhoea
Little firm, spherical masses	Constipation (irritable colon syndrome, overuse of laxatives)
Narrow ribbon-like stool	Spastic bowel or rectal narrowing or stricture
Clay coloured	Obstructive jaundice or presence of Barium sulphate
Reddish stool	Blood from lower gastrointestinal tract, beets consumption or BSP use
Black, tarry stool	Bleeding from upper GIT, Iron, bismuth or charcoal consumption
Green stool	Ingestion of spinach, etc, calomel, presence of biliverdin, seen in patients taking anti-biotics orally
Parasites	Parasitic infestation (discussed later)

c. Black or very dark brown colour may be due to drugs such as iron, charcoal, and bismuth, to foods such as cherries, or to an unusually high proportion of meat in the diet.
d. Light-coloured stool with little odour may be due to diets high in milk and low in meat
e. Claylike colour may be due to a diet with excessive fat intake or barium used in X-ray examination
f. Red colour may be due to a diet high in beet or use of drugs such as BSP
g. Drug-induced colour changes are given below:
   - Black—iron salts, bismuth salts, charcoal
   - Green—mercurous chloride, indomethacin, calomel
   - Green to blue—dithiazanine
   - Brown staining—anthraquinones
   - Red—phenolphthalein, pyruvinium pamoate, tetracyclines in syrup, BSP
   - Yellow—santonin
   - Yellow to brown—senna
   - Light—sitosterols
   - Whitish discolouration—antacids
   - Orange red—phenazopyridine
   - Pink to red to black—anticoagulants (excessive dose) salicylates causing internal bleeding.

Pus: Patients with chronic ulcerative colitis and chronic bacillary dysentery frequently pass large quantities of pus with the stool that has to be examined microscopically.

It may also occur in localised abscesses or fistulas communicating with sigmoid rectum or anus. Large amounts of pus NEVER accompany amoebic colitis. No inflammatory exudate is seen in the watery stools of patients with viral gastroenteritis.

Mucus: Even in slightest quantity is abnormal.

Remarks	*Causes*
Translucent gelatinous mucus clinging to the surface of the formed stool.	Spastic constipation or mucous colitis. In emotionally disturbed patients and may result from excessive straining.
Bloody mucus clinging to stool mass.	Neoplasm, inflammation of rectal canal.
Mucus with pus and blood.	Ulcerative colitis, bacillary dysentery, ulcerating carcinoma of the colon, and more rarely, acute diverticulitis or intestinal tuberculosis.
Copious mucus, up to 3-4 litres of mucus per day.	Villous adenoma of the colon (may lead to dehydration and hypokalaemia).

Odour and pH

Normal values

Characteristic odour varies with the pH of stool; normal pH is neutral or weakly alkaline.

The pH is dependent on bacterial fermentation and putrefaction in the bowel. Substances called indole and skatole, formed by intestinal putrefaction and fermentation, are mainly responsible for the odour of normal stools.

Interfering Substances

Carbohydrate fermentation changes pH to acid. Protein breakdown changes the pH to alkaline.

Blood: Blood in stools should never be ignored, however, slight the quantity may be. Bleeding in the upper GIT may give black-tarry appearance to stools while that arising from lower GIT may give red colour or be seen as frank blood.

Causes

Upper GI Tract:
- Peptic ulcer—gastric or duodenal
- Erosive gastritis.
- Atrophic gastritis.
- Oesophageal varices.
- Mallory-Weiss syndrome.
- Hiatus hernia.
- Oesophagitis.

Small and large bowel:
- Meckel's diverticulum.
- Polyps.
- Infectious diarrhoeas.
- Inflammatory bowel disease (Crohn's disease, ulcerative colitis)
- Diverticular disease.
- Vascular malformations.
- Carcinoma.

Rectum and anus:
- Haemorrhoids.
- Anorectal fissure.

Drugs: Associated with increased GIT blood loss.
- Salicylates.
- Steroids.
- Rauwolfia derivatives.
- Indomethacin.
- Colchicine.

Loss of more than 50-75 ml of blood from the upper GIT generally imparts a dark red to black colour and a tarry consistency to the stool. Persistence of tarry appearance for two or three days suggests loss of at least 1000 ml of blood. Smaller increases in blood content may not alter appearance of the stool. Such stools are said to contain "OCCULT BLOOD" (usually associated with GIT neoplasm).

Interfering Factors

Drugs such as salicylates, steroids, indomethacin, colchicine, iron (used in massive therapy), and rauwolfia derivatives are associated with increased gastrointestinal bleeding in normal persons and with even more pronounced bleeding when disease is present. Gastrointestinal bleeding tests may be falsely positive in the undermentioned circumstances:

- Meat in diet contains haemoglobin and enzymes that can give false-positive tests for up to 4 days after eating. The guaiac method does not require meat-free diet due to lesser sensitivity.
- Vitamin C taken in quantities greater than 500 mg per day may cause false-negative test for occult blood in stool.
- Drugs that may cause a false-positive test for occult blood include:
  - Boric acid
  - Bromides
  - Colchicine
  - Iodine
  - Inorganic iron
  - Oxidising agents
- Testing method must be followed exactly or the results are not reliable:
  - Use an aliquot from centre of formed stool
  - Time reaction exactly
  - Liquid stools may cause false-negatives with filter paper methods.

Tests for Occult Blood

These tests are based upon a little understood chemical reaction in which the reagent is oxidised by hydrogen peroxide at low pH (acid added) and catalysed by the presence of haeme—the intact iron containing porphyrin ring.

All iron haeme derivatives are active. Free iron and free porphyrin rings are not active. The most important substance, which contains the active 'haeme' besides haemoglobin, is myoglobin contained in muscle fibres.

The ideal test for screening should be sensitive enough to react to a significant amount of blood without reacting to the minute amounts of blood present in the faeces of normal people on a normal diet (especially if nonvegetarian). It should also be specific enough not to react with substances in diet or in common medicines and at the same time be simple, easy, rapid and inexpensive to perform.

Commonly used reagents
1. Gum gauicum.
2. Orthotolidine.
3. Benzidine (carcinogenic).
4. Phenolphthalein.

Benzedine Test

Benzedine test is an extremely sensitive test and can give false-positives in people on abundant meat diet.

Only 1-2% people with significant bleeding will show a negative test (false-negative). False-positives may be overcome in some cases by boiling the emulsion of faeces for 1-2 minutes and then repeating the test.

Method

Benzidine reagent consists of 4 gm benzidine base/ 100 ml of glacial acetic acid. It is stable for about 4 months. Emulsify pea-sized bit of faeces in 5 ml of water. Mix 1 ml emulsion and 1 ml of reagent in test tube and add several drops of 3% H_2O_2. Positive reaction is indicated by the appearance of a blue colour in the mixture and is reported as follows:

Trace —Faint blue colour after 1 minute.
1+ —Definite blue-green slowly.
2+ —Green-blue rapidly.
3+ —Blue almost immediately.
4+ —Dark blue immediately

Guaiac Test

This is less sensitive. Has 5% false-positive in patients on nonvegetarian diet and 3-5% false-negatives. It is a better screening test. With loss of 20-30 ml of blood, all tests will be positive.

Method

Guaiac reagent consists of–1 gm guaic in 5 ml of 95% ethanol (stable in brown bottle for a month in a refrigerator).

To an emulsion of faeces—or better yet, a small smear of faeces on a piece of filter paper add 2-3 drops of gum guaiac solution, 2-3 drops of glacial acetic acid and 2-3 drops of 3% H_2O_2.

Positive tests are reported as:

Trace –Faint blue-green in 1 minute.
1+ —Light blue slowly.
2+ —Clear blue rapidly
3+ —Deep blue almost immediately
4+ —Deep blue immediately.

Orthotolidine

This test has an intermediate sensitivity and is replacing other tests, though, not in India.

Reagents

Mix:
Orthotolidine barium peroxide 200 mg.
Glacial acetic acid 5 ml.
(Stable only for one day)

Method

- Using a clean applicator stick, smear the stool on a small square of filter paper.
- Pipette a few drops of the reagent on to the filter paper.
- After exactly 30 seconds, examine for a blue colour.

Result

A blue green colour appearing within 30 seconds means a positive test.

COMMERCIALLY AVAILABLE KIT OCCULT BLOOD (HEMOSPOT®) Courtesy: Tulip Group of Companies

Summary

Faecal occult blood is a term used to describe the presence of blood in the faeces. Blood is present in the faeces due to bleeding from the gastrointestinal tract. Small increases in blood content may not alter the appearance of the stool and such stools are said to contain "occult blood", detection of which can be most useful in uncovering and localising disease. Haemoglobin levels of 5 mg/dl or more are diagnostically significant.

Screening for occult blood is especially important because over one half of all cancers (excluding skin) are those of the gastrointestinal tract. Early diagnosis and treatment of patients with colonic cancer results in a relative good prognosis for survival.

Hemospot test is useful in the detection of bleeding caused by gastrointestinal disorders such as colitis, polyps, diverticulitis, colorectal cancer and hookworm infestation.

Faecal occult blood tests are recommended for use in:

1. As an aid to routine physical examinations.
2. Routine hospital testing.
3. Screening for gastrointestinal bleeding from any source including colorectal cancer.

Reagents

1. Hemospot test cards consisting of a filter paper impregnated with the guaiac resin (reactive surface).
2. Developer solution consists of stabilised hydrogen peroxide solution, which is ready to use.
3. Positive control.

Reagent Storage and Stability

Store the reagent at 20-30°C, in a cool place away from direct sunlight, fluorescent light, UV rays and moisture. Do not refrigerate.

The shelf life of the reagents and test cards is mentioned on the kit/developer solution label.

Principle

If blood is present in the stool sample, the haematin in the haemoglobin molecule catalyses the release of oxygen from the hydrogen peroxide, which in turn oxidises the colourless phenolic components of gum guaiac to coloured quinones.

During test, after the addition of the developer solution to the reactive surfaces of the result window, the reaction area turns blue if occult blood is present in the sample. If the reaction area does not change colour, then it indicates that there is no occult blood present in the sample.

Note

1. *In vitro* diagnostic reagent for laboratory or professional use only. Not for medicinal use.
2. The kit contains hydrogen peroxide solution, which may be irritating. Avoid contact with eyes, skin and clothing. In case of contact, flush with large quantities of water.
3. Do not expose the test cards and developer solution to direct sunlight, fluorescent light and UV rays.

Quality Control

Positive control provided with the kit should be run occasionally to validate the performance of the test cards and reagent.

PREPARATION AND SAMPLE COLLECTION

Preparation of the Patient

1. As for all occult blood tests, certain medications such as aspirin, indomethacin, phenylbutazone, reserpine, corticosteroids and nonsteroidal anti-inflammatory drugs can induce gastrointestinal bleeding and cause false-positive results. These medications should be temporarily discontinued with the consent of the physician for 7 days prior to testing and during the test period.
2. Vitamin C when taken in amounts greater than 250 mg per day has been shown to induce false-negative results. Rectal medications (suppositories) and iron containing medications may also interfere with these tests and should be discontinued two days before and during the test period with the consent of the physician.
3. For at least 2 days before and during the test period, all raw meat and red meat should be avoided. Raw broccoli, cauliflower, radishes and turnips may cause false-positive results, hence should be avoided.

Sample Collection

1. A clean dry detergent free glass or plastic container of a suitable size is ideal for collection of the specimen. Urine should not be passed simultaneously into the collection container. Clean pieces of plastic are convenient for transferring stool from the collection container to the transport vessel.
2. The stool samples should be collected from different areas of the formed stool (samples from the outside of stool are most likely to reflect the condition of the lower colon, while specimens taken from inside of the stool are more likely to reflect conditions of the upper gastrointestinal tract) and also provides a more representative sample to be tested.
3. The two test fields provided in Hemospot facilitate detection and localising the source of bleeding. Because bleeding may be intermittent, it is preferable to collect specimens from different bowel movements, preferably consecutive ones.

Material Provided with the Kit

1. Hemospot test cards
2. Dropper bottle containing developer solution
3. Sample applicators
4. Positive control.

Additional Material Required

Gloves, stop watch, rust free needle/pin.

Test Procedure

1. Pierce the nozzle of the developer solution with a rust free sharp pin or needle.
2. Retrieve the required number of test cards to perform the desired number of tests.

3. Label the cards with correct patient identity.
4. Open the sample application windows labelled A and B respectively, to expose the reactive surfaces of the test card.
5. By using the sample applicator provided in the kit, spread a very thin layer of stool on the reactive surfaces on the window A; similarly, on window B; from a different part of the stool.
6. Wait until the smeared sample has *dried completely.*
7. *Turn over the test card.*
8. Open the result window and add one drop of developer to fields RA and RB (the reverse side of the sample smeared on the sample application windows) respectively.
9. Observe for colour change *exactly at two minutes.*
10. Even if one of the field's has a blue colour, the test is positive for occult blood.

Interpretation of Results

- No blue colour indicates absence of occult blood in the stool.
- Trace blue colouration indicates presence of approximately 5 mg/dl of occult blood in the stool.
- Strong blue colouration indicates significantly more than 5 mg/dl of occult blood in the stool.

Remarks

1. Stool samples collected during menstrual bleeding, constipation-induced bleeding, bleeding haemorrhoids or when rectal medication is used may cause positive results.
2. Hands, collection containers and test area should be kept free of blood as they may cause false-positive results.
3. Certain medications may induce gastrointestinal bleeding and cause false-positive reactions, hence should be avoided during and prior to the testing period.
4. Diet containing exogenous peroxidases may induce false-positive results.
5. Dosages of vitamin C more than 250 mg per day will cause a false-negative result.
6. If the test is developed before the sample smear dries completely on the test card, the results obtained may not be accurate.
7. Only use the sample applicators provided in the kit for applying the samples.

Faecal Fat

Normal value

In a normal diet, fat in the stool will be up to 20% of total solids.

Lipids measured as fatty acids: 2-5 gm/24 hr.

It is raised in malabsorption syndromes, the commonest example being steatorrhoea.

Faecal fat quantitation can be done by:

1. Gravimetric method.
2. Isotopic techniques, (radioisotopes).
3. Electrical capacitance method.
4. Titrimetric method of Van de Kamer.

Titrimetric Method

Fats and fatty acids are converted to soap by boiling with alcoholic potassium hydroxide. After cooling, excess hydrochloric acid is added to convert soaps to fatty acids. These are extracted with petroleum ether. An aliquot is evaporated, taken up in neutral alcohol, and titrated with sodium hydroxide. Fats are calculated as fatty acids.

Electrical Capacitance Method

This has replaced the titrimetric method now. An aliquot of faecal suspension is extracted with solvent consisting chiefly of chlorinated benzenes. The extract is filtered and its electrical capacitance is measured and compared with standards of triolein similarly treated.

Interpretation

To quantitate fat excretion, there must be known dietary intake and timed stool collection. The usual technique involves a diet containing 100 gm of fat daily, with a 3-day stool collection to measure total fat excretion. Excretion of more than 6 gm per day is abnormal and values may range from 50 gm or more.

Faecal fat increase occurs in:

- Enteritis and pancreatic diseases when there is lack of lipase

- Surgical removal of a section of intestine
- Malabsorption syndromes
- In chronic pancreatic disease, fat is more than 10 gm/24 hr.
- A stool specimen high in fat content will have a pasty appearance and can be detected by gross examination

Interfering Factors

1. Increased neutral fat may occur under the following conditions:
   - with use of rectal suppositories
   - with ingestion of castor oil or mineral oil
   - with ingestion of dietetic low calories mayonnaise
2. Barium interferes with test results.

Other Methods of Assessing Malabsorption

Glucose tolerance test: The GTT curve becomes flat since adequate amounts of orally given glucose are not absorbed, whereas in the same patient if glucose is given parenterally, a normal curve is obtained.

Protein loss: Protein loss estimation is not necessary for diagnosing protein-losing enteropathy.

Proteins within the intestine are reduced enzymatically to their component amino acids, which are then reabsorbed. If mucosal abnormalities prevent reabsorption or if protein leakage exceeds reabsorptive capacity, hypoproteinaemia may result. The faecal protein excretion can be documented by administering isotopically labelled albumin or povidone (PVP) rather than by chemical analysis of faeces.

MICROSCOPIC EXAMINATION OF STOOL SPECIMENS

Stool specimens should be fresh and must not be contaminated with detergents or disinfectants, etc.

Having described the gross appearance, proceed on for microscopic examination for cells and parasites as follows:

1. Place a small piece of stool on a slide and mix with saline until smooth. Cover with a coverslip. If the specimen contains mucus, examine preferably without saline. The mucus is put on the slide and covered with a coverslip.
2. Examine under 10x and 40x objectives, with a reduced condenser aperture.
3. Report the presence of:
   - Large numbers of pus cells or muscle fibers.
   - Red blood cells.
   - Free living amoebae, flagellates or ciliates.
   - Eggs and larvae.
   - Cysts.
   - Yeast cells.

Parasitic amoebae, flagellates, ciliates, eggs, larvae and cysts are usually reported as the number seen in the entire preparation as follows:

- Scanty (rare): 1 to 3.
- Few (1+): 4 to 10.
- Moderate number : (2+) 10 to 20.
- Many (3+): 20 to 40.
- Very many (4+): over 40.

Cells are usually reported as the number seen per high power field as in urine deposit.

Use of Saline

Normal (0.85%) saline is used for routine examination of stool specimens, as it is isotonic with living organisms. Use fresh uninfected saline.

Use of Iodine

Iodine is used to examine the nuclear structure of cysts, the preparation is made in the same way as for saline.

Using an iodine solution, the chromatin granules and karyosome of nuclei stain brown. The glycogen vacuole stains brown and the chromatid bars remain unstained. The solution used is called Dobells's iodine.

- Iodine :1.0 gm.
- Potassium iodide :2.0 gm.
- Distilled water :50 ml.

Iodine should not replace saline for routine use, as it kills living material, and would therefore make it impossible to detect motility of amoebae, flagellates, ciliates and larvae. In addition iodine makes the chromatid bars of *E. histolytica* difficult to see.

Use of 1% Eosin

This provides a pink background against which the cysts and amoebae stand out as clear unstained objects.

Use of Sargeaunt's Stain

This is used to stain the chromatid bars of cysts, and is of value especially for *E. histolytica*.

The nuclear structure stains pale green, the chromatid bars stain deeper green.

The stain consists of:
- Malachite green : 0.2 gm.
- 95% Ethanol : 3 ml.
- Distilled water : 100 ml.

This stain can only be used after a formol ether stool concentration method, because the use of ether appears to be necessary for the staining reaction.

Stool Concentration Methods

Where heavy infestation is present, this method is not needed.

Concentration Methods may be Used

1. To see whether treatment of the parasites has been successful.
2. To find ova of *S. mansoni* or *Taenia* if few or for other ova and cysts if they have not been seen on routine examination (being very few) and are suspected to be present.
3. To examine stool specimens from patients who do not come from an area where a particular parasite is found.

Flotation Concentration Methods

In flotation methods, the stool is mixed with a solution, e.g. zinc or magnesium sulphate, which has a high specific gravity so that the parasitic contents float to the surface.

Zinc Sulphate Concentration Method

This method can be used to concentrate cysts, larvae and most helminth eggs, except those of *P. westermani, F. buski, C. sinensis* and *D. latum* and other operculated eggs and also *Schistosoma* eggs which do not float.

Reagents

Zinc sulphate solution of sp. gravity 1.180 is needed. Prepared by dissolving 33 gm of chemical in 100 ml of distilled water.

Method

1. Mix a small piece of stool with about 10 ml of water or saline, in a bottle or tube.
2. Sieve the suspension into a beaker, through a strainer with small holes.
3. Pour the contents of the beaker into a centrifuge tube.
4. Centrifuge at 2000-3000 rpm/min for 1 minute.
5. Pour off the supernatant fluid.
6. Resuspend the deposit in clean water and add enough water to fill the tube.
7. Mix well and re-centrifuge.
8. Pour off the supernatant fluid.
9. Resuspend in zinc sulphate solution, fill the tube with the solution.
10. Centrifuge at high speed for 1 minute.
11. Transfer the contents from the surface of the tube to a slide, using a bacteriological wire loop. This surface film must be removed immediately.
12. Add small drops of saline and mix.
13. Cover with a coverslip.
14. Examine under 10x and 40x objectives.

Sedimentation Concentration Methods

In sedimentation methods, the parasites are not floated but deposited, usually by centrifuging.

Simple Sedimentation Method

A small piece of stool is mixed with saline in a tube or bottle and sieved through a strainer. The sieved contents are centrifuged and the supernatant fluid poured off. The deposit is resuspended in more saline, mixed, and centrifuged. This is repeated until the supernatant fluid is clear. The deposit is examined directly on a slide.

By this simple method, parasitic cysts, eggs, and free-living parasites can be concentrated.

Formol-saline Ether Sedimentation Method

This method gives a good concentration of parasitic contents and is recommended for routine work. This method, however, cannot be used to concentrate free-living forms as formalin kills the parasites.

Reagents

10% formol-saline
- Saline 450 ml.
- Conc. formaldehyde solution 50 ml (40% w/v)
- Add the formaldehyde solution to the saline and mix well.

Method

1. Mix a small piece of stool in about 10 ml of 10% formol-saline, in a tube or bottle.
2. Sieve the suspension into a beaker through a strainer with small holes.
3. Pour about 6 ml of the sieved suspension into a centrifuge tube.
4. Add about 3 ml of ether.
5. Mix well and immediately centrifuge at 3,000 rpm/min for 1 minute.
6. Four layers are seen (Fig. 7.1)
   a. An upper layer of ether.
   b. Middle layer of stool particles
   c. A lower layer of formol-saline.
   d. The deposit in which parasitic contents will be found.
7. Using an applicator stick, separate the middle layer from the sides of the tube and pour this away together with the ether and formol-saline.
8. Resuspend the deposit by tapping the bottom of the tube with the finger.

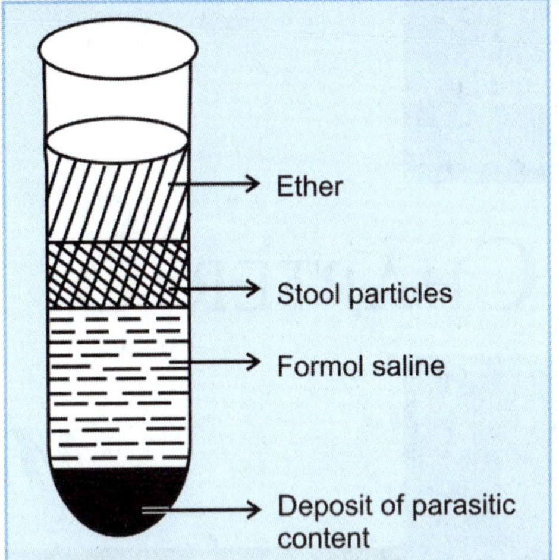

Fig. 7.1: Various layers as seen after centrifugation

9. Transfer the deposit to a slide using a pasteur pipette.
10. Cover with a coverslip and examine under 10x and 40x objectives with a reduced condenser aperture. For the identification of cysts; iodine, eosin, or Sargeaunt's stain can be used.

CHAPTER 8

Medical Parasitology

MEDICAL PARASITES

Parasitism is a category of association of living things in which one partner (the parasite) maintains itself at the expense of the energy of the other (the host). By definition, medical parasitology, then, would include even viruses and bacteria, but it is restricted to those animal parasites, chiefly protozoa and helminths, that produce a state of disease in man or are closely related to others that do. Microbial human parasites are included, for convenience, in the field of microbiology (discussed elsewhere), and with the specialised subspecialities of virology, bacteriology, and mycology.

Importance of Morphologic Identification

Recognition and differentiation of the animal parasites of man, often involving separation of pathogenic from very similar nonpathogenic (harmless) forms, need precise knowledge of their morphology. Proficiency in this part of laboratory work is gained by extensive practical experience with properly collected and processed clinical specimens. The diagnosis and differentiation of protozoal diseases, whether intestinal or systemic, often present unusual problems. Differentiation of intestinal amoebae demands particular care, especially to distinguish the nonpathogenic small race (*Entamoeba hartmanni*) from the very similar larger form (*E. histolytica*) that is responsible for amoebiasis.

The following pages present medical parasitology in tabular and pictorial forms.

INTESTINAL PROTOZOA OF MAN

Infections worldwide prevalence depends on sanitation level and degree of natural or acquired resistance. *Entamoeba histolytica* is found often in Indian rural and urban population. The intestinal protozoans present a serious threat in tropical rather than temperate climates, but usually much less common than asymptomatic infection. Incidence of *Giardia lamblia* varies with age, most common in children, relatively rare in adults. *Balantidium coli* is comparatively rare but may be common where

Table 8.1A: Tabulated life cycle of common human intestinal pathogenic protozoans

Parasite	*Enters man*	*Infective form*	*Life cycle in man*		*Exit*	*Reservoir host*
Entamoeba histolytica	Orally by contamination	Cyst	Becomes trophozoite in intestine	May invade mucosa or body organs, chiefly liver	Cyst or trophozoites in faeces (latter not infective)	Man
Giardia lamblia	-do-	-do-	-do-	Duodeuum and bile passages		Man
Balantidium coli	-do-	-do-	-do-	Many invade mucosa of large intestine.	-do-	Man, pig, monkey.

sanitary conditions are very poor. Only these three commonly accepted forms are considered in Tables 8.1A and B. Pathogenicity of other species is rare or questionable.

Nonpathogenic protozoa are commonly found in the faeces of man and should be differentiated from the recognised pathogenic forms. The commoner organisms: amoebaes—*Entamoeba hartmanni, E. coli, Endolimax nana, Dientamoeba fragilis, Iodamoeba butschilii;* flegellates—*Chilomastix mesnili, Trichomonas hominis.* Their main importance is that they are a sign of environmental pollution with fresh faeces and may elicit unnecessary treatment or inaccurate diagnosis.

Table 8.1B: Intestinal protozoal diseases of man

Disease and aetiology	*Possible clinical features*	*Laboratory diagnosis*
Amoebiasis ***E. histolytica***	Flask-shaped ulcers in mucosa of large intestine which appear as pinpoint dots on surface with mild inflammation but may produce extensive undermining below surface. Localised in caecum and whole large intestine, especially on flexures and sigmoid colon. *Blood:* Leukocytosis, anaemia. Eosinophilia rare in uncomplicated protozoal infections. *Symptoms:* Dysentery, bloody diarrhoea, sometimes followed by constipation; abdominal pain, gas distension; poor appetite, weight loss, headache, nervous manifestations, local tenderness. *Complications:* Liver abscess (single or multiple) with liver enlargement and congestion. Pain, swelling, leukocytosis, anaemia, fever. Lung abscess primary or, more commonly secondary to liver abscess. Peritonitis—bacterial with usual manifestations. Ulcerations and abscesses of other organs or tissues, manifestations depending upon site infected. (Incubation period: acute, 8-10 days, chronic, 2 months to years.)	Examine faeces by smear, concentration, culture. Abscess and ulcer material (as for faeces) Amoebic serology. (ELISA method)
Giardiasis ***G. lamblia***	Duodenitis, perhaps choledochitis. Mucosal inflammation possible mechanical and toxic interference with absorption of vitamin A and fats, resulting in diarrhoea and steatorrhoea.	Examine faeces by smear, concentration
Balantidiasis ***B. coli***	Limited to large intestine where parasites localise, with pathology and symptoms that may resemble amoebic dysentery. Most cases asymptomatic with high natural resistance; acute or chronic disease. Epidemic outbreaks may occur with cases of extensive ulceration.	Examine faeces by smear, concentration, culture.

Entamoeba histolytica
Morphology

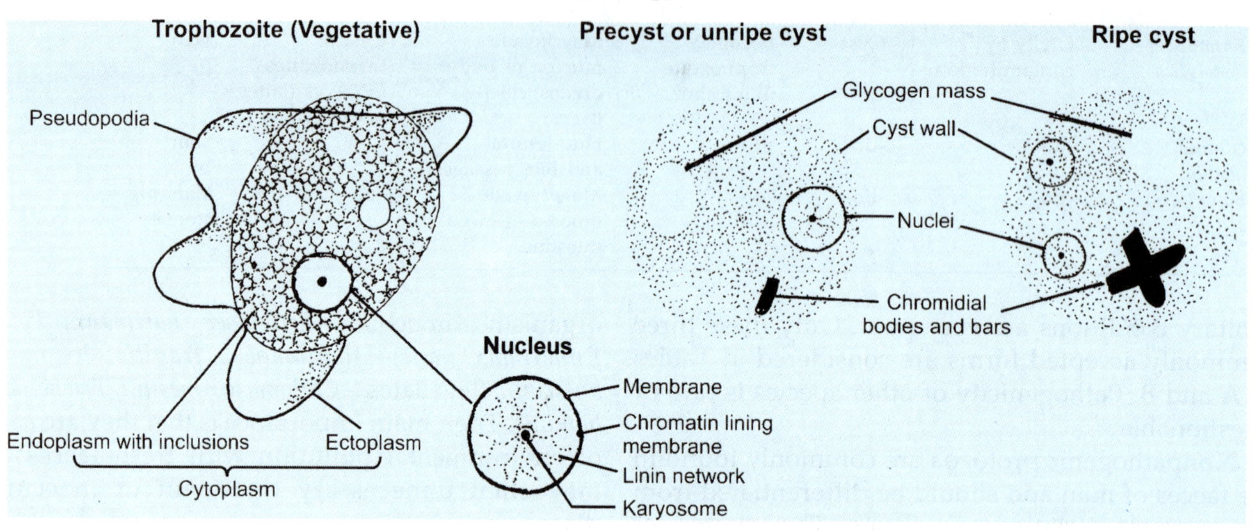

Unstained preparations

E.histolytica | *E.coli*

Trophozoite

E.histolytica		*E.coli*
Granular	Cytoplasm	Conspicuously granular
Clear finger-like	Pseudopodia	Blunt
Active purposeful	Movement	Sluggish not purposeful
Generally invisible	Nucleus	Ring refractile granules with eccentric karyosome
Red blood cells	Inclusions	Vacuoles, crystals, vegetable cells, bacteria, NO RBCs

15-60 μ

Precyst and unripe cyst

E.histolytica		*E.coli*
Granular	Cytoplasm	Granular
May be refractile ring	Nucleus	Visible as refractile ring
Rod-like refractile chromidial bars Glucogen masses	Inclusions	May be slender refractile chromidial bars Glycogen masses

Ripe cyst

E.histolytica		*E.coli*
Round	Shape	Round
Refractile	Wall	Conspicuous refractile double outline
Difficult to see (1-4)	Nuclei	1-8 refractile nuclei with eccentric karyosomes
Refractile chromidial bars often	Inclusions	Only rudimentary slender chromidial bars

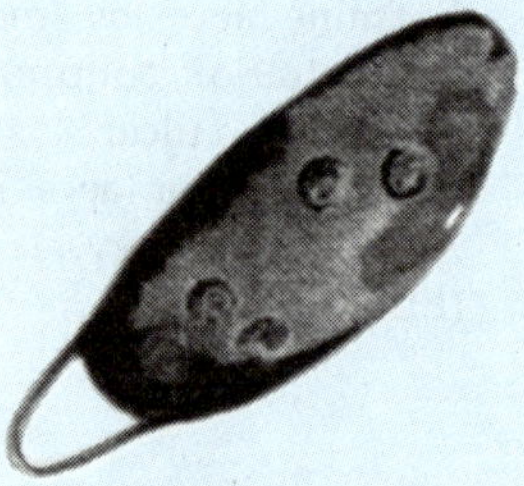

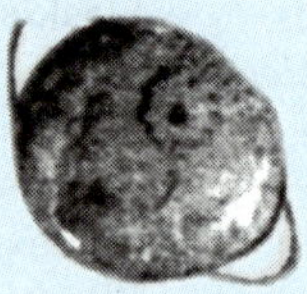

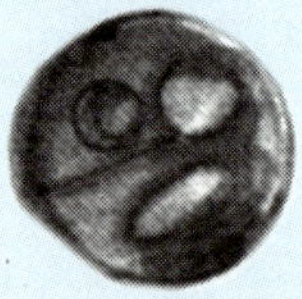

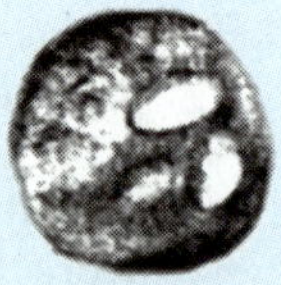

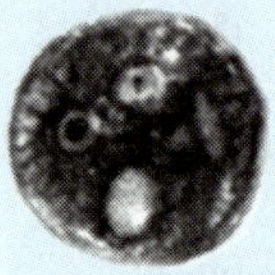

35-20 μ 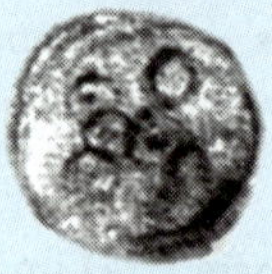 | 10-33 μ

Note: Small race <10 μ. May be commensal *(E.hartmanni)*
Large race cysts >10 μ Pathogenic

Morphology (Contd...)

E.histolytica		*E.coli*
Iodine preparations		
Trophozoite		
Finely granular yellow green	Cytoplasm	Conspicuous granularity
Red cells (yellow)	Inclusions	Bacteria etc. No. RBC
Yellow ring with centre yellow dot (karyosome)	Nucleus	Nuclear membrane with eccentric karyosome easily recognised
Precyst		
Brown, diffuse	Glycogen	Brown, compact
As above	Cytoplasm, Nucleus	As above
Stained by Iron Haematoxylin		
Trophozoite		
Purplish brown Faintly granular	Cytoplasm	Greyish blue Coarsely granular
RBC black	Inclusion	Vacuoles black, as are bacteria etc.
Lined with minute granules	Nucleus membrane	Thick plaques of black chromatin
Small black central dot	Karyosome	Eccentric black dot or plaque
Trace only seen	Linin network	More conspicuous may have chromatin plaques
Precyst		
Round	Shape	Round
As trophozoite	Cytoplasm nucleus	As trophozoite
Black chromidial bodies or bars	Inclusions	May have slender black chromidial bars
Glycogen (dissolved) replaced by vacuoles		Glycogen (dissolved) replaced by vacuoles
Cyst		
Grey-blue	Cytoplasm	Greyish blue, granular
As precyst, less conspicuous or absent	Inclusions	As precyst, less conspicuous or absent In 2 nuclei stage glycogen vacuoles may be dumb bell shaped
Unstained, hyaline	Wall	Unstained, hyaline
As trophozoite 1-4	Nuclei	As trophozoite 1-8

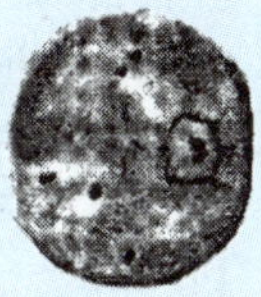

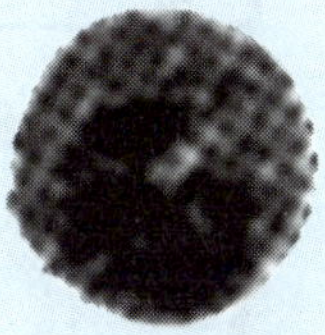

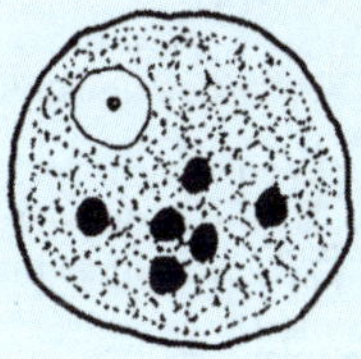

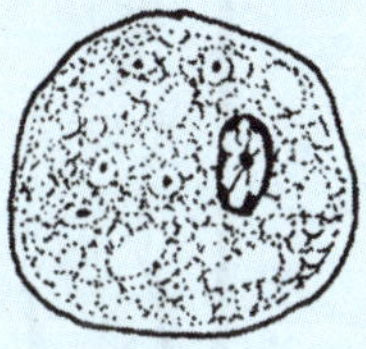

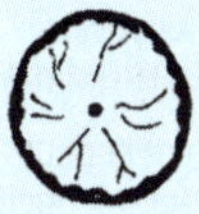

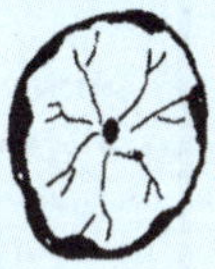

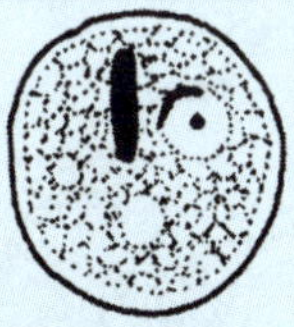

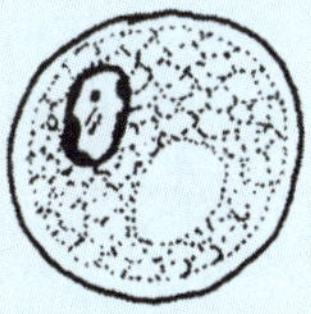

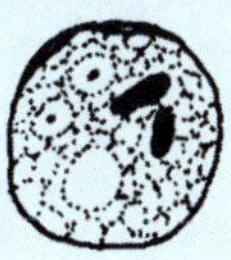

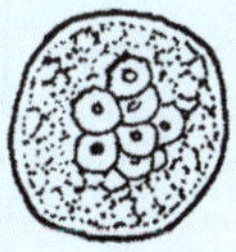

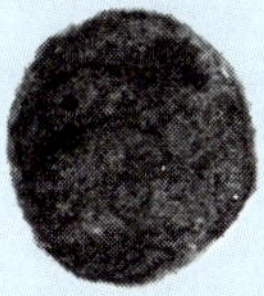

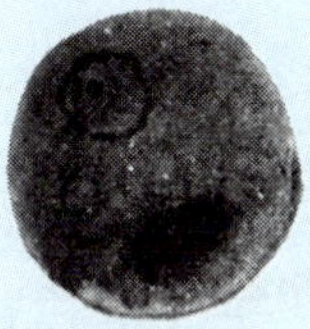

Entamoeba histolytica (causing amoebiosis) Life Cycle

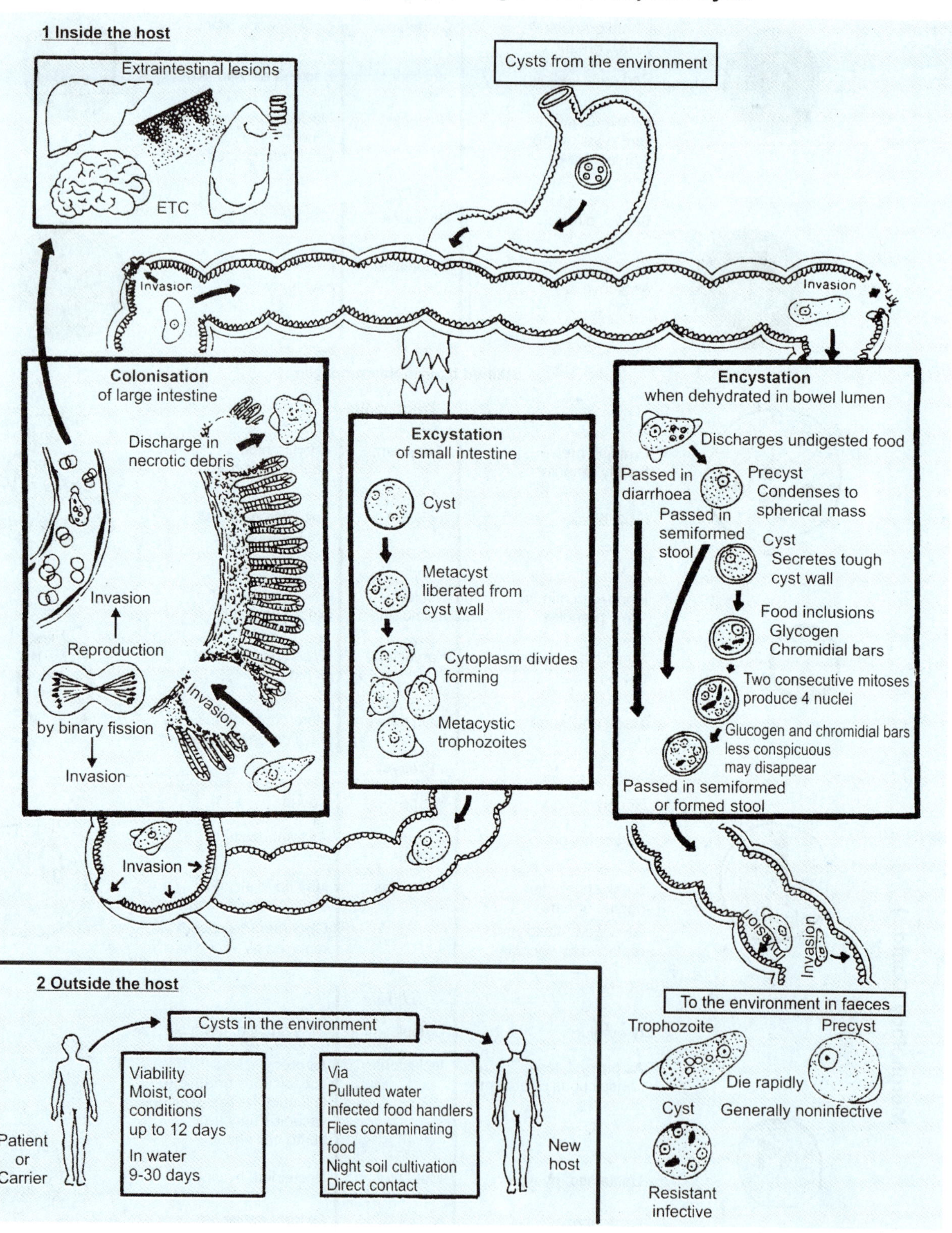

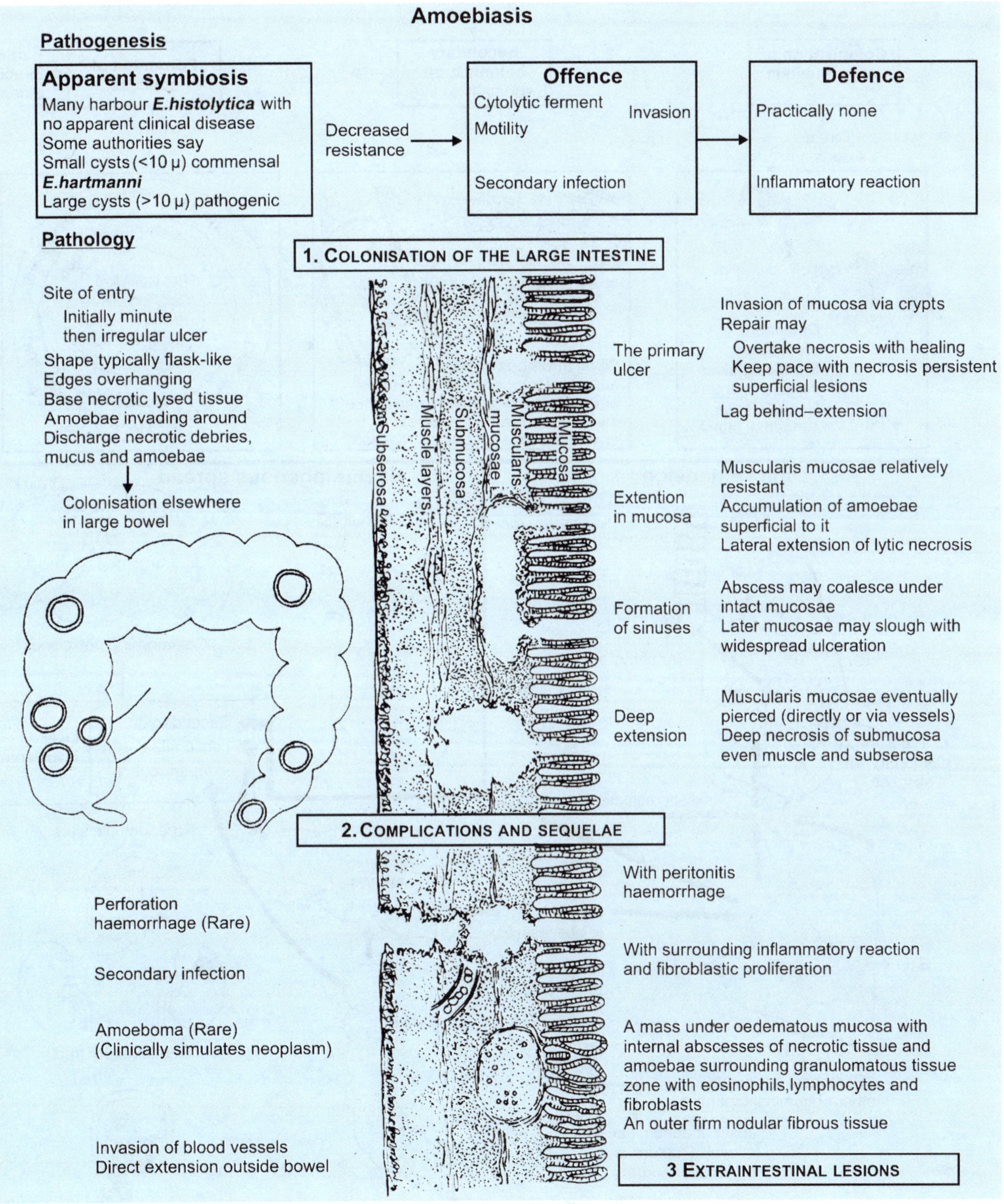
Amoebiasis
Pathogenesis
Apparent symbiosis
Many harbour E.histolytica with no apparent clinical disease
Some authorities say
Small cysts (<10 μ) commensal
E.hartmanni
Large cysts (>10 μ) pathogenic
Decreased resistance
Offence
Cytolytic ferment
Motility
Secondary infection
Invasion
Defence
Practically none
Inflammatory reaction
Pathology
1. COLONISATION OF THE LARGE INTESTINE
Site of entry
Initially minute
then irregular ulcer
Shape typically flask-like
Edges overhanging
Base necrotic lysed tissue
Amoebae invading around
Discharge necrotic debries, mucus and amoebae
Colonisation elsewhere in large bowel
Subserosa
Muscle layers
Submucosa
Muscularis mucosae
Mucosa
The primary ulcer
Invasion of mucosa via crypts
Repair may
Overtake necrosis with healing
Keep pace with necrosis persistent superficial lesions
Lag behind–extension
Extention in mucosa
Muscularis mucosae relatively resistant
Accumulation of amoebae superficial to it
Lateral extension of lytic necrosis
Formation of sinuses
Abscess may coalesce under intact mucosae
Later mucosae may slough with widespread ulceration
Deep extension
Muscularis mucosae eventually pierced (directly or via vessels)
Deep necrosis of submucosa even muscle and subserosa
2. COMPLICATIONS AND SEQUELAE
Perforation
haemorrhage (Rare)
With peritonitis
haemorrhage
Secondary infection
With surrounding inflammatory reaction and fibroblastic proliferation
Amoeboma (Rare)
(Clinically simulates neoplasm)
A mass under oedematous mucosa with internal abscesses of necrotic tissue and amoebae surrounding granulomatous tissue zone with eosinophils,lymphocytes and fibroblasts
An outer firm nodular fibrous tissue
Invasion of blood vessels
Direct extension outside bowel
3 EXTRAINTESTINAL LESIONS

***Pathology of Amoebiasis* (Contd...)**

Extraintestinal Lesions

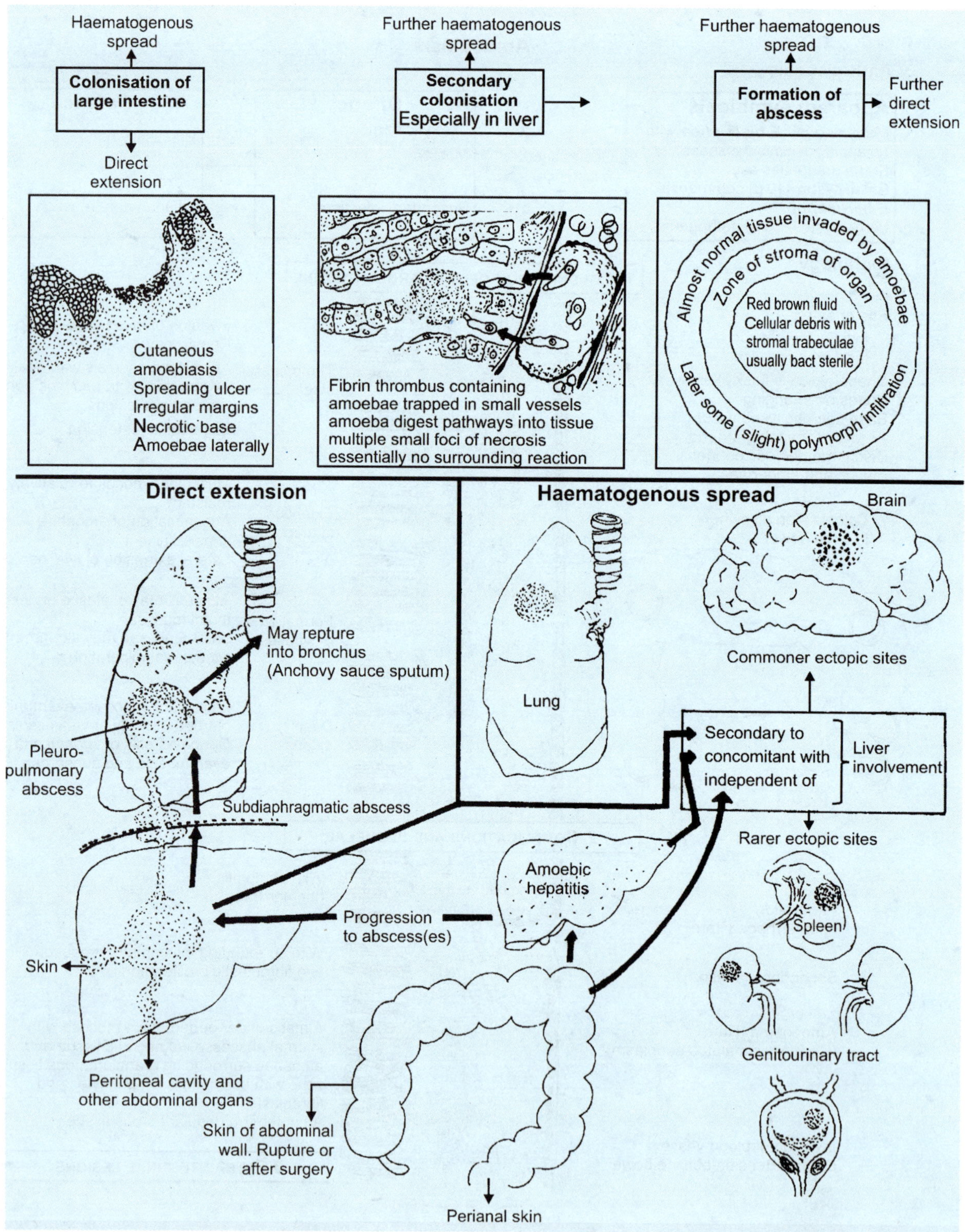

The Intestinal Flagellates

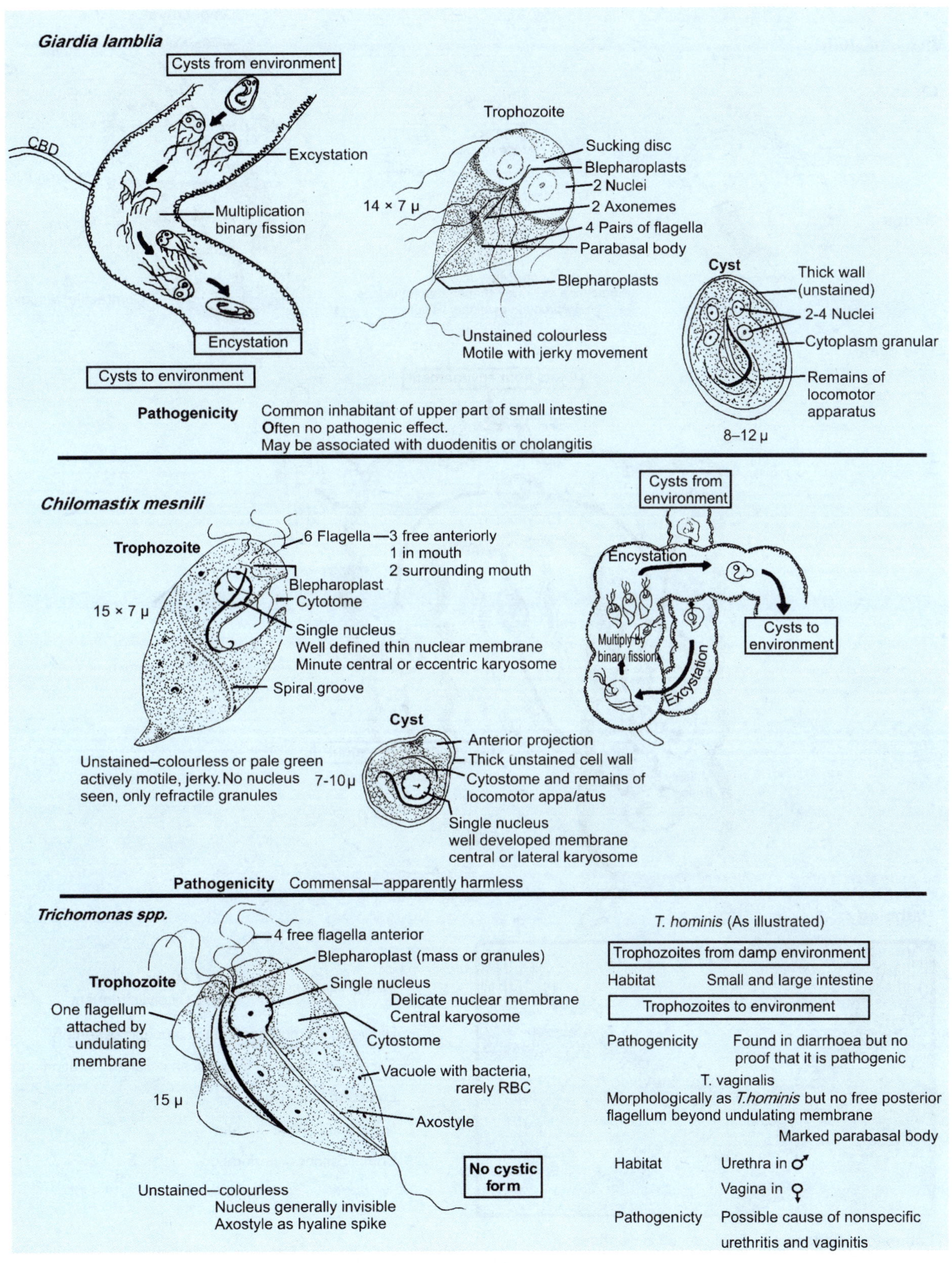

Balantidium coli (causing balantidiasis)

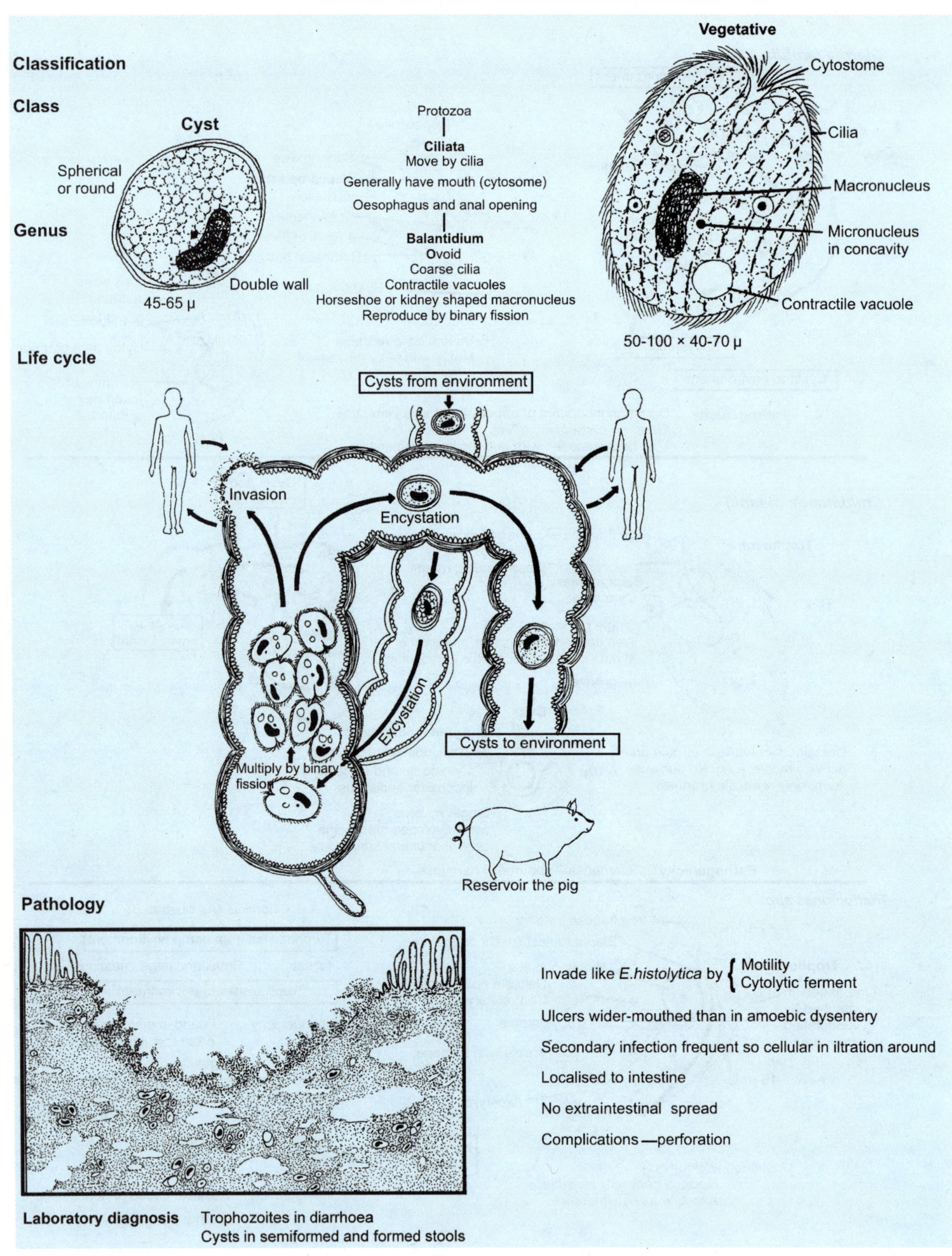

The Nonpathogenic Intestinal Amoebae

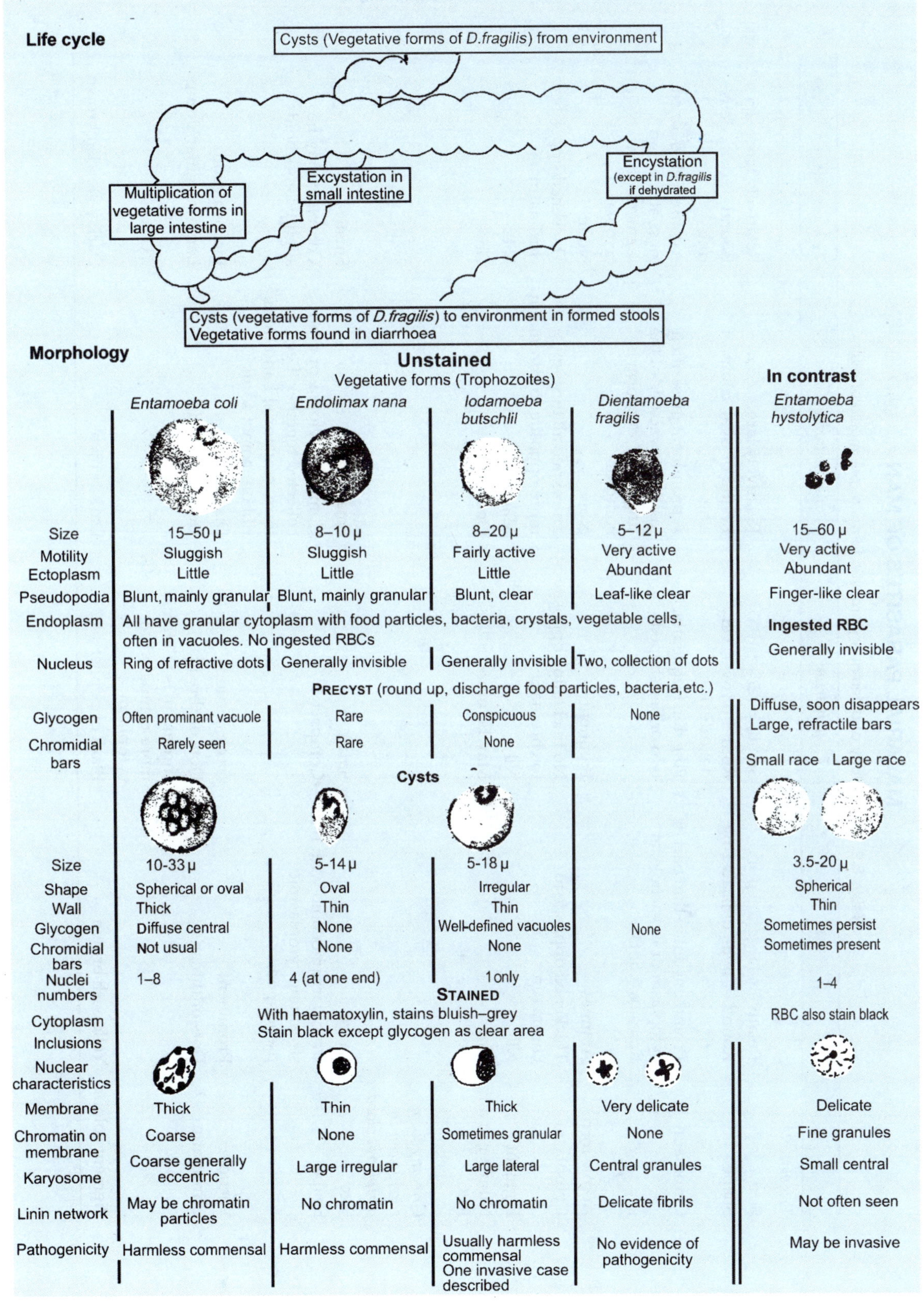

Morphology

	Entamoeba coli	*Endolimax nana*	*Iodamoeba butschlii*	*Dientamoeba fragilis*	In contrast *Entamoeba hystolytica*
Unstained – Vegetative forms (Trophozoites)					
Size	15–50 μ	8–10 μ	8–20 μ	5–12 μ	15–60 μ
Motility	Sluggish	Sluggish	Fairly active	Very active	Very active
Ectoplasm	Little	Little	Little	Abundant	Abundant
Pseudopodia	Blunt, mainly granular	Blunt, mainly granular	Blunt, clear	Leaf-like clear	Finger-like clear
Endoplasm	All have granular cytoplasm with food particles, bacteria, crystals, vegetable cells, often in vacuoles. No ingested RBCs				Ingested RBC
Nucleus	Ring of refractive dots	Generally invisible	Generally invisible	Two, collection of dots	Generally invisible
PRECYST (round up, discharge food particles, bacteria,etc.)					
Glycogen	Often prominant vacuole	Rare	Conspicuous	None	Diffuse, soon disappears
Chromidial bars	Rarely seen	Rare	None		Large, refractile bars
Cysts					Small race / Large race
Size	10-33 μ	5-14 μ	5-18 μ		3.5-20 μ
Shape	Spherical or oval	Oval	Irregular		Spherical
Wall	Thick	Thin	Thin		Thin
Glycogen	Diffuse central	None	Well-defined vacuoles	None	Sometimes persist
Chromidial bars	Not usual	None	None		Sometimes present
Nuclei numbers	1–8	4 (at one end)	1 only		1–4
STAINED					
Cytoplasm	With haematoxylin, stains bluish–grey				RBC also stain black
Inclusions	Stain black except glycogen as clear area				
Nuclear characteristics					
Membrane	Thick	Thin	Thick	Very delicate	Delicate
Chromatin on membrane	Coarse	None	Sometimes granular	None	Fine granules
Karyosome	Coarse generally eccentric	Large irregular	Large lateral	Central granules	Small central
Linin network	May be chromatin particles	No chromatin	No chromatin	Delicate fibrils	Not often seen
Pathogenicity	Harmless commensal	Harmless commensal	Usually harmless commensal One invasive case described	No evidence of pathogenicity	May be invasive

MALARIAL PARASITES OF MAN

Table 8.2: Morphology of different erythrocytic forms of plasmodia of man

	P. vivax	*P. falciparum*	*P. malariae*	*P. ovale*
Trophozoite				
Size	Relatively large, 2.5 μ	Small; < 1.5 μ	Relatively large, 2.5 μ	Relatively large, 2.5 μ
Shape	Round or oval, delicate ring	Round or oval, very delicate ring	Round or oval, compact ring	Round or oval, dense ring
Chromatin	Prominent dot in thin part of cytoplasm or in vacuole; at times two dots	Fine dot; frequently two or bar shaped	A prominent mass often inside the vacuole of the ring. 'Bird' eye form is common	A dense well-defined mass at the thin segment of the cytoplasm
Accole form	At times	Frequent	None	None
Cytoplasm	Thickened opposite to chromatin	No thickening opposite to chromatin	Thicekned all through, more opposite to chromatin	Thickened opposite to chromatin
Pigment	Nil	Nil	May be present	Nil
Number in an RBC	One	May be more	One	One
Growing form rarely seen in peripheral blood				
Size	Large	Small	Small	Small
Shape	Irregular; amoeboid with fine streaming cytoplasmic pseudopodia	Compact	Compact; cytoplasm more collected together; Egg form, equatorial band form, ribbon, comet form	Compact; may be slightly amoeboid
Vacuole	Prominent	Inconspicuous	Disappears early	Inconspicuous
Chromatin	Dots or threads	Dots or threads; chromatin is relatively more compared to cytoplasm	Dots or threads	Large irregular clumps
Pigment colour	Yellowish brown	Black or pepper-like	Dark brown	Dark yellowish brown

Contd...

Contd...

	P. vivax	*P. falciparum*	*P. malariae*	*P. ovale*
Microgametocyte (male)				
Size	Large (10 to 12 μ); fills enlarged RBC	Large (8 to 10 $\mu \times 2$ to 3 μ); larger than RBC	Smaller than size of a normal RBC	About the size of normal RBC
Shape	Round or oval, compact	Kidney or bean shaped; ends bluntly rounded	Round; compact	Round; compact
Cytoplasm	Light blue	Pinkish blue	Reddish blue (stains badly)	Pale blue
Chromatin	Fibril in skin; large, diffuse; stains poorly; lies across equator, surrounding area unstained	Fine granules; scattered through 1/3 of the body of the parasite lie amongst pigment granules, stains lightly in the central part	Fibril in skin; medium, diffuse; arranged in zone like bands, surrounding area unstained	As in *P. vivax*
Pigment	(i) Fine granular (ii) Light brown to yellow brown (iii) Scattered throughout cytoplasm	(i) Fine granular (ii) Blackish (ii) Scattered throughout	(i) Coarse granular (ii) Dark brown (iii) Scattered and also aggregated in chunks and masses	
Macrogametocyte (female)				
Size	Large (12 to 14 μ; larger than male); fills enlarged RBC	Larger (10 to 12 $\mu \times 2$ to 3 μ) larger than male; larger than RBC	Smaller than size of RBC	Size of RBC
Shape	Round or oval	Crescent shaped; ends sharply rounded or pointed	Round; compact	Round; compact
Cytoplasm	Deep blue	Deep blue	Deep blue	Deep blue
Chromatin	Condensed into compact mass; eccentric in position often surrounded by a halo	Condensed into a small deep staining compact mass; in position lies in the midst of pigment (no halo)	As in *P. vivax*	As in *P. vivax*
Pigment	(i) Yellow brown (ii) Aggregated in small masses (iii) Arranged at periphery or wreath-like	(i) Black (ii) Granular or small clumps (iii) Arranged round the chromatin masses	(i) Dark brown (ii) and as in *P. vivax*; abundant pigment—pigmented parasite	(i) Dark yellow brown; (ii) and as in *P. vivax*

Trichomonas vaginalis, known only in the trophozoite stage, inhabits the human vagina and urethra of male and female. Produces vaginitis with severe itching and mucopurulent discharge in small proportion of cases. *T. vaginalis* is worldwide in distribution, occurring in 10-40% of women examined. It is mainly transmitted by coitus but may also be transferred by recently contaminated toilet articles. The male is the chief agent of spread, although he seldom suffers symptoms. Treatment of the female, however, should always include treatment of her sexual partner.

Morphology of Malarial Parasites Stained by Leishman or Giemsa

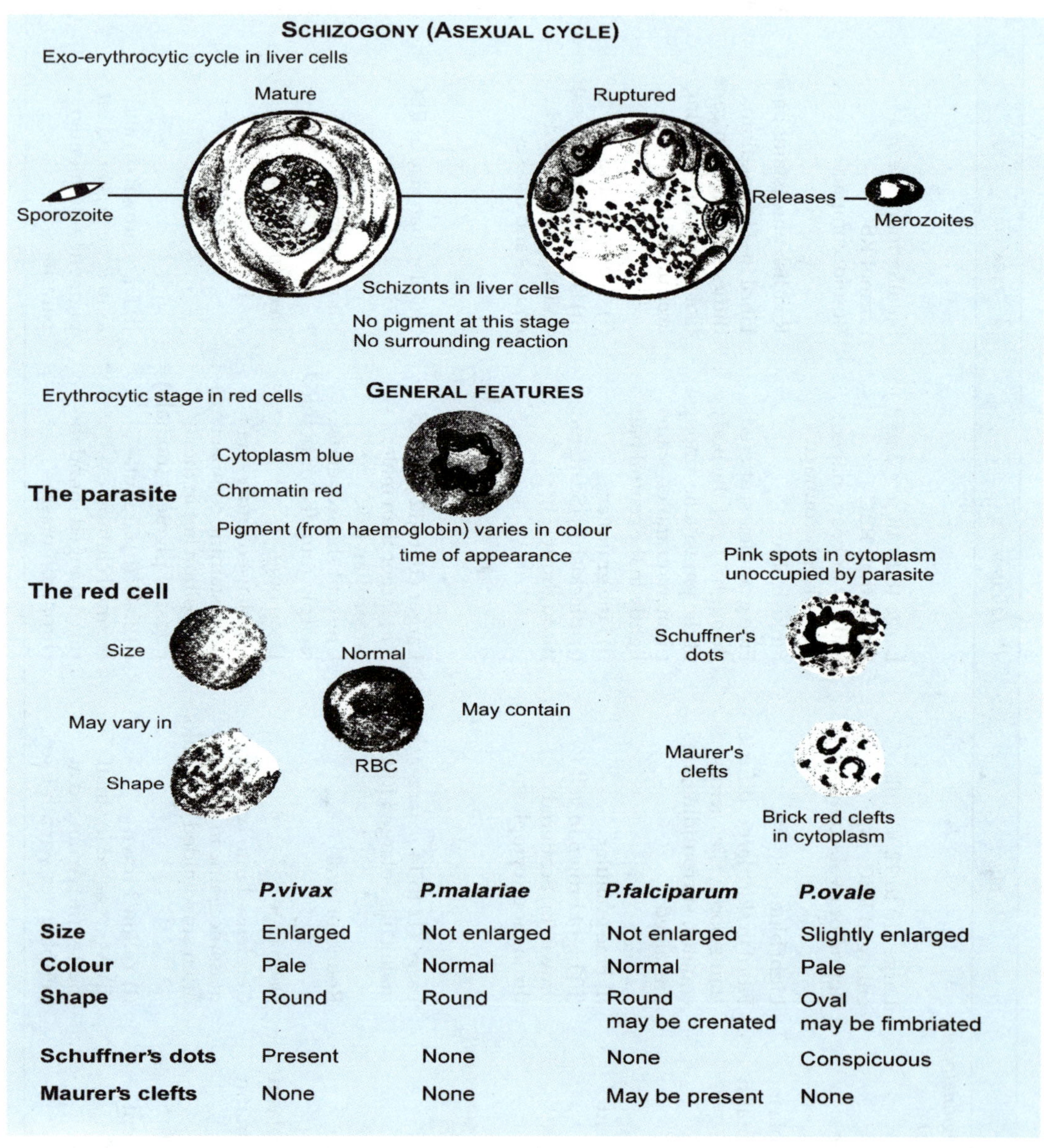

	P.vivax	*P.malariae*	*P.falciparum*	*P.ovale*
Size	Enlarged	Not enlarged	Not enlarged	Slightly enlarged
Colour	Pale	Normal	Normal	Pale
Shape	Round	Round	Round may be crenated	Oval may be fimbriated
Schuffner's dots	Present	None	None	Conspicuous
Maurer's clefts	None	None	May be present	None

Morphology of Malarial Parasites

Stages in Thin Films

Ring forms (Early trophozoites)

	P.vivax	*P.malariae*	*P.falciparum*	*P.ovale*
Size	Up to 1/3 Red cell	Up to 1/3	Up to 1/5	Up to 1/3 Red cell
Shape	Delicate ring	Compact ring	Very delicate ring	Delicate ring
Chromatin	Fine dot sometimes two	One mass often inside ring	Fine dots frequently two	Dense, well defined mass
Accole forms	Sometimes	None	Frequent	None
Pigment	None at this stage	May be present	None at this stage	None at this stage

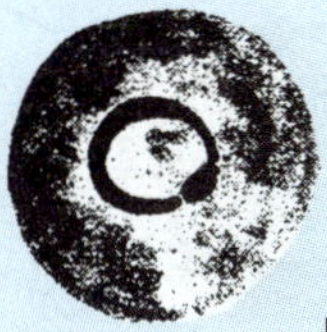

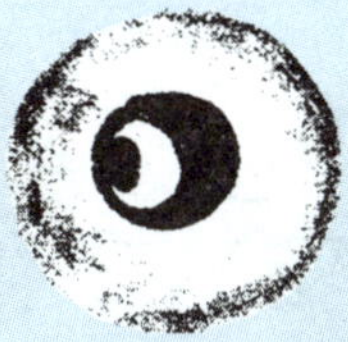

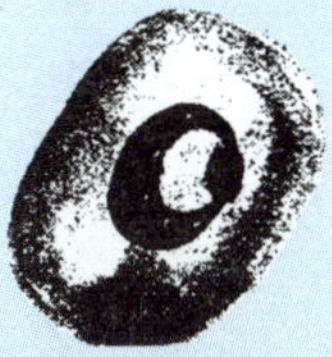

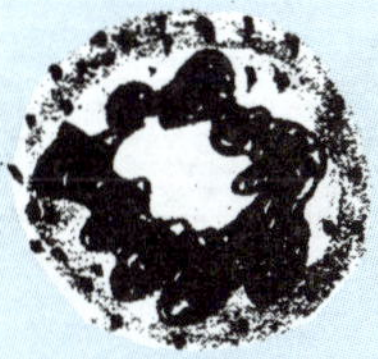

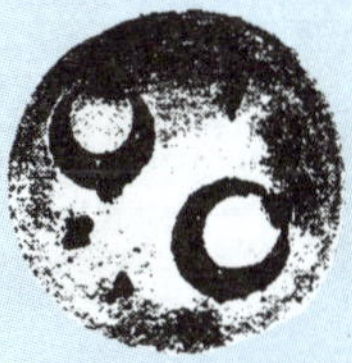

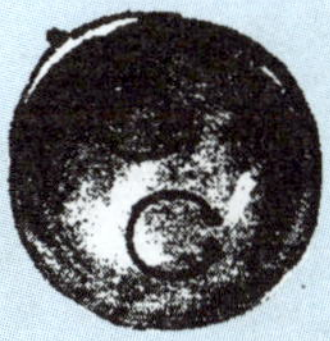

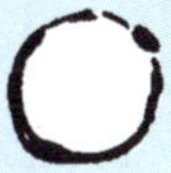

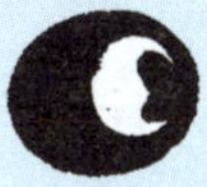

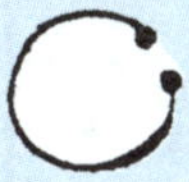

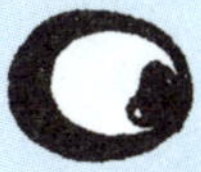

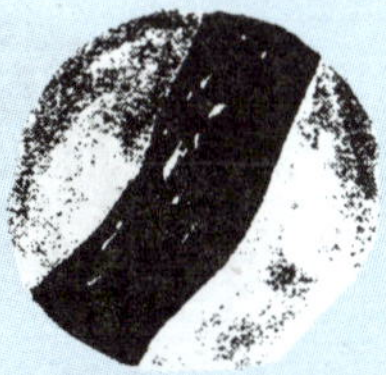

Developing trophozoites

		P.vivax	*P.malariae*	*P.falciparum* (Rarely seen in peripheral blood)	*P.ovale*
Size		Large	Small	Small	Small
Shape		Very irregular	Compact, often band forms	Compact	Compact
Vacuole		Prominent	Inconspicuous	Inconspicuous	Inconspicuous
Chromatin		Dots or threads	Dots or threads	Dots or threads	Large irregular clumps
Pigment	**Texture**	Fine	Coarse	Coarse	Coarse
	Colour	Yellow brown	Dark Brown	Black	Dark yellow brown
	Quantity	Medium	Abundant	Medium	Medium
	Distribution	Scattered fine particles	Scattered clumps and rods	Aggregated in two clumps	Scattered coarse particles

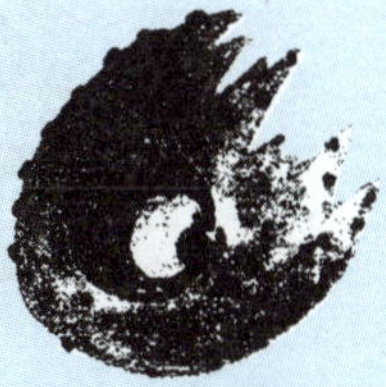

Morphology of Malarial Parasites (Contd....)

IMMATURE SCHIZONTS

	P.vivax	*P.malariae*	*P.falciparum* (Rarely seen in peripheral blood)	*P.ovale*
Size	Almost fills red cells	Almost fills red cells	Almost fills red cells	Almost fills red cells
Shape	Somewhat amoeboid	Compact	Compact	Compact
Chromatin	Numerous irregular masses	Few irregular masses	Numerous irregular masses	Few irregular masses
Pigment	Scattered	Scattered	Scattered	Scattered

MATURE SCHIZONTS

	P.vivax	*P.malariae*	*P.falciparum* (Rarely seen in peripheral blood)	*P.ovale*
Size	Fills red cells	Nearly fills red cells	Nearly fills red cells	Fills ¾ of red cells
Shape	Segmented	Segmented daisy head	Segmented	Segmented
Merozoites Range	14–24	6–12	8–32	6–12
Mean	16	8	24	8
Size	Medium	Large	Small	Large
Pigment	Aggregated in centre (Yellow brown)	Aggregated in centre (Dark brown)	Aggregated in centre (Black)	Aggregated in centre (Dark yellow brown)

Morphology of Malarial Parasites (Contd....)

	P.vivax	*P.malariae*	*P.falciparum*	*P.ovale*
	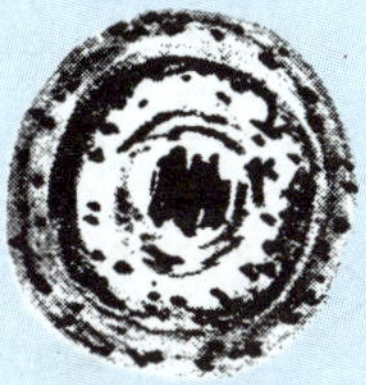	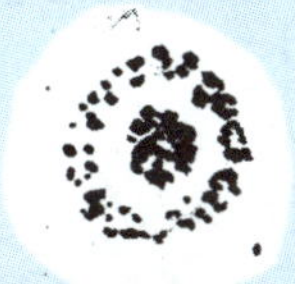 **MICROGAMETOCYTES**	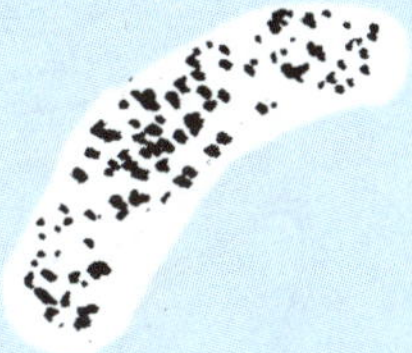	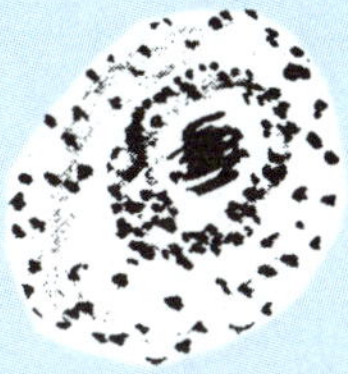
Time of appearance	3–5 days	7–14 days	7–12 days	12–14 days
Number in bloodstream	Many	Scanty	Many	Scanty
Size	Fills enlarged red cell	Smaller than red cell	Larger than red cell	Size of red cell
Shape	Round or oval compact	Round compact	Kidney shaped bluntly round ends	Round compact
Cytoplasm	Pale blue	Pale blue	Reddish blue	Pale blue
Chromatin	Fibrils in skin with surrounding unstained area	As for ***P.vivax***	Fine granules scattered throughout	As for ***P.vivax***
Pigment	Abundant brown granules throughout	As for ***P.vivax***	Dark granules throughout	As for ***P.vivax***
		MACROGAMETOCYTES		
Time of appearance	3–5 days	7–14 days	7–12 days	12–14 days
Number in bloodstream	Many	Scanty	Many	Scanty
Size	Fills enlarged red cell	Smaller than red cell	Larger than red cell	Size of red cell
Shape	Round or oval compact	Round compact	Crescentic–sharply rounded or pointed ends	Round compact
Cytoplasm	Dark blue	Dark blue	Dark blue	Dark blue
Chromatin	Compact peripheral mass	As for ***P.vivax***	Compact masses near centre	As for ***P.vivax***
Pigment	Small masses round periphery	As for ***P.vivax***	Black granules round nucleus	As for ***P.vivax***

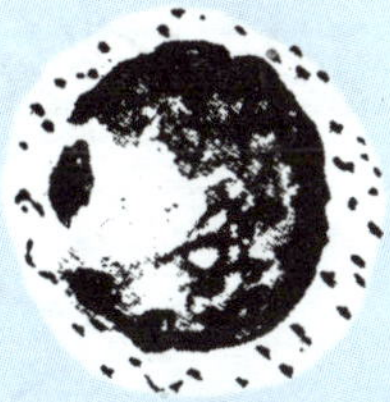

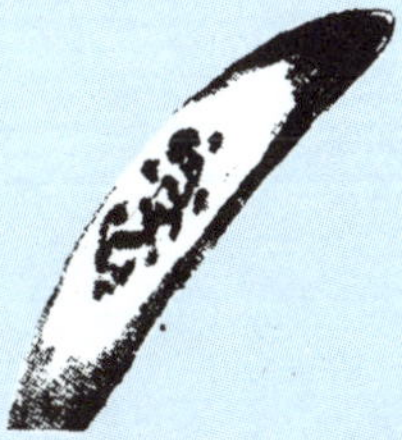

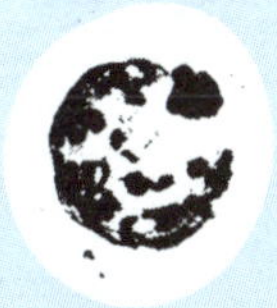

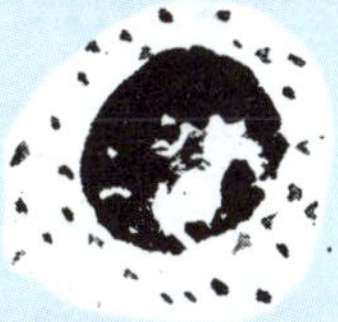

Life Cycle of Malarial Parasites

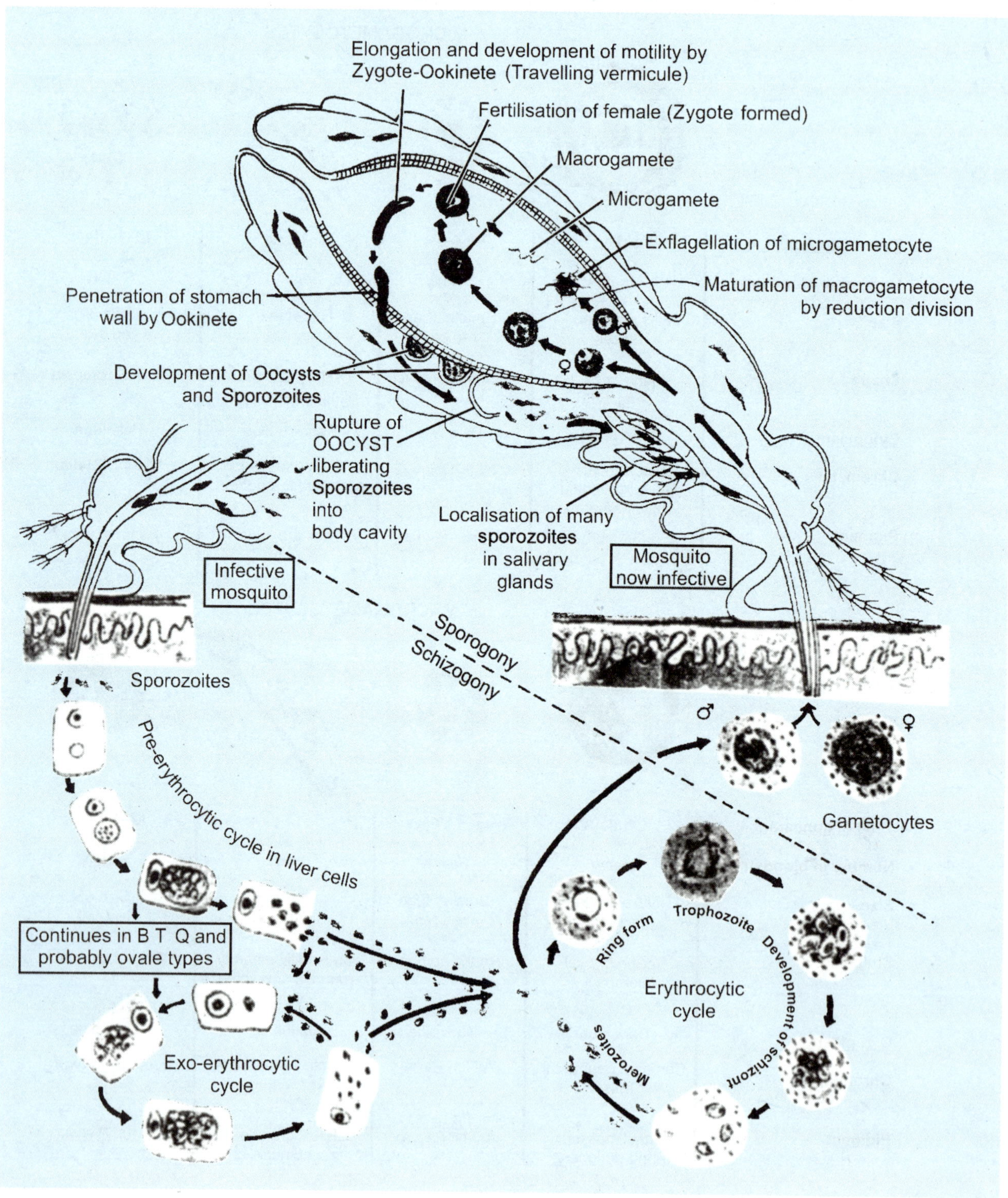

The Pathogenesis of Malaria

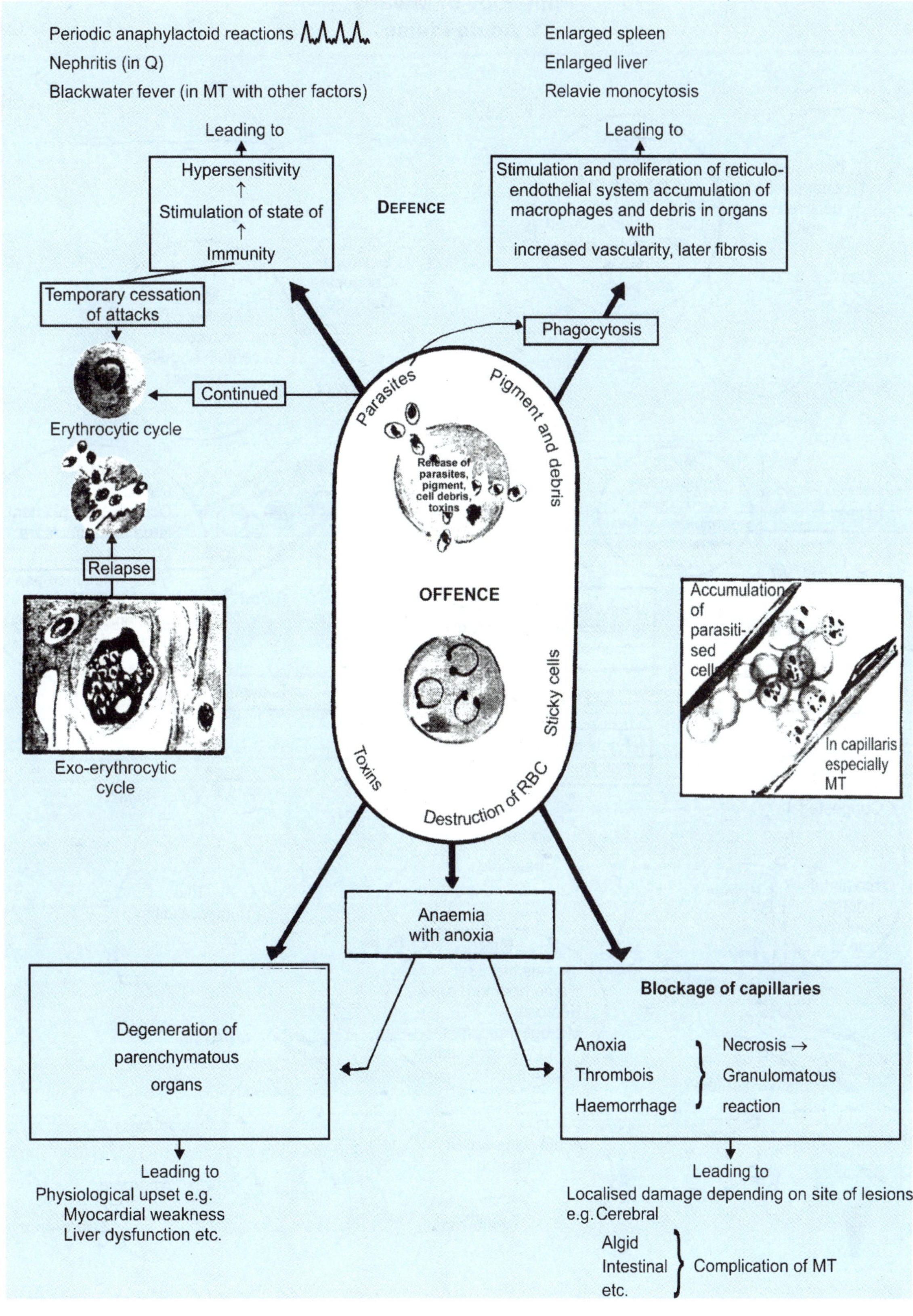

Pathology of Malaria
1. Acute Phase

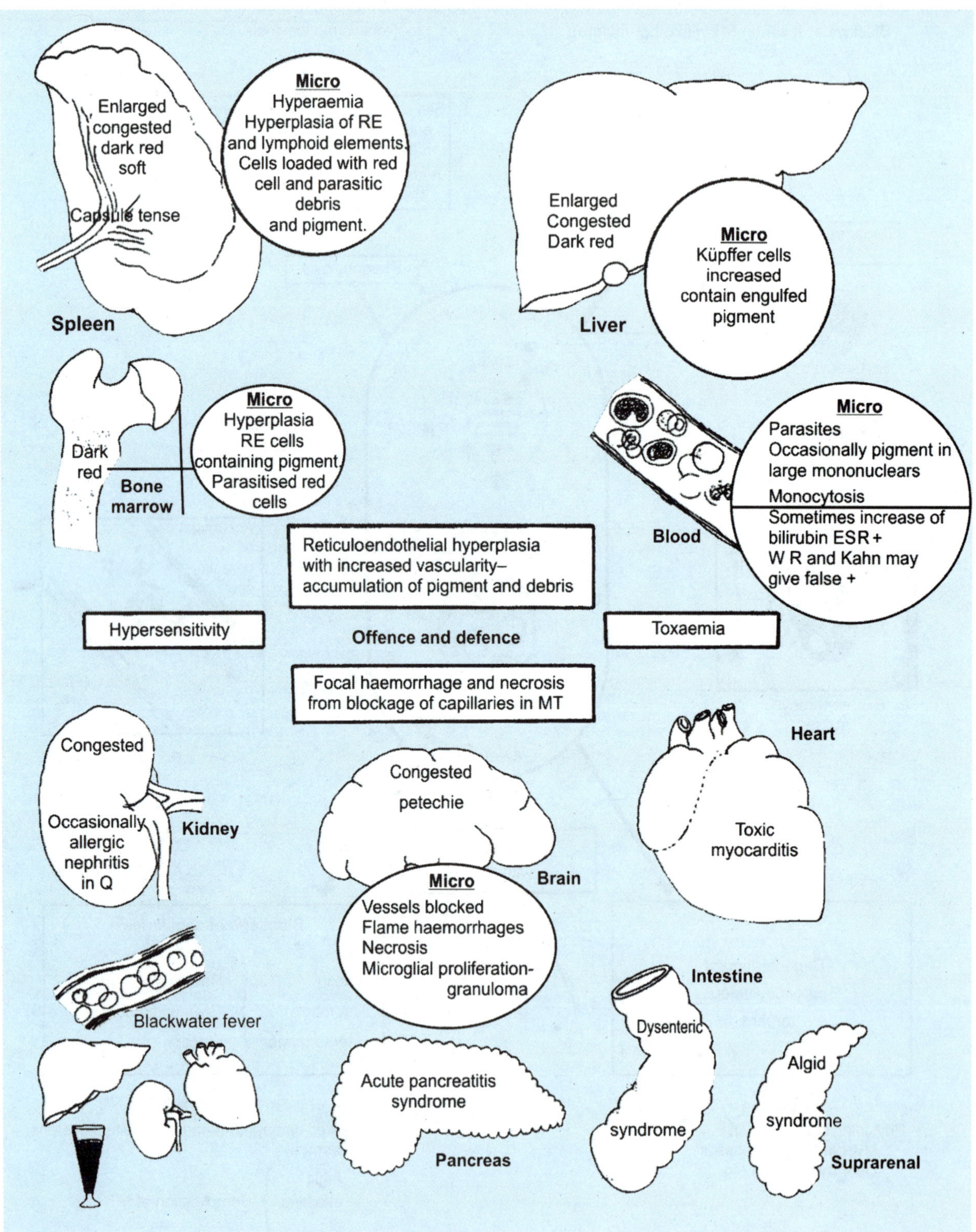

Pathology of Malaria
2. Chronic Phase

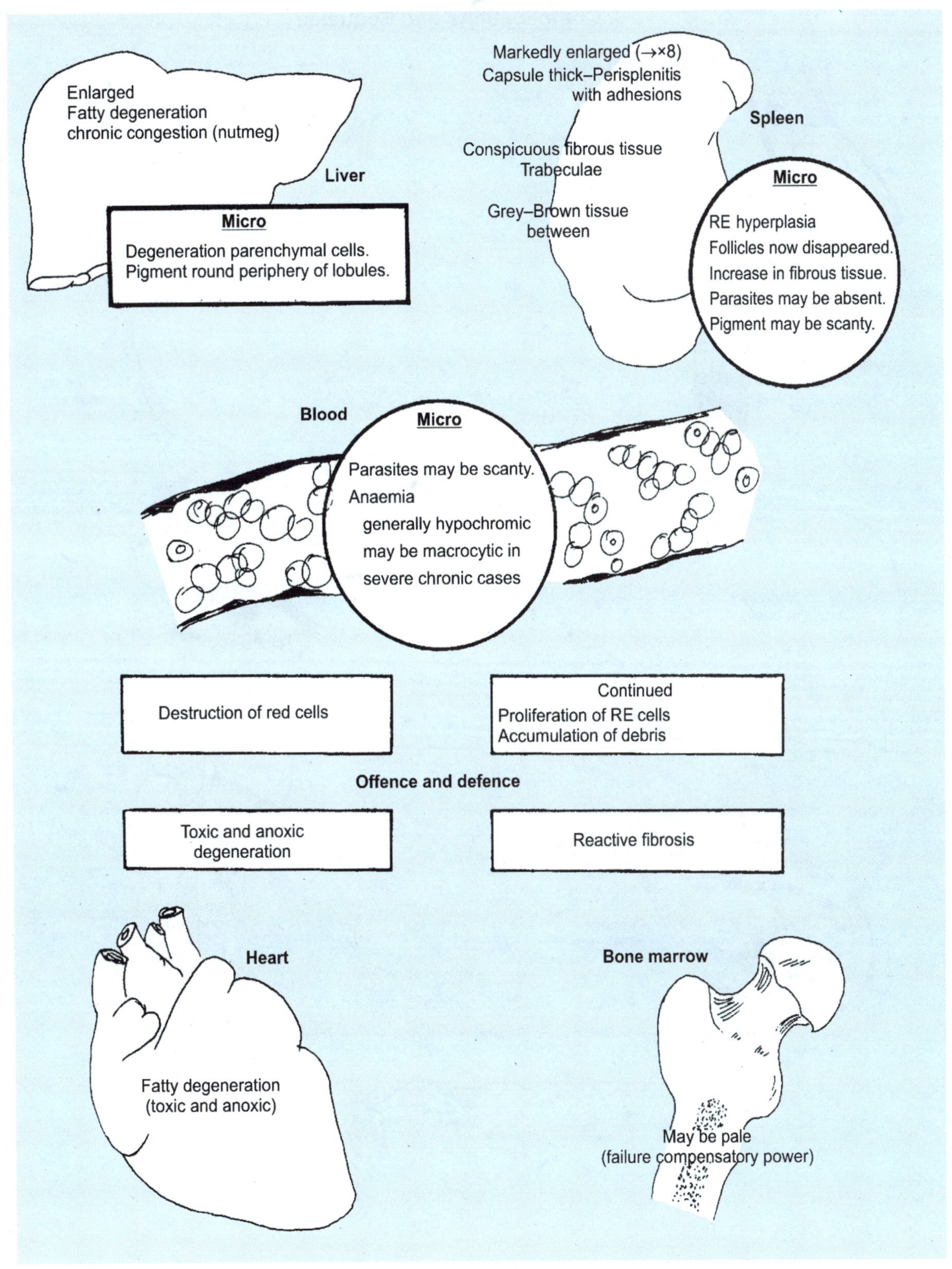

Pathology of Malaria
3. Complications and Sequelae

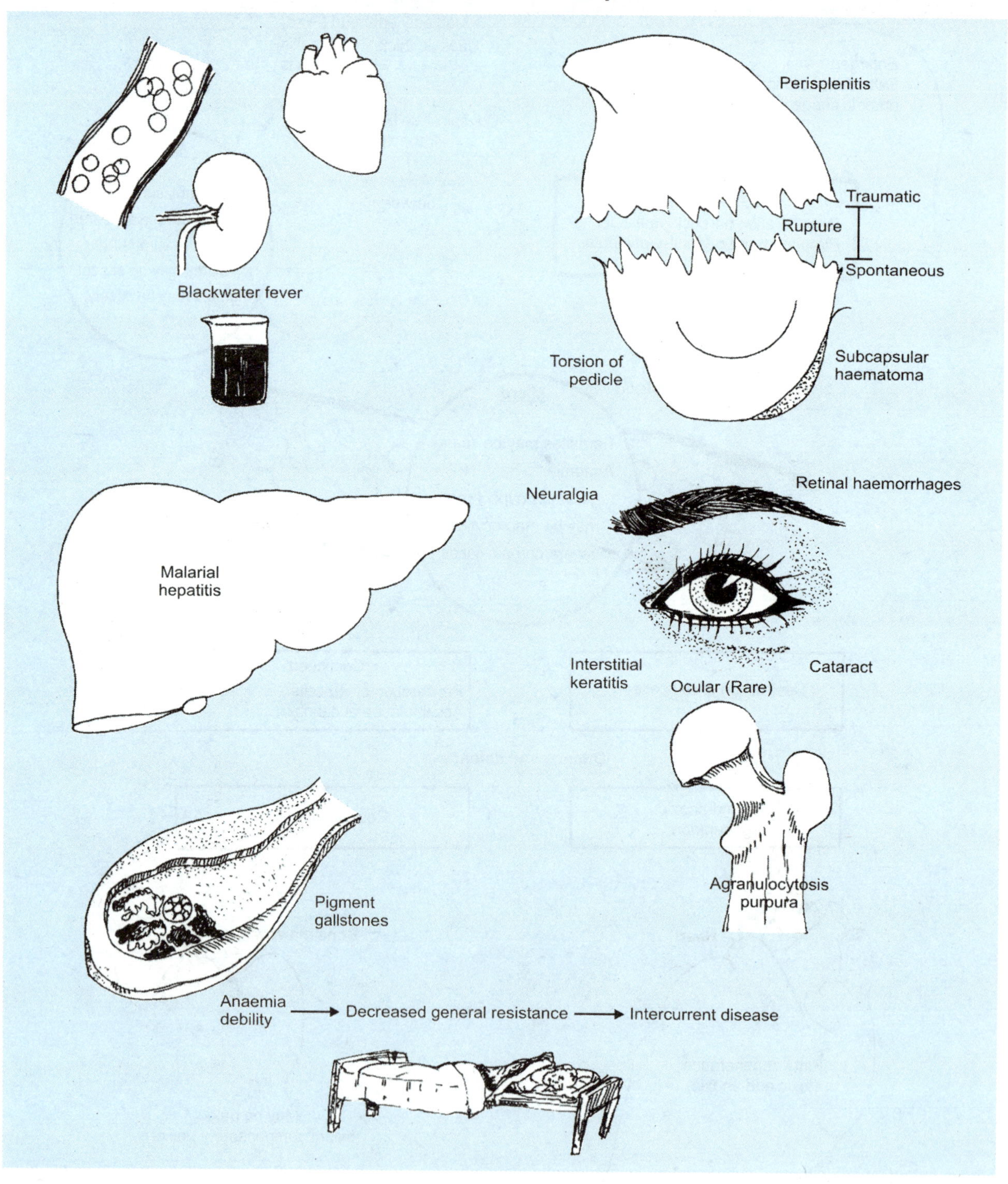

Pathology of Malaria
4. Blackwater Fever

Acute haemolytic attacks in MT malarias; associated with taking of quinine; numerous theories as to mechanism

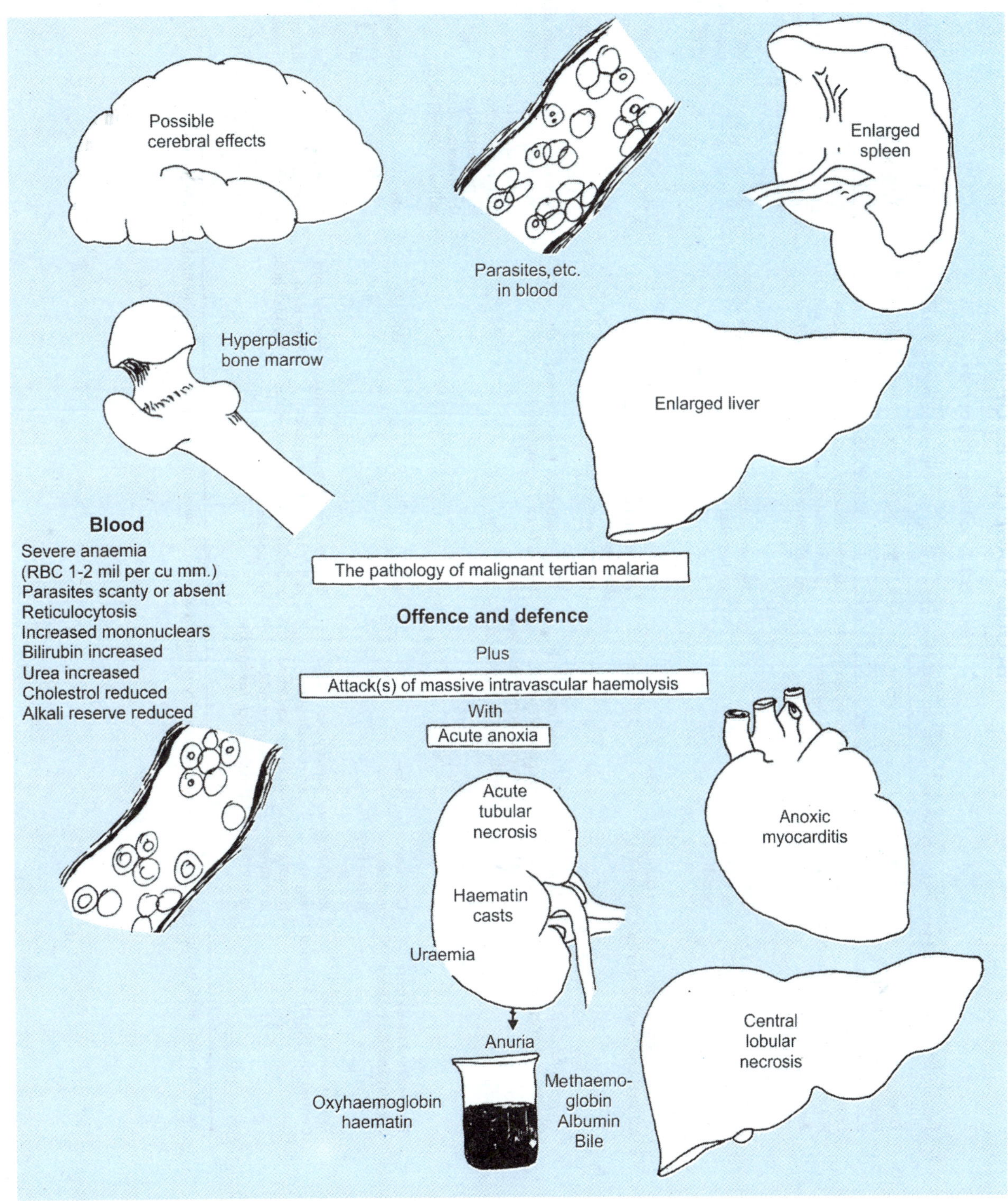

BLOOD FLAGELLATES OF MAN

Table 8.3: Blood flagellates of man

Prevalence depends upon presence of vertebrate reservoirs and proper insect hosts and varies with human habitation, habits, and agricultural practices.

Parasite and distribution	*Fly host*	*Enters man*	*Life cycle in man*	*Exit*	*cycle in fly*	*Reservoir host*[*]
Leishmania donovani Asia, Africa, tropical South America, Middle East, Mediterranean basin	*Phlebotomus* or Lutzomyia (Sandfly)	Plug of promastigotes (leptomonad) injected with bite of fly	Become amastigotes (leishmania or LD bodies) in RES macrophages	Sucked into fly with blood of host	Become promastigotes (leptomonads) in the intestine of fly	Man, dogs, foxes or other carnivores, wild rodents
Leishmania tropica Asia, South and Central America, Middle East, Europe	*Phlebotomus* or Lutzomyia (Sandfly)	-do-	Become amastigotes in endothelial cells of skin	-do-	-do-	Man, various wild rodents, possibly dogs
Leishmania brasiliensis Central and South America	*Lutzomyia* (Sandfly)	-do-	Become amastigotes in endothelial cells of skin and secondarily in mucous membranes of nasopharynx	-do-	-do-	Man, various wild rodents, possibly dogs
Trypansoma gambiense Central and West Africa	*Glossina palpalis* (tsetse fly)	Fly bites; metacyclic trypomastigotes (trypanosomes) injected with saliva	Trypomastigotes in lymph and blood; later in spinal fluid	-do-	Become epimastigotes (crithidia) and then metacyclic trypomastigotes in the intestine and salivary glands of fly	Man, domestic animals
Trypanosoma rhodesiense Central and East Africa	*Glossina morsitans* (tsetse fly)	-do-	-do-	-do-	-do-	Man, wild game animals (antelopes)
Trypanosoma cruzi Central and South America	*Panstrongylus megistus* (kissing bug) and other reduvid bugs	Metacyclic trypomastigotes in faeces scratched into skin or rubbed into mucous membrane of eye	Become amastigotes in tissue cell (particularly cardiac muscle) and trypomastigotes in bloodstream	Sucked into bug with blood of host	Become epimastigotes and then metacyclic trypomastigotes in the hind intestine of bug.	Man, dogs, cats, foxes, armadillo, opossum, rodents

[*]Varies in each area, in India and Africa, the dog apparently is not involved in *L. donovani* transmission. RES = Reticuloendothelial system.

Table 8.4: Blood flagellate diseases of man

Disease and aetiology	*Clinical features*	*Laboratory diagnosis*
Kala-azar (visceral leishmaniasis) *L. donovani* ,	Chronic febrile disease, causing hyperplasia and then blockage of the reticuloendothelial system, particularly spleen and liver. Irregular fever (may spike twice a day) with chills, sweating, diarrhoea, oedema, cachexia, leukopenia, anaemia. Splenomegaly and leukopenia characteristic. (Incubation period: 2-9 months.) Untreated cases usually end fatally; with proper treatment, fatality is under 5%.	Blood: Thick and thin smears, culture in NNN or Tobie's diphasic blood agar. CF test diagnostic; nonspecific tests such as Napier and Chopra serum tests for screening; skin tests for past infection. Nasal scrappings, lymph node biopsy, sternal marrow and splenic or hepatic aspirate. Stained smears, culture, inoculation of hamsters.
Oriental sore (cutaneous leishmania- of ulcer): Stained sis) *L. tropica*	Endothelial cells and lymphoid tissue of skin parasitised. Itching red papule→ scaling→ crusted ulcer → ulcer enlargement →healing. May be multiple [Incubation period: several days to months, depending on strain, (1) dry (urban), relatively benign, slowly ulcerating form; or (2) moist (rural) acute, rapidly ulcerating zoonotic form.]	Ulcer curettings (from margin, not centre smears, culture.
American leishmaniasis (espundia, forest yaws, uta; mucocutaneous leishmaniasis)*L. brasiliensis*	Initial ulcers similar to oriental sore, but this enlarges, producing weeping 'saucer' ulceration. Destructive and deforming secondary lesions occur at mucocutaneous junctions, particularly of nasopharynx. Produces fever, pain, malaise, and anaemia (Incubation period: indeterminate). Initial lesion—few days, complications—months to years. Nutrition probably very important in severity.	Ulcer curettings (from margin not centre, of smear): Stained smears, culture.
Sleeping sickness West African (*Trypanosoma gambiense*) East African (*Trypanosoma rhodesiense*)	Local lesion at fly bite followed by fever, adenitis, rash, transitory oedemas. May fulminate (*T. rhodesiense*) or go on to meningoencephalitis and meningomyelitis, with mental and physical wasting leading to coma and death (*T. gambiense*). (Incubation period: *T. gambiense*, 1-3 weeks; *T. rhodesiense*, 1-2 weeks.)	Blood: Thick and thin smears, concentration, culture. Spinal fluid sediment smears. Lymph node fluid: Smears and culture

Contd...

Contd...

Chagas' disease *T. cruzi*	Acute, usually in children: Febrile illness with generalised adenopathy lasting a few months; placental infection common. Chronic cardiac involement, particularly of right ventricle, consisting of degeneration of cardiac muscle. Patient seldom lives beyond age 50. Megacolon or megaoesophagus a sequel. Anaemia. Romana's sign (palpebral oedema) most probably an allergy to insect bite (Incubation period: 1-2 weeks)	Blood: Thick and thin smears only in initial phases. Culture. Xenodiagnosis. Complement fixation most reliable serologic test

* Direct blood film stain positive except in heavy infections; buffy coat smear or culture better.*

The basis of serum biochemical tests for Leishmaniasis

These tests assess alterations in serum proteins particularly serum gamma globulin. The positive results are obtained after 2 to 3 months or more.

Napier's aldehyde test: When serum of the patient is treated with formaldehyde, it causes flocculation and opacity. To 1 ml of patient's serum, add 2 drops of formaldehyde—if flocculation and opacity occur within 10 minutes, the test is strongly positive. If this change occurs in about 2 hours time, it is labelled as weakly or doubtful positive.

Chopra's antimony test: Dilute patient's serum 10 times with normal saline. To 1 ml of diluted serum, add 2 drops of 4% urea stibamine solution. Immediate appearance of flocculum and turbidity indicates a positive test.

For exact determination of individual classes of gamma globulins, immunoturbidometric or nephalometric techniques may be used. However for screening purposes and normal routine clinical testing, the given above tests are quite satisfactory.

ELISA techniques are ideal.

Leishmaniasis

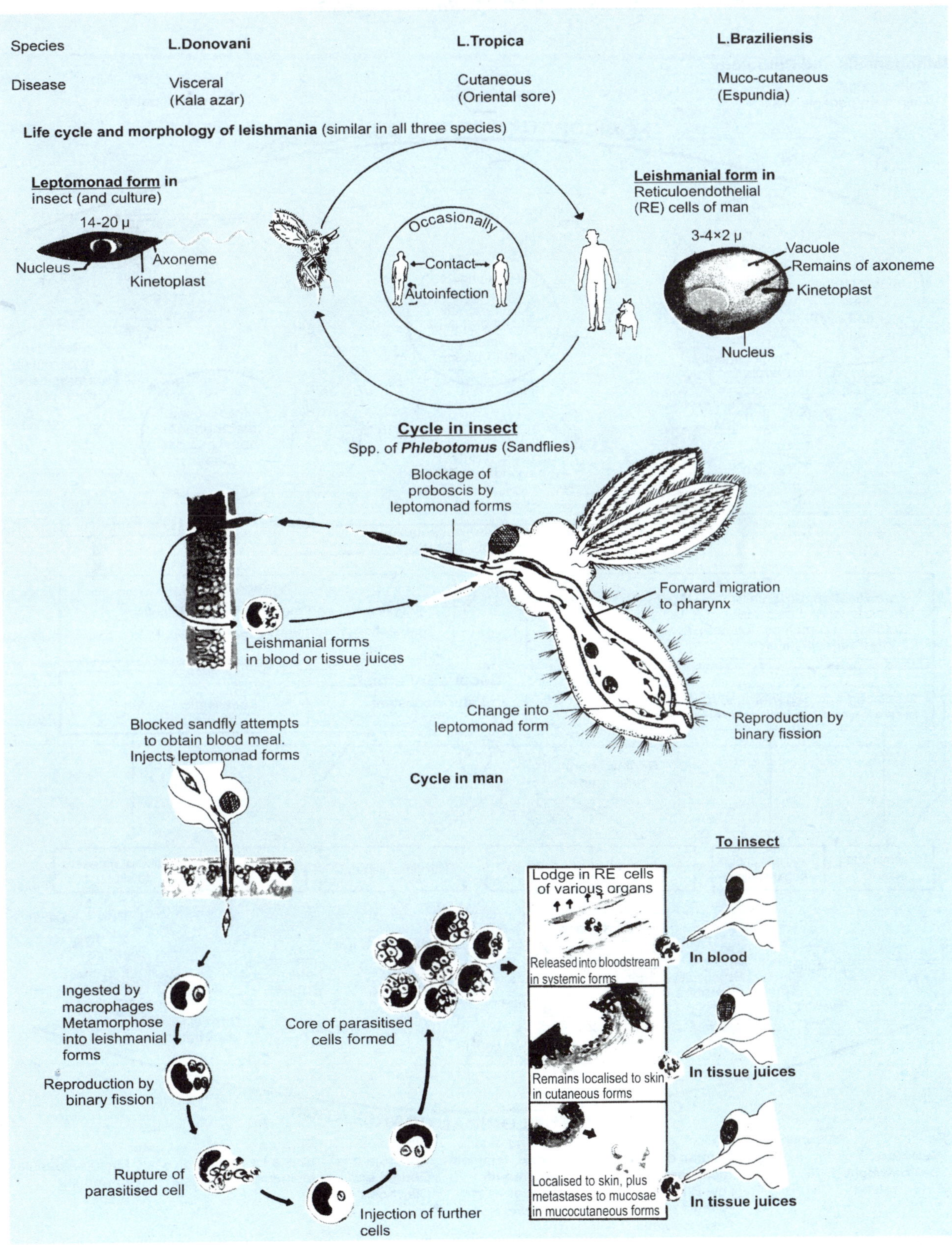

Visceral Leishmaniasis (Kala Azar)
Caused by *Leishmania donavani*

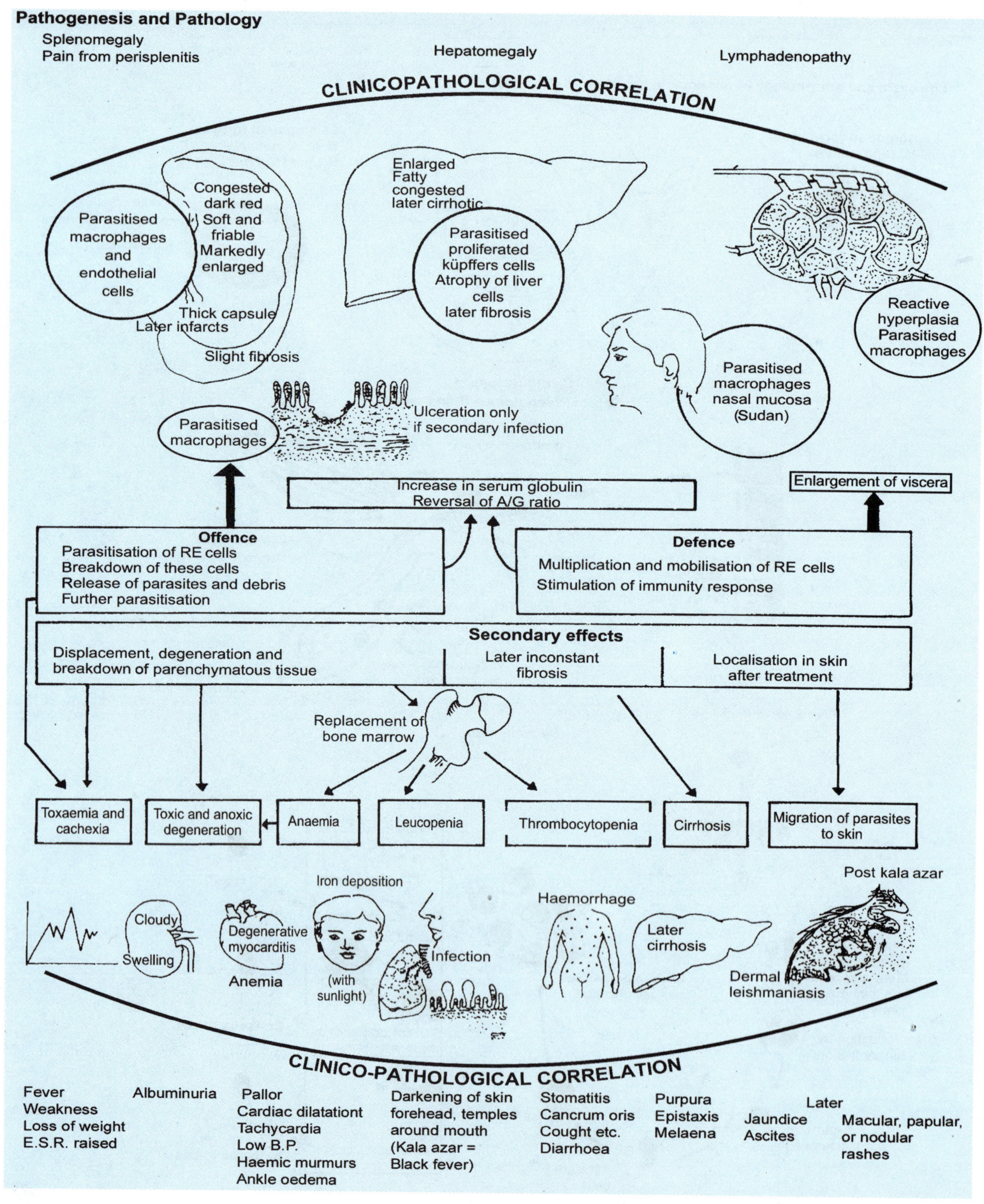

Cutaneous Leishmaniasis (Oriental Sore, Chiclero's disease, Uta, etc.) Caused by *Leishmania tropica*

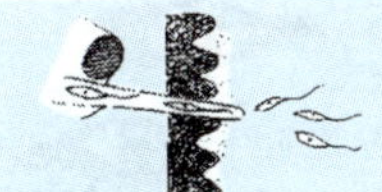

Blocked sandfly injects leptomonad forms

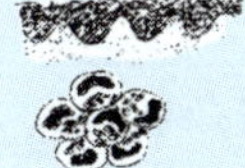

Core of cells parasitised by LD bodies formed

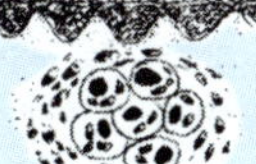

Acanthosis cellular infiltration

Remains localised to skin

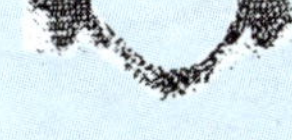

Pressure necrosis and ulceration

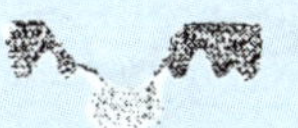

Secondary injection

Ulcer with sharp cut edges and surrounding induration

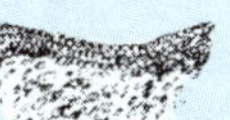

Granulation

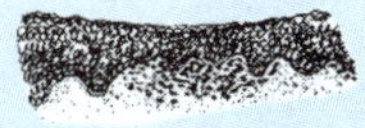

Healing (2-12 months) with depressed pigment scar

Mucocutaneous Leishmaniasis (Espundia)

Caused by Leishmania braziliensis

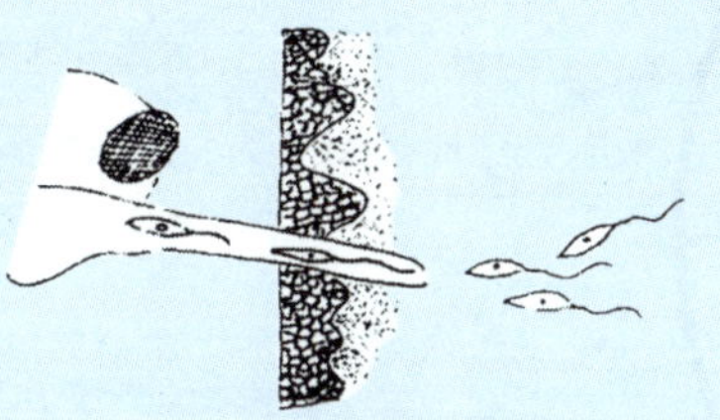

Blocked sandfly injects leptomonad forms

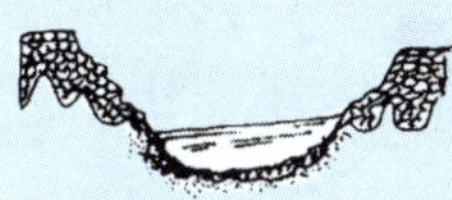

Cutaneous manifestations like oriental sore but often weeping ulcers

→

Spread to mucosae of mouth-nose, larynx, pharynx, ear

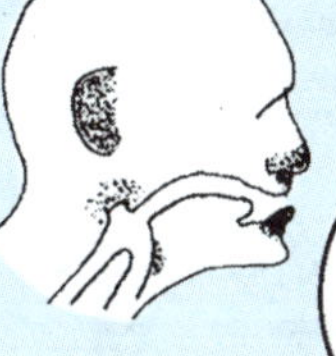

Parasitised cell
Inflammatory infiltration
Necrosis
Later reactive fibrosis

Secondary effects in loose mucosal tissues

Oedema and capillary involvement Interference with local blood supply Necrosis–Extensive destruction	Secondary infection Deep erosion locally Spread of infection to lungs or elsewhere	Healing with fibrosis

Leading to

Extensive disfiguring lesions

General constitutional upset (fever, pain, anaemia)

Bronchopneumonia and septicaemia

Diagnosis of leishmaniasis

Visceral

1. Demonstration of parasite by Stained film, Culture (NNN), Animal inoculation (Hamsters) In
   - Blood
   - Bone marrow
   - Lymph node juice
   - Nasal scrapings (Sudan)
   - Spleen puncture } not free from danger
   - Liver puncture } not free from danger

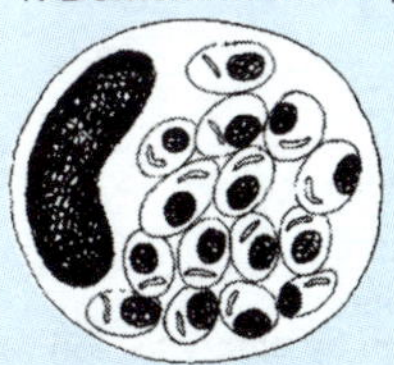

2. Serological tests

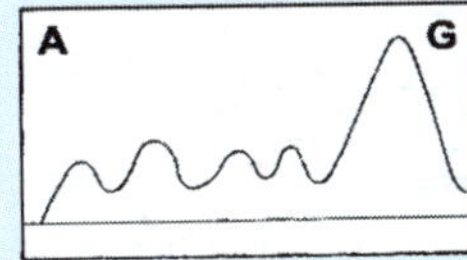

Specific — CFT (antigen, Leishmania cultures)

Nonspecific — Depending on reversal A G ratio
- Formal gel (Napier)
- Aldehyde (Chopra)
- Euglobulin precipitation (Sia)
- Electrophoresis

Cutaneous and Mucocutaneous

1. Demonstration of parasite by Stained film, Culture, Animal inoculation In
   - Serum from indurated edge of ulcer
   - Biopsy of margin ulcer
   - Mucosal scraping in mucocutaneous type
2. Intradermal test (Montenegro). Antigen culture of appropriate Leishmania
3. Serological tests in mucocutaneous type

Trypanosomiases
African type: Sleeping Sickness

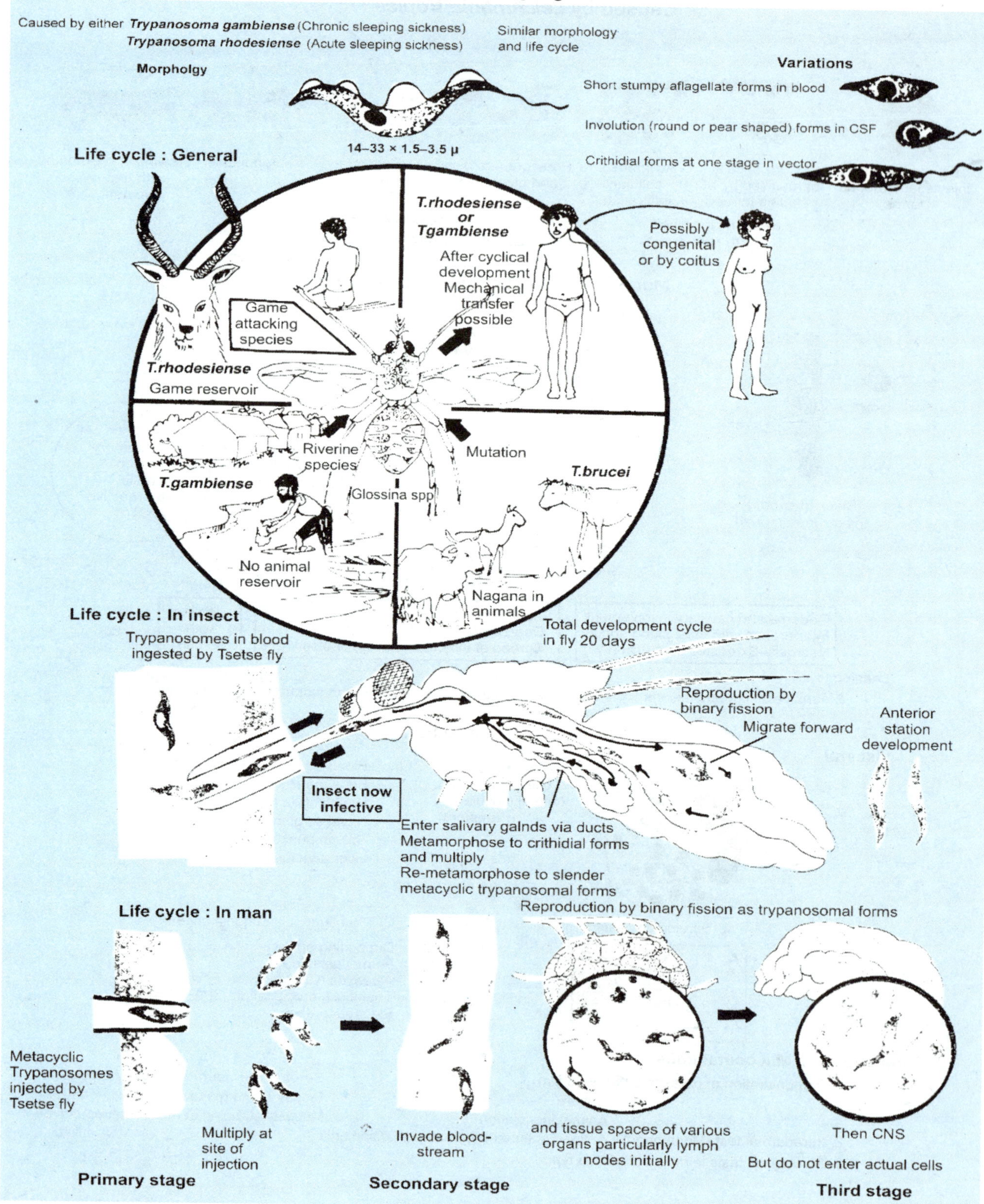

African Trypanosomiasis (Sleeping sickness) (Contd...)

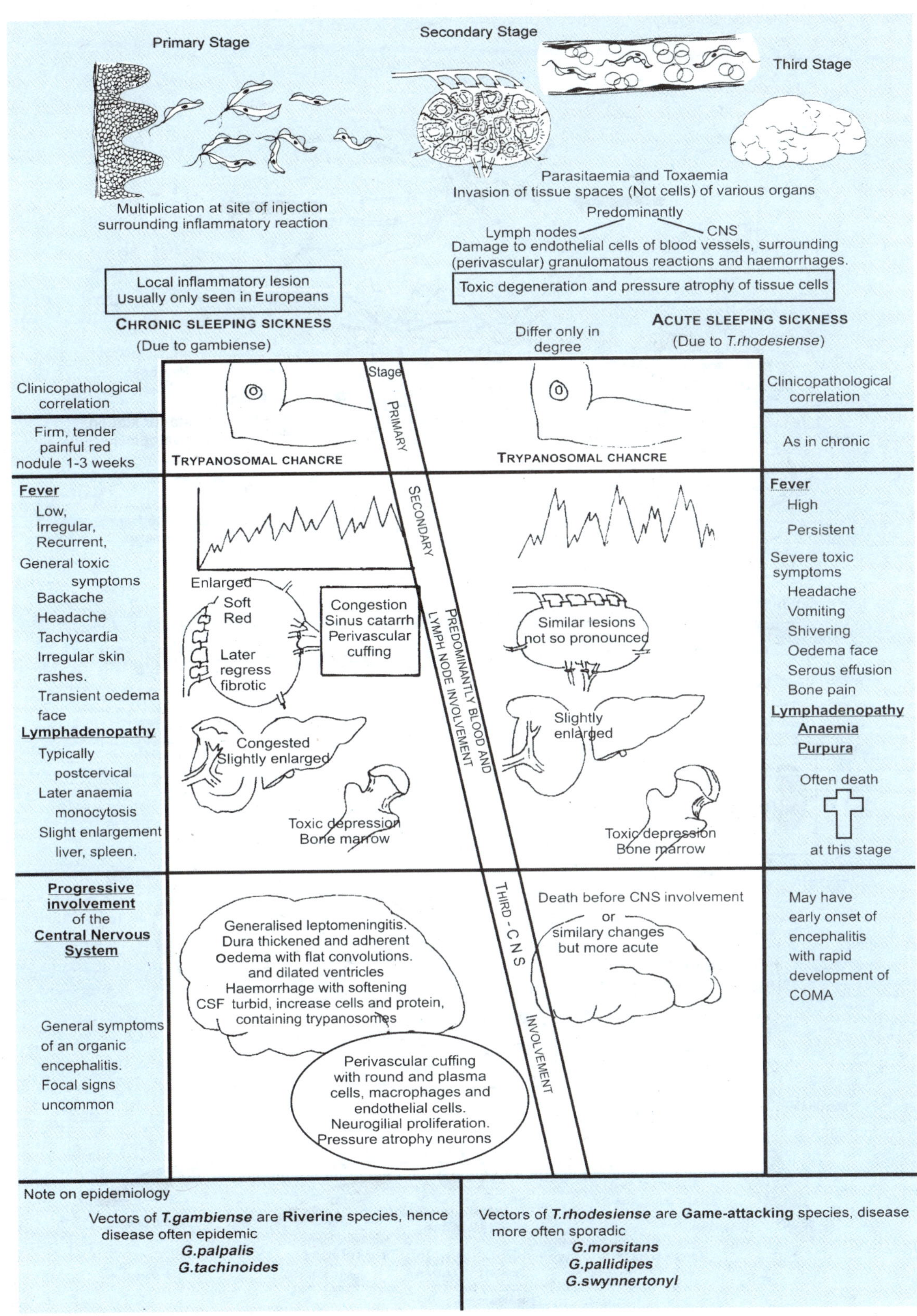

Note on epidemiology

Vectors of ***T.gambiense*** are **Riverine** species, hence disease often epidemic	Vectors of ***T.rhodesiense*** are **Game-attacking** species, disease more often sporadic
G.palpalis	***G.morsitans***
G.tachinoides	***G.pallidipes***
	G.swynnertonyl

Trpanosomiasis South AmericanType: Chaga's Disease

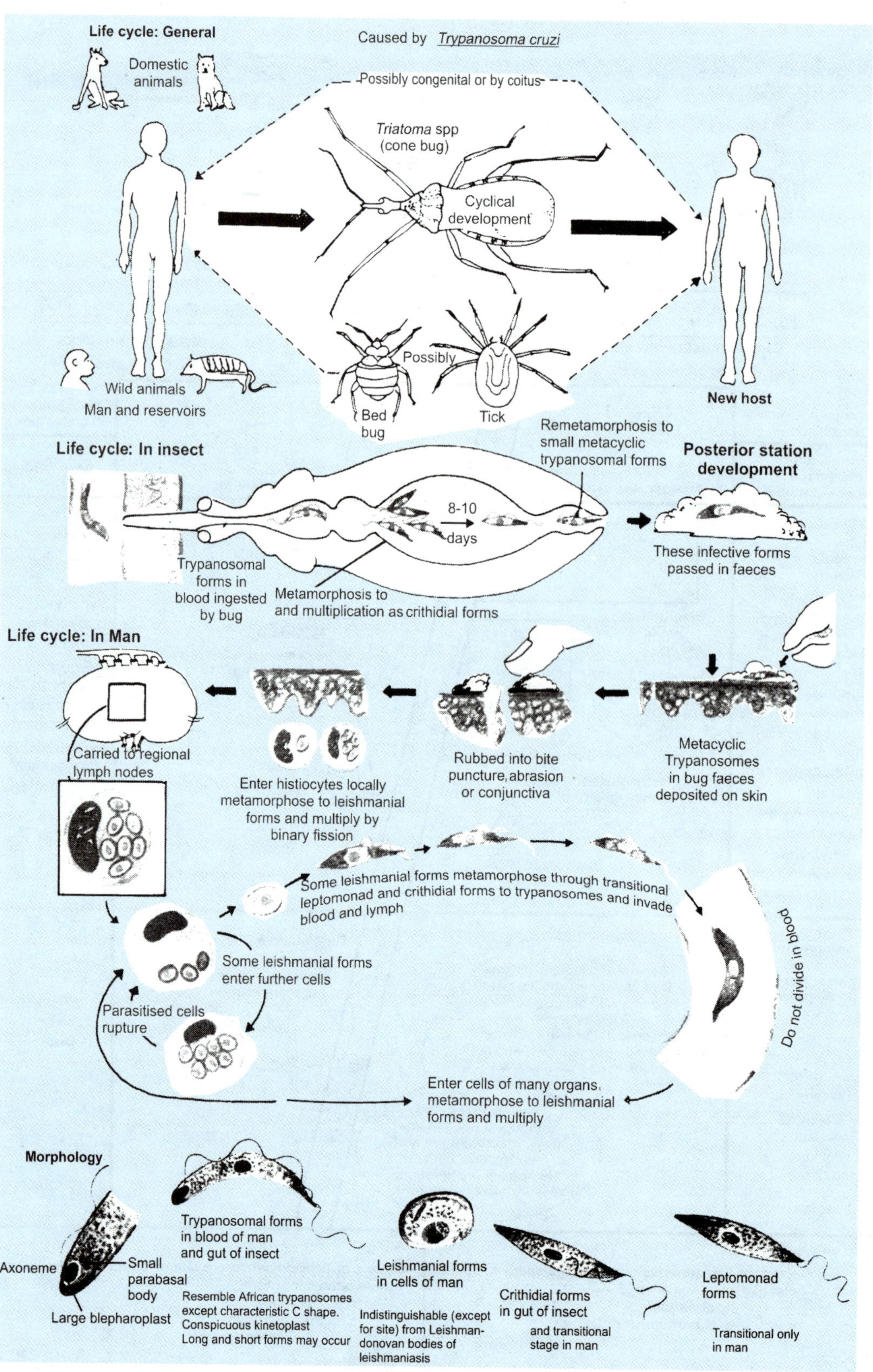

South American Trypanosomiasis (Chaga's Disease) (Contd..)

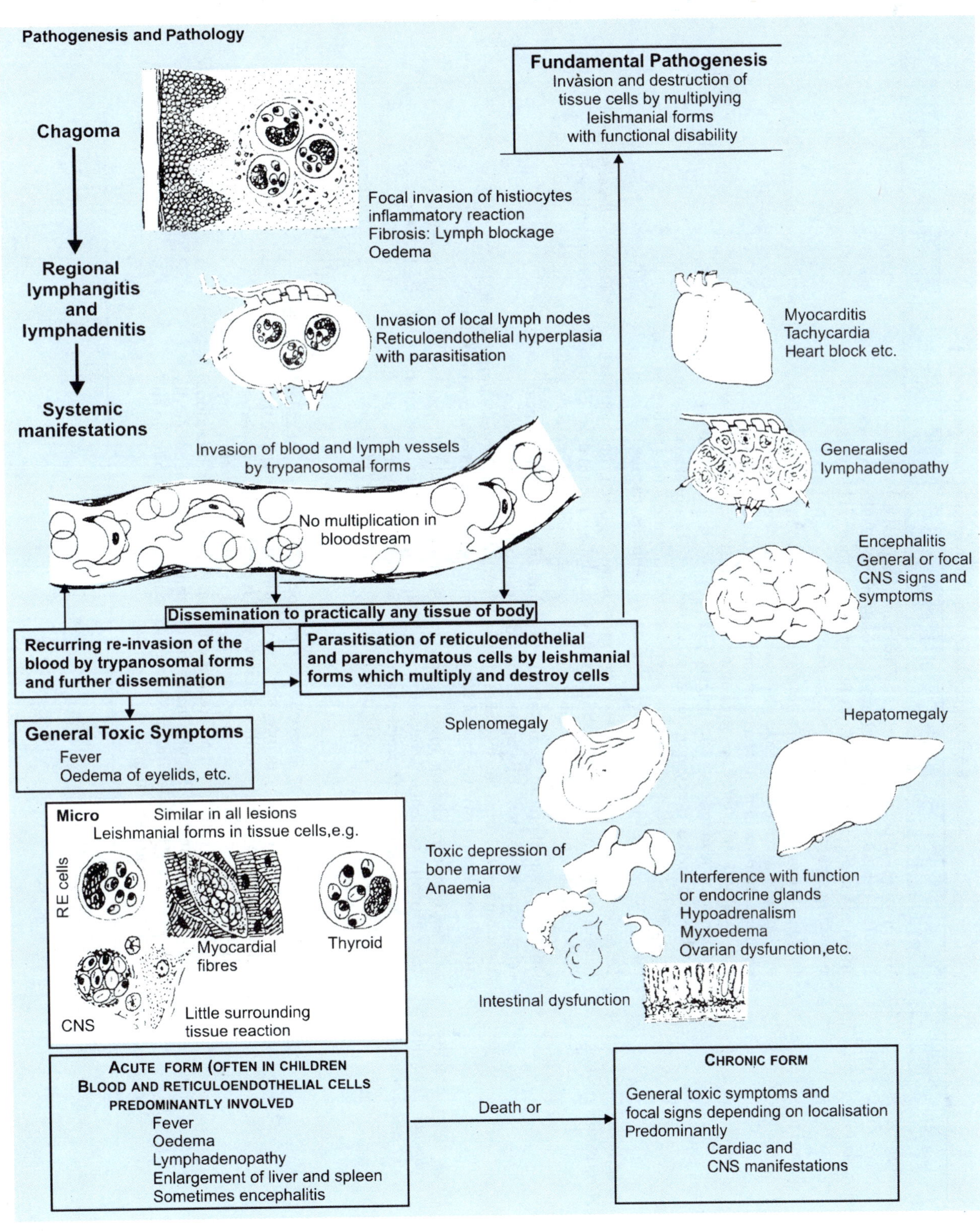

COMMON INTESTINAL ROUNDWORMS OF MAN–PATHOLOGY

Table 8.5: Common intestinal roundworms of man pathology

Disease and aetiology	*Clinical features*	*Laboratory diagnosis*
Enterobiasis Pinworm infection *Enterobius vermicularis*	Symptomless to perianal itching and irritation. Vaginal itch when female worms leave anus and enter genital passage. Nervousness, insomnia in persistent or heavy infection, especially from biting finger-nails after scratching infected rectal area.	Cellulose (Scotch) tape swab
Trichuriaisis *Trichuris trichiura*	Depend on worm load. Symptomless to chronic debilitating diarrhoea and anaemia, with damage to physical and mental development. Lower right quadrant pain is quite a common complaint. Chronic diarrhoea, bloody stools, and tenesmus in heavier infections. Weight loss, wasting, rectal prolapse in massive trichuriasis, especially in children. Worms visible attached to mucosa under sigmoidoscopy in heavy infections, mucosa hyperaemic, friable, oedematous, stools are mucoid and sticky with sreaks of blood, numerous Charcot-Leyden crystals, eosinophils, trichuris eggs.	Faeces: Direct smear, concentration.
Ascariasis *Ascaris lumbricoides*	*Larvae* (migratory phase): Rarely pneumonitis with cough, haemoptysis, haemorrhages, lung consolidation, focal eosinophilic inflammation. Eosinophilia (usually under 30%) during larval migration, falls rapidly afterwards. *Adults* (intestinal phase): Symptomless to serious intestinal mechanical complications (pancreatitis, appendicitis, diverticulitis) especially after disturbance of worms causing obstruction or perforation; metabolic complication (malabsorption, nutritive drain). Nausea, vomiting, aggravation of malnutrition.	Faeces: Direct smear, concentration.
Hookworm infection *Ancylostoma duodenale* *Necator americanus*	*Larvae* (migratory phase): Intense skin invasion may produce "ground itch", pruritic vesicular lesions followed by lung reactions (less intense than in ascariasis); cough, tracheal irritation, eosinophilia. Nausea, vomiting, dyspnoea may result from larvae of *Ancylostoma* (Wakana disease in Japan). *Adults* (intestinal phase): Hypochromic, microcytic anaemia is the chief clinical feature, varies with intensity and duration of infection, iron intake nutritive state, age and condition of patient. Hypoproteinaemia, oedema, trophic skin disorders, growth reduction, and mental retardation may follow. Allergic urticaria, diarrhoea, abdominal pain in heavy infections. Intestinal malfunction through malabsorption and possible metabolic disturbance probably of significant importance, particularly in children and undernourished populations.	Faeces: Direct standardised smear to count eggs or examine after concentration, cultivation of faeces on filter paper strips in test tubes (Harada-Mori technique).

Contd...

Contd...

Strongyloidiasis *Strongyloides stercoralis*	*Larvae:* Invasion of skin may cause "ground itch," similar to hookworm. Malaise and cough, pulmonary infiltration may occur; high eosinophilia with larvae in focal lesions in colon, abdominal lymph nodes, liver, lungs following autoreinfection. *Adults:* Alternate diarrhoea and constipation; inflammation of intestinal mucosa; may be haemorrhage and microulceration with watery, mucoid diarrhoea, colicky abdominal pain, tenderness, flatulence. Heavier. infections produce atrophy of mucosa, ulcerous enteritis, oedema, and fibrosis of intestinal wall. Extreme cases (usually after autoreinfection) with rapid deterioration, asthenia, anorexia, and death or chronic invalidism. Intestinal malfunction with impaired protein digestion and fat absorption may produce a condition similar to sprue.	Faeces: Larvae (not eggs) in direct smear, concentration. Cultivation of faeces on filter paper strips in test tubes (Harada-Mori technique).

EXTRAINTESTINAL ROUNDWORM INFECTION OF MAN-LARVAL WORM PATHOLOGY

Table 8.6: Externaintestinal roundworm infections of man-larval worm pathology

Disease and aetiology	*Clinical features*	*Laboratory diagnosis*
Trichinosis *Trichinella spiralis*	*Adults* (intestinal phase): Irritate and inflame the intestinal mucosa, vomiting, diarrhoea, pain. *Larval migration and penetration* (1-6 weeks after infection) Muscular rheumatic pains, oedema of the eyes, face and hands. Irregular persistent sweating and fever; difficulty with breathing, swallowing, and speech; rash and high eosinophilia (50-90%). *Larval encystment:* (muscle phase) (after 6 weeks) Cachexia, toxic oedema, skin eruptions, anaemia, dehydration, and gradual subsidence of muscular pains. Fatalities usually occur 4-6 weeks after ingestion of heavily infected pork by nonimmune individuals. Using a home-butchered hog implicated.	Biopsy material: Examination by compression of tissue between glass slides or by digestion. Intradermal test, complement fixation, bentonite flocculation and latex agglutination tests.
Cutaneous larva migrans *Ancylostoma braziliense* and other nonhuman hookworms, species of animal *Strongyloides, Gnathostoma spinigerum,* and possibly other nematodes.	Intracutaneous violently itching, serpiginous tunnels, which are caused by wandering of hookworm larvae unable to complete normal penetration, migration, and development. Worms move about in the area of initial penetration, producing irregular papulovesicular lesions. Dry crust may form with local eosinophilia and cellular infiltration. This condition usually is transitory but larvae may also penetrate to deeper tissues; produce pulmonary infiltration and be recovered in sputum. The larvae may last several weeks to months, moving at intermittent periods of 1-3 cm/day.	Clinical signs sufficient. No worms identified except in experimental animals.
Visceral larva migrans: *Toxocara canis, T. cati* (dog, cat ascarids); also *Ancylostoma caninum, A. braziliense, Capillara hepatica, possibly Ascaris lumbricoides* var suum and filariae of the genus *Dirofilaria,* other animal nematodes.	Chiefly in children aged 1-4, often benign, asymptomatic; later there may develop 20-90% eosinophilia and hepatomegaly. Fever, cough, joint and muscle pains, anorexia, weight loss, nervousness, abdominal pain, pneumonitis, splenomegaly all reported. Symptoms vary with number and location of larvae and patient's allergic response. Chief result of wandering of larvae is indication of a series of focal eosinophilic inflammations succeeded by granulomatous reactions. Endophthalmitis reported in young adolescents who apparently harboured larvae in their tissues from childhood.	Heavy infections show larvae and eosinophilic granulomatous lesions in liver biopsy. Chiefly a clinical diagnosis (persistent eosinophilia, hepatomegaly, hyperglobulinaemia and frequent pneumonitis); haemagglutination technique useful for confirmation

Plasmid Nematodes (Contd...)
Hookworms

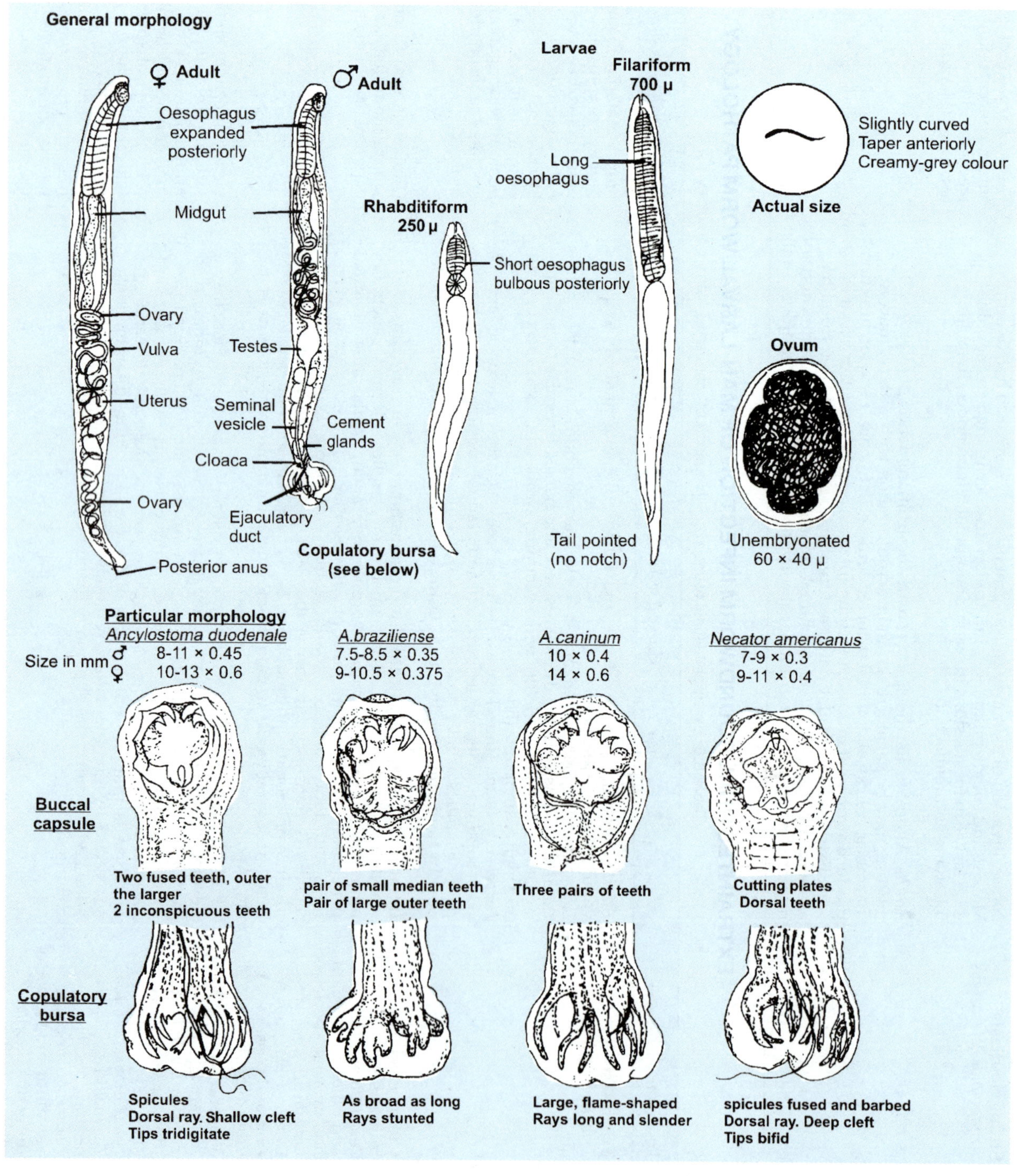

Enterobius vermicularis (thread, pin or seat worm) Syn. oxyuris vermicularis

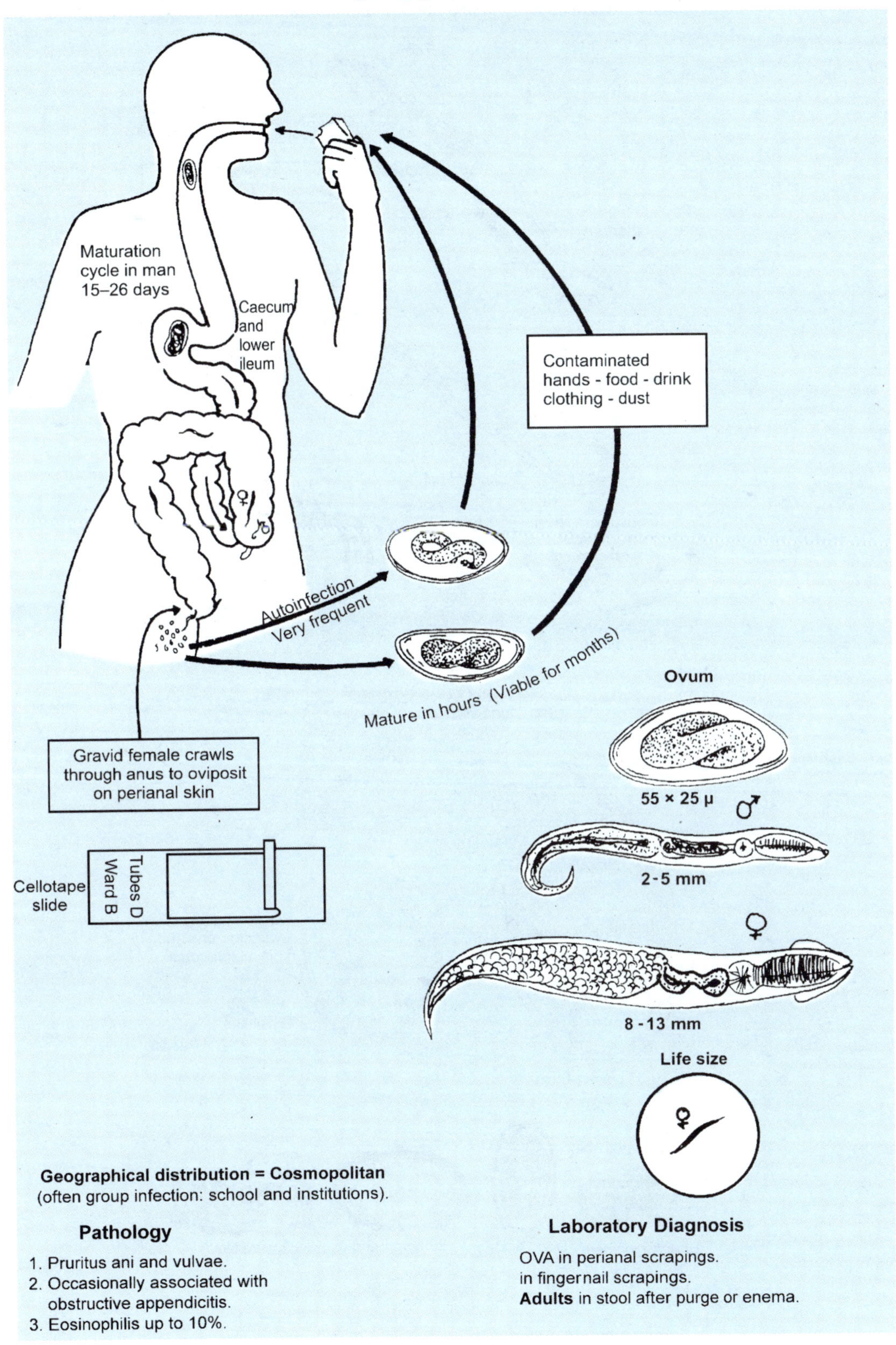

Geographical distribution = Cosmopolitan
(often group infection: school and institutions).

Pathology

1. Pruritus ani and vulvae.
2. Occasionally associated with obstructive appendicitis.
3. Eosinophilis up to 10%.

Laboratory Diagnosis

OVA in perianal scrapings.
in fingernail scrapings.
Adults in stool after purge or enema.

Plasmid Nematodes (contd...)
Enterobius vermicularis

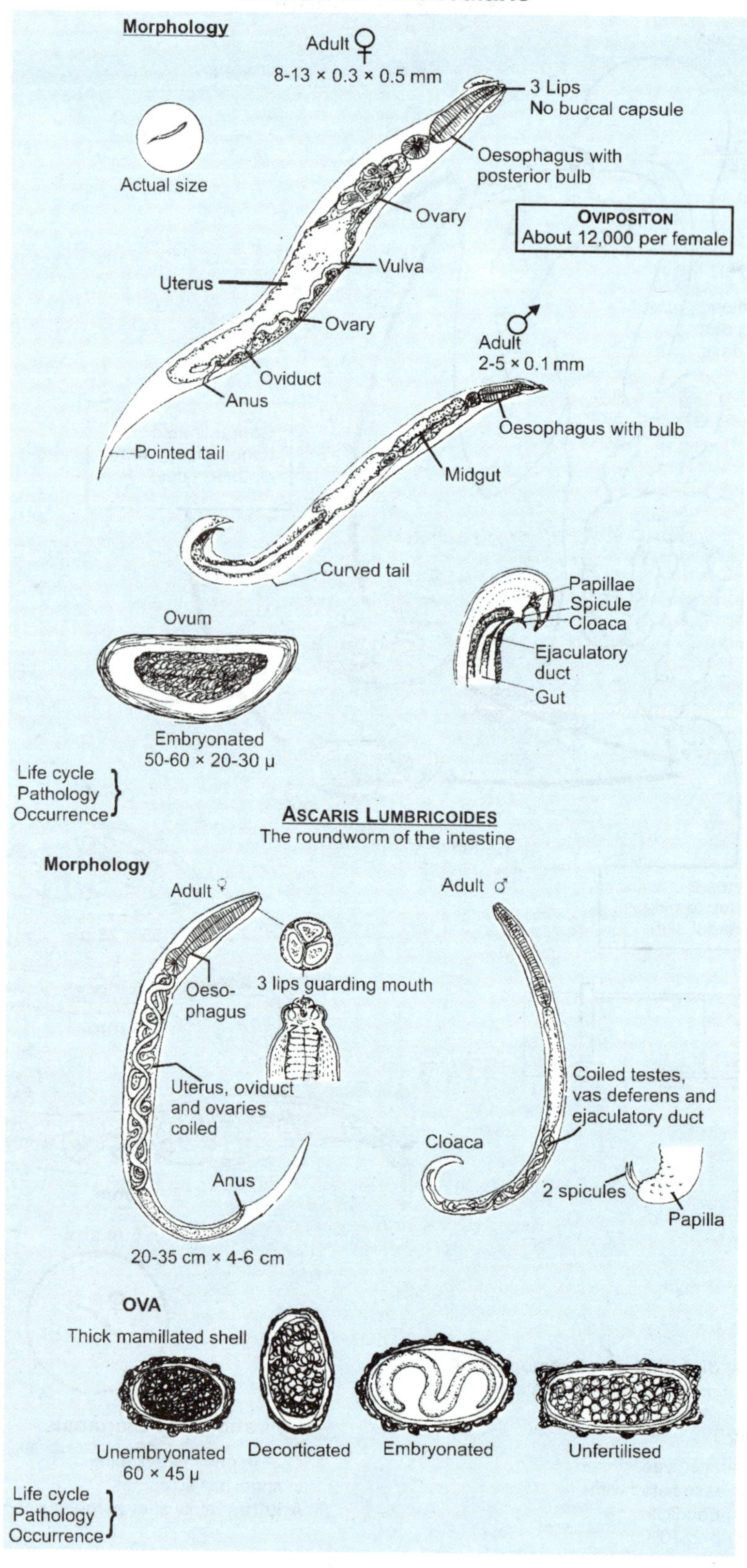

Ascaris lumbricoides (The roundworm)

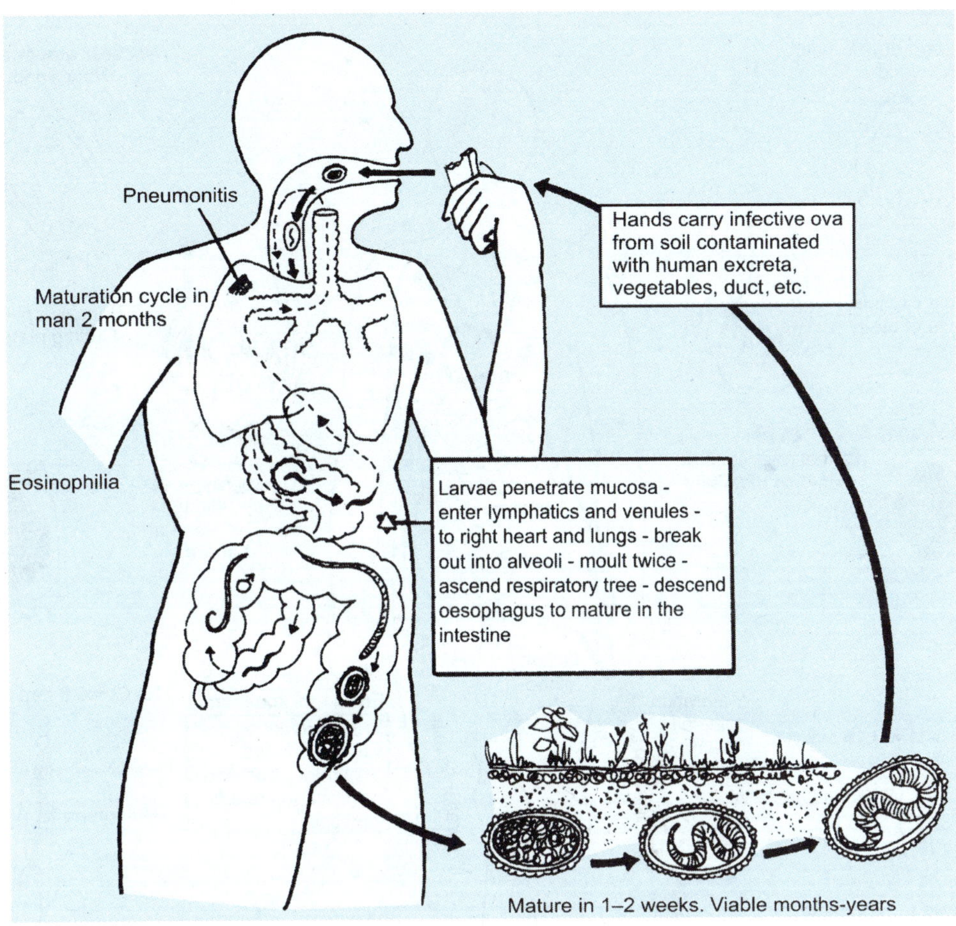

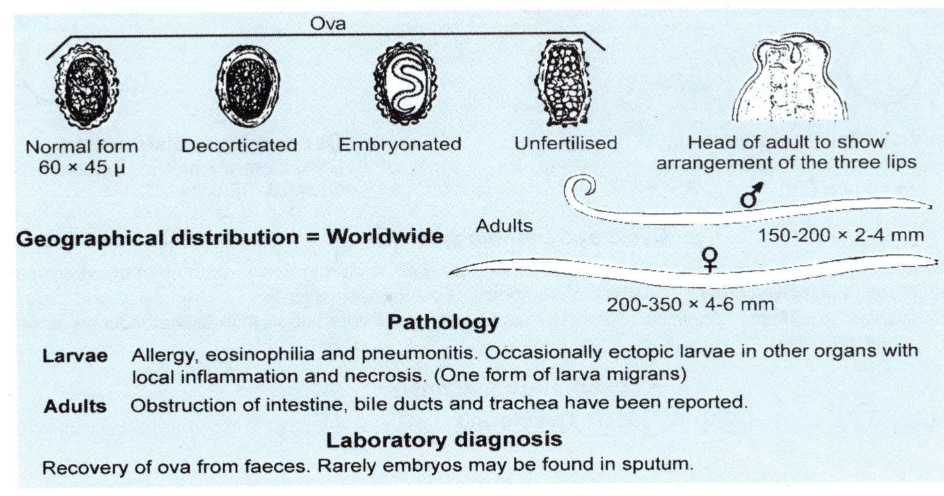

Geographical distribution = Worldwide

Pathology

Larvae Allergy, eosinophilia and pneumonitis. Occasionally ectopic larvae in other organs with local inflammation and necrosis. (One form of larva migrans)

Adults Obstruction of intestine, bile ducts and trachea have been reported.

Laboratory diagnosis

Recovery of ova from faeces. Rarely embryos may be found in sputum.

The hookworms

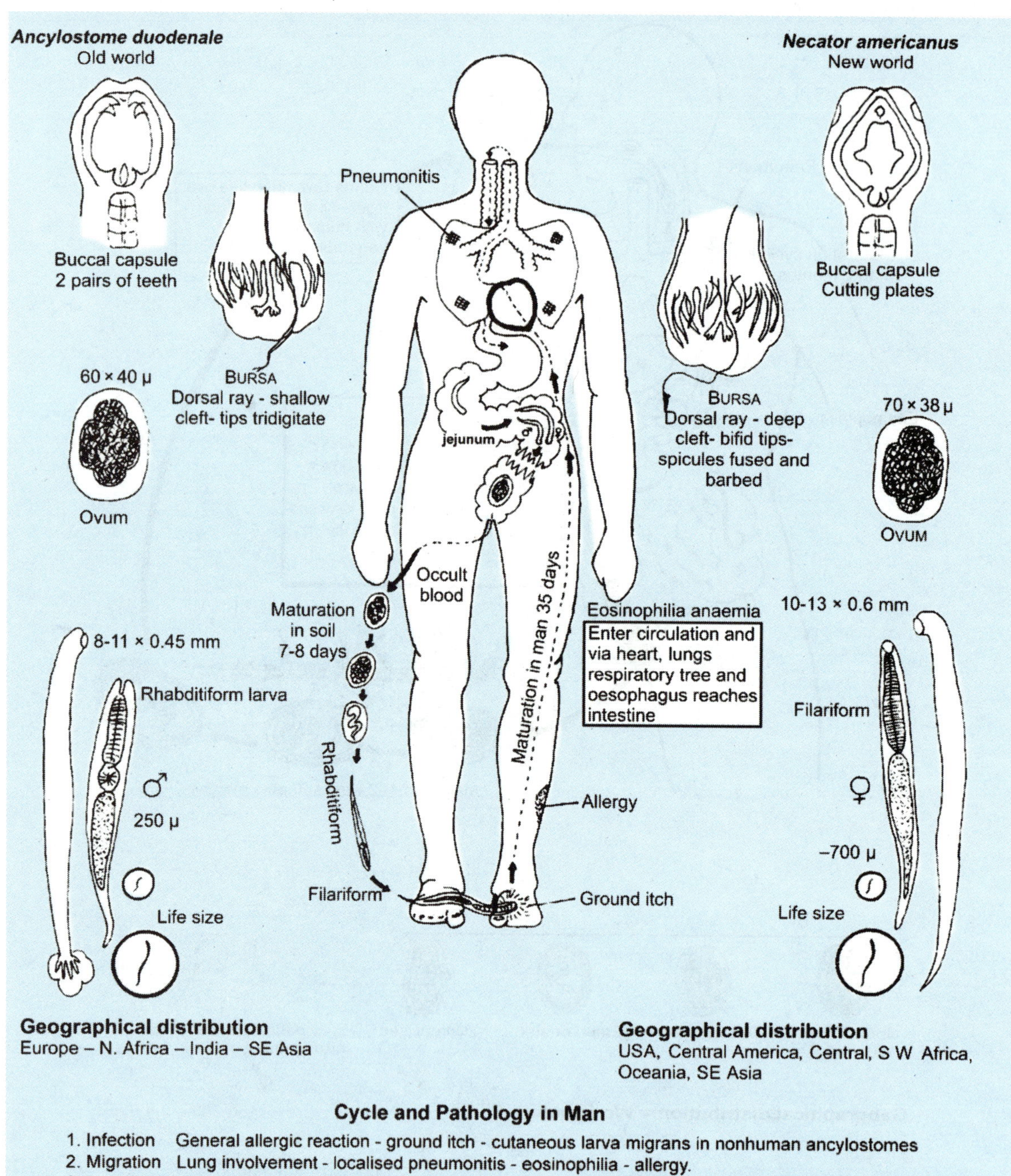

Geographical distribution
Europe – N. Africa – India – SE Asia

Geographical distribution
USA, Central America, Central, S W Africa, Oceania, SE Asia

Cycle and Pathology in Man

1. Infection General allergic reaction - ground itch - cutaneous larva migrans in nonhuman ancylostomes
2. Migration Lung involvement - localised pneumonitis - eosinophilia - allergy.
3. Localisation in jejunum - ingestion of blood by parasites - occult bleeding from intestinal mucosa- anaemia (and sequelae).

Laboratory Diagnosis

Ova in stools

TISSUE ROUNDWORMS OF MAN, CHIEFLY FILARIAE

Table 8.7: Tissue roundworms of man—chiefly filariae, life cycle

Parasite and distribution	*Intermediate host*	*Mode of human infection*	*Site of worm maturation*	*Larvae found in*	*Exit*	*Larval development in*	*Reservoir host*
Wuchereria bancrofti ***Brugia malayi*** Tropics and subtropics	Culex, aedes, anopheles, Mansonia, and other mosquitoes	Filariform larvae actively leave mosquito at time of biting, usually enter skin via puncture	In lymph vessels and nodes	Bloodstream (nocturnal periodicity)* certain strains sub- or non-periodic	Microfilariae taken up by insect when biting	Thoracic muscles; larvae migrate to proboscis (8-15 days)	For B. *malayi*- Cats, dogs monkeys
Loa loa Tropical Africa	Chrysops (deer or mangrove flies)	Probably same	In subcutaneous tissues	Bloodstream (diurnal periodicity)	Same	Abdomen, larvae migrate to proboscis	Primates?
Onchocerca volvulus Tropical Africa Venezuela, and mountainous portions of central Africa	Simulium (buffalo gnat)	Probably same	Same, host reaction, produces nodule around cluster of adults	Subcutaneous tissue; eye (no periodicity)	Same	Thoracic muscles; larvae do not concentrate in proboscis	Man
Dracunculus medinensis Africa, India, Far and Middle East, Indonesia	Cyclops (water flea)	Infected cyclops accidentally ingested in water	Digested out of cyclops, than worm migrates into tissues; mature female passes to skin (may be 1 m long)	Adult female in skin causes host to form blister near head of worm. Blister then filled with larvae, bursts when skin immersed in water, discharging larvae. New blister later forms as female moves to new site		Cyclops feeds on larva, which penetrates gut, develops in haemocoel (18-21 days).	Man

*Periodicity of microfilarial appearance in peripheral blood. May be nocturnal in circulating blood from 8 pm, after which microfilariae confined to pulmonary capillaries.

Table 8.8: Tissue roundworms of man—chiefly filariae, pathology

Disease and aetiology	*Clinical features*	*Laboratory diagnosis*
Bancroft's filariasis *W. bancrofti* **Malayan filariasis** *B. malayi*	Filariae in afferent lymph nodes (of lower extremities, male genitalia, vulva, mammary gland) may cause inflammation followed by intensely fibrotic reaction involving whole area in a mass of scar tissue. Pain, fever, chills, toxaemia, eosinophilia. Chronic stage (after disappearance of microfilariae) varies from microscopic lesion to lymph varicosity to marked elephantiasis. High eosinophilia and superficial lymphadenopathy in Malayan filariasis. Pathology probably a general and focal sensitisation response.	Blood: Thick and thin smears, concentration. Intradermal test gives useful group filaria reaction, indirect haemagglutination, fluorescent antibody tests.
Loiasis *Loa loa*	Fugitive swelling ("Colabar swelling") in skin due to local oedema and skin reaction against migrating adult worm. The latter commonly moves across surface of eyeball or under skin at bridge of nose (best times for removal with local anaesthesia). Eosinophilia with occasional proteinuria produced.	Microfilariae in nodule aspirate or skin snip; repeated skin snips may be required; scapular cutane-
Onchocerciasis *O. volvulus*	Small cutaneous fibrous skin nodules with filariae entwined in centre. Microfilariae in nodule, in neighbouring tissue, or in normal skin far from nodules, rarely in blood. Skin reactions particulary common in Africa; reduction of elastic fibres, depigmentation, progressive thickening, pruritus, papulovesicular lesions or hyperkeratotic patches with microfilariae in scrapings. Eosinophilia and transient urticaria during incubation. Ocular involvement leading to blindness, a common result of prolonged infection. Conjunctiva and vitreous humour with numerous microfilariae. Pathology due to mechanical action, toxins, hypersensitive response of patient; ocular symptoms after 7-9 years.	ous region area of choice, manifestations: eosinophilia ocular lesions, pruritus may follow diethylcarbamazine (Hetrazan) therapy
Dracontiasis *D. medinensis*	Asymptomatic until reddish papular lesion appears, usually on legs. Lesion forms blister bearing head of female worm and numerous larvae. Blister bursts when immersed in water, releasing larvae. Urticaria, pruritus, allergic symptoms, eosinophilia. Accidental rupture of worm may produce intense inflammatory reaction with secondary infection.	Local lesion with head of worm and larvae in blister. X-ray reveals calcified worm; reflected light shows worm under skin. Intradermal test

Eosinophilic lung describes a host allergic response to migration of microfilariae that are trapped in lungs, producing an allergic, asthma-like response. Probably, caused by human filariae or closely related species, as completion of worm development and microfilariae production required. Diagnosed by clinical signs, eosinophilia (3000 or more absolute count, usually over 35%), high haemagglutination or complement fixation titre that drops following Heterazan therapy, elevated ESR, mottled lung lesions visible under X-ray.

Plasmid Nematodes (contd...)
The Filarial worms

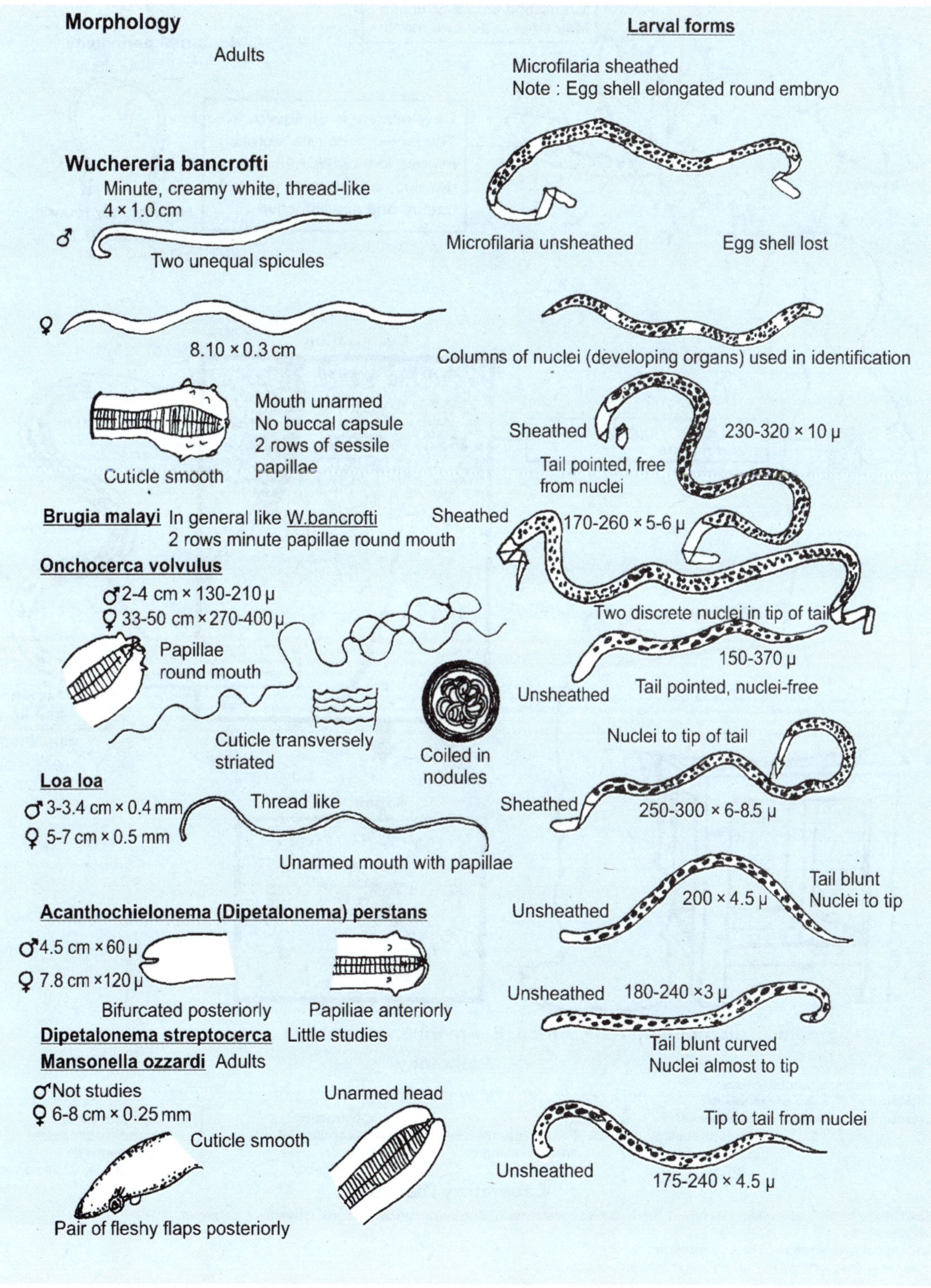

Wuchereria bancrofti

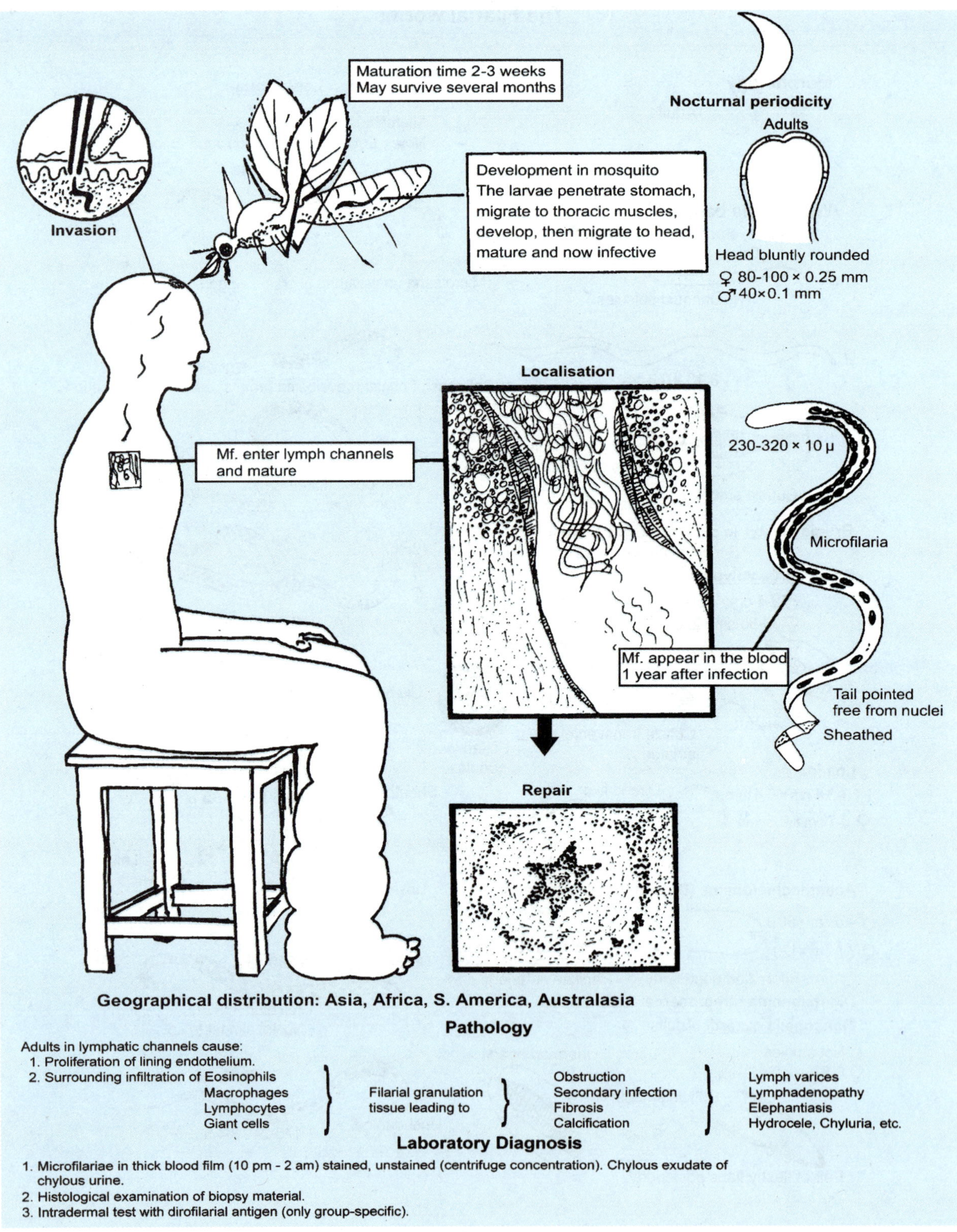

Phasmid Nematodes (Filarial Worms) (contd...)

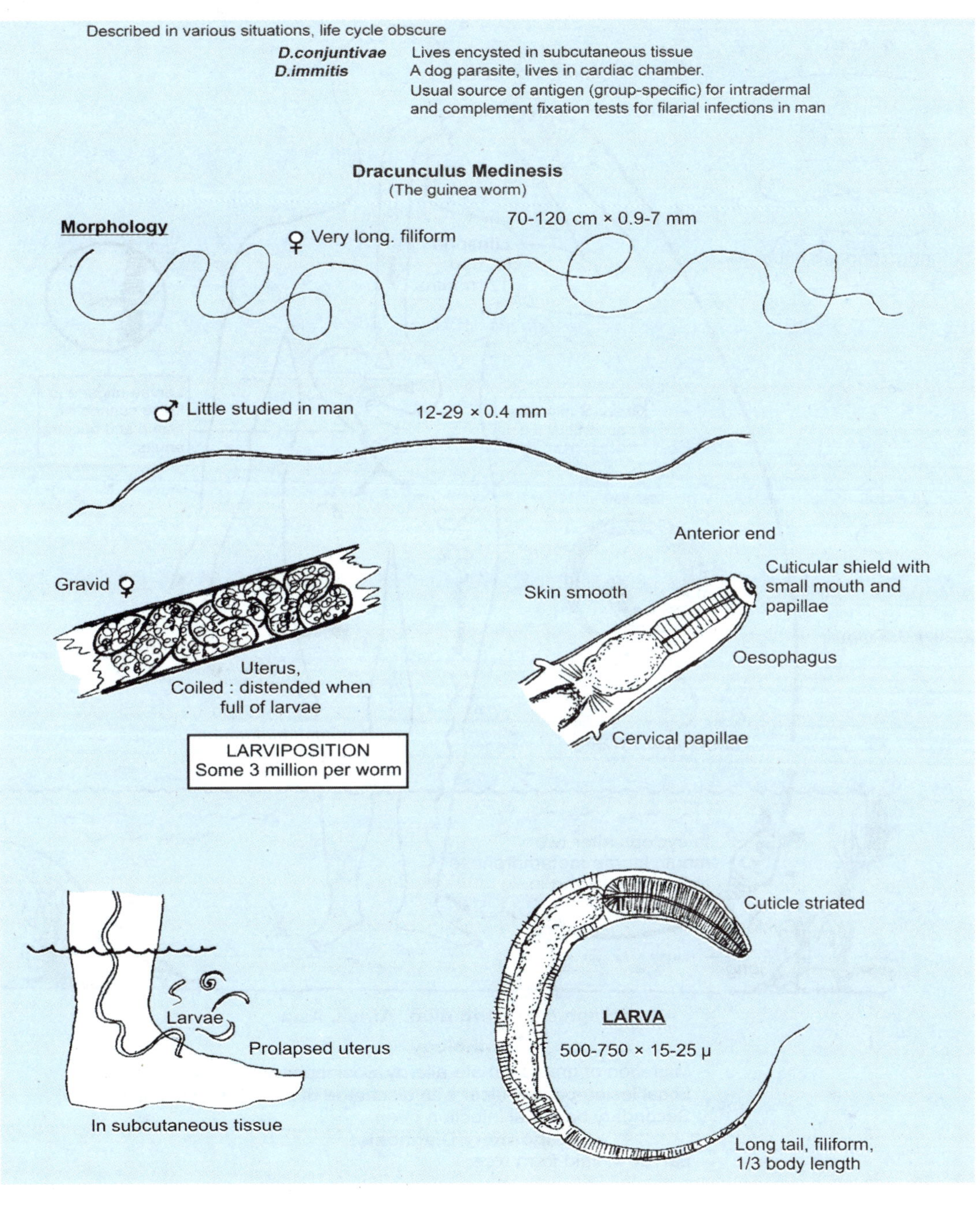

Dracunculus medinensis (The Guinea Worm)

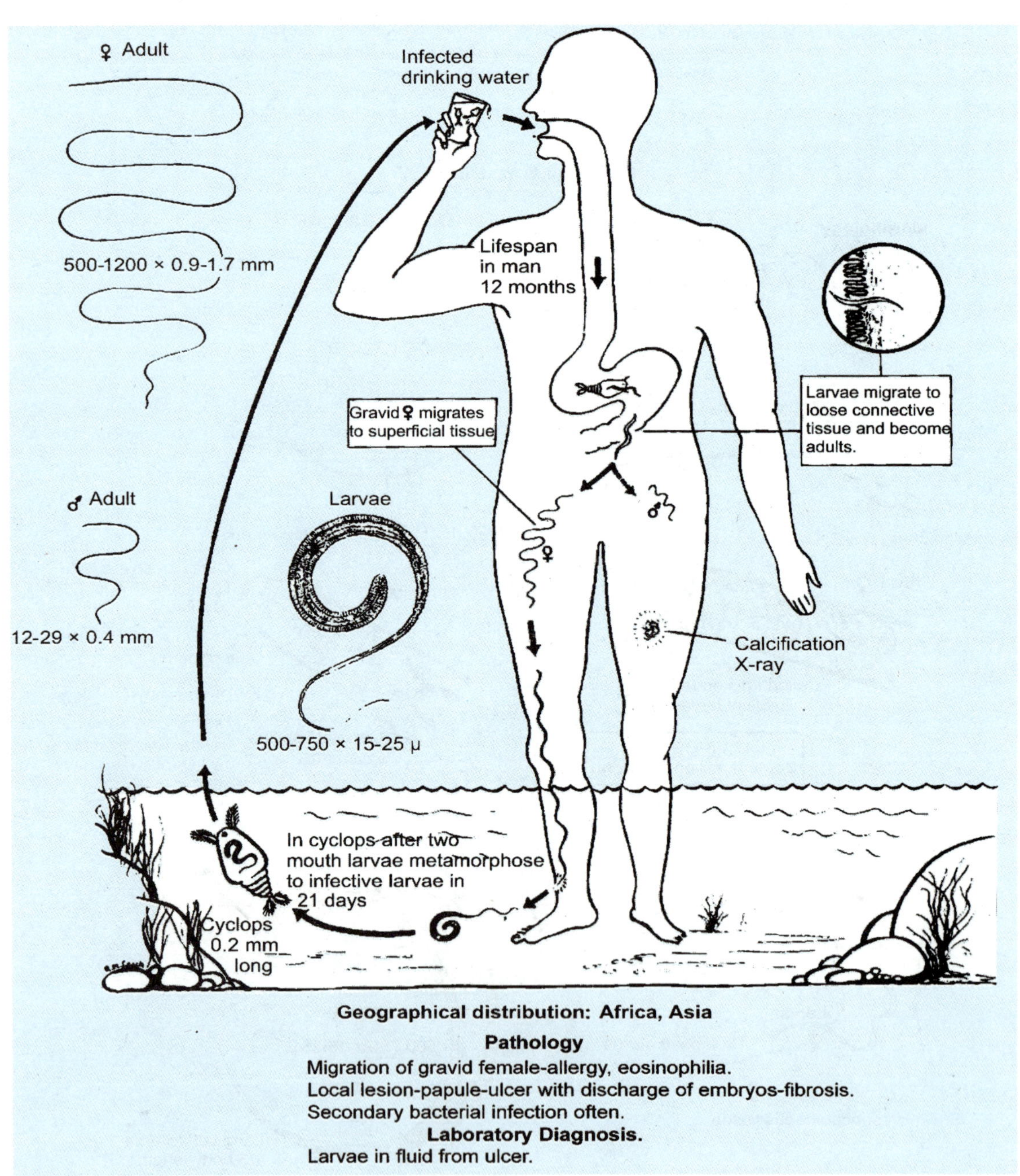

Geographical distribution: Africa, Asia

Pathology

Migration of gravid female-allergy, eosinophilia.
Local lesion-papule-ulcer with discharge of embryos-fibrosis.
Secondary bacterial infection often.

Laboratory Diagnosis.

Larvae in fluid from ulcer.

TAPEWORMS OF MAN

Table 8.9: Tapeworms of man

Diphyllobothrium latum, 80-100% in highly endemic areas; *Taenia saginata* commonest of the large tapeworms; *Hymenolepis nana*, probably quite common. *Echinococcus granulosus*, 3-16% in some endemic areas; *Taenia solium*, where pork is eaten raw.

Parasite and distribution	*Infection*	*Cycle in intermediate route*	*Host fate*	*Cycle in definitive maturation of worm*	*Host exit*	*Summary of hosts*
Taenia saginata (beef tapeworm) worldwide	Ingestion of egg (cattle)	Egg hatches in intestine; *Oncosphere* released, penetrates intestine, enters blood-stream of vertebrate	Encysts in muscles or organs, forms a *cysticercus* larva (bladderworm) in cattle called *cysticercus bovis*	Man ingests cysticercus in raw beef: scolex attaches to duodenum, becomes adult in 6-12 months	Gravid segments per anus	*Definitive:* Man *Intermediate;* Cattle buffalo, giraffes. llamas, goats
Taenia solium (pork tapeworm) worldwide	Ingestion of egg (hogs, man); autoreinfection	-do-	Similar to *T. saginata*, cysticercus larva (in hogs) called *C. cellulosae*	As for *T. saginata*, but infection source is under-cooked pork	-do-	*Definitive:* Man *Intermediate:* Pigs, man (autoreinfection)
Echinococcus granulosus (hydatid worm) Sheep raising areas	Ingestion of egg (sheep, accidental ingestion in man)	-do-	Forms *hydatid cyst* with thousands of infective scoleces in fluid, although cysts may also be sterile. Chiefly in liver, also in lungs rarely in brain	Sheep, dogs ingest hydatid sand (infective scoleces) from hydatid cyst in sheep carcass. Worms attach to canine intestinal wall; become adult	Eggs in faeces	*Definitive:* Dogs, all canids; rarely cats. *Intermediate:* Sheep, hogs, cattle, man
Hymenolepis nana (dwarf tapeworm) worldwide	Ingestion of egg by man or rodent (direct cycle) or by various insects (indirect cycle)	Egg hatches in intestine; oncosphere released. In man, it invades villus; in insect it penetrates gut and enters haemocoele	*Cysticercoid* larva containing scolex of future adult worm, formed either in villus of human host or haemocoele of insect	In man, larva leaves villus, attaches to small intestine, becomes adult. If infected insect ingested, cysticercoid digested out, hatches, attaches, grows to adult in 10-12 days. Cysticercoid derived either from insect or direct egg-to-cercoid cycle in man can produce infection	Eggs in faeces	Man, rats and mice, gerbils in Africa. Common tapeworm of man; possibly distinctive strain in man and rodents
Diphyllobothrium latum (fish or broad tapeworm) Orient, Latin America, Great Lakes, Northern Europe	Water flea ingests swimming embryo (coracidium) hatched from egg in water	Hooked embryo penetrates gut wall, develops into *procercoid* larva in haemocoele	Freshwater fish eats water flea; larva digested out in intestine, penetrates to muscles or organs, becomes third stage larva (*plerocercoid* or *sparganum*)	Man ingests fish with sparganum; larva liberated in intestine, attaches to intestinal wall, becomes adult	Eggs in faeces into water	*Definitive:* Fish-eating mammals *Intermediate:* Water fleas (Diaptomus), then various fresh-water fish.

Table 8.10: Tapeworm diseases of man

Disease and aetiology	*Clinical features*	*Laboratory diagnosis*
Hymenolepiasis *Hymenolepis nana*	Symptomless to systemic toxaemia depending on worm load. Eosinophilia, nervous manifestations, with or without diarrhoea, and pain. Heavy worm load, probably following autoreinfection, may produce convulsions, insomnia, dizziness.	Faeces: Direct smear or concentration to show eggs.
Taeniasis saginata *Taenia saginata*	Abdominal and hunger pains, chronic indigestion, weight loss, persistent diarrhoea or alternating with constipation; nervous manifestations. Eosinophilia.	Faeces: Not reliable. Recovery of gravid segments which actively crawl from anus; can be found in underwear or bed linen. Segments or eggs may be rare in faeces.
Taeniasis solium *Taenia solium*	*Intestinal:* Same as *T saginata.* *Cysticercosis:* Symptoms may vary with number of larvae and site in tissues. Foreign body response and inflammation, followed by fibrosis and necrosis of parasite, later calcification. Shows affinity for CNS, symptoms resemble brain tumour, epilepsy, and other disorders. Chief sites: Subcutaneous tissues, eye, brain.	Faeces: Recovery of gravid segments. Recovery of larvae by biopsy from infected tissue. Detection of calcified larvae by X-ray.
Hydatid disease *Echinococcus granulosus* *E. multilocularis*	*E. granulosus* produces unilocular cysts, 80-90% in liver and lungs. The host becomes sensitised following escape of fluid through fissures. Pressure symptoms. Anaphylactic shock may occur upon rupture. Cachexia results from secondary metastases, pulmonary or cerebral emboli may occur. Manifestations resemble cholelithiasis or renal, hepatic or intestinal colic, sometimes of long standing. *E. multilocularis* produces uncontrolled, untreatable metastases in liver with final destruction of most of parenchyma.	Cyst contents in urine. Sputum: Direct smear. Serology: Complement fixation, bentonite flocculation, haemaggultination, intradermal tests. X-rays for pulmonary cysts or calcified cysts elsewhere. Clinical history and picture of great value.
Diphyllobothriasis (fish tapeworm disease); *Diphyllobothrium latum*	Symptomless to systemic toxaemia. Pain, Weight loss, diarrhoea, eosinophilia. Severe macrocytic anaemia, similar to pernicious anaemia, found in some cases. Worm competes with host for vitamin B_{12}.	Faeces: Direct smear or concentration to show eggs.

Cestoda
Cyclophyllidean Tapeworms of Man

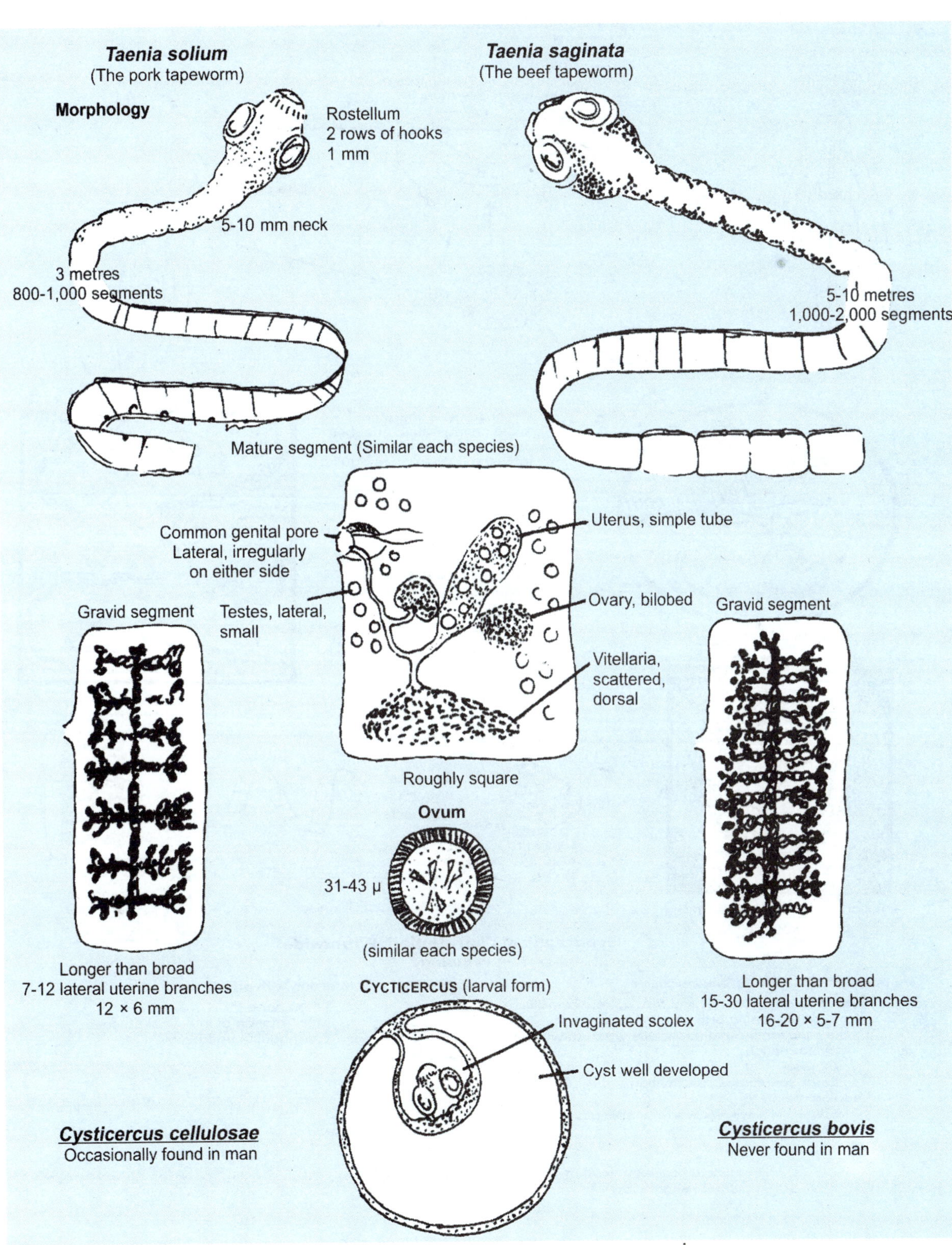

Taenia solium
(The Pork Tapeworm)

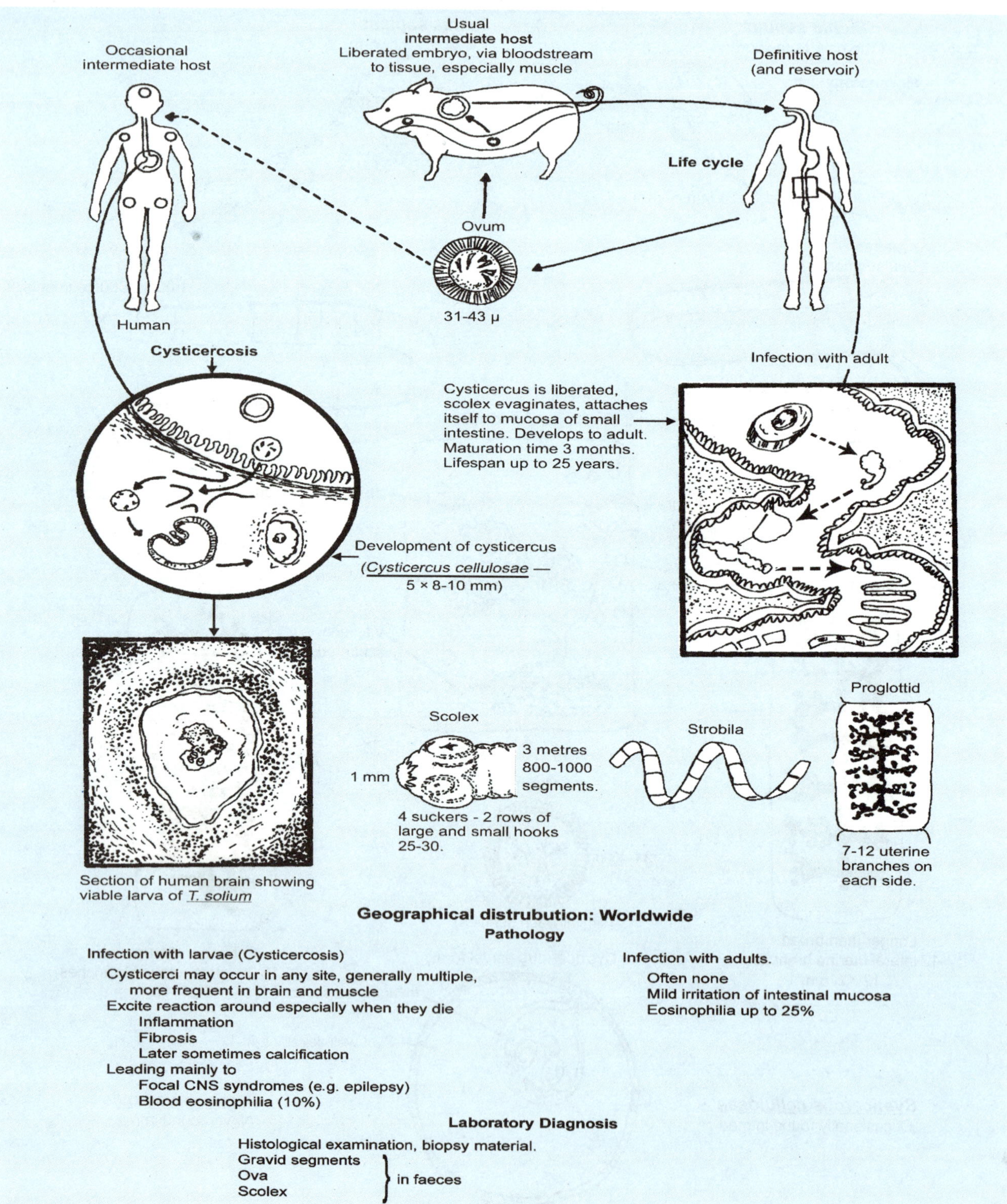

Taenia saginata
(The Beef Tapeworm)

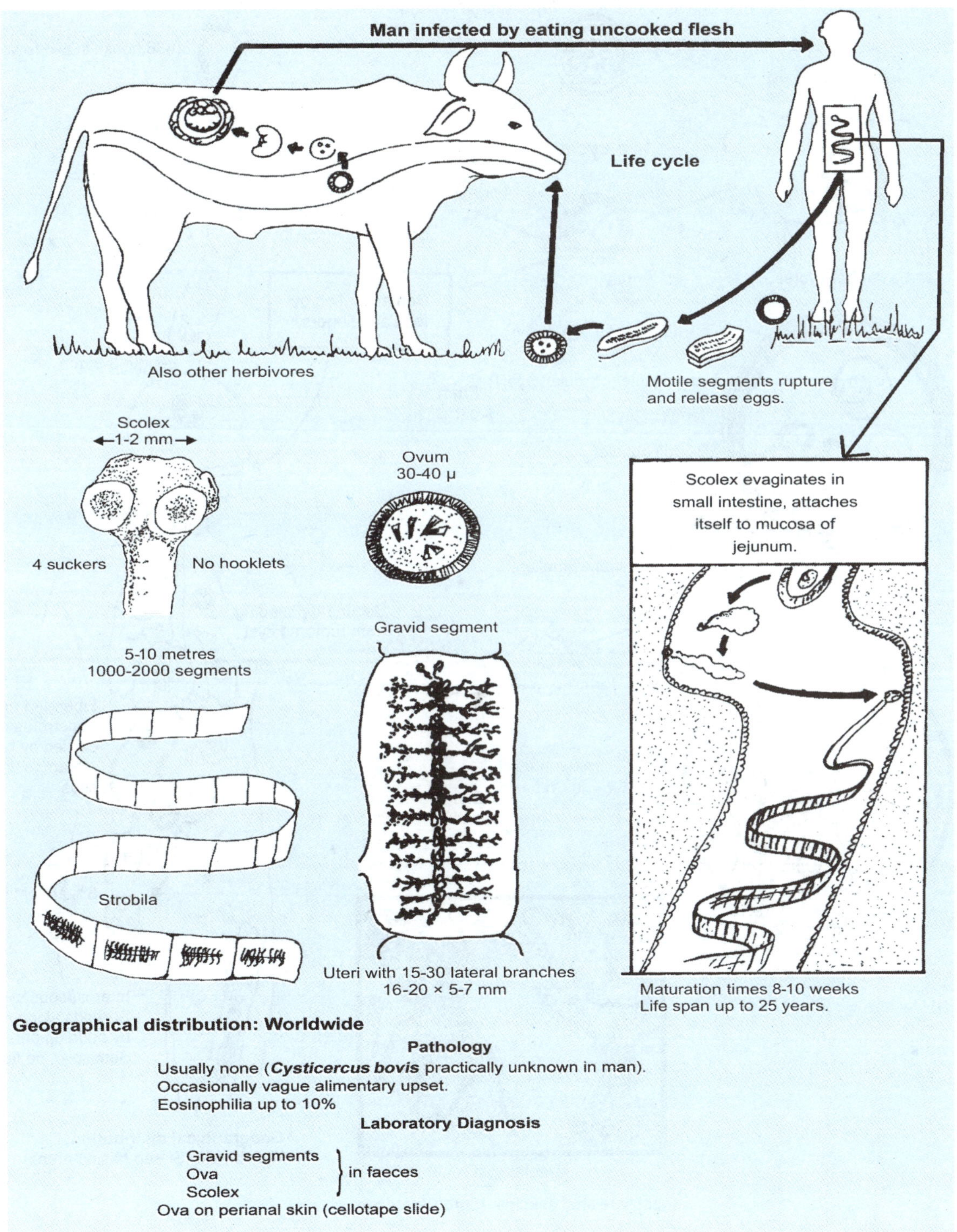

Echinococcus granulosus
(Causing Hydatid Disease)

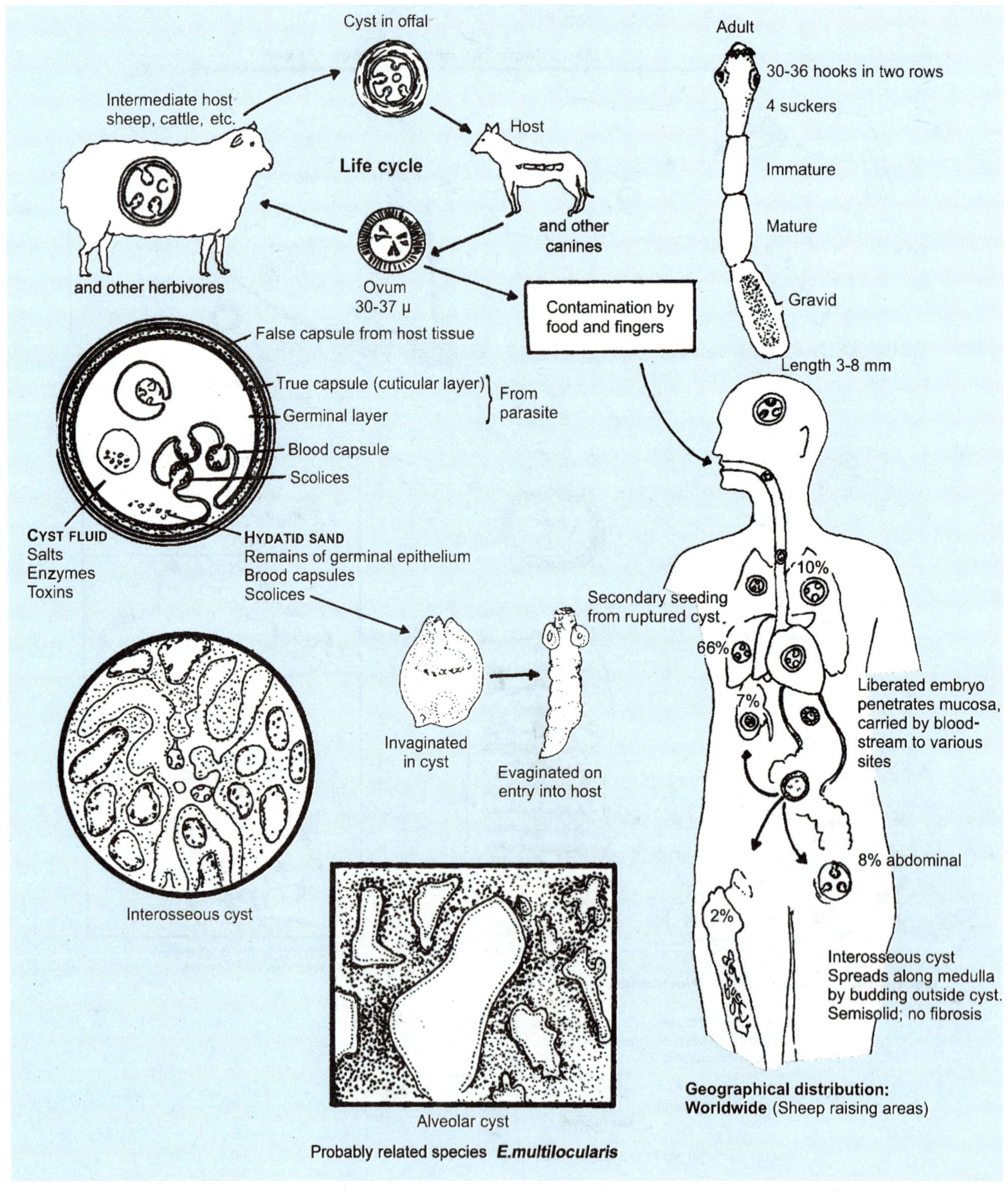

Dwarf Tapeworms
Hymenolepsis Nana

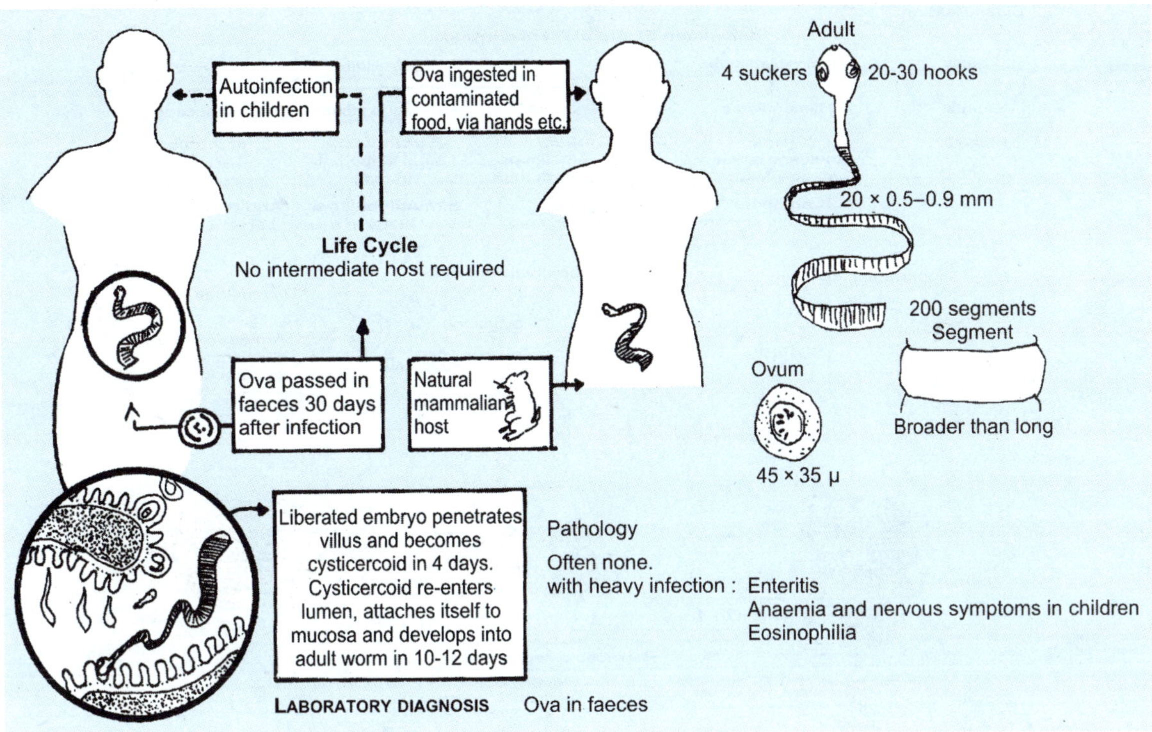

Hymenolepis diminuta

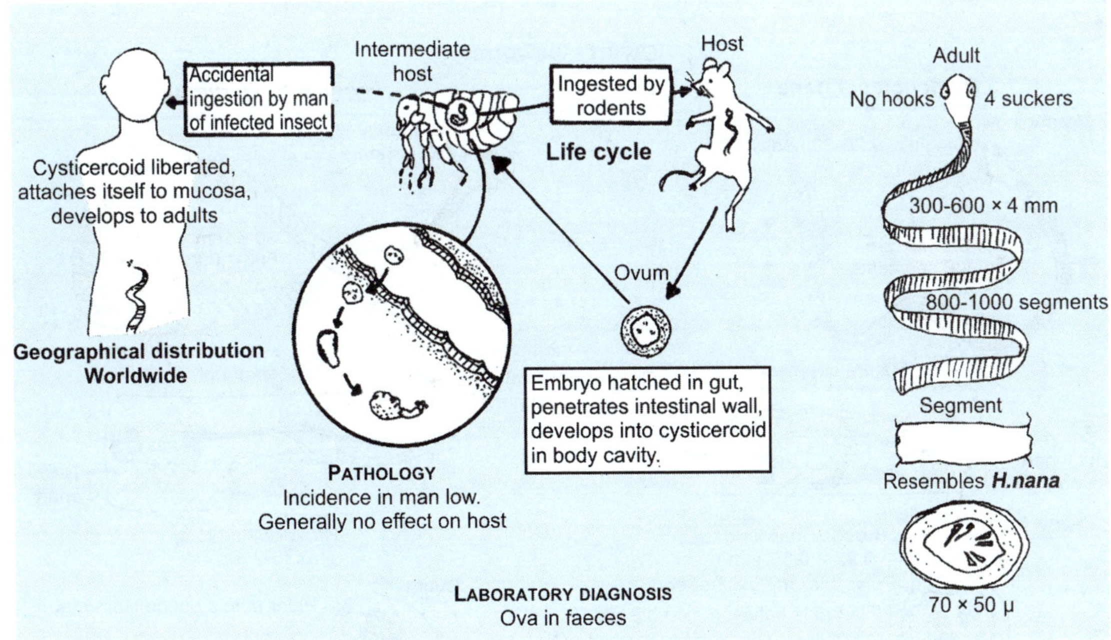

B. Occasionally infect man

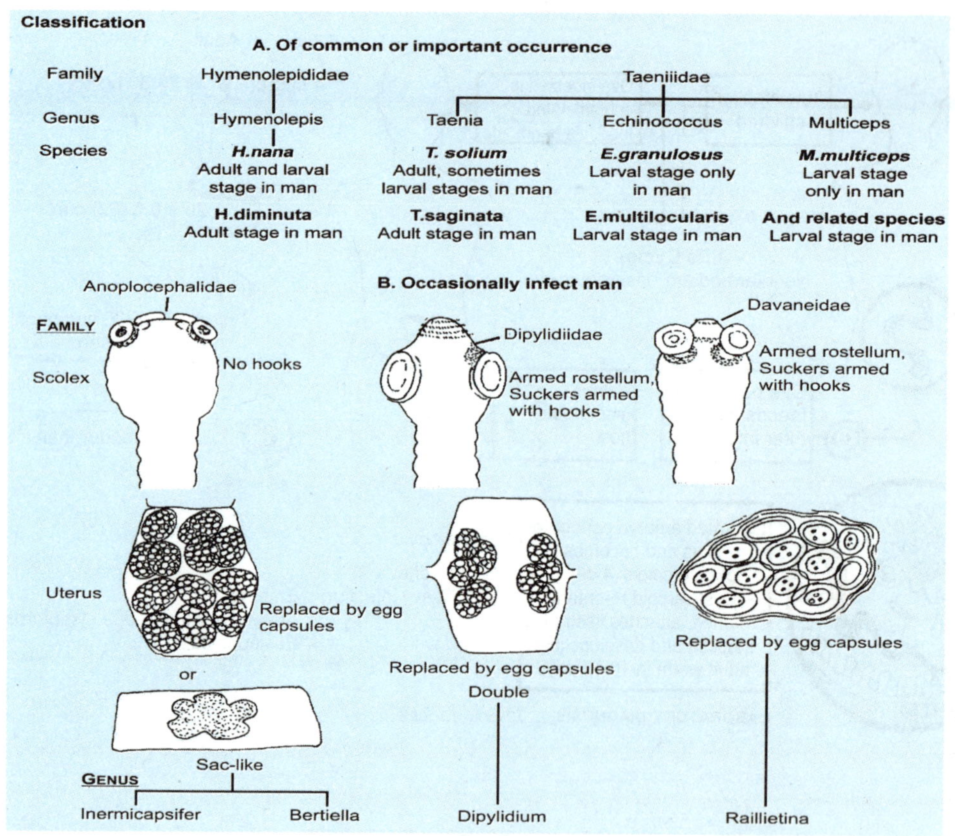

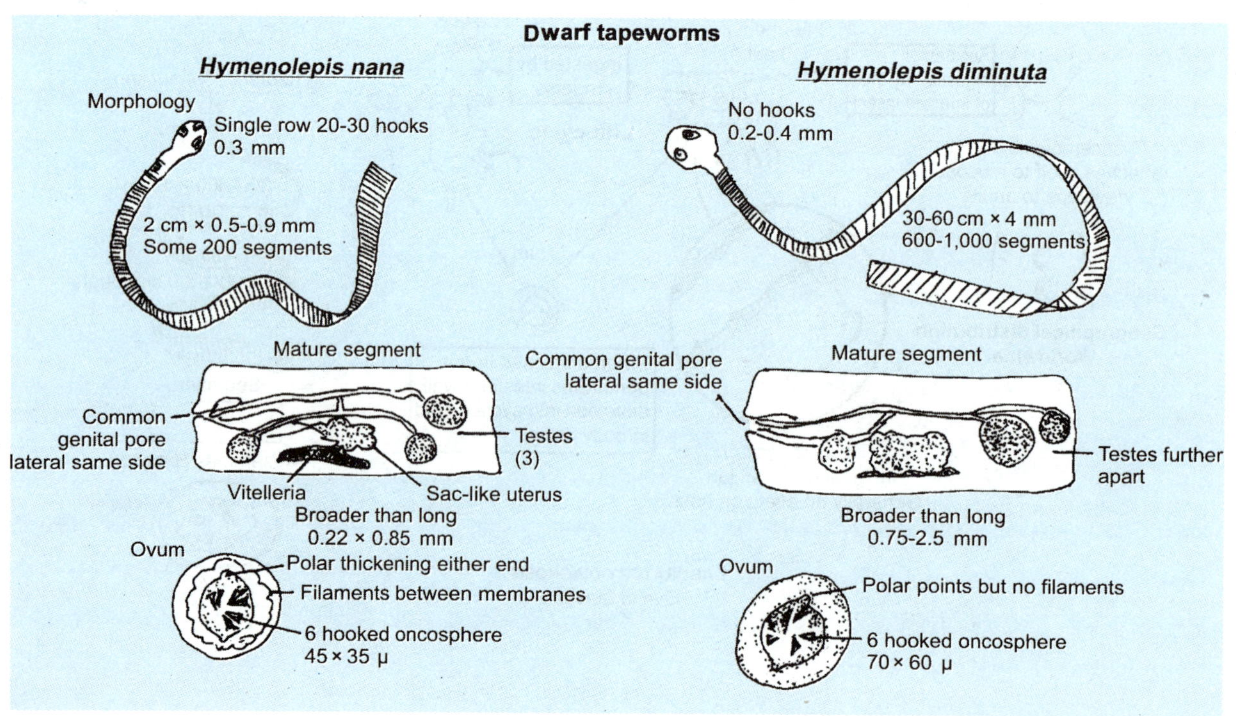

Cestoda (General Morphology) (contd...)

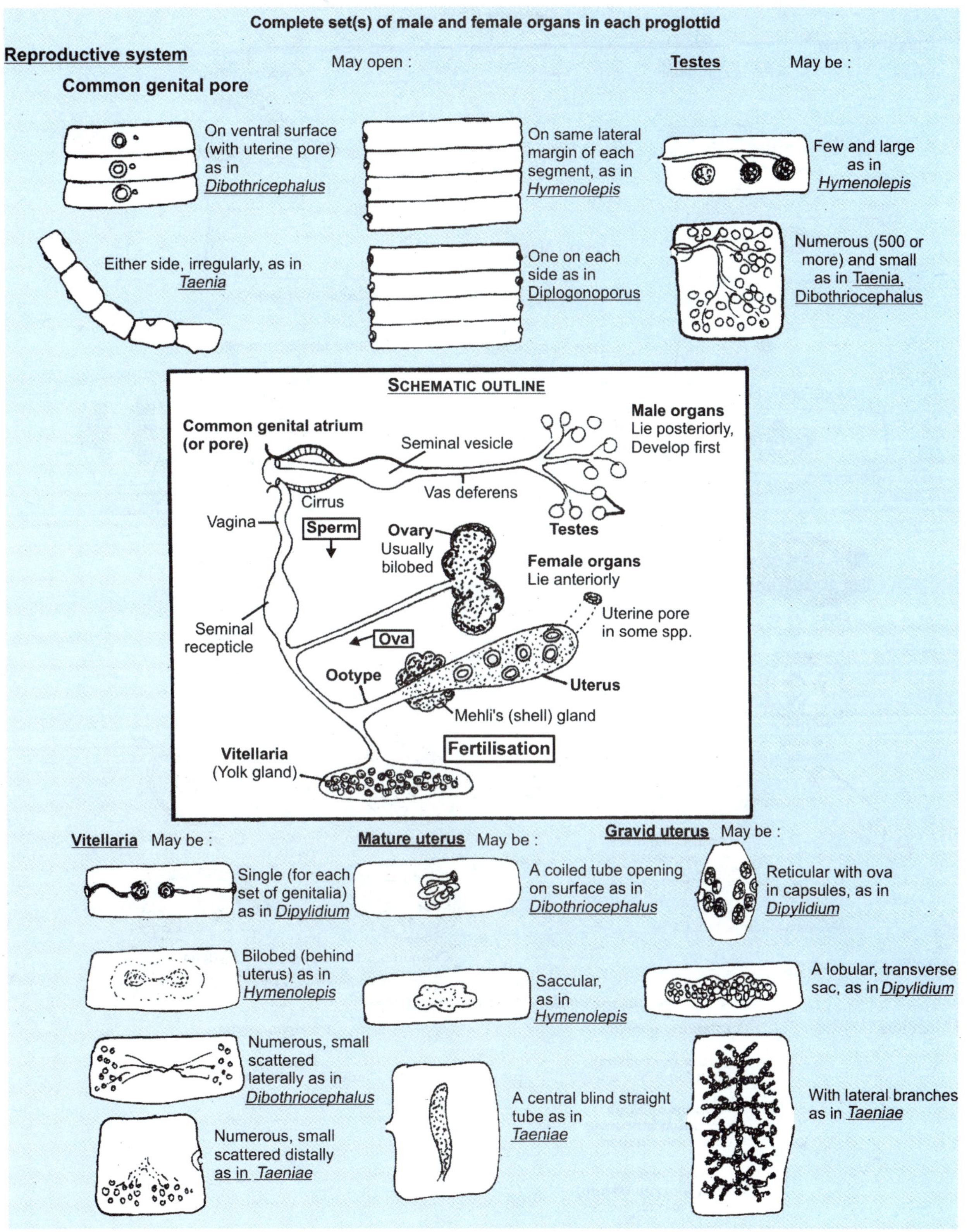

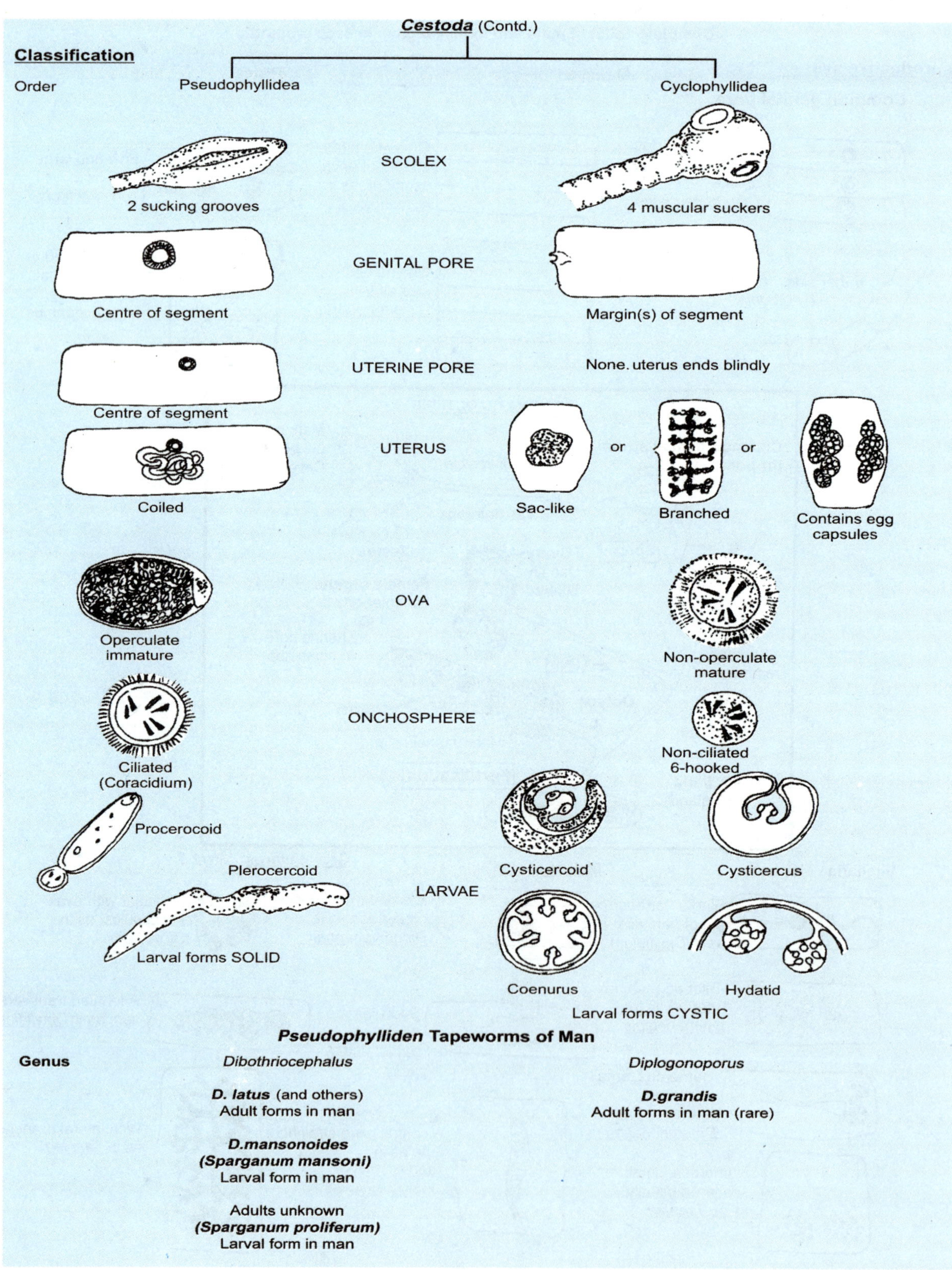
Cestoda (Contd.)
Classification
Order
Pseudophyllidea
Cyclophyllidea
SCOLEX
2 sucking grooves
4 muscular suckers
GENITAL PORE
Centre of segment
Margin(s) of segment
UTERINE PORE
Centre of segment
None. uterus ends blindly
UTERUS
Coiled
Sac-like
or
Branched
or
Contains egg capsules
OVA
Operculate immature
Non-operculate mature
ONCHOSPHERE
Ciliated (Coracidium)
Non-ciliated 6-hooked
Procerocoid
Plerocercoid
Cysticercoid
Cysticercus
LARVAE
Larval forms SOLID
Coenurus
Hydatid
Larval forms CYSTIC
Pseudophylliden Tapeworms of Man
Genus
Dibothriocephalus
Diplogonoporus
D. latus (and others)
Adult forms in man
D.grandis
Adult forms in man (rare)
D.mansonoides
(Sparganum mansoni)
Larval form in man
Adults unknown
(Sparganum proliferum)
Larval form in man

FLUKES OF MAN

Table 8.11: Flukes of man

Parasite and *Distribution*	*Enters man*	*Definitive host* *Habitat*	*Exit*	*Intermediate host cycle* *outside man*	*Reservoir host*
Schistosoma haematobium Middle East, Africa, Egypt is classical focus	Cercaria penetrates skin	Vesical and pelvic venous plexuses draining urinary bladder	Terminal spined large egg in urine or faeces (rare)	Egg hatches to release swimming miracidium in water. Invades appropriate snail (Clonorchis egg ingested by snail)	Man, monkeys
Schistosoma mansoni Africa, Latin America, Carribean Islands	-do-	Branches of inferior mesenteric veins draining rectum and sigmoid colon	Lateral spined large egg in faeces	In snail tissues each miracidium becomes a sporocyst, which forms a number of embryos (sporocysts or rediae, depending on species) which in turn produce many cercariae	Man, baboons, monkeys, oppossums, wild rats
Schistosoma japonicum Japan, East Asia, Philippine Islands	-do-	Same as for *S. mansoni* but occurs chiefly in superior mesenteric veins draining small intestine	Round small spined eggs in faeces	Cercariae swarm from snail	Man, horses, pigs, sheep, goats, cows, dogs, cats, water-buffaloes, rodents
Fasciolopsis buski East and South Asia	Ingested metacercaria on water plant or other vegetation	Small intestine, attached to intestinal wall		Encyst on water plants *(Fasciola and Fasciolopsis)* or invade fish *(Clonorchis)* crayfish or crab *(Paragonimus)* or directly penetrate human skin *(Schistosoma)*	Man, pigs
Fasciola hepatica Worldwide, sheep and cattle raising areas		Major bile ducts after migrating from intestine through peritoneal cavity, liver capsule, and parenchyma	Egg in bile to faeces	-do-	Sheep, cattle, other herbivores, man an accidental host
Clonorchis sinensis South Asia, immigrants in America	Ingested metacercaria in raw fish	Bile ducts migrating from intestine through ampulla of Vater	-do-	-do-	Man, dogs, cats, fish-eating mammals
Paragonimus westermani	Ingested metacercaria in crayfish, crab	Encysted in lungs, pleural and peritoneal cavities, liver, migrating from intestine through peritoneal cavity	Egg in sputum or faeces	-do-	Man, wildcats, foxes, wolves, dogs, rats, pigs, weasels.

Table 8.12: Fluke diseases of man

Disease and aetiology	*Clinical features*	*Laboratory diagnosis*
Schistosomiasis or bilharziasis *Schistosoma haematobium mansoni japonicum*	*Initial:* Skin penetration by cercariae producing itching, erythema, petechiae, usually a hypersensitisation following repeated exposures. Eosinophilia in later case, with fever *Maturation of worms:* Fever, hepatomegaly with tenderness, oedema, diarrhoea; eosinophilia variable. *Adult worms:* Systemic and histologic changes due mainly to granulomatous reaction against eggs acting as foreign bodies. Symptoms vary with duration, frequency, and severity of exposure and degree of host reaction, itself related to age, nutrition and concurrent infections. Generally with bowel and vesical disturbances, lasting for months to years. *Chronic disturbances:* Portal hypertension with resulting oesophageal varices; liver and intestinal or bladder granulomata and fibrosis. Thickening and calcification in bladder wall (*S. haematobium*), thickening of small intestine (*S japonicum*), Prolapse of rectum (*S. mansoni*), loss of gut motility, local tissue and organ dysfunction.	Urine: Direct smear for eggs, sedimentation and hatching of miracidia in diluted urine for *S. haematobium*, prefer—ably in last portion of urine passed. Faeces: Direct smear; concentration for *S. mansoni* or japonicum eggs. Rectal biopsy and sigmoidoscopy (*S. haematobium*). Blood: Precipitin (circumoval or CHR) test.
Fasciolopsiasis *Fasciolopsis buski*	Localised inflammation of jejunum or duodenum, followed often by ulceration at sites of worm attachment. Diarrhoea with foul-smelling stools; abdominal pain. In severe infections eosinophilia, ascites, anorexia, nausea, vomiting, toxaemia, prostration.	Faeces: Direct smear, sedimentation.
Fascioliosis *Fasciola hepatica*	Worm migrations cause tissue necrosis and fibrosis. Bile duct damage resembles that for Clonorchis. Picture like any biliary derangement (gallbladder, choledochus involvement). Eosinophilia. Infection runs a chronic course of many years.	Faeces: Direct smear, sedimentation. Duodenal drainage; complement fixation, skin tests.
Clonorchiasis *Clonorchis sinensis*	Similar hepatic involvement, large numbers of parasites cause diarrhoea, jaundice, cachexia, eosinophilia. Proliferation and desquamation of biliary epithelium, dilatation, and thickening of the wall occur, severe symptoms of liver dysfunction, recurring jaundice with hepatomegaly may follow. Long continued chronic course common.	Direct smear, sedimentation; eggs in biliary drainage.
Paragonimiasis *Paragonimus westermani*	*Lung:* Parasites are embedded, usually in pairs, in subpleural cysts (eggs act as foreign bodies) with inflammation, eosinophilia and fibrous capsule formation. Chronic cough with fever, brown sputum, haemoptysis, severe chest pain, bronchial pneumonia or pleural fluid common. May enter any organ and produce local symptoms, e.g. abdominal pain, diarrhoea, CNS involvement. Similar lesions in other tissues.	Sputum: Direct smear. Faeces: Direct smear, sedimentation; complement fixation, etc.

FASCIOLA HEPATICA
(The sheep liver fluke)

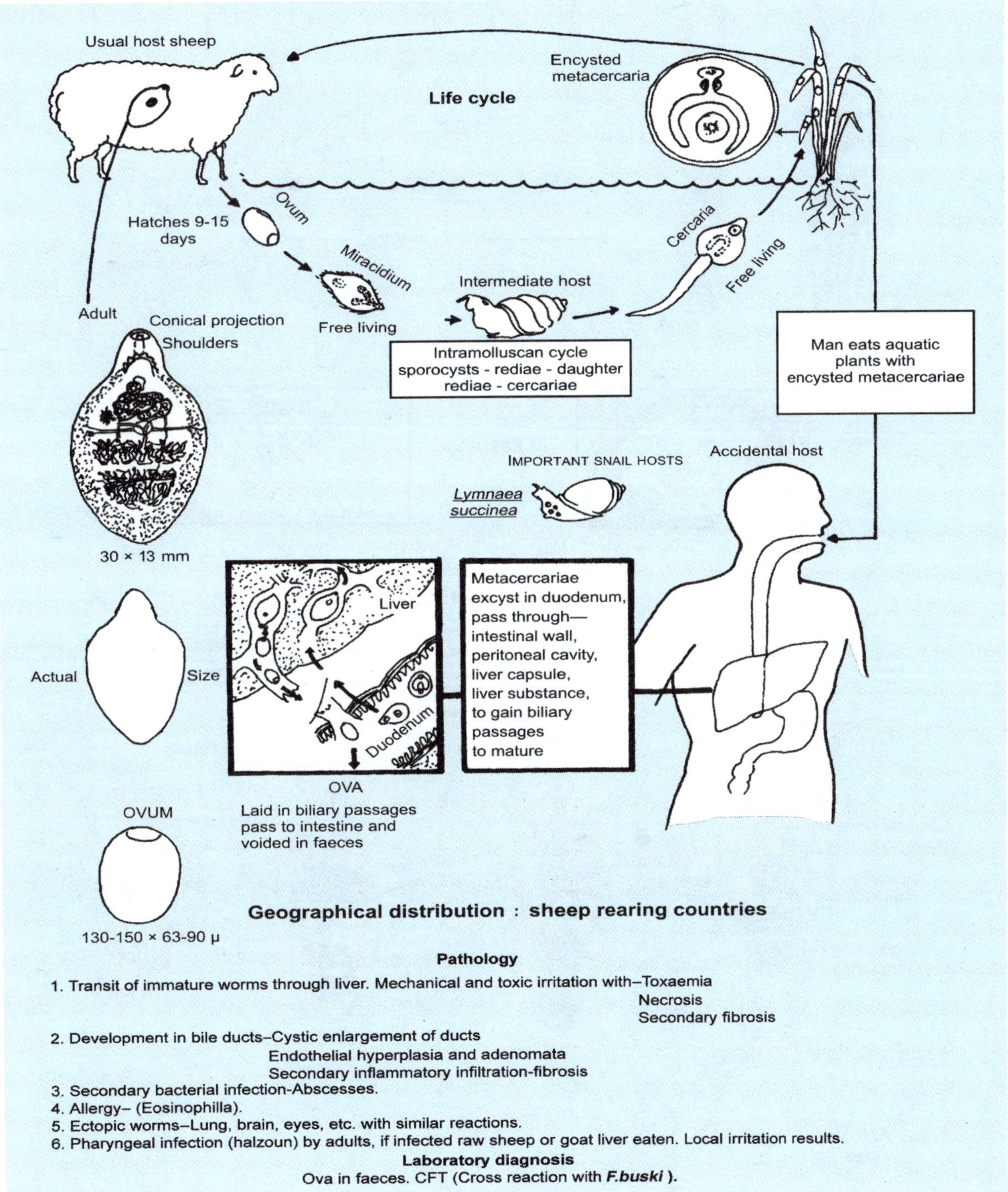

Morphology of Adults and Larvae Cestoda (Contd...)

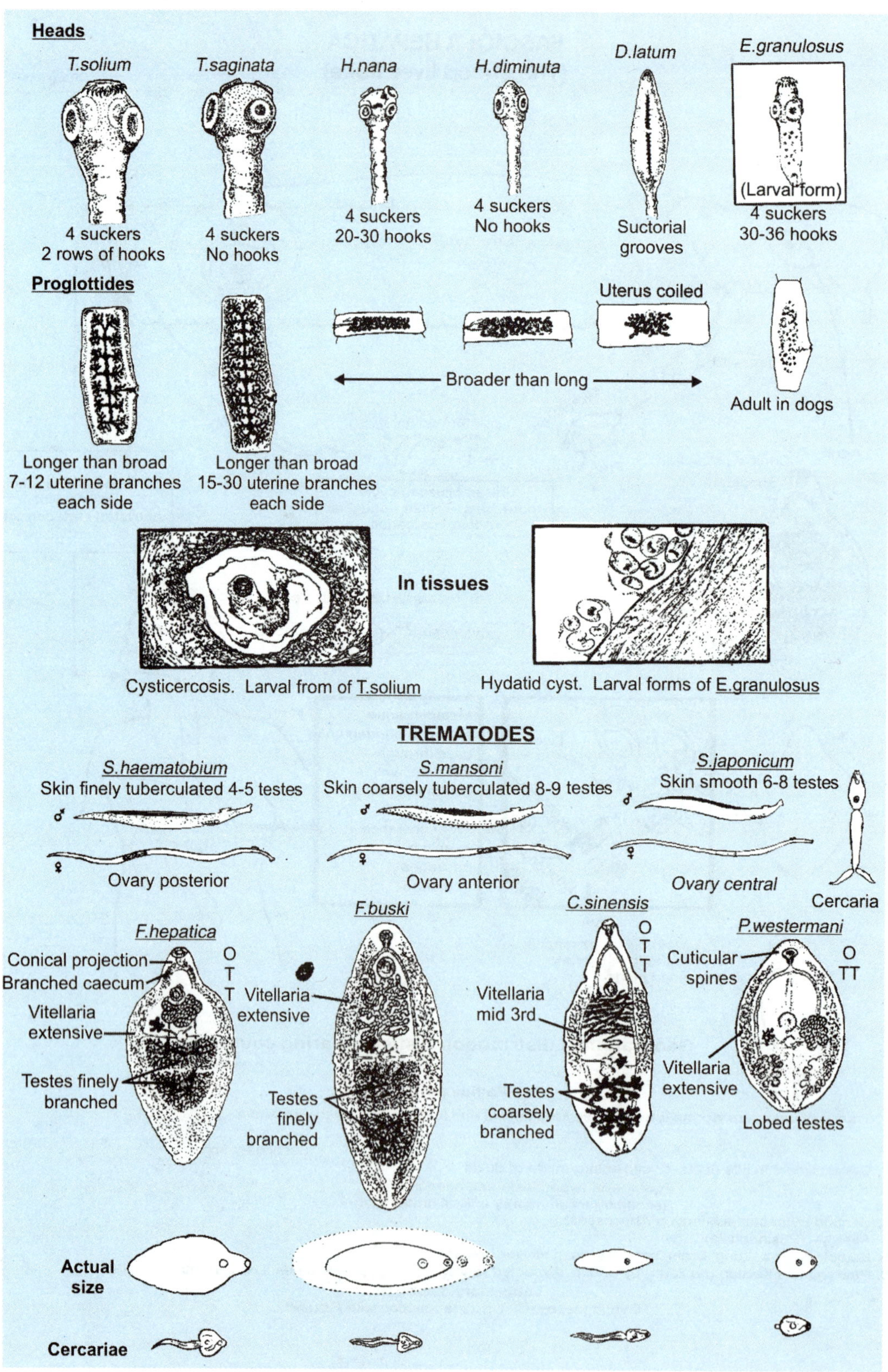

RECAPITULATION

The Amoebae of the Intestinal Canal

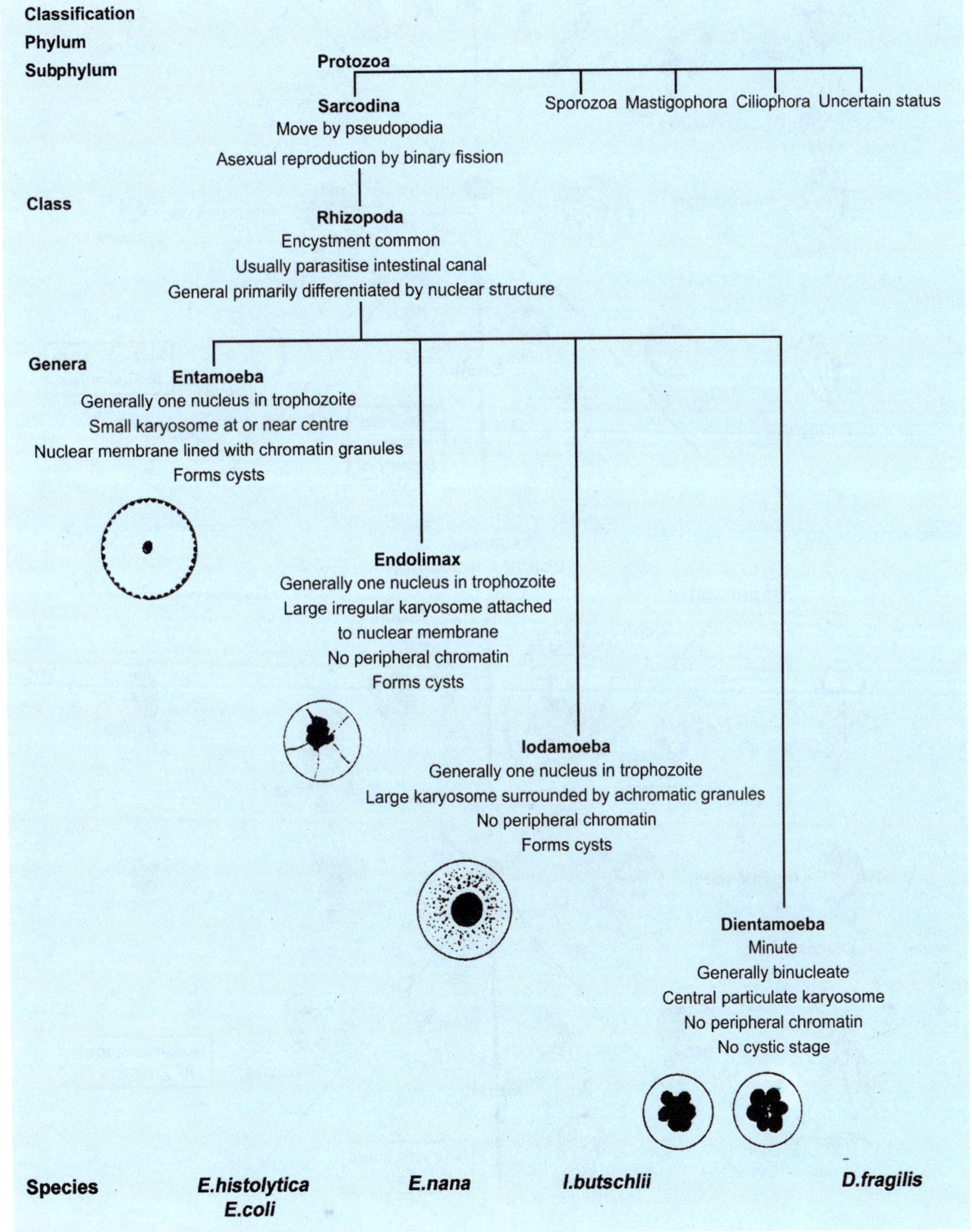

Recapitulation
Protozoa inhabiting the intestine

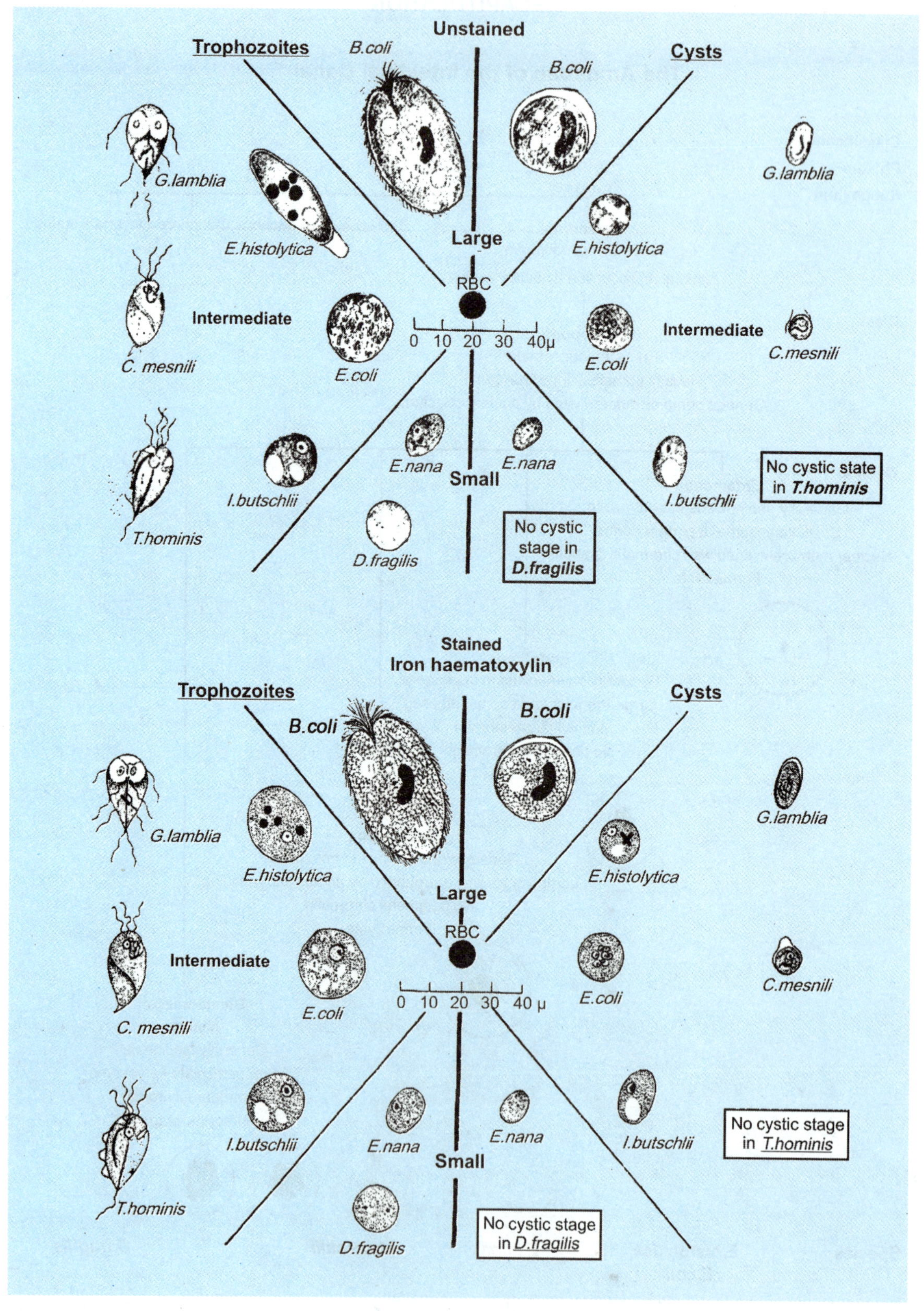

The Body Fluid and Tissue Flagellates (Causing Leishmaniasis and Trypanosomiasis)

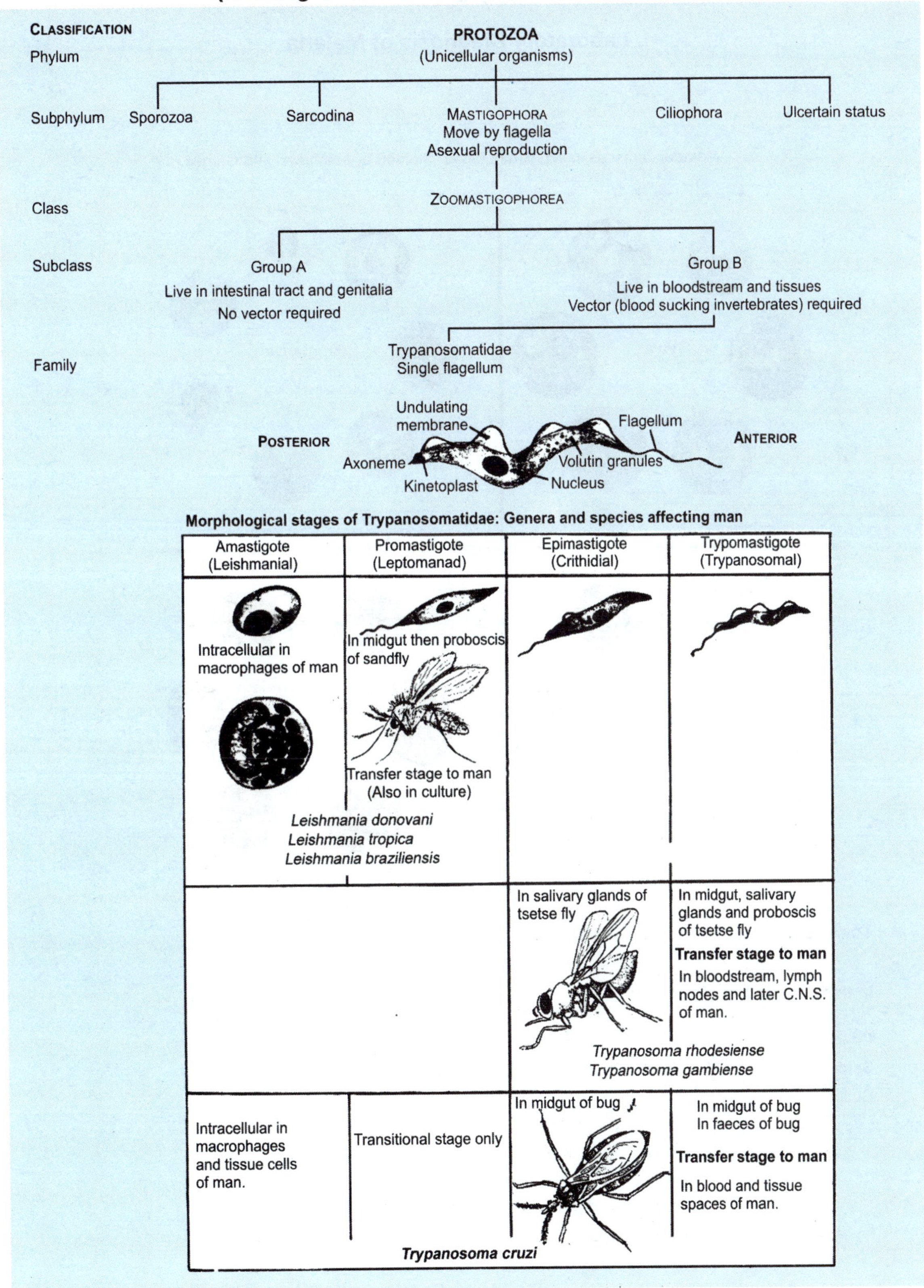

Laboratory Diagnosis of Malaria

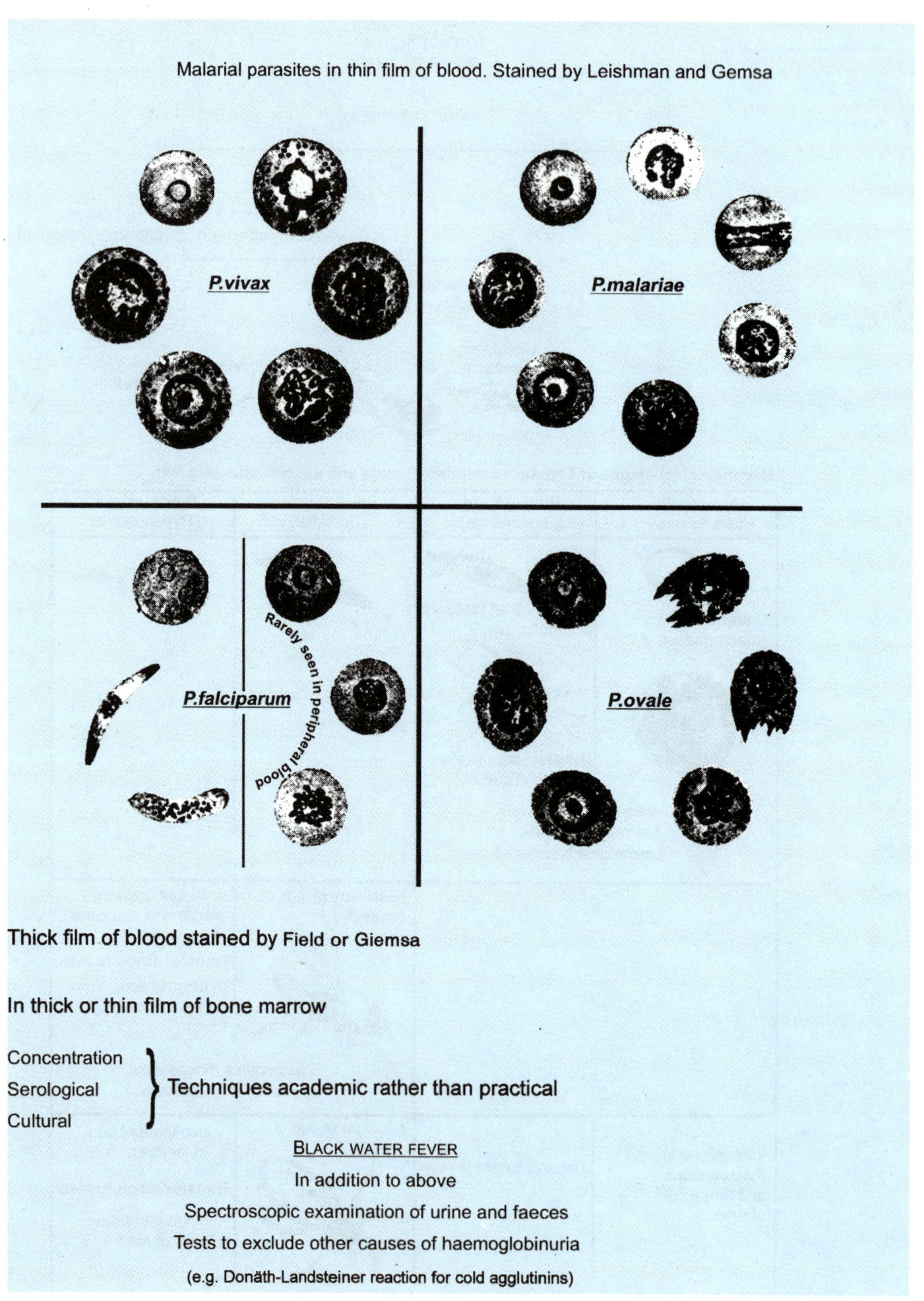

Malaria
Species identification in the mosquito—pigment in oocysts

Oocysts	*P.vivax*	*P.malariae*	*P.falciparum*	*P.ovale*
Length of cycle in days	9	15-21	10	15
Size in μ	10-46	5-44	8-60	9-37
Pigment				
Colour	Greenish brown	Dark brown or nearly black	Blackish	Dark brown or nearly black
Texture	Fine	Medium coarse	Very coarse	Medium coarse
Number of grains	50-100	30	10-20	50-60
Pattern				
Days				
3	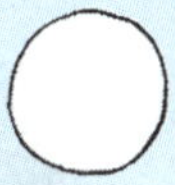 None			
4–5	Typical Prince of Wales feather design	Distributed, some clumping	Concentrated at periphery in double row often	Concentrated at periphery in semicircles or dotted lines
7–10	Obscured by nuclei	Increased clumping	Mainly obscured	Most clearly defined, dotted line often crosses
After 10		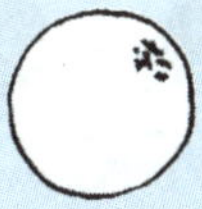 If visible, clumped at periphery	Seldom visible	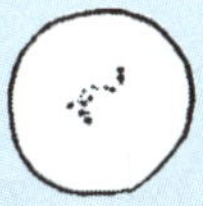 Mainly obscured
Recapitulation of distinctive features	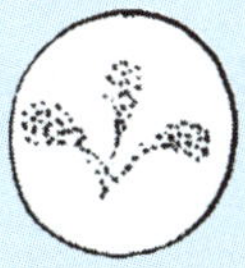 Prince of Wales feather design	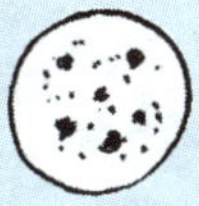 Distributed then clumped	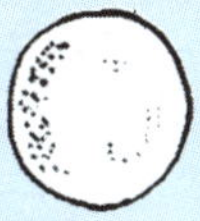 Peripheral in rows	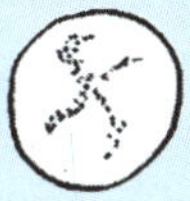 Semicircular or crossed line design

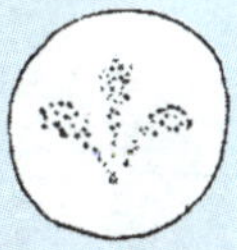

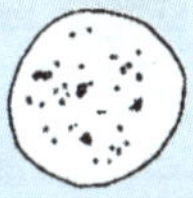

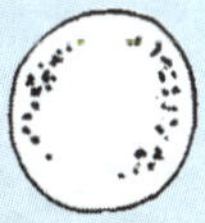

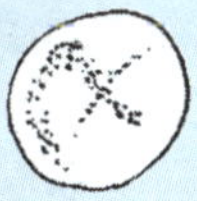

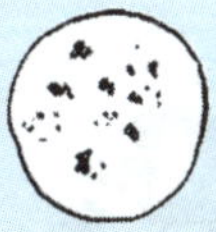

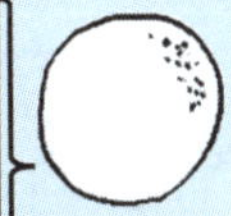

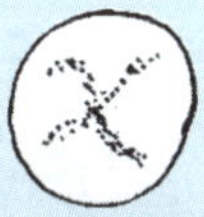

Recapitulation
Morphological Differentiation

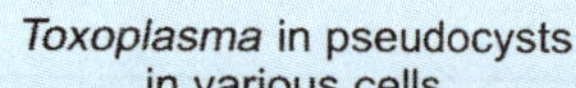

Toxoplasma in pseudocysts in various cells

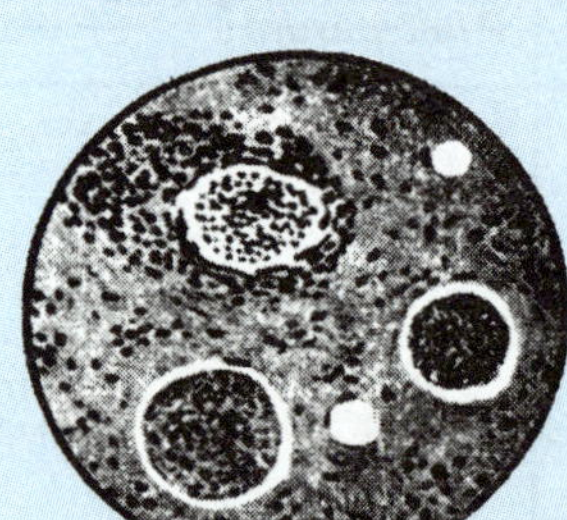

Exoerythrocytic schizonts of *Plasmodium* in liver cells

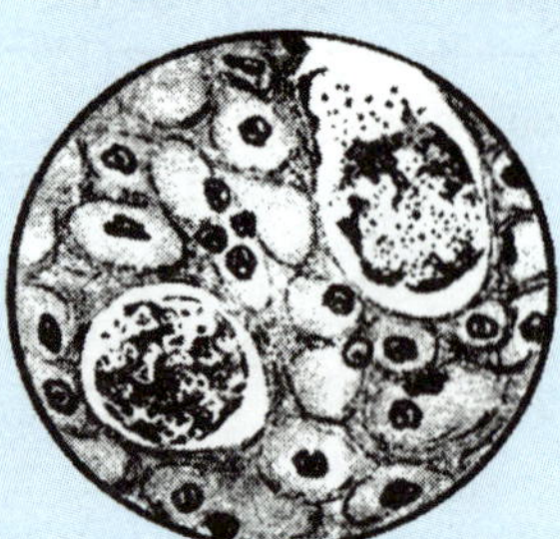

Sarcocystis lindemanni in human muscle

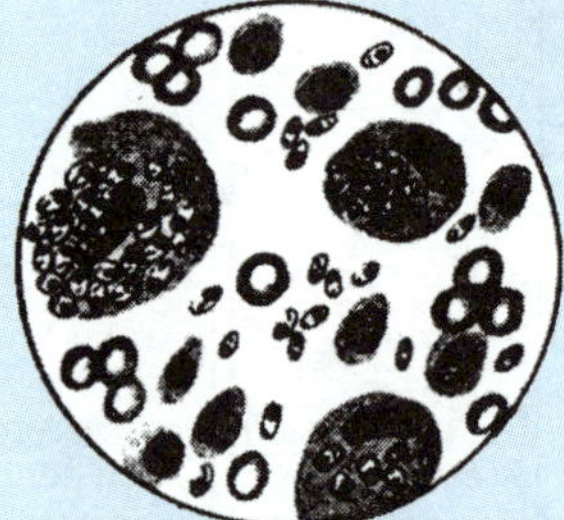

Leishman donovan bodies in RE cells in visceral leishmaniasis

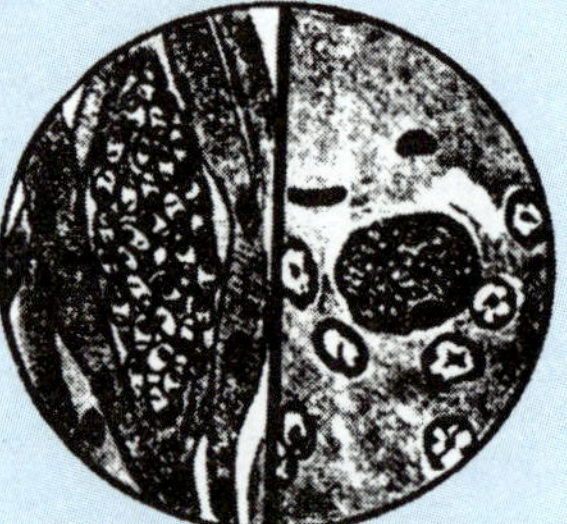

Leishmanial forms of *Trypanosoma cruzi* in myocardial and CNS cells

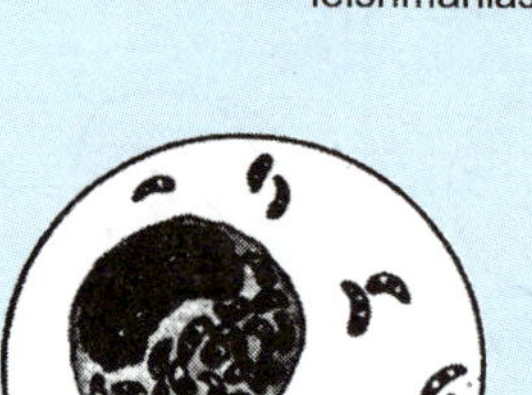

Toxoplasma gondii NOT in blood

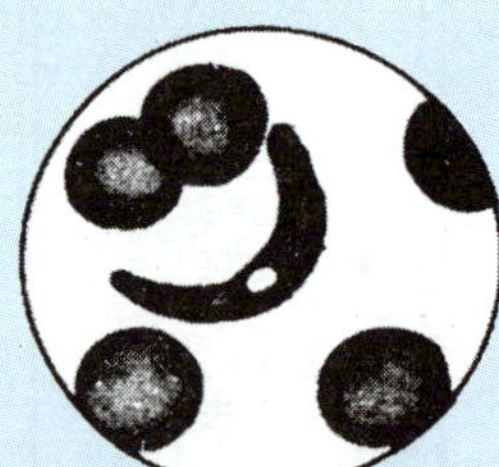

Ookinete of *Plasmodium* in mosquito's stomach

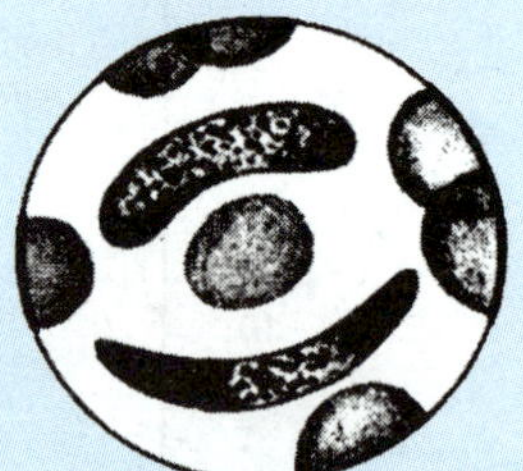

Gametocytes of *P.falciparum* in blood

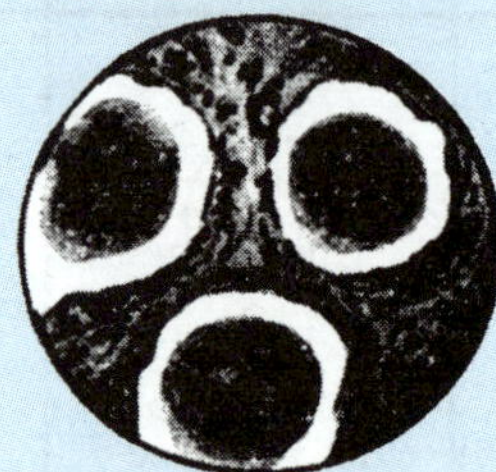

Pneumocystic carinii in lung

Recapitulation

RECAPITULATION

THE ESSENTIAL DIFFERENCES BETWEEN:

	African trypanosomiasis (Sleeping sickness)	South american trypanosomiasis (Chagas' disease)	Visceral leishmaniasis (Kala azar)
Caused by	*Trypanosoma gambiense* or *Trypanosoma rhodesiense*	*Trypanosoma cruzi*	*Leishmania donovani*
Vector	*Glossina spp.* (Tsetse flies)	*Triatomida spp.* (Cone-nosed bugs)	Phlebotomus spp. (sandiflies)
CYCLE IN VECTOR	Anterior station development	Posterior station development	Anterior station development
Stage ingested	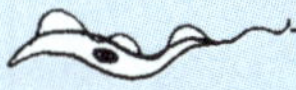 Trypanosomal	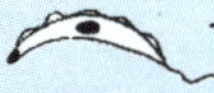 Trypanosomal	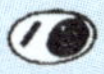 Leishmanial
Then	Multiply and move forward Enter salivary glands via duct 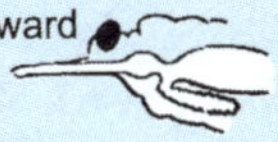 Metamorphose to crithidia 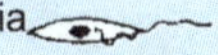 multiply Metamorphose to metacyclis Trypanosomes 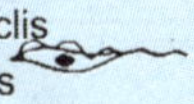	Metamorphose to crithidia 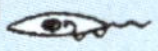 Multiply Move backward Metamorphose to metacyclic Trypanosomes 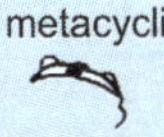	Metamorphose to leptomonad 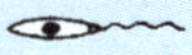 Multiply Move backward Block proboscis
	INFECTIVE : INJECTED IN SALIVA	**INFECTIVE : PASSED IN BUG FAECES**	**INFECTIVE : INJECTED FROM PROBOSCIS**
CYCLE IN MAN Form injected	Metacyclic Trypanosome	Metacyclic Trypanosome	Leptomonad
	NONE - remain as Trypanosomes	Enter histiocytes locally and become Leishmanial 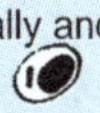	Enter histiocytes locally and become Leishmanial
Multiplication (all by binary fission)	As TRYPANOSOMES in BLOOD and tissue spaces 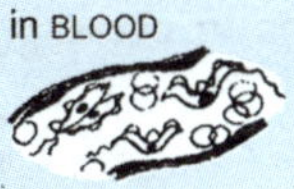	As Leishmandal forms in cells 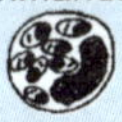	As Leishmanial forms in macrophage cells 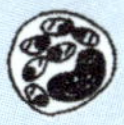
Then	Remain in bloodstream as Trypanosomes	Carried to regional nodes: some Leishmanial forms infect further histiocytes: some metamorphose 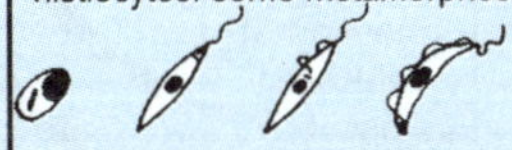 through transitional Leptomonad and Crithidial forms to gain blood as Trypanosomes. Do not multiply as such but disseminated, enter further tissue cells, metamorphose to Leishmanial forms and multiply	Further dissemination as Leishmanial forms ONLY
PATHOGENESIS	Circulating, multiplying Trypanosomes cause Parasitaemia and Toxaemia, damaging tissues	Parasitisation and destruction of all types of tissue cell Circulating Trypanosomes produce toxaemia	Parasitisation and destruction of RE cells
PATHOLOGICAL EFFECTS	Mainly general toxaemia lymphadenopathy CNS involvement	General toxaemia Local functional disability of whichever tissues invaded, especially lymph nodes, heart, CNS	General toxaemia from breakdown of RE cells Proliferation of RE cells (mainly spleen, liver, bone marrow, lymph nodes) No CNS involvement
CLINICO-PATHOLOGICAL CORRELATION	Acute *(T.rhodesiense)* Fever and severe toxaemia Chronic *(T.gambiense)* Fever Lymphadenopathy Encephalitis	Fever Enlarged nodes, spleen and liver Protean manifestations depending on localisation in tissues especially Cardiac CNS syndromes	Fever Anaemia Enlarged liver and spleen

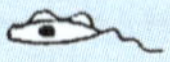

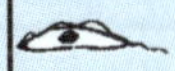

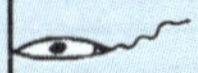

Neomatoda (Contd....)

Life cycle in general

A. NO INTERMEDIATE HOST REQUIRED

OUTSIDE MAN	INFECTION BY	INSIDE MAN	SPECIES
Embryonated ova to environment	Ingestion	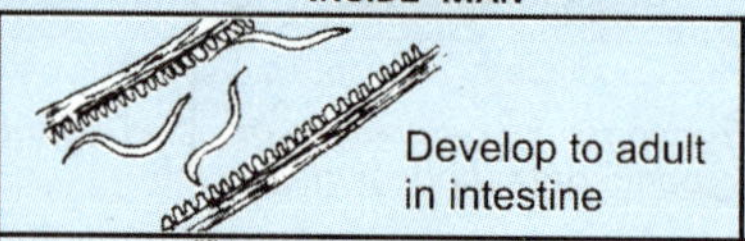 Develop to adult in intestine	*Enterobius vermicularis*
Non-embryonated ova to environment		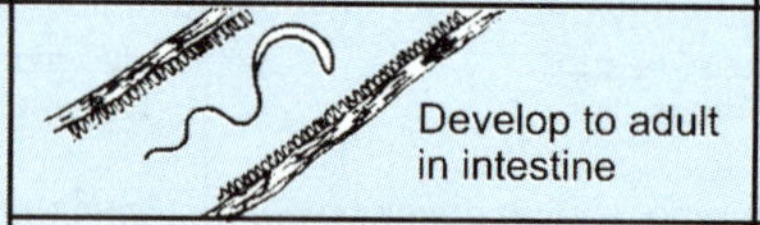 Develop to adult in intestine	*Trichuris trichiura*
Mature in damp soil	Ingestion	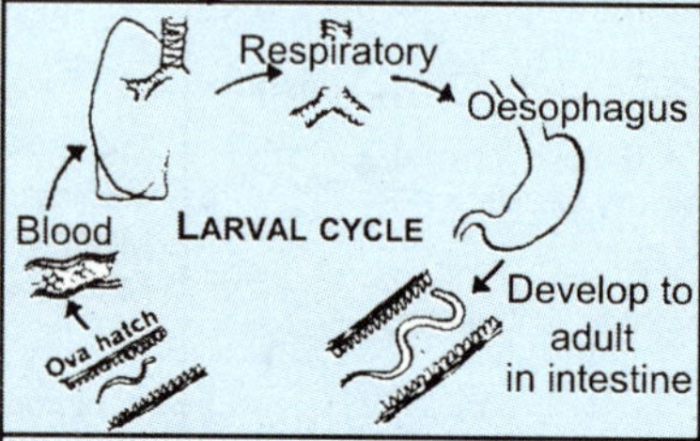 Respiratory → Oesophagus Blood LARVAL CYCLE Ova hatch Develop to adult in intestine	*Ascaris lumbricoides* *Toxocara* spp. in animals. Larval stage only in man
Mature, Hatch Encyst on vegetation	Ingestion encysted	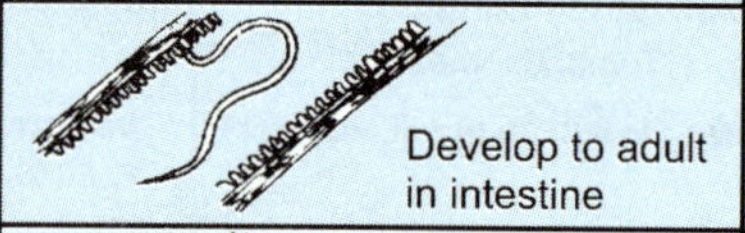 Develop to adult in intestine	*Trichostrongylus* spp *Haemonchus contortus*
Mature and ↓ Hatch in damp soil	Piercing skin	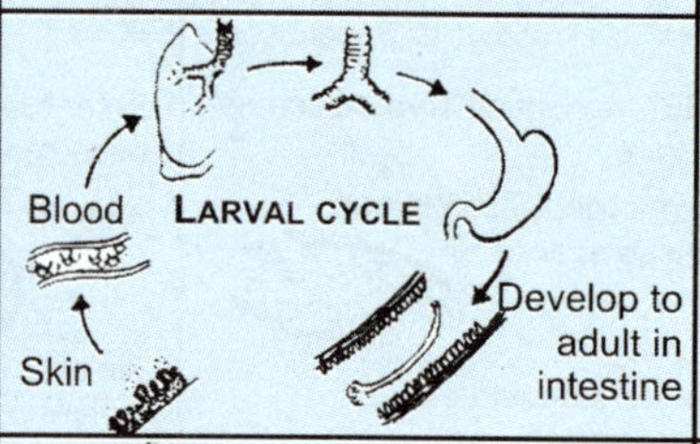 Blood LARVAL CYCLE Skin Develop to adult in intestine	Hookworms Ancylostoma *duodenale* *A. braziliense* (human strains) necator *americanus*
OVA LAID IN TISSUES In liver	Ingestion of infected tissue	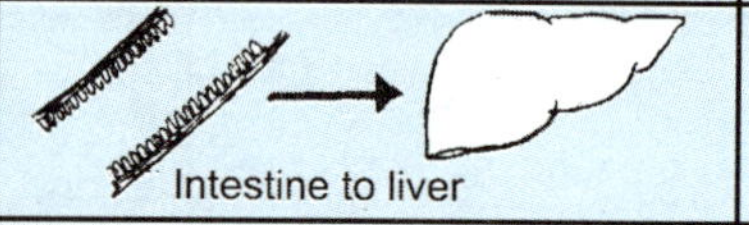 Intestine to liver	*Strongyloides stercoralis*
In intestinal wall Larvae to gut lumen Larvae re-enter host Larvae to environment Infect new host Become free living Larvae from free cycle	Piercing mucosa or anal skin Piercing skin Piercing skin	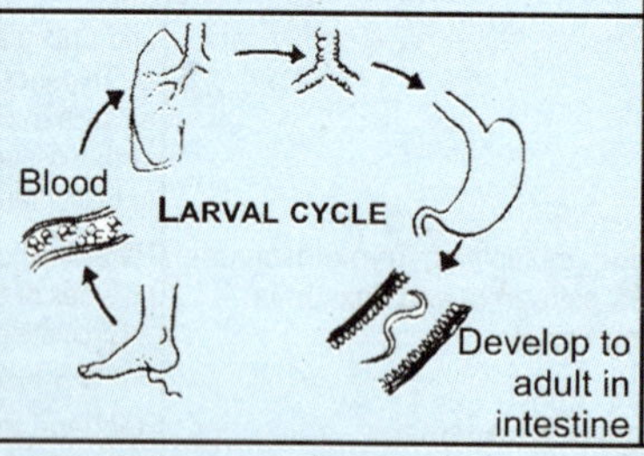 Blood LARVAL CYCLE Develop to adult in intestine	*Strongyloides stercoralis*

B. INTERMEDIATE HOST(S) REQUIRED

OUTSIDE MAN	INTERMEDIATE HOST	INFECTION OF MAN BY		SPECIES
EMBRYONATED OVA TO ENVIRONMENT	Ingested by beetles Larvae Hatch and encyst	Ingestion of infected beetles	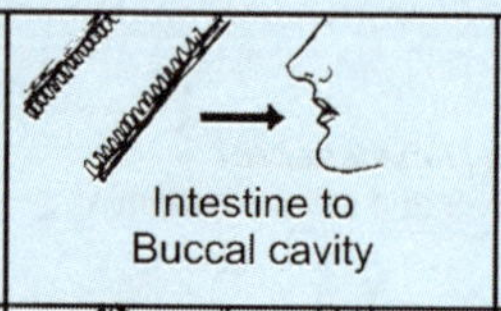 Intestine to Buccal cavity	*Gongylonema pulchrum*
Hatch in soil	Ingested by earthworms	Ingestion of earthworms	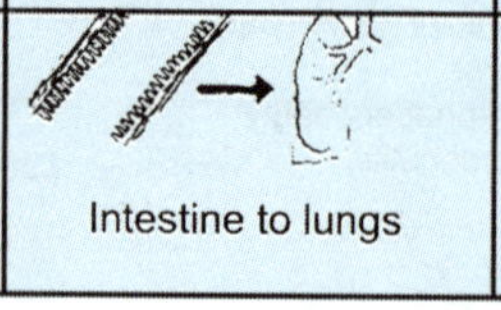 Intestine to lungs	*Metastrongylus elongatus*

Cestoda (Contd....)

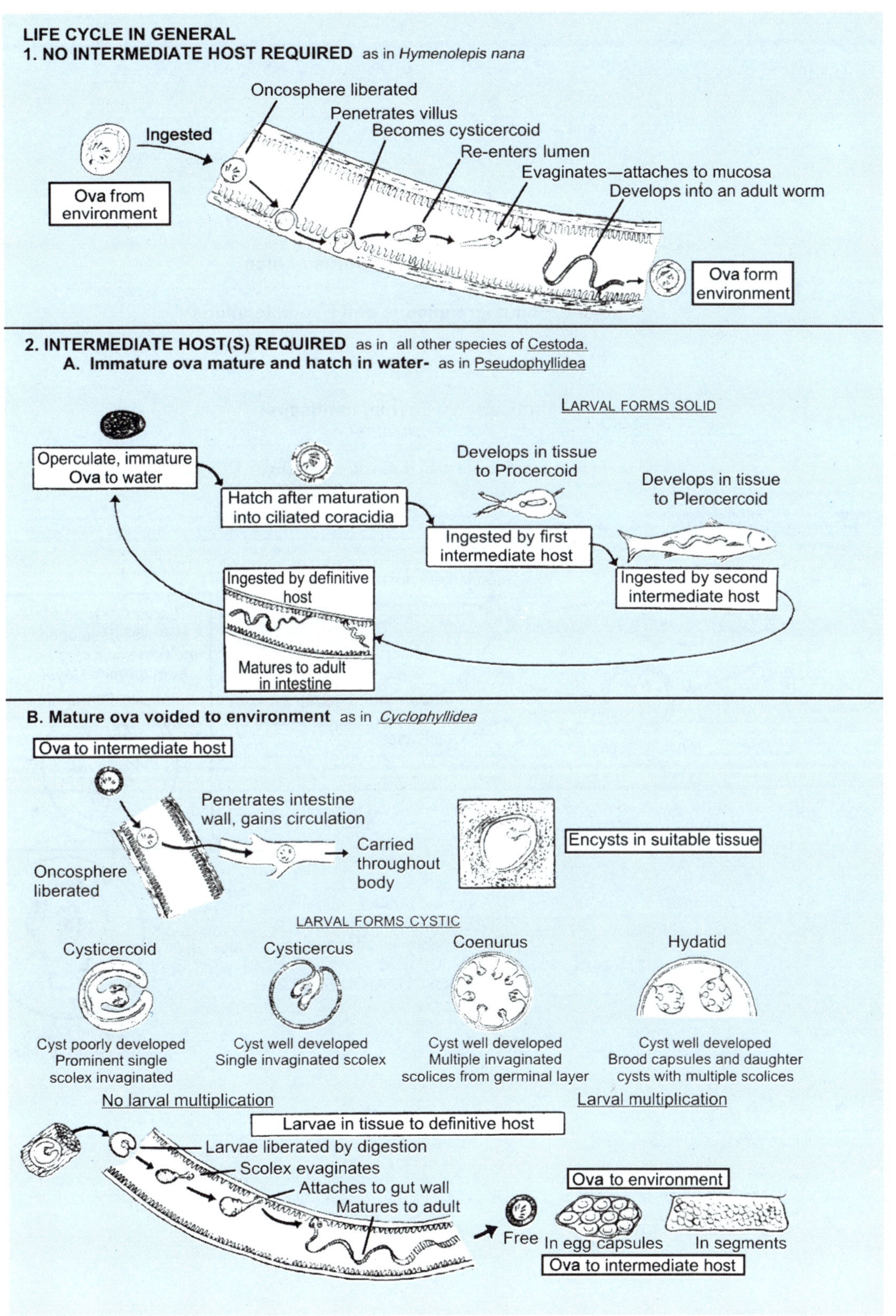

Cyclophyllidean tapeworms of man

Echinococcus granulosus and E.multilocularis

Larval stage (Hydatid and alveolar cysts) only in man
See plates 18-19

Multiceps (or Taenia) multiceps)
(The gid worm)

Larval stage only described in man, causing COENURUS CEREBRALIS

Life cycle

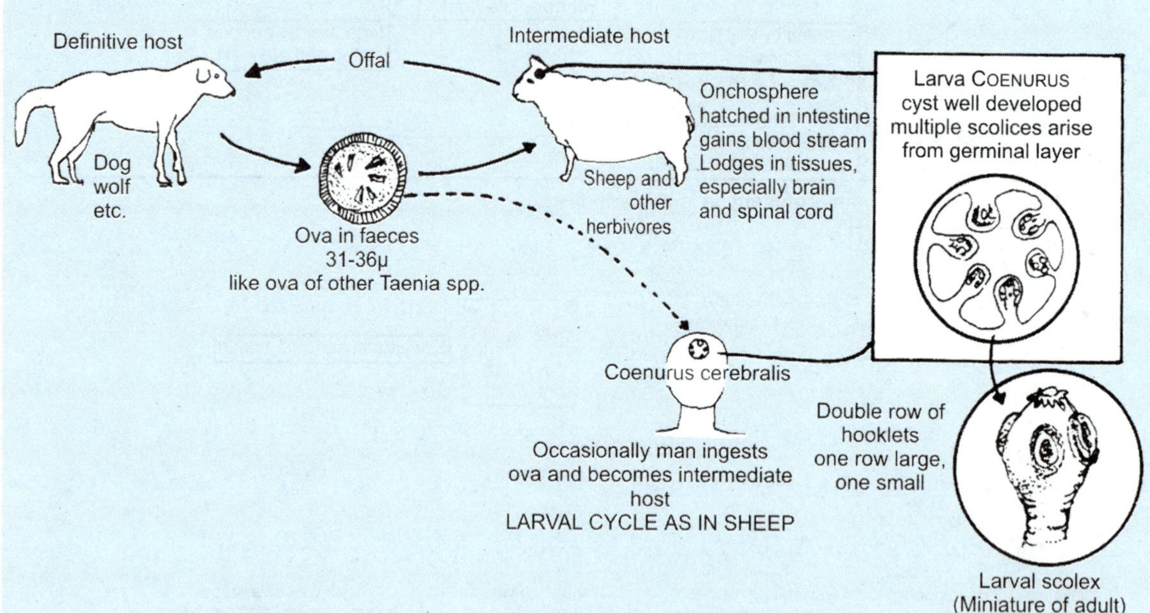

Recapitulation
Pathogenesis and Pathology of Worm Infections

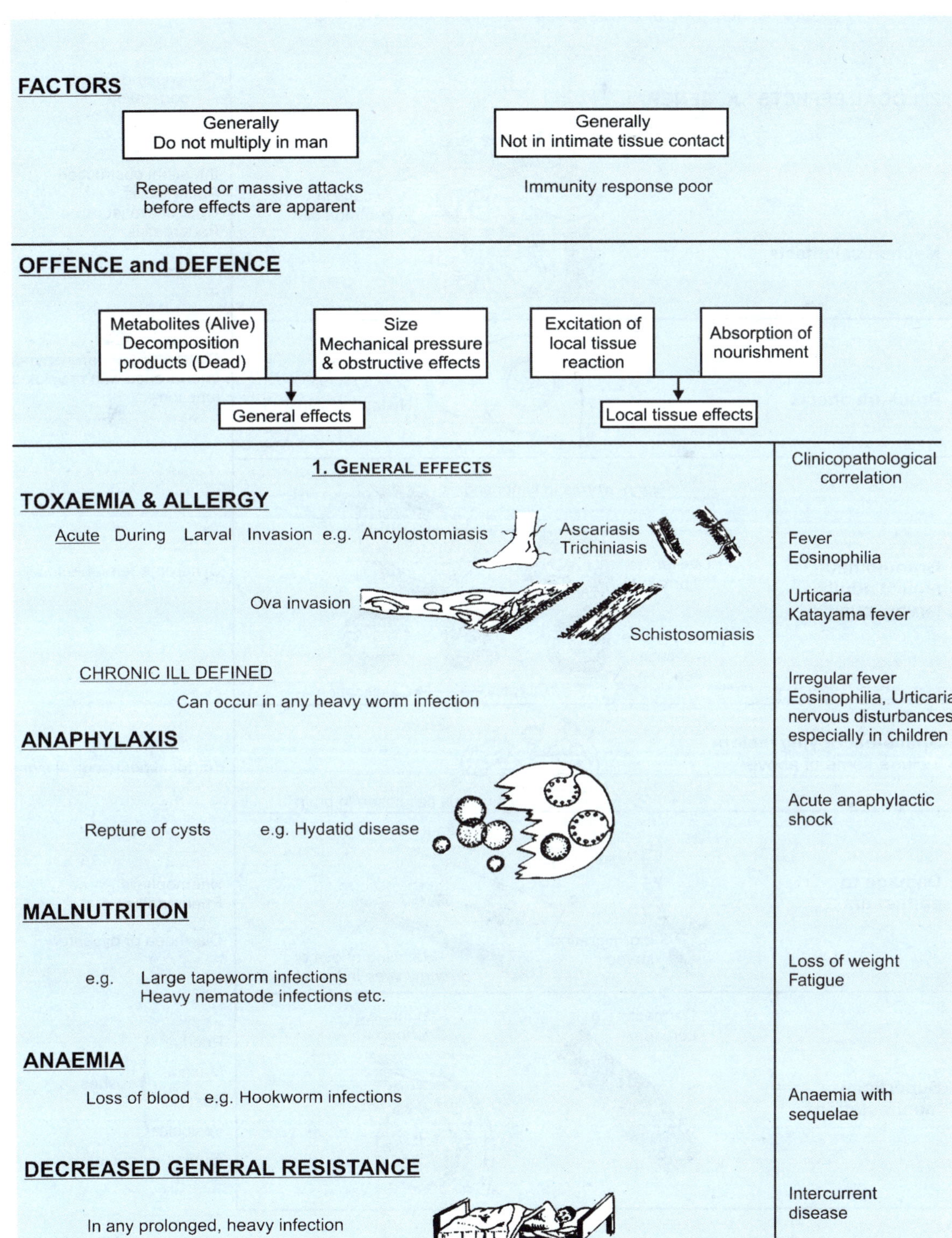

Recapitulation (Contd....)

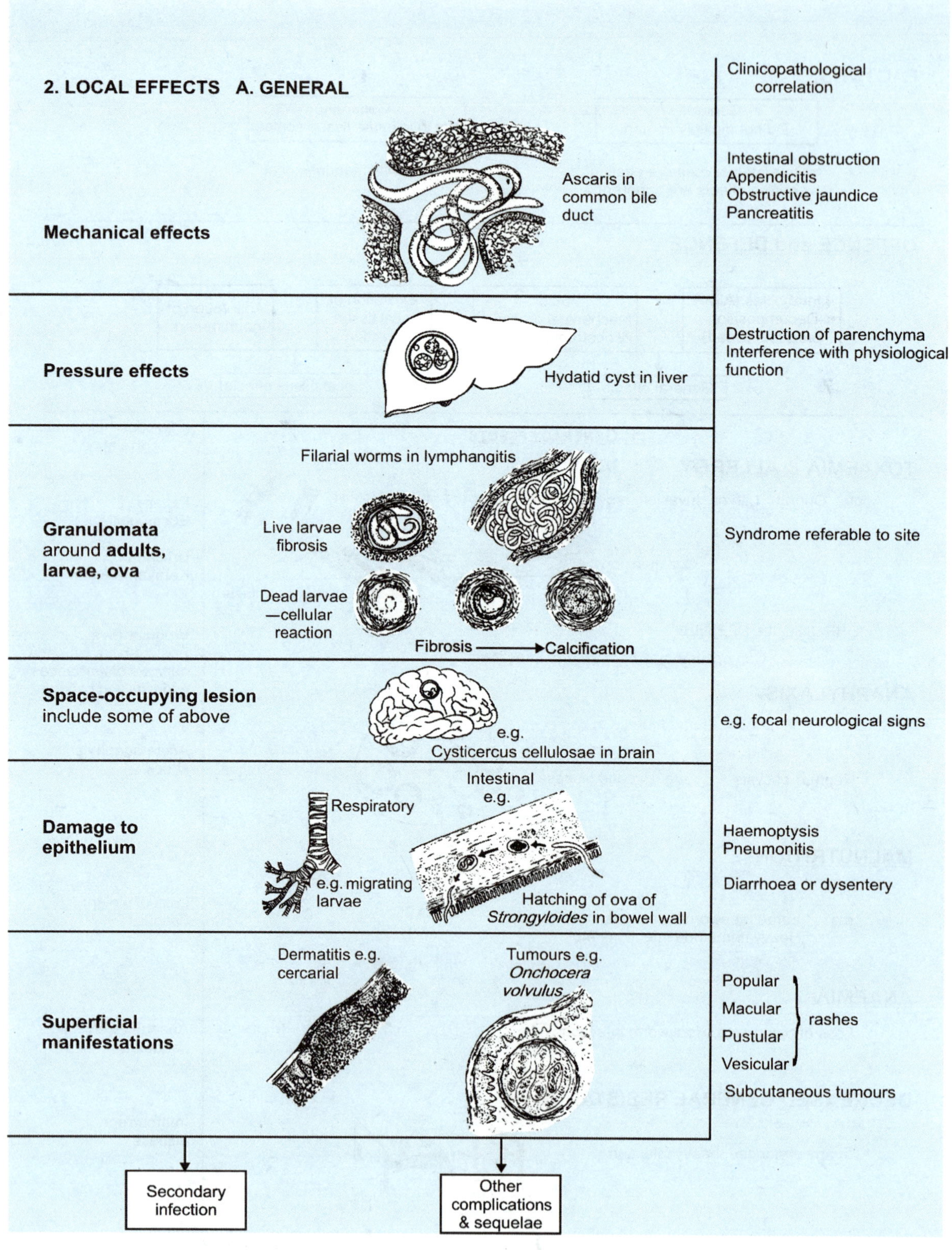

Recapitulation (Contd....)

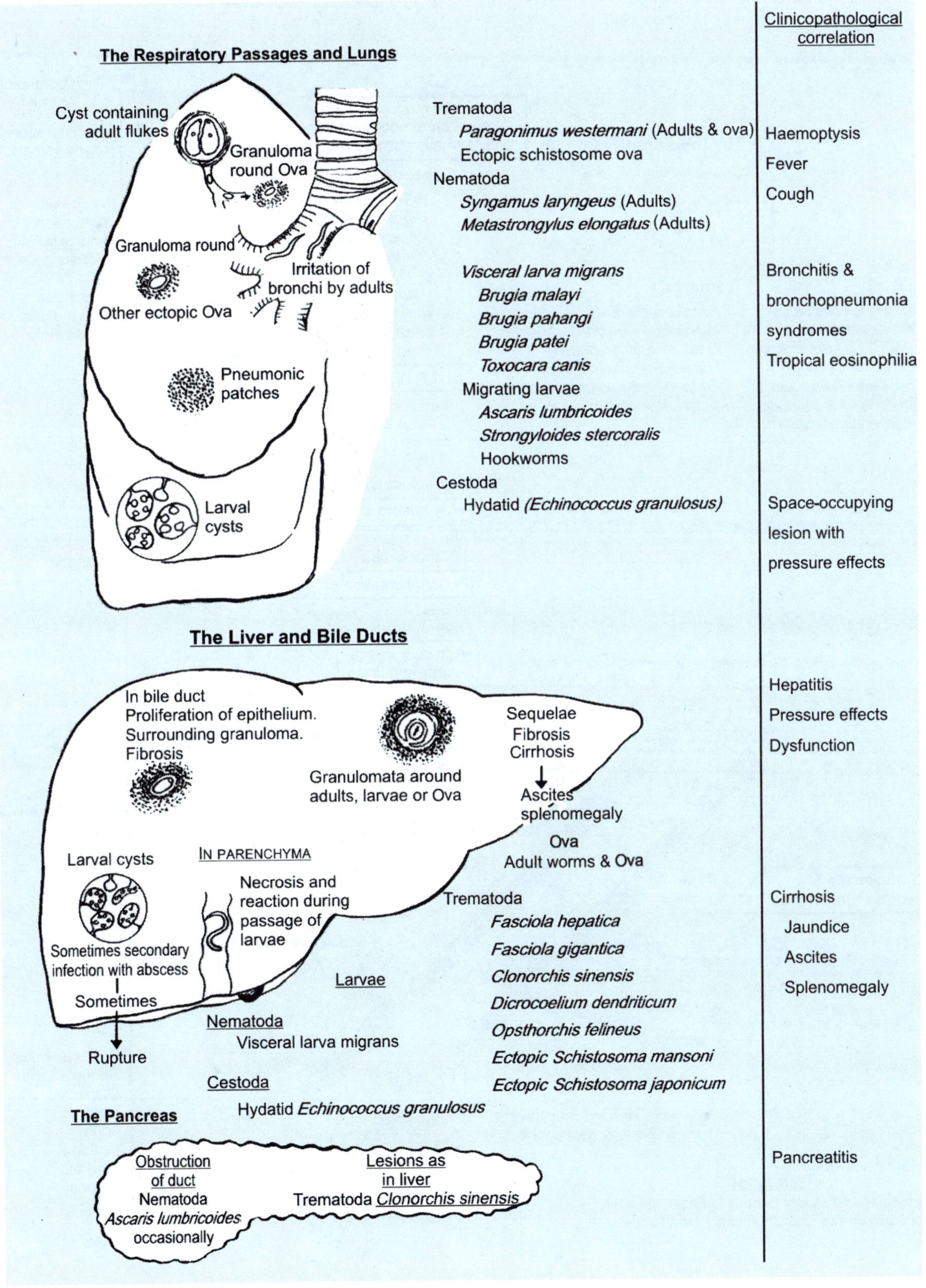

Recapitulation (Contd....)

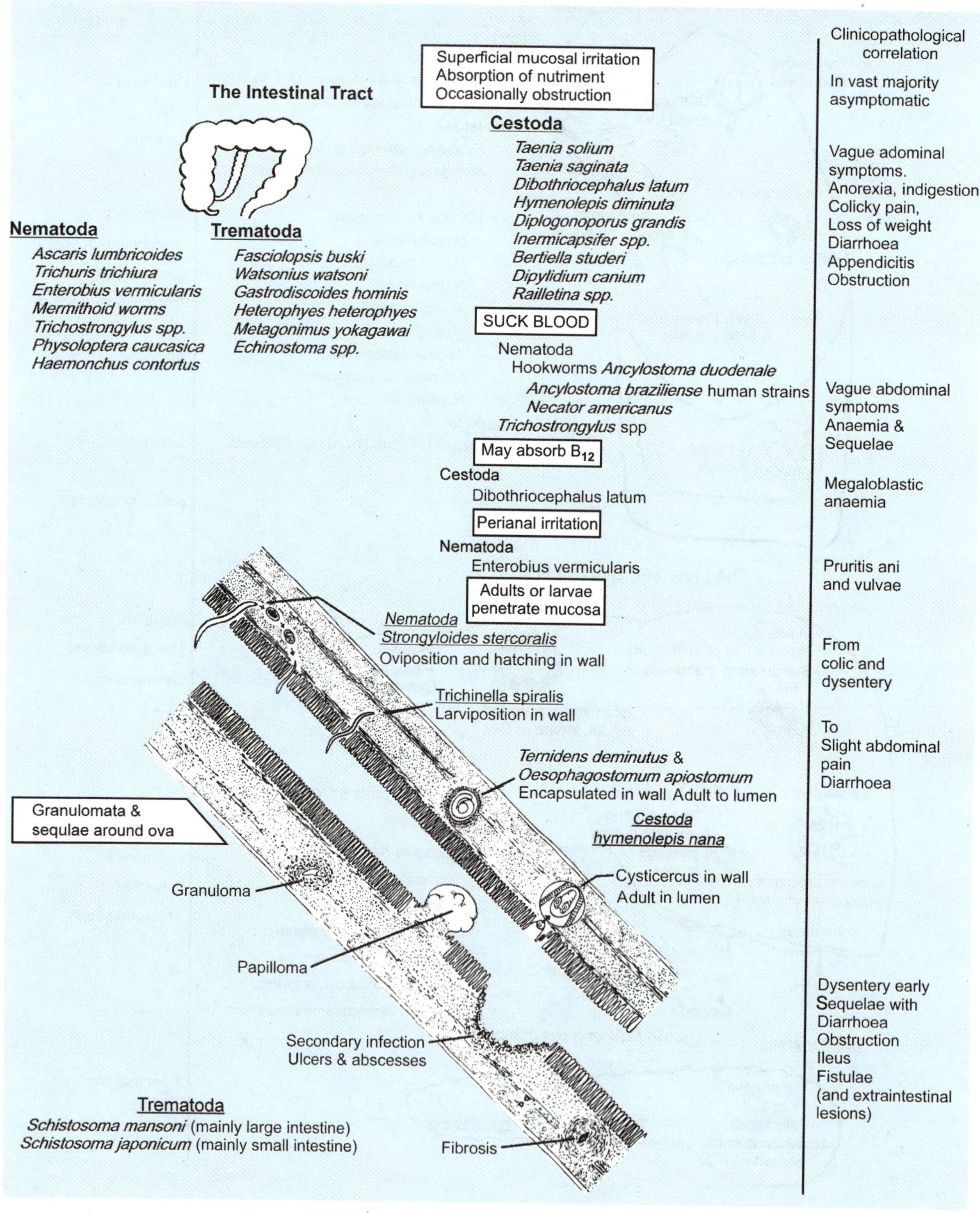

Recapitulation (Contd....)
Local effects of worm infections

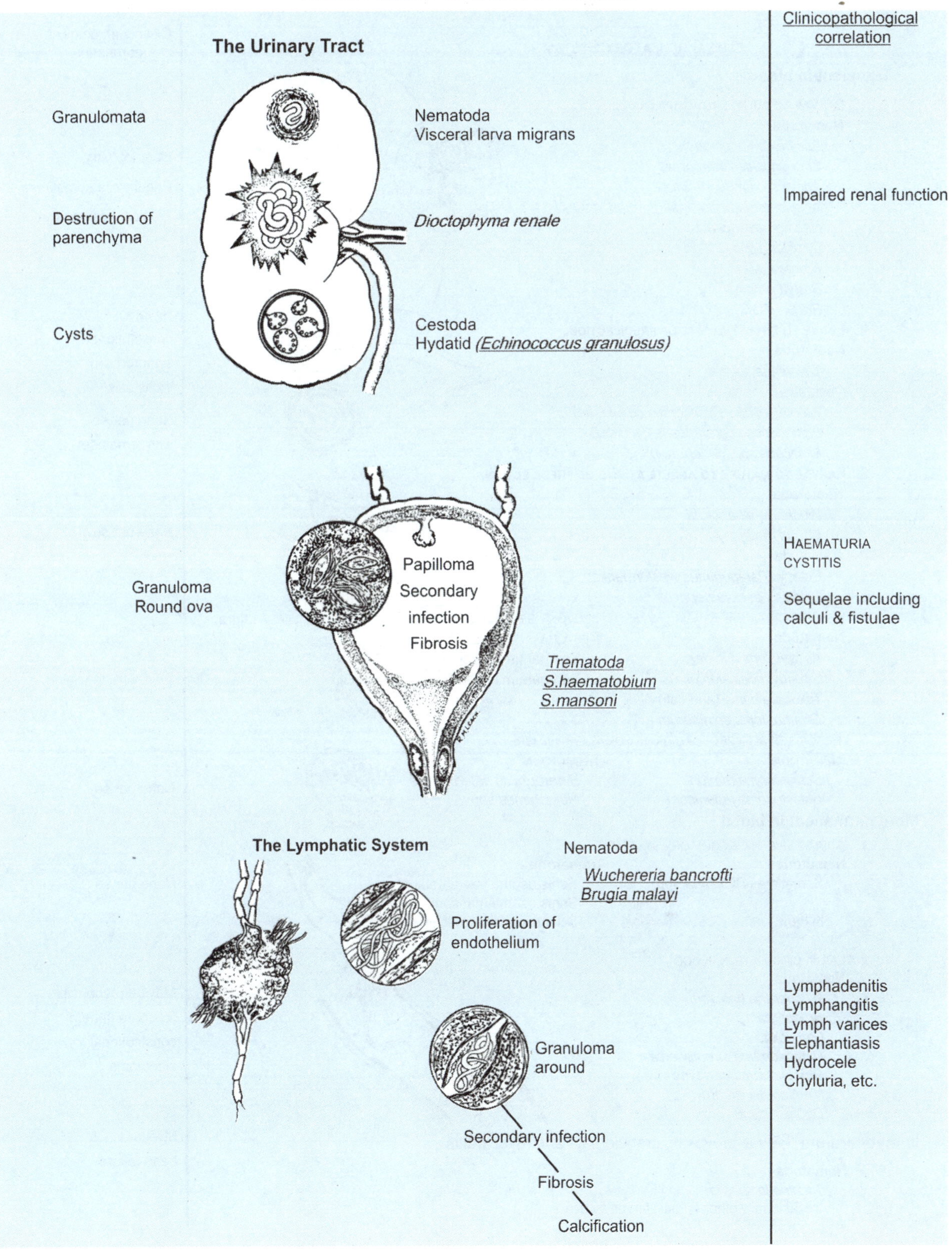

Recapitulation (Contd....)
Local effects of worm infections

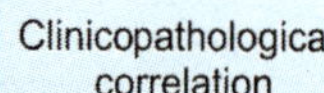

Clinicopathological correlation

THE CIRCULATORY SYSTEM

Transient in blood

1. LARVAE TO PULMONARY CAPILLARIES

Nematoda

Ascaris lumbricoides
Strongyloides stercoralis
Ancylostoma duodenale
Ancylostoma braziliense (human strains)
Necator americanus
Dirofilaria spp
Brugia malayi
Brugia pahangi
Brugia patei

Clinicopathological correlation: Haemoptysis; Pneumonia sometimes; Tropical eosinophilia

2. LARVE TO ENCYST AT SITE OF PREDILECTION

Nematoda

Trichinella spiralis

Cestoda

Taenia solium (Cysticercus cellulosae)
Echinococcus granulosus (Hydatid)
Multiceps spp. (Coenurus)

Clinicopathological correlation: Severe constitutional symptoms in trichinosis; None per se with remainder

3. LARVAE TO MATURE TO ADULTS AT SITE OF PREDILECTION

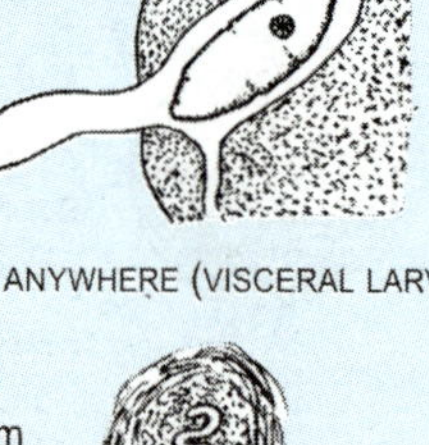

Nematoda

Wuchereria bancrofti
Brugia malayi

Trematoda

Ectopic *Paragonimus westermani*
Ectopic *Fasciola hepatica*

Clinicopathological correlation: None per se

4. ECTOPIC OR ANIMAL STRAIN LARVAE TO PROVOKE GRANULOMATA ANYWHERE (VISCERAL LARVA Migrans)

Nematoda

Ascaris lumbricoides
Strongyloides stercoralis
Toxocara canis (and cati)
Gnathostoma spinigerum

CESTODA

Sparganum mansoni
Sparganum proliferum

Clinicopathological correlation: None per se; None per se

5. ECTOPIC OVA TO PROVOKE GRANULOMATA ANYWHERE

NEMATODA

Schistosoma manoni
Schistosoma japonicum

TREMATODA

Heterophyes heterophyes
Metgonimus spp

Clinicopathological correlation: None per se

More permanent in blood

1. ADULTS LIVE IN CIRCULATORY SYSTEM

Nematoda

Sometimes *Dirofilaria* spp.

in heart

Trematoda

Schistosoma haematobium
Schistosoma mansoni
Schistosoma japonicum

Clinicopathological correlation: None per se

2. LARVA CIRCULATE IN BLOOD

Nematoda

Wuchereria bancrofti
Brugia malayi
Loa Loa
Dipetalonema streptocerca
Dipetalonema perstans
Mansonella ozzardi
Dirofilaria spp.

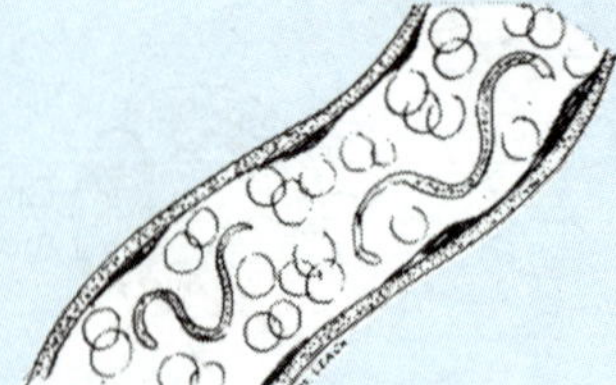

Clinicopathological correlation: May be responsible for some general constitutional symptoms

In myocardium Larvae provoking granulomata and myocarditis

Nematoda

Trichinella spiralis
Occasionally other ectopic larvae to ova

Clinicopathological correlation: Myocarditis & heart failure

Recapitulation (Contd....)

Local effects of worm infections, continued.

Clinicopathological correlation

The Skin and Subcutaneous Tissue

Penetration by Invading Larvae

Nematoda
- *Strongyloides stercoralis*
- *Ancylostoma duodenale*
- *A. braziliense* (human strains)
- *Necator americanus*

— Petechial dermatitis, Swimmer's itch

- A. braziliense (animal strains)
- A. caninum — Cutaneous larva migrans

— Creeping eruption

Trematoda
- Schistosoma spp. (human strains) — Little effect
- Schistosoma spp. (animal strains) — Cercarial dermatitis

Nematoda
- Filarial larvae *Wuchereria bancrofti*, *Brugia malayi* — None per se, or slight dermatitis

Site of Predilection of Adult

Fleeting swelling

Fibrosis around

Dermatitis from MF

Inflammation

Presents through skin

Nematoda
- *Loa Loa* — Calabar swelling
- *Onchocerca volvulus* — Fibrotic tumour, MF dermatitis
- *Dracunculus medinesis* — Ulcer

Nematoda
Gnathostoma spinigerum
(Visceral larva migrans)

Cestoda
Sparganum mansoni
Sparganum proliferum

— Swelling, Irritation, Infection

Cestoda
Cysticercus cellulosae
(Taenia solium)

Irritation by Adult

Nematoda
Enterobius vermicularis — Pruritis ani and vulvae

The Muscle and Bone

Nematoda
Trichinella spiralis
may calcify

CESTODA
- *Cysticercus cellulosae (Taenia solium)* — Pain and swelling
- *Sparganum spp.*
- HYDATID *(Echinococcus granulosus)* — Pain and spontaneous fractures

Recapitulation
Morphology of adults and larvae Nematodes

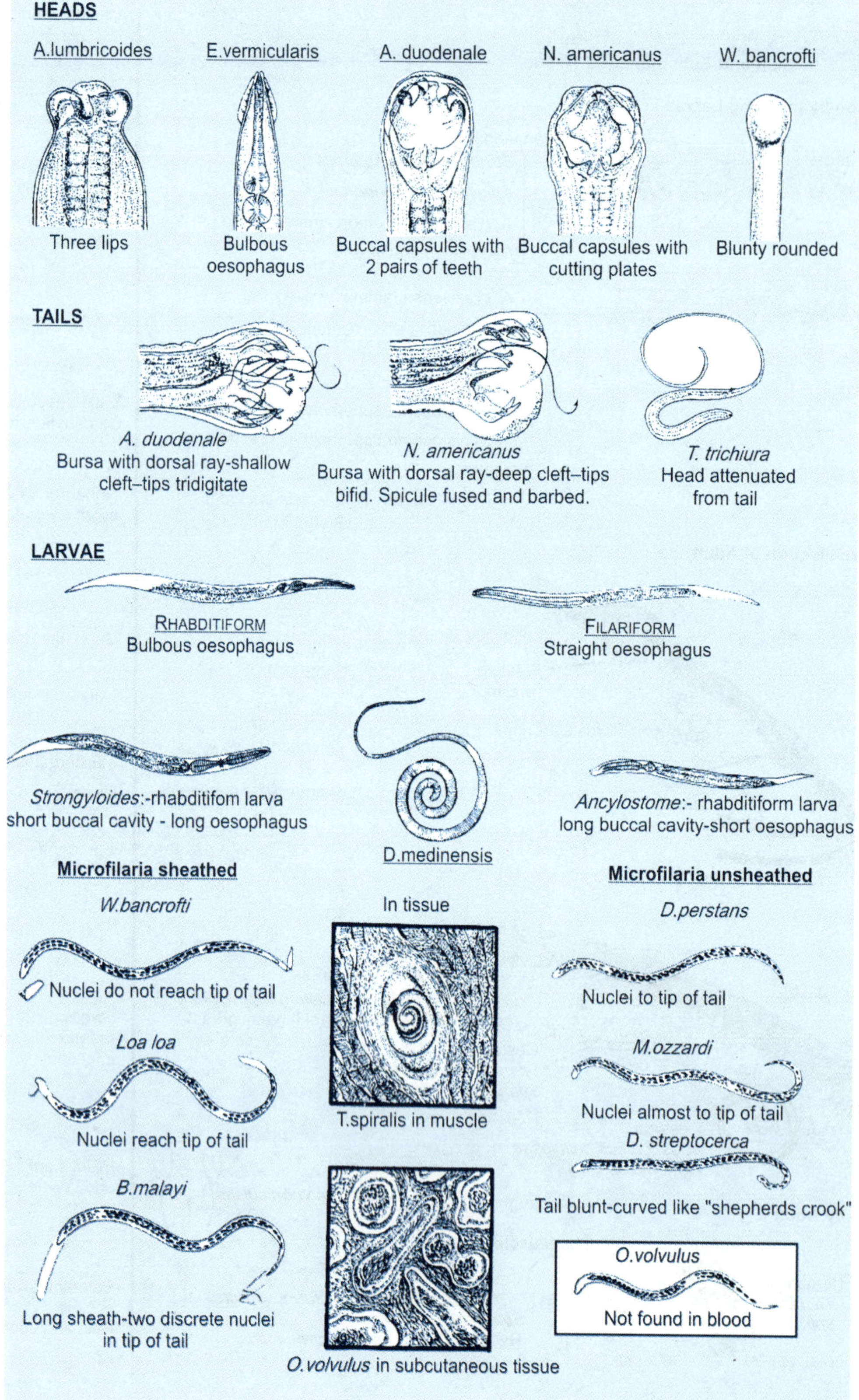

Recapitulation
Ova

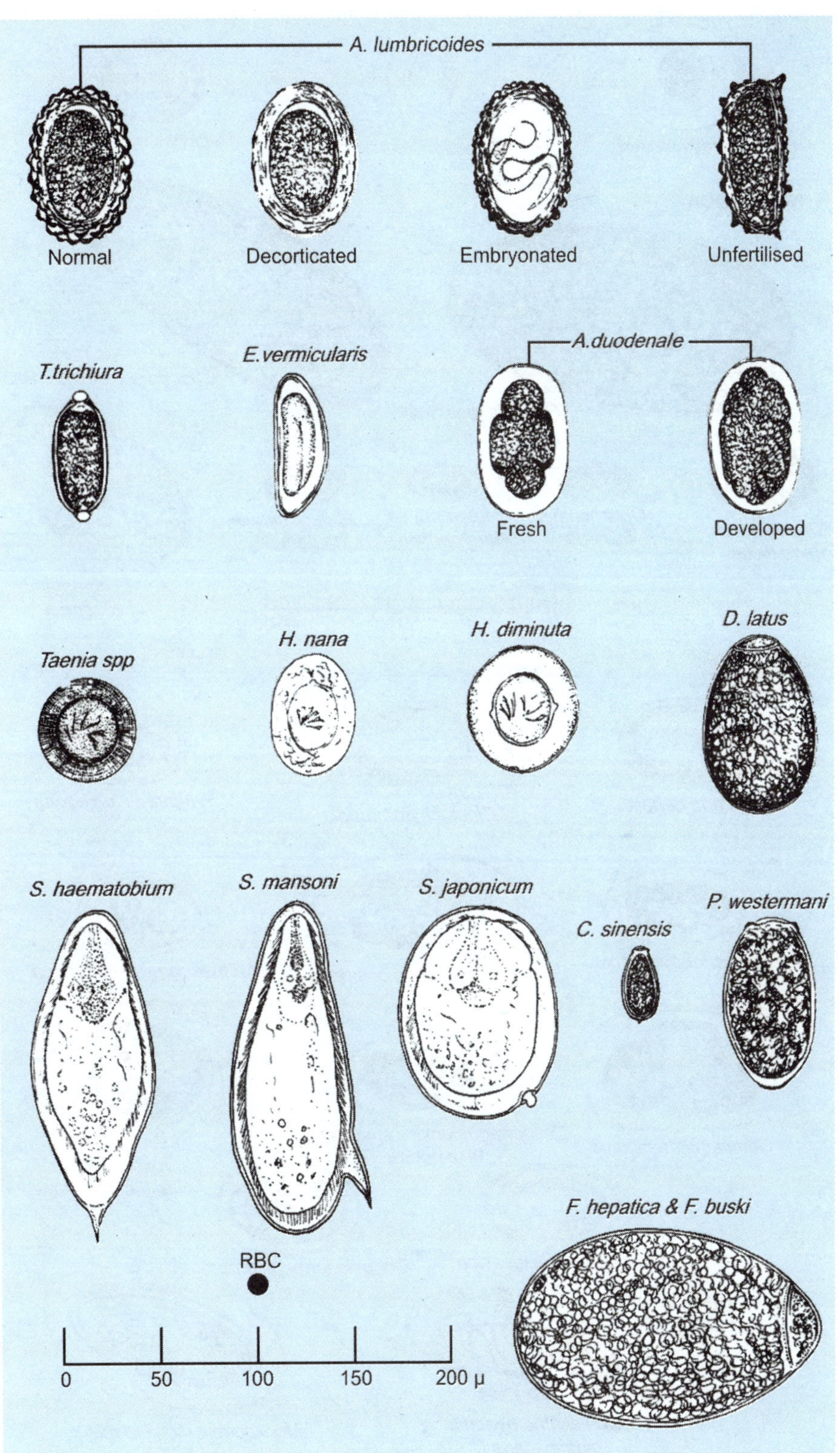

Recapitulation
Ova of the less common or less important worms

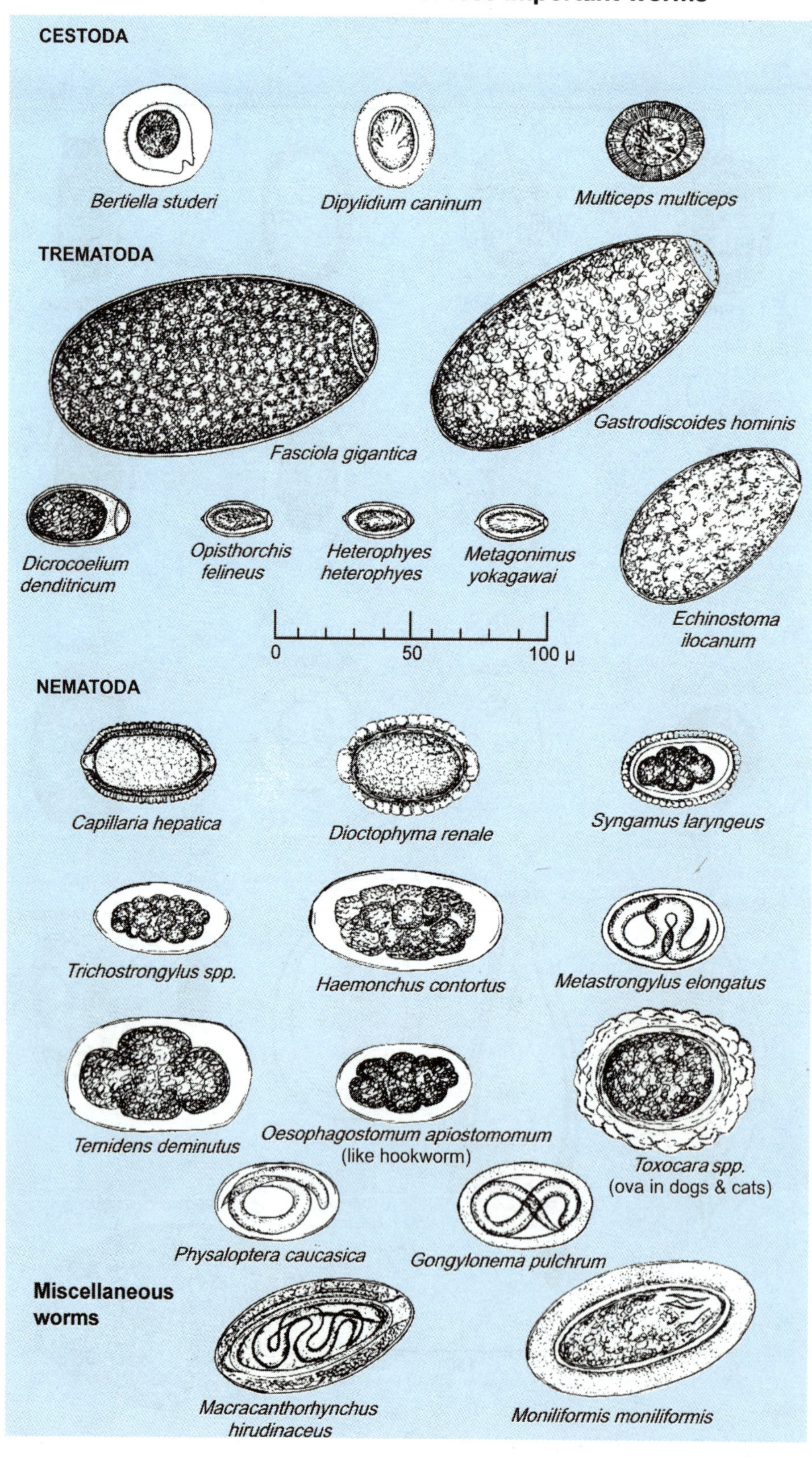

LABORATORY EXAMINATION FOR PARASITES

Preservation and Shipment of Specimens to be Examined for Trophic and Encysted Protozoa

PVA (Polyvinyl Alcohol) Method of Brooke and Goldman

Excellent for amoeba, especially if permanent slides are required. For collection of field specimens and for mass surveys, the Merthiolate-Iodine-Formatin (MIF) method is recommended.

1. *Reagent*—Modified Schaudinn's solution is prepared by mixing 5 ml of glacial acetic acid, 1.5 ml of glycerol and 93.5 ml of Schaudinn's solution (2 parts saturated aqueous mercuric chloride and 1 part 95% ethyl alcohol).
   Heat the above solution to 75°C; while stirring, slowly add 5 gm polyvinyl alcohol (PVA) powder. This final solution should be clear and free of lumps after cooling. It is used at room temperature, and lasts several months.
2. *Preparation of specimens*
   a. One specimen should be sent without above fixative to be used for detection of protozoan cysts and helminthic ova. This specimen can be used for temporary or permanent smears or for concentration procedures.
   b. Second specimen is prepared by thoroughly mixing with 3 or more parts of fixative in a small vial. To prepare slides, a small amount of this faecal mixture (recent or months old) is spread thinly over about one-third of the slide. After drying for 3 or more hours at 37°C or overnight at room temperature, the smear is stained by the iron haematoxylin method. This procedure is particularly suitable for the preservation and staining of the trophic forms of intestinal protozoa. To obtain satisfactory stained faecal smears containing cystic stages, the excess clear PVA solution is decanted from the vial and a small amount of the remaining fixed faecal material is placed on a piece of facial tissue or toilet paper. The excess PVA solution is allowed to absorb for 5-10 minutes, leaving a moist faecal residue. Gently scrape up a small amount of the residue with the sharp edge of a broken applicator stick and smear with gentle brushing strokes on a slide. Drop smear immediately into 70% alcohol to which iodine has been added to produce a portwine colour, and stain by the iron haematoxylin method. To ensure satisfactory preparation of both types smears are recommended.

MIF (Merthiolate—Iodine-Formalin) Method of Sapero and Lawless

This is now the standard method for mass surveys, collection of bulk material, or parasitologic field studies. Faecal specimens are fixed and stained immediately, and can be examined at any time within several months of collection. This method is particularly good for protozoa.

1. *Reagents*: MIF stock solution is made from 250 ml distilled water, 200 ml of tincture of merthiolate, 25 ml of formaldehyde, 5 ml of glycerol. Store in brown bottle. Lugol's solution (5% iodine in 10% potassium iodide in distilled water), not over 1-week old, forms the second solution.
2. *Preparation of specimens*: For each specimen to be collected, have ready 2.35 ml MIF stock solution in a Kahn test tube with cork stopper and 0.15 ml Lugol's solution in a second Kahn tube with a rubber stopper. Combine the 2 solutions just before adding the faecal specimen. Break up about 0.25 gm faeces into the combined solution, mix thoroughly, and stopper well (may be examined immediately on a slide, 1 drop faecal preparation and 1 drop distilled water; or stored in a well-stoppered tube, where the stain will be retained for several months).

ROUTINE STOOL EXAMINATION AND CONCENTRATION METHODS HAVE BEEN DEALT WITH ELSEWHERE

Negative Stain Direct Faecal Smear Examination

Prepare normal faecal smear in saline to which 1-2 drops of 1% isotonic eosin are added. Background material and dead parasites turn uniformly pink. Stain will not penetrate living trophozoites, causing them to stand out markedly as clear, translucent organisms against a pink background. A rapid and useful procedure.

Isotonic eosin, 1%, and brilliant cresyl blue, 0.2%, makes a good vital stain, causing living material to appear as shiny pale blue-green objects on the pink background.

Kato Cellophane Thick Smear Technique (Kato and Miura, 1954)

This method permits rapid examination of a large number of samples (up to 70/hour) for eggs of the common helminths. It is not suitable for protozoa or minute helminths or for highly fibrous or gaseous samples.

Materials

1. Wettable cellophane of medium thickness (40-50 μm), cut in strips 22 × 30 mm.
2. Glycerine-malachite green solution: 100 ml pure glycerine, 100 ml water, 1 ml 3% aqueous malachite green.

The cellophane strips should be soaked in the glycerine mixture for at least 24 hours before use.

Procedure

1. Place 50-60 mg faeces (4 mm cube) on a clean slide.
2. Cover with a glycerine-soaked cellophane strip, press to spread faeces in an even layer. Faeces need not be spread to all areas of cellophane; a circumference equal to the width of the strip is sufficient.
3. Allow to stand at room temperature for 1 hour (or 20-30 minutes at 40°C in a dry incubator). This dries and clears the specimen. (Do not overydry, as gas bubbles will form and air cells will surround the eggs).
4. Examine the entire film under low poor magnification.

Heidenhain's Iron Haematoxylin Staining Method for Intestinal Protozoa

Iron haematoxylin is generally accepted as the most reliable stain for nuclear detail in amoebae and for accurate laboratory diagnosis. It also provides a permanent stain preparation. However, it requires critical care and individual slide destaining (to be done carefully), a major handicap in routine handling of specimens by clinical laboratories. The trichrome stain has therefore superseded iron haematoxylin staining for routine diagnosis, though for critical definition, iron haematoxylin is still unsurpassed. Both iron haematoxylin and trichrome can be used for either PVA-fixed or nonpreserved material.

Staining Solutions

1. *Schaudinn's fixative*—described earlier.
2. *Haematoxylin stain* (stock solution)—Dissolve 100 gm haematoxylin powder in 100 ml absolute ethanol. Let stand several weeks for maturation. For use, 5 ml of ripened hematoxylin is added to 95 ml distilled water.
3. *Mordant*—Dissolve 5 gm ferric ammonium sulphate in 10 ml distilled water and filter.

Procedure

1. Make thin faecal smear on a clean glass slide with toothpick, applicator, or stiff haired paste brush.
2. Before drying occurs, immerse slide in Schaudinn's fluid with acetic acid added, heated to 45°C. Fix for 5-15 minutes at this temperature or for 30 minutes at room temperature (omit this step for PVA-fixed specimens).
3. Staining in Coplin jars—

70% alcohol	15 minutes
70% iodine alcohol	5 minutes
70% alcohol	2 minutes
50% alcohol	2 minutes
Tap water (running)	2 minutes
Distilled water	Rinse
5% aqueous iron-alum (mordant)	5 minutes at 30°C
Distilled water (2 changes)	Rinse
0.5 % haematoxylin	10 minutes
Differentiate in 1% aqueous iron-alum	Usually 3-5 minutes
Tap water (running)	15-20 minutes
50% alcohol	2 minutes
70% alcohol	2 minutes
95% alcohol	5 minutes
Isopropyl alcohol	2 changes of 5 minutes
Carbol-xylol	5 minutes
Xylol (2 changes)	5 minutes each

Mount in xylol-balsam, xylol-Damar or DPX mountant with a cover glass of No. 1 thickness.

Gomori's Trichrome Stain

Preferred permanent stain for routine diagnosis.

Staining Solution

To 100 ml distilled water, add 0.6 gm Chromotrope 2 R, 0.3 gm light green SF, 0.7 gm phosphotungstic acid, and 1 ml glacial acetic acid.

Procedure

Prepare slides as for haematoxylin staining. (Omit steps 1 and 2 for PVA-fixed specimens).

1. Immerse in Schaudinn's fixative	30 minutes at room temperature
2. 70% alcohol (wash)	15 minutes
3. 70% iodine alcohol	10 minutes
4. 70% alcohol (wash)	2 changes of 5 minutes
5. Trichrome stain	20 minutes
6. Acidified 90% alcohol (1% acetic acid)	2 dips
7. 95% alcohol	2 changes of 5 minutes
8. Carbol-xylene	2 minutes
9. Xylene	2 minutes

10. Mount immediately as for haematoxylin preparations.

Cultivation of Intestinal Protozoa

Numerous types of special media have been developed for the cultivation of the intestinal amoebae and flagellates as well as for the ciliate *Balantidium coli*. Among these are Boeck-Drbohlav-Locke-egg serum medium, Nelson's egg yolk infusion-liver extract medium, and Dobelle's medium which contains serum, egg albumin and starch. The parasite (*E. histolytica*) grows in 24 to 36 hours at 37°C. The morphological character of the colony is quite typical of the species.

THE CULTIVATION OF FREE-LIVING JUVENILES OF ANCYLOSTOMA DUODENALE AND STRONGYLOIDES STERCORALIS is done on sterilised sand or charcoal paste. Samples of soil or feces containing ova are mixed with equal quantity of sterilised fine sand or animal charcoal and water to make a thick paste. The paste is kept on a filter paper in a petridish and covered with lid. It is kept at 25 to 30°C for several days. The free-living juveniles collect in the water of condensation.

Urine

Collect urine in a clean, dry container, avoiding faecal contamination. Study centrifuged sediment. Trophozoites of *Trichomonas vaginalis*, unhatched eggs of *Schistosoma haematobium*, and intact scoleces or hooklets of *Echinococcus granulosus* may appear in the urine. Viable *S. haematobium* eggs will hatch only after dilution of urine.

Sputum

Examine for parasites as a direct smear under a cover glass. If the sputum is thick, bloody, or pus-laden, mix with equal volume 1-2% sodium hydroxide. Stir, let settle, and study sediment. Larvae of *Strongyloides stercoralis*, scoleces of *Echinococcus granulosus*, eggs of *P. westermani*, or migrating nematode larvae may be present in the sputum. Charcot-Leyden crystals and eosinophils can also be observed in wet mounts or after wet fixation and staining.

Gastric Washings: For night-swallowed sputum will often yield *Paragonimus* eggs or migrating nematode larvae better than will sputum or faeces (owing to less detritus).

Duodenal aspirates: These are useful for nematode eggs and are particularly helpful for eggs of *Clonorchis* and other bile-dwelling parasites.

Spinal Fluid

Examine centrifugate directly under the microscope. Make smears, stain with Giemsa's stain and examine. Culture some of the sediment, as for blood. Inoculate guinea pigs or mice if necessary.

Vaginal Secretions

Wet preparation may be examined directly for *Trichomonas vaginalis*. Cultures can also be made.

Graham Cellulose Tape Technique for Diagnosis of Enterobiasis

With the help of a tongue depressor, press the adhesive side of a small strip or loop of cellulose tape (e.g. Scotch tape) over the anal and perianal surfaces, preferably at night. Then place tape with adhesive side down in a drop of toluene on a microscopic slide. Examine for eggs or worms which have adhered to the tape.

BLOOD

Combined Thin and Thick Films

Making Films

Cleanse finger, ear lobe, heel, or toe (of children) thoroughly with spirit and allow to dry. Prick skin deeply to cause a few drops of blood to flow freely. On one end of a meticulously clean slide free of fingerprints or oil film, make a thin smear as for a blood count. For the preparation of the thick film, deposit a large drop of blood at the other end of the slide and spread it out evenly with the corner of another slide to a diameter of about 20 mm. The film should not be too thick since it may crack and peel when dry. Dry the slide in a flat position so that the distribution of blood will be even. Protect from dust and insects, avoid excessive heat. Allow to dry in air for at least 8-12 hours or for 2 hours in an incubator at 37°C. Keep free from dust or contamination with excreta of flies or roaches. Stain as soon as practicable, freshly stained material gives distinctly superior results.

Staining Films

Fix thin-filmed end of slide in methanol for 2-3 minutes. *The thick films must not be fixed.* Immerse slides for 30 minutes in a mixture of 1 drop of concentrated Giemsa's stain to each ml of phosphate-buffered distilled water (pH 7.2). Wash off with buffered water and dry in air. Examine with oil immersion objective. Haematoxylin or methylene blue stain is preferred for microfilariae since nuclear detail and sheaths (if present) stain more distinctly.

Concentration of Microfilariae

Haemolyse 10 ml or more of citrated blood with 50 ml of a 2% solution of a saponin in physiologic saline. Centrifuge and examine the sediment. Chylous urine and scrotal aspirates should always be centrifuged to attempt recovery of microfilariae.

Bone Marrow Smear

For a proper diagnosis of kala azar, bone marrow smear obtained by sternal puncture is essential. The Leishman's stain or Giemsa's stain are used for this purpose. Microscopic examination under oil immersion show the presence of intracellular oval bodies containing blue-stained cytoplasm and pink-stained rod-like kinetoplast.

Serological Tests

Serum samples obtained from the patients are used for following tests in certain parasitic infections:

1. *Precipitation:* It is done for trichinelliasis, hydatid disease and cysticercosis.
2. *Flocculation test*: Slide flocculation tests are useful for trichinelliasis and schistosomiasis.
3. *Complement fixation test*: This test is used in several parasitic infections for detecting complement fixing antibodies, but this is of special value in cases of schistosomiasis, trichinelliasis, hydatid disease, nonpulmonary paragonimiasis, and toxoplasmosis.
4. *Fluorescent antibody test (FAT)*: This test is applied to demonstrate the presence of parasites or their specific antibodies in tissue or in the blood of the patient, e.g. *Toxoplasma gondii* and *Entamoeba histolytica.*
5. ELISA tests now are available for most parasitic infestations.
6. Immunochromatography technique based kit.

Intradermal Tests

These are done to demonstrate allergic state in certain parasitic diseases. The antigen of the suspected parasite is injected intradermally and in positive cases, wheal or induration results. These tests are useful for hydatid disease (Casoni's test), trichinelliasis, filariasis, chronic schistosomiasis and toxoplasmosis.

Casoni's Test

It was first developed by Casoni in 1911. Intradermal injection of 0.2 ml on flexor aspect of right arm of a fresh sterile hydatid fluid (sterilised by Seitz filter) produces within half an hour in all positive cases a large wheal (5 cm in diameter) with multiple pseudopodia, it fades in an hour.

A delayed reaction appears after 18 to 24 hours characterised by oedema and induration 5-6 cm surrounding the site of injection. A negative reaction does not exclude echinococcal infection. The test usually becomes positive 8-12 weeks after infection and remains positive after surgical removal of cyst from the patient.

Hydatid fluid from human cases (removed operatively) or from animals (obtained from a slaughter house) is used as an antigen. While 0.2 ml of antigen is injected to one arm, sterile normal saline 0.2 ml is injected in the other arm for control.

Muscle Biopsy for *Trichinella spiralis*

Small pieces of deltoid, biceps, or gastrocnemius muscle are removed from the vicinity of their tendinous attachment under local anaesthesia.

1. Microscopically examine small pieces of muscle compressed between 2 glass slides for encysting or encysted larvae.

2. Digest muscle in artificial gastric juice (pepsin and hydrochloric acid) and examine sediment for motile larvae.

OVERVIEW OF MALARIA AND ITS DIAGNOSIS

Introduction

Malaria is widespread, especially in hot, humid tropical and subtropical countries of the world. It is most common between 23.5° North latitude and 23.5° South latitude, which include regions of Africa, Asia, South America, Central America, the Caribbean and some isolated parts of North America (Fig. 8.1).

Globally, approximately 300 million new cases occur every year, of which 2.7 million are fatal.

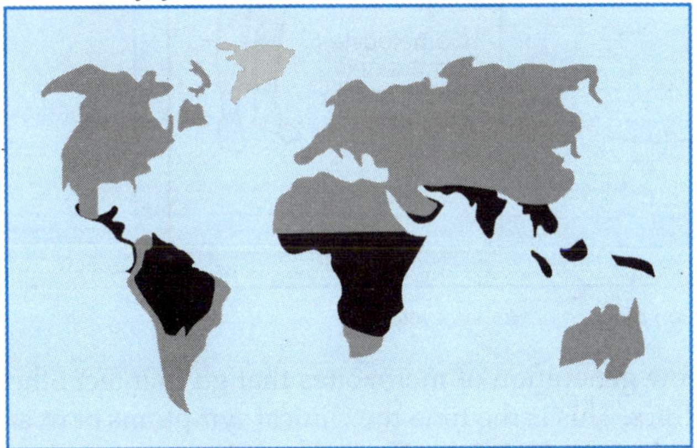

Fig. 8.1 : Geographical distribution of malaria infection

Malaria in humans is caused by the four species of the *Plasmodium* parasites; *P. vivax, P. falciparum, P. malariae* and *P. ovale.*

The tropical zone is the endemic home of all malaria parasites. *P. malariae* is a parasite of the subtropic zone. *P. vivax* is the prevalent species in the temperate zone. The distribution of *P. ovale* has been reported mainly from East Africa, West Africa and from the Philippines in Asia.

Plasmodium falciparum is the most common species in tropical areas and is transmitted primarily during the rainy season. This species is the most dangerous, accounting for half of all clinical cases of malaria and 90 percent of deaths from the disease. *P. vivax* is the most widely distributed parasite, existing in temperate as well as tropical climates. *P. malariae* can also be found in temperate and tropical climates but is less common than *P. vivax*.

P. ovale is a relatively rare parasite, restricted to tropical climate and is found primarily in eastern Africa.

Climatic changes, human migration and drug resistance are the key factors that affect the rapid spread of malaria all over the world.

Historical Perspectives

The word *malaria* (*mal* = bad; *aria* = air) is based on the association between the bad air of marshes (where the anopheline mosquito vector breeds) and human infection by malaria parasites, *Plasmodium* species. Malaria has afflicted humankind since millenia and continues to do so till today. Examination of the primate malarias suggests that human plasmodia have evolved together with their hosts from the plasmodia of primates. This hypothesis is supported by the remarkable similarities between several primate malarial parasites (*Plasmodium reichenowi, P. cynomolgi* and *P. brasilianum*) and their human counterparts (*P. falciparum, P. vivax* and *P. malariae* respectively).

In terms of recorded history, the earliest references to malaria are descriptions of splenomegaly with fever from China in the *Nei Ching Canon of Medicine* in 1700 BC and from Egypt in the *Ebers Papyrus* in 1570 BC. Hippocrates clearly recognised the syndrome of malaria and its relationship to marshes. Literary references to malaria appear in Homer's *Iliad* and in the works of Chaucer and Shakespeare. Incidentally, that malarial parasite infects RBCs, was discovered by Ross (a British researcher) in India itself.

Today, malaria remains an overwhelming problem in tropical developing countries (with 300 to 500 million cases and 2 to 3 million deaths per year) and a potentially life-threatening complication for travellers to the tropics.

Malaria Life Cycle

Plasmodium parasites undergo many stages of development, and their life cycle is completed in two hosts, viz; humans and mosquitoes (Fig. 8.2). The parasites are transmitted to humans by female mosquitoes of the genus *Anopheles.* About 60 of the 390 species of *Anopheles* mosquito transmit the malaria parasite. Of these, only a dozen species are important in the transmission of malaria worldwide. Usually, just one or two species play a role in malaria transmission in a particular region where the disease is prevalent. Malaria transmission begins when a female mosquito bites a human already infected with the malaria parasite. The mosquito ingests blood

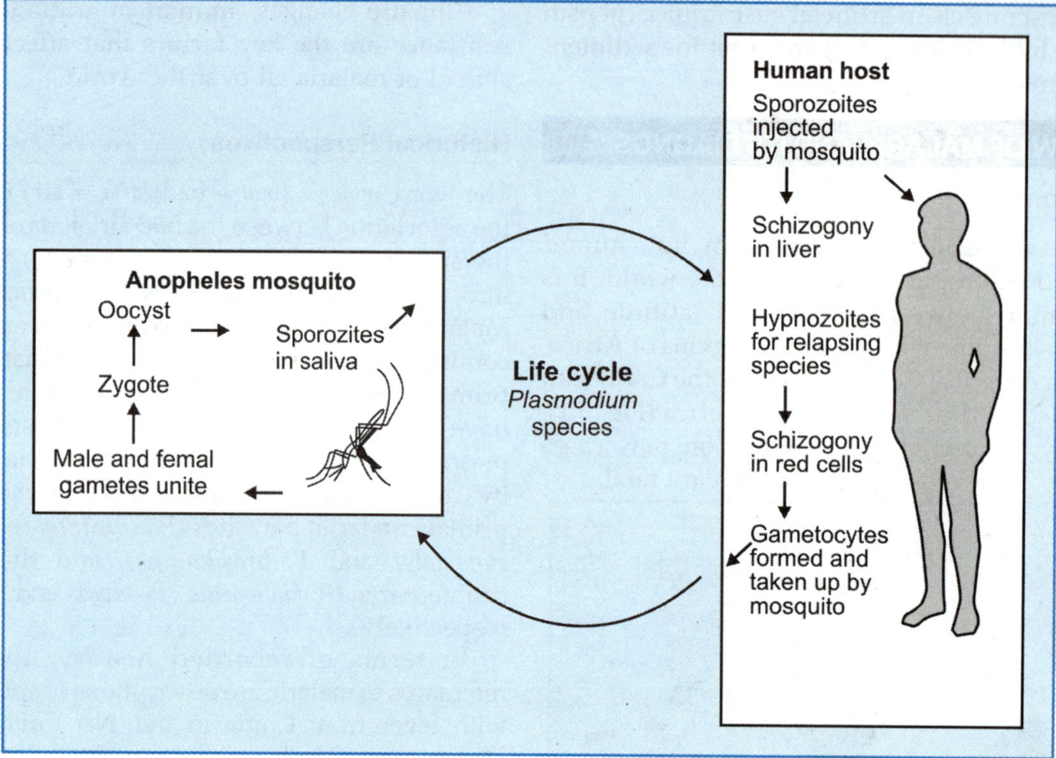

Fig. 8.2: Diagrammatic representation of *Plasmodium* life cycle

containing immature male and female gametes (sex cells) of the malaria parasite. Inside the mosquito's stomach, the gametes quickly mature. A male gamete fuses with a female gamete to produce a cell known as zygote. The zygote enters the wall of the mosquito's gut and develops into an oocyst. The oocyst multiplies to produce thousands of cells known as sporozoites. The sporozoites leave the wall of the gut and migrate to the mosquito's salivary glands. The mosquito phase of the malaria parasite's life cycle is normally completed in 10 to 14 days. This development process occurs more slowly in areas with cooler temperatures. Sporozoite development of *P. falciparum* is slowed down particularly by low temperatures, preventing transmission of this parasite in temperate climates except during summer.

When the infected mosquitobites another human, sporozoites in the mosquito's saliva are transferred to the blood of the human. Sporozoites travel through the blood to the liver. In liver cells, over the course of one to two weeks, the sporozoites divide repeatedly to form 30,000 to 40,000 merozoites. The merozoites leave the liver to enter the bloodstream, where they invade RBCs. Inside these blood cells, the merozoites multiply rapidly until they force the red cells to burst, releasing into the bloodstream a new generation of merozoites that go to infect other RBCs. This is the time the clinical symptoms of overt malaria in the infected individuals become apparent. Some merozoites divide to form gametocytes, i.e. immature male and female gametes. If another mosquito bites the human and ingests these gametocytes, the life cycle of the malaria parasite begins again.

Malaria and *Plasmodium* Species

Out of the total occurrence of malaria cases globally, it is estimated that about 40% are caused by *P. falciparum*, about 50% caused by *P. vivax*, about 7-8% caused by *P. malariae* and the rest by *P. ovale*.

In India, it is estimated that about 60% of the infections are due to *P. vivax* and 40% of the infections are due to *P. falciparum*. *P. malariae* in India is said to be responsible for less than 1% infections. In India, it is also estimated that about 4-8% of the malaria infections are of the mixed type, involving more than one parasite, usually *P. vivax* and *P. falciparum*.

The *P. ovale* has an exoerythrocytic cycle in the liver, similar to the *P. vivax* and the hypnozoites situated in the liver can cause a relapse.

P. malariae does not have an exoerythrocytic cycle like the *P. vivax* and *P. ovale* and in this sense is similar to *P. falciparum*. However, malaria caused by *P. malariae* is of a benign type, whereas the one caused by *P. falciparum* is severe and of the malignant type.

P. falciparum malaria (due to the mortality and morbidity associated with it) and *P. vivax* (due to the morbidity and high infection and relapse rates) are still considered to be the "Big Two" and logically have also become the targets for prevention, eradication, diagnosis and treatment.

DISTRIBUTION OF MALARIAL DISEASE BY AGE AND SEX

South and East Asia and the Western Pacific

In most of this region, including the Mekong countries, China, Indonesia, the Philippines, India, and Sri Lanka, the incidence of malarial infection is spread throughout life. The incidence of *P. falciparum* tends to peak broadly between 10-40 years of age and that of *P. vivax* more sharply and earlier, when the patient is aged approximately 2-15 years. Point prevalence of either species in the age groups at highest risk tends to be approximately 0.3-3%. In the economically most productive age group of people approximately 15-50 years of age, the risk of malarial infection in boys and men relative to girls and women is between 1.3:1 and 2.5:1 and this is due to differences in occupation that place men at a higher risk of exposure to infection.

A major exception to the said generalisation concerning malaria risk is the situation of pregnant women, who are at a generally higher risk of developing malarial disease and at 3 times the risk of developing severe malaria than nonpregnant women or men of the same age when they become infected with *P. falciparum*. The risk of acquiring even *P. vivax* has been found to be greater in the pregnant than nonpregnant state, although there is no associated risk of severe complications during pregnancy.

Within the Pacific region, the islands of Papua New Guinea, the Solomon Islands, and the Vanuatu Islands have much higher levels of malaria transmission, and the above mentioned generalisations do not apply. Peak prevalences of *P. vivax* lie between 1-15 years, much as elsewhere in the region, whereas peak prevalences of *P. falciparum* fall between 5-20 years of age. Within the age groups at highest risk, however, the point prevalence of both *P. vivax* and *P. falciparum* are very much greater than elsewhere in the region, generally 5-50% for either species. Differences between sexes in risk of malaria are probably less marked than in the other countries of the region.

Eastern Mediterranean

Malaria transmission rates are, with the exception of those in Sudan, relatively low throughout this region, and the incidence of malaria and risk of death from malaria can be expected to be spread throughout life, but mainly in early adulthood and middle age. For occupational reasons, the risks of malaria and of death from malaria can be expected to be several times greater in men than in women.

North and South America

Transmission intensities of malaria are generally low to moderate in this region, and incidence of malaria can generally be expected to be spread throughout life in most settings, with the peaks occurring in early adulthood. In a few areas, namely French Guiana, Guyana, and Surinam, transmission intensities are relatively very high (mainly *P. falciparum*); the incidence of malaria can be expected to be highest in early childhood and low in adolescence and adulthood. Elsewhere, transmission intensities are low (mainly *P. vivax*), and point prevalence is generally much less than 1%. Risk of malaria spreads throughout life, but young and middle-age adults are at the highest risk—especially men, who, for occupational reasons, may be at 2-3 times the risk of acquiring malaria infection than women.

Africa

Ninety per cent of global mortality on account of malaria occurs in Africa, mainly in children and pregnant women.

Among the 4 species of malaria parasite that infect humans, *P. vivax* and *P. falciparum* vie for greatest prevalence in the world today. Of these 2 species, *P. falciparum* is justifiably regarded as the greater menace because of the high levels of mortality with which it is associated, its widespread resistance to antimalarial drugs, and its dominance on the world's most malarious continent. However, malaria due to *P. vivax* has also placed huge burdens on the health, longevity and general prosperity of large sections of the human population.

Clinical Malaria

Incubation Time

The time interval between mosquito bite and development of malaria is 8-14 days except in *P. malariae* (35 days).

Typical Presentations

Initially, the symptoms in patients resemble those of a minor viral illness such as: lack of sense of well being, headache, fatigue, abdominal discomfort, muscular aches followed by fever and nausea/ vomiting.

These may be followed by typical malaria picture such as fever spikes (sudden rise and fall in temperature), chills and rigours.

Cold Stage

As the temperature begins to rise, there is intense headache and muscular discomfort. The patient feels cold, clutches blankets and curls up shivering and uncommunicative (the rigour). Within minutes, the limbs begin to shake and teeth chatter, and the temperature climbs rapidly to a peak. This phase usually lasts for 10-30 minutes but can last up to 90 minutes.

Hot stage

By the end of rigour there is peripheral vasodilatation and the skin feels hot and dry. The temperature is high.

Sweating

Profuse sweat then breaks out. It lasts for up to 2-4 hours. The patient is soaked in sweat and the temperature falls. The blood pressure is relatively low (vasodilation). The patient feels exhausted and may sleep. Defervescence usually takes 4-8 hours. Fever is irregular at first with temperature exceeding 39°C, however, it may rise up to 40°C.

If the Infection is Left Untreated

- Fever recurs every third day in *P. vivax* and *P. ovale* infection establishing a 2-day cycle (tertian).
- Spike occurs every three days (quartan) in *P. malariae* infection, i.e. fever every fourth day.
- The pattern of fever in *P. falciparum* infection is erratic.

  Paroxysms with rigours are more common in *P. vivax* and *P. ovale* than in *P. falciparum* and *P. malariae* malaria. True rigours are unusual in naturally acquired falciparum malaria.
- As the infection continues, the spleen and liver enlarge (hepatosplenomegaly) and anaemia develops. The patient loses weight. If no treatment is given the natural infection stabilizes for several weeks or months and then gradually resolves.

Relapse

Relapse is the return of a disease after its apparent cessation. Both *P. vivax* and *P. ovale* have a tendency to relapse after resolution of a primary infection. Relapses occur weeks or months after the primary infection.

Recrudescence

Recrudescence is the recurrence of symptoms after temporary abatement. The chief distinction between a recrudescence and relapse is the time interval, a recrudescence occurring after a few days or weeks, a relapse after some weeks or months. *P. falciparum* is the usual cause of recrudescence infection and these arise 2-4 weeks following treatment.

COMPLICATIONS IN MALARIA

Severe Falciparum Malaria

Severe, often life-threatening malaria is nearly always caused by *P. falciparum.* The following conditions have been proposed as manifestations of severe falciparum malaria by a working group convened by the World Health Organization (WHO):

1. **Cerebral malaria:** The clinical symptoms of cerebral malaria are coma, convulsions, severe anaemia (particularly in children), muscle tone may be increased or decreased, fever, jaundice (adults), enlarged liver and spleen, retinal hemorrhage on ophthalmoscopy. Untreated cerebral malaria is probably uniformly fatal. Overall mortality in treated cerebral malaria in reported studies average 15% in children and 20% in adults (but up to 50% in pregnant women).
2. **Hypoglycaemia**
   - May be asymptomatic.
   - May present as further deterioration in the level of coma.

3. **Pulmonary oedema**
   - Hyperventilation (respiratory distress).
4. **Acute renal failure**
   - Common complication of malaria in adults living in areas of low or unstable transmission.
   - Oliguria or polyuria.
   - Jaundice.
   - Bleeding tendency.
5. **Metabolic acidosis**
   - Hyperventilation with increased inspiratory effort.
   - Hypotension.
6. **Blackwater fever:** It is a condition where:
   - After several bouts of falciparum malaria, particularly if there has been inadequate treatment, there is occasionally an abrupt onset of massive intravascular haemolysis with fever, chills and prostration.
   - The haemoglobin escapes into the urine turning it black, if the urine is acidic. Hence, the designation—Blackwater fever.
7. **Algid malaria** It is a malarial condition where:
   - There may be subnormal temperature, weakness, prostration, feeling cold, vomiting, loose motions, rapid respiration and oliguria.
   - Death may occur but the patient is conscious till the end.
   - It could be due to adrenal crisis, absorption of endotoxin from the gut or cachectin-tumour necrosis factors from endotoxin activated macrophages.
8. **Malaria in pregnancy**
   - There is increased risk of severe falciparum malaria in the second and third trimesters of pregnancy.
   - In areas of reduced or diminished transmission, it is an important cause of foetal death and results in high maternal mortality.
   - In areas of intense transmission, it may be associated with low birth weight. The infected mothers may be asymptomatic.
9. **Malaria in children:** The majority of childhood malaria infections present with fever and malaise. In addition to the clinical features mentioned for adults, malaria in children may lead to convulsions, coma, hypoglycaemia, metabolic acidosis and severe anaemia.

In highly endemic areas, the patient may be infected with one, two or even more species of the malaria parasite.

Tropical splenomegaly syndrome (TSS) is often the result of chronic malaria and has its own attendent complications.

Differentiating Features of the "Big Two" (*P. vivax* and *P. falciparum* malaria)

S. No.	*P. vivax*	*P. falciparum*
1	*P. vivax* is relatively **benign** and rarely produces serious complications or death.	*P. falciparum* on the other hand, is associated with **serious complications**, e.g. cerebral malaria, jaundice, renal failure, etc. including high mortality.
2	In *P. vivax*, **relapse occurs** due to persistence of inactive forms (hypnozoites) in liver tissues which periodically invade bloodstream producing clinical malaria.	*P. falciparum* does not have any dormant form in liver and once the infection is cured, there is **no relapse.**
3	In *P. vivax* malaria, less than 1% of **RBCs** are parasitised.	In *P. falciparum*, the number of **RBCs** involved may go up to 35%.
4	Mainly the young RBCs are infected.	Infects young and old erythrocytes alike.
5	The **gametocytes** (sexual stage) —male and female mature in **peripheral blood** and are sucked up by the female *Anopheles* mosquito for completion of their life cycle.	For maturation of gametocytes, *P. falciparum* **must invade deeper circulation.** The blood capillaries of internal organs get clogged with infected RBCs thus obstructing flow of blood. Also some biochemical changes take place which damage the organs.
6	Gametocytic stage persists in the peripheral blood for 2 days.	Gametocytes persist in the blood for **30-60** days or more.

Drug-Resistant Malaria

- Literally speaking, drug-resistant malaria means malaria caused by a *Plasmodium* species that is resistant to the usual antimalarial drugs.
- Although chloroquine-resistant strains of *P. vivax* have been described, drug resistance poses a serious clinical problem only with *P. falciparum*, which accounts for over 70% of cases and much of the mortality associated with human malaria.

Indian Scenario of Drug-Resistant Malaria

- Of the two plasmodia which cause malaria in India, incidence of drug resistance is more common with *P. falciparum*.
- Occasionally, *P. vivax* may also be drug resistant and this occurs specially as a result of improper treatment and inadequate dosage.
- Originally, both the *Plasmodia—vivax* and *falciparum*—were sensitive to chloroquine, but, in recent years, more and more *P. falciparum* are developing resistance against chloroquine.
- To overcome this problem of chloroquine resistance, sulphadoxine, and pyrimethamine combinations were used. But very soon, some strains of falciparum developed resistance to this combination also.
- *P. falciparum* resistant to traditional drugs like Quinine have also been reported.

- Incidence of drug-resistant malaria in India will be difficult to know because in many cases it may not be recorded.
- Resurgence of *P. falciparum* resistant to chloroquine has been reported from several regions of India. Earlier reports indicated chloroquine resistance to *P. falciparum* in North Eastern parts of the country with new foci of drug resistance being added gradually.

However, for all practical purposes, drug resistant malaria in the Indian context means malaria caused by strains of *P. falciparum* which are resistant to chloroquine.

Clinical and Laboratory Diagnosis of Malaria

Several approaches have been adopted to detect malaria.

Clinical Diagnosis

Clinical diagnosis is still the most widely used approach in the developing world, particularly in rural areas and in the peripheral health care system that lack laboratory facilities. Inhabitants of endemic areas are sometimes familiar with the symptomatology and frequently, self-diagnose malaria. Though pure clinical diagnosis is inexpensive to perform, since the malaria symptoms are non-specific and mimic other febrile illnesses, diagnosis and treatment of malaria on clinical basis alone is unreliable and should be supported by laboratory test results as far as possible.

Microscopic Diagnosis

Microscopy of thin and thick blood smears for detecting malarial parasites with nonspecific chemical stains is still the frontline and established method for the laboratory diagnosis and confirmation of malaria.

Well-prepared and well-stained blood films read by careful and experienced microscopists is still considered as the gold standard for detecting and identifying malarial parasites. In the hands of an expert and skilled technician, microscopy can detect as low as 10 parasites per μl of blood. Apart from being helpful in speciation, morphological alterations can be read to assess the parasitaemia, as well as efficacy and response to chemotherapy. While microscopy is relatively inexpensive, it does suffer from a few important shortcomings, such as:

- In field conditions, typical microscopic procedures may not be able to detect parasitaemia under 100/μl of blood.
- Microscopy is labour-intensive and each slide may take about 60 minutes from blood collection to being read and may involve delay in providing results.
- Reliable microscopy results are dependent absolutely on individual microscopist's skills, techniques, microscopes and reagents which vary inherently, especially in the rural and peripheral areas, where the aforesaid variables may not be controlled well.
- Paradoxically, microscopy which is a 'gold standard' can be an unreliable tool that may lead to doubtful results.
- **Delay in providing results**, inherent variability of the method and risk of unreliability may infact revert the clinicians back to pure clinical diagnosis of the disease.

In view of the limitations of pure clinical diagnosis and the microscopic methods, a need has been felt for specific, simpler and rapid tests for laboratory diagnosis of malaria. Preferably, tests that are versatile enough to be used in:

- A cross section of laboratory settings
- Field conditions
- Simple to perform
- Independent of technician skill
- Rapid enough to accord the benefit of malaria laboratory results for diagnosis and treatment.

Key Factors Affecting Diagnosis and Treatment of Malaria

- Microscopic detection suffers from variability assay arising out of microscopist's skill, techniques, reagents and equipment.
- At least one hour needs to be spent by an expert microscopist to rule out negative smear results.
- Issues of due diligence *vs* urgency.
- Ability to speciate correctly.
- Patient history/especially travel details.
- Knowledge of the malaria species endemic to the area of travel and where the infection was contracted.
- Clinical picture of the patient.
- Rule out overlapping febrile illness.
- Drug regimen required for adequate effective treatment.
- Drug regimen required to prevent relapse/recrudescence.

- Geographical/drug resistance patterns.
- Follow-up of the patient to assess clearance of parasitaemia, rule out drug resistance, establish efficacy of treatment.

Rapid Diagnostic Tests for Malaria

Considering the expertise and skill that is required to detect and speciate malaria microscopically, there has been a pressing need to have sensitive and specific diagnostic tests to serve as simple and rapid tools for onsite diagnosis. Research efforts have been targeted specifically at this task. Advancements in protein purification, monoclonal antibody production as well as nitrocellulose membrane technology have lead to design and development of specific diagnostic platforms fulfiling this aim, in the form of rapid diagnostic tests, also popularly known as RDTs.

Isolation of Malaria Parasite Antigen

The discovery and isolation of many specific malarial parasite antigens from the blood of infected individuals and the development of corresponding antibodies raised and directed against these target parasite antigens have led to the development of several diagnostic platforms for the specific and rapid detection of malarial infection. The two most important antigenic markers targeted for detection by the rapid diagnostic tests are:

- Histidine-rich protein-II (HRP-II).
- Parasite lactate dehydrogenase (pLDH).

Antibodies to the Antigenic Markers of Malaria

To date, the following monoclonal antibodies have been raised to detect malarial specific antigens in human blood:

- Antibodies to HRP-II specific for *P. falciparum* malaria.
- Antibody to pLDH specific to *P. falciparum* malaria.
- Antibody to pLDH specific to *P. vivax* malaria.
- Antibodies to pan malaria pLDH co-specific to all four malarial species *P. vivax, P. falciparum, P. ovale* and *P. malariae*.

While antibodies specific to parasitic aldolase enzyme have also been raised, however, due to the poor sensitivity of the resultant test system, the use of aldolase has not found favour with manufacturers or users lately, as a marker for malaria.

Antibodies to HRP-II (*P. falciparum* specific antigen) and antibodies to *P. falciparum* specific pLDH and antibodies to pan pLDH (co-specific to pLDH for all malarial species) have been, in recent times, the back bone for assay design of all malaria rapid diagnostic tests being used currently.

Recently, development of monoclonal antibodies to *P. vivax* specific pLDH have opened up a new avenue for a better and more advanced assay design for the immunodiagnosis of malaria RDTs.

The malaria RDTs are grouped in terms of "generations" from the point of view of their ability to speciate between the different malarial infections.

First Generation Rapid Diagnostic Tests for Malaria

P. falciparum specific Histidine-Rich Protein-II (Pf. HRP II)-based Assays

HRP-II is a water-soluble protein produced by trophozoites and young (but not mature) gametocytes of *P. falciparum.*

The amount of Pf. HRP-II increases throughout the intraerythrocytic cycle of the infection, with the largest amount being released during schizont rupture. On an average, 9-12 days after the mosquito bite, Pf. HRP-II is found in the circulation coinciding with the overt clinical malarial symptoms.

Pf. HRP-II based assays, which are well formulated, achieve sensitivity and specificity for *P. falciparum* malaria detection well in excess of 99% as compared to expert microscopy.

The test runs on a 5 μl whole blood sample. Results are obtained within 15 minutes. These 'first generation' tests are in intensive use by various international organisations for RBM programmes, NGOs and laboratarians globally.

These tests are available in a cassette as well as a dipstick format.

Principle of Pf. HRP-II Based Assays

Pf. HRP-II utilises the principle of immunochromatography. As the test sample flows through the membrane assembly of the dipstick or device, after placing the clearing buffer, the coloured anti-Pf. HRP-II antibody-colloidal gold conjugate (monoclonal) complexes with the Pf. HRP-II in the lysed sample.

This complex moves further on the membrane to the test region where it is immobilised by the anti-Pf. HRP-II (monoclonal) antibody coated on the membrane leading to formation of a pink coloured band which confirms a positive test result.

Absence of this coloured band in the test region indicates a negative test result. The unreacted conjugate and unbound complex if any, moves further on the membrane and is subsequently absorbed at the soak pad. Antirabbit antibodies coated on the membrane at the control region, react with the rabbit IgG travelling along with the unreacted/unbound complex, forming a pink band. This control band serves to validate the test performance (Fig. 8.4) .

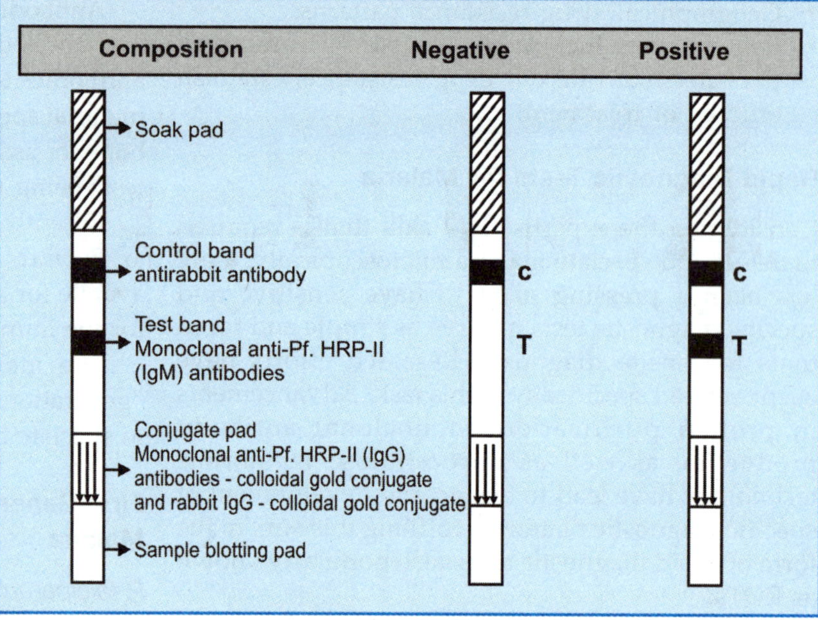

Fig. 8.4: Principle of HRP-II RDT.

Plasmodium Lactate Dehydrogenase (pLDH)

pLDH is a soluble intracellular metabolic glycolytic enzyme that is expressed at high levels by blood stage parasites. All the four human malaria parasites produce a specific and unique pLDH activity as well as co-specific pLDH activity that follows the level of parasitaemia in patient plasma as measured by microscopy.

pLDH is a good antigenic marker for active malarial infection. A panel of monoclonal antibodies raised against pLDH; when used in the right combination in the RDT, is capable of distinguishing and binding specifically pLDH isoforms from either *P. falciparum* or *P. vivax,* allowing pLDH-based malaria detection assays to correctly speciate *P. falciparum* from *non-P. falciparum* malaria in lysed whole blood samples. Antibody to pan malaria antigen, that is cospecific to pLDH from all malarial parasites *(P. vivax, P. falciparum, P. malariae.* and *P. ovale)* has also being utilised in the development of RDTs for malaria.

Principle of pLDH-Based Assays

1. HRP-II + pan pLDH Combination RDT

HRP-II + pan pLDH combination RDT for malaria utilises the principle of immunochromatography. As the test sample flows through the membrane assembly of the dipstick/device after addition of the clearing buffer, the coloured monoclonal anti-HRP-II/anti-pan specific pLDH colloidal gold conjugate antibody complexes with the HRP-II/pLDH in the lysed sample.

This complex moves further on the membrane to the test region where it is immobilised by the monoclonal anti-HRP-II/anti-pan specific pLDH antibody coated on the membrane leading to formation of purple coloured band/s which confirms a positive test result. While both bands appear at the test region in falciparum positive samples, only one band appears in nonfalciparum malaria positive samples.

Absence of this coloured band/s in the test region indicates a negative test result. The unreacted conjugate and unbound complex if any, move further on the membrane and are subsequently immobilised by antirabbit antibodies coated on the membrane at the control region, forming a purple band. This control band serves to validate the test performance (Fig. 8.5).

2. Pf. pLDH + pan pLDH Combination RDT

Pf. pLDH + pan specific pLDH combination are usually two-component systems comprising of a conjugate well and a test membrane dipstick and is based on the principle of immunochromatography. The conjugate well contains an indicator-tagged monoclonal antibody to pLDH, dried onto its surface. The anti-pLDH antibody is specific to all the isoenzymes LDH of the genus *Plasmodium* (pan pLDH).

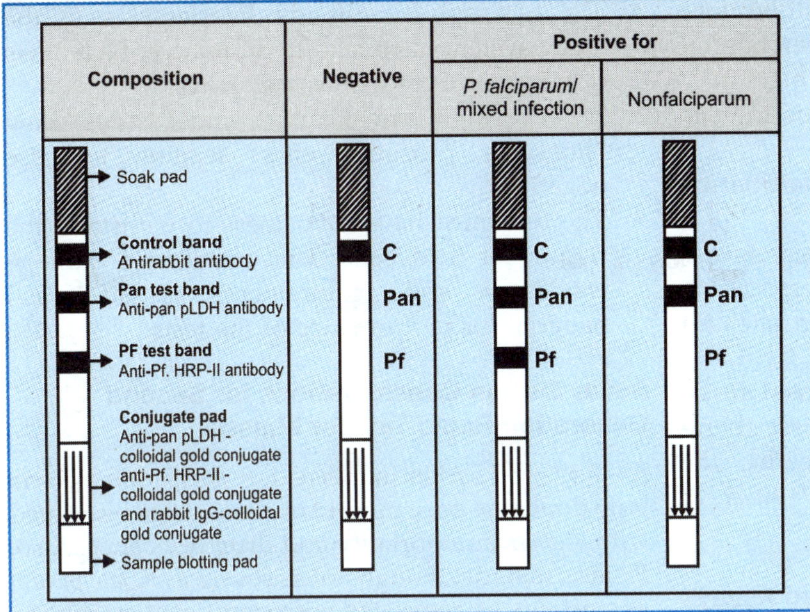

Fig. 8.5: Principle of HRP-II + pan pLDH RDT

The membrane assembly contains three regions each coated with monoclonal anti-pLDH specific to *P. falciparum;* monoclonal anti-pan pLDH and anti-mouse antibodies respectively.

The blood sample is added to the conjugate wells along with the lysing buffer. pLDH if present in the sample reacts with the anti-pLDH conjugate in the well and rises up the membrane dipstick where it is captured by anti-Pf. specific pLDH and/or anti-pan specific pLDH, causing the appearance of a coloured band at the respective regions.

Absence of band(s) at this region indicates a negative test result. The unreacted conjugate reacts with the antimouse antibodies at the control region and serves to validate the test performance (Fig. 8.6).

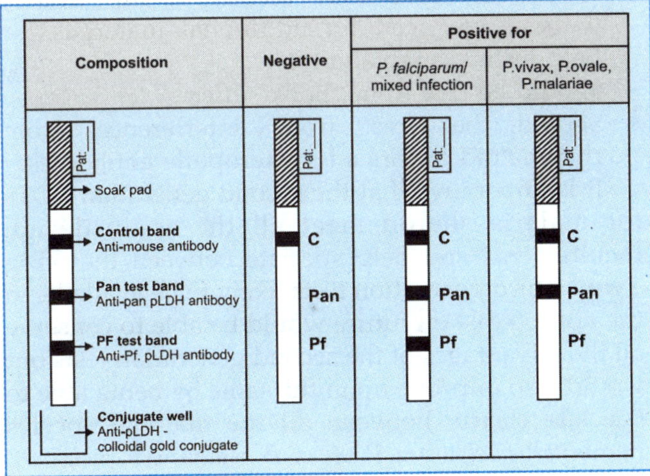

Fig. 8.6: Principle of Pf. pLDH + pan pLDH RDT

Limitations of First Generation Rapid Diagnostic Tests for Malaria

The stand alone rapid tests for *P. falciparum* malaria test based on HRP-II detection achieve excellent sensitivity and specificity, as reported in the published literatures, for the detection of *P. falciparum* malaria. However, they do suffer from the following limitations:

- The detection is limited to *P. falciparum* malaria only.
- These tests remain positive for 7-14 days following successful antimalarial therapy, even though these patients no longer have clinical symptoms or parasitaemia.
- Since HRP-II is secreted only in asexual erythrocytic schiozogony stage, the immunochromatographic tests that detect the presence of Pf. HRP-II would give a negative reaction if mature gametocytes are present due to the absence of the antigenemia (Pf. HRP-II).

On the other hand, tests for the detection of *P. falciparum* and differentiation of nonfalciparum malaria test based on *P. falciparum* specific pLDH and pan malaria cospecific pLDH have the following limitations:

- When the patient specimen is positive for *P. falciparum* malaria, the pan malarial band is also positive.
- Differentiation between *P. falciparum* infection and mixed infection is not possible.

- Speciation under microscopy must still be done for correct therapy, especially in hyperendemic areas where mixed infection rates are high.
- When *P. falciparum* band is negative and the pan band is positive
- The correct interpretation is "nonfalciparum malaria".
- In the absence of speciation under microscope, the presence of pan band has to be interpreted in the context of prevalence and infection rates for the other nonfalciparum species.
- *P. falciparum* negative samples still need to be speciated under microscopy for correct therapeutic decision to pinpoint as to whether the positivity of the pan band is due to *P. vivax, P. ovale* or *P. malariae.*

Experience with HRP-II and pLDH-Based Assays for the Detection of *P. falciparum* Malaria

Currently, first generation malaria tests based on stand alone detection of HRP-II for *P. falciparum* malaria and pLDH. *P. falciparum* and pan pLDH (nonfalciparum) combination tests are being used extensively for the detection of malaria globally. Experience of users in field settings as well as in reference labs as published in international journals of repute, have brought out a few important characteristics of antibodies to HRP-II vis-a-vis antibodies to pLDH for *P. falciparum* detection. These reports are summarised in "Summary of International Reports".

The general conclusions emerging out of the aforesaid reports are as follows:

- Tests for *P. falciparum* malaria based on detection of HRP-II have been on an overall basis found to have superior sensitivity as compared to tests based on *P. falciparum* specific pLDH.
- The detectability of *P. falciparum* infections with lower parasitaemia is better with HRP-II-based systems as compared to pLDH-based test systems.
- The tests utilising pan pLDH antibodies for detection of *P. vivax* malaria have a relatively poor sensitivity for *P. vivax* infection.
- Tests using similar antibodies to the malarial antigen may have different sensitivities and specificities probably due to overall system design competence amongst manufacturers.
- The heterophile antibody interferences in the assay system have lead to an unacceptable level of false positives with some assays.
- At very high parasitaemia, some assays show "hook or prozone" effect leading to false negatives.
- The test must have robustness to withstand the rigours of field conditions in terms of storage conditions and requirements of additional material for performance of the tests.

Assay Design Considerations for Second Generation Rapid Test for Malaria

As discussed earlier in this text, *P. falciparum* malaria is no doubt the most morbid of all malarias associated with significant mortality and drug resistance. Also, *P. vivax* malaria, though not as severe as *P. falciparum* in mortality, is associated with significant morbidity. Together, 90% of the malarial infections are caused by these two parasites leading to tremendous economic burden due to lost mandays and cost of therapy.

Thus, it is imperative that any advancements in rapid diagnostic tests of malaria should ideally speciate all four malarial species and if not, at least the **"Big Two"** that is *P. falciparum* and *P. vivax.*

Thus, a second generation test for malaria should:

- Speciate and differentiate between *P. falciparum* and *P. vivax* malaria.
- Should have good clinical sensitivity for *P. falciparum* and *P. vivax* malaria.
- Should also be able to monitor success of anti-malarial therapy.
- Should be stable at ambient temperatures, without the need for additional materials for field testing adaptability.
- Should be free from "hook" effect.
- Should be free from interference from rheumatoid factors and heterophile antibodies.

It is imperative that the second generation RDTs for malaria should meet all the assay design requirements and help speciate between the **"Big Two"**. Third generation tests likely to be available in the not-too distant future would be able to conserve all the advantages of the second generation tests but would also improve upon the same by being able to speciate clearly between all the malarial species namely; *P. falciparum, P. vivax, P. ovale* and *P. malariae..*

Until such time, the choice and use of available formats of rapid diagnostic tests for malaria detection should be based on adequate evaluation of the existing health delivery systems as well as the species prevalence rates. Employment of the type of laboratory diagnosis for malaria, including the use of RDTs should be based on the following criteria:

- Prevalence rates of various species.
- Areas of epidemic malaria and in situation which call for rapid confirmation of the infection.
- Inadequate laboratory services (inexperienced and/or nonexpertise laboratory technicians).

Rapid Diagnostic Tests for Malaria: Formats—Pros and Cons

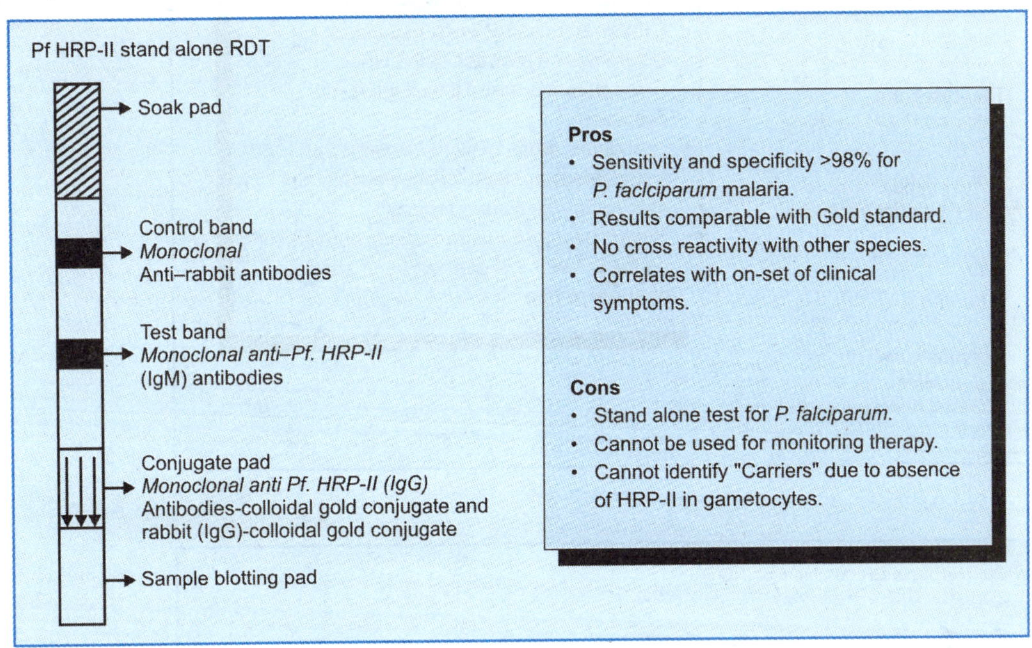

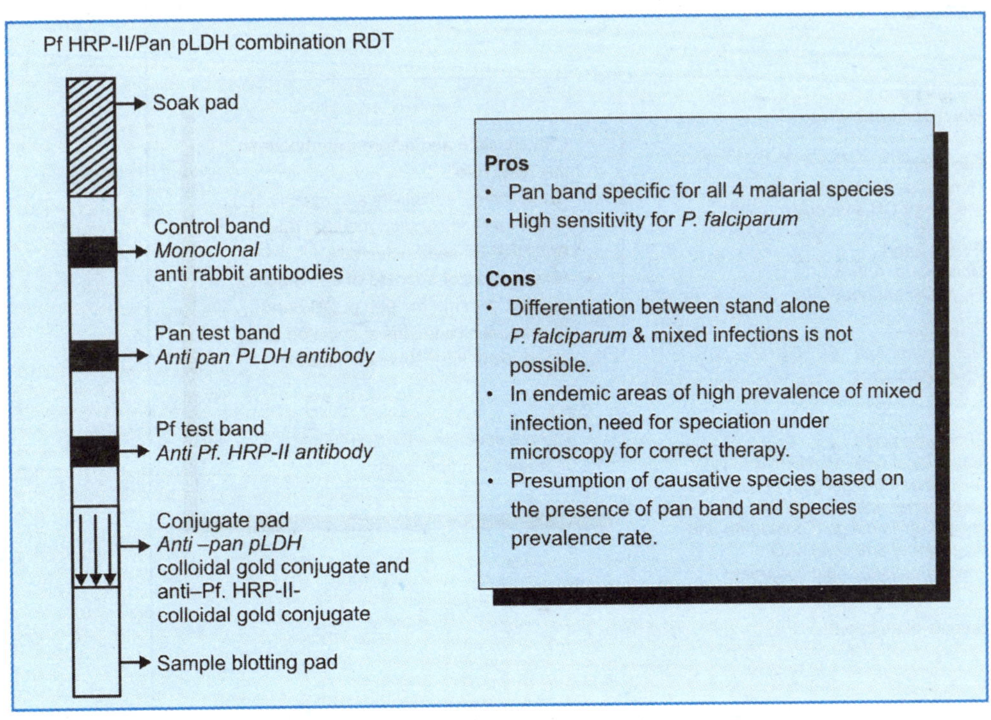

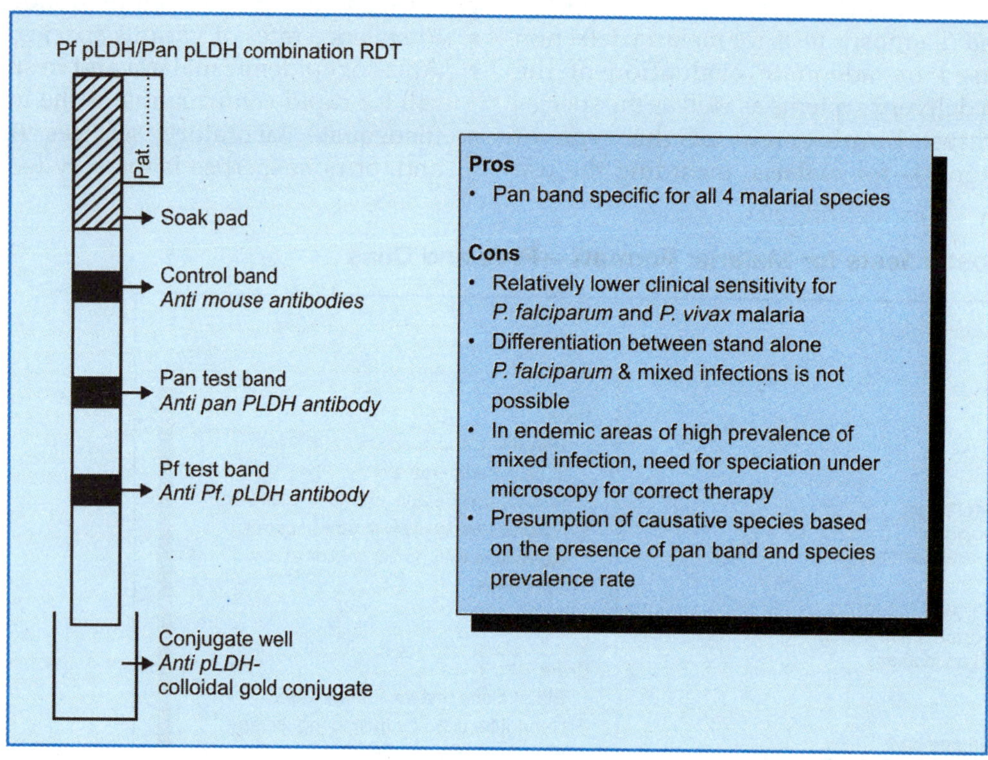
Pf pLDH/Pan pLDH combination RDT
Pat.
Soak pad
Control band
Anti mouse antibodies
Pan test band
Anti pan PLDH antibody
Pf test band
Anti Pf. pLDH antibody
Conjugate well
Anti pLDH-
colloidal gold conjugate
Pros
• Pan band specific for all 4 malarial species
Cons
• Relatively lower clinical sensitivity for P. falciparum and P. vivax malaria
• Differentiation between stand alone P. falciparum & mixed infections is not possible
• In endemic areas of high prevalence of mixed infection, need for speciation under microscopy for correct therapy
• Presumption of causative species based on the presence of pan band and species prevalence rate

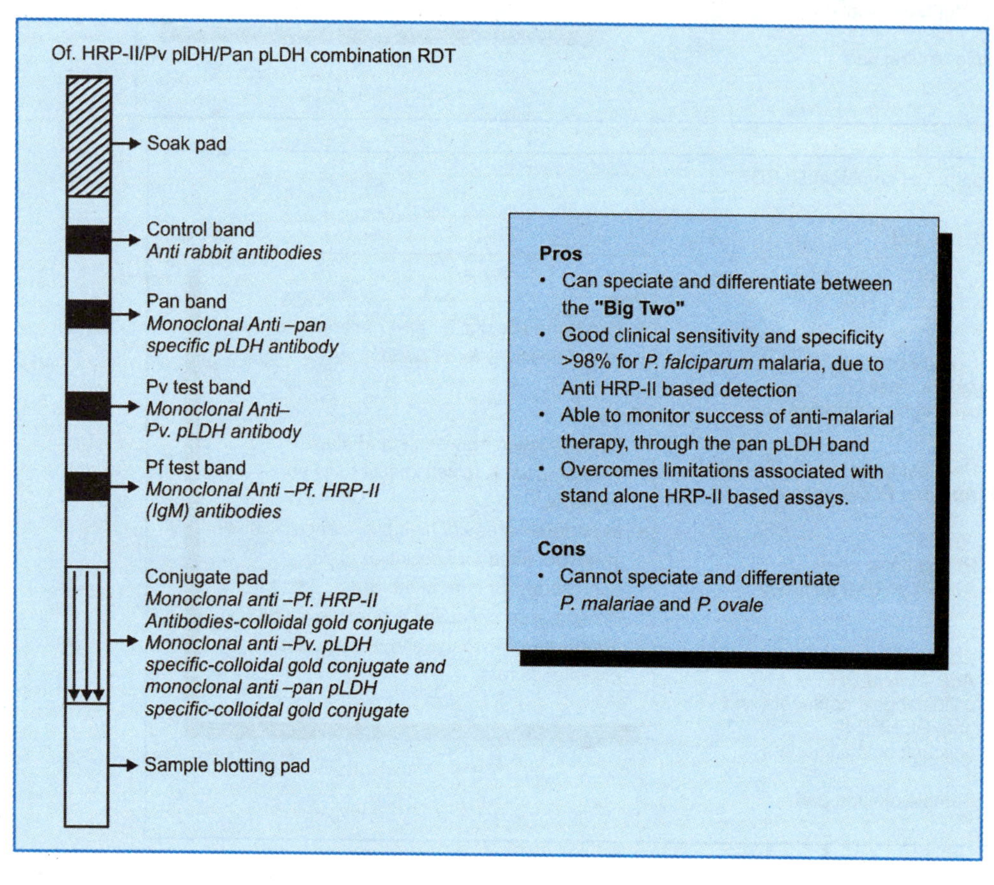
Of. HRP-II/Pv plDH/Pan pLDH combination RDT
Soak pad
Control band
Anti rabbit antibodies
Pan band
Monoclonal Anti –pan
specific pLDH antibody
Pv test band
Monoclonal Anti–
Pv. pLDH antibody
Pf test band
Monoclonal Anti –Pf. HRP-II
(IgM) antibodies
Conjugate pad
Monoclonal anti –Pf. HRP-II
Antibodies-colloidal gold conjugate
Monoclonal anti –Pv. pLDH
specific-colloidal gold conjugate and
monoclonal anti –pan pLDH
specific-colloidal gold conjugate
Sample blotting pad
Pros
• Can speciate and differentiate between the "Big Two"
• Good clinical sensitivity and specificity >98% for P. falciparum malaria, due to Anti HRP-II based detection
• Able to monitor success of anti-malarial therapy, through the pan pLDH band
• Overcomes limitations associated with stand alone HRP-II based assays.
Cons
• Cannot speciate and differentiate P. malariae and P. ovale

- Excessive time lag for diagnosis.
- Mobile clinics/on-field health workers.
- Severe and complicated malaria cases in which peripheral parasitaemia may be absent but wherein the rapid tests may be expected to provide evidence of antigenaemia.
- In malaria patients, a prompt and accurate diagnosis is the key to effective disease management. The two diagnostic approaches currently used most often, however, do not allow a satisfactory diagnosis of malaria. Clinical diagnosis, the most widely used approach, is unreliable because the symptoms of malaria are very nonspecific. Microscopic diagnosis, the established method for laboratory confirmation of malaria, presents technical and personnel requirements that cannot be met, particularly in facilities at the periphery of the health care system. In addition, delays in the provision of the microscopy results to the clinician mean that decisions on treatment may be taken without the benefit of the results.

Thus, the recent introduction of rapid diagnostic tests (RDTs) for malaria is of considerable interest.

It is expected that with the availability of second generation and third generation RDTs, detection, speciation and diagnosis of malaria would be simple and easier, leading to swift detection and treatment of malaria globally.

Management of Malaria

Management of clinical malaria (febrile episode)		*Prevention of relapse (for P. vivax)*
Uncomplicated	Complicated	
P. vivax / P. falciparum	*P falciparum*	
Chloroquine Sulphadoxine + Pyrimethamine Quinine sulphate (Tab)	Quinine Dihydrochloride inj. Halofantrine tabs Artemether/Artesunate/ Artemether/ Mefloquine	Primaquine

Management of Drug-resistant Malaria

Patients not seriously ill (Can take oral medications)	**Patients critically ill (Cannot take oral medications)**
Sulphadoxine/Pyrimethamine combination Quinine. Artemisinin and related compounds Mefloquine Amodiaquine (use limited because of severe hepatotoxicity)	Quinine diydrochloride inj. Artemether injection

General Prophylactic Drugs Used

- Chloroquine
- Chloroquine + Proguanil
- Mefloquine
- Doxycycline

Drugs in various combinations are used for treatment and prevention of further transmission of parasites. Many vaccines are also under clinical trials, to impart immunity against malarial infections.

CHAPTER 9

Clinical Haematology

The blood consists of a fluid of complicated and variable composition, the plasma, in which are suspended erythrocytes (red blood cells—RBCs), leucocytes (white blood cells—WBCs) and platelets. By using an anticoagulant, the formed elements can be separated from plasma. When blood coagulate, the fluid that remains after separation of the clot is called serum. Serum = Plasma—fibrinogen. The techniques of haematology are concerned mainly with the cellular formed elements of blood, their number or concentration, the relative distribution of various types of cells and the structural or biochemical abnormalities that promote disease.

WAYS OF OBTAINING BLOOD

Capillary or Peripheral Blood

For haematologic exercises, venous blood obtained from a vein is better. However, for total and differential blood counts and for haemoglobin estimation, blood can be taken by pricking: (i) the lobe of the ear, (ii) the palmar surfaces of the tip of the finger, (iii) in infants, from the plantar surface of the (a) heel or (b) the great toe. The puncture should be about 3 mm deep. An oedematous or a congested part should not be used. If the area to be punctured is cold and cyanotic, warm it by massaging or else erroneous results may be obtained. Clean the site with spirit or alcohol, let dry and puncture. Wipe off the first drop of blood, never press out blood. Having obtained the requisite amount of blood, let the patient apply slight pressure over the area with sterile swab (see Fig. 9.1).

Venous Blood (Venipuncture)

Reassure the patient about what is to be done. Inspect the veins, use a tourniquet if needed(see Fig. 9.2). Use a syringe of a size according to the amount of blood required. Needles of gauge less than 22 should be used and be 1 to 1½ inches long. Instead of a tourniquet, one can use a sphygmomanometer cuff, apply pressure that is midway between systolic and diastolic pressure. Ask the patient to open and close his fist several times. Take aseptic precautions, and puncture the vein. Sometimes, it may be difficult to obtain blood at the first instance, in such a case,

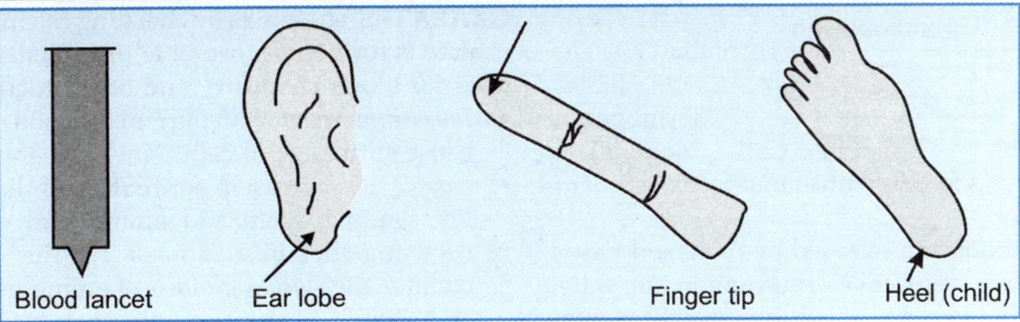

Fig. 9.1: Sites for obtaining-blood skin puncture

first the skin around the vein is punctured and then the vein is punctured, the moment needle enters the vein, blood flows back into the syringe. If still blood has not been obtained withdraw the needle and in many instances blood would be obtained. Having withdrawn blood, loosen the tourniquet and ask the patient to open his fist. Let the patient apply a sterile gauze piece with gentle pressure over the area. The patient should apply pressure gently with three fingers. Why three fingers? Simply because the site of skin puncture is not the same as the site of venipuncture. Make sure that the bleeding has stopped before the patient leaves. In infants blood may be secured from femoral or external jugular vein. Wash the syringe after dispensing the blood in the right container. Transfer blood from syringe into the container gently (not through the needle).

Complications

Immediate: Haematoma and syncope. Haematomas can be avoided by applying adequate gentle pressure at the site and for syncope a physician should be brought to take care. In any case, let the patient lie down if he or she is already not and raise the foot end. Some patients with a bleeding tendency may overbleed.

Late local complications: Thrombosis of the vein. Rarely thrombophlebitis may occur. Apply *Thrombophob*® if it happens.

Late-general complications: Transmission of serum hepatitis, AIDS by using contaminated needle and syringe.

Clinical Alert

1. If oozing from the puncture site is difficult to stop, elevate area and apply a pressure dressing. Stay with the patient until bleeding stops.
2. Never draw blood for any laboratory test from the same extremity that is being used for IV fluids, IV medications or blood transfusion.
3. In patients with leukaemia or agranulocytosis and in others with lowered resistance, the finger-prick and ear lobe puncture are more likely to cause infection than venipuncture. If capillary sample is necessary in these patients, the cleansing agent should remain in contact with the skin for 7 to 10 minutes. Alcohol is not bactericidal, povidone-iodine (*Betadine*®) is the cleansing agent of choice on leukaemic patients.

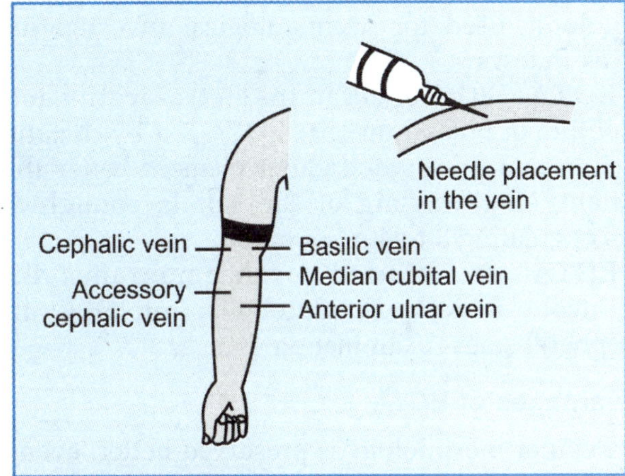

Fig. 9.2: Sites for obtaining blood by venipuncture from forearm

ANTICOAGULANTS

On letting blood stand, it clots after some time. Anticoagulants are agents that prevent clotting when mixed with blood in an appropriate proportion. The common pathway of the clotting mechanism is represented as under:

Prothrombin —Thromboplastin / Ca^{++}→ Thrombin

Fibrin ← Fibrinogen
(insoluble) Thrombin + Ca^{++} (soluble)

Fibrin with blood cells with entrapped constituents comprise a clot.

The thromboplastin released by damaged tissue, or platelets converts inactive prothrombin into active thrombin in the presence of calcium ions. Thrombin converts soluble fibrinogen into insoluble fibrin clot in the presence of calcium ions. Anticoagulants commonly used for haematological investigations are as follows.

EDTA (Ethylenediamine tetra-acetic acid, disodium or potassium salt). EDTA acts by chelating calcium and preserves cellular element better than oxalates. Eight(8) mg of the salt is enough for anticoagulating 3 to 4 ml of blood.

— EDTA can be used for haemograms, ESR (Wintrobe's method), platelet count, DLC and peripheral smear examination.

Advantages of EDTA

- Cellular morphology is preserved better, even 2-3 hours after blood collection
- As platelet clumping is prevented, EDTA is a better anticoagulant for platelet counts
- EDTA 2K salt is recommended for CBC, is more water soluble (1.5 $\pm$ 0.25 mg/ml of blood).

Disadvantages of EDTA

- When in excess, EDTA shrinks RBCs and leucocytes. If in excess of 2 mg/ml:
  - — PCV is significantly reduced
  - — MCHC is proportionately increased
  - — Platelets swell and disintegrate, therefore, a fallaciously high platelet count may be obtained
- It cannot be used for coagulometry applications

Making EDTA Bulbs

Four (4) gm of disodium or dipotassium salt is added to 100 ml of deionised water. About 0.2 ml of this solution is added to chemically clean vials, the vials are later kept in an incubator or hot air oven till complete liquid dries up (may take 1-2 hours at 60-80°C). White layer of anticoagulant can be seen at the bottom. This bulb is for 3-4 ml of blood, as it contains 8 mg of EDTA per vial.

OXALATES These acts by chelating calcium, calcium oxalate is formed as insoluble precipitate. These are used for blood chemistry and haematocrit.

- *Potassium oxalate* (2-3 mg/ml of blood) but it may cause shrinkage of cells. Not used anymore.
- *Double oxalate* used for ESR and haematocrit. Potassium oxalate and ammonium oxalate are used together in a ratio of 2:3, this is done to counter the swelling effect of ammonium oxalate and shrinking effect of potassium oxalate on the RBCs.
  - — *Double oxalates can be used for*
    - Hemoglobin, TLC, RBC count, ESR by Wintrobe's method and PC estimation.
  - — *Disadvantages*
    - Leucocytic morphology is not well preserved and hence not suitable for peripheral smear studies
    - The calcium chelated is precipitated in calcium oxalate which is a toxic substance, it is never to be used for blood banking applications

Making Double Oxalate Bulbs

Prepare double oxalate solution as follows:

1. Potassium oxalate 1.6 gm.
2. Ammonium oxalate 2.4 gm.
3. Deionised water 100 ml. Mix well, 0.2 ml of the solution will contain 8 mg of the oxalates which prevent clotting of about 3 to 4 ml of blood.
4. **Trisodium citrate** is used for ESR and some coagulation studies. This too acts by chelating calcium. For ESR, ratio is 1:4; while for coagulation studies ratio is 1:9. 1 part of 3.8% trisodium citrate and 4 or 9 parts of blood respectively.
5. **Heparin** (powder or liquid) acts by inhibiting thrombin and other stages of clotting factor activation.
6. **Special anticoagulants** include ACD (acid-citrate-dextrose) used in blood banking and fluoride and oxalate for sugar estimations. Other blood banking anticoagulants are also used.

WHEREVER POSSIBLE, THE NECESSARY TESTS, INVESTIGATIONS AND PREPARATION OF BLOOD FILMS SHOULD BE DONE IMMEDIATELY

If this is not possible, refrigerate the sample at 4°C. Before taking blood from the venous blood containers, invert them gently several times (60) or else unacceptable deterioration in precision may ensue.

Anticoagulated Blood Storage and Blood Cell Morphology

Peripheral Smears (anticoagulated or direct blood used and stored at 25 ± 5°C). Unfixed smears.

- Up to 60 minutes: No worthwhile notable change
- Up to 3 hours Few changes may be visible
- Up to 12-18 hours: Neutrophils are affected
  - — Lobes may get separated
  - — Cytoplasmic borders may appear ragged with small intracytoplasmic vacuolation
- Mononuclear cells may show cytoplasmic vacuolation, nuclear disintegration or budding
- RBCs do not change for up to 6 hours at room temperature (25 ± 5°C) but longer periods may cause progressive crenation and sphering.

EDTA Blood

- On storing EDTA blood, the following changes may occur:

— MCV increases
— Osmotic fragility increases
— Sedimentation rate gradually decreases
— TLC and platelet counts decrease
— Reticulocyte count decreases within 6 hours
— Haemoglobin remains unchanged if the sample does not get infected.

Diagnostic Alerts

- Perform all investigations as soon as the blood sample is taken
- Never freeze the sample. On storing the sample at 4°C, the deterioration rate slows down
- Perform all counts within 2 hours of blood collection
- Excessive EDTA in the sample will significantly lower TLC within 1-2 hours
- Leucocytic degenerative changes will affect automated differential counts
- A refrigerated sample must always be brought to room temperature before being used. All samples must be mixed gently, preferably by rotation, for at least 2 minutes before testing.

BLOOD COLLECTION SYSTEM

Whatever be the reason for obtaining blood, in the interest of the patient and your own interest, it is ideal and necessary to use sterile disposable blood collection systems, viz., disposable syringes or the Vacutainers. These are meant for single use and are to be discarded (never to be used again). New in our country, but established all over the world and being used for decades, is the Vacutainer blood collection system manufactured by *Becton Dickinson* (BD).

The Vacutainer system consists of a needle, a needle holder and a glass/plastic vacuum tube instead of the syringe barrel and plunger. Once the vein is punctured, the Vacutainer tube appropriately in contact with the needle, the requisite quantity of blood flows automatically into the Vacutainer tube so that the need to pull the plunger out is obviated. Vacutainer is simple to use, quicker, cleaner and safer. It offers—leakproof tubes, standardisation of specimen quality at high level, opportunity to rationalise laboratory procedures and innovative, high technology tubes. Appropriate anticoagulants, and other additives are pre-added in appropriate quantities so that all that is required is clean venipuncture. Containers also available for collecting blood from infants with the help of a skin puncture, these are called Microtainers. The blood so collected is adequate for micro or dry chemistries. From a single venipuncture, blood can be collected in separate Vacutainers (for different purposes—EDTA or oxalate-fluoride or citrate Vacutainers) meant for different purposes and very easily identified by the colour of their caps. The Vacutainer system is a cleaner system, as blood does not come in contact with atmosphere as it flows straight from the vein through the sterile needle into the sterile tube. The process of transferring blood from syringe to different bulbs is eliminated. Contamination from fallen blood is entirely removed. The incidence of haemolysis is significantly reduced because the major cause of it—the transfer of blood from the syringe to container—is eliminated. In haematology, because of the instant contact between blood and anti-coagulant minimises microclot formation. Furthermore, all Vacutainer tubes are sterile, guaranteeing the biological integrity of the sample—a particularly important factor with ESR determinations and coagulation studies, which can be seriously distorted by microbial growth in the citrate solution. The maximum benefit is derived by the laboratory personnel (by use of Vacutainers) though the physician is assisted only indirectly in the form of quality reports. Also available are Vacutainer culture systems, where blood is injected into the culture media directly without even coming in contact with atmosphere.

Table 9.1 gives colour codes for the Vacutainer systems and in all cases different volume containers are available—from 2 to 15 ml.

HAEMOGLOBIN (Hb)

Haemoglobin is the main constituent of the RBCs and carries out the important function of transportation of oxygen from lungs to various parts of the body. To a lesser extent, it transports back carbon dioxide from the body to the lungs. When fully saturated, each gram of haemoglobin holds approximately 1.34 ml of oxygen. The red cell mass of an adult contains approximately 600 gm of haemoglobin, capable of carrying 800 ml of oxygen.

HAEMOGLOBIN ESTIMATION

Sahli's method: (Sahli's haemoglobinometer) (Fig. 9.3):

This is based on conversion of haemoglobin to acid haematin, which has a brown colour. Fill haemoglobin tube till 20 mark with N/10 HCl. To this, add blood sucked till the specific mark (20 μl) on the haemoglobin pipette and wait for 5-45 minutes. During this time keep stirring the mixture of acid-blood in the tube. Add distilled water until a match is obtained with the brown glass standard (comparator) provided. Read the lower level of fluid meniscus on gm% side of the tube. Report haemoglobin in gm/100 ml of blood. If haemoglobin is less than 2 gm%, take double the quantity of blood and divide the result by 2. If haemoglobin concentration is extremely high dilute blood with equal amount of normal saline, take the reading and multiply by 2. This method, however, does not estimate carboxyhaemoglobin, methaemoglobin and sulphhaemoglobin. Non-haemoglobin substances (protein, lipids) in plasma and cell stroma may influence the colour of blood diluted with acid. It is, therefore, not a very satisfactory method.

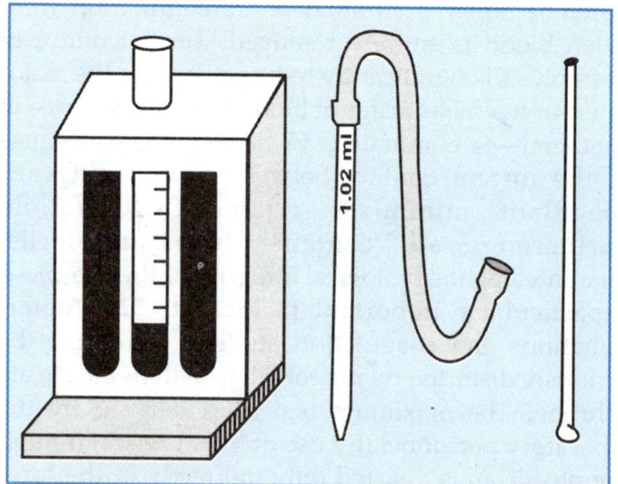

Fig. 9.3: Sahli's haemoglobinometer, middle: Hb pipette, right: Stirrer

Cyanmethaemoglobin Method

(DRABKIN'S SOLUTION AND THE STANDARD AVAILABLE FROM CORAL CLINICAL SYSTEMS, GOA)

Drabkin's Reagent

In 1000 ml of deionised water are mixed:
- — Potassium ferricyanide: 400 mg
- — Potassium dihydrogen phosphate: 280 mg
- — Potassium cyanide: 100 mg
- — Nonidet (nonionic detergent): 1 ml

This reagent can be stored in a polythene container. Concentrated stock solutions can also be prepared and diluted accordingly when needed.

Pipette carefully and take care not to discard cyanide solutions into sinks or receptacles containing acid (to prevent formation of hydrocyanic acid). To 5 ml of Drabkin's solution, add 20 μl of blood. Mix well. Read in a photocolourimeter at 540 nm (green filter).

For this procedure, certified standard haemoglobin solution may be obtained from reputable laboratory supply firms. By diluting the known standard haemoglobin solution, a graph (linear) may be obtained by plotting the known Hb concentration against the colorimetric optical density reading so that in future the corresponding haemoglobin value can directly be read off from the calibration curve after knowing the optical density of a particular unknown blood sample.

Sheard-Sanford Oxyhaemoglobin Method

Mix 20 ml of 0.1% sodium carbonate and 0.1 ml of blood or aliquots of these (e.g., 4 ml diluent for 20 ml blood); read optical density in photometer at 540 nm within 30 minutes. Photometer calibration should be based on blood iron determination or oxygen capacity determination.

Table 9.1: Vacutainer colour codes and their usage

Stopper colour code	*Additive*	*Used for*	*Remarks*
1. Grey and red	Inert polymer Barrier material	Chemistry tubes	Serum separation
2. Yellow and red	None	Chemistry	Clot activator tubes
3. Red	None	Chemistry	Silicone coated interior
4. Red/orange green	None	Chemistry	-
5. Yellow	None	Chemistry	Silicon-coated interior
6. Royal blue	None/heparin/ EDTA	Toxicology and nutrition studies e.g., trace elements, heavy metals, etc.	
7. Brown	Sodium heparin	Lead determination	
8. Yellow black	Thrombin (NIH)	For stat procedures as thrombin hastens clotting and therefore quick serum separation	
9. Grey	Sod. fluoride/ Iodoacetic lithium salt potassium oxalate/ potassium oxalate- NaF/EDTA-NaF/ Thymol NaF	For glucose estimation	
10. Green	Sodium heparin Lithium heparin Ammonium heparin	For chemistry or cytology	
11. Blue	Sodium citric acid	For coagulation studies	
12. Lavender	EDTA	For haematology studies	
13. Yellow	ACD solution A ACD solution B ACDP solution Alsever's solution	For blood banking For blood banking	
14. Green	Na heparin	LE cell preparation	Prelabelled
15. Grey/Black	Gives citrate Blood a ratio of 1:4	For ESR estimation by Westergren's method	Prelabelled
16. Blue	Ammonium oxalate and potassium oxalate in a ratio of 6:4	For ESR estimation by Wintrobe's methods	Prelabelled
17. Yellow	Sodium polyane tholesulphonate 0.35% in 0.85% sodium chloride	For microbiology	Prelabelled

Other Methods

Alkali haematin method

It does not estimate foetal haemoglobin and is no longer used in routine haemoglobinometry.

Gasometric method

Van Slyke's oxygen capacity method. It is an indirect method, which estimates the amount of haemoglobin from the amount of oxygen it absorbs. This method is very complicated for routine clinical work.

Specific gravity method

The normal specific gravity of blood ranges from 1.048 to 1.066. The average for men is 1.057 and for women it is 1.053. From specific gravity of the unknown sample, its haemoglobin is calculated. This is a very rapid and an uncomplicated method and finds its main use in screening potential blood donors for anaemia.

Chemical Methods

Obsolete. Haemoglobin is estimated by finding the iron content.

Sodium Lauryl Sulphate Method

Available from Coral Clinical Systems, Goa

This is a KCN-free reagent where SLS substitutes KCN. The colour complex formed is SLS-Hb which is read at 540 nm. The greatest advantage being that *ALL FORMS OF Hb ARE CONVERTED.* The method is relatively free from interferences due to lipemia and presence of WBCs. Linearity is superior to that of Cyanmeth Hb method.

Normal Haemoglobin Values

Men	15.5±2.5 gm/dl	14-18 gm%
Women	14.0±2.5 gm/dl	11.5-16.5 gm%
Infants full term cord blood	16.5±3.0 gm/dl	13.5-19.5 gm%
Children, 1 year	12.0±1.0 gm/dl	11.0-13.0 gm%
Children, 10-12 years	13.0±1.5 gm dl	11.5-14.5 gm%

According to current WHO specification for male 13.2 gm/dl and for female up to 11.7 gm/dl Hb are said to be normal. For children from 3 months to puberty. normal is 10.7 gm/dl.

THE LOWER LIMIT OF ANAEMIA

It is defined as reduction in the concentration of haemoglobin in the peripheral blood below the normal for the age and sex of the patient.

Diurnal variations: Hb values are highest in the morning and lowest in the evening. A change in the Hb must be 1.5 gm% or more to be considered definitely significant.

Causes of Anaemia

1. *Blood loss.*
   - Acute post-haemorrhagic anaemia
   - Chronic post-haemorrhagic anaemia
2. Impaired red cell formation.
   a. *Disturbance of bone marrow due to deficiency of substances essential for erythropoiesis*
      - Iron deficiency anaemia
      - Megaloblastic macrocytic anaemias due to deficiency of Vitamin B_{12} or folic acid
      - Anaemia associated with scurvy

   b. *Disturbance of bone marrow function not due to deficiency of substances essential for erythropoiesis.*
      - Anaemia associated with
        - infection
        - renal failure
        - liver disease
        - disseminated malignancy
      - Aplastic anaemia
      - Anaemia associated with bone marrow infiltration, e.g., leukaemia, malignant lymphoma, multiple myeloma, myelosclerosis
      - Anaemia associated with myxoedema and hypopituitarism
      - Sideroblastic anaemias
      - Congenital dyserythropoietic anaemias
3. *Increased destruction of red cell (haemolytic) anaemia.*
   a. Haemolysis due to corpuscular defects (intracorpuscular or intrinsic abnormality)
   b. Haemolytic anaemia due to abnormal haemolytic mechanisms (extracorpuscular or extrinsic defect).

POLYCYTHEMIA

RAISED HAEMOGLOBIN VALUE FOR THE AGE AND SEX OF THE PATIENT IS CALLED POLYCYTHAEMIA. Of course, one has to refer to other parameters as well.

Polycythemia (Erythrocytosis) Refers to

- increase in Hb
  - above 18 gm% in males
  - above 16.5 gm% in females

In addition, there is:

- Increase in red cell count:
  - above 6 million/cu mm in males
  - above 5.5 million/cu mm in females
- increase in haematocrit (PCV)
  - above 55% in males
  - above 47% in females

Causes

Primary: Polycythaemia vera (neoplastic)

Secondary

1. *Associated with hypoxia*
   a. Cardiovascular disease, usually congenital resulting in significant venous admixture
   b. Pulmonary disease resulting in:
      - Impaired gas perfusion
      - Perfusion of poorly aerated lung
      - Pulmonary arteriovenous fistula
   c. High altitude residence
   d. Hypoventilation associated with obesity (Pickwickian syndrome)
   e. Haemoglobin variants with increased affinity for oxygen
   f. Heavy smoking
   g. Methaemoglobinaemia (rarely)
2. *Due to inappropriate erythropoietin increase in*
   a. Benign/malignant tumours of
      - Kidney
      - Liver
      - CNS
      - Uterus
      - Ovary.
   b. Renal disease (besides malignancies)
      - Hydronephrosis
      - Vascular impairment
      - Cysts.
3. *Associated with adrenocortical steroids or Androgens*
   a. Adrenal hypercorticism (all types)
   b. Virilising tumours
   c. Androgens used therapeutically (rarely corticoids)
4. *Associated with chronic chemical exposure:*
   a. Nitrites, sulphonamides, other substances producing methaemoglobin and sulphaemoglobin.
   b. Cobalt, shellac components, various alcohols.
5. *Relative*
   a. Stress or spurious polycythemia
   b. Dehydration: water deprivation, vomiting
   c. Plasma loss: burns, enteropathy.

HAEMATOCRIT/PACKED CELL VOLUME (PCV)

Definition

Haematocrit is the volume of red cells expressed as a percentage of the volume of whole blood in the sample. The venous haematocrit is almost same as that obtained from a skin puncture. Dried heparin, EDTA or double oxalate are satisfactory anticoagulants.

Methods

1. Using Wintrobe's tube
2. Using microhaematocrit capillaries

Wintrobe's Tube

Fill the Wintrobe's tube till the 100 mark on top with a Pasteur pipette ensuring that there are no air-bubbles in the blood column. Centrifuge this tube for 15 minutes at 3500 rpm (or longer at lower speeds) until packing is complete. After centrifuging, the blood is separated into 3 layers, a column of red blood cells at the bottom, a narrow middle layer—buffy coat of WBCs and platelets and the topmost fluid column of plasma. The percentage of the height of the column of blood occupied by packed red cells constitutes the haematocrit. Roughly, the haematocrit value is three times the haemoglobin concentration.

Sources of error

1. Inadequate mixing of blood
2. Irregularity of the bore of the tube
3. Incomplete packing.

Microhaematocrit

This method is in common use in most well-equipped laboratories. Capillary tubes coated with anticoagulant can be filled with blood obtained from finger puncture or from a venipuncture or with blood already anticoagulated. One end of the filled capillary tube is sealed with sealing wax (e.g. Plasticine) or the empty end is sealed with heat. The sealed tube is centrifuged for 3 minutes in a special high-speed centrifuge. By reading the packed cell height and the total height of the entire specimen, the haematocrit can be determined. Special reading devices are available.

Values: If the red cells are of normal size (normocytic), and the red cell count is 5 million, the haematocrit is about 45%.

Men—Range 42-52% Average = 47%
Women—Range 37-47% Average = 42%

Interpretation

Causes of reduced haematocrit—causes of anaemia
Causes of raised haematocrit—causes of polycythemia.

If packed cell volume has been determined by Wintrobe's tube, one can obtain some more information.

Buffy coat: A buffy coat of thickness 1 mm approximately corresponds to a total leucocyte count of about 10,000. Absent or minimal buffy coat implies leucopenia, a thickness more than 1 mm implies leucocytosis. In addition, in subleukaemic leukaemia, a film can be made from the buffy coat where a greater concentration of WBCs will be available, and identification of atypical cells would become easier and less time consuming. Another advantage is for performing LE cell or phenomenon test, for which also WBCs can be picked up from the buffy coat. The platelets form a very thin layer above the white cells, the coat is pinkish white but is of no use clinically, one has to do platelet counts if necessary.

Plasma layer: The topmost layer of plasma can give important clues by observing its colour. Its normal colour is pale yellow or straw.

Yellow—jaundice

Pink—haemolysis

Creamy white—hyperlipidaemia, especially chylomicrons

Brown—methaemalbuminaemia.

BLOOD CELL COUNTS

WBC

A white cell count (TLC) estimates the total number of white cells in a cubic millimetre of blood. It is important in the diagnosis of disease, especially when accompanied by a differential white cell count.

The diluting fluid: WBC diluting fluid contains a weak acid to lyse the RBCs and a stain for staining the nucleus of WBCs, e.g. Turke's fluid

Glacial acetic acid	1.5 ml
1% aqueous solution of Gentian violet	1.0 ml
Distilled water	98.0 ml

(A pinch of thymol may be added to the diluting fluid to prevent growth of moulds).

Counting Chamber

The chamber normally used for cell counts is the improved Neubauer's chamber which has an area of 9 sq/mm and a depth of 0.1 mm.

Other counting chambers can also be used including the Burker's chamber which has the same area and depth as the improved Neubauer (Fig. 9.4) and the Fuchs-Rosenthal ruled chamber which has the same area but a double depth of 0.2 mm.

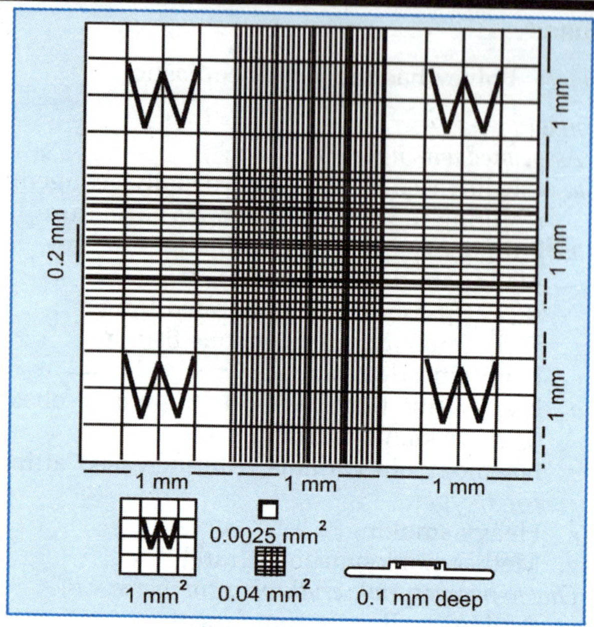

Fig. 9.4: Improved Neubauer's chamber *(Counting area)*

Methods

1. Using a WBC pipette (Fig. 9.5) of a haemacytometer draw well mixed venous blood or capillary blood and fill till the 0.5 mark. Clean the tip of the tube. Now draw WBC diluting fluid till the 11 mark (or to 0.38 ml of diluting fluid add 0.02 ml of blood with a Hb pipette).

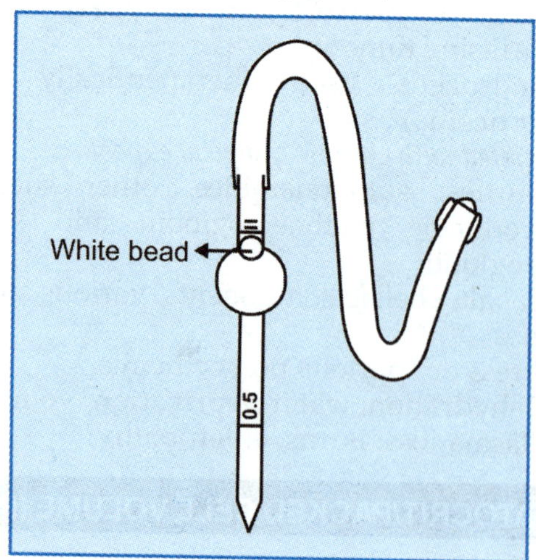

Fig. 9.5: WBC pipette

2. Mix the fluid and blood mixture gently, avoiding bubbling.
3. Place the coverslip on the counting chamber at the right place.

Shake the fluid-blood mixture and transfer the mixture using a fine bore Pasteur pipette on to the counting chamber (called charging the chamber), taking care that the mixture does not overflow. If it does overflow, wash and dry the chamber to be recharged again.

Allow the cells to settle to the bottom of the chamber for 2 minutes. See that fluid does not get dried up. (For preventing this, take a petridish, place a wet filter paper at its bottom, now place the charged chamber gently and close off the dish for about 2 minutes).

For counting, clean the under part of the chamber if it was left in the petridish and place it on the stage of the microscope. Using 10x or low power objective, count the WBCs uniformly in the four larger corner squares (as indicated in the diagram). Cells present on the outermost lines should be counted on one side and those present on the line opposite should not be counted.

Calculate the number of cells per cubic millimetre of blood as follows:

$$\frac{\text{Cells counted} \times \text{blood dilution} \times \text{chamber depth}}{\text{Area of chamber counted}}$$

$$= \text{number of cells counted} \times \frac{20 \times 10 \text{ (depth factor)}}{4}$$

$$= \text{number of cell counted} \times 50$$

(Dilution factor is 20 for there is no mixing of cells till first 1 mark of the WBC pipette, hence 0.5 parts of blood are present in 10 parts of the diluting fluid-dilution factor, then, is 10/0.5 = 20).

Falsely high counts occur due to:

1. Blood taken from an area where there was haemoconcentration.
2. Not wiping away the blood on the outside of tip of the pipette.
3. Blood drawn above the mark in the pipette (happens usually when the rubber mouthpiece is too short).
4. Diluting fluid not taken till the requisite mark.
5. Improper mixing.
6. Uneven distribution in the counting chamber.
7. Extraneous material present (yeast, dirt, etc).
8. Errors in calculation.

Falsely low counts occur due to:

1. Dilution of the blood with tissue fluid due to oedema or squeezing.
2. Delay in counting (this does not affect RBCs as much as WBCs, which are reduced by about 15% in 24 hours).
3. Blood not drawn up to the requisite mark.
4. Diluting fluid taken in excess of the requisite mark.
5. Saliva in the mouthpiece running into the upper end of the pipette causing further dilution.
6. Improper mixing.
7. Uneven distribution in the counting chamber.
8. Uniform systematic counting not done.
9. Cells lost through haemolysis (in RBC count-for instance).
10. Errors in calculation.
11. Clumping of cells or coagulation of the blood.

Causes of raised and reduced leucocyte counts would be presented with differential leucocyte counts, since raised or lowered total counts are usually accompanied by abnormal differential counts.

Correcting the white cell count for nucleated red cells: From peripheral smear, find out the number of nucleated red cells per 100 WBCs counted.

Calculation

$$\frac{\text{Number of nucleated RBCs}}{100 + \text{number of nucleated RBCs}} \times \text{TLC}$$

= Nucleated RBC/cu mm

Corrected count = TLC–Nucleated RBC count.

RBCs

Diluting Fluid

This should be isotonic so that RBCs are not haemolysed. Normal saline can be used but it may cause crenation of the RBCs and allow rouleaux formation.

One can use:

1. Sodium citrate 3 gm
   Formalin 1 ml
   Distilled water to 100 ml
   (Cheap and good) Or
2. Hayem's fluid
   Mercuric chloride 0.5 gm
   Sodium chloride 1.0 gm
   Sodium sulphate 5.0 gm
   Distilled water to 200 ml.

   (Needs to be made frequently and in hyperglobulinaemia one may set precipitation of protein so RBC clumping may occur. Mercuric chloride acts as an antiseptic).

Method

Draw blood to the 0.5 mark in the RBC pipette (Fig. 9.6). Wipe tip clean and draw diluting fluid to the 101 mark. Shake for 3 minutes. Charge the chamber. Count the RBCs using 40x objective in the 80 smallest squares as indicated in the diagram of the chamber.

RBC count =

$$\frac{\text{No of cells counted} \times \text{Dilution factor} \times \text{Depth factor}}{\text{Area counted}}$$

Where Dilution is 1 in 200, Depth is 1/10 mm

Area counted is $\frac{80}{400} = \frac{1}{5}$ sq mm.

$$\frac{\text{Number counted} \times 200 \times 10}{1/5}$$

= Number counted × 10,000

Interpretation

RBC counts are low in anaemia and high in polycythaemia, the causes of these have already been discussed.

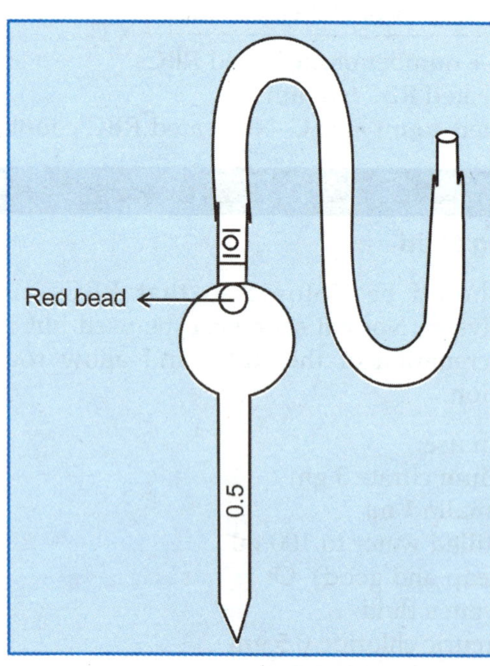

Fig. 9.6: RBC pipette

PLATELETS

Preferably, use venous blood for platelet counts. Finger prick may cause clumping of platelets. In small children, however, this clumping can be prevented by thinly smearing Vaseline over the area to be punctured (make sure that there has been no clotting of bood).

The blood is diluted in 1% ammonium oxalate stored refrigerated at 4°C. which haemolyses the RBCs (prepared by dissolving 1 gm of ammonium oxalate in 100 ml of distilled water).

Method

- Fill blood and diluent (in this case 1% ammonium oxalate) as described for the RBC count and using the RBC pipette. If platelet count is low, a WBC pipette can be used instead.
- Charge the chamber with the help of the pipette employed.
- Using 40x objective with reduced condenser aperture, count the platelets in the same squares as indicated for RBC counting.
- Calculate as (if RBC pipette used)

$$\frac{\text{Cells counted} \times \text{blood dilution} \times \text{chamber depth factor}}{\text{Area of chamber counted}}$$

= N × 200 × 5 × 10
= N × 10000

However, if a WBC pipette is employed, the appropriate formula and method should be used. Platelet counts are made in the small 5 RBC squares only.

Platelet count = N × 20 × 5 × 10 or N × 1000
Normal platelet counts = 1.5-3.5 lakhs/cu mm.

Rees-Ecker Method for Platelet Count

Various components of the diluting fluid used have various functions, e.g. citrate prevents coagulation while formaline fixes the platelets and prevents their clumping together. Here, no attempt is made to lyse RBCs. Platelets are identified by their size, shape and dark colour. Brilliant cresyl blue (the dye used) provides the background during cell counting. This dye does not stain the platelets and, therefore, is not essential for the counting procedure.

Diluting fluid

Consists of:

Trisodium citrate	3.8 gm
Neutral formaldehyde	0.2 ml

Brilliant cresyl blue	0.1 gm
Deionised water	100 ml

Dissolve the ingredients in 100 ml volumetric flask, filter, centrifuge, transfer to a well-stoppered bottle and keep at 2-8ºC (refrigerate). This fluid if not contaminated will stay good indefinitely. Filter aliquot of the diluting fluid immediately before use.

ALL GLASSWARE MUST BE SCRUPULOUSLY CLEAN. DIRT OR DUST PARTICLES CAN RESEMBLE AND MAY BE COUNTED AS PLATELETS.

Procedure

- Take 3.98 ml of diluent (freshly filtered) into a test tube.
- Add to the diluent 0.02 ml (20 μl) of well-mixed anticoagulated blood. With the help of a Sahli pipette, wipe out the outer tip of the pipette before dilution. Wash out the contents in the pipette into the diluent tube 3-4 times.
- Immediately mix the diluent with the specimen for at least 5 minutes or so.
- Employ the Sahli's pipette for charging either side of the chamber.
- Keep the charged haemocytometer inside a moist chamber (can be a petridish with a moistened or wet filter paper — on which the chamber can be kept). Let stay for about 15 minutes. This permits the platelets to settle down, and the moistened chamber does not allow evaporation of the fluid.
- Place the haemocytometer on the stage of the microscope, focus the RBC counting area under low magnification. Now move to the corner square of the red cell area carefully to high dry objective.
- Platelets are bluish and must be distinguished from debris. They are oval, round, or comma-shaped, refractile bodies that vary in size normally from 1 to 5 microns.
- Count the platelets in the finely ruled centre area (1 mm^2) of each side of the chamber. Take the average counts of two sides.
  (In the new improved Neubauer ruling, there are 25 small squares and each of these contain 16 smallest squares. The area covered by the 25 squares is equal to 1 sq mm.)

Platelet count/ml or cu mm =

$$\frac{\text{Number of platelets counted} \times \text{dilution}}{\text{Volume of fluid.}}$$

Where
volume of fluid for the 1 sq mm area = 1 × 0.1 = 0.1 ml (cu mm)

Dilution = 200

So platelet count/cu mm =

$$\frac{\text{Number of platelets counted} \times 200}{0.1}$$

= Number of platelets counted × 2000

Rough Estimation of Platelets Count from Stained thin Smear

A well-prepared peripheral blood smear can be used to check the results of direct counting. Determine the ratio of platelets to red cells on a thin blood smear used for differential leukocyte count. If the average number of platelets is 8 to 25 in 10 fields, it is reported to be adequate, and if it is 0 to 5, it is reported as inadequate.

Causes of Thrombocytopenia

1. *Causes of platelet production failure:*
   Selective megakaryocyte depression.
   - Drugs
   - Chemicals
   - Viral infections.

   Part of general bone marrow failure.
   - Aplastic anaemia
   - Leukaemia
   - Myelosclerosis
   - Marrow infiltration, e.g. in carcinoma, lymphoma
   - Multiple myeloma
   - Megaloblastic anaemia.
2. *Increased destruction of platelets*
   - Acute or chronic ITP (idiopathic thrombocytopenic purpura)
   - Secondary immune thrombocytopenia (post-infection, SLE, CLL, and lymphomas)
3. *Abnormal distribution of platelets*
   - Splenomegaly.
4. *Dilutional loss*
   - Massive transfusion of old blood to bleeding patients.

Raised Platelet Count (Thrombocytosis)

Can occur as a part of generalised myeloproliferative disorder, e.g., CML or following acute haemorrhage.

ERYTHROCYTE INDICES

These can be calculated from:

a. Haematocrit
b. Haemoglobin concentration and
c. Red cell counts.

1. *The mean cell volume (MCV)*

$$\text{MCV} = \frac{\text{Packed cell volume}}{\text{Red cell count per litre}} \times 10^{15}\ \text{fl.}$$

Normal values

Adults 76-96 fl.
Infants, full term cord blood Avg. 106 fl.
Children, 1 year 76-87 fl.
Children 10-12 years 76-93 fl.
MCV is reduced in microcytic anaemias
MCV is raised in macrocytic anaemias

2. *The mean cell haemoglobin (MCH)*

$$\text{MCH} = \frac{\text{Haemoglobin in gm/L}}{\text{Red cell count per ml}}\ \text{pg.}$$

Normal MCH in adults is from 27 to 32 pg.
MCH is reduced in hypochromic anaemias.

3. *The mean cell haemoglobin concentration (MCHC)*

$$\text{MCHC} = \frac{\text{Hb in gm\%}}{\text{PCV}} \times 100 = 31\text{-}35\ \text{gm\%}$$

This too, is low in hypochromic anaemias.

COMPLETE BLOOD COUNT (CBC), BLOOD

Normal Values

		SI Units
Haematocrit (HCT)		
Adult females	37-47%	0.37-0.47 L/L
Pregnant		
Trimester 1	35-46%	0.35-0.46 L/L
Trimester 2	30-42%	0.30-0.42 L/L
Trimester 3	34-44%	0.34-0.44 L/L
Postpartum	34-44%	0.34-0.44 L/L
Adult males	40-54%	0.40-0.54 L/L
Children		
Newborn	42-68%	0.42-0.68 L/L
3 months	29-54%	0.29-0.54 L/L
1 year	29-41%	0.29-0.41 L/L
3 years	31-44%	0.31-0.44 L/L
10 years	34-45%	0.34-0.45 L/L

Contd...

Contd...

Haemoglobin (HGB)		
Adult females	12-16 g/dl	7.4-9.9 mmol/L
Pregnant		
Trimester 1	11.4-15.0 g/dl	7.1-9.3 mmol/L
Trimester 2	10.0-14.3 g/dl	6.2-8.9 mmol/L
Trimester 3	10.2-14.4 g/dl	6.3-8.9 mmol/L
Postpartum	10.4-15.0 g/dl	6.4-9.3 mmol/L
Adult males	14.0-18.0 g/dl	8.7-11.2 mmol/L
Panic low level	<5g/dl	<3.1 mmol/L
Panic high level	>18 g/dl	>11.2 mmol/L
Children		
Newborn		
Day 1	15.5-24.5 g/dl	9.6-15.2 mmol/L
Days 2-3	19.0 g/dl	11.8 mmol/L
Days 4-8	14.3-22.3 g/dl	8.9-13.8 mmol/L
Days 9-13	16.5 g/dl	10.2 mmol/L
2-8 weeks	10.7-17.3 g/dl	6.6-10.7 mmol/L
3-5 months	9.9-15.5 g/dl	6.1-9.6 mmol/L
6-11 months	11.8 g/dl	7.3 mmol/L
1-2 years	9.0-14.6 g/dl	5.6-9.0 mmol/L
3-9 years	9.4-15.5 g/dl	5.8-9.6 mmol/L
10 years	10.7-15.5 g/dl	6.6-9.6 mmol/L
11-15 years	13.4 g/dl	8.3 mmol/L
Panic levels	<5g/dl	<3.1 mmol/L
	>18 g/dl	>11.2 mmol/L
Red Blood Cell (RBC) Count		
Adult females	4.0-5.5 million/µl	4.0-5.5 ´ 10^{12}/L
Pregnant		
Trimester 1	4.0-5.0 million/µl	4.0-5.0 × 10^{12}/L
Trimester 2	3.2-4.5 million/µl	3.2-4.5 × 10^{12}/L
Trimester 3	3.0-4.9 million/µl	3.0-4.9 × 10^{12}/L
Postpartum	3.2-5.0 million/µl	3.2-5.0 × 10^{12}/L
Adult males	4.5-6.2 million/µl	4.5-6.2 × 10^{12}/L
Children		
Newborn		
Day 1	4.1-6.1 million/µl	4.1-6.1 × 10^{12}/L
Days 2-8	5.1 million/µl	5.1 × 10^{12}/L
Days 9-13	5.0 million/µl	5.0 × 10^{12}/L
2-8 weeks	3.8-5.6 million/µl	3.8-5.6 × 10^{12}/L
3-5 months	3.8-5.2 million/µl	3.8-5.2 × 10^{12}/L
6-11 months	4.6 million/µl	4.6 × 10^{12}/L
1-2 years	3.6-5.5 million/µl	3.6-5.5 × 10^{12}/L
3 years	4.5 million/µl	4.5 × 10^{12}/L
4 years	4.0-5.2 million/µl	4.0-5.2 × 10^{12}/L
5 years	4.6 million/µl	4.6 × 10^{12}/L
6-10 years	4.7 million/µl	4.7 × 10^{12}/L
11-15 years	4.8 million/µl	4.8 × 10^{12}/L
Mean Cell Volume (MCV)		
Adults	82-98 μ^3	82-98 fl
Children		
Newborn		
Day 1	106 μ^3	106 fl
Days 2-3	105 μ^3	105 fl

Contd...

Contd...

Days 4-8	103 μ^3	103 fl
Days 9-13	98 μ^3	98 fl
2-8 weeks	90 μ^3	90 fl
3 months	82 μ^3	82 fl
4-5 months	80 μ^3	80 fl
6-11 months	77 μ^3	77 fl
1 year	78 μ^3	78 fl
2 years	77 μ^3	77 fl
3 years	79 μ^3	79 fl
4-10 years	80 μ^3	80 fl
11-15 years	82 μ^3	82 fl
Mean Cell Haemoglobin (MCH)		
Adults	26-34 pg	1.61-2.11 fmol
Children		
Newborn		
Day l	38 pg	2.36 fmol
Days 2-3	37 pg	2.30 fmol
Days 4-8	36 pg	2.23 fmol
Days 9-13	33 pg	2.05 fmol
2-8 weeks	30 pg	1.86 fmol
3 months	28 pg	1.73 fmol
4-5 months	27 pg	1.67 fmol
6-11 months	26 pg	1.61 fmol
1-2 years	25 pg	1.55 fmol
3 years	26 pg	1.61 fmol
4-10 years	27 pg	1.67 fmol
11-15 years	28 pg	1.73 fmol
Mean Cell Haemoglobin Concentration (MCHC)		
Adults	31-38%	19.2-23.58 mmol/L
Children		
Newborn		
Day 1	36%	22.34 mmol/L
Days 2-8	35%	21.72 mmol/L
Days 9-13	34%	21.10 mmol/L
2-8 weeks	33%	20.48 mmol/L
3-5 months	34%	21.10 mmol/L
6-11 months	33%	20.48 mmol/L
1-2 years	32%	19.86 mmol/L
3 years	35%	21.72 mmol/L
4-15 years	34%	21.10 mmol/L
White Blood Cell (WBC) Count		
Adult females	4500-11,000/µl	4.5-11.0 × 10^9/L
Pregnant		
Trimester 1	6600-14.100/µl	6.6-14.1 × 10^9/L
Trimester 2	6900-17,100/µl	6.9-17.1 × 10^9/L
Trimester 3	5900-14,700/µl	5.9-14.7 × 10^9/L
Postpartum	9700-25,700/µl	9.7-25.7 × 10^9/L
Adult males	4500-11,000/µl	4.5-11.0 × 10^9/L
Children		
Newborn	9000-30,000/µl	9.0-30.0 × 10^9/L
3 months	5700-18,000/µl	5.7-18.0 × 10^9/L
1 year	6000-17,500/µl	6.0-17.5 × 10^9/L

Contd...

Contd...

3 years	5700-16,300/µl	5.7-16.3 × 10^9/L
10 years	4500-13,500/µl	4.5-13.5 × 10^9/L
White Blood Cells Differential		
GRANULOCYTES		
Segmented		
Neutrophil (Segs)	54-62%	0.54-0.62
Adults	3800/µl or mm^3	3800 × 10^6/L
Children		
Birth	8400/µl or mm^3	8400 × 10^6/L
12 hours	12,100/µl or mm^3	12,100 × 10^6/L
24 hours	8870/µl or mm^3	8870 × 10^6/L
1 week	4100/µl or mm^3	4100 × 10^6/L
2 weeks	3320/µl or mm^3	3320 × 10^6/L
1-2 months	2750/µl or mm^3	2750 × 10^6/L
4 months	2730/µl or mm^3	2730 × 10^6/L
6 months	2710/µl or mm^3	2710 × 10^6/L
8 months	2680/µl or mm^3	2680 × 10^6/L
10 months	2600/µl or mm^3	2600 × 10^6/L
12 months	2680/µl or mm^3	2680 × 10^6/L
2 years	2660/µl or mm^3	2660 × 10^6/L
4 years	3040/µl or mm^3	3040 × 10^6/L
6 years	3600/µl or mm^3	3600 × 10^6/L
8-14 years	3700/µl or mm^3	3700 × 10^6/L
1&-20 years	3800/µl or mm^3	3800 × 10^6/L
Band		
Neutrophils (Bands)	3-5%	0.03–.05
Adults	620/µl or mm^3	620 × 10^6/L
Children		
Birth	2540/µl or mm^3	2540 × 10^6/L
12 hours	3460/µl or mm^3	3460 × 10^6/L
24 hours	2680/µl or mm^3	2680 × 10^6/L
1 week	1420/µl or mm^3	1420 × 10^6/L
2 weeks	1200/µl or mm^3	1200 × 10^6/L
1 month	1150/µl or mm^3	1150 × 10^6/L
2 months	1100/µl or mm^3	1100 × 10^6/L
4-10 months	1000/µl or mm^3	1000 × 10^6/L
12 months	990/µl or mm^3	990 × 10^6/L
2 years	850/µl or mm^3	850 × 10^6/L
4 years	710/µl or mm^3	710 × 10^6/L
6 years	670/µl or mm^3	670 × 10^6/L
8 years	660/µl or mm^3	660 × 10^6/L
10 years	645/µl or mm^3	645 × 10^6/L
12-14 years	640/µl or mm^3	640 × 10^6/L
16-20 years	620/µl or mm^3	620 × 10^6/L
Eosinophils	1-4%	0.01-0.04
Adults	200/µl or mm^3	200 × 10^6/L
Children		
Birth	400/µl or mm^3	400 × 10^6/L
12-24 hours	450/µl or mm^3	450 × 10^6/L
l week	500/µl or mm^3	500 × 10^6/L
2 weeks	350/µl or mm^3	350 × 10^6/L
1 month-l yr	300/µl or mm^3	300 × 10^6/L
2 years	280/µl or mm^3	280 × 10^6/L
4 years	250/µl or mm^3	250 × 10^6/L

Contd...

Contd...

6 years	230/µl or mm³	230 × 10⁶/L
8-20 years	200/µl or mm³	200 × 10⁶/L
Basophils	(M) 0.75%	0-0.0075
Adults	40/µl or mm³	40 × 10⁶/L
Children		
Birth-24 hours	100/µl or mm³	100 × 10⁶/L
1 week-8 years	50/µl or mm³	50 × 10⁶/L
10-20 years	40/µl or mm³	40 × 10⁶/L
MONOCYTES	2-10%	0.02—0.1
Adults	300/µl or mm³	300 × 10⁶/L
Children		
Birth	1050/µl or mm³	1050 × 10⁶/L
12 hours	1200/µl or mm³	1200 × 10⁶/L
24 hrs-1 wk	1100/µl or mm³	1100 × 10⁶/L
2 weeks	1000/µl or mm³	1000 × 10⁶/L
1 month	700/µl or mm³	700 × 10⁶/L
2 months	650/µl or mm³	650 × 10⁶/L
4 months	600/µl or mm³	600 × 10⁶/L
6-8 months	580/µl or mm³	580 × 10⁶/L
10-12 months	550/µl or mm³	550 × 10⁶/L
2 years	530/µl or mm³	530 × 10⁶/L
4 years	450/µl or mm³	450 × 10⁶/L
6 years	400/µl or mm³	400 × 10⁶/L
8-12 years	350/µl or mm³	350 × 10⁶/L
14 years	380/µl or mm³	380 × 10⁶/L
16-18 years	400/µl or mm³	400 × 10⁶/L
20 years	380/µl or mm³	380 × 10⁶/L
LYMPHOCYTES	20-40%	0.20–0.40
Adults	2500/µl or mm³	2500 × 10⁶/L
Children		
Birth-12 hrs	5500/µl or mm³	5500 × 10⁶/L
24 hours	5800/µl or mm³	5800 × 10⁶/L
1 week	5000/µl or mm³	5000 × 10⁶/L
2 weeks	5500/µl or mm³	5500 × 10⁶/L
1 month	6000/µl or mm³	6000 × 10⁶/L
2 months	6300/µl or mm³	6300 × 10⁶/L
4 months	6800/µl or mm³	6800 × 10⁶/L
6 months	7300/µl or mm³	7300 × 10⁶/L
8 months	7600/µl or mm³	7600 × 10⁶/L
10 months	7500/µl or mm³	7500 × 10⁶/L
12 months	7000/µl or mm³	7000 × 10⁶/L
2 years	6300/µl or mm³	6300 × 10⁶/L
4 years	4500/µl or mm³	4500 × 10⁶/L
6 years	3500/µl or mm³	3500 × 10⁶/L
8 years	3300/µl or mm³	3300 × 10⁶/L
10 years	3100/µl or mm³	3100 × 10⁶/L
12 years	3000/µl or mm³	3000 × 10⁶/L
14 years	2900/µl or mm³	2900 × 10⁶/L
16 years	2800/µl or mm³	2800 × 10⁶/L
18 years	2700/µl or mm³	2700 × 10⁶/L
20 years	2500/µl or mm³	2500 × 10⁶/L

Contd...

Contd...

Platelets		
Adults	150,000–400,000/µl or mm³	150–400 × 10⁹/L
Panic/Levels	<30,000/µl or mm³	<30 × 10⁹/L
	>1,000,000/µl or mm³	>1000 × 10⁹/L
Children		
Newborn	100,000-300,000/µl or mm³	100-300 × 10⁹/L
3 months	260,000/µl or mm³	260 × 10⁹/L
1-10 years	250,000/µl or mm³	250 × 10⁹/L
Panic/Levels	<20,000/µl or mm³	<20 × 10⁹/L
	> 1,000,000/µl or mm³	>1000 × 10⁹/L

Complete Blood Count (CBC)

CBC includes—TLC, DLC, RBC count, haemoglobin, haematocrit, RBC indices, platelet count and a peripheral smear examination.

ERYTHROCYTE SEDIMENTATION RATE (ESR)

This is the rate at which erythrocytes sediment on their own weight when anticoagulated blood is held in a vertical column, it is expressed as the fall of RBCs in mm at the end of first hour (starting point—when the tube or pipette was filled with blood).

Methods

Westergren's Method

1. Westergren's pipette (open at both ends) is about 30 cm long with a bore diameter of about 2.5 mm (Fig. 9.7).
2. The lower 20 cm are marked from 0 (top) to 200 (bottom).
3. Anticoagulant used is 3.8% trisodium citrate solution. One part of anticoagulant is added to 4 parts of blood.
4. The pipette accepts about 1 ml of blood. Fill the pipette by sucking till the 0 mark and clamp it vertically in the Westergren's rack.
5. Read the upper level of red cells exactly after 1 hour.

This is a better method than Wintrobe's since the reading obtained is magnified as the column is lengthier.

Normal Values

Males—0 to 5 mm at the end of 1st hour.

Females—0 to 7 mm at the end of 1st hour.

Wintrobe's Method

1. The Wintrobe's tube (Fig. 9.8) is about 11 cm long, bore diameter is 2.5 mm and the bottom 10 cm are graduated.
2. Graduations are from zero (top) to hundred (bottom) for ESR and zero (bottom) to hundred (top) for PCV.
3. EDTA blood is used and the tube is filled till zero mark on top with the help of a Pasteur pipette.
4. Set it up vertically and read exactly after 1 hour.
5. As has already been said that this tube can also be used for PCV estimation.

Normal Values
Males—0 to 9 mm at the end of 1st hour.
Females—0 to 20 mm at the end of 1st hour.

Microsedimentation (Landau) Method

Capillary blood can be taken.

Materials Required

1. 5.0 gm/dl sodium citrate solution.
2. Landau pipette: This pipette resembles RBC pipette. It is graduated from 0 to 50 mm.
3. Landau pipette stand.
4. Suction device for drawing blood into the pipette.
5. Capillaries for blood collection.

Procedure

1. Attach Landau pipette to the suction device.
2. Draw 5.0 gm/dl citrate up to first line on the stem.
3. Now draw by suction device up to second mark on the stem (avoid air bubbles).
4. Wipe excess blood on the external side of the pipette.
5. Draw citrate solution and blood into the bulb of the pipette. Mix the contents thoroughly.
6. Force back the mixture into the stem of the pipette.
7. Set the upper level of the mixture of the zero mm mark at the top.
8. Detach the suction device.
9. Place the pipette in vertical position on the stand, set time to one hour.
10. Note the reading (the distance red cells have fallen or the extent of plasma column) after one hour.

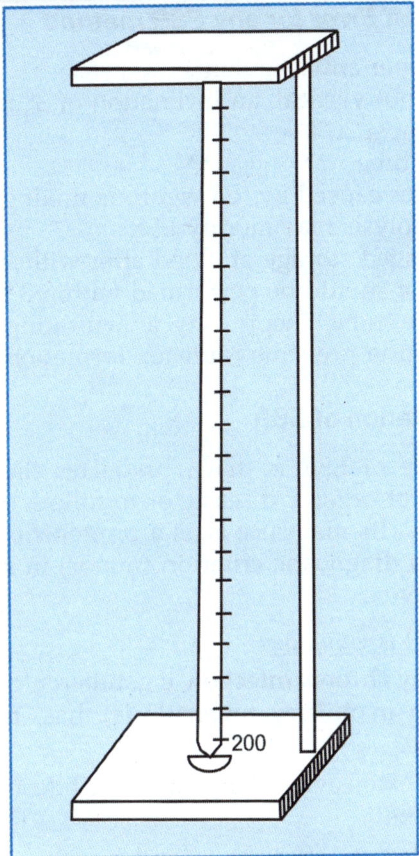

Fig. 9.7: Westergren's ESR ipette with stand

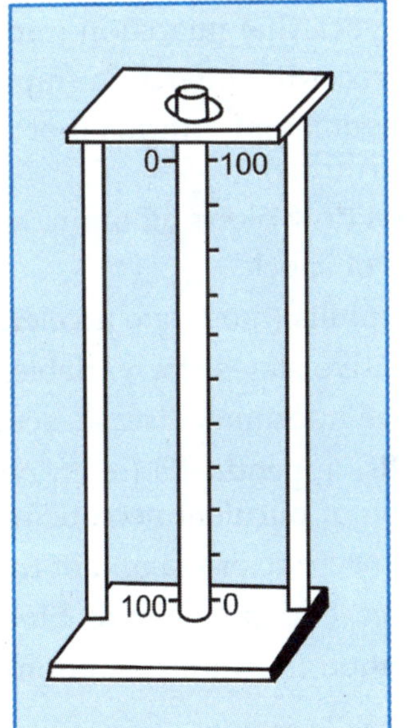

Fig. 9.8: Wintrobe's ESR tube with stand

Normal Values

Male: 0-5 mm after Ist hour
Female: 0-8 mm after Ist hour

Sources of Error for any ESR method

1. Improper anticoagulant.
2. Tube not vertical, an inclination of 3° raises ESR by almost 30%.
3. Dirty tube.
4. Bubbles caused by too vigorous mixing.
5. Haemolysis may modify ESR.
6. Prolonged storage of blood after withdrawing it, the test should be performed within 3 hours.
7. Pipette/tube kept on a vibrating surface (vibration prevents rouleaux formation).

Interpretation of ESR

The value of ESR is that it indicates the possible presence of organic disease, or to follow the course of disease. Its main use is as a prognostic tool. It is used as a diagnostic criterion (minor) in rheumatic fever only.

Rapid ESR is found in:

1. In any chronic infection, e.g. tuberculosis (maximum in miliary tuberculosis), has prognostic value.
2. Any extensive inflammation, cell destruction or toxaemia.
3. Pregnancy, after the second month.
4. Puerperium, returns to normal within 2 months.
5. Active myocardial infarction (rapid rise).
6. Acute myocardial infarction (rapid rise).
7. Active rheumatoid arthritis (not much elevated in osteoarthritis).
8. Nephrosis (low blood albumin, anaemia).
9. All types of shock.
10. Active syphilis (moderate acceleration).
11. Postoperative states (for variable periods).
12. Any active infectious disease, acute or chronic.
13. Salpingitis, appendicitis (often normal), due to absorption of purulent necrotic material.
14. Infected, necrotic or malignant tumours.
15. Liver disease (depends upon blood proteins).
16. Menstruation (slight acceleration).

Slow ESR is usually seen in:

1. Newborn infants.
2. Polycythaemia.
3. Congestive heart failure.
4. Allergic states.
5. Sickle cell anaemia (poikilocytosis).

Factors that play a role in ESR:

1. *Plasma factors:*
   - An accelerated ESR is favoured by elevated levels of fibrinogen, and to a lesser extent, of globulins (α and β globulins are more effective than γ globulin).
   - These plasma factors cause increased formation of rouleaux which due to more weight sediment more rapidly than do single cells.
   - Albumin retards sedimentation.
   - Extreme increase in plasma viscosity slows down ESR.
   - Cholesterol accelerates and lecithin retards the ESR.
2. *Red cell factors:*
   - Anaemia is responsible for accelerated ESR. The change in erythrocyte-plasma ratio favours rouleaux formation.
   - Microcytes sediment more slowly and macrocytes somewhat more rapidly than normocytes. The sedimentation rate is directly proportional to the weight of the cell aggregate and inversely proportional to the surface area.
   - Poikilocytosis retards ESR because abnormal shape hampers rouleaux formation.
3. *Anticoagulants:*
   - Sodium citrate and EDTA do not effect ESR but oxalates and heparin may.

Stages in ESR:

1. First 10 minutes—is the period of aggregation. Rouleaux formation occurs at this stage and sedimentation is slow.
2. Next 40 minutes—is period of fast settling, during this period rate of fall is constant.
3. Last 10 minutes—is the final period of packing.

Interfering Factors

1. The blood sample should not be allowed to stand for more than 2 hours before the test is started because rate will increase.
2. In refrigerated blood the sedimentation rate is greatly increased. Refrigerated blood should be allowed to return to room temperature before the test is performed.
3. *Factors leading to reduced rates:*
   - High blood sugar
   - High albumin level
   - High phospholipids
   - Decreased fibrinogen level of the blood in newborns

- Certain drugs (see below)

4. *Drugs*
   a. That increase ESR levels
      - Dextran
      - Methyldopa
      - Methysergide
      - Oral contraceptives
      - Penicillamine
      - Theophylline
      - Trifluperidol
      - Vitamin A
   b. Those that decrease levels
      - Ethambutol
      - Quinine
      - Salicylates
      - Drugs that cause a high blood glucose level (cortisone and ACTH)

BLOOD FILM EXAMINATION

Preparation of a Thin Blood Film

A thin blood film is made by spreading a drop of blood evenly across a clean grease-free slide, using a smooth edged spreader.

Making of Spreaders (Fig. 9.9)

- Select a slide which has smooth edges
- Using a glass cutter and a ruler, mark off 4 equal divisions, each measuring 19 mm
- Break off at each division to give 4 spreaders.

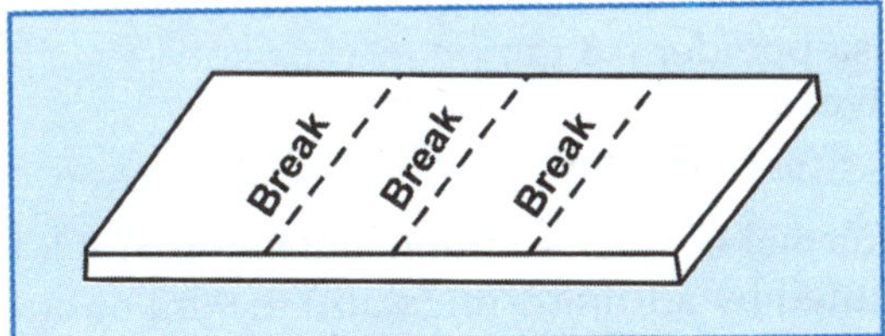

Fig. 9.9: Making a spreader

For anaemic blood, a rapid smearing is needed; whereas for thick concentrated blood, smearing should be done slowly. A well-spread smear shows no lines extending across or downwards through the film and the smear should be tongue shaped (Fig. 9.10).

Making Thick Smears

While the thin smears are used for describing blood cells, the thick smears are used for detecting malarial parasites and microfilariae. A large drop of blood is taken on the centre of a slide and with the aid of a needle or slide corner spread the drop over 1/2 an inch square area. When dry, the thickness should be such that printed matter can be seen through it.

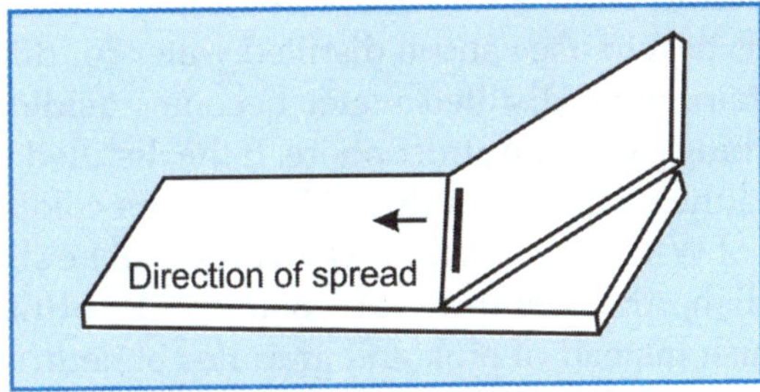

Fig. 9.10 (A): Direction of spread

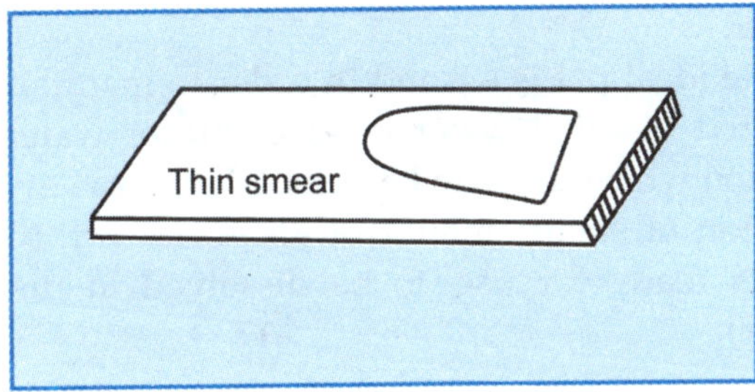

Fig. 9.10 (B): A thin peripheral blood smear

Fixing of Blood Films

Before staining, the blood films need to be fixed with acetone-free methyl alcohol for ½ to 1 minute in order to prevent haemolysis when they come in contact with water while staining them with aqueous (water-based) stains or when water has to be added subsequently. Alcohol denatures the proteins and hardens the cell contents. For Wright's stain and Leishman's stain, no prefixation is required as these contain acetone-free methyl alcohol; but for Giemsa's stain, prefixation is a must because the alcohol content is only 5% in the ready-to-use stain.

Staining of Blood Films

Blood cells have structures that are acidophilic and some basophilic structures, so they vary in their reaction (pH). The nuclei are basophilic and stain blue. The highly basophilic (acidic) basophil granules also stain blue. Haemoglobin (being basic) stains acidophilic or red.

Stains that are made up of combinations of acid and basic dyes are called Romanowsky stain and various modifications are available, e.g. Wright's, Leishman's, Giemsa's, and Jenner's stains. Most use methylene blue as the basic stain, though toluidine blue is used in some. Most use eosin as the acid stain, though Azure I and Azure II are also used.

The dried film can stay for a couple of days in hot dry weather, but gets bad if they are not fixed in hot and humid climate that exists in India.

It is best to use neutral distilled water for diluting the stain. Stale distilled water becomes acidic after absorbing CO_2 from atmosphere. If the distilled water is alkaline RBCs stain a dirty bluish green colour, the parts of WBC which should stain blue will be slightly purplish, the granules of eosinophils bluish or greenish instead of pink and granules of neutrophils overstained. If the water is acidic RBCs stain bright orange and nuclei of the white cells a very pale colour.

The ideal pH is 6.8 and in order to maintain this buffered distilled water is used. Buffer water is a solution which tends to keep its original pH even on addition of small amount of alkali or acid. (Buffer tablets ready for use, to be dissolved in distilled water).

Buffer solution used in the laboratory

Solution No. I
- NaOH (sodium hydroxide) 8 gm.
- Distilled water 1000 cc.

Solution No. II
- KH_2PO_4(Potassium dihydrogen phosphate) 27.2 gm.
- Distilled water 1000 cc.

Take 23.7 cc of solution I, add to it 50cc of solution II, add 20 cc of the above mixed solution to 1000 cc of distilled water. This has a pH of 6.8.

Stain Preparation and Staining

Wright's Stain

Wright's stain (powder) 0.2 gm.
Acetone free methyl alcohol 100cc
Let stand this solution for a few days.

If the WBC granules do not stand out clearly, try out a 0.25 or 0.3% solution.

Method

Cover the slide with stain for 1-2 minutes taking care that it does not dry on the slide. Now dilute this with equal amount of buffer water (if the stain is ripe, a scum or film with a metallic sheen will form on the surface of the diluted stains on the slide). The diluted stain is allowed to act for 3-5 minutes and then flooded off with buffer or tap water. The stain should never be poured off or a precipitate of the stain will be deposited on the slide. Should this occur, it can sometimes be removed by flooding the slide with undiluted stain for 10-15 seconds and then washing it off again by flooding the slide once more with buffered water.

Leishman's Stain

Powdered Leishman's stain 0.15 gm.
Acetone-free methyl alcohol 133 ml.

All the stain should be dissolved (better if the stain crystals are well ground before), keep the stain in a glass stoppered bottle. Do not filter.

Method

Like that for Wright's stain but with double dilution of the buffer water; (i) Pour few drops (about 8) on the slide. Wait for 2 minutes, (ii) Add double the amount (16 drops) of buffered water. Mix by rocking and not by blowing and wait for 7-10 minutes, (iii) The stain is flooded off with distilled water and this should be complete in 2-3 seconds. Longer washing will remove stain, and (iv) Stand in a rack to drain and air dry. A fan will expedite the process.

Giemsa's Stain

Giemsa powder 0.3 gm
Glycerine 25.0 ml
Acetone free methyl alcohol 25.0 ml.

This makes stock solution and before use it has to be diluted by adding 1 ml (stain) to 9 ml of buffered distilled water.

Method

The blood film is fixed with methyl alcohol for 3-5 minutes and dried. Pour on diluted stain and keep for 15 minutes or longer. Wash off with tap water or neutral distilled water and dry.

Staining of Thick Films

Thick films have to be dehaemoglobinised before staining with one of the previously mentioned stains. The slide is kept in distilled water for 10 minutes, then taken out, dried and stained with any of the stains already mentioned. They must not be fixed before staining, or the water will not haemolyse the cells. The stains commonly used are Field's stain and Simeon's stain.

Field's Stain

Field's stain A

Methylene blue 0.8 gm
Azure I 0.5 gm
Disodium hydrogen phosphate (anhydrous) 5.0 gm
Potassium dihydrogen phosphate anhydrous 6.25 gm
Disttiled water 500 ml

Field's stain B

Eosin (yellow eosin, water soluble) 1.0 gm
Disodium hydrogen phosphate (anhydrous) 5.0 gm
Potassium dihydrogen phosphate (anhydrous) 6.25 gm
Distilled water 500 ml.

Grind all solids well and dissolve in the said solvent, keep the stains for 4 hours for ripening and filter before use. Keep the stains in covered jars. The depth of the solution should be about 3 inches, the level should be maintained by adding more of the stain solution.

Method

1. Dip the film for one second in solution A.
2. Remove from solution A and immediately rinse by waving very gently in clean water for a few seconds, until the stain ceases to flow from the film and the glass of the slide is free from stain.
3. Dip for one second in solution B.
4. Rinse by waving gently for 2-3 seconds in clean water.
5. Place vertically in a rack to drain and dry.

Simeon's Modification of Boye's and Sterenal's Method

This stain can be used instead of Leishman's or Wright's stain when methyl alcohol is not available to prepare them.

Solution I

Eosin pure 1 gm
Distilled water 1000 ml

Solution II

a. Medicinal methylene blue 1 gm, Distlilled water 75 ml } dissolve completely

b. Potassium permanganate 1.5 gm, Distilled water 75 ml } dissolve completely

1. Mix (a) and (b) in a flask. A massive precipitate is formed.
2. The flask is kept in a water bath at boiling point for half an hour during which time the precipitate re-dissolves.
3. Filter. The stain is now ready for use, it needs no further dilution.

Method for Staining Thin Films

1. Fix the smear by immersion into rectified spirit—1 minute.
2. Rinse with tap water—4 seconds.
3. Immerse into solution I—10 seconds.
4. Rinse with tap water—4 seconds.
5. Immerse into solution II—15 seconds.
6. Rinse with tap water—4 seconds.
7. Immerse again into solution I—5 seconds.
8. Rinse with tap water—4 seconds.
9. Allow to dry in an upright position.

Procedure for Staining Thick Smears

1. Dehaemoglobinise by immersion into tap water, if necessary.
2. Immerse in Sterenel's blue (solution II)—6 seconds.
3. Wash in tap water.
4. Immerse in eosin solution (solution I)—12 seconds.
5. Wash in tap water, allow it to dry in air. Examine under microscope.
   The stains are useful for screening purposes.

Mounting and Preservation of Films

Unstained films cannot be preserved well. Due to hardening of plasma, they do not stain well after some time. Stained films if left unmounted tend to fade away rapidly. Canada balsum should not be used as it decolourises the smear. Gurr's neutral mounting medium is quite satisfactory. Use only thin coverslips for mounting.

RAPID DIAGNOSTICS

Automation in Haematology

Various kinds of systems are available—some that offer 5 parameters to those providing 18 parameters.

Instruments from 2 acclaimed manufactures are discussed below.

1. Sysmex range: (From Transasia Biomedicals Pvt. Ltd., Transasia House, G-7, MIDC, Andheri East, Mumbai - 400 093). Transasia provides the sysmex line of top quality haematology analysers. Accuracy, precision and reliability are assured through continued research, advanced engineering, and reliable quality assurance programmes. Extensive testing and evaluation have resulted in functionally designed instrument systems that are easy to operate and maintain and the programme continues, guaranteeing instrumentation as advanced as the company itself (Towa Medical Electronics Co. Ltd., Japan). Three models are described below:
   a. *Sysmex K-1000:* 18-parameter, automated haematology analyser. Optimising utility through micro-sample, speed, and simplicity. Eight parameters analysing WBC, RBC, HCT, HGB, MCV, MCH, MCHC, PLT. Test results are printed by built-in thermal graphic printer. Three histograms for WBC, RBC and PLT plus 10 analytical parameters for W-SCR (LYMPH%), W-MCR (MXD%), W-LCR (NEUT%), W-SCC (LYMPH#), W-MCC (MXD#). W-LCC (NEUT#), RDW-CV, or RDW-SD, PDW, MPV and P-LCR. Sysmex NE-1500 is fully automated and gives 23 parameters, 5 histograms and one scattergram.
   b. *Sysmex F-800:* 15-parameter, semi-automated haematology instrument system. Eight parameters analysing WBC, RBC, HGB, HCT, MCV, MCH, MCHC and PLT plus 7 haematology parameters for LYMPH%, MO+GR%, LYMPH#, MO+GR#, RDW-CV, PDW and MPV. Three histograms for WBC, RBC and PLT. Sysmex K-800 is 8-parameter, automated haematology analyser.
   c. *ERMA PC-607:* 7-parameter analysing RBC, HGB, WBC, HCT, MCV, MCH and MCHC with histogram facility. (Manufactured by ERMA INC., Tokyo, Japan)
   d. *ERBA haematology reagents:* Complete range of haematology reagents and controls for use with blood cell counters and analysers are available from Transasia.
2. **Hemacomp** (From Bayer India Ltd, Sayajipura, Ajva Road, Baroda - 390 006).

Model Hemacomp-5M and 10 provide 5 and 10 haematology parameters respectively. The 5M provides RBC, WBC, Hb, HCT and MCV. The system has a large, easily visible LED display and a built-in printer. It is equipped with self-test programme, has an automatic cleaning procedure and gives error codes for easy troubleshooting. **SEAC Hemacomp 10** provides RBC, WBC, Hb, HCT, MCV, MCH, MCHC, PLT, MPV, PCT.

- LCD display of histograms and printout of all parameters on preformated paper.
- RBC, WBC, PLT histogram magnification for accurate analysis.
- Calibration in memory
- Complete self-control facility
- Automatic platelet threshold adjustment
- Automatic wash cycle after every analysis
- Double transducers for speed and convenience
- Easy to operate
- Highly reliable and accurate
- High throughput capacity, 80 samples an hour
- Self-diagnostic capability
- Enhanced automation through automatic diluter
- Standard RS-232 for computer interfacing optional.

DEVELOPMENT OF BLOOD CELLS SITES OF BLOOD FORMATION

Normal Sites

Foetus: Less than 2 months—yolk sac.

From 2-7 months: Liver, with minimal haemopoiesis in spleen.

After 3 months: Haemopoiesis starts in bone marrow.

Full-term infant: Bone marrow is the only site for production of granulocytes and monocytes. Occurs mainly in the spleen, lymph nodes and other lymphoid tissues, though liver and bone marrow produce these in much less numbers.

After birth: Same as above except that the monocytes are provided by the bone marrow, spleen and lymphoid tissues contribute minimally.

Abnormal Sites

Extramedullary haemopoiesis (myeloid metaplasia): In certain disorders the foetal organs revert to their old function supported by the reticulum cells which retain their potential haemopoietic activity. This occurs when bone marrow cannot any further fulfil the requirements or demand imposed upon it, e.g. in

- Growing children with haemolysis
- Myelosclerosis
- Secondary carcinoma of the bone.

DEVELOPMENT OF BLOOD CELLS (Chart 9.1)

Blood formation has to undergo three stages:

1. Multiplication of precursor cells (1% of all marrow cells are in dividing phase).
2. Gradual maturation (both structural and functional).
3. Release into the peripheral circulation. The exact release mechanism is ill understood, granulocytes achieve this by their motility and RBCs by diapedesis.

ERYTHROPOIESIS

Erythroblast is a nucleated red cell.

Normoblast implies normal (reaction) erythropoiesis.

Normoblastic maturation involves:

- Reduction in cell size.
- Ripening of cytoplasm, i.e. haemoglobinisation.

Maturation time from pronormoblast to RBC is 7 days. Mitotic division occurs till the intermediate normoblast stage.

Pronormoblast: 12-20 µm, large nucleus surrounded by a rim of deep basophilic cytoplasm and has a perinuclear halo. Nucleus is round and has several nucleoli.

Early normoblast: 10-16 µm, nucleus still large, chromatin coarser and deeply staining nucleoli disappear.

Intermediate normoblast: 8-14 µm, nucleus smaller, haemoglobinisation commences, cytoplasm takes an acidophilic tint, chromatin becomes coarser and very deeply staining.

Late normoblast: 8-10 µm, cytoplasm is acidophilic, nucleus becomes much smaller, later it becomes pyknotic and is eccentrically placed, ultimately it is lost by extrusion.

Reticulocyte: Flat, non-nucleated, disc shaped, slightly larger than mature RBC. It shows diffuse pale basophilia which appears in the form of a reticulum with supravital stains (brilliant cresyl blue or new methylene blue). In 1-2 days, it loses its basophilia and becomes a mature erythrocyte.

Control of erythropoiesis: Erythropoietin (formed in kidneys) is released in response to lowered tissue oxygen tension.

Erythropoietin is a glycoprotein and stimulates primitive cell differentiation to pronormoblasts. It affects the rate of multiplication and maturation. It acts up to early normoblast stage and also affects the rate of haemoglobinisation.

Erythropoietin levels are reduced in:

- Acute starvation.
- Hypophysectomy.
- Transfusion-induced polycythaemia.

Erythropoietin levels are increased in:

- All anaemias except those of renal origin.
- Aplastic anaemia.
- Polycythaemia.

LEUCOPOIESIS

The Myeloid Series

Specific granules are developed at the myelocyte stage which determine the nature of the mature cell.

Development of a Mature Neutrophil

Maturation involves:

1. Development of specific granules.
2. Loss of basophilia of the cytoplasm.
3. Nuclear ripening till the segmented stage.
4. Ability to be motile and to phagocytose.
   (Mitotic division occurs till the myelocyte stage only).

Myeloblast: 15-20 µm has a large round or oval nucleus, evenly stained chromatin in strands or granules with reticular appearance, 1-6 nucleoli. The cell is peroxidase negative.

Promyelocyte: It is like myeloblast except that it contains azurophilic granules which are peroxidase positive. Nuclear chromatin becomes condenser and nucleoli are less well defined.

Metamyelocyte: Specific neutrophilic granules appear, nucleus shows no nucleoli. N:C ratio reduces, cytoplasm is pale pink, chromatin thicker and deeply stained.

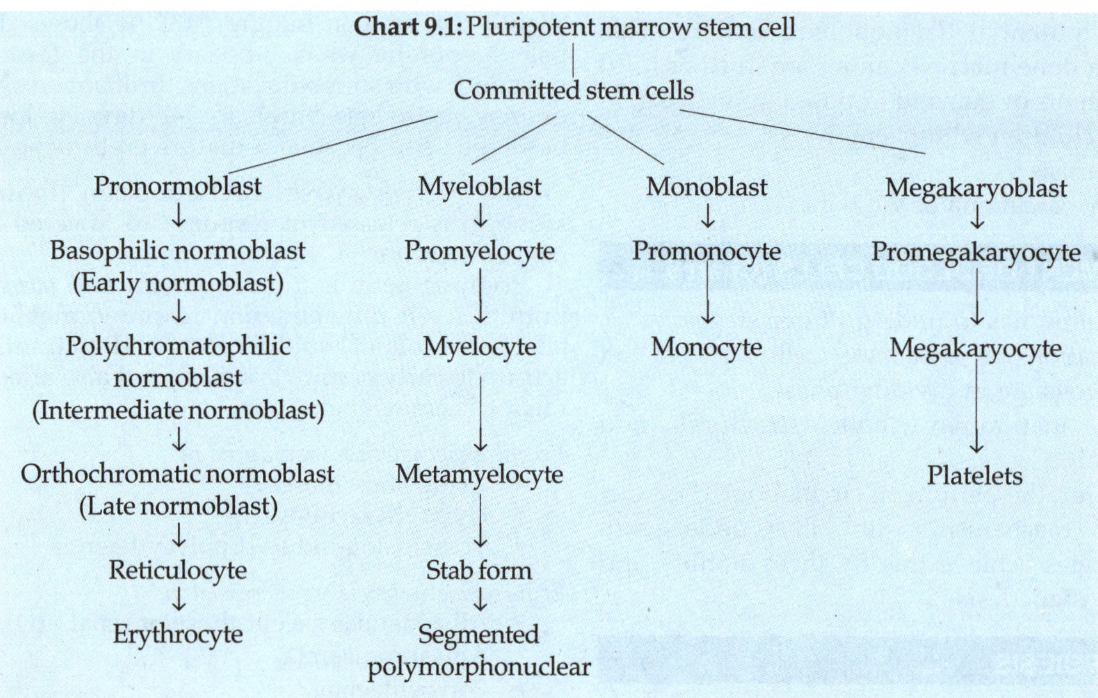

Chart 9.1: Pluripotent marrow stem cell

Metamyelocyte: Nucleus is smaller and indented, cytoplasm is pink with neutrophilic granules (purplish).

Band or stab form: Cell becomes still smaller, nucleus has a deep indentation, chromatin is coarsely clumped. Cytoplasm is pink with purplish granules.

Segmented neutrophil: 12-14 µm in size, nucleus shows 2-5 lobes, chromatin in dark purple clumps, cytoplasm has numerous, fine, evenly distributed purplish granules. In female at least 6 neutrophils/ 500 should show drumsticks.

The mature eosinophil: 16 µm in size, granules are acidophilic and larger. Nucleus is bilobed and is not masked by granules.

The mature basophil: It usually has a bilobed nucleus, but the nucleus is masked by about 10 large basophilic granules.

Lymphocytic Series

Lymphoblast: 15-20 µm in size, resembles myeloblast, cytoplasm is agranular and moderately basophilic. Nuclear chromatin gives fine reticular appearance with up to 2 nucleoli. It is peroxidase negative.

Large lymphocyte: 12-16 µm in size, has abundant pale sky blue cytoplasm with a few purplish red granules seen in about 33% of the cells.

Small lymphocyte: 9-12 µm in size, has scanty cytoplasm. Nucleus is usually round and shows heavily clumped chromatin.

Monocytic Series

Monoblast: It resembles myeloblast.

Promonocyte: Up to 20 µm in size, has a large convoluted nucleus, chromatin is seen in skein like strands. Cytoplasm is dull grey-blue and may contain a few azurophilic granules.

Monocyte: 15-20 µm in size, has abundant dull grey-blue cytoplasm with a ground glass appearance and may show vacuolation and fine azurophilic granules. It has a kidney-shaped nucleus.

THROMBOPOIESIS

Megakaryoblast: 20-30 µm in size, has a large, oval or kidney-shaped nucleus with several nucleoli. It possesses relatively small amount of agranular cytoplasm.

Promegakaryocyte: 30 µm in diameter, cytoplasm is intensely basophilic with fine azurophilic granules. Nucleus may show mild lobulation and chromatin appears denser.

Megakaryocyte: 30-90 µm in diameter, it contains a single multilobulated or indented nucleus. Nuclear lobes may vary from 4-16 in number. Cytoplasm is bulky, light blue with fine azurophilic granulation. The margin is irregular and may show fragmentation or budding, precursor of circulating platelets.

Mature platelet: 1-4 µm. It is formed by fragmentation of megakaryocytic pseudopods. In circulation they acquire a discoid shape. Cytoplasm stains light blue and contains purple reddish granules which may be clumped centrally.

Control of platelet production: Perhaps by a humoral factor called thrombopoietin, acts by a feedback mechanism.

EXAMINATION OF A BLOOD FILM

Method

1. *Mount:* Cover the slide using a neutral mounting medium.
2. *Low power field examination:* Look for:
   - Quality of film
   - Number, distribution and staining of WBCs.
   - RBCs examination, select an area where they just touch each other without overlapping, i.e. between tail and body of the film.
3. *High power field examination:*
   Assess RBC
   - size.
   - shape
   - haemoglobin concentration
4. *Oil immersion examination:* Assess atypical cells and note fine details, e.g. inclusion bodies.

ALWAYS NOTE

RBCs

Size: Normocytes, microcytes, macrocytes, anisocytosis (variation in size).

Shape: Abnormal shape oval, pencil, tear, pear, oat and sickle-shaped cells, fragmented cells, target cells, spherocytes, crenated cells, burr cells, acanthocytes, stomatocytes (poikilocytes).

Haemoglobin: Normochromic, hypochromic.

Immature forms: Polychromatic, stippled or nucleated red cells.

Inclusion bodies: Howell-Jolly bodies, Cabot rings, Pappenheimer bodies, malarial parasites, etc.

Arrangement: Autoagglutination, excess rouleaux formation.

WBCs

Number: Normal, increased, decreased.

Abnormal or immature forms: Immature forms, hypersegmented macropolycytes, abnormal forms.

Platelets

Number: Normal, increased, decreased.

Form: Abnormalities of size and shape, present in groups or lying scattered.

Differential Leucocyte Count (DLC)

For differential leucocyte counts, choose an area where the morphology of the cells is clearly visible. Ensure that there is no tailing of the WBCs or else a false DLC may be obtained. Do differential count by moving the slide as shown in order to include central and peripheral areas of the smear.

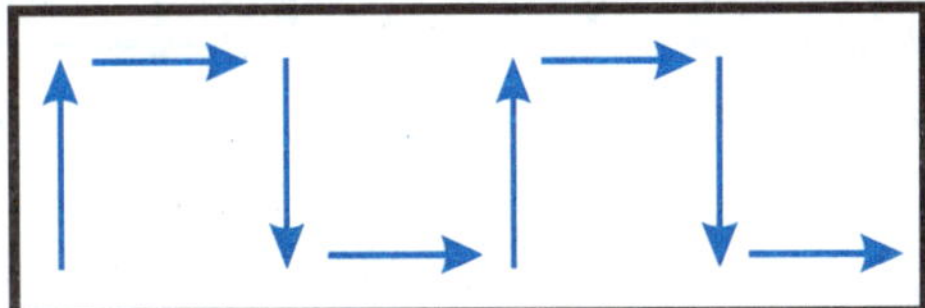

While doing DLC, look for vacuolation, toxic granulation, size and maturity of the WBCs. Count at least 100 cells and give percentage of the cells seen. Counting becomes easier if 100 squares are made on a paper and the letters P for neutrophil, L for lymphocyte, M for monocyte, E for eosinophil and B for basophil can be entered in each square. Another easier way is using Laboratory cell counter (Fig. 9.11).

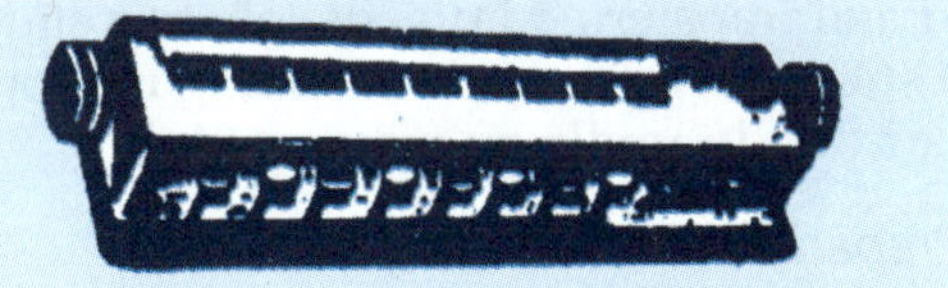

Fig. 9.11: Nine unit laboratory cell counter

BONE MARROW EXAMINATION

Bone marrow can be obtained by using Salah's, Klima's or Jamshidi's marrow aspiration needles. Not more than 0.2 ml of bone marrow should be taken out at one time.

If blood or dry taps have occurred on 2 different occasions, a trephine biopsy should be performed.

For aspiration of bone marrow, Klima's needle is better as the guard has no chances of getting slipped and hence dangers of puncturing substernal structures are less.

Before entering the site of puncture, take all aseptic precautions, i.e. cleaning with spirit, iodine and spirit again. *The various sites for obtaining bone marrow are:*

In adults:

- Sternal aspiration.
- Anterior iliac crest.
- Vertebral spinous processes.
- Posterior superior iliac spine.

In children:

- Tibia, superior medial surface of the tibia, inferior to the medial condyle and medial to the tibial tuberosity.
- Posterior iliac crest.
- Calcaneum.

BONE MARROW EXAMINATION AND REPORTING

Marrow Film Preparation

Delay in marrow film preparation should NOT be there. Get rid of blood by using a capillary pipette leaving the greyish marrow particles behind. Make a smear as has been described for peripheral blood. The smear should be 3 to 5 cm long and should not be more than 2 cm wide. The particles should be dragged behind but not squashed. A trail of cells is left behind. Criteria of a good preparation—presence of both particles and free marrow cells in the smear.

Imprints

Another way is imprint method. The marrow particle is picked and transferred immediately to a slide and made to stick to it by a gentle smearing motion. The slide is air dried rapidly by waving.

Crush Preparation

Marrow particles in a small drop of aspirate are placed on a slide near one end. Another slide is carefully placed over the first. Slight pressure is exerted to crush the particles, and the slides are separated by pulling them apart in a direction parallel to their surfaces. Dry the smears immediately. The appearance of fat (irregular holes) on the smear implies that marrow has been obtained.

1. Good fixation is essential.
2. Any of the previously mentioned stains can be used for staining bone marrow films.

Examination

The examiner should be informed of the clinical picture before he or she examines the marrow films. An impression can be formed by examining various fields on the different stained slides prepared. Start with 10x through 40x, to oil immersion, now actually make a differential count of large number of cells (300 to 1000) and calculate the percentage of each type of cell.

The procedure given below is recommended for studying the marrow films:

1. Naked eye inspection of the slides to select the smear containing particles.
2. With 10x objective, survey the particles whether they are normoplastic, hypoplastic or hyperplastic.
3. Select a cellular area (usually in the tail portion of the film around particles), study the cytologic details by high power—40x and oil immersion—100x objectives.

Note the undermentioned points:

Cellularity: Normo/hypo/hyperplastic marrow particles. Cellularity is better defined by studying histologic sections of aspirated particles, though crude estimates can be given on films. The normal cellularity of the marrow varies with age being more in infants and least in elderly individuals.

Next look for *reaction of erythropoiesis,* whether it is normoblastic, megaloblastic or micronormoblastic. Look for maturity of leukopoietic cells. The M:E ratio is based on a count of 500 to 1000 marrow cells. In the normal adult the reaction is normoblastic leukopoietic maturity is normal and *ME ratio* is about 3 or 4:1. The ME ratio at birth is 1.85:1; during the first two weeks, it reaches its peak of 11:1. It then gradually drops to the (years 1 to 20) average of 3:1.

Look for megakaryocytes, their number, size, nuclear lobulations, functioning capacity.

Megakaryocytes with budding or cloud-like appearance at the periphery are functioning ones. *In addition, if suspected, look for metastatic cells, increased number of normal or abnormal (myeloma) plasma cells, cells containing unduly large amounts of lipid, carbohydrate, etc.—storage disease. One may also see haemoparasites* in the marrow especially *LD bodies of Kala- azar.*

BONE MARROW ASPIRATION ANALYSIS

Normal Values

Red marrow contains connective tissue, fat cells, and hematopoietic cells. Yellow marrow contains connective tissue and fat cells. Interpretation of cell count and histopathology by a haematologist, pathologist, or oncologist is required.

Response to staining: Iron stain for haemosiderin: 2+. *Periodic Acid-Schiff (PAS) glycogen reactions:* Negative.

Sudan black B (SBB) granulocyte: Negative.

DIFFERENTIAL CELL COUNT

	Adult (%)	*Child (%)*	*Infant (%)*
Basophils	0.1	0.06	0.07
Eosinophils	3.1	3.6	2.6
Haemocytoblasts	0.1-1.0		
Lymphocytes (all stages)	2.7-24	16	49
Megakaryocytes	0.03-0.5	0.1	0.05
Plasmacytes	0.1-1.5	0.4	0.02
Promyelocytes	0.5-8.0	1.4	0.76
Reticulum cells	0.1-2.0		
Undifferentiated cells	0.0-0.1		
Neutrophils, total	56.5	57.1	32.4
Metamyelocytes	9.6-24.6	23.3	11.3
Neutrophilic	10-32		
Eosinophilic	0.3-3.7		
Basophilic	0-0.3		
Monocytes (all stages)	0-2.7		
Myeloblasts	0.1-5.0	1.2	0.62
Myelocytes	4.2-15	18.4	2.5
Neutrophilic	5.0-20		
Eosinophilic	0.1-3.0		
Basophilic	0-0.5		
Segmented granulocyte	6.0-12.0	12.9	3.6
Neutrophilic	7.0-30		
Eosinophilic	0.2-4.0		
Basophilic	0-0.7		
Band cells	9.5-15.3	0	14.1
Neutrophilic	10-35		
Eosinophilic	0.2-2.0		
Basophilic	0.3		
Erythroid series			
Normoblasts, total	25.6	23.1	8.0
Pronormoblasts	0.2-4.0	0.5	0.1
Basophilic normoblasts	1.5-5.8	1.7	0.34
Polychromatophilic normoblasts	5.0-26.4	18.2	6.9
Orthochromic normoblasts	3.6-21	2.7	0.54
Promegaloblasts	0		
Basophilic megaloblasts	0		
Polychromatic megaloblasts	0		
Orthochromic megaloblasts	0		

M:E ratio: (Myeloid:Erythroid is the ratio of WBCs to nucleated RBCs.)

Adult	6:1-2:1
Birth	1.85:1
2 weeks	11:1
1-2 months	5.5:1
1 1-20 years	2.95:1

Usage: Helps to distinguish primary and metastatic tumours. Assists in the identification, classification, and staging of neoplasias. Aids evaluation of the progress and/or response to the treatment of neoplasias. Assists in the definitive diagnosis of blood disorders. Culture of an aspirated sample can aid in the identification of infections such as histoplasmosis or tuberculosis. Histologic examination aids in the diagnosis of carcinoma, granulomas, lymphoma, or myelofibrosis. Iron stain showing decreased haemosiderin levels may indicate iron deficiency and SBB stain differentiates acute granulocytic leukaemia from acute lymphocytic leukaemia.

Increased eosinophils: Bone marrow carcinoma, eosinophilic leukaemia, lymphadenoma, myeloid leukaemia and pernicious anaemia (relapse).

Increased lymphocytes: Aplastic anaemia, hypoplasia of the bone marrow, infectious lymphocytosis or mononucleosis, lymphatic leukaemoid reactions, lymphocytic leukaemia (B-cell and T-cell), lymphoma, macroglobulinaemia, myelofibrosis and viral infections.

Increased megakaryocytes: Acute haemorrhage, ageing, chronic myeloid leukaemia, hypersplenism, idiopathic thrombocytopenia, infection, megakaryocytic myelosis, myelofibrosis, pneumonia, polycythaemia vera and thrombocytopenia.

Increased plasma cells: Agranulocytosis, amyloidosis, aplastic anaemia, carcinomatosis, collagen disease, hepatic cirrhosis, Hodgkin's disease, hypersensitivity reactions, infection, irradiation, macroglobulinaemia, malignant tumour, multiple myeloma, rheumatic fever (acute), rheumatoid arthritis, serum sickness, syphilis and ulcerative colitis.

Increased granulocyte: Hypoplasia of the bone marrow, infections, myelocytic leukaemia, myelocytic leukaemoid reaction and myeloproliferative syndrome.

Increased normoblasts: Anaemia (iron deficiency, haemolytic, megaloblastic), blood loss (chronic), erythema, erythroid-type myeloproliferative disorders, hypoplasia of the bone marrow and polycythaemia vera.

Increased M:E ratio above 7:1 Decreased haematopoiesis, erythroid hypoplasia, infection, leukemoid reactions, and myeloid leukaemia.

Increased diffuse bone marrow hyperplasia: Myeloproliferative syndromes and pancytopenia reactions.

Decreased megakaryocytes: Anaemia (aplastic, pernicious), bone marrow hyperplasia (with carcinomatous or leukaemic deposits), cirrhosis, irradiation (excessive), and thrombocytopenia purpura. Drugs include benzene, chlorothiazides, and cytotoxic drugs.

Decreased granulocytes: Agranulocylosis, hyperplasia of the bone marrow, and ionising radiation.

Decreased normoblasts: Anaemia (aplastic, hypoplastic), folic acid or vitamin B_{12} deficiency.

Decreased M:E ratio below 2:1 Agranulocylosis, anaemia (iron deficiency, normoblaslic, pernicious, posthaemolytic, posthaemorrhagic), erythroid activity (increased), hepatic disease, myeloid formation (decreased), polycythaemia vera, sprue, and steatorrhoea.

Decreased diffuse bone marrow hypoplasia: Ageing, cellular infiltrations, dengue fever, myelofibrosis, myelosclerosis, myelotoxic agents, osteoporosis, rubella, and viral infections.

Description: Bone marrow is the soft, organic, sponge-like material contained in the medullary cavities, long bones, some haversian canals, and within the spaces between trabeculae of cancellous bone. It is composed of red and yellow marrow, with the chief function being production of erythrocytes, leucocytes, and platelets. Only the rusty, red marrow produces blood cells. The yellow marrow is formed of connective tissue and fat cells, which are inactive. During infancy and childhood, bone marrow is primarily red marrow, and in the adult, 50% is red marrow. The bone marrow aspiration procedure obtains a sample of bone marrow by needle. A stained blood smear of the sample is evaluated for bone marrow morphology and examination of blood cell erythropoiesis, cellularity, differential cell count, bone marrow iron stores, and M:E ratios.

Indications for Bone Marrow Aspiration

Absolute Indications

- Megaloblastic macrocytic anaemia.
- Aleukaemic or subleukaemic leukaemia.

Diagnostic Importance

- Multiple myeloma.
- Aplastic anaemia.
- Gaucher's disease.

Confirmatory Importance

- Leukaemias of all types.
- Haemolytic anaemia.
- Idiopathic thrombocytopenic purpura.
- Idiopathic granulocytopenia.
- Leishmaniasis.
- Disseminated lupus erythematosus (LE cells).
- Metastatic disease.
- Myeloproliferative disorders.
- Lipid storage.
- Sideroblastic anaemia.
- Iron deficiency anaemia.
- Lymphoma (staging).

(Bone marrow may be obtained from one person for transplantation into another).

In many cases one may just obtain blood (*blood tap*) or nothing at all (*dry tap*). Under these conditions, a *bone marrow biopsy* has to be performed. It can be obtained with *Jamshidi's needle* or with *Sacker-Nordins bone biopsy trephine.*

Bone biopsy may be needed in
- Malignant lymphoma.
- Metastatic carcinoma.
- Sarcoidosis.
- Tuberculosis.
- Brucellosis.
- Histoplasmosis.
- Storage disorders.
- Aplastic anaemia.
- Myelofibrosis.
- Acute leukaemias.

Contraindications

- Haemophilia.
- Bleeding diathesis.
- Infection at site of puncture.

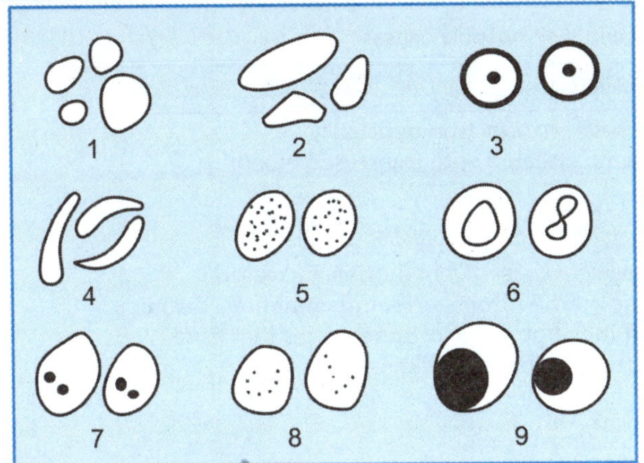

Fig.9.12: Morphological alterations in RBCs: (1) Anisocytosis, (2) Poikilocytosis, (3) Target cells, (4) Sickle cells, (5) Basophilia, (6) Cabot's rings, (7) Howell-Jolly bodies, (8) Reticulocytes (large basophilic), (9) Normoblasts

Morphological Types of Red Blood Cells

Usually anaemias are described on two grounds:
- The average cell volume (MCV)
- The average haemoglobin concentration (MCHC).

Three main types of anaemias are recognised:
1. The *normocytic anaemias*, in which MCV is within normal range (76-96 fl). Most normocytic anaemias are also normochromic (i.e. MCHC is between 30-35 gm%) but in some, mild hypochromia may occur. For size of an RBC, compare its size with that of a small lymphocyte. As for haemoglobinisation normally only a small area of central pallor is seen (central 1/3 rd).
2. The hypochromic, microcytic anaemias, in which the MCV is reduced (less than 76 fl) and MCHC is also reduced (less than 30 gm%).
3. The macrocytic anaemias in which the MCV is increased (greater than 96 fl). Most macrocytic anaemias are normochromic; but in some, a mild hypochromia may occur.

RBC MORPHOLOGY, BLOOD

Normal Values

Microscopic interpretation is required.

Colour	Uniformly normochromic
Size	6-8 μ only slight size variation
Shape	Round, biconcave disc
Stained appearance	Mature erythrocytes stain uniformly and contain a normal concentration of haemoglobin with an area of central pallor.
Nucleus	Absent
Nuclear remnants	Absent
Cellular inclusions	Absent
Acanthocytes	Absent
Crescent bodies	Absent
Drepanocytes	Absent
Echinocytes	Absent
Leptocytes	Absent
Poikilocytes	Absent
Schizocytes	Absent
Spherocytes	Absent
Stomatocyte	Absent
Cabot rings	Absent
Heinz bodies	Absent
Siderocytes	Absent

CLASSIFICATION OF VARIATION FROM NORMAL

Abnormal RBCs/HPF	*Score*	*Interpretation*
3-6	1+	Slight
7-10	2+	Moderate
11-20	3+	Marked
>20	4+	Very marked

Usage

Detection of blood dyscrasias; and differentiation of anaemias, leukaemia, and thalassaemia (Table 9.2).

RETICULOCYTE COUNT

Reticulocytes. These are immature red cells which still contain the remains of ribonuclear protein. Their number in peripheral blood increases following increased erythroid activity in the bone marrow. This may occur when there is reduction in number of red cells in the peripheral blood, e.g. by haemorrhage or abnormal haemolysis. The reticulocyte count is of value in pernicious/megaloblastic anaemias, for improvement is indicated by a rise in reticulocytes in the peripheral blood.

Normal Values

Comprises 1-2% of the total RBC count

		SI Units
Adult females	0.5-2.5%	$0.005\text{-}0.025 \times 10^{-3}$
Adults males	0.5-1.5%	$0.005\text{-}0.015 \times 10^{-3}$
Cord blood	3.0-7.0%	$0.030\text{-}0.070 \times 10^{-3}$
Newborn	1.1-4.5%	$0.011\text{-}0.045 \times 10^{-3}$
Neonates	0.1-1.5%	$1.010\text{-}0.015 \times 10^{-3}$
Infants	0.5-3.1%	$0.005\text{-}0.031 \times 10^{-3}$
Children >6 months	0.5-4.0%	$0.005\text{-}0.040 \times 10^{-3}$

Table 9.2: Various RBC abnormalities and their possible causes

Description of abnormalities of RBC colour	*Possible causes of abnormal RBC colour*
Anisochromia is demonstrated by variable staining intensities indicating unequal haemoglobin content due to multiple populations of red blood cells (RBCs).	*Anisochromatism:* Iron-deficiency anaemia treated with transfused blood
Hyperchromia is demonstrated by the presence of cells having a smaller than normal area of central pallor, causing the cells to take on excessive staining and demonstrate higher than normal pigmentation. Increased amounts of these cells are called hyperchromatism.	*Hyperchromatism:* Dehydration, increased bone marrow iron stores, inflammation (chronic), and in the presence of spherocytes that have increased cell wall thickness
Hypochromia is demonstrated by the presence of cells having a larger than normal area of central pallor, causing the cells to stain weakly and appear to have less than normal pigmentation. Increased amounts of these cells is called hypochromatism.	*Hypochromatism:* Anaemia (iron deficiency) and decreased haemoglobin concentration
Polychromatophils are cells that are stainable with many types of stains, such as stains with both an acid and base component. They are demonstrated by a bluish-pink tinge caused by the presence of both haemoglobin stained by acid and cytoplasmic ribonucleic acid (RNA) stained by the basic component. Both the larger-than-normal cell size and the presence of cytoplasmic RNA indicate that polychromatophils are reticulocytes (newly made RBCs). Increased amounts of polychromatophils is called polychromatosis and occurs in accelerated RBC production.	*Polychromatosis:* Haemorrhage, haemolysis, reticulocytosis, and therapy for iron deficiency anaemia or pernicious anaemia
Description of abnormalities of RBC shape	*Possible causes of abnormal RBC shape*
Acanthocytes are cells with irregular, thorny, spiculated membrane surface projections containing bulbous, rounded ends. They result from an irreversible defect in the lipid content of the RBC membrane. The presence of acanthocytes is called acanthocytosis.	*Acanthocytosis:* Abetelipoprotenaemia (most common cause), alcoholic cirrhosis, haemolytic anaemia (induced by pyruvate kinase deficiency), hepatic disease, postsplenectomy, and retinitis pigmentosa. Drugs include heparin calcium and heparin sodium.
Crescent bodies (achromocytes) are cells with a faint quarter-moon shape caused by RBC rupture	*Achromocytosis:* Any condition that increases the fragility of RBCs (i.e., sickle cell anaemia, reduced oxygen supply) ,
Drepanocytes/sickle cells are cells formed in the shape of a sickle with a point at one end. The presence of these cells is called drepanocytosis.	*Drepanocytosis:* Anaemia (haemolytic, sickle cell) and haemoglobin SC disease
Echinocytes/burr cells/crenated: RBCs have a cell surface with 10-30 uniformly distributed, blunt spicules. Echinocytes may be commonly due to pH changes due to faulty drying during smear preparation, but certain physiologic conditions, including a reversible defect in the lipid content of the RBC membrane, have been associated with their presence. The presence of these cells is called echinocytosis.	*Echinocytosis:* Bile acid abnormalities, blood loss (acute), burns (extensive), carcinoma of the stomach, disseminated intravascular coagulation (DIC), gastric ulcers (bleeding), increased free fatty acids, microangiopathic haemolytic anaemia, pyruvate kinase deficiency, renal failure, thrombotic thrombocytopenic purpura, and uraemia. Drugs include barbiturates, heparin calcium, heparin sodium, and salicylates.

Contd...

Contd...

Elliptocytes/ovalocytes have a cigar shape, which distinguishes them from the more oval shape of the ovalocytes. They are normal constituents of mature RBCs. Higher than normal amounts of these cells are called elliptocytosis.	*Elliptocytosis:* Anaemias (iron deficiency, pernicious, sickle cell), hereditary elliptocytosis, leukaemia, megaloblastic haematopoiesis, and thalassaemia
Leptocytes/target cells have an increased ratio of surface to volume, often due to a shape that looks like a cup, bell, or hat. They have a colourless centre and are thinner and lighter staining than normal RBCs due to abnormally low amounts of haemoglobin. When stained, the depth of the "cup" collapses, causing a bulls-eye appearance. The presence of leptocytes is termed leptocytosis.	*Leptocytosis:* Anaemia (iron deficiency, sickle cell), cellular dehydration, cirrhosis, haemoglobin C disease, haemoglobin SC disease, hepatitis, jaundice (obstructive), postsplenectomy and thalassaemia
Poikilocytes occur in varying shapes, ranging from slightly irregular to dumbbell-like, pear-shaped or teardrop-shaped. Defective bone marrow production causes poikilocytosis, a general term used to describe the presence of cells demonstrating variation from the normal shape of the RBC.	*Poikilocytosis:* Anaemia (iron deficiency, haemolytic, megaloblastic. pernicious), myelofibrosis, myeloid metaplasia, and thalassaemia
Schizocytosis/schistocytes are RBCs with adhesions of spiral and triangular RBC fragments due to haemolysis, haemoglobinopathies, or erythrocytic mechanical damage from fibrin strands. The presence of these cells is called schizocytosis.	*Schizocytosis or Schistocytosis:* Anaemia (acute haemolytic, microangiopathic haemolytic), burns (severe), disseminated intravascular coagulation (DIC), prosthetic heart valves, pyruvate kinase deficiency, renal graft rejection, uraemic-haemolytic syndrome, valve prosthesis and valvular stenosis
Spherocytes are cells that are globe-like rather than biconcave, with an abnormally small dimple. They are thicker than normal, with many fine-needle-like projections. Spherocytes lack an area of central pallor (due to an increased mean corpuscular haemoglobin concentration) and have a smaller surface area relative to their size. Spherocytes are caused by mechanical fibrin strand damage to circulating RBCs. The presence of spherocytes is called spherocytosis.	*Spherocytosis:* ABO haemolytic disease of the newborn, accelerated reticuloendothelial RBC destruction, anaemia (haemolytic), following blood transfusion, hereditary spherocytosis, and thermal injury of the cell membrane
Stomatocytes are cup-shaped RBCs with an abnormal area of central pallor that may be oval or rectangular elongated, or slitlike. These cells are produced by antibodies or hydrocytosis. The presence of these cells is called stomatocytosis.	*Stomatocytosis:* Alcoholism, cirrhosis, erythrocyte sodium pump defect, hepatic disease (obstructive), hereditary spherocytosis, hereditary, stomatocytosis, and Rh null cells

Description of abnormalities of RBC size	*Possible causes of abnormalities of RBC size*
Anisocytosis is a general term that describes any variation in the size of the RBC.	*Anisocytosis:* Anaemias (iron deficiency, pernicious), folic acid deficiency, following blood transfusion of normal cells into an abnormal RBC population, leukaemia, newborns, and reticulocytosis

Contd...

Contd...

Macrocytes are large erythrocytes having a diameter > 8 μ, a mean corpuscular volume > 96 μ, and higher than normal haemoglobin content. They are usually increased due to stress erythropoiesis. Increased amounts of macrocytes are called macrocytosis.	*Macrocytosis:* Anaemia (haemolytic, pernicious), folic acid deficiency, following haemorrhagic states, hepatic disease, hyperthyroidism, idiopathic steatorrhea, newborns, reticulocytosis, and thalassaemia
Microcytes have a RBC diameter <6 μ, a mean corpuscular volume <76 μ, and mean corpuscular haemoglobin concentration <27%. Increased amounts of microcytes are called microcytosis.	*Microcytosis:* Anaemia (from chronic haemorrhage, iron deficiency), haemoglobinopathies, hereditary spherocytosis, and thalassaemia

Description of abnormalities of RBC content of structure	*Possible causes of abnormal RBC structure or content*
Agglutination: Clumping together of RBCs is an immune mechanism caused by antibody formation.	*Agglutination:* Invading antigen(s)
Basophilic stippling is demonstrated by the presence of minute basophilic granules that cause a bluish / purple colour when reticulocytes are stained. They are caused by ribosomal aggregation that occurs as smears are prepared. Small amounts of basophilic stippling normally occur as the smears are dried. Increased amounts occur in conditions in which RNA has aggregated in the cells.	*Increased basophilic stippling:* Alcoholism, anaemia (megaloblastic, sickle cell), heavy metal intoxication (bismuth, lead, mercury, and silver), haemorrhage (gastrointestinal), leukaemia, and thalassaemia
Cabot's rings are cells containing mitotic spindle remnants appearing as fine, threadlike filaments of bluish purple colour in the shape of a single ring or a double ring (figure-eight shape).	*Presence of Cabot's rings:* Anaemia (severe, pernicious), lead poisoning, myelofibrosis, and myeloid metaplasia
Heinz bodies are denatured particles of haemoglobin attached to the RBC membrane that appear when stained with cresyl blue or new methylene blue. Heinz bodies usually indicate abnormal erythrocyte stability due to haemolytic conditions or haemoglobinopathies.	*Presence of Heinz bodies:* Alpha-thalassaemia, anaemia (haemolytic), glucose-6-phosphate dehydrogenase deficiency, haemoglobinopathies, methaemoglobinaemia, and postsplenectomy. Drugs include analgesics, antipyretics, chlorates, phenacetin, phenothiazines. phenylacetamide, phenylhydrazine phenylamine, primaquine phosphate, resorcinol, and sulphapyridine
Howell-Jolly bodies are nuclear fragments contained in red cells that stain purple or violet. They are normally present in immature RBCs and in mature erythrocytes before they pass through the splenic circulation. In conditions causing increased RBC production, erythrocytes contain higher than normal amounts of these bodies.	*Presence of Howell-Jolly bodies:* Anaemia (haemolytic, megaloblastic), leukaemia, splenic absence (congenital or surgical removal), and splenic atrophy

Contd...

Contd...

Platelets on RBCs appear as a halo that resists staining and can be easily confused with RBC inclusion bodies.	
Rouleaux formation is demonstrated by a cellular configuration in stacks or rolls. Increased rouleaux formation may be caused by increased fibrinogen or globulins in the blood. Rouleaux formation is decreased by the presence of abnormally shaped RBCs, which inhibits adherence of the cells in a stacked shape. Rouleaux formation may also result from a delay in slide preparation.	*Increased rouleaux formation:* Hyperfibrinogenaemia, macroglobulinaemia, and multiple myeloma *Decreased rouleaux formation:* Hereditary spherocytosis
Siderocytes/Pappenheimer bodies are cells with mitochondrial concentrations of ferritin (nonhaemoglobin iron) deposits. These cells stain as purple-bluish granules only in the presence of iron stains such as Prussian-blue reactions. Pappenheimer bodies are noniron basophilic granules contained in the iron-protein matrix and stain positive for iron in the presence of noniron stains. Ferritin is normally absent in RBCs. During haemoglobin formation in the premature infant and newborn, siderocyte free-iron granules commonly occur in developing normoblasts and reticulocytes. The presence of siderocytes is called siderocytosis.	*Siderocytosis/Pappenheimer bodies:* Anaemia (chronic haemolytic, congenital spherocytic, dyserythropoietic, megaloblastic, pernicious, refractory, sideroblastic), burns (severe), haemochromatosis, infection, lead poisoning, postsplenectomy, and thalassaemia

Staining

Ribonuclear protein is a living material which requires special staining, using a supravital stain such as brilliant cresyl blue. Methyl alcohol destroys ribonuclear protein; and hence, it cannot be seen in Romanowsky stained preparation. In Romanowsky stained films, they appear as larger cells showing polychromasia.

Stain

1% Brilliant cresyl blue
Brilliant cresyl blue 1 gm.
Sodium chloride 0.7 gm.
Sodium citrate 0.6 gm.
Distilled water 100 ml.

Store in dark bottle under refrigeration, filter before use (new methylene blue can also be used instead of BCB).

Method

- Place I volume of filtered stain in small test tube.
- Place I volume of capillary or venous blood and mix.
- Incubate at room temperature or at 37°C for 10-30 minutes.
- Remix the tube contents and spread 1 drop of the stained blood on a slide making a thin film.

When dry, examine with the oil immersion lens. Count systematically at least 500 cells, including in this the number of reticulocytes. Reticulocytes appear larger than mature cells and contain irregular dark purple granules or fine threads of ribonuclear material, calculate the percentage of reticulocytes.

Interpretation: Reticulocyte counts are low in ineffective erythropoiesis, e.g. myelosclerosis, aplastic anaemia, megaloblastic anaemia, thalassaemia, erythroleukaemia and sideroblastic anaemia. Reticulocytosis occurs after blood loss or effective therapy for certain kinds of anaemia, e.g., therapy of iron deficiency or megaloblastic macrocytic anaemia. Reticulocytosis also occurs in haemolytic anaemias.

RED CELL FRAGILITY TEST

Screening test: One needs 0.45% sodium chloride solution and haemocytometer for counting red cells. Blood is drawn to the 0.5 mark in 2 red cell pipettes.

Red Blood Cell Abnormalities seen on stained Smear (In brief)

Descriptive term	*Observation*	*Importance*
Macrocytosis	Cell diameter > 8 μm MCV > 96 fl.	Megaloblastic anaemias, severe liver disease Hypothyroidism
Microcytosis	Cell diameter < 6 μm MCV < 76 fl. MCHC < 27	Iron deficiency anaemia Anaemia of chronic disease Thalassaemia
Hypochromia	Increased zone of central pallor	Reduced Hb content
Polychromatophilia	Presence of red cells not fully haemogolobinised	Reticulocytosis
Poikilocytosis	Variability of cell shape	Sickle cell disease Microangiopathic haemolysis Leukaemias Extramedullary haematopoiesis Marrow stress of any cause
Anisocytosis	Variability in cell size	Reticulocytosis Transfusing normal blood into microcytic or macrocytic cell population
Leptocytosis	Hypochromic cells with small central zone Hb (target cells)	Thalassaemias Iron deficiency anaemia, obstructive jaundice
Spherocytosis	Cells without central pallor, loss of biconcave shape MCHC high	Loss of membrane relative to cell volume. Hereditary spherocytosis. Accelerated RBC destruction by reticuloendothelial system
Schistocytosis	Presence of cell fragments in circulation	Increased intravascular mechanical trauma Microangiopathic haemolysis
Acanthocytosis	Irregularly spiculated surface	Irreversibly abnormal membrane lipid content Liver disease Abetalipoproteinaemia
Echinocytosis	Regularly spiculated cell surface	Reversible abnormalities of membrane lipid content. High plasma free fatty acids, bile acid abnormalities. Effects of barbiturates, salicylates, etc.
Stomatocytosis	Elongated, slit-like zone of central pallor	Hereditary defect in membrane sodium metabolism Severe liver disease
Elliptocytosis	Oval cells	Hereditary anomally, usually harmless.

The first is diluted to the 101 mark with Hayem's (RBC diluting fluid) and the second with 0.45% sodium chloride solution. Both pipettes are shaken for 2 minutes and counts made from both pipettes, the percentage of cells haemolysed in the 0.45% saline solution is thus determined. Less than 30% of normal erythrocytes are haemolysed by this technique. An abnormal increase in red cell fragility, as in congenital haemolytic icterus will cause haemolysis of more than 70% of the cells.

Quantitative Test

Principle: Tubes containing solution of varying concentration of saline buffered to pH 7.4 are used. Heparinised or defibrinated blood is added to each tube in a proportion of 1 to 100 and the degree of haemolysis in each is noted using a photoelectric colourimeter. The result may be reported as a graph or stating the concentration at which haemolysis begins and that at which it is complete.

Reagents

A stock solution of buffered sodium chloride (AR) osmotically equivalent to 10% NaCl, is made up as follows. NaCl 180 gm, Na_2HPO_4 27.31 gm and $NaH_2PO_4 2H_2O$ 4.86 gm are dissolved in distilled water and the final volume adjusted to 2 litres. This solution will keep for months in a well-stoppered bottle. In preparing solutions for use it is convenient to make first a 1% solution from the 10% stock solution by dilution with distilled water. Dilutions equivalent to 0.85, 0.75, 0.65, 0.60, 0.55, 0.45, 0.40, 0.35, 0.30, 0.20 and 0.10 per cent NaCl are convenient test concentrations. Intermediate concentrations such as 0.475% and 0.525% are useful in critical work.

If the test is performed very occasionally, smaller volumes of the solutions may be made up as given at the bottom of this page.

Method

Use: Heparinised or defibrinated blood, oxalated and citrated blood may change the tonicity which is not desirable.

Add 0.05 ml of blood to each tube containing 5 ml of the different concentrations of saline. Mix well and let the tubes stand at room temperature for 30 minutes. Remix and centrifuge for 5 minutes at 2000 rpm and measure the amount of haemolysis in each tube in a photoelectric colorimeter with green filter. The supernatant from 0.85% NaCl is used as the blank because there is no haemolysis in this concentration (normal) of saline. The supernatant from the 0.1% NaCl is used to estimate 100% lysis (the supernatant can easily be decanted into the cuvette of the colorimeter). The depth of colour should be such that the reading on the colourimeter scale for complete lysis does not exceed 50 (optical density 0.5). If necessary, the supernatant may be diluted with an equal volume of 0.1% NaCl or the initial proportion of blood may be 1:200 instead of 1:100. With a good colorimeter, as little as 1% haemolysis may be detected.

The blood added should be exactly 0.05 ml. It can be done by using capillary automatic pipettes. Alternatively straight glass pipettes graduated till 0.05 ml may be used. Less time consuming and far less accurate method is to add one drop of blood to each tube.

Factors affecting osmotic fragility tests

In carrying out osmotic fragility tests by any method three variables capable of markedly affecting the results must be controlled, quite apart from the accuracy with which the saline solutions have been made up. These are; (i) the relative volumes of blood and saline, (ii) the final pH of the blood-saline suspension, and (iii) the temperature at which the tests are carried out.

Interpretation

Spherocytes, being already round are unable to swell very much and therefore, rupture even when a small amount of water has entered the cell. Haemolysis may thus commence even at 0.75% and may be complete at 0.4% (a feature of spherocytosis). On the other hand, target cells seen in thalassaemias and iron deficiency anaemia cells can swell a great deal before they rupture because they are relatively flat. Fragility is, therefore, said to be decreased.

Clinical Implications

A. *Increased fragility (> 0.5%) occurs in*
   1. Hereditary spherocytosis
   2. Haemolytic jaundice
   3. Autoimmune anaemia (ABO and Rh) incompatibility
   4. Chemical poisons
   5. Burns.

B. *Decreased fragility (< 0.3%) occurs in*
   1. Obstructive jaundice
   2. Thalassaemia
   3. Sickle cell anaemia
   4. Iron-deficiency anaemia
   5. Polycythaemia vera

Distilled water drop	18	17	16	15	14	13	12	11	10	9	8	7
1% NaCl	9	10	11	12	13	14	15	16	17	17	17	18
Nacl%	0.28	0.32	0.36	0.40	0.44	0.48	0.52	0.56	0.60	0.64	0.68	0.72

6. Liver disease
7. Splenectomy (following)

Decreased fragility indicates that red cells are excessively flat. Occurs in iron deficiency anaemia, thalassaemia, and sickle cell disease.

QUALITATIVE ASSESSMENT OF G6PD DEFICIENCY

Methaemoglobin Reduction Test

Reagents

1. Sodium nitrite 1.25 gm in 100 ml distilled water.
2. Glucose 5 gm in 100 ml distilled water.
3. Methylene blue 150 mg in 100 ml distilled water.

Method

Withdraw 6 ml of blood and add to 1.2 ml of ACD solution.

Label three test tubes as A, B and C, add as follows:

a. To tube A, add:
   0.1 ml sodium nitrite solution
   0.1 ml glucose solution
   0.1 ml methylene blue solution
   2 ml blood.

b. To tube B, add:
   0.1 ml sodium nitrite solution
   0.1 ml glucose solution
   2 ml blood.

c. To tube C, add 2 ml of blood only.

Mix well and keep the tubes A, B and C at 37°C for 3 hours. Mix again and aerate at 1, 2, and 3 hours (hourly intervals).

Take three test tubes each containing 10 ml of distilled water.

To one, add 0.1 ml of mixture of A.
To second, add 0.1 ml of mixture of B.
To third, add 0.1 ml of contents from C.
Wait for 10 minutes.

Test tube with distilled water and contents from C should always be red.

Test tube with distilled water and solution from B should always be brown.

Interpretation

Test tube with distilled water and solution from A.

- if this is red—there is no G6 PD deficiency
- if brown like B—full expression of deficiency of G6 PD
- if between red and brown—intermittent expression of G6PD deficiency.

Ageing red cells are especially susceptible to oxidative challenge by drugs, systemic infection, metabolic acidosis and other stress. Oxidative stress induces rapid intravascular destruction of susceptible cells, leading to haemoglobinaemia, haemoglobinuria and a sudden drop of haematocrit.

Young cells have higher G6PD content than the older ones, regardless of the genetic variant that is present. If the enzyme has defective activity, older cells are preferentially destroyed during a mild to moderate haemolytic phase. Reticulocytes released to replace lost cells have high enzyme levels. False-negative test results often occur if blood is examined just after a haemolytic episode, because the non-haemolysed remaining cells are, by definition, those with adequate enzyme levels. Newly generated reticulocytes have still higher levels, and this can affect the results for 3 to 10 days after the episode.

Drugs that haemolyse G6PD deficient cells are those that either act as direct oxidants themselves or produce peroxide activity. Primaquine, an anti-malarial drug is notable in this respect. Many sulpha drugs, quinine derivatives, nitrofurans and antipyretic-analgestic drugs can induce haemolysis in G6PD deficient patients. Susceptibility seems to vary among different individuals. The presence of coexisting fever, metabolic disease, or hepatic or renal failure increases likelihood that symptoms will emerge.

COMMERCIALLY AVAILABLE KIT FOR G6PD ASSESSMENT: G-SIX TEST FOR SCREENING AND QUANTITATION OF G6PD DEFICIENCY Courtesy: Tulip Group of Companies

Summary

Glucose-6-Phosphate-Dehydrogenase (G6PD) deficiency is one of the most common human enzyme deficiency in the world. During G6PD deficiency, the red cells are unable to regenerate reduced nicotine adenine dinucleotide phosphate (NADPH), a reaction that is normally catalysed by the G6PD enzyme.

Since the X chromosome carries the gene for G6PD enzyme, this deficiency mostly affects the males. The two major conditions associated with G6PD deficiency are haemolytic anaemias and neonatal jaundice, which may result in neurological complications and death. Screening and detection of G6PD deficiency helps in reducing such episodes, through appropriate selection of treatment, patient counselling and abstinence from disease precipitating drugs such as antimalarials and other agents.

Reagents

G-SIX test is a ready to use, three component reagent system of the detection of G6PD deficiency in human blood using the WHO recommended methemoglobin reduction method. The test system contains three vials *P, *T and *N predispensed with appropriate reagents along with Quantitation graph paper.

Each batch of the reagent undergoes rigorous quality control at various stages of manufacture for its sensitivity and performance.

Storage and Stability

a. Ideally, the product should be stored at 2-8°C. It may also be stored between 20-25°C in a cool dark place away from light and moisture.
b. The shelf-life of the reagent system is as per the expiry date mentioned on the G-SIX carton.

Principle

The G-SIX test is based on the principle of reduction of methaemoglobin by G6PD activity of the red cells under test. The rate of reduction is proportional to the G6PD activity of the red cells under test. During the test procedure, the test sample is processed in triplicate so as to simultaneously also derive positive and normal reference controls. During screening method, the colour of the test sample is compared visually to the reference controls in order to arrive at the diagnostic conclusion. Quantitation of the percentage of G6PD deficiency can also be done spectrophotometrically.

Note

Laboratory reagent for professional use only. Not for medicinal use.

Sample Collection and Preparation

1. The test requires minimum 3 ml of fresh whole blood sample collected in EDTA or Heparin only. The samples must be used within one hour of collection, since the G6PD enzyme actively decreases on storage at 2-8°C.
2. Blood samples may be collected in ACD and can be stored up to 7 days at 2-8°C before performing the test.
3. No special preparation of the patient is required prior to sample collection by approved techniques.
4. If the haematocrit of the sample is less than 30%, enough plasma should be removed from the sample to bring back the PCV to 40% ± 5%.

Additional Material Required

1. 5 ml capacity clean and clear glass test tubes of same diameter and height.
2. Incubator at 37°C.
3. 0.05 ml, 1 ml, 5 ml clean precision pipettes, spectrophotometer with 490 nm filter or colourimeter with blue green filter.
4. Timer.
5. Test tube stand.
6. Distilled/Deionized water.

Screening Test Procedure

1. Open the pack of the reagent vials *P (for test reference),*T (for test reference) and N (for normal reference). Mark patients ID on the three vials. Use immediately upon opening.
2. Add 1 ml of the blood sample under test to each of the vials *P, *T and *N and mix well by gentle inversion.
3. Recap the vials tightly using the screw cap (the plug may be discarded) and place them vertically in an incubator which has already been stabilised at 37°C.
4. Incubate undisturbed, at 37°C, for 3 hours.
5. Meanwhile set up three 5 ml test tubes on a test tube stand and dispense 5 ml distilled/deionised water into each of these tubes.
6. Label these reference tubes as **PR, TR** and **NR** respectively and mark patient ID on each tube, (if more number of samples are being run simultaneously set up equivalent number of such distilled/deionised water tube sets).

7. Remove the vials after 3-hour incubation and mix gently.
8. Uncap the incubated test vials*P,*T and *N and dispense exactly 50 µl (0.05 ml) of the well-mixed incubated samples using different pipettes into the corresponding appropriately labelled distilled water reference tubes **PR**, **TR** and **NR**.
9. Mix evenly by gentle inversion.
10. Observe and compare the colour of tube **TR** with **PR** and **NR** against light to interpret the results.
11. The test results must be interpreted within three hours of the preparation of tubes **PR**, **TR** and **NR** for screening test and within 30 minutes for the quantitative procedure.

Quantitative Procedure

1. Set the spectrophotometer filter on 490 nm.
2. Dispense/aspirate required amount of **NR** as obtained in point no. 9 of screening procedure into the cuvette. **NR** serves as blank.
3. Similarly read the OD of **PR** and place the corresponding value on the G-SIX quantitation graph paper, which equates to 100% deficiency on the Y-axis.
4. Make a straight line joining the blank value (0.00) and the OD of **PR**.
5. Read the OD of **TR** and place it on the graph paper.
6. Find out the %G6PD deficiency, corresponding to the OD value of **TR** on the Y axis of the graph paper.

Interpretation of Results

Screening Test

Normal Sample	: Tube **TR** has a clear red colour, matching with the normal reference tube **NR.**
G6PD Deficient Sample (Full Expression)	: The test tube **TR** has a brown colour matching with the positive reference tube **PR.**
G6PD Deficient Sample (Intermediate females)	: The tube **TR** has intermediate colour as compared to positive reference tube **PR** and negative reference tube **NR** depending on the degree of expression of the deficiency trait.

Quantitative Test

Class of deficiency	*% of G6PD deficiency*	*Clinical relevance*
CLASS I	Complete	Chronic, congenital nonspherocytic, anaemia without drugs/oxidative stress
CLASS II	90% or more	Acute haemolytic crisis induced by oxidative drugs
CLASS III	40%-90%	Oxidative drugs/infection induces self-limiting haemolysis without previous haematologic disorder
CLASS IV	Less than 40%	Associated with milder clinical conditions, depending on the variant involved

% G6PD deficiency of up to 20% as obtained by G-SIX test, corresponds to the normal range of 4.5 - 13.5 U/g Hb activity.

Remarks

1. Do not expose the reagents during storage or during test to direct sunlight. Before performing the test, if the reagent vials show any moisture or condensation on the inner walls; they must be discarded, use another set for conducting the test.
2. The reagent vials should be used immediately after opening.
3. Young red cells have a higher G6PD content than the older ones, regardless of the genetic variant that is present. If the enzymes have defective activity, older cells are preferentially destroyed during mild-to-moderate haemolytic phase. Since reticulocytes released to replace lost cells have high enzyme levels, false-negative results may occur if blood is tested immediately after a haemolytic episode.
4. The blood should be tested within an hour of collection as recommended. Delay in testing may give rise to false-positives.
5. It is extremely important that the 5 ml test tubes used for postincubation sample dilution are free from acids or alkalies as this may interfere with end colour stability.
6. Transfer of correct samples to the correctly labelled reference tubes **PR**, **TR** and **NR** is extremely vital for achieving correct results.

7. Vitamin C supplements or a large dietary intake of vitamin C may interfere with the reaction.
8. The positive reference **PR** must be a brown colour. The negative reference must have a cherry pink to cherry red colour. These colours must be achieved to validate test run and correct transfer of incubated samples to correct and corresponding reference tubes.
9. If the positive and negative reference tubes (**PR** and **TR**) have a different colour than expected the test must be re-run. It must be noted however, that the test reference will show varying colours from red to brown depending upon the degree of G6PD deficiency in the sample.

Clinical Implications

1. A decreased level is associated with G6PD deficiency, which is a sex-linked disorder. Affected males inherit the abnormal gene from their mothers who are almost always asymptomatic carriers. In some cases of this disorder, there is lifelong haemolysis; but more commonly, the condition is asymptomatic and results only in susceptibility to acute haemolytic episodes that may be triggered by drugs such as primaquine, sulphonamides, and antipyretics, by ingestion of fava beans, or by viral or bacterial infections.
2. The major types of G6PD deficiency are
   a. Type A, found in blacks
   b. Mediterranean type, found in both Caucasians and Orientals such as Greeks, Sardinians and Sephardic Jews.
   c. Rare, congenital nonspherocytic anaemia
   d. Nonimmunologic haemolytic disease of the newborn.
3. G6PD levels are increased in:
   a. Pernicious anaemia
   b. Werlhof's disease
   c. Hepatic coma
   d. Hyperthyroidism
   e. Myocardial infarction
   f. Chronic blood loss
   g. Other megaloblastic anaemias.

EXAMINATION OF FOETAL HAEMOGLOBIN

Qualitative Method

Peripheral blood film staining method. (Acid elution technique).

Always use freshly prepared smears

- Fix in 80% ethanol for 10 minutes.
- Take 37.7 ml of citric acid solution prepared (21 gm of citric acid by dissolving, in 100 cc of distilled water) in a jar kept at 37°C.
- To this, add 12.2 ml of $Na_2H\ PO_4$ solution (prepared by dissolving 57.6 gm of $Na_2H\ PO_4 \cdot 12H_2O$ (in 1000 cc of distilled water).
- In this mixture keep the slide for 30 minutes.
- Wash with distilled water.
- Stain with 1% eosin solution for 5 minutes.

Interpretation

Normal red cells will appear as ghost cells. Foetal haemoglobin containing cells will appear as bright red cells.

Quantitative Method

STEP A

Preparation of haemolysate

1. Take 8 cc of EDTA blood, centrifuge it for 15 minutes, remove the plasma.
2. To the RBCs sediment, add normal saline and fill the centrifuge tube to 4/5th of it. Mix thoroughly and centrifuge for 20 minutes. Remove the saline and repeat the said process at least twice more.
3. To the packed RBCs, add equal quantity of distilled water and half the quantity of toluene. Mix them throughly and keep in the deep freezer for one hour.
4. Remove from the freezer chest. Thaw it and centrifuge it for 30 minutes. Now there will be 3 zones in the tube.
5. Pass a pipette to the haemolysate zone through the side of the test tube without disturbing the upper two zones, suck up the haemolysate.
6. Check the hemoglobin of the haemolysate and adjust to 8-10 gm%. This haemolysate can be stored at –20°C for 6 months and can be used for quantitative (alkali denaturation method) estimation of foetal haemoglobin or for haemoglobin electrophoresis.

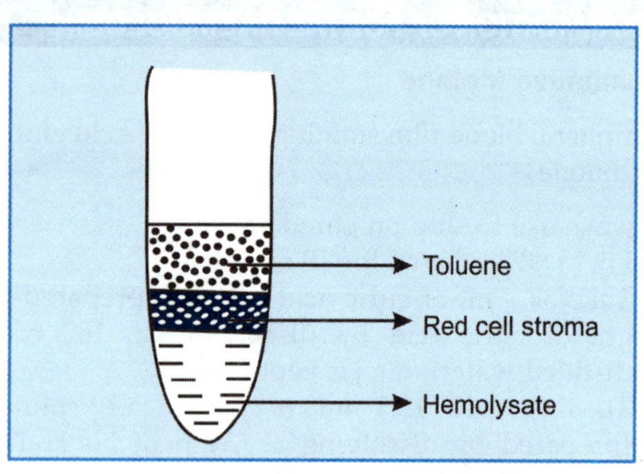

Fig. 9.13: Preparation of hemolysate

STEP B

Quantitative alkali denaturation method for estimation of foetal haemoglobin

1. Take 9.5 ml of Drabkin's solution in a test tube, add 0.5 ml of haemolysate. Cyanmet-haemoglobin (Hi CN) is formed. Mix well.
2. Transfer 2.8 ml of HiCN solution in a tube and keep at 20°C. To this, add 0.2 ml of 1.2N-NaOH solution. Mix rapidly—incubate for 2 minutes at 20°C. Add 2 cc of saturated solution of ammonium sulphate. Mix again and let stand for 5-10 minutes. Filter through Whatman filter paper number 3.
3. Prepare the total haemoglobin by adding 0.4 ml of the original HiCN solution to 6.5 ml of distilled water.
4. Using Drabkin's solution as blank at 540 nm, read the total haemoglobin and filtrate.
5. The optical density should fall between 0.05 and 0.5. If it is beyond 0.5, dilute the hemolysate with distilled water and repeat the said procedure.
6. Calculate as

Haemoglobin F percentage of HbF

$$= \frac{\text{OD of filtrate}}{\text{OD of total haemoglobin}} \times \frac{100}{10}$$

HbF and HbS concentration as percentage of total Hb concentration in various disorders is given below:

Disorder	*HbF%*	*HbS%*
Normal	< 1% (in adults)	not present
Sickle cell trait (AS)	normal	30-40%
Sickle cell anaemia (SS)	1-20%	75-95%
HbS β thalassaemia		
[Sβ⁺ (some β chains present)]	2-10%	60-85%
[Sβ° (no β chains present)]	5-30%	76-90%
HbS-C (SC)	1-5%	50-55%
HbS-D (SD)	1-5%	95% (S+D)
β Thalassaemia major	10-98%	—
α Thalassaemia	reduced	—

Normal Values

Adults	0-2% of total haemoglobin
Children	
Newborn	< 60-90% of total haemoglobin
1-5 months	< 75% of total haemoglobin
6-12 months	< 5% of total haemoglobin
1-20 years	< 2 % of total haemoglobin

TESTS FOR SICKLING

Sickle cells are abnormal forms resulting from the presence of abnormal haemoglobin, which in the deoxidised state undergoes a hydrophobic-bond dependent polymerisation. Rigid threads or rods of S haemoglobin result, with consequent production of the rigid sickle cells. Sickling occurs in 10% of blacks, but only a few of these have anaemia.

Methods

1. *Moist cover slip preparation:* Cover a small drop of fresh blood on a slide with a coverslip, seal with petrolatum, paraffin or nail polish, keep at warm room temperature and examine for sickling every 12 hours up to 72 hours. To find percentage of circulating sickling forms, draw 4 ml of blood into a syringe containing 1 ml of 10% formalin, examine wet preparation.
2. *Daland and Da Silva method:* Acceleration of removal of oxygen from haemoglobin by use of reducing substances.

   Reagents

   Sodium bisulphite or ascorbic acid, 2 gm, in 100 ml water (to be made fresh each time).

   Method

   Use capillary blood, oxalated or defibrinated. Mix 2 drops of either reagent with one drop of blood on a glass slide. Cover, and seal coverslip with petrolatum or nail polish. If no sickling appears in 4 hours, the test is negative.

   Positive test: 10% or more red cells show sickled forms.

3. *Dithionite tube test:* The red cells are lysed, haemoglobin deoxygenated, and the β-globin chains are displaced to provide the molecular steric fit characteristic of sickling of S and no S haemoglobins. The test solution becomes turbid if sickling haemoglobins are present.

Reagents

Stock solution

$KH_2 PO_4$	160.48 gm
$K_2H PO_4$	281.18 gm

Distilled water to 1 litre.

Working solution

Stock buffer	800 ml
$Na_2S_2O_4$	60 gm
Saponin (5%) solution	20 ml
Distilled water to	1000 ml

Method

Add 20 μl (0.02 ml) of well mixed whole blood (EDTA anticoagulated) to 2 ml dithionite working solution in a 12 × 75 mm test tube. Mix by inverting and allow to remain at room temperature for 5-6 minutes. Examine for opacity by holding the tube 2.5-3 cm from a sheet of black newsprint.

Interpretation

Turbidity (newsprint not visible) indicates the presence of sickling haemoglobin. Clear solution indicates a negative test. A positive test (turbidity) indicates the presence of any of the haemoglobins S (SS or AS), C (Harlem), C (Georgetown), Barts and perhaps Alexandra. All positive tests should be followed by haemoglobin electrophoresis. Hemoglobin S can be separated from other haemoglobins by the urea-dithionite test.

4. *Urea-dithionite test:*

Reagents

To 50 ml of working solution (above: from previous test), add 6 gm of urea. Mix until dissolved.

Method

Add 20 μl (0.02 ml) whole blood to 2 ml of urea-dithionite solution in a 12 × 75 mm test tube. Mix by inverting tube and allow to remain at room temperature for 5 minutes. Read with tube 2.5-3 cm away from newsprint background.

Interpretation

Turbidity produced by the sickled liquid crystal system of haemoglobin S in dithionite is dispersed in the urea-dithionite by the urea, which breaks the hydrophobic bonds essential to sickling.

Haemoglobin	*Dithionite*	*Urea-dithionite*
SS, AS and C (Harlem)	Turbid	Clear
Nonsickling C (Georgetown), Barts, Alexandra	Turbid	Turbid

Refer to table given under HbF estimation for percentage of HbS in various disorders.

The presence of HbA guards, to a modest extent, against tactoid (polymerisation) formation, HbF exerts a very strong protective effect. It is probable that the cells of patients with sickle cell disease undergo intravascular sickling and unsickling many times as they circulate. Repeated shape changes, however, stresses the cell membrane and causes the loss of small membrane fragments. This reduces the ratio of surface to volume, making the cell less flexible and less responsive to physical changes. Some cells gradually loose their mechanical and osmotic resistance and undergo intravascular dissolution, whereas others are removed early by reticuloendothelial system. Red cells in HbS disease experience a chronically shortened lifespan.

The likelihood of sickling increases with low oxygen tensions, lowered pH and increased body temperature. HbS protects against *Plasmodium falciparum*infection. Sickle cell anaemia rarely becomes clinically apparent before 6 months of age because protective amounts of HbF remain in cell; for the same reason, it is difficult to screen newborns for HbS disease.

QUANTITATIVE ESTIMATION OF G6PD G-SIX KIT (KINETIC METHOD)FOR THE DETERMINATION OF G6PDH ACTIVITY IN RBC'S. (FOR IN VITRO DIAGNOSTIC USE ONLY) Courtesy: Tulip Group of Companies

Summary

Glucose-6-Phosphate-Dehydrogenase (G6PDH) deficiency is one of the most common human enzyme deficiencies in the world. During G6PD deficiency, the red cells are unable to regenerate reduced Nicotineamide adenine dinucleotide phosphate (NADPH), a reaction that is normally catalyzed by the G6PD enzyme. Since the X chromosome carries the gene for G6PD enzyme, this deficiency mostly affects the males.

The two major conditions associated with G6PD deficiency are hemolytic anemia's and neonatal jaundice, which may result in neurological complications and death. Screening and detection of G6PD deficiency helps in reducing such episodes, through appropriate selection of treatment, patient counseling and abstinence from disease precipitating drugs such as anti malarials and other agents.

Principle

G6PDH in the RBC's is released by a lysing agent present in the reagent. The G6PDH released catalyzes the oxidation of Glucose 6 phosphate with the reduction of NADP to NADPH. The rate of reduction of NADP to NADPH is measured as an increase in absorbance, which is proportional to the G6PDH activity in the sample.

$$\text{G-6-P} + \text{NADP} \xrightarrow{G\text{-}6\text{ - }PDH} \text{Gluconate-6 - P} + \text{NADPH} + \text{H}$$

Normal Reference Values

G6PDH Activity (U/g Hb.) : 4.6 to 13.5 at 30°C/6.4 to 18.7 at 37°C

(U/10^{12} RBC's) : 146 to 376 at 30° C/ 202 to 522 at 37°C

It is recommended that each laboratory establish its own normal range representing its patient population.

Contents	5 x 1 test	5 x 5 tests
L1 : G6PDH Reagent	5 x 1 ml	5 x 5.5 ml
L2 : Starter Reagent	10 ml	50 ml

Storage/stability

Contents are stable at 2-8°C till the expiry date mentioned on the labels.

Reagent Preparation

Reconstitute G6PDH reagent (L1) with D.W. as per the volume mentioned on the label. This working reagent is stable for 6 hours at R.T. and at least 3 days when stored at 2-8°C.

The Starter Reagent (L2) is ready to use.

Sample Material

Fresh whole blood sample collected in EDTA, Heparin or ACD. Red Cell G6PDH in whole blood is reported to be stable for 7 days at 2-8°C, but is unstable in hemolysates. Freezing is not recommended.

Procedure

Wavelength/filter : 340 nm
Temperature : 30°C/37°C
Light path : 1 cm

Addition Sequence	S (ml)
G6PD Working Reagent (L1)	1.0
Whole Blood	0.01
Mix well & incubate for 5 -10 min. at R.T. and add Substrate Reagent	2.0

Mix well & incubate for 5 min. at 30°C/37°C and read the initial absorbance A0 and repeat the absorbance reading after every 1, 2 and 3 minutes. Calculate the mean absorbance change per minute (ΔA/min).

If the G6PDH activity is very low, the absorbance change per minute will also be very low. In such cases read the initial absorbance A1 and read another absorbance A2 exactly 5 min. later. Calculate the mean absorbance change per minute (ΔA /min.)

$$\Delta A/\text{min.} = \frac{A2 - A1}{5}$$

Calculations

$$\text{G6PDH Activity (U/1012 RBC)} = \Delta A \times \frac{47780}{\text{RBC Count } (/\text{mm}^3)}$$

$$\text{G6PDH Activity (U/gHb)} = \Delta A \times \frac{4778}{\text{Hb (g/dl)}}$$

Temperature Conversion Factors

Assay Temperature	Desired Reporting Temperature 25°C	30°C	37°C
25°C	1.00	1.32	1.82
30°C	0.76	1.00	1.39
37°C	0.55	0.72	1.00

Notes

Since the activity of G6PDH is reported in Hb. concentration or RBC count the same should be determined before performing the assay. RBCs are well preserved when collected in ACD and such samples give an accurate count, for samples collected in Heparin counts become unreliable after 2 days and in such cases results are best reported in Hb. concentration.

Copper and Sulphate ions inhibit the G6PDH activity; hence use of good quality D.W for reconstitution of L1 and properly cleaned glassware is essential.

Young red cells have a higher G6PD content then the older ones, regardless of the genetic variant that is present. If the enzymes have defective activity, older cells are preferentially destroyed during mild to moderate hemolytic phase. Since reticulocytes released to replace lost cells have high enzyme levels, falsely elevated results may occur if blood is tested immediately after a hemolytic episode.

Normally the activity contributed by WBC, platelets or serum is very small. In cases of severe anemia, leucocytosis, or very low G6PDH levels, the use of a sample after removing the Buffy Coat is recommended.

LABORATORY DIAGNOSIS OF DISORDERS RELATED TO RBCs

LABORATORY DIAGNOSIS OF IRON DEFICIENCY ANAEMIA

Peripheral Blood

MCV < 76 fl.
MCH < 27 pg.
MCHC < 30 gm%
RBC count—normal

Peripheral Smear

1. Anisocytosis, microcytic red cells
2. Poikilocytosis, pencil-shaped cells and target cells
3. Hypochromia, ring or pessary cells
4. Few polychromatophils
5. Reticulocyte count is variable
6. RBC osmotic fragility is slightly decreased
7. Haematocrit low, plasma appears paler
8. Radiochromium—^{51}Cr studies show reduced red cell span; however, TLC, DLC and platelets have normal lifespan.

Bone Marrow

1. Micronormoblastic erythroid hyperplasia
2. Predominantly intermediate normoblasts are seen
3. Cytoplasm is decreased and shows differential staining
4. Cytoplasm matures so slowly that nucleus may be pyknotic, while cytoplasm is still polychromatic
5. Bone marrow iron is reduced or absent.
   [Perl's reaction done on fixed bone marrow slide shows absent/reduced free iron (blue particles) and lack of siderotic granules in normoblasts.]

Serum Biochemistry

1. Serum iron is reduced (15-16 μg%).
2. Total iron binding capacity is raised (up to 550 μg%).
3. Unsaturated iron-binding capacity is also raised.
4. Percentage saturation is reduced to about 10%.
5. Red cell protoporphyrin increased (no iron available to form haemoglobin.

Normal Values for Iron Metabolism

Serum iron (Fe): 60-170 μg%
Total iron-binding capacity (TIBC): 300-360 μg%
% Saturation: 20-45%
Serum ferritin:12-300 μg/L.

Laboratory Findings in Iron Deficiency

Blood Count

Microcytic, hypochromic red cells if Hb < 12 gm% (men), < 10 gm% (women)
Degree of Hb reduced, RBC count diminished depends on severity. Leukopenia may occur.
Platelets increased in number with active bleeding.
Reticulocytes lower than expected for degree of anaemia.

Bone Marrow

Erythroid hyperplasia.
Micronormoblastic reaction.
Stainable iron is reduced

Other

Serum iron is reduced, iron-binding capacity is increased % saturation is diminished
Serum ferritin < 10 ng%.
Free erythrocyte protoporphyrin increased
RBC survival time slightly increased

Causes of Iron Deficiency Anaemia

Blood Loss

Uterine (menorrhagia, metrorrhagia)
Chronic gastrointestinal blood loss, e.g. in

- Oesophageal varices
- Hiatus hernia
- Peptic ulcer
- Chronic aspirin ingestion
- Carcinoma of:
  - stomach
  - colon
  - caecum
  - rectum
- Ulcerative colitis
- Haemorrhoids
- Diverticulosis
- Hookworm infestation (anaemia with eosinophilia).

Other causes of chronic blood loss

- Haematuria
- Repeated epistaxis
- Haemoptysis

Increased Requirements

- Prematurity (decreased iron stores)
- Growth (iron deficiency anaemia is commonest in children 6-24 months of age)
- Females in reproductive age group:
  - Menstruation
  - Pregnancy
  - Lactation

Impaired Absorption

- Achlorhydria (especially in middle-aged females) achlorhydria → iron deficiency anaemia
- Gastrectomy (HCl not available)
- Gastroenterostomy (Inflammed anastomosis or intestinal hurry hence no time for absorption).

Inadequate Intake

- Improper feeding in infants and young children
- Poverty
- Dietary fads
- Anorexia (nervosa, of pregnancy or malignancies)

LABORATORY DIAGNOSIS OF MEGALOBLASTIC MACROCYTIC ANAEMIAS

Peripheral Blood Findings in Vitamin B_{12} or Folic Acid Deficiency

1. Anaemia with macro (ovalo) cytosis.
2. Anisopoikilocytosis.
3. RBCs may show:
   - Howell-Jolly bodies
   - Cabot's rings
   - Basophilic stippling.
4. MCV > 96 fl.
5. Moderate leucopenia due to neutropenia.
6. Hypersegmented neutrophils, i.e. more than 3 neutrophils having more than 5 nuclear lobes/ 100 neutrophils.
7. Macropolycytes (large neutrophils).
8. Mild, usually asymptomatic thrombocytopenia.

Bone Marrow

Dyserythropoiesis

1. Megaloblasts (larger normoblasts with large open sieve-like nucleus) a constant feature.
2. Late megaloblast
   - has an eccentric, indented lobulated nucleus
   - may show Howell-Jolly bodies.
3. Dissociation of cytoplasmic-nuclear maturation (haemoglobinisation occurs faster than the nuclear maturation).
4. Mitoses common, may be abnormal, i.e. tri-or quadripolar.
5. Maturation arrest, promegaloblasts and early megaloblasts constitute 50% of the erythroblasts.

WBC Series

1. Large atypical cells.
2. Giant metamyelocytes.
3. Absolute number of granulocytes increases but is not evident because of simultaneous erythroid hyperplasia.

Megakaryocytes

1. Number is variable, occasionally diminished
2. Have deep basophilic cytoplasm
3. Hypersegmented nuclei.

Special Tests for Diagnosing Vitamin B_{12} Deficiency

1. Serum Vitamin B_{12} assay
2. Increased urinary excretion of methylmalonic acid
3. Radioactive Vitamin B_{12} absorption test.

Serum Vitamin B_{12} Assay

- Microbiological
- Radioisotope assay

a. *Microbiological*
   Organisms used:
   - *Euglena gracilis*
   - *Lactobacillus leichmanii*

   Test serum

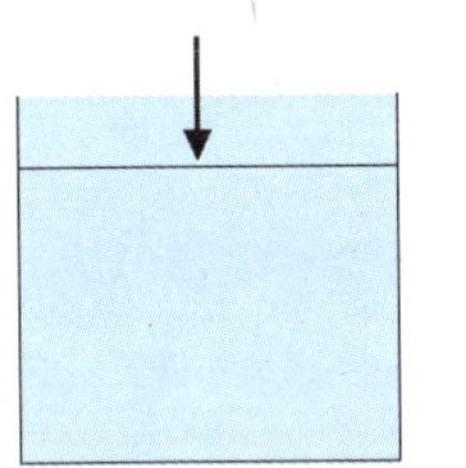

Microorganism + all necessary growth factors except vitamin B_{12}

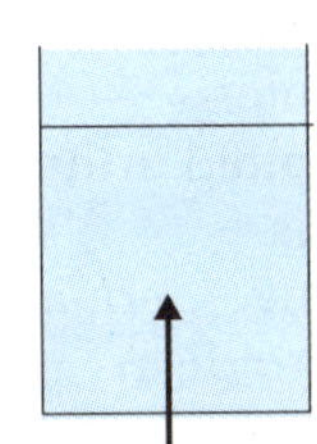

Microorganism + all necessary growth factors + known amount of vitamin B_{12}

Both the tubes are inoculated and later the turbidity developed due to growth of the microorganism is measured and serum vitamin B_{12} level is deduced.

- Using *E. gracilis,* normal values are 160-925 ng/L (mean = 475 ng/L).
- A value < 100 ng/L implies frankly megaloblastic anaemia.

b. *Radiosotope assay*
   Test serum + Vitamin B_{12} labelled with ^{57}Co
   1. Vitamin B_{12} binding protein or intrinsic factor.
   2. Separate free and bound form
   3. Compare with Standards
      — Normal values = 200-300 ng/L

Radioactive Vitamin B_{12} Absorption Test

Principle: Ability to absorb ^{57}Co-labelled vitamin B_{12} orally, if simultaneous administration of intrinsic factor improves absorption, it implies lack of intrinsic factor.

Absorption of radioactive vitamin B_{12} can be measured in 5 ways

1. Radioactivity in faeces.
2. Radioactivity in urine (Schilling test).
3. External counting over liver (chief storage organ).
4. Whole body counting.
5. Estimation of plasma radioactivity.

Schilling Test

1. Give 1 mg unlabelled vitamin B_{12} parenterally.
2. Give 1 μg labelled vitamin B_{12} orally.
3. Within 24 hours 1/3rd of absorbed radioactive vitamin B_{12} is flushed out in urine.
4. Normal excretion is > 10% of oral dose.
5. Pernicious anaemia patients excrete < 5%.
6. If the test is normal no further testing necessary.
7. If it is abnormal—repeat the said procedure with simultaneous oral administration of intrinsic factor.
8. If excretion increases, it implies lack of intrinsic factor. If it does not, then there is some defect in absorption.
   (Repeat test can be done 48 hours later).

Recent variant of Schilling test

- Give orally
  - Free ^{58}Co-labelled vitamin B_{12} and
  - ^{57}Co-labelled intrinsic factor bound vitamin B_{12}
- Estimate amounts in urine.
- If ^{57}Co-labelled vitamin B_{12} is excreted more, there is deficiency of intrinsic factor.

Causes of Vitamin B_{12} Deficiency

1. *Reduced intake*—nutritional deficiency.
2. *Impaired absorption*
   Gastric causes
   - Adult pernicious anaemia
   - Congenital lack of IF.
   - Total or partial gastrectomy.

   Intestinal causes
   - Chronic tropical sprue.
   - Intestinal stagnant loop syndrome, e.g. jejunal diverticulosis, blind loops, strictures.
   - Crohn's disease and ileal resection.

- Congenital selective malabsorption with proteinuria.
- Fish tapeworm infestation.
- Severe pancreatitis.
- Coeliac disease.
- Therapy with metformin or phenformin.

Special Tests for Diagnosing Folate Deficiency

Serum Folate Assays

1. *Microbiological:* As for vitamin B_{12} except that *Lactobacillus casei* is used here. Normal values = 6-21 μg/L
2. *Radio-isotope assay*-As for vitamin B_{12} except that Cow's milk is used here as the binding protein. Value < 4 μg/L implies megaloblastic, macrocytic anaemia.
   (Normal red cell folate 160-640 μg/L)

FIGLU Test

Folate is essential for conversion of histidine to glutamic acid. Formiminoglutamic acid (FIGLU) is an intermediate product. In folate deficiency FIGLU is increased which appears in urine. This test, however, is not very specific.

Radioactive Folic Acid Test-Like Schilling Test

dU Suppression test (for both Vit. B_{12} and FA deficiency)

1. Short term *in vitro* bone marrow cultures are used.
2. In normoblastic cultures, added deoxyuridine enters DNA thymine pathway and supresses the subsequent incorporation of subsequently added tritiated thymidine in DNA.
3. In Vit B_{12} and folic acid deficiency the added deoxyuridine causes less suppression, but the defect can be corrected by supplying the missing vitamin.

Causes of Folic Acid Deficiency

Nutritional

- Especially old age
- Poverty
- Scurvy
- Partial gastrectomy
- Goat's milk anaemia

Malabsorption

- Tropical sprue
- Coeliac disease
- Partial gastrectomy
- Extensive jejunal resection
- Crohn's disease

Increased Demand

Physiological

- Pregnancy
- Lactation
- Prematurity

Pathological

1. Haematological diseases
   - Haemolytic anaemias
   - Myeloproliferative disorders
   - Myelosclerosis
   - Sideroblastic anaemia
   - Multiple myeloma
2. Various carcinomas
3. Inflammatory diseases
   - Crohn's disease
   - Tuberculosis
   - Rheumatoid arthritis
   - Psoriasis
   - Exfoliative dermatitis
4. Hyperthyroidism
5. Excess urinary loss
   - Active liver disease
   - Congestive heart failure
6. Anticonvulsant drug therapy and oral contraceptives
7. Mixed
   - Liver disease
   - Alcoholism.

Laboratory Findings in Megaloblastic Anaemias

Blood Counts

Severe anaemia (Hb may fall up to 3 gm%).
Macrocytosis (MCV 100-140 fl), with anisocytosis.
Ovalocytes, and macro-ovalocytes numerous.
WBCs, platelets often low in number
Hypersegmented neutrophils > 3%
Reticulocytes disproportionately low vis-a-vis degree of anaemia.

Bone Marrow

Marked erythroid hyperplasia.
Megaloblastic nuclear appearance in all 3 cell lines.
Storage iron normal or increased

Blood Chemistry

Bilirubin increased (indirect)
Serum iron increased
Increased LDH, with LDH-1 > LDH-2.

Other Studies

Schilling test abnormal (pernicious anaemia).
Antibodies to gastric cells, intrinsic factor (pernicious anaemia).
Serum RBC levels of vitamin B_{12} reduced (vitamin B_{12} deficiency).
Urine methylmalonate increased (vitamin B_{12} deficiency).
Urine FIGLU - (folic acid deficiency).

Causes of Bone Marrow Megaloblastosis

1. Vitamin B_{12} deficiency
2. Folic acid deficiency
3. Folic acid antagonists
4. Inhibitors of purine or pyrimidine synthesis
5. Alcoholism
6. Genetically determined enzyme defects:
   a. Lesch-Nyhan syndrome
   b. Orotic aciduria
7. Cytotoxic drugs
8. Liver disorders
9. Myxoedema
10. Sideroblastic anaemia
11. Multiple myeloma
12. Widespread neoplastic disease
13. Metastatic deposits in bone marrow.

LABORATORY DIAGNOSIS OF HAEMOLYTIC ANAEMIAS CAUSES AND CLASSIFICATION OF HAEMOLYTIC ANAEMIAS

Intracorpuscular Defects

Hereditary or congenital
  Membrane defects
    Hereditary spherocytosis
    Hereditary elliptocytosis
    Hereditary stomatocytosis
Haemoglobin defects
  Haemoglobinopathies
  Sickle cell disease
  Hb CDE, etc.
  Unstable haemoglobin disease
Thalassaemias
  β Thalassaemia major
  Hb H disease
Enzyme defects
  Nonspherocytic congenital haemolytic anaemia due to phosphokinase deficiency or other EM pathway enzyme defects. Due to G6PD deficiency or other pentose phosphate pathway enzyme defects.
Drug-induced haemolytic anaemia—Favism
Acquired
  Paroxysmal nocturnal haemoglobinuria.

Extracorpuscular Defects

Acquired

Immune mechanism
- Autoimmune haemolytic anaemia.
  Warm antibody type
  Cold antibody type
- Haemolytic disease of the newborn
- Incompatible blood transfusion
- Drug-induced hemolytic anaemia.

Non immune mechanism
- Mechanical haemolytic anaemia
- Cardiac haemolytic anaemia
- Microangiopathic haemolytic anaemia
- March haemoglobinuria.

Miscellaneous

- Haemolytic anaemia due to direct action of drugs / chemicals
- Haemolytic anaemia due to infection (*Clostridia welchii*)
- Haemolytic anaemia due to burns
- Lead poisoning.

Evidences of Haemolysis

Increased Breakdown of Haemoglobin

- Jaundice and hyperbilirubinaemia
- Reduced plasma haptoglobin and haemopexin
- Increased plasma LDH

- Increased urinary urobilinogen
- Increased fecal urobilinogen
- Haemoglobinuria and haemoglobinemia
- Methaemalbuminaemia
- Haemosiderinuria

} evidences of intravascular haemolysis

Compensatory Erythroid Hyperplasia

- Reticulocytosis, Erythroblastemia
- Macrocytosis, polychromasia
- Erythroid hyperplasia of bone marrow (reversal of M:E ratio)
- Skeletal X-ray (Widening of marrow space)
- Radiological changes in skull and tubular bones (in congenital haemolytic anaemias only).

Damage to Red Cells

- Spherocytosis
- Fragmentation of red cells
- Heinz bodies.

Demonstration of Shortened Lifespan of Red Cells

Normal plasma haptoglobin level = 1-1.5 gm/L. Levels are assessed by rapid latex agglutination test. Levels under 1 gm/L imply two to three times haemolysis or the half-life of red cells is 17 days or less. Normal plasma haemopexin level is = 0.5-1 gm/L. Its concentration is measured by radial immunodiffusion technique. In most intravascular haemolysis, its levels are diminished.

LABORATORY DIAGNOSIS OF HEREDITARY SPHEROCYTOSIS

Blood Picture

- Anaemia with spherocytosis (Hb 9-12 gm%)
- Osmotic fragility, reticulocyte count (5-7%) and serum bilirubin (indirect) are raised.
- Negative Coombs' test
- Autohaemolysis after 48 hr at 37°C—10-50% (normal $\leq$ 4%)
- Glucose or ATP addition abolishes autohemolysis.

Peripheral Smear

- Spherocytes
- Polychromatophils.
- Platelets diminished in number if splenomegaly present
- MCV normal or reduced
- MCH normal
- MCHC often increased (34-40%)
- Reticulocyte count raised (5-20%).
- There can be pancytopenia in aplastic crisis.
- ^{51}Cr autologous red cell life reduced with excessive counting over spleen (the main pitting organ).

Chemistry

Bilirubin slightly (indirect) increased
Urine urobilinogen increased
Haptoglobin reduced.

LABORATORY DIAGNOSIS OF HEREDITARY ELLIPTOCYTOSIS

- In peripheral smear, ovalocytes, are > 50% usually.
- Both MCV and MCH are normal.
- Osmotic fragility may be raised in anaemic patients.

LABORATORY DIAGNOSIS OF ENZYME DEFICIENCY RELATED ANAEMIAS

G6PD Deficiency

Blood Picture

- Polychromasia
- Basophilic stippling
- Spherocytosis ±
- Heinz bodies, 1-2, after commencement of therapy.

Besides methemoglobin reduction test already described, other tests which can be done are:

1. Brilliant cresyl blue (BCB) reduction test.
2. Heinz body test.
3. Fluorescent spot test: NADPH autofluoresces in long wave ultraviolet light.
4. Enzyme assays.

LABORATORY DIAGNOSIS OF AUTOIMMUNE HAEMYLOTIC ANAEMIA (AIHA)

Laboratory Diagnosis of Warm Antibody AIHA

Blood Picture

- Haemolytic anaemia.
- Positive direct antiglobin (Coombs') test

- Monocytosis in peripheral smear ± erythrophagocytosis.
- Variable total leucocyte count TLC.
- Blood withdrawn often shows autoagglutination because RBCs, are heavily coated with immunoglobulins.
- Red cell and serum folate levels are diminished.

Immunology

- Autoantibodies demonstrated *in vitro* in most cases.
- Antibody is found on red cell surface and in serum (surface antibodies are revealed by direct Coombs' test)
- IgA immunoglobulin deficiency.

Laboratory Diagnosis of Cold Antibody AIHA

This has 2 forms:
- Cold haemagglutinin disease (CHAD)
- Paroxysmal cold haemoglobinuria (PCH)

CHAD

Blood picture
- Anaemia
- Red cell agglutination of peripheral (smear) blood (avoidable by raising temperature to 37°C).
- Reticulocytosis.
- Hyperbilirubinaemia
- Positive (direct) Coombs' test (because of C_3d on red cell surface as shown by specific antiglobulin sera).

PCH

- Donath Landsteiner antibody test, chill the blood, take back to 37°C, haemolysis occurs.
- Positive Coombs' (direct) test only during the attack.

LABORATORY DIAGNOSIS OF PAROXYSMAL NOCTURNAL HEMOGLOBINURIA

Blood Picture

- Anaemia, macrocytosis, polychromasia.
- Reticulocytosis, moderate leucopenia, mild thrombocytopenia.
- HbF occasionally raised.
- Hyperbilirubinaemia.
- Neutrophil alkaline phosphatase score is low, but normal in aplastic cases.
- Hypercoagulability.
- Direct Coombs' test ±.

Further Investigations:

- Haemoglobinuria.
- Haemosiderinuria.
- Serological tests.

1. *Ham's serum test:* Patient's red cells will undergo lysis in compatible acidified serum at 37°C (serum may be patient's own). About 10-50% lysis implies a positive test with patient's own serum.
2. *Sucrose haemolysis test:* Isotonic solution of low ionic strength if causes haemolysis of more than 10% cells—indicates diagnosis of PNH.

LABORATORY DIAGNOSIS OF LEAD POISONING

Blood Picture

- Basophilic stippling in peripheral smear and bone marrow.
- Normocytic, normochromic or microcytic, hypochromic anaemia.
- Polychromasia, slight reticulocytosis and erythroblastemia.
- Osmotic fragility of red cells is decreased.
- TLC is usually normal.

Bone Marrow

- Stippling of erythroblasts.
- Sideroblastosis.

Urine

Increased excretion of coproporphyrin and ALA.

LABORATORY DIAGNOSIS OF HAEMOGLOBIN STRUCTURE AND SYNTHESIS DISORDERS

Clinical finding
Ethnic origin of patient
Any family history
Preliminary blood studies
] suggest haemoglobinopathy
↓
Haemoglobin electrophoresis confirms

SPECIAL TESTS

Tests Depending on Physicochemical Properties

- Sickle test, Hb solubility tests—HbS
- Intracellular Hb Crystals—HbC
- HbH inclusions—Thalassaemia
- Heinz bodies
- Heat instability test
- Isopropanol precipitation test—Unstable Hb
- Oxygen dissociation studies—High O_2 affinity Hb
- Alkali denaturation, acid elution test—HbF.

Haemoglobin Electrophoresis

The apparatus consists of two basic units:

1. The electrophoresis trough
2. The voltage and amperage regulator.

There are two troughs on either side containing the appropriate fluid.

The paper strips or agar gel covered slides are placed in the centre of the instrument, and either end is connected to the respective trough with the help of wet filter paper strips—with one end dipping in the fluid and the other touching the gel or paper strip. This kind of connection is made on both the sides. The haemolysate is applied gently with the help of coverslip (broken) to get about 0.5-1 cm size. The positive and negative points are connected to the electrophoresis trough and then it is covered. Electrophoresis is allowed to continue for a specific time. The agar gel slides are dipped in amido black and left overnight for destaining in dilute acetic acid solution. The haemoglobin bands become clearly visible, the agar slide can be left for drying and a permanent record obtained. Having used the apparatus once, change the anode and cathode terminals for use next time. Most electrophoresis troughs are provided with water cooling systems, attach the inlet tube to a slow water stream from a tap and the outlet water to be drained into a waste sink.

Cellulose acetate electrophoresis done at pH = 8.6

Agar gel electrophoresis, using citrate buffer done at pH = 6.0

The mobilities seen are presented Fig. 9.14a:

(For further precise quantitations, electrophoresis can be done on starch gel or starch block)

After obtaining the bands, one needs to know densities of the bands obtained. Systronics provides, autoscanning and computing densitometer 205.

Autoscanning and Computing Densitometer 205

Densitometer 205 is microprocessor based, designed to quantify electrophoretically separated bands. The embedded software allows quantification of serum protein pattern by default, and any other multiband pattern (e.g. haemoglobin, lipoprotein, etc.) in an N-BAND mode. Postscan facilities like base line shifting, deletion of area, selection of minimas make the unit practically very useful and enhance its application in research-oriented studies.

A special 'PC LINK 205' software (optional) links the Densitometer 205 to a PC. With this, densitograms can be conveniently stored/recalled/displayed/edited/compared on a CRT monitor using the keyboard of the PC (Fig. 9.14b).

Features

- Quantification of five classical bands of serum protein by default.
- N-Band (2-15) to quantify any pattern.
- Accepts any multiband pattern on a transparent dry media.
- Postscan EDIT facilities.
- Patient identification with date and time.
- Hard copy of densitogram and/or computed values.
- Optional 'PC-LINK 205' software.

Minimum System Configuration

- Systronics Densitometer 205.
- 80 column dot-matrix printer (EPSON compatible).

System Configuration with 'PC-:LINK 205' Software

- Systronics Densitometer 205.
- 80 column dot-matrix printer (EPSON compatible).
- Systronics PC-LINK 205 software.
- PC (286, 386, 486 or Pentium) with VGA/EGA colour monitor.

Technical Specifications

Optical

Wavelength Range: 400-700 nm.

Filters: 520 nm, 600 nm, (interference) and white light; another up to 5 filters optional.

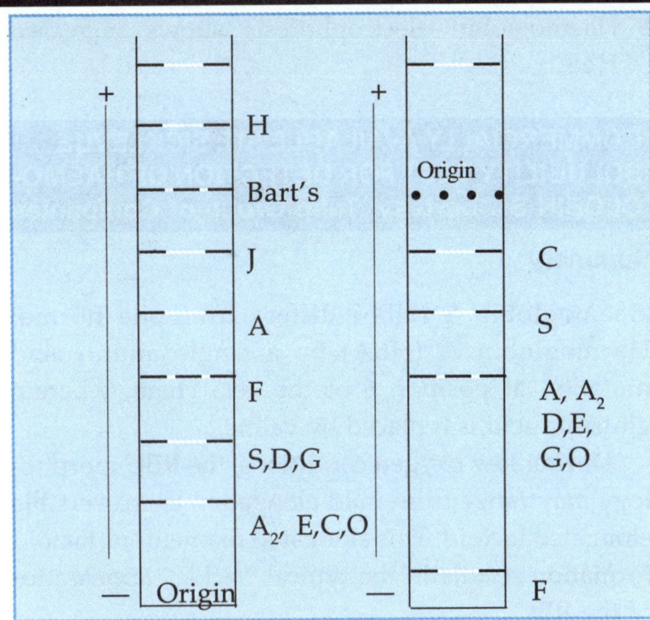

Fig. 9.14A

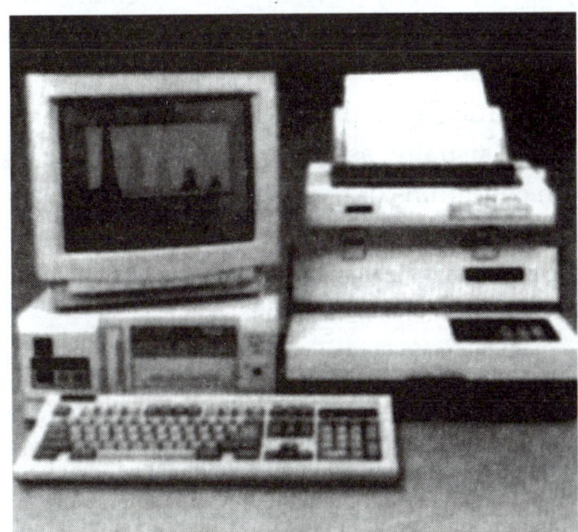

Fig. 9.14B: Densitometer 205 linked to a PC with 'PC-LINK 205' software through RS232C interface

Light source: 6 V, 6 W tungsten lamp.
Slit size (projected): 0.5 mm × 7 mm.
Detector: Silicon photodiode.
Density range: 0 to 2 OD.

Mechanical

Scanning Length: 120 mm, programmable in steps of 0.1 mm.
Scanning speed: 40 mm per minute.
Carriage movement: X-axis: automatic
Y-axis: manual.

Scanning resolution: 10 readings per mm.
Max. pattern size: L-120 mm, W-50 mm, H-5 mm

Electronics

Microprocessor: 8085 (Intel)
Display: (1) segment LED display for set-up/programming interface.
(2) 80-column dot-matrix printer for display of:
a. Densitogram (with graduated X and Y axes to facilitate editing),
b. Computed values,
c. Patient ID No.,
d. Date and time.

Computing and Editing

Input of date: & programme keys: 11 numerical and 13 functional soft-touch
Computations: Proportional fraction in % and values with reference to total for:
1. Five classic bands serum proteins (by default).
2. N-band (2 to 15, selectable)

Editing:
1. Baseline shifting
2. Deletion of area.
3. Selection of minimas (rejection or introduction)

Printed Records

1. 5-band Serum: Protein mode
(a) Proportional fraction % of Albumin, Alpha-1, Alpha-2, Beta, Gamma
(b) Protein values of Albumin, Alpha-1, Alpha-23, Beta, Gamma with reference to total protein value.
(c) Albumin/globulin ratio.

OR

N-Band Mode:	(a) Proportional fraction % of N-bands.
	(b) Values with reference to total.
2. Patient ID No:	Up to 999.
3. Date & time:	D/M/Y/ & Hr/Min.

Power

230 V ± 10%, 50 Hz.

Optional Accessories

i. RS 232 interface to communicate with external computer
ii. 'PC-LINK 205', Software

LABORATORY DIAGNOSIS OF SICKLE CELLS TRAIT

1. Sickling tests (positive).
2. Solubility tests for HbS (positive).
3. Hb electrophoresis

LABORATORY DIAGNOSIS OF SICKLE CELL ANAEMIA

Blood Picture

1. Anaemia—moderate to marked; normocytic, normochromic (MCV and MCH are normal).
   - anaemia occurs because of reduced RBC lifespan to about 8 days and in part due to ineffective erythropoiesis.
   - haemolytic and aplastic crises further reduce Hb concentration.
   - irreversibly sickled cells (ISC) have a life of 2 days.
   - osmotic fragility is decreased.
2. ESR is decreased, sickling prevents rouleaux formation.
3. There is moderate to marked anisopoikilocytosis.
4. Serum and red cell folate values are decreased.
5. There is evidence of intravascular haemolysis.
6. Sickle and solubility tests are positive.
7. There is irregular distribution of HbF (acid elution test).
8. Haemoglobin electrophoresis shows increased HbS.

COMMERCIALLY AVAILABLE KIT: SICKLEVUE SOLUBILITY TEST FOR DETECTION OF HAEMOGLOBIN S Courtesy: Tulip Group of Companies

Summary

Haemoglobin S (HbS) differs from the normal Haemoglobin A (HbA) by a single amino acid mutation at position 6 of the beta chain, wherein glutamic acid is replaced by valine.

During low oxygen conditions, the RBC morphology may range from mild elongation to irreversible elongated tactoid. This elongated filamentous tactoid formation results in the typical "sickle" appearance of the RBC.

Individuals with sickle cell anaemia (homozygous S/S) may have early mortality with vascular occlusions of multiple organ systems, severe haemolytic anaemia and hypoxia.

Individuals with the sickle cell trait (heterozygous A/S) are usually asymptomatic. However, under certain conditions of reduced oxygen tension such as hypoxia during anaesthesia, fight in poorly pressurised airplanes, sever pneumonia, they can experience a sickle cell crisis.

Reagents

a. *SICKLEVUE reaction tubes*: Prefilled with sodium dithionite.
b. *Phosphate buffer*: A concentrated, ready-to-use solution containing a red cell lysing agent.

Reagent Storage and Stability

Store the reagents at RT (15-30°C). *Do not refrigerate or freeze.*

Do not expose to light for excessive periods. Best stored as supplied in the kit.

The shelf-life of the reagents is as per the expiry date mentioned on the SICKLEVUE carton.

Principle

SICKLEVUE is based on the solubility difference between HbS and HbA in concentrated phosphate buffer solution. RBCs under test are lysed by a powerful haemolytic agent and the released haemoglobin is then reduced by sodium dithionite in a concentrated phosphate buffer.

In the presence of sodium dithionite, HbS precipitates causing turbidity of the reaction mixture. Under the same conditions, HbA, as well as most other haemoglobins, are soluble.

HbS when reduced in the phosphate buffer forms a turbid solution, which is easily visualised. Normal HbA and most other haemoglobins remain in solution resulting in a clear suspension.

Note

1. Reagent for laboratory use only.
2. Do not pipette by mouth.
3. Phosphate buffer does not contain preservatives. Aseptic conditions should be followed to avoid contamination. However, as a powerful haemolytic agent is included in the composition, avoid contact with skin or mucosa. Wash hands after use.
4. The reagent can be damaged due to microbial contamination or on exposure to extreme temperatures.
5. Use reagent of same lot numbers. Do not interchange reagent of different lot numbers.

Sample Collection and Preparation

No special preparation of the patient is necessary prior to specimen collection by approved techniques. Collect whole blood in EDTA, heparin, sodium citrate or ACD anticoagulant. Though fresh blood samples are preferable, the sample can be stored at 2-8°C for upto 24 hours, in case of delay in testing.

Materials Provided with the Kit

Reagent Pack

SICKLEVUE reaction tubes, phosphate buffer and result reading card.

Additional Material Required

2 ml pipettes, Micropipette (20 nl), test tube rack, stop watch, laboratory centrifuge.

Test Procedure

Bring all reagents and samples to room temperature before use.

Screening Method

1. Retrieve the required number of SICKLEVUE reaction tubes, as the number of samples to be tested.
2. Label the reaction tubes appropriately and set on a test tube rack.
3. Add 2 ml of the buffer to each of the reaction tubes, using the pipette. Alternately, fill up the tubes by pouring the buffer up to the 2 ml marking.
4. Mix well and allow to stand for 5 minutes at RT.
5. With the help of a micropipette, add 20 μl of whole blood sample.
6. Mix and allow to stand for 10 minutes.
7. To read the results, place the tubes into the slots of the Result Reading Card provided.
8. Read the turbidity in the tubes by holding the tubes against a dim illumination and viewing the horizontal black lines printed on the viewing card, below the 2 ml marking, through the solution, in the SICKLEVUE tube.

Differentiation Method

To differentiate between sickle cell trait (Hb AS) and sickle cell anaemia (Hb SS).

1. If positive results are obtained during the screening method, take a fresh SICKLEVUE Reaction tube and repeat the test procedure as in Screening Method with 100 μl of whole blood sample.
2. Centrifuge the reaction tube at 1200 g for 5 minutes in a laboratory centrifuge.
3. Allow the centrifuge to stop without braking and carefully remove the reaction tubes without disturbing the contents.
4. Observe the pattern formed in the reaction tubes.

Interpretation of Results

Screening Method

a. A turbid solution (horizontal black lines on the Result Reading Card are barely visible or cannot be seen) indicates a positive test for sickle cell haemoglobinopathies.

b. A clear solution (horizontal black lines on the Result Reading Card are clearly visible) indicates a negative test result.

Differentiation Method

a. Hb SA-Hb S forms a red precipitate at the top and soluble Hb if present forms a red colour solution below this precipitate.
b. Hb SS-A red precipitate at the top and solution is colourless. If substantial amount of Hb F is present, the solution may be pink.
c. All other Hb yield clear red solutions.

Remarks

1. All positive results should be confirmed on electrophoresis.
2. Severe anaemia can cause false negative results. If the haemoglobin concentration is 8 gm % or less the sample volume for testing should be doubled to 40 μl.
3. Blood samples from patients with multiple myeloma, cryglobulinaemia and other dysglobulinaemias may give false-positive results.
4. It is recommended that the performance of reagents should be verified with known positive and negative controls.
5. As with all tests, the result of the test should be correlated with clinical findings to arrive at the final diagnosis.

LABORATORY DIAGNOSIS OF UNSTABLE Hb HAEMOGLOBINOPATHY

Blood Picture

1. Mild to severe anaemia.
   - peripheral blood
   - anisopoikilocytosis
   - punctate basophilia, polychromasia.
   - reticulocytosis.
2. MCH is reduced
3. Red cell life is 20-30 days.

Special Tests

1. *Demonstration of Heinz bodies:* Preformed Heinz bodies cannot be shown by supravital staining except in 50% of splenectomised patients. Sterile incubation of affected red cells at 37°C for 24 hours leads to Heinz body formation.
2. *Heat instability test:* Incubate a fresh hemolysate with phosphate or tris buffer at 50°C for 1 hour—precipitation implies presence of unstable Hb.
3. *Isopropanolol precipitation test:* Incubate fresh haemolysate with isopropranolol tris buffer at 37°C for 1 hour, precipitation denotes presence of unstable Hb.
4. *Haemoglobin electrophoresis:* Abnormal Hb band (at pH = 8.6) in 50% cases.

THALASSAEMIAS (REDUCED SYNTHESIS RATE)

Are of two types
- α, affecting mainly α chain
- β, affecting mainly β chain

In β Thalassaemia

There is reduced β chain production hence reduced HbA leading to microcytic, hypochromic anaemia. Total Hb is maintained by increase in γ and δ chains so HbA_2 and HbF increase. Because of lack of β chains, α chains accumulate in cells forming aggregates → causing ineffective erythropoiesis.

In α Thalassaemia

Level of HbA, A_2 and F are equally depressed leading on to microcytic, hypochromic anaemia. In the absence of normal chains, β or γ chains increase and form HbH (β_4) or Hb Bart's (γ_4.)

Laboratory Diagnosis of β Thalassaemia Minor

Blood Picture

Hb is normal, MCV and MCH. MCHC is normal.

Peripheral Smear Shows

- Microcytic, hypochromic cells; target cells.
- Basophillic stippling, reticulocytosis (up to 6%).
- Osmotic fragility is decreased.
- Evidence of haemolysis.

Hb Electrophoresis

HbA_2 increased, slight increase in HbF.

Laboratory Diagnosis of β Thalassaemia Major

Blood Picture

(resembles iron deficiency anaemia)
- Marked microcytosis with hypochromia.
- Moderate degree of anisopoikilocytosis, tear drop cells.

- Target cells are prominent.
- All; MCV, MCH and MCHC are diminished.
- Normoblasts (intermediate/late) in peripheral smear.
- Granular inclusions in cytoplasm, represent α-chain aggregates which can be shown by methyl violet.
- Polychromasia and moderate degree of punctate basophilia.
- Reticulocytosis (10%).
- Leucocytosis (5,000-40,000) with shift to the left (immature forms seen).
- Platelet count normal but decreases with splenomegaly.
- Osmotic fragility decreased, the curve has a tail because of a few very fragile cells.
- Evidences of intravascular haemolysis.

Bone Marrow

- Erythroid hyperplasia
- Micronormoblastic reaction.
- Increase in early and intermediate normoblasts.
- Methyl violet positive inclusion bodies and PAS positive glycogen (PAS-periodic acid Schiff's reagent).
- Sideroblastosis, often ring sideroblasts.

Hb Pattern on Electrophoresis

- HbF (10-98%) estimated also by acid elution and alkali denaturation tests.
- HbA (very little or absent).
- HbA_2 (variable).

Laboratory Diagnosis of α Thalassaemia

Hb-H Disease

Blood picture
- Marked microcytosis with hypochromia.
- Target cells, fragmented cells and normoblasts in peripheral blood.
- Reticulocytosis, basophilic stippling.
- Numerous HbH inclusions.

Hb Pattern (electrophoresis)
- HbH = 5-25%
- Remainder is HbA, A_2 and F.

Demonstration of HbH inclusions: With a redox dye e.g., brilliant cresyl blue (BCB) or new methylene blue (NMB); HbH being relatively unstable, precipitates and the red cells appear pitted with numerous inclusions (golf-ball appearance).

Haemoglobin electrophoresis: At pH 8.6, both HbH and Hb Bart's are fast moving, they migrate in front of HbA towards anode.

Hb Bart's—Hydrops Foetalis

Blood picture:
- Marked anisopoikilocytosis with hypochromia.
- Polychromasia.
- Target cells and normoblasts.

Hb pattern
- Hb Bart's 80-90%.
- Some HbH and Hb Portland.
- No HbA, A_2 or F.

LABORATORY DIAGNOSIS OF APLASTIC ANAEMIA

Blood Picture

- RBC morphology is usually normal (polychromasia, normoblasts and stippling usually NOT SEEN).
- Sometimes macrocytosis, mild aniso-poikilocytosis.
- Hb and PCV are diminished to about 7 gm% and 20% respectively.
- Red cell osmotic fragility is normal.
- Leucopenia—neutropenia, polymorphs are qualitatively and quantitatively abnormal, show coarse granules.
  - absolute lymphocytopenia but relative lymphocytosis.
  - neutrophil alkaline phosphatase count is increased.
- Thrombocytopenia—bleeding time is increased.
- Clot retraction time is increased.
- Coagulation parameters are abnormal.
- Serum iron is increased.
- Radio-iron bone marrow uptake is reduced.
- Red cell life may be decreased.
- Plasma erythropoietin level is raised.

Bone marrow may be:
- Aplastic
- Hypoplastic
- Normal or
- Patchily hypercellular
  Aspiration
  - blood tap or dry tap
  - is hypoplastic (there is both myeloid and erythroid hypoplasia).
  - fat cells are increased.

- plasma cells and reticulum cells are prominent.
- megakaryocytes are diminished in number.
- WBCs may show maturation arrest.
- developing granulocytes are abnormal and may show:
  - abnormal granulation or.
  - vacuolisation.
- bone marrow iron may be normal or increased.

Hence the diagnosis is based upon:

- Pancytopenia
- Rapid ESR.
- No immature cells in peripheral smear
- Bone marrow is aplastic/hypoplastic (if 2 consecutive aspirations have been unsuccessful do a bone marrow trephine biopsy).

Classification and Causes of Aplastic Anaemia

1. *Primary*
   - idiopathic (cause unknown).
2. *Secondary*
   - to effects of chemical/physical agents on bone marrow.
3. *Miscellaneous*
   - Familial hypoplastic anaemia (Fanconi's syndrome).
   - Aplastic anaemia associated with
     - infective hepatitis (1-2%)
     - pancreatic insufficiency
     - paroxysmal nocturnal haemoglobinuria (PNH).
4. *Pure red cell aplasia*
   - Congenital (Diamond Blackfan type).
   - Acquired
     - with thymoma.
     - without thymoma.

(In both primary and secondary aplastic anaemia clinical and haematological features are similar).

Primary type is less common

Secondary type occurs due to:

- Chemicals
  - Industry
  - Domestic
  - Drugs
- Physical
- Ionising radiation.

Drugs

Especially those which have an amino group near a benzene ring.

Bone marrow depression depends upon:

- Dosage and period of treatment
- Idiosyncracy, susceptibility and hypersensitivity to the drug.

Drugs which Regularly Cause Aplastic Anaemia

- Anticancer drugs.

Drugs which Occasionally Cause Bone Marrow Depression

(Either because of idiosyncracy or hypersensitivity)

- *Antiepileptics*
  - phenylhydantoin
  - mesantoin
  - paradione.
- *Antibacterials*
  - chloramphenicol
  - sulphas
  - streptomycin
  - chlorotetracycline
  - INH
- *Tranquillisers*
  - chlordiazepoxide
  - chlorpromazine
- *Antidiabetics*
  - tolbutamide
  - chlorpropamide
- *Antirheumatics*
  - oxyphenylbutazone
  - phenylbutazone
  - indomethacin
  - gold salts
  - aspirin
  - colchicine.

(Commonest drugs—phenyl and oxyphenyl-butazone and chloramphenicol).

Chemicals

- Benzene
- Lindane
- TNT
- DDT

Physical Agents

- Ionising radiation is most-dangerous (e.g. X-ray, γ rays, neutrons).
- Particles have a limited range and hence cause effects only on entering the body.

PANCYTOPENIA

Reduction in number of the three blood cells types RBCs, WBCs and platelets.

Blood Picture

Hb < 13.5 gm% in males
< 11.5 gm% in females
TLC < 4,000 cells/cu mm,
Platelet count < 1.5 lakh/cu mm.

Causes

- Subleukaemic leukaemia.
  Refractory anaemia with medullary myeloblastosis.
- Aplastic anaemia.
- Pancytopenia with hyperplastic bone marrow.
- Bone marrow infiltration or replacement.
- Hypersplenism.
- Megaloblastic macrocytic anaemia.
- Systemic lupus erythematosus.
- Disseminated tuberculosis.

NORMAL WHITE CELL VALUES AND PHYSIOLOGICAL VARIATIONS

Normal total leucocyte count = 4,000-11,000 cells/cu mm.

TLC undergoes minor physiological and diurnal variations. It increases slightly in the afternoon 'afternoon tide'. Various stimuli that may increase the count are:
- food intake
- physical exercise
- emotion
- pregnancy and following parturition.

Pathological Variations in White Cell Counts

Neutrophilia

Infections
- Pyogenic bacteria
  - Staphylococcal
  - Streptococcal
  - Pneumococcal
  - Meningococcal
  - Gonococcal
- Nonpyogenic
  - acute rheumatic fever
  - diphtheria
  - scarlet fever
  - acute poliomyelitis
  - cholera
- Herpes zoster
- Mycobacterial
- Fungal
- Spirochetal
- Parasitic

Metabolic disorders—due to varied causes leading to
- acute yellow atrophy of liver
- uraemia
- diabetes
- acidosis
- gout
- eclampsia.

Neoplasms
- Myeloproliferative disorders
- Myeloid leukaemia
- Lymphomas
- Polycythemia vera
- Myelosclerosis
- Other malignancies
  - Carcinomas (metastatic or otherwise)
  - Sarcomas.

Conditions causing cell necrosis or destruction:
- acute haemolysis (especially intravascular, type)
- infarctions
- drug intoxication
  - nephrotoxins
  - hepatotoxins

Various drugs/chemicals implicated are:
- phenacetin
- digitalis
- quinine
- organic arsenicals
- lead
- mercury
- carbon monoxide

Trauma and haemorrhage
- haemorrhage
  - acute haemorrhage (especially internal haemorrhage)
- trauma
  - operative
  - fractures
  - crush injuries
  - burns.

Cardiac disorders—paroxysmal tachycardia.

Collagen diseases
- polyarteritis nodosa
- acute phases of:
  - rheumatoid arthritis
  - dermatomyositis.

Miscellaneous
- serum sickness
- acute anoxia
- spider venom poisoning
- histiocytosis-X.

Eosinophilia

Allergic states
- asthma
- hay fever
- exfoliative dermatitis
- erythema multiforme
- urticaria
- food sensitivity
- angioneurotic oedema
- serum sickness
- drug allergy.

Parasitic diseases

Intestinal
- hookworm
- roundworm
- tapeworm.

Tissue form
- *Toxocara*
- *Trichina*
- *Strongyloides*
- *Echinococcus*
- *Filariasis*
- *Malaria*

Skin disorders
- pemphigus
- dermatitis herpetiformis
- psoriasis
- scabies
- prurigo.

Drug administration
- liver extracts
- penicillin
- streptomycin
- chlorpromazine.

Neoplasms
- Myeloproliferative
  - eosinophilic leukaemia
  - chronic myeloid leukaemia
  - polycythaemia
- Others
  - Hodgkin's lymphoma
  - multiple myeloma
  - metastatic and necrotic tumours
  - occult abdominal tumour.

Miscellaneous
- familial eosinophilia
- eosinophilic granulomatosis (visceral larva migrans)
- eosinophilic syndrome
- scarlet fever
- polyarteritis nodosa
- tropical eosinophilia
- pernicious anaemia
- postsplenectomy
- post-transfusion mononucleosis
- idiopathic neutropenia.

Lymphocytosis

Acute infections
- infectious mononucleosis
- infectious lymphocytosis
- pertussis
- mumps
- chickenpox
- rubella
- infective hepatitis
- convalescent stage of many acute infections
- toxoplasmosis
- influenza

Chronic infections
- brucellosis
- tuberculosis
- syphilis (secondary)

Endocrine disorders
- thyrotoxicosis
- adrenocortical insufficiency
- hypopituitarism
- myaesthenia gravis

Neoplasms
- non-Hodgkin's lymphomas
- chronic lymphatic leukaemia
- lymphosarcoma
- multiple myeloma.

Monocytosis

Infections
- Bacterial
  - brucellosis

- tuberculosis
- subacute bacterial endocarditis
- typhoid fever
- recovery stage of an acute infection

- Rickettsial
  - rocky mountain spotted fever
  - typhus
- Protozoan
  - malaria
  - kala-azar
  - trypanosomiasis
  - oriental sore
- Viral
  - infectious mononucleosis

Neoplasms

- monocytic leukaemia
- Hodgkin's and other lymphomas
- myeloproliferative disorders
- multiple myeloma
- carcinomatosis

Collagen diseases

- rheumatoid arthritis
- SLE

Miscellaneous

- chronic ulcerative colitis
- regional enteritis
- sarcoidosis
- lipid storage disease
- haemolytic anaemia
- hypochromic anaemia
- recovery from agranulocytosis

Basophilia

- chronic myeloid leukaemia
- myelosclerosis
- polycythaemia vera
- hypersensitivity states
- myxoedema
- iron deficiency anaemia (some cases)
- haemolytic and toxic anaemias of long standing
- pre-leukaemia (some cases).

Morphologic Forms of Lymphocytes

Virocyte

(also called stress lymphocytes, Downey type cells, or atypical lymphocytes)

1. These are small atypical cells that appear in viral diseases such as mononucleosis, viral hepatitis, viral pneumonia, and viral upper respiratory tract infections.
2. These may also be found in numerous nonviral conditions:
   a. Fungoid and protozoid nonviral conditions
   b. Autoimmune states
   c. Allergic reactions
   d. After transfusions and tissue graft
3. When seen in stress response, these are called stress lymphocytes.
4. May be found in apparently healthy children
5. Up to 10% of all lymphocytes, can be considered normal

Transformed Lymphocytes

1. *Examples*
   a. Lymphocyte cells that may be seen in macroglobulinemia
   b. Turk cells and Reider cells that are seen in acute lymphatic leukaemia
   c. Vacuolated lymphocytes that are seen in lipidosis
2. Culturing of lymphocytes in laboratory:
   a. Stimulates small lymphocytes to transform into large atypical cells which produce immunoglobulin.
   b. Transformation response is impaired in culturing of lymphocytes from patients with:
      - Hodgkin's disease.
      - Lymphatic leukaemia
      - Lymphocytosis
      - Agammaglobulinaemia.
   c. Transformation response increased in sarcoidosis
3. Other uses of transformation test are to determine histocompatibility of recipient and donor for tissue grafts:
   a. Lymphocytes from donor not related to recipient stimulates the production of up to 3% of transformed lymphocytes in recipient.
   b. Lymphocytes from sibling react less strongly
   c. No reaction occurs on cultures from fraternal twins.

Arneth Count

Neutrophils can be divided into five main groups according to the number of lobes in their nuclei.

Group 1 One lobe, even if it shows indentation and thinning out at one or more places.

Group 2 Two lobes connected by one thin filament.

Group 3 Three lobes connected by two thin filaments.

Group 4 Four lobes connected by three thin filaments.

Group 5 Five or more lobes connected by four or more thin filaments.

Using the above mentioned classification, count 100 neutrophils and the number in each group is to be expressed as percentage. Usual normal values:

Group	1	2	3	4	5
Number	5	35	42	16	2

Interpretation: In acute infections there is rapid turnover of neutrophils and in the process younger neutrophils with lesser number of lobes are released into circulation, thus increasing the number of cells in groups 1 and 2 (shift to the left).

In macrocytic megaloblastic anaemias, the neutrophil production rate is slow, hence cells with hypersegmented nuclei are released into circulation (shift to the right).

However, Arneth count is now no longer in use.

Arneth Index

The percentage of cells in groups 1, 2 and ½ of 3 is about 60 (normal range 51-65). Only 2-5% fall in group 1.

Neutropenia and Agranulocytosis

Discussed elsewhere.

Lymphopenia

- Severe pancytopenia
- Congestive heart failure
- Adrenocorticosteroid therapy (transient)

Eosinopenia

Drug/hormone therapy

- Adrenocortical steroids
- Adrenaline
- Ephedrine
- Insulin

Response to stress

- Acute infections
- Traumatic shock
- Surgical operations
- Severe exercise
- Burns
- Acute emotional stress
- Exposure to cold

Endocrine diseases

- Cushing's disease
- Acromegaly
- Pheochromocytoma

Miscellaneous

- Aplastic anaemia
- DLE.

Basophilopenia

- Neutrophil leucocytosis or leukaemoid reaction associated with:
  - infection
  - neoplasia
  - tissue necrosis
  - acute anaemia
- Allergic conditions
- Hyperthyroidism
- Myocardial infarction
- Cushing's syndrome
- Following prolonged corticosteroid therapy.

LEUKAEMOID REACTIONS

Excessive leucocytic response to a stimulus and/or immature cell spilling over in peripheral blood.

Neutrophilic

- Haemolytic crises
- Haemorrhage
- Hodgkin's disease
- Infections
  - tuberculosis
  - other bacterial infections
  - congenital syphilis
- Burns
- Eclampsia
- Mustard gas poisoning
- Vascular thrombosis and infarction
- Marrow replacement and myeloid metaplasia.

Lymphocytic

- Infectious lymphocytosis
- Infectious monocytosis
- Pertussis
- Varicella
- Tuberculosis

Eosinophilic

- Visceral larva migrans

BONE MARROW PLASMACYTOSIS

Acute infections
- Rubella
- Rubeola
- Varicella
- Infective hepatitis
- Scarlet fever

Chronic infections
- Tuberculosis
- Syphilis
- Fungal

Allergic states
- Serum sickness
- Drug reactions

Collagen—vascular disorders
- Acute rheumatic fever
- Rheumatoid arthritis
- SLE

Neoplasms
- Disseminated carcinoma
- Hodgkin's disease
- Multiple myeloma

Others
- Cirrhosis of liver.

WHITE BLOOD CELLS

Neutropenia and Agranulocytosis

Neutropenia is reduction in number of circulating neutrophils below 2500 cells/cu mm.

Blood Picture of Drug-Induced Neutropenia

- Neutropenia with no anaemia or thrombocytopenia.
- In some cases there may be lymphopenia and monocytopenia also.
- Neutrophils may show toxic and degenerative changes.
- ESR is usually raised.

Bone Marrow

- Absence of granulocytic precursors with normal erythropoiesis and a normal number of megakaryocytes (sometimes depleted).
- Toxic granulation in developing granulocytes.
- Granulocytic hyperplasia implies recovery.

Causes of Neutropenia

Drugs

1. *Drugs that cause aplastic anaemia.*
2. *Drugs that induce selective neutropenia.*
   Antipyretic, analgesics—Amidopyrine.
   Antithyroid drugs—Thiouracil, methimazole, carbimazole.
   Antihistamines—Promethazine, chlorpheniramine, mepyramine etc.
   Tranquillisers and antidepressants —Chlorpromazine, meprobamate, imipramine, amitryptiline, etc.
   Antibacterials—Tetracycline, streptomycin, ristocetin, salazopyrin, sodium methicillin, etc.
   Anticoagulants—Phenindione, dicoumarol.
   Antituberculars—Isoniazid, PAS, thiacetazone.
   Antimalarials—Primaquine, amodiaquin.
   Miscellaneous—Procainamide, penicillamine, metronidazole, etc.

OTHER CAUSES OF NEUTROPENIA

1. *Chronic idiopathic neutropenia (agranulocytosis)*-neutrophil count = 500-2000 cells/cu mm—absolute or relative lymphocytosis.
2. *Infections*
   - Acute viral
     - rubeola
     - hepatitis.
   - Bacterial
     - typhoid
     - brucellosis

   Rickettsial
   Protozoan—malaria
   All grave infections
   - bacteraemia
   - miliary tuberculosis.
3. *Marrow aplasia* All causes of aplastic anaemia.

4. *Due to known cause or myelophthisis*
   - Leukaemia
   - Neoplasia
5. *Nutritional deficit*
   - Folic acid } Megaloblastic macrocytic anaemia
   - Vitamin B_{12}
6. *Hypersplenism:* Congestive or infiltrative
7. *Miscellaneous*
   - SLE
   - Anaphylaxis
   - Antileucocyte antibodies
   - Immunodeficiencies
   - Pancreatic exocrine deficiency
   - Cyclic neutropenia (familial/sporadic)

Symptomatic neutropenia occurs usually in aplastic anaemia, drug-induced neutropenia, hypersplenism and idiopathic neutropenia, and acute leukaemia.

LABORATORY DIAGNOSIS OF INFECTIOUS MONONUCLEOSIS

Blood Picture

- There is both absolute and relative lymphocytosis, large numbers of them atypical.
- Haemoglobin value and platelet counts are normal.
- Initial leucopenia due to reduction in number of neutrophils, the neutrophil alkaline phosphatase count is often low.
- Lymphocytosis is maximum at about the tenth day.
- Lymphocytosis (atypical) as described by Downey and Mckinley
  Type I—Monocytoid lymphocytes
  Type II—Plasmacytoid lymphocytes
  Type III—Blastoid lymphocytes.
- ESR is raised in 50% cases.
- Wasserman reaction may be positive in 3-10% cases.
- ELISA test is also available.

Paul Bunnel Test for Heterophile Antibody

This is based upon the presence of antisheep red cell haemagglutinins in unusually high titres in the sera of these patients. It is positive in about 80-90% of cases. It remains positive for a variable period of time. In addition to the said antibodies, at least 2 other types of agglutinin for sheep red cells occur in human serum. They are:

1. an antibody present in low titres in normal persons and in malignant lymphomas. This antibody is absorbed by guinea pig kidney but not by ox cells.
2. an antibody occurring following the injection of horse serum and in serum sickness. This is absorbed both by guinea pig kidney and ox cells.

This antibody of infectious mononucleosis is not absorbed by guinea pig kidney but is absorbed by ox cells.

LUPUS ERYTHEMATOSUS (LE) CELL/PHENOMENON

Method

1. Draw 5-10 ml of venous blood. Place in a 50 ml flask containing 20-30 glass beads 3-5 mm in diameter or clear metal paper clips. Swirl or shake gently for 10-15 minutes to defibrinate the blood.
2. Let stand 15 minutes (preferrably at 37°C).
3. Transfer blood and a few beads to a test tube or container and mix on a rotator or by inverting for 30 minutes.
4. Let stand at room temperature (preferrably at 37°C) for 1 hour.
5. Centrifuge at 2000-3000 rpm for 5-10 minutes.
6. Transfer the buffy coat to Wintrobe's haematocrit tube and centrifuge again for 5-10 minutes.
7. Transfer the buffy coat and an equal volume of plasma to a small tube, mix well, and prepare smears. Dry rapidly and stain with Giemsa's or Leishman's stain.
8. Examine smears for clumps of platelets and neutrophilic leucocytes where the typical LE cell is most likely to be found. Look for neutrophils containing ingested homogeneous blue to magenta coloured bodies (LE cell) or a group of neutrophils encircling (garlanding) such a body (LE phenomenon).

It should be differentiated from 'tart cell' in which though neutrophil may show an inclusion that is not homogeneous and is of the same colour and appearance of their nuclei.

Interpretation: Positive LE cells in blood are found in
- Systemic lupus erythematosus (70-80%)
- Rheumatoid arthritis (10%)
- Occasionally other collagen disorders

- Malaria
- Drug induced, e.g. hydralazine and procainamide.

CLASSIFICATION OF ACUTE MYELOMONOCYTIC LEUKAEMIAS

FAB Classification

M1. *Myeloblastic leukaemia without maturation:* Nongranular blasts with occasional Auer rods or azurophilic granules, 3% or more are myeloperoxidase positive; no maturational changes

M2. *Myeloblastic leukaemia with maturation:* Maturation to promyelocytic stage: 50% of marrow cells are blasts or promyelocytes, later stages variably present, often with bilobed nuclei, Pelger-Huet anomaly or decreased granulation.

M3. *Hypergranular promyelocytic leukaemia:* Predominent cell is heavily granulated promyelocytes; bundles of Auer rods common in cytoplasm or free on smear.

M4. *Myelomonocytic leukaemia:* Promonocytes plus monocytes comprise 20% of nucleated cells in marrow, blood or both; myeloblasts plus promyelocytes are 20% of marrow cells; monocytic cells have strong nonspecific esterase reaction inhibited by fluoride; esterase activity in myelocytic cells persists after fluoride exposure.

M5. *Monocytic leukaemia:* Granulocytic cells less than 10% differentiated and poorly differentiated subtypes depend on degree of maturation; esterase reaction inhibited by sodium fluoride.

M6. *Erythroleukaemia:* Marrow has 50% erythropoietic forms, often with bizarre morphology or megaloblastic changes (show PAS+ve granules), myeloblasts and promyelocytes 30% or more; abnormal megakaryocytes present.

LABORATORY DIAGNOSIS OF LEUKAEMIAS

Cytochemical Methods for Staining Leucocytes

Neutrophil Alkaline Phosphatase (Kaplow's Method)

Principle: The enzyme, located in the neutrophil specific granules, is exposed to the substrate (α naphthol phosphate) in the presence of a diazonium salt (fast blue or fast violet) at an alkaline pH, 9.5. The substrate is hydrolysed by the enzyme, releasing a phosphate and an aryl naphthol amide. The latter is immediately coupled to the diazonium salt, forming an insoluble azo dye.

Reagents

Fixative: 10% formalin in absolute methanol. To 10 ml 37% formal dehyde, add 90 ml absolute methanol. Store at 10 to 20°C.

Buffer stock: 0.2 M propanediol. Dissolve 21 gm of 2-amino-2 methyl-1, 3-propanediol in distilled water and dilute to 1000 ml. Store at 4°C.

Working: 0.05 M propanediol pH 9.4 to 9.6. Add 70 ml 0.1 N HCI to 250 ml of stock buffer and dilute to 1000 ml with distilled water. Store at 4°C.

Substrate mixture: Dissolve 5 mg of naphthol AS-BI phosphate or naphthol AS-MX phosphate or naphthol AS phosphate in 0.2 to 0.3 ml dimethyl

FAB Classification of lymphoblastic leukemias

Observation	*L1*	*L2*	*L3*
Consistency of appearance	Homogeneous	Heterogeneous	Homogeneous
Cell size	Uniformly small	Large, but variable	Uniformly large
Nuclear shape	Regular, little clefting	Irregular, clefted, indented	Regular, rounded
Nucleoli	None or inconspicuous	One or more large	One or more, prominent
Amount of cytoplasm	Scant	Variable, often abundant	Abundant
Other findings	T d T* usually	T d T usually Myeloperoxidase negative	May have B cell markings

*(T d T—Terminal deoxynucleotidyl transferase)

formamide in a dry flask and add 60 ml of 0.05 M propanediol buffer and 40 mg of fast blue salt RR, BB, or BBN (or fast red violet LB). Shake well, filter into a Coplin jar and use immediately.

Counterstain: Mayer's hematoxylin. Add 1 gm. hematoxylin to 500 ml distilled water. Heat just to boiling and add another 500 ml distilled water. Add 0.2 gm sodium iodate and 50 gm of aluminium potassium sulphate. Shake well, filter and store in brown bottle at room temperature.

Procedure

Use freshly made blood films. If venous blood is used, heparin should be the anticoagulant, as the enzyme activity diminishes rapidly in EDTA.

Fix air dried blood films in 10% formal methanol for exactly 30 seconds at 0 to –10°C.

Wash in gently running tap water for 30 to 60 seconds.

Air dry slides, then place them in substrate mixture for exactly 10 minutes. Wash in gently running tap water again for 30 to 60 seconds.

Counterstain for 6 to 8 minutes in filtered Mayer's haematoxylin.

Wash in running tap water for 2 minutes. Air dry. Positive controls are run with each batch of slides. Women in last trimester of pregnancy are good controls, because their scores are high normal or somewhat increased.

Scoring procedure: Examine 100 mature neutrophils in the thin part of the film, where red cells barely touch each other and score each as follows:

Unstained cells	0
Cells stained faintly diffusely, or a few discrete granules	1
Cells with moderate number of granules	2
Cells with granules filling the cell	3
Cells staining deeply, almost obscuring the nucleus	4

Adding the scores for 100 cells can give a possible range of 0 to 400. The normal range with this method is 20 to 100.

The NAP scores are raised in:

- bacterial infections
- myocardial infarction
- trauma
- diabetic acidosis
- polycythaemia vera
- myelosclerosis
- following corticosteroid therapy
- during pregnancy
- use of oral contraceptives.

The NAP scores are lowered in:

- chronic myeloid leukaemia } always
- paroxysmal nocturnal haemoglobinuria } always
- idiopathic thrombocytopenic purpura] sometimes
- infectious mononucleosis] sometimes
- pernicious anaemia relapse] sometimes
- collagen disorders and refractory anaemias] sometimes
- hypophosphataemia] sometimes

Peroxidase (Myeloperoxidase, Kaplow's Method)

Principle: In the presence of hydrogen peroxide, peroxidase in leucocyte granules oxidises benzidine from a colourless form to blue or brown derivative which is localised at the site of the enzyme.

Reagents

Fixative: Mix 10 ml of 37% formal dehyde with 90 ml of absolute ethanol:

Incubation mixture	
Ethanol 30% (v/v) in water	100 ml
Benzidine dihydrochloride	0.3 gm
Zn SO_4. $7H_2O$, 0.132M (3.8% w/v)	1.0 ml
Sodium acetate ($Na_2C_2H_3O_2$. $3H_2O$)	1.0 gm
3% hydrogen peroxide	0.7 ml
Sodium hydroxide, 1.0 N	1.5 ml
Safranin O	0.2 gm

Reagents are mixed in the stated order. A precipitate forms after adding zinc sulphate but dissolves after other reagents are added. The pH is not critical between 5.8 and 6.5. The mixture is filtered and may be kept in a closed container and reused for a period of several months.

Procedure

Freshly made films or imprints are used. Peroxidase is unstable in the light, but unfixed films are satisfactory for as long as 3 weeks if kept in the dark. Heparin/oxalate/EDTA can be used as an anticoagulant.

Place slides in fixative for 60 seconds at room temperature. Wash in gently running tap water.

Place slides in incubation mixture for 30 seconds at room temperature. Wash in gently running tap water for 30 to 60 seconds.

Allow slides to dry, and examine under the microscope.

The slides may be counterstained with Wright's stain or with 1% aqueous cresyl violet if greater nuclear detail is wanted.

Interpretation

Peroxidase activity is indicated by blue granules in the cytoplasm. The nucleus and background cytoplasm stain red.

In neutrophilic series peroxidase becomes positive in late myeloblasts and on till mature neutrophil. In eosinophils specific granules contain peroxidase. Basophils, lymphocytes and erythroid cells do not stain. Monocytes stain less intensely than do neutrophils, and the granules are smaller.

Peroxidase reaction is used in differentiating acute myeloblastic leukaemia (+ve) from acute lymphoblastic leukaemia (–ve). It parallels Sudan Black B reaction; Auer rods are positive with both.

Peroxidase activity may be absent in some toxic neutrophils in infection.

PERIODIC ACID-SCHIFF (PAS) REACTION

Principle: Periodic acid (HIO_4) is an oxidising agent that converts hydroxy groups on adjacent carbon atoms to aldehydes. The resulting dialdehydes are combined with Schiff's reagent to give a red-coloured product. A positive reaction is, therefore, seen with polysaccharides, mucopolysaccharides, and glycoproteins.

Reagents

- Fixative: Mix 10 ml of 37% formaldehyde with 90 ml of absolute ethanol.
- Periodic acid, 5 gm, is dissolved in 500 ml of distilled water. Stored in dark bottle and is good for 3 months.
- Schiff's reagent: Dissolve 5 gm of basic fuchsin in 500 ml of hot distilled water and filter after it has cooled. Saturate with sulphur dioxide gas by bubbling for 1 hour. Extract the solution with 2 gm. of activated charcoal for a few seconds in a hood and immediately filter through Whatman No. 1 filter paper into a dark bottle. The solution is kept for 2 to 3 months.
- Harris haematoxylin.

Procedure

- Place air-dried blood and marrow films or imprints in fixative for 10 minutes. Wash briefly with tap water.
- Control slides are exposed to digestion with saliva (diastase) for 30 minutes. Place slides in periodic acid for 10 minutes. Wash briefly with tap water and blot dry.
- Immerse slides in Schiff's reagent for 30 minutes.
- Rinse slides in several changes of sulphur-dioxide water for 20 to 30 minutes.
- Wash for 5 to 10 minutes in tap water and counterstain with Harris haematoxylin for 10 minutes.

Interpretation

In blood cells a positive PAS reaction usually indicates presence of glycogen. This is shown by digestion with diastase and consequent loss of staining.

Neutrophils react at all stages of development, the most strongly in the mature stage (similarly for eosinophils). The glycogen is not in the granules but in the background cytoplasm. Myeloblasts contain a few small PAS-positive granules. Monocytes have a faint staining reaction in the form of fine granules. Lymphocytes may contain a few small or large granules. Normoblasts are normally PAS negative.

In erythroleukaemia and in thalassaemia some of the erythroid precursors are PAS positive. In acute lymphoblastic leukaemias, the lymphoblasts often contain large coarse clumps of PAS-positive material (block positivity).

Sudan Black B Stain (Sheehan and Storey)

Principle: Sudan Black B stains phospholipids and other lipids. It appears to stain both azurophilic and specific granules in neutrophils, whereas the peroxidase is found only in azurophilic granules. In early forms, late myeloblasts and early promyelocytes, the Sudan Black B reaction is therefore, parallel to the peroxidase in its utility in separating acute lymphoblastic from acute myeloblastic leukaemia.

Reagents

Stock solution of stain: Dissolve 0.3 gm of Sudan Black B powder in 100 ml ethyl alcohol.

Buffer solution: Dissolve 16 gm crystalline phenol in 30 ml ethyl alcohol. Add this to a solution of 0.3 gm hydrated disodium hydrogen phosphate ($Na_2HPO_4 \cdot 12H_2O$) dissolved in 100 ml distilled water.

Working stain solution
Add 40 ml buffer solution to 60 ml stock stain solution. Filter using suction. This is stable for approximately 2 months.

Procedure

- Fix air dried films in formalin vapour for 10 minutes. Slides need not be freshly made.
- Wash slides in running tap water for 10 minutes.
- Place slides in working stain solution (in Coplin jar) for 60 minutes.
- Wash slides with 70% ethyl alcohol for 2 to 3 minutes to remove excess dye.
- Wash slides in tap water for 2 minutes.
- Allow slides to dry. Counterstain slides with Wright's stain or haematoxylin.

Interpretation

Cytoplasmic granules stain faintly in neutrophil precursors and strongly in mature neutrophils with a brown black colour. Eosinophilic granules are brown but often show a central pallor. Monocytes have scattered fine brown-black granules. Lymphocytes and lymphoblasts are negative, but at least some myeloblasts contain Sudan Black positive granules.

The peroxidase and Sudan Black B reactions show roughly similar patterns in the various cell types. These techniques are most useful in distinguishing myeloblasts from lymphoblasts when large numbers of primitive blast forms are present in acute leukaemias.

Nonspecific Esterase

Alpha-Naphthol Acetate Esterase (Yam *et al*).

Reagents

Fixative: Buffered formalin and acetone.

Formaldehyde, 37%; 25 ml, Na_2 HPO_4, 20 mg, KH_2PO_4 100 mg; distilled water, 30 ml; acetone 45 ml.

Buffer Sorensen's phosphate buffer (M/15. pH=7.6)

Incubation mixture: Add in the following manner
- Buffer 44.5 ml.
- Hexazotised parasanilin 3.0 ml
- Alpha-naphthol acetate 50 gm dissolved in 2.5 ml ethylene glycol monomethyl ether
- Filter mixture through Seitz filter
- Harris haematoxylin.

Procedure

Place air dried blood or marrow films in fixative for 30 seconds at 4°C. Wash in running tap water.

Place slides in incubation mixture for 60 minutes. Wash in running tap water.

Counterstain with Harris haematoxylin for 10 minutes.

Interpretation

Alpha-naphthol acetate esterase activity is found in monocytes but not in neutrophils or neutrophil precursors, other granulocytes or lymphocytes. It may be found, however, in activated or atypical lymphocytes, in lymphocytes in imprints of active lymphoid tissue, and probably in the poorly differentiated lymphocytes of some lymphomas.

ACUTE LEUKAEMIAS, LABORATORY DIAGNOSIS

Routine Haematologic Investigations

- A normocytic, normochromic anaemia.
- The white cell count may be decreased, normal or increased up to 2 lakh/cu mm.
- Thrombocytopenia occurs in most cases, often extremely low in AML.

Blood Film Examination

Shows variable numbers of blast cells. In AML the blasts may show Auer rods and other abnormal cells may be present, e.g. promyelocytes, myelocytes, agranular neutrophils, pseudopelger cells, myelomonocytic cells. In erythroleukaemia many normoblasts may be seen but these may be seen in smaller numbers in the other forms. The differentiating features of various blast cells have been discussed elsewhere. In leukaemias one may see typical and atypical blasts.

Bone marrow is hypercellular with a marked proliferation of leukaemic blast cells which typically amount to over 75% of the marrow cell total. In ALL marrow may be difficult to aspirate due to increased reticulin fibre.

Differentiation of ALL from AML

In most cases the clinical features and morphology on routine stains separate ALL from AML. In ALL blasts show no differentiation whereas in AML some evidence of differentiation, to granulocytes is often seen in the blasts of their progeny. Special cytochemical staining techniques just described are needed when cells are undifferentiated.

Cytochemistry	*ALL*	*AML*
Peroxidase	—	+ (including Auer rods)
Sundan Black B	—	+
Nonspecific esterase	—	+ (in monocytic types)
PAS	+ (coarse)	+ (fine)
Acid phosphatase	(T cell ALL)	—

Other Investigations

Tests for disseminated intravascular coagulation (DIC) are positive in promyelocytic leukaemia. Lumbar puncture shows raised spinal fluid pressure, it contains leukaemic cells in patients with meningeal leukaemia.

CHRONIC MYELOID LEUKAEMIA

Laboratory Investigations

Diagnostic Features

- Leucocytes usually > 50,000/cu mm and sometimes > 5 lakh/cu mm.
- A complete spectrum of myeloid cells in the peripheral blood. The levels of neutrophils and myelocytes exceed those of blast cells and promyelocytes.

Additional Features

- Philadelphia chromosome on cytogenetic analysis of blood or bone marrow.
- Bone marrow is hypercellular with granulopoietic predominance (especially myelocytes).
- Neutrophil alkaline phosphatase score invariably low.
- Increased circulating basophils.
- Normocytic, normochromic anaemia.
- Platelet count is usually increased but may be normal or decreased.
- Serum vitamin B_{12} and vitamin B_{12} binding capacity are increased.
- CML is said to be undergoing blast transformation when percentage of myelocytes and promyelocytes exceeds 20% in peripheral smear or 30% in bone marrow.

CHRONIC LYMPHOCYTIC LEUKAEMIA (CLL)

Laboratory Findings

- Leucocytosis. The absolute lymphocyte count is above 5000/cu mm and in the majority of patients it is 30-3000 × 10^9/L. Between 70 and 99% of white cells on blood film appear as mature lymphocytes. Smudge or smear cells are also present.
- Normocytic, normochromic anaemia in later stages.
- Thrombocytopenia occurs in many patients.

Bone marrow aspiration: Shows lymphocytic replacement of normal marrow elements. Lymphocytes comprise 25-95% of all the cells.

Reduced concentration of serum immunoglobins: They are found in most cases, particularly with advanced disease.

Leukaemia can be differentiated from leukaemoid reaction: By taking into consideration the clinical picture, neutrophil alkaline phosphatase score (high or normal in leukaemoid reaction but low in leukaemia). In addition, cytochemical stains may be used for differentiation.

PARAPROTEINAEMIAS

Causes

- Multiple myeloma,
- Macroglobulinaemia,
- Malignant lymphoma,
- Chronic lymphocytic lymphoma,
- Benign monoclonal gammopathy,
- Chronic cold haemagglutinin disease.
- Rarely with carcinomas.

MULTIPLE MYELOMA

Multiple myeloma (can be solitary myeloma called plasmacytoma in extramedullary sites) is a neoplastic proliferation of plasma cells. Characterised by lytic bone lesions, plasma cell (myeloma cell) accummulation in the bone marrow and the presence of monoclonal protein in serum and in about half the cases in urine also.

Laboratory Diagnosis

1. In about 98% cases monoclonal protein occurs in serum and/or urine.
   Incidence of serum paraprotein
   IgG 66%
   Ig A 33%
   Ig M or
   Ig D 1%
   The normal immunoglobulins are depressed.
   The Bence-Jones proteins found in urine are free light chains, either kappa or lambda of the same type as serum paraprotein.
2. The bone marrow shows more than 10% plasma, cells and often with abnormal 'myeloma cells'.
3. 60% of patients have osteolytic areas
   20% show generalised bone rarefaction or osteoporosis which may cause pathological fractures.
   20% show no such lesions.
   Most often two of the three diagnostic features stated above are present.

Other Laboratory Findings

1. Normochromic, normocytic anaemia is usual. Marked rouleaux formation is seen. Neutropenia and thrombocytopenia seen in advanced cases. There may be myeloma cell spillover in the peripheral blood or there may be (very rare) plasma cell leukaemia. Leucoerythroblastic changes (immature cells of both myeloid and erythroid series in the peripheral blood) are occasionally found.
2. About half the cases have raised serum calcium levels and elevated serum alkaline phosphatase.
3. ESR is markedly raised.
4. Renal damage leads to raised blood urea and serum creatinine levels.
5. Serum albumin is low.

The monoclonal peak (M peak, spike) is found by immunological and electrophoretic techniques. Immunoglobulins IgG, IgM and IgA can be measured quantitatively by using immunoturbidometric or nephalometric kits available for estimation of the immunoglobulins IgG, IgM and IgA separately.

POLYCYTHAEMIA VERA

Laboratory Diagnosis

1. Raised red cell count, haematocrit and haemoglobin.
2. Anisocytosis and poikilocytosis in late stages.
3. Neutrophilic leucocytosis (50% cases), in some cases basophilia.
4. Raised platelet count (50% cases).
5. Reticulocyte count raised.
6. Raised neutrophil alkaline phosphatase score.
7. Increased vitamin B_{12} binding capacity.
8. Bone marrow is hypercellular (generalised hypercellularity), with prominent megakaryocytes. Storage iron diminished Reticulin diminished (late stages).
9. Serum uric acid may be raised, serum iron—histamine levels (blood and urine)—arterial oxygen saturation normal (92%).

MYELOSCLEROSIS

Laboratory Diagnosis

1. Anaemia is usual.
2. At the onset, white cell and platelet counts are frequently high but later leucopenia and thrombocytopenia are common.
3. A leucoerythroblastic blood picture is seen. The red cells characteristically show 'tear drop' poikilocytes.
4. Bone marrow is usually unobtainable by aspiration. A trephine biopsy may show a hypercellular marrow with an increase in reticulin pattern. Increased megakaryocytes are frequently seen. In some cases there is increased bone formation.
5. Low serum folate, raised serum vitamin B_{12}, and raised vitamin B_{12} binding capacity, increased neutrophil alkaline phosphatase.
6. High serum urate, LDH and hydroxybutyrate dehydrogenase levels reflect the increased but largely ineffective turnover of haemopoietic cells.
7. Extramedullary haemopoiesis may be documented by radioiron studies, by liver biopsy or splenic aspiration.

HODGKIN'S DISEASE

This is a neoplastic disorder of lymphoreticular tissue and four morphologic types are known, viz.

1. Lymphocyte predominance (5-13%).
2. Nodular sclerosis (40-50%).
3. Mixed cellularity (35-40%).
4. Lymphocyte depletion (5-10%).

Laboratory Findings in Hodgkin's Disease

Early in course

- Mild normocytic, normochromic anaemia; from depressed erythropoiesis.
- Moderate leucocytosis, with eosinophilia up to 10%.
- Normal or increased platelet count.
- Increased ESR.
- Decreased serum iron and iron-binding capacity; normal or ↓ marrow iron.
- Decreased cell-mediated immunity, antibody activity normal.

Later in disease

- Lymphopenia.
- More severe anaemia.
- Coombs' positive haemolysis (relatively rare).
- Thrombocytopenia.
- Mild hypoalbuminaemia, hyperglobulinaemia.
- Hyercalcaemia.
- Hyperuricaemia.
- Low serum zinc, high serum copper.

Chapter 10

Clinical Haematology Bleeding Disorders

PLATELETS, COAGULATION AND BLEEDING DISORDERS: LABORATORY INVESTIGATIONS

Platelet Count—Dealt in depth elsewhere

CAPILLARY FRAGILITY TEST OF HESS

(Rumpel-Leede Sign, Tourniquet Test)

1. Inflate sphygmomanometer cuff around arm at 80 mm of Hg pressure for 5 minutes.
2. Look for petechiae in an area 5 cm in diameter just below the elbow.
3. Under normal circumstances the number of petechiae should be less than 5, more than 5 indicate a positive test.

A positive test may be found in reduced capillary resistance (or increased capillary fragility) as in nonthrombocytopenic purpura and scurvy. It may also be positive in thrombocytopenia when the platelet count is below approximately 70,000/cu mm of blood.

Clinical Implications

1. Increased petechiae formation occurs most commonly in thrombocytopenia and less commonly in: (i) thrombasthenia, (ii) vascular purpura, (iii) senile purpura, and (iv) scurvy.
2. The number and size of petechiae are roughly proportional to the bleeding tendency and possibly to the degree of thrombocytopenia. However, the test can be positive because of capillary fragility in the presence of normal platelet count.
3. Results will be normal in coagulation disorders and vascular disorders.

Interfering Factors

1. *Menstruation:* Capillary fragility is normally increased before menstruation.
2. *Infectious disease:* Capillary fragility is increased in measles and influenza.
3. *Age:* Women over 40 with decreasing estrogen levels may have a positive test that is not indicative of a coagulation disorder.
4. *Re-administration:* Repetition of test on same arm within 1 week of the first test may lead to error.
5. *Variation:* Results may vary because of differences in texture, thickness, and temperature of the skin.

BLEEDING TIME

The duration of bleeding from a standard puncture wound of the skin is a measure of the function of platelets as well as the integrity of the vessel wall.

Duke's Method

Requirements

1. Stop watch.
2. Lancet.
3. Filter paper.
4. Glass slide.
5. Alcohol sponges.

Method

1. Clean the lobe of the ear or tip of a finger with alcohol and let dry.
2. For ear—glass slide is placed behind the ear lobe and held firmly in place. This provides a firm site for incision.
3. Pierce the lobe of the ear by a firm stroke against the glass slide (or pierce the finger-tip). Discard the glass slide if ear lobe has been incised. Start the stop watch when the stab was made.
4. Bleeding of the wound should be allowed to proceed without pressure and the blood is allowed to drop on the filter paper. The paper should be moved so that each drop will fall on a fresh area. When bleeding slows, the wound is touched gently with a fresh area of the filter paper at 30 second intervals. When blood no longer stains the filter paper, the watch is stopped and the time recorded.

Normal values: The normal range is upto 6 minutes. Between 6 and 10 minutes, the results are borderline. Over 10 minutes is definitely abnormal.

Precautions

1. In children heel should be used.
2. In suspected cases of a bleeding disorder, the bleeding may not be controlled easily from the ear lobe hence, fingertip puncture wounds are better.
3. The area to be punctured should not be congested.
4. The size and depth of the wound may vary if one does not have a standardised technique.
5. If bleeding persists for more than 15 minutes it should be stopped by placing a dry gauge sponges over the site and applying finger pressure (the filter paper used to collect the drops of blood can be dried and saved as a record of the procedure).

Ivys's Method

(Preferred because of greater ease of standardisation)

Method

1. Cleanse the inner aspect of the forearm with spirit and let dry.
2. Place a blood pressure cuff on the upper arm, inflate at 40 mm Hg, and maintain the same throughout the test.
3. Select an area on the forearm—Volar aspect which is devoid of superficial veins. Stretch the skin laterally between the thumb and forefinger and hold in a taut position.
4. Take a cork, through which a no. 11 surgical blade has been inserted with the tip extending 3 mm beyond the cork surface (both cork and blade should have been sterilized before), the blade should be withdrawn from the cork and autoclaved before being used again.
5. Hold the cork with the thumb and forefinger of the free hand, and with the heel of the hand resting on the patient's arm, quickly make two skin punctures (actually they are small incisions) in the selected area. It is important that the surface of the cork meet the skin to ensure a 3 mm deep incision. Holding the skin taut prevents the test area from being depressed when the blade enters the skin.
6. Timing is begun as soon as the incisions are made and bleeding starts.

7. Using the edge of a piece of a filter paper to collect the blood, gently touch paper to the drop of blood which forms over the wound every 30 seconds. Do not rub or remove the clot. Do not touch the skin. Any disruption of formed fibrin or clot will prolong the bleeding time.
8. The bleeding time is reported when no blood stain is seen on the filter paper after a gentle touch. It is reported in intervals of 30 seconds. One can measure both wounds and average them, or take the reading of the last one to stop bleeding.

Normal values are 1 to 6 minutes. More than 6 minutes should be taken as abnormal.

Interpretation

1. Results of duplicate tests performed on the same individual should agree within 2 to 3 minutes at most.
2. Bleeding time is prolonged
   - when platelet count < 100,000/mm^{3}.
   - in patients on aspirin therapy.
   - in acquired fibrinogen disorders.

(If the platelets are young even in a thrombocytopenia patient, the bleeding time may not be raised as young platelets have enhanced hemostatic capabilities).

When platelet counts are low, one can calculate the expected bleeding time with the following formula.

$$\text{Bleeding time} = 30.5 \times \frac{\text{Platelet count/cu mm}}{3850}$$

A bleeding time longer than that calculated from platelet numbers alone, suggests defective platelet function in addition to reduced number. It is also possible to detect above-normal hemostatic capacity in cases in which active young platelets comprise the entire population of circulating platelets.

Clinical Implications

1. Bleeding time is prolonged when the level of platelets is decreased or when the platelets are qualitatively abnormal, as in
   a. thrombocytopenia.
   b. platelet dysfunction syndromes.
   c. decrease or abnormality in plasma factors such as von Willebrand's factor and fibrinogen.
   d. abnormalities in walls of the small blood vessels—vascular defects.
   f. severe liver disease.
   g. leukemia.
   h. aplastic anaemia.
   i. DIC disease.
2. Bleeding time can be either normal or prolonged in von Willebrand's disease. It will definitely be prolonged if aspirin is administered prior to testing.
3. A single prolonged bleeding time does not prove the existence of haemorrhagic disease because a larger vessel may have been punctured. The puncture should be done twice (on the contralateral side) and the average of the bleeding times can be taken.

Interfering Factors

1. The normal range may vary when the puncture is not of standard depth and width.
2. Touching the incision during the test will break off any fibrin particles and prolong the bleeding time.
3. Heavy alcohol consumption (as in alcoholics) may cause bleeding time to be increased.
4. Prolonged bleeding time will result from the ingestion of 10 gm of aspirin up to 5 days before the test.
5. Other drugs that may cause the bleeding time to be increased include
   - Dextran
   - Streptokinase—streptodornase
   - Mithramycin
   - Pantothenyl alcohol

Patient Preparation

1. Explain the purpose and procedure of the test to patient.
2. Warn patient not to consume aspirin for 5 days prior to test.
3. Advise patient not to consume alcohol in any form.

COAGULATION TIME

Capillary Tube Method of Wright

Blood is collected in about a dozen capillary tubes from a finger prick made after aseptic precautions. The tubes are sealed with plasticine and immersed in water bath at 37°C. After 4 minutes remove the first tube from the bath and expel the blood in it with one end immersed in a dish containing water. Repeat this every 30 seconds with the other tubes till the blood is expelled in a worm clot and note the time.

(An alternative way of determining the end point is to break the capillary tubes every 30 seconds until a clot is seen between the two broken ends). By these methods the normal clotting time is 5 to 10 minutes at 37°C and longer if performed at room temperature. This test should be avoided as tissue thromboplastin contaminates the oozing blood and hence, false reports may be obtained.

Lee and White's Method

Principle: Whole blood, when removed from the vascular system and exposed to a foreign surface, will form a solid clot. Within limits the time required for the formation of the solid clot is a measure of the coagulation system.

Requirements

1. Stop watch.
2. Equipment for collection of blood.
3. Clean, dry glass test tubes (10 x 75 mm).
4. Water bath (37°C).

Method

1. Make a clean venipuncture with as little trauma to (or time spent passing through) the connective tissue between skin and vein as possible. One may routinely or in selected cases use the two syringe technique, whereby one rinses the needle of all interstitial tissue fluid by drawing back 1 cc. of blood after entering the vein. Then remove the first syringe from the needle and quickly place on a second clean and dry syringe and draw back blood for the test.
2. Timing is begun when the blood first enters the syringe. The second syringe in the 'Two syringe' technique.
3. Draw 3-5 ml of blood and withdraw the syringe and needle. Disconnect the needle. Place approximately 1 ml of blood in each of three (10 × 75 mm) test tubes.
4. Place the tubes in a stand so that they remain upright and undisturbed, at room temperature for 10 minutes. If a 37°C water bath is available one may do the entire test at 37°C, and shorter clotting times will be found (if the test has been done at 37°C, do not wait for more than 5 minutes).
5. After 10 minutes (or 5 minutes) take the first of the tubes and gently tip it every 30 seconds to test for clotting. Do not tip it further than necessary to get the information.
6. When the first tube is clotted (can be inverted without blood running down the edge of the tube), record the time and start the tipping of the second tube every 30 seconds until it is also found to be clotted. Then do the same with the third tube (tipping is intended to allow one to ascertain when blood is clotted—not as a means of hastening clotting or of assuring mixing of the blood).
7. The time recorded for the clotting of the third tube is taken as the clotting time (the purpose of the first two tubes is to tell one when to start looking in the third tube, since the agitation of tipping does hasten the clotting).

   Some choose to tip the tubes in rotation (at 37°C) every 15 seconds, or tip all tubes at once, and average the results of the three tubes.

Normal Values

Normal times depend on method used. Normal range at 37°C is usually 5 to 10 minutes. Normal times at room temperature will vary with the degree of temperature present and the method used. If one uses the method which waits 10 minutes before starting to tip, then normal values may go as high as 22 to 25 minutes, especially in the cool season. Values shorter than 10 minutes should be suspected and the test repeated using the two-syringe technique to rule out contamination by tissue fluid (in the heat of April, May or June in our country blood will clot before 10 minutes without having been contaminated by tissue fluids). If one uses the method which waits 5 minutes before tippings begins, normal result are between 8 to 18 minutes. Longer than 20 minutes is abnormal. If clotting occurs in less than 7 minutes, the test should be repeated using two-syringe technique.

Precautions and Errors

1. The venipuncture must be without trauma to avoid contamination with tissue thromboplastin.
2. If all three tubes are clotted at 10 minutes (or 5 minutes) when one starts to tip the first tube, the test is unsatisfactory and should be repeated. If blood was drawn by single syringe technique, the most likely explanation is contamination, of

the blood by tissue thromboplastin. If a two-syringe technique is used, it suggests that the patient's blood is hypercoagulable.

3. Vigorous agitation of the tubes will significantly shorten the coagulation time. So tipping should really be very gentle just to see if the blood has clotted.

Clinical Implications

1. Severe deficiencies of any of the coagulation factors must be present before the coagulation time will be prolonged. Fibrinogen for example, needs to be decreased to 50 mg/100 ml or less before the coagulation time is affected, the normal range of fibrinogen is 200 to 400 mg/100 ml.
2. When prothrombin is diminished to a level of 30 per cent of normal, there will be a small change in coagulation time.
3. Prolonged coagulation time will be noted in afibrinogen and marked hyperheparinemia.

Interfering Factors

1. *Quality of venipuncture:* The venipuncture must be carefully done because either tissue thromboplastin obtained as a contaminant when the venipuncture is done, or haemolysed red blood cells suctioned when the blood is drawn, can cause a marked shortening of the coagulation time. The time required for a severe haemophiliac's blood to clot can be shortened from 1 hour to a normal value when a poor venipuncture is done.
2. *Type of test tube:* The coagulation time will be lengthened to 20 to 40 minutes if plastic or silicone coated test tubes are used.
3. *Drugs:* Increased coagulation time may be seen with
   - Mithramycin.
   - Tetracyclines.
   - Anticoagulants.
   - Azathioprine.
   - Carbenicillin.

   Decreased coagulation time may be seen with
   - Corticosteroids.
   - Epinephrine.

CLOT RETRACTION

Principle

When whole blood is allowed to clot spontaneously, the initial coagulum is composed of all elements of the blood. With time the coagulum reduces in mass and fluid serum is expressed from the clot. This is due to an action of platelets on the fibrin network.

Requirements

1. Equipment for collecting blood
2. Clean, dry plain glass graduated centrifuge tube
3. Timer
4. Water bath 37°C.

Method

1. 5 ml blood is obtained with a standard two-syringe technique and transferred to the centrifuge tube.
2. Incubate it at 37°C in vertical position.
3. Record degree of retraction after 1, 2, and 4 hours. It may be necessary to loosen the clot gently from the wall of the test tube if contraction is not apparent at the end of 1 hour. The degree and rate of retraction should be noted. Note also any digestion of clot or discolouration of serum.

Clot retraction is directly related to platelet count, hence, it is impaired in thrombocytopenia, but is normal in hemophilia. In the method just described, one can remove the clot by using a hooked long needle and the volume of serum left behind can be measured. The percentage of clot can be calculated from the initial 5 ml of blood taken. In normal individuals, the clot percentage is about 50 per cent at the end of one hour of the original blood volume taken.

Interpretation

- Patients with qualitative or quantitative platelet disorders have samples with scant serum and a soft, plump, poorly demarcated clot.
- The clot is small and serum voluminous if the patient has a low hematocrit.
- Patients with polycythemia have poor clot retraction because the large numbers of captured red cells separate fibrin stands and interfere with platelet contraction.

- If fibrinogen levels are low, the initial clot is so fragile that the delicate strands rupture and red cells spill out into the serum when retraction begins.
- Serum contamination by red cells is especially striking if fibrinolysis is abnormally brisk, as often happens with reduced fibrinogen levels. Sometimes in these cases, the incubated tube contains only cells and plasma with no fibrin clot at all.

Errors

1. When fibrinogen is reduced in amount, the clot may be very small and retraction may be interpreted as normal even though it is inadequate.
2. In the presence of active fibrinolytic activity, the clot may dissolve.
3. In normal blood the exuded serum will be clear and free of RBC's. The presence of significant number of RBC's in the serum suggests fibrinolytic activity.
4. With a low hematocrit value, the mass of the clot will be proportionately small and may give enormously high values.

HEPARIN THERAPY

Protocols and Blood Coagulation tests

1. Heparin combines in the blood with an alpha globulin (heparin cofactor) for a potent antithrombin.
2. The intravenous injection of heparin will give an immediate anticoagulant effect, so it is used when rapid effects are desired.
3. Because of heparin not remaining in the blood very long, the clotting time is measured before each injection.
4. The coagulation time is ordinarily maintained at two to two and one half times the normal limit.
5. To evaluate the effect of heparin, the blood is tested for coagulation time.
   a. Before therapy is started for baseline
   b. 1 hour before next dose is administered
   c. Dependent upon the status of patient during heparin therapy (signs of bleeding).
6. Protamine sulphate is the antidote for heparin overdose and haemorrhage.

QUALITY ASSURANCE FOR ROUTINE HAEMOSTASIS LABORATORY

Introduction

Coagulation tests for the routine assay parameters in laboratories are fairly simple to perform and master.

The performance of basic tests require simple apparatus such as waterbath, test tubes, pipettes and stop watch and/or automatic clot timer. And it's precisely for this reason that these techniques appear deceptively easy.

There are a number of pre test variables that effect the accuracy and precision of coagulation results. These may relate to collection techniques, processing of samples, selection and preparation of reagents. In order to achieve optimum and reproducible results the impact of variables needs to be understood and controlled so as to reduce variability and errors and improve accuracy and reproducibility. Various variables that impact the results are discussed, along with the basis that leads to such recommendation.

Preparation of Patients

- Although no special preparation of patients is required prior to approved techniques it is preferable that patients are not heavily exercised before blood collection. Fasting patients or patients on a light non-fatty meal are preferable.
  - Patients who are fasting or on a light non-fatty meal prior to blood collection provide samples with desirable lower opacity this improves the sensitivity of clot detection especially when photooptical instruments are being used.
  - Turbid, icteric, lipemic or grossly haemolysed samples generate erroneous results due to varying opacity.

Sample Collection Techniques (Phlebotomy)

- Blood should be withdrawn without undue venous stasis and without frothing into a plastic syringe with a short needle of 19 to 20 SWG.
- The venepuncture must be a 'clean' one and incase of difficulty with a new syringe and needle another vein should be tried. The tourniquet should not be placed too tightly or for extended lengths of time. Patting the venepuncture site should also be avoided.

- Distribute blood into test tubes (preferably plastic) after detaching the needle from the syringe. Do not delay mixing blood with anticoagulant by gentle inversion of the tube.
  - 'Clean' venepuncture is essential to avoid formation of microclots at the site of venepuncture and consumption of factors, which will lead to artificially prolonged results.
  - Usage of short bigger bore needle allows free flow of blood within the syringe and reducing blood contact with metal surface. With smaller bore longer needles blood will remain in contact with metal surface for longer time. This will lead to initiation of clotting or partial consumption of factors being assayed leading to erroneous results during test procedures.
  - Frothing when distributing the blood into anticoagulant tube should be avoided because frothing induces microclot formation.

Sample Preparation

- The anticoagulant of choice for most coagulation procedures is sodium citrate or preferably buffered sodium citrate.
  Sodium citrate is an ideal anticoagulant since Factor V and Factor VII are more stable in citrate. These factors are more labile in sodium oxalate. Heparin neutralizes thrombins action on fibrinogen.
- The recommended molarity of sodium citrate for coagulation studies is 0.109M, which equates to 3.2 per cent of tri sodium citrate.
- Use of buffered sodium citrate is preferred over plain sodium citrate solution.
  - After collection of blood in citrate during centrifugation for preparation of PPP or PFP the pH of the solution shifts releasing carbon dioxide (CO_2). This shift in pH affects the labile Factor V leading to erroneous results during test. Use of appropriately formulated buffered citrate overcomes this phenomenon.
  - When samples are collected in 3.8 per cent citrate (129 mm) the prothrombin time of samples especially with patients receiving oral anticoagulants give prolonged results. Also the ISI of thromboplastins is lowered. It is for this reason 3.2 per cent citrate is recommended universally instead of 3.8 per cent for increasing accuracy of test results.
- The optimum ratio of citrate to blood is 1 part of anticoagulant to 9 parts of blood.
  - When the molarity of citrate is accurate the anticoagulant supplied in this amount and ratio is sufficient to bind all the available calcium in the collected sample so as to prevent clotting. A shift in this ratio leads to erroneous results as follows:
  - *More blood less citrate:* The chelating activity of citrate will not be sufficient to bind the calcium present in the sample. This will lead to formation of clots, consumption of factors and subsequent prolongation of results during test.
  - *More citrate less blood :* Excess citrate remaining in the blood sample would consume the calcium from the reagents thereby giving prolonged results.
- The optimum concentration of Calcium chloride to be used for APTT test should be 0.02 M
  - The concentration of 0.02 M $CaCl_2$ replaces the calcium necessary to activate the intrinsic coagulation cascade. This ultimately generates thrombin from prothrombin via the coagulation cascade.'
  - Appropriate volumes of $CaCl_2$ should be aspirated for the days work. Prewarmed $CaCl_2$ should always be discarded at the end of the working day.
- The standard ratio of blood to anticoagulant of 9:1 is for normal hematocrit or PCV.
  - For occasional patients with PCV less than 20 per cent (e.g., Microcytic hypochromic anaemia) and greater than 50 per cent (e.g., Polycythemia vera) the anticoagulant to blood ratio must be readjusted using the following formula,
    $C = 1.85 \times 10^{-3}$ (100-H) V
    C = Volume of sodium citrate in ml
    V = Volume of whole blood–Sodium citrate in ml
    H = Hematocrit in percentage
  - When the PCV is higher than 55 per cent the patient blood contains so little plasma that excess unutilized anticoagulant remains and is available to bind reagent calcium to prolongation of test results.
  - On the other hand, if the PCV is less than 20 per cent the patient blood contains excess of plasma but less of anticoagulant and the chelating activity of citrate will not be sufficient to bind the calcium present in sample. This will

lead to formation of clots *in vitro*, consumption of factors and prolongation of results.

Sample Processing and Storage

- Containers for collection and processing of plasma should be ideally made out of plastic or siliconized glass tubes. They should be scrupulously clean and dry.
  - — The containers should be ideally made out of plastic and not from glass as scratched glass surfaces can activate *in vitro* the coagulation mechanism within the sample due to contact with silica. While plastic tubes overcome this problem they should be free from leavening chemicals used by the plastic industry during moulding. These chemicals usually have an inhibitory effect. Scrupulous washing and drying overcomes this problem.
  - — All the containers used for collection, storage and test should be free from detergents, acids and alkalies. These chemicals have a varying effect on pH. Change in pH effects factor stability. Detergents inhibit reactive characteristics of the sample/ reagent mixture.
  - — Ideally the cleaning of glassware used in coagulation tests should be the responsibility of one individual and should be handled separately from routine laboratory glassware. Alternatively disposable labware should be used.
- The specimen to be tested for coagulation studies must be used preferably immediately.
  - — As most of coagulation factors are time as well as temperature labile it is of utmost importance that they should not be subjected to high temperatures and tests be performed as early as possible, preferably immediately.
  - — If specimen are held at 22°C to 24°C then they must be tested within 2 hours and if the specimen are held at 2°C to 4°C then they must be tested within 3 hours.
  - — Plasma samples held at 4°C to 8°C for prolonged periods may undergo cold activation leading to erroneous results.
  - — Samples obtained for factor assays and tests for fibrinolysis should be stored in crushed ice if a delay in testing is anticipated.
  - — Citrated blood for platelet aggregation studies should remain in capped tubes at RT (20°C to 25°C) before testing.
- The sample collected must be stored tightly capped.
  - — The samples collected must be stored tightly capped. If the tubes are not capped the samples will absorb atmospheric CO_2 leading to shift in pH to an unacceptable range. This hampers factor stability and accuracy of results.
  - — Centrifugation speed and time are of absolute importance in coagulation studies. The PT test uses PPP while the APTT test uses PFP.
  - — Excessive centrifugation may destroy clotting factors due to the heat generated during centrifugation.
  - — Under centrifugation would lead to the presence of platelets in plasma sample which could lead to activation of clotting mechanism *in vitro* which leads to erroneous results.
  - — Normally centrifugation for 15 minutes at approximately 1500 g yields PPP (platelet poor plasma) and centrifugation at approximately 2000 g for 15 minutes yields PFP (platelet free plasma). The 'g' is a function of length of rotor head and RPM. It is for this reason each laboratory must calibrate its own equipment to achieve satisfactory samples depending on test performed and kind of plasma sample required.

Buffered 3.2% Citrate Solution (Profact) Courtesy: Tulip Group of Companies

Ready to use 3.2 per cent Buffered Citrate solution for coagulation assays and ESR by Westergren method.

Summary

Accurate coagulation testing is dependant on numerous preanalytical variables, which may affect the results of routine coagulation assays. To improve the precision and accuracy of laboratory testing, it is important to identify these variables and control their potential effect on results.

Preanalytical variables pertinent to routine coagulation testing can be classified into three major categories: specimen collection, specimen processing and specimen storage and transport. 3.2 per cent citrate is also the anticoagulant of choice for performing ESR by Westergren method.

Reagent

Laboratory reagent. Ready to use solution.

Profact is a unique ready to use 3.2 per cent buffered Tri sodium Citrate solution formulated for collection of blood for routine coagulation assays. PROFACT can be used for sample preparation in the following clot based assays such as PT, APTT, TT, Quantitative estimation of fibriogen, test for factor deficiency, test for lupus anticoagulants, Protein C and Protein S tests. PROFACT can also be used for collection of blood to perform ESR by Westergren method.

Principle

3.2 per cent Tri-sodium Citrate is the anticoagulant of choice for coagulation studies. When anticoagulated blood is centrifuged for preparing PPP for routine coagulation assays, the centrifugation process leads to release of carbon dioxide (CO_2). The end result being shift in pH, which has an adverse impact on the results of clot-based assays. PROFACT incorporates 3.2 per cent Trisodium Citrate in a unique protective solution, which arrests shift in pH due to the release of carbon dioxide during centrifugation. Also labile factor V and VIII are well preserved and the results of clotbased assays are more accurate.

Also PROFACT incorporating 3.2 per cent citrate is the anticoagulant of choice for ESR by Westergren method.

Storage and Stability

Store the reagent at 2 to 8°C.
Stability of unopened vial: 12 months from the date of manufacturing.
Stability of opened vial: 90 days from the date of opening, provided it is not contaminated.

Material Required But Not Provided

Sterile and clean 0.5/1 ml micropipettes, micropipette tips or glass blow out pipettes, ESR tube.

SAMPLE COLLECTION AND PREPARATION

For Coagulation assays

Though no special preparation of the patient is required prior to sample collection by approved techniques, it is preferable that patients are not heavily exercised before blood collection. Fasting or only light non-fatty meals prior to blood collection provides sample with a desirable low opacity.

Withdraw blood without undue venous or frothing into a plastic syringe fitted with a short needle of 19 to 20 SWG. The venepuncture must be a 'clean' one and if there is any difficulty, take a new syringe and try another vein. Transfer the blood into tubes containing PROFACT, after detaching the needle from the syringe. Do not delay mixing blood with PROFACT. Avoid foam formation during mixing. Mix exactly nine parts of freshly collected blood with one part of PROFACT. For occasional patients with haematocrit less than 20 per cent or greater than 50 percent, this ratio must be readjusted to ensure valid results. Centrifuge immediately for 15 minutes at 1500 to 3000 rpm (approximately 1500 g) on a laboratory centrifuge and transfer the plasma into a clean test tube. It should be ensured that the plasma is free from platelets (PPP). Cap the test tubes to prevent deterioration of samples. Plasma must be tested preferably immediately. However, if the specimen is held at 22 to 24°C then they may be tested within 2 hours and if the specimen is held at 2 to 4°C then they may be tested within 3 hours. Also plasma samples obtained after collection with PROFACT may be stored at –20°C for 2 to 3 weeks before testing.

For ESR by Westergren Method

For performing the test, venous blood is mixed accurately in the proportion of 1 part of PROFACT and 4 parts of whole blood.

The sedimentation rate is reduced in stored blood, hence the test should be carried out within 4 hours of collecting the blood, and a delay upto 6 hours is permissible provided that the blood is kept at 4°C.

Precautions

1. Take every possible aseptic precaution to minimize contamination while drawing the reagent.
2. Avoid dipping contaminated pipettes/micropipette tips in the reagent vial. Ideally pour the required quantity for the days work into another sterile clean vial.
3. Recap and replace the reagent vial immediately back at 2 to 8°C.

Remarks

1. Since most of the routine coagulation assays use PPP each laboratory must calibrate the necessary force and time required during centrifugation to yield PPP.
2. Incorrect mixture of blood and PROFACT is a potential source of error both in coagulation assays and ESR estimation.

3. If the reagent vial develops turbidity, do not use the reagent as this would lead to erroneous results.

Calibration of instruments/equipments

- Waterbaths or heating blocks calibrated and preset at 37°C ± 0.5°C are an important requirement to achieve accuracy and reproducibility.
  - The whole process of the coagulation tests is based on a series of enzymatic reactions which are dependent on pH, ionic strength and the temperature of the reaction process. A correct temperature at 37°C ± 0.5°C is critical as most of the reagent systems are standardized at this temperature. Day to day shift in reaction temperature of equipment will introduce uncontrolled variation into test conditions. Therefore, temperature of all equipments must be calibrated daily and diligently to avoid erroneous results and ensure accuracy and reproducibility.
  - Sample/reagent dispensing mechanisms must be accurate and precise.
  - Well-calibrated dispensing mechanisms are required for all coagulation- based tests to accurately dispense samples as well as reagents. Any shift in ratio or individual volumes of the sample and or reagent can lead to shortening or prolongation of results.
  - Straight 0.1 and 0.2 ml glass pipettes are usually satisfactory, provided they are scrupulously clean and dry.
  - Automatic micropipettes which are able to deliver the required volumes are replacing the glass pipettes, provided these pipettes are-calibrated frequently. The use of clean disposable tips places this system at an advantage over the older mechanisms.

Storage of Reagents

- Usually reagent manufacturers recommend aspiration of adequate reagent for the days use in a thoroughly clean and dry tube instead of intermittent aspiration from reagent vials at the time of test.
  - Most coagulation reagents are extremely delicate reagents. For them to maintain their sensitivity and performance the reagent formulations must maintain reagent integrity over the usage period. Repeated intrusions into the reagent vial exponentially increases the chances of reagent contamination and destruction of reagent formulations and integrity. Undried and or contaminated pipettes, tips, glassware are usually the main culprits. Such contaminated reagents perform suboptimally.
  - The reagent vials must be immediately stored back to the recommended storage temperatures after the aspiration of the days requirement separately so that the remaining reagent remains at optimal temperature for future use. Keeping unused reagents at higher ambient temperatures during the day causes steady deterioration of the reagent due to thermal stress.
- The recommended storage temperature for reagents should be strictly complied to.
  - Most of the liquid stable or reconstituted reagents such as PT and APTT are colloidal suspensions of lipoproteins and or phospholipids. Subjecting them to elevated temperatures through repeated freeze- thaw cycles stresses the colloidal system. Especially detrimental are the effects of freezing (below 2°C). After freezing the reagent colloidal suspension undergoes an irreversible change and precipitates out or present itself as a particulate mass. Such reagents give erroneous results.
- Bringing reagents/samples to room temperature should be a two step process.
  - When enough reagent is aspirated out for the days testing as recommended the reagent and samples stored at 2 to 8°C should be first allowed to'attain room temperature (25°C to 30°C) and then they should be subsequently brought to the optimal test temperature of 37°C ± 0.5°C.
  - When reagents samples from 2 to 8°C are directly brought to 37°C the required time of 3 to 5 minutes may not be sufficient for the reagent samples to attain a homogeneous temperature of 37°C within the recommended time. This affects the reaction kinetics leading to erroneous results.

End Point Reading

- Reading of endpoint of clotbased tests varies from user to user.
  - Usually when manual techniques are followed the definition of "end point" is important.

Ideally the end point tests should be read "as soon as the first fibrin strand is visible and the gel clot formation begins".

- When some users use a fully formed gel clot as an end point, there is a variation of 1 to 3 seconds between the end points as recorded by the ideal method and user based variation.
- It is advisable to have well illuminated background for reading the clotbased end points. Since user variations based on proficiency continue to influence results, it is advisable not change personnel involved in coagulation tests off and on.

- Manufacturers instructions must be followed meticulously when instrument based or automatic clot detection systems are used.
  - Each clot detection system works on a different principle such as electro mechanical, turbidimetric or photo-optical. Each system of clot detection has its requirements for optimum functioning. Special care must be taken while using optical instruments for clot detection since reagent induced turbidity can influence the results dramatically. Usually low turbidity reagents are preferred for manual as well as instruments based clot detection.

Drug/Clinical Conditions Influencing Patient Results

- Drugs/clinical conditions influence results of patients coagulation studies.
  - PT tests are influenced on administration of following drugs

PT may be shortened
DRUGS

- Antihistamines
- Butabarbital
- Phenobarbital
- Caffeine
- Oral contraceptives
- Vitamin K

PT may be prolonged
DRUGS

- Corticosteroids
- EDTA
- Asparaginase
- Clofibrate
- Erythromycin
- Ethanol
- Tetracycline
- Aspirin
- Anticoagulants such as warfarin, heparin

APTT tests are influenced on administration of following drugs.

APTT may be shortened
Drugs

- Oral contraceptives
- Conjugated estrogen
- Therapy

APTT may be prolonged
Drugs

- Diphenylhydantoin
- Heparin
- Warfarin
- Naloxone
- Radiographic agents

Thrombin Time Test is prolonged in the following clinical conditions.

Clinical Conditions

- Normal newborn infant
- Systemic lupus erythematosus
- Macroglobulinemia
- Presence of exogenous /endogenous circulating anticoagulants
- Hepatic diseases
- Toxemia of pregnancy
- Multiple myeloma

MNPT and INR

- MNPT is a critical requirement in the derivation of INR.

  MNPT is a critical requirement in the derivation of INR. Ideally each laboratory must derive its own MNPT from 20 or more normal patients for a given PT reagent and Lot under use. This corrects within laboratory test variables that influence PT results.

  By definition INR represents the PT ratio which would have been obtained for a particular patient sample as if the WHO reference thromboplastin itself (ISI=1.0) had been used in the PT determination.

  $INR = [R]^{[ISI]}$

$$INR = \left[\frac{\text{Patient PT in seconds}}{\text{Mean of the normal range}}\right]^{ISI}$$

A PT ratio is obtained by dividing the patient PT in seconds by the **"Mean of the normal range"** (MNPT). This ratio is then "normalized" by raising the results to the power of the ISI of the PT reagent used.

If "normal control plasmas" are used in place of patient plasma for arriving at the MNPT it can effect the evaluation of the patients level of anti coagulation. For example:

Reagent ISI=2.5	Test Day1	Test Day 2	Test Day 3
Patient PT (sec)	16.0	16.0	16.0
Normal Control			
(10.4-12.3 sec)	11.5	10.4	12.3
INR Formula	$16.0^{2.5}$	$16.0^{2.5}$	$16.0^{2.5}$
$[R]'^{SI}$	11.5	10.4	12.3
Resulting INR	2.27	2.89	1.92

If the control time is greater than the mean normal range (MNPT), the PT ratio for any patient PT will be smaller, potentially leading to over coagulation. If the control time is lesser than MNPT the ratio for any patient PT will be greater, leading to under coagulation.

On the other hand, MNPT for a particular laboratory using the same combination of methodology, reagent and instrument would remain constant.

Quality Control Aspects

- Quality of water used for reconstituting lyophilized coagulation reagents must be good.
  — The water used for reconstitution of lyophilized coagulation reagents should be atleast distilled twice and kept separately labelled for "coagulation studies". The reagents employed for coagulation studies are extremely delicate and inability to use good quality distilled water could lead to incorporation of metallic impurities in. the reagent formulation as well as change in pH. Such changes can alter reaction kinetics and overall stability and performance of reagents.
- Quality assurance for coagulation based reagents must be performed preferably on a daily basis.
  — Each laboratory should test coagulation reagents with normal and abnormal control plasma specimens at the beginning of each days work to verify instruments, temperature calibration and also reagent performance.

If the control results fall within the stated limits, the test results are considered valid.

But if the results fall outside the stated control limits then the reagents, control and equipments are checked and the problem should be corrected.

Control results should be recorded and analyzed after regular intervals to ascertain the long term validity of results.

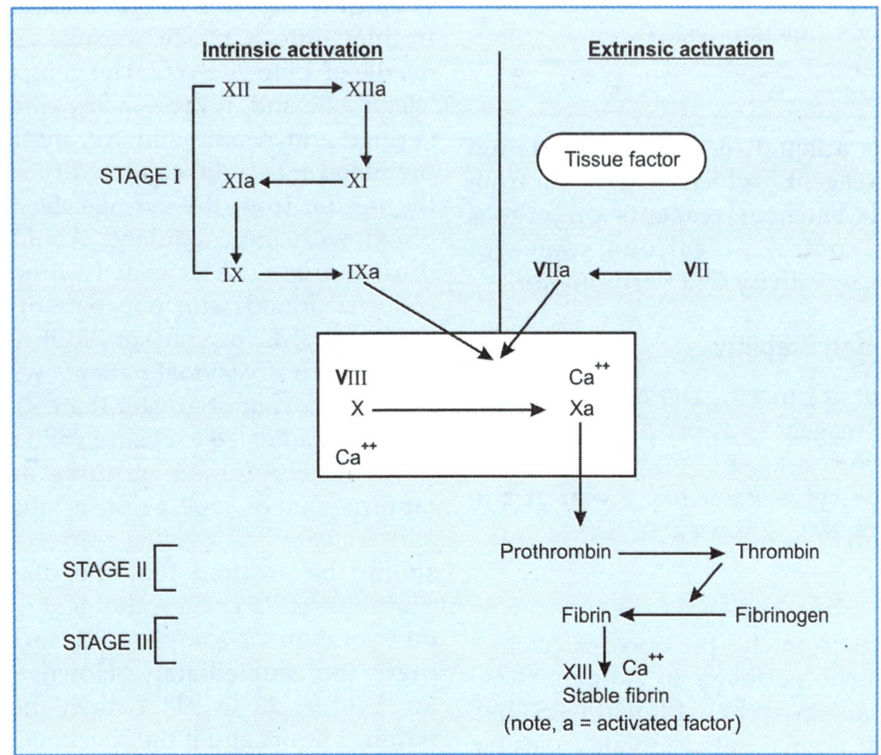

CLOTTING MECHANISM-CASCADE SYSTEM

(PROTHROMBIN TIME) (QUICK ONE-STAGE METHOD) LIQUIPLASTIN®
(Coutesy: Tulip Group of Companies)

Thromboplastin Reagent for Prothrombin Time (PT) Determination

Summary

The arrest of bleeding depends upon primary platelet plug formed along with the formation of a stable fibrin clot. Formation of this clot involves the sequential interaction of series of plasma proteins in a highly ordered and complex manner and also the interaction of these complexes with blood platelets and materials released from the tissues.

Tissue thromboplastin, in the presence of calcium, is an activator, which initiates the extrinsic pathway of coagulation, which includes plasma coagulation factors VII, X, V, Prothrombin and Fibrinogen. During oral anticoagulant therapy most of these factors are depressed, as also during the deficiencies of clotting factor activity which may be hereditary or acquired.

Prothrombin Time determination is the preferred method for presurgical screening, determination of congenital deficiency of factors II, V, VII and X and for monitoring of patients on oral anticoagulant therapy and as a liver function test.

Reagent

LIQUIPLASTIN® is a liquid ready to use **Calcium Thromboplastin Reagent,** which is derived from rabbit brain. Each batch of reagents undergoes rigorous quality control at various stages of manufacture for its sensitivity and performance.

Reagent Storage and Stability

(a) Store the reagent at 2 to 8°C. **DO NOT FREEZE.** (b)The shelf life of reagent is as per the expiry date mentioned on the reagent vial label. The uncontaminated reagent is stable for: **1 year at 2 to 8°C, 1 week at 18 to 25°C, 2 days at 37°C.**

Principle

Tissue Thromboplastin in the presence of calcium activates the extrinsic pathway of human blood coagulation mechanism. When LIQUIPLASTIN® reagent is added to normal anticoagulated plasma, the clotting mechanism is initiated, forming a solid gel clot within a specified period of time. The time required for clot formation would be prolonged if there is a deficiency of factors/factor activity in the extrinsic pathway of the coagulation mechanism.

Note

(1) In vitro diagnostic reagent for laboratory and professional use only. Not for medicinal use. (2) LIQUIPLASTIN® reagent is not from human source hence, contamination due to HBsAg and HIV is practically excluded. (3) LIQUIPLASTIN® reagent contains 0.01per cent Thimerosal as preservative. (4) It is **very important** that clean and dry micropipette tips be used to dispense the reagent. (5) **Avoid exposure** of the reagent to elevated temperatures and contamination. **Immediately** replace cap after use and store at recommended temperatures **only.**

Sample Collection and Preparation of PPP

Though no special preparation of the patient is required prior to sample collection by approved techniques, it is preferable that patients are not heavily exercised before blood collection. Fasting or only light non-fatty meals prior to blood collection provide samples with a desirable lower opacity. Withdraw blood without undue venous stasis or frothing into a plastic syringe fitted with a short needle of 19 to 20 SWG. The veinpuncture must be a 'clean' one and, if there is any difficulty, take a new syringe and needle and try another vein. Transfer the blood into anticoagulated tubes, after detaching the needle from the syringe. Do not delay mixing blood with anticoagulant. Avoid foam formation during mixing. Mix exactly nine parts of freshly collected blood with one part of trisodium citrate (0.11 mol/l, 3.2 percent) or PROFACT available from TULIP; For occasional patients with hematocrit less than 20 per cent or greater than 50 percent, this ratio must be readjusted to ensure valid results. Centrifuge immediately for 15 minutes at 1500-3000 rpm (approximately 1500 g) on a laboratory centrifuge and transfer the plasma into a dean test tube. It should be ensured that the plasma is free from platelets (PPP). Cap the test tubes to prevent deterioration of samples. **Plasma must be tested preferably immediately.** However if the specimen are held at 22 to 24° C then they may be tested within 2 hours and if the specimen is held at 2 to 4°C then they may be tested within 3 hours.

Additional Material Required for Manual and Calibration Curve Methods

12 × 75 mm test tubes (plastic tubes are preferred), 0.1 ml and 0.2 ml precision pipettes, Stop watch, Water bath or heating block at 37° C, Fresh normal plasmas for establishing MNPT.

TEST PROCEDURE

Manual Method

1. Aspirate from the reagent vial enough reagent for immediate testing requirements in a thoroughly clean and dry test tube (Plastic test tubes are preferred).
2. Bring this reagent to room temperature before prewarming at 37° C for testing purposes.
3. Recap the reagent vial and replace immediately to 2-8° C.
4. To a 12 × 75 mm tube add 0.1 ml of plasma and place the tube in a water bath for 3 to 5 minutes at 37° C.
5. To the tube **forcibly** add 0.2 ml of LIQUIPLASTIN[8] reagent (prewarmed at 37° C for atleast 3 minutes) and simultaneously start a stop watch. Shake the tube gently to mix contents.
6. Gently tilt the tube back and forth and stop the stopwatch **as soon as the first fibrin strand is visible and the gel/clot formation begins.** Record the time in 'seconds'.
7. Repeat steps 4-6 for a duplicate test on the same samples.
8. Find the average of the duplicate test values. This is the Prothrombin Time (PT). **If a coagulation instrument is being used to perform the tests, the instrument manufacturers instructions must be strictly adhered to.**

CALCULATION OF RESULTS

Manual Method

The result may be reported directly in terms of the mean of the double determination of PT of the test plasma in 'seconds'.
or as a ratio'R':

$$R = \frac{\textbf{Mean of the patient plasma PT in seconds}}{\textbf{MNPT for the reagent}}$$

Or as International Normalized Ratio (INR), INR = $(R)^{ISI}$ 'where ISI = International Sensitivity Index of the reagent (Refer reagent vial label).'

It is recommended by the WHO that MNPT should be established for each lot of PT reagents by each laboratory, since PT results are dependent on the combination of reagent lot, instrument and technique followed at each laboratory. Usually plasma from at least 20 normal healthy individuals should be used to establish the MNPT. The average of such PT results in seconds = MNPT.

Expected Values

Normal values using LIQUIPLASTIN® are between 10 and 14 seconds. Between manual and Turbo densitometric instrument results a variation of 1 to 2 seconds may be expected. For photo-optical instruments, it is recommended that each laboratory must establish their own normal range. It is mandatory that each laboratory must establish its own MNPT for each lot of LIQUIPLASTIN®.

Oral Anticoagulant Therapeutic Range : INR = 2.0-3.5

Remarks

(1) It is recommended that controls with known factor activity should be run simultaneously with each test series to validate test run. (2) Incorrect mixture of blood and Trisodium citrate, insufficient prewarming of plasma and reagent, contaminated reagents, glassware, etc. are potential source of errors. (3) Oxalated plasma may induce prolonged clotting times. (4) Since the PT test functions correctly only at 37° ± 0.5° C, temperature of all equipment must be calibrated daily. (5) Clotting time of patients on anticoagulant therapy depends upon the type and dosage of anticoagulant and also the time lag between the specimen collected and the last dose. (6) Turbid , icteric, lipemic or grossly hemolysed samples may generate erroneous PT results. (7) Glasswares and cuvettes used in the test must be scrupulously clean and free from even traces of acids / alkalies or detergents. (8) Plasma samples held at 4-8° C may undergo 'cold activation' leading to a marked shortening of the PT. (9) The PT may be shortened during acute inflammatory conditions which are accompanied by increase in Fibrinogen levels and also by agents such as antihistamines, butabarbital, phenobarbital, caffeine, oral contraceptives and vitamin K. The PT may be prolonged by corticosteroids, EDTA, oral contraceptives, asparaginase, clofibrate, ethanol,

tetracycline, aspirin and anticoagulants such as heparin and warfarin. (10) It is important that each laboratory express the results in terms of INR for patients on oral anticoagulant therapy for the clinician to adjust the dosage based on INR. (11) Since the test uses platelet poor plasma, each laboratory must calibrate the necessary force and time required during centrifugation to yield the PPP. Contamination of plasma with excess platelets could falsely elevate levels of some of the factors. (12) Homogenisation of LIQUIPLASTIN® reagent suspension before use is important to achieve accurate and consistent results.

SENSITIVE THROMBOPLASTIN REAGENT FOR PROTHROMBIN TIME (PT) DETERMINATION (ISI=1.0)

Summary

The arrest of bleeding depends upon primary platelet plug formed along with the formation of a stable fibrin clot. Formation of this clot involves the sequential interaction of series of plasma proteins in a highly ordered and complex manner and also the interaction of these complexes with blood platelets and materials released from the tissues. Tissue Thromboplastin, in the presence of calcium, is an activator, which initiates the extrinsic pathway of coagulation, which includes plasma coagulation factors VII, X, V, Prothrombin and Fibrinogen. During oral anticoagulant therapy most of the Vitamin K-dependent factors such as II, VII, IX, X, Protein C and Protein S are depressed, as also during the deficiencies of clotting factor activity which may be hereditary or acquired. Prothrombin Time determination is the preferred method for presurgical screening, as a liver function test, determination of congenital deficiency of factors II, V, VII and X and for monitoring of patients on oral anticoagulant therapy.

Reagent

UNIPLASTIN is a novel, highly-sensitive, low opacity, ready to use liquid calcified Thromboplastin Reagent, which is derived from rabbit brain. Each batch of reagent undergoes rigorous quality control at various'stages of manufacture for its sensitivity and performance.

Reagent Storage and Stability

(a) Store the reagent at 2 to 8°C. DO NOT FREEZE, (b) The shelf life of the reagent is as per the expiry date mentioned on the reagent vial label. The uncontaminated reagent is stable for: 1 year at 2-8°C, 1 week at 18-25°C, 2 days at 37°C.

Principle

Tissue Thromboplastin in the presence of calcium activates the extrinsic pathway of human blood coagulation mechanism. When UNIPLASTIN reagent is added to normal citrated plasma, the dotting mechanism is initiated, forming a solid gel clot within a specified period of time. The time required for clot formation would be prolonged if there is acquired or congenital deficiency of factors/factor activity in the extrinsic pathway of the coagulation mechanism or reduction in the activity of Vitamin K-dependent clotting factors during oral anticoagulant therapy.

Note

(1) In vitro diagnostic reagent for laboratory and professional use only. Not for medicinal use. (2) UNIPLASTIN reagent is not from human source, hence contamination due to HBsAg and HIV is practically excluded. (3) Reagent contains 0.01per cent Thimerosal as preservative. (4) It is very important that scrupulously clean and dry micropipette tips be used to aspirate/dispense the reagent. (5) Avoid exposure of the UNIPLASTIN reagent to elevated temperatures, contamination and undue stress due to high and low temperature exposure cycles. Immediately replace reagent cap after use and store at recommended temperatures only. (6) On prolonged storage at 2-8°C the thromboplastin suspension has a tendency to settle down. Homogenise the reagent by resuspending before use.

Additional Material Required

12 x 75 mm test tubes (plastic tubes are preferred), 0.1 ml and 0.2 ml precision pipettes, Stop watch, Water bath or heating block at 37° C, Fresh normal plasmas for establishing MNPT.

Sample Collection and Preparation of PPP

Though no special preparation of the patient is required prior to sample collection by approved techniques, it is preferable that patients are not heavily exercised before blood collection. Fasting or only light non-fatty meals prior to blood collection provide samples with a desirable lower opacity. Withdraw blood without undue venous stasis or frothing into a plastic syringe fitted with a short needle of 19 to 20 SWG. The veinpuncture must be a 'clean' one and, if there is any difficulty, take a new syringe and needle and try another vein. Transfer the blood into anticoagulated tubes, after detaching the needle from the syringe. Do not delay mixing blood with anticoagulant. Avoid foam formation during mixing.

Mix exactly nine parts of freshly collected blood with one part of Trisodium citrate (0.11 mol/l, 3.2 percent). For occasional patients with hematocrit less than 20 per cent or greater than 55 percent, this ratio must be readjusted to ensure valid results. Centrifuge immediately for 15 minutes at 1500-2000 rpm (approximately 1500 g) on a laboratory centrifuge and transfer the plasma into a clean test tube. It should be ensured that the plasma is free from platelets (PPP). Cap the test tubes to prevent deterioration of samples. Plasma must be tested preferably immediately. However, if the specimen are held at 22 to 24°C then they may be tested within 2 hours and if the specimen is held at 2 to 4°C then they may be tested within 3 hours.

TEST PROCEDURE

Manual Method

1. Bring the reagent vial to room temperature (20 to 30°C). Mix the contents of the vial to homogenise the suspension completely.
2. Aspirate from the reagent vial enough reagent for immediate testing requirements in a thoroughly clean and dry test tube (Plastic test tubes are preferred).
3. Prewarm the reagent and bring to 37°C before use in test procedure (5-10 minutes may be required depending on the reagent volume to attain 37°C before testing).
4. Recap the reagent vial and replace immediately to 2 to 8°C.
5. To a 12 × 75 mm tube add 0.1 ml of plasma (PPP) and place the tube in a waterbath for 3 to 5 minutes at 37°C.
6. To the tube forcibly add 0.2 ml of UNIPLASTIN reagent (prewarmed at 37°C for atleast 3 minutes) and simultaneously start a stopwatch. Shake the tube gently to mix contents.
7. Gently tilt the tube back and forth and stop the stopwatch as soon as the first fibrin strand is visible and the gel/clot formation begins. Record the time in 'seconds'.
8. Repeat steps 4 to 6 for a duplicate test on the same sample.
9. Find the average of the duplicate test values. This is the Prothrombin Time (PT).

If a coagulation instrument is being used to perform the tests, the instrument manufacturers instructions must be strictly adhered to.

CALCULATION OF RESULTS

Manual Method

The results may be reported directly in terms of the mean of the double determination of PT of the test plasma in 'seconds'.
Or as a ratio 'R':

$$R = \frac{\text{Mean of the patient plasma PT in seconds}}{\text{MNPT for the reagent}}$$

Or as International Normalized Ratio (INR), INR = $(R)^{ISI}$, where ISI = International Sensitivity Index of the reagent (Refer reagent vial label).

It is recommended by the WHO that MNPT should be established for each lot of PT reagents by each laboratory, since PT results are dependent on the combination of reagent lot, instrument and technique followed at each laboratory. Usually plasma from atleast 20 normal healthy individuals should be used to establish the MNPT. The average of such PT results in seconds = MNPT.

Expected Values

Normal values using UNIPLASTIN are between 11-15 seconds. Between manual and Turbo densitometric instrument results a variation of 1-2 seconds may be expected. For photo optical instruments, it is recommended that each laboratory must establish their own normal range. It is mandatory that each laboratory must establish its own MNPT for each lot of UNIPLASTIN.

Oral Anticoagulant Therapeutic range: INR = 2.0-3.5

Remarks

(1) It is recommended that controls with known factor activity should be run simultaneously with each test series to validate test run. (2) Incorrect mixture of blood and Trisodium citrate, insufficient prewarming of plasma and reagent, contaminated reagents, glassware, etc. are potential source of

errors. (3) Oxalated plasma may induce prolonged clotting times. (4) Since the PT test functions correctly only at 37 ± 0.5°C , temperature of all equipment must be calibrated daily. (5) Clotting time of patients on anticoagulant therapy depends upon the type and dosage of anticoagulant and also the time lag between the specimen collected and the last dose. (6) Turbid, icteric, lipemic or grossly hemolysed samples may generate erroneous PT results. (7) Glasswares and cuvettes used in the test must be scrupulously clean and free from even traces of acids/alkalies or detergents. (8) Plasma samples held at 4 to 8°C may undergo 'cold activation' leading to a marked shortening of the PT. (9) The PT may be shortened during acute inflammatory conditions which are accompanied by increase in Fibrinogen levels and also by agents such as antihistamines, butabarbital, phenobarbital, caffeine, oral contraceptives and vitamin K. The PT may be prolonged by corticosteroids, EDTA, oral contraceptives, asparaginase, clofibrate, erythromycin, ethanol, tetracycline, aspirin and anticoagulants such as heparin and warfarin. (10) It is important that each laboratory express the results in terms of INR for patients on oral anticoagulant therapy for the clinician to adjust the dosage based on INR. (11) Since the test uses platelet poor plasma, each laboratory must calibrate the necessary force and time required during centrifugation to yield the PPP. Contamination of plasma with excess platelets could falsely elevate levels of some of the factors. (12) Homogenisation of UNIPLASTIN reagent suspension before use is important to achieve accurate and consistent results.

THROMBOPLASTIN REAGENT FOR PROTHROMBIN TIME (PT) DETERMINATION (Lyophilised reagent, ISI=1.0) Courtesy: Tulip Group of Companies

Summary

The arrest of bleeding depends upon primary platelet plug formed along with the formation of a stable fibrin clot. Formation of this clot involves the sequential interaction of series of plasma proteins in a highly ordered and complex manner and also the interaction of these complexes with blood platelets and materials released from the tissues. Tissue Thromboplastin, in the presence of calcium, is an activator, which initiates the extrinsic pathway of coagulation, which includes plasma coagulation factors VII, X, V, Prothrombin and Fibrinogen. During oral anticoagulant therapy most of the Vitamin K dependent factors such as II, VII, IX, X, Protein C and Protein S are depressed, as also during the deficiencies of clotting factor activity which may be hereditary or acquired. Prothrombin Time determination is the preferred method for presurgical screening, as a liver function test, determination of congenital deficiency of factors II. V, VII and X and for monitoring of patients on oral anticoagulant therapy.

Reagent

LYOPLASTIN is a sensitive, lyophilized calcified thromboplastin reagent which is derived from rabbit brain.

Each batch of reagent undergoes rigorous quality control at various stages of manufacture for its sensitivity and performance.

Storage and Stability

(a) Store the reagent at 2-8° C. DO NOT FREEZE, (b) The shelf life of the reagent is as per the expiry date mentioned on the reagent vial label, (c) The reconstituted LYOPLASTIN reagent can be used for 10 days when stored at 2-8°C provided it is not contaminaled.(d) It is strongly recommended that enough reconstituted reagent should be retrieved for the days use and the unused reagent should be immediately replaced to 2-8°C.

Principle

Tissue thromboplastin in the presence of calcium activates the extrinsic pathway of human blood coagulation mechanism. When LYOPLASTIN reagent is added to normal citrated plasma, the clotting mechanism is initiated, forming a solid gel clot within a specified period of time. The time required for clot formation would be prolonged if there is acquired or congenital deficiency of factors/factor activity in the extrinsic pathway of the coagulation mechanism or reduction in the activity of vitamin K dependent clotting factors during oral anticoagulant therapy.

Note

(1) In vitro diagnostic reagent for laboratory and professional use only. Not for medicinal use. (2) LYOPLASTIN reagent is not from human source, hence contamination due to HBsAg and HIV is practically excluded. (3) It is very important that

scrupulously clean and dry micropipette tips be used to aspirate / dispense the reagent. (4) Avoid exposure of the LYOPLASTIN reagent to elevated temperatures, contamination and undue stress due to high and low temperature exposure cydes. Immediately replace reagent cap after use and store at recommended temperatures only.

Additional Material Required

12 × 75 mm test tubes (plastic tubes are preferred), 0.1 ml and 0.2 ml precision pipettes, 1 ml precision pipette, distilled water, stop watch, water bath or heating block at 37° C, fresh normal plasmas for establishing MNPT.

Reagent Preparation

Bring the LYOPLASTIN reagent to room temperature (25-30° C) prior to reconstitution. LYOPLASTIN reagent is reconstituted with 3 ml de-ionized, distilled water as follows : (a) Add accurately 3 ml of distilled water to the lyophilized LYOPLASTIN reagent, (b) Gently mix to dissolve, (c) Keep for 10 minutes and mix again gently ensuring complete resuspension of the lyophilized reagent. Avoid froth formation, (d) Thorough mixing should be ensured before withdrawing material every time for test purposes.

Sample Collection and Preparation of PPP

Though no special preparation of the patient is required prior to sample collection by approved techniques, it is preferable that patients are not heavily exercised before blood collection. Fasting or only light non-fatty meals prior to blood collection provide samples with a desirable lower opacity. Withdraw blood without undue venous stasis or frothing into a plastic syringe fitted with a short needle of 19 to 20 SWG. The veinpuncture must be a 'clean' one and, if there is any difficulty, take a new syringe and needle and try another vein. Transfer the blood into anticoagulated tubes, after detaching the needle from the syringe. Do not delay mixing blood with anticoagulant. Avoid foam formation during mixing.

Mix exactly nine parts of freshly collected blood with one part of Trisodium citrate (0.11 mol/l, 3.2 percent) or PROFACT available from TULIP, Cat No. 670020. For occasional patients with haematocrit less than 20 per cent or greater than 55 percent, this ratio must be readjusted to ensure valid results. Centrifuge immediately for 15 minutes at 1500-2000 rpm (approximately 1500 g) on a laboratory centrifuge and transfer the plasma into a clean test tube. It should be ensured that the plasma is free from platelets (PPP). Cap the test tubes to prevent deterioration of samples. Plasma must be tested preferably immediately. However if the specimen are held at 22-24° C then they may be tested within 2 hours and if the specimen is held at 2-4°C then they may be tested within 3 hours.

TEST PROCEDURE

Manual Method

(1) Aspirate from the reagent vial enough reagent for immediate testing requirements in a thoroughly clean and dry test tube. (Plastic test tubes are preferred). (2) Bring the reagent to room temperature before prewarming at 37°C for testing purpose. (3) Recap the reagent vial and replace immediately to 2-8°C. (4) To a 12 x 75 mm tube add 0.1 ml of plasma (PPP) and place the tube in a waterbath for 3 to 5 minutes at 37°C. (5) To the tube forcibly add 0.2 ml of LYOPLASTIN reagent (prewarmed at 37°C for atleast 3 minutes) and simultaneously start a stopwatch. Shake the tube gently to mix contents. (6) Gently tilt the tube back and forth and stop the stopwatch as soon as the first fibrin strand is visible and the gel/clot formation begins. Record the time in 'seconds', (7) Repeat steps 4-6 for a duplicate test on the same sample. (8) Find the average of the duplicate test values. This is the Prothrombin Time (PT). If a coagulation instrument is being used to perform the tests, the instrument manufacturers instructions must be strictly adhered to.

CALCULATION OF RESULTS

Manual Method

The results may be reported directly in terms of the mean of the double determination of PT of the test plasma in 'seconds'.
Or as a ratio 'R':

$$R = \frac{\text{Mean of the patient plasma PT in seconds}}{\text{MNPT for the reagent*}}$$

Or as International Normalized Ratio (INR), INR $= (R)^{ISI}$, where ISI = International Sensitivity Index of the reagent (Refer reagent vial label).

*It is recommended by the WHO that MNPT should be established for each lot of PT reagents by each laboratory, since PT results are dependent on the combination of reagent lot, instrument and technique followed at each laboratory. Usually plasma from atleast 20 normal healthy individuals should be used to establish the MNPT. The average of such PT results in seconds = MNPT.

Expected Values

Normal values using LYOPLASTIN are between 11-15 seconds. Between manual and Turbo densitomeltric instrument results a variation of 1-2 seconds may be expected. For photo-optical instruments, it is recommended that each laboratory must establish their own normal range. It is mandatory that each laboratory must establish its own MNPT for each lot of LYOPLASTIN.

Oral anticoagulant therapeutic range : INR = 2.0-3.5

Remarks

(1) It is recommended that controls with known factor activity should be run simultaneously with each test series to validate test run. (2) Incorrect mixture of blood and Trisodium citrate, insufficient prewarming of plasma and reagent, contaminated reagents, glassware, etc. are potential source of errors. (3) Oxalated plasma may induce prolonged clotting times. (4) Since the PT test functions correctly only at 37 $\pm$ 0.5° C. temperature of all equipment must be calibrated daily. (5) Clotting time of patients on anticoagulant therapy depends upon the type and dosage of anticoagulant and also the time lag between the specimen collected and the last dose. (6) Turbid, icteric, lipemic or grossly hemolysed samples may generate erroneous PT results. (7) Glasswares and cuvettes used in the test must be scrupulously clean and free from even traces of adds/alkalies or detergents. (8) Plasma samples held at 4-8°C may undergo 'cold activation' leading to a marked shortening of the PT. (9) The PT may be shortened during acute inflammatory conditions which are accompanied by increase in Fibrinogen levels and also by agents such as antihistamines, butabarbital, phenobarbital, caffeine, oral contraceptives and vitamin K. The PT may be prolonged by corticosteroids, EDTA, oral contraceptives, asparaginase, clofibrate, erythromycin, ethanol, tetracycline, aspirin and anticoagulants such as heparin and warfarin. (10) It is important that each laboratory express the results in terms of INR for patients on oral anticoagulant therapy for the clinician to adjust the dosage based on INR. (11) Since the test uses platelet poor plasma, each laboratory must calibrate the necessary force and time required during centrifugation to yield the PPP. Contamination of plasma with excess platelets could falsely elevate levels of some of the factors. (12) Homogenisation of LYOPLASTIN reagent suspension before use is important to achieve accurate and consistent results.

Clinical Implications

Conditions accompanied by an increased prothrombin time (PT) include

- Prothrombin deficiency
- Vitamin K deficiency
- Haemorrhagic disease of the newborn
- Liver disease (eg; alcoholic hepatitis)
- Anticoagulant therapy
- Biliary obstruction
- Salicylate intoxication
- Hypervitaminosis A
- DIC disease

Interfering Factors

1. *Diet*: Excessive amounts of green, leafy vegetables will increase body's absorption of vitamin K.
2. *Alcohol*: PT is increased due to liver disease.
3. *Diarrhoea and vomiting*: These increase PT.
4. *Quality of venipuncture*: It is important that a clean and careful venipuncture is done, otherwise the PT can be shortened.
5. Many drugs can alter PT.

Clinical Alert

1. If PT is excessively prolonged, vitamin K is given intramuscularly. Ordinarily, intramuscular injections are contraindicated during anticoagulant therapy because large painful haematomas may form at the injection site. As values get into danger zones, assess carefully for bleeding, including: (i) craniotomy checks, (ii) lung auscultation (especially of upper lobes), and (iii) occult blood in the urine.
2. Patients who are being monitored by PT for long-term anticoagulant therapy should not take any drugs unless absolutely necessary.

3. When unexpected changes in anticoagulant doses are needed to maintain a stable PT, or when there is a consistent change in PT, a drug interaction should be suspected.
4. Blood for PT should be drawn for a base line and prior to administration of anticoagulants.
5. Protamine sulphate is the antidote for heparin.

MONITORING ORAL ANTICOAGULANT THERAPY

Introduction

Since the introduction of the one stage prothrombin time test by Dr Armand Quick in 1935, there have been various attempts to standardize the methodology and reporting of results using the prothrombin time reagents.

Oral anticoagulant therapy with 4-hydroxy coumarin vitamin K antagonists, such as Warfarin are commonly used for the treatment and prevention of thromboembolic episodes. Most physicians also prefer to monitor the oral anticoagulant therapy using the Prothrombin time test.

Since the individual thromboplastin reagent preparations differ significantly in their sensitivities to the deficiencies of the vitamin K-dependant coagulation factors, the use of 'seconds' or 'PTFR' (Ratio) as a reporting format has led to confusion amongst clinicians. In order to correctly dose deserving patients with oral anticoagulant drugs so as to achieve the dual goal of adequate anti-coagulation and reduce the risk of bleeding simultaneously, the WHO introduced a method for monitoring patients stabilized on oral anticoagulant therapy using International Normalized Ratio (INR).

The INR normalizes the PT ratio to an International reference preparation of thromboplastin. The therapeutic ranges expressed in terms of INR values for common clinical conditions requiring oral anticoagulant treatment and monitoring have been determined by double blind clinical trials.

The INR method of reporting PT results has helped to ensure that a uniform intensity of oral anticoagulant therapy is used world-wide, independent of the influences of varying sensitivity of the thromboplastins used for obtaining the test result using PT reagents.

Relevance and Use of the Prothrombin Time Test

The prothrombin time test is used to detect coagulation disorders and specifically the activity of the factors of the extrinsic pathway namely II, V, VII, X and fibrinogen. The classical extrinsic pathway is initiated by the release of tissue thromboplastin (Tissue Factor) which is exposed to the blood when there is a damage to the blood vessel. Circulating factor VII forms a complex with tissue thromboplastin and calcium in the presence of phospholipids. This complex activates factor X to Xa. Factor Xa catalyses prothrombin (Factor II) to thrombin (lla). Thrombin converts fibrinogen (Factor I) to fibrin (Fig. 10.1).

The factors of the extrinsic pathway namely II, V, VII and X are synthesized in the liver parenchymal cells from precursor proteins. These classical vitamin K-dependant plasma clotting factors undergo a conformational change in the presence of Ca^{+2} ions. This is a necessary requirement for these vitamin K-dependant factors (II, V, VII, X) for binding to their co-factors on phospholipid surfaces and exerting their coagulant activity.

Within the liver parenchymal cells the inactive precursor proteins of three key vitamin K-dependant factors i.e. VII, IX and X are carboxylated. These carboxylated proteins then function as active factors with coagulant activity.

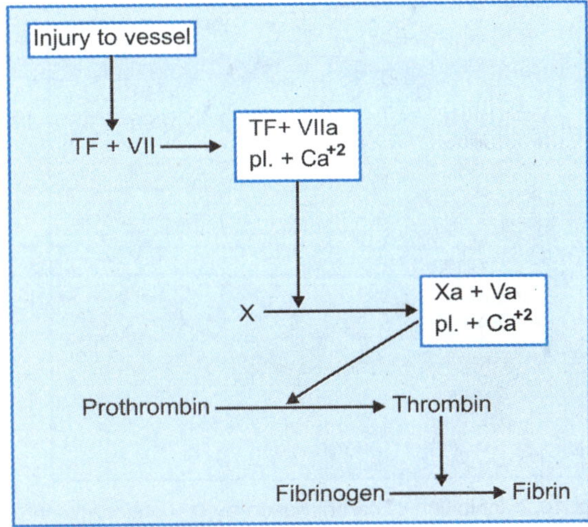

Fig. 10.1: Classical extrinsic pathway

Oral Anticoagulant Agents

The clinical effectiveness of oral anticoagulants has been well established based on results of numerous well designed trials for a variety of indications.

Oral anticoagulants are effective and used for:

- Prevention of primary and secondary venous thromboembolism.
- Prevention of systemic arterial embolism in patients with mechanical prosthetic heart valves or with atrial fibrillation.

- Prevention of acute myocardial infarction in patients with peripheral arterial disease.
- Prevention of stroke and recurrent infarction

Warfarin sodium a 4-hydroxy coumarin derivative is the most common vitamin K antagonist used for oral anticoagulant therapy. Acenocoumarol, phenprocoumon are the other derivatives, which are also used for achieving oral anticoagulation in patient groups. The use of indandione derivatives such as phenindione has been discontinued largely due to their relative hepatic toxicity.

All the 4-hydroxy coumarin derivatives, as far as known today, have the same mode of action, but exhibit different pharmacokinetics and are metabolized differently.

Pharmacology of Oral Anticoagulants

The oral anticoagulants such as Warfarin inhibit the process of carboxylation by interfering in the inter-conversion of vitamin K epoxide (Fig. 10.2).

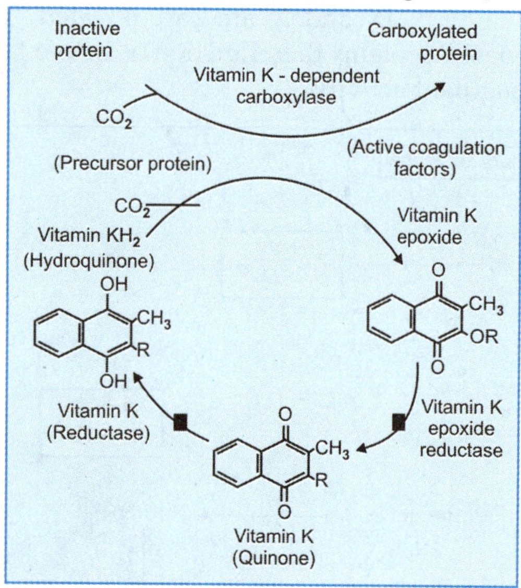

Fig. 10.2: Inhibition of carboxylation by oral anticoagulants

This inhibition results in a decreased ability of the liver to effectively carry out post-translational conversion of glutamyl residues (glu) on the inactive precursor proteins to α-carboxyglutamyl (gla) residues. The gla residues impart these proteins the ability to exert their coagulant action (as factors) in a Ca^{+2} dependant fashion.

It is now known that the fully functional carboxylated proteins i.e. factors, contain a normal complement of 10 to 13 gla residues.

It has been estimated that when the number of gla residues on the carboxylated proteins reduce from 10-13 to 9, it results in a 30 per cent reduction in their coagulant activity, while reduction to less than 6 residues results in a loss of more than 95 per cent of the coagulant activity of the factors.

This inhibition in the cyclic conversion of vitamin K also results in the production and secretion of proteins that are partially carboxylated or des-carboxylated. These are dysfunctional factors.

PIVKA'S

As the effect of oral anticoagulants take effect, the process of conversion of the precursor proteins to active factors through carboxylation is inhibited. The partially carboxylated or des-carboxylated, biologically inactive proteins appear in plasma. On the other hand, the plasma concentration of biologically active factors VII, IX, X decreases (Fig. 10.3).

This pool of partially carboxylated proteins are as a group known as PIVKA's. (Protein induced by vitamin K absence/or antagonism). Since PIVKA's are biologically inactive, they do not participate in the haemostatic control mechanism *in vivo.* PIVKA's also do not play a role in bleeding complications of anticoagulated patients.

However, the most important practical consequence of the PIVKA effect is that it is an important confounding factor in the standardization of thromboplastins used for monitoring oral anticoagulant therapy. PT reagents derived from rabbit or human tissues or from recombinant technology have varying sensitivity to PIVKA's.

The Role of PT Test in Monitoring Effects of Oral Anticoagulant Therapy

The PT is the method of choice for monitoring oral anticoagulant therapy, as it is responsive to the depression of the vitamin K-dependant clotting factors of the extrinsic pathway. Rate of depression of the individual clotting factors is determined by their biological half life. Factor VII falls most rapidly followed by factors IX, X and II. As the active clotting factor levels begin to fall, the PT results start to prolong. Factor V and Fibrinogen are not affected by oral anticoagulants.

On the other hand upon withdrawal of the oral anticoagulant therapy (as may be required to review the effects of over anticoagulation) these factors return to normal levels in the reverse order and so do the PT results (Fig. 10.4).

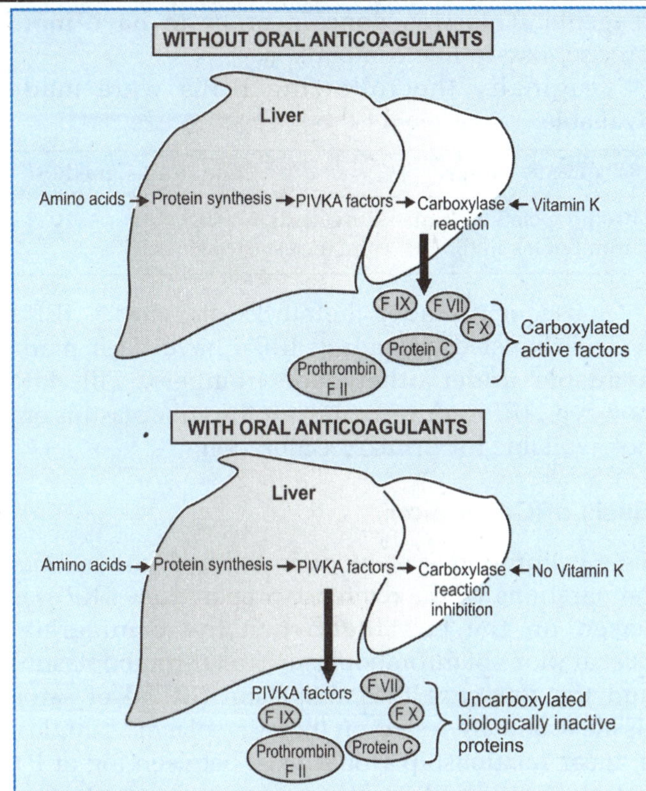

Fig. 10.3: Without oral anticoagulants, with oral anticoagulants

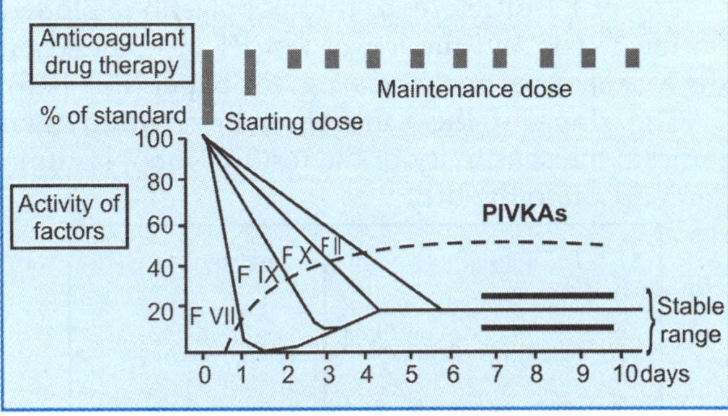

Fig. 10.4: Course of anticoagulant therapy

Problems in monitoring Oral Anticoagulant therapy

Historically the Prothrombin time (PT) results are reported in "seconds" or as a percentage of coagulant activity or as ratio (PTR). Physicians use sufficient oral anticoagulant drugs to maintain the PT ratio at 1.5 to 2.0 or 1.3-2.0 times the median value of the normal range. The problem with this approach is that it fails to take into account the variation in sensitivity or "responsiveness" of different PT reagents.

PT ratio (PTR)

For example: For a given reduction in the plasma levels of the clotting factors, more responsive PT reagents (A) results in greater prolongation of the PT in 'seconds' as compared to an unresponsive PT reagent (B).

Practically this translates into different PT times (seconds) or ratios for the same patient sample, when tested using reagent A or B. For example

Factors Influencing Anticoagulant Effects of Warfarin

GUT	PLASMA
Anticoagulant Effect	**Anticoagulant Effect**
Potentiated • Low vitamin K intake • Reduced vitamin K absorption in fat malabsorption	*Unchanged* • Displacement of warfarin from albumin binding does not influence anticoagulant effect of coumarins
Anticoagulant Effect Counteracted • Increased vitamin K intake • Reduced absorption of warfarin by cholestyramine	

Liver

Anticoagulant *Effect Potentiated*	**Cimetidine** *Omprazole*	**Hypermetabolic States:**
		• Pyrexia
• Drugs	Thyroxine	Thyrotoxicosis
Phenylbutazone	Ketoconazole	*Anticoagulant Effect*
Metronidazole	Fluconazole	*Counteracted*
Sulfinpyrazone	Isoniazid	• Drugs:
Trimethoprim	Piroxicam	Barbiturates
Sulfamethoxazole	Tamoxifen	Rifampicin
Disulfiram	Quinidine	Griseofulvin
Amiodarone	VitaminE	Carbamazepine
Erythromycin	(megadoses)	Penicillin
Anabolic steroids	Phenytoin	Alcohol
Clofibrate	Liver disease	

Haemostatic Plug

Impaired Haemostatic Plug Formation	**Impaired Platelet Function:**
Impaired Coagulation: • Reduced vitamin K dependant coagulation factors • Reduction in concentration of other coagulation factors • Other anticoagulants (heparin, ancrod)	**Thrombocytopenia** • Aspirin • Other nonsteroidal anti inflammatory drugs • Ticlopidine • Moxalactam • Carbencicillin and high doses of other penicillins

Lab	Reagent	FNP Normal	Test	PTR	Therapeutic ratio
X	Reagent A	12.0	30	2.5	1.5-2.0
Y	Reagent B	12.0	18	1.5	1.5-2.0

This patient appears over anticoagulated when tested with reagent (A) and just about adequately anti coagulated when tested with reagent (B).

Percent Activity

The other method of reporting PT results is as a percentage of coagulation activity. First a dilution of normal plasma is made. Then the normal dilution curve is plotted using these dilutions. Then the patients clot time is converted to per cent activity of factors from the dilution curve.

Since the dilutions of normal plasma do not contain PIVKA's and Thromboplastins vary in their sensitivity to PIVKA's, the accuracy of the normal dilution curve has been rightly challenged.

Thromboplastins based on their tissue origin and method of preparation vary markedly in their responsiveness to depression of vitamin K-dependant factors and PIVKA's. Therefore, PT results reported using different reagents are not interchangeable between laboratories when the older system such as seconds, ratios or percentage activity are used to report PT results.

Standardization of Prothrombin Time Reagents and Reporting System

In view of the aforesaid variations in the reagent sensitivities an attempt to standardize PT test results was initiated internationally. By mid 1970 a number of regulatory and advisory groups such as WHO (World Health Organization), ICTH (International Committee for Thrombosis and Haemostasis) and ICSH(International Committee for Standardization in Haematology) started work towards standardization of PT for monitoring oral anticoagulant therapy.

The first step was the preparation of IRP's (International Reference Preparations) of thromboplastins by the WHO. This was done to have an accurate reference reagent which could serve as a standard for calibrating responsiveness/ sensitivity of commercial thromboplastin reagents.

The various IRP's were made from thromboplastins derived from various animal tissues in use for manufacture of commercial thromboplastin (PT) reagents. This was done in order to have more precise, like-to-like comparison.

Originally the following IRP's were made available:

IRP's Tissue source	Code	Assigned ISI
Thromboplastin (Human combined)	67/40	1.0
Thromboplastin (Bovine combined)	68/434	1.0

Subsequently after the stocks of primary IRP's were exhausted secondary IRP's have been made available under other code numbers. Till date however, IRP's for recombinant thromboplastins are not available for primary calibration.

Basis of Calibration

This calibration system of individual commercial preparations vs. the reference preparations (IRP's) is based on the fact that when the commercial preparations of thromboplastin (test thromboplastin) and the reference thromboplastin (IRP's) of same tissue origin are tested on the same plasma samples, a linear relationship would exist between log of PT ratios obtained with reference and test thromboplastins.

Log of PT of reference thromboplastin is plotted on the Y-axis and the log of test PT are plotted on the X-axis respectively on a log/log paper (Fig. 10.5).

The slope of the calibration line would then indicate the sensitivity of the test thromboplastin in comparison to the IRP.

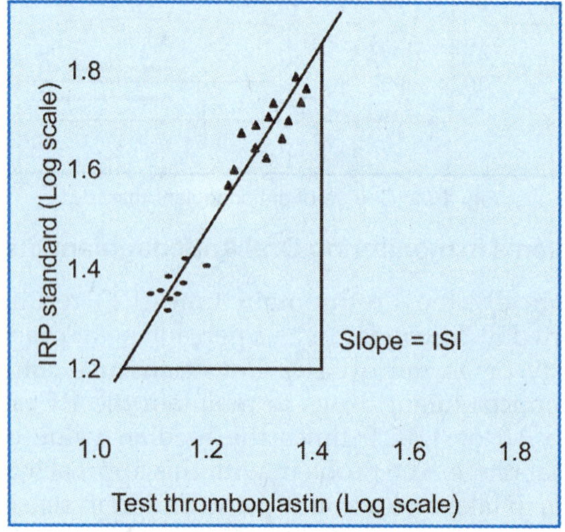

Fig. 10.5: Calibration of Test Thromboplastin vs. WHO IRP
▲ Samples from patients stabilised on oral anticoagulant for minimum 6 weeks.
• Normal patient population samples.

The ISI (International Sensitivity Index) indicates the sensitivity of test thromboplastin in comparison to the international reference preparation. When the calibration line has a slope =1.0, the test thromboplastin equates to the IRP in sensitivity or responsiveness.

The ISI in practical terms is a measure of the responsiveness (prolongation of PT values) of a given thromboplastin to the reduction of the vitamin K-dependant coagulation factors. The lower the ISI (more close it is to 1.0) the more sensitive is the thromboplastin.

The recommended calibration methodology includes normal plasma samples as well as plasma from patients on oral anticoagulant therapy containing PIVKA's. Hence, the assignment of sensitivity also corrects for thromboplastin sensitivity to PIVKA's.

This method for standardization of PT reagent sensitivity based on "ISI" was the first step towards eliminating reagent based variability in expression of PT results.

Manufacturers assign ISI value for each lot of thromboplastin by the WHO recommended methods to assist laboratorians in calculation of the INR (International Normalized Ratio).

The INR Method of Reporting Results

By definition INR represents the PT ratio which would have been obtained for a particular patient sample as if the WHO reference thromboplastin itself (ISI=1.0) had been used in the PT determination.

$INR = [R]^{ISI}$

$$INR = \left[\frac{\text{Patient PT in seconds}}{\text{Mean of the normal range}}\right]^{ISI}$$

A PT ratio is obtained by dividing the patient PT in seconds by the **"Mean of the normal range"**(MNPT). This ratio is then "normalized" by raising the results to the power of the ISI of the PT reagent used. Lower the ISI of the reagent used, closer will be the INR to the observed PT ratio. Ideally, when the ISI of the reagent is 1.0 then the INR is a simple PT ratio since $(R)^{1.0} = R$.

Currently many coagulation instruments are available that can perform this exponential calculation by entering the ISI of the reagent in use. Alternatively a table is provided by reagent manufacturers for reading off "INR" directly for the given patient PT ratio, corresponding to the ISI value of the reagent used. For example,

INR Conversion Table

ISI

Ratio ↓ R	1.00	1.05	1.10	1.15	1.20	1.25	1.29
1.0	1.00	1.00	1.10	1.00	1.00	1.00	1.00
1.1	1.10	1.11	1.11	1.12	1.12	1.13	1.13
1.2	1.20	1.21	1.22	1.23	1.24	1.26	1.27
1.3	1.30	1.32	1.33	1.35	1.37	1.39	1.40
1.4	1.40	1.42	1.45	1.47	1.50	1.52	1.54
1.5	1.50	1.53	1.56	1.59	1.63	1.66	1.69
1.6	1.60	1.64	1.68	1.72	1.76	1.80	1.83
1.7	1.70	1.75	1.79	1.84	1.89	1.94	1.98
1.8	1.80	1.85	1.91	1.97	2.02	2.08	2.13
1.9	1.90	1.96	2.03	2.09	2.16	2.23	2.29
2.0	2.00	2.07	2.14	2.22	2.30	2.38	2.45
2.1	2.10	2.18	2.26	2.35	2.44	2.53	2.60
2.2	2.20	2.29	2.38	2.48	2.58	2.68	2.77
2.3	2.30	2.40	2.50	2.61	2.72	2.83	2.93
2.4	2.40	2.51	2.62	2.74	2.86	2.99	3.09
2.5	2.50	2.62	2.74	2.87	3.00	3.14	3.26
2.6	2.60	2.73	2.86	3.00	3.15	3.30	3.43
2.7	2.70	2.84	2.98	3.13	3.29	3.46	3.60
2.8	2.80	2.95	3.10	3.27	3.44	3.62	3.77
2.9	2.90	3.06	3.23	3.40	3.59	3.78	3.95
3.0	3.00	3.17	3.35	3.54	3.74	3.95	4.13
3.1	3.10	3.28	3.47	3.67	3.89	4.11	4.30
3.2	3.20	3.39	3.59	3.81	4.04	4.28	4.48
3.3	3.30	3.50	3.72	3.95	4.19	4.45	4.67
3.4	3.40	3.61	3.84	4.09	4.34	4.62	4.85
3.5	3.50	3.73	3.97	4.22	4.50	4.79	5.03
3.6	3.60	3.84	4.09	4.36	4.65	4.96	5.22
3.7	3.70	3.95	4.22	4.50	4.81	5.13	5.41
3.8	3.80	4.06	4.34	4.64	4.96	5.31	5.60
3.9	3.90	4.17	4.47	4.78	5.12	5.48	5.79
4.0	4.00	4.29	4.59	4.92	5.28	5.66	5.98
4.1	4.10	4.40	4.72	5.07	5.44	5.83	6.17
4.2	4.20	4.51	4.85	5.21	5.60	6.01	6.37
4.3	4.30	4.63	4.98	5.35	5.76	6.19	6.58
4.4	4.40	4.74	5.10	5.50	5.92	6.37	6.76
4.5	4.50	4.85	5.23	5.64	6.08	6.65	6.96
4.6	4.60	4.96	5.36	5.78	6.24	6.74	7.16
4.7	4.70	5.03	5.49	5.93	6.40	6.92	7.36
4.8	4.80	5.19	5.62	6.07	6.57	7.10	7.56
4.9	4.90	5.31	5.74	6.22	6.73	7.29	7.77
5.0	5.00	5.42	5.87	6.37	6.90	7.48	7.97
5.1	5.10	5.53	6.00	6.51	7.06	7.66	8.18
5.2	5.20	5.65	6.13	6.66	7.23	7.85	8.39
5.3	5.30	5.76	6.26	6.81	7.40	8.04	8.60
5.4	5.40	5.88	6.39	6.95	7.57	8.23	8.81
5.5	5.50	5.99	6.52	7.10	7.73	8.42	9.02
5.6	5.60	6.10	6.65	7.25	7.90	8.61	9.23
5.7	5.70	6.22	6.78	7.40	8.07	8.81	9.44
5.8	5.80	6.33	6.91	7.55	8.24	9.00	9.66
5.9	5.90	6.45	7.05	7.70	8.41	9.20	9.87
6.0	6.00	6.56	7.18	7.85	8.59	9.39	10.09

Recommended therapeutic ranges for oral anticoagulant therapy

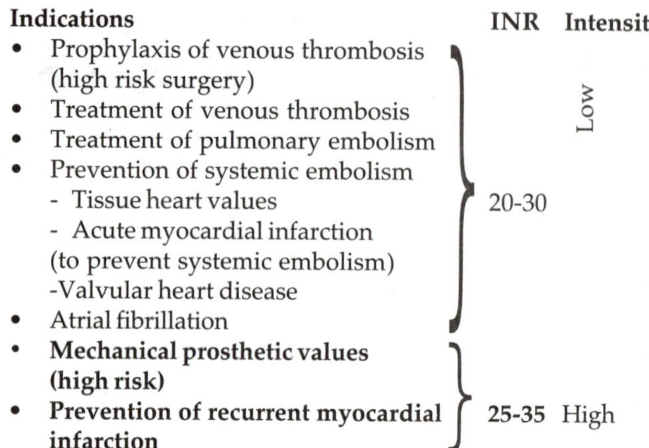

Indications	INR	Intensity
• Prophylaxis of venous thrombosis (high risk surgery) • Treatment of venous thrombosis • Treatment of pulmonary embolism • Prevention of systemic embolism - Tissue heart values - Acute myocardial infarction (to prevent systemic embolism) -Valvular heart disease • Atrial fibrillation	20-30	Low
• **Mechanical prosthetic values (high risk)** • **Prevention of recurrent myocardial infarction**	**25-35**	High

Other Factors Influencing The INR

The variability in the responsiveness of the PT reagents, is corrected through the "ISI" calibration, however, three additional technical factors influence The INR:

- Derivation of MNPT
- Magnitude of difference in the ISI value of test thromboplastin and IRP(ISI=1.0)
- Method of clot detection employed during PT test

MNPT

MNPT is a critical requirement in the derivation of INR. Ideally each laboratory must derive its own MNPT from 20 or more normal patients for a given PT reagent and Lot under use. This corrects within laboratory test variables that influence PT results. If "normal control plasmas" are used in place of patient plasma for arriving at the MNPT it can effect the evaluation of the patients level of anticoagulation. For example,

Reagent ISI=2.5	**Test Day 1**	**Test Day 2**	**Test Day 3**
Patient PT (sec)	16.0	16.0	16.0
NormalControl (10.4-12.3 sec)	11.5	10.4	12.3
INR Formula $[R]^{ISI}$	$16.0^{2.5}$	$16.0^{2.5}$	$16.0^{2.5}$
Resulting INR	2.27	2.89	1.92

If the control time is greater than the mean normal range (MNPT), the PT ratio for any patient PT will be smaller, potentially leading to over coagulation. If the control time is lesser than MNPT the ratio for any patient PT will be greater, leading to under coagulation.

On the other hand MNPT for a particular laboratory using the same combination of methodology, reagent and instrument would remain constant.

ISI value of PT used and Method of Clot Detection

INR looses some precision when comparisons are made with thromboplastins with markedly different ISI values as against the IRP (ISI=1.0) and different methods of clot detection, e.g. manual, mechanical, optical, etc.

Therefore, manufacturers must provide ISI values adapted to the method used for clot detection. Also the reagent used for reporting results should be ideally as close to 1.0 as possible.

Practical Considerations for Warfarin Therapy

Oral administration of Warfarin results in a rapid absorption of the drug, however, an observable anticoagulant effect is delayed. This delay is due to the time required for des-γ-carboxylated (dysfunctional) vitamin K-dependant factor to replace the normal clotting factors.

Depending on the dose the delay may range from 1 to 7 days.

The early anticoagulant effect is mainly caused by the loss of fully carboxylated procoagulant factor VII which has a half life of approximately 5 hours.

However, these oral anticoagulant reagents also cause suppression in the synthesis of **natural anticoagulant protein C and protein S.** Due to this, in the early phase of initiation of oral anticoagulant therapy there is a potential for initial prothrombotic effect. This event underlines the syndrome of coumadin induced skin necrosis, especially in patients with hereditary deficiencies of protein C and protein S.

Therapy can begin with an anticipated maintenance dose (e.g. 5 mg/day). A small loading dose of about twice the average maintenance dose may also be used initially. This dosage achieves a steady state anticoagulant effect in 5-7 days. The use of a large loading dose (e.g., 20-40 mg) has little benefit. Such dosing not only produces a marked factor VII deficiency (which alone may not protect against thrombosis) but also an acquired protein C deficiency, which could produce a prothrombotic state.

If the need for antithrombotic effect is more urgent, heparin should be given as indicated. Heparin is then discontinued when INR is in the therapeutic range.

Considerations for frequency of Laboratory tests for monitoring oral anticoagulant therapy

PT monitoring of patients initially should be performed daily for the first 5 days and 2 to 3 times a week for the first 1 to 2 weeks. Depending on the stability of the PT results from the third week onwards the frequency of monitoring may be further reduced to every 4-8 weeks. While some patients on long term Warfarin therapy have unexpected fluctuations in dose response, some have unexplained requirement for increase in dosage.

The unexpected fluctuations in dose response could be due to: change in diet, undisclosed concomitant drug use, poor patient compliance, surreptitious self-medication, alcohol consumption, intermittent illness or unsuspected changes in the responsiveness of the PT reagent used to perform the PT test.

Management of patients with high INR values with or without bleeding complications

INR	Recommendations
INR> 3.5 but <6.0 patient not bleeding	Rapid reversal not indicated, omit Warfarin for a few doses and resume warfarin at lower dose when, NR reaches therapeutic range
INR>6.0 but < 10.0 patient not bleeding	If rapid reversal required give 1-2 mg sc vit.K • reduction of INR will occur in 8 hrs • back in therapeutic range in 24 hrs • If INR remains high at 24 hrs additional dose of 0.5mg vit.K may be given. • Warfarin can be resumed at lower dose when INR returns to therapeutic range
INR > 10.0 patient not bleeding	Give 3 mg sc. vit.K • INR will be reduced substantially by 6 hrs • Check INR at 6 hrs • vit.K can be repeated if necessary
INR > 20.0 or patient bleeding	• Give 10 mg sc.vit.K supplemented with FFP or prothrombin complex. • Check INR every 6 hrs • Administration of Vit. K inj. may be repeated every 12 hrs • In case of life threatening bleeding or serious warfarin overdose replacement with prothrombin complex concentrate is indicated, supplemented with iv. Vit. K 10 mg; repeated as necessary depending on INR

Advantages of the INR system

- Major advantage of the INR system is that it helps alleviate confusion in the interpretation of PT results. Usually laboratory changes like change in thromboplastin and/or equipments could go unnoticed by the attending physicians. the INR remains constant even with such changes.
- INR system affords comparison of PT results between laboratories.
- INR system provides a more accurate and convenient means of monitoring patients who travel extensively.
- INR therapeutic ranges for different clinical conditions are based on international collaborative studies. Usage of standardized dosage reduces the risk of thrombotic episodes or secondary bleeding.

Disadvantages of the INR system

- The prothrombin time test is always a part of the preoperative screening panels. It is also frequently used to evaluate other haemostatic disorders such as liver disease, DIC, LA, hereditary factor deficiencies and acquired vitamin K deficiency. Since these disorders have been excluded from the derivation of the ISI, INR has a diagnostic and therapeutic value mainly applicable for patients stabilized on oral anticoagulants. Therefore, laboratories may prefer to report both the INR and patients time in seconds depending on clinical application.

- The INR systems effectiveness would still depend on the calibration of the coagulation instruments as well as thromboplastin reagents used.
- Derivation of the correct MNPT and use of the mean normal range in each laboratory.
- Usage of thromboplastin reagents with ISI of preferably 1.0 or as close to 1.0 as possible.
- The correct use of the formula to compute the INR.
- Uniform understanding of the INR system by clinicians as well as laboratorians.

PROTHROMBIN DETERMINATION (Two stage method)

Principle

Prothrombin in the presence of optimal procoagulants and calcium will form thrombin. The amount of thrombin formed can be calculated by determining the dilution of plasma that will clot a standard fibrinogen reagent in a specific period of time. The amount of thrombin formed is a measure of the amount of prothrombin present in the starting sample.

The test consists of two stages. In the first stage, prothrombin is incubated with a standard mixture containing thromboplastin, calcium, a buffer and a source of procoagulants. In the second stage, samples of the incubating mixture are added to a standard fibrinogen solution and the clotting time is determined.

Results

1. The object of the procedure is to determine the dilution of plasma from which will evolve one unit of thrombin under optimal conditions. A unit of thrombin is defined as that amount which will form a clot of 1 ml of fibrinogen in 15 seconds under standard conditions.
2. If varying amounts of thrombin are added to standard amounts of fibrinogen the clotting time of the mixture is an index of the thrombin concentration within a specific range. When thrombin concentrations are plotted against clotting times, the results describe a hyperbolic curve. With thrombin concentrations between 0.80 and 1.34 units, there is good correlation between thrombin concentration and clotting time. With greater amounts of thrombin, there is little change in the speed of clotting, with relatively large changes in thrombin concentration. With lesser amounts of thrombin, small changes in thrombin concentration result in large changes in the speed of clotting.

APTT/PTTK Cephaloplastin Reagent For Partial Thromboplastin Time (APTT) Determination Using Ellagic Acid As Activator

Summary

The arrest of bleeding depends upon primary platelet plug formed along with the formation of a stable fibrin clot. Formation of this clot involves the sequential interaction of a series of plasma proteins in a highly ordered and complex manner and also the interaction of these complexes with blood platelets and materials released from the tissues. Activated Partial Thromboplastin Time is prolonged by a deficiency of coagulation factors of the intrinsic pathway of the human coagulation mechanism such as factor XII, XI, IX, VIII, X, V, II and Fibrinogen. Determination of APTT helps in estimating abnormality in most of the clotting factors of the intrinsic pathway including congenital deficiency of factor VIII, IX, XI and XII and is also a sensitive procedure for generating heparin response curves for monitoring heparin therapy.

Reagent

LIQUICELIN-E® is a liquid ready to use activated cephaloplastin reagent for the determination of Activated Partial Thromboplastin Time. It is a phospholipid preparation derived from rabbit brain with ellagic acid as an activator.

Each batch of reagent undergoes rigorous quality control at various stages of manufacture for its sensitivity and performance.

Reagent Storage and Stability

(a) Store the reagent at 2-8°C. **DO NOT FREEZE,** (b) The shelf life of the reagent is as per the expiry date mentioned on the reagent vial label. The reagent is stable for: **1 year at 2-8°C, 1 week at 18-25°C, 2 days at 37°C.**

Principle

Cephaloplastin activates the coagulation factors of the intrinsic pathway of the coagulation mechanism in the presence of calcium ions. APTT is prolonged by a deficiency of one or more of these clotting factors of the intrinsic pathway and in the presence of coagulation; inhibitors like heparin.

Note

(1) In vitro diagnostic reagent for laboratory and professional use only. Not for medicinal use. (2) LIQUICELIN-E, reagent is not from human source hence, contamination due to HBsAg and HIV is practically excluded. (3) Reagent contains 0.01 per cent Thimerosal as preservative. (4) It is **very important** that clean and dry micropipette tips be used to dispense the reagent. (5) **Avoid exposure** of the reagent to elevated temperatures and contamination. **Immediately** replace cap after use and store at recommended temperatures **only.**

Sample Collection and Preparation

No special preparation of the patient is required prior to sample collection by approved techniques. Withdraw blood without undue venous stasis and without frothing into a plastic syringe fitted with a short needle of 19 to 20 SWG. The veinpuncture must be a 'clean' one and, if there is any difficulty, take a new syringe and needle and try another vein. Transfer the blood into tubes, after detaching the needle from the syringe.

Mix exactly nine parts of freshly collected blood with one part of Trisodium citrate (0.11 mol/l, 3.2 percent) or PROFACT available from TULIP; Centrifuge immediately for 15 minutes at 3000 rpm (approximately 2000 g) and transfer the plasma into a clean test tube. **Plasma must be tested within three hours of blood collection.** For heparin determination, platelet deficient plasma should be used, hence higher centrifugation time is required.

FNP Collection

Prepare a plasma pool (FNP) of freshly collected blood from atleast five normal healthy donors and process as above. Plasma must be tested within three hours of blood collection.

Additional Material Required

(a) 12 x 75 mm test tubes (b) 0.1 ml, 0.2 ml and 2.0 ml precision pipettes (c) Stop watch (d) Water bath or heating block 37° C (e) FRESH NORMAL POOLED PLASMA (f) $CaCl_2$ (0.02 mol/l)

*AVAILABLE FROM TULIP DIAGNOSTICS.

TEST PROCEDURE

Manual Method

(1) Before use, the reagent should be mixed well by gentle swirling. Do not shake. (2) Aspirate from the reagent vial enough reagent for the immediate testing requirement in a thoroughly clean and dry test tube. Bring this reagent to room temperature before prewarming at 37°C for testing purposes. (3) Separate test tubes containing LIQUICELIN-E* and TULIP calcium chloride solution should be brought to 37°C. (Depending on volume, approximately 5 to 10 minutes required). Do not incubate the test plasma. (4) To a 12 x 75 mm test tube, add 0.1 ml test plasma and 0.1 ml LIQUICELIN-E[8]. Shake tube briefly to mix the reagent and plasma, place tube at 37°C for 3 to 5 minutes. (5) Following incubation period, add forcibly 0.1 ml prewarmed calcium chloride into the plasma and LIQUICELIN-E® mixture, simultaneously start a stop watch. Shake tube briefly to mix contents, keep at 37°C for 20 seconds. (6) Following 20 seconds incubation, remove the tube, gently tilt back and forth until a gel clot forms, stop the watch, record time. (7) Repeat steps 2-4 for a duplicate test using the same test plasma. (8) Find the average from the duplicate test values. This is the Activated Partial Thromboplastin Time (APTT of patient plasma). (9) Similarly repeat steps 2-4 twice, and record duplicate values using FNP in place of test plasma (APTT of FNP).

If a coagulation instrument is being used to perform the tests, the instrument manufacturers instructions must be strictly adhered to.

Calibration Curve Method (For determination of heparin concentration):

1. Dilute heparin (as used for treatment) with physiological saline to a concentration of 10 U/ml.
2. Mix 0.2 ml of 10 U/ml diluted heparin with 1.8 ml of FNP to give a heparin standard of 1 U/ml concentration.
3. Dilute the heparin standard as prepared above (1 U/ml) with FNP as follows :

Test tube No.	1	2	3	4	5	6	7
Heparin standard (1 U/ml) in ml	0.5	0.4	0.3	0.2	0.1	0.1	-
FNP in ml	-	0.1	0.2	0.3	0.4	0.9	0.5
Heparin concentration (U/ml)	1	0.8	0.6	0.4	0.2	0.1	0.0

4. Pipette 0.1 ml each of the seven heparin dilutions into clean test tubes.
5. Add 0.1 ml LIQUICELIN-E® reagent to each test tube.
6. Mix well and incubate each test tube at 37°C for exactly 3 minutes before testing.
7. **Forcibly** add 0.1 ml calcium chloride (prewarmed at 37°C) to each test tube, one by one and simultaneously start the stopwatch.
8. Gently tilt the tube back and forth and stop the stopwatch as the first fibrin strand is visible and the gel/clot formation begins. Record the time in seconds.
9. Repeat steps 4-8 for each dilution for duplicate test, and find the average of the duplicate test values.
10. Plot the mean of the double determination in 'seconds', against each heparin concentration using LIQUICELIN-E® graph paper.
11. Clotting times (APTT) of test specimens can be interpolated against the heparin concentration to determine the heparin concentration of the sample in U/ml.

CALCULATION AND REPORTING OF RESULTS

Manual Method

a. The result may be reported directly in terms of the mean of the double determination of the APTT of the test plasma.

OR

b. As a ratio R as follows:

$$R = \frac{\text{APTT of patient plasma (in seconds)}}{\text{APTT of FNP (in seconds)}}$$

Calibration Curve Method

Heparin concentration in the test sample can be directly obtained from the LIQUICELIN-E® calibration curve by interpolating the test plasma clotting time against the heparin concentration in U/ml.

Expected Values

Normal values using LIQUICELIN-E® reagent are between 21 and 29 seconds at 3 minutes activation time. Between manual and turbo-densitometric instrument results a variation of 1-2 seconds may be expected. For photo optical instruments, it is recommended that each laboratory must establish their own normal range.

Remarks

(1) Due to inter and intra-laboratory variations users must establish their own normal population range as well as normal and abnormal range. (2) It is recommended that controls with know factor activity should be run simultaneously with each test series routinely. (3) Incorrect mixture of blood and Trisodium citrate, insufficient prewarming of plasma and reagent, contaminated reagents, glassware, etc. are potential source of errors. (4) Incorrect dilutions of heparin is also a potential source of error. (5) Oxalated plasma may induce prolonged clotting times. (6) Clotting time of patients on anticoagulant therapy depends upon the type and dosage of anticoagulant and also the time lag between the specimen collected and the last dose. (7) Abnormalities of coagulation factor VII, factor XIII and platelets are not detected by this test procedure. (8) For automated equipment it is strongly recommended that the equipments manufacturers methodology is strictly adhered to. (9) In heparin monitoring time of collection of blood sample is important since the *in vivo* half life of heparin is approximately 1.5 hours. When it is administered intravenously it has an immediate anti-coagulant effect but its efficacy decreases rapidly with time. (10) Platelet factor IV, a heparin-neutralising factor can be released due to platelet aggregation or damage. In order to prevent this phenomenon *in vitro* the specimen should be collected with a minimum of trauma. (11) Decrease in APTT time is observed in males under estrogen therapy and oral contraceptive administration in females.

SOYABEAN CEPHALOPLASTIN REAGENT FOR PARTIAL THROMBOPLASTIN TIME (APTT) DETERMINATION USING ELLAGIC ACID, AS AN ACTIVATOR CELIN-SE. (Courtesy: Tulip Group of Companies)

Summary

The arrest of bleeding depends upon primary platelet plug formed along with the formation of a stable fibrin clot. Formation of this clot involves the sequential interaction of a series of plasma proteins in a highly ordered and complex manner and also the interaction of these complexes with blood platelets and materials released from the tissues. Activated partial thromboplastin time is prolonged by a deficiency of coagulation factors of the intrinsic pathway of the human coagulation mechanism such as factor XII, XI, IX. VIII, X, V, II and fibrinogen. Determination of APTT helps in estimating abnormality in most of the clotting factors of the intrinsic pathway including congenital deficiency of factor VIII, IX, XI and XII and is also a sensitive procedure for generating heparin response curves for monitoring heparin therapy.

Reagent

CELIN-SE is a liquid ready to use activated cephaloplastin reagent for the determination of activated partial thromboplastin time. It is a phospholipid preparation derived from soyabean with ellagic acid as an activator. Each batch of reagent undergoes rigorous quality control at various stages of manufacture for its sensitivity and performance.

Reagent Storage and Stability

(a) Store the reagent at 2-8°C. **DO NOT FREEZE** (b) The shelf life of the reagent is as per the expiry date mentioned on the reagent vial label. The reagent **is stable for: 1 year at 2°C,1 week at 18-25°C, 2 days at 37°C.**

Principle

Cephaloplastin activates the coagulation factors of the intrinsic pathway of the coagulation mechanism in the presence of calcium ions. APTT is prolonged by a deficiency of one or more of these clotting factors of the intrinsic pathway and in the presence of coagulation inhibitors like heparin.

Note

(1) In vitro diagnostic reagent for laboratory and professional use only. Not for medicinal use. (2) CELIN-SE reagent is not from human source, hence contamination due to HBsAg and HIV is practically excluded. (3) It is **very important** that dean and dry micropipette tips be used to dispense the reagent. (4) **Avoid exposure** of the reagent to elevated temperature and contamination. **Immediately** replace cap after use and store at recommended temperatures **only.**

Sample Collection and Preparation

No special preparation of the patient is required prior to sample collection by approved techniques. Withdraw blood without undue venous stasis and without frothing into a plastic syringe fitted with a short needle of 19 to 20 SWG. The veinpuncture must be a 'clean' one and, if there is any difficulty, take a new syringe and needle and try another vein. Transfer the blood into tubes, after detaching the needle from the syringe. Mix exactly nine parts of freshly collected blood with one part of trisodium citrate (0.11 mol/l, 3.2 percent) or PROFACT available from TULIP; Centrifuge immediately for 15 minutes at 3000 rpm (approximately 2000 g) and transfer the plasma into a dean test tube. **Plasma must be tested within three hours of blood collection**. For heparin determination, platelet deficient plasma should be used, hence higher centrifugation time is required.

FNP Collection

Prepare a plasma pool (FNP) of freshly collected blood from at least five normal healthy donors and process as above. Plasma must be tested within three hours of blood collection.

Additional Material Required

(a) 12 × 75 mm test tubes (b) 0.1 ml, 0.2 ml and 2.0 ml and 2.0 ml precision pipettes (c) Stop watch (d) Water bath or heating block at 37°C (e) FRESH NORMAL POOLED PLASMA (f) $CaCl_2$ (0.02 mol/l)*
*Available from Tulip Diagnostics.

TEST PROCEDURE

Manual Method

1. Before use, the reagent should be mixed well by gentle swirling. Do not shake.
2. Aspirate from the reagent vial enough reagent for the immediate testing requirement in a thoroughly clean and dry test tube. Bring this reagent to room temperature before prewarming at 37°C for testing purposes.
3. Separate test tubes containing CELIN-SE and TULIP Calcium chloride solution should be brought to 37°C. (Depending on volume,

approximately 5 to 10 minutes required). Do not incubate the test plasma.

4. To a 12 x 75 mm test tube, add 0.1 ml test plasma and 0.1 ml CELIN-SE. Shake tube briefly to mix the reagent and plasma, place tube at 37°C for 3 to 5 minutes.
5. Following incubation period, add forcibly 0.1 ml prewarmed calcium chloride into the plasma and CELIN-SE mixture, simultaneously start a stop watch. Shake tube briefly to mix contents, keep at 37°C for 20 seconds.
6. Following 20 seconds incubation, remove the tube, gently tilt back and forth until a gel clot forms, stop the watch, record time.
7. Repeat steps 2-4 for a duplicate test using the same test plasma.
8. Find the average from the duplicate test values. This is the activated partial thromboplastin time (APTT of patient plasma).
9. Similarly repeat steps 2-4 twice, and record duplicate values using FNP in place of test plasma (APTT of FNP).

If a coagulation instrument is being used to perform the tests, the instrument manufacturers instructions must be strictly adhered to.

Calibration Curve Method (For determination of heparin concentration):

1. Dilute heparin (as used for treatment) with physiological saline to a concentration of 10 U/ml.
2. Mix 0.2 ml of 10 U/ml diluted heparin with 1.8 ml of FNP to give a heparin standard of 1 U/ml conoentration.
3. Dilute the heparin standard as prepared above (1U/ml) with FNP as follows:

Test tube No.	1	2	3	4	5	6	7
Heparin standard (1 U/ml) in ml	0.5	0.4	0.3	0.2	0.1	0.1	-
FNP in ml		0.1	0.2	0.3	0.4	0.9	0.5
Heparin concentration (U/ml)	1	0.8	0.6	0.4	0.2	0.1	0.0

4. Pipette 0.1 ml each of the seven heparin dilutions into clean test tubes.
5. Add 0.1 ml CELIN-SE reagent to each test tube.
6. Mix well and incubate each test tube at 37°C for exactly 3 minutes before testing.
7. **Forcibly** add 0.1 ml calcium chloride (prewarmed at 37°C) to each test tube, one by one and simultaneously start the stop-watch.
8. Gently tilt the tube back and forth and stop the stopwatch as the first fibrin strand is visible and the gel/clot formation begins. Record the time in seconds.
9. Repeat steps 4-8 for each dilution for duplicate test, and find the average of the duplicate test values.
10. Plot the mean of the double determination in 'seconds' against each heparin concentration using CELIN-SE graph paper.
11. Clotting times (APTT) of test specimens can be interpolated against the heparin concentration to determine the heparin concentration of the sample in U/ml.

CALCULATION AND REPORTING OF RESULTS

Manual Method

a. The result may be reported directly in terms of the mean of the double determination of the APTT of the test plasma.

OR

b. As a ratio R as follows:

$$R = \frac{\text{APTT of Patient Plasma (in seconds)}}{\text{APTT of FNP (in seconds)}}$$

Calibration Curve Method

Heparin concentration in the test sample can be directly obtained from the CELIN-SE calibration curve by interpolating the test plasma clotting time against the heparin concentration in U/ml.

Expected Values

Normal values using CELIN-SE reagent are between **23 and 33 seconds** at 3 minutes activation time. Between manual and Turbo densitometric instrument results a variation of 1-2 seconds may be expected. For photo optical instruments, it is recommended that each laboratory must establish their own normal range.

Remarks

(1) Due to inter and intra-laboratory variations users must establish their own normal population range as well as normal and abnormal range. (2) It is recommended that controls with know factor activity

should be run simultaneously with each test series routinely. (3) Incorrect mixture of blood and tri-sodium citrate, insufficient prewarming of plasma and reagent, contaminated reagents, glassware, etc. are potential source of errors. (4) Incorrect dilutions of heparin is also a potential source of error. (5) Oxalated plasma may induce prolonged clotting times. (6) Clotting time of patients on anticoagulant therapy depends upon the type and dosage of anticoagulant and also the time lag between the specimen collected and the last dose. Abnormalities of coagulation factor VII, factor XIII and platelets are not detected by this test procedure. (8) For automated equipment it is strongly recommended that the equipments manufacturers methodology is strictly adhered to. (9) In heparin monitoring time of collection of blood sample is important since the *in vivo* half life of heparin is approximately 1.5 hours. When it is administered intravenously it has an immediate anti-coagulant effect but its efficacy decreases rapidly with time. (10) Platelet factor IV, a heparin-neutralising factor can be released due to platelet aggregation or damage. In order to prevent this phenomenon *in vitro* the specimen should be collected with a minimum of trauma. (11) Decrease in APTT time is observed in males under estrogen therapy and oral contraceptive administration in females.

Recalcification solution

Application	For use with APTT reagent
Reagent	Ready to use Liquid, 0.02 M
Storage/Stability	Room Temperature (20-25°C) ,12 months

CLINICAL IMPLICATIONS OF APTT

1. The APTT is prolonged in all coagulation defects of stage I (includes platelet activity and thromboplastin).
2. The APTT is usually prolonged in Willebrand's disease and is accompanied by a consistently diminished factor VIII level.
3. The APTT and PT will detect 95 per cent of coagulation abnormalities. When APTT is performed in conjunction with a prothrombin time (PT), a further clarification of coagulation defects is possible. For example, a normal PT and abnormal APTT means that the defect lies in the first stage of the clotting mechanism.

Causes of Prolonged APTT

- Haemophilia.
- Vitamin K deficiency.
- Liver disease.
- Presence of circulating anticoagulants.
- DIC disease (chronic or acute).

Shortened APTT occurs in

- extensive cancer, except when liver is involved
- immediately after acute haemorrhage.
- very early stages of DIC.

Circulating Anticoagulants

Usually occurs as an inhibitor of a specific factor (e.g., Factor VIII). Most commonly seen in the development of anti-factor VIII or anti-factor IX in 5 to10 per cent of haemophiliacs. Anticoagulants that develop in the treated haemophiliac are detected by prolonged APTT. Circulating anticoagulants also can be detected in some cases

- Following repeated plasma transfusions.
- Drug reactions.
- Tuberculosis.
- Chronic glomerulonephritis.
- Systemic lupus erythematosus.
- Rheumatoid arthritis.

NORMAL AND ABNORMAL CONTROL PLASMAS FOR COAGULATION ASSAYS Plasmatrol H-I/II® (Courtesy: Tulip Group of Companies)

Summary

Tulip PLASMATROL H-I and PLASMATROL H-II are two level human plasma controls that are suitable for use as normal and abnormal control plasma for PT, APTT, TT and fibrinogen testing using clot based methods. Coagulation controls provide a means of day to day quality control in the hemostasis laboratory for control of accuracy and precision.

Reagent

PLASMATROL is a stabilized and freeze dried preparation of selected human plasma with values determined and assigned for specific clot based tests, which are lot specific. The plasma controls are assaysed using Tulip coagulation reagents.

Reagent Storage and Stability

Unopened vials should be stored at 2-8°C and are stable upto the expiry date mentioned on the vial labels. After reconstitution the shelf life of the control plasma is 3 hours at 25-30°C and 8 hours when stored at 2-8°C.

Principle

The properties of the control plasma are similar to those of pooled fresh plasmas. Since the plasma controls have assigned values, when substituted in place of a sample, in clotbased coagulation assays, they can be used for laboratory quality assurance.

Note

1. In vitro diagnostic reagent for laboratory and professional use only. NOT FOR MEDICINAL USE.
2. The source material used for preparation of the reagent is screened by third generation assays for HBsAg, HCV and HIV antibodies and are found to be non-reactive. However, handle the material as if it is infectious, as no known test method can assure that infectious agents are absent.

Preparation of the Reagent

1. Reconstitute the control plasma with exactly 1 ml of bi-distilled water. Avoid using water containing preservatives.
2. Re-stopper the vial and allow to stand until, the hydration is complete (usually 5-7 minutes).
3. Mix by gently swirling and inversion, avoiding froth formation. Do not shake.
4. Allow to stand and equilibrate for a further 15 minutes before use.
5. Use the reconstituted plasma within 3 hours of reconstitution.

Test Procedure

1. Use the reconstituted PLASMATROL controls in the same manner as freshly prepared titrated Platelet Poor Plasma from a patient.
2. Use the procedure as laid out in the UNIPLASTIN, LIQUIPLASTIN®, LIQUICELIN-E®, FIBROSCREEN, FIBROQUANT pack inserts.

Expected Values

1. The expected value of specific assays are provided on the assay value sheet accompanying each kit, and are lot specific.
2. The expected values are obtained using replicate assay of each manufactured lot of PLASMATROL, manually and using mechanical coagulometers such as HEMOSTAR, HEMOSTAR XF.
3. The individual laboratory values should fall within the expected values.
4. It must however be noted that each laboratory should establish its own normal values and reference range according to GLP.

Remarks

1. When used appropriately, PLASMATROL controls are subjected to the limitations of the assay system deployed.
2. If proper values are not obtained it may indicate problems with one or more variables of the assay system.
3. Stability of the reagent is dependent on storage and handling conditions. Since these can vary between laboratories, each laboratory should determine the stability of the reagent under usual operating conditions.
4. Incorrect mixing of control plasma and reagent, insufficient preparation of plasma/reagent, contaminated reagents and glassware, etc. are a potential source of error.
5. Due to inter-laboratory variations in techniques, standardization of test procedures and calibration of equipments, some variation from assigned mean values may be expected.

FIBROSCREEN THROMBIN TIME TEST FOR QUALITATIVE ESTIMATION OF FIBRINOGEN

Courtesy: Tulip Group of Companies

Summary

At present there are known to be at least eleven factors in circulating blood, which are required for normal haemostasis. Deficiency in any of these factors viz. Factors I, II, V, VII, VIII, IX, X, XI and XIII results in a notable haemorrhagic condition, and the severity of the bleeding is proportional to the degree of deficiency. In order to treat the haemorrhagic condition, it is important to identify and quantify the deficient factor.

FIBROSCREEN reagent is one such test reagent, which can identify the deficiency of Factor I (Fibrinogen). The reagent is used as a source of thrombin to determine the qualitative reactivity of fibrinogen.

Reagent

FIBROSCREEN reagent is a lyophilised preparation of bovine thrombin of 50 NIH/ml. Reconstitute with 1 ml of distilled water; wait for 5 minutes, do not shake and mix gently by swirling till the solution attains homogeneity. Further keep aside for 10 minutes to attain equilibrium. Gently swirl the vial while drawing the reagent for use. Once reconstituted it is ready to use reagent for the thrombin time test.

Storage and Stability

1. Store the unopened reagent vials at 2-8°C. DO NOT FREEZE.
2. The shelf life of the reagent is as per the expiry date mentioned on the reagent vial label and carton label.
3. Once reconstituted the FIBROSCREEN reagent is stable for 6 days when stored at 2-8°C and for 4 hours at room temperature (20- 25°C), provided it is not contaminated. Extreme care has to be taken to maintain aseptic precautions while reconstituting, retrieving and handling reagents to prevent contamination. The FIBROSCREEN reagent vial must be replaced at 2-8°C immediately upon retrieving the reagent for the day's work.

Principle

When a known quality and concentration of FIBROSCREEN reagent is added to citrated plasma, by observing the time required for clot formation and the quality of clot formed, a qualitative estimation of fibrinogen in the sample can be obtained.

Note

1. *In vitro* diagnostic reagent for laboratory and professional use. Not for medicinal use.
2. The reagent contains 0.1 per cent sodium azide as preservative.
3. FIBROSCREEN thrombin reagent is not from a human source, hence contamination due to HBsAg, HIV and HCV is practically excluded.
4. It is very important that absolutely clean and dry micropipettes be used to aspirate and dispense the reagent.
5. Avoid exposure of the reagent to elevated temperatures, direct light and contamination. Immediately replace cap after use and store at recommended temperature.

Quality Control

A known normal control should be run in parallel with each batch of tests. This control may be TULIP plasma coagulation control PLASMATROL-I or freshly drawn normal plasma.

Sample Collection and Preparation

No special preparation of the patient is required prior to sample collection by approved techniques. Withdraw blood without undue venous stasis and without frothing into a plastic syringe fitted with a short needle of 19 to 20 SWG. The venepuncture must be a 'clean' one and, if there is any difficulty, take a new syringe and needle and try another vein. Transfer the blood into tubes, after detaching the needle from the syringe. Mix nine parts of freshly collected blood with one part of sodium citrate (0.109-M mol/l, 3.2 percent). Centrifuge immediately for fifteen minutes at 3000 rpm (approximately 2000 g) and transfer the plasma into a clean test tube. Plasma must be tested within 3 hours of collection.

Additional Material Required

10 ×75 mm glass test tubes, 0.2 ml precision pipettes, stop watch, distilled water, fresh plasma.

Procedure

Bring all the reagents and samples to room temperature before testing.

Manual method

Testing should be done in duplicate at room temperature (20-25°C).

1. To a clean and dry 10 x 75 mm test tube add 0.2 ml of plasma to be tested and 0.2 ml of the reconstituted FIBROSCREEN reagent.
2. Start a stopwatch simultaneously with the addition of the FIBROSCREEN reagent.
3. Shake the tube gently to mix the contents and then tilt the tube back and forth.
4. Note the time at the first appearance of the clot and for the remaining portion of 60 seconds for consistency and character of the clot formed.

Interpretation of Results

Normal plasma begins to show clot formation within 15 seconds after FIBROSCREEN reagent has been added. Because time of clot formation may be influenced by additional factors in the test system, estimation of approximate concentration of fibrinogen cannot be made from the initial clotting time alone but must be also made from observations of the consistency and character of the clot at 60 seconds. At 60 seconds, samples with normal fibrinogen levels will form a firm clot that adheres to the walls of the test tube when the tube is inverted. If either of these parameters are not met, (i.e. clotting time below 15 seconds or formation of a firm adhering clot after inversion of the test tube) abnormality (less than 100 mg percent) of the fibrinogen reactivity should be suspected. In such cases quantitative estimation of fibrinogen using FIBROQUANT is strongly recommended.

Expected Values

A normal value using FIBROSCREEN reagent is the formation of a solid gel clot in 5-15 seconds, which adheres to the test tube wall on inversion at 60 seconds.

Remarks

1. Fibroscreen thrombin time remains normal in deficiencies of factor XIII (fibrin stabilizing factor).
2. Fibrin gels may form in plasma with a fibrinogen concentration below normal. However, these gels are not firm, extrude considerable serum, and tend to slide on the side walls of the tilted test tube. Careful comparison of such gels with the firm clot with normal plasma used as a control will eliminate the possibility of confusion.
3. Fibroscreen thrombin time test is usually performed first before any specific assays are attempted, when a prolongation of (PT and APTT) cannot be explained.

Interpretation of first line tests:

TEST				CONDITION
PT	APTT	TT	Platelet count	
N	N	N	N	Disorder of platelet function, factor XIII deficiency, disorder of vascular haemostasis, normal haemostasis.
Long	N	N	N	Factor VII deficiency, Early oral anticoagulation.
N	Long	N	N	Factor VIII: C, IX, XI, XII, Prekallikrein, HMWK deficiency, von Willebrand's disease, Circulating anticoagulant.
Long	Long	N	N	Vitamin K deficiency, Oral anticoagulants factorV, VII and II deficiency.
Long	Long	N	N	Heparin, Liver disease, Fibrinogen deficiency, hyperfibrinolysis.
Long	Long	N	N	Thrombocytopenia.
Long	Long	N	Low	Massive transfusion, Liver disease.
Long	Long	Long	Low	DIC, Acute liver disease.

N-Normal

FIBRINOGEN ESTIMATION-QUANTITATIVE

FIBROQUANT, REAGENT FOR QUANTITATIVE ESTIMATION OF FIBRINOGEN (Courtesy Tulip Group of Companies)

Summary

At present there are known to be atleast eleven factors in circulating blood, which are required for normal haemostasis. Deficiency in any of these factors viz., factors I, II, V, VII, VIII, IX, X, XI and XIII, results in a notable hemorrhagic condition, and the severity of the bleeding is proportional to the degree of deficiency. In order to treat the hemorrhagic condition, it is important to identify and quantify the deficient factor.

Fibrinogen (Factor I) is a high molecular weight glycoprotein synthesized in the liver, which plays an important role in haemostasis. For normal haemostasis to occur in response to injury or tissue damage, a sufficient concentration of fibrinogen must be present in plasma. Fibrinogen is converted into fibrin by the action of thrombin and is a key component of clot formation.

FIBROQUANT kit contains lyophilized thrombin and fibrinogen calibrator to determine the quantitative reactivity of fibrinogen. Since the reagent system contains heparin-neutralizing substances, heparin levels upto 0.4 IU/ml does not interfere with test results.

When used as a front line test with PT, APTT, platelet count and thrombin time, fibrinogen assay helps in investigating acute haemostatic failure.

Reagent

FIBROQUANT kit contains:

1. Thrombin reagent, which is a lyophilized preparation from bovine source ~50 NIH units per vial.
2. Fibrinogen calibrator, which is a lyophilized preparation of human plasma equivalent to stated amount of fibrinogen on a mg basis (refer FIBROQUANT graph paper supplied with each kit for the value of each lot).
3. Owren's buffer, ready to use (pH 7.35).

Storage and Stability

1. Store the unopened reagent vials at 2-8°C. DO NOT FREEZE.

2. The shelf life of the reagents is as per the expiry date mentioned on the reagent vial labels.
3. Once reconstituted the FIBROQUANT thrombin reagent is stable for 6 days when stored at 2-8°C and for 4 hours at room temperature (20-25°C), provided it is not contaminated. Extreme care has to be taken to maintain aseptic precautions while reconstituting, retrieving and handling reagents to prevent contamination. The reagent vial must be replaced to 2-8°C immediately upon retrieving the reagent for the day's work.
4. The reconstituted FIBROQUANT fibrinogen calibrator is stable for 6 hours at 2-8°C and for 2 hours at room temperature (20-25°C).

Principle

The addition of thrombin coagulates fresh citrated plasma. The coagulation time is proportional to the fibrinogen concentration. This allows the estimation of plasma fibrinogen by functional clotting assay.

Note

1. *In vitro* diagnostic reagent for laboratory and professional use. Not for medicinal use.
2. The individual reagents contain 0.1 per cent sodium azide as preservative.
3. FIBROQUANT thrombin reagent is not from a human source hence, contamination due to HBsAg, HIV and HCV is practically excluded.
4. Fibrinogen calibrator provided in the FIBROQUANT kit is from a human source, which was tested and found to be non-reactive for HBsAg, HCV and HIV. However, no known test methods can assure that infectious agents are absent. Handle all human products as potentially infectious.
5. It is very important that absolutely clean and dry micropipettes be used to aspirate and dispense the reagent.
6. Avoid exposure of the reagent to elevated temperatures, direct light and contamination. Immediately replace the cap after use and store at recommended temperature.

Quality Control

A known normal control should be run in parallel with each batch of tests. This control may be TULIP plasma coagulation control PLASMATROL-I or freshly drawn normal plasma.

Sample Collection and Preparation

No special preparation of the patient is required prior to sample collection by approved techniques. Withdraw blood without undue venous stasis and without frothing into a plastic syringe fitted with a short needle of 19 to 20 SWG. The venepuncture must be a 'clean' one and, if there is any difficulty, take a new syringe and needle and try another vein. Transfer the blood into tubes, after detaching the needle from the syringe. Mix nine parts of freshly collected blood with one part of sodium citrate (0.109 mol/l, 3.2 percent). Centrifuge immediately for fifteen minutes at 3000 rpm (approximately 2000 g) and transfer the plasma into a clean test tube. Plasma must be tested within 3 hours of collection.

Additional Material Required

10 × 75 mm glass test tubes, 0.2 ml and 0.1 ml precision pipettes, Stop watch, water bath at 37°C, distilled water, automated, semiautomated/mechanical/optical instrument if applicable.

Procedure

Bring all the reagents and samples to room temperature before testing.

A. Procedure for fibrinogen Calibration Curve Preparation

- The FIBROQUANT thrombin reagent vial must be **reconstituted exactly with one ml of distilled water;** wait for 5 minutes, do not shake but gently swirl the vial till the solution attains homogeneity. Further keep the vial aside for 10 minutes to attain equilibrium. Once reconstituted it is ready to use for the fibrinogen test.
- The FIBROQUANT fibrinogen calibrator vial must be **reconstituted with exactly one ml of distilled water;** wait for 5 minutes, do not shake, gently swirl the vial till the solution attains homogeneity. Further keep the vial aside for 10 minutes to attain equilibrium. This is the fibrinogen calibrator stock solution.

- Dilute fibrinogen calibrator stock solution with Owrens buffer as follows:

Test tube no.	I	II	III
Owrens buffer	NIL	0.8 ml	0.9 ml
Fibrinogen calibrator	0.2 ml	0.2 ml	0.1 ml
Dilution (calibrator)	NIL	1.5	1:10

1. Pipette 0.2 ml of each fibrinogen calibrator dilution into clean test tubes and prewarm for 3 minutes at 37°C.
2. Add 0.1 ml of reconstituted thrombin reagent (pre-warmed at 37°C for one minute) and simultaneously start stopwatch.
3. Stop the stop watch at the first appearance of the fibrin web, as the gel clot begins to form and record the time in seconds.
4. Repeat steps 1 to 3 for a duplicate test one each calibrator dilution.
5. Plot the average of the duplicate test values on TULIP FIRBRINOGEN graph paper*.
6. Connect the points, which should produce a straight line.
7. The calibration curve may be extended beyond the lowest and highest point.
***The calibration curve is valid only for the same lot of FIBROQUANT thrombin reagent**

B. Test Procedure for Sample

1. Prepare a 1:10 dilution of plasma specimen with Owrens buffer solution.
2. To a 10 × 75 mm test tube at 37°C add 0.2 ml of 1:10 dilution of plasma sample to be tested.
3. Incubate at 37°C for one minute.
4. To the test tube add 0.1 ml of FIBROQUANT thrombin reagent (prewarmed at 37°C for one minute) and start the stopwatch simultaneously.
5. Stop the stopwatch at the first appearance of the fibrin web, as the gel clot begins to form and record the time in seconds.
6. Repeat steps 1-5 for a duplicate test.
7. If at the sample dilution of 1:10 the observed clotting time is usually between 8 and 25 seconds, the fibrinogen content is normal (Fibrinogen content between 150 and 400 mg/dl). Assay results can be read off directly from the graph paper provided with the FIBROQUANT kit for the fibrinogen concentration.
8. If the fibrinogen content is high the clotting time will be less than 8 seconds. In such cases repeat the test at 1:20 dilution of the sample or 1:30 dilution of the sample. The results read off the graph will be multiplied by a factor 2 or 3 for the respective dilution.
9. Conversely, if fibrinogen content is low, the clotting time will be over 25 seconds. Repeat the assay at 1:5 dilution, or if necessary at 1:2 dilution. In this case the results read off the graph will be divided by a factor of 2 or 5 for the respective dilutions.

This procedure can also be performed on an automated/semiautomated mechanical/optical instrument but the equipment manufacturers methodology should be strictly adhered to.

Remarks

1. Significant levels of heparin and elevated levels of fibrinogen degradation products (FDP) in the patient plasma can cause falsely low fibrinogen results.
2. Insufficient pre-warming of plasma and reagent or contaminated glassware may cause erroneous results.
3. EDTA should not be used as an anticoagulant.
4. Use reagents of the same lot for performing the test.
5. Do not interchange reagents from different lots.

FIBRINOLYTIC ACTIVITY

The three methods presented below are measures of fibrinolytic activity in general and are influenced by many factors. These serve as screening procedures, but the specific contribution of the various factors must be determined by other means. The lack of suitable standards makes quantitative measurements unavailable for most diagnostic laboratories.

EUGLOBULIN LYSIS TIME

Principle

Euglobulin fraction of plasma contains fibrinogen and all the plasminogen activator and plasminogen of plasma but only traces of the anti-plasmins. The lysis of a fibrin clot formed by the addition of thrombin is a measure of the fibrinolytic activity.

Requirements

1. Equipment for collection of blood
2. Centrifuge
3. Topical thrombin
4. Serological pipettes
5. Carbon dioxide. A tank of CO_2 fitted with a valve to allow control of the rate of flow.

Method

1. Blood is collected in the usual manner and mixed immediately with 0.11 M sodium citrate in a ratio of 1 part citrate solution to 9 parts blood.
2. Plasma is obtained by centrifugation.
3. 0.4 ml plasma is placed in a test tube and 7.6 ml. distilled water is added.
4. CO_2 is bubbled into the solution through a capillary tube for 30 seconds.
5. The precipitate which forms is collected by centrifugation at about 3,000 rpm for 15 minutes.
6. The precipitate is dissolved in 1 ml M/15 phosphate buffer, pH 7.2.
7. To the euglobin in phosphate buffer, 0.1 ml thrombin (topical thrombin diluted to 100 units per ml with saline) is added. The solution is mixed.
8. Clotting should be rapid. After clotting has occurred, the tube is placed in water bath (37°C) and observed for lysis of clot, which is the end-point.

Result

In normal plasma a period of 2 to 4 hours is required for euglobin clot lysis to occur. (The technique should be standardized in each laboratory).

DILUTE BLOOD CLOT LYSIS TIME

Principle

Plasmin inhibitors lose activity on dilution to a greater extent than fibrinolytic activity. Whole blood is diluted with a buffer solution and clotted by the addition of thrombin. The clot is observed for lysis of the clot.

Requirements

1. Equipment for collection of blood sample
2. Test tube
3. Timer
4. Phosphate buffer, pH-7.4. To 1000 ml distilled water, 9.47 gm Na_2HPO_4 is added and dissolved. This is mixed with 250 ml distilled water containing 3.02 gm $KH_2 PO_4$
5. Topical thrombin (or any other make) diluted to 100 units per ml with normal saline.

Method

1. Tubes containing 1.70 ml buffer and 0.1 ml. thrombin solution are placed in an ice bath.
2. Collect blood sample in standard manner using a syringe that can deliver accurately 0.2 ml aliquots of blood.
3. Add 0.2 ml blood to each of two tubes containing buffer and thrombin and mix.
4. Clotting should occur promptly.
5. Tubes are placed in refrigerator (4°C) for 30 minutes and then transferred to a water bath at 37°C.
6. The clots are observed for lysis. The endpoint is fragmentation rather than complete dissolution of the clot.

Result

Blood from a normal subject should not lyse in less than 6 to 10 hours. The test is qualitative. If results indicate rapid lysis of the clot, more quantitative methods are necessary.

FDPs

A QUALITATIVE AND SEMIQUANTITATIVE LATEX SLIDE TEST FOR DETECTING CROSS LINKED FIBRIN DEGRADATION PRODUCTS IN HUMAN PLASMA. Courtesy: Tulip Group of Companies

Summary

During coagulation sequence of reactions occur in the body in response to variety of external and or internal stimuli. The enzymatic cascade reaction terminates in the conversion of FIRBRINOGEN to FIBRIN, by the enzyme THROMBIN.The fibrin gel is then converted to a stable fibrin clot by thrombin activated Factor XIII.

Finally, the fibrin network is dissolved by the enzyme PLASMIN to generate cross-linked fibrin degradation products (XL FDP). D dimer comprising of two D fragments cross linked together, is the smallest plasmin resistant molecular unit present within XL FDP. Detection of D dimer is invaluable as a diagnostic marker for thrombotic conditions such as DIC, DVT and PE. D dimer levels can also be used to monitor thrombolytic therapy with tPA and with streptokinase, thrombotic complications in pregnancy, acute myocardial infarction, sickle cell crisis, severe septic infections, liver disease, DIC accompanying snake bite and prognosis and response to therapy in cancer.

Reagent

1. **XL FDP reagent**: A uniform suspension of polystyrene latex particles coated with mouse monoclonal anti D-dimer Antibody (DD-3B6/22). The reagent is standardized to detect XL FDP $\geq$ 200 ng/ml.
2. **Positive control,** reactive with XL FDP latex reagent.
3. **Negative control,** non-reactive with XL FDP latex reagent.
4. **Phosphate buffer,** for performing semi quantitative test.

   All the reagents contain 0.1 per cent sodium azideas preservative.

   Each batch of reagents undergoes rigorous quality control at various stages of manufacture for its specificity, sensitivity and performance.

Reagent Storage and Stability

1. Store the reagent at 2-8°C. DO NOT FREEZE.
2. The shelf life of the reagent is as per the expiry date mentioned on the reagent vial labels.

Principle

XL FDP slide test for detection of cross-linked fibrin degradation products is based on the principle of agglutination. The test specimen (plasma) is mixed with XL FDP latex reagent. The sensitivity of the reagent is ~ 200 ng/ml, below which samples are negative and above which samples give a positive agglutination reaction.

The cross-linked fibrin degradation products, D dimer, D dimer E, and high molecular weight derivatives are all recognized by TULIP XL FDP reagent incorporating the monoclonal antibodies. No binding was found to the fibrinogen degradation products XYD and E to 20 mg/L or to fibrinogen upto 1000 mg/L.

Note

1. *In vitro* diagnostic reagent for laboratory and professional use only. Not for medicinal use.
2. The reagents contains 0.1 per cent sodium azide as preservative. Avoid contact with skin and mucosa. On disposal flush with large quantities of water.
3. All the reagents derived from human source have been tested for HBsAg and Anti HIV antibodies and are found to be non-reactive. However, handle the material as if infectious.
4. The reagent can be damaged due to microbial contamination or on exposure to extreme temperature conditions. It is recommended that the performance of reagent be verified with positive and negative controls supplied with the kit.
5. Shake the XL FDP latex reagent vial before use to disperse the latex particles uniformly and improve test readability.
6. Only a clean and dry glass slide must be used. Clean the slide with distilled water and wipe dry.

Sample Collection and Preparation

No special preparation of the patient is required prior to sample collection. Plasma samples are recommended for use with XL FDP test. Fresh EDTA, citrate or heparinised anticoagulated plasma specimens are suitable for performing the test.

Sample storage:	20-25°C	-8 hours
	2-8°C	-4 days
Frozen	(-20°C)	-2 months

Thaw frozen specimens at 37°C and centrifuge plasma before testing.

KIT Composition

1. XL FDP latex reagent, positive control, negative control, PBS buffer.
2. Glass slide with six reaction circles, disposable sample dispensing dropper, mixing sticks, rubber teat, package insert.

Additional Material Required

Stop watch, test tubes high intensity direct light source.

Test Procedure

Bring all the reagents and sample to room temperature before performing the test.

Qualitative Method

1. Pipette one drop of plasma specimen onto the glass slide using the disposable dropper provided with the kit. Hold the dropper exactly in vertical position to dispense the drop accurately.
2. Add one drop of XL FDP latex reagent adjacent to the drop of plasma specimen, taking care to hold the dropper in a vertical position while dispensing the drop. Do not let the dropper tip touch the plasma specimen on the slide.
3. Using a mixing stick, mix the plasma and latex reagent uniformly over the entire circle.
4. Immediately start a stop watch, rock the slide gently, back and forth, and observing for agglutination macroscopically at three minutes.
5. Do not read the test result beyond three minutes.

Semi-quantitative Method

1. Using PBS buffer solution prepare serial dilutions of the plasma sample 1:2,1:4,1:8,1:16,1:32 and so on.
2. Pipette each dilutions of plasma specimen on to the separate reaction circles.
3. Add one drop of XL FDP latex reagent to each drop of diluted plasma specimen on to the slide. Do not let the dropper tip touch the diluted plasma specimen on the slide.
4. Immediately start the stop watch. Rock the slide gently, back and forth, observing for agglutination macroscopically at three minutes.

Interpretation of Results

Qualitative Method

- Agglutination is a positive result indicating D dimer level above 200 ng/ml.
- No agglutination is a negative result indicating absence of clinically significant D dimer levels in the plasma specimen.

Semi-quantitative Method

Agglutination in the highest plasma dilution corresponds to the approximate amount of D dimer level in ng/ml.

To calculate D dimer level in ng/ml in the sample, use the following formula,

D dimer level (ng/ml) = $200 \times d$

d = highest dilution of plasma showing agglutination during the semi-quantitative test of the sample.

NB: Activation of the coagulation system with subsequent microvascular fibrin deposition and lysis has been reported in diverse clinical conditions such as trauma, surgery, inflammation and malignancy. Elevated levels of plasma XL FDP may be expected to occur in such conditions.

Remarks

1. D dimer half-life is approximately 6 hours in circulation of individuals with normal renal function. Patients with stabilized clots and not undergoing active fibrin deposition and plasmin activation may not give detectable D dimer elevations.
2. In PE, the larger the clot size, higher the expected level of circulating D dimer. Conversely, the amount of D dimer released from very small clots may be diluted by the circulation and may not give a detectable increase.
3. Fibrinolysis is a highly regulated process and in delicate dynamic balance. In case of hereditary, acquired deficiency and dysfunction of fibrinogen, the rate of fibrinolysis will be altered there by not giving a detectable D dimer level.
4. As with any laboratory test, detection of elevated levels of XL FDP in a specimen should be correlated with clinical findings.

SCREENING TESTS FOR DIAGNOSIS OF PROCOAGULANT DEFICIENCY

Principle: Most of the coagulation disorders can be classified on the basis of the prothrombin time used in conjunction with the partial thromboplastin time. The effect of $BaSO_4$-adsorbed normal plasma on the results of the abnormal test is of diagnostic importance.

Requirements

1. All reagents and equipment necessary for the prothrombin time and partial thromboplastin time.
2. $BaSO_4$-treated normal plasma.

Method

1. The plasma under study is tested in the usual manner by both the prothrombin time and the partial thromboplastin time.
2. Mix equal volumes of the test plasma and normal control plasma. About 0.5 ml of the mixture is needed.
3. Mix equal volumes of the test plasma and $BaSO_4$-treated normal plasma. About 0.5 ml of the mixture is needed.
4. Determine the prothrombin time and the partial thromboplastin time each of the mixtures.

Results

1. If both the prothrombin time and the partial thromboplastin time are normal, it is doubtful that clinically significant coagulation disorder is present.
2. If the normal plasma fails to correct an abnormal prothrombin time or partial thromboplastin time, it is likely that the patient has a circulating anticoagulant.
3. If normal plasma corrects either the prothrombin time or the partial thromboplastin time, the presumptive diagnosis is as indicated in the table.
4. Factor XII deficiency will have a pattern similar to that of factor VIII deficiency. The correct diagnosis can be further elucidated by the lack of a real bleeding tendency in the factor XII deficiency. Definite diagnosis can be established only by having samples of plasma known to be specifically deficient in factor VIII and factor XII. Failure of correction of the patient's partial thromboplastin time by plasma known to be deficient in factor VIII establishes the diagnosis of hemophilia. Likewise, failure of correction of the patient's partial thromboplastin time by plasma known to be deficient in factor XII establishes the diagnosis of Hageman trait.
5. Factor XI deficiency may have a pattern similar to that of factor VIII or factor IX deficiency. The correct diagnosis can be further elucidated by the sex-linked recessive transmission of factor VIII or factor IX deficiency. Definitive diagnosis can be established only by having available sample of plasma known to be deficient in factors VIII, IX, and XI. Failure of correction of the patient's partial thromboplastin time by plasma known to be deficient in factor XI establishes the diagnosis of factor XI deficiency.

The two-stage prothrombin method is needed to distinguish a true deficiency of prothrombin from the pattern indicated for factor X deficiency.

A severe deficiency of fibrinogen will have a pattern similar to that of factor V deficiency. A quantitative method for fibrinogen is required to determine the fibrinogen level.

For delving further into details of coagulation disorder diagnosis, spectral diagnostics provides kits for estimation of —antiplasmin, antithrombin III, A2, antitrypsin, factor II reagent, factor V reagent, factor VII reagent, factor VIII reagent, factor VIII R:AG antiserum, factor IX, factor X reagent, factor XIII, fibrinogen reagent,—macroglobulin, PTT reagent, thrombin reagent, thrombin coagulase and *Staphylococcus* clumping test.

LABORATORY DIAGNOSIS OF VASCULAR BLEEDING DISORDERS

Hess's test is positive in these

Causes and classification

1. *Hereditary*
   - Hereditary haemorrhagic telangiectasia
2. *Acquired*
   - Simple easy bruising
   - Senile purpura
   - Purpura of infections
   - Henoch-Schonlein syndrome

Prothrombin		*Partial thromboplastin time*		*Presumptive diagnosis*
Test plasma alone	Test plasma $+BaSO_4$ plasma	Test plasma alone	Test plasma $+BaSO_4$ plasma	Deficiency of factor
Long	Normal	Long	Normal	V
Long	Long	Normal	Normal	VII
Normal	Normal	Long	Normal	VIII
Normal	Normal	Long	Long	IX
Long	Long	Long	Long	X

- Scurvy
- Steroid purpura.

LABORATORY DIAGNOSIS OF PLATELET DISORDERS

IDIOPATHIC THROMBOCYTOPENIC PURPURA (ITP)

1. Platelet count is usually 10-50 x 10^9/L.
2. The blood film shows reduced numbers of platelets, those present are often large.
3. The bone marrow usually shows increased number of megakaryocytes.
4. Sensitive tests can demonstrate antiplatelet IgG, either alone or with complement, on the platelet surface or in the serum in most patients.
5. Autologous platelet survival studies with ^{51}Cr or DF^{32}P-labelled platelets may be used to show reduced platelet survival. In severe cases, the mean platelet survival may be reduced to one hour.
6. Hess's test may be positive in some cases.

DRUG INDUCED IMMUNE THROMBOCYTOPENIA

1. Thrombocytopenia. Platelet count is often <14 x 10^9/L.
2. Bone marrow may show normal or increased numbers of megakaryocytes.
3. Drug-dependent antibodies against platelets may be demonstrated in sera of some patients. Drugs usually incriminated are:
   - Quinine
   - Quinidine
   - Sulphonamides
   - PAS
   - Rifampicin
   - Stibophen
   - Digitoxin, etc.

DISSEMINATED INTRAVASCULAR COAGULATION (DIC)

1. In acute cases blood may not clot due to gross fibrinogen deficiency.
2. Platelet count is low.
3. Fibrinogen screening tests, titres or assays indicate deficiency.
4. Thrombin time is prolonged.
5. High levels of serum fibrin/fibrinogen degradation products, are found in serum and urine.
6. Prothrombin time and Partial Thromboplastin time are prolonged.
7. Factor V and factor VIII activity is diminished.
8. Due to microthrombi causing mechanical hemolytic anaemia, RBCs may show crenation and poikilocytosis.

Causes of DIC

1. *DIC may be caused by entry of procoagulant material into circulation, e.g.* in
   - amniotic fluid embolism
   - premature placental separation
   - widespread mucin secreting adenocarcinoma
   - severe falciparum malaria
   - hemolytic transfusion reaction
   - promyelocytic leukemia and
   - some snake bites.
2. *DIC may also be initiated by extensive endothelial damage and collagen exposure,* e.g. in
   - endotoxemia
   - gram negative and meningococcal septicemia
   - septic abortion
   - certain viral infections (purpura fulminans)
   - severe burns and
   - hypothermia
3. *Massive intravascular platelet aggregation can also precipitate DIC as occurs in some*
   - bacterial and viral infections
   - immune complexes may have a direct effect on platelets.

FUNCTIONAL PLATELET DISORDERS

Platelet reactions in the hemostatic process

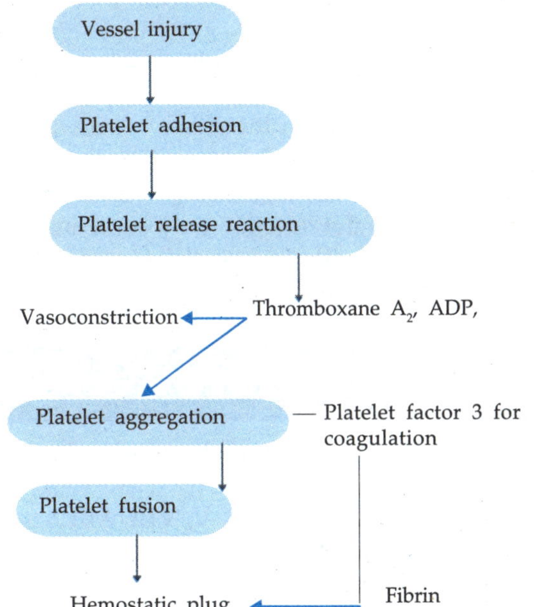

Laboratory Diagnosis

1. Platelet count normal.
2. Prolonged bleeding time.
3. Abnormal platelet aggregation studies with ADP, adrenaline, collagen and ristocetin.
4. Abnormal adhesion studies and nucleotide pool measurement.
5. Factor VIII clotting assay (for von-Willebrand's disease).

Abnormal platelet function should be suspected in cases where bleeding is prolonged despite a normal platelet count. Various causes included in this are as follows:

Hereditary Disorders

1. Platelet storage pool disease: There is defective release of ADP and 5HT due to an intrinsic deficiency in the number of dense granules.
2. Thrombasthenia (Glanzmann's disease): There is failure of primary platelet aggregation.
3. Bernard-Soulier syndrome: Platelets are larger than normal, lack surface glycoprotein and fail to make phospholipid available or to adhere to vessel walls.
4. von Willebrand's disease: There is defective platelet adhesion as well as coagulation factor VIII deficiency.

Acquired Disorders

1. Aspirin therapy: may lead to abnormal bleeding time although purpura is rare. Aspirin leads to impaired thromboxane-A_2 synthesis. So, there is failure of the release action aggregation with ADP and adrenaline.
2. Hyperglobulinemia: interferes with platelet adherence, release and aggregation.
3. Myeloproliferative disorders: Intrinsic abnormalities of platelet function may occur in patients with essential thrombocythemia and other myeloproliferative disorders.

LABORATORY DIAGNOSIS OF COAGULATION DISORDERS

Some properties of the coagulation factors are given below.

1. *Fibrinogen group*: Factors, I, V, VIII, XIII.
   - Thrombin interacts with them all
   - Activity lost in coagulation process (not present in serum)
   - Increase during inflammation, in pregnancy and women on oral contraceptives
   - V and VII lose activity in stored plasma
   - Liver parenchyma synthesis (except factor VIII).
2. *Prothrombin group:* Factors II, VII, IX and X.
   - Activated form contains an active serine centre
   - Liver parenchymal cell synthesis
   - All except prothrombin (II) are not consumed during coagulation (present in serum)
   - Dependent on vitamin K for synthesis
   - Stable, well preserved in stored plasma.
3. *Contact group*: Factors XI, XII.
   - Activated forms contain an active serine centre
   - Not dependent on vitamin K for synthesis
   - Stable, well preserved in stored plasma.

Factor VIII is most important as far as coagulation disorders are concerned. Its structure is as follows:

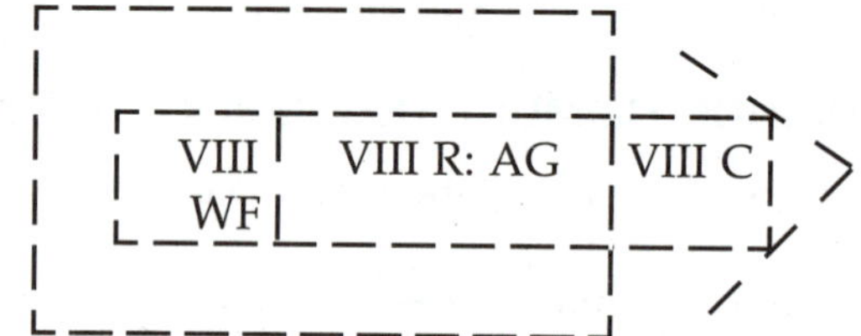

VIII C = Part has coagulant activity.
VIII R: AG = Factor VIII Related Antigen, effects platelet function also.
VIII WF = von Willebrand factor
(VIII C does not function in the absence of other parts)

In hemophilia A the VIII C portion is defective so there is lack of clotting activity but platelet function is normal.

In von Willebrand's disease VIII R: AG is missing so there is abnormal platelet function alongwith lack of clotting activity (VIII C portion does not function alone).

LABORATORY DIAGNOSIS OF HEMOPHILIA

- Activated partial thromboplastin time raised.
- Whole blood coagulation time prolonged in severe cases.
- Factor VIII clotting assay (VIII C) lowered.
- Immunological methods show normal VIII R: AG.
- Bleeding time and prothrombin time tests are normal
- Carrier females have half the clotting activity (VIII-C) expected for the level of VIII R: AG.

Christmas Disease (Hemophilia B)

- Activated partial thromboplastin time prolonged.
- Whole blood clotting time raised (in severe cases).
- Factor IX clotting assay diminished.
- Both bleeding time and prothrombin time tests are normal.

vON WILLEBRAND'S DISEASE

- Prolonged bleeding time.
- Low levels of factor VIII clotting activity (VIII C).
- Low levels of factor VIII related protein VIII R:AG.
- Defective platelet aggregation with ristocetin. The aggregation response to other agents (collagen, thrombin, adrenaline) is normal.
- In some patients there is defective retention of platelets in glass bead columns.

HEMORRHAGIC DISEASE OF NEWBORN

- The prothrombin time and activated partial thromboplastin time are both prolonged.
- The platelet counts and fibrinogen levels are normal with absent fibrin degradation products.

LUPUS ANTICOAGULANTS: BASIC CONCEPTS AND LABORATORY DIAGNOSIS

General Background

Lupus anticoagulants (LA) were first described in the year 1952 by Conley and Hartmann in two patients suffering from Systemic Lupus Erythematosus (SLE). It was given the name "Lupus" since it was initially recognized in patients with SLE and the name "Anticoagulant" because the two patients diagnosed as SLE developed bleeding complications. It is now clear that Lupus anticoagulant is also encountered in patients without SLE and is associated mainly with thrombosis rather than abnormal bleeding.

Patients with Lupus anticoagulants but without SLE can be categorised as follows:

- Patients presenting with venous and arterial thrombotic events for which no underlying cause may be apparent.
  Patients seeking medical attention for other disorders, discovered because of prolonged results with APTT in routine pre-operative evaluation of haemostasis status.
- Patients receiving drugs namely procainamide, chlorpromazine, quinidine, hydralazine and interferon
- Patients with a recent acute viral infection
- Patients with HIV infection

Though the terminology 'Lupus Anticoagulant' is a misnomer, it is still extremely popular and hence ISTH (International Society of Thrombosis and Haemostasis) has recommended the continued usage of the same. LA is neither a syndrome nor a disease but a laboratory phenomenon detected by prolonged results with phospholipid dependant clotbased assays.

Anti-Phospholipid Antibody-Lupus Anticoagulants

Anti-phospholipid antibody is an autoantibody directed against phospholipids, an important extracellular body constituent. Among the various types of anti-phospholipid antibodies, clinically important are Lupus anticoagulants (LA) and anti-Cardiolipin antibodies (ACL).

The clinical importance of LA and ACL is associated with their high frequency of occurrence in patients with unexplained thrombotic events in APS (Anti-phospholipid Syndrome).

Although LA and ACL may be found concurrently in patients with recurrent thromboemblic disease, they are not necessarily connected to each other. Recent studies have suggested that LA and ACL are separate antibody subgroups with different phospholipid binding characteristics.

Lupus anticoagulants are antibodies (IgG or IgM or both) that prolong phospholipid dependant coagulation assays by binding to the epitopes of the anionic phospholipid portion of the prothrombinase complex.

Prothrombinase is a complex of Factor Xa, Factor Va, anionic phospholipid and calcium, which converts prothrombin to thrombin in the coagulation pathway (Fig. 10.6).

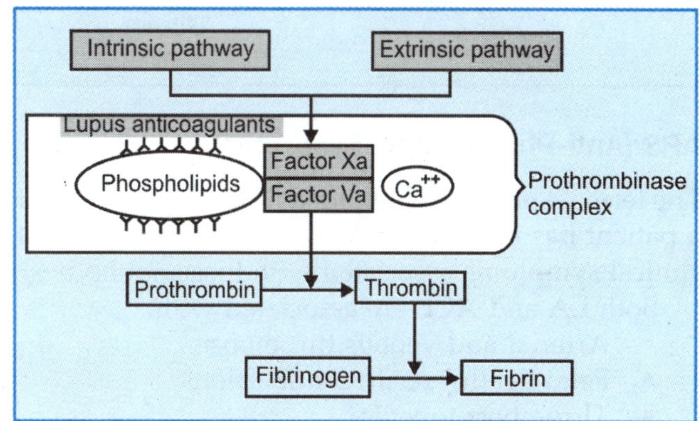

Fig. 10.6: LA section on prothrombinase complex

In vitro, Lupus anticoagulants prolong phospholipid dependant coagulation assays and exert their inhibitory effect probably by:

- Binding to epitopes of anionic phospholipids on the prothrombinase complex
- Blocking the calcium-mediated binding of Factor Xa and Factor Va to the phospholipids
- Reduce the conversion of prothrombin to thrombin, which leads to the prolongation of assay time

On the other hand, anti-Cardiolipin antibodies (ACL) are IgG or IgM or IgA class of antibodies directed against a complex consisting of β-2 Glycoprotein (β-2 GPI) bound to cardiolipin, an anionic phospholipid. The anti-Cardiolipin antibodies are usually detected by solid phase immunoassays such as ELISA based methods and employ cardiolipin and (β-2 GPI (as a cofactor) on the solid phase.

Lupus anticoagulants v/s anti-Cardiolipin antibodies

Parameters	*Lupus Anticoagulants*	*Anti-Cardiolipin antibodies*
Family	Anti-phospholipid	Anti-phospholipid
Autoantibody class	IgG or IgM	IgG or IgM or IgA
Autoantibody directed against	Anionic Phospholipids	Anionic Phospholipids
Phospholipid Binding Characteristics	Bind with anionic phospholipids on the prothrombinase complex	Binds to complesx of anionic phospholipid, cardiolipin and β-2 GPI
Method of Detection	Phospholipid dependent coagulation assays	ELISA/ immunoasays
Diagnostic relevance	Thrombosis, Recurrent fetal loss, Thrombocytopenia	Thrombosis, Recurrent fetal loss, Thrombo-cytopenia

APS (Anti-Phospholipid Syndrome)

The term "Anti-phospholipid syndrome" means that a patient has LA and/or ACL in addition to typical clinical symptoms associated with these antibodies.

Both LA and ACL are associated with:

- Arterial and venous thrombosis
- Fetal death/ recurrent abortions
- Thrombocytopenia

In **"Primary anti-phospholipid syndrome"**, no underlying identifiable disease is present for the thrombotic condition. In primary APS, the antibodies persist in the body regardless of therapeutic intervention.

In **"Secondary anti-phospholipid syndrome"**, an underlying disease/cause is present such as:

- An autoimmune disorder (e.g.: SLE)
- Malignancy
- Infection (bacterial or viral)
- Inflammation
- Drugs (e.g., chlorpromazine, procainamide, quinidine, hydralazine, interferon)

In the secondary syndrome, the APA's usually decline with successful management of the underlying disease; especially in autoimmune disease such as SLE.

Clinical findings with LA

Patients with Lupus anticoagulants usually present one of these clinical conditions:

Clinical Manifestations	*General Findings*
Venous thrombosis	• Deep venous thrombosis • Pulmonary embolism
Arterial thrombosis	• Myocardial infarction • Gangrene • Stroke
Thrombocytopenia	• Reduced Platelet count
Repeated abortions	• Intrauterine growth retardation • Intrauterine death of fetus
Neurologic symptoms	• Migraine • Chorea
Cutaneous symptoms	• Widespread cutaneous necrosis • Distal cutaneous ischaemia • Livedo reticularis • Leg ulcers

Clinically recognition of Lupus anticoagulants is important in the management of patients, with or without SLE, who experience unusual thrombotic events or thrombotic events at a younger age than expected.

In patients with SLE or related autoimmune disorders there is a definite increased incidence of thrombocytopenia associated with the presence of the Lupus anticoagulants.

Another major clinical manifestation associated with Lupus anticoagulant is fetal loss or a history of recurrent first trimester abortions, second or third trimester intrauterine death. The probable mechanism by which fetal loss occurs can be attributed to thrombosis of placental vessels and placental infarction. The recurrent abortions can occur in patients with or without SLE.

In summary, the patient groups that need to be tested for LA are:

- Patients experiencing unexplained recurrent thrombotic events
- Patients presenting with thrombotic events at a younger age than expected
- Patients with SLE
- Pregnant patients with recurrent abortions or intrauterine death of fetus
- Patients seeking medical attention for other disorders, accidentally discovered by prolonged APTT time in routine pre-operative haemostasis status

Pathophysiological Mechanism of Thrombosis

A strong correlation exists between the occurrence of Lupus anticoagulants and high incidence of thrombotic disease. The exact pathophysiological mechanism accounting for the frequency of thrombosis in patients with Lupus anticoagulants is not clear but various studies suggest that there is more than one mechanism causing thrombosis in LA patients (Fig. 10.7).

The probable mechanisms of thrombosis can be attributed as follows:

- Since a number of patients with Lupus anticoagulants and thrombosis have some degree of thrombocytopenia, platelet activation is thought to play an important role in arterial thrombosis. In patients with Lupus anticoagulants and concomittant Antithrombin III or Protein C deficiency, there is an increased risk of venous thrombosis.
- In patients with SLE, the mechanism of thrombosis is probably mediated by autoantibodies that affect the endothelial cell function.
- In normal population, the vessel wall provides a non thrombogenic surface, as PGI_2 (Prostacyclin) secreted by the endothelial cells is a potent vasodilator and inhibits platelet aggregation. In some patients it has been observed that the Lupus anticoagulant interfere with the secretion of PGI_2 from the vessel walls. Thus an impaired synthesis or deficient release of PGI_2 from endothelial cells could account for an increased risk of thrombosis.
- Other possible mechanisms by which Lupus anticoagulants might mediate thrombosis include,
  - Inhibition of Protein C activation thereby resulting in impaired degradation of Factor Va by activated Protein C
  - Decreased fibrinolytic activity
  - Prekallikrein inhibition
  - Inhibition of antithrombin III activity

LUPUS ANTICOAGULANTS AND BLEEDING COMPLICATIONS

Bleeding complications in patients with Lupus anticoagulants is a rare phenomenon. But recent studies indicate that a subset of patients with LA were associated, interestingly, with bleeding complications. A reason for this rare phenomenon remained obscure until some workers demonstrated that patients with LA presenting bleeding complications also exhibited prothrombin deficiency.

As per their observations, the probable mechanism of LA interaction with prothrombin molecule can be summarised as follows:

- Lupus anticoagulants bind to epitope of prothrombin molecule not actively involved in the coagulation pathway.
- The LA-prothrombin complex so formed is cleared rapidly from the circulation giving rise to prothrombin deficiency, which results in bleeding complcations.

The aforesaid phenomenon was coined as "Hypoprothrombinemia—Lupus anticoagulant" syndrome. Studies point out that clinically it may also be important to evaluate the prothrombin time when screening patients for LA.

Phospholipid Dependence of Lupus Anticoagulants

It is now clear that Lupus anticoagulants are immunoglobulins of IgG class or IgM class or both, that prolong phospholipid dependant clotbased assays. The phospholipid dependence of Lupus anticoagulants in the *in vitro* assay systems has been extensively studied and convincing evidence of the same may be summarised as follows:

- The Lupus anticoagulants react against negatively-charged phospholipids and are able to inhibit the binding of Factor X and prothrombin to

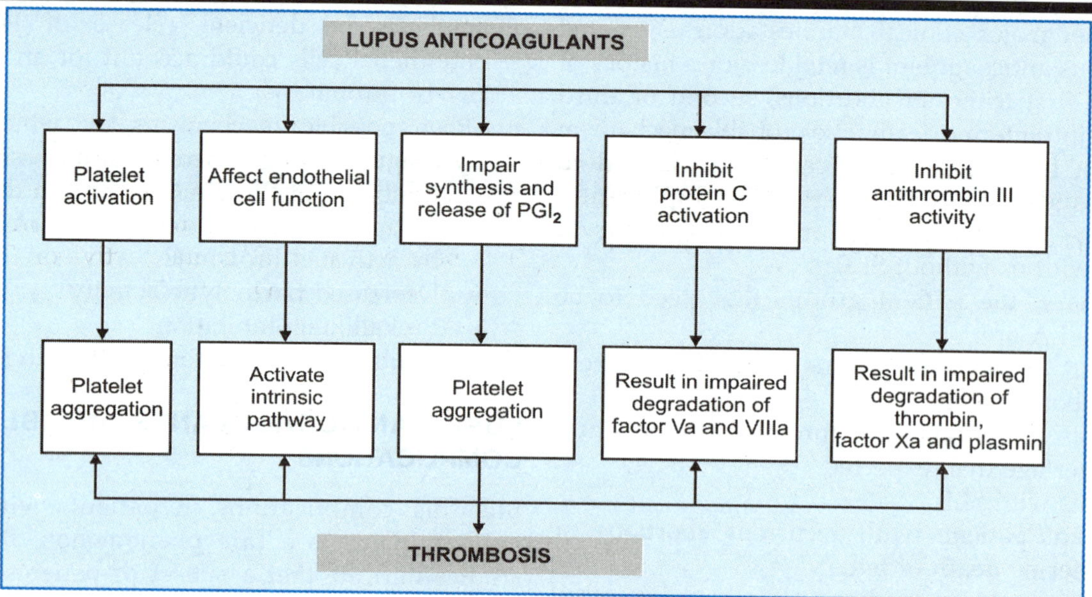

Fig. 10.7: LA and Thrombosis

the procoagulant phospholipid surface, thereby accounting for prolongation of phospholipid dependant clotbased assays (Fig. 10.8).

- Reducing the phospholipid component of clotting mixture potentiates the Lupus anticoagulants effect. Thus, the most sensitive tests for detecting the phospholipid inhibitor contain limited amount of phospholipids.
- Increasing the procoagulant phospholipid in clotting mixture diminishes the effect of anticoagulant (neutralization effect) and corrects the abnormal clotting time so observed initially. This confirms the phospholipid dependancy of Lupus anticoagulants.

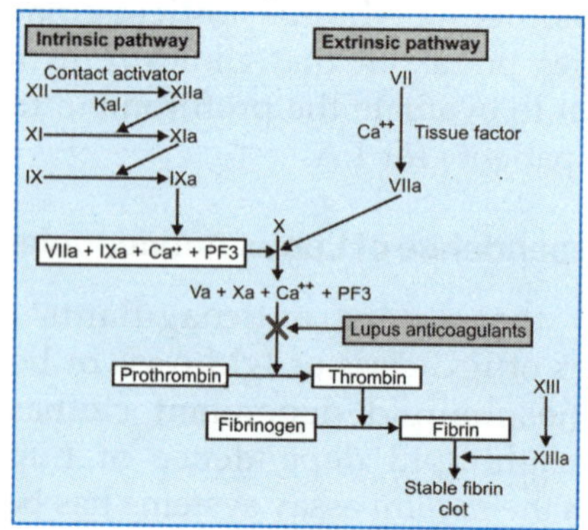

Fig. 10.8: In vitro LA action

Laboratory Diagnosis of Lupus Anticoagulants

In the past a number of different tests have been proposed and used for the diagnosis of Lupus anticoagulants.

The traditional screening methods used for the laboratory diagnosis of Lupus anticoagulants can be broadly classified as follows:

- Immunological assays
- Clot-based assays incorporating phospholipids in the reagent system

Immunological Assays

Patients with Lupus anticoagulants may also show the presence of other anti-phospholipid antibodies. The most frequent finding is the presence of anti-Cardiolipin antibodies. The commonly employed method is the ELISA technique where the solid phase is coated with cardiolipin and β-2 GPI (as a cofactor). The ELISA method detects IgM, IgG and IgA class of anti-Cardiolipin antibodies. An important point to note is that Lupus anticoagulants and anti-Cardiolipin antibodies differ in their phospholipid binding characteristics, hence detection of anti-Cardiolipin antibodies is not specific for the presence of Lupus anticoagulants though they can be present in the same patient.

CLOT-BASED ASSAYS

APTT (Activated Partial Thromboplastin Time)

Since Lupus anticoagulants bind to the phospholipid complex they do prolong phospholipid based coagulation assays. Logically the activated partial thromboplastin time (APTT) is prolonged and this property has been used for the detection of LA using APTT reagents.

In the context of LA detection, the APTT test has certain shortcomings:

— An important variable related to the suitability of APTT reagents in the detection of Lupus anticoagulants is the composition of phospholipids used in the reagent system. Different reagents have varying sensitivity for the presence of Lupus anticoagulants on the basis of their phospholipid composition.
  The APTT test is affected by the presence of specific inhibitors to Factor VIII, IX and XI. In order to rule out the presence of inhibitors usually mixing studies are performed. In mixing studies a 1:1 or 1:4 (Normal plasma: Patient plasma) is used. Failure to correct the prolongation of clotting time using the mixing studies indicates the presence of Lupus anticoagulants.

— The APTT test is also the test of choice for monitoring heparin therapy. This reduces the specificity of the APTT to LA. The presence of heparin can be ruled out by using a thrombin time test. If thrombin time test shows normal values, then the sample does not contain heparin. But if the thrombin time test is abnormal, then heparin neutralisation test has to be used which includes protamine sulphate. In this test, various concentrations of protamine sulphate are added to plasma before the addition of thrombin reagent. When protamine sulphate neutralises all the heparin present, the clotting time reverts to normal value.

TTI (Tissue Thromboplastin Inhibition Test)

The Tissue Thromboplastin Inhibition test utilizes a dilute PT reagent. The results are expressed as ratio of patient values to normal control values.

The TTI test is affected by numerous variables.

— Choice of "Normal" reference plasma is the most critical variable, because depending on the laboratory the choice of reference plasma could be a lyophilized plasma, a frozen plasma pool or fresh plasma. The ratio of patient to normal can change according to the choice of "normal" plasma.

— Species and tissue origin of thromboplastin can affect the test results as different sources of thromboplastin have varying sensitivity and responsiveness.

— Some IgM Lupus anticoagulants do not prolong the TTI test.

KCT (Kaolin Clotting Time)

KCT is similar to APTT, the difference being that KCT reagent is devoid of phospholipids and incorporates Kaolin as contact activator. The test is performed on a range of mixture of normal and patient's plasma. Different patterns of response are obtained indicating the presence of Lupus anticoagulants or the deficiency of one or more coagulation factors.

The KCT test though sensitive is not specific for LA, additionally:

— It cannot be automatized

— The test shows prolonged results with Factor VIII, IX, XI & XII deficiency or corresponding inhibitors

— The test is also highly-sensitive for the presence of heparin.

PNP (Platelet Neutralization Procedure)

In PNP test platelets substitute the phospholipid extract of the APTT reagent. The platelets have the ability to adsorb the Lupus anticoagulant and this property is used in the PNP test.

If a sample shows initial prolonged time with APTT reagent, then it is further tested with dilute APTT reagent incorporating platelet substitute. Since platelets have the ability to adsorb LA, a reduced clotting time with dilute APTT reagent indicates the presence of LA. But if an inhibitor is directed against specific coagulation factor, the clotting time continues to show prolonged values.

The PNP test though useful did not gain wide usage:

— Due to limited stability the platelet preparations loose their activities on storage hence do not show reproducible results.

— They cannot differentiate between Lupus anticoagulants and Factor VIII inhibitors.

Hexagonal Phase Phospholipids

The hexagonal phospholipid neutralisation assay is a dilute APTT reagent, which contains phospholipids in hexagonal steric configuration. The principle of this method is same as the PNP test.

The major drawback of this test is that hexagonal phospholipids do not occur *in vivo*. Hence, the authenticity of this test principle for detecting the presence of Lupus anticoagulants has been recently challenged.

Recommendations and Criteria for the Diagnosis of Lupus Anticoagulants

The Lupus Anticoagulant/Anti-phospholipid Antibody subcommittee of ISTH (International Society of Thrombosis and Haemostasis) first published its recommendations and criteria for diagnosis of Lupus anticoagulants in 1991.

Subsequently, the subcommittee further reviewed:

- Important advances in the understanding of Lupus anticoagulants
- New assays for the identification of Lupus anticoagulants
- New information concerning the technical aspects of test performance.
- In 1995, the subcommittee published the revised recommendations and criteria for the laboratory diagnosis of Lupus anticoagulants.

Current Recommendations of the ISTH

- Both patient and normal plasma should be as platelet free as possible; the platelet count should be less than 10 x 10^9/l. This applies for testing on fresh plasmas, preparation of frozen samples and preparation of pooled normal plasma. Filtration appears to be an excellent method for the preparation of platelet free plasma for LA testing but may interfere with testing of other coagulation factors. Ultracentrifugation may be performed carefully to avoid formation of platelet debris. Alternately atleast a two step centrifugation of properly collected blood at the correct speed is also acceptable.
- Two or more tests should be used to screen for diagnosis of LA. At least one of these tests should be based on a low phospholipid concentration e.g.
  - — dRVVT
  - — KCT
  - — dAPTT
  - — dPT

  The assays should represent different principle for example, a dRVVT and a dAPTT.
- Inhibitor activity should be documented by the effect of patient plasma on pooled normal plasma. This step can be incorporated into the initial screening procedure. The sensitivity and specificity of the ratio of patient to normal plasma should be established before it is used routinely.
- A diagnosis of a LA should not be made on the basis of multiple abnormal screening assays and mixing studies alone. Confirmatory studies need to be performed to document the phospholipid dependence of the inhibitor.
- Confirmatory assay should be based in the method giving an abnormal screening assay. For example, if the dRVVT is abnormal, then a confirmatory assay based on the dRVVT should be used.
- Routine clotting tests, such as PT and APTT, should be performed to evaluate the possibility of other coagulation disorders that may interfere with the LA methodology. If the chosen method for screening or confirmation is known to be sensitive to heparin, a thrombin time may be helpful in ruling out its presence.
- Solid phase assays for anti-phospholipid antibodies such as ELISA (e.g. anti-Cardiolipin antibodies) although frequently positive in patients with LA's should not be considered as a confirmatory procedure for LA activity.
- Factor assays should be performed whenever there is suspicion of a specific factor deficiency or inhibitor. Two or more dilutions of the patient plasma should be evaluated in any factor assay.
- The term Lupus anticoagulant should be retained until the pathophysiology of these inhibitors is more fully delineated.

Based on these recommendations, a flow chart (Fig. 10.9) was established thereby assisting the laboratorians to establish a routine approach in the diagnosis of LA's and improve testing standards in the detection of LA's.

Scientific Subcommittee Criteria for the Laboratory Diagnosis of Lupus Anticoagulants

In order to make a diagnosis of LA; the test sample should show each of the following:

- Prolongation of at least one phospholipid dependant clot-based assay.
- Evidence of inhibitory activity shown by the effect of patient plasma on pooled normal plasma.
- Evidence that the inhibitory activity is dependant on concentration of phospholipids. This may be achieved by addition or alteration of phospholipids/ hexagonal phase phospholipids/ platelet/platelet vesicles in the test system.

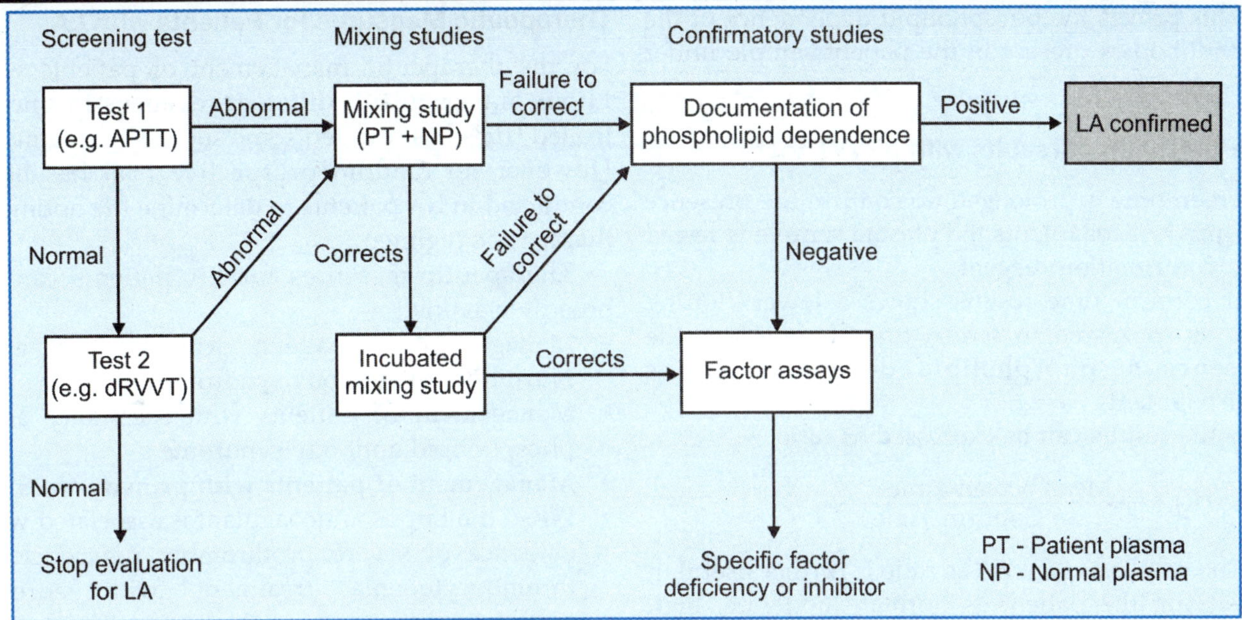

Fig. 10.9: Flow chart for laboratory diagnosis of LA

- LA's must be carefully distinguished from other coagulopathies that may give similar laboratory results or may occur concurrently with LA's. Specific factor assays and the clinical history may be helpful in differentiating LA's from these other possibilities.

dRVVT: The test of choice for screening and confirmation of LA

The dilute Russell's viper venom time test (dRVVT) first became popular following publication by Thiagarajan et al. in 1986. Dr. Exner further simplified and standardised this method subsequently. In general dRVVT based tests comprise of:

— Screening reagent, containing limited amount of phospholipids with RVV (Russell's Viper Venom)

— Confirmation reagent, containing additional phospholipids with same amount of Russell's Viper Venom, to confirm the presence of phospholipid dependant Lupus anticoagulants.

Principle of dRVVT for LA detection

Russell's Viper Venom directly activates Factor V and Factor X in presence of phospholipids and calcium ions, bypassing Factor VII of the extrinsic pathway and the contact and antihaemophilic factors of the intrinsic pathway (Fig. 10.10).

In normal plasma, in the absence of Lupus anticoagulants, Factor V and Factor X is directly activated by Russell's Viper Venom, which in presence of phospholipids and calcium ion leads to clot formation.

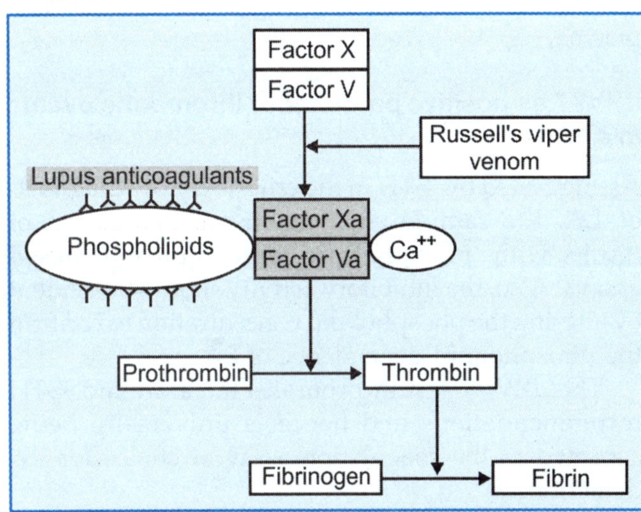

Fig. 10.10: Principle of the dRVVT test

In patients with LA, autoantibodies bind the epitopes of reagent phospholipids thereby preventing the activation of prothrombinase complex. This results in a prolongation of clotting time with screening reagent. The confirmation reagent incorporates additional phospholipids to neutralise the LA. Once LA are neutralised the clot formation proceeds relatively uninterrupted achieving a lower clotting time.

This proves the phospholipid dependence of the autoantibodies present in the patient sample under test.

Interpretation of results with dRVVT test

If Screen time is prolonged, to confirm the presence of lupus anticoagulants the plasma sample is tested with confirmation reagent.

If confirm time results shows a lower clotting time as compared to screen time, it indicates the presence of phospholipid dependant Lupus Anticoagulants.

Also the results can be expressed as ratio,

$$\text{Ratio (R)} = \frac{\text{Mean Screen Time}}{\text{Mean Confirm Time}}$$

The results expressed, as ratio is further useful in classifying the patient as normal, moderate, high and very high LA.

If results of the ratio are borderline, mixing studies may be done further with the sample specimen. The mixing studies should be carried out with a 50:50 mixture of test plasma and normal plasma.

dRVVT as positive predictor of thrombotic events in APS

As suggested by ISTH in the criteria for the diagnosis of LA, the sample should show prolongation of results with **phospholipid-dependant clot-based assays.** Also, the inhibitory activity should be evident by altering the phospholipid concentration to confirm the phospholipid dependence of LA.

The dRVVT test incorporates the aforesaid ISTH recommendations and hence is universally being accepted as the coagulation assay of choice for LA detection.

The assay utilizes screening and confirmation reagent thereby:

- Indicating the phospholipid dependence of LA
- Achieving maximum sensitivity for the presence of LA.

The clinical value of any diagnostic assay is directly proportional to its positive and negative predictive value. dRVVT in independent studies has proven to be 100% specific for presumed thrombotic events, miscarriage and pulmonary hypertension as compared to solid phase immunoassays which had lower clinical relevance (83%).

Therapeutic Measures for Patients with LA

For the therapeutic management of patients with Lupus anticoagulant, different regimens in uncontrolled trials has resulted some success in treatment. However no random prospective trial has been conducted in LA patients to determine the optimum therapeutic regimen.

Therapeutic measures for LA patients can be broadly classified as,

- Management of patients with primary anti-phospholipid antibody syndrome
- Management of patients with secondary anti-phospholipid antibody syndrome
- **Management of patients with primary 'APS'**
- When the Lupus anticoagulant is associated with evidence of severe prothrombin deficiency or thrombocytopenia treatment with adrenal corticosteroids is indicated.
- Presence of Lupus anticoagulant and thrombosis is guided by the fact that recurrence is common. Hence for patients presenting with venous thrombosis, long term anticoagulation (probably for life) with oral anticoagulants is indicated. For arterial thrombosis low dose aspirin is indicated.
- In management of pregnant patients with or without SLE and Lupus anticoagulants the exact regimen to be used till date is not clear. Initially some workers reported successful pregnancy out comes in patients with LA by treating with prednisolone and low dose aspirin. However long term, high dose corticosteroids during pregnancy are associated with significant side effects namely:
  - — severe preclampia
  - — infections
  - — gestational diabetes
  - — osteoporosis

Recently some workers have suggested the use of low dose aspirin and low dose heparin with some success in pregnancy outcomes. Thus, different therapeutic regimens in uncontrolled trials have resulted in some success, but no careful randomised trials have yet been conducted to arrive at an optimum and safe therapeutic regimen that can be universally adapted.

- **Management of Patients with Secondary 'APS'**
- When the Lupus anticoagulant is present in patients with an underlying autoimmune disease,

management with appropriate immunosuppressive therapy is indicated.

dRVVT for Screening and Confirmation of Lupus Anticoagulants LADS, (Courtesy: Tulip Group of Companies)

Summary

Lupus Anticoagulants (LA) are autoantibodies against the anionic phospholipid portion of prothrombinase. Prothrombinase is a complex of factor Xa, factor Va, phospholipid and calcium ions involved in the conversion of prothrombin to thrombin in the coagulation pathway. The autoantibodies produced are of lgG class or IgM class or cloth. As these type of antibodies were first detected in-patients with systemic lupus erythematosus (SLE) they were named LA. LA's prolong phospholipid-dependent tests such as the activated partial thromboplastin time (APTT) and kaolin clotting time (KCT). The name anticoagulant is a misnomer since patients do not have a bleeding tendency. Instead there is a clear association of thrombc-embolism. LA is also an important cause at recurrent abortions in women. Since these antibodies are also found in-patients with SLE (Systemic lupus erythematosus), detection of LA is important in management of patients with or without SLE experiencing unusual thrombotic events and habitual abortions.

The dilute Russell's Viper Venom test (dRVVT) was first introduced by Thiagarajan et al in 1986. dRVVT is a simple, sensitive and specific assay for detection of LA. Since Russell's Viper Venom activates factor X directly, dRVVT is more specific for LA than APTT. Results are affected neither by contact factor abnormalities nor by factor VIII, factor XI deficiencies or corresponding inhibitors.

Principle

Russell's Viper Venom directly activates factor X in the presence of phospholipid and calcium ions, bypassing factor VII of the extrinsic pathway and the contact and antihaemophilic factors of the intrinsic pathway. In normal plasma in the absence of lupus anticoagulants, factor X is directly activated by Russell's Viper Venom, which in presence of phospholipid and calcium ion leads to clot formation. In-patients with LA, autoantibodies bind the epitopes of reagent phospholipids thereby preventing the activation of prothrombinase complex. This results in a prolongation of clotting lime with SCREEN reagent. The CONFIRM reagent incorporates additional phospholipids to neutralize LA, thereby achieving a lower clotting time, thus proving the phospholipid dependence of the autoantibodies.

Reagents Provided with the Kit

TULIP'S LA Detection System comprises of a 3-reagent set for screening and confirmation of Lupus anticoagulants. LA SCREEN (Reagent 1) and LA CONFIRM (Reagent 2) are lyophillised preparations containing Russell's Viper Venom enriched with phospholipid at different concentrations, sufficient for performing 10 assays. Both LA SCREEN and LA CONFIRM reagents contain 0.01 per cent thimerosal as preservative. Calcium Chloride (Reagents 3, 0.025M) contains heparin neutralizing substance, making the reagent system insensitive to the presence of heparin upto 0.4 U/ml. Calcium chloride reagent is intended for use with LA SCREEN and LA CONFIRM reagents, the quantity being 2.5 ml sufficient for performing 20 assays.

Note

Since SCREEN and CONFIRM reagents of the same lot are optimized as a system, it is important that reagents from the same lot are used for accurate and reproducible results.

Storage and Stability

(1) Store the reagent at 2-8° C. DO NOT FREEZE. (2) The shelf life of the reagents is as per the expiry date mentioned on the reagent vial label. (3). Reconstituted reagents can be used for 5 days when stored at 2-8°C, provided it is not contaminated and handled aseptically. (4) It is strongly recommended that enough reconstituted reagents should be retrieved for the days use and the unused reagent should be immediately replaced to 2-8°C.

Additional Material Required

10 mm × 75 mm glass test tubes, water bath at constant temperature of 37ºC, stop watch, 100 μl precision pipettes, scrupulously clean and dry micropipette tips, distilled water, 1ml precision pipette.

Reagent Preparation

Bring the LA SCREEN reagent and LA CONFIRM reagent to room temperature (25-30°C) prior to reconstitution. LA SCREEN reagent and LA CONFIRM reagent are reconstituted with 1 ml de-ionized, distilled water each as follows: (1) Add 1 ml of distilled water to the lyophilized LA SCREEN reagent and LA CONFIRM reagent. (2) Gently mix to dissolve. (3) Keep for 15-20 minutes at room temperature (20-30°C) and mix again gently ensuring complete re-suspension of the lyophilized material. (4) Thorough mixing should be ensured before withdrawing material every time for test purposes.

Sample Preparation

Mix nine parts of freshly collected patient's blood with one part of Trisodium citrate (3.2 percent). Buffered citrate containing 0.05M HEPES buffer (pH 7.0) in a plastic or siliconized tubes is preferable (such as PROFACT). Centrifuge as soon as possible after collection at $\geq$1500 g for 15 minutes to obtain PPP. Store in capped tubes at 4°C, and use within 4 hours of collection. If the samples are to be frozen for subsequent testing, the plasma must be centrifuged again or filtered through a 0.2 μm filter to remove platelets (to below $20 \times 10^9/l$) as these can otherwise shorten the SCREEN TIME.

- Clotted samples should be discarded.
- Erroneous results may also occur in-patients with abnormal haematocrits, as the plasma to citrate concentration in these samples is not optimal.

Test Procedure

Bring all reagents to room temperature (25-30°C) before prewarming at 37°C for testing purpose.

(1) Aspirate enough quantity of reagent from Calcium Chloride reagent vial for immediate testing requirements in a thoroughly clean and dry test tube. Incubate the tube at 37°C for 10 minutes. (2) Place 0.1 ml of LA SCREEN reagent in a clean and dry test tube (ensure thorough mixing before withdrawing material for testing purpose). (3) To this tube add 0.1 ml of plasma (PPP). Shake the tube gently to mix the contents and incubate for 1 -2 minutes at 37°C. (4) Finally to this tube add 0.1 ml of Calcium chloride (prewarmed at 37°C for 10 minutes) and simultaneously start the stopwatch. (5) Stop the stop-watch as soon as the clot formation begins. Record the time in seconds. (6) This is the SCREEN TIME for the plasma specimen. If SCREEN TIME is less than 45 seconds it indicates absence of LA and there is no need to perform CONFIRMATORY test (7) When the SCREEN TIME is more than 45 seconds repeat the test procedure for the sample using CONFIRM reagent. Repeat the steps 2 to 6 for testing sample plasma specimen using LA CONFIRM reagent.

It is important that SCREEN TIME and CONFIRM TIME on a sample are performed simultaneously for comparative studies.

It is recommended that sample should be run in duplicate with SCREEN and CONFIRM reagents and the mean time may be used for arriving 1 at the results.

Interpretation of Results

The normal expected values for SCREEN TIME is 28-45 sec.

The normal expected values for CONFIRM TIME is 28-40 sec.

TULIP'S LA Detection system is based upon the ratio of clotting time using LA SCREEN reagent and clotting time of the same sample using LA CONFIRM reagent

$$\text{Ratio(R)} = \frac{\text{Mean Screen Time}}{\text{Mean Confirm Time}}$$

Ratio (R)	*R<1.3*	*R = 1.5-1.8*	*R = 1.8-2.4*	*R>2.4*
Interpretation of results	Normal	Moderate LA	High LA	Very High LA

If results are borderline, (ratio of 1.3-1.4) mixing studies may be done further wilh the sample specimen. These tests should be carried out on a 50:50 mixture of test plasma and normal plasma.

Interpretation of results with mixing studies

LA SCREEN (Reagent 1)		LA CONFIRM (Reagent 2)		
				Interpretation of Resutts
Patient plasma	50:50 mixture of patient and normal plasma	Patient plasma	50:50 mixture of patient and normal plasma	
N		N	N	LA absent
Ab.N	Ab.N	N	N	LA present
Ab.N	N	Ab.N	N	Factor deficient
Ab.N	Ab.N	Ab.N	N	LA + factor deficient
Ab.N	Ab.N	Ab.N	Ab.N	Other inhibitor

N- Normal, Ab.N- Abnormal

- Prolonged Screen Time and Confirm Time are also obtained with plasma samples of patients with factor II, V and X deficiencie as well on warfarin therapy. These defects correct on addition of normal plasma. In such cases individual assays of factor II, V and X sould be performed.
- Plasma sample that has LA along with factor deficiencies remains abnormal in SCREEN TIME, showing only partial correction of the defect on mixing. Such plasma yields abnormal CONFIRM TIME only in neat plasma due to factor deficiency and not the LA.
- If normal plasma corrects neither the screen time nor the confirm time then an inhibitor against any of the factors II, V and may be suspected and should show an abnormal PT result also.

Remarks

1. Each laboratory should use known platelet depleted normal (also available with TULIP) and abnormal LA control plasmas (also available with TULIP) with each test series for validation of results.
2. Each laboratory should establish the acceptable control values and normal range.
3. Incorrect mixture of blood and Trisodium citrate, insufficient prewarming of plasma and reagent contaminated reagents, glassware, etc. are potential sources of error.
4. Since the LA test functions optimally at 37°C ± 0 5°C, temperature of all equipment must be calibrated daily.
5. Glasswares and cuvettes used in the test must be scrupulously clean and free from even traces of acids/alkalies or detergents.
6. Since the test uses platelet poor plasma, each laboratory must calibrate the necessary force and time required during centrifugation to yield PPP. Contamination of plasma with excess platelets could lead to erroneous results.
7. It is recommended that results of the tests should be correlated with clinical findings to arrive at the final diagnosis.
8. Thorough mixing and homogenization of reconstituted LA SCREEN and LA CONFIRM reagent suspension before use is important to achieve accurate and consistent results.

LA REFERENCE PLASMA FOR LA TEST (Courtesy: Tulip Group of Companies)

Summary

LA reference plasma has been specifically formulated for calibration and quality control of reagents used for dRVVT based LA detection test. In routine basis, it is often difficult to get abnormal LA samples. Thus LA reference plasma would help each laboratory determine its acceptable control values and reference range with reference plasma of known values.

Reagent

LA reference plasma is a freeze-dried plasma preparation with known values expressed as ratio of SCREEN TIME to CONFIRM TIME for dRVVT based LA test.

Each lot of LA reference plasma is assayed using TULIP LA Detection System reagents along with platelet depleted fresh normal plasma.

Principle

Russell's viper venom directly activates factor X in the presence of phospholipid and calcium ions, bypassing factor VII of the extrinsic pathway and the contact and antihemophilic factors of the intrinsic pathway. In normal plasma in the absence of lupus anticoagulants, factor X is directly activated by Russell's Viper Venom, which in presence of phospholipid and calcium ion leads to clot formation. With LA reference plasma, autoantibodies bind the epitopes of reagent phospholipids thereby preventing the activation of prothrombinase complex. This results in a prolongation of clotting time with SCREEN reagent. The CONFIRM reagent incorporates additional phospholipids to neutralize LA, thereby achieving a lower clotting time.

Reagent Storage and Stability

1. Unopened vials should be stored at 2-8°C and are stable upto the expiry date mentioned on the vial labels.
2. If the reconstituted LA reference plasma is kept at 20-30°C it should be used within 3 hours.
3. If the reconstituted reference plasma is to be frozen for subsequent testing, the shelf life of LA reference plasma is 48 hours at –20°C.

Note

1. In vitro diagnostic reagent for laboratory and professional use only. NOT FOR MEDICINAL USE.
2. Thorough mixing and homogenization of reconstituted reagent is advisable for achieving accurate and consistent results.

Preparation of the Reagent

1. Bring the LA reference plasma vial to room temperature prior to reconstitution.
2. Reconstitute the LA reference plasma with 0.5 ml of sterile distilled water.
3. Gently mix the reagent at an interval of 1 minute for 5 minutes.
4. Let the reconstituted plasma stand for 10 minutes to attain equilibrium.
5. The reconstituted reagent so obtained can be used for testing purpose immediately.

Test Procedure

1. Use the reconstituted LA reference plasma in the same manner for testing patient sample using dRVVT based LA test.
2. Platelet depleted fresh normal control plasma should also be used concurrently for testing purpose.
3. For estimation of ratio of SCREEN TIME to CONFIRM TIME refer package insert of TULIP LA Detection System.

Remarks

1. Incorrect mixing of LA reference plasma and reagent, insufficient prewarming of plasma/reagent, contaminated reagents and glassware etc. are a potential source of error.
2. Due to inter-laboratory variation in techniques, standardization of test procedure and calibration of equipment, some variation from the assigned may be expected.

AUTOMATION IN COAGULATION ANALYSIS HEMOSTAR

Sleek, user-friendly coagulation analyser based on turbo-phototometric detection of clotbased assays. Hemostar has 10 in-built incubation positions for Sample and 1 location for reagents (Fig. 10.11).

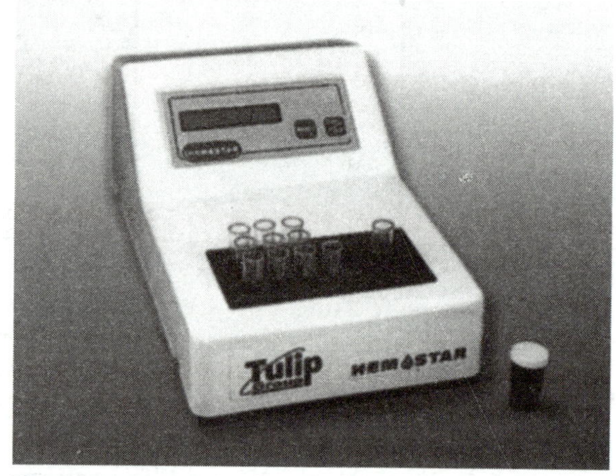

Fig. 10.11: Hemostar *(Courtesy: Tulip group of companies)*

- It allows the user to make all baisc tests for the analysis of plasmatic hemostatic phase, e.g. Quick, test (PT), aPTT, TT, Fibrinogen, defective factors, etc.
- It is a totally open instrument to be used with all kinds of quality reagents, simply by following the producers instructions.
- It includes a magnetic stirrer system in order to mix well the reagents and plasma.
- Optical group: Made up of a Wolfram lamp at low voltage and long self life, an optical light pass, the reaction cell holder and a solid state photocell which registers all absorption changes produced.
- Thermostatic block: Thermostated device at 37° C ± 0.1°C with magnetic stirrer motor built-in
- Screen: Four digit indicator with tenth of second precision, thermostatic block control temperature LED (37°C) and two operation keys, the chronometer can be used seperately to control incubation time.

- Tests: Quick Test (PT), aPTT, TT, Fibrinogen, deficiency factors, etc.
- Power requirements: AC 220 V. 50 Hz 120 VA
- Dimensions: 180 × 300 × 140 nm
- Weight: 2, 3 kg

Technical Features

System	• Automatic Single channel Coagulometer based on Turbo-photometric clot detection system.
Measurement	• Opto-mechanical measuring system. • Automatic start of measurement on addition of reagent/sample for precise result. • On screen digital chronometer to measure tenth of a second accurately.
Sensitivity	• Highly-sensitive in all measuring range because of Opto-mechanical measuring system (combination of optical controls with mechanical movement of magnetic stirrers).
Incubator	• Inbuilt Incubator (solid state) fixed at 37°C. • Incubator lodges 10 reaction cuvettes and one reaction vial.
Testing Mode	• PT, APTT, TT, Fibrinogen and Factor Assays.
General	
Lamp Source	Low voltage tungsten lamp
Detector	IR detector.
Motor	For stirring action of magnetic stirrer.
Display	Back illuminated LCD with single row and 14 characters.
Power supply	220V, 50 Hz/60 Hz.
Power consumption	50VA.
Serial output	RS 232 standard.
Working temperature	15° to 35°C.
Dimensions	18 × 30 × 40 cm.
Weight	2.2 Kgs.

HEMOSTAR XF

Single channel coagulometer with turbo-photometric clot detection principle with an Opto-mechanical which improves sensitivity of detecting weak fibrin polymers. Hemostar XF has 10 open locations which enables to perform PT, APTT, TT, Fibrinogen assays and factors assays. This walk away plug and play system has been designed to make complicated clotting analysis of hemostasis system into a simple error free task (Fig. 10.12).

- Single-channel coagulometer, fully-controlled by built-in microprocessor.
- Turbophotometric detection of fibrin polymer formation (clots)
- Solid state thermostat set at 37°C
- Keyboard for programming and data entry.
- Digital control and results display.
- Integral printer for easier transcription of results
- Enables performance of all types of hemostasis plasma phase studies and particularly: QUICK, a PPT, TT, FIRBRINOGEN, FACTOR STUDIES.

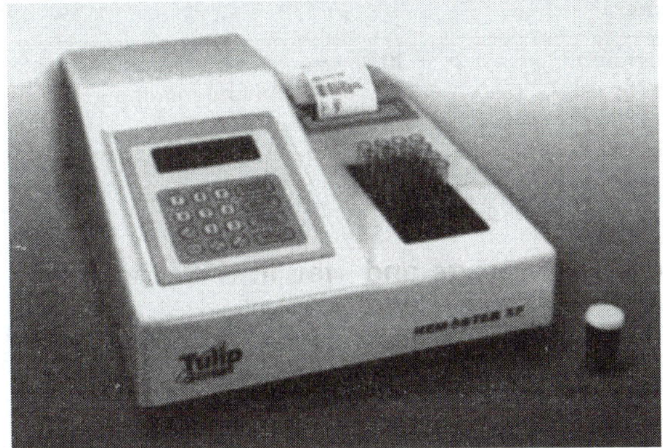

Fig. 10.12: Hemostar XF *(Courtesy: Tulip group of companies)*

- Optics: Low voltage photometry lamp
- Truncated cone reading cell
- Photofeed detection
- Magnetic stirrer motor
- Thermostat: Metal block thermostatted to 37°C ± 0.1°C by solid state elements
- Capacity for 10 cells and a reagent bottle
- Programming: The CLOT 1A has a permanent memory for programming the parameters for each coagulation technique. These parameters remain stored in the memory until they are off reprogrammed, even when the unit is switched
- The keypad enables the user to sequentially access the programming and speeds up date entry during routine use of the instrument
- The digital display functions as a programming and results monitor
- Results: Displayed on the screen and in printout form, containing all parameters and the relevant identification number
- Size: 30 × 35 × cm
- Weight: 3,700 kg
- Power supply: 220 V 50 Hz 100 VA

Technical Features

System	• Microprocessor controlled automatic Single channel Coagulometer based on Turbo-photometric clot detection system.
Measurement	• Opto-mechanical measuring system. • Automatic start of measurement on addition of reagent/ sample for precise result. • On screen digital chronometer to measure tenth of a second accurately.
Sensitivity	• Highly-sensitive in all measuring range because of Opto-mechanical measuring system (combination of optical controls with mechanical movement of magnetic stirrers).
Incubator	• Inbuilt Incubator (solid state) fixed at 37°C. • Having 19 incubation positions.
Testing Mode	• PT, APTT, TT, Fibrinogen and Factor Assays.

General	
Programming	10 Locations for programming parameters.
Key board	Key board for programming and data entry.
Printer	Built in quiet thermal printer for direct reporting of result in INR, per cent Activity, PTR and APTT ratio.
Serial output	RS 232 standard.
Lamp Source	Low voltage tungsten lamp
Detector	IR detector.
Motor	For stirring action of magnetic stirrer.
Display	Back illuminated LCD with 4 rows of 20 characters.
Working temperature	15° to 35° C.
Power supply	220V, 50 Hz, 60 Hz.
Power consumption	100VA.
Dimensions	31 × 15 × 35 cm.
Weight	3.7 kgs.

CoaLAB 6000

Fully-automated compact and versatile bench top coagulation analyser for clotting assays based on the patented Turbodensitometric principle of clot detection. CoaLAB 6000 is engineered to operate in random access mode for PT, APTT and fibrinogen with an option for batch and stat mode. CoaLAB 6000 has the agility for throughput of 130 PT tests per hour. CoaLAB is an ideal coagulation analyser designed to simplify complicated coagulation analysis into a walkway task for laboratories with high and medium throughput (Fig. 10.13).

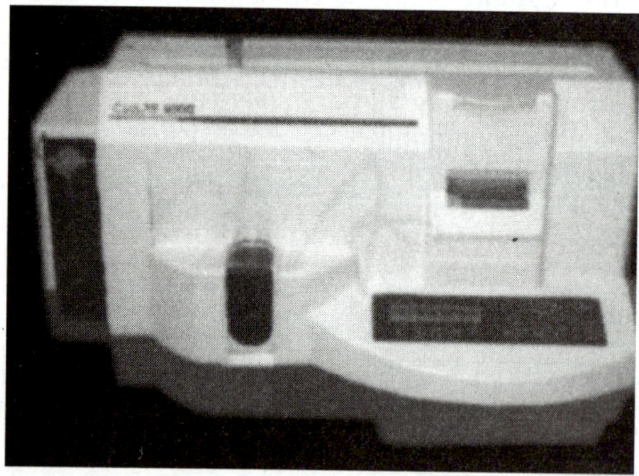

Fig. 10.13: CoaLAB 6000 *(Courtesy: Tulip group of companies)*

Compact

- Bench Top coagulation analyser
- Built-in Computer with display and keypad
- Internal Thermal Printer
- On board waste box for used cartridges

Versatile

- Single and double determination adjustable
- Primary and secondary tubes can be used
- All reagent positions can be stirred
- On or off switch option allowing real time or patient oriented printing of results
- Stat-Program
- Automatic reagent level control
- All Test parameters can be re-programmed and/or changed by the user

User Friendly

- Easy installation of the analyser
- Optimal user guidance through routine software
- Easy method change via chip cards
- Optimized cuvette cartridge consumption
- Pre-programmed method settings and evaluation procedures for: PTT, aPTT and fibrinogen assays
- Updating and/or upgrading via chipcards

Technical Specifications

CoaLAB 6000 : Fully Automated coagulation analyser for clotting assays

Measuring principle : Turbodensitometric. This optomechanical principle is able to measure lipemic and turbid plasma samples and reagents containing kaolin.

Measuring station : 6 measuring channels (parallel working mode)

Loading station : 18 sample positions (for primary and special cups) 6 reagent positions (for 4 ml/10 ml vials) at room temperature. All reagent positions can be stirred. 6 positions for cuvette cartridges, each cartridge includes 6 cuvettes.

Cuvette : Cuvette cartridges with 6 cuvettes including mixers, reagent vials, sample-cups. Test volume: max, 250μl

Traverse : Movement into 2 directions X-Z, for pipetting and transport of plasma and reagent Pipettor heated to 37°C. A level sensor detects the presence of liquid.

Dilutor	: 250μl syringe, 1 pipetting tube
System liquid	: Distilled water for washing and cleaning of pipettor
Washing solution	: Special washer to avoid carry-over of Thrombin.
Display	: Alphanumeric LCD-Display, 2 lines, 20 characters each.
Operating mode	: Random access mode for PT/aPTT and fibrinogen, batch mode selectable
Throughput	: >120 PT Tests/hour
Printer	: Built-in thermal printer
Printout	: Patient and result oriented (selectable)
Barcode reader	: Optional, for fast introduction of patient/sample numbers.
Interfaces	: 1 × RS232 C Host/Service, 1x Barcode Scanner
Power supply	: 100-240 V, 57-63 Hz, 150 VA
Dimensions	: 72 × 45 ×55 cm (~28.3 × 17.7 × 21.7 in)
Weight	: 17 Kg (~ 35 pounds)
Software features	: Optimal user guidance through routine software. Method menu for PT, aPTT and fibrinogen. Additional assays evaluated on the analyser: Factor II, V, VII, VIII, IX, X, XII and Thrombin Time. Documentation of all test parameters, e.g. calibration curves, date, time, conversions of percent, g/l, mg/dl, Ratio, INR and incubation time can automatically be loaded via ChipCARD. Easy method change via ChipCARD Two software languages (German/English) on board Consecutive award of sample/patient ID's or by optional barcode scanner or manually by user External service and research program.
Special features	: Single and double determination adjustable On board waste box for used cartridges, for hygienic disposal of used cuvette cartridges. Plasma or reagent start (can be configured) Optimized cuvette cartridge consumption to avoid waste of unused cuvettes. On or off switch option allowing "real time" or patient oriented printing. User oriented result management (print-out, LCD and Host). Advanced paper feed button. Wide range power supply 100 - 240 V, 47-63 Hz
Safety features	: Easy installation of analyser ("plug and play") Highlighted Status/Error Messages in printout. Special check of liquid level in washing station. Optimized liquid check at pipettor. Optimized cuvette cartridge guidance. Software controlled cuvette cartridge detection. Acoustic status signals of analyser for convenient user information. Easy change of analyser tubings.

CHAPTER 11

Blood Banking (Immunohaematology)

The ABO and Rh are the major (clinically significant) blood group antigens though almost 400 of them have been recognised. Given below are the more important blood group systems:

1. ABO, 2. Rhesus, 3. Dell, 4. Duffy, 5. Kidd, 6. Lutheran, 7. Lewis, 8. P 9. MNS, 10.I. (All of the above if mismatched can cause hemolytic transfusion reaction and 1 to 6 can be responsible for hemolytic disease of the newborn).

BLOOD GROUP ANTIBODIES

Naturally Occurring Antibodies

Under normal circumstances, the newborn has no ABO antibodies. However, after 10-20 weeks later, moderate amount of antibodies are present which appear without any specific antigenic stimulies. So these are called naturally occurring antibodies. Anti-A and Anti-B are important examples of this class. They are IgM Immunoglobulins, they react optimally at room temperature, they are also called cold antibodies. They are complete antibodies in serological behaviours, because these antibodies readily agglutinate the red cells carrying the corresponding antigen in saline.

Immune Antibodies are produced in response to immunisation either by transfusion or pregnancy. They are usually IgG antibodies, they react best at body temperature-37°C and are called warm antibodies. Rh antibody (anti-D) is important immune antibody. They are often called incomplete antibodies as they do not cause agglutination of red cells with corresponding antigen in saline. These antibodies cause only sensitisation or coating of the red cells.

In 1900, Karl Landsteiner discovered the blood groups ABO and classified blood into A, B and O groups. A fourth blood group 'AB' was discovered by Landsteiner's associates, Von Decastello and Struli in 1902.

The four blood groups are determined by the presence or absence of blood group antigens (agglutinogens) on red blood cells and accordingly an individual's group is A, B, AB or O (O denotes absence of A or B antigens). In addition, it has been shown that corresponding to antigen A and B, there are naturally occurring antibodies anti-A and anti-B (agglutinins) in the plasma/serum of individuals whose red cells lack the corresponding antigen. Group A individuals have anti-B, group B individuals have anti-A, group O individuals have both anti-A and anti-B and group AB individuals have no agglutinins in plasma/serum.

Table 11.1: The ABO antigens and corresponding antibodies

Antigen on RBC	*Antibody in Plasma/serum*	*Blood group*
A	anti-B	A
B	anti-A	B
AB	none	AB
None	anti-A and anti-B	O

It was further shown that Group A could be subdivided into two principal subgroups A1 and A2. On the basis of this, ABO system is divided in six main groups A1, A2, B, A1B, A2B and O.

GENETICS OF ABO SYSTEM

ABO system follows mendelian law of inheritance. The locus for ABO grouping is a chromosome 9 which is occupied by one of three major allelic genes namely A, B and O. Each individual has a pair of chromosomes (one from each parent). The A and B genes are dominant, while O gene is recessive, thus, not detected directly and accordingly absence of A and B antigens on red cells indicates 'O' blood group.

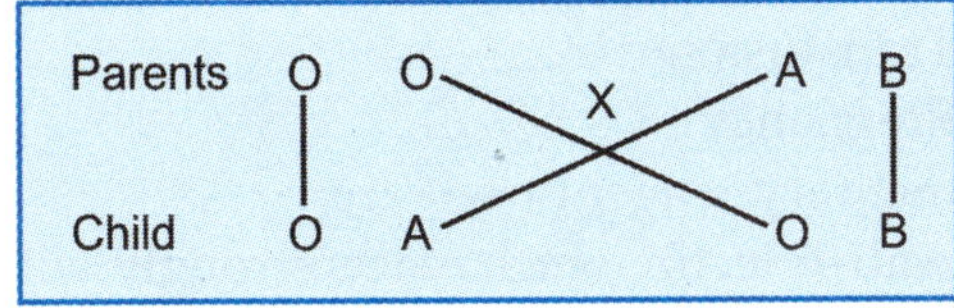

Fig. 11.1: The possible Phenotypes and Genotypes in ABO group system

Biochemistry

The expression of A and B genes appears to be dependent on another gene called H gene. H gene is inherited, independent of A, B and O genes. H gene is expressed both as homozygous (HH) and heterozygous (Hh). When no H gene is inherited, a (hh) phenotype results which is extremely rare. This is commonly called Bombay group. Bombay group individuals are homozygous for hh gene.

Table 11.2: The possible Phenotypes and Genotypes in ABO group system

Phenotypes	Genotypes
A_1	A_1A_1, A_1A_2-A_1O
A_2	A_2A_2.A_2O
B	BB, BO
A_1B	A_1B
A_2B	A_2B
O	OO

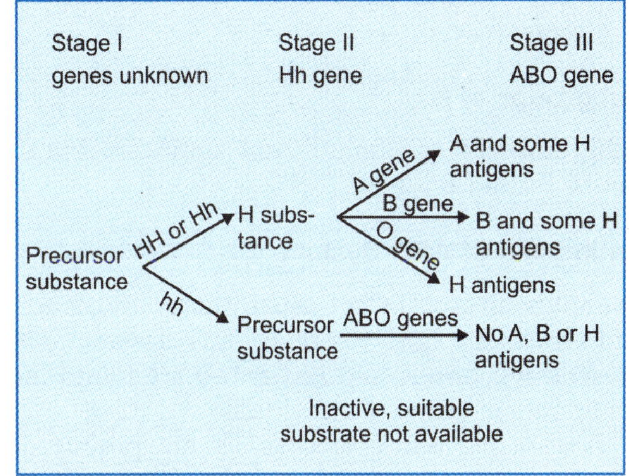

Fig. 11.2: Stages in production of blood group determinants of red cells

As shown in Fig. 11.2 there is a basic precursor substance which is converted to H Substance by an Enzyme L. Fucosyl transferase (a product of H gene).

H substance is next acted upon by A and/or B gene specified transferase enzyme and is converted to A and/ or B antigens. The 'O' gene is an amorph (no gene product) and thus, group 'O' cells enter only H substance.

The persons with genetic configuration of 'hh' cannot act on the precursor substance and the precursor substance remains unaltered. Since no H substance is produced, the ABO genes remain inactive and there is no conversion to A, B or H antigen (These are the persons called Bombay Group).

SUBGROUPS OF A AND AB

Anti-A serum very seldom differentiates between A_1 and A_2. For this reason we use human anti-A_1 and Lectin anti-A which agglutinate A_1 and A_1B cells but not A_2 and A_2B cells. About 20% of persons with A antigen in A or AB group are A_2 or A_2B.

It is not necessary to classify group A patient or donors as A_1 or A_2 except when the individual serum contains anti-A_1. Anti-A_1 occurs in the serum of 1-8% of A_2 group persons and 22-35% of A_2B group persons.

Anti-A1 causes discrepancies between ABO cell and serum groupings and may cause crossmatch incompatibilities, but it is considered clinically significant if it reacts at 37°C.

Subgroups weaker than A_2 occur infrequently. They are characterised by declining number of 'A' antigens on red cells and reciprocal increase in H reactivity. Weaker variants of A are A_3, Ax, Am and A intermediate.

Subgroups of B

Subgroups of B are clinically not significant, but they can be Bx and Bm type.

Antibodies of ABO System

The antibodies in ABO are usually naturally occurring and are mostly IgM. However, IgG classes are also present. IgG anti-A and IgG anti-B are found more commonly in group O individuals.

Anti-A and anti-B are usually not produced in infants up to age of 3-6 months. However, they reach a maximum titre by 5-10 years and then gradually become weaker as the individual ages. The antibodies found in the serum of infants at birth are almost of maternal origin. The serum grouping of a newborn is, therefore, not recommended.

Anti-H

Anti-H very rarely occurs as cold reactive agglutinin in individuals with very low levels of H antigens on their cells and have little clinical significance. However, anti-H found in Bombay blood group (Oh) is an all antibody and is clinically significant. It occurs as a hemolysin and agglutinates cells at 37°C.

ABO TESTING PROCEDURES

- For demonstration of true ABO group of an individual, it is important to do both cell grouping (forward typing) and serum grouping (reverse typing). Both forward and reverse typing must match to confirm the true ABO type of an individual.
- Serum should always be added before adding the cells and examine each tube after serum has been added to ensure that none has been left.
- ABO grouping test should be done at room temperature, or below. Testing at 37°C weakens reaction.
- Tubes, slides and microplates should be labelled properly.

ABO Antibody Reagents

The development of monoclonal antibodies obtained from cultures of cells secreting antibodies called hybridomas has made available a new source of ABO typing reagent. Before the advent of hybridoma technology, the ABO grouping reagent were derived from human donors with or without immunisation and are called polyclonal reagent. The monoclonal reagent anti-A, anti-B and Anti AB have significant advantage over earlier traditional polyclonal reagent in terms of specificity, potency, consistency and should be free from virus such as HIV and hepatitis.

Red Cells Reagents

The red cells used in ABO grouping are pooled A cells, B cells and O cells. The cells should be washed in saline to remove serum or plasma. The supernatant of last wash should be clear. Use 2-4% cell suspension for tube, microplate typing and 30-40% for slide typing.

Group 'O' cells are used in serum grouping to detect antibodies other than anti-A or anti-B in some donors. These antibodies are not naturally occurring and are called irregular antibodies. They occur due to immunisation either by:

- Transfusion
- Pregnancy

Supplementary reagent used are:

- Anti-A lectin which reacts strongly with A individuals.
- Anti-H reacts selectively with ABO group according to H substance. Group O individuals which contain only H react strongly with anti-H while A, B contains very little H and thus, reacts very weakly or negatively with anti-H. Other supplementary reagent that may be used to resolve the discrepancies of ABO grouping may include.

- Group A_2 Cells
- Group O reagent screen cells.

Group O reagent Screen Cells

Group O reagent screen cells contain red cells with various antigen specificities. These 2 or 3 group O cells are"complimentary to each other to provide antigens for detection of most of clinically significant antibodies. They are used to rule out ABO typing discrepancy caused by cold antibodies.

Preparation of Red Cell Suspensions

Depending upon the specific technique employed, 2,5,10 or 50% red cell suspensions are required. These can be prepared by transferring freshly obtained blood from a skin puncture into saline or suspending in saline the packed red cells obtained from citrated or oxalated blood. Preservative anticoagulant solutions are also available that permit preservation of red cells for one month or longer. This is most useful for controls and panel cells of known antigenic composition (reagent red cells). Most frequently, suspensions are made by gently breaking up blood clots with an applicator stick and transferring the red cell aggregates into saline or other suspending media.

Method (for 2% suspension)

1. To about 5 ml of normal saline, add several drops of whole blood (fresh, citrated, oxalated or fragments of clots).
2. Centrifuge, in order to pack the red cells.
3. Withdraw the supernatant fluid as completely as possible.
4. Add 0.1 ml of packed red cells to a test tube containing 4.9 ml of normal saline and mix well. This represents a 2% suspension of red cells in saline.

All red cell suspensions must be refrigerated when not in use. They are unsuitable if they show hemolysis and should be used within 12 hours of preparation.

Blood grouping sera should meet the following requirements

1. It should have titre of recommended potency.
2. It should be free of cold agglutinins.
3. It should be free of so-called irregular agglutinins.
4. It should not form rouleaux when mixed with red cells.
5. It should be clear, of normal colour (except when a dye is added for identification), and free of cells or any other particles, not hemolysed, icteric or chylous.
6. It should be free of complement.
   Anti-A serum (minimum titer with A_1 cells 256)*
   Anti-B serum (minimum titer with B cells 256)**
   Anti-AB serum (serum of group O) (minimum titer 256 with A_1 and B cells)
   Anti-A_1 reagent (absorbed anti-A serum, plant lectins)
   Anti-Rh (D) serum (minimum titer 32)
   Anti-A serum is coloured blue
   Anti-B serum is coloured yellow

ANTI-A, ANTI-B, ANTI-A,B

Blood Grouping Antisera for Slide and Tube Tests (FromTulip's Erybank Range)

Summary

Human red blood cell antigens can be divided into four groups A, B, AB and O depending on the presence or absence of the corresponding antigens on the red blood cells. Approximately 41% of the Caucasian population have the A-antigen, 9% have the B antigen, 4% have both A and B antigens, while the remaining have neither A nor B antigen.

Reagents

Erybank anti-A, anti-B and anti-A,B are ready to use reagent prepared from human serum. These reagent of the immunoglobulin class IgM are a pool of specific human serum obtained from certified selected donors who are found to be negative for HBsAg and anti HIV antibody. Each batch of reagent undergoes rigorous quality control at various stages of manufacture for its specificity, avidity and performance.

Reagent Storage and Stability

a. Store the reagent at 2-8°C. Do not freeze.
b. The shelf life of the reagent is as per the expiry date mentioned on the reagent vial label.

Principle

Human red blood cells possessing A and / or B antigen will agglutinate in the presence of antibody directed towards the antigen. Agglutination of red blood cells with anti-A, anti-B and anti-A,B reagent is a positive test result and indicates the presence of the corresponding antigen. Absence of agglutination of red blood cells with anti-A, anti-B and anti-A,B reagent is a negative test result and indicates the absence of corresponding antigen.

Note

1. *In vitro* diagnostic reagent for laboratory and professional use only. Not for medicinal use.
2. Erybank reagent are from human source and the source material used in its manufacture is tested by approved techniques and found negative for HBsAg and HIV, HCV antibodies.
3. The reagent contains sodium azide 0.1% as preservative. Avoid contact with skin and mucosa. On disposal flush with large quantities of water.
4. Extreme turbidity may indicate microbial contamination or denaturation of protein due to thermal damage. Such reagent should be discarded.

Sample Collection and Preparation

No special preparation of the patient is required prior to sample collection by approved techniques. Samples should be stored at 2-8°C if not tested immediately. Do not use haemolysed samples. Anticoagulated blood using various anticoagulants should be tested within the below mentioned time period:

EDTA or heparin	: 2 days
Sodium citrate or sodium oxalate	: 14 days
ACD or CPD	: 28 days

Clotted whole blood should be tested within 14 days.

Additional Material Required for Slide and Tube Tests

Glass slide (50 × 75 mm), Test tubes (10 × 75 mm), Pasteur pipettes, Isotonic saline, Centrifuge, Timer, and Mixing sticks.

Test Procedure

Bring reagent and samples to room temperature before testing.

Slide Test

1. Place one drop of Erybank reagent anti-A or anti-B or anti-A,B on a clean glass slide.
2. To each reagent drop, add one small drop of whole blood.
3. Mix well with a mixing stick uniformly over an area of approximately 2.5 cm^2.
4. Rock the slide gently back and forth.
5. Observe for agglutination macroscopically at two minutes.

Tube Test

1. Prepare a 2-3% suspension of the red cells to be tested in isotonic saline.
2. Place one drop of Erybank anti-A, anti-B, anti-A, B into correspondingly labelled test tubes.
3. Pipette into each of the test tubes, one drop of the test red cell suspension and mix well.
4. Centrifuge for 1 minute at 1000 rpm (125 g) or 20 seconds at 3400 rpm (1000 g) or incubate at room temperature for 20-30 minutes.
5. Gently resuspend the cell button, observing for agglutination macroscopically.

INTERPRETATION OF RESULTS

Slide and tube tests

Agglutination is a positive test result and indicates the presence of A and/or B antigen.

Do not interpret peripheral drying or fibrin strands as agglutination.

No agglutination is a negative test result and indicates the absence of A and/or B antigen.

Remarks

1. In the tube test procedure, it is recommended that tubes with negative reactions should be recentrifuged and results read again after 5 minutes so that weak antigens are not overlooked.
2. Anti-A, lectin can be used to differentiate between A, and A_1 subgroups.
3. A_3 cells demonstrate a mixed field agglutination.
4. Certain weaker subgroups of A and B may produce weak reactions with anti-A, B.
5. As undercentrifugation or overcentrifugation could lead to erroneous results, it is recommended that each laboratory calibrate its own equipment and determine the time required for achieving the desired results.

ANTI-A, ANTI-B, ANTI-A, B

Monoclonal Blood Grouping Antibodies for Slide and Tube Tests (From Tulip's Eryclone Range)

Summary

Monoclonal antibodies are derived from hybridoma cell lines, created by fusing mouse antibody producing B lymphocytes with mouse myeloma cells. Each hybridoma cell line produces homogeneous antibodies of only one immunoglobulin class, which are identical in their chemical structure and immunological activity. Human red blood cell antigens can be divided into four groups A, B, AB and O depending on the presence or absence of the corresponding antigens on the red blood cells. Approximately 41% of the Caucasian population have the A antigen, 9% have the B antigen, 4% have both A and B antigens, while the remaining have neither A nor B antigen.

Reagent

Eryclone® anti-A, anti-B and anti-A,B are ready-to-use reagent prepared from supernatants of mouse hybridoma cell cultures. These antibodies of immunglobulin class IgM are a mixture of several monoclonal antibodies of the same specificity but having the capability of recognising different epitopes of the human red blood cell antigens A and B. Each batch of reagent undergoes quality control at various stages of manufacture for its specificity, avidity and performance.

Reagent Storage and Stability

1. Store the reagent at 2-8°C. Do not freeze.
2. The shelf life of reagent is as per the expiry date mentioned on the reagent vial label.

Principle

Human red blood cells possessing A and / or B antigen will agglutinate in the presence of antibody directed towards the antigen. Agglutination of red blood cells with anti-A, anti-B, anti-A,B reagent is a positive test result and indicates the presence of the corresponding antigen. Absence of agglutination of red blood cells with anti-A, anti-B, anti-A,B reagent is a negative test result and indicates the absence of the corresponding antigen.

Note

1. *In vitro* diagnostic reagent for laboratory and professional use only. Not for medicinal use.
2. The reagent contains sodium azide 0.1% as preservative. Avoid contact with skin and mucosa. On disposal fiush with large quantities of water.
3. Extreme turbidity may indicate microbial contamination or denaturation of protein due to thermal damage. Such reagent should be discarded.
4. Eryclone® reagent are not from human sources, hence, contamination due to HBsAg and HIV is practically excluded.

Sample Collection and Preparation

No special preparation of the patient is required prior to sample collection by approved techniques. Samples should be stored at 2-8°C if not tested immediately. Do not use haemolysed samples. Anticoagulated blood using various anticoagulants should be tested within the below mentioned time period:

EDTA or Heparin : 2 days
Sodium citrate or Sodium oxalate : 14 days
ACD or CPD : 28 days

Clotted whole blood should be tested within 14 days.

Additional Material Required for Slide and Tube Tests

Glass slides (50 × 75 mm), Test tubes (12 × 75 mm), Pasteur pipettes, Isotonic saline, Centrifuge, Timer, and Mixing sticks.

Test Procedure

Bring reagent and samples to room temperature before testing.

Slide Test

1. Place one drop of Eryclone® anti-A or anti-B or anti-A,B reagent on a clean glass slide.
2. To each reagent drop, add one small drop of whole blood.
3 Mix well with a mixing stick uniformly over an area of approximately 2.5 cm^2.
4. Rock the slide gently, back and forth.

5. Observe for agglutination macroscopically at two minutes.

Tube Test

1. Prepare a 2-3% suspension of the red cells to be tested in isotonic saline.
2. Place one drop of Eryclone® anti-A, anti-B, anti-A, B into correspondingly labelled test tubes.
3. Pipette into each of the test tubes, one drop of the test red cell suspension and mix well.
4. Centrifuge for 1 minute at 1000 rpm (125 g) or 20 seconds at 3400 rpm (1000 g) or incubate at room temperature for 30 minutes.
5. Gently resuspend the cell button, observing for agglutination macroscopically.

INTERPRETATION OF RESULTS

Slide and Tube tests

Agglutination is a positive test result and indicates the presence of A and/or B antigen. Do not interpret peripheral drying or fibrin strands as agglutination. No agglutination is a negative test results and indicates the absence of A and/or B antigen.

Remarks

1. (a) Eryclone® anti-A, anti-B and anti-A,B reagent do not show a reaction with crypt antigens (T, Tn, Tk activated cells) (b) Eryclone® anti-B is truly negative reacting with acquired B characteristics.
2. In the tube test procedure, it is recommended that tubes with negative reactions should be recentrifuged and results read again after 5 minutes so that weak antigens are not overlooked.
3. As undercentrifugation or overcentrifugation could lead to erroneous results, it is recommended that each laboratory calibrates its own equipment and determine the time required for achieving the desired results.
4. Results of forward grouping obtained by using anti-A, anti-B, anti-A, B reagent should always be reconfirmed by performing reverse grouping with known red cells.
5. It is strongly recommended that red cells with known ABO characteristics should be occasionally run, preferably on a daily basis so as to control reagent performance and validate test results.
6. After usage, the reagent should be immediately recapped and replaced to 2-8°C storage.

ANTI-A1 LECTIN

Dolichos Biflorus Lectin for Slide and Tube Tests (From Tulips Erybank Range)

Summary

Human red blood cells possessing the A antigen can be broadly subdivided into two main subgroups namely A_1 and A_2 based on their reaction with A_1 lectin. A_2 subgroups comprises of weaker subgroups of A such as A_1, A_2, A_3, A_4, A_5, A_6, A_0, etc.

Group A red blood cells which agglutinate with Anti-A_1 lectin are classified as subgroup A_1, whereas red blood cells which do not agglutinate with Anti-A_1 lectin are classified as subgroup A_2. It is estimatd that about 80% of the group A population are A_1 and the remaining A_2 or weaker. Anti-A_1 lectin is especially useful in selecting blood for an A_2 or A_2B recipient whose blood may contain Anti-A_1 antibodies.

Reagent

Erybank® anti-A_1 lectin is a ready to use purified extract of *Dolichos biflorus* seeds that is carefully calibrated to differentiate most A_1 cells from A_2 cells. It contains a phytohaemagglutinin which is virtually specific for A_1 antigen on the human red blood cells.

Each batch of reagent undergoes rigorous quality control at various stages of manufacture for its specificity, avidity and titre.

Reagent Storage and Stability

a. Store the reagent at 2-8°C. Do not freeze.
b. The shelf life of the reagent is as per the expiry date mentioned on the reagent vial label.

Principle

Human red blood cells possessing A_1 antigen well agglutinate in the presence of seed extract (lectins) containing phytohaemagglutinin specifically directed towards it.

Agglutination of red cells with erybank® anti-A_1 lectin is a positive test result and indicates the presence of A_1 antigen. No agglutination with Erybank® anti-A_1 lectin is a negative test result and indicates the absence of the A_1 antigen. Red blood cells that are positive with anti-A reagent and negative with A_1 lectin are classified as A_2.

Note

1. In vitro diagnostic reagent for laboratory and professional use only. Not for medicinal use.
2. The reagent contains sodium azide 0.1% as preservative. Avoid contact with skin and mucosa. On disposal flush with large quantities of water.
3. Extreme turbidity may indicate microbial contamination/reagent deterioration. Such reagent should be discarded.

Sample Collection and Preparation

No special preparation of the patient is required prior to sample collection by approved techniques. Samples should be stored at 2-8°C, if not tested immedicately. Do not use haemolysed samples. Anticoagulated blood using various anticoagulants should be tested within the below mentioned time period:

EDTA or Heparin	:	2 days
Sodium citrate or sodium oxalate	:	14 days
ACD or CPD	:	28 days

Clotted whole blood should be tested within 14 days.

Additional Material Required for Slide and Tube Tests

Glass slides (50 × 75 mm), test tubes (12 × 75 mm), pasteur pipettes, isotonic saline, centrifuge, timer, mixing sticks.

Test Procedure

Bring all reagent and samples to room temperature before testing.

Slide Test

1. Prepare a 10% suspension of the red blood cells to be tested in isotonic saline.
2. Place on drop of erybank® anti-A_1 lectin on a clean glass slide.
3. Pipette two drops of the cell suspension on the slide.
4. Mix well with a mixing stick uniformly over an area of approximately 2.5 cm^2.
5. Rock the slide gently, back and forth.
6. Observe for agglutination macroscopically at one minute.

Tube Test

1. Prepare a 5% suspension of the red cells to be tested in isotonic saline.
2. Place one drop of Erybank® anti-A_1 lectin into a labelled test tube.
3. Pipette into the test tube, one drop of the test red cell suspension.
4. Centrifuge for 1 minute at 1000 rpm (125·g) or 20 seconds at 3400 rpm (1000 g).
5. Gently resuspend the cell button, observing for agglutination macroscopically.

INTERPRETATION OF RESULTS

Slide and Tube Tests

Agglutination is a positive test result and indicates the presence of A_1 antigen. Do not interpret peripheral drying or fibrin strands as agglutination. No agglutination is a negative test result and indicates the absence of A_1 antigen.

Remarks

1. A_1 antigen is not fully expressed on the red blood cells of newborns below one year of age, hence, false negative results may occur.
2. It is strongly recommended that known A_1 and A_2 cells should be occasionally run, preferably on a daily basis to control reagent performance and validate test results.
3. A_1 A_2 (A_{int}) cells may agglutinate moderately with Erybank®. Anti-A_1 lectin. These should be tested further with Anti-H lectin to confirm A_{int} cells.
4. As undercentrifugation or overcentrifugation can lead to erroneous results, it is recommended that each laboratory calibrate its own equipment and determine the time required for achieving the desired result.

ANTI-H LECTIN

Ulex Europaeus Lectin for Slide and Tube Tests (From Tulip's Erybank Range)

Summary

The H antigen is a basic blood group antigen present in human beings. There is considerable variation in the H antigen content in different individuals of the same ABO group, but the general pattern indicates their strength as O>A_2>A_2B>B>A_1>A_1B. Water-soluble H substance can also be demonstrated in saliva or body fluids of individuals who are secretors. Human red blood cells that do not agglutinate with Anti-H lectin are classified as Bombay phenotype (Oh). The Bombay phenotype is more common in India than other parts of the world and the estimated gene frequency of Oh phenotype in Bombay is 0.0066%.

Reagent

Erybank Anti-H lectin is a ready-to-use purified extract of *Ulex europaeus* seeds. It contains a phytohaemagglutinin which is virtually specific for the H antigen on human red blood cells. Erybank Anti-H lectin is used for recognition of the H antigen on human red blood cells. It is useful, especially for assessing the H secretor status of group 'O' individuals and also in differential grouping of A_{int} subgroup along with anti-A lectin.

Reagent Storage and Stability

a. Store the reagent at 2-8°C. Do not freeze.
b. The shelf life of the reagent is as per the expiry date mentioned on the reagent vial label.

Principle

Human red blood cells possessing the H antigen will agglutinate in the presence of seed extract (lectins) containing phytohaemagglutinin specifically directed towards it. Water-soluble H substance present in saliva neutralises anti-H lectin. Agglutination of red blood cells/neutralization of Anti-H lectin by saliva is a positive test result and indicates the presence of H substance on/in the red cell/saliva respectively. No agglutination/neutralisation of Anti-H lectin is a negative test result and indicates the absence of H substance on/in the red cell/saliva respectively.

Note

1. *In vitro* diagnostic reagent for laboratory and professional use only. Not for medicinal use.
2. The reagent contains sodium azide 0.1% as preservative. Avoid contact with skin and mucosa. On disposal flush with large quantities of water.
3. Extreme turbidity may indicate microbial contamination/reagent deterioration. Such reagent should be discarded.

Sample Collection and Preparation

For recognition of H antigen on human red blood cells

No special preparation of the patient is required prior to sample collection by approved techniques. Samples should be stored at 2-8°C, if not tested immediately. Do not use haemolysed samples. Anticoagulated blood using various anticoagulants should be tested within the below mentioned time period:

EDTA or heparin	:	2 days
Sodium citrate or sodium oxalate	:	14 days
ACD or CPD	:	28 days

Clotted whole blood should be tested within 14 days.

For Assessing Secretor Status in Human Saliva

a. Collect about 2 ml of fresh saliva in a glass tube and incubate in a boiling water bath for 10 minutes.
b. Centrifuge at 3400 rpm (1000 g) for 10 minutes.
c. Use the clear supernatant immediately for the study or freeze immediately if to be tested later.

Additional Material Required for Slide and Tube Tests

Glass slides (50 × 75 mm), Test tubes (10 × 75 mm), Pasteur pipettes, Isotonic saline, Centrifuge, Timer, Mixing sticks, Red blood cells positive for H antigen, Red blood cells negative for H antigen, Saliva positive for H antigen, Saliva negative for H antigen.

Procedure

Bring all reagent and samples to room temperature before testing.

Slide Test

1. Place one drop of Erybank Anti-H lectin on a clean glass slide.
2. Add one drop of whole blood to be tested on the slide and mix well with a mixing stick uniformly over an area of approximately 2.5 cm^2.

3. Rock the slide gently, back and forth.
4. Observe for agglutination macroscopically at two minutes.

Tube Test

1. Prepare a 5% suspension of the red cells to be tested in isotonic saline.
2. Place one drop of Erybank Anti-H lectin into a test tube.
3. Pipette into the test tube, one drop of the test red cell suspension and mix well.
4. Centrifuge for 1 minute at 1000 rpm (125 g) or 20 seconds at 3400 rpm (1000 g).
5. Gently resuspend the cell button, observing for agglutination macroscopically.

Tube Test (Secretor Status)

1. Place two drops of anti-H lectin into two clean glass tubes.
2. Pipette two drops of saliva into the tubes and mix well.
3. Incubate at room temperature for ten minutes.
4. Add one drop of negative and positive cell suspensions into the tubes, mix well and incubate at room temperature for five minutes.
5. Mix well and centrifuge for one minute at 1000 rpm (125 g) or 20 seconds at 3400 rpm (1000 g).
6. Gently resuspend the cell button, observing for agglutination macroscopically.

INTERPRETATION OF RESULTS

Slide and Tube Tests

Agglutination is a positive test result and indicates the presence of H antigen. No agglutination is a negative test result and indicates the absence of H antigen and the red cells being of Bombay phenotype (Oh).

Tube Test (Secretor Status)

Agglutination of the red cells indicates that the anti-H has not been neutralised and the patient is a non-secretor. No agglutination of the red cells indicates the anti-H has been neutralized and the patient is a secretor.

Remarks

1. Do not interpret peripheral drying or fibrin strands as agglutination.
2. It is recommended that known negative and positive cells must be included as controls with each test series.
3. As undercentrifugation or overcentrifugation could lead to erroneous results, it is recommended that each laboratory calibrate its own equipment and the time required for achieving the desired results.

OTHER REQUIREMENTS

1. Normal saline solution.
2. Bovine or human albumin (22% or 30%).
3. Reagent red blood cells: Suspensions of red cells in which presence or absence of significant blood group antigens has been determined may be collected periodically from suitable donors or be purchased commercially wherever available.
4. Enzymes: Bromelin, ficin, papain, trypsin.

PHYSIOLOGICAL SALINE SOLUTION FOR SEROLOGICAL APPLICATIONS (FROM TULIP'S ERYBANK RANGE) (SODIUM CHLORIDE 0.9% W/V)

Summary

In blood group serology, for detection of either antigens or antibodies, physiological saline (0.85% to 0.9% w/v) is being extensively used. However, it is important that the physiological saline used should be compatible with red blood cell membrane integrity.

Reagent

Erybank natrium chloride 0.9% w/v solution is standardised for its serological applications. Reagent contains 0.1% sodium azide as preservative.

Principle

Red blood cell lysis or shrinkage is observed in case of diluents used which contain very low salt concentration or very high salt concentration respectively. So optimal salt concentration is very essential to maintain the red cell membrane integrity. Sodium chloride with 0.9% w/v concentration is observed as the optimal salt concentration. It is routinely used as diluent for serological applications.

Note

1. Store the reagent at RT, it also can be stored at 4-8°C.

2. The reagent contains 0.1% sodium azide as preservative.
3. Avoid contact with skin and mucosa. On disposal flush with large quantities of water.

Uses

1. The reagent is used for the suspension of red blood cells.
2. The reagent is used as a diluent for the antibodies.
3. Washing of red blood cells.
4. Making dilutions of reagent or samples for testing.

BOVINE SERUM ALBUMIN 22% SOLUTION FOR SEROLOGICAL APPLICATIONS (From Tulip's Erybank Range)

Summary

Bovine serum albumin is mainly used to enhance the reactivity of blood grouping and typing antibodies in direct agglutination tests. bovine albumin also enhances the reactivity and sensitivity of indirect antiglobulin test which is used for compatibility testing, antibody screening, identification and titration.

Reagent

Erybank® bovine serum albumin is manufactured from selected raw bovine serum, its protein concentration and pH adjusted to 22% and 7.1 (± 0.1) respectively. Its conductivity is controlled specifically for serological applications.

Reagent Storage and Stability

1. Store the reagent at 2-8°C. Do not freeze.
2. The shelf life of the reagent is as per the expiry date mentioned on the reagent vial label.

Principle

Agglutination of antibody coated red cells depends upon the class and type of antibody involved and the characteristics of the reaction medium such as ionic strength and pH. Incomplete antibodies of IgG class, especially those with Rh specificity, agglutinate red cells if the zeta potential between the red cells is adjusted by addition of colloids and salts such as bovine serum albumin (BSA). Addition of BSA enhances such immunological reactions and increases test sensitivity.

Note

1. *In vitro* diagnostic reagent for laboratory and professional use only. Not for medicinal use.
2. The reagent contains sodium azide 0.1% as preservative. Avoid contact with skin and mucosa. On disposal flush with large quantities of water.
3. Extreme turbidity may indicate microbial contamination or denaturation of protein due to thermal damage. Such reagent should be discarded.

Sample Collection and Preparation

No special preparation of the patient is required prior to sample collection by approved techniques. Samples should be stored at 2-8°C if not tested immediately. Do not use haemolysed samples. Donor units can be tested up to the end of their dating. For the indirect antiglobulin test, serum from fresh clotted whole blood should be used.

Additional Material Required for Compatibility Testing

Test tubes (10 × 75 mm), 0.2 ml serological pipettes, Pasteur pipettes, Human red blood cells with specific antigen reacting with the antibody to be titrated, Centrifuge, Incubator, Isotonic saline, Anti-humanglobulin reagent such as Eryclone® Anti-human globulin reagent, Coomb's control cells (Refer Eryclone® anti-human globulin pack insert), AB neutral human serum.

BROAD-SPECTRUM COMPATIBILITY TEST

Major Cross match Procedure

Initial Phase

1. Label two test tubes as A (for albumin) and B (for saline), depending upon the number of donors to be cross matched, as many pairs of such labelled tubes would be required.
2. Prepare a 5% suspension of the red cells to be tested in isotonic saline.
3. Pipette two drops of recipient serum in both the labelled test tubes.
4. Pipette one drop of donor red cells in both the labelled test tubes and mix well.
5. Only to the albumin tube (A), add two drops of Erybank® bovine serum albumin reagent and mix well.

6. Centrifuge both the tubes for one minute at 1000 rpm (125 g) or for 20 seconds at 3400 rpm (1000 g).
7. First observe for haemolysis. Resuspend the cell button and observe for agglutination macroscopically.
8. Proceed to incubation phase.

Incubation Phase

1. Incubate the saline tube at room temperature and the albumin tube at 37°C for fifteen minutes.
2. First observe for haemolysis. Resuspend the cell button and observe for agglutination macroscopically.
3. Proceed to the antiglobulin phase.

Antiglobulin Phase

1. Only the albumin tubes (A) are tested in the antiglobulin phase.
2. Wash the mixture of red blood cells and serum thoroughly with isotonic saline for a minimum of three times. Decant completely after the last wash
3. Place two drops of Eryclone® anti-human globulin reagent into the test tube containing the sedimented cells and mixwell.
4. Centrifuge for one minute at 1000 rpm (125 g) or 20 seconds at 3400 rpm (1000 g).
5. Very gently, resuspend the cells and observe for agglutination macroscopically.

Antibody Titration Test

1. a. Prepare a 5% suspension of red blood cells with specific antigen reacting with antibody to be titrated, in Erybank® bovine serum albumin reagent .
   b. Also, prepare a 5% suspension of patient red cells in Erybank® bovine serum albumin reagent.
2. Label ten test tubes (1 to 10) and make progressive dilutions of the patients serum as indicated below:
   a. Pipette 0.1 ml of AB neutral serum into each test tube except the first tube.
   b. Pipette 0.1 ml of the patient serum into first two tubes only.
   c. After mixing the contents of the second tube thoroughly, transfer 0.1 ml of the mixture to the third tube. Continue the serial dilution by transfer up to tube No. ten. Discard 0.1 ml of the mixture from the last tube.
3. To tubes No. One through to Nine, add one drop of albumin suspended selected red blood cells, (as prepared in point No. 1 (a) above) and mix well.
4. To tube No. ten, add one drop of patient's red cells suspended in albumin (as prepared in point No.1 (b) above) and mix well.
5. Incubate all the tubes at 37°C for a minimum of fifteen minutes.
6. Centrifuge all the tubes for one minute at 1000 rpm or 20 seconds at 3400 rpm (1000 g).
7. Very gently, resuspend the cell buttons and observe for agglutination macroscopically.
8. Antiglobulin test should be performed on all tubes which do not show a very strong agglutination.

INTERPRETATION OF RESULTS

Compatibility Test

In all phases of the compatibility test, if no agglutination or haemolysis is observed, then the patient and the donor may be considered compatible. If haemolysis or agglutination at any point till the completion of the antiglobulin phase is observed, the patient and donor are considered incompatible.

Antibody Titration Test

The end point of the titration is the reciprocal of the dilution in the last tube showing agglutination.

Remarks

1. If plasma is used in the indirect antiglobulin test, the complement-dependent antibodies may not be detected due to the absence of calcium.
2. To all negative test results, after the antiglobulin test phase, one drop of Coomb's control cells should be added. If the Coomb's control cells do not agglutinate, then the compatibility test must be repeated.
3. Red blood cells showing a positive direct antiglobulin test should not be used for the indirect antiglobulin test.
4. Bovine serum albumin will not bring about agglutination of red cells by all IgG blood grouping typing antibodies.
5. As undercentrifugation or overcentrifugation can lead to erroneous results, it is recommended that each laboratory calibrates its own equipment

and determine the time required for achieving the desired results.

6. After usage, the reagent should be immediately recapped and replaced at 2-8°C storage.

CONCENTRATED ISO-OSMOTIC PHOSPHATE BUFFERED SALINE FOR SEROLOGICAL APPLICATIONS (Osmosol from Tulip)

Summary

The pH of reaction medium is an important factor in antigen-antibody interaction. It has been observed that irrigation/infusion saline solution of low pH, isotonic saline autoclaved and stored in plastic containers could severly compromise the sensitivity and specificity of antiglobulin test when used as wash solutions/resuspension medium in immunohaematological procedures. Hence, careful consideration should be given to the source, pH and storage container of isotonic saline solutions intended for use in immunohaematological procedures. Usage of buffered isotonic phosphate saline such as Osmosol maintains the pH at 7.0-7.2 thereby improving the sensitivity and specificity of tests employed in immunohaematological procedures.

Reagent

Osmosol is a concentrated 20X buffered isotonic phosphate saline useful for preparing iso-osmotic saline preparation, especially for immunohaematological use. Inclusion of sodium azide in the final formulation prevents contamination during use.

Reagent Storage and Stability

Store the reagent at room temperature. Once opened, store at 2-8°C.

The shelf life of the concentrated Osmosol reagent is as per the expiry date mentioned on the reagent vial label.

Upon dilution, the isotonic buffered saline solution so obtained is stable for at least a month provided it is not contaminated during use.

Principle

Osmosol with osmolarity similar to blood serum or plasma, incorporating phosphate buffer maintains red blood cell membrane integrity and optimum pH of the reaction medium for antigen-antibody reaction during immunohaematological tests thereby improving the sensitivity and specificity of the test.

Note

1. *In vitro* diagnostic reagent for laboratory and professional use only. Not for medicinal use.
2. The reagent contains 0.2% sodium azide as preservative. Avoid contact with skin and mucosa. On disposal flush with large quantities of water.
3. Extreme turbidity may indicate contamination. Such reagent must be discarded.

Additional Material Required

Distilled water for blood bank use, pH paper capable for reading pH at 6.5-7.5 or pH meter, sterile and scrupulously clean glasswares for preparing the isotonic buffered saline solution.

Method of Preparation

1. Invert the contents of Osmosol vial into a scrupulously clean, sterile glass jar/bottle. Make the volume to 500 ml with distilled water. Gently mix the contents. Alternatively, if lesser quantity of isotonic buffered saline is required then dilute 1 part of concentrated Osmosol with 19 parts of distilled water. The glasswares used for preparing the isotonic buffered saline should be sterile and scrupulously clean.
2. Check the pH of isotonic buffered saline. The pH of the isotonic buffered saline should be in the range 6.9-7.2.
3. The isotonic buffered saline so obtained is ready-to-use for washing and preparing red blood cell suspension, dilution medium for antibodies in serological applications.

Remarks

1. Erroneous test results can occur from microbial or chemical contamination of buffered saline. The final reagent so obtained should be a clear solution.
2. Isotonic buffered saline obtained from Osmosol should not cause haemolysis of red blood cells, gel formation with serum under test. Any observable change in serum or cellular elements, the reagent must be discarded.
3. Occasionally, it is recommended that the pH of the isotonic buffered saline obtained from

Osmosol should be checked before using for serological applications. The pH should be in the range 6.9-7.2. Any change in pH value out of the specified range, the reagent should be discarded.

4. The isotonic buffered saline obtained from Osmosol should be strictly stored in scrupulously clean, sterile beakers/glass wares and not in plastic containers.
5. The 20x concentrated Osmosol vial may show fine particulate appearance if stored at 2-8°C. This can be ovecome by gently warming the concentrated solution to 25°C, before dilution.

MEDIA FOR COLLECTION AND PRESERVATION OF REAGENT RED CELLS

1. *Modified Alsever's solution:*
   Dextrose—2.05 gm
   Sodium citrate—0.8 gm
   Citric acid—0.05 gm
   Sodium chloride—0.45 gm
   Distilled water—100 ml
   (Expected pH = 6.1)
2. *Serum lactose solution*:
   Lactose—10 gm
   Dextrose—1.53 gm
   Sodium citrate—1.38 gm
   Citric acid—0.5 gm
   Distilled water—100 ml

This 100 ml solution is mixed with 100 ml of serum from a person of group AB (serum must be free of irregular and cold agglutinins).

Precautions

Antisera must be refrigerated when not in use. Reagent s and blood specimens for hemagglutination test must be handled aseptically since bacterial contamination may cause both, falsely negative and falsely positive results. Positive and negative controls must be run daily with all antisera.

RED CELL PRESERVING SOLUTION FOR SEROLOGICAL APPLICATIONS (Erywell from Tulip)

Summary

In blood group serology, known red cell panels are of immense value in confirming the results of forward grouping, antibody screening and detection of rare phenotypes. A red cell preserving solution is utilized to preserve the red cells of interest. Erywell red cell preservation solution is formulated specifically for enhanced preservation of red cells carrying clinically important phenotype or genotype, which are required for routine immunohaematological practice.

Reagent

Laboratory reagent. Ready-to-use solution.

Erywell red cell preserving solution is a standardized Alsever's solution for maintaining red cell integrity and survival.

Principle

Red blood cell shrinkage and loss of antigenic properties are observed on storage. To preserve the red cells for a longer time and ensure enhanced usage life for serological procedures, the Erywell solution supplies the necessary nutrients, salts and preservatives for maintaining red cell integrity and antigenic properties useful during serological procedures.

Storage and Stability

Store the reagent at 2-8°C.
Stability of unopened vial: 12 months from the date of manufacturing.

Additional Material Required

1. Freshly collected red blood cells in EDTA di-potassium salt (1.5 mg/ml of whole blood)
2. Test tubes 12 × 100 mm, scrupulously clean and dry
3. 10 ml pipettes, scrupulously clean and dry
4. 500 μl micropipette and micropipette tips
5. Freshly prepared normal saline (0.9% NaCl)
6. Table centrifuge
7. Sterile 10 ml vials

Procedure

a. Quick method for whole blood preservation

1. Collect 5 ml whole blood in EDTA di-potassium salt (1.5 mg/ml of whole blood). Add equal volume of Erywell solution to it. Gently mix the solution.
2. Before using the red cells prepared by the quick method, it is recommended to wash the red cells three times with normal saline before use for testing purpose.

b. Preparation of 2/3/5% stabilized Red Blood cell suspension in Erywell solution

1. Collect 2 ml of freshly drawn venous blood in a clean and dry test tube containing 3 mg of EDTA di-potassium salt.
2. Add 5 ml of normal saline solution and mix well.
3. Centrifuge the tube at 3000 rpm for 2-3 minutes to form a red cell button.
4. Discard the supernatant.
5. Resuspend the red cell button in normal saline solution.
6. Centrifuge the tube at 3000 rpm for 2-3 minutes.
7. Repeat the washing of the red cells (steps 4 and 5) one more time in normal saline.
8. After the centrifugation, remove the supernatant without disturbing the red cell button.
9. Now resuspend the red cell button in 5 ml of Erywell solution.
10. Centrifuge the tube at 3000 rpm for2-3 minutes.
11. After the centrifugation, remove the supernatant without disturbing the red cell button.
12. Take 0.2/0.3 ml of packed red cells from the above cell button and resuspend them in 10 ml of Erywell solution for preparation of 2/3% red cell suspension. To obtain a 5% red cell suspension resuspend 0.5 ml of packed red cells from the above cell button in 10 ml of Erywell solution.
13. Store the red cell suspension in a sterile 10 ml vial.
14. The red cell suspension so obtained is ready-to-use for testing.

Storage

1. The whole blood preserved in Erywell solution prepared by the quick method can be stored up to 4 weeks at 2-8°C.
2. The ready-to-use 2-3-5 % stabilized red blood cell suspension in Erywell solution should be stored at 2-8°C and can be utilized for weeks from the date of preparation.

Precautions

1. Store Erywell at 2-8°C with cap tightly closed.
2. Do not contaminate the solution as it may subsequently effect the stability of red cell suspension.
3. Glassware used to retrieve Erywell red cell suspension should be scrupulously clean and sterile.

ABO GROUPING

Slide ABO Grouping Test

1. Prepare a 10% suspension in saline of the red cells to be tested.
2. Mark the left slide of a clean glass slide 'anti-A' and the right side 'anti-B'.
3. Add to the left side a drop of anti-A grouping serum and to the right side a drop of anti-B grouping serum.
4. Next to the antisera drops, place 1 drop of 10% saline suspension of unknown red cells. The contents on the left and right sides should not get mixed up.
5. With one-half of an applicator stick, mix the red cell suspension with the anti-A serum; and with the other half-mix the red cell suspension with the anti-B serum.
6. Gently rock the slide back and forth and observe the mixture for one minute unless agglutination occurs earlier.
7. It is necessary to confirm the slide grouping by testing the unknown serum with the known red cell suspensions of groups A, B, and O as indicated for six-tube method. (Instead of 10% saline suspension, citrated/ oxalated blood or direct blood from skin puncture may be taken. Slow and weak agglutinations may occur in A subgroups).

Six-tube Method (Fig. 11.3)

1. Separate the serum from red cells or clot of unknown specimen.
2. Prepare a two per cent suspension in saline of the red cells of the unknown specimen.
3. For each specimen-six test tubes are labelled showing in addition to proper identification of the unknown specimen the undermentioned information: Tube 1, anti-A; tube 2, anti-B; tube 3, anti-AB; tube 4, A; tube 5, B; tube 6, O.
4. Place 1 drop of anti-A serum in tube 1, 1 drop of the anti-B serum into tube 2, and 1 drop of the anti-A, B serum into tube 3.
5. Add two drops each of the serum of the unknown specimen to tubes 4, 5, and 6.

6. Add one drop each of the 2% red cell suspension in saline of the unknown specimen to tubes 1, 2, and 3.
7. To tube 4, add 1 drop of a 2% red cell suspension in saline of group A cells; to tube 5, add 1 drop of a 2% red cell suspension in saline of group B cells; and to tube 6, add 1 drop of a 2% suspension of red cells in saline of group O cells.
8. Mix the contents of all tubes by shaking the test tube rack.
9. Depending on the speed necessary for completing the test, one of the two alternatives may be chosen: (i) the test tubes may be left at room temperature for at least 2 hours, or (ii) after 2 to 3 minutes, the tubes may be centrifuged (1 minute at 1500 rpm in a clinical centrifuge).
10. After incubation or centrifugation, the red cell suspensions are redispersed by tapping the tubes. Presence of agglutination is checked with the naked eye, with the scanning lens of a microscope and if the results are doubtful or negative, microscopically (10x objective) after placing a drop on a slide.

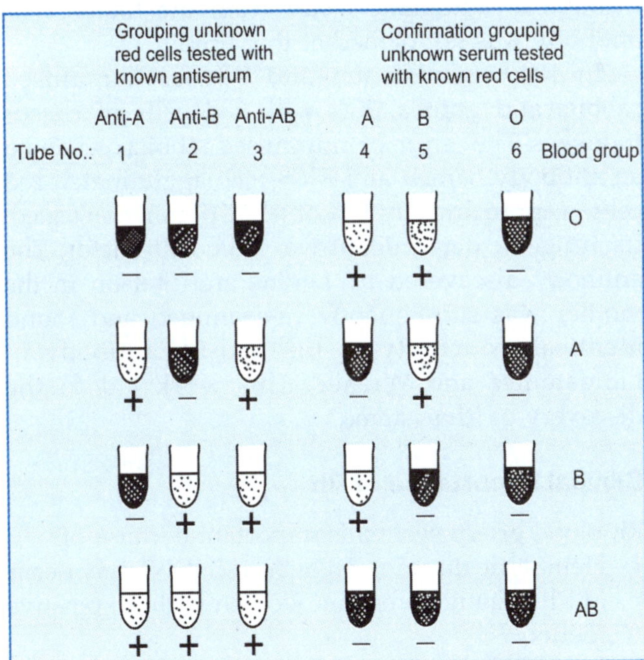

Fig. 11.3: ABO blood grouping—tube method

Interpretation

The results of an ABO grouping test can be accepted as valid only if the findings obtained in the first three test tubes with known antisera agree with those obtained in the second three test tubes with known red cell suspensions; this second, part of the test is called confirmation, check or reverse grouping. Given on previous page are the result in the four main ABO groups in such tests when both the unknown red cells and unknown serum are tested. Agglutination is indicated by the +sign, –sign indicates no agglutination.

Absent or weak agglutination with the unknown serum may be simulated by hemolysis of the known red cells, this suggests the presence of hemolytic anti-A or anti-B antibody. The assumption that hemolysis is due to anti-A or anti-B must be confirmed by repeating the test with the serum after its inactivation in a water bath at 56°C for 30 minutes—use of the inactivated serum is expected to result in agglutination instead of hemolysis.

If discrepancies in the two parts of ABO grouping are observed, the test should be redone. If a second test reveals the same discrepancy, the following possibilities are to be considered:

1. Cold agglutinins may cause agglutination of the known cells by the unknown serum regardless of its ABO group. Confirm this by testing the unknown serum with its own red cells at 4°C for 1 to 2 hours. Under those conditions cold agglutinins produce agglutination, which disappears after transfer of the specimen to a water bath at 37°C for 5 to 10 minutes.
2. Agglutination of the unknown red cells by known antisera that conflict with the results obtained in the confirmation grouping may be due to coating of the red cells by autoantibodies. Confirmation of this phenomenon is obtained by performing on the unknown red cells the direct antiglobulin test and obtaining positive results. In order to obtain in such cases a reliable ABO grouping, the red cells should be washed several times with large amounts of isotonic saline solution, following which they are more likely to give adequate result.
3. Unexpected agglutination obtained with the unknown serum may reflect presence of irregular agglutinins, such as Rh antibodies, which react with the corresponding blood factor in the suspensions of the known red cells.
4. Discrepancies in the two parts may sometimes be present due to A subgroup. In which anti-A_1 serum, anti-A_2 serum, and A_1 and A_2 reagent red cells are used for confirmation.

5. Serum of newborn and young infants may not contain the isoagglutinins expected from the reactivity of their red cells; hence, in infants, the use of unknown serum is not a reliable method. Much less frequently isoagglutinins may be absent in older children and adults due to hypo or agammaglobulinemia or for unknown reasons.

Briefly the reasons can be described as:

a. Improper identification of specimen.
b. Improper techniques like:
   - Failure to add proper reagent
   - Incorrect cell to serum ratio
   - Failure to identify hemolysis
   - Incorrect reading, recording or interpretation of test results.
c. Failure of equipment.
d. Poor standardised or stored reagent
e. Patients Problems
   - Patient may fail to express ABO antigens on red cells, e.g.
     1. Age (newborn or old age)
     2. Disease states, i.e. leukemia or lymphomas.
     3. This leads to false negative results.

- Acquired B-antigen can occur
  1. Gram-negative septicaemia.
  2. Carcinoma colon

  This may cause false positive reaction.
- Rouleaux formation: This is an aggregation of red cells in the form of piles of coins and can be misinterpreted as agglutination.
- Acquired antibodies, e.g. anti-A_1, in A_2 persons anti-H in Bombay phenotype, cold autoantibodies, unexpected all antibodies
- Absence or weakening of antibodies, e.g. immune deficiency states. Agammaglobulinaemias, etc.

Solving Problems of Discrepancies

Once a discrepancy is detected in ABO cells and serum grouping, repeat the test before additional investigations are carried out. Quality assurance of reagent, correct technique, careful observation and interpretation of results resolve many problems.

Repeat Preliminary Procedures

1. Obtain a fresh blood sample from donor unit or patient to rule out discrepancy due to contamination or unidentified samples.
2. Wash the cells 3-4 times in normal saline to rule out rouleaux formation and prepare 2-5% cell suspension.
3. Perform direct antiglobulin test on the cells, to detect if cells are coated with antibody as in HDN and AIHA.
4. Retest the cells with fresh and potent anti A, anti-B, anti-AB, anti-A or anti-H as appropriate for individual problem.
5. Test the serum against appropriate A_1, A_2 and B cells. Group O cells and autologous cells should be used as controls to detect alloagglutinins and autoagglutinins.
6. Use group O cord cells if anti-I is suspected.

RH BLOOD GROUP SYSTEM

It had been suspected for a long time that cause of many transfusion reactions was due to specific differences in blood other than the four main blood groups originally described by Landsteiner. In 1939, Levine and Stetson described an antibody in the serum of a group O mother who delivered stillborn foetus and subsequently developed symptoms of hemolytic transfusion reaction when transfused with her husband's group O blood. They noted that the responsible antibody developed in the mother through an antigenic factor from the foetus. The antibody was not named at that time.

In 1940, Landsteiner and Wiener immunised rabbits and guinea pigs with red cells of rhesus monkeys. The serum of immunised rabbits contained an antibody named anti-Rh which agglutinated red cells in approximately 85% of white population tested. Its antigenic determinant was called Rh factor. The antibody discovered by Levine and Stetson in the mother was subsequently re-examined and found identical in activity as the anti-Rh antibody of Landsteiner and Wiener. This work led to the discovery of Rh system.

Clinical Importance of Rh

Rh blood group system is important because of:

1. Hemolytic disease of newborn (HDN) may occur in Rh negative pregnant women with Rh positive foetus.
2. Rh antibodies may develop in Rh negative patient if given Rh positive blood.

Present Status and Nomenclature

The genes of the Rh system are present a chromosome 1. There are three pairs of genes called Cc, Dd, and

Ee but only five antigens (C, c, D, E, e) as there is no antigen produced by the 'd' gene. Rh gene travels in the set of three, e.g. CDC, CDE, CDE, etc. with one set being received from each parent. There are thus, eight possible chromosomes each of which carry genes for three factors (Table 11.3).

Table 11.3: The eight basic chromosomes of fisher and race

DCe(R_1)	dce(r)
DcE(R_2)	dCe(r′)
Dce (R_0)	dcE (r″)
DCE(R_z)	dCE (r^y)

Any two chromosomes, one from each parent may be inherited by an individual so that 36 different genotypes are possible Table 11.4 gives the most common genotypes.

Out of various gene combinations as shown in Table 11.4, it is presence or absence of D gene which is most important. When a person inherits 'D' antigen its red cells react with anti-D and these are called Rh-D Positive. If a person does not inherit D antigen, the red cells do not react with anti-D and thus, called Rh-D Negative.

Table 11.4: Common genotypes

DCe/dce	(R_1r)	dce/dce (rr)
DCe/DCe	(R_1R_1)	
DCe/DcE	(R_1R_2)	
DcE/dce	(R_2r)	dcE/dce (r″r)
DCe/DCe	(R_1R_0)	
DcE/DcE	(R_2R_2)	
Dce/dce	(R_0r)	
DCe/dcE	(R_1r″)	
DCe/dCe	(R_1r′)	dCe/dce (r′r)

Rh D^u Antigen

It is defined as weakened expression of the normal D antigen i.e. there are fewer than normal D antigens per red cells. There are two grades of D^u:

High grade D^u

Low grade D^u

High grade D^u red cells are agglutinated by certain anti-D sera while low grade D^u are mostly detected by (Anti Human Globulin) AHG test.

It has been shown that D^u positive bloods may immunize the Rh negative patient resulting in the formation of anti-D antibodies, hence, it is important to exclude D^u individuals from Rh negative blood donor list.

Rh Antibodies

Rh antibodies are usually immune IgG type but may be IgM or even IgA. Most Rh antibodies result from exposure to Rh positive red cells, either due to pregnancy or transfusion in individuals who lack the corresponding antigen.

Auto Rh antibodies may be found in individual with warm autoimmune hemolylic anaemia and anti-e is the most commonly found antibody.

Reagents for Rh(D) Grouping

Both polyclonal and monoclonal reagent are available in different combinations.

I. Polyclonal human and D serum
   a. Anti-Rh(D) serum for saline or rapid tube test (high protein medium).
      This contains macromolecular additives and gives rapid reliable results.
   b. Anti-D for saline tube test
      1. Anti-D-IgM
      2. Anti-D-IgG

II. Monoclonal Anti-D Reagents
   1. IgM anti-D monoclonal Reagent
   2. IgG anti-D monoclonal Reagent
   3. IgM and IgG (Blend) anti-D monoclonal reagent
   4. Blend of IgM monoclonal and IgG polyclonal reagent.

The IgM anti-D monoclonal is highly specific, saline reacting working well at room temperature and at 37°C. It is good for emergency slide test, or immediate spin tube test as well as routine Rh-D typing, but IgM anti-D are unreliable for detecting weak D by antiglobulin test, while IgM and IgG (Blend) monoclonal reagent or IgM anti-D monoclonal and IgG anti-D (polyclonal) blend can be used for weak D testing by antiglobulin test.

RH(D) GROUPING PROCEDURES

Rh(D) grouping is done along with ABO grouping using same techniques as used for ABO grouping:

1. Slide or Tile Method
2. Tube Method
3. Microplate Method.

Slide Testing

Slide test is not recommended for routine test because it is not reliable especially for weak reactive cells.

Method

1. Place one drop of anti-Rh (D) on a labelled slide.
2. Place one drop of 22% albumin on another labelled slide to serve as control.
3. Put one drop of 40-50% red cells on both the slides.
4. Mix the cell suspension and reagent, using a clean stick for each slide and spread the mixture evenly on the slide over area of 15 mm diameter.
5. Place both slides on a view box (lighted), till gently and continuously for two minutes. Observe for agglutination.

A positive test has agglutination with anti-Rh(D) in the 'test' and a smooth suspension of cells in control. A negative test has smooth suspension of cells in both 'test' and 'control.

Tube Method

1. Place one drop of anti-Rh(D) serum in a tube labelled test
2. Place one drop of 22% albumin in a tube labelled 'control'.
3. Add 1 drop of 2-5% cell suspension in plasma or serum in each tube.
4. Mix well and keep at 37°C for 1 hour (sedimentation method).
   In case of emergency, incubate the tube for 10 minutes at 37°C and then centrifuge at 1000 rpm for 1 min (spin tube).
5. Gently resuspend the cell button and observe for agglutination. All negative results must be confirmed under microscope.

Interpretation

A positive test has agglutination with anti-Rh(D) in the test and a smooth suspension of cells in the control. A negative test has smooth suspension of cells in both 'test' and 'control'.

Testing for D^u

Method

1. Take one drop of anti-Rh(D) serum in a clean labelled test tube.
2. Place one drop of appropriate control in a labelled tube.
3. Add 1 drop of 2-5% cell suspension to be tested to both the tubes.
4. Mix and incubate both the tubes at 37°C for 15-30 minutes.
5. Centrifuge at 1000 rpm for 1 minute.
6. Gently resuspend the cell button and examine for agglutination. If there is strong agglutination of cell in 'test' tube, then sample is Rh(D) positive and there is no need to proceed with antiglobulin phase of test.
7. If no agglutination or doubtful reaction is observed, wash the cells 3-4 times with saline and decant the last washing.
8. Add 1-2 drops of antiglobulin reagent (Coomb's), mix gently and centrifuge at 1000 rprn for 1 minute.
9. Resuspend the cell button gently and examine for agglutination and record the results.
10. If the test is negative, the reaction can be confirmed by adding known IgG sensitised cells, recentrifuge and re-examine for agglutination. Presence of agglutination confirms the test result.

Interpretation

Agglutination in the 'test' tube and none in negative control tube constitutes a positive test result and blood is accordingly labelled Rh-D^u positive.

ANTI-D (Rho)

Human (IgG) Polyclonal Blood Typing Antibodies for Slide and Modified Tube Tests (From Tulip's Erybank Range)

Summary

Polyclonal antibodies are derived from hyperimmune human serum containing Anti-D (Rho) antibodies directed towards the human D (Rho) antigen. Human red blood cells are classified as RhoD positive or RhoD negative depending on the presence or absence of the D antigen on them. Approximately 85% of the Caucasian population is RhoD positive. The D^u phenotype is a variant of the D antigen and is recognised by performing the antiglobulin test.

Reagent

Erybank anti-D polyclonal is a ready-to-use high-protein reagent prepared from pools of hyperimmune human serum containing antibodies directed towards the human D (Rho) antigen. These antibodies of the immunoglobulins class IgG are a mixture of several polyclonal antibodies of the same specificity but having the capability of recognising different epitopes of the human red blood cell antigen D (Rho).

Each batch of reagent undergoes rigorous quality control at various stages of manufacture for its specificity, avidity and titre. The reagent is suitable for slide and modified tube tests.

Reagent Storage and Stability

1. Store the reagent at 2-8°C. Do not freeze.
2. The shelf life of the reagent is as per the expiry date mentioned on the reagent vial label.

Principle

Human red blood cells possessing D antigen will agglutinate in the presence of antibody directed towards the antigen. Agglutination of red blood cells with Erybank Anti-D polyclonal reagent is a positive test result and indicates the presence of D antigen. No agglutination with anti-D reagent is a negative test result and indicates absence of D antigen. All negative test results should be further tested for D^u by performing the D^u test procedure as described later.

Note

1. *In vitro* diagnostic reagent for laboratory and professional use only. Not for medicinal use.
2. Erybank Anti-D polyclonal reagent is from human source and the source material used in its manufacture is tested by approved techniques and found negative for HBsAg and HIV, HCV antibodies.
3. The reagent contains sodium azide 0.1% as preservative. Avoid contact with skin and mucosa. On disposal flush with large quantities of water.
4. Extreme turbidity may indicate microbial contamination or denaturation of protein due to thermal damage. Such reagent should be discarded.

Sample Collection and Storage

No special preparation of the patient is required prior to sample collection by approved techniques. Samples should be stored at 2-8°C if not tested immediately. Do not use haemolysed samples. Anticoagulated blood using various anticoagulants should be tested within the below mentioned time period:

EDTA or Heparin	: 2 days
Sodium citrate / Sodium oxalate	: 14 days
ACD or CPD	: 28 days

Clotted whole blood should be tested within 14 days.

Additional Material Required for Slide and Tube Tests

Glass slides (50 × 75 mm), Test tubes (10 × 75 mm), Pasteur pipettes, Isotonic saline, Centrifuge, Timer, Mixing sticks, Rl viewing box with 40-45°C surface temperature, Eryclone anti-human globulin (Coomb's) reagent, EryconeRh-hr control.

TEST PROCEDURE

Slide Test

1. Place one drop of Erybank Anti-D polyclonal reagent on a clean prewarmed glass slide (40-45°C surface temperature)
2. Add one equal drop of whole blood.
3. Mix well with a mixing stick uniformly over an area of approximately 2.5 cm^2.
4. Rock the slide gently, back and forth.
5. Observe for agglutination macroscopically at two minutes.

Tube Test

1. Prepare a 5% suspension of the red cells to be tested in isotonic saline.
2. Place one drop of Erybank Anti-D polyclonal reagent into a labelled test tube.
3. Pipette into the test tube, one drop of the 5% cell suspension and mix well.
4. Centrifuge for 1 minute at 1000 rpm (125 g) or 20 seconds at 3400 rpm (1000 g).
5. Gently resuspend the cell button, observing for agglutination macroscopically.

D^u Test Procedure

1. Prepare a 5% suspension of the red cells to be tested in isotonic saline.
2. Place one drop of Erybank anti-D polyclonal reagent into a labelled test tube.
3. Pipette into the test tube one drop of the 5% cell suspension and mix well. Incubate at 37°C for 15 minutes.
4. Wash the contents of the tube thoroughly, at least three times, with isotonic saline and decant completely after the last wash.

5. Add two drops of Eryclone Anti human globulin reagent and mix well.
6. Centrifuge for 1 minute at 1000 rpm (125 g) or 20 seconds at 3400 rpm (1000 g).
7. Very gently, resuspend the cell button and observe for agglutination macroscopically.

INTERPRETATION OF RESULTS

Slide and Tube Tests

a. Agglutination with reagent and no agglutination with control is a positive test result and indicates the presence of D antigen. Do not interpret peripheral drying or fibrin strands as agglutination. No agglutination with reagent and control is a negative test result and indicates absence of D antigen.
b. Agglutination in Rh-hr (negative) control indicates the presence of autoantibodies or rouleaux formation. In such cases, it is recommended that the determination of Rh factor should be made in a saline reacting anti-D such as RHOFINAL anti-D (IgM + IgG).
c. Cord cells, heavily sensitized with anti-D, may give a false negative immediate spin test result.

D^u Test Procedure

a. Agglutination with reagent and no agglutination with control indicate the presence of D^u antigen. No agglutination with reagent and control indicates absence of D^u antigen.
b. Mixed field agglutination in D^u test on red cells from a recently delivered woman may indicate a mixture of maternal Rh negative and fetal Rh positive blood.
c. Red cells demonstrating a positive direct antiglobulin test cannot be accurately tested for D^u antigen.

Remarks

As undercentrifugation or overcentrifugation could lead to erroneous results, it is recommended that, each laboratory calibrates its own equipment and the time required for achieving the desired results.

ANTI-D (Rho) (IgM)

Monoclonal Blood Typing Antibodies for Slide and Tube Tests (From Tulip's Eryclone Range)

Summary

Monoclonal antibodies are derived from hybridoma cell lines, created by fusing mouse antibody producing B lymphocytes with mouse myeloma cells or are derived from a human B cell line through EBV transformation. Each hybridoma cell line produces homogeneous antibodies of only one immunoglobulin class, which are identical in their chemical structure and immunological activity.

Human red blood cells are classified as RhoD positive or RhoD negative depending on the presence or absence of D antigen on them. Approximately 85% of the Caucasian population is Rh positive. The D^u phenotype is a variant of D antigen and is recognised by performing the antiglobulin test.

About 60% of the traditional D^us, now classified as weak or partial D's may react with Eryclone anti-D (IgM) in slide tests and about 90% may be detected by the tube technique.

Reagent

Eryclone Anti-D (IgM) is a ready-to-use reagent, prepared from supernatants of cell cultures with antibody producing B lymphocytes obtained through EBV transformation and is a blend of monoclonal antibodies of immunoglobulin class IgM. These antibodies are a mixture of several monoclonal antibodies of the same specificity but having the capability of recognising different epitopes of human red blood cell antigen D (Rho).

Eryclone Anti-D (IgM) does not detect all weak and partial D's. For the confirmation of negative reactions with Eryclone Anti-D (IgM) further testing with an incomplete Anti-D of IgG class is strongly recommended to confirm the presence or absence of weak/partial D's.

Each batch of reagent undergoes rigorous quality control at various stages of manufacture for its specificity, avidity and performance.

Reagent Storage and Stability

a. Store the reagent at 2-8°C. Do not freeze.
b. The shelf life of the reagent is as per the expiry date mentioned on the reagent vial label.

Principle

Human red blood cells possessing D antigen will agglutinate in the presence of antibody directed towards the antigen. Agglutination of red blood cells with Eryclone anti-D (IgM) reagent is a positive test result and indicates the presence of D antigen.

No agglutination with the reagent is a negative test result and indicates the absence of D antigen. All negative test results should be further tested for D (presence of weak / partial D's) by performing the D^u test procedure using an incomplete Anti-D of IgG class, as described later.

Note

1. *In vitro* diagnostic reagent for laboratory and professional use only. Not for medicinal use.
2. Eryclone Anti-D (IgM) reagent is not from human source, hence, contamination due to HBsAg and HIV is practically excluded.
3. The reagent contains sodium azide 0.1% as preservative. Avoid contact with skin and mucosa. On disposal flush with large quantities of water.
4. Extreme turbidity may indicate microbial contamination or denaturation of protein due to thermal damage. Such reagent should be discarded.

Sample Collection and Storage

No special preparation of the patient is required prior to sample collection by approved techniques. Samples should be stored at 2-8° C if not tested immediately. Do not use haemolysed samples. Anticoagulated blood using various anticoagulants should be tested within the below mentioned time period:

EDTA or heparin	:	2 days
Sodium citrate or sodium oxalate	:	14 days
ACD or CPD	:	28 days.

Clotted whole blood should be tested within 14 days.

Additional Material Required for Slide and Tube Tests

Glass slides (50 × 75 mm), Test tubes (10 × 75 mm), Pasteur pipettes, Isotonic saline, Centrifuge, Timer, Mixing sticks, Eryclone anti-human globulin (Coomb's) reagent, Eryclone anti-D (IgG) or Rhofinal anti-D (IgM + IgG)

Test Procedure

Bring reagent and samples to room temperature before testing.

Slide Test

1. Place one drop of Eryclone Anti-D (IgM) reagent on a clean glass slide
2. Pipette one equal drop of whole blood on the slide.
3. Mix well with a mixing stick uniformly over an area of approximately 2.5 cm.
4. Rock the slide gently, back and forth.
5. Observe for agglutination macroscopically at two minutes.

Immediate Spin Tube Test

1. Prepare a 5% suspension of the red cells to be tested in isotonic saline.
2. Place one drop of Eryclone anti-D (IgM) reagent into a labelled test tube.
3. Pipette into the test tube one drop of the 5% cell suspension and mix well.
4. Centrifuge for 1 minute at 1000 rpm (125 g) or 20 seconds at 3400 rpm (1000 g).
5. Gently resuspend the cell button, observing for agglutination macroscopically.

D^u Test Procedure

1. Prepare a 5% suspension of the red cells to be tested in isotonic saline.
2. Place one drop of any incomplete anti-D (IgG class) reagent such as Eryclone anti-D (IgG) into a labelled test tube.
3. Add to the test tube one drop of the 5% cell suspension and mix well. Incubate at 37°C for 15 minutes.
4. Wash the contents of the tube thoroughly, at least three times, with isotonic saline and decant completely after the last wash.
5. Add two drops of Eryclone anti-human globulin reagent and mix well.
6. Centrifuge for 1 minute at 1000 rpm (125g) or 20 seconds at 3400 rpm (1000g).
7. Very gently, resuspend the cell button and observe for agglutination macroscopically.

INTERPRETATION OF RESULTS

Slide and Tube tests

a. Agglutination is a positive test result and indicates the presence of D antigen. Do not interpret peripheral drying or fibrin strands as agglutination. No agglutination is a negative test result and indicates the absence of D antigen.

b. Cord cells heavily sensitized with anti-D may give a false negative immediate spin test result.

D^u Test Procedure

a. Agglutination indicates the presence of D^u antigen (Presence of weak/partial D's). No agglutination indicates the absence of D^u antigen (Absence of weak/partial D's).
b. Mixed field agglutination in the D^U test on red cells from a recently delivered woman may indicate a mixture of maternal RhoD negative and fetal RhoD positive blood.
c. Red cells demonstrating a positive direct antiglobulin test cannot be accurately tested for D^u antigen (Presence of weak/partial D's).

Remarks

As under centrifugation or overcentrifugation could lead to erroneous results, it is recommended that each laboratory calibrate its own equipment and determine the time required for achieving the desired results. It is strongly recommended that as a routine quality control measures known RhoD positive and RhoD negative red cells be occasionally run, preferably on a daily basis so as to control reagent performance and validate test results. After usage the reagent should be immediately recapped and replaced at 2-8°C storage.

ANTI-D (Rho) (IgG)

Monoclonal Blood Typing Antibodies for Slide and Modified Tube Tests (From Tulip's Eryclone Range)

Summary

Monoclonal antibodies are derived from hybridoma cell lines, created by fusing mouse antibody producing B lymphocytes with mouse myeloma cells or are derived from a human B cell line through EBV transformation. Each hybridoma cell line produces homogeneous antibodies of only one immunoglobulin class, which are identical in their chemical structure and immunological activity.

Human red blood cells are classified as Rho(D) positive or Rho(D) negative depending upon the presence or absence of D(Rho) antigen on them. Approximately 85% of the Caucasian population is Rho(D) positive. The D^u phenotype is a variant of D(Rho) antigen and is recognised by performing the antiglobulin test.

Reagent

Eryclone® anti-D(Rho) (lgG) is a ready-to-use high-protein reagent, prepared from supernatants of cell cultures with antibody producing B lymphocytes obtained through EBV transformation. These antibodies of the immunoglobulin class IgG are a mixture of several monoclonal antibodies of the same specificity but having the capability of recognising different epitopes of the human red blood cell antigen D (Rho).

Each batch of reagent undergoes rigorous quality control at various stages of manufacture for its specificity, avidity and performance.

Reagent Storage and Stability

1 Store the reagent at 2-8°C. Do nor freeze.
2 The shelf life of reagent is as per the expiry date mentioned on the reagent vial label.

Principle

Human red blood cells possessing the D(Rho) antigen will agglutinate in the presence of antibody directed towards the antigen. Agglutination of red blood cells with Eryclone® anti-D(Rho) (lgG) reagent is a positive test result and indicates the presence of D(Rho) antigen. No agglutination with anti-D(Rho) (lgG) reagent is a negative test result and indicates the absence of D (Rho) antigen. All negative test results should be further tested for D^u (Presence of weak/partial D's) by performing the D^u test procedure as described later.

Note

1. *In vitro* diagnostic reagent for laboratory and professional use only. Not for medicinal use.
2. Eryclone® anti-D (Rho) (IgG) reagent is not from human source, hence, contamination due to HBsAg and HIV is practically excluded.
3. The reagent contains sodium azide 0.1% as preservative. Avoid contact with skin and mucosa. On disposal flush with large quantities of water.
4. Extreme turbidity may indicate microbial conta-

mination or denaturation of protein due to thermal damage. Such reagent should be discarded.

Sample Collection and Preparation

No special preparation of the patient is required prior to sample collection by approved techniques. Samples should be stored at 2-8°C if not tested immediately. Do not use haemolysed samples. Anticoagulated blood using various anticoagulants should be tested within the below mentioned time period

EDTA or Heparin	: 2 days
Sodium citrate or sodium oxalate	: 14 days
ACD or CPD	: 28 days.

Clotted whole blood should be tested within 14 days.

Additional Material Required for Slide and Tube Tests

Glass slides (50 × 75 mm), Test tubes (10 × 75 mm), Pasteur pipettes, Isotonic saline, Centrifuge, Timer, Mixing sticks, Eryclone® anti-human globulin (Coomb's) reagent, Eryclone® Rh-hr control.

Test Procedure

It is recommended that a negative control be run simultaneously with each RhoD test sample using Eryclone® Rh-hr control because invalid positive results may be obtained as with all high-protein blood typing reagent, especially with samples having autoantibodies or abnormal serum proteins.

Bring reagent and samples to room temperature before testing.

Slide Test

1. Place one drop of Eryclone®anti-D (Rho) (lgG) reagent on a clean prewarmed glass slide (40-45°C surface temperature).
2. Add one equal drop of whole blood.
3. Mix well with a mixing stick uniformly over an area of approximately 2.5 cm^2.
4. Rock the slide gently, back and forth.
5. Observe for agglutination macroscopically at two minutes.

Tube Test

1. Prepare a 5% suspension of the red cells to be tested in isotonic saline.
2. Place one drop of Eryclone® anti-D (Rho) (lgG) reagent into a labelled test tube.
3. Pipette into the test tube, one drop of the 5% cell suspension and mix well. Incubate at 37°C for 15 minutes.
4. Centrifuge for 1 minute at 1000 rpm (125 g) or 20 seconds at 3400 rpm (1000 g).
5. Gently resuspend the cell button, observing for agglutination macroscopically.

D^u Test Procedure

1. Prepare a 5% suspension of the red cells to be tested in isotonic saline.
2. Place one drop of Eryclone® Anti-D (Rho) (lgG) reagent into a labelled test tube.
3. Pipette into the test tube one drop of the 5% cell suspension and mix well. Incubate at 37°C for 15 minutes.
4. Wash the contents of the tube thoroughly, at least three times, with isotonic saline and decant completely after the last wash.
5. Add two drops of Eryclone®anti-human globulin reagent and mix well.
6. Centrifuge for 1 minute at 1000 rpm (125 g) or 20 seconds at 3400 rpm (1000 g).
5. Very gently, resuspend the cell button, observing for agglutination macroscopically.

INTERPRETATION OF RESULTS

Slide and Tube tests

a. Agglutination with reagent and no agglutination with Rh-hr control is a positive test result and indicates the presence of the D(Rho) antigen. Do not interpret peripheral drying or fibrin strands as agglutination. No agglutination with reagent and control is a negative test result and indicates absence of the D(Rho) antigen.
b. Agglutination in Rh-hr (negative) control indicates the presence of autoantibodies or rouleaux formation. In such cases, it is recommended that the determination of Rh factor should be made with a saline reacting anti-D such as RHOFINAL® anti-D (IgM + IgG).
c. Cord cells heavily sensitized with anti-D(Rho) may give a false negative immediate spin test result.

D^u Test Procedure

a. Agglutination with reagent and no agglutination with control indicates the presence of D^u antigen (weak/partial D's). No agglutination with reagent and control indicates absence of the D^u antigen.

b. Mixed field agglutination in the D^u test on red cells from a recently delivered woman may indicate a mixture of maternal Rho(D) negative and fetal Rho(D) positive blood,
c. Red cells demonstrating a positive direct antiglobulin test cannot be accurately tested for D^u antigen (weak/partial D's).

Remarks

1. As undercentrifugation or overcentrifugation could lead to erroneous results, it is recommended that each laboratory calibrates its own equipment and determine the time required for achieving the desired results.
2. It is strongly recommended that as a routine quality control measure known Rho(D) positive and Rho(D) negative red cells be occasionally run, preferably on a daily basis so as to control reagent performance and validation of test results.
3. After usage the reagent should be immediately recapped and replaced to 2-8°C storage.

ANTI-D (Rho) (IgM + IgG)

Monoclonal Blood Typing Antibodies for Slide and Tube Tests (Rhofinal from Tulip)

Summary

Monoclonal antibodies are derived from hybridoma cell lines, created by fusing mouse antibody producing B lymphocytes with mouse myeloma cells or are derived from a human B cell line through EBV transformation. Each hybridoma cell line produces homogeneous antibodies of only one immunoglobulin class, which are identical in their chemical structure and immunological activity. Human red blood cells are classified as Rho(D) positive or Rho(D) negative depending on the presence or absence of Rho(D) antigen on them. Approximately 85% of the Caucasian population is Rho(D) positive. The D^u phenotype is a traditional definition to describe the weak/partial D's that can be detected with Rhofinal® anti-D (Rho) (lgM + IgG). About 60% of the D^us(weak/partial D^us) may react with Rhofinal® anti-D (Rho) (IgM + IgG) in slide tests and about 90% may be detected by the tube technique.

Reagent

Rhofinal® anti-D (Rho) (lgM +IgG} is ready-to-use reagent, prepared from supernatants of cell cultures with antibody producing B lymphocytes obtained through EBV transformation and is a blend of monoclonal antibodies of immunoglobulin class IgM and IgG. These antibodies are a mixture of several monoclonal antibodies of the same specificity but having the capability of recognising different epitopes of the human red blood cell antigen D (Rho).

Rhofinal® Anti-D (Rho) (IgM + IgG) is a blend of IgM and IgG class of Anti-D (Rho) monoclonals, a characteristic which accords versatility to the reagent. It gives an avid saline reacting slide/tube test reagent the capability of detecting D^u (weak/partial D's) in the anti human globulin phase. Each batch of reagent undergoes rigorous quality control at various stages of manufacture for its specificity, avidity and performance.

Reagent Storage and Stability

1. Store the reagent at 2-8°C. Do not freeze.
2. The shelf life of the reagent is as per the expiry date mentioned on the reagent vial label.

Principle

Human red blood cells possessing D(Rho) antigen will agglutinate in the presence of antibody directed towards the antigen. Agglutination of red blood cells with Rhofinal® anti-D (Rho) (IgM-IgG) reagent is a positive test result and indicates the presence of D(Rho) antigen. No agglutination with Rhofinal® anti-D (Rho) (IgM + IgG) reagent is a negative test result and indicates the absence of D(Rho) antigen. All negative test results should be further tested for D^u (weak/partial D's) by performing the D^u test procedure, as described later.

Note

1. *In vitro* diagnostic reagent for laboratory and professional use only. Not for medicinal use.
2. Rhofinal® anti-D (Rho) (lgM+IgG) reagent is not from human source, hence, contamination due to HBsAg and HIV is practically excluded.
3. The reagent contains sodium azide 0.1% as preservative. Avoid contact with skin and mucosa. On disposal flush with large quantities of water.

4. Extreme turbidity may indicate microbial contamination or denaturation of protein due to thermal damage. Such reagent should be discarded.

Sample Collection and Preparation

No special preparation of the patient is required prior to sample collection by approved techniques. Samples should be stored at 2-8°C if not tested immediately. Do not use haemolysed samples. Anticoagulated blood using various anticoagulants should be tested within the below mentioned time period:

EDTA or Heparin	:	2 days
Sodium citrate or sodium oxalate	:	14 days
ACD or CPD	:	28 days

Clotted whole blood should be tested within 14 days.

Additional Material Required for Slide and Tube Tests

Glass slides (50 × 75 mm), Test tubes (12 × 75 mm), Pasteur pipettes, Isotonic saline, Centrifuge, Timer, Mixing sticks, Eryclone® anti-human globulin (Coomb's) reagent.

Test Procedure

Bring reagent and samples to room temperature before testing.

Slide Test

1. Place one drop of Rhofinal® anti-D (Rho) (lgM+lgG) on a clean glass slide.
2. Pipette one equal drop of whole blood on the slide.
3. Mix well with a mixing stick uniformly over an area of approximately 2.5 cm^2.
4. Rock the slide gently, back and forth.
5. Observe for agglutination macroscopically at two minutes.

Tube Test

1 Prepare a 5% suspension of the red cells to be tested in isotonic saline.
2. Place one drop of Rhofinal® anti-D (Rho) (IgM + IgG) reagent into labelled test tube.
3. Pipette into each of the test tube one drop of the 5% cell suspension and mix well.
4. Centrifuge for 1 minute at 1000 rpm (125 g) or 20 seconds at 3400 rpm (1000 g).
5. Gently resuspend the cell button, observing for agglutination macroscopically.

D^u Test procedure

1. Prepare a 5% suspension of the red cells to be tested in isotonic saline.
2. Place one drop of Rhofinal® anti-D (Rho) (lgM+lgG) reagent into labelled test tube.
3. Add to the test tube, one drop of the cell suspension and mix well. Incubate at 37°C for 15 minutes.
4. Wash the contents of the tube, at least three times, with isotonic saline and decant completely after the last wash.
5. Add two drops of Eryclone® anti-human globulin reagent and mix well.
6. Centrifuge for 1 minute at 1000 rpm (125 g) or 20 seconds at 3400 rpm (1000 g).
7. Very gently, resuspend the cell button and observe for agglutination macroscopically.

INTERPRETATION OF RESULTS

Slide and Tube tests

a. Agglutination is a positive test result and indicates the presence of the D (Rho) antigen. Do not interpret peripheral drying or fibrin strands as agglutination. No agglutination is a negative test result and indicates absence of the D (Rho) antigen.
b. Cord cells heavily sensitised with anti-D(Rho) may give a false negative immediate spin test result.

D^u Test Procedure

a. Agglutination with the reagent and no agglutination with the control indicates presence of the D^u antigen (weak/partial D's). No agglutination with reagent and control indicates absece of the D^u antigen (weak/partial D's).
b. Mixed field agglutination in the D^u test on red cells from a recently delivered woman may indicate a mixture of maternal Rho(D) negative and fetal Rho(D) positive blood.
c. Red cells demonstrating a positive direct antiglobulin test cannot be accurately tested for D^u antigen (weak/partial D's).

Remarks

1. As undercentrifugation or overcentrifugation could lead to erroneous results, it is recommended that each laboratory calibrates its own equipment and determine the time required for achieving the desired results.
2. It is strongly recommended that as a routine quality control measure known Rho(D) positive and Rho(D) negative red cells be occasionally run, preferably on a daily basis so as to control reagent performance and validation of test results.
3. After usage, the reagent should be immediately recapped and replaced at 2-8°C storage.

BLOOD GROUP TESTING IN MICROPLATES

The microplates consist of 12 × 8 = 96 wells. We can do 12 groups in one plate.

Anti-A	®	O	O	O	O	O	O	O	O	O	O	O
Anti-B	®	O	O	O	O	O	O	O	O	O	O	O
Anti-AB	®	O	O	O	O	O	O	O	O	O	O	O
Anti-D1	®	O	O	O	O	O	O	O	O	O	O	O
Anti-D2	®	O	O	O	O	O	O	O	O	O	O	O
A Cell	®	O	O	O	O	O	O	O	O	O	O	O
B Cell	®	O	O	O	O	O	O	O	O	O	O	O
O Cell	®	O	O	O	O	O	O	O	O	O	O	O

In the first 5 wells we do direct blood grouping (cell grouping) and in remaining 3 wells we do serum grouping.

a. For all microtitration techniques, the cell suspension required is 2% (so we prepare 2% cell suspension of patient/donor cell and also 2% suspension of A cell, B cell, O cells (pooled).
b. Antisera used in microtitre plates are also diluted. Roughly we dilute anti-A and anti-B seras as 1:20 dilution and anti-D as 1:10 (Dilution of antisera depends on the titration of anti-A, anti-B and anti-D. We select the best dilution at which the reaction occurs).

Procedure

1. In the first 5 wells put one drop each of Diluted (as described above) anti-A, anti-B, anti-AB, anti -D1, and anti-D2 (i.e. anti-D of two different companies).
   +
   Add 1 drop of patient/donor red cell suspension (2%).
2. In the next three wells (reverse grouping) put one drop each of A cell, B cell and O cell
   +
   Add one drop of patient serum.
3. Incubate the tubes at RT for 60 minutes.
   In emergency cases, centrifuge the plates at 1000 rpm for 3-4 minutes and see for agglutination.

Results: In negative reaction, the red cells trail from the centre of the well; and in positive reaction, cells remain in the centre or fall in discrete button to the bottom of well.

ANTIHUMAN GLOBULIN TEST

Historical Perspective

The first step towards a rational approach to blood transfusion became possible with Landsteiners discovery in 1901 of the ABO blood group system. Nearly half a century later, the next advance occurred with the introduction of serological techniques permitting the detection of incomplete antibodies, which are nonagglutinating immunoglobulin G (IgG) antibodies that sensitize red blood cells. In 1945, Coomb's et al described the use of anti human globulin test for the detection of weak and non-agglutinating antibodies in serum. Further in 1946, Coomb's et al described the use of anti human globulin test to detect *in vivo* sensitization of red blood cells in babies suffering from haemolytic disease of the newborn. Although the test initially was of great value in investigating Rh_o (D) haemolytic disease of the newborn, it was not long before its versatility for the detection of other IgG blood group antibodies became evident.

Although Coomb's and his coworkers were instrumental in introducing the anti human globulin test to blood group serology, the principle of the test had in fact been described by Moreschi in 1908. Moreschi studies involved the use of rabbit anti goat antiserum to agglutinate rabbit red blood cells that were sensitized with low non-agglutinating dose of goat anti rabbit red cell serum.

Later, in 1957, Dacie et al published data regarding the importance of anti human complement activity. Further, in 1960, many reports were published indicating the need for anti human complement activity in anti human globulin serum to allow the detection of antibodies in the indirect test. Though many of the antibody specificities mentioned in these reports are now considered of little clinical significance; however, one specificity that was consistently mentioned and is still considered to be clinically significant was Anti-Jk[a]. Further it was also shown that the presence of anti human complement activity would enhance the reaction of some antibodies namely Anti-Fy[a] and Anti-K.

Preliminary Notes: Antigen and antibody related to blood group serology

Antigens are foreign substances, which initiate an immune response in human body and react specifically with antibodies. Blood group antigens that are located on the surface of red blood cells when transferred to another individual are almost certain to carry antigens not possessed by the recipient. These foreign antigens then initiate an immune response and production of antibodies *in vivo.* Antibodies are counter agents produced as a defence mechanism when foreign antigen enters human body. With respect to blood group serology, it means that blood group antibodies are specific and are formed against red blood cell antigens not possessed by the recipient.

Antibody Nomenclature with Respect to Blood Group Serology

Red blood cell antibodies may be naturally occurring or immune in nature. Naturally occurring antibodies are produced because of the exposure of human body to certain bacteria and plant substances whose antigenic structure resembles blood group antigens. Naturally occurring antibodies are most often IgM class of antibodies.

Immune antibodies (alloantibodies) are antibodies present in an individual due to transfusion or pregnancy. Immune antibodies most often are IgG class of antibodies, sometimes IgM or a mixture of IgM and IgG class of antibodies.

IgM Class Antibodies

IgM antibodies are pentamers in which five polypeptide sub units are held together by disulphide bonds and joined by J chain. IgM antibodies do not cross the placenta but are most effective in activating complement (Fig. 11.4).

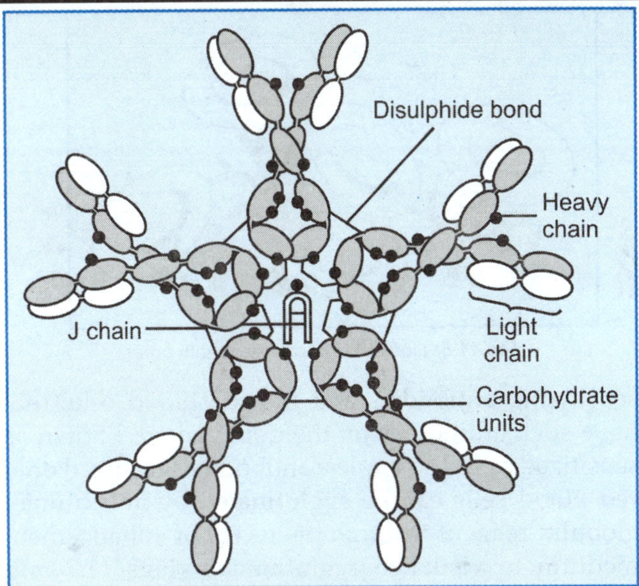

Fig. 11.4: Illustration of IgM molecule

Sialic acid present on the red cell membranes impart to the cells, a net negative charge. As a result mutual repulsive force exists between red blood cells known as zeta potential and the red blood cells are separated by a distance. In blood group serology IgM antibodies are termed as complete antibodies because of their ability to directly bridge the distance between two red blood cells in spite of the zeta potential and bring about visible agglutination. IgM antibodies are able to bridge this distance and bring about visible agglutination (Fig. 11.5).

IgG Class Antibodies

IgG antibodies are monomers with two heavy chains and two light chains. IgG is the only immunoglobulin that can cross the placental barrier, a fact which explains the role of IgG antibodies in haemolytic disease of the newborn. Four subclasses of IgG are present and they vary widely in their ability to activate complement (Fig. 11.6). IgG3 molecules are highly effective in activating complement, IgG1 moderately activate complement, IgG2 slightly activate complement and IgG4 do not activate complement.

IgG antibodies are also known as incomplete antibodies because they cannot bridge the distance between two red blood cells and bring about direct agglutination like the IgM immunoglobulins. Antibodies that do not agglutinate red blood cells directly are termed as incomplete antibodies or

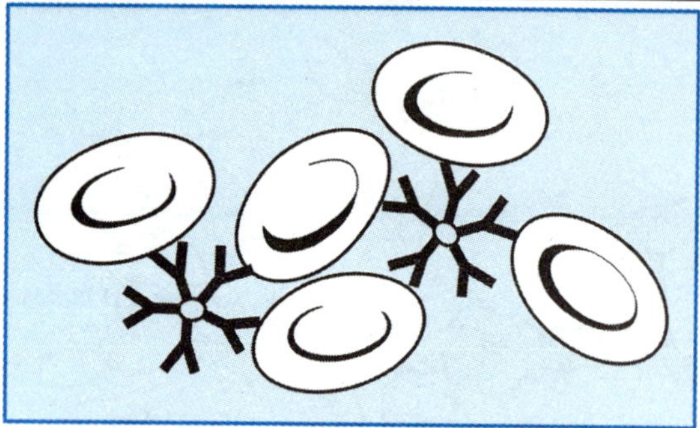

Fig.11.5: Illustration of complete antibodies

sensitizing antibodies and the red blood cells that have such antibodies on their surface are known as sensitized cells. Incomplete antibodies sensitized onto red blood cells can be agglutinated by anti human globulin reagent through the usage of enhancement medium to visualize agglutination (Figs 11.7 and 11.8).

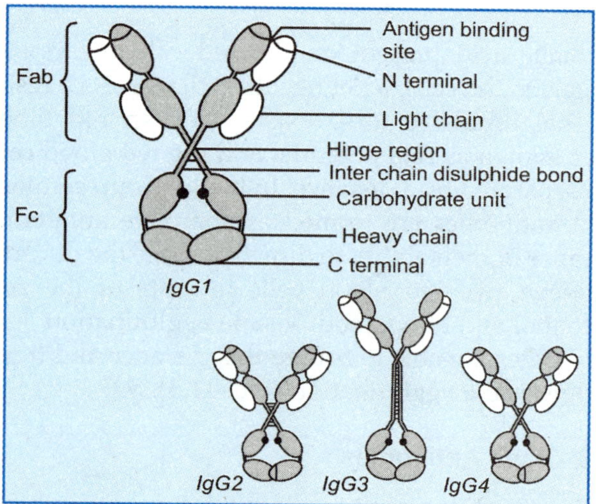

Fig. 11.6: Structure of four subclasses of IgG

Role of Enhancement Medium

An enhancement medium can either be a protein (e.g. bovine serum albumin) or enzymes (e.g. papain, bromelin, ficin) or low ionic salt solution (LISS) or charged molecules (polybrene) that reduce zeta potential, enhance antibody uptake, enhancement in agglutination reactions (Fig. 11.9).

In order to clearly understand antibody enhancement methods, it is important to consider the basic aspect of haemagglutination reactions. Agglutination is a reversible chemical reaction and occurs probably in two stages:

Stage 1: Sensitization, i.e. attachment of antibody to red blood cell membrane antigen.

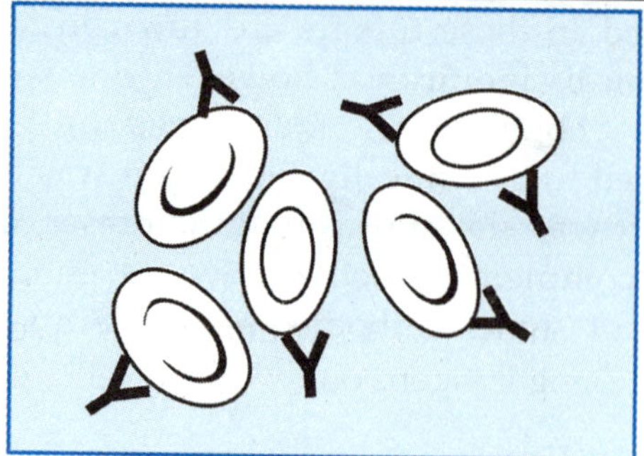

Fig. 11.7: Illustration of red blood cells sensitized with incomplete antibodies

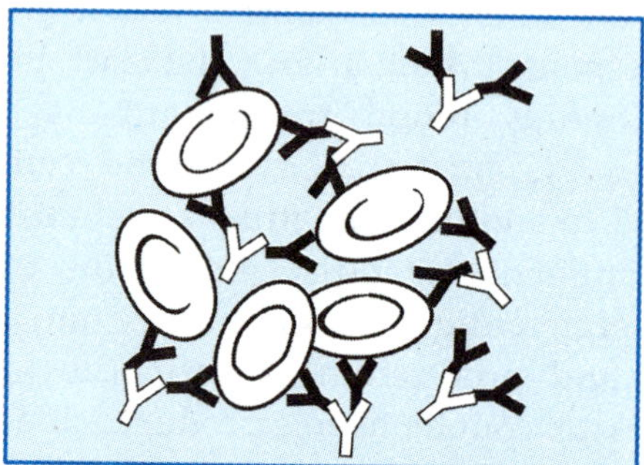

Fig. 11.8: Illustration of IgG sensitized red blood cells agglutinated by AHG reagent

Stage 2: Formation of bridges between the sensitized red blood cells to form lattice (crosslinking) to visualize agglutination.

Thus, various factors that affect these two stages can be manipulated to enhance agglutination.

ENHANCEMENT TECHNIQUES

Albumin Additives

Bovine serum albumin (BSA), a dipolar protein has been used routinely for many years as an enhancement medium. The enhancement effect of albumin is attributed to its influence on the second stage of agglutination by reducing the net negative charge on the red blood cell membranes thereby potentiating agglutination. Bovine serum albumin is available as solutions of 22% or 30% concentration.

Enzymes

Treating red blood cells with certain enzymes enhances agglutination of antibodies with red blood cell antigens. Most commonly used enzymes in immunohaematological procedures are papain, bromelin and ficin which belong to thiol protease class of enzymes.

Proteolytic enzymes reduce the red blood cell surface charge by cleaving sialic acid molecules on red blood cell membrane, lowering the zeta potential and enhance agglutination. Enzyme treatment also causes spicule formation on the red blood cell membrane. This greatly increases the potential number of contact points for antibodies to react with corresponding antigens on red blood cell membrane.

The reaction of Anti-P, Lewis and Kidd blood group antibodies are stronger with enzyme treated red blood cells. Another important observation is that Lewis and Kidd blood group antibodies may lyse enzyme-treated red blood cells.

Positively Charged Molecules

In the presence of positively charged polymers, such as hexadimethrine bromide (Polybrene®), protamine sulphate and poly-L-lysine, normal red blood cells exhibit spontaneous aggregation. Thus, any red blood cells sensitized with antibody will exhibit enhanced agglutination.

The action of these charged molecules may be due to neutralization of negative charge contributed by sialic acid and release of water molecules that cover red blood cell membrane thereby enhancing agglutination.

Polybrene® generally is added to red blood cells that have been incubated with antibody at low ionic strength and low pH.

Polyethylene Glycol (PEG)

PEG is a water-soluble polymer used as an additive to increase antibody uptake. Its action is to remove water molecule that takes up more space around the red blood cell membrane, thereby enhancing antibody uptake and reaction strength.

LISS (Low Ionic Salt Solution) and LISS additives

LISS (approximately 0.03 M) greatly increases stage 1 uptake of antibody to red blood cells, as compared to normal saline (approximately 0.17 M). To prevent lysis of red blood cells at such a low ionic strength, a non-ionic substance, such as glycine, is incorporated in LISS.

LISS additives may sometimes contain macromolecules (e.g. BSA) in addition to ionic salts and buffers. Addition of macromolecules to LISS reduces ionic strength with shortened incubation times.

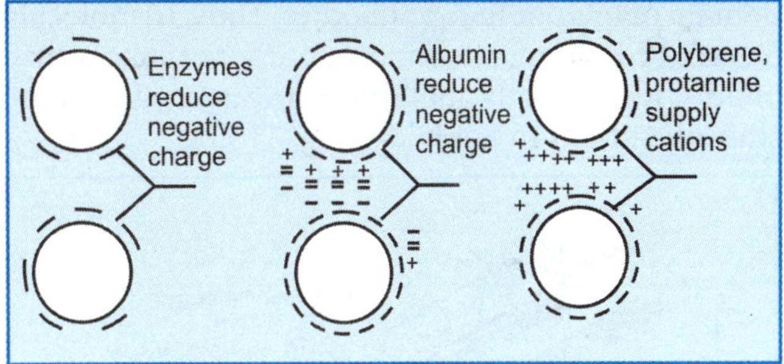

Fig. 11.9: Illustration of antibody enhancement

COMPLEMENT

An observable phenomenon that may result from red blood cell antigen-antibody interaction is haemolysis. This requires co-operation of another defense mechanism of body known as the complement system. Complement is the name given to a set of approximately twenty serum proteins, which in response to antigenic stimulus react with one another in a sequential cascade.

The most important complement component is C3b, which can be activated either by the classical (Fig. 11.10) or the alternate pathway. The antigen-antibody interactions activate the classical pathway that is of great significance in blood group serology.

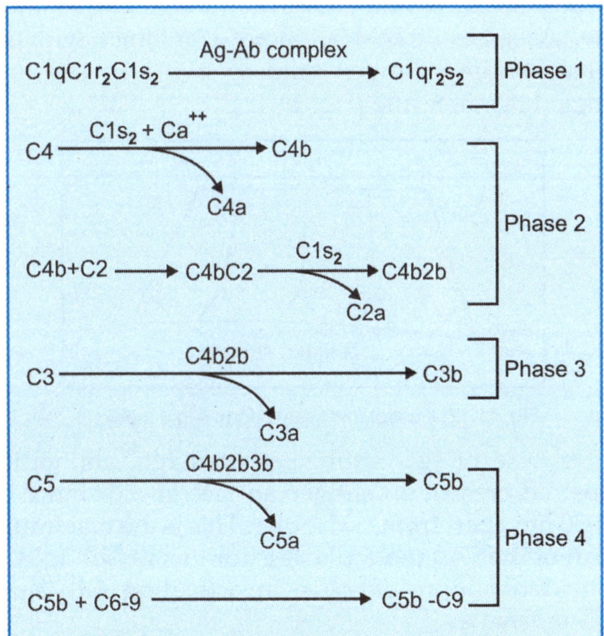

Fig. 11.10: Activation of classical complement pathway

Immunoglobulin Requirements for Activation of Classical Pathway

The mode of activation of classical pathway is through binding of C1q to CH2 domain of IgM or to the CH2 domain of IgG1 or IgG_3 antibodies. The C1q molecule has six Fc-binding sites and in order to make a firm bond with antibody molecule, at least two of these sites must bind to antibody (Fig. 11.11).

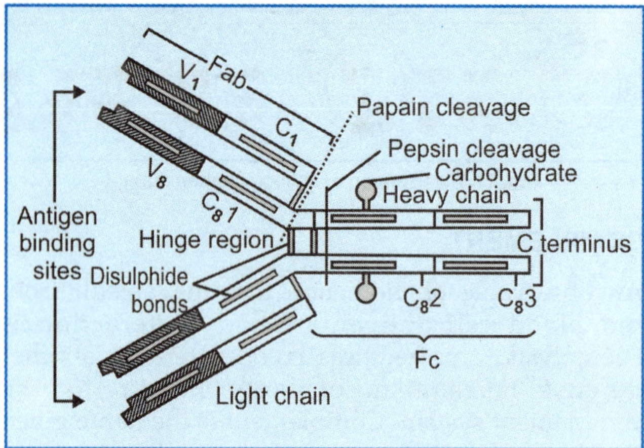

Fig. 11.11: Illustration of immunoglobulin molecule

In case of IgM antibodies, when the molecule is in planar or star form, there is only a single binding site for C1q, as a result it cannot bind firmly and activate C1q. However, when combined with antigen, IgM molecule usually assumes staple form with the F(ab) at right angle with Fc. The distortion produced by this movement exposes an additional C1q binding site. As a result IgM antibody combined with its corresponding antigen bind to two C1q sites on single IgM molecule (Fig. 11.12).

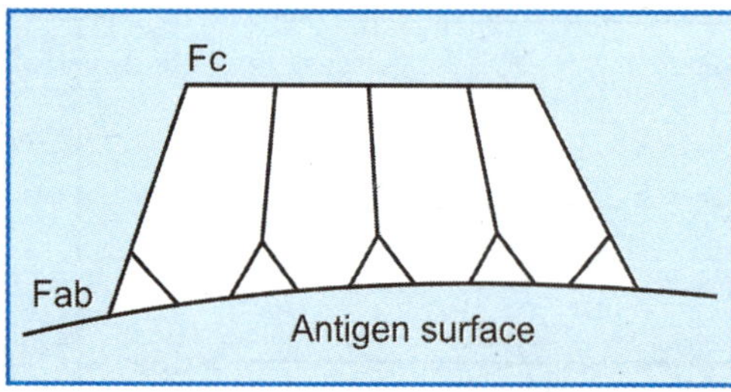

Fig. 11.12: Illustration of staple form—IgM molecule

In case of IgG antibodies, two IgG antibodies must be present on antigen surface at a distance of 20-30 nm apart from each other. This is the maximum span of the C1q molecule. It is for this reason IgM is considered more effective in activating C1q than IgG molecule.

An important point to note is that all examples of immune anti-D fail to activate complement. The reason being that the D antigenic sites are too far apart from each other on the red blood cell surface. As discussed, two IgG molecules must be at a distance of 20-30 nm apart from each other so as to activate C1q. Since D antigenic sites are too far apart from each other, the bound IgG molecules cannot activate C1q.

Complement Binding Antibodies (Table 11.5)

Complement components may attach to red blood cells *in vivo* or *in vitro* via one of the probable mechanisms.

- Complement binding alloantibody (blood group antibodies present in an individual due to transfusion or pregnancy) specific for red blood cell antigen may cause sensitization of complement component on red blood cell surface due to transfusion.

Complement-binding alloantibodies when present in low concentrations bring about the attachment of complement component up to the C3 stage, but produce little or no haemolysis. Further activation of C3 occurs only when complement is powerfully activated due to high concentration of antibodies, leading to the generation of large amount of C3b. Certain antibodies such as Anti-Jk^a are seldom lytic but invariably activate complement thereby leading to the deposition of complement components on the red blood cell surface.

Table 11.5: Complement binding by human red cell antibodies

System	*Antibody*	*Readily detectable haemolysis*	*Positive antiglobulin test (anti-complement)*
ABO	anti-A		
	anti-B	many	many
	anti-A, B		
	anti-A-	none	very few
	anti-HI	none	few
	anti-H^t	all	all
Lewis	anti-Le^a	some	all
	anti-Le^b	few	many
P-	anti-P_1	few	few
	anti-PP_1P^k	all	all
	anti-P (auto-)	all	all
	anti-P (allo-)	many	all
li	anti-l auto-	many	many
	anti-1		
Sd	anti-Sd^a	none	some
Rh	anti-D	none	none
	anti-c, E, etc.	none	none
K	anti-K	none	many
Fy	anti-Fy^a	none	many
Jk	anti-Jk^a	few	all
MNSs	anti-M, -N	none	none
	anti-S,-s	none	some
Lu	anti-Lu^a,-Lu^b	none	none
Di	anti-Di^a	few	few
Xg	anti-Xg^a	none	many

- About 10-20% of patient with warm AIHA (Autoimmune haemolytic anaemia) demonstrate *in vivo* sensitization with complement component C3.
- In cold haemagglutinin disease, the cold reactive autoantibody can react with red blood cell antigens at temperature up to 32°C range (thermal amplitude 10-32°C). When the patient is exposed to cold temperature, red blood cell is sensitized with autoantibody, which activates complement. If the red blood cells escape haemolysis, they return to the central circulation where the temperature is 37°C and the autoantibody dissociates from the cells, leaving complement component C3d firmly bound to the red blood cell membrane.

Basic Concepts of Anti-human Globulin Testing

Two major class of antibodies react with red blood cell antigens namely the complete antibodies and the incomplete antibodies.

Complete antibodies, or saline agglutinins will agglutinate red blood cells suspended in saline, which are usually IgM class of antibodies.

Incomplete antibodies do not react in saline but require special techniques to agglutinate red blood cells; which are IgG class of antibodies.

After combining with their corresponding antigen, blood group antibodies have the ability to activate complement. Thus, sensitization of incomplete antibodies or complement component can occur either *in vivo* or *in vitro*. Anti-humanglobulin reagent is used to detect IgG or complement sensitized red blood cells.

For detecting *in vivo* antibody or complement sensitization, DAT (Direct Antiglobulin Test) is used; whereas for detecting *in vitro* antibody or complement sensitization, IAT (Indirect Antiglobulin Test) is used.

Anti-human Globulin Reagents

Polyspecific Anti-human globulin (Coomb's) Reagent: The term 'polyspecific' reagent refers to reagent system containing blend of antibodies for more than one antigen, i.e. blend of Anti-human IgG, Anti-human C3b, Anti-human C3d. Polyspecific reagent may be a blend of:

- Polyclonal Anti-human IgG, polyclonal Anti-human C3b, polyclonal Anti-human C3d.
- Polyclonal Anti-human IgG, monoclonal Anti-human C3b, moncolonal Anti-human C3d.
- Polyclonal Anti-human IgG, monoclonal Anti-human C3d.

ICSH Recommendations for Polyspecific Anti-human Globulin Reagents

ICSH has recommended certain specifications, which a commercially available Anti-human globulin reagent should comply:

- The reagent should only agglutinate red blood cells sensitized with antibodies and/or coated with significant levels of complement components.
- The potency of Anti-human IgG component should be evaluated by serological titration (chequer board titration).
- A polyspecific reagent should contain Anti-human C3c and Anti-human C3d at controlled levels to avoid false positive reactions or a suitable potent monoclonal Anti-human C3d. It should contain little or no Anti-human C4 activity. The assessment of these qualities requires red cells specifically coated with complement components for evaluating the serological potency.
- All the evaluations should be done in parallel with international reference reagent.

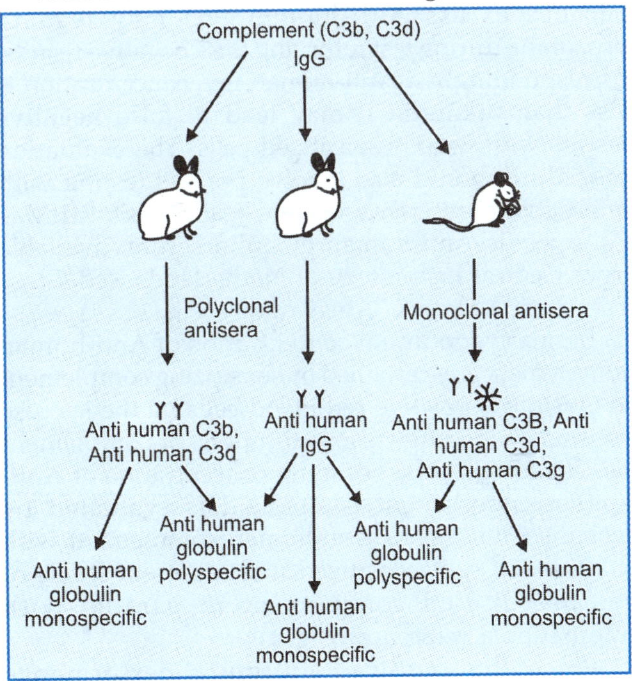

Fig. 11.13: Anti-human globulin manufacture

Polyclonal Anti-human IgG is usually prepared in rabbits, though when large volumes of antibody are required, sheep or goats may be used. In production of polyclonal Anti-human IgG, animals are hyperimmunised to produce high titer, high avidity Anti-human IgG class antibodies. After achieving the desired specificity and titer, the animals are bred for the production batch of reagent (Fig. 11.13).

With monoclonal antibodies, the hybrid clones are screened for antibodies with the required specificity and affinity. The antibody secreting clones may then be propagated in culture or by innoculation into mice, in which case the antibody is collected in ascites. Monoclonal anti human complement may be either IgM or IgG class of antibodies.

Thus, separate blends of Anti-human IgG and Anti-human complement antibodies are made, and each pool is then adsorbed with A, B and O red blood cells to remove heterospecific antibodies. The total antibody content of each pool is determined and then pools are analysed by titration method to calculate the optimum antibody dilution for Anti-human IgG component and Anti-human complement component.

Optimum concentration of Anti-human IgG component is ascertained by chequer board titration method. In chequer board titration dilutions of Anti-human IgG are reacted with various dilutions of anti-D IgG sensitized cells. This is a critical step because excess Anti-human IgG may lead to prozoning during test returning false negative results, correspondingly if Anti-human IgG concentration is less than optimum it may lead to false negative results with weakly sensitized cells. The evaluation procedure should also involve parallel testing with international reference reagent (e.g. WHO. RIIIM—Polyspecific Anti-human globulin serum, available from Central Laboratory of Netherlands Red Cross Transfusion Service, Amsterdam) (Fig. 11.14).

Similarly, optimum concentration of Anti-human complement is ascertained by sensitizing complement to O Rh_o (D) positive red blood cells by the sucrose method, preparing various dilutions of complement sensitized cells. The optimum concentration of Anti-human complement component is evaluated by reacting dilutions of Anti-human complement with dilutions of cells sensitized with different levels of serially diluted complement in parallel with international reference reagent.

Once the required optimum performance characteristic for each component is ascertained, reagent blend of Anti-human IgG and Anti-human complement antibodies is prepared and run as a system in parallel with the international reference reagent. Thus, the final product is one that contains optimum concentration of Anti-human IgG and Anti-human complement antibodies for broad-spectrum reactivity.

Monospecific Coomb's Reagent

Monospecific reagent for use in anti human globulin test are prepared by similar procedure, however, the reagent contains antibody of only one specificity.

- Monospecific Anti-human IgG reagent contains only polyclonal Anti-human IgG
- Monospecific Anti-human C3b reagent contains only polyclonal Anti-human C3b or monoclonal Anti-human C3b.
- Monospecific Anti-human C3d reagent contains only polyclonal Anti-human C3d or monoclonal Anti-human C3d.

DIRECT ANTI-HUMAN GLOBULIN TEST (DAT)

DAT is used to detect *in vivo* sensitization of red blood cells with immunoglobulin, complement or both. A positive DAT, with or without shortened red blood cell survival, may result from:

- Autoantibodies to intrinsic red blood cell antigens.
- Alloantibodies in recipients circulation reacting with antigens on recently transfused donor red blood cells.
- Alloantibodies in donor plasma, plasma derivatives or blood fractions, which react with antigens on red blood cells of transfusion recipients.
- Alloantibodies in maternal circulation, which cross placenta and sensitize foetal red blood cells (HDN).
- Antibodies directed against certain drugs, which bind to red blood cell membranes (e.g. Penicillin).
- Adsorbed proteins, including immunoglobulins, which attach to abnormal membranes or red blood cells modified by therapy with certain drugs, notably those of cephalosporin group.
- Complement components or rarely IgG bound to red blood cells after administration of drugs such as quinidine and phenacetin may induce drug antidrug interaction.

- Non-red blood cell immunoglobulins associated with red blood cells in patient with hypergammaglobulinaemia or recipients with high dose of intravenous gammaglobulin.
- In-patient with organ transplantation, passenger lymphocytes of donor origin produce antibodies directed against ABO or other antigens on the recipient's cells, causing a positive DAT.
- Patients receiving ALG (antilymphocyteglobulin) or ATG (antithymocyte globulin) of animal origin may develop a positive DAT within a few days, apparently related to high titer heterophile antibodies in these products and the presence of corresponding antibodies in animal-derived AHG sera.

MAJOR APPLICATIONS OF DAT IN BLOOD GROUP SEROLOGY

Haemolytic Disease of the Newborn (HDN)

In HDN foetal red blood cells *in vivo* are sensitized with IgG alloantibody of maternal origin thereby demonstrating a positive DAT with cord red blood cells. The most commonly observed HDN is due to Rh_o (D) incompatibility between mother and foetus.

If the father is Rh_o (D) positive and the mother is Rh_o (D) negative and during first pregnancy their progeny inherits Rh_o (D) positive red blood cell antigens. During parturition, the foetal red blood cells can enter mother's circulation providing antigenic stimulus for the production of anti-D antibodies. These anti-D antibodies normally will not have any effect during the first Rh-incompatible pregnancy unless the mother has anti-D antibodies by previous incompatible blood transfusions.

During subsequent pregnancy, for the same couple, if the foetus is Rh_o (D) positive again, the anti-D antibodies will be activated along with the presence of anti-D antibodies from the first pregnancy already in the circulation. Since the IgG antibodies cross the placental barrier, these circulating anti-D will sensitize and destroy foetal Rh_o (D) positive cells. This process is demonstrated by a positive DAT on cord red blood cells (Fig. 11.15).

Transfusion Reactions

A patient will demonstrate positive DAT, if serum contains antibodies against red blood cell antigens of donor red blood cells. Likewise antibody present in donor plasma may also react with recipient red blood cells thereby demonstrating positive DAT.

Other Immune Haemolytic Diseases

A positive DAT may be observed due to acquired haemolytic anaemia probably because of autoantibodies directed against individual's own intrinsic red blood cell antigens.

Dilutions of IgG sensitized cells

Dilutions of AHG	N		16		32		64		128		256		512		1024		2048		4096	
N	3.5	3.5	3.5	3.5	3.5	3.5	2.5	3.5	2.5	2.5	1.0	1.0	1.5	1.5	1.0	1.5	1.0	1.5	G^{r}	2.0
1:2	3.5	3.5	3.5	3.5	3.5	3.5	3.5	3.5	2.0	2.0	2.0	2.0^{s}	1.5	1.0^{s}	1.5	1.0^{s}	2.0	2.5	1.0	1.0
1:4	3.5	3.5	3.5	3.5	3.5	3.5	2.5	3.0	1.5	2.0	1.5	1.5	1.0^{s}	1.0^{s}	1.0^{s}	1.0	1.0^{s}	1.0	1.0^{w}	1.0^{w}
1:8	3.5	3.5	3.5	3.5	3.0^{s}	3.0^{s}	2.0^{w}	3.0	1.5	1.5	1.0^{s}	1.5	1.0^{s}	1.5	1.0^{s}	1.0	1.0^{w}	1.0^{s}	1.0^{w}	1.0
1:16	3.5	3.5	3.5	3.0^{s}	3.0^{s}	2.5	2.0	2.0	1.5	1.5	1.5	1.5	1.0^{s}	1.0^{s}	1.0^{s}	1.0^{s}	1.0^{w}	1.0	1.0^{w}	1.0
1:32	3.5	3.5	2.0	3.5^{s}	3.0^{s}	2.5	2.0	2.0^{w}	2.0	1.0^{s}	1.5	1.0^{s}	1.0^{s}	1.0	1.0	1.0	1.0^{w}	0.5	1.0^{w}	Gr
1:64	3.5	3.5	2.0^{s}	2.0	2.0	2.0	2.0	1.5	1.0^{s}	1.0^{s}	1.0^{s}	1.0^{s}	1.0^{s}	1.0^{w}	Gr	0.5	0.5	0.5	Gr	---

□ W.H.O. R III M ■ Commercially available polyspecific AHG

Fig. 11.14: Chequer board titration results

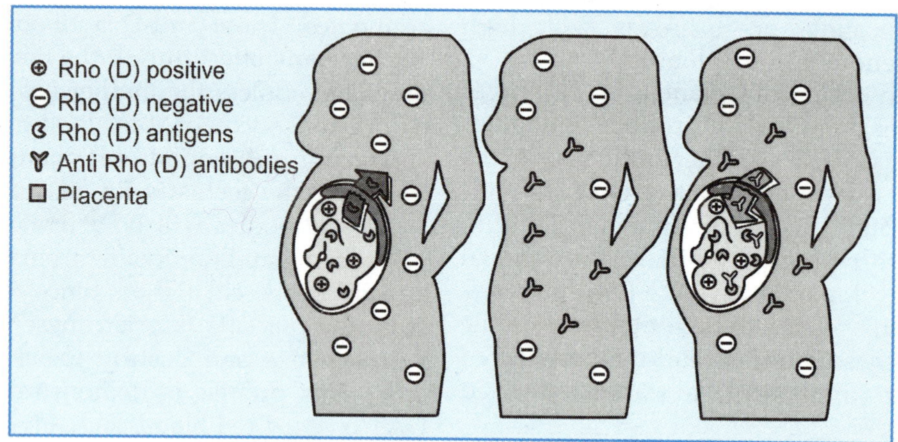

Fig. 11.15: Illustration of HDN

Classification of Autoimmune Haemolytic Anaemia

- Warm Autoimmune Haemolytic Anaemia (WAIHA)
  - Primary (idiopathic)
  - Secondary (to conditions such as lymphoma, SLE, carcinoma, drug therapy)
- Cold Agglutinin Syndrome (CAS)
  - Primary (idiopathic)
  - Secondary (to conditions such as lymphoma, *Mycoplasma pneumoniae*, infectious mononucleosis)
- Mixed type Autoimmune Haemolytic Anaemia
  - Primary (idiopathic)
  - Secondary (to conditions such as SLE, lymphoma)
- Paroxysmal Cold Haemoglobinuria (PCH)
  - Primary (idiopathic)
  - Secondary (to conditions such as syphilis, viral infections)
- DAT Negative Autoimmune Haemolytic Anaemia
  - Primary (idiopathic)
  - Secondary (to conditions such as lymphoma, SLE)

Drug-induced Haemolytic Anaemia

Also, certain drugs namely penicillin, procainamide, cephalosporins may also be associated with immune red blood cell destruction thereby demonstrating a positive DAT (Fig. 11.16).

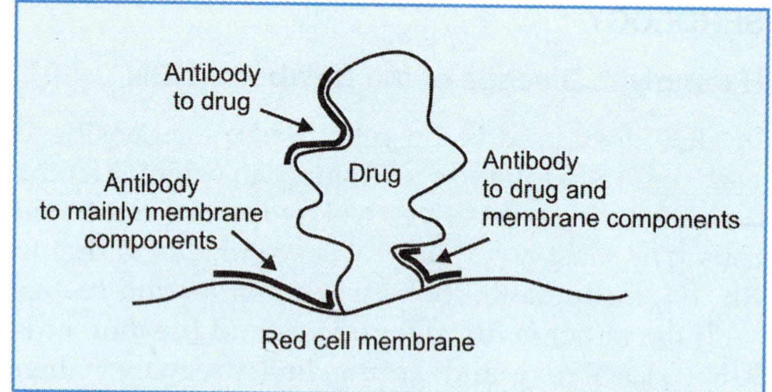

Fig. 11.16: Illustration of drug-induced antibody reactions

Importance of Serological Studies in DAT Positive Results (Table 11.6)

As per AABB technical manual, three investigation approaches are helpful in evaluation of positive DAT:

- Test the DAT positive red blood cells with Monospecific Anti-human IgG and Monospecific Anti-human C3d reagent to characterize type of proteins sensitized with red blood cell membrane,
- Test serum/plasma to detect and identify clinically significant antibodies to red blood cell antigens.
- Test eluate prepared from sensitized red blood cells with a panel of reagent red blood cells to define whether the sensitized protein is immunoglobulin or complement component. Elution frees antibody from sensitized red blood cells and recovers antibody in usable form. When only complement is sensitized, eluates are frequently non-reactive.

Table 11.6: Probable serological findings with DAT positive—AIHA / drug induced haemolytic anaemia

Parameter	*WAIHA*	*CAS*	*Mixed type AIHA*	*PCH*	*Drug-induced AIHA*
DAT positive result	IgG / IgG + C3/ C3	Mostly C3	IgG + C3	Mostly C3	IgG / IgG + C3
Immunoglobulin Type	IgG (sometimes IgA or IgM rarely alone	IgM	IgG, IgM	IgG	IgG
Eluate	IgG	Non reactive	IgG	Non reactive	IgG
Serum	• May react by IAT • May haemolyze enzyme treated red cells at 37°C • Mostly agglutinate enzyme treated red cells at 37°C • May agglutinate untreated red cells at 20°C • Rarely agglutinate untreated cells at 37°C	• IgM haem-agglutinating antibody reactive at 4°C usually react at 30°C in albumin	• IgG IAT reactive antibody • IgM haem-agglutinating antibody usually react at 30-37°C in saline, also may react at 4°C saline	• IgG biphasic haemolysin (Donath Landsteiner antibody)	• IgG antibody similar to WAIHA
Specificity	Usually Rh specificity	Usually Anti-1 but can be Anti-i rarely Anti-Pr	Usually specificity unclear, can be Anti-I, Anti-i or other cold agglutinin specificities	Anti-P (non-reactive with p and P^k red cells	Specificity often Rh related

INDIRECT ANTI-HUMAN GLOBULIN TEST (IAT)

In IAT procedures, serum or plasma is incubated with red blood cells, washed to remove unbound globulins. Agglutination that occurs after addition of Anti-humanglobulin reagent indicates reaction between antibody in the serum and antigen present on the red blood cell membrane.

Applications of IAT

IAT determines *in vitro* sensitization of red blood cells and is used in the following situations:

- Detection of incomplete antibodies to potential donor red blood cells, pregnant women, blood donors.
- Identification of antibody specificity using a panel of red blood cells with known antigenic profile.
- Determination of red blood cell phenotype using known antisera (e.g. D^u testing)
- Titration of incomplete antibodies.

PROBABLE SOURCES OF ERROR IN ANTI-HUMAN GLOBULIN TESTING

False Negative Results

- Neutralization of anti-human globulin Reagent
- Failure to wash cells adequately to remove all serum/plasma. Fill tube at least three fourth full of saline for each wash.

- If increased serum volumes are used, routine wash may be inadequate. Wash additional times more than three or four wash phases.
- Contamination of Anti-human globulin reagent by extraneous protein. Do not use finger or hand to cover tube. Contaminated droppers or wrong reagent dropper can neutralize entire vial of Anti-human globulin reagent.
- High concentration of IgG paraproteins in test serum (cryoglobulin). Wash additional times more than three or four wash phases.

- Interruption in testing
  - Bound IgG may dissociate from red blood cells or leave too little IgG to detect or may neutralize Anti-human globulin reagent. Perform the test immediately.
  - Agglutination of IgG coated cells will weaken. Centrifuge and read immediately.
- Improper reagent storage
  - Anti-human globulin reagent may loose reactivity if frozen. Reagent may become bacterially contaminated. Store at the recommended storage condition.
  - Excess heat or repeated freeze/thaw cycles may cause loss of reactivity of Anti-human globulin reagent. Replace the reagent back to the recommended storage condition.
- Improper procedure
  - Overcentrifugation may pack cells so tightly that agitation required to resuspend cells breaks up agglutinates. Undercentrifugation may not be optimal for agglutination. The optimum centrifugation speed should be ascertained for each centrifuge.
  - Failure to add test serum, enhancement medium or Anti-human globulin reagent may lead to negative test result. Follow the manufacturer's' instructions meticulously.
  - Too heavy red cell concentration may mask weak agglutination. Too light suspension may be difficult to read.
  - Improper/insufficient serum-cell ratio.
- Complement
  - Rare antibodies, notably Anti-Jk^a and Anti-Jk^b may only be detected when polyspecific Anti-human globulin reagent is used and active complement is present.
- Saline
  - Low pH of saline solution can decrease sensitivity of Anti-humanglobulin test. Optimal wash solution for most antibodies is pH 7.0-7.2. It has been observed that commercially available infusion saline/saline stored in plastic containers can seriously compromise the sensitivity of anti human globulin test. Saline stored in plastic containers and further autoclaved leads to leaching of certain chemicals which shifts the pH to the acidic side and impacts the sensitivity of anti human globulin test. Preferably, use phosphate buffered saline as wash solution or suspending medium.
  - Some antibodies may require saline to be at specific temperature to retain antibody on red blood cell. Use 37°C or 4°C saline.

False Positive Results

- Particles or Contaminants
  - Dust or dirt in glassware may cause clumping of cells. Fibrin or precipitates in test serum may similarly produce cell clumps that mimic agglutination.
- Improper procedure
  - Overcentrifugation may pack cells so tightly that they do not easily disperse and appear positive.
  - Centrifugation of test with polyethylene glycol or positively charged polymers prior to washing may create clumps that do not disperse.
- Cells with positive DAT result
  - Cells that are positive by DAT will also be positive in any indirect antiglobulin test. In such cases, antibodies should be eluted from the sensitized cells.
- Complement
  - Complement components, primarily C4, may bind to cells from clots or from CPDA-1 donor segments during storage at 4°C and occasionally at higher temperature. For DATs, use red blood cells anticoagulated with EDTA, ACD or CPD.
  - Samples collected in scratched glass tubes can lead to spurious activation of complement.
  - Complement may attach to cells in specimens collected from infusion lines used to administer dextrose-containing solutions. Strongest reactions are seen when large bore needles are used or when sample volume is less than 0.5 ml.

Coomb's Control Cells/Complement Coated Cells

Coomb's control cells should be used routinely in direct and indirect anti-human globulin test. Coomb's control reagent is anti-D IgG sensitized, washed and made up to a 5% suspension. Coomb's control cells are used for:

- Procedural validation of tests employing Coomb's reagent. Coomb's control cells are added after performing anti-human globulin test. To a negative result after addition of Coomb's control cells, agglutination indicates that AHG was indeed added and that it has not been neutralized.
- Functional validation of Coomb's reagent. The performance of Coomb's reagent can be validated as a quality control measure on routine basis.

Similarly, complement-coated cells can also be prepared *in vitro*. Thus, complement-coated cells can also be used for functional validation of Coomb's reagent.

Now with commercially available red blood cell stabilizing solution, the Coomb's control cells and complement-coated cells can be prepared *in situ* and stored in cell stabilizing solution for long-term storage and use.

INDIRECT ANTI-HUMAN GLOBULIN TEST FOR THE DETECTION OF RED BLOOD CELL ANTIBODIES

Saline Phase Indirect Anti-human Globulin Test

Specimen

Serum or plasma may be used. Preferably, freshly collected serum should be used.

Reagents

1. Normal saline
2. Polyspecific AHG or Monospecific Anti-human IgG reagent
3. Coomb's control cells
4. Donor cells/reagent red blood cells

Procedure

1. To properly labeled test tubes add two drops of serum.
2. Add one drop of reagent red blood cells or donor red blood cells as a 2 to 5% saline suspension to each tube and mix well.
3. Centrifuge for 15 to 20 seconds at approximately 900 to 1000 g. Observe for haemolysis and/or agglutination. Grade and record the results.
4. Incubate at 37°C for 30 to 60 minutes.
5. Centrifuge for 15 to 20 seconds at approximately 900 to 1000 g and observe for haemolysis and/or agglutination. Grade and record the results.
6. Wash the red blood cells three or four times with saline and completely decant after the final wash.
7. Add AHG reagent to the cell button according to the manufacturer's instruction's. Mix well.
8. Centrifuge for 15 to 20 seconds at approximately 900 to 1000 g and observe for reaction. Grade and record the results.
9. Confirm the validity of negative tests by adding Coomb's control cells.

ALBUMIN PHASE INDIRECT ANTI-HUMAN GLOBULIN TEST

Specimen

Serum or plasma may be used. Preferably, freshly collected serum should be used.

Reagents

1. Normal saline
2. Bovine albumin (22% or 30%)
3. Polyspecific AHG or Monospecific Anti-human IgG reagent
4. Coomb's control cells
5. Donor cells/reagent red blood cells

Procedure

1. To properly labeled test tubes add two drops of serum.
2. Add an equivalent volume of 22% or 30% bovine albumin (unless manufacturers directions state otherwise).
3. Add one drop of 2 to 5% saline suspended reagent or donor red blood cells to each tube and mix.
4. Incubate at 37°C for 15 to 30 minutes.
5. Centrifuge for 15 to 20 seconds at 900 to 1000g. Observe for haemolysis and/or agglutination. Grade and record the results.
6. Wash the cells three or four times with saline and completely decant after final wash.
7. Add AHG to cell button according to the manufacturers instruction. Mix well.
8. Centrifuge and observe for reaction. Grade and record the results.
9. Confirm the validity of negative tests by adding Coomb's control cells.

LISS PHASE INDIRECT ANTI-HUMAN GLOBULIN TEST

Specimen

Serum or plasma may be used. Preferably, freshly collected serum should be used.

Reagents

1. Normal saline
2. LISS
3. Polyspecific AHG or Monospecific Anti-human IgG reagent
4. Coomb's control cells
5. Donor cells/reagent red blood cells

Procedure

1. Wash reagent or donor red blood cells three times in normal saline and completely decant saline after last wash.
2. Resuspend the cells to a 2-5% suspension in LISS.
3. To properly labeled test tube, add two drops of serum.
4. Add two drops of LISS suspended red blood cell suspension and incubate according to manufacturers direction. Typically, this is 10 to 15 minutes at 37°C.
5. Centrifuge according to manufacturers direction.Typically, this is 15 to 30 seconds at 900 to 1000 g and observe for haemolysis and agglutination by gently resuspending the cell button. Grade and record results.
6. Wash the cells three or four times with saline and completely decant after final wash.
7. Add AHG to cell button according to the manufacturers instruction. Mix well.
8. Centrifuge for 15 to 20 seconds at 900 to 1000 g and observe for reaction. Grade and record the results.
9. Confirm the validity of negative tests by adding Coomb's control cells.

PEG-ENHANCED INDIRECT ANTI-HUMAN GLOBULIN TEST

Specimen

Serum or plasma may be used. Preferably, freshly collected serum should be used.

Reagents

1. Normal saline
2. PEG (20% in PBS)
3. Polyspecific AHG or monospecific Anti-human IgG reagent
4. Coomb's control cells
5. Donor cells/reagent red blood cells

Procedure

1. For each sample to be tested, mix 2 drops of test serum, 4 drops of 20% PEG in PBS, and 1 drop of 2-5% red blood cell suspension.
2. Incubate according to manufacturers directions. Typically, this is 15 minutes at 37°C.
3. Do not centrifuge.
4. Wash the cells four times with saline and completely decant after the final wash.
5. Add AHG to cell button according to the manufacturers instruction. Mix well.
6. Centrifuge for 15 to 20 seconds at 900 to 1000 g and observe for reaction. Grade and record the results.
7. Confirm the validity of negative tests by adding Coomb's control cells.

LIM (LOW IONIC MEDIUM-POLYBRENE) INDIRECT ANTI-HUMAN GLOBULIN TEST

Specimen

Serum or plasma may be used. Preferably, freshly collected serum should be used.

Reagents

1. Normal saline
2. Low ionic Medium (LIM): To a 500 ml volumetric flask, add 25 g of dextrose and 1 g of Na_2 EDTA $2H_2O$. Fill flask to 500 ml mark with distilled water.
3. Polybrene® (Commercially available)
4. Resuspending medium: 0.2 M trisodium Citrate, 5% dextrose; Working solution made by mixing 60 ml of 0.2 M trisodium citrate with 40 ml of 5% dextrose
5. Washing solution (for anti human globulin Testing): 0.01 M trisodium citrate
6. Polyspecific AHG or monospecific Anti-human IgG reagent
7. Coomb's control cells
8. Donor cells/reagent red blood cells

Procedure

1. Prepare 1% suspension of donor or reagent red blood cells in the serum used for testing.
2. Add 1.0 ml of LIM solution. Mix and incubate for 1 minute at room temperature.
3. Add 0.1 ml of 0.05% Polybrene to each tube and mix.

4. Centrifuge according to manufacturer's directions. Typically, this is 10 seconds at 900 to 1000 g and decant the supernatant fluid. Do not resuspend cell button.
5. Add 0.1 ml of resuspending solution. Shake tube gently and observe for persistent agglutination. If strength of agglutination is weak, examine the test and a known negative control macroscopically. Do not recentrifuge.
6. If desired, the anti-human globulin test may be performed as follows:
   a. Add 0.05 ml of resuspending solution to each tube and mix well.
   b. Wash the cells three times with 0.01 M trisodium citrate solution.
   c. Add two drops of AHG reagent to the cell button and mix.
   d. Centrifuge for 15 seconds at 900 to 1000 g. Read and record the results.
   e. Add Coomb's control cells to each negative tube.

Interpretation of Results for anti-human globulin Tests

1. Agglutination/haemolysis after incubation at 37°C constitutes a positive test.
2. The presence of agglutination after addition of AHG reagent constitutes a positive test.
3. Anti-human globulin tests are considered negative when no agglutination is observed after initial centrifugation and positive result with Coomb's control cells. If after addition of Coomb's control cells a negative result is observed, then the test is invalid and must be repeated.
4. For the LIM (Low Ionic Medium-Polybrene) procedure, agglutination that persists after addition of resuspending solution indicates a positive result.

Controls

1. The procedure used for the detection of unexpected antibodies in transfusion testing should be checked daily with weak antibodies.
2. When LIM technique is used, test an unknown serum against reagent red blood cells, an inert serum should be tested against a random cell sample for comparative purposes.

Notes

1. The incubation time and volume and concentration of red cells incubated are those given in literature. In all cases, the manufacturer's package insert should be strictly adhered to.
2. For the PEG procedure:
   a. Omit centrifugation after 37°C incubation, as red blood cells will not resuspend readily.
   b. Use monospecific anti human IgG rather than polyspecific AHG to avoid unwanted positive reactions due to C3-binding antibodies.
3. LISS additive and PEG solutions are available from various commercial sources. Manufacturers instruction should be followed when using these reagent.

PAPAIN—ONE-STAGE ENZYME TECHNIQUE / TWO-STAGE ENZYME TECHNIQUE

Specimen

Serum to be tested. Preferably, freshly collected serum should be used.

Reagent

1. Reagent red blood cells
2. Polyspecific AHG or Monospecific Anti-human IgG reagent
3. Coomb's control cells
4. Donor cells/reagent red blood cells

Procedure for One-stage Enzyme Technique

1. To an appropriately labeled test tube, add two drops of serum.
2. Add two drops of 2-5% saline suspension of reagent red blood cells.
3. Add two drops of papain solution and mix well.
4. Incubate at 37°C for 30 minutes.
5. Centrifuge for 15-20 seconds at 900-1000 g and gently resuspend the cells, observe for agglutination. Grade and record the results.
6. Wash the cells four times with saline and completely decant after the final wash.
7. Add AHG to cell button according to the manufacturer's instruction. Mix well.
8. Centrifuge for 15-20 seconds at 900-1000 g and observe for reaction. Grade and record the results.
9. Confirm the validity of negative tests by adding Coomb's control cells.

Procedure for Two-stage Enzyme Technique

1. Add one drop of washed packed cells and one drop of papain reagent to appropriately labeled tube.
2. Incubate at 37°C for 30 minutes.
3. Wash the papain treated three times with isotonic saline and prepare 2-5% cell suspension.
4. To an appropriately labeled test tube, add one drop of papain-treated red blood cell suspension and two drops of serum under test.
5. Mix well and incubate at 37°C for 30 minutes.
6. Centrifuge for 15-20 seconds at 900-1000 g and gently resuspend the cells, observe for agglutination. Grade and record the results.
7. Wash the cells four times with saline and completely decant after the final wash.
8. Add AHG to cell button according to the manufacturer's instruction. Mix well.
9. Centrifuge for 15-20 seconds at 900-1000 g and observe for reaction. Grade and record the results.
10. Confirm the validity of negative tests by adding Coomb's control cells.

ANTIBODY TITRATION STUDIES

Antibody Titration for Characterizing Type of Antibody in Serum

Specimen

Serum (antibody) to be titrated.

Reagents

1. Red blood cells that express the antigen(s) corresponding to the antibody specificity(ies), in a 2-5% saline suspension. Uniformity of cell suspensions is very important to ensure comparability of results.
2. Normal saline (Dilutions may be made with 6% albumin if desired).

Procedure

The master dilution technique for titration studies is as follows:

1. Label ten test tubes according to the serum dilution (e.g. 1 in 1,1 in 2, etc.).
2. Deliver one volume of saline to all test tubes except the first.
3. Add an equal volume of serum to each of the first two tubes (undiluted and 1 in 2).
4. Using a clean pipette, mix the contents of the 1 in 2 dilution several times, and transfer one volume into the next tube (1 in 4 dilution).
5. Continue the same process for all dilutions, using a clean pipette to mix and transfer each dilution. Remove one volume of diluted serum from the final tube and save it for use if further dilutions are required.
6. Label ten 10 × 75 mm or 12 ×75 mm tubes for the appropriate dilutions.
7. Using separate pipettes for each dilution, transfer two drops of each diluted serum into the appropriately labeled tubes, and add one drop of red blood cell suspension.
8. Mix well and test by serologic technique appropriate to the antibody.
9. Examine test results macroscopically, grade and record the reactions. The prozone phenomenon may cause reactions to be weaker in the more concentrated serum preparations than in higher dilutions; to avoid misinterpretation of results, it may be preferable to examine first the tube containing the most dilute serum and proceed through the more concentrated samples to the undiluted specimen.

Interpretation

1. Observe the highest dilution that produces 1 + macroscopic agglutination. The titer is the reciprocal of the dilution. If there is agglutination in the tube containing the most dilute serum, the endpoint has not been reached, and additional dilutions should be prepared and tested.
2. In comparative studies, a significant difference in titer is three or more dilutions. Variations in technique and inherent biologic variability can cause duplicate tests to give results that differ by one dilution in either direction.
3. Titer values alone can be misleading, without additional evaluation of strength of agglutination.

The observed strength of agglutination can be assigned a number and the sum of these numbers for all tubes in a titration study represents the score. The arbitrarily assigned threshold for significance in comparing scores is a difference of 10 or more between different test samples (Table 11.7).

Table 11.7: Examples of Antibodies Tilers, Endpoint and Scores

	Reciprocal of serum Dilution											
	1	2	4	8	16	32	64	128	256	512	Titer	Score
Sample 1 Strength:	3+	3+	3+	2+	2+	2+	1+	±	±	0	64(256)	
Score:	10	10	10	8	8	8	5	3	2	0		64
Sample 2 Strength:	4+	4+	4+	3+	3+	2+	2+	1+	±	0	128(256)	
Score:	12	12	12	10	10	8	8	5	3	0	80	
Sample 3 Strength:	1+	1+	1+	1+	±	±	±	±	±	0	8(256)	
Score:	5	5	5	5	3	3	3	2	2	0	33	

Notes

Titration is a semiquantitative technique and technical variables greatly affect the results. Hence, care should be taken to achieve the most uniform possible practices.

1. Careful pipetting is essential. Pipettes with disposable tips that can be changed after each dilution is recommended.
2. Optimal time and temperature of incubation, time and force of centrifugation must be used consistently.
3. The age, phenotype and concentration of test red blood cells influence the results. When the titers of several antibody containing sera are to be compared, all should be tested against red blood cells (preferably freshly collected) from the same donor. If this is not possible, the tests should use a pool of reagent red blood cells from donors of the same phenotype. When a single serum is to be tested against different red blood cell samples, all samples should be collected and preserved in the same manner, and diluted to the same concentration before use.
4. Completely reproducible results are virtually impossible to achieve. Comparisons are valid only when specimens are tested concurrently. In prenatal testing of sequential serum samples to detect changing antibody activity, samples should be frozen for comparison with subsequent samples. Each new sample should be tested in parallel with the immediately preceding sample. In tests with a single serum against different red blood cell samples, material from the master dilution must be used for all tests.
5. Measurements are more accurate with large volumes than with small volumes, a master dilution technique gives more reliable results than individual dilutions for a single test. The volume needed for all planned tests should be calculated and an adequate quantity of each dilution prepared.

Antibody Titration Studies for Early Detection of Haemolytic Disease of the Newborn

Specimen

Serum for titration (containing potentially significant unexpected antibodies to red blood cell antigens, 1 ml). If possible, test the current sample in parallel with the most recent previously submitted (preceding) sample from the current pregnancy.

Materials

1. Anti-human IgG reagent
2. Dilute bovine albumin (approximately 6% w/v), optional: 22% (w/v) bovine albumin, 1 ml; isotonic saline, 3 ml.
3. Micropipettes or equivalent: 0.1 - 0.5 ml delivery, with disposable tips.
4. Red blood cells: Group O reagent red blood cells with double dose expression of antigen to which the serum contains antibody (use R_2R_2 RBCs when titrating anti-D); wash three times and dilute to a 2% red blood cell suspension with isotonic saline.

Quality Control

1. Test the preceding sample in parallel with the current sample.
2. Prepare dilutions using separate pipette for each tube. Failure to do so will result in falsely high titers due to carry-over.
3. Confirm all negative reactions with Coomb's control cells.

Procedure

1. Using 0.5 ml volumes, prepare serial dilutions of serum in saline or 6% albumin. The initial tube should contain undiluted serum and the doubling dilution range should be from 1 in 2 to 1 in 2048 (total of 12 tubes).
2. Place 0.1 ml of each dilution into appropriately labeled 10 or 12 × 75 mm test tubes.
3. Add 0.1 ml of red blood cell suspension to each dilution.

4. Gently agitate the contents of each tube; incubate at 37°C for 1 hour.
5. Wash the tubes four times with saline; completely decant the final wash supernatant.
6. To the cell buttons thus obtained, add Anti-human IgG according to the manufacturer's direction.
7. Centrifuge as for haemagglutination tests.
8. Examine the results macroscopicaly; grade and record the reactions.
9. Add one drop of Coomb's control cells to all negative tests; recentrifuge and examine the tests macroscopically for mixed field agglutination; repeat antibody detection tests when tests with Coomb's control cells are nonreactive.

Results

The titer is reported as the reciprocal of the highest dilution of serum at which 1 + agglutination is observed. A titer greater than or equal to 16 is considered significant and may warrant monitoring for HDN by cordocentesis, high resolution ultrasound, or examination of the amniotic fluid for bilirubin pigmentation.

Notes

1. Titration studies should be performed upon initial detection of the antibody; save an aliquot of the serum (frozen at -20°C or colder) for comparative studies with the next submitted sample.
2. When the titer is less than 16 and the antibody specificity has been associated with HDN, it is recommended that repeat titration studies be performed every 2-4 weeks, beginning at 18 weeks of gestation; save an aliquot of the serum (frozen at -20°C or colder) for comparative studies with the next submitted sample.
3. When the decision has been made to monitor the pregnancy by an invasive procedure such as amniocentesis, no further titrations are warranted.
4. Each institution should develop a policy to ensure some degree of uniformity in reporting and interpreting antibody titers.
5. For antibodies to low incidence antigens, consider using paternal red blood cells.
6. Do not use enhancement techniques (albumin, PEG, LISS) or enzyme treated red blood cells, because elevated titers may be obtained.
7. LISS should not be used as diluent in titration studies; nonspecific uptake of globulins may occur in serum-LISS dilutions.
8. Failure to obtain the correct results may be caused by incorrect technique, notably; failure to use separate pipette tips for each dilution or failure to mix thawed frozen serum.

Use of Sulfhydryl Reagents to Distinguish between IgM and IgG Antibodies

Specimen

Two ml of serum to be tested

Reagents

1. Phosphate buffered saline at pH 7.3.
2. About 0.01 M dithiothreitol (DTT) prepared by dissolving 0.154 g of DTT in 100 ml of pH 7.3 PBS Store at 2-8°C.

Procedure

1. Dispense 1 ml of serum into each of two test tubes.
2. To one tube, labeled as control, add 1 ml of pH 7.3 PBS.
3. To the other tube, labeled as test, add 1 ml of 0.01 M DTT.
4. Mix and incubate at 37°C for 30-60 minutes.
5. Test the antibody activity in each sample by titration against red blood cells of appropriate phenotype (Table 11.8).

Table 11.8: Effect of Dithiothreitol on Blood Group Antibodies

	Dilution					
Test sample	1/2	1/4	1/8	1/16	1/32	Interpretation
Serum + DTT	3+	2+	2+	1+	0	IgG
Serum + PBS	3+	2+	2+	1+	0	
Serum + DTT	0	0	0	0	0	IgM
Serum + PBS	3+	2+	2+	1+	0	
Serum + DTT	2+	1+	0	0	0	IgG + 1gM*
Serum + PBS	3+	2+	2+	1+	0	

* May also indicate only partial inactivation of IgM

Notes

1. Sulfhydryl reagent used at low concentration may weaken antigens of Kell system. For investigation of antibodies in Kell system, it may be necessary to use alkylation with iodoacetic acid, followed by dialysis.
2. Gelling of serum or plasma sample may be observed during treatment with DTT. This can occur if the DTT has been prepared incorrectly,

and has a concentration above 0.01 M. Gelling may also occur if serum and DTT are incubated too long. An aliquot of the sample undergoing treatment can be tested after 30 minutes of incubation, if the activity thought to be due to IgM has disappeared, there is no need to incubate further. Gelled samples cannot be tested for antibody activity because overtreatment with DTT causes denaturation of all serum proteins.

ELUTION TECHNIQUES

Citric Acid Elution Method

Specimen

Packed DAT positive red blood cells washed six times with saline.

Reagents

1. Elution solution: Citric acid (monohydrate), 1.3 g, KH_2PO_4 0.65 g saline to 100 ml, store at 4°C.
2. Neutralizing solution: Na_3PO_4, 13.0g; distilled water to 100 ml; store at 4°C.
3. Supernatant saline from final wash of the red blood cells to be tested.

Procedure

1. Chill all reagent to 4°C in ice bath before use.
2. Place 1 ml of packed red blood cells in a 13 × 100 mm test tube.
3. Add 1 ml of eluting solution and note the time.
4. Stopper the tube and mix by inversion for 90 seconds.
5. Remove the stopper and promptly centrifuge the tube at 900-1000 g for 45 seconds.
6. Transfer supernatant fluid to a clean test tube and add 5-6 drops of neutralizing solution; save red blood cells for use in adsorption studies if needed.
7. Check pH; adjust it, if necessary, to pH 7.0 by adding more neutralizing solution.
8. Centrifuge at 900-1000g for 2-3 minutes to remove precipitate that forms after neutralization. Harvest the supernatant eluate and test it in parallel with supernatant saline from final wash.

Notes

1. Once the red blood cells have been rendered DAT-negative, they may be tested for the presence of blood group antigens, except those of the Kell blood group system. Expression of antigens in the Kell system is markedly weakened after citric acid treatment.
2. Citric acid modified red blood cells may also be treated with protease and used in autologous adsorption studies.

COLD ACID ELUTION

Specimen

Packed DAT positive red blood cells washed six times with saline.

Reagents

1. Glycine-HCl (0.1 M, pH 3.0), prepared by dissolving 3.75 g of glycine and 2.922 g of sodium chloride in 500 ml of distilled water. Adjust pH to 3.0 with 12N HCl. Store at 4°C.
2. Phosphate buffer (0.8 M, pH 8.2), prepared by dissolving 109.6 g of Na_2HPO_4 and 3.8 g of KH_2PO_4 in approximately 600 ml of distilled water. Adjust pH, if necessary, with either 1N NaOH or 1N HCl. Dilute to a final volume of 1 titre with distilled water. Store at 4°C.
3. Normal saline, at 4°C.
4. Supernatant saline from final wash of red blood cells to be tested.

Procedure

1. Place the red blood cells in 13 × 100 mm test tube and chill them in an ice bath for 5 minutes before adding glycine-HCl.
2. Add 1 ml of chilled saline and 2 ml of chilled glycine-HCl to 1 ml of washed red blood cells.
3. Mix and incubate the tube in an ice bath for 1 minute.
4. Quickly centrifuge the tube at 900-1000 g for 2-3 minutes.
5. Transfer the supernatant eluate into a clean test tube, and add 0.1 ml of pH 8.2 phosphate buffer for each 1 ml of eluate.
6. Mix and centrifuge at 900-1000 g for 2-3 minutes.
7. Transfer the supernatant eluate into a clean test tube, and add test in parallel with the supernatant saline from the final wash.

Notes

1. Keep glycine in ice bath during use, to maintain correct pH.
2. Phosphate buffer will crystallize during storage at 4°C. Redissolve it at 37°C before use.

3. Addition of phosphate buffer restores neutrality to the acidic eluate. Unneutralized acidity may cause haemolysis of the reagent red blood cells used in testing the eluate. The addition of 22% bovine albumin (one part to four parts of eluate) may reduce such haemolysis.

Glycine-HCl/EDTA Elution

Specimen

Packed DAT positive red blood cells washed six times with saline

Reagents

1. Disodium EDTA (10% w/v): Na_2EDTA, 2 H_2O,10 g, distilled water 100 ml.
2. Glycine-HCl (0.1 M at pH 1.5): Glycine 3.754 g; NaCl 2.922 g; distilled water 500 ml; adjust to pH 1.5 with 12 N HCl; store at 4°C.
3. TRIS base: Hydroxymethyl aminomethane, 12.1g; distilled water 100 ml.
4. Supernatant saline from final wash of the red blood cells to be tested.

Procedure

1. Mix 4 ml of glycine-HCl and 1 ml of EDTA in 16 × 100 mm test tube.
2. Immediately add 1 ml of washed red blood cells and mix well.
3. Incubate at room temperature for 1-2 minutes.
4. Centrifuge the tube at 900-1000 g for 2-3 minutes.
5. Transfer the supernatant eluate into a clean test tube and adjust to pH 7.5 with 1 M TRIS base.
6. Mix and centrifuge at 900-1000 g for 2-3 minutes.
7. Transfer the supernatant eluate into a clean test tube, and test it in parallel with the supernatant saline from the final wash.

Notes

1. Once the red blood cells have been rendered DAT-negative, they may be tested for the presence of blood group antigens, except those in the Kell system. Treatment with glycine-HCl/EDTA denatures Kell system antigens.
2. Red blood cells modified with glycine-HCl/EDTA may be treated with protease and used in autologous adsorption studies.

Heat Elution

Specimen

Packed DAT positive red blood cells washed six times with saline.

Reagents

1. Six per cent bovine albumin, prepared by diluting 22% or 30% bovine albumin with saline.
2. Supernatant saline from final wash of the red blood cells to be tested.

Procedure

1. Mix equal volumes of washed packed cells and 6% bovine albumin in 13 × 100 mm test tube.
2. Place the tube at 56°C for 10 minutes. Agitate the tube periodically during the incubation period.
3. Centrifuge the tube at 900-1000 g for 2-3 minutes, preferably in a heated centrifuge.
4. Immediately transfer the supernatant eluate into a clean test tube, and test in parallel with supernatant saline from final wash.

Donath-Landsteiner Test

Specimen

Serum separated from freshly collected blood sample maintained at 37°C.

Reagents

1. Freshly collected normal serum, to use as a source of complement.
2. 50% suspension of washed group 0 red blood cells that express the P antigen.

Procedure

1. Label three sets of three 10 × 75 mm test tubes as follows: A1-A2-A3; B1-B2-B3; C1-C2-C3.
2. To tubes 1 and 2 of each set, add 10 volumes of the patient's serum.
3. To tubes 2 and 3 of each set, add 10 volumes of fresh normal serum.
4. To all tubes, add one volume of 50% suspension of washed P-positive red blood cells and mix well.
5. Place the three 'A' tubes in a bath of melting ice for 30 minutes, and then at 37°C for 1 hour.
6. Place the three 'B' tubes in a bath of melting ice, and keep them in melting ice for 9 minutes.

7. Place the three 'C' tubes at 37°C, and keep them at 37°C for 90 minutes.
8. Centrifuge all tubes, and examine the supernatant fluid for haemolysis.

Interpretation

The Donath-Landsteiner test is considered positive when the patient serum, with or without added complement, causes haemolysis in the tubes that were incubated first in melting ice and then at 37°C (i.e. tubes A1 and A2), and there is no haemolysis in any of the tubes maintained throughout at 37°C or in melting ice. The A3, B3 and C3 tubes serve as a control for complement activity and should not manifest haemolysis.

Notes

1. The biphasic nature of the haemolysin associated with PCH requires that serum be incubated with cells at cold temperature and then at 37°C.
2. Active complement is essential for demonstration of the antibody. Because patient with PCH may have low levels of serum complement, fresh normal serum should be included in the reaction medium as a source of complement.
3. To avoid loss of antibody by cold autoadsorption before testing, the patient's blood should be allowed to clot at 37°C, and the serum separated from the clot at this temperature.

Chequer Board Titration for Quality Control of Anti-IgG Potency in Polyspecific AHG Reagent and Evaluation of Complement Potency with Complement-coated Cells

Reagents and materials required for chequer board titration

1. Anti-D IgG reagent with albumin titer 256-512.
2. Polyspecific AHG reagent
3. Freshly collected O Rh_o D positive cells
4. Normal saline
5. 12 ×100 mm and 12 × 75 mm Test tubes
6. Pipettes 1 ml and 5 ml
7. Table centrifuge
8. Timer
9. Water bath or laboratory incubator

Reagent Preparation Procedure

Preparation of 3% cell suspension

1. Collect 2 ml of freshly drawn venous blood in a clean 12 × 100 mm test tube with suitable anticoagulant.
2. Centrifuge at 3000 rpm for 2-3 minutes to form a cell button.
3. Discard the supernatant.
4. Resuspend the cell button in 5 ml of normal saline.
5. Centrifuge at 3000 rpm for 2-3 minutes.
6. Repeat the washing of cells (steps 4 and 5) twice more so that the cells are washed three times.
7. After the final centrifugation, remove the supernatant without disturbing the cell button.
8. Take 0.75 ml of packed cells and resuspend them in 24.25 ml of normal saline to get a 3% cell suspension.

Dilutions of anti-D (IgG) reagent

1. Take a set of ten, 12 × 100 mm test tubes and number them from 1 to 10.
2. Add 2 ml of normal saline to each of the tubes from tube number 2 to 10.
3. Add 2 ml each of anti-D (IgG) reagent to tube number 1 and 2.
4. Mix the content of tube number 2 and transfer 2 ml of diluted reagent to tube number 3 with the help of pipette.
5. Continue this serial dilution till tube number 10.
6. Discard 2 ml of diluted reagent from tube number 10.

CELL SENSITIZATION

1. To each of the above dilutions of anti-D (IgG), add 2 ml of well mixed freshly prepared 3% cell suspension.
2. Mix well all the tubes and cover them with aluminium foil.
3. Incubate the tubes at 37°C for 30 minutes, with periodic mixing.
4. Centrifuge the tubes at 3000 rpm for 2-3 minutes.
5. Remove the supernatant and resuspend the cell button in 5 ml of normal saline.
6. Centrifuge at 3000 rpm for 2-3 minutes.
7. Repeat the washing (Step 4 and 5) at least four times.
8. Resuspend the cell button from each tube in 2 ml of normal saline to get a 3% suspension of sensitized cells.

Note

Thorough washing of sensitized cells (after incubation) is very important as even slight traces of free anti-D IgG can lead to false negative results.

Dilutions of Anti-human Globulin Reagent

1. Take a set of six, 12 × 100 mm test tubes and number them from 1 to 6.
2. Add 2.5 ml of normal saline to each of the tubes from tube number 2 to 6.
3. Add 2.5 ml of Polyspecific AHG reagent to tube number 1 and 2.
4. Mix the content of tube number 2 and transfer 2.5 ml of the diluted reagent to tube number 3.
5. Continue this serial dilution till tube number 6.
6. Discard 2.5 ml of diluted reagent from tube number 6.

Preparation of Complement-Coated Cells

Reagents and material required:

1. LISS solution
2. Buffered saline
3. O group red blood cells 50% suspension
4. Inert O group serum
5. Test tubes 12 × 100 mm
6. Table centrifuge
7. Water bath or laboratory incubator

Preparation of 50% Cell Suspension of O Group Red Blood Cells

1. Collect 1 ml of freshly drawn venous blood in a clean 12 × 100 mm test tube containing suitable anticoagulant.
2. Centrifuge the tube at 3000 rpm for 2-3 minutes to form cell button.
3. Discard the supernatant.
4. Resuspend the cell button in 5 ml of buffered saline.
5. Centrifuge at 3000 rpm for 2-3 minutes.
6. Repeat the washing of cells (steps 4 and 5) twice more so that the cells are washed three times.
7. After the final centrifugation, remove the supernatant without disturbing the cell button.
8. Add 1 ml of buffered saline to the packed red blood cells to get a 50% O group red cell suspension.

Collection of inert O group serum

1. Collect 2 ml of freshly drawn venous blood in a clean 12 × 100 mm test tube.
2. Immediately centrifuge at 3000 rpm for 2-3 minutes.
3. Collect 0.5 ml of serum in a clean test tube.

Sensitization of O group red blood cells

1. Place 8.5 ml of LISS into a 20-25 ml container.
2. Add 0.5 ml of fresh inert O group serum to it.
3. Mix well and add 1 ml of 50% O group red cell suspension.
4. Mix thoroughly and incubate at 37°C for 30 minutes with occasional further mixing.
5. Centrifuge at 3000 rpm for 2-3 minutes to form a cell button.
6. Discard the supernatant and resuspend the cell button in 20 ml buffered saline.
7. Centrifuge at 3000 rpm for 2-3 minutes.
8. Repeat the washing of cells (steps 6 and 7) three more times so that cells are washed four times.
9. After the final centrifugation, remove the supernatant without disturbing the cell button.
10. Add 14.5 ml of buffered saline to packed red blood cells to obtain 2-3% suspension of complement-coated cells.

Chequer Board Titration

1. Take a set of sixty, 12 × 75 mm test tubes, number and arrange them as shown below in the table 11.9:

Table 11.9: Chequer board titration

Dilution of AHG	3% Rho (D) + ve senstitized cells								
N	1:2	1:4	1:8	1:16	1:32	1:64	1:128	1:256	1:512
N									
1:2									
1:4									
1:8									
1:16									
1:32									

2. Add 0.2 ml each of N (neat) AHG in the respective tubes.
3. Similarly add dilutions of AHG in their respective tubes (horizontal rows).

4. Referring to Table 11.9, add 0.2 ml each of 2% suspension of sensitized cells with anti-D (IgG) dilutions in their respective tubes (vertical rows).
5. Mix well all the tubes.
6. Centrifuge the tubes at 3000 rpm for 20 seconds.
7. Gently dislodge the cell button and observe for agglutination.
8. Chart the results in Table 11.9.

Table 11.10: Complement potency titration

Dilution of AHG	2% cell suspension of complement coated Cells
N	
1:2	
1:4	
1:8	
1:16	
1:32	

1. Add 0.2 ml neat AHG reagent.
2. Similarly add dilutions of AHG in respective tubes.
3. Referring to Table 11.10, add 0.2 ml each of 2% suspension of complement-coated cells to all the tubes containing AHG reagent with dilutions.
4. Mix well all the tubes.
5. Centrifuge the tubes at 3000 rpm for 20 seconds.
6. Gently dislodge the cell button and observe for agglutination.

Preparation of Coomb's Control Cells

Reagents and materials required:

1. Anti-D (IgG)
2. Freshly collected O Rh_o (D) positive cells
3. Normal saline
4. Test tubes 12 × 100 mm
5. Pipettes 1 ml and 5 ml
6. Table Centrifuge, timer.
7. Water bath or laboratory incubator.

Procedure

Since commercially available anti-D (IgG) reagent have albumin titer of 256-512, diluting anti-D (IgG) reagent 1:40 to 1:50 in normal saline is enough to achieve sensitization with O Rh_o(D) positive cells:

1. Take equal volume of 1:40 to 1:50 diluted anti-D (IgG) in a 12 × 75 mm test tube and 3% cell suspension of O Rh_o (D) positive cells.
2. Mix well and incubate at 37°C for 30 minutes. Periodic mixing during 30 minutes interval ensures thorough sensitization.
3. Remove the supernatant and resuspend the cell button in 5 ml of normal saline.
4. Centrifuge at 3000 rpm for 2-3 minutes.
5. Repeat the washing (steps 3 and 4) at least four times.
6. Resuspend the cell button in normal saline to obtain a 3% suspension of Coomb's control cells.

ANTI-HUMAN IgG MONOSPECIFIC COOMB'S REAGENT FOR DIRECT AND INDIRECT ANTI-GLOBULIN TEST (From Tulip's Erybank Range)

Summary

Generally, antibodies involved in transfusion reactions are of two types namely the complete and incomplete, whereas the complete antibodies agglutinate red cells in saline medium, the incomplete type of antibodies sensitizes red cells without agglutination.

In the direct antiglobulin tests, Anti-human globulin reagent is used to detect antibodies adsorbed to the red blood cells *in vivo*. After direct antiglobulin testing with a polyspecific reagent reveals globulins, anti-human IgG monospecific coombs reagent is used to characterize the coating proteins.

In the indirect antiglobulin tests, anti-human globulin reagent is used to detect antibodies adsorbed to red blood cells *in vitro*. Anti-human IgG monospecific coombs reagent is used in indirect antiglobulin testing to distinguish patterns of reactivity in a single serum containing complement-binding and noncomplement-binding antibodies.

Anti-human IgG monospecific coombs reagent is useful for antibody detection, antibody identification and umbilical cord red blood testing.

Reagent

Erybank® anti-human IgG monospecific Coomb's reagent is a ready-to-use reagent containing antibodies reactive with human gamma globulins. Each batch of reagent undergoes rigorous quality control at various stages of manufacture for its specificity, avidity and titre.

Reagent Storage and Stability

1. Store the reagent at 2-8°C. Do not freeze.

Reactions of Common Erythrocyte Antibodies

Antibody For	*Saline Medium*	*Albumin Medium*	*AHG Test*	*Enzyme Test*	*In Vitro Hemolysis*	*Optimal C⁰* 4	24	37
H, l	M	S	F	S	S	M	S	F
A, B, A, B	M	F	F	M	S	M	S	F
Lu^a	M	S	F	F	N	M	S	M
Lu^b	S	S	M	F	N	R	S	M
M, N	M	S	S	F	N	M	M	F
P_1	M	S	S	S	F	M	S	F
PP_1P^k	M	M	M	M	M	S	M	M
Le^a, Le^b	M	S	S	M	S	M	S	F
S, s	S	S	M	S	N	F	S	M
K, k, Js^a Js^b	F	S	M	F	N	F	S	M
C, D, E, c, e,	S	S	M	M	N	F	S	M
Fy^a, Fy^b	F	F	M	F	N	N	F	M
Jk^a, Jk^b	F	S	M	M	F	N	S	M

*M = Most (>20%), S = Some (5-20%), F = Few (1-5%), R = Rare (<1%), N = Not reported.

2. The shelf life of the reagent is as per the expiry date mentioned on the reagent vial label.

Principle

Normal human red blood cells, in presence of antibody directed towards the antigen they possess, may fail to agglutinate and become sensitized. This may be due to the particular nature of antigen and antibody involved. Erybank® Anti-human IgG monospecific Coomb's reagent would react with red cells sensitized with gamma globulins and cause agglutination of red blood cells.

Note

1. *In vitro* diagnostic reagent for laboratory and professional use only. Not for medicinal use.
2. The reagent contains sodium azide 0.1% as preservative. Avoid contact with skin and mucosa. On disposal flush with large quantities of water.
3. Extreme turbidity may indicate microbial contamination or denaturation of protein due to thermal damage. Such reagent should be discarded.
4. Erybank® anti-human IgG monospecific Coomb's reagent is not from human source, hence, contamination due to HBsAg and HIV is practically excluded.

Sample Collection and Storage

No special preparation of patient is required prior to sample collection by approved techniques. Do not use haemolysed samples.

For Direct Antiglobulin Test

Blood drawn into EDTA is preferred but oxalated, citrated or clotted whole blood may be used. The blood sample should be tested as soon as possible after collection and should not be stored.

For Indirect Antiglobulin Test

Serum not more than 48 hours old should be used for testing purpose.

ADDITIONAL MATERIAL REQUIRED

For Direct Antiglobulin Test

Test tubes (12 × 75 mm), Pasteur pipettes, centrifuge, isotonic saline, Coomb's control cells, optical aid.

For Indirect Antiglobulin Test

Test tubes (12 × 75 mm), Pasteur pipettes, centrifuge, incubator (37°C), isotonic saline, Erybank® bovine serum albumin, reagent red blood cells for antibody detection and antibody identification, Coomb's control cells, optical aid.

Procedure

Bring reagent to room temperature before testing.

Direct Antiglobulin Test

1. Prepare a 5% suspension of red blood cells to be tested in isotonic saline.
2. Pipette on drop of the cell suspension into a test tube.

3. Fill the tube with fresh isotonic saline and centrifuge for 30 seconds at 3400 rpm (1000 g).
4. Decant and repeat this washing at least thrice.
5. Add two drops of Erybank®, anti-human IgG monospecific Coomb's reagent and mix well.
6. Centrifuge for one minute at 1000 rpm (125 g) or for 20 seconds at 3400 rpm (1000 g).
7. Very gently, resuspend the cell button observing for agglutination macroscopically.
8. To all negative results, add one drop of Coomb's control cells and observe for agglutination.

Indirect Antiglobulin Test for Antibody Identification

1. Prepare 5% suspension of reagent red blood cells to be tested in isotonic saline.
2. Pipette two drops of serum to be tested in an appropriately labelled test tube.
3. Pipette one drop of 5% reagent red blood cell suspension and mix well.
4. If required, add two drops of Erybank® bovine serum albumin reagent and mix well and incubate at 37°C for fifteen minutes.
5. If enhancement medium is not being used, incubate the tube at 37°C for 30 minutes.
6. After incubation, wash the cells thoroughly with isotonic saline for minimum three times. Decant completely after last wash.
7. Add two drops of Erybank® anti-human IgG monospecific Coomb's reagent into the test tube containing the sedimented cells and mix well.
8. Centrifuge for one minute at 1000 rpm (125 g) or 20 seconds at 3400 rpm (1000 g).
9. Very gently, resuspend the cell button and observe for agglutination macroscopically.

INTERPRETATION OF RESULTS

Direct Antiglobulin Test

Agglutination of red blood cells is a positive result and indicates presence of human IgG on the red blood cells.

No agglutination is a negative test result and indicates absence of human IgG on red blood cells.

Indirect Antiglobulin Test

Agglutination of red blood cells is a positive result and indicates presence of antibody against the antigen in the serum under test.

No agglutination of red blood cells is a negative result and indicates absence of antibody against the antigen in the serum under test.

Remarks

1. To all negative test results, after the antiglobulin test, one drop of Coomb's control cells should be added. If Coomb's control cells do not agglutinate then the test must be repeated.
2. Red blood cells showing a positive direct antiglobulin test cannot be used for the indirect antiglobulin test.
3. It is recommended that Anti-IgG activity of anti-human IgG monospecific Coomb's reagent be tested from time to time preferably on a daily basis using Coomb's control cells as a positive control.
4. All glassware used in the test should be scrupulously clean, dry and free from contamination with human serum.
5. Contaminated bovine serum albumin, saline or glassware may inactivate anti-human IgG monospecific Coomb's reagent .
6. Use of various drugs and certain diseases (such as megaloblastic anaemia) are known to be associated with a positive direct antiglobulin test.
7. Cord cells obtained from a newborn exhibiting haemolytic disease of the newborn, especially due to ABO incompatibility may give false negative results.
8. Erybank® anti-human IgG monospecific Coomb's reagent is free from anti-T activity.
9. As undercentrifugation or overcentrifugation could lead to erroneous results, it is recommended that each laboratory calibrate its own equipment and determine the time required for achieving the desired results.

ANTIHUMAN GLOBULIN REAGENT

For Direct and Indirect Antiglobulin Tests (Eryclone® from Tulip)

Summary

Generally antibodies involved in transfusion reactions are of two types, namely the complete and the incomplete, whereas the complete antibodies agglutinate red cells in saline medium, the incomplete type of antibody sensitizes red cells without agglutination. Usually, IgM class of antibodies and IgG_1 and IgG_3 type of IgG antibodies fix complement.

Cell lysis, *in vivo* is mediated through the complement system and the complement component C_3b is further acted upon to produce C_3d.

In the direct antiglobulin tests, Anti-human globulin reagent is used to detect antibodies adsorbed to the red blood cells *in vivo*. In the indirect antiglobulin tests, Anti-human globulin reagent is used to detect antibodies adsorbed to the red blood cells *in vitro*. Anti-human globulin reagent is useful for compatibility testing, antibody detection, antibody identification, umblical cord red blood testing and detection of the D^u variant of the human red blood cell antigen D(Rho).

Reagents

Eryclone® Anti-humanglobulin is a balanced ready-to-use blend of highly purified immunoglobulins. It contains Anti-human IgG antibodies and antibodies reactive with human complement components C_3b and C_3d. These anti-complement antibodies are IgM class monoclonals and they impart the necessary sensitivity to the reagent. Each batch of reagent undergoes rigorous quality control at various stages of manufacture for its specificity, avidity and titre.

Reagent Storage and Stability

a. Store the reagent at 2-8°C. Do not freeze.
b. The shelf life of the reagent is as per the expiry date mentioned on the reagent vial label.

Principle

Normal human red blood cells, in presence of antibody directed towards the antigen they possess, may fail to agglutinate and become sensitized. This may be due to the particular nature of the antigen and antibody involved. Eryclone® anti-human globulin reagent would react with red cells sensitized with gammaglobulins or components of human complement involved and cause agglutination of the red blood cells.

Note

1. *In vitro* diagnostic reagent for laboratory and professional use only. Not for medicinal use.
2. The reagent contains sodium azide 0.1% as preservative. Avoid contact with skin and mucosa. On disposal flush with large quantities of water.
3. Extreme turbidity may indicate microbial contamination or denaturation of protein due to thermal damage. Such reagent should be discarded.
4 Eryclone® reagent are not from human sources, hence, contamination due to HBsAg and HIV is practically excluded.

Sample Collection and Storage

No special preparation of the patient is required prior to sample collection by approved techniques. Do not use haemolysed samples.

For direct antiglobulin test: Blood drawn into EDTA is preferred but oxalated, titrated or dotted whole blood may be used. The blood sample should be tested as soon as possible after collection and should not be stored.

For indirect antiglobulin test: Serum, not more than 48 hours old, should be used. Donor units may be tested up to the end of their dating.

Preparation of Coomb's Control Cells

1. Dilute Eryclone® anti-D (IgG)/Erybank® anti-D (polyclonal) reagent 1: 50 in isotonic saline.
2. Prepare a 5% suspension of group 'O' RhoD positive cells in isotonic saline.
3. Mix equal volumes of diluted anti-D reagent (as in 1 above) and 5% suspension of 'O' RhoD positive cells (as in 2 above) and incubate at 37°C for 15 minutes.
4. Decant and wash thoroughly with isotonic saline at least thrice.
5. Resuspend in isotonic saline to make a 5% suspension of coombs control cells.

Additional Material Required

For direct antiglobulin test: Test tubes (10 × 75 mm), Pasteur pipettes, Centrifuge, Isotonic saline, Coomb's control cells, Optical aid.

For indirect antiglobulin test and compatibility test: Test tubes (10 × 75 mm), Pasteur pipettes, Erybank® bovine serum albumin, Centrifuge, Incubator (37°C), Isotonic saline, Coomb's control cells, Optical aid.

Procedure

Bring reagent to room temperature before testing.

Direct Antiglobulin Test

1. Prepare a 5% suspension of the red cells to be tested in isotonic saline.
2. Pipette one drop of the cell suspension into a test tube.
3. Fill the tube with fresh isotonic saline and centrifuge for 30 seconds at 3400 rpm (1000g).
4. Decant and repeat this washing at least thrice.
5. Add two drops of Eryclone® anti human globulin reagent and mix well.
6. Centrifuge for one minute at 1000 rpm (125 g) or for 20 seconds at 3400 rpm (1000 g).
7. Very gently, resuspend the cell button observing for agglutination macroscopically.
8. To all negative antiglobulin tests add one drop of Coomb's control cells and observe for agglutination.

INDIRECT ANTIGLOBULIN TEST

Major Cross-match Procedure

Initial Phase

1. Label two test tubes as A (for albumin) and B (for saline), depending upon the number of donors to be crossmatched, as many pairs of such labelled tubes would be required.
2. Prepare a 5% suspension of the red cells to be tested in isotonic saline.
3. Pipette two drops of recipient serum in both the labelled test tubes.
4. Pipette one drop of donor red cells in both the labelled test tubes and mix well.
5. Only to the albumin tube (A), add two drops of Erybank® bovine serum albumin reagent and mix well.
6. Centrifuge both the tubes for one minute at 1000 rpm (125 g) or for 20 seconds at 3400 rpm (1000 g).
7. First observe for haemolysis. Resuspend the cell button and observe for agglutination macroscopically.
8. Proceed to incubation phase.

Incubation Phase

1. Incubate the saline tube at room temperature and the albumin tube at 37°C for fifteen minutes.
2. First observe for haemolysis. Resuspend the cell button and observe for agglutination macroscopically.
3. Proceed to the antiglobulin phase.

Antiglobulin Phase

1. Only the albumin tubes (A) are tested in the antiglobulin phase.
2. Wash the mixture of red blood cells and serum thoroughly with isotonic saline for minimum of three times. Decant completely after the last wash.
3. Place two drops of Eryclone® Anti-human-globulin reagent into the test tubes containing the sedimented cells and mix well.
4. Centrifuge for one minute at 1000 rpm (125 g) or for 20 seconds at 3400 rpm (1000 g).
5. Very gently, resuspend the cell button and observe for agglutination macroscopically.

INTERPRETATION OF RESULTS

Direct Antiglobulin Phase

Agglutination of the red blood cells is a positive test result and indicates the presence of human IgG or components of complement on the red blood cells.

No agglutination is a negative test result and indicates the absence of human IgG or components of complement on the red blood cells.

Indirect Antiglobulin Phase

In all phases of the compatibility test, if no agglutination or haemolysis is observed, then the patient and the donor may be considered compatible. If haemolysis or agglutination at any point till the completion of the antiglobulin phase is observed, the patient and the donor are considered incompatible.

Remarks

1. If plasma is used in the indirect antiglobulin test, the complement-dependent antibodies may not be detected due to the absence of calcium.
2. To all negative test results, after the antiglobulin test phase, one drop of Coomb's control cells should be added. If Coomb's control cells do not agglutinate then the compatibility test must be repeated.
3. In the indirect antiglobulin test procedure an auto control tube (individual's cells in his own serum) should be run.
4. Red blood cells showing a positive direct antiglobulin test cannot be used for the indirect antiglobulin test.

5. It is recommended that Anti-IgG activity of the anti-human globulin reagent be tested from time to time preferably on a daily basis using Coomb's control cells as a positive control.
6. All glassware used in the test should be scrupulously clean dry and free from contamination with human serum.
7. Contaminated bovine serum albumin, saline or glassware may inactivate Anti-humanglobulin reagent.
8. Use of various drugs and certain diseases (such as megaloblastic anaemia) are known to be associated with a positive direct antiglobulin test.
9. Cord cells obtained from a newborn exhibiting haemolytic disease of the newborn, especially due to ABO incompatability may give false negative results.
10. Eryclone® Anti-human globulin reagent does not contain anti-C_4 and is free from anti-T activity.
11. As undercentrifugation or overcentrifugation could lead to erroneous results, it is recommended that each laboratory calibrate its own equipment and determine the time required for achieving the desired results.

PREPARING COOMB'S CONTROL CELLS (AGTROL® FROM TULIP, STARTER PACK)

Summary

Anti-human globulin reagent is used in blood group serology for performing compatability testing, antibody screening, antibody detection and detection of D^u red cell type. Usage of Coomb's control cells is advocated for functional validation of anti-human globulin reagent and procedural validation of tests employing anti-human globulin reagent.

Reagent

Agtrol starter pack for preparing Coomb's control cells contains.

1. Ready-to-use, standardized-prediluted anti-D (IgG) monoclonal antibody reagent
2. Red blood cell preserving solution for serological applications

Each batch of reagent undergoes rigorous quality control at various stages of manufacture for its performance characteristics.

Reagent Storage and Stability

Store the reagent at 2-8°C. Do not freeze.

The shelf life of the reagent is as per the expiry date mentioned on the reagent vial label.

Principle

Human 'O' Rho(D) positive cells in presence of Agtrol prediluted monoclonal reagent do not agglutinate but are sensitized with IgG antibodies. After processing, these sensitized red blood cells are resuspended in red blood cell preserving solution for long-termstorage and use. When anti-human globulin reagent is added to these sensitized cells the incomplete anti-D (IgG) antibodies are agglutinated by the anti-human IgG component. The agglutination reaction validates the serological activity of the anti-human globulin reagent and confirms that the anti-human globulin reagent was added in the test procedure.

Note

1. In vitro diagnostic reagent for laboratory and professional use only. Not for medicinal use.
2. Agtrol anti-D reagent is not from human source, hence, contamination due to HBsAg and HIV is practically excluded.
3. Agtrol anti-D reagent and red cell preserving solution contains 0.1% sodium azide as preservative. Avoid contact with skin and mucosa. On disposal flush with large quantities of water.
4. Extreme turbidity in both Agtrol anti-D IgG and red blood cell preserving solution reagent may indicate microbial contamination. Such reagent must be discarded.

Sample Collection and Storage

No special preparation is required prior to sample collection by approved techniques. Samples should be stored at 2-8°C if not tested immediately. Do not use heamolysed samples. Anticoagulated blood using various anticoagulants should be tested within the below mentioned time period:

- EDTA or heparin:2 days
- Sodium citrate or sodium oxalate:14 days
- ACD or CPD-28 days, clotted whole blood should be used within 14 days.

Additional Collection and Storage

Test tubes (12 × 75 mm), Pasteur pipettes, isotonic saline/isotonic buffered saline (available from

Tulip:Osmosol, Cat. No.280025), anti-human globulin reagent (Available from Tulip: Eryclone® anti-human globulin reagent, Cat.No: 160002, 160005), Rho (D) positive red blood cells, Incubator at 37°C, laboratory centrifuge, optical aid.

Procedure

Bring all the reagent to room temperature (25-30°C) before testing.

Preparation and Validation of Coomb's Control Cells

Preparation of 5% Coomb's control cell suspension

1. Collect fresh O Rho(D) positive red blood cells preferably with citrate as an anticoagulant.
2. Wash 1 ml of freshly collected O Rho(D) positive red blood cells with isotonic saline at least three times.
3. After the third wash, thoroughly decant the supernatant. To the cell button, add 5 ml of Agtrol anti-D (IgG) reagent and gently resuspend the red blood cells.
4. Incubate the mixture at 37°C for 15 minutes.
5. After incubation, wash the sensitized red blood cells thoroughly at least 4 to 5 times with isotonic saline.
6. Decant the supernatant thoroughly after the last wash. Resuspend the cell button gently with about 1-2 ml of Agtrol red blood cell preserving solution. The complete resuspended red cells should be added back to the balance Agtrol red blood cell preserving solution in the dropper vial. A stabilized suspension of 5% Coomb's control cells is thus, obtained. Label appropriately with the date of preparation.
7. Store the Coomb's control cells at 2-8°C. **Use within 4 weeks of preparation.**

Validation of prepared 5% Coomb's control cell suspension

1. Add one drop of Coomb's control cells into a test tube.
2. Add two drops of anti-human globulin reagent and mix well.
3. Centrifuge for 1 minute at 1000 rpm or 20 seconds at 3400 rpm.
4. Very gently, resuspend the cell button and observe for agglutination macroscopically.

Use of Coomb's Control cells

Validation of Anti-human globulin reagent

1. Add one drop of Coomb's control cells into a test tube.
2. Add two drops of anti-human globulin reagent and mix well.
3. Centrifuge for 1 minute at 1000 rpm or 20 seconds at 3400 rpm.
4. Very gently, resuspend the cell button and observe for agglutination macroscopically.

Confirmation of negative Antiglobulin test reactions

1. Add one drop of Coomb's control cells to the samples negative during Direct or Indirect Antiglobulin test.
2. Centrifuge for 1 minute at 1000 rpm or 20 seconds at 3400 rpm.
3. Very gently, resuspend the cell button and observe for agglutination macroscopically.

Interpretation and Results

Agglutination reaction indicates that the anti-human globulin reagent is functional and the test is valid. No agglutination indicates that the anti-human globulin reagent does not have sufficient activity and the test is invalid.

Remarks

1. As undercentrifugation or overcentrifugation could lead to erroneous results, it is recommended that each laboratory calibrates its own equipment and determine the time required for achieving the desired results.
2. Erroneous results may also occur due to improper red blood cell concentration, improper temperature while performing the test.
3. Store the Coomb's control cells at 2-8°C with cap tightly closed.
4. Do not contaminate the prepared Coomb's control cell suspension as it may subsequently effect the stability.
5. Glassware used to retrieve the Agtrol reagent and Coomb's control cell suspension should be scrupulously clean and sterile.

LOW IONIC SALT SOLUTION FOR SEROLOGICAL APPLICATIONS (TULISS FROM TULIP)

Summary

The antigen-antibody interaction in blood group serology is dependent on antigen density, concentration of antibody, pH, ionic concentration of reaction medium and temperature. Reducing the ionic concentration of the reaction medium especially enhances the uptake of weak antibodies by the red blood cell antigens. Usage of low ionic salt solution is helpful in detection of weak antibodies during crossmatch techniques, antibody screening and antibody identification.

Reagent

Tuliss is a buffered low ionic salt solution of appropriate sodium chloride molarity useful in serological applications such as antibody detection and crossmatch techniques.

Reagent Storage and Stability

1. Store the reagent at 2-8°C. Do not freeze.
2. The shelf life of the reagent is as per the expiry date mentioned on the reagent vial label.

Principle

In blood group serology, the ionic concentration of reaction medium is largely dependent on the concentration of sodium and chloride ion contributed by isotonic saline. When optimum concentration of antibody is present, antigen-antibody interaction occurs even though the sodium and chloride ions are present in sufficient quantity. But when weak antibodies are present, sodium and chloride ions may interfere with binding of antibody to the antigens present on the red blood cell membarane. By lowering the ionic concentration of salt, the ionic strength is reduced which increases the rate of antibody uptake by red blood cells.

Note

1. *In vitro* diagnostic reagent for laboratory and professional use only.
2. The reagent contains 0.1 % sodium azide as a preservative. Avoid contamination with skin and mucosa. On disposal flush with large quantity of water.
3. Do not freeze or expose the reagent to elevated temperatures. After usage immediately replace the reagent vial back to 2-8°C.
4. Marked turbidity may indicate reagent deterioration or contamination, such reagent should not be used. Do not use the reagent beyond expiry date.

Sample Collection and Storage

No special preparation is required prior to sample collection by approved techniques. Samples should be stored at 2-8°C if not tested immediately. Do not use heamolysed samples. Anticoagulated blood using various anticoagulants should be tested within the below mentioned time period:

EDTA or heparin : 2 days
Sodium citrate or sodium oxalate : 14 days
ACD or CPD : 28 days

Clotted whole blood should be used within 14 days.

Additional Material Required

Test tubes (12 × 75 mm), Pasteur pipettes, laboratory centrifuge, incubator (37°C), isotonic saline/isotonic buffered saline (Available from Tulip: Osmosol Cat No. 280025), donor red blood cells and recipient serum for crossmatch, reagent red blood cells for antibody detection, anti-human globulin reagent for crossmatch and antibody detection (Available from Tulip: Eryclone® anti-human globulin reagent Cat. No. 160002, 160005), optical aid.

Procedure

Bring all the reagent to room temperature (25-30°C) before testing.

Indirect Antiglobulin Test for Cross Match

Initial phase

1. Wash donor red blood cells three times in isotonic saline. Decant the supernatant completely after last wash.
2. Finally wash the donor blood red cells with Tuliss. A final wash with Tuliss is recommended to reduce the effect of residual isotonic saline on the final ionic concentration of the test medium.
3. Prepare a 2-3% donor red blood cells suspension in Tuliss.
4. To an approximately labelled test tube, add two drops of recipient serum.
5. Add two drops of Tuliss suspended donor red blood cells.
6. Centrifuge the tube at 1000 rpm for 30 seconds.
7. First observe for heamolysis. Resuspend the cell button and observe for agglutination macroscopically.

Incubation Phase

1. Incubate the tube containing the mixture of donor red blood cells and recipient serum at 37°C for 10 minutes.
2. First observe for haemolysis. Resuspend the cell button and observe for agglutination macroscopically.
3. Proceed to the antiglobulin phase.

Antiglobulin Phase

1. Wash the mixture of donor red blood cells and recipient serum thoroughly with isotonic saline minimum for three times. Decant completely after the last wash.
2. Place two drops of anti-human globulin reagent into the test tube and mix well.
3. Centrifuge at 1000 rpm for 30 seconds.
4. Very gently, resuspend the cell button and observe for agglutination macroscopically.

For Antibody Detection

Initial Phase

1. Wash red blood cells three times in isotonic saline. Decant the supernatant completely after last wash.
2. Finally wash the reagent red blood cells with Tuliss. A final wash with Tuliss is recommended to reduce the effect of residual isotonic saline on the final ionic concentration of the test medium.
3. Prepare a 2-3% reagent red blood cell suspension in Tuliss.
4. To an approximately labelled test tube, add two drops of serum to be tested.
5. Add two drops of Tuliss suspended reagent red blood cells.
6. Centrifuge the test tube at 1000 rpm for 30 seconds.
7. First observe for haemolysis. Resuspend the cell button and observe for agglutination macroscopically.

Incubation Phase

1. Incubate the tube containing the mixture of donor red blood cells and recipient serum at 37°C for 10 minutes
2. First observe for haemolysis. Resuspend the cell button and observe for agglutination macroscopically.
3. Proceed to the antiglobulin phase.

Antiglobulin phase

1. Wash the mixture of reagent red blood cells and serum thoroughly with isotonic saline minimum for three times. Decant completely after the last wash.
2. Place two drops of anti-human globulin reagent into the test tube and mix well.
3. Centrifuge at 1000 rpm for 30 seconds.
4. Very gently, resuspend the cell button and observe for agglutination macroscopically.

INTERPRETATION OF RESULTS

Crossmatch

In all phases of the compatibility test, if no agglutination or haemolysis is observed, then the patient and donor may be considered to be compatible. If haemolysis or agglutination at any point till the completion of the antiglobulin phase is observed, the patient and donor are considered to be incompatible.

Antibody Detection

Agglutination or haemolysis indicates that the antibody has reacted with the corresponding red blood cell antigen. No agglutination or haemolysis indicates the absence of corresponding antibody.

Remarks

1. As undercentrifugation or over-centrifugation could lead to erroneous results, it is recommended that each laboratory calibrate its own equipment and determine the time required for achieving the desired results.
2. Erroneous results may also occur due to improper red blood cell concentration, improper incubation time or temperature while performing the test.
3. The ionic strength of the test system is dependant on the amount of serum used. Alteration of the ionic strength of Tuliss procedure by addition of excess human serum will increase the ionic strength and decrease the sensitivity of the test system.
4. The performance of Tuliss reagent should be periodically evaluated with a known LISS enhanced antibody and the corresponding antigen for positive result and red cell lacking the corresponding antigen for negative result.

5. To all negative test results after the antiglobulin test phase, one drop of Coomb's control cells should be added. If Coomb's control cells do not agglutinate, then the test must be repeated.
6. Low ionic strength media have been used to enhance many antigen-antibody reactions. However, not all antibodies are reactive in a LISS test system. Some weakly reactive IgM antibodies of ABO system may not be detected in the system employing low ionic strength media.

STABILIZED, ACTIVATED PAPAIN ENZYME SOLUTION FOR SEROLOGICAL APPLICATIONS (Liquipap from Tulip)

Summary

Enzyme treatment enhances the reactivity of red blood cells with certain antibodies of Rh, Kidd, Lewis and P systems. Certain clinically significant antibodies of Rh and Kidd systems can be detected only with enzyme treated cells. Traditionally, papain needs to be prepared fresh for use and long-term storage at 20°C is recommended. This leads to frequent reagent preparation, lot to lot variation of and strict quality control to assess adequate and correct performance. Stabilized papain solution overcomes this limitation. Thus, an activated, stabilized papain enzyme solution is useful in detecting clinically significant antibodies for specific serological studies. Proteolytic activity of papain destroys blood group antigens notably M, N, S, Fy^a and Fy^b, a property which may be useful for the identification and separation of mixed antibodies.

Reagent

Liquipap is a stabilized ready-to-use papain reagent useful for serological applications such as antibody screening, antibody detection and crossmatch techniques.

Reagent Storage

1. Store the reagent at 2-8°C. Do not freeze.
2. The shelf life of the reagent is as per the expiry date mentioned on the reagent vial label.

Principle

The sialic acid molecules present in the red cell membrane impart a net negative charge to the surface of the red cell. Due to the negative charge a repulsive force exists between two red blood cells, which is termed as the 'zeta potential'. Proteolytic enzymes, such as papain, reduce the red blood cell surface charge by cleaving the sialic acid molecules from the polysaccharide chains on the red blood cell membrane. Also, the enzyme treatment causes spicule formation on the red cell thereby exposing the red blood cell antigens on the surface. This dual action of reduction in the 'zeta potential' and exposure of the red blood cell antigens on the surface enhances the agglutination reaction.

Note

1. *In vitro* diagnostic reagent for laboratory and professional use only. Not for medicinal use.
2. The reagent contains 0.1% sodium azide as a preservative. Avoid contamination with skin and mucosa. On disposal flush with large quantities of water.
3. Do not freeze or expose the reagent to elevated temperatures. After usage, immediately replace the reagent vial back to 2-8°C.
4. Marked turbidity may indicate reagent deterioration or contamination, such reagent should not be used. Do not use the reagent beyond expiry date.

Sample Collection and Preparation

No special preparation is required prior to sample collection by approved techniques. Serum samples may be stored at 2-8°C up to 3 hours if not tested immediately. Do not use haemolysed samples.

Red blood cells used for detecting antibodies should preferably be fresh.

Additional Material Required

- Test tubes (10 × 75 mm), Pasteur pipettes, laboratory centrifuge, incubator (37°C), isotonic saline/isotonic buffered saline (Available from Tulip: Osmosol Cat. No.280025), donor red blood cells and recipient serum for cross-match, reagent red blood cells for antibody detection, optical aid.

Procedure

Bring all the reagent to room temperature (25-30°C) before testing.

One-stage test

A. For cross-match

1. Wash the donor red blood cells to be tested at least three times in isotonic saline.
2. Prepare 2 to 3% red blood cell (donor) suspension in isotonic saline.
3. To an appropriately labelled test tube, add two drops of recipient serum to be tested and two drops of donor red blood cell suspension. Mix the contents thoroughly but gently.
4. Immediately add two drops of Liquipap reagent.
5. Incubate at 37°C for 15 to 30 minutes.
6. Centrifuge at 1000 rpm for 2 minutes,
7. Gently resuspend and observe for agglutination and/or haemolysis macroscopically and microscopically.

B. For antibody detection

1. Wash the reagent red blood cells to be tested at least three times in isotonic saline.
2. Prepare 2 to 3% reagent red blood cell suspension to be tested in isotonic saline.
3. To an appropriately labelled test tube, add two drops of serum to be tested and two drops of reagent red blood cell suspension under test.
4. Mix the contents and immediately add two drops of Liquipap reagent .
5. Incubate at 37°C for 15 to 30 minutes.
6. Centrifuge at 1000 rpm for 2 minutes.
7. Gently resuspend and observe for agglutination and/or haemolysis macroscopically and microscopically.

Alternatively, a two-stage test using Liquipap reagent can also be performed as follows.

Two stage test

A. For Cross match

1. Wash the donor red blood cells three times in isotonic saline.
2. To an appropriately labelled test tube, add one drop of washed packed cells (donor) and one drop of Liquipap reagent.
3. Incubate the test tube at 37°C for 15 to 30 minutes.
4. Wash the Liquipap-treated donor red blood cells at least three times with isotonic saline.
5. Prepare Liquipap treated 2 to 3% red blood cell suspension of donor in isotonic saline.
6. To an appropriately labelled test tube, add one drop of Liquipap treated 2 to 3% donor red blood cell suspension.
7. Add two drops of recipient serum to be tested.
8. Mix well and incubate at 37°C for 30 minutes.
9. Centrifuge at 1000 rpm for 2 minutes.
10. Gently resuspend and observe for agglutination and/or haemolysis macroscopically and microscopically.

B. For antibody detection

1. Wash the reagent red blood cells to be tested three times in isotonic saline.
2. To an appropriately labelled test tube, add one drop of washed packed reagent red blood cells under test and one drop of Liquipap reagent.
3. Incubate the test tube at 37°C for 15 to 30 minutes.
4. Wash the Liquipap treated reagent red blood cells under test at least three times with isotonic saline.
5. Prepare Liquipap treated 2 to 3% reagent red blood cell suspension under test in isotonic saline.
6. To an appropriately labelled test tube, add one drop of Liquipap treated 2 to 3% reagent red blood cell suspension under test.
7. Add two drops of serum to be tested.
8. Mix well and incubate at 37°C for 30 minutes.
9. Centrifuge at 1000 rpm for 2 minutes.
10. Gently resuspend and observe for agglutination and/or haemolysis macroscopically and microscopically.

Interpretation of Results

Agglutination and/or haemolysis indicates an antibody directed against the antigen present on the red blood cell under test.

No agglutination and/or haemolysis indicates absence of enzyme reactive antibodies directed against the antigen present on the red blood cell under test.

Remarks

1. As undercentrifugation or over-centrifugation could lead to erroneous results, it is recommended that each laboratory calibrate its own equipment and determine the time required for achieving the desired results.
2. Erroneous results may also occur due to improper red blood cell concentration, improper incubation time or temperature while performing the test.

3. All enzyme preparations are subject to some loss of potency, it is therefore, recommended to check the reagent performance with known negative control (neutral AB serum) and positive control (Coomb's control cells) on a regular basis.
4. The ability of papain to denature IgG molecule renders the one-stage technique less sensitive though it is a convenient method for use in crossmatch techniques.
5. Papain is not suited for the detection of Anti-M, N-S-Duffy since the corresponding antigens are destroyed during the proteolytic action of papain enzyme.
6. Liquipap reagent is a colourless to pale yellow clear solution. Repeated exposure to elevated temperatures may impart a dark colour to the reagent. In such cases, the reagent performance must be assessed closely before use.
7. Usage of isotonic buffered saline while performing the test ensures in maintaining the optimum pH of the reaction milieu for antigen antibody reaction.
8. Alternatively, LISS (Low ionic strength solution) can be used while performing the test. LISS lowers the ionic concentration of the reaction milieu thereby potentiating the rate of antibody uptake by the antigen present on the red blood cell membrane.
9. It is recommended to run a control with each assay series.

BLOOD TRANSFUSION

The procedures described earlier in this chapter are done mainly for providing appropriate blood for transfusion, i.e. the donor's blood should be compatible in all ways with the recipient's blood.

BLOOD DONORS

Most individuals can give blood without any ill effects, as a matter of fact, without any symptoms at all. The donors may be volunteers or paid donors. Blood transfusion should always be a safe, harmless procedure, therefore, the donors must be screened. Two basic principles govern the transfusion services:

1. The donor should not be harmed in any way.
2. The recipient should equally be safe, i.e. the transfusion should be absolutely safe for the recipient.

Donor Screening

1. *Identification:* Identify the donor name, address and other pertinent information. No donor should donate twice in three months' period. Preferably, the donors should be between the ages 18 and 60 years.

2. *History:* The questions should be guided about the present state of health; recent illness, if any; operations, if any; if the donor has ever been transfused; (for woman) if she ever gave birth to children who developed jaundice shortly after birth; if they have had malaria, jaundice, syphilis, tuberculosis; if they have heart disease, diabetes, etc. Donors may give wrong information on two accounts: (i) They want to donate blood for want of money. (ii) They do not want to donate blood for they are afraid of doing so. Hence, a battery of tests to be done becomes necessary.

3. *Physical examination:*
   - Temperature reading, (exclude those having fever).
   - Blood pressure should be normal or only slightly raised. Disqualify those who have moderate to marked hypertension.
   - Pulse should be normal without any irregularities.
   - Auscultate the chest for any respiratory or cardiac disorder. Discard individuals with respiratory/cardiac problem.
   - Pregnant women should not donate if they are anaemic.
   - Finding of any venereal disease should outrightly disqualify the donor until he receives adequate treatment and gets rid of his problem.

4. *Haemoglobin*: The donors should not be anaemic. It is best to disqualify anybody having Hb < 12 gm % but keeping in view our health, dietetic, and economic structure up to 10 gm % can, however, be accepted, weighing the urgency of the demand for blood. As given in the hematology section specific gravity by copper sulphate method is adequate for screening donors' Hb.

5. *Malarial parasite*: Malarial blood can cause transfusion malaria if it is transfused. Screen all donors by making thick and thin smears of their

blood. In some chronic malaria patient, no parasites may be seen on the peripheral smear examination but a unit of their blood would pass on enough parasites to the recipient.

6. *Microfilaria*: Screening for microfilaria should be done both by making a wet, coverslip mount of a drop of fresh blood (looking for the shipping movement of the microfilaria) and also on the direct and stained films used for searching malarial parasites. All microfilaria harbouring donors are rejected.

7. *Icteric index*: This is the easiest method of measuring and quantitating the amount of measuring and quantitating the amount of pigment (mostly bilirubin) in the blood. Serum hepatitis is one of the most dreaded complications of transfusion. If a person has had jaundice during the last 5 years or is having it—he should be disqualified as a donor. History might be difficult to obtain and hence, liver function tests may be necessary where there is even slightest of doubt. The simplest and quickest to perform is icteric index, a measurement of the level of bilirubin, expressed in units based upon a comparison of the colour of the serum and the colour of a standard dilute solution of potassium dichromate. If the Icterus index is > 6 units, the donor should not be allowed to donate.

A major complication of transfusing blood from a Hepatitis B/C patient or carrier is the *transmission* of the disease to the recipient.

Now ELISA techniques are available.

8. *Serology*: VDRL/Kahn's tests should be performed on blood of all donors. The blood positive for this test may pass on live spirochetes to the recipient. Weighing the need of blood even such a positive sample may be transfused and the recipient given a course of penicillin. In no case should any drug be put into the transfusion bottle. It is known that *Treponema pallidum* can not survive for more than 48-72 hours with the condition of storage of anticoagulated blood in a refrigerator at 4°C. Within that time they are all dead. Hence, blood which has been stored as mentioned above cannot transmit syphilis since there would be no viable organisms remaining. A new syphilis patient' blood may be VDRL/Kahn's negative even though his blood would contain the spirochetes, hence, some believe in storing all blood for 48-72 hours before allowing it to be transfused. It is a good practice to indicate to the doctor who has requisitioned the blood, date and time of procuring that unit of blood.

9. *Grouping and typing of donor*: This has already been dealt with at great length earlier in this chapter.

10. *Antibody Screening*: Ideally an indirect Coombs' test should be done on every donor to screen for atypical, incomplete antibodies.

11. AIDS screening is a MUST.

(Information regarding kits—refer to Serology chapter)

Drawing of Blood

1. Have the donor lie down.
2. Under aseptic conditions, do a veni-puncture with a fairly large needle on the donor set-15 or 16 gauge needle, for gravity flow collection method. The bottle is kept below the level of arm and has an airway so that air may escape while the bottle gets filled with blood.
3. Where vacuum bottles are available a smaller gauge needle can be used. Do not puncture such a bottle.
4. Plastic bags containing the preservative fluid are already collapsed and hence, need no airway.
5. A unit of blood may mean different volumes at different centres. A standard unit is 420 ml of blood and 80 ml of ACD or CPD solution, i.e. a total 500 ml.
6. While the blood is being drawn swirl the bottle gently to allow the ACD to act.
7. Flow of blood is usually hastened by: (i) having a blood pressure cuff on the arm above the needle, inflated to a pressure of 40-50 mm Hg and (ii) asking the patient to gently flex the fingers or clench and unclench his fist to assist the flow of the blood into the vein from which it is being taken.
8. When the full amount of donation has been collected, draw the needle from the bottle and put 5 to 10 ml samples into 2 or 3 sterile, dry tubes, each with the same number as that of the large blood transfusion bottle.

9. Now the needle from the vein and the blood pressure cuff can be removed.
10. Immediately apply pressure with cotton at the area, preferrably with the arm held straight up in an extended position. Have the donor hold it for minimum 3 to 5 minutes.
11. Close the bottle immediately after sterilizing the rubber cover.
12. Once closed do not open and enter the bottle until the requisitioning doctor inserts the giving set. Be sure the bottle is completely and correctly labelled Number, Name, Group, Type, Date, etc. Double check this.
13. Do not let the donor get up immediately. Let the donor's body adjust to the loss of this blood. Offering a nourishing drink and snacks to the donor is indeed a very good way of saying thanks to the donor. Encourage him to drink little extra water for a few hours after the donation.
14. The preservative have been mentioned in the foregoing pages.
15. Store the donated blood at 4-6°C (37-42°F) in a refrigerator that should solely be used for keeping the blood transfusion bottles only. If this blood is kept constantly at the required temperature—a duration of 21 days may be allowed to lapse between collection and transfusion of the blood. If storage conditions are less ideal, then it is best to shorten the storage time to about 14 days (after this duration it should not be transfused).

ADVERSE DONOR REACTIONS

Problems with Blood Flow

Occasionally, venepuncture is unsuccessful or the vein may develop spasm after venepucture so that blood flow is not maintained

If this happens:

1. Do not try to probe around in the vein, as this can result in a haematoma and discomfort for the donor.
2 Remove the needle and discard the pack as it will be contaminated.
3 Never resite the needle in the same arm.
4 Reassure the donor, giving a full explanation for the unsuccessful venepuncture in order to retain their confidence, and apologize.

If the donor consents, a further venepuncture on the other arm may be attempted, provided that a suitable vein is located. No more than a total of 350/450 ml of blood should be withdrawn from both sides.

If there is a failure to maintain a blood flow during the collection, the person who has performed the venepuncture should be informed immediately. Slowing of the flow rate may be due to:

- Reduced cuff pressure: Check that cuff pressure has been maintained
- Occlusion of the lumen of the needle by the vein wall: Rotating the needle may help
- Positioning of the lumen of the needle on a valve within the vein: Try to re-establish the flow by withdrawing the needle gently or even by slight rotation of the needle

Before doing any of these things:

1. Explain that there is a problem with the blood flow and ask whether the donor is experiencing any discomfort.
2. Remove the swab and check that there is no haematoma present.
3. If there are no other apparent problems, proceed with adjusting the needle.
4. Avoid excessive manipulation of the needle or squeezing the donor tubing as small clots may form which will then be released into the circulation.

A failure to re-establish a blood flow will result in a partial collection. This should be marked on the donor's record form and the donor should be given an explanation and apology, if the collection is too slow, the donation should be discontinued. This should be recorded on the donor's record form.

Haematoma

Haematoma can be prevented by good venepuncture technique and application of adequate pressure following donation.

If a haematoma is noted:

1. Stop the donation.
2. Apply firm pressure until the venepuncture site stops oozing blood.
3. Apply an anti-inflammatory cream in a circular motion over the area and cover it with a small; plaster or swab dressing, then apply a pressure bandage.

4. Reassure the donor, explaining what has happened and the reason for the bruise, and then apologize.
5. Ask the donor to keep the paster on for 24 hours and the bandage on for 2 to 4 hours. If they feel that it is too tight and stopping their circulation, it should be loosened.
6. Tell the donor that they can use their arm normally, but should not lift any heavy objects. Also, tell them that they can take painkillers for moderate discomfort, but that if the area becomes unduly painful, they should contact the transfusion centre or their own doctor.
7. Record details of the haematoma on the donor's record form.

Accidental Puncture of the Artery

This is an uncommon complication of blood donation, and one should be able to recognize it immediately by a very fast flow of bright red blood.

If accidental puncture of the artery occurs

1. Discontinue the donation immediately and apply hard pressure to the puncture site immediately after the withdrawal of the needle. Raise the limb above heart level.
2. Maintain pressure for a minimum of 15 minutes.
3. When the bleeding has stopped, apply a pressure bandage and tell the donor to keep this on for 4 to 6 hours.
4. Reassure the donor, giving a full explanation of what has happened, and apologize.
5. Record the appropriate information on the donor's record form.
6 Do not allow the donor to leave until they are feeling well and after the most senior member of the donor clinic staff has discharged them.
7. If you suspect that tissue bleeding may still be continuing, refer the donor to the nearest hospital or health centre. If the donor lives near the donor clinic, ask him to come back for assessment the following day.

Mild, Moderate or Severe Reactions

Most people can tolerate the withdrawal of 350 or 450 ml of blood without any ill-effects. Others experience reactions ranging in severity from a feeling of uneasiness' to obvious shock-like symptoms, fainting or even generalized convulsions. These reactions can occur at any time—during the donor selection process, during donation, in the resting or refreshment area or even hours following a donation.

There is a psychological element to most reactions, so a friendly, cheerful atmosphere at the session can often reduce donor anxiety and perhaps prevent any adverse reactions. Donor reactions do sometimes occur, however, and can be categorized as follows:

Mild: Vasovagal symptoms without loss of consciousness.

Moderate : A progression of symptoms associated with a mild donor reaction resulting in unconsciousness.

Severe : Any of the above, accompanied by convulsions (uncommon).

Mild Donor Reactions

The signs of mild donor reactions include :

— anxiety
— increased respiration
— rapid pulse
— pallor and mild sweating
— dizziness / continuous yawning
— nausea / vomiting

When Mild Donor Reactions Occur

1. Discontinue the donation.
2. Raise both of the donor's legs and lower the head to improve the blood supply. If a donor is vomiting, turn him on one side to avoid accidental inhaling of vomitus.
3. Loosen or remove tight clothing.
4. Keep the donor cool by opening windows or switching on a fan.
5. Have a suitable receptacle available at the bed-side in case the donor vomits.
6. Allow a sufficient rest period.
7. Offer a cold drink.
8. Once the donor has recovered, assist him from the bed to the refreshment area where another cold drink should be given.
9. Reassure and talk to the donor throughout all these stages. Explain that this type of reaction is common and does not mean that they are now physically 'unwell'.
10. Record the reaction on the donor's record form.
11 Advise the donor that, if symptoms persist, they should report to the blood bank or consult a doctor.

12. Ensure that the donor is fully recovered before leaving the session and has been seen by a trained member of staff.

Moderate Donor Reactions

The signs of moderate donor reactions include:
— loss of consciousness (fainting)
— repeated periods of unconsciousness
— a slow pulse which may be difficult to feel because of poor volume
— shallow respirations.

When moderate donor reactions occur

1. Discontinue the donation.
2. Raise both of the donor's legs and lower the head.
3. Ensure that the donor is examined by a medical officer or a senior nurse.
4. Loosen or remove tight clothing.
5. Keep the donor cool by opening windows or switching on a fan.
6. Have a suitable receptacle available at the bedside in case the donor vomits.
7. Check the pulse rate regularly. The appearance of the donor and the pulse rate are a good guide to the donor's condition.
8. If possible, remove the donor to another room for privacy and to prevent other donors from seeing what is happening.
9. If there is no other room available, put screens around the donor.
10. Ensure that someone remains with the donor.
11. Reassure and talk to the donor throughout all these stages. It may be necessary to advise the donor not to donate in future.
12. Record the reaction on the donor's record form.
13. Ensure that the donor rests for some time and is fully recovered before leaving.
14. Advise the donor that if symptoms persist, they should contact their doctor of the nearest hospital.
15. Ensure that the donor is discharged by a senior member of staff.
16. Where feasible, arrange transport home for the donor.

Severe Donor Reactions

A faint may be accompanied by convulsions. Convulsions may be preceded by all the signs and symptoms of a vasovagal attack or they may occur without warning. Convulsions vary in severity from loss of consciousness accompanied by a slight twitching of extremities to a grandmal: type seizure with incontinence of urine or faeces. A medical officer or trained nurse must be called immediately.

Faints are common but convulsions are very uncommon. If the correct procedure for donor screening has been carried out through the medical history and health check convulsions should not occur. Most convulsions stop within a few minutes, but they are often very upsetting for other donors so staff not actively involved in looking after a convulsing donor should distract and reassure other donors.

When Generalized Convulsions Occur

1. Turn the donor to a lateral position to maintain a clear airway.
2. Gently restrain the donor to prevent and injury.
3. Put screens around the donor to maintain privacy.
4. Check the pulse rate frequently.
5. Ensure that the donor is examined by a medical officer.
6. Loosen tight clothing.
7. Keep the donor cool by opening windows or switching on a fan.
8. If a convulsion lasts longer than five minutes, this is a medical emergency and a medical officer must be in attendance. Valium may be given intravenously under the direction of the medical officer. IM Valium is unaffected in these circumstances.
9. Reassure the donor and explain what has happened.
10. Tactfully advise the donor not to donate blood again.
11. Record the incident:
    — on the donor's record form.
    — in the Blood Bank incident book.
12. Recheck the donor's medical history and record of the predonation health check to identify whether there were any indications that a convulsion might occur.
13. Advise the donor that they should contact their doctor or the nearest hospital.
14. Ensure that the donor rests for some time and is fully recovered before leaving the session.
15. Ensure that the donor is discharged by a medical officer or a very senior member of staff.

16. Inform the donor's own doctor about the incident.
17. Arrange transport home for the donor when fully recovered and ensure that they are escorted or arrange for their transfer to hospital.

Hyperventilation

Hyperventilation is a rapid overbreathing which lowers the carbon dioxide content of blood. In turn, this leads to muscle spasms. Talking to the donor to reassure him and relieve anxiety should prevent hyperventilation.

If hyperventilation occurs:

1. Instruct the donor to breathe quietly and slowly, but not deeply.
2. If this fails to relieve muscle spasms, instruct the donor to rebreathe expired air into a paper bag.
3. Explain what is happening and reassure the donor.

Accidents

There may be a risk of injury to the head or body if a donor faints and falls

When head injuries or other injuries requiring medical attention occur:

1. Always ensure that the donor is examined by a medical officer or senior nurse.
2. If there is any doubt about the donor's condition, arrange for his transfer to hospital with a doctor or qualified nurse as escort.
3. **Record the incident:**
   - on the donor's record form.
   - on an accident form (this should also be filled in if a member of staff is involved in an accident)
   - in the Blood Bank incident book.

If the Injury is of a Minor Nature:

1. Ensure that the donor rests for some time and is fully recovered before leaving, unless transfer to hospital has been arranged.
2. Ensure that the donor is discharged by a senior member of staff who should decide whether the donor's own doctor should be informed.
3. Advise the donor that if he feels unwell, he should contact his doctor or the nearest hospital.

COMPATIBILITY TESTING

The Cross-Match

The final green signal for allowing blood transfusion is compatibility between the donor's and recipient's blood. This is done *in vitro* in the laboratory/blood bank. A compatibility test is mandatory before all transfusions.

Cross matching is done in two parts: (i) the major cross-match and (ii) the minor cross-match. In the former the donor's cells are mixed with the patient's serum and in latter the patient's cells are mixed with the donor's serum (Fig. 11.17).

Saline Cross-Match

Saline suspension of the cells is mixed with serum. This is done at room temperature and only complete, saline active, 'cold' antibodies will be detected.

The Open Slide Method

1. Label one tube with patient's name or number (number is preferrable as there may be many patient with the same name).
2. Label another tube with the donor's name or number—one for each bottle of blood to be crossmatched.
3. Half-fill each tube with saline.
4. Label one slide for each cross-match. Draw a line in the middle to separate the two sides. Put the patient's number on the left side and mark it 'P' on that side. This is the major side which uses the patient's (P) serum. Put the donor's number on the right side and identify it further by marking it 'D'. This is the minor side, which uses the donor's (D) serum. Draw two circles one on each side with a glass marking pencil (Fig. 11.16).

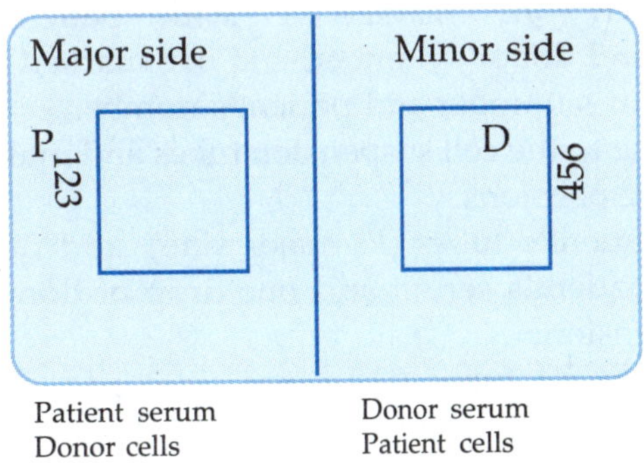

Fig. 11.17: Cross Matching

5. Make 5% red cell suspension in each of the labelled tubes—patient's and the donor's bloods. (Get the donor cells and serum from one of the 'pilot' tubes filled at the end of the donation of

blood). Do not enter the bottle of ACD blood for this purpose unless absolutely necessary. If you do enter the bottle, you have almost inevitably introduced bacteria —even if you have been careful–and that blood should be used immediately or not at all.

6. To the patient's (P), major side of the slide, add one drop of patient's serum and one drop of the donor's cell suspension
7. To the donor's (D), minor side of the slide, add one drop of donor's serum and one drop of the patient's cell suspension.
8. Mix by gently rotating the slide and incubate at room temperature for 10-15 minutes. (Drying will make the results difficult to interpret. Drying can be retarded if the slides are kept in a petridish).
9. Examine both macroscopically and microscopically for agglutination (by gently rotating and tipping the slide).

This is a simple and a rapid method. However, incompatibilities due to weak saline agglutinins and all incomplete immune antibodies will not be detected. The period of incubation should not be reduced or else agglutination may not occur. Almost all ABO group incompatibilities will be detected by this method. Rh incompatibilities will never be detected.

Saline Tube Method

1. Label one tube for the patient's 2-5% saline cell suspension. Label one tube for each donor's saline cell suspension. Label two tubes for each cross-match—one marked P with patient's number and donor's number, and one marked D with donor's number and patient's number.
2. Add saline to the cell suspension tubes and make the cell suspensions.
3. To the patient's tubes (P. major side), add one drop of patient's serum and one drop of donor cell suspension.
4. To the donor's tubes (D. minor side) add one drop of donor's serum and one drop of patient cell suspension.
5. Mix the cells and sera by gently tapping the tubes.
6. Let stand at room temperature for 30 minutes.
7. Examine for agglutination both macroscopically and microscopically.

This method needs a longer incubation period but has the advantage of detecting weak reactions more often. However, it still will only detect complete agglutinins—not immune antibodies of the Rh type.

Immediate-spin and Thermal Incubation Modification

1-5. as in the previous method.

6. After 2-3 minutes at room temperature, centrifuge at 500 to 1000 rpm for 2 minutes.
7. Remove and examine macroscopically, holding the bottom of the tube over a concave mirror (a microscope mirror is good enough) so that you can observe the button of cells at the bottom when you tap the tube gently to resuspend the cells. If the cells, show agglutination, check them microscopically by placing a drop on a slide. This indicates incompatibility and the cross-match result can be recorded. If the cells resuspend without any clumps, then proceed to the next step.
8. Incubate the tube for 60 minutes at 37°C.
9. Examine the cells for agglutination, both, macroscopically and microscopically. Centrifugation brings the cells into close proximity and hastens agglutination where it is going to occur—the immediate spin. Incubation at 37° C may detect some complete warm antibodies active in saline but missed in room temperature incubations.

Albumin Tube Method

1. Set up the tubes as for saline method.
2. Incubate the cells and serum for 60 minutes at 37°C—thermal saline incubation.
3. Allow a drop of albumin to run down the inside of each cross-matching tube so that it forms a layer between the cells and serum (human/bovine albumin, 22-30%).
4. Incubate at 37°C for an additional 30 minutes.
5. Dislodge the cells gently and look for agglutination microscopically. This method will pick up some incompatibilities not detected in saline due to incomplete, immune antibodies, such as Rh antibodies.

Coomb's' Cross-Matching

1. Wash the patient's and donor's cells three times in saline. Then make 5-10% suspension of each in saline.

2. To labelled patient's tubes (P. major side) add 2 drops of patient's serum and 2-4 drops of donor cell suspension.
3. To labelled donor's tube (D. minor side) add 2 drops of donor's serum and 2-3 drops of patient cell suspension.
4. Incubate tubes at 37°C for one hour.
5. Centrifuge, decant the serum and wash the cells thrice in saline.
6. Add Coombs' serum to each tube and after letting stand for 5 minutes at room temperature, centrifuge at 500-1000 rpm for 2 minutes.
7. Examine the cells macroscopically and microscopically.

The Coombs' serum in the cross-match as in the indirect Combs' test, will detect the presence of incomplete, immune antibodies such as Rh antibodies and show any Rh incompatibility. Remember that not all Rh negative persons have anti-Rh (D) antibodies—in fact only very few do—so that not all cross-matches of Rh-negative recipients with Rh-positive donors—or *vice versa*—will be incompatible. Transfusion of the blood may be perfectly safe. However, the Rh-positive transfused cells may sensitize the recipient so that he or she develops anti-Rh antibodies. On subsequent cross-matches (after 2-3 weeks), an incompatibility would be demonstrated. Thus, where Rh-negative individuals have been previously transfused, it is important to do a more sensitive cross-match, since there is a good chance that the previous transfusion may have been with Rh-positive blood.

It is obvious that cross-matching of bloods of the same groups generally gives a compatible result (major and minor). Cross-matching of O group blood with any other group gives a compatible major side (hence, O group people are called universal donors) but always gives an incompatible minor side. Any group of blood may be given to AB group of patient with a compatible major cross-match (universal recipients) but again there is an incompatible minor cross-match.

Given on next page are the diagrammed results of the cross-matching of the different groups of blood (+ = agglutination, — = no agglutination).

Blood which shows a major incompatiblity should never be transfused (in the patient's body the 'major side' would be the full plasma volume—about 2,500 ml of antibodies and the transfused donor cells—200-250 ml). The minor cross-match is important but not as important as the major side, (in the patient's body, the minor side would be the donor plasma volume 250-300 ml—of antibodies and the large number of his own cells—about 2500 ml. The donor plasma becomes diluted in the much larger volume of the patient's plasma, and thus, the donor antibodies become diluted and dispersed so that although a few cells may be coated or agglutinate, there is no major reaction). In an emergency, therefore, it is possible to use blood which is minor incompatible (but major compatible) without leading to transfusion reaction. Sometimes however, one can get into difficulty by transfusing blood which shows a minor incompatibility as given below.

High titre of donor antibodies: If the titre (amount) of antibodies in the donor blood is very high, then even if there is dilution of the donor's plasma in the patient's plasma, the antibodies may still be present in significant numbers to cause agglutination, hemolysis and result in a reaction. O donors with high titre are said to be dangerous universal donors.

Method of Cross-Matching Universal Donor Blood

1. Do major cross-match as described (Fig. 11.18).
2. Make a 1 : 100 dilution of donor serum in saline.
3. Use this diluted serum for a minor cross-match.
4. If there is no agglutination on minor side using the 1 : 100 diluted serum, then this a low titre (< 1:100) plasma and can safely be transfused as long as too many bottles of such blood are not needed.
5. If there is agglutination on the minor side, it means that this is high titre (> 1 : 100) plasma and should better not be used especially if more than one unit is required (for AB patient, it is possible to use A, B, or O donor blood. Whichever is given, it should be crossmatched in this way).

Factors Leading to False Results

1. Auto-agglutination.
2. Cold antibodies.
3. Bacterial contamination.
4. Drying.

If Still an Unexpected Incompatibility is Obtained:

1. Test for autoagglutination.
2. Test for cold antibodies.
3. Regroup the patient and donor cells.

4. Back-type (serum type) the patient and donor serum.
5. Repeat the cross-match by tube technique.
6. Check the records to see if patient's present grouping is correct.
7. Ask for a fresh patient specimen if necessary.

CHOICE OF MATERIAL FOR TRANSFUSION

1. Shock due to hemorrhage or decreased blood volume: Whole blood fresh, stored or preserved.
2. Shock resulting from trauma, burns, or infection: Plasma liquid, frozen or dried; plasma substitutes.
3. Chronic anaemia: Whole blood or resuspended red blood cells.
4. Leukopenia: Large amounts of fresh whole blood. Leukocyte concentrates.
5. Prothrombin factor deficiency not corrected by vitamin K: Fresh whole blood.
6. Hemophilia: Factor VIII (AHF) cryoprecipitate concentrate. Factor IX complex concentrate. Whole blood or plasma administered within 6 hours of collection.
7. Thrombocytopenia: Platelet transfusion with fresh (< 3 days old) platelets.

BLOOD AND ITS PRODUCTS

Whole blood: In most instances whole blood is requisitioned by the concerned physician/surgeon, except in certain circumstances when a special preparation may be asked for.

Fresh Blood

Stored bank blood contains nearly all of the substances required in a usual transfusion therapy. A few labile substances are lost.

1. *Platelets*: These stick to the rubber and glass surfaces and also die soon or become nonfunctional. If platelets are needed, fresh blood is necessary.
2. *WBC's*: These die fairly rapidly. On occasions where the patient is suffering from severe leukopenia with infection, a transfusion of fresh blood provides viable leukocytes which help to fight the infection but which do not raise the WBC count.

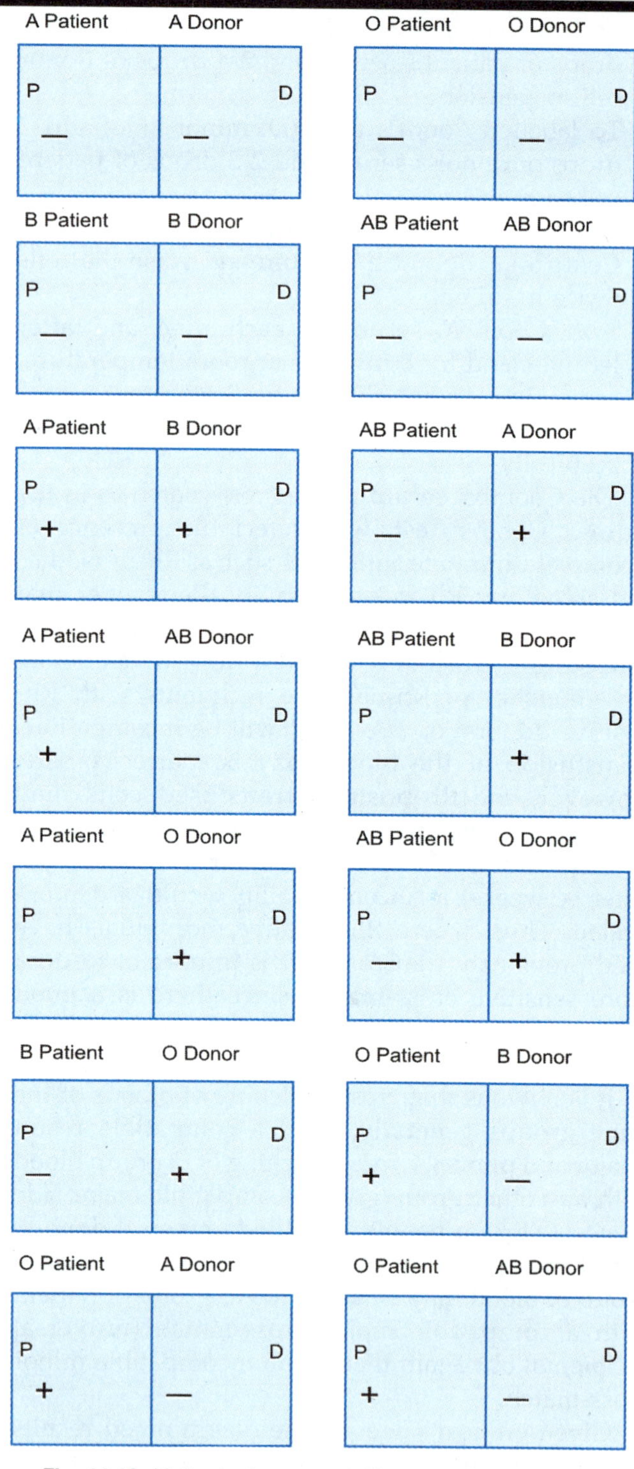

Fig. 11.18: Method of cross-matching universal donor blood

3. *Factor VIII*: Antihemophilic globulin. Patients with hemophilia should be transfused with fresh blood if they need transfusion to help stop bleeding, since AHG disappears rapidly from stored blood.

4. *Other labile factors:* Can be provided by giving frozen or dried plasma.

Packed Cells

Sedimented cells: The bottle kept in the refrigerator shows at bottom settled cells and above it the plasma. In chronic anaemia one may want to transfuse just the packed cells. This can be prepared by aspirating the plasma into a separate sterile bottle, leaving the cells in original bottle. Lable the plasma bottle with the date, the bottle number and the group and type of the blood from which it is obtained, aspirate a small amount of plasma into a 'pilot' tube for later cross-matches.

The packed cells should be transfused within 4 hours. Aspirate plasma only when someone comes to collect it, this ensures that the packed cells would be used immediately.

Plasma

The ACD plasma aspirated from the sedimented cells may be stored for months at 4-6°C and is safe for transfusion. If the plasma becomes cloudy or shows floating granules (bacterial colonies)—suck little bit of it from the top, do a hanging drop and Gram stain of the same—discard if it is found contaminated. Minor cross-matching should be done with the patient's red cells and the donor's plasma. Plasma may be used as:

1. *Liquid plasma:* It should contain 5% dextrose to prevent precipitation of fibrin at room temperature. The prothrombin titre diminishes rapidly after 72 hours. Liquid plasma may be kept at room temperature for 3 years. Hepatitis virus is attenuated or destroyed in plasma that has remained at room temperature for 6 months.
2. *Frozen plasma:* Plasma frozen within 72 hours after blood is drawn may be stored indefinitely at –20°C (–4°F). Reliquefy at 37°C (98.6°F) in a water bath and use promptly. Frozen plasma retains its full content of labile constituents (prothrombin, complement, antibodies). Hepatitis virus is also preserved, frozen plasma should therefore not be used unless no other substitute for blood is available.
3. *Dried plasma*: Plasma dried after freezing within 72 hours after blood is drawn is stable at room temperature for 5 years if kept in an airtight container. Reliquefy with 0.1% solution of citric acid and administer within 1 hour. Dried plasma retains its full content of labile constituents. Hepatitis virus is preserved too.

BLOOD TRANSFUSION COMPLICATIONS

Complications Appearing Early

1. Hemolytic reaction:
   — immediate or
   — delayed.
2. Reactions due to infected blood.
3. Allergic reactions to white cells, platelets or proteins.
4. Pyrogenic reactions (febrile reactions)
   - Pyrogens may come from the bottle, tubing, or the blood itself. Precaution should be taken that equipment, solutions, etc. used should be absolutely sterile.
   - Bacterial contamination too would lead to pyrogenic reaction.
5. Circulatory overload.
6. Air embolism.
7. Thrombophlebitis.
8. Hyperkalemia.
9. Citrate toxicity.
10. Clotting abnormalities (after massive transfusion).

Complications Appearing Late

1. Disease transmission, e.g.
   - Hepatitis B/C
   - Syphilis
   - Malaria
   - Cytomegalovirus
   - AIDS
2. Transfusional iron-overload
3. Immune sensitisation.

INVESTIGATIONS IN A CASE OF TRANSFUSION REACTION

The occurrence of a transfusion reaction should be immediately reported to the blood supplying laboratory or bank.

The reporting authority should send

1. A post-transfusion blood sample
2. A post-transfusion urine sample
3. A pre-transfusion blood sample
4. If the blood has been discontinued, the bottle and the tubing intact should also be sent.

The laboratory or the bank providing the blood should already have

1. the patient's original cross-match specimen (these should be preserved for at least 48 hours after dispatching the blood or its products).
2. the donor's pilot tube/bottle (also to be preserved for 48 hours as mentioned above)
3. all the laboratory/bank records.

Proceed as Mentioned Below

1. Inspect the post-transfusion urine sample for the presence of haemolysis—hemoglobinuria. Centrifuge the specimen to see if the red colour stays in the supernatant (hemoglobinuria) or goes down with the sediment (hematuria).
2. Centrifuge the post-transfusion blood specimen. Inspect the serum for the presence of hemolysis. If hemolysis has been established report it to the concerned physician/surgeon so that he may treat the patient as a case of haemolytic transfusion reaction.

   To establish the cause of hemolysis:
3. Regroup and retype the original donor pilot blood sample, the original patient's cross-match sample, the blood in the blood bottle or tubing.
4. Group and type the new patient's pretransfusion blood sample (if available—and post-transfusion specimen).
5. Recross-match—if available use combined saline and Coombs' cross-matches—the donor blood with the original patient specimen.
6. Cross-match the donor blood with the new patient specimen.
7. Make hanging drop preparation and Gram stain of blood in tubing or blood bottle looking for bacteria. Culture the blood in the bottle or tubing.
8. Schumm's test—a spectroscopic examination of plasma for the bands which are typical of methemalbumin—found when there has been intravascular hemolysis.

Interpretation of Results

1. If there was no evidence of hemolysis in the blood and no free hemoglobin in the urine, the patient has not had a hemolytic reaction, but a pyrogenic/allergic reaction.
2. If there is evidence of haemolysis in the blood and hemolysis in the urine (haemoglobinuria), a haemolytic transfusion reaction has occurred.
3. If the recross-matching shows incompatibility, then the first cross-match was done or recorded in error.
4. If the recross-match with the original patient specimen is compatible, but the cross-match with the new patient specimen is incompatible, the mistake lies in mistaken identification of the patient, either when the first sample for cross-match was done, or at the time of giving the transfusion.
5. If the saline cross-matches are compatible but the Coombs' cross-matches are incompatible then the problem lies with an immune antibody incompatibility—the most common being the Rh incompatibility.

LABORATORY DIAGNOSIS OF HEMOLYTIC DISEASE OF THE NEWBORN

Laboratory findings at birth:

1. *Cord blood:*
   - variable anaemia (Hb<18 gm%)
   - reticulocytosis
   - hyperbilirubinaemia
   - positive direct Coombs' test
   - baby is Rh positive.
2. *The mother:*
   - is Rh negative and
   - has a high plasma titre of anti-D.

Chapter 12

Cerebrospinal and Other Body Fluids

CEREBROSPINAL FLUID

Cerebrospinal fluid (CSF) is formed primarily in ventricular choroid plexuses by a combination of both, active process and ultracentrifugation. Concentrations of sodium, chloride, magnesium and glutamine are greater in CSF than in plasma, while concentrations of glucose, potassium, calcium, cholesterol, uric acid, iron, thyroxine and zinc are lower in CSF.

Normal Values for Lumbar CSF in Adults

Pressure	70-150 mm of water column (patient lying on side)
Volume	90-150 ml
Specific gravity	1.006-1.008
Total solids	0.85-1.70 gm%
Cells	0-8 lymphocytes/cu mm Neutrophils and erythrocytes absent
Protein	20-50 mg%
Of this	
albumin is	50-70%
α_1 globulin is	3-9%
α_2 globulin is	4-10%
β globulin is	10-18%
γ globulin is	3-9%
fibrinogen is	Absent
Sodium	144-154 mEq/L
Potassium	2.0-3.5 mEq/L
Chloride	118-132 mEq/L
pH	7.3-7.4
Creatinine	0.5-1.2 mg%

Cholesterol	0.2-0.6 mg%
Glucose	50-80 mg%
Glutamine	6-16 mg%
Iron	1-2 mg%
Thyroxine	0.1-0.2 mg%
Urea	6-16 mg%
Uric acid	0.5-4.5 mg%

Lumbar Puncture

Lumbar puncture needle is a long needle with a stylette inside. Lumbar puncture is usually performed at L_3-L_4 or lower to avoid damage to the spinal cord. In small children the conus medullaris extends lower than in adults, so puncture should be performed at L_4-L_5 or lower.

Indications

1. Detection and diagnosis of suspected meningitis, subarachnoid haemorrhage, encephalitis, central nervous system (CNS) syphilis, spinal cord tumour or multiple sclerosis.
2. Differential diagnosis of cerebral infarction *vs* intracerebral hemorrhage (almost 80% of latter show blood or xanthochromia).
3. Introduction of anaesthetics, radiographic contrast media or drugs.
4. Treatment of elevated CSF pressure in selected patients with benign intracranial hypertension.
5. Removal of exudate or blood from subarachnoid space.

The procedure should be done with a stylette inside to avoid implantation of skin which may form dermoid cyst in the spinal canal. A manometer and three-way stopcock should be attached to the needle, so that initial pressure can be accurately measured and CSF removed under control.

Complications of Lumbar Puncture

1. Production of cerebellar pressure cone in patients with increased intracranial pressure.
2. With spinal cord tumour, progression of paresis to paralysis may follow lumbar puncture.
3. Introduction of infection by:
   - passing the needle through superficial or deep sepsis in the lumbar region.
   - improperly sterilised equipment.
   - poor technique.
   - development of dermoid cyst if lumbar puncture is performed without the stylette.
   - postpuncture headache resulting from leakage of CSF (incidence can be decreased by using a small bore needle and keeping the patient horizontal for 24 hours).
4. In infants death due to asphyxiation caused by restraint or tracheal obstruction from pushing the head forward.

Elective lumbar puncture should be performed in the morning rather than late afternoon or evening.

CSF Rhinorrhoea and Otorrhoea

Fluid coming through ear or nose may be CSF. Confirmation can be done by inserting a glucose-oxidase strip into nose or ear for 5 minutes: a 2+ or 3+ reaction, indicates glucose present, is considered evidence of CSF rhinorrhoea or otorrhoea (30% false positives). Normal concentration of glucose in nasal secretions is 10 to 25 mg%. If the test is inconclusive, cotton may be placed in the nasopharynx and radioactive iodinated serum albumin (RISA) injected into the lumbar subarachnoid space, the cotton is left in place for 12 hours and then counted for gamma radiation.

CSF Pressure

If the opening pressure exceeds 180, reassure the patient and straighten the leg, back and neck and to make sure there is no breath holding or abdominal or jugular compression. If the pressure then falls to normal, it is probable that the initial elevation was artefactual. CSF pressure is directly related to pressure in the jugular and vertebral veins, which communicate with the intracranial dural sinuses and spinal dura. Hence, CSF pressure is decreased with circulatory collapse and increased with congestive heart failure, obstruction of the superior vena cava, straining, breath holding, or pressure against the abdomen (e.g. obese patients in lying position).

Pathologically increased pressure is usually due to:

- inflammation of the meninges
- a space-occupying lesion (SOL), such as a tumour, abscess, cerebral-oedema or intra-cerebral haemorrhage.

If the initial pressure exceeds 200 mm. CSF, not more than 1-2 ml of fluid should be removed, a 25 to 50% fall in pressure after removing 1-2 ml suggests cerebellar herniation or spinal cord compression above the puncture site. STOP removing CSF. Observe the patient for several hours. Usually, three 2 ml samples are taken in sterile tubes and labelled sequentially.

If initial pressure is normal and there is clinical suspicion of subarachnoid block, Queckenstedt's test may be done: Normally if both jugular veins are manually compressed, CSF pressure rapidly returns to normal when compression ceases. With sinus thrombosis, obstruction at the foramen magnum, or a mass lesion in the spinal canal, the rise of CSF pressure may be decreased/delayed—this is a positive Queckenstedt's test. In such cases, normal variations in pressure due to respiration will be diminished/absent but straining or abdominal compression should result in increased CSF pressure (due to vertebral vein congestion) if the needle is placed correctly.

Almost 80% of patients with cord compression have a positive Queckenstedt's test. Lesions responsible for cord compression include:

- herniated intervertebral disc
- vertebral fracture
- extradural abscess
- adhesions due to pachymeningitis
- neoplasms (primary or metastatic) involving vertebrae, meninges, or spinal cord.

CSF

Gross Examination

Normal CSF is crystal clear.

Evaluate colour by holding the CSF tube beside a distilled water tube against a clean white paper. If a pale yellow or pink colour is noted—centrifuge the sample at high speed for 5 minutes and examine the supernatant visually. Xanthochromia (pale pink to pale orange or yellow colour in supernatant) is usually graded from 1 to 4 and may be due to:

- CSF protein > 100 mg%.
- traumatic tap with lysis of erythrocytes due to detergent in needle or sample tube.
- bilirubinaemia (both conjugated bilirubin in adults and unconjugated bilirubin in neonates may pass the blood-CSF barrier.
- intracerebral or subarachnoid haemorrhage.
- contamination of CSF by iodine/merthiolate used to disinfect the skin.
- carotenaemia.
- melanin in CSF due to meningeal melanosarcoma.

Two to twelve hours after a subarachnoid haemorrhage, pale orange xanthochromia appears in CSF in 90% cases. Yellow xanthochromia due to conversion of haemoglobin to bilirubin within two to four days. The orange xanthochromia of oxyhaemoglobin usually disappears in four to eight days, while yellow xanthochromia due to bilirubin typically persists for 12-40 days. Gross blood due to subarachnoid haemorrhage may disappear within 24 hours, but generally persists for 7-14 days.

Turbidity in CSF may result from large numbers of leucocytes or bacteria and varies from slight opalescence typical in tuberculous meningitis to the grossly purulent appearance in some cases of pyogenic meningitis. Turbidity is usually graded from O (crystal clear) to 4+ (newsprint cannot be seen though the tube).

Clotting in CSF may be seen grossly in:

- traumatic tap
- markedly elevated CSF protein or
- moderately elevated CSF protein in association with tuberculous meningitis (cobweb coagulum).

Cell Counts

Diluting the Fluid

1. Draw Unna's polychrome methylene blue to the '1' mark in a RBC pipette and fill pipette to '101' mark with spinal fluid. This colours white cells blue and red cells yellow.
2. Turbid fluid: When many cells are present (as in turbid or purulent fluid), better counts are obtained with a WBC pipette and WBC diluting fluid.
3. Bloody fluid: When significant numbers of red cells are present in the fluid, the possiblity of traumatic bleeding should be considered. Fresh RBCs are intact with a smooth round margin. Older cells have crenated appearance.

Count

Count 9 large squares in the counting chamber for both RBCs and WBCs—the total multiplied by 1.1 gives the number of cells per cubic mm.

Differential count: Centrifuge the CSF and make smears from the sediment. Stain and count as for a blood smear.

Various types of cells in CSF

Large number of polymorphs → pyogenic meningitis due to:

- *Neisseria meningitidis*
- *Haemophilus influenzae*
- Pneumococci
- Streptococci
- Staphylococci
- Coliforms.
- Sometimes in viral meningitis or aseptic meningeal reaction.
- Rarely in intracerebral haematoma, fungal meningitis, RISA injection, or following lumbar puncture with detergent-contaminated needles.

Mixed reaction (*neutrophils, lymphocytes and monocytes*) *occurs in*:

- Subacute bacterial meningitis
- Tuberculous meningitis
- Mycotic meningitis
- Viral meningoencephalitis.

Monocytic and/or lymphocytic reaction is seen in:

- Viral meningoencephalitis
- Multiple sclerosis
- Tuberculous } meningitis
- Fungal } meningitis
- Syphilitic } meningitis

Blasts may be seen in leukaemic cell infiltrates in the meninges.

Abnormal malignant/benign cells in certain CNS neoplasms.

Globulin test: These are valueless if the spinal fluid is bloody.

1. *Pandy's test*: Place 1-2 ml of a saturated solution of phenol in a small test tube and add 1 drop of spinal fluid. Cloudiness against a black background indicates increased amounts of globulin. Report as O, +, ++, +++ or ++++.
2. *Ross Jones test*: Carefully layer 0.5 ml clear spinal fluid over 1 ml of saturated solution of ammonium sulphate. A thin white ring appearing at the juncture of the liquids, which disappears on mixing, indicates a 1+ reaction. Heavy cloudiness persisting after mixing is a 4+ reaction.

Total proteins (Quantitative method of Dennis and Ayer): Place 1.2 ml of clear spinal fluid, 0.8 ml of distilled water, and 2 ml of 5% sulphosalicylic acid in a small test tube and mix by inversion. Let stand for 5 minutes, then read in a colorimeter against a known standard protein suspension (make known suspension by mixing 2 ml of a standard protein solution with 2 ml of 5% sulphosalicylic acid). If the unknown is too heavy with protein, dilute and compare. Consider dilution factor in the calculation.

$$\frac{\text{Transmission standard}}{\text{Transmission unknown}} \times 50 = \text{mg of protein/100 ml of fluid}$$

CSF electrophoresis shows prodominantly albumin.

In adults, levels of 60-75 mg% are considered slightly increased, levels of 75 to 150 mg% moderately increased and beyond 150 mg% are markedly increased.

Increase in CSF protein may occur with any lesion causing injury to cerebral tissue or blood-brain barrier; viral, tuberculous, mycotic, syphilitic or bacterial meningoencephalitis, polyneuritis, intracerebral haemorrhage, degenerative disease, or aseptic meningeal reaction. Brain tumours cause variable increases, depending upon their location—gliomas deep in the pons or cerebrum may be associated with normal levels, while acoustic neuromas in tumours of the corpus callosum usually cause marked increase in CSF protein. Other causes include diabetic neuropathy, myxoedema, heavy metal intoxication, isopropanol intoxication, hypercalcaemia and diphenylhydantoin (Dilantin) intoxication. Multiple sclerosis causes minimal increase in CSF protein; whereas, cerebral thrombosis, subdural haematoma and aseptic and viral meningitis usually are associated with normal CSF protein.

Conditions that Elevate CSF Protein

Mild elevation, to 300 mg%:

Viral meningitis, neurosyphilis, subdural haematoma, cerebral thrombosis, brain tumour, multiple sclerosis (rarely > 100 mg%).

Electrophoretic evidence of IgG:

Multiple sclerosis, subacute sclerosing panencephalitis, neurosyphilis.

Moderate or pronounced elevation:
Acute bacterial meningitis, tuberculous meningitis, spinal cord tumour, cerebral haemorrhage, intracranial tumour, Guillain-Barré syndrome (ascending polyneuritis).

The term albuminocytologic dissocation refers to increased CSF protein with normal or near normal CSF cell count—classically seen in Guillain-Barré syndrome, but it may also occur in subarachnoid block, brain tumour, multiple sclerosis, cerebral thrombosis and various types of polyneuritis.

Froin's syndrome refers to CSF changes which may occur with subarachnoid block at or below the foramen magnum—markedly increased total protein (often > 500 mg%), xanthochromia (owing to increased protein) and spontaneous clotting.

Protein electrophoresis of CSF
Proteins larger than 9S (sedimentation coefficient) do not diffuse rapidly into the CSF, unless there is injury to the blood-CSF barrier.

Monoclonal increase can be shown in some myeloma cases. Multiple sclerosis causes increased IgG in CSF. Besides multiple sclerosis, diffuse or discrete pathologic gamma bands can be seen in:

- subacute sclerosing leucoencephalitis
- advanced neurosyphilis
- primary lateral sclerosis
- viral encephalitis
- fungal meningitis
- monoclonal gammopathy
- myelopathy due to vitamin B_{12} deficiency.

Lange's Colloidal Gold Test

Colloidal gold test
Though obsolete, it can be of great use if electrophoresis cannot be done. It is an empirical way of evaluating CSF protein fractions.

In the Lange's method, progressive dilutions of CSF are added to 10 test tubes containing colloidal gold solution (Fig. 12.1). Precipitation causes the brilliant red colloidal gold colour (0) to change to—

reddish blue	(1+)
purple	(2+)
deep blue	(3+)
pale blue	(4+)
colourless	(5+)

The highest CSF concentration is reported on the left with progressively decreasing concentrations to the right. Normal fluids cause either no reaction or slight precipitation in the middle dilutions, e.g. 0001210000.

A first zone curve is found in about 50% of patients with multiple sclerosis as well as in general

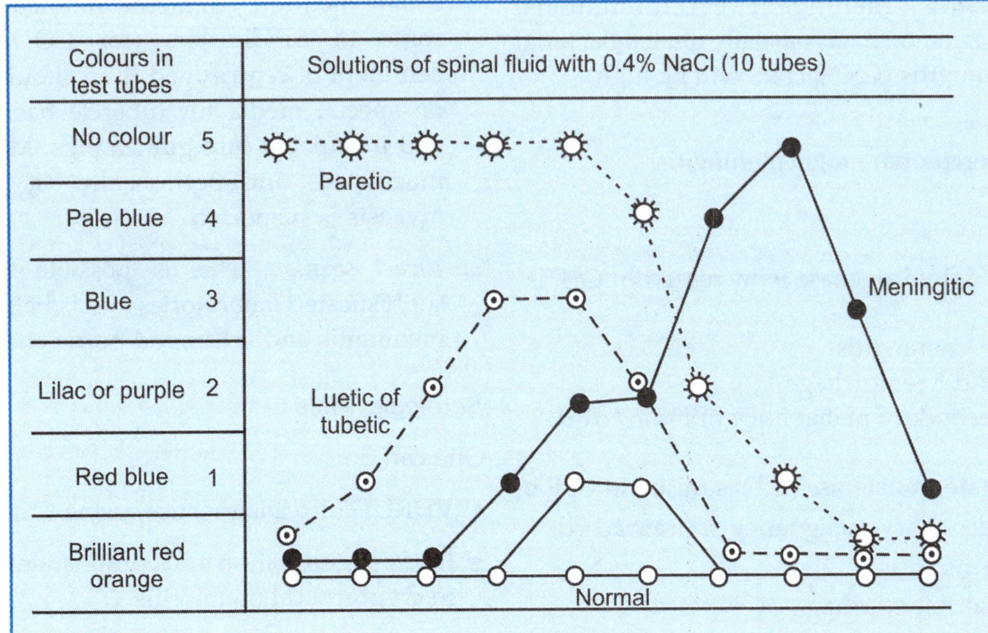

Fig. 12.1: Lange's colloidal Gold test

paresis of insane. It may also be seen in encephalitis, postinfections, encephalomyelopathy, sarcoidosis, haemorrhage, aseptic meningeal reaction, polyneuritis, and meningeal carcinoma. A typical series would be 5554210000 (Fig. 12.1).

A midzone curve or end zone curve is nonspecific and may be found in any CSF with high protein content.

Glucose

Normally, CSF glucose is about 60-80% of corresponding blood levels, or 50-80 mg%. Usually CSF glucose less than 40 mg% is considered decreased. Possible causes include:

- Systemic hypoglycaemia
- Bacterial / tuberculous / fungal meningitis
- Meningeal carcinomatosis / leukaemia infiltration
- Sarcoidosis involving CNS
- Subarachnoid haemorrhage
- Viral meningitis including mumps meningo-encephalitis.

Conditions that Effect the CSF Glucose

No significant change
Viral meningitis, neurosyphilis, brain or cord tumour, cerebral thrombosis, multiple sclerosis, polyneuritis.

Moderate reduction
CNS leukaemia, meningeal carcinomatosis, subarachnoid haemorrhage, partially treated bacterial or fungal meningitis (CSF lactate will be high).

Marked reduction
Bacterial / tuberculous / fungal meningitis.

Enzymes

LDH: Lactate dehydrogenase is increased in CSF in

- bacterial } meningitis
- viral } meningitis
- subarachnoid haemorrhage
- primary / secondary malignancy of brain / cord.

SGOT: Aspartate transferase (AT) is raised in CSF in

- primary / secondary malignancy of brain / cord
- bacterial meningitis
- intracerebral haemorrhage
- subarachnoid haemorrhage.

CPK: Raised CSF-CPK (creatine phosphokinase) is found in

- brain infarct
- multiple sclerosis
- brain tumours
- demyelinating disease and
- polyneuropathies.

Bacteriologic Examination

Smears and cultures for bacteria should be made of all fluids when indicated.

1. *Smears*: Make smears directly if fluid is very turbid, otherwise from sediment of centrifuged CSF. All smears should be stained with Gram's stain. If no characteristic bacteria are found, do an acid-fast stain and search for mycobacteria (AFB) stain should also be done if a pellicle forms on standing. An India ink preparation is required for *Cryptococcus*. Immunofluorescent stains can be used for *Haemophilus influenzae* and some other organisms.
2. *Cultures*: Cloudy fluid should be streaked on chocolate agar, Sabouraud's agar, and agar plates and inoculated into blood broth and thioglycollate medium. All media are incubated at 37°C, some in candle jars (for CO_2 atmosphere). Sediment of centrifuged fluid should be cultured on special media for tubercle bacilli and fungi and inoculated into guinea pigs. Mice should be inoculated intraperitoneally if coccidioidomycosis is suspected.
3. *Virus isolation*: This is possible only in very sophisticated laboratories and is helpful in aseptic meningitis and arthropod-borne encephalitis.

Serologic Tests

One can do:

- VDRL (Tulip Diagnostics) using CSF in syphilis.
- Latex agglutination and complement fixation tests in cryptococcal meningitis.

Table 12.1: CSF in differential diagnosis

Disease	*Initial pressure mm H_2O column*	*Appearance*	*Cells/cu mm*	*Protein mg%*	*Glucose mg%*	*Colloidal gold*	*Remarks*
Normal	70-150	crystal clear	0-8, lympho's	20-50	50-80	0000110000	In fasting afebrile individuals
Acute purulent meningitis	↑	Opalescent to purulent clot	500-20,000 mostly poly's	50-1000+	0-45	Variable	Organism in sediment or clot, culture positive
Tuberculous meningitis	↑	Opalescent fibrin web, pellicle	10-500 mostly lympho's	45-500+	0-45	Variable	Sugar and chloride values falling progressively
Early, acute syphilitic meningitis	↑	Clear to turbid, occasional clot	25-2000 mostly lympho's	45-400+	15-75	Ist / midzone curve	Often +ve serologic test in CSF & blood
Late CNS syphilis	↑	Normal	Normal or ↑	Normal or ↑	Normal	Depending on activity	Often +ve serologic test in CSF
Aseptic meningeal reaction (brain or extradural abscess, thrombosis, etc.)	Usually normal	Clear or turbid, often xanthochromic	↑	Normal or ↑	Normal	Variable	CSF culture negative
Acute poliomyelitis	Usually normal	Usually clear and colourless	↑	↑	45-100	Normal or midzone	
Viral encephalitis (arthropod borne)	Normal or ↑	Normal	0-100, mostly	Normal or increased	45-100	Variable	Proved by serologic tests
Viral meningoencephalitis	Normal or ↑	Normal	0-2000 + mostly lympho's	Normal or ↑	Normal	Variable	Proved by virus isolation and serologic tests
Postinfectious encephalitis	Usually ↑	Normal	Slightly ↑	Normal or increased	Increased	Variable	
Traumatic (bloody) tap	Normal	Bloody	Many fresh RBCs	↑	Normal	Normal	Most blood in Ist tube, least blood in last tube

Contd...

Contd...

Cerebral haemorrhage: ventricular, subarachnoid	Slightly ↑	Bloody, supernatant yellow	Many RBC's crenated or fresh	↑	Variable	Normal	Blood present in all specimens equally
Subdural haematoma	Usually ↑	Clear/yellow	Normal	Normal or ↑	Variable	Normal	
Brain tumour	Usually ↑	Clear/xan-thochromic	Normal or increased	Usually ↑	Normal or increased	Variable	If papilloedema is present lumbar puncture is contraindicated
Spinal cord tumour (Subarachnoid block)	Normal or low	Often xan-thochromic	Normal or ↑	Usually ↑	Normal or increased	Variable	Little fluid obtained
Multiple sclerosis	Low	Normal	Normal or increased	Normal or increased	Normal	Normal, Ist or midzone	50% cases have normal CSF
Uremia	Usually	Normal	Normal or ↑	Normal or ↑	Normal or ↑	Variable	CSF NPN is high
Diabetic coma	Low	Normal	Normal or ↑	Normal	Increased	Normal	May have spasticity, weakness, convulsions

SYNOVIAL FLUID (SF)

Normally, about 1 ml of SF is present in each large joint: knee, ankle, hip, elbow, wrist, and shoulder Table 12.3).

Clinical indications for aspiration include:

- Arthritis of unknown aetiology, manifested by effusion.
- Possible infectious arthritis, with or without effusion, to obtain material for culture.
- Effusions of known aetiology, to relieve pain or to allow mobility.

Aspiration must be done under absolute aseptic conditions. Since effusion often exists when aspiration is indicated, 10-20 ml of fluid may usually be obtained. The specimen is collected in 3 to 4 sterile tubes.

1. Plain tube for gross examination, evaluation of viscosity, and mucin clot test.
2. EDTA tube for cell counts and microscopic study.
3. A sterile, plain or preferably heparinised tube (precludes clot formation) for microbiologic study.
4. Appropriate tube(s) for serologic or chemical examinations: Plain tube for serologic tests or enzyme assays, heparinized tube for total protein, oxalate fluoride tube for glucose.

Viscosity: When normal fluid drips from a syringe, a tenacious 'string' at least 4 cm long forms with each drop. This provides an estimate of whether viscosity is normal, decreased (string less than 4 cm in length), or markedly decreased (string less than 1 cm in length).

Another method for evaluating viscosity is to see how far a drop of fluid can be stretched between the thumb and index finger before breaking: fluids with very low viscosity will behave like water. Decreased viscosity reflects decreased hyaluronate in the synovial fluid.

Mucin clot test (Ropes' Test): This is done by adding 1 ml of synovial fluid to 20 ml of 5% (v/v) acetic acid in a small breaker. Normally, a compact large clot will form, surrounded by clear solution, this is graded as 'good'. If a soft clot forms in a turbid solution, this is graded as fair. A friable clot with cloudy surrounding fluid is graded as 'poor' or 'fragile'. No clot formation, with flakes in a cloudy suspension, is graded as 'very poor'. Good

Table 12.2: Grades of syphilitic spinal fluid

Investigation	*Grade I*	*Grade II*	*Grade III*
Serology	—	±	++
Number of WBCs/cu mm	5-25	25-100	70-100
Protein increase	+	++	+++
Colloidal gold curve	0000000000	0023454310	5555554310

Table 12.3.

Synovial fluid		*SI Units*
Appearance	Clear or colourless to pale yellow	
Crystals	Absent	
Glucose		
Transudate	≤ 10 mg/dl lower than blood glucose (whole blood adult norm 60-89 mg/dl, child norm 51-85 mg/dl)	
Edxudate	Lower than whole blood levels	
Lactate dehydrogenase		
Transudate	≤ Client's serum LD (serum adult norm 45-90 U/L, child norm 60-170 U/L)	
Exudate	> Client's serum LD	
pH	7.4	
Specific gravity		
Transudate	< 1.016	< 1.016
Exudate	> 1.016	> 1.016
Total protein		
Transudate	1-3 g/dl	10-30 g/L
Exudate	> 3 g/dl	> 30 g/L
Volume	< 4 ml	
Viscosity	High	
White blood cells		
Transudate	< 100/mm^3	< 100 × 10^9/L
Exudate	> 1000/mm^3	> 1000 × 10^9/L

clots do not break up when agitated, while poor clots break up into small shreds. This procedure actually is an estimate of synovial hyaluronate and not mucin, which is absent in joint fluid.

Microscopic Examination

Total and differential counts as for CSF. But the usual leucocyte diluent with 1% glacial acetic acid precipitates synovial fluid hyaluronate and is unsatisfactory, instead methylene blue in saline can be used. If the fluid is very turbid, use saline dilution or digestion with hyaluronidase (2 ml SF incubated with 150 IU hyaluronidase for 1 hr at 37°C) may be helpful. Differential count can be done from EDTA sample (sediment) that has been centrifuged, a film made and stained as for peripheral blood.

LE cells are frequently seen in stained SF from patients with systemic lupus erythematosus (SLE). Sometimes, they can be seen in cases of rheumatoid arthritis. Large phagocytes containing neutrophils may be found in SF and are called 'Reiter cells', they are nonspecific and may be present in effusions of varying aetiology. RA cells or 'Ragocytes' are neutrophils containing 0.5 to 1.5 inclusions better seen with phase contrast microscopy. They are seen in 94% cases of rheumatoid joint fluids but are non-specific for they can also be found in septic arthritis, gout, etc.

Both wet preparation (a drop of SF put on a slide and coverslipped) and stained films should be studied for crystals, using polarised light to detect monosodium urate (MSU) or calcium pyrophosphate dihydrate (CPPD). MSU crystals appear birefringent and needle or rod shaped; while CPPD crystals will appear birefringent and rhomboid or rod shaped. MSU crystals are found in acute/chronic gout joints. CPPD crystals are found in pseudogout or chondrocalcinosis.

Immunologic Studies

Sero-negative rheumatoid arthritis may have a positive joint fluid, but this is not very specific. Decreased synovial fluid complement (under 30% of serum level) occurs in rheumatoid arthritis and SLE (Table 12.4).

PLEURAL FLUID

The pleural surfaces are normally moistened by 1 to 10 ml of fluid derived by ultrafiltration of plasma.

Normal protein concentration of this fluid is 1-2 gm% with no fibrinogen.

Pleural Fluid		SI Units	
Appearance	Clear, slightly amber		
Cholesterol			
Transudate	< 60 mg/dl	< 1. 55 mmol/L	
Exsudate	> 60 mg/dl	> 1. 55 mmol/L	Glucose
Transudate	Approximates whole blood levels (whole blood adult norm 60-89 mg/dl, child norm 51-85 mg/dl)		
Exudate	Lower than whole blood levels		
Lactate dehydrogenase			
Transudate	< Client's serum LD (serum adult norm 45-90 U/L, child norm 60-170 U/L)		
Exudate	> Client's serum LD		
pH	7.4		
Specific gravity			
Transudate	< 1.016	< 1.016	
Exudate	> 1.016	> 1.016	
Total protein			
Transudate	< 2.5 g/dl	<25 g/L	
Exudate	> 3 g/dl	> 30 g/L	
Volume	< 25 ml		
White blood cells			
Transudate	< 100/mm^3	< 100 ×	010^9/L
Exudate	> 1000/mm^3	> 1000 × 10^9/L	

Abnormal pleural fluid accumulation, or pleural effusion may be caused by

1. Increased capillary permeability due to inflammation; this typically is associated with increased pleural fluid protein (over 3 gm%).
2. Decreased plasma colloid osmotic pressure due to hypoproteinaemia, this typically is associated with pleural fluid protein, about 1 gm%.
3. Increased hydrostatic pressure due to increased systemic and/or pulmonary venous pressure, as in congestive heart failure. Pleural fluid protein concentration is variable in these cases.
4. Decreased lymphatic drainage due to tumour, inflammation, or fibrosis involving mediastinal lymph nodes (also systemic venous hypertension). This typically is associated with increased pleural fluid protein (over 3 gm%).

Indications for Thoracentesis

1. Effusion of unknown aetiology.
2. Effusion of known aetiology causing symptoms.
3. Intrapleural instillation of drugs for treatment of infection or malignancy.
4. Haemothorax or empyema (to prevent organization).

Complications of thoracentesis may include:

1. Haemopneumothorax due to lung laceration.
2. Mediastinal shift or pulmonary oedema (if large amounts are aspirated at one time).

Do not remove more than 1 litre of fluid at one time. Collect pleural fluid in three sterile anticoagulated EDTA tubes labelled sequentially: Ist tube for culture and Gram's stain, the rest for cell counts, differential counts, total protein, glucose, cytology, etc. If malignancy or tuberculosis is suspected, several hundred ml of anticoagulated fluid should be given for examination.

Gross Examination

Haemorrhagic fluids can be distinguished from traumatic tap by noting the colour of aspirate in the successive tubes filled with fluid. In traumatic tap the later tubes become clearer.

Haemorrhagic pleural fluid can be found in

- intrapleural malignancy (60% cases)
- pancreatitis
- pulmonary infarction
- pleural infection
- closed chest trauma
- tuberculosis
- postmyocardial infarction syndrome
- congestive heart failure occasionally
- hepatic cirrhosis.

Haemothorax can be distinguished from hemorrhagic effusion. Similar PCV of fluid and blood implies haemothorax. Cloudy, turbid fluid is usually due to large numbers of leucocytes associated with septic/nonseptic inflammation.

Milky fluid: Pseudochylous effusion may occur in:

- tuberculosis
- rheumatoid arthritis, etc.

True chylothorax is rare, occurs due to leakage of thoracic duct contents, is creamy fluid with consistency of milk, which clears and decreases in volume with alkalinisation and ether extraction.

Pleural fluid should be *observed for clotting* in plain tube or after adding $CaCl_2$ to EDTA fluid tube. Presence of fibrinogen suggests damage to capillary walls caused by inflammation or neoplasm.

Table 12.4: Synovianalysis in arthritis

	Appearance	*Viscosity*	*White Cells*	*Mucin clot*	*Protein (Avg-gm%) Total*	*Globulin*	*Remarks*
Normal	Straw-coloured, clear, cloudy	High	200-600/25% poly's	Good	1.36	0.05	
Traumatic	Yellow to bloody	High	± 2000/30% poly's	Good	4.27		
Osteoarthritis	Yellow, clear	High	± 1000/20% poly's	Good	3.08	0.75	Cartilage fibrils
Rheumatic	Yellow, slightly cloudy	Low	± 10,000/50% poly's	Good	3.74	1.07	
Systemic lupus erythematosus	Straw-coloured, slightly cloudy	High	± 5000/10% poly's	Good			
Gout	Yellow to milky cloudy	Low	± 12,000/60% poly's	Fragile	4.18	1.54	Urate crystals
Tuberculous arthritis	Yellow, cloudy	Low	± 25,000 50-60% poly's	Fragile	5.3	2.0	Tubercle bacilli
Septic arthritis	Greyish or bloody, turbid	Low	± 80,000/90% poly's	Fragile	5.64	2.45	Bacteria
Rheumatoid arthritis	Yellow to greenish, cloudy	Low	± 15,000 65% ± poly's	Fragile	4.74	1.79	Rheumatoid factor

Microscopic Examination

This should be done as has been told in CSF examination (TLC and DLC). A WBC count over 1000/cu mm or over 50% of neutrophils, suggests inflammation (septic or non-septic). A high percentage of lymphocytes (> 50%) suggests tuberculosis, lymphoma or carcinoma.

Sometimes lymphocytic effusion may be seen in:
- cardiopulmonary disease
- cirrhosis
- SLE
- infectious mononucleosis
- subacute bacterial pulmonary infection.

RA cells may sometimes be seen in rheumatoid pleural effusions. *LE cells* may be seen in *SLE.*

Eosinophilic pleural effusions may be seen in:
- convalescent pneumonia
- pneumothorax
- pulmonary infarction
- hypersensitivity diseases
- asthma
- Loeffler's syndrome
- periarteritis
- parasitic diseases.

Immature blood cells may be seen in
- chronic myeloid leukaemia
- myeloid metaplasia (extramedullary haemopoiesis).

Chemical Examination

Pleural effusions are classified as transudates or exudates with the former having protein content less than 3 gm% and the latter more than 3 gm%.

Normal pleural fluid glucose is about equal to whole blood glucose. Blood glucose changes are reflected in pleural fluid after a lag period of 1 to 3 hours. A pleural fluid glucose concentration 30-40 mg% less than whole blood suggests bacterial infection (including tuberculosis), nonseptic inflammation (especially rheumatoid pleuritis), or malignancy. In contrast to rheumatoid disease, the effusions due to SLE typically have normal glucose concentrations.

Microbiologic Examination

All effusions should be examined for bacteria by Gram's stain and culture. The possibility of tuberculosis should always be considered with idiopathic pleural effusions.

PERICARDIAL FLUID (PF)

The pericardial sac under normal circumstances contains 20-50 ml of clear, straw-coloured fluid. A rapid abnormal accumulation of 200 ml may produce cardiac tamponade, while gradual accumulation of 1000 ml or more may be relatively asymptomatic.

Normal

Pericardial fluid		*SI Units*
Apperance	Clear to pale yellow	
Glucose		
Transudate	Approximate whole blood levels (Whole blood adult norm 60-80 mg/dl, Whole blood child norm 51-85 mg/dl)	
Exudate	Lower than whole blood levels	
Lactate dehydrogenase		
Transudate	≤ Client's serum LD (serum adult norm 45-90 U/L, serum child norm 60-170 U/L)	

Indications for Pericardial Fluid Aspiration

1. Acute or chronic cardiac tamponade
2. To confirm diagnosis and establish cause for pericardial effusion of unknown aetiology.

Complications of the (blind) pericardial fluid aspiration:

1. Cardiac arrhythmias, especially ventricular fibrillation.
2. Infection of pleural spaces by purulent pericardial fluid.
3. Laceration of an atrium or coronary artery.
4. Pneumothorax.
5. Inadvertent injection of air into the cardiac chamber.

Pericardial fluid aspiration: This should be in 3 sterile tubes at least—EDTA tube for gross and microscopic examination, plain or heparinised tube for microbiologic examination, and heparinised tube for chemical examination. Aspiration should be done under CT scan guidance.

Gross Examination

Gross appearance of PF may be clear, cloudy, blood-tinged, grossly bloody, milky (chylous or pseudochylous) or similar to gold paint.

Increased amounts of normal-appearing pericardial fluid may be found in:

- congestive heart failure
- early stages of inflammation
- some patients with idiopathic (viral) pericarditis.

Cloudy appearance may be associated with:

- septic/nonseptic inflammation (bacterial, rheumatoid or rheumatic)
- chronic effusions of any aetiology
- myoxoedema
- idiopathic
- postmyocardial infarction syndrome.

Blood-tinged pericardial fluid is seen in:

- traumatic tap, but it clears on aspirating more fluid.

Grossly bloody fluid may be caused by:

- idiopathic haemorrhagic pericarditis (? viral)
- postmyocardial infarction syndrome
- postpericardiectomy syndrome
- tuberculosis
- rheumatoid arthritis
- systemic lupus erythematosus
- metastatic carcinoma
- bacterial pericarditis
- leaking aortic syndrome → (haemopericardium→ acute cardiac tamponade (haemopericardium has a PCV similar to that of peripheral blood).

Milky pericardial fluid (unusual) may be due to:

- true chylopericardium
- chronic pericarditis from any cause, e.g.
  - bacterial
  - fungal
  - tuberculous
  - rheumatoid pericarditis
  - rheumatic
  - myoxoedema

Microscopic Examination

Total and differential counts done as for CSF. Increased leucocytes with preponderance of neutrophils are characteristic of bacterial pericarditis but may also be seen in viral pericarditis or chronic postmyocardial infarction syndrome. A high percentage of lymphocytes suggests tuberculous pericarditis.

Microbiologic Examination

Cultures for bacteria, fungi, and tuberculosis should be performed in all effusions of unknown aetiology.

Chemical Examination

Pericardial fluids should be classified as transudates or exudates.

Transudates are typically seen in

- congestive heart failure
- hypoproteinemic states
- myoxoedema
- viral pericarditis
- early septic/nonseptic inflammation

PERITONEAL FLUID

Normally, the peritoneal cavity contains less than 100 ml of clear, straw-coloured fluid.

Peritoneal fluid		*SI Units*
Appearance	Clear or pale yellow	
Albumin	Negative	
Alkaline phosphatase		
Adult female	76-250 U/L	
Adult male	90-239 U/L	
Ammonia	< 50 g/L	
Cholesterol		
Transudate	< 46 mg/dl	< 1.19 mmol/L
Exudate	> 46 mg/dl	> 1.19 mmol/L
Glucose	60-100 mg/dl	3.3-6.1 mmol/L
Transudate	Lower than whole blood levels (Whole blood adult norm 60-89 mg/dl, child norm 51-85 mg/dl)	
Lactic acid	10-20 mg/dl	1.1-2.3 mmol/L
Lactate dehydrogenase		
Transudate	≤ Client's serum LD (serum adult norm 45-90 U/L, child norm 60-170 U/L)	
Exudate	> Client's serum LD	
pH	7.4	7.4
Specific gravity		
Transudate	< 1.016	< 1.016
Exudate	> 1.016	> 1.016
Total protein		
Transudate	< 2.5 g/dl	< 25 g/L
Exudate	> 3 g/dl	> 30 g/L
Volume	< 100 ml	
White blood cells		
Transudate	< 100/mm^3	< 100 × 10^9/L
Exudate	> 1000/mm^3	> 1000 × 10^9/L

Indications for abdominal paracentesis

To be done under ultrasound guidance.

1. Ascites of unknown aetiology.
2. Symptomatic ascites, e.g. dyspnoea.
3. Possible ruptured viscus or intra-abdominal haemorrhage due to trauma.
4. Acute abdominal pain of unknown aetiology.
5. Postoperative hypotension and pain of unknown aetiology.
6. Instillation of cytotoxic drugs in ascites due to malignancy.

(The chief complication of abdominal paracentesis is intestinal perforation, perforation of other viscera is rare. If aspiration reveals gross blood or intestinal contents—laparotomy must be done).

Gross Examination

Colour of Peritoneal Fluid

Pale yellow to amber in:

- congestive heart failure
- hepatic vein obstruction
- cirrhosis
- nephrotic syndrome.

Similar appearance in:

- ruptured urinary bladder

Turbid fluid suggests peritonitis due to:

- appendicitis
- pancreatitis
- strangulated/infarcted intestine
- torn/ruptured bowel due to trauma/primary bacterial infection.

Blood-tinged or grossly bloody fluid may be seen in:

- ruptured spleen
- ruptured liver

- torn mesenteric vessels (trauma)
- aortic aneurysm rupture
- splenic artery, leaking aneurysm
- hepatic vessel rupture
- haemorrhagic pancreatitis
- peritoneal laceration following muscular effort
- traumatic tap—clears as more fluid is aspirated.

Greenish in:
- perforated duodenal ulcer
- perforated intestine
- cholecystitis
- perforated gallbladder
- acute appendicitis
- (biliary peritonitis is usually rapidly fatal).

Milky fluid is due to chylous ascites, various causes are:
- lymphoma
- carcinoma
- tuberculosis
- parasitic infestations
- adhesions
- hepatic cirrhosis
- nephrotic syndrome.

(If surgical treatment is not indicated, elimination of dietary long-chain fatty acids will decrease accumulation of chylous fluid in abdomen, pericardium or pleural cavity).

Microscopic Examination

In peritoneal fluid TLC > 500/cu mm or RBC count > 100,000/cu mm are considered abnormal. Increased TLC, chiefly neutrophils, typically occur with acute peritonitis from any cause and may be the only evidence of intestinal rupture due to blunt trauma. A high incidence of lymphocytes should suggest the possibility of tuberculous peritonitis, but may also be found with chylous ascites.

Cytology examination with Papanicolaou stained films should be done. Sometimes, differentiation between reactive shed mesothelial cells and true neoplastic cells may be difficult.

Microbiologic Examination

Gram's stain and AFB stain should be done as usual. Cultures should also be done to know the actual pathogenic organism and its sensitivity.

Chemical Examination

Ascitic transudate is seen in:
- congestive heart failure
- constrictive pericarditis
- hepatic vein obstruction
- cirrhosis
- nephrotic syndrome.

An acid pH of the peritoneal fluid should suggest perforated peptic ulcer.

With pancreatitis the fluid amylase level is raised.

Elevated ammonia levels in peritoneal fluid above 3 gm/ml are NOT found in pancreatitis and suggest intestinal necrosis, perforation, or urinary extravasation.

Jejunal and ileal fluids have very high alkaline phosphatase (100-10,000 times serum level).

Ascitic fluid LDH is raised in:
- malignancy of peritoneum
- haemorrhagic peritoneal fluid of any aetiology.

Differential diagnosis of peritoneal transudate Vs. aspirated urine: Simultaneous measurements of creatinine and urea nitrogen on blood and peritoneal fluid are helpful. High levels of peritoneal fluid urea and creatinine with normal serum levels suggest inadvertent aspiration from the urinary bladder. High levels of peritoneal fluid urea and creatinine with elevated urea but normal creatinine in peripheral blood suggest rupture of the urinary bladder, since urea diffuses more rapidly than creatinine across the peritoneal surface.

AMNIOCENTESIS AND AMNIOTIC FLUID ANALYSIS, DIAGNOSTIC

Normal Value

Routine Analysis

Colour: Colourless, straw-coloured, or clear to milky.

		SI Unit
Acetylcholinesterase	Negative	
Alpha$_1$-Fetoprotein		
12 weeks' gestation	≤42 μg/ml	
14 weeks' gestation	≤35 μg/ml	
16 weeks' gestation	≤29 μg/ml	
18 weeks' gestation	≤20 μg/ml	
20 weeks' gestation	≤18 μg/ml	
22 weeks' gestation	≤14 μg/ml	
30 weeks' gestation	≤3 μg/ml	
35 weeks' gestation	≤2 μg/ml	
40 weeks' gestation	≤1 μg/ml	

Contd...

Contd...

Normal values may also be reported in multiples of the median (MOM) or 0.5-3.0 MOM.

Bilirubin		
Trimester 1, 2	≤ 0.074 mg/dl	≤ 1.2 μmol/L
40 wks' gestation	≤ 0.024 mg/dl	<0.4 μmol/L
Calcium	4 mEq/L	4 mmol/L
Carbon dioxide	16 mEq/l,	16 mmol/L
Chloride	102 mEq/L	102 mmol/L
Creatinine		
≤ 27 weeks' gestation	0.8-1.1 mg/dl	72-99 μmol/L
30-34 weeks' gestation	1.1-1.8 mg/dl	99-162 μmol/L
35-40 weeks' gestation	1.8-4.0 mg/dl	162-360 μmol/L
Oestriol		
Trimester 1, 2	≤ 9 ug/dl	<309 μmol/L
Term	≤59 ng/dl	<2023 μmol/L
Glucose	30 mg/dl	2 mmol/L
Lecithin		
≤35 weeks' gestation	6-9 mg/dl	
≥ 35 weeks' gestation	15-20 mg/dl	
Lecithin/sphingomyelin (L/S) Ratio		
Immaturity	≤ 1.5	
Borderline maturity	1.5-1.5	
Maturity	2.0-4.0	
Postmaturity	≥4.1	
Meconium	Negative	
pH		
Trimester 1, 2	7.12-7.38	7.12-7.38
Term	6.91-7.43	6.91-7.43
Potassium	4.9 mEq/L	4.9 mmol/L
Sodium	133 mEq/L	133 mmol/L
Sphingomyelin	4-6 mg/dl	
Total protein	2.5 g/dl	25 g/L
Urea		
Trimester 1, 2	12-24 mg/dl	
Term	19-42 mg/dl	
Uric acid		
Trimester 1, 2	2.76-4.68 mg/dl	0.17-2.8 mmol/L
Term	7.67-12.13 mg/dl	0.46-0.72 mmol/L

Abnormalities that may be found upon Routine Analysis

Abnormal Colour	*Possible Cause*
Yellow	Due to foetal bilirubin, erythroblastosis foetalis
Green	Due to meconium, breech presentation, foetal death, defaecation, distress, hypoxia, intrauterine growth retardation, postmaturity, vagal stimulation
Red	Due to presence of blood, intrauterine haemorrhage
Port wine	Acute foetal distress, abruptio placentae
Brown	Oxidised haemoglobin, maternal tissue trauma, foetal death, foetal maceration

Abnormal Bilirubin			*SI Units*
Foetal involvement	0.10-0.28 mg/dl	= 1+	1.6-4.5 μmol/L
Later foetal involvement	0.29-0.36 mg/dl	= 2+	4.7-5.8 μmol/L
Foetal distress	0.47-0.95 mg/dl	= 3+	7.6-15.4 μmol/L
Foetal death	>0.95 mg/dl	= 4+	> 15.4 μmol/L

Abnormal Creatinine		
35-40 weeks' gestation: Large muscle mass, possible diabetes	> 2 mg/dl	> 180 μmol/L
Low birthweight	<2 mg/dl	< 180 μmol/L

Increased alpha$_1$-fetoprotein: Anencephaly, cystic fibrosis, duodenal atresia, oesophageal atresia, foetal bladder *neck* obstruction with hydronephrosis, foetal death, meningomyelocele, multiple pregnancy, nephrosis (congenital), neural tube defects, spina bifida, omphalocele, and Turner's syndrome.

Increased bilirubin: Anencephaly, erythroblastosis foetalis, haemolytic disease of the newborn, hydrops foetalis, intestinal obstruction, and Rh sensitisation.

Positive acetylcholinesterase: Neural tube abnormalities that allow cerebrospinal fluid (which contains acetycholinesterase) to leak into the amniotic sac.

Positive meconium: Foetal distress.

Decreased alpha$_1$-fetoprotein: Not applicable.

Decreased bilirubin: Not clinically significant,

Decreased creatinine: Foetal lung immaturity.

Chromosome analysis: Interpretation required.

Description

Detection of foetal jeopardy or genetic disease and determination of foetal maturity. *Amniocentesis* is a 20-30 minute procedure in which an aspiration of amniotic fluid is taken transabdominally and usually performed after week 12 of gestation. In routine analysis, amniotic fluid is examined for levels of calcium, chloride, carbon dioxide, creatinine, oestriol, glucose, pH, potassium, sodium, protein, urea, uric acid, culture, and or genetic defects, chromosomal studies, detection of foetal jeopardy or distress (via colour, bilirubin) and to measure lung maturity (via L/S ratio) and age (via creatinine) of the foetus. *Alpha$_1$-alpha-fetoprotein* is a globulin protein secreted by the yolk sac and by foetal liver cells during hepatic cell multiplication. Highest amounts are found during pregnancy and in hepatic cancer, Measurement is usually performed from week 16 to 20 to help identify foetal neural abnormalities, gastroesophageal atresia, and nephrosis. *Chromosome analysis* of amniotic fluid cells is performed by examining karyotyped cells for genetic abnormalities such as Down syndrome, Tay-Sachs disease, and other inborn errors of metabolism. Aminiotic fluid is examined for colour and bilirubin level for purposes of detecting foetal jeopardy or distress due to hemolysis of foetal red blood cells. Erythroblastosis foetalis occurs when maternal antibodies attack foetal RBCs, causing foetal anaemia. This occurs when the mother's blood contains the Rh factor that reacts with foetal erythrocyte antigens. The test is usually performed at gestation week 24 or later and can help determine the need for intrauterine foetal blood transfusion.

Risks

Bleeding, intrauterine death, premature labour, spontaneous abortion.

Contraindications

Abruptio placentae, incompetent cervix, placenta previa, and a history of premature labour.

Preparation

1. Obtain an aminocentesis tray, surgical scrub solution, a light-protected container, and providone-iodine solution. Also, obtain RhoGAM for Rh-negative mothers.
2. Obtain maternal vital signs. Auscultate baseline foetal heart tones.
3. Note the estimated date of conception and week of gestation on the laboratory requisition.
4. Procedure should be performed in a darkened room if the specimen will be tested for bilirubin.
5. *See patient and family teaching.*

Procedure

1. The position of the foetus and a pocket of amniotic fluid are determined using ultrasound and palpation, with the mother in a supine position.
2. The mother's abdominal area is cleansed with surgical scrub solution and povidone-iodine and allowed to dry.
3. The aspiration site is draped, demarcating a sterile field.
4. The mother is instructed to place her hands behind her head, and the aspiration site is anaesthetised with 1 ml of 1 or 2 % lidocaine intradermally and subcutaneously.
5. A 20 to 22-gauge, 5-inch-long spinal needle with a stylete is inserted through the abdominal wall into the intrauterine cavity, and the stylete is withdrawn.
6. About 10-15 ml of amniotic fluid is aspirated through the spinal needle into a syringe, and the needle is withdrawn. Use a 20-ml amniotic fluid sample for direct genetic analysis for the four most common mutations responsible for Tay-Sachs disease.

Postprocedure Care

1. Apply a dry sterile dressing to the aspiration site.
2. Inject 5 ml of amniotic fluid into a light-protected (foil-covered or amber) test tube to test for bilirubin. Inject 10 ml of amniotic fluid into a sterile, siliconised glass container or a polystyrene container for culture and genetic and other studies (AFP). Specimens to be transported to another site for testing should be packed in a cool, insulated container to maintain a temperature of 2-5°C. Freezing temperatures should be avoided.
3. Obtain the mother's vital signs. Auscultate foetal heart tones for changes from the baseline.
4. The mother should rest on her right side for 15-20 minutes after the procedure.
5. RhoGAM may be prescribed for Rh-negative mothers.
6. Transport the amniotic fluid specimen to the laboratory immediately and refrigerate.

Patient and Family Teaching

1. Empty your bladder immediately prior to the procedure if gestation is 21 weeks or more. You must have a full bladder during the procedure if gestations is 20 weeks or less.
2. It is important to lie motionless throughout the procedure. You may experience a strong contraction with the needle insertion.
3. Chromosome analysis results may take up to 4 weeks.

4. Inform the patient with abnormal genetic findings of choices regarding pregnancy and pregnancy termination. Also, refer the patient for genetic counselling prior to future attempts to become pregnant.
5. After the procedure, notify the physician for cramping, abdominal pain, unusual vaginal drainage/fluid loss, fever, chills, dizziness, or more or less than the usual amount of foetal activity.

Factors that Affect Results

1. Reject frozen or clotted specimens.
2. Inadvertent aspiration of maternal urine can be ruled out by testing the specimen for blood urea nitrogen (BUN) and creatinine. Urine BUN is >100 mg/dl, whereas amniotic fluid is well under 100 mg/dl. Urine creatinine is usually 0.80 mg/dl, whereas amniotic fluid creatinine is usually ≤4 mg/dl.
3. Nonsiliconised glass containers for routine analysis may result in cell adherence on the sides of the container.
4. Amniotic fluid testing must be performed within 3 days of collection.
5. Amniocentesis should be performed between weeks 24 and 28 when checking for haemolytic disease of the newborn and Rh sensitisation.
6. Falsely low bilirubin levels may result from failure to protect the specimen from light.
7. Specimens contaminated with blood should be tested for foetal haemoglobin to determine whether the blood is of maternal or foetal origin. Foetal blood contamination results in falsely high bilirubin levels. Foetal or maternal blood will interfere with measurements of foetal lung maturity and amniotic fluid constituents that are also constituents of plasma, such as protein, potassium, and glucose.
8. Creatinine levels are affected by maternal creatinine clearance and maternal creatinine levels. A concurrent maternal serum creatinine should be drawn. Maternal serum to amniotic fluid creatinine should be about 2:1.
9. Elevated AFP results may be caused by contamination of the specimen with foetal blood.
10. Small and closed neural tube defects may not cause elevated AFP levels.
11. Accurate L/S ratio measurement is not possible if the specimen is contaminated with blood (foetal or maternal) or meconium.

Other Data

1. Direct karyotyping of placental villi samples obtained by needle aspiration has been found to yield faster results than amniotic fluid chromosome analysis.
2. Chromosomal aberration has been found in 4.6% of foetuses in women over 38 years old, the most common being trisomy 21 (62%), Klinefelter's syndrome (11%), and Edward's syndrome {(trisomy 18) (11%)}.
3. For diamniotic twin pregnancies, each amniotic sac should be sampled.
4. A 1995 study suggested that early amniocentesis is feasible from 11 weeks of gestation and "can be performed for the usual indications" as an alternative to chorionic villus sampling. In the future, results will be available in less than 1 week using cytogenetic techniques.
5. Prenatal cystic fibrosis profile may be performed by polymerase chain reaction.

CHAPTER 13

Semen Analysis

SEMEN ANALYSIS

Semen examination is an integral part of the evaluation of infertility. As a result of its relative simplicity, semen examination is often requested before the more complicated and expensive examination of the female. Repeat examination should be done if once it is found to be of normal.

Semen consists of spermatozoa suspended in seminal plasma. Spermatozoa comprise about 5% of semen volume (derived from testis). Approximately 60% of the semen volume is derived from the seminal vesicles. This viscid, neutral, or slightly alkaline fluid is often yellow or even deeply pigmented because of its high flavin content. Prostate contributes 20% of the volume of semen. This milky fluid is slightly acidic, with a pH of about 6.5 largely because of its high content of citric acid. The prostatic secretion is also rich in proteolytic enzymes and acid phosphatase. These proteolytic enzymes are believed to be responsible for the coagulation and liquefaction of semen. Less than 10-15% of semen volume is contributed by epididymidis, vasa deferentia, bulbourethral and urethral glands.

Collection

A 3 days period of abstinence is recommended before collecting the semen sample. Prolonged abstinence from intercourse should be avoided. The most satisfactory specimen is that collected in the laboratory by masturbation. If specimen will be delivered in a condom, the condom should first be cleaned and washed thoroughly, dried and then used. During transportation of the specimen, it should not be exposed to extremes of temperature and in no case the delay after collection till submission to the laboratory be more than 2 hours.

Gross Examination

Physical Characteristics

Freshly ejaculated semen is a highly viscid, opaque, white or grey-white coagulum which may have a distinct musty or acrid odour. After 10 to 20 minutes, the coagulum will spontaneously liquefy to form a translucent, turbid, viscous fluid which is mildly alkaline, with a pH of about 7.7. The pH may be slightly acidic in congenital aplasia of the vasa deferentia and seminal vesicles. Increased or decreased turbidity is not of much significance, except when increased turbidity is because of leucocytes associated with an inflammatory process in some parts of the reproductive tract.

All the parameters mentioned above should be checked for in every specimen received. Also important is the volume of the ejaculate.

Viscosity: Can be assessed by pouring semen, if it falls drop by drop, its viscosity is normal. Increased viscosity is important if it compromises the sperm motility.

Liquefaction: of the specimen should be complete within 30 minutes. It is important to distinguish persistent viscosity from delayed liquefaction.

Volume: The normal semen volume averages 3.5 ml, with a usual range of 1.5 to 5.0 ml. Paradoxically increased semen volume is more often (causes reduced sperm count) associated with infertility. Less volume may result in poor penetration of the cervical mucus. Semen volume does not vary significantly with the period of abstinence.

Microscopic Examination

Sperm Counts

Diluting fluid consists of:

Sodium bicarbonate 5 gm
Formalin neutral 1 ml
Distilled water 100 ml.

Counting can be done with WBC pipette. Following liquefaction draw semen till '0.5' mark, dilute with the diluting fluid till 11 mark. Mix properly. Charge the chamber, let stand for 2 minutes (sperms settle down). The spermatozoa in 4 sq mm (four large squares) are counted. Multiply this number by 50,000 to get the number of sperms per millilitre of semen. When seminal viscosity is markedly increased, a mucolytic agent prior to pipette dilution can be added in equal volume (1:1 dilution) and then the final count be multiplied by 2. Normal sperm count range is 60 to 150 million/ml with an average of 100 million/ml. Counts of less than 20 million/ml are considered distinctly abnormal.

Motility: Active motility is a must for normal spermatozoa as they have to migrate from cervix to the fallopian tubes where fertilisation of the ovum occurs. A drop of liquefied semen should be kept on a prewarmed slide and coverslipped. The coverslip should be ringed by petrolatum. Count at least 200 spermatozoa, the whole depth of the fluid should be screened and the nonmotile sperms settled at the bottom be included also to assess motility. The percentage of sperms showing actual progressive motion should be recorded. Normal semen contains more than 70% motile sperms. Semen should be considered abnormal if fewer than 60% of spermatozoa show progressive motion in specimens examined within 3 hours of collection.

Sperm Morphology (Fig. 13.1)

This is assessed by performing differential count of morphologically normal and abnormal spermatozoa types on stained smears (Fig. 13.1). Smears are made on slides as for blood smears. Place the smear immediately in a fixative 95% ethanol (v/v) or 50% (v/v) ethanol ether before drying has occurred. The most suitable stain is Papanicolaou. Air dried smears can be stained by Mayer's haematoxylin [air dried smears in 10% (v/v) formalin for 1 minute; water rinse; Mayer's haematoxylin 2 minutes; water rinse; air dry], but this is not a very satisfactory method. Other staining techniques include Giemsa, basic fuchsin and crystal violet. Basic fuchsin and crystal violet need heat fixing.

At least 200 spermatozoa should be examined under oil immersion and the percentage of abnormal forms noted. Normal semen has fewer than 30% abnormal forms. In addition to sperm morphology, the presence of RBCs, WBCs and epithelial cells should be noted. Differentiate immature germinal cells from macrophages or leucocytes. Numerous granules and globules are normally present in the semen.

Chemical Examination of Semen

Fructose: This is the main sugar of semen and reduced levels of seminal fructose correspond well with diminished androgen deficiency. There is an inverse relationship between fructose level and sperm count. A low fructose concentration is the result of a low

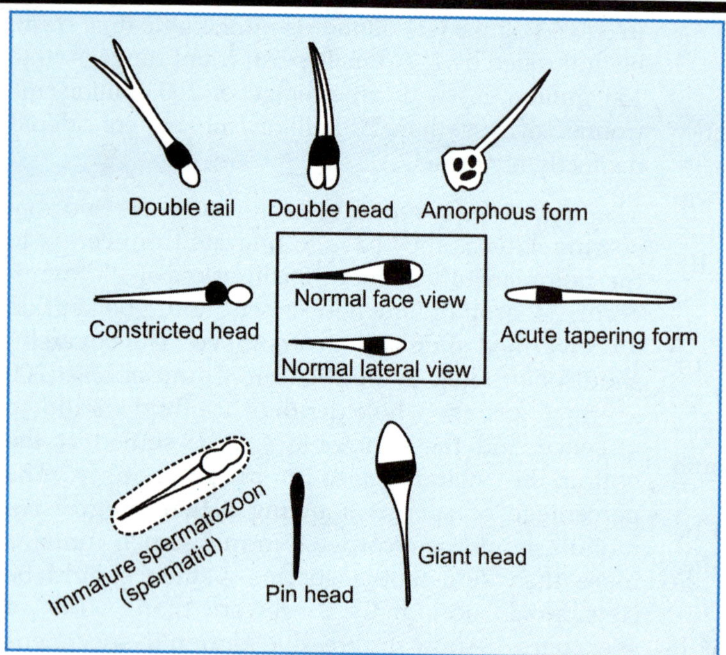

Fig. 13.1: Morphological forms of spermatozoa

testosterone level or seminal vesical insufficiency. Resorcinol method is quite simple and inexpensive.

This principle of the test being that fructose heated with resorcinol in an acidic medium produces a red precipitate. The reaction involves the conversion of fructose to hydroxymethyl furfural that condenses with resercinol to form the real precipitate.

Reagent

Resorcinol 50 mg
Conc. Hydrochloric acid 33 ml.
Dissolve and make to 100 ml with distilled water.

Method

- Take 5 ml of resorcinol reagent in a test tube (15 ml)
- Add 0.5 ml of seminal fluid
- Bring the solution to the boil (take care—the test tube opening should not be facing you)
- Examine the solution and report as mentioned below.

Reporting

Negative: No change in colour seen.

Positive: Red coloured precipitate forms within 30 seconds. Check the positive reaction with 0.5% aqueous fructose solution. 2% glucose can evoke similar test result, but such quantities of glucose are not seen in semen.

Other Tests of Semen

Postcoital (Sims-Huhner) test: Optimum time ovulatory phase at midcycle. The woman reports within 8 hours after coitus. Mucus is aspirated from the endocervical canal and sent to the laboratory.

Measure the volume of the mucus. Evaluate Spinn-Barkeit (refers to tenacity of the mucus). Grasp a portion of mucus with forceps and note the distance which it can be drawn before breaking. A good spinnbarkeit which should prevail at midcycle, is at least 10 cm. A drop of mucus is then placed on a microscope slide, covered with a coverslip and examined for the presence of sperms. An estimate of the number of sperms per high power field with percentage of motile forms should be reported. At the same time, look for WBCs, RBCs and *Trichomonas*.

Antibodies to Spermatozoa

These can be produced in the male himself or in female. Role of spermatozoal antibodies in infertility is now an established fact in experimental studies, but information pertaining to human spermatozoa is equivocal. Most clinical correlative studies thus far have utilised sperm agglutination tests. The method Franklin and Dukes employed makes use of serum and semen. Results were read (for sperm agglutination) macroscopically after a 4-hour incubation at 37°C. Some medical diagnostic companies provide kits also for assessing antibodies to sperms. These kits can be obtained from Spectral Diagnostics, Delhi (See appendices for address).

CHAPTER 14

Sputum Examination

Tracheobronchial secretions are often collectively referred to as sputum. Sputum is constituted by plasma, water, electrolytes and mucin. As it comes out, it is contaminated by nasal and salivary secretions, and normal bacterial flora of the oral cavity. Under appropriate immunologic or inflammatory stimulus, mast cells, eosinophils and plasma cells may contribute to the secretions. Sputum is viscoelastic, i.e. some of the properties of a liquid. Chemical composition reveals sputum is 95% water and only 5% solids. The solid content increases with inflammation. It also shows exfoliation of lining cells.

Specimen Collection

1. Before collecting or expectorating sputum, the mouth should be prerinsed and this removes contaminants from oral cavity especially.
2. For most examinations, a first morning specimen is best as it represents the pulmonary secretions accumulated overnight.
3. To obtain a good specimen, patient's cooperation and understanding is essential. Usually, no problem arises with adults. Children are problematic sometimes. The undermentioned methods can be used for them:
   a. A nasopharyngeal swab may be taken which is quite representative of the bronchial pathogens.
   b. A cough plate is held before the child's mouth and the child is urged to cough.
   c. Cough swab method gives the most representative, noncontaminated sputum sample. The child's mouth is held open by using a tongue depressor. Epiglottis is visualised and is touched with a swab to induce cough. Material expelled from trachea is (coughed) deposited on the swab, which can then be plated on appropriate culture media.

d. In patients who are uncooperative or cannot produce adequate sputum, induction should be tried. Commonly used inductants are 10% sodium chloride, acetylcysteine and sterile or distilled water aerosols. In persons with a history of bronchospasmodic disorders, bronchodilators should be given after inductants are used. Acetylcysteine breaks the disulphide bonds which maintain the gel structure of mucus. Acetylcysteine can be given in an aerosol form with a bronchodilator.

The specimen should be collected in a sterile disposable, impermeable container with a screw cap.

SPUTUM EXAMINATION

Transfer the specimen in a sterile petridish placed against a dark background. Wooden applicator sticks can be used to spread it thinly and can be seen with the naked eye or by using a hand lens.

Macroscopic Examination

Volume: A 24-hour volume of sputum is measured in patients with chronic bronchitis, lung abscesses or bronchial asthma. A rising volume or decreasing volume indicates worsening and improvement respectively.

Consistency and Appearance

Sputum may be described as serous (liquid), mucoid, purulent, bloody or combinations of these, e.g. seropurulent, mucopurulent.

A normal sputum is clear and watery and any opalescence is because of cellular material suspended in it. In pulmonary oedema sputum is serous, frothy and blood tinged. Most opaque particles are masses of pus and epithelium. Other materials seen in the sputum can be Curschmann's spirals, Dittrich's plugs, casseous material, bronchial casts, or food substances.

Colour: Normal sputum is clear and colourless. A *Yellow colour* indicates pus and epithelial cells as seen in a pneumonic process.

Greenish tint implies *Pseudomonas* as the aetiologic agent.

Rust coloured sputum is due to decomposed haemoglobin and is seen in pneumococcal pneumonia or pulmonary gangrene, whereas a *bright red* sputum is found in recent haemorrhage which can follow acute cardiac infarction, pulmonary infarction, neoplasm invasion and rupture of a vessel.

Odour: Normal sputum is odourless. Suppurative pulmonary disorders such as lung abscesses, cavitary tuberculosis or gangrene produce most putrid odours. A ruptured subphrenic or liver abscess may impart a faecal odour.

Other Findings

1. *Cheesy masses:* Fragments of necrotic pulmonary tissue seen in pulmonary gangrene or tuberculosis.
2. *Bronchial casts:* These are branching tree-like casts of bronchi and their size depends upon the size of bronchi from which they have been expectorated. These can be seen in untreated lobar pneumonias, fibrinous bronchitis. To recognise these casts, they have to be floated on water against a black background.
3. *Broncholiths* (lung stones): These are formed due to calcification of necrotic/infected tissue within a larger bronchus or cavity. The central core of these may be a foreign body or a fungus growth. Though rare, but when seen, chronic tuberculosis should be kept in mind.
4. *Dittrich's plugs:* They are seen in putrid bronchitis and bronchiectasis. When expectorated, they are usually solitary of a variable size. When crushed, they are found to be made of cellular debris, fatty acid crystals, fat globules, and bacteria. These plugs are seen most commonly in chronic bronchitis, bronchiectasis and bronchial asthma.
5. *Foreign bodies:* These are usually objects inhaled by a child. Usually, substances inhaled are peanuts and buttons. Radiologically, they are difficult to see.
6. *Parasites:* Various parasites that can be seen in sputum are *Ascaris lumbricoides, Echinococcus granulosus, Toxocara canis* and *Paragonimus westermani.*

Microscopic Examination

Having done the macroscopic examination, transfer the suspicious looking particles to a clear slide and examine unstained if necessary (one may come across Curschmann's spirals, elastic fibres, fungus and myelin globules). The remaining portion of the sputum is cultured. Smears made on clear slides should be air dried, fixed over a flame and then stained with Gram's stain/Ziehl-Neelsen stain. Wright's stain can be done for blood cells and buffered crystal violet for epithelial cells. Pap's stain is best for studying cytology of sputum (Fig. 14.1).

If cells characteristic of the bronchopulmonary tree are not seen—consider the specimen as inadequate and discard it even for culture. The presence of squamous cells signifies the specimen as being more representative of the oral cavity than the bronchopulmonary tree.

The basal cells are about the size of a lymphocyte with scanty cytoplasm. Columnar bronchial epithelial cells may or may not be ciliated, the nonciliated ones are of the goblet type. The presence of alveolar macrophage is the best indication that the material being examined has arisen from the lower respiratory tract, these cells often show anthracotic pigment which is not of any significance.

Blood cells are best seen by the usual peripheral smear stains. Neutrophils predominating imply an acute pyogenic infection, lymphocytes are predominant in tuberculosis and eosinophils are usually seen in bronchial asthma. Erythrocytes in large numbers indicate exudation or haemorrhage.

Sputum Culture

Each specimen received should be plated on blood agar, chocolate agar, MacConkey's agar and thioglycollate broth.

COMMON RESPIRATORY DISORDERS

Mycobacteria

A culture should always be performed in a previously undiagnosed case of respiratory tuberculosis. In a fulminant form the sputum is mucopurulent and shows RBCs, caseous and necrotic materials. Elastic fibres in the necrotic tissue indicate pulmonary tissue destruction (e.g. blood vessels; alveoli and bronchi from which they can be derived) and can be seen in abscesses, bronchiectasis, or malignancy. Most often, they are seen in advanced cases of tuberculosis. Within the caseous material, acid-fast bacilli (AFB) can usually be demonstrated. Sputum induction gives a higher recovery rate of tubercle bacilli. The slides can be stained with auramine-rhodamine (AR) stain and/or Ziehl-Neelsen (ZN) stain. AR stain shows nonviable bacilli also (ZN does not); so for prognostic evaluation, all AR positive specimens should be stained with ZN also. AR staining is superior to ZN because:

a. AFB have more affinity for AR dye
b. The entire smear can be screened as the low power (X 10) objective is used and
c. The black background in fluorescent microscopy makes the bacilli stand out sharper to allow more rapid and accurate slide screening.

Mycotic (Fungal) Disease

Respiratory fungal disease often mimics either inflammatory or neoplastic disease in clinical symptoms and X-ray findings. A first morning specimen is preferred as it represents the overnight secretions of the tracheobronchial tree. Place the specimen in a sterile container and view against a dark background. Fungi are usually seen as tiny flecks or particles which appear yellow or grey in colour and more dense than the surrounding sputum.

Make a direct mount with 10% sodium hydroxide and examine under low and high power. If no fungi are seen, the specimen can be concentrated by using 4% NaOH or the enzyme pancreatin. Confirm microscopic finding by cultures.

Pathological Fungi

Actinomyces israelii

Not a true fungus, is a gram-positive organism that grows slowly with branching filaments. It is a commensal but becomes invasive. Macroscopically it appears as yellow (sulphur) granules less than 1 mm in diameter. Microscopically, they are gram-positive mycelial filaments surrounded by a sheath of eosinophilic matter which imparts a club-shaped appearance to the ends of these filaments.

Nocardia asteroides

Are like *A. israelii* but lack the clubbed ends. The filaments are gram-positive, bacilliform in shape and in some stains are partially acid fast. It may, however, be a saprophyte in the upper respiratory tract. Its repeated presence is diagnostic of pulmonary nocardiosis.

Cryptococcus neoformans

Direct examination with India ink is advocated. The organism appears as a single budding blastospore, 2

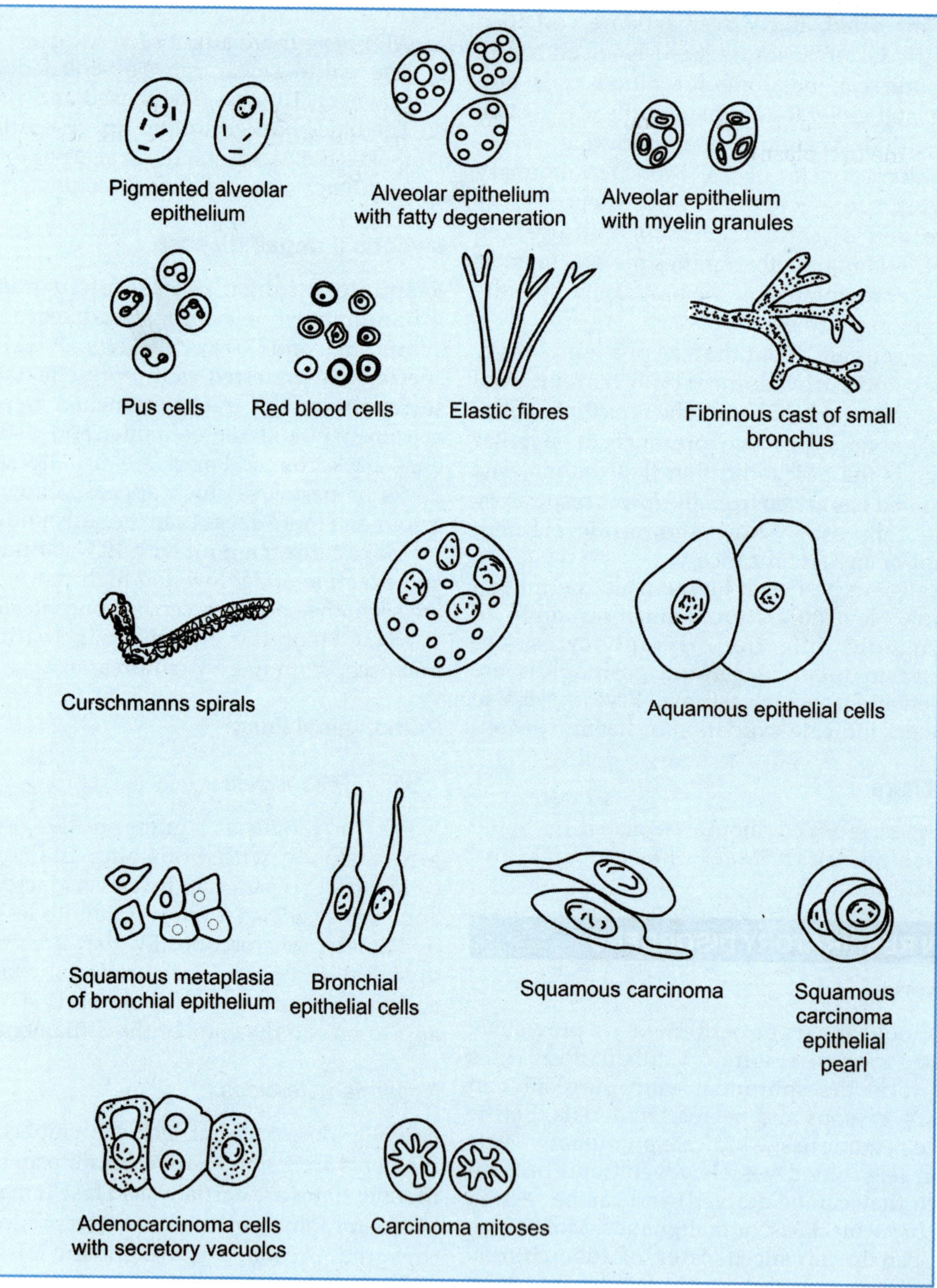

Fig. 14.1: Microscopic structures that may be seen in sputum

to 20 μ in diameter and is surrounded by a capsule from 3 to 5 μ in diameter.

Histoplasma capsulatum

Sputum staining with Wright's / Giemsa's stain reveals macrophages with characteristic intracellular small yeast cells in the cytoplasm.

Coccidiodes immitis

Examine sputum by wet direct mounts. The organism appears as a spherule, 5-200 μ in diameter and is filled with endospores. In the chronic cavity hyphae may be seen.

Blastomyces dermatidis

Infection beginning from lungs may spread haematogenously. In direct wet mounts, the organisms appear as 8-15 μ diameter spherules without a capsule. Budding may be seen with a characteristic sputum. No mycelium occurs in sputum.

Candida albicans

Is a throat commensal but overgrows with excessive use of antibiotics and immunosuppressants and becomes pathogenic (keep in mind that they can grow very well on sputum *in vitro* also). The report should indicate the number of organisms seen per field. On direct mount, they appear as 4 μ diameter, thin-walled organisms singly, in pairs, or in small clusters. Budding forms and pseudomycelia may be seen. The organisms stain intensely positive with Gram's stain.

Aspergillus fumigatus

Are like *C. albicans,* the organism appears often as a sputum contaminant.

Phycomycetes

Mucormycosis rarely causes pulmonory lesions and occur more commonly in diabetics. Direct wet mount may show huge (15 μ diameter) aseptate hyphae. Isolation on culture is a must.

Bronchial Asthma

The sputum is usually white and mucoid and contains no blood or pus unless an underlying infection is present.

Various findings seen are:

1. *Eosinophilia:* Sputum has eosinophilic staining properties (attributed to increased accumulation of serum proteins), not seen in chronic bronchitis.
2. *Bronchial epithelial cells:* These often occur singly and show hydropic change with poorly defined original morphology. During acute phases, these cells gather in larger clusters, display a vacuolated cytoplasm with ciliated border—known as Creola bodies. In addition, one may see hypersecretory goblet cells singly / clustered.
3. *Charcot-Leyden crystals:* Seen almost only in the sputum of bronchial asthma cases. The crystals are colourless, pointed hexagons and variable in size (may look needle shaped). These are derived from disintegration of eosinophils, hence they stain strongly with eosin.
4. *Blood cells:* Mostly eosinophils are seen, infection brings with it a neutrophilic response. Monocytes and histiocytes appear in significant numbers during the recovery phase.
5. *Creola bodies:* Almost exclusively seen in sputum of bronchial asthma cases. Their appearance is a poor prognostic sign.
6. *Curschmann's spirals:* Are characteristic of bronchial asthma sputum but may be seen in other respiratory disorders. Macroscopically, they can sometimes be recognised by the naked eye and appear as yellow-white, mucoid, wavy threads frequently coiled into little balls. Their length may exceed 1.5 cm. Microscopically, they show a central thread around which mucus is wrapped, supported by a fibril network.

Bronchiectasis

The production of mucopurulent sputum is one of the cardinal signs of bronchiectasis and the amount expectorated varies with the posture. Morning cough is typical. Characteristically, the sputum is putrid, grey green in colour (50-250 ml / day), at times blood tinged. On sitting, the sputum separates into three layers: (i) upper frothy layer, which later subsides, (ii) a middle turbid mucous layer and (iii) a bottom layer of pus cells and various organisms. The microscopic examination of bottom layer discloses bronchial epithelial cells, fatty crystals, bacteria and occasionally Dittrich's plugs. When crushed, they emit a foul odour.

Chronic Bronchitis

This may be catarrhal or cellular. Macroscopically the sputum is tenacious, white and mucoid in appearance. Intercurrent infections make it purulent yellow-green in colour. The average volume expectorated is about 60 ml/day. A decreasing volume implies improvement. In early chronic bronchitis, large numbers of histiocytes and monocytes indicate a stable phase, during exacerbation these cells disappear. When entering remission, these cells reappear. Leucocytes and epithelial cells are increased during active disease and diminished in number with recovery. Presence of necrotic tissue/elastic fibres indicates abscess formation or bronchiectasis. Examination of the Gram's stain usually reveals the presence of mixed organisms. Active phase is accompanied by raised sputum LDH levels. When bacterial resistance to antibiotic therapy is developing, increased LDH activity may be observed before clinical deterioration. Therefore, appropriate changes in antibiotics may be made sooner rather than waiting for culture or clinical signs. In addition, DNA levels also rise during infections. Levels fall as improvement is noted.

Lung Abscess

Only when it ruptures into a bronchus—it leads to sputum production. The aetiologic agent usually isolated are *Klebsiella, Haemophilus, Staphylococcus aureus, Streptococcus haemolyticus.* Following rupture, a large amount of bloody, creamy, foul smelling pus is suddenly and violently expectorated. More often than not, mixed organisms are present. A search for tubercle bacilli or malignant cells must also be made.

Pneumonia

Early diagnosis can be established by a Gram's stain of the sputum. Sputum should be homogenised for a more even distribution of pathogenic organisms on gram's stain. Of the gram-positive pneumonias, the main pathogen is *Diplococcus pneumoniae,* rarely are staphylococci and streptococci involved.

In pneumococcal pneumonia, the sputum characteristics change with the stage of the disease. Early lobar pneumonia sputum is scanty and transparent with occasional blood flecks. In red hepatisation stage the sputum becomes rustly red in colour, tenacious and mucopurulent. Microscopically, many intra- and extracellular organisms, epithelial cells, leucocytes and red cells are seen. During resolution stage, the sputum becomes more abundant, less tenacious and assumes the appearance as seen in chronic bronchitis. Reappearane of rusty character should indicate further progression or involvement of the opposite lung. Daily sputum Gram's stains should be performed on these patients for two reasons: (i) to follow the effect of treatment, and (ii) to rule out secondary infection.

In staphylococcal pneumonia, a yellow purulent, voluminous sputum is present. On Gram's stain, large numbers of staphylococci and neutrophils are seen.

Gram-negative pneumonias are often caused by *Klebsiella, Haemophilus, Pseudomonas* and *Escherichia coli*. With the exception of foul green sputum seen in *Pseudomonas* infections, no classic macroscopic findings are present in these sputums. As a group, sputums in the various gram-negative pneumonias are purulent and foul smelling. Putrid sputums may be associated with anaerobic organisms and should be cultured accordingly.

In Gram's stain, *Haemophilus* is often missed as safranin does not stain it well but methylene blue stain permits easier recognition of *H. influenzae.*

Pneumoconiosis

1. In *anthrasilicosis* angular black granules will be both intra- and extracellular but are not pathognomonic as they can be seen in urban dwellers and smokers.
2. In *asbestosis,* dumbbell-shaped asbestos needles in clusters is diagnostic. Numerous multinucleated giant cells and histiocytes may also be seen.
3. In *silicosis* the particles are detected by polarisation microscopy. The crystals appear sharp, elongated, and fragmented. Numerous neutrophils, macrophages, and multinucleated giant cells may be observed.
4. In *byssinosis* also, polarised light can be used to demonstrate the crystals. They appear as rectangular, prism-shaped crystals that shine brightly with polarised light.

Pulmonary Embolism

Pulmonary embolism causing infarction reveals bright red blood in a very tenacious, mucoid background. As the infarction resolves, the sputum becomes progressively darker in colour. Microscopic examination shows erythrocytes, macrophages with denatured haemoglobin in the cytoplasm. Bacterial superinfection occurs at this stage.

Heart Disease

In certain types of heart disease the sputum has characteristic findings.

In acute oedema, the sputum is abundant, frothy and pink (up to 1 litre may be brought out in a day). Microscopically, it shows numerous RBCs and large hyaline masses (protein in nature). In mitral heart disease the sputum is tenacious and blood is present, either in streaks or in dark masses mixed with mucus.

In chronic congestive heart failure, the sputum is frothy and rust coloured. Microscopy reveals the presence of RBCs and heart failure cells. In fresh unstained sputum, these cells appear as round colourless bodies filled with various sized granules of yellow to brown pigment. This pigment (haemosiderin) can be demonstrated by staining with 10% potassium ferrocyanide for a few minutes and then with 0.1 N HCl. Haemosiderin pigment stains a blue colour.

Viral Infections

Viruses are responsible for 70 to 90% of all respiratory infections. Preparation of sputum specimens for viral examination is similar to sputum cytology for malignant cells. Instead of examining for malignant changes in cells, the presence of inclusion bodies is looked for.

The inclusion bodies of herpes simplex and adenovirus are intranuclear. Herpes simplex is easier to identify and the changes are seen in the young columnar or squamous exfoliated cells. These mononuclear cells along with giant cells develop intranuclear eosinophilic inclusion bodies surrounded by a halo.

Eosinophilic intracytoplasmic inclusions are seen in parainfluenza and measle virus infections, while basophilic intracytoplasmic inclusions are present in respiratory syncytial and cytomegalic viral infections.

Pulmonary Alveolar Proteinosis

Lung biopsy is confirmatory but microscopic examination of the sputum shows an increase of hypertrophic, hyperplastic alveolar cells with a granular protein deposit in the background.

Cytologic Examination in Malignancy

Cytologic sputum examination forms an extremely important diagnostic test and gives a 50% yield in positive cases. The most ideal specimen is the single, early morning, 'deep cough' sputum and should be collected on 3 or 5 consecutive mornings. The samples (unfixed) should be submitted to the laboratory fresh. Examine the fresh specimen and select the tissue flecks and bloody areas for smearing onto a clean slide. The accepted criterion for a satisfactory sputum sample is the presence of alveolar macrophages. Four slides are prepared for examination and stained with the Papanicolaou stain. If multiple sputum collections are impractical, the most reliable sample then is the postbronchoscopy sputum specimen.

Central bronchogenic carcinoma gives the highest percentage positive results in sputum examination, although peripheral carcinomas and metastatic carcinomas may sometimes yield positive results.

CHAPTER 15

Pregnancy Tests

Pregnancy test is a misnomer as most of the methods employed measure human chorionic gonadotrophin (hCG) and not the presence of foetus. hCG is a glycoprotein produced by trophoblastic cells beginning about 10 days after conception. hCG is a dimer—the subunits are nonspecific (shared with LH, FSH and TSH), the β subunits are unique to hCG.

Five weeks after last menstrual period (*LMP*), *hCG begins to rise rapidly in urine and attains peak levels at 10 weeks of gestation.*

For laboratory confirmation of early pregnancy, hCG is the most logical measurement (for evaluation of foetal distress during the third trimester, oestriol is more useful).

BIOASSAYS

1. **Aschheium and Zondek test (1928):** Over a 2 day period give multiple injections of urine to 5 immature female mice about 1 day old, weighing 5 to 7 gms each. Sacrifice all animals four days after the first injection. Examine their ovaries for corpus luteum formation. This test is reliable but too long and time consuming for general clinical use.

2. **Friedman test (1931):** A mature female rabbit is injected intravenously with urine; at 48 hours the ovaries are examined for corpora lutea and hemorrhagic follicles (The rabbits used should be isolated for 30 days before use to avoid false-positive results).

3. **Bellerby test (1934).** Female South African clawed toads, *Xenopus laevis*, deposit eggs within 24 hours following injection with hCG. Since large doses of hCG are required, concentration by alcohol precipitation or kaolin adsorption is necessary for adequate sensitivity.

4. **Rat ovarian hyperaemia test of Frank and Berman:** Two immature female rats weighing 45 to 60 gms each are given two injections of urine/serum and sacrificed 24 hours later using carbon monoxide. Positive result is indicated by ovarian hyperemia due to capillary dilatation associated with thecal cell hyperplasia.

5. **Tests using male toad/male frog:** Galli-Mainini used male toad *Bufo arenarum,* while Wiltberger and Miller used male frog *Rana pipiens*: 4 to 6 hours after injection with hCG, these animals release sperm which can be detected microscopically. For adequate sensitivity concentration is required.

Normal Values of hCG (Serum/Plasma)

hCG		*SI Units*
Males	< 5.0 mIU/ml	< 5.0 IU/L
Females		
Nonpregnant	< 5.0 mIU/ml	< 5.0 IU/L
< 1 week gestation	5-50mIU/ml	5-50 IU/L
2 weeks gestation	50-500 mIU/ml	50-500 IU/L
3 weeks gestation	100-10,000 mIU/ml	100-10,000 IU/L
4 weeks gestation	1000-30,000 mIU/ml	1000-30,000 IU/L
5 weeks gestation	3500-115,000 mIU/ml	3500-115,000 IU/L
6 to 8 weeks gestation	12,000-27,000 mIU/ml	12,000-27,000 IU/L
12 weeks gestation	15,000-220,000 mIU/ml	15,000-220,000 IU/L

Comments

With all bioassays, drugs excreted in the urine may cause decreased sensitivity and false-negative tests or even death of the animal. Quinidine, barbiturates, laxatives, antihistamines, sulphonamides, salicylates, antibiotics, ergot and morphine derivatives may cause interference. So, the patient should discontinue all medication 3 to 4 days prior to the test. High concentrations of urinary electrolytes (especially K^+), bacteria and unspecified endogenous substances, all of these may cause false-negative reactions.

Toxic substances may be removed partially or completely from urine by: (i) dialysis in cellophane tubing for 30 to 60 minutes under running water, (ii) acidification with 0.1 N hydrochloric acid to a pH of about 6.0, (iii) extraction with ether, or (iv) absorption with kaolin. False-positive reactions may be caused by high titres of LH and/or FSH due to menopause or primary ovarian failure, as well as number of drugs, especially phenothiazines, prochlorperazine, and promazine.

Concentration of hCG is often expressed in animal units. There are rat units, mouse units, male and female toad and frog units, etc. These units are difficult to compare. More accurate is the international unit (IU) of hCG, related to specific gonadotrophic activity of 0.1 mg of a dried standard kept at the National Institute for Medical Research, London. This is the amount of activity sufficient to cause cornification of the vaginal epithelium of immature rats.

IMMUNOLOGIC METHODS

1. *Haemagglutination inhibition test*
2. *Latex particles agglutination inhibition test*
3. *Radioimmunoassays for the β-subunit of hCG* (this is by far the most sensitive and specific method available).
4. ELISA/Immunochromatography.

Most routine pregnancy tests have a sensitivity of about 0.7-1.0 IU/ml. ELISA tests have sensitivity of upto 20 mIU/ml. Kits available from Ranbaxy and Tulip/Orchid Diagnostics.

Immunologic Tests for Pregnancy

If purified hCG is injected into an animal, a specific hCG-neutralising antibody will be formed. Several tests for the presence of hCG in urine depend on the specificity of an antigen-antibody reaction.

Before proceeding with the test, perform the heat coagulation test for proteinuria, if positive—a false positive pregnancy test can be anticipated. The test is done in one of the two main ways, which differ in the carrier used for the external source of hCG. In one method, the patient's urine—1 drop—is mixed with 1 drop of an antiserum. The mixture is then incapable of reacting with the hCG carried on a suspension of latex particles which is added next and no agglutination now occurs.

If the test urine does not contain hCG, the added antiserum will not be neutralised, when the hCG-coated latex principle suspension is added, the still active anti-serum will react with the hCG on the particles causing them to agglutinate. A positive result is thus shown by an even suspension of the latex particles, a negative result, by clumping. This, then, is a latex agglutination inhibition test (False-positive results may occur in proteinuria). In some methods the latex particles are coated with hCG antibody, hence, the reversal of readings and interpretations should be considered, i.e. agglutination implying a positive result.

In the other type of method, performed in a tube, the external hCG, of the system is carried on red cells, which are said to be sensitized to hCG. The test urine is mixed with anti-hCG serum, and then with a suspension of sensitized red cells. If the urine contains hCG the anti-hCG serum will be neutralized and the sensitized red cells will be unaffected, they fall to the bottom of the tube, forming a well-defined ring. This is a positive reaction. If the urine does not contain hCG, the still active antiserum will agglutinate the hCG-sensitized red cells, which will form an evenly dispersed layer on the bottom of the test tube. Thus the test can be regarded as a hemagglutination inhibition test. This is not affected by proteinuria.

Both procedures may be performed with dilutions of urine in order to assess the 24 hour output of hCG in the follow up for placental-trophoblastic tumors. The hemagglutination test is easier to read and the slide test requires less time and less equipment. The use of known positive and negative controls is strongly recommended for both methods. Latest methods using ELISA (enzyme-linked immunosorbent-assay) are being marketed, these are more sensitive tests.

SLIDE TEST FOR PREGNANCY (Foretel® from Tulip Group of Companies)

Latex Agglutination Inhibition Method

Summary

Human chorionic gonadotrophin (hCG), a hormone produced by viable placental tissue during pregnancy, is excreted in urine approximately 20 days after the last menstrual period. The levels of hCG rise rapidly reaching peak levels after 60 to 80 days and then the hCG levels fall suddenly and eventually plateau out.

The hCG molecule consists of two combined dissimilar subunits namely, alpha and beta. The alpha subunit is practically identical to the alpha subunit of leutenising hormone (LH), follicle stimulating hormone (FSH), thyroid stimulating hormone (TSH) and the pituitary glycoprotein hormone. The beta subunit of hCG, by virtue of its unique amino acid sequence and content, confers biological and immunological specificity to the entire hCG molecule.

The appearance of hCG in urine soon after conception and its rapid rise in concentration make it an ideal marker for detection and confirmation of pregnancy. However, elevated hCG levels are frequently associated with trophoblastic and non-trophoblastic neoplasms; these conditions should be considered before a diagnosis of pregnancy can be made.

FORETEL slide test for pregnancy employs monoclonal antibodies specific to the beta subunit of hCG.

Reagents

1. Anti-beta human chorionic gonadotrophic antibody (mouse monoclonal); The antibodies are adjusted to provide a sensitivity of about 0.3 IU/ml of hCG.
2. Suspension of polystyrene latex particles to which hCG has been chemically coupled. Each batch of reagents undergoes rigorous quality control at various stages of manufacture for its specificity, sensitivity and performance.

Reagent Storage and Stability

a. Store the reagents at 2-8°C. Do not freeze.
b. The shelf life of the reagents is as per the expiry date mentioned on reagent vial labels.

Principle

FORETEL slide test for pregnancy utilises the principle of latex agglutination inhibition. The urine specimen to be tested is first mixed with the antibody reagent containing antibodies directed against the beta subunit of hCG. Then hCG coupled latex reagent is added and the mixture is allowed to react. When the urine specimen is from a non-pregnant woman and does not contain hCG, the anti-beta hCG monoclonal antibodies will be free to react with latex coupled hCG causing agglutination. When the urine specimen is from a pregnant woman and contains atleast 0.3 IU/ml of hCG, the anti-beta hCG monoclonal antibodies will be neutralised and will not react with latex coupled hCG antigen. Hence no agglutination will be observed.

Note

1. In vitro diagnostic reagent for laboratory and professional use only. Not for medicinal use.
2. The reagents contain sodium azide, 0.1 percent as preservative. Avoid contact with skin and mucosa. On disposal flush with large quantities of water.

3. The reagents can be damaged due to microbial contamination or on exposure to extreme temperatures. It is recommended that the performance of reagents should be verified by testing with known positive and negative urine controls.
4. Use reagents of the same lot numbers. Do not interchange reagents to different lot numbers.
5. Do not interchange vial droppers.
6. Shake the latex antigen vial well before use to disperse the latex particles uniformly and improve test readability.
7. Only a clean and dry glass slide must be used. Clean the slide with distilled water and wipe dry. Do not use detergents, soaps or organic solvents to clean the slide.

SAMPLE COLLECTION AND PREPARATION

Qualitative Method

Though random urine specimens can be used, first morning urine specimen is preferable. Specimens should be collected in clean glass or plastic containers free of detergents. Specimens should be tested immediately preferably within 12 hours of collection. Should a delay in testing occur, add thimerosal (0.001 percent) or sodium azide (0.01 percent) to the specimen and store at 2—8°C upto 72 hours. Do not use grossly contaminated specimens and if the specimen is cloudy or bloody, centrifuge at 1000 rpm (125 g) for one minute and use clear supernatant for testing.

Semi-quantitative Method

Specimens collected over a 24 hour period should be pooled in a clean detergent free container and refrigerated at 2 — 8°C. Thimerosal (0.001%) or sodium azide (0.01%) are recommended as urine preservatives.

MATERIAL PROVIDED WITH THE KIT

Reagent Pack

Anti-beta human chorionic gonadotropic antibody (mouse monoclonal), hCG latex antigen.

Accessories Pack

Glass slide with three reaction circles, pipettes for dispensing urine specimen, mixing sticks, rubber teats.

Additional Material Required

Positive and negative urine controls, isotonic saline, a high intensity direct light source, stop watch.

Test Procedure

Bring all reagents and samples to room temperature before use.

Qualitative Method

1. Place one drop of urine (specimen or control) on the glass slide using a disposable pipette provided with the kit. Deliver the drop vertically.
2. Add one drop of anti-beta hCG antibody to the drop of urine on the slide. Deliver the drop vertically.
3. Using a mixing stick, mix the antibody and urine uniformly over the entire circle for 30 seconds.
4. Add one drop of latex reagent to the mixture. Mix uniformly over the entire circle. Do not let the dropper tip touch the liquid on the slide.
5. Immediately start a stop watch. Rock the slide gently back and forth, observing for agglutination macroscopically at three minutes.

Semi-quantitative Method

1. Measure and record the total volume of patient urine collected over a 24 hour period.
2. Using isotonic saline, prepare progressive dilutions from an aliquot of collected urine specimen. (1:2,1:4,1:8 and so on.)
3. Perform the qualitative test procedure using each dilution as specimen.

INTERPRETATION OF RESULTS

Qualitative Method

Agglutination is a negative test result indicating the absence of detectable levels of hCG.

No agglutination is a positive test result indicating the presence of detectable levels of hCG.

Semi-quantitative Method

No agglutination in the highest urine dilution corresponds to the amount of hCG/ml. To calculate the concentration of hCG in the specimen, use the following formula, hCG = S × D

where, S = sensitivity of the test, i.e. 0.3 IU/ml

D = highest dilution of urine showing no agglutination.

For determining 24 hour hCG concentration, use the following formula, hCG 24 hours = S × D × V where, V = volume of 24 hours urine specimen.

Remarks

1. Patient specimens, in pathological conditions such as a hydatiform mole or choriocarcinoma or testicular tumor, may contain hCG and produce a positive test result not necessarily indicating a pregnancy.
2. Values of hCG greater than 250 IU/ml, 110 days after LMP, suggest the presence of a pathological condition such as a hydatiform mole or choriocarcinoma.
3. Use only urine as test specimen. Do not use serum.
4. It is recommended that results of the tests should be correlated with clinical findings to arrive at the final diagnosis

SLIDE TEST FOR PREGNANCY (Foresight—from Tulip Group of Companies)

Direct Latax Agglutination Method

Summary

Human Chorionic Gonadotrophin (hCG), a hormone produced by viable placental tissue during pregnancy, is excreted in urine approximately 20 days after the last menstrual period. The levels of hCG rise rapidly reaching peak levels after 60 to 80 days and then the hCG levels fall suddenly and eventually plateau out.

The hCG molecule consists of two combined dissimilar subunits namely, alpha and beta. The alpha subunit is practically identical to the alpha subunit of leutinising hormone (LH), follicle stimulating hormone (FSH) and thyroid stimulating hormone (TSH). The beta subunit of hCG, by virtue of its unique amino acid sequence and content, confers biological and immunological specificity to the entire hCG molecule.

The appearance of hCG in urine soon after conception and its rapid rise in concentration makes it an ideal marker for detection and confirmation of pregnancy. However, elevated hCG levels are frequently associated with trophoblastic and non-trophoblastic neoplasms, these conditions should be considered before a diagnosis of pregnancy can be made. Foresight slide test for pregnancy employs monoclonal antibodies specific to the beta subunit of hCG.

Reagent

1. Foresight latex reagent: A uniform suspension of polystyrene latex particles coated with beta hCG specific mouse monoclonal antibodies.
2. Positive control, reactive with the Foresight latex reagent.
3. Negative control, non-reactive with the Foresight latex reagent.

Each batch of reagent undergoes rigorous quality control at various stages of manufacture for its specificity, sensitivity and performance.

Reagent Storage and Stability

Store the reagent at 2-8°C. Do not freeze.

The shelf life of reagent is as per the expiry date mentioned on the reagent vial label.

Principle

Foresight slide test for pregnancy utilises the principle of DIRECT LATEX AGGLUTINATION. The urine specimen to be tested is mixed with the latex reagent coated with beta hCG specific mouse monoclonal antibodies and mixture is allowed to react. When the urine specimen is from a pregnant woman and contains at least 0.2 IU/ml of hCG, it reacts with latex reagent coated with anti-beta hCG causing agglutination.

When the urine specimen is from a non-pregnant woman and does not contain hCG it does not react with the latex reagent coated with beta hCG specific monoclonal antibodies and hence no agglutination is observed.

Note

1. *In vitro* diagnostic reagent for laboratory and professional use only. Not for medicinal use.
2. Reagent contains 0.1 percent sodium azide as preservative. Avoid contact with skin and mucosa. On disposal flush with large quantities of water.
3. The reagent can be damaged due to microbial contamination or on exposure to extreme temperatures. It is recommended that the performance

of the reagent should be verified by testing with known positive and negative urine controls.

4. Do not interchange vial droppers/caps.
5. Shake the latex reagent vial well before use to disperse the latex particles uniformly and improve test readability.
6. Only a clean and dry glass slide must be used. Clean the slide with distilled water and wipe dry. Do not use detergents, soaps, or organic solvents to clean the slide.
7. Accessories provided with the kit only must be used for optimum results.

SPECIMEN COLLECTION AND PREPARATION

Qualitative Method

Though random urine specimens can be used, first morning urine specimen is preferable. Specimens should be collected in clean glass or plastic containers free of detergents. Specimens should be tested immediately preferably within 12 hours of collection. Should a delay in testing occur, add thimerosal (0.001%) or sodium azide (0.01%) to the specimen and store at 2-8°C upto 72 hours. Do not use grossly contaminated specimens and if the specimen is cloudy or bloody, centrifuge at 1000 rpm (125 g) for one minute and use clear supernatant for testing.

Semi-quantitative Method

Specimens collected over a 24 hour period should be pooled in a clean detergent free container and refrigerated at 2-8°C. Thimerosal (0.001%) or sodium azide (0.01%) are recommended as urine preservatives.

Material Provided with the Kit

Latex reagent coated with beta hCG-specific mouse monoclonal antibodies, Positive control, negative control, glass slide with three reaction circles, Pipettes for dispensing urine specimen, mixing sticks, rubber teats.

Additional Material Required

Isotonic saline, A high intensity direct light source, stopwatch.

Test Procedure

Bring reagent and urine specimen to room temperature before testing.

Qualitative Method

1. Place one drop of urine (specimen or control) on the glass slide using the disposable pipette provided with the kit. Deliver the drop by holding the dropper vertically.
2. Even for dispensing controls, the use of sample dispensing pipettes is recommended.
3. Add one drop of latex reagent to the specimen. Mix uniformly over the entire circle. Do not let the dropper tip touch the liquid on the slide.
4. Immediately start the stopwatch. Rock the slide gently back and forth, observing for agglutination macroscopically at two minutes.

Semi-quantitative Method

Measure and record the total volume of patient's urine collected over a 24 hour period. Using isotonic saline, prepare progressive dilutions from an aliquot of collected urine specimen (1:2,1:4,1:8 and so on). Perform the qualitative test procedure using each dilution as specimen.

INTERPRETATION OF TEST RESULTS

Qualitative Method

Agglutination is a positive test result and indicates presence of detectable levels of hCG in the specimen indicating pregnancy. No agglutination is a negative test result and indicates absence of detectable levels of hCG.

Semi-quantitative Method

To calculate the concentration of hCG in the specimen, use the following formula:

$$hCG = S \times D$$

where, S = Sensitivity of the test i.e. 0.2 IU/ml

D = Highest dilution of urine under test showing agglutination

Remarks

1. Patient specimen, in pathological conditions such as hydatidiform mole or choriocarcinoma, may contain hCG and produce a positive test result not necessarily indicating a pregnancy.
2. During the first trimester of a normal pregnancy, hCG levels as high as 160-180 IU/ml may be obtained.
3. Values of hCG greater than 250 IU/ml, 110 days after L.M.P., may suggest the presence of

pathological condition such as hydatidiform mole or choriocarcinoma.

4. Foresight is designed to detect hCG levels attained during the course of a normal pregnancy. As in case of similar pregnancy tests, prozoning may occurwith hCG levels above 260 lU/ml.
5. Use only urine as test specimen. Do not use serum.
6. It is recommended that results of the tests should be correlated with clinical findings to arrive at the final diagnosis.
7. If the result is negative and pregnancy is still suspected, the test should be repeated with a fresh specimen collected after a week.

ELISA PREGNANCY TEST (Vectra from Tulip Group of Companies)

Introduction

Vectra pregnancy test is a rapid, visual, qualitative, enzyme immunoassay for the determination of human chorionic gonadotrophin (hCG), a marker for pregnancy in urine/serum.

Summary

Human chorionic gonadotrophin (hCG) is a glycoprotein hormone secreted by the synciotrophoblastic cells of placenta, after fertilization. In normal pregnancy, hCG can be detected approximately 6 to 8 days after conception. Following conception approximately after 6 to 8 days, hCG is released and its concentration doubles approximately every 1.7 days. The levels of hCG rise rapidly reaching peak levels after 60 to 80 days.

The appearance of hCG soon after conception and its subsequent rise in concentration makes it an ideal marker for early detection and confirmation of pregnancy. However elevated hCG levels are frequently associated with trophoblastic and non-trophoblastic neoplasms and hence these conditions should be considered before a diagnosis of pregnancy can be made.

Vectra enzyme immunoassay for pregnancy detects the presence of hCG in urine/serum specimens, qualitatively, at concentrations of 25 mlU/ml of hCG and above in about 10 minutes.

Principle

Vectra pregnancy test utilises the principle of sandwich enzyme immunoassay, with a unique mono antibody combination specific against hCG present in urine/serum.

The patient urine/serum specimen is allowed to react with the monoclonal antibody directed against hCG, coated on the microtiter wells and the monoclonal antibody- enzyme conjugate complex. If hCG is present in the test specimen, antibody-hCG-antibody-enzyme complex will be formed on the surface of the microtiter well. Washing the well under running tap water will clear off the unbound complex and the unreacted conjugate. Incubating the well with substrate reagent results in development of blue colour. The intensity of the blue colour is proportional to the concentration of hCG present in the urine/serum specimen. Visual comparison of the intensity of the blue colour with test specimen well as against the positive control well indicates the concentration of hCG greater than or equal to 25 mlU/ml of hCG in the test specimen.

REAGENTS AND MATERIAL SUPPLIED

Reagents for performing the test:

1. Sealed pouches containing breakable microtiter wells predispensed with monoclonal anti-hCG antiserum (8 wells/pouch).
2. Enzyme conjugate containing monoclonal anti-hCG antibody peroxidase conjugate.
3. Substrate reagent containing tetra-methyl benzidine in appropriate buffer.
4. Negative control serves to validate the test procedure.
5. Positive control provides colour equivalent to 25 mlU/ml of hCG.

Materials for performing the test:

- Well holder.
- Disposable sample droppers.

Additional Material Required

- Sample collection container.
- Timer/stop watch.
- Flowing tap water.
- Absorbent paper/tissue.

Storage and Stability

The kit must be stored at 2-8°C till the duration of shelf life as indicated on the carton label and the respective individual kit component labels.

Note

1. For *in vitro* diagnostic use only. Not for medicinal use.
2. Since reagents from the same lot are optimized as a system, it is important that reagents of the same lot are used for performing the test.
3. Foil pouches may be cut open carefully from the sealed end. In case of less number of microtiter wells being used, replace back the unused wells into the foiled pouch and seal appropriately for future use. Protect the wells from direct exposure to moisture.
4. Do not interchange reagent bottle caps.
5. Once the test is performed, immediately replace the kit at 2-8°C.
6. Avoid exposure of the substrate solution to direct light during use or storage.
7. Do not use the kit beyond expiry date.
8. Addition sequence of samples and reagents must be observed meticulously for achieving accurate results.

Specimen Collection

Though random urine specimens can be used, first morning urine specimen is preferable as it contains the highest concentration of hCG. Specimens should be collected in clean glass or plastic containers. If testing is not immediate, the urine specimens may be stored at 2-8°C for up to 72 hours. Turbid specimens should be centrifuged or allowed to settle and only the clear supernatant should be used for testing.

Test Procedure

1. Bring all reagents to room temperature before testing. Also refrigerated specimens must be brought to room temperature prior to testing.
2. Cut open the foiled pouch to retrieve the required number of microtiter wells.
3. Place the required number of microtiter wells on the well holder.
4. Tighten the vial cap of all the reagent bottles provided with the kit in clockwise direction to pierce the dropper bottle nozzle.
5. Dispense two drops of urine/serum sample to be tested using the dropper provided with the kit to the appropriate microtiter wells.
6. Add two drops each of POSITIVE AND NEGATIVE control into the appropriate wells.
7. Add one drop of ENZYME CONJUGATE to the test, positive and negative control wells.
8. Incubate for 5 min. at room temperature.
9. Empty the entire content of the wells into the sink by flicking off the liquids.
10. Wash the wells under running tap water (or distilled water) 6 times by filling and emptying the wells. Take care to avoid well to well contamination from water overflow during rinsing.
11. Blot dry after the last wash.
12. Add two drops of SUBSTRATE REAGENT into each well.
13. Incubate for 5 min. at room temperature.
14. Visually compare the development of blue colour in test well as against the positive control well against a white background.

Interpretations of Results

Positive Results- Wells showing blue colour equal to or more intense than the positive control well indicates a positive result.

Negative Results- Wells showing no colour at the end of final incubation of 5 min. indicates that the concentration of hCG is less than 25 mIU/ml or a negative result.

Remarks

1. A number of conditions other than pregnancy including trophoblastic and non-trophoblastic neoplasms such as hydatidiform mole, choriocarcinoma etc. can cause elevated levels of hCG. Such clinical conditions must be ruled out before a diagnosis of pregnancy can be made.
2. Highly dilute urine specimens and specimens from early pregnancy may not contain representative levels of hCG. If pregnancy is still suspected, repeat the test with first morning urine after 48 to 72 hours.
3. As with all diagnostic tests, the results must be correlated with clinical findings.
4. Avoid air bubble formation during addition of reagents, positive and negative control, urine sample to be tested while performing the test.

5. A slight blue tinge in the test well with a intensity lesser than the positive control well indicates insufficient washing and should be considered negative.
6. It is recommended to run positive and negative control simultaneously with each assay run.

Perspectives on membrane-based rapid diagnostic tests and detection of hCG using these tests

PERSPECTIVES ON MEMBRANE-BASED RAPID DIAGNOSTIC TESTS AND DETECTION OF hCG USING THESE TESTS

Index

- What are the principles of membrane-based Rapid Diagnostic Tests?
- What are the components of membrane-based Rapid Diagnostic Tests and how are they constructed?
- What are the limitations and effects of various components on the performance of membrane-based Rapid Diagnostic Tests?
- How does the nitrocellulose membrane affect the sensitivity of Rapid Diagnostic Tests?
- Why are colloidal gold sol particles commonly employed in the detector reagent in membrane-based Rapid Diagnostic Tests?
- Why are variations in band appearance commonly observed in membrane-based Rapid Diagnostic Test employed for antigen detection.
- What is the role of sample pad in membrane-based rapid diagnostic tests?
  What is the role of soak pad in membrane-based rapid diagnostic tests?
- Why do "Faint Ghost Bands" appear at the test region if the device is left out on the work table?
- How do we interpret "Broken Bands" at the test/control region?
- What is pregnancy testing?
- What is human Chorionic Gonadotrophin (hCG)?
- What are the levels of hCG observed during normal pregnancy?
- What is the effect of antibody pair used in the membrane-based rapid diagnostic pregnancy tests for detection of hCG?
- What are the implications of sensitivity and specificity on membrane-based Rapid Diagnostic Tests for pregnancy?
- What is the clinical significance of hCG?
- What is the ideal specimen to be employed for pregnancy testing?
- Why are discrepant results observed during problem pregnancies?
- During which conditions other than pregnancy are detectable levels of hCG observed?
- How do procedural errors affect Rapid Diagnostic Tests?

The need for a rapid, reliable, simple, sensitive *in vitro* diagnostics assay for use at point-of-care, have lead to the commercialisation of *in vitro* rapid diagnostic tests based on the principle of immunochromatography.

Rapid diagnostic tests are membrane-based immunoassays that allow visual detection of an analyte in liquid specimens. In clinical assays, specimens such as urine whole blood, serum or plasma, saliva and other body fluids may be employed.

What are the principles of membrane-based Rapid Diagnostic Tests?

Currently available Rapid Diagnostic Tests comprise of a base membrane such as nitrocellulose. A detector reagent (antigen/antibody-indicator complex) specific to the analyte, impregnated at one end of the membrane. A capture reagent is coated on the membrane at the test region.

When the specimen is added to the sample pad, it rapidly flows through the conjugate pad. Analyte if present in the specimen, binds to the detector reagent. As the specimen passes over the test band to which the capture reagent is coated, the analyte-detector reagent complex is immobilised. A coloured-band proportional to the amount of analyte present in the sample, develops. The excess unbound detector reagent moves further up the membrane and is immobilised at the control band.

What are the components of membrane-based Rapid Diagnostic Tests and how are they constructed?

Rapid Diagnostic Tests consists of:

1. Sample pad
2. Detector reagent/conjugate: Antigen/antibody-indicator complex specific to the analyte, impregnated in the conjugate pad but remains unbound
3. Test band: Coated on nitrocellulose membrane; specific to the analyte
4. Control band: Usually anti-detector antibodies coated on the membrane, serves to validate the test results (Fig. 15.1).

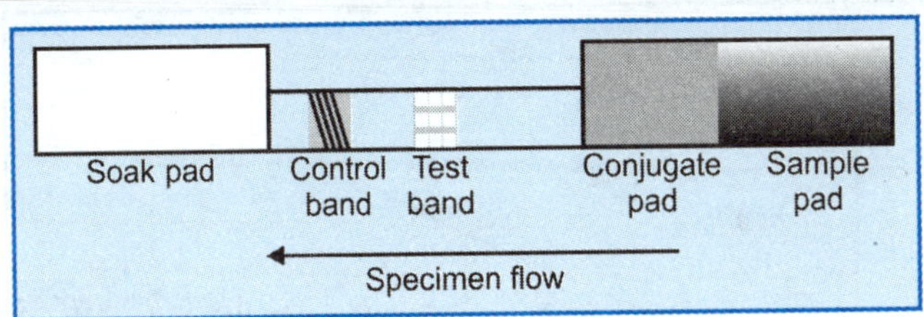

Fig. 15.1: Construction of rapid diagnostic tests

Currently immunochromatography tests are available in two formats; "Lateral flow" and "Transverse flow or Flow through". The lateral flow are available in device or dipstick format. The lateral flow formats are commonly employed where rapid detection of pregnancy, drug abuse, infectious disease or parasitology is required, and serve as qualitative screening assay at laboratories, physician's office or at homes due to their simplicity and ease of performance. The flow through format is less common as the assay requires greater operator involvement. However, some of these assays enable semi-quantitative estimation of the analyte by visual comparison with an in-built reference.

Regardless of the format used, the desired specificity, sensitivity and assay performance depends upon reliable formulation and proper assay assembly.

What are the limitations and effects of various components on the performance of membrane-based Rapid Diagnostic Tests?

This section highlights the role of various components of Rapid Diagnostic Tests and their effect on attaining the desired performance characteristics.

How does the nitrocellulose membrane affect the sensitivity of Rapid Diagnostic Tests?

Rapid Diagnostic Tests are fabricated on a solid support membrane, usually made of nitrocellulose. Membranes employed in Rapid Diagnostic Tests are porous. Depending upon the porosity, some membranes are better suited for applications with certain specimens than others. This is because, the pore size of the membrane has significant effect on the capture reagent binding properties and the lateral flow rate. The combined effects of these two-phenomenon in turn determine the sensitivity and performance of the test assay.

Pore size and capture reagent binding properties

It has been observed that as the pore size decreases the effective surface area available for binding of capture reagent increases. Greater effective surface area available for binding, results in optimal coating of the capture reagent, which is essential for attaining the desired sensitivity of the assay.

Pore size and lateral flow rate

It has also been observed that as the pore size increases, the lateral flow rate increases. However slower flow rate increases the effective concentration (concentration required for interaction) of the analyte, since a slower flow rate allows the analyte and the capture reagent to be in close proximity for a longer time. As it is well known, immunological reactions are time-dependent and prolonged exposure of the analyte with the capture reagent allows better interaction and thus results in increased sensitivity. The flow rate is important when the analyte is present in low concentrations, such as borderline samples. The relationship between lateral flow rate and effective analyte concentration is: effective analyte concentration

$$\alpha = \frac{1}{(\text{flow rate})^2}$$

Thus, it is important to optimize the membranes such that Rapid Diagnostic Tests can achieve rapid results which are also reliable and accurate

Why are colloidal gold sol particles commonly employed in the detector reagent in membrane-based Rapid Diagnostic Tests?

Interpretation of results in rapid diagnostic Tests depends upon the development of a signal at the stipulated time. A signal is generated when capture reagent-analyte-detector reagent complex is formed. The detector reagent/conjugate consists of an antibody or antigen bound to the indicator. The indicator imparts colour to the signal, enabling visual interpretation of results.

Coloured latex particles, colloidal gold sol particles, dyes, enzymes and carbon particles are some of the indicators used in immunochromatographic assays. However, stability, protein-binding properties, particle size are critical factors that determine their use in immunochromatographic assays. The most popular indicators used in immunochromatographic assays is the colloidal gold sol particle.

Colloidal gold sol particles as indicator

Homogenous colloidal gold sol particles are inert and can couple with antibody/antigen, which is stable in dried as well as in liquid form. All the above mentioned parameters are determined by the particle shape and size of colloidal gold.

Effect of shape of colloidal gold sol particles on stability

Colloidal gold sol particles have a net negative charge called "Zeta Potential". This Zeta Potential maintains the minimal distance between two particles resulting in long term stability. Ideally, colloidal gold sol particles should be spherical in shape, since this shape allows uniform distribution of Zeta Potential at the surface. In case of non-homogenous particles, the Zeta Potential is not uniformly distributed thus the particles may come together to form aggregates. These aggregates may permanently get impregnated into the conjugate pad, or during the test assay may deposit on the nitrocellulose membrane leading to discrepant results. Such non-homogenous colloidal gold is usually blue/black in colour.

Effect of shape of colloidal gold sol particles on sensitivity

Spherical, homogenous colloidal gold sol particles also allow uniform coating of the detector reagent at their surface. Whereas non-homogenous colloidal gold sol particles do not allow uniform coating of detector reagent, resulting in decreased assay sensitivity and specificity.

Effect of size on colour of colloidal gold sol particles

It has been observed that as the colloidal gold sol particles increase in size, the colour turns from light pink to cherry-red to red-purple to blue-black to grey-black. Darker coloured particles are preferred in Rapid Diagnostic Tests since darker colours allow easy interpretations of results. However, as the colloidal gold sol particles increase in size, these particles are less stable and aggregate together. Secondly due to the steric hindrance, the larger colloidal gold sol particles tend to dwarf the coated antigen/antibody making interaction with the analyte difficult (Fig. 15.2).

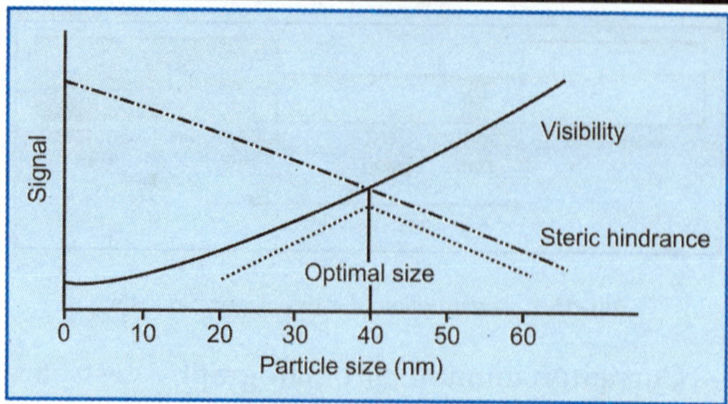

Fig. 15.2: Graph of particle size v/s signal colour of colloidal gold sol

Ideally, the colloidal gold sol used in immunochromatographic assays is ~ 40 nm in size and imparts a cherry-red colour, which enables optimal visualization of results against a clear white background and is stable in dry and liquid form. However, purple coloured colloidal gold sol particles if properly stabilized, can also be used in Rapid Diagnostic Tests.

Why are variations in band appearance commonly observed in membrane-based Rapid Diagnostic Tests employed for antigen detection?

The sensitivity/specificity of Rapid Diagnostic Tests primarily depends upon the detector and capture reagent pair. Ideally, the detector reagent should be specific to one epitope of the analyte and the capture reagent specific to another epitope of the same analyte, thereby enabling two-site sandwich immunoassay. To illustrate the same please refer to the diagram below (Fig. 15.3):

For higher analyte sensitivity, manufacturers of commercial Rapid Diagnostic Tests for antigen detection depend on the use of various combinations of capture reagents at the test and control band. Avid capture reagents have a high affinity for the analyte. When the sample containing the analyte reaches the avid capture reagent at the test band, due to high affinity, the avid reagent at the edge of the band captures most of the analyte. Thus resulting in a distinct thin coloured line at the edge of the test band.

On the other hand, use of less avid capture reagent (lesser affinity for the analyte) results in capture of the analyte uniformly across the test or control band. Thus broader bands are generated by less avid antibodies.

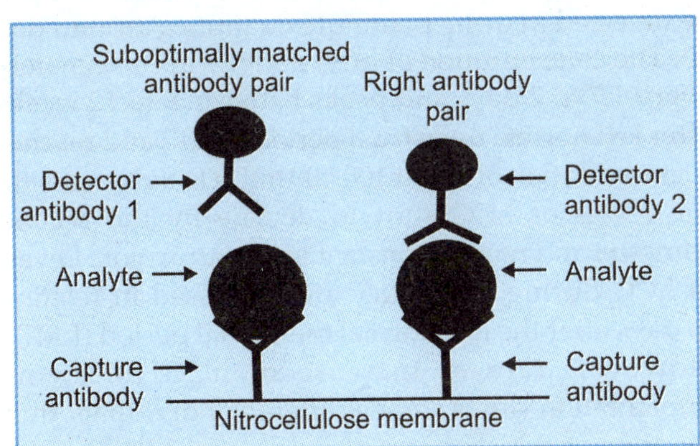

Fig. 15.3: Two-site sandwich immunoassay

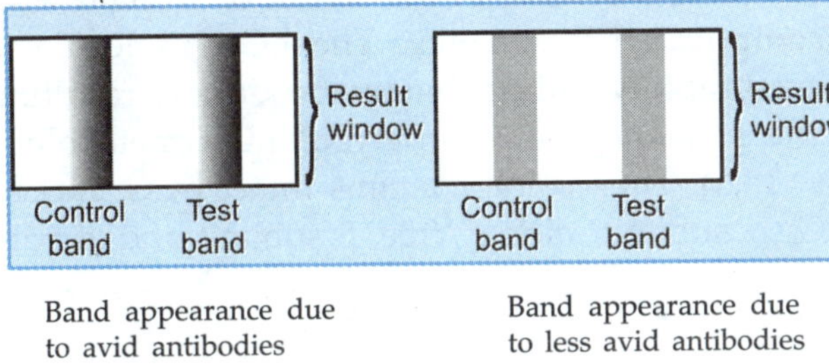

Band appearance due to avid antibodies

Band appearance due to less avid antibodies

Fig. 15.3A: Band appearance Vs and antibodies

Variations in band appearance in different assays is due to use of varying avidity of the antibodies at the test/control band (Fig. 15.3A).

What is the role of sample pad in membrane-based Rapid Diagnostic Tests

Rapid Diagnostic Tests enable detection of the analyte in several specimen such as urine, whole blood, serum or plasma. However, the pH, viscosity, ionic concentration, turbidity, total protein content may vary from specimen to specimen. Variations in these factors can cause alterations in the colloidal gold particles or the capture reagent leading to non-specific results. For example, highly turbid specimens can cause invalid results since the particles from the specimen may block the membrane preventing sample flow. Urine specimen becomes acidic on storage due to bacterial growth. Due to a shift in the pH, the colloidal gold particles come together to form aggregates which may interfere in the performance of the test.

Rapid Diagnostic Tests incorporating serum as specimen may give false positive results due to the presence of Heterophillic Antibodies. These antibodies have multispecificity and bind the capture reagent to the detector reagent leading to false positive results. Use of Rapid Diagnostic Tests incorporating Heterophillic Blocking Reagents (HBR) is recommended to avoid this interference. A sample pad with a bed volume of minimum retention capacity facilitates transfer of the entire specimen dispensed. This not only ensures minimal wastage of specimen but the excess specimen can be used to wash away unbound conjugate from the test region for better visualization of results.

Thus use of sample pad that allows incorporation of buffer salts, stabilizers and HBR, to a large extent eliminates variation in pH, ionic concentration and interference of heterophillic antibodies.

What is the role of soak pad in membrane-based Rapid Diagnostic Tests?

Use of a soak pad with high bed volume is preferred in rapid diagnostic Tests because the total volume of specimen that enters the test assay can be increased. This increased volume can be used to dislodge the conjugate as well as wash away the unbound/unreacted conjugate from the test region contributing to clearer background and better visualization of results.

Why do "Faint Ghost Bands" appear at the test region if the device is left out on the work-table?

A common phenomenon observed in the device format is appearance of faint ghost bands at the test region after some time. After completion of the test, if the device is exposed to warm ambient temperatures, evaporation occurs from the result window. Due to evaporation, the excess sample along with unreacted/unbound conjugate from the soak pad flows back to the reaction area. This unreacted or unbound conjugate may then get deposited on the test band resulting in appearance of a **"Faint Ghost Band"** after some time (Fig. 15.4).

Result must be recorded at the end of the recommended reaction time for correct Interpretation.

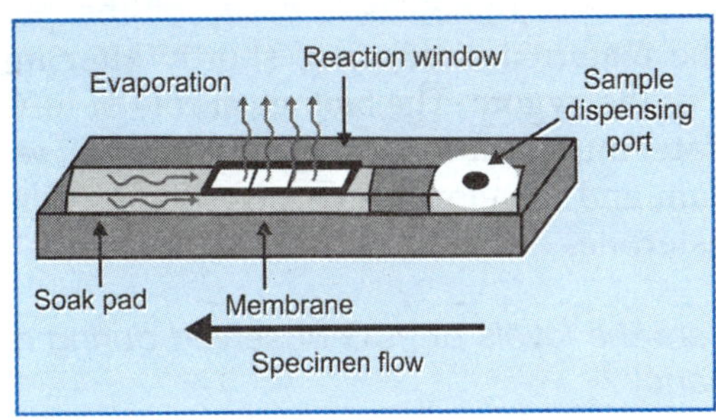

Fig. 15.4: Appearance of "Faint Ghost Band"

How do we interpret "Broken Bands" at the test/control region?

To prevent evaporation of the specimen from the test window, the membrane of the device is laminated with the help of a thin transparent tape. Sometimes, during the process of lamination, air pockets may be formed between the membrane and the tape. These air pockets, prevent uniform sample flow, which may result in appearance of broken bands at the test/control region.

However, appearance of even a broken and at the test region indicates positive results.

In the following section we shall discuss the role of hCG as a marker for diagnosing pregnancy and certain conditions that may give discrepant results.

What is pregnancy testing?

Presence of human Chorionic Gonadotrophin (hCG) and its subunits in urine/serum is an important marker in diagnosis of early pregnancy and determining problem pregnancies. Most pregnancy tests employed today, are based on two-site sandwich immunoassay that utilize polyclonal/monoclonal antibodies raised against different epitopes on the hCG molecule.

What is human Chorionic Gonadotrophin (hCG)?

Human Chorionic Gonadotrophin (hCG) is a complex glycoprotein hormone consisting of two dissimilar polypeptide subunits, α and β, linked non-covalently. The a subunit of hCG is similar to that of the other pituitary glycoprotein hormones; Luteinizing Hormone (LH), Follicle Stimulating Hormone (FSH) Thyroid Stimulating Hormone (TSH). It is the (β subunit that provides the differentiating characteristics of hCG from LH, FSH and TSH. hCG is secreted by the synctiotrophoblastic tissue of the placenta into the maternal circulation, shortly after implantation of the zygote. The biological role of hCG is to facilitate implantation of the zygote as well as maintain and develop the corpus luteum to secrete progesterone.

What are the levels of hCG observed during normal pregnancy?

In a normal 28-days menstrual cycle, with ovulation occurring at day 14, serum hCG can be detected within 24 hours post implantation, whereas hCG can be detected in urine in minute quantities around day 23. The concentration of hCG doubles approximately every 1.7 to 2 days and peaks between 8 to 12 weeks after last normal menstrual period (LMP) and reaches a concentration of about 100,000 mIU/L. Subsequently the levels of hCG start to decline by the second trimester and remain constant until parturition. Levels of hCG during pregnancy are expressed in relation to days after the last normal menstrual period (LMP). However, rate of increase of hCG following implantation varies among different individuals, thus the time at which a test becomes positive may also vary. During the 1st trimester, 96-98% hCG circulates as an intact molecule in the serum of women with uncomplicated pregnancy. The hCG molecule is cleaved rapidly and cleared by the kidneys resulting in the formation of a variety of hCG metabolites (Fig. 15.5). Thus urine contains intact hCG, nicked hCG, α subunit, nicked/free β subunit and β core fragment.

What is the effect of antibody pair used in the membrane-based Rapid Diagnostic Pregnancy Tests for detection of hCG?

Anti-hCG antibodies used in the detector or capture reagent are specific to certain epitopes on the hCG molecule. Different species of antibodies detect different epitopes of hCG molecule. Since, different antibodies are used by different manufactures, thus different brands do not recognize the same epitope of the hCG molecule. Secondly, since hCG and its metabolites are present in the maternal circulation and in the urine, depending on the epitope specificity of the antibody pair used as the detector or capture reagent, different brands may detect either intact hCG, nicked hCG, a subunit, nicked/ free b subunit or b core fragment. This can result in discrepancies between brands in few cases of hCG detection.

What is the clinical significance of hCG?

In normal, healthy women of child-bearing age, elevated levels of hCG are associated with pregnancy. However, certain other clinical conditions such as trophoblastic diseases and non-trophoblastic disease such as hydatidiform mole, choriocarcinoma, testicular tumor are associated with high levels of hCG and its dissociated or degraded subunits in the

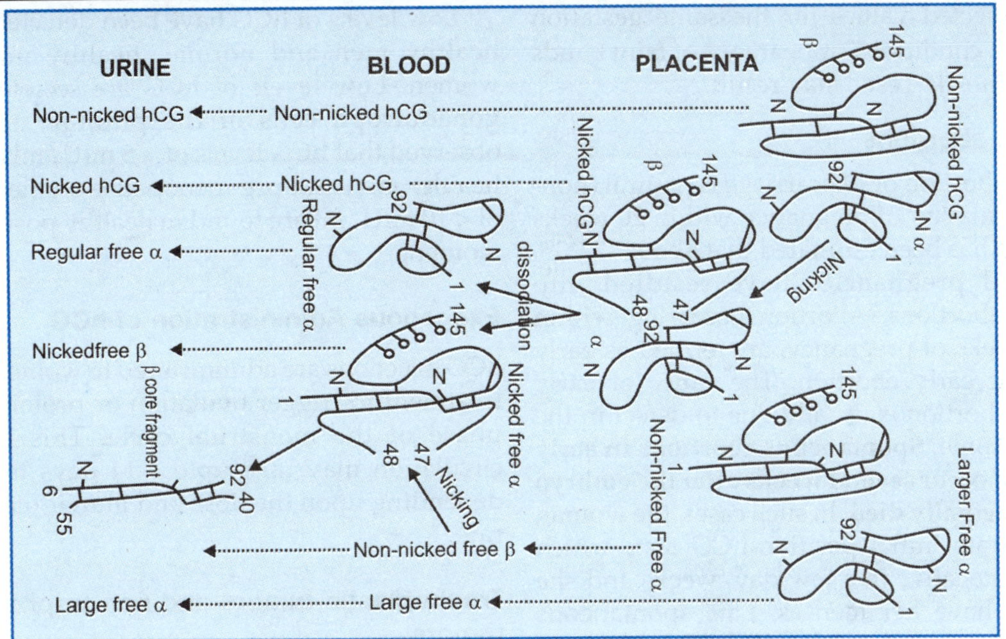

Fig. 15.5: hCG and its metabolites during pregnancy
Adapted from-Immunoassay of human Chorionic Gonadotrophin, free subunits, and metabolites" LA. Cole; Clinical Chemistry, 43:12; 2233-2243; 1997

patient's circulation. Thus the clinical significance of measuring hCG and its subunits are:

1. To diagnose early pregnancy.
2. To monitor pregnancy prognosis.
3. Diagnose and monitor trophoblastic tumors.

What are the implications of sensitivity and specificity on membrane-based Rapid Diagnostic Tests for Pregnancy?

An ideal pregnancy test is one, which can detect and is sensitive to the lowest levels of hCG in the patient's urine/serum. On an average hCG levels of 25-100 mIU/ml are reached on the first day of missed period. The ideal cut-off of pregnancy test should be adjusted so as to detect hCG levels greater than 10 mIU/ml, since, it has been observed that hCG levels of < 10 mIU/ml may be found in healthy non-pregnant women and even normal, healthy men. Since the a subunit of hCG is similar to that of LH, FSH and TSH, Rapid Diagnostic Tests for pregnancy should be specific to the β subunit of hCG only, ensuring no false positive reactions due to cross reactivity with other hormones.

What is the ideal specimen to be employed for pregnancy testing?

Urine is the most widely used specimen for pregnancy assays. However, hCG can be detected in serum within 24 hours post implantation. Thus serum as a specimen can be used for early detection of hCG and monitoring fertility treatment. Concentration of hCG in urine specimens depends on time of urine collection, volume of urine excreted, fluid intake where as the level of hCG is uniformly distributed in serum and hence it can be collected at any time of the day. hCG is a very stable molecule if preserved or kept in blood or serum, however hCG dissociates at a much faster rate when left in urine. Since urine facilitates bacterial growth it may drastically alter the pH, ionic concentration as well as increase turbidity of the specimen, which may affect the hCG concentration.

Why are discrepant results observed during problem pregnancies?

Abnormal pregnancies such as ectopic pregnancies, threatened abortions, spontaneous abortions and early pregnancy loss are associated with low levels of hCG and its subunits.

Ectopic Pregnancy

Implantation of the zygote outside the uterus is known as ectopic pregnancy. It has been observed that during ectopic pregnancies the hCG levels are below the expected values for the same gestation period. In such conditions, appearance of faint bands in Rapid Diagnostic Tests, may result.

Spontaneous abortions

Spontaneous abortion or Miscarriage is natural (non-induced) termination of pregnancy within 20 weeks of gestation. It has been estimated that about 15-20% of recognized pregnancies have resulted into spontaneous abortions. Abortion occurring within the first 16 weeks of pregnancy, are termed as early miscarriage or early abortion. The cause of early spontaneous abortion is usually due to defect in the foetal chromosome. **Spontaneous abortions in early pregnancy can occur several weeks after the embryo or foetus has actually died.** In such cases, the woman may demonstrate initial positive hCG tests which may be come negative in a few day/weeks and she may still not have her menses. Late spontaneous abortions occur between the 17th-20th week of pregnancy. The main causes are often related to the mother's state of health. The probable causes are severe malaria infection, Rh incompatibility, hormonal imbalance, Venereal diseases, chronic diabetes, high blood pressure, abnormalities of the immune system or abnormalities of the uterus or cervix.

Early Pregnancy Loss

Early pregnancy loss is a clinical condition where in the embryo fails to implant into the uterus or it is rejected by uterus in the form of a normal or slightly heavy menses. This occurs during the 2nd week after implantation of the embryo. Thus most women are unaware that they had an early pregnancy loss hCG levels rise during the first week post implantation as in the case of a normal pregnancy, peak at second week of implantation (28th day from LMP) and then rapidly decline with the occurrence of bleeding along with foetal loss. An hCG assay, if performed during the 1st or 2nd day of missed period (28th-29th day from LMP) would indeed give a positive result due to the presence of hCG. However, negative results are obtained if the test assay is repeated after an interval of 1 to 2 days, i.e around the 31st day after LMP.

During which conditions other than pregnancy are detectable levels of hCG observed?

Detectable levels of hCG has been observed in the following cases:

Normal, healthy men and normal, healthy non-pregnant women.

Low levels of hCG have been detected in normal, healthy men and normal, healthy non-pregnant women. Low levels of hCG are secreted from the gonadotroph cells of the pituitary. It has been observed that hCG levels of = 5 mlU/ml are found in healthy men and pre-menopause women and levels of < 10 mlU/ml are found in healthy post menopause women.

Exogenous Administration of hCG

hCG injections are administered to women on fertility treatment to trigger ovulation or prolong the luteal phase of the menstrual cycle. This hCG in the circulation may take upto 5-14 days to be cleared depending upon the dose and individual's clearance rate.

Trophoblastic tumors and non-trophoblastic tumors

Trophoblastic tumors such as trophoblastic neoplasm, hydatidiform mole, choriocarcinoma have been shown to secrete variable ratios of intact hCG and its metabolites. Also non-trophoblastic diseases such as testicular/ovarian and bladder cancers are associated with high levels of hCG and its subunits. Thus prior to performing a hCG test, trophoblastic and non-trophoblastic disease conditions should be ruled out as these conditions.

Phantom hCG-like immuno-reactivity

Certain trypsin-like molecules, cholera toxin or certain bacterial secretions produce phantom hCG-like immuno-reactivity in serum, which may then interfere in the serum based test assay. Serum dilution can rule out this phenomenon.

After normal delivery

Low levels of hCG have been found in the maternal circulation after a normal delivery. However, persistence of low hCG levels may indicate an underlying pathological condition such as retained pieces of the placenta.

How do procedural errors affect Rapid Diagnostic Tests? Improper storage conditions

As recommended in the manufacturers pack insert, all reagents should be stored at the recommended temperature 2-30°C. Exposing the reagents to excess freeze-thaw can result in deterioration of the detector and capture antibodies, leading to invalid results.

Procedural Errors

All specimens/reagents should be brought to room temperature prior to testing. In Rapid Diagnostic pregnancy Tests, the reaction time between antigen and antibody is short (5 to 15 minutes), thus the sensitivity of the test assay depends upon the temperature of the assay. As such, the antigen-antibody reactions are optimized at RT Hence it is important that the device/dipstick be brought to RT prior to testing.

Dropper and Drop Size

Always use the droppers provided with the kit to dispense the sample specimen while performing the test. Secondly, it is important to hold the dropper vertically straight, perpendicular to the sample pad/ sample dispensing port. Variation in the force required to dispense the liquid and the angle at which the dropper is held leads to variations in the drop size. This may affect the sensitivity of the test assay, especially in borderline samples. It is important that exactly the recommended drop size should be used for correct assay performance.

Excess Sample Volume Dispensed

Adding excess sample in no way improves the performance of the test. The excess sample added, cannot be absorbed by the sample pad and thus flows out through the sides of the device. Sometimes, the excess sample may flow out along with the conjugate. The amount of the conjugate left in the device is insufficient to perform the assay, leading to invalid results. Secondly, once the specimen flows through the device, the soak pad cannot retain the excess volume of the sample, which then may flow out through the sides of the device or may also flow back to the membrane along with unreacted/ unbound conjugate. This unreacted/unbound conjugate may then deposit onto the membrane resulting in apparently discrepant results.

Damage in Packing

Check the device/dipstick pouch for pinholes and observe any colour change in the desiccant (should be bluish). Once opened, the test is to be performed immediately. Prolonged exposure of the nitrocellulose membrane to the surroundings can lead to absorption of moisture. The water molecules fill up the pores preventing sample-detector reagent flow, through the device/dipstick.

Reading results at the recommended time

Since the test band completion in an immuno-chromatographic test is based on the membrane capillary action, the detector-analyte complex travels onto the test (capture) band. In routine, depending upon the analyte concentration the test band formation starts rapidly enough. However when borderline concentration at the limit of assay sensitivity are encountered, the test band appearance is delayed. Sometimes to the extent of reaching the time of completion of the test itself. It is thus recommended to retest such samples subsequently by recollecting the sample instead of reporting the results based on reading the test beyond the recommended assay time.

Understanding the limitations of rapid diagnostic test, sample and procedure related limitations, would aid the laboratory personnel minimize erroneous reporting and trouble shoot confidently for confident result reporting.

DIPSTICK ICT PREGNANCY TEST (CLUE FROM ORCHID BIOMEDICAL SYSTEMS)

Clue one step pregnancy test is a rapid, self-performing, qualitative, two-site sandwich immunoassay for the determination of human chorionic gonadotrophin (hCG), a marker for pregnancy, in urine specimens.

Summary

Human chorionic gonadotrophin (hCG), a glycoprotein hormone secreted by viable placental tissue during pregnancy, is excreted in urine approximately 20 days after the last menstrual period. The levels of hCG rise rapidly reaching peak levels after 60 to 80 days.

The appearance of hCG in urine soon after conception and its rapid rise in concentration makes it an ideal marker for the early detection and confirmation of pregnancy. However elevated hCG levels are frequently associated with trophoblastic and non-trophoblastic neoplasms and hence these conditions should be considered before a diagnosis of pregnancy can be made.

Clue one step pregnancy test detects the presence of hCG in urine specimens, qualitatively, at concentrations as low as 10 mIU/ml in less than five minutes.

Principle

Clue on step pregnancy test utilizes the principle of Immunochromatography, a unique two site immunoassay on a membrane. As the test sample flows through the membrane assembly of the dipstick, the coloured anti-hCG-colloidal gold conjugate complexes with the hCG in the sample. This complex moves further on the membrane to the test region where it is immobilized by the anti-hCG coated on the membrane leading to formation of a pink-coloured-band which confirms a .positive test result. Absence of this coloured-band in the test region indicates a negative test result. The unreacted conjugate and unbound complex if any move further on the membrane and are subsequently immobilized by the anti-mouse antibodies coated on the membrane at the control region, forming a pink band. This control band serves to validate the test results.

REAGENTS AND MATERIALS SUPPLIED

Each individual pouch contains :

1. Dipstick: Membrane assembly predispensed with anti-hCG antiserum-colloidal gold conjugate and anti-hCG antiserum and anti-mouse antiserum at the respective regions.
2. Desiccant pouch.

Storage and Stability

The sealed pouches in the test kit may be stored between 4-30°C till the duration of the shelf life as indicated on the pouch.

Note

1. For *in vitro* diagnostic use only. Not for medicinal use.
2. Do not use beyond expiry date.

Specimen Collection and Preparation

Though random urine specimens can be used, first morning urine specimen is preferable as it contains the highest concentration of hCG. Specimens should be collected in clean glass or plastic containers. If testing is not immediate, the urine specimens may be stored at 2-8°C for up to 72 hours. Turbid specimens should be centrifuged or allowed to settle and only the clear supernatant should be used for testing.

Test Procedure and Interpretation of Results

1. Collect urine specimen in a clean test tube. Ensure that only sufficient quantity of the specimen is collected to allow submerging the red area of the dipstick (About 1 cm high).
2. Bring the sealed pouch to room temperature, open the pouch and remove the dipstick. Once opened, the dipstick must be used immediately.
3. Dip the red area of the dipstick in the urine specimen submerging only the red area.
4. Observe for the release of the colloidal gold complex on the membrane. This would be seen as a pink moving front on the membrane and could take 10 to 15 seconds to appear depending upon the sample.
5. Remove the dipstick and place horizontally on a flat surface. Alternatively the dipstick may be left to stand in the specimen for the entire duration of the test ensuring only the red area is left submerged in the specimen.
6. At the end of five minutes read the results as follows:

   Negative: Only one pink-coloured-band appears on the dipstick.

   Positive: Two distinct pink-coloured bands appear on the dipstick.
7. The test should be considered invalid if neither the test band nor the control band appears. Repeat the test with a new dipstick ensuring sufficient dip time as mentioned in point no. 4.

Limitation of the Test

1. A number of conditions other than pregnancy including trophoblastic and non-trophoblastic neoplasms such as hydatidiform mole, choriocarcinoma, etc. cause elevated levels of hCG. Such clinical conditions must be ruled out before diagnosis of pregnancy can be made.
2. Highly dilute urine specimens and specimens from very early pregnancy may not contain representative levels of hCG. If pregnancy is still suspected, repeat the test with first morning urine after 48-72 hours.
3. As with all diagnostic tests, the results must be correlated with clinical findings.

PERFORMANCE CHARACTERISTICS

1. Sensitivity

Clue one step pregnancy test detects the presence of hCG in urine specimens, qualitatively, at concentrations as low as 10 mlU/ml. Concentrations of about 100 mlU/ml of hCG are reached by the first day of the missed menstrual period in normal pregnancy. Thus **clue** one step pregnancy test is able to detect pregnancy at very early stages.

2. Specificity

Healthy men and healthy non-pregnant women do not have detectable levels of hCG by **clue** one step pregnancy test. Homologous hormones and other potentially interfering substances spiked beyond peak physiological concentrations did not cross react with **clue** one step pregnancy test.

3. Accuracy

The results obtained by **clue** one step pregnancy test correlated very well when run in parallel with other commercially available tests for pregnancy, using known positive and negative specimens.

DEVICE ICT PREGNANCY TEST (CLUE, FROM ORCHID BIOMEDICAL SYSTEMS)

Introduction

Clue one step pregnancy test is a rapid, self-performing, qualitative, two site sandwich immunoassay for the determination of human chorionic gonadotrophin (hCG), a marker for pregnancy, in urine specimens.

Summary

Human chorionic gonadotrophin (hCG), a glycoprotein hormone secreted by viable placental tissue during pregnancy, is excreted in urine approximately 20 days after the last menstrual period. The levels of hCG rise rapidly reaching peak levels after 60 to 80 days.

The appearance of hCG in urine soon after conception and its rapid rise in concentration makes it an ideal marker for the early detection and confirmation of pregnancy. However elevated hCG levels are frequently associated with trophoblastic and non-trophoblastic neoplasms and hence these conditions should be considered before a diagnosis of pregnancy can be made clue one step pregnancy test detects the presence of hCG in urine specimens, qualitatively, at concentrations as low as 10 mlU/ml in less than five minutes.

Clue: One step pregnancy test detects the presence of hCG in urine specimens qualitatively at concentrations as low as to ml U/ml in less than five months.

Principle

Clue one step pregnancy test utilizes the principle of Immunochromatography, a unique two site immunoassay on a membrane. As the test sample flows through the membrane assembly within the test device, the coloured anti-hCG-colloidal gold conjugate complexes with the hCG in the sample. This complex moves further on the membrane to the test region where it is immobilized by the anti-hCG coated on the membrane leading to formation of a pink-coloured-band which confirms a positive test result. Absence of this coloured-band in the test region indicates a negative test result. The unreacted conjugate and unbound complex if any move further on the membrane and are subsequently immobilized by the anti-mouse antibodies coated on the membrane at the control region, forming a pink band. This control band serves to validate the test results.

REAGENTS AND MATERIALS SUPPLIED

Each individual pouch contains :

1. Test device: Contains membrane assembly predispensed with anti-hCG antiserum-colloidal gold conjugate and anti-hCG antiserum and anti-mouse antiserum at the respective regions.
2. Disposable plastic dropper.
3. Desiccant pouch.

Storage and Stability

The sealed pouches in the test kit may be stored between 4-30°C till the duration of the shelf life as indicated on the pouch.

Note

1. For *in vitro* diagnostic use only. Not for medicinal use.
2. Do not use beyond expiry date.

Specimen Collection and Preparation

Though random urine specimens can be used, first morning urine specimen is preferable as it contains the highest concentration of hCG. Specimens should be collected in clean glass or plastic containers. If testing is not immediate, the urine specimens may be stored at 2-8°C for up to 72 hours. Turbid specimens should be centrifuged or allowed to settle and only the clear supernatant should be used for testing.

Test Procedure and Interpretation of Results

1. Bring the sealed pouch to room temperature, open the pouch and remove the device. Once opened, the device must be used immediately.
2. Dispense two drops of urine specimen into the sample well'S' using the dropper provided. Refrigerated specimens must be brought to room temperature prior to testing.
3. At the end of five minutes read the results as follows:

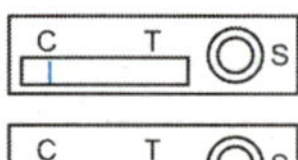

Negative: Only one coloured-band appears on the control region 'C'.

Positive: In addition to the control bands, a distinct coloured-band also appears on the test region T.

4. The test should be considered invalid if neither the test band nor the control band appear. *Repeat the test with a new device.*
5. Although, depending on the concentration of hCG in the specimen, positive results may start appearing as early as 30 seconds, negative results must be confirmed only at the end of five minutes.

Limitation of Tests

1. A number of conditions other than pregnancy including trophoblastic and non-trophoblastic neoplasms such as hydatid form mole, choriocarcinoma, etc. cause elevated levels of hCG. Such clinical conditions must be ruled out before a diagnosis of pregnancy can be made.
2. Highly dilute urine specimens and specimens from very early pregnancy may not contain representative levels of hCG. If pregnancy is still suspected, repeat the test with first morning urine after 48-72 hours.
3. As with all diagnostic tests, the results must be correlated with clinical findings.

PERFORMANCE CHARACTERISTICS

1. Sensitivity

Clue one step pregnancy test detects the presence of hCG in urine specimens, qualitatively, at concentrations as low as 10 ml Ul/ml. Concentrations of about 100 mlU/ml of hCG are reached by the first day of the missed menstrual period in normal pregnancy. Thus **clue** one step pregnancy test is able to detect pregnancy at very early stages.

2. Specificity

Healthy men and healthy non-pregnant women do not have detectable levels of hCG by **clue** one step pregnancy test. Homologous hormones and other potentially interfering substances spiked beyond peak physiological concentrations did not cross react with **clue** one step pregnancy test.

3. Accuracy

The results obtained by **clue** one step pregnancy test correlated very well when run in parallel with other commercially available tests for pregnancy, using known positive and negative specimens.

ICT TECHNIQUES FOR URINE/SERUM SAMPLE

For routine pregnancy testing, urine is the most preferred specimen, requiring no specialized skills for collection, processing and storage. However, during problem pregnancies and bad obstetrics cases, levels of hCG in urine are very low. Due to factors such as fluid intake, time of collection of specimen, urine may not contain representable amounts of hCG, thereby affecting the sensitivity of membrane-based one step assays.

ADVANTAGES OF SERUM TESTING

- During normal pregnancies, hCG is present as an intact molecule in maternal serum.
- Serum hCG levels can be detected within 24 hours post-implantation
- Serum specimens facilities early pregnancy detection.
- hCG is uniformly distributed in serum and is not affected by fluid intake and can be collected at any time of the day.
- hCG is a very stable molecule when stored in serum.

DIPSTICK ICT, URINE/SERUM PREGNANCY TEST (GRAVI CHECK FROM ORCHID BIOMEDICAL SYSTEMS)

Introduction

Gravi Check, One Step Pregnancy Test is a rapid, self-performing, qualitative, two site sandwich immunoassay for the/ruination of human Chorionic Gonadotrophin (hCG), a marker for pregnancy, in urine/serum specimens.

Summary

Human Chorionic Gonadotrophin (hCG), a glycoprotein hormone is secreted by viable placental tissue during pregnancy. The appearance of hCG in urine/serum soon after conception and its rapid rise in concentration makes it an ideal marker for the early detection and confirmation of pregnancy. However elevated hCG levels are frequently associated with trophoblastic and non-trophoblastic neoplasms and hence these conditions should be considered before a diagnosis of pregnancy can be made.

Gravi Check

One Step Pregnancy Test detects the presence of hCG in urine/serum specimens, qualitatively, at concentrations as low as 10 mlU/ml.

Principle

Gravi Check, One Step Pregnancy Test utilizes the principle of **Immunochromatography**, a unique two site immunoassay on a membrane. As the test sample flows through the membrane assembly of the dipstick, the coloured anti-hCG-colloidal gold conjugate complexes with the hCG in the sample. This complex moves further on the membrane to the test region where it is immobilised by the anti-hCG coated on the membrane leading to formation of a coloured-band which confirms a positive test result. Absence of this coloured-band in the test region indicates a negative test result. The unreacted conjugate and unbound complex if any move further on the membrane and are subsequently immobilised by the anti-rabbit antibodies coated on the membrane at the control region, forming a coloured band. This control band serves to validate the test results.

Reagents and Materials Supplied

Each individual pouch contains:

1. Test dipstick: Comprising of membrane assembly predispensed with anti-hCG antisera-colloidal gold conjugate, rabbit IgG colloidal gold conjugate and anti-hCG antiserum and anti-rabbit antiserum at the respective regions.
2. Desiccant pouch.

Storage and Stability

The sealed pouches in the test kit may be stored between 4-30°C till the duration of the shelf life as indicated on the pouch.

Note

1. For *in vitro* diagnostic use only. *NOT FOR MEDICINAL USE.*
2. Do not use beyond expiry date.

SPECIMEN COLLECTION AND PREPARATION

Urine as Sample

Though random urine specimens can be used, first morning urine specimen is preferable as it contains the highest concentration of hCG. Specimens should be collected in clean glass or plastic containers. If testing is not immediate, the urine specimens may be stored at 2-8°C for up to 72 hours. Turbid specimens should be centrifuged or allowed to settle and only the clear supernatant should be used for testing.

Serum as Sample

No special preparation of the patient is necessary prior to specimen collection by approved techniques. Though fresh serum is preferable, serum specimens may be stored at 2-8°C for up to 24 hours, in case of delay in testing. Do not use hemolysed or contaminated specimens. Turbid specimens should be centrifuged or allowed to settle and only the clear supernatant should be used for testing.

TEST PROCEDURE AND INTERPRETATION OF RESULTS

1. Collect urine/serum specimen in a clean test tube. Ensure that only sufficient quantity of the specimen is collected to allow submerging the orange area of the dipstick (About 1 cm high).

2. Bring the sealed pouch to room temperature, open the pouch and remove the dipstick. Once opened, the dipstick must be used immediately.
3. Dip the orange area of the dipstick in the urine/ serum specimen submerging only the orange area.
4. For urine samples: Dip the dipstick in the urine sample for 10-15 seconds and place horizontally on a flat surface. Alternatively the dipstick may be left to stand in the specimen for the entire duration of the test ensuring only the orange area is left submerged in the specimen. **At the end of five minutes**, read the results as overleaf. For serum samples: Leave the dipstick in the specimen for entire duration of the test ensuring only the ora) submerged in the specimen. Read the results **at the end of fifteen minutes** as follows:

   Negative: Only one coloured-band appears on the dipstick.

   Positive: Two distinct coloured bands appear on the dipstick.
5. The test should be considered invalid if neither the test band nor the control band appears. Repeat the test with a new dipstick ensuring sufficient dip time.

Limitations of the Test

1. A number of conditions other than pregnancy including trophoblastic and non-trophoblastic neoplasms such as hydatidiform mole, chorio-carcinoma, etc. cause elevated levels of hCG. Such clinical conditions must be ruled out before a diagnosis of pregnancy can be made.
2. Highly dilute urine specimens and specimens from very early pregnancy may not contain representative levels of hCG. If pregnancy is still suspected, repeat the test with first morning urine after 48-72 hours after the initial test.
3. As with any assay employing animal antibodies, presence of cross-reacting heterophilic anti-bodies may yield discrepant results.
4. As with all diagnostic tests, the results must be correlated with clinical findings.

PERFORMANCE CHARACTERISTICS

1. Sensitivity

Gravi Check, One Step Pregnancy Test detects the presence of hCG in urine/serum specimens, qualitatively, at concentrations as low as 10 mlU/ml. Concentrations of about 100 mlU/ml of hCG are reached by the first missed menstrual period in normal pregnancy. Thus **Gravi Check,** One Step Pregnancy Test is able to detect pregnancy at very early stages.

2. Specificity

Healthy men and healthy non-pregnant women do not have detectable levels of hCG by the One Step Pregnancy Test. Homologous hormones and other potentially interfering substances spiked beyond peak physiological concentrations did not cross react with **Gravi Check** , One Step Pregnancy Test.

3. Accuracy

The results obtained by **Gravi Check,** One Step Pregnancy Test correlated very well when run in parallel with other commercially available tests for pregnancy, using known positive and negative specimens.

DEVICE ICT URINE/SERUM PREGNANCY TEST (GRAVI CHECK FROM ORCHID BIOMEDICAL SYSTEMS)

Introduction

Gravi Check, One Step Pregnancy Test is a rapid, self-performing, qualitative, two sites sandwich immunoassay for the determination of human Chorionic Gonadotrophin (hCG), a marker for pregnancy, in urine/serum specimens.

Summary

Human Chorionic Gonadotrophin (hCG), a glycoprotein hormone is secreted by viable placental tissue during pregnancy. The appearance of hCG in urine/serum soon after conception and its rapid rise in concentration makes it an ideal marker for the early detection and confirmation of pregnancy. However elevated hCG levels are frequently associated with trophoblastic and non-trophoblastic neoplasms and hence these conditions should be considered before a diagnosis of pregnancy can be made.

Gravi Check, One Step Pregnancy Test detects the presence of hCG in urine/serum specimens, qualitatively, at concentrations as low as 10 ml U/ml.

Principle

Gravi Check, One Step Pregnancy Test utilises the principle of Immunochromatography, a unique two site immunoassay on a membrane. As the test sample flows through the membrane assembly of the device, the coloured anti-hCG-colloidal gold conjugate complexes with the hCG in the sample. This complex moves further on the membrane to the test region where it is immobilised by the anti-hCG coated on the membrane leading to formation of a coloured-band which confirms a positive test result. Absence of this coloured-band in the test region indicates a negative test result. The unreacted conjugate and unbound complex if any move further on the membrane and are subsequently immobilised by the anti-rabbit antibodies coated on the membrane at the control region, forming a coloured band. This control band serves to validate the test results.

Reagents and Materials Supplied

Each individual pouch contains:

1. Test device: Comprising of membrane assembly predispensed with anti-hCG antisera - colloidal gold conjugate, rabbit IgG colloidal gold conjugate and anti-hCG antiserum and anti-rabbit antiserum at the respective regions.
2. Disposable plastic dropper
3. Desiccant pouch.

Storage and Stability

The sealed pouches in the test kit may be stored between 4-30°C till the duration of the shelf life as indicated on the pouch.

Note

1. For *in vitro* diagnostic use only. *NOT FOR MEDICINAL USE.*
2. Do not use beyond expiry date.

SPECIMEN COLLECTION AND PREPARATION

Urine as Sample

Though random urine specimens can be used, first morning urine specimen is preferable as it contains the highest concentration of hCG. Specimens should be collected in clean glass or plastic containers. If testing is not immediate, the urine specimens may be stored at 2-8°C for up to 72 hours. Turbid specimens should be centrifuged or allowed to settle and only the clear supernatant should be used for testing.

Serum as Sample

No special preparation of the patient is necessary prior to specimen collection by approved techniques. Though fresh serum is preferable, serum specimens may be stored at 2-8°C for up to 24 hours, in case of delay in testing. Do not use hemolysed or contaminated specimens. Turbid specimens should be centrifuged or allowed to settle and only the clear supernatant should be used for testing.

Test procedure and Interpretation of Results

1. *Bring the sealed pouch to room temperature,* open the pouch and remove the device. Once *opened, the device must be used immediately.*
2. Dispense two drops of urine/serum specimen into the sample well 'S' using the dropper provided. Refrigerated specimens must be brought to room temperature prior to testing.
3. Read the results **at the end of five minutes** for urine samples and **at the end of fifteen minutes** for serum samples as follows:

   C T S **Negative:** Only one coloured-band appears on the control region 'C'.

   C T S **Positive:** In addition to the control band, a distinct coloured-band also appears on the test region.
4. The test should be considered invalid if no band appears. Repeat the test with a new device.
5. Although, depending on the concentration of hCG in the specimen, positive results may start appearing as early as 30 to 60 seconds, negative results must be confirmed only at the end of the stipulated time.

Limitation of the Test

1. A number of conditions other than pregnancy including trophoblastic and non-trophoblastic neoplasms such as hydatidiform mole, choriocarcinoma etc. cause elevated levels of hCG. Such clinical conditions must be ruled out before a diagnosis of pregnancy can be made.
2. Highly dilute urine specimens and specimens from very early pregnancy may not contain representative levels of hCG. If pregnancy is still suspected, repeat the test with first morning urine after 48-72 hours after the initial test.

3. As with any assay employing animal antibodies, presence of cross-reacting heterophilic antibodies may yield discrepant results.
4. As with all diagnostic tests, the results must be correlated with clinical findings.

PERFORMANCE CHARACTERISTICS

1. Sensitivity

Gravi Check, One Step Pregnancy Test detects the presence of hCG in urine/serum specimens, qualitatively, at concentrations as low as 10 ml U/ml. Concentrations of about 100 mIU/ml of hCG are reached by the first missed menstrual period in normal pregnancy. Thus **Gravi Check**, One Step Pregnancy Test is able to detect pregnancy at very early stages.

2. Specificity

Normally, healthy men and healthy non-pregnant women do not have detectable levels of hCG by **Gravi Check**, One Step Pregnancy Test. Homologous hormones and other potentially interfering substances spiked beyond peak physiological concentrations did not cross react with **Gravi Check**, One Step Pregnancy Test.

Accuracy: The results obtained by **Gravi Check**, One Step Pregnancy Test correlated very well when run in parallel with other commercially available tests for pregnancy, using known positive and negative specimens.

ALTERED LABORATORY RESULTS IN NORMAL PREGNANCY

Test	*Alteration*	*Demonstrated or possible reason*
Hematology		
Hb	Falls but not lower than 11 gm%	Plasma volume expands more than RBC mass
WBC	Mild neutrophilia; no lymphocytosis	Similar response seen in stress, strenuous exercise
Platelets	Slight decrease or no change	Plasma volume expansion
Reticulocytes	Rise to 2-5%	Need to increase RBC mass
Blood volume	Rises by 40-50%	Increase in plasma and red cells
Serum iron	Falls modestly, even if stores are adequate	Loss to foetal blood supply; Increased plasma volume; Supplementation is desirable
Iron binding capacity	Increases	Estrogen—induced increase in Protein synthesis
Folate levels	Serum concentration falls; RBC concentration should be constant	Foetal use; estrogen associated folate block. Supplementation desirable
ESR	Increases markedly	Elevated fibrinogen levels
Coagulation		
Fibrinogen	Rises about 50%	? Acute phase reaction
PT & PTT	Normal or slightly shortened	Increased factor levels affect tests relatively little
Plasminogen	Increases	?
Antithrombin III	Decreases moderately	Comparable effect seen with therapy
Fibrin degradation products	Increased slightly	? Effect of increased plasminogen and decreased antithrombin III ? Effect of fibrin deposition in placenta

Contd...

Contd...

Chemistry		
Serum albumin	Decreases by as much as 1 gm%	Increased degradation, hemodilution
Immunoglobulins	Ig G, Ig A drop	? degradation ? Altered immunologic responsiveness
Serum alkaline phosphatase	↑ by 200-300%	Placental alkaline phosphatase in serum
Serum cholesterol	↑ 30-40%	? Effect of placental hormones
Serum free fatty acids	↑ 50-60%	? Effects of placental hormones, altered insulin reactivity
Serum creatinine	↓	Hemodilution; ↑ Glomerular filtration rate (G F R)
Plasma bicarbonate	↓ 10-15%	Compensation for chronic hyperventilation
Urine glucose	Mild glycosuria with normal blood sugar levels	Lowered renal threshold
Renal function	GFR increases, Concentrating capacity ↓	Mobilization of retained fluid
Endocrine		
Thyroid Total & Free T_4 Total & free T_3	↑ and normal respectively ↑ and normal respectively	
ACTH	Markedly ↓ in early months	?
Serum total cortisol	↑	Estrogen—associated rise in binding protein
Serum testosterone	↑	? ↑ ovarian synthesis
Parathormone	↑	?
Aldosterone	Progressive ↑	Altered plasma volume, renal sodium load
Renin—angiotensin	↑ in latter half	With ↑ Na or ↑ blood pressure, level decreases.

Chapter 16

Examination of Gastrointestinal Contents

NORMAL SALIVA—CONSTITUENTS

Constituents

Volume secreted/24 hours	1000–1500 ml
pH	6.3 to 6.85
pH in mouth is usually	7.5-8.0
Specific gravity	1.002 to 1.008
Total solids	0.5 gm%
Sodium	17.4 (8.7 to 24) mEq/L
Potassium	14.1 (13-16) mEq/L

Gastric Constituents

Digestive enzymes/factors

Pepsin and hydrochloric acid (for protein digestion).

Renin for curdling milk, and gastric lipase—a weak lipolytic ferment.

Normal Gastric Constituents in Infants and Children

The stomach of neonates secretes small amounts of pepsin, renin, and free acid. Almost 4% of otherwise normal children have achlorhydria, this percentage gradually rises with age (30% have achlorhydria at age 60 years and above). During the first year of life, the volume of the residuum is 2-5 ml (pH = 2.6-3.0). Both these rise to adult levels at 15-20 years of age.

Abnormal Gastric Constituents

These may include the following:

1. Blood: An important abnormal finding.
2. Food remnants many hours after eating.
3. Large amounts of mucous or bile.
4. Sarcinae, pyogenic bacteria, lactobacilli, yeast cells.
5. Tissue fragments, large amounts of epithelium.
6. Parasites and ova.
7. Organic acids, e.g. lactic acid, seen in absence of hydrochloric acid.
8. Tubercle bacilli, in pulmonary tuberculosis, by swallowing of sputum containing *Mycobacterium tuberculosis.*

ROUTINE GASTRIC JUICE EXAMINATION

Gross Examination

1. *Amount:* Normal fasting content is 50-100 ml.
2. *Colour:*
   a. Blood is red or the colour of coffee ground if acid haematin is formed.
   b. Fresh bile is yellow; old bile is green.
   c. In stasis, food colours may persist.
3. *Odour:*
   a. Normal is sour or slightly rancid.
   b. Faecal in intestinal obstruction.
   c. Ammoniacal in uraemia
4. *Character:* Let stand, note the three layers:
   a. Top—Mucous
   b. Middle—Opalescent fluid
   c. Bottom—Bread-like residue.
5. *Reaction:* Acidic—normal pH.
6. *Rate of secretion:*
   a. Mean values for basal rate of secretion of acid

Age (years)	*mEq/L*
20-49	2.5
50-59	2.0
> 60	1.5

   b. Mean values for 12-hour nocturnal secretion in a normal person
      Volume—580 ml
      Free acid—29 mEq/L or
      16.85 mEq/12 hours.

Chemical Examination

1. *Blood:* May be due to one of the causes of haematemesis, or may be due to trauma of passing a tube. Do guaiac or benzidine tests.
2. *Qualitative test for free HCI (Topfer's test):* To 5 drops of gastric juice in evaporating dish, add 1 or 2 drops of 0.5% alcoholic solution of dimethylaminoazobenzene (Topfer's reagent). Cherry-red colour occurs with HCl.

NORMAL GASTRIC CONSTITUENTS IN ADULTS

Constituents	*Normal residuum*	*Appetite juice (post seeing/ smelling/ tasting of food)*
Water (%)	99.02	99.45
Total solids (%)	0.98	0.55
Organic solids (%)	0.53	0.41
Inorganic solids (%)	0.45	0.14
Specific gravity	1.006-1.009	1.007
pH	0.9-1.5	0.9-1.5
Total acidity (mEq/L)	10-50	20-100
Free HCI (mEq/L)	0-30	25-50
Chlorides (g%)	0.5-0.6	
Total nitrogen (avg: 66 mg%)	51-75	
NPN	20-30	
Urea nitrogen (in mg%)	1.3-4	
Total sulphur (in mg%)	7	
Total phosphorus (in mg%)	5	5
Amino acid N (in mg%)	3-9	3-9
Ammonia N (in mg%)	2-3	2-3

3. *Titration for Acid*

   Method

   Transfer 5 ml of gastric juice to an evaporating dish add 20 ml water. Add 3 drops of Topfer's reagent and 3 drops of phenolphthalein, and titrate with N/10 NaOH until the last trace of red colour disappears. This is the amount of NaOH needed to neutralise the free HCI—this value multiplied by 20 equals the mEq/L of free HCl. Carry on titrating until red colour of phenolphthalein reappears. The total number of ml of NaOH used (in both titrations) multiplied by 20 equals the mEq/L of total acidity.

   Comments

   In the fasting state, gastric contents ordinarily contain 0-15% HCl. For gastric juice, the maximum concentration of HCl is about 0.160 or 160 mEq of HCl/L. The free rather than total acid primarily determines the pH, which usually varies in fasting contents from 2.0-1.0, and this pH range corresponds to an HCl normality (normality = mEq/L/1000) of about 0.05–0.10. If the normality drops to 0.01 or so, the pH may be about 3.0, and it takes very little amount of food or any other diluent to bring the pH to 7.0.

4. *Lactic acid (Kelling's Test):* Seen usually in achlorhydria only. Add 2 drops of 10% ferric chloride to one test tube full of water, mix, and divide into 2 test tubes. Add 1 ml of gastric juice to one tube and compare. Lactic acid gives canary yellow colour. Much lactic acid (over 0.1%) suggests gastric carcinoma.

Microscopic Examination

Place one drop of sediment on a slide and coverslip it. Look for undigested food particles, blood, mucous, bacteria, tissue fragments, parasites, sarcinae, yeasts. Lactobacilli are large nonmotile rods which stain brown with Gram's stain and form lactic acid, they occur in stasis in the absence of HCl.

Exfoliative cytologic preparations of fresh gastric washings should be used in the search for gastric neoplasms.

GASTRIC TEST MEALS

Procedures

If the test is to be performed in the morning, give nothing orally after supper the previous night.

Tubeless Gastric Analysis

This test employs azure-A resin as the indicator (Diagnex Blue Test).

Azure-A carbacrylic resin dissociates in the presence of acid to yield free azure A, which is then excreted in the urine. In the absence of free acid in the stomach, no azure-A will be released and hence none will appear in the urine.

The test meal consists of caffeine with sodium benzoate to stimulate gastric secretion and azure-A resin granules as the indicator substance. Urine is analysed for azure-A by a simple colorimetric method. On getting up in the morning, urine is micturated and discarded. Nil orally till the completion of the test. The gastric stimulant, either 500 mg caffeine sodium benzoate or 50 mg Histalog is taken with a glass of water or else histamine or Histalog can be administered subcutaneously. One hour later, patient urinates and discards the sample. Immediately thereafter, 2 gm of azuresin are ingested with half glass of water. Two hours later, the patient urinates and saves the entire sample. The sample is diluted to 300 ml with water and a 10 ml aliquot is placed in each of 3 test tubes. Two of the tubes serve as colour controls and to each of these approximately 300 mg of L-ascorbic acid is added. This reduces the azure-A to a colourless form. The tubes are then placed in a comparator block containing azure-A standards of 0.3 mg/300 ml and 0.6 mg/300 ml. If the colour of the test urine is more intense than that of 0.6 mg standard, the test is completed and the patient is presumed to secrete hydrochloric acid. If the colour of the test urine is less than that of 0.6 mg standard, a drop of solution containing 195 mg $CuSO_4 \cdot 5H_2O$ in 100 ml of 18% HCl (Diagnex blue reagent) is added to each of the three urine tubes. All 3 tubes are placed in a boiling water bath for 10 minutes. After cooling at room temperature for 2 hours, the colour development is again compared to the standard solutions. The results are reported as less than 0.3 mg, to 0.6 mg, or greater than 0.6 mg.

Interpretation

This is strictly a qualitative test. An excretion of greater than 0.6 mg azure-A in 2 hours is considered to be indicative of HCl secretion, while values less than 0.3 mg are considered presumptive evidence of anacidity. Values between 0.3 and 0.6 mg represent borderline secretion.

Basal Gastric Secretion

This represents the response of the stomach to endogenous stimuli which are continually present in the interdigestive or fasting state.

The minimum requirements include the following:
1. The patient must be in the fasting state and free from the sight or odour of food.
2. All medications influencing gastric secretion must be withheld for 24 hours.
3. The patient must be removed from environmental situations evoking untoward psychological reactions such as fear, anger, or depression.

The 1 hour morning aspiration has replaced the cumbersome and inherently less precise 12-hour nocturnal aspiration.

Method

1. Following a 12-hour overnight fast, the patient is intubated. Water may be taken until 8 hours prior to intubation.
2. The residual volume of gastric secretion is measured and qualitatively examined.
3. Continuous aspiration is begun, preferably manually with a syringe. Segregate the aspirate into 15-minute samples. Usually, the first 1 or 2 samples are discarded to allow the patient to adjust to the intubation procedure. Subsequent to this adjustment period, four 15-minute samples are taken.
4. If the basal secretion study is to be followed by the augmented histamine test, a suitable dose of antihistamine be given parenterally 30 minutes before completing the collection of basal secretion.
5. For each 15 minutes sample, the volume, pH, and titrable acidity are measured and the acid output calculated. The sum of the acid outputs in the 4 samples, expressed in milliequivalents, represents the 1-hour basal acid output.

Interpretation

The mean basal acid output reported for normal males ranges from 1.3 to 4.0 mEq/hour. Lower values occur in females and with ageing. Somewhat lower values are reported in most large series for gastric carcinoma and benign gastric ulcer and distinctively higher values for duodenal ulcer or jejunal ulcer following partial gastrectomy with gastrojejunostomy. Extremely high acid output is present in patients with the Zollinger-Ellison syndrome.

Augmented Histamine Test (AHT)

A dose of 0.04 mg per kg body weight is the optimum dosage that can be given, and any further increase in dosage does not increase the gastric acid output. All parietal cells capable of acid secretion are stimulated by histamine, functioning parietal cell mass. The AHT or the analogous Histalog test are now established as definitive tests for the diagnosis of anacidity.

The side effects of histamine are overcome by previous administration of antihistamine. A history of bronchial asthma or urticaria, the presence of severe cardiac, pulmonary or renal disease and paroxysmal hypertension or other possible signs and symptoms of phaeochromocytoma are contraindications to the performance of this test.

Method

1. Following a 12-hour fast, basal secretion is collected for 1 hour as previously described.
2. Thirty minutes before completion of the basal secretion collection, a suitable dose of antihistamine is given I/M, e.g. 10 mg chlorpheniramine maleate or 50 mg diphenhydramine hydrochloride.
3. After the conclusion of the basal secretion study, histamine acid phosphate is administered subcutaneously in a dose of 0.04 mg per kg body weight.
4. Gastric contents are then collected in 15 minute samples for 1 hour.
5. The volume, pH and titrable acidity are measured for each sample and the acid output is calculated. From these, the 1-hour or maximal acid output in mEq is computed.

Interpretation

The maximum rate of acid secretion is characteristically attained within 15 minutes after histamine injection and is maintained for approximately 30 minutes. By 60 minutes after histamine injection, acid secretion usually falls to the basal level. The maximum output, representing the sum of the acid.

The upper limit of normal is 30 mEq HCl secreted in the 30-minute period between 15 and 45 minutes after the histamine injection. Values higher than the stated upper normal limit are usually found in duodenal ulcer and Zollinger-Ellison syndrome. Anacidity in the augmented histamine test is most commonly found in adults with pernicious anaemia or gastric carcinoma, it has also been reported in other conditions, e.g. hypochromic anaemia, rheumatoid arthritis, steatorrhoea, aplastic anaemia, myxoedema, nutritional megaloblastic anaemia and the asymptomatic relatives of patients with pernicious anemia.

The basal and AHT are used as determining factors for gastrectomy or vagotomy. It has been suggested that an increased functioning parietal cell mass evidenced by an elevated maximal acid output indicates the need for gastric resection. Whereas, raised basal secretion with normal or only slightly elevated maximal secretion is taken as an indication for vagotomy.

Histamine Infusion Test

The use of a slow I/V infusion of histamine allows measurement of acid output in a sustained steady state.

Advantages

1. It obviates the need for doing both basal and augmented histamine tests
2. The greater acid output achieved in the sustained steady state facilitates the detection of low levels of acid output
3. This is a highly reproducible test and
4. The slow histamine infusion has lesser side effects.

Method

1. The patient is intubated following a 12-hour overnight fast.
2. A basal hour collection is obtained.
3. Thirty minutes before completion of the basal hour, a suitable dose of antihistamine is given intramuscularly.
4. After completion of the basal hour, an I/V infusion of histamine in physiologic saline is begun and the dose rate is adjusted to deliver 0.04 mg of histamine phosphate per kg body weight per hour.
5. The infusion is continued until four 15-minute steady state samples have been collected. The initiation of the steady state is evident from the plateau reached in volume output and usually requires about 30 to 45 minutes to obtain after the start of the infusion.
6. Each sample of the basal hour and steady state is analysed for volume, pH and titrable acidity.

Interpretation

The normal values of acid output in mEq/hour for males is 16 to 32 and for females 18-25. The values are markedly higher in duodenal ulcer patients.

Histalog Test

Histalog (3 β-aminoethyl pyrazole dihydrochloride, Betazole), an analogue of histamine can be used instead of histamine.

Advantage: Lesser side effects and obviation of the need to give antihistamine.

The augmented Histalog dosage is 1.7 mg/kg given I/M. The test is similar as AHT except that: (i) no antihistamine is needed, and (ii) eight instead of four 15-minute post-Histalog samples are collected.

The peak acid secretion in Histalog test is reached in the second to fifth 15-minute period. The peak secretory rate may last for 45 to 90 minutes.

Insulin Hypoglycaemia Test

Acid secretion is stimulated by hypoglycaemia caused by insulin administration. The major stimulus is transmitted via vagus nerve and can be removed by vagotomy.

Hypoglycaemic response—for about 30 minutes after insulin injection there is a slight depression of gastric secretion.

The predominant effect during the remainder of the first 2 hours consists of marked enhancement of gastric secretion.

The final effect is manifested after 2 hours and is also stimulatory to gastric secretion (the second phase is via the vagus and the third is humoral via the adrenocortical hormones—hence the second but not the third stage can be abolished by vagotomy).

Method

1. Following a 12-hour overnight fast the patient is intubated. A 2-hour basal secretion is obtained in 15-minute samples.

2. Blood samples for glucose estimation are obtained upon completion of the basal secretion study and at 30, 60 and 90 minutes after insulin injection.
3. Insulin is given I/V either at a fixed dosage of 15 or 20 units or at a calculated dosage of 0.20 units per kg of body weight (keep a 50 ml syringe filled with 50%-w/v-glucose solution readily available to counteract any serious hypoglycaemic effects).
4. Gastric secretion is collected in 15-minute samples for 2 hours after insulin.
5. For each basal and postinsulin gastric sample, the volume and titrable acidity are determined, and the acid output is computed.

Interpretation

This test is valid only if the blood glucose falls below 50 mg% at some point of the test, which will usually be 30 minutes after insulin administration. Validity of the test also depends upon the capability of the stomach to secrete hydrochloric acid. Hence if no acid is present in either the basal or postinsulin periods, it is necessary to perform an augmented histamine test in an attempt to evoke acid secretion. If the stomach is truely anacidic, no conclusion can be drawn regarding the completeness of vagotomy, but the question of simple peptic ulceration is then effectively excluded.

The patient can be considered completely vagotomised if the acid output in the greater of the two postinsulin hours is less than the greater of the two basal hours. Incomplete vagotomy is likely if the acid output in the 2-hour postinsulin period exceeds that of the 2-hour basal period by more than 0.5 mEq. Incomplete vagotomy is also suggested by an acid output of greater than 2 mEq in either basal hour. In incomplete vagotomy if acid output is elevated in the first postinsulin hour—the prognosis is bad in the sense that recurrence may occur; whereas, elevation in the second hour is less likely to be followed by a recurrence.

Gastrin Secretory Test

One mg of gastrin (prepared from gastric antra of Swine) per kg of body weight can be given subcutaneously or else a single 50 gm I/V injection can be given. Most subjects will show a maximum output beginning about 20 minutes after gastrin injection and will maintain this level of acid output for 20 to 40 minutes. The response is quite rapid with I/V administration, with peak levels occurring in 5 to 10 minutes.

Pentagastrin (a synthetic pentapeptide with gastrin nucleus) can be used instead of gastrin, the results are reproducible and without the side effects of histamine.

Miscellaneous Investigations

Mycobacterial culture: Individuals having pulmonary tuberculosis but cannot produce sputum or in children who cannot effectively expectorate, this method of aspirating and culturing the gastric contents is quite useful. It is essential that the gastric contents be collected in the early morning prior to eating or drinking and preferably immediately upon awakening before increased gastric motor activity has largely emptied its contents. The sample withdrawn should be immediately submitted for culturing.

Exfoliative cytology: For diagnosing gastric carcinomas—gastric cytology, gastroscopy and roentgenography—can be used, but the most discriminating information is provided by exfoliative cytology (chymotrypsin can be used to facilitate the exfoliation of cells by liquefying the mucous coating). Diagnosis rate is almost 90%.

EXAMINATION OF DUODENAL CONTENTS

Duodenal Drainage

Indications

1. For diagnosis of liver or biliary tract disease. Drainage may be done to help diagnose exacerbations of chronic infections early so that they can be controlled.
2. For other diagnostic purposes relating to parasites, pancreatic enzyme etc.
3. For therapeutic drainage in cholangitis or biliary obstruction.

Method for Diagnostic Drainage

1. Give nothing orally after midnight.
2. In the morning intubate (Rehfuss or Levintube) to a length of 50 cm (29 inches). Withdraw gastric specimen.

3. With the patient erect or lying on his right side before the fluoroscope, feed and massage tube into middle third of the duodenum. Now aspirate duodenal contents for 5-30 minutes and label "A", this evacuation specimen is of little value for bile study.
4. Slowly inject 50 ml of warm 33% magnesium sulphate through the tube to relax sphincter of Oddi. Clamp tube for 5 minutes then drain for 30 minutes and level "B". Gallbladder bile is first dark, then lighter. If no "B" bile is obtained, inject another 50 ml of magnesium sulphate. If still unsuccessful, inject 30 ml of olive oil.
5. During the final period of 30 minutes, try to collect yellow hepatic bile. Label it "C".

Examination for Diagnosis

1. Note density, colour, and flocculi in all 3 specimens. Test for bile, blood, reaction, and ferments as necessary.
2. Microscopy: This is important in detecting early cholelithiasis (gallsand). Note pus cells, bacteria, cellular elements and crystals.
3. Giardia or other parasites may be present.
4. Culture for bacteria, especially typhoid bacilli.

Interpretation

1. Absence of dark "B" bile indicates loss of gallbladder function. No bile may appear in common duct obstruction.
2. In cholelithiasis, many cholesterol and calcium bilirubinate crystals appear in "B" and "C" bile. The cholesterol crystals may be perfect or atypical or may be mixed with cellular detritus. The calcium bilirubinate comes as yellow or reddish particles the size of a pinhead.
3. In biliary tract inflammation, there is much yellow cellular and bacterial material in "B" and "C" bile.
4. Blood may be grossly visible in advanced carcinoma.

COMPOSITION OF BILE

Gross and Chemical Characteristics

a. Volume per 24 hours: 700-1000 ml
b. Specific gravity: Hepatic duct—1.010, gallbladder—1.026 to 1.032.
c. *Total Solids*

	Hepatic duct (gm%)	*Gallbladder (gm%)*
Bile salts	1.8	8.7
Fatty acids and lipids	0.24	1.8
Cholesterol	0.16	0.87

d. pH : Hepatic duct, 7.5 (6.2-8.5); gallbladder, 6.0 (5.6-8.0)
e. Sodium : 134-156 mEq/L
f. Potassium : 3.9-6.3 mEq/L
g. Chloride : 83-110 mEq/L
h. Bicarbonate : 38 mEq/L

PANCREATIC FUNCTION TESTS

Composition of Pancreatic Juice

Obtain specimen by duodenal drainage, it is mixed with bile. The flow of pancreatic juice is stimulated by an injection of secretin. Secretin is a hormone normally produced by upper intestinal mucosa in response to the presence of acid. The flow of pancreatic juice begins 5 minutes after a meal, is at its height in 2-3 hours, lasts 6-8 hours in all.

Gross and Chemical Characteristics of Pancreatic Juice

a. Volume per 24 hours: 500-800 ml.
b. Specific gravity: 1.007.
c. Total solids: 1.5-2.5 g%.
d. Alkalinity: pH is 7.0-8.2; 10 ml of pancreatic juice = 10-13 ml of 0.1 N NaOH and is more effective than bile or succus entericus in neutralising acid gastric juice.
e. Bicarbonate: 70-100 mEq/L.
f. Sodium: 100-150 mEq/L.
g. Potassium: 2-8 mEq/L.
h. Chlorides: 50-95 mEq/L.

Digestive Enzymes

Proteolytic Enzymes

1. Trypsin is a pancreatic protease. There are 100-200 units/L. It is much more active than pepsin. The inactive trypsinogen secreted is activated by enterokinase or by trypsin itself. Trypsin hydrolyses proteins at peptide bonds.

2. *Chymotrypsin:* Two forms, A and B are secreted and are activated by trypsin. Its action is like that of trypsin.
3. *Collagenase:* It digests collagen and is the one that initiates tissue destruction in necrotising pancreatitis.
4. *Elastase:* Digests elastin, which is the most resistant of all body proteins to lytic agents.

Peptidases

1. *Carboxypeptidase:* The active enzyme removes amino acids one by one from the carboxyl ends of the peptide chains.
2. *Aminopeptidase:* The active enzyme removes amino acids one by one from the ends of the peptide chains bearing the free amino groups.

Nucleases

Ribonuclease and deoxyribonuclease are secreted in probably more than one or perhaps several forms, they hydrolyse the respective nucleic acids.

Amylolytic Enzymes

Amylase: Alpha amylase attacks the alpha-1-4-glucosidic bonds of starches breaking them down to the disaccharide maltose.

Lipolytic Enzymes

1. *Lipase:* It partially hydrolyses neutral fats, splitting off one fatty acid at a time, thus forming diglycerides and monoglycerides along with liberated free fatty acids. Its optimum pH range is 7 to 9. This enzyme is activated by biliary contents. It shows optimal activation when the substrate is in emulsified form rather than in true solution form. The emulsifying action of bile salts and bile acids is very helpful for optimal enzymic action.
2. *Lecithinase* (phospholipase) Phospholipases A and B act in succession. Both of these remove fatty acids, the end products formed from lecithin and cephalin are glyceryl phosphoryl choline, glyceryl phosphoryl ethanolamine and glyceryl phosphoryl serine.

Acute Pancreatitis

Acute pancreatic necrosis (acute haemorrhagic pancreatitis) has over 50% mortality rate. It is known to be related to gallstones, alcoholism, trauma, infection (mumps), renal transplantation, various metabolic disorders, e.g. hyperlipidaemia, uraemia and hyperparathyroidism.

Serum amylase estimation has been widely used in the diagnosis of acute pancreatitis. Serum amylase activity rises within hours following an episode. Values over 5 times the upper limit of normal are suggestive of the diagnosis. Values may return to normal within 5 days following a mild oedematous attack. Persisting elevated values longer than this suggest continuing necrosis or possible pseudocyst formation. The urine amylase activity rises promptly, often within several hours of the rise in serum activity. Values over 1000 units per hour (in urine) or higher are seen, almost exclusively in patients with acute pancreatitis.

Amylase activity in blood (or in peritoneal fluid in certain conditions) may be raised to 1000 Somogyi units in various (nonpancreatic) disorders as: (i) intestinal obstruction, strangulation, or perforation, (ii) following upper abdominal surgery, (iii) ruptured ectopic pregnancy, (iv) mumps, (v) renal insufficiency, and (vi) following morphine administration. Values over 5000 units suggest a diagnosis of acute pancreatic necrosis.

Chronic Pancreatitis (Cirrhosis of Pancreas)

There is variable degree of fibrosis and atrophy in the pancreatic parenchyma. Diagnosis as in the case of acute pancreatitis, depends in part on determination of amylase activity in serum and urine.

Carcinoma of Pancreas

Serum amylase may be elevated but is of little diagnostic importance.

LIPASE

This is an esterase acting on ester linkages in triglycerides. Bile salts and calcium enhance its activity. Lipase occurs predominantly in the pancreas, but small amounts are produced in the gastric and small bowel mucosa.

Principle (Lipase estimation in serum)

The classic method of serum lipase determination is that of Cherry and Crandall using olive as substrate, overnight incubation (24 hours), and titration of lib erated fatty acids with sodium hydroxide, using phenolphthalein as indicator. Normal range of values is up to 1.5 units in serum.

The method given above takes a long time and if the report is to be given on emergency basis—a rapid (20-minute incubation) specific turbidimetric method is available. The disadvantage of this method is spuriously high results obtained in the presence of jaundice. By this method, values above 10 units are doubtful, above 19 units definitely abnormal.

Interpretation

Acute pancreatitis: Serum lipase activity rises slower than that of amylase, sometimes as late as 24 to 48 hours after onset, often peaking on the fourth day. It may remain elevated longer than the serum amylase. Even though it is less sensitive than the serum amylase, it provides confirmatory evidence for the diagnosis when positive. Elevation in patients with mumps strongly suggests significant pancreatic as well as salivary gland involvement by the disease.

Chronic pancreatitis: Serum lipase estimation is of relatively little value in the diagnosis of chronic pancreatitis.

Pancreatic carcinoma: Serum lipase is elevated more often in patients with pancreatic carcinoma than is serum amylase, although not with sufficient frequency to make it of much value diagnostically.

SECRETIN TEST

A double lumen tube, providing for separate aspiration of gastric and duodenal contents, is passed into the duodenum, using fluoroscopic guidance and maintaining constant aspiration of gastric contents. Duodenal contents are aspirated until clear. The patient is then given I/V one unit of secretin per kg of body weight, and pancreatic secretion entering the duodenum is collected for 80 minutes. The aspirate is examined for volume, bicarbonate content, and amylase activity.

The test is not employed for the diagnosis of acute pancreatic necrosis (it would be hazardous). Patients with chronic pancreatitis are unable to secrete juice of high bicarbonate content (less than 90 mEq/L). As in the case of chronic pancreatitis, this test may assist in diagnosis of pancreatic carcinoma tumours of head of pancreas tend to depress the overall volume flow (lower limit of normal—2 ml per kg body weight per 80 minutes). In carcinoma body of pancreas half the patients may show normal volume, carcinoma of tail does not affect the volume.

Patients with ductal obstructive lesion may exhibit elevation of serum amylase during and following the test, normally there is no elevation of serum amylase activity. The pattern of increased volume with decreased bicarbonate and normal amylase has been associated with haemochromatosis. Rarely, an increase in the amylase with normal bicarbonate concentration and volume flow has been noted in patients with nutritional and metabolic pancreatic fibrosis as well as in pancreatitis associated with inflammatory disease of the intestines. In some patients of pancreatic ductal obstruction, levels may rise.

Tumours of the head of the pancreas associated with jaundice must be differentiated from nonsurgical cholestatic liver disease, from carcinoma, obstructing stone, or other obstructing pathologic lesions of the common bile duct, and from ampullary carcinoma.

Duodenal aspirate containing cholesterol crystals or calcium bilirubinate pigment and pus, especially when associated with a normal secretin test, suggests gallstone aetiology. However, a duodenal aspirate containing calcium bilirubinate pigment is not specific for cholelithiasis. Unremittent jaundice, alcoholic duodenal fluid and stools, consistently negative urine urobilinogen tests, and less than 5 mg faecal urobilinogen per 24 hours, associated with a normal secretin test, suggest carcinoma of the common bile duct or gallbladder. Intermittent jaundice and presence of blood in the aspirate suggest carcinoma of the duodenal papilla, especially when associated with an abnormal secretin test. Cytologic examination of aspirate may be helpful in the diagnosis of carcinoma, as are the results of enzyme and volume outputs.

OTHER LABORATORY TESTS IN ACUTE PANCREATITIS

- Leucocytosis in patients with acute pancreatitis (up to 30,000/cu mm).
- Haemoconcentration, so raised haemoglobin.
- Serum levels of lecithinase A, trypsin and deoxyribonuclease activity are also elevated.
- A falling serum calcium points to the more serious form of pancreatitis as does turbidity of serum.
- In alcohol-related pancreatitis serum bilirubin may rise.
- Transient hyperglycaemia may also occur.

MISCELLANEOUS TESTS FOR CHRONIC PANCREATITIS

Various tests for malabsorption can be done

- Serum carotenoid level.
- Glucose tolerance test.
- Three-day faecal fat determination.
- Gross and microscopic examination of stool.
  - ^{131} I triolein test.
  - D-xylose test.

SWEAT ELECTROLYTES PILOCARPINE IONTOPHORESIS

Pilocarpine is iontophoresed into the skin to stimulate locally increased sweat gland secretion. The resulting sweat is absorbed by filter paper, diluted with distilled water and analysed for sodium and chloride contents. The method is painless and reliable. Total body sweating is hazardous in cystic fibrosis patients.

Diagnostic Application of Sweat Testing

Fibrocystic disease of pancreas (Mucoviscidosis)

This is a familial, Mendelian recessive disease characterised by abnormal secretion by the various exocrine glands of the body, including pancreas, salivary glands, peritracheal, peribronchial and peribronchiolar glands, lacrimal glands, sweat glands, mucosal glands of small intestine and even the bile ducts.

Laboratory diagnosis depends largely upon demonstration of increased sodium and chloride in the sweat, found in almost 99% of patients. Screening tests for sweat chloride have also been used and depend upon hand imprints on silver nitrate containing agar or paper. The sweat chloride precipitates with silver, and the intensity of the print is roughly proportional to the sweat chloride precipitation. However, chemical estimation of sweat chloride is more accurate.

In adult males values of sweat chloride up to 70 mEq/L and in females up to 65 mEq/L are normal.

Normal values in children

Chloride	*Sodium*
Below 50 mEq/L: normal	Below 70 mEq/L: normal
50-60 mEq/L: equivocal	70-90 mEq/L: equivocal
Over 60 mEq/L: abnormal	Over 90 mEq/L: abnormal

Chapter 17

The Endocrine System

INTRODUCTION

The sciencc concerned with the structure and functions of the endocrine glands and the diagnosis and treatment of disorders of the endocrine system is called endocrinology. This term comes from the Greek words *'endo'* (within), *'crine'* (to secrete) and *'logos'* (study of).

The endocrine system consists of glands situated in different areas of the body as shown in Fig. 17.1. Each gland produces different hormones, which regulate the activity of other organs and tissues in the body. These hormones are released directly into the blood flowing through the gland. This is in contrast to exocrine glands, which release hormones down a tube or duct.

Glands are functional units of hormone-secreting cells located in various regions of the body making up the endocrine system. Each gland has specific functions that help to maintain the normal internal environment and promote the survival of the organism. Although there are some diffuse endocrine tissues, as in the gastrointestinal epithelium, there are several major glands or control centres within the endocrine system.

PITUITARY GLAND

The pituitary gland, which lies in a small depression in the sphenoid bone of the skull called the sella turcica, has often been termed the *'Master Gland'* because many of the hormones it releases affect the release of other hormones. However, the pituitary is really not the master. It is controlled by a brain region called the hypothalamus via the release of releasing factors into a special blood vessel network (hypothalamic-hypophyseal portal system) that feeds the pituicytes. These releasing factors then cause or inhibit the release of pituitary hormones which

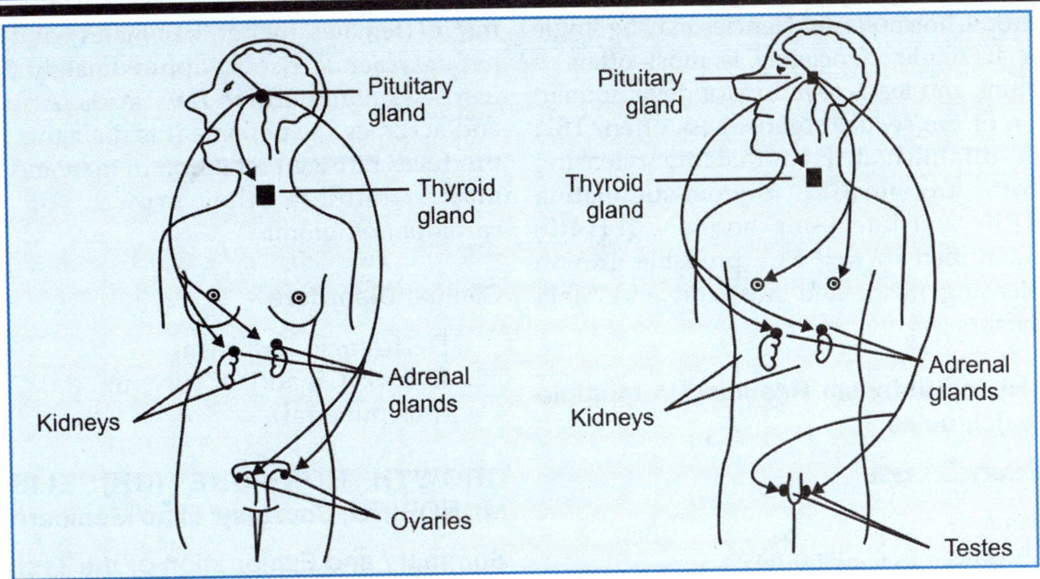

Fig. 17.1: Endocrine glands

travel via the circulatory system to the target organ (Fig. 17.2).

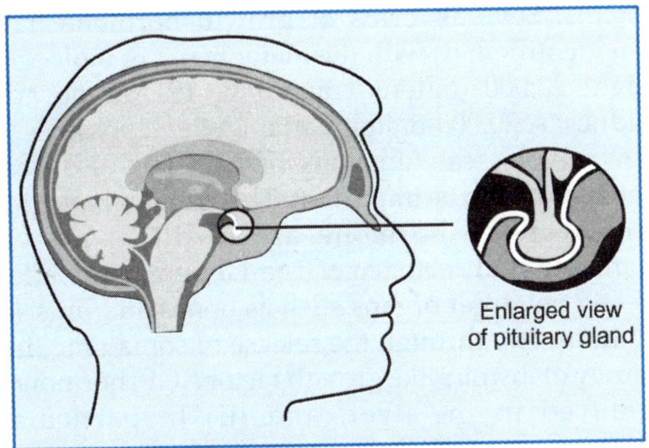

Fig. 17.2: Pituitary gland

Anatomically and functionally the pituitary can be divided into three portions.

Anterior Pituitary (Adenohypophysis)

Six peptide hormones are secreted by the adenohypophysis:

- Growth hormone (somatotrophin, GH)
- Corticotrophin (ACTH)
- Thyroid-stimulating hormone (TSH)
- Follicle-stimulating hormone (FSH)
- Luteinising hormone (LH)
- Prolactin (PRL)

All except growth hormone and prolactin regulate the activities of other glands. Somatotrophin, PRL and ACTH are polypeptide hormones and LH, FSH, and TSH are glycoproteins having very similar structures.

The ACTH is an anterior pituitary hormone that stimulates cortisol and androgen production by the adrenal gland. Diurnal variation of ACTH are typical, with peak levels occurring from 0600 to 0800 hrs. and trough levels occurring from 1800 to 2300 hrs.

Hormones Secreted by the Pituitary Gland

Anterior pituitary	*Posterior pituitary*	*Intermediate lobe*
Growth hormone	Oxytocin	MSH
TSH	ADH	
FSH		
LH		
ACTH		
Prolactin		

The regulation of hormones elaborated by the endocrine glands is complex and varied. The tropic hormones of the anterior pituitary are regulated by CNS factors (hypothalamic-releasing hormones) as well as by products of their target organs. A delicate balance is thus maintained. Antidiuretic hormone (ADH) is regulated by osmotic pressure and volume. Parathormone is controlled by calcium and phosphorus concentrations, norepinephrine and epinephrine by direct neural stimuli; and insulin secretion by blood glucose concentrations. The MSH secretion is inhibited by glucocorticoids and causes skin pigmentation when cortisol is absent.

Clinical tropic hormone deficiencies may be single or multiple. If single, deficiency is most often of gonadotrophins and leads to failure of development or involution of the sexual organs. Less often, TSH or ACTH is diminished. Hypothalamic-releasing factors for corticotrophin (CRF), thyroid-stimulating hormone (TRF), and luteinising hormone (LH-RF) have been identified as well as a probable growth hormone-releasing factor and prolactin and MSH inhibitory factors.

Causes of Hypopituitarism Resulting in Multiple or Single Deficiencies

Intrinsic Pituitary Disease

1. Neoplasms:
   - Chromophobe adenomas
   - Craniopharyngiomas
   - Carcinoma
   - Metastatic carcinoma
2. Histiocytosis
3. Infections
4. Metabolic disorders, e.g. hemochromatosis
5. Vascular disorder:
   - Infarction (postpartum necrosis)
   - Intracerebral vascular malformation

Extrinsic Pituitary Disorders

1. Surgical, heavy particle, or other forms of pituitary ablation
2. Hypothalamic neoplasms or metastatic deposits.

ANTERIOR LOBE

GROWTH HORMONE (GH)

Growth hormone has no specific target tissue. All cells of the human body are affected by this hormone. It is very important in the growing child, but it remains essential to many bodily functions throughout life. The GH has effects on the growth of bone and cartilage, protein metabolism, RNA formation, electrolyte balance, fat and glucose metabolism.

Actions

The GH stimulates growth of all nonendocrine tissues in the body and may affect secretions of the medulla and pancreas. Normal plasma levels are less than 3 ng/ml (females, higher than males), and after insulin hypoglycaemia rise to approximately 25 ng/ml. It increases nonesterified fatty acids. Also, in diabetic and acromegalic patients it is diabetogenic. The GH produces nitrogen retention in man and monkeys. It may stimulate the growth of malignant carniopharyngioma.

Clinical Disorders

1. **Deficiency:** Dwarfism
2. **Excess:** Gigantism (prepubertal), acromegaly (postpubertal).

GROWTH HORMONE (GH) ELISA (FROM MONOBIND, Courtesy: Lilac Medicare)

Summary and Explanation of the Test

Growth hormone (hGH, somatotrophin), secreted from the anterior pituitary, is a polypeptide with two intrachain disulfide bridges, which circulates free or bound to number of different GH-binding proteins. Several forms of growth hormone have been identified: (i) with the major being of molecular weight 22,000 daltons containing 191 amino acid residues. A 20,000-dalton variant, which posseses all known biological functions of GH, has also been demonstrated to be important. The primary biological actions of the hormone are in direct growth promoting and lactogenic. The GH exerts its effect directly on target organs such as bones and muscles and indirectly through the release of somatomedins, a family of insulin-like growth factor (IGF) hormones, produced in the liver, and (ii) In particular, somatotrophin C (IGF-1) is essential for bone growth during childhood.

The clinical usefulness of the measurement of GH in children has been well established in ascertaining linear bone growth along the epiphyseal plate. Abnormal elevated levels lead to gigantism, while complete absence slows the rate of growth to one-third to one-half of normal. In adults, the epiphyseal growth plates have fused; GH excess gradually produces acromegaly, a coarse thickening of the bones of the skull, hands and feet.

In this method, GH calibrator, patient specimen or control is first added to a streptavidin coated well. Biotinylated monoclonal and enzyme-labeled antibodies (directed against distinct and different epitopes of GH) are added and the reactants mixed. Reaction between the various GH antibodies and native GH forms a sandwich complex that binds with the streptavidin coated to the well.

After the completion of the required incubation period, the enzyme-growth hormone antibody bound conjugate is separated from the unbound enzyme-growth hormone conjugate by aspiration or decantation. The activity of the enzyme present on the surface of the well is quantitated by reaction with a suitable substrate to produce color.

The employment of several serum references of known growth hormone levels permits the construction of a dose response curve of activity and concentration. From comparison to the dose response curve, an unknown specimen's activity can be correlated with growth hormone concentration.

PRINCIPLE

Immunoenzymometric Assay

The essential reagents required for an immunoenzymometric assay include high affinity and specificity antibodies (enzyme and immobilised), with different and distinct epitope recognition, in excess, and native antigen. In this procedure, the immobilisation takes place during the assay at the surface of a microplate well through the interaction of streptavidin coated on the well and exogenously added biotinylated monoclonal anti-GH antibody.

Upon mixing monoclonal biotinylated antibody, the enzyme-labeled antibody and a serum containing the native antigen, reaction results between the native antigen and the antibodies, without competition or steric hindrance, to form a soluble sandwich complex. The interaction is illustrated by the following equation:

$$^{Enz}Ab_{(p)} + Ag_{GH} + {}^{Btn}Ab_{(m)} \underset{k_{-a}}{\overset{Ka}{\rightleftharpoons}} {}^{Enz}Ab_{(p)}\text{-}Ag_{GH}\text{-}{}^{Btn}Ab_{(m)}$$

$^{Btn}Ab_{(m)}$ = Biotinylated monoclonal antibody (excess quantity)

Ag_{GH} = Native antigen (variable quantity)

$^{Enz}Ab_{(p)}$ = Enzyme labeled polyclonal antibody (excess quantity)

$^{Enz}Ab_{(p)}\text{-}Ag_{GH}\text{-}{}^{Btn}Ab_{(m)}$ = Antigen-antibodies sandwich complex

k_a = Rate constant of association

k_{-a} = Rate constant of dissociation

Simultaneously, the complex is deposited to the well through the high affinity reaction of streptavidin and biotinylated antibody. This interaction is illustrated below:

$$^{Enz}Ab_{(p)}\text{-}AgGH\text{-}{}^{Btn}Ab_{(m)} + Streptavidin_{c.w.} \Rightarrow \text{immobilized complex}$$

$Streptavidin_{c.w.}$ = Streptavidin immobolised on well

Immobilised complex = sandwich complex bound to the solid surface

After equilibrium is attained, the antibody-bound fraction is separated from unbound antigen by decantation or aspiration. The enzyme activity in the antibody-bound fraction is directly proportional to the native antigen concentration. By utilising several different serum references of known antigen values, a dose response curve is generated from which the antigen concentration of an unknown is ascertained.

REAGENTS FOR 96-WELL MICROPLATE

A. Growth Hormone Calibrators —1.0 ml/vial

Six (6) vials of references for GH antigen in human serum at levels of 0(A), 0.5(B), 2.5(C), 10(D), 25(E) and 50(F) ng/ml. Store at 2-8°C. A preservative has been added.

B. Enzyme (HRP)—Polyclonal antibody Conjugate and Biotinylated Monoclonal antibody—11 ml/vial

One (1) vial containing horseradish peroxidase (HRP)-labeled affinity purified rabbit antibody, biotinylated monoclonal mouse IgG in buffer, dye, and preservative. Store at 2-8°C.

C. Streptavidin-coated Microplate—96 wells

One 96-well microplate coated with streptavidin and packaged in an aluminum bag with a drying agent. Store at 2-8°C.

D. Wash Solution Concentrate—20 ml

One (1) vial containing a surfactant in phosphate buffered saline. A preservative has been added. Store at 2-30°C.

E. Substrate A ~7.0 ml/vial

One (1) bottle containing tetramethylbenzidine (TMB) in buffer. Store at 2-8°C.

F. Substrate B–7.0 ml/vial

One (1) bottle containing hydrogen peroxide (H_2O_2) in buffer. Store at 2-8°C.

G. Stop Solution - 6.0 ml/vial

One (1) bottle containing a strong acid (1N HCl). Store at 2-30°C.

Note 1: Do not use reagents beyond the kit expiration date.

Note 2: Opened reagents are stable for sixty (60) days when stored at 2-8°C.

FOR IN VITRO DIAGNOSTIC USE

Not for Internal or External Use in Humans or Animals

Precautions

All products that contain human serum have been found to be nonreactive for hepatitis B surface antigen, HIV 1 and 2 and HCV antibodies by FDA required tests. Since no known test can offer complete assurance that infectious agents are absent, all human serum products should be handled as potentially hazardous and capable of transmitting disease. Good laboratory procedures for handling blood products can be found in the Center for Disease Control/ National Institute of Health, "Biosafety in Microbiological and Biomedical Laboratories," 2nd Edition, 1988, HHS.

Specimen Collection and Preparation

The specimens shall be blood serum in type and the usual precautions in the collection of venipuncture samples should be observed. For accurate comparison to established normal values, a fasting morning serum sample should be obtained. The blood should be collected in a plain redtop venipuncture tube without additives or gel barrier. Allow the blood to clot. Centrifuge the specimen to separate the serum from the cells.

Samples may be refrigerated at 2-8°C for a maximum period of five (5) days. If the specimen(s) cannot be assayed within this time, the sample(s) may be stored at temperatures of –20°C for up to 30 days. Avoid repetitive freezing and thawing. When assayed in duplicate, 0.100 ml of the specimen is required.

MATERIALS

Provided

1. Six (6) vials of growth hormone human serum calibrators.
2. One (1) vial of combined biotinylated monoclonal antibody and enzyme labeled polyclonal reagent.
3. One 96-well streptavidin coated microplate.
4. One (1) bottle of wash buffer concentrate.
5. One (1) bottle of substrate A.
6. One (1) bottle of substrate B.
7. One (1) bottle of stop solution.
8. Instructions.

Required but not Provided

1. Pipette(s) capable of delivering 50 μl and 100 μl volumes with a precision of better than 1.5 per cent.
2. Dispenser(s) for repetitive deliveries of 0.100 ml and 0.300 ml volumes with a precision of better than 1.5 per cent (optional).
3. Microplate washer or a squeeze bottle (optional).
4. Microplate reader with 450 nm wavelength absorbance capability.
5. Container(s) for mixing of reagents (see-below).
6. Absorbent paper for blotting the microplate wells.
7. Plastic wrap or microplate cover for incubation steps.
8. Vacuum aspirator (optional) for wash steps.
9. Timer
10. Storage container for storage of wash buffer
11. Distilled or deionised water.

Reagent Preparation

1. Working Reagent 1—Wash buffer: Dilute contents of wash concentrate to 1000 ml with distilled or deionised water in a suitable storage container. Store at room temperature.

2. Working Reagent 2—Substrate Solution—Prepare before use: Determine the amount of reagent needed and prepare by mixing equal portions of Substrate A and Substrate B in a suitable container. For example, add 1 ml of A and 1 ml of 8 per two (2) eight well strips (A slight excess of solution is made). Use within one (1) hour of preparation for maximum performance of the assay.

Test Procedure

Before proceeding with the assay, bring all reagents, serum references and controls to room temperature.

1. Format the microplates' wells for each serum reference, control and patient specimen to be as-

sayed in duplicate. Replace any unused microwell strips back into the aluminum bag, seal and store at 2-8°C.

2. Pipette 0.050 ml (50 μl) of the appropriate serum reference, control or specimen into the assigned well.
3. Add 0.100 ml (100 μl) of the biotinylated/enzyme-labeled antibodies to each well. It is very important to dispense all reagents close to the bottom of the coated well.
4. Swirl the microplate gently for 20-30 seconds to mix and cover.
5. Incubate 60 minutes at room temperature.
6. Discard the contents of the microplate by decantation or aspiration. If decanting, tap and blot the plate dry with absorbent paper.
7. Add 300 μl of wash buffer (see reagent preparation section), decant (tap and blot) or aspirate. Repeat two (2) additional times for a total of three (3) washes. An automatic or manual plate washer can be used. Follow the manufacturer's instruction for usage. If a squeeze bottle is employed, fill each well depressing the container (avoiding air bubbles) to dispense the wash. Decant the wash and repeat two (2) additional times.
8. Add 0.100 ml (100 μl) of working substrate solution to all wells (see reagent preparation section). Always add reagents in the same order to minimise reaction time differences between wells.
9. Incubate at room temperature for fifteen (15) minutes.
10. Add 0.050 ml (50 μl) of stop solution to each well and swirl the microplate gently for 15-20 seconds to mix. Always add reagents in the same order to minimise reaction time differences between wells.
11. Read the absorbance in each well at 450 nm in a microplate reader. The results should be read within thirty (30) minutes of adding the stop solution.

Note: For assaying specimens with concentration greater than 50 ng/ml, pipete 25 μl of the specimen and 25 μl of the 0 serum calibrator into the sample well (this maintains a uniform protein environment). Multiply the result by 2 to obtain the human growth concentration of the specimen.

Quality Control

Each laboratory should assay controls at levels in the low, normal and elevated range for monitoring assay performance. These controls should be treated as unknowns and values determined in every test procedure performed. Quality control charts should be maintained to follow the performance of the supplied reagents. Pertinent statistical methods should be employed to ascertain trends. The individual laboratory should set acceptable assay performance limits. Other parameters that should be monitored include the 80, 50 and 20 per cent intercepts of ths dose response curve for run-to-run reproducibility. In addition, maximum absorbance should be consistent with past experience. Significant deviation from established performance can indicate unnoticed change in experimental conditions or degradation of kit reagents. Fresh reagents should be used to determine the reason for the variations.

Results

A dose response curve is used to ascertain the concentration of growth hormone levels in unknown specimens.

1. Record the absorbance obtained from the printout of the microplate reader as outlined in Example 1.
2. Plot the absorbance for each duplicate serum reference versus the corresponding GH concentration in ng/ml on linear graph paper (do not average the duplicates of the serum references before plotting).
3. Draw the best-fit curve through the plotted points.
4. To determine the concentration of GH for an unknown, locate the average absorbance of the duplicates for each unknown on the vertical axis of the graph, find the intersecting point on the curve, and read the concentration (in ng/ml) from the horizontal axis of the graph (the duplicates of the unknown may be averaged as indicated). In the following example, the average absorbance (0.873) intersects the dose response curve at (12.8 ng/ml) GH concentration (Fig. 17.3).

Note: Computer data reduction software designed for IEMA assays may also be used for the data reduction.

Example 1

Well	Serum references	Absorbance		
1	0.0 ng/ml	0.01		
2	0.0 ng/ml	0.009		
3	0.5 ng/ml	0.047		
4	0.5 ng/ml	0.046		
5	2.5 ng/ml	0.195		
6	2.5 ng/ml	0.195		
7	10.0 ng/ml	0.737		
8	10.0 ng/ml	0.724		
9	25.0 ng/ml	1.525		
10	25.0 ng/ml	1.505		
11	50.0 ng/ml	2.234		
12	50.0 ng/ml	2.253		
Well	**Unknown I. D.**	**O.D.**	**Avg. O.D.**	**Value**
13	Unknown #1	0.846		
14	Unknown #1	0.899	0.873	12.8 ng/ml

The data presented in Example 1 and Figure 17.3 are for illustration only and should not be used in lieu of a dose response curve prepared with each assay.

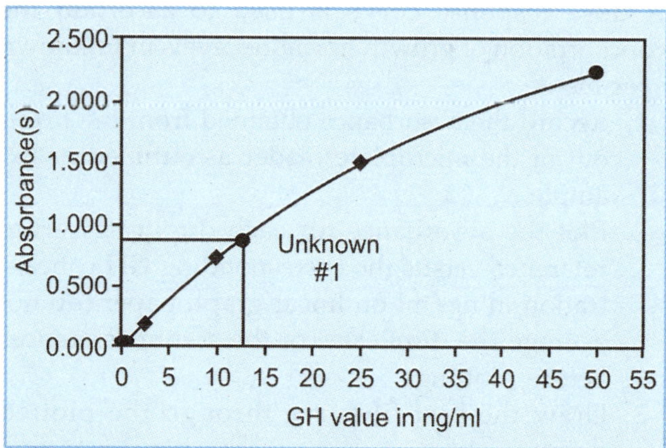

Fig. 17.3: GH value deduction

LIMITATIONS OF PROCEDURE

A. Assay Performance

It is important that the time of reaction in each well is held constant for reproducible results. Pipetting of samples should not extend beyond ten (10) minutes to avoid assay drift. If more than one (1) plate is used, it is recommended to repeat the dose response curve.

Addition of the substrate solution initiates a kinetic reaction, which is terminated by the addition of the stop solution. Therefore, the addition of the substrate and the stopping solution should be in the same sequence to eliminate any time deviation during reaction.

Plate readers measure vertically. Do not touch the bottom of the wells.

Failure to remove adhering solution adequately in the aspiration or decantation wash step(s) may result in poor replication and spurious results.

Sample(s) that are contaminated microbiologically should not be used in the assay. Highly lipaemeic or haemolysed specimen(s) should similarly not be used.

Each component in one assay should be of the same lot number and stored under identical conditions.

This immunoassay has been designed so that the high dose "hook effect" is not an issue for elevated samples. Specimens with concentrations between 50 ng/ml and 1000 ng/ml will read greater than the 50 ng/dl standard and should be diluted and reassayed.

Patients on hGH replacement may develop antibodies to hGH that may interfere in the assay and cause falsely low values. Genetic variants or degradation products may alter antibody binding characteristics and affect final results. Such samples may display discordant results on different assays that utilised antibodies, which recognise different epitopes.

B. Interpretation

If computer controlled data reduction is used to interpret the results of the test, it is imperative that the predicted values for the calibrators fall within 10 per cent of the assigned concentrations.

Growth hormone secretion follows a circadian rhythm characterised by discontinuous pulsatile discharge bursts with intervening periods during the day when GH level s are undetectable. The highest levels, in two major bursts, are usually attained within one or two hours after the onset of sleep. Other physiological stimuli of growth hormone are stress, exercise, high-protein meals and hypoglycaemia.

Hyperglycemia inhibits growth hormone secretion. Age is an important factor in growth hormone concentrations. At birth, GH is high and generally declines with age with the exception of a burst during the growth phase of adolescence. Women typically have a 50 per cent higher level than their age-matched males.

Since growth hormone concentration is pulsatile and sporadic during the course of the day (coupled with its short half-life), single serum random levels do not yield clinically useful information. To overcome this problem, provocative tests are utilised that employ physiological or pharmacological stimuli to induce the secretion or inhibition of GH. For these reasons, the determination of growth hormone alone is not sufficient to assess clinical status.

Expected Ranges of Values

Because of the pulsatile and sporadic nature of growth hormone secretion, reference intervals for basal values are without meaning. However, normal levels rarely have been reported above 50 ng/ml. The well rested, fasting (12 hours) subjects should have GH values of 20 ng/ml or less.

With this caveat in mind, 75 apparently healthy adults were assayed the hGH immunoassay. The results are depicted below.

Expected values for the GH IEMA test system (in ng/ml)

	N	*Mean*	*Range*
Specimens	75	2.8	0-17

Provocative tests for hGH response are normally used to access the function of the anterior pituitary. Stimulatory procedures measure the secretion ability of the anterior pituitary to release hGH. Children suspected of growth retardation are common subjects for stimulatory testing. Several dynamic tests are available to induce GH release: exercise (3), L-dopa administration (4), insulin tolerance test (5), and arginine infusion (6). Each laboratory should assess the normal response, but a peak GH release in excess of 8 ng/ml is probably normal in all cases.

Inhibitory testing measure the suppression of hGH release from the anterior pituitary. Inhibitory tests are useful in ascertaining growth hormone excess and the resulting conditions of gigantism and acromegaly. The glucose tolerance test is a dynamic test to measure growth hormone excess. The failure of hGH levels to fall below 1 ng/ml within 60-120 minutes suggests excess hGH secretion.

It is important to keep in mind that establishment of a range of values which can be expected to be found by a given method for a population of "normal" persons is dependent upon a multiplicity of factors: the specificity of the method, the population tested and the precision of the method in the hands of the analyst. For these reasons, each laboratory should depend upon the range of expected values established by the manufacturer only until an in-house range can be determined by the analysts using the method with a population indigenous to the area in which the laboratory is located.

Deficiency: In children, careful attention to growth records and X-ray of the skull and hands (especially of wrists) for bone age, looking primarily for retarded bone age. Hypopituitarism must be differentiated from isolated growth hormone deficiency, where normal pubertal development occurs. Other causes of short stature must be considered, e.g. constitutional causes, hypogonadism, hypothyroidism, and gonadal dysgenesis. Eunuchoid habitus eventually emerges only in the hypogonadal disorder. Normal plasma levels are less than 3 ng/ml, after insulin hypoglycaemia the level rises to approximately 10-25 ng/ml within 60 minutes. Caution should be used in the dose of insulin administered. If hypopituitarism is suspected, doses of 0.05 units/kg are recommended; the dose can be increased if insufficient hypoglycaemia is achieved. The infusion of arginine 0.5 gm/kg for 30 minutes, can also increase GH levels to greater than 10 ng/ml in 60-90 minutes. This test has the advantage of not producing hypoglycaemia. Absence of a normal response to these provocative tests is diagnostic.

Excess: Growth records, changes in soft tissue mass, enlargement of sella turcica, increased sweating, tufting of phalanges, vertebral overgrowth and spur formation, and organomegaly are all useful indications of GH excess. Serial studies of visual fields are essential. While increases in BMR and serum phosphorus concentration are helpful, the diagnosis is established by the level of GH and its response to suppressive manoeuvres. Serum GH levels are greater than 10 ng/ml and are not suppressed after oral glucose loads. The availability of serum GH levels makes possible the evaluation of surgical or radiologic treatment.

Clinical Disorders

1. Deficiency: Dwarfism
2. Excess: Gigantism (prepubertal)
   Acromegaly (postpubertal)

Interfering Factors

1. Increased levels are associated with use of oral contraceptives and estrogens.
2. Decreased levels are associated with obesity and use of corticosteroids.

CORTICOTROPHIN (ACTH)

Actions

This stimulates production of all adrenocortical hormones (transient stimulatory effect on aldosterone) and causes hyperplasia of adrenal cortex. In the adrenal it promotes increased protein synthesis, accelerates glycolysis and increases steroidogenesis. Extra-adrenal actions include mobilisation of nonesterified fatty acids from fat depots. Normally, the amount of circulating ACTH is controlled by the levels of cortisol in the blood, individual biorhythms and stress.

Methods of Evaluation

The X-ray of sella turcica should be taken, study basal excretion of 17-hydroxycorticosteroids, assess diurnal variation patterns, study plasma cortisol levels. *Corticotrophin lack is indicated by:*

1. Failure of adrenocortical function
2. Low 24-hour urinary excretion of 17 ketosteroids and 17-hydroxycorticosteroids, which increase stepwise in response to daily corticotrophin administration
3. Failure of hydroxycorticosteroid excretion to increase following administration of metyrapone, which blocks the production of cortisol and results in increase of corticotrophin production by the intact hypophysis.
4. Normal or slightly reduced aldosterone excretion
5. Plasma ACTH levels—normally barely detectable are markedly increased in adrenal insufficiency and Cushing's disease.

		SI units
0800 hours, peak	25-100 pg/ml	25-100 ng/L
1800 hours, trough	0-50 pg/ml	0-50 ng/L

Clinical Disorders

Increased Addison's disease, ectopic ACTH syndrome, pituitary adenoma, pituitary Cushing's syndrome, primary adrenal insufficiency, and stress. Drugs include amphetamine sulphate, calcium gluconate, corticosteroids, oestrogens, ethanol, lithium carbonate, and spironolactone (corticotrophin-like substances elaborated by malignant tissue, particularly in the lung, pancreas or prostate, may also lead to Cushing's disease).

Decreased Primary adrenocortical hyperfunction (due to tumour or hyperplasia) and secondary hypoadrenalism.

OTHER ANTERIOR PITUITARY HORMONES TSH

This hormone stimulates the synthesis and secretion of thyroid hormones. It is a glycoprotein hormone controlled by feedback from thyroid hormones.

The TSH controls production and release of T3 and T4 at three levels:

- The entry of I- into the follicle.
- The entry of Tg bound T3 and T4 from follicular space into the lumen.
- The release of T3 and T4 from Tg with the help of protease enzyme.

FSH

The target organs for FSH are the testes, in men, and the ovaries in women. The hormone stimulates the germinal epithelium in the testes to cause and facilitate the making of sperm. In women it stimulates the growth and development of the follicle. It stimulates the production of testosterone in men and oestrogen and progesterone in women. Its release from the pituitary is governed by a negative feedback mechanism involving these steroids.

LH

The male target organ is the testes and the testosterone producing interstitial cells of Leydig in particular. In women the target of LH is the developing follicle within the ovary where it is necessary for ovulation to occur and a corpus luteum to develop.

LH, FSH—Recommendations for Testing

- Irregular menstrual periods—amenorrhoea.
- Primary and secondary hypogonadism in male and female
- When a female complains of masculinising features or a male complains of feminine features
- Infertility cases

- IVF centres—assisted conception
- Monitor LH, FSH levels after LHRH stimulation
- LH/FSH ratio is a useful parameter in diagnosis of PCO
- FSH is a good indicator in menopause
- In children where they seem to grow faster than their age or otherwise (precocious and delayed puberty)

PROLACTIN

This hormone is involved in breast development and lactation. In concert with oestrogen, it prepares the mammary gland for lactation and then causes the synthesis of milk. Secretion is regulated by a release inhibiting factor and suckling may cause the release of prolactin from the pituitary. It steadily increases during pregnancy, reaching 200 ng/ml in the 3rd trimester and returns to normal in nonlactating women 2-3 weeks postpartum. In lactating women 6 months postpartum. It also increases with breast stimulation, exercise, sleep, and stress.

Prolactin—Recommendations for Testing

- Diagnosis of hyperprolactinaemia and monitoring the effectiveness of treatment.
- When a male complains of impotence, decreased libido.
- Female complains of irregular menstrual cycle—amenorrhoea.
- Pituitary tumour (microadenoma or macroadenoma).
- Used alone or with LH and FSH for detecting pituitary dysfunction.

INTERMEDIATE LOBE (PARS INTERMEDIA)

In the adult human this lobe is diminished with poor vascular and neural connections such that secretion is not facilitated. Cells in the pars intermedia may secrete MSH (melanocyte-stimulating hormone) which stimulates the activity of melanocytes in the skin.

POSTERIOR PITUITARY (NEUROHYPOPHYSIS)

This portion of the pituitary is really an extension of the hypothalamus. Neurons with their cell bodies in the hypothalamus and their terminal portions in the neurohypophysis release two hormones. Antidiuretic hormone (ADH) and oxytocin are stored there within the terminal processes of neurons until the signal to release them is received.

ADH

It is also known as vasopressin. In the presence of ADH, the kidneys reabsorb more water from the forming urine within renal tubules. Without ADH the kidney tubules are almost completely impermeable to water such that a very dilute urine is excreted (diabetes insipidus). The ADH has a direct effect on vascular smooth muscle causing vasoconstriction and an increase in blood pressure when present in large doses. They are stimulated by a high blood osmolarity (increased concentration) causing the release of ADH. The hormone then causes the kidney tubules to reabsorb more water to return osmolarity to normal. Volume receptors also play a role when they sense a low blood pressure. Alcohol inhibits ADH secretion.

Normal Values

Serum osmolarity	*ADH level*	*SI units*
270-280 mOsm/kg	<1.5 pg/ml	<1.4 pmol/L
280-285 mOsm/kg	<2.5 pg/ml	<2.3 pmol/L
285-290 mOsm/kg	1-5 pg/ml	0.9-4.6 pmol/L
290-295 mOsm/kg	2-7 pg/ml	1.9-6.5 pmol/L
295-300 mOsm/kg	4-12 pg/ml	3.7-11.1 pmol/L

The ADH elaboration is initiated by increase in the extracellular fluid osmotic pressure, by direct nervous system stimulation of the hypothalamus; and, to a minor degree, by extracellular fluid volume. It is formed by the neurosecretory cells in the supraoptic and paraventricular nuclei of the hypothalamus, and travels along axons to the posterior lobe, where it is stored. Lesions at any of these sites interfere with ADH release to the body.

Clinical Disorders

A. *Deficiency of ADH:* ADH deficiency produces diabetes insipidus if the anterior pituitary is still functioning.

B. *Excess ADH:* Inappropriate ADH secretion syndrome.

Methods of Evaluation

Deficiency

Study for intracranial lesion (lumbar puncture, skull film, EEG), STS, chest X-ray (metastases), bone marrow examination (multiple myeloma, eosinophilic granuloma). However, 45 per cent are classified as idiopathic. Differentiate diabetes insipidus (10 to 15 per cent cases) by administration of vasopressin. The simple measurement of a urine volume of more than 5 litres/day is strong presumptive evidence of deficiency.

1. *Water restriction:* Though quite simple, careful supervision is necessary so that losses of 3 to 5 per cent of body weight are avoided. Greater care has to be exercised in children. Volume and concentration (specific gravity or mOsm/kg) are determined at each voiding. Urine flow should reach less than 0.5 ml/minute, and urine concentration should be greater than 800 mOsm/kg (specific gravity 1.020).
2. *Hypertonic saline test* (Carter-Robbins test, Hickey-Hare test): This test is used to differentiate psychogenic polydipsia from diabetes insipidus. Here again caution is needed, since dehydration may cause vasomotor collapse in patients with diabetes insipidus. Administration of hypertonic saline solution may be hazardous in cardiac or renal disease.
   Antidiuretic therapy is stopped until urine output reaches its original level. The patient may be cautiously dehydrated for 8-12 hours or this step may be omitted. Just before the test, the patient drinks 20 ml of water per kg of body weight in 1 hour. Urine is collected at 15-minute intervals. When the urine flow exceeds 5 ml/min, 2.5 per cent saline solution is given IV at a rate of 0.25 ml/kg body weight/min for 45 minutes.
   In normal subjects and in psychogenic polydipsia, a marked reduction in urinary flow will occur during the saline infusion or during the two 15-minute intervals immediately following it.
   In 85 to 95 per cent of patients with true diabetes insipidus, the urine flow does not decrease with the saline infusion, but administration of 0.1 unit of vasopressin will inhibit diuresis in the absence of renal disease.
3. *Response to vasopressin:* This test also differentiates diabetes insipidus from vasopressin-resistant polyuria due to other causes, e.g.
   a. Potassium depletion
   b. Hypercalcaemia
   c. Chronic renal disease
   d. Congenital nephrogenic diabetes insipidus
   e. After renal transplantation
   f. Sjögren's syndrome
   g. Obstructive uropathy.

   Urine volume and specific gravity and symptoms of polyuria and polydipsia are observed before and after repeated subcutaneous injections of 0.2 ml (4 units) vasopressin every 3 or 4 hours day and night for 24 hours, or before and after a 1 hour of infusion of aqueous vasopression (5 mu/minute).
   Patients with chronic nephritis or vasopressin-resistant diabetes insipidus experience no relief of symptoms during test period. In diabetes insipidus or psychogenic polydipsia, symptoms may improve, urine volume may decrease, urine specific gravity may increase to 1.015 or more, and urine osmolality may rise above serum osmolality.
4. *Nicotine stimulation:* Various side effects (nausea, vomiting, sweating) limit the usefulness of this test. Give 0.5-1 mg IV of nicotine base to non-smokers and doses as high as 3 mg IV to habitual smokers undergoing water diuresis. The normal response to intravenous nicotine is secretion of vasopressin, 80 per cent reduction in urine flow, and rise in osmolality. Responsiveness to nicotine but not to hypertonic saline stimulus suggests that osmoreceptor centres are functionally separate from vasopressin sensory centres.

Syndrome of Inappropriate ADH Secretion (SIADH)

Hyponatraemia is a frequently observed laboratory finding in severely ill patients. The recognition of SIADH is critical to their management. Findings consist of hyponatraemia, normal BUN, urinary sodium loss, competent circulatory system, and increased urinary osmolality. These findings are similar to the observations made after exogenous administration of ADH to man. This syndrome is seen most frequently in pulmonary neoplasms, but it is reported in CNS disorders, tuberculous meningitis, head trauma, pneumonia, intrathoracic tumours, myxoedema, acute intermittent porphyria, sickle cell anaemia, cerebral thrombosis and postoperative ADH release after morphine or barbiturates. Neoplastic tissue in some cases has been shown to possess ADH activity.

Oxytocin: A major role of this hormone is the stimulation of smooth muscle cells in the pregnant uterus. When labour begins, stretching of the cervix and vagina stimulates a reflex production and release of oxytocin. Oxytocin then travels in the blood to the uterus where it causes more forceful contraction of the smooth muscle. This hormone is also involved in lactation. It causes milk ejection by acting on the smooth muscle surrounding the milk producing cells. Again, its production and release is mediated by a neural reflex, the suckling reflex. Emotion, anxiety and pain can inhibit oxytocin release.

FEEDBACK MECHANISM

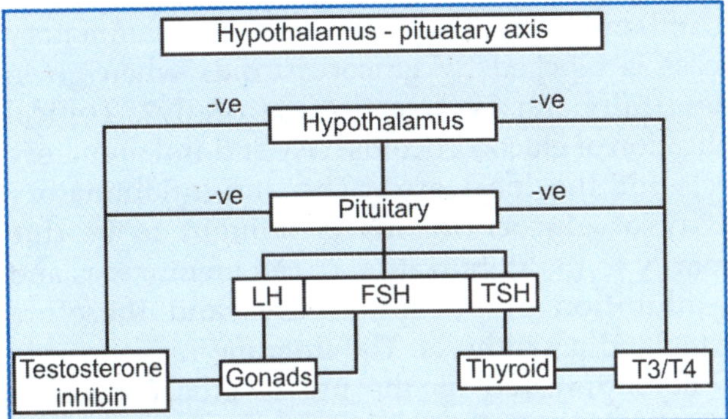

Disorders of the Pituitary System

It is of two types:
Underproduction of hormones—hypopituitarism.
Overproduction of hormones—pituitary adenoma (micro and macro adenoma)

The effects of these disorders vary with the hormone and the target organ of action.

1. **TSH Disorders**
   Hypothyroidism: Secondary or subclinical hypothyroidism.
   Hyperthyroidism: TSH-secreting tumour leading to Hyperthyroidism.
2. **Prolactin Disorders**
   Hyperprolactinaemia: Consistently elevated serum prolactin (PRL>20 ng / ml) in the absence of pregnancy or postpartum lactation.
   Aetiology: Prolactinoma, acromegaly, Cushing's disease, lactotroph hyperplasia, empty sella syndrome, other pituitary tumours, hypothalamic disease, pharmocologic agents, macroprolactinaemia.
3. **Gonadotrophin Disorders**
   Excess and reduced production of gonadotrophs manifests as fertility disorders. The hormones control gametogenesis in males and females at different levels together with negative feedback mechanism of the hypothalamus.
4. **Growth Hormone Disorders**
   The symptoms of GH deficiency in adults are subtle, consisting of decreased muscle strength and exercise tolerance and a reduced sense of well-being (e.g., diminished libido, social isolation). Patients with GH deficiency have increased body fat, particularly intra-abdominally, and decreased lean body mass compared with normal adults. Some patients have decreased bone mineral density, which may improve with GH replacement.

HYPOTHALAMUS

Anterior pituitary functions are controlled by the region of the brain called the hypothalamus via the secretion of releasing and inhibiting factors. Specialised neurons in the hypothalamus, controlled by feedback and other communication methods release factors that cause the release of hormones from the anterior pituitary. The pituitary trophic hormones then control the release of other hormones from a target gland. With the exception of prolactin, release promoting factors are more important to the release of pituitary hormones.

- Somatostatin (inhibits GH release),
- Prolactin-inhibiting factor (PIF, dopamine),
- LH-releasing factor (LHRF),
- FSH-releasing factor (FSHRF),
- Prolactin-releasing factor (PRF),
- Corticotrophin-releasing factor (CRF),
- Thyrotrophin-releasing hormone (TRH)

These hormones control the release of anterior pituitary hormones. The release of these factors is controlled by feedback from the target organ hormone to maintain the proper hormonal balance.

ADRENAL (SUPRARENAL) GLAND

The suprarenal glands are located on top of each of the kidneys. The adrenal cortex (outer portions) produces four major groups of hormones:

- **Glucocorticoids:** Cortisol, Cortisone.
- **Androgens:** Androstenedione, Dihydroepiandrostenedione (DHEA).
- **Mineralocorticoids:** Aldosterone, Deoxycorticosterone, Corticosterone.
- **Oestrogens and Progesterones.**

The *adrenal medulla* is actually an extension of the nervous system. The adrenal medulla produces norepinephrine and epinepherine (adrenaline) that are released in response to stress or a fright.

Mineralocorticoids

The major mineralocorticoid, which is secreted almost independently of ACTH from the pituitary, is aldosterone. Aldosterone secretion is controlled mostly by the levels of potassium and sodium in serum and a blood pressure control system called the renin-angiotensin system. Aldosterone has the opposite effect on serum levels of potassium as it is lost in the urine in exchange for sodium in the renal tubules. Salivary and sweat glands are also influenced by aldosterone to save sodium and the intestine increases the absorption of sodium in response to aldosterone.

Clinical Relevance

1. Elevated levels occur in primary aldosteronism as in:
   - Aldosterone-producing adenoma.
   - Adrenal cortical hyperplasia.
   - Glucocorticoid remediable hyperaldosteronism.
2. Elevated levels also occur in secondary aldosteronism when aldosterone output is elevated due to external stimuli or because of greater activity in the renin angiotensin system as in:
   - Salt depletion.
   - Potassium loading.
   - Large doses of ACTH.
   - Cardiac failure.
   - Hepatic cirrhosis with ascites.
   - Nephrotic syndrome.
   - Barter's syndrome.
   - Postsurgical syndrome.
   - Hypovolaemia and haemorrhage.

GLUCOCORTICOIDS

The major glucocorticoid is cortisol. Cortisol has important actions in the control and metabolism of carbohydrates, lipids, and proteins and assists in the metabolic reaction to stress, especially chronic stress. It causes glucose to be liberated from the liver by increasing glucose production from fatty acids (by-products of lipid breakdown) and amino acids. Cortisol causes the tissues to take up less glucose from the blood and mobilises fat breakdown. The net effect is to increase serum glucose concentrations which is protective for the brain in that it cannot use any other fuel source than glucose. It also stimulates protein breakdown for glucose formation in all tissues except the liver where it stimulates protein synthesis.

Cortisol Abnormalities

Excess
Cushing's syndrome
Deficiency
Congenital adrenal hyperplasia

At high concentrations (greater than physiologic), glucocorticoids (such as hydrocortisone or prednisone) are useful for the treatment of allergies and inflammation. Each step of the inflammatory process is blocked by glucocorticoids when given systemically (an IV injection or orally). Topical application of glucocorticoids have anti-inflammatory effects for the local area. The anti-inflammatory activity of glucocorticoids is thought to be due primarily to the stabilization of cell membranes and the inhibition of phospholipases and therefore prostaglandin synthesis. The immune response can also be suppressed by the use of glucocorticoids. Eosinophils and lymphocytes decrease in the circulation affecting both cellular and humoral immunity. The glucocorticoids are used for many other conditions including asthma, renal diseases, rheumatic disorders such as lupus and inflammatory bowel disease.

Adrenal Medulla

The adrenal medullary hormones are catecholamines—epinephrine and norepinephrine, the parent compound from which epinephrine is formed by addition of a methyl group.

Epinephrine is sympathomimetic, increases cardiac output and rate, systolic blood pressure, blood glucose, hepatic glycogenolysis, basal metabolic rate, sweating and causes mydriasis and skin-vessel constriction. By contrast, norephinephrine causes bradycardia, peripheral vasoconstriction and rise in diastolic blood pressure, and has much less prominent metabolic effects.

Clinical Disorders

Deficiency: Hypotension. Idiopathic spontaneous hypoglycaemia (failure of epinephrine response to hypoglycaemia).

Excess: Paroxysmal or persistent hypertension, headache, sweating, tachycardia, and elevated blood glucose.

THYROID

The thyroid is a large endocrine organ that functions mostly to control metabolism. It is located in the neck between the trachea and larynx and is bilobed with a connecting isthmus (Fig. 17.4).

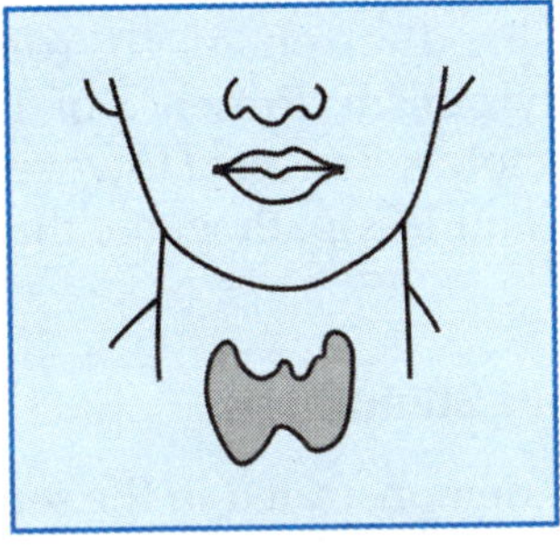

Fig. 17.4: Thyroid gland anatomical position

The gland is composed of many tiny follicles, that are in effect, each a separately functioning gland with a single-layer epithelial lining. Each follicle accumulates a storage form of the circulating thyroid hormones, thyroglobulin. Thyroglobulin is a large protein molecule that contains multiple copies of the amino acid tyrosine. The thyroid hormones are very simple modifications of the amino acid tyrosine. Both T4 and T3 enter cells and bind to an intracellular receptors whereby they increase the metabolic capabilities of the cell. Thyroid hormones are necessary for normal growth and development. They have metabolic effects on protein synthesis, lipid metabolism and carbohydrate metabolism.

Also produced by parafollicular cells within the thyroid is the polypeptide hormone calcitonin. It functions in calcium maintenance to decrease the levels of calcium in the blood. When serum calcium levels are excessive, calcitonin is released. It inhibits bone resorption (by inhibiting osteoclast activity), allows the loss of calcium in the urine and, therefore, decreases calcium in the blood. It opposes the action of parathyroid hormone and has been used clinically for the treatment of osteoporosis.

Markers of the gland

Hormones	T3, T4, FT3, FT4
Structural	Tg–(thyroglobulin)
Antibodies	Anti-Tg, Anti-TPO
Carrier protein	TBG (thyroxine-binding globulin)
Pituitary marker	TSH (thyroxine-stimulating hormone)

Role of Carrier Protein

The hormone synthesised in the gland is transported to various parts by carrier proteins.

TBG: Thyroxine-binding globulin protein is the major carrier protein. It has more affinity to T4 than T3.

TBPA: Thyroxine-binding pre-albumin, binds to T3 than T4.

Thyroxine-binding Globulin (TBG) Test

Almost all the thyroid hormones in the bloodstream are bound to proteins, and these thyroxine-binding proteins play an important role in regulating the free thyroxine (FT4) in the circulation. Thyroxine-binding globulin (TBG) is by far the most important determinant of the overall binding of T4. A measure of TBG should provide a good approximation of the thyroxine-binding function of the blood. This can be a valuable aid in clarification of many clinical conditions. The TBG test is a direct measurement of the total thyroxine-binding capacity of the specific thyroxine-binding interalpha (alpha1-alpha2) globulin in serum.

Free Hormones

Some portions of the hormone remain, unbound to the carrier protein. These are called **free hormones:**

Hormone	Bound %	Free %	Carrier protein
T3	97	3	TBPA
T4	99.7	0.3	TBG

Free T3 and Free T4 are the "Physiologically active hormones"

Measurement of these hormones is more relevant in clinical conditions where the levels of total hormones does not correlate.

Feedback Mechanism

Thyroid hormones have a negative feedback on the pituitary. Whenever the concentrations of T3 and T4 are high, the release of TSH is inhibited from the pituitary. When the thyroid hormones levels are low, it is stimulated. But this need not be true always (Fig. 17.5).

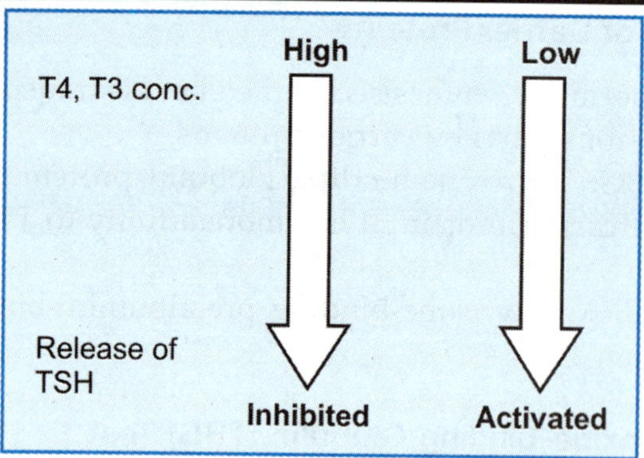

Fig. 17.5: Thyroid hormones feedback mechanism

Neonatal Thyroxine

Newborn infants normally have circulating levels of T4 that are considerably higher than normal adults; but within the first week of life, the values would have decreased markedly. Failure or extreme deficiency of T4 production occurs at a frequency of approximately 1 in 4000 live births. If this deficiency is left untreated, growth deficit, neurologic impairment and mental retardation (cretinism) result. Such infants are characterized by low circulating levels of T4 and, in thyroid gland failure (primary hypothyroidism), by very high levels of TSH. The disorders are markedly affected by the stage of development during which the defect arises. Later-phase development results in transient abnormalities, especially in premature infants, whereas permanent disorders result from early-stage defects.

Since early diagnosis on clinical grounds is difficult and since initiation of treatment before three months of age appears to be necessary to prevent neurologic defects, neonatal screening for hypothyroidism has become a key test in neonatal patient management.

Anti-TPO (Thyroid Peroxidase Antibodies)

The TPOs are autoantibodies directed against the enzyme peroxidase. Because the antibodies bind to the microsomal part of the thyroid cells, they are known as thyroid microsomal antibodies.

Clinical Application

- TPO antibody tests are used to distinguish between different types of goiters.
- It is positive in Hashimoto's disease whereas in nontoxic goiter, it is normally negative.
- Twenty percent of patient's thyrotoxic patients have high titers of TPO antibodies.
- The presence of TPO and elevated TSH is a predictor of future hypothyroidism.

Anti-Tg (Anti-Thyroglobulin Antibodies)

Antibodies are produced against Thyroglobulin. These autoantibodies gradually destroy the thyroid tissue and prevent the production of thyroid hormones, causing hypothyroidism. Presence of Tg antibodies indicates Hashimoto's disease. However, they are less often present and less pathogenic than TPO.

LATS (Long-Acting Thyroid Stimulator)

In 1956, Adams and Purces demonstrated in the sera of some hyperthyroid patients the existence of a thyroid-stimulating factor which had a longer acting effect than TSH. The name applied to this factor was long-acting thyroid stimulator (LATS). It does not appear to have its origin in the pituitary and has been classified as a 7S g-globulin. The LATS is now considered to be a thyroid autoantibody. Since it may persist for years following total thyroidectomy, the nature of the antigen is unknown. It is considered one of a group of thyroid-stimulating immunoglobulins. These antibodies are stimulators and do not destroy thyroid tissue as do the antithyroglobulin and antimicrosomal antibodies. The presence of certain HLA antigens (HLA-B8 and HLA-DR3) indicated an approximate fourfold increase in risk for Graves' disease.

Clinical Significance

The frequent finding of LATS in the sera of patients with malignant exophthalmos and Graves' disease makes its detection an important part of thyrodiagnostic evaluations. The LATS has been overwhelmingly associated with a complex of symptoms known as Graves' disease. Studies showed that positive LATS findings in patients without Graves' disease are "low positive". In patients with active Graves' disease or patients who are presently in remission, "low" as well as unequivocally "high" results are found. Infants born of mothers with Graves' disease may also suffer from this illness because of the transplacental passage of LATS from the maternal to fetal circulation. Fortunately, prenatal testing can warn the physician of this potential threat; under alert management such infants will recover since the LATS will undergo metabolic destruction.

Disorders of the Gland

- **Hypothyroid**—Low levels of thyroid hormones.
  Primary Hypothyroidism—Where the low levels of thyroid hormones are due to failure of the thyroid gland.
  Secondary Hypothyroidism—Where the low levels of thyroid hormones are caused by failure of the hypothalamic-pituitary system to produce TRH or TSH or both.
  Subclinical Hypothyroidism—Elevated TSH levels in the absence of any clinical symptoms.
- **Hyperthyroid**—High levels of thyroid hormones.
  Autoimmune disease—Graves' disease.
  Thyroiditis—Inflammation of the thyroid gland.
  Tumours in the Thyroid—T3 toxicosis, T4 toxicosis.
- Due to a high dose of T4 therapy.
- Induced in patients with goiters if iodine is administered.
- **Nonthyroidal Illness (NTI)**—Abnormal thyroid hormones due to other disorders. Severe illness or injury can induce changes in thyroid hormone levels. In seriously ill patients TSH, T3 and T4 levels may decrease, and a severe decrease often signifies that the patient is dying.

Clinical Manifestations

Overactivity (Hypothyroidism)	*Underactivity (Hyperthyroidism)*
1. Nervousness, increased activity	Decreased energy, physical and mental stability
2. Weight loss without loss of appetite	Weight gain but decreased appetite
3. Warm moist skin	Dry rough skin
4. Tachycardia	Bradycardia
5. Increased bowel movements, diarrhoea	Constipation, disturbed equilibrium
6. Muscle weakness, Osteoporesis	

Tests for Thyroid Function

Generally recommended in:

- Abnormal weight loss or gain.
- Typical symptoms of hypothyroidism—tiredness, lethargy, intolerance to cold.
- Constipation, bradycardia, increased menstruation.
- In children—if they fail to grow normally. If ability to comprehend is less and mental growth is found to be insufficient. If puberty is delayed.
- Symptoms of hyperthyroidism—tiredness, hot, tachycardia, short of breath, increased appetite but lose weight, muscular atrophy, characteristic features of protruding, starring eyes and enlarged thyroid gland.
- Infertility

Different markers of thyroid function are tested in combination for assessment of thyroid status.

- Total tri-iodothyronine (T3)
- Total thyroxine (T4)
- Thyrotrophin (TSH) (by ultra-sensitive method)
- Free tri-iodothyronine (FT3)
- Free thyroxine (FT4)
- Anti-thyroglobulin (Anti-Tg) antibody
- Anti-thyroid peroxidase (Anti-TPO) or Anti-microsomal antibody
- T-uptake

Information to be taken before sample collection

The answers to the following questions will aid in the accurate diagnosis of the patient:

- Whether male or female?
- Age?
- Symptoms?
- Is the patient on treatment—Replacement therapy (thyroxine, cytomel), antithyroid drug?
- Does the patient suffer from any other illness—HIV, hepatitis, tumour, and nephrotic syndrome?
- Has the patient had any major surgery, trauma, stress?
- Is the patient hospitalised?
- Is the patient on any other drugs—oral contraceptives, estrogens, androgens, anabolic steroids, glucocorticoids, propranolol, dopamine, and metaclopromide?
- Family history—Does anyone in the patient's family suffer from autoimmune disorders?
- Does the patient suffer from Autoimmune or connective tissue disorder.
- Has the patient had any neck/whole body irradiation?
- If the patient is a female—Does she have a regular menstrual cycle? Pregnant or Postmenopausal?
- Geographical location—Does the patient come from an iodine deficient/excess region?

Tests for FT3/FT4 are gaining more importance in the diagnosis of thyroid disorders. All limitations of total T3, total T4 due to bound proteins is overcome by free T3 and free T4. FT3 and FT4 are considered to be the "**physiologically active hormones**".

FT3, FT4—Recommendations for Testing

Generally recommended in

- Monitoring treatment—thyroid replacement or suppression.
- Hospitalized patients, where patients may show symptoms of non-thyroidal illness.
- Pregnant women suffering from thyroid disorders.
- Patients known to take certain drugs which will interfere with total T3 and total T4 test results.
- Elderly patients.
- Particularly if a patient's thyroid function test does not correlate with clinical history.

Free Thyroxine Index (FTI)

An estimate (index) related to free T4 levels in serum can be calculated as the product of a T4 result and a T3 uptake ratio (T3UR) test. The reasoning is based on the premise that the T3UR result is inversely proportional to unsaturated thyroxine-binding globulin (UTBG) in serum, and that free T4 varies directly with total T4 and inversely with UTBG levels.

Thus: FT4 Index = T4 (total)× T3UR.

Results may be expressed in any arbitrary terms and may even be related to actual FT4 levels by calculation, using actual values for FT4,T4, and T3UR on a number of normal specimens. It has been observed that the FT4 index is not as discriminatory as the actual estimation of FT4 by equilibrium dialysis. In particular, aberrant results may occur in patients whose TBG is abnormal and in patients whose concentration of TBG is markedly increased or decreased.

T3 Uptake Ratio (T3UR)

(An Index of the Unsaturated Thyroxine-binding Globulin Fraction of Serum)

The test has nothing to do with the actual T3 serum level in spite of its name which, unfortunately, is sometimes abbreviated to "T3 test". It must be emphasized that the T3 uptake ratio and the true T3 (T3 by EIA) are entirely different tests.

Clinical Significance

The T3 uptake ratio, in conjunction with the T3 measurement in serum, is used as a screening test of thyroid function.

Pregnancy: Elevated T3 values are to be expected in euthyroid patients. TBG and unsaturated TBG are both increased in normal pregnancy. This appears towards the end of the first trimester and is caused by increased estrogen secretion. In such patients low-T3UR test values are to be expected because of the increase in unsaturated TBG. This is important because the normally expected low-T3UR values are not found in certain cases of habitual threatened abortions as well as in pregnancy complicated by hyperthyroidism.

High or low-T4 in a euthyroid individual: In rare cases this is caused by a hereditary abnormality in the level of TBG. Thus, in a eumetabolic person with hereditary absence of TBG, a low-T3 will be found and the T3UR test value will be high; the converse applies to the person with a hereditary excess of TBG.

A normal T3 in a hypothyroid patient: This can occur when the unsaturated TBG is elevated.

PARATHYROID

The four parathyroid glands lie on top of the thyroid gland in separate nodes spread out to the four quadrants of the thyroid. Parathyroid hormone is under direct feedback control of circulating levels of calcium. If calcium levels fall, then parathyroid hormone is released. As calcium levels rise, release of the hormone is reduced. Parathyroid hormone acts on bones, the kidneys and the intestines to reabsorb calcium.

Hyperparathyroidism: Increased levels of parathyroid hormone. It is usually rare and occurs as a result of tumour. It is leads to osteitis cystica fibrosis.

Hypoparathyroidism: Low levels of parathyroid hormone can result due to trauma or removal during thyroid surgery.

PANCREAS

The pancreas is a mixed exocrine and endocrine gland. The exocrine portion makes many of the digestive enzymes necessary for gastrointestinal function. The endocrine portion is comprised of discrete islands of cells called the islets of Langerhans. Cells within the islets produce two hormones that regulate the concentration of glucose in the blood.

Insulin

It is a small protein (MW 6000 Daltons) and is composed of two chains (A and B) held by disulphide bonds. It is secreted only by the β-cells of the pancreas. The α-cells of the pancreas secretes glycogen.

Insulin is secreted in a precursor form, *Proinsulin.* This is cleaved to release *Insulin and C-Peptide.* C-peptide is the connecting peptide between the A and B chains of insulin. All the three—Proinsulin, Insulin and C-peptide are found in the blood. Estimation of these is important in different conditions (Fig. 17.6).

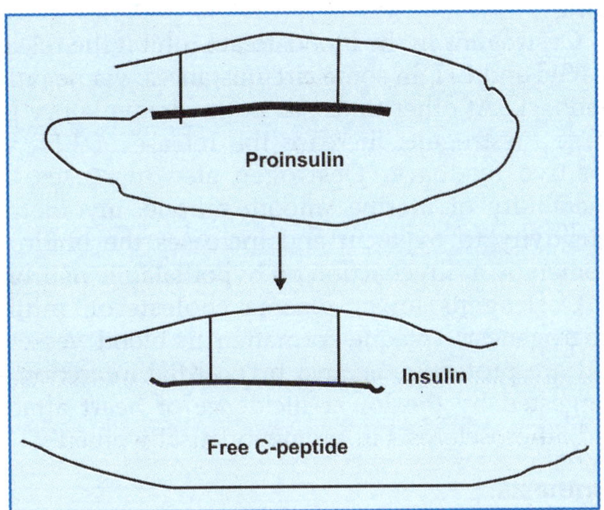

Fig. 17.6: Proinsulin and cleaved products

Functions of Insulin

- Reduces blood sugar level by stimulating uptake of sugar by various tissues.
- Stimulates liver to store glucose in the form of glycogen.
- Promotes synthesis of fatty acids in liver.
- Stimulates uptake of amino acids, contributing to overall anabolic effect.
- Increase the permeability of many cells to potassium, magnesium and calcium ions.

Clinical relevance of C-peptide

Indicators of β-cell function than peripheral insulin concentration.

Primary indicator for evaluation of fasting hypoglycaemia.

Condition	*Insulin*	*C-peptide*
Insulinoma	Increased	Increased
Insulin producing β-cell tumours	Normal	Increased
Hypoglycaemia (injected / exogenous)	Increased	Decreased

Anti-Insulin Antibodies

Antibodies against insulin hormone have been observed in many conditions. These can be against endogenous or exogenous insulin. It is found in Type 1 diabetes. These are developed under insulin therapy. There are two types of antibodies.

Against endogenous insulin: Antibodies against insulin, produced in the body (human insulin).

Against exogenous insulin: Antibodies against insulin, taken by medication—insulin injection (bovine, porcine and recombinant human insulin).

Both types are present in the body. Detection of both these types are important.

Glucagon is a small protein produced by alpha cells within the islets that cause the level of blood glucose to increase. Its release is controlled by blood levels of glucose. As levels fall, glucagon release is increased causing the release of stored glucose and the synthesis of glucose until levels are increased and glucagon release is then reduced via negative feedback. Glucagon opposes the metabolic actions of insulin. This opposition plus the negative feedback control of glucose levels maintain very tight control on blood glucose levels.

TESTES

Testosterone is the principal hormone of the testes and is synthesised from cholesterol by the Leydig cells. The secretion of testosterone is under the control of LH from the pituitary. The LH secretion is decreased by increased levels of testosterone in the blood via negative feedback. Testosterone develops and maintains the male secondary sex characteristics, is anabolic and growth promoting and participates in the formation of sperm. It also causes aggressive behaviour and increased libido. Body hair is increased by androgens while scalp hair is decreased.

Like other steroids, testosterone enters cells and binds to an intracellular receptor and then causes the production of mRNA coding for proteins that manifest the changes induced by testosterone. In some target tissues a form of testosterone, DHT, is produced that has greater stability in combination with the receptor and, therefore, produces a longer lasting effect. The DHT is needed for the maturation of the accessory glands and external genitalia, while testosterone is more important in the growth of muscle mass, development of the internal genitalia and maintenance of the male libido and sex drive.

Another hormone produced by the testes is the polypeptide hormone, *inhibin*, produced by the Sertoli cells. It inhibits FSH secretion by a direct action on the pituitary.

Androgen Abnormalities

Androgen Excess

Males

- Children—precocious puberty
- Adults—infertility

Females

- Hirsuitism and virilisation
- Pseudohermaphroditism

Androgen Deficiency

Males

- Improper growth—eunuchoid features
- Disappearance of body hair
- Muscular atrophy
- Infertility
- Testicular feminisation

Females

- Generally low in females.

OVARY

The ovaries produce the steroid hormones (oestrogens and progesterone) that cause the development of secondary sexual characteristics and develop and maintain the reproductive function in the female. Specifically, the oestrogens are secreted by the theca interna cells and the granulosa cells of the ovarian follicle, the corpus luteum and the placenta. The LH from the anterior pituitary binds to receptors on theca interna or granulosa cells to cause the production of estradiol from cholesterol or a downstream precursor androstenedione that is passed from the thecal cells to the granulosa cells. Progesterone is secreted mostly by the corpus luteum and the placenta, but some are made by the developing follicle. Negative feedback from progesterone decreases LH secretion and large doses can prevent ovulation.

Oestradiol is the most potent and major secreted oestrogen although oestrone and estriol can be found in circulation as well. Like other steroid hormones, oestrogens enter target cells, combine with a nuclear receptor and cause the production of mRNAs that, when translated into proteins, modify cell function. Oestrogens are metabolised by the liver and secreted in bile where some are reabsorbed back into the body. Metabolites of oestradiol are excreted in the urine.

Oestrogens in the bloodstream inhibit the release of FSH and LH, in some circumstances, via negative feedback. At other times, as in the preovulatory LH surge, oestrogens increase the release of LH, via positive feedback. Oestrogen also increases the excitability of uterine smooth muscle, myometrial sensitivity to oxytocin and increases the libido in women by a direct action on hypothalamic neurons.

Oestrogens lower plasma cholesterol, inhibit atherogenesis (plaque formation in blood vessels), and are protective against myocardial infarction as suggested by the lower incidence of heart attacks and atherosclerosis in premenopausal women.

Synthesis

Pregnant women: Placenta (mainly Oestriol- E_3)

Nonpregnant women: Ovaries (mainly Oestradiol- E_2)

Oestrogen Abnormalities

Excess

- Menstrual irregularities
- Amenorrhoea
- Hermaphroditism
- Hashimoto's thyroiditis
- Addison's disease
- Turner's syndrome

Deficiency

- Tumour of the ovary
- Hirsutism
- Infertility

Progesterone has the principal targets of the uterus, breasts and the brain. It promotes the development of breast tissue, causes changes in the endometrial lining during the luteal phase of the cycle, decreases the excitability of myometrial cells and decreases uterine sensitivity to oxytocin.

Progesterone Abnormalities

Excess

- Congenital adrenal hyperplasia
- Hirsutism
- Amenorrhoea
- Infertility

Deficiency

- Menstrual irregularities
- Hermaphroditism
- Corpus luteum deficiency

PINEAL GLAND

The pineal gland can be found deep in the brain at the top of the third ventricle where it is close communication with the cerebrospinal fluid. In the adult, the pineal gland can often be seen in X-rays of the brain because of the accumulation of radiopaque calcium phosphate and carbonate into small granules called pineal sand. The cells of the pineal gland secrete the hormone *melatonin* in a diurnal cycle (the amount changes throughout a 24-hour period) where the amount remains low during the daylight hours but increases during the dark hours. This diurnal variation is controlled by norepinephrine from sympathetic nervous input that is regulated by the light-dark cycle in the environment.

Although some people use melatonin supplements to treat insomnia, this effect has not been proven in scientific trials. There have been reports of increased insomnia and depression as well as other side effects associated with its use.

HORMONES AND FERTILITY

Disturbance in the hormonal system is a major cause of male and female fertility problems.

The brain plays a key role in regulating the hormones that affect the development of sperm (spermatogenesis) in males and regulation of menstrual cycle (ovulation) in females. The process begins when the hypothalamus (a part of the brain) emits a substance (gonadotrophin-releasing hormone, or GnRH) that stimulates the pituitary gland, located at the base of the brain. The pituitary gland then emits LH (luteinising hormone) and FSH (follicle-stimulating hormone). These stimulate testicular development and sperm production in males and regulate the menstrual cycle and release of ovum in females.

The LH and FSH also regulate the production of steroid hormones responsible for male and female sexual characteristics.

MALE FERTILITY

The Four Factors of Male Fertility

Pretesticular Function (Hormones)

Disturbances in the hormonal system cause about 10 per cent of male fertility problems.

Testicular Function

Testicular failure represents about 55 per cent of male fertility problems.

To respond to hormone stimulation properly, the testicles, or testes, must be capable of producing sperm (spermatogenesis).

Post-testicular Function

Tubal obstruction including vasectomy accounts for about 6 per cent of male infertility.

The post-testicular system of ducts must be capable of storing and delivering sperm. Sperm delivery system problems include obstruction or interruption of the tubes as a result of congenital malformation, disease, surgery, or trauma.

Ejaculatory Disturbance, Impotence, and Sexual Problems

Ejaculatory disturbances, impotence, and sexual problems may prevent the delivery of sperm.

These disorders represent about 10 per cent of male fertility problems.

Problems associated with male infertility

Problem %	Infertile population
Hormone:	
Endocrine	9
Hyperprolactinemia (elevated prolactin)	10-40
Congenital adrenal hyperplasia	1
Stress	?
Sperm production:	
Varicocoele	40
Testicular failure	14
Smoking, heat, drugs	?
Sperm delivery:	
Obstructed ducts	7
Congenital obstruction / absence of ducts	2
Erection, orgasm, ejaculation:	
Sexual problems	5
Ejaculation problems	2

THE MALE HORMONE SYSTEM

The Hypothalamus and Pituitary Start the Action

Approximately every ninety minutes a specialised area in the brain (hypothalamus) secretes GnRH (gonadotrophin-releasing hormone). GnRH signals the pituitary gland, located at the base of the brain, to produce LH (luteinising hormone) and FSH (follicle-stimulating hormone). The LH tells the testes to secrete the male hormone testosterone. Testosterone stimulates the sexual desires and develops and maintains male secondary sex characteristics such as hair growth and deep voice. Together, testosterone and FSH stimulate the testes to produce sperm (spermatogenesis). The body's ability to make and regulate these hormones is vital for maintaining virility and sperm production (see Fig. 17.7).

Feedback Hormones from Testicles

There are feedback hormones—testosterone and inhibin—that keep a check and balance on GnRH, LH, and FSH levels. Once the Leydig cells in the testicles produce enough testosterone, the hormone control systems cut back on GnRH and LH production. When the Sertoli cells, which respond to FSH stimulation, produce enough inhibin, the pituitary cuts back FSH production.

Where Can Things Go Wrong?

Fertility Factor: The Hormone Balancing Act
Several things can go wrong with the hypothalamus—pituitary endocrine system:

- The brain can fail to pulse GnRH properly.
- The pituitary can fail to produce enough LH and FSH to stimulate the testes.
- The testes' Leydig cells may not produce testosterone in response to LH (pituitary) stimulation.
- The body may produce other hormones and chemical compounds which interfere with sex-hormone balance.

Any one of these conditions can impair sperm production.

An Overview of Hormonal Treatment

If the pituitary hormones (LH and FSH) are low, but the hypothalamus and pituitary gland are working fine, then clomiphene citrate (cc) is administered to stimulate the hypothalamus to pulse GnRH at regular intervals. When the hypothalamus properly releases GnRH, the pituitary gland will respond by producing LH and FSH. If clomiphene citrate does not improve LH and FSH levels, then one can suspect that your pituitary gland may be malfunctioning.

If the pituitary cannot manufacture the missing sex hormones, one has to take hormone supplements — hCG or Pergonal (LH + FSH).

DIAGNOSING AND BEATING SPECIFIC HORMONAL PROBLEMS

Hyperprolactinaemia

Hyperprolactinaemia (elevated prolactin) can be difficult to diagnose because FSH, LH, and testosterone levels will be normal. We find elevated prolactin, a hormone associated with nursing mothers, in 10 to 40 per cent of infertile males. Mild prolactin elevation produces no symptoms; however, greater elevations can reduce sperm production, impair sex drive, and cause impotence. Hyperprolactinaemia responds well to bromocriptine. A prolactin-secreting tumour will also respond to bromocriptine; however, surgery and/or radiation therapy may be necessary.

Hypothyroidism

Found in 1 per cent of infertile men, hypothyroidism (low thyroid hormone) can cause poor semen quality, poor testicular function, and/or disturbances in sex drive. The person will be lethargic, intolerant of cold, and overweight. Because the pituitary gland is trying its best to stimulate the unresponsive thyroid gland, the pituitary-produced TSH (thyroid-stimulating hormone) level will be elevated. Elevated prolactin levels, frequently found with this disorder, may cause impotence.

Correcting the diet or beginning thyroid hormone replacement therapy should elevate sperm count to previous levels.

Congenital Adrenal Hyperplasia

Found in 1 per cent of infertile males, congenital adrenal hyperplasia may be suspected when a semen analysis shows a low sperm count, an increased number of immature sperm cells, sperm with long tapered heads, and low motility. These abnormalities occur when the pituitary is suppressed by increased levels of adrenal androgens. Men with this disease may also have hypertension (high blood pressure) and oedema (water retention). Early onset of the disease may result in ambiguous genitalia at birth or reaching puberty at an early age. Adult onset may be characterised by infertility, high blood pressure, and/or water retention.

Cortisone replacement therapy will lower the androgens and allow the pituitary to function normally. Therefore, indirectly, cortisone replacement therapy will elevate sperm count.

Hypogonadotrophic Hypopituitarism

Hypogonadotrophic hypopituitarism is a spectrum of diseases with a complicated name that means low (hypo-) pituitary gland output of LH and FSH. Other stages of this disease are called isolated gonadotrophin defect and panhypopituitarism, in which the entire (pan-) pituitary gland is affected.

These diseases arrest sperm development and cause the progressive loss of germ cells from the testes. In addition, the seminiferous tubules and Leydig cells (which produce testosterone) also deteriorate. If the condition persists for a long time, there will be no sperm production at all. When the disease is associated with a pituitary tumour, elevated prolactin levels may also cause impotence.

Panhypopituitarism

Complete pituitary gland failure (panhypopituitarism) lowers growth hormone, ACTH level, thyroid-stimulating hormone (TSH), and LH and FSH levels. Person having this rare disease will have multiple symptoms that include impotence, decreased sex drive, loss of secondary sex characteristics, and normal or undersized testicles. Hypothyroidism (low thyroid hormone) will cause to gain weight, be intolerant of cold, and feel lethargic. If the disorder began early enough in your life it may even cause dwarfism. The hormonal deficiency is often caused by a tumour, surgery, or trauma to the pituitary gland.

Kallmann's Syndrome

Kallmann's syndrome is a congenital hypothalamic dysfunction. A person born with this unusual condition will have underdeveloped testicles and possibly a harelip, cleft palate, color blindness, and/or the inability to smell. Affected men have varying

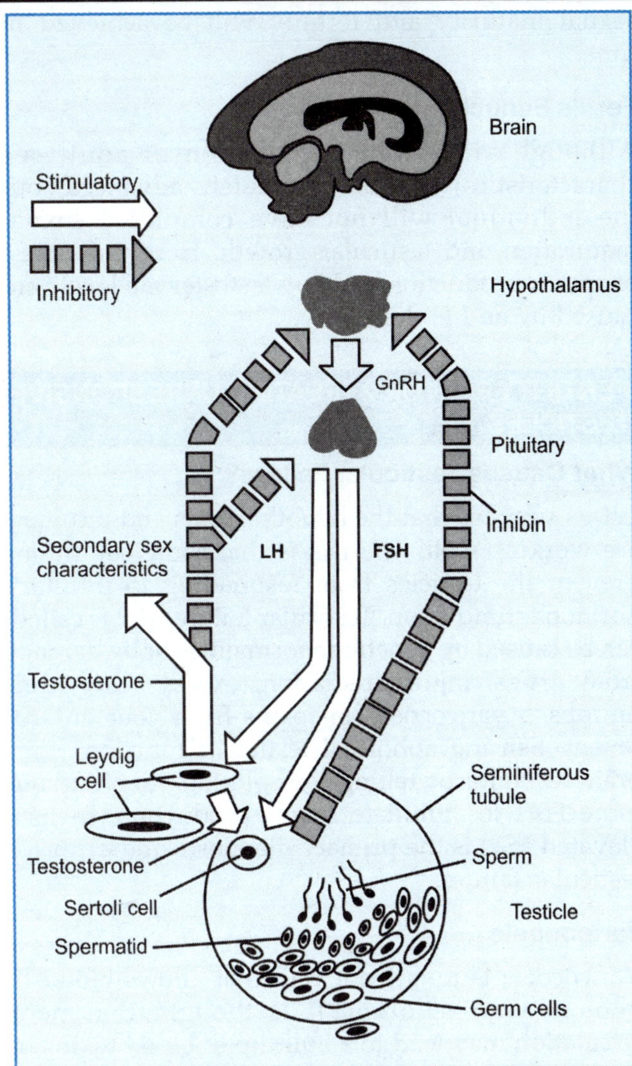

Fig. 17.7: Male hormones, feedback and effects

degrees of sexual infantilism (prepuberty) and no sperm production. Since the hypothalamus fails to stimulate the pituitary adequately, FSH, LH, and testosterone levels are low.

Kallmann's syndrome is treated similarly to hypogonadotrophic hypopituitarism. Although at first it seems hopeless, men afflicted with Kallmann's syndrome can achieve normal puberty and eventually become fertile.

Delayed Puberty

Individuals with isolated pituitary growth hormone deficiency do not sexually mature until their mid to late twenties. Hormone supplements can make them look virile, but until they go through puberty, they would not be fertile. The LH/FSH and/or hCG injections can bring on puberty, although if left alone, sexual maturity and fertility will be achieved in time.

Fertile Eunuch

Although virilisation (acquisition of adult sex characteristics) will be moderately advanced, but the individual will not have completed sexual maturation and testicular growth. Here, the arrest of sperm production and low testosterone levels are caused by an LH deficiency.

FERTILITY FACTOR 2 TREATING UNRESPONSIVE TESTICLES

What Causes Testicular Failure?

Let us suppose that the hypothalamus and pituitary are working well. The fact is that some conditions prevent the testicles from responding to pituitary hormone stimulation. Testicular failure, as it is called, can be caused by genetic abnormalities or by damage from drugs, injury, radiation, excess heat, adult mumps, a varicocoele, or toxins from your environment. Sensing abnormal testicular function, your brain responds by telling your pituitary to pump out more FSH to stimulate sperm production. In fact, elevated FSH is the primary diagnostic indicator for testicular failure.

Varicocoele

Varicocoele is a varicose vein that allows blood to pool in your scrotum. It is thought that poor circulation may lead to a buildup of blood toxins or increase your scrotal temperature. Either of these conditions may result in infertility.

Cryptorchidism

Undescended testicles occur in 8 out of 1,000 boys. Hence, it causes infertilty.

Infection

Mumps, tuberculosis, brucellosis, gonorrhoea, typhoid, influenza, smallpox, and syphilis can cause the testes to atrophy. With some of these infections, LH and testosterone (virility) levels may remain normal. However, if FSH is high, then prognosis for testicular recovery is poor.

Torsion

Torsion of the testis and/or blood vessels supplying the testis (spermatic cord) is a common problem that threatens fertility.

Klinefelter's Syndrome

Each cell in a normal man's body has only one Y (male) and one X (female) chromosome. People with Klinefelter's syndrome, however, have one Y and two X chromosomes in each cell. In the beginning stages of this rare disorder FSH is only slightly elevated, indicating minimal testicular failure. However, eventually all other active testicular structures will atrophy, including germ cells, tubules, Leydig cells, and Sertoli cells; the testes themselves actually shrink. After testicular failure occurs (causing FSH levels to rise dramatically), improving fertility is impossible.

Cushing's Syndrome

Cushing's syndrome occurs when the adrenal gland secretes excessive amounts of cortisol. People with this rare disorder will have a moon-shaped face and will suffer from water retention, obesity, impotence, feminized characteristics, loss of sex drive, and infertility. The condition may be due to an adrenal tumour or to excessive stimulation of the adrenal gland by ACTH (adrenocorticotrophic hormone) from the pituitary. If ACTH is high, either the pituitary is overactive or an ACTH-secreting pituitary tumour is present (called Cushing's disease). Elevated adrenal androgens suppress LH and FSH production and spermatogenesis. Cortisone replacement therapy will reduce cortisol levels and restore natural LH, FSH, and sperm production. If a tumour is present, surgery and/or radiation therapy is required.

Germ Cell Aplasia (Sertoli Cell Only)

Germ cell aplasia (Sertoli cell only) is an inherited condition. Testes have normal Leydig cells, no germ cells. Because their Leydig cells continue to produce testosterone, these men remain virile, but they cannot produce sperm. Germ cell aplasia can also be caused by exposure to large doses of radiation and prolonged exposure to toxic substances.

Testicular Enzyme Defects

Testicular enzyme defects prevent the testes from responding normally to hormonal stimulation. These rare genetic defects can cause multiple genital abnormalities, incomplete virilization, small testes, and low or no sperm production. The LH and FSH will both be high, since the brain is doing its best to stimulate the unresponsive testicles.

FEMALE FERTILITY

The Five Female Fertility Factors

Fertility Factor—1: Ovulation

Any woman complaining of very heavy menstrual flow, very light menstrual flow, no menstrual flow, irregular cycles, breast discharge, or scanty or overabundant body hair growth is telling that she may not be ovulating. This may be due to an intrinsic malfunction of her reproductive organs or hormones or to a systemic disease causing other body chemistry problems.

Fertility Factor—2: Sperm-Mucus Interaction

Normally, the cervical mucus forms an impervious plug that keeps foreign materials, including sperm, from entering the uterus. Once each month, responding to oestrogen, the cervical mucus becomes clear, thin, and stringy so sperm can swim through the cervix into the uterus.

Fertility Factor—3: Fertilisation

Fertilisation depends on the sperm's ability to penetrate the outer layers of the egg and transfer its genetic information.

Fertility Factor—4: Tubal Factor

Other clues uncovered during the physical examination may point to transport problems. Abdominal adhesions can prevent the egg from entering the fallopian tube as well as impede its passage through the tube. Endometriosis can cause adhesions and impair ovulation.

Depending on their size and location, fibroids and ovarian cysts can also interfere with egg transport. These conditions will usually respond to surgery.

Fertility Factor—5: Embryo Implantation

The egg or (if the egg is fertilized) the embryo has to successfully implant in the woman's uterus. Sometimes, during the physical examination one can detect obvious causes for miscarriage such as congenitally malformed reproductive organs, an abnormally shaped cervix or a cervix distorted by previous surgical procedures.

FEMALE HORMONE SYSTEM

What is Ovulation?

Ovulation is a fascinating harmony performed by several different "players"—the hypothalamus, pituitary gland, and ovary. The hypothalamus maintains the hormonal "tempo" by regularly pulsing GnRH (gonadotrophic-releasing hormone). These pulses stimulate the pituitary gland to produce LH (luteinising hormone) and FSH (follicle-stimulating hormone).

The pituitary gland plays the chorus—a pattern repeated from month to month in a beautifully precise rhythm. Each month the pituitary secretes FSH to stimulate the development and growth of over one thousand eggs. This phase in the ovulation cycle is known as the follicular phase. At puberty, a woman has about half a million primitive germ cells. Only four or five hundred, however, will ever reach maturity. Due to some mysterious mechanism, which we do not yet understand, usually each month only one of the thousand developing eggs becomes dominant and grows to maturity. This egg, or ovum, is cradled within the ovary in a tiny, fluid-filled capsule called the follicle.

During the follicular phase of the cycle, LH acts on the ovary's theca cells to initiate oestrogen production by the granulosa cells. The oestrogen makes the follicle even more responsive to FSH, which further stimulates follicular growth and development of the egg. As the follicle expands toward the surface of the ovary, the egg increases in size nearly forty times. The ovary tells the pituitary when it needs more or less FSH to finish the job of egg maturation by making a feedback hormone called inhibin (folliculostatin).

Shortly before ovulation, the genetic material (nucleus) in the egg divides (meiosis) to half the number of chromosomes in the cell. If the egg is fertilised, a second meiotic division leaves the ovum with twenty-three chromosomes—a perfect complement to the sperm's twenty-three. To form an egg, the female germinal cell divides twice, as does the male germinal cell. During female germ cell divisions, however, the "surviving" ovum jealously hoards the bulk of cellular material (nutrients) and casts off the excess genetic material (polar bodies). The egg or (if the egg is fertilized) the embryo survives on these nutrients until the embryo successfully implants in the woman's uterus.

Oestrogen also stimulates the uterine lining (endometrium) to become thick, lush, and filled with nutrients for the embryo. The cervical mucus responds to elevated oestrogen by becoming clear, watery, and stringy. Normally, impervious to sperm, at midcycle the mucus welcomes the sperm and promises easy passage toward the egg.

When your oestrogen level peaks at midcycle, the pituitary "knows" that the egg is ready to embark on its journey. The pituitary responds to the oestrogen peak by producing a surge of LH, which releases the egg within eighteen to thirty-six hours. The outer wall of the ovary dissolves away from the bulging follicle; and within two to three minutes, the ovum escapes into the woman's abdominal cavity. Surrounded by a sticky protective layer of cells (cumulus oophorus), the egg gently floats toward the fallopian tube. The expelled follicular fluid stimulates the fimbriated end of the fallopian tube to reach toward the ovum, grasp the ovary, and vacuum up the egg. The muscles and tiny hairs (cilia) lining the fallopian tube gently coax the egg on its three-to-four-day journey through the narrow passage. For conception to occur during this cycle, the sperm must fertilise the egg in the fallopian tube within twelve hours of ovulation.

During the egg's journey, the ruptured follicle begins an amazing transformation into the corpus luteum. Stimulated by LH from the pituitary gland, this yellow-pigmented, glandular, ovarian structure enlarges to make up nearly a third of the ovary. During the luteal phase (latter half of the cycle), the corpus luteum produces progesterone, a hormone that prepares the uterine lining for implantation of the embryo. Progesterone also acts on your body's temperature-regulating mechanism by raising basal body temperature (BBT) approximately one-half degree. Thus, shortly after ovulation, you will see a rise on your BBT chart. If fertilisation does not take place, the corpus luteum deteriorates. Oestrogen and progesterone levels decline rapidly in the week or so prior to menstruation. Deprived of these hormones, the endometrium atrophies and menstrual flow begins. At the site of the original follicle, the corpus luteum degenerates and leaves a minute piece of scar tissue as a reminder of its brief existence. If fertilisation takes place, a corpus luteum of pregnancy forms to maintain the uterine lining (endometrial bed) and support the implanted fertilised ovum (conceptus) (see Fig. 17.8).

The hypothalamus, pituitary, and ovary must all work in perfect harmony. When they do not, the most obvious symptom is abnormal menses.

Cyclical Changes in the Menstrual Cycle

What makes One have a Period?

Normally, each month oestrogen and progesterone stimulate the growth of the uterine lining. When the progesterone-producing corpus luteum deteriorates toward the end of the cycle, "progesterone withdrawal bleeding" occurs: you have a period. Waves of vasoconstriction (blood vessel spasms) restrict the blood supply to the endometrium and thus provoke the onset of menses. At the conclusion of menses, clotting factors seal off exposed bleeding sites, and resumed oestrogen production begins restoring the endometrium.

CLUES FROM THE MENSTRUAL HISTORY

The Three Types of Menstrual Patterns

The Regular Menstrual Period

The critical point about this category is that the period is regular from month to month, beginning like clockwork every twenty-five days or every thirty-five days, for example. If the periods are regular, then she is probably ovulating. The consistently irregular menstrual cycle, however, where one month she begins menstruating after twenty-five days, the next month after thirty-four, and the next in thirty, may indicate that she has a fertility problem. If a woman reports a regular menstrual history, one should look at other areas of the reproductive system for a breakdown in the fertility formula (see Fig. 17.9).

Irregular Menstrual Periods or Amenorrhea for Six or More Months

This is the most common complaint found with fertility problems. The woman's menstrual periods occur infrequently and at unpredictable intervals. Some women, even report that at some point their periods stopped altogether. Because these women are capable of menstruating (as demonstrated by their history), there is a good chance that with the proper treatment ovulation and a regular menstrual cycle will resume.

Nonexistence of the Menstrual Period

Women who have never menstruated may have genetic abnormalities, congenitally deformed reproductive organs, delayed puberty, or a pituitary malfunction. If by the age of sixteen a woman has not started menstruating, she should be concerned. It is important to diagnose the problem early and to determine if such women will respond to hormonal therapy or surgical correction.

CLUES FROM PHYSICAL EXAMINATION

The Physical Examination

During the physical examination, the doctor looks for evidence that the woman is are ovulating, that her mucus allows sperm to reach the egg in good shape, and that the fertilized egg can successfully implant and grow in your uterus. A number of things may go wrong during this process. The sperm may not be able to journey through inhospitable cervical mucus or, having reached the egg, they may be unable to penetrate its surface. The egg may get lost in the body cavity and never find its way into the fallopian tube. Fallopian tubes, damaged by infection or trapped in adhesions, may not be capable of moving the egg toward the uterus. The growing, fertilised egg may become entangled in webs of intratubal adhesions caused by infection and develop into an ectopic pregnancy. Or the uterine lining may fail to nourish the early embryo. Once the doctor determines where these processes are breaking down, he has a good chance of restoring her fertility.

During the physical examination, the doctor would look for evidence of systemic disease: jaundiced (yellow) skin and eyes are indicative of liver disease; tenderness in the middle of the back and water retention (oedema) may indicate kidney malfunction.

The body build and secondary sex characteristics may provide additional clues to hormonal imbalance. Undersized breasts, scanty pubic hair, and underdeveloped hips all suggest a female hormone deficiency. An enlarged clitoris and abnormal hair growth such as a mustache may suggest excess male hormones. Rarer conditions such as ambiguous genitalia (not clearly male or female) and duplicate reproductive organs may point to genetic or enzyme defects that can interfere with ovulation. Although breast size, body conformation, and hair distribution are not conclusive evidence, they may corroborate suspicions created by other clues.

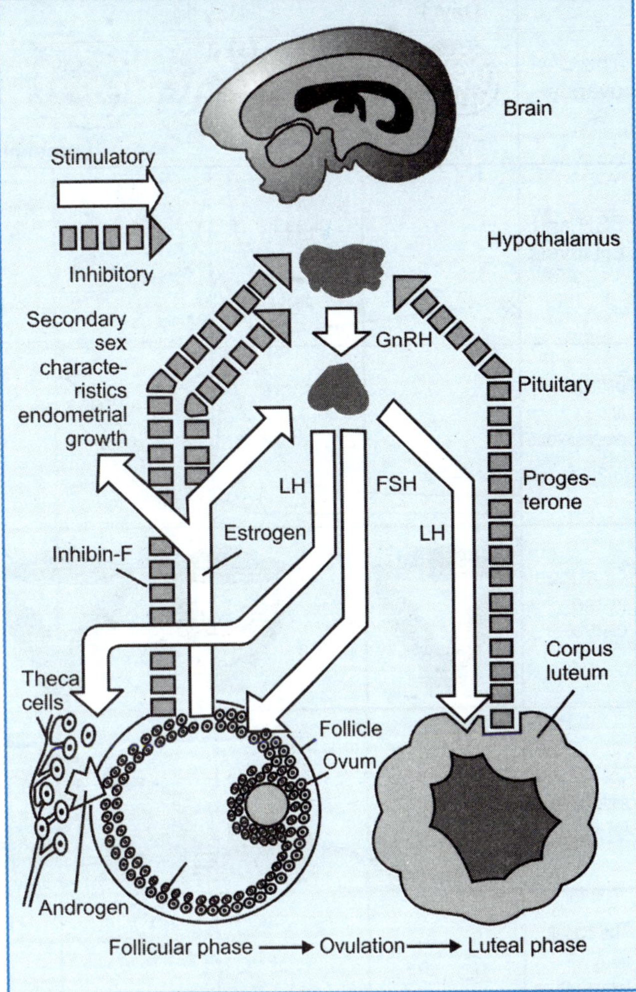

Fig. 17.8: Female hormone system

Based on the menstrual history and physical examination, the doctor will recommend a number of tests to confirm this diagnosis.

Diagnostic Approaches for Irregular Menstrual Periods or Amenorrhea

Several basic tests will help determine why your periods are abnormal.

Pregnancy Test

This may seem surprising, but pregnancy is the single most common reason for women reporting that their periods have stopped. Always conduct a pregnancy test to rule out the possibility of pregnancy.

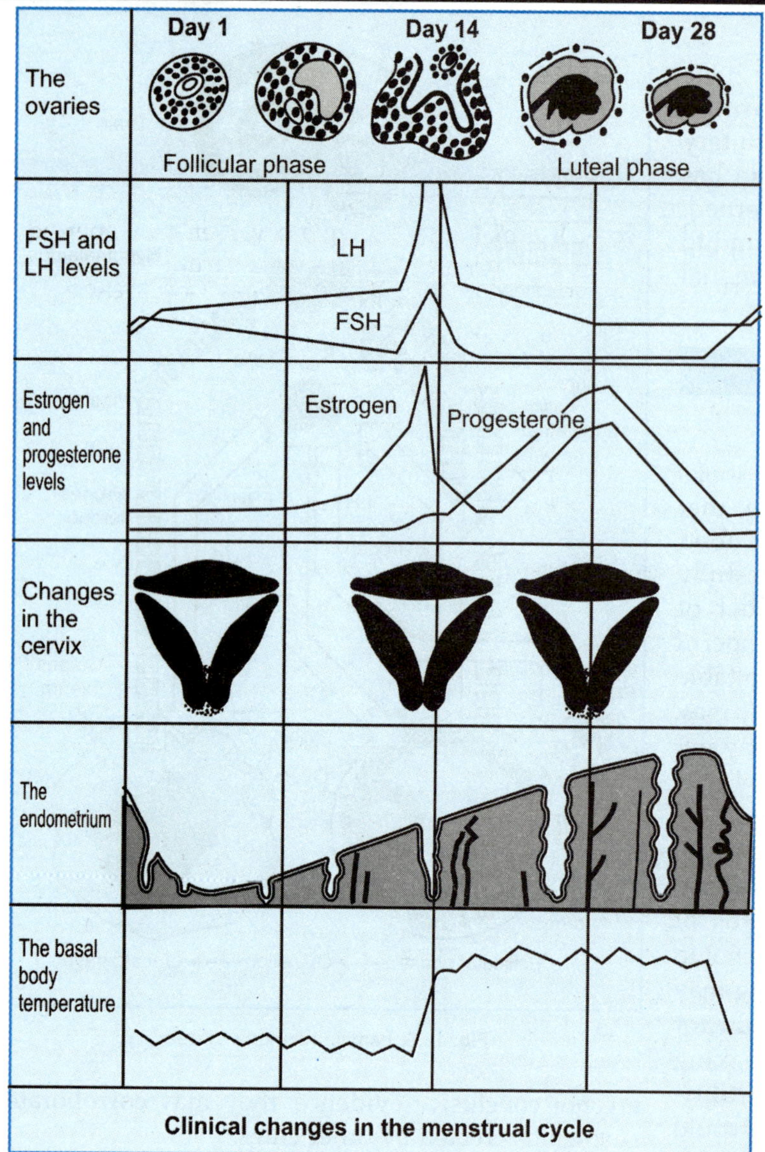

Fig. 17.9: The Menstrual Cycle

Progesterone Withdrawal Test

The progesterone withdrawal test will confirm if the uterus is capable of menstruating. If it is, then the cause of menstrual irregularity lies with the hormonal systems. If the uterus cannot "bleed," then the problem lies with the uterus itself.

The doctor can bring period either by giving you oral progesterone over a five- or ten-day period or by giving a progesterone injection. After taking the progesterone, the period should begin within fourteen to twenty days.

Positive Response to Progesterone Withdrawal

If progesterone withdrawal causes the period to start up, then a number of things are clear.

First, we know that the ovaries are producing enough oestrogen to build up the uterine lining. We also know that the uterus is capable of responding to oestrogen and progesterone stimulation. Since the uterus is functioning normally, the fertility problem lies somewhere in the hormonal system.

Second, the failure to menstruate is because of failure to ovulate. For some reason, the pituitary is not producing the LH spike necessary to release the ovum from the follicle.

Two conditions must exist before the pituitary will release an LH surge: the follicles growing in the ovaries must release enough oestrogen to signal the pituitary that it is time to release the LH surge—in other words, that at least one egg has reached maturity. And the pituitary gland must be capable of generating the LH spike.

One can suspect that your hypothalamus just isn't prodding your pituitary well enough. If the follicles do not grow to maturity, there will never be enough oestrogen to trigger the LH spike to release the egg and thus ovulate. A pituitary malfunction can cause the same problem.

Negative Response to Progesterone Withdrawal

Most women will "bleed" in response to progesterone withdrawal. However, if one dose not, it is possible that the oestrogen supply is not adequate to stimulate uterine lining growth. If the uterus is normal, taking oestrogen to prime the growth of the uterine lining should guarantee that one will have a period after progesterone withdrawal. So repeat the progesterone withdrawal after oestrogen stimulation.

If the oestrogen/progesterone-stimulated cycle fails to produce a "bleed," it means that the uterus cannot respond to oestrogen and progesterone stimulation: we can pinpoint the uterus as the problem.

Positive Withdrawal to Oestrogen/Progesterone Stimulation

When one has a period after taking oestrogen and progesterone, we know that the uterus is capable of menstruating. The reason she had not been menstruating is that her ovaries were not producing adequate amounts of oestrogen. At this stage in the diagnostic procedures, we do not know for certain why the ovaries are not producing oestrogen, but several possibilities exist:

1. The ovaries are not capable of producing estrogen,
2. The hypothalamus is not stimulating the pituitary to release FSH and LH, which control follicular development and oestrogen production,
3. The pituitary is unable to produce adequate amounts of LH and FSH,
4. Other hormonal imbalances are tricking your pituitary into "thinking" that it is doing a good job when, in fact, it is not.

Since oestrogen stimulation is vital for the growth of the uterine lining, one should measure oestrogen hormone levels to confirm this diagnosis before venturing into new diagnostic territories. In addition, measure FSH level to rule out ovarian failure. (A high FSH level indicates that the ovaries have been severely damaged or have run out of eggs.)

DETECTING OVARIAN FAILURE

Ovarian failure occurs when the ovaries are severely damaged or when they run out of eggs. When this happens, the pituitary gland tries to force the ovary to manufacture oestrogen and to ovulate by working overtime to produce FSH. The pituitary gland's signals fall on deaf ears, though, because the damaged ovaries cannot respond to the extra FSH stimulation.

Ovarian failure may be caused by a number of conditions including infection, chemical toxins, medications, radiation exposure, tumour, surgery, immunologic dysfunction and genetic abnormalities.

DIAGNOSING ANOVULATION

Once uterine abnormalities and ovarian failure are ruled out, we confirmed that the periods are irregular because of not ovulating (anovulation). For some reason, the pituitary is not sending adequate amounts of LH and FSH to the ovaries.

Symptoms of Anovulation

Although a few anovulatory women will have normal periods, most will have a few or no periods at all (amenorrhoea). Prolonged or heavy periods (menorrhagia), spotting during the middle of the cycle (metrorrhagia), and prolonged spotting may also occur. Women with anovulatory menstrual periods do not experience the typical menstrual discomforts often found in ovulatory women: breast soreness, mood changes, or cramping. The anovulatory woman's BBT chart will be flat (monophasic) and her cervical mucus will fern, indicating that progesterone (produced by the corpus luteum that forms after ovulation) never opposes the oestrogen stimulation.

Tests Used to Determine the Cause of Anovulation

In the next phase of testing, the doctor will try to determine why the pituitary gland is not stimulating the ovaries to ovulate. He needs to answer a number of questions:

- Is the hypothalamus not "beating the drum" by producing regular pulses of GnRH?
- Is the pituitary gland damaged?
- Is the pituitary gland getting misleading feedback messages about ovarian function?

Several tests will give me the additional answers he needs.

Hormonal Tests for Diagnosing the Cause of Anovulation

Prolactin Pituitary Hormone

Excessive prolactin can suppress pituitary output (LH and FSH) and can act directly on the ovary to suppress follicular growth.

Thyroid Hormone

Hyper- and hypothyroidism can interfere with hormonal metabolism (the rate at which hormones are used up by the body) and with the delicate hormonal balance between the pituitary and ovary. In addition, through an intriguing mechanism, hypothyroidism may contribute to excess prolactin production.

FSH and LH Pituitary Hormones

Elevated FSH almost always indicates ovarian failure. If FSH and LH are depressed, suspect one of three things: that a faulty hormonal feedback mechanism is inappropriately telling the pituitary to cut back production; that the hypothalamus is not "beating the drum" to stimulate the pituitary to function; or that a pituitary inadequacy prevents the gland from functioning normally.

Adrenal Androgens (DHEAS and Testosterone)

In the presence of excessive hair (hirsutism) or male secondary sex characteristics (enlarged clitoris or ambiguous genitalia), elevated male hormone (testosterone), elevated DHEAS, or elevated adrenal androgens may indicate a congenital enzymatic defect, polycystic ovaries, or a tumour in the pituitary gland, adrenal gland, or ovary. Testosterone or adrenal androgens can suppress ovulation as well as cause a number of other problems discussed later.

Conditions that can Interfere with Ovulation and Menstruation

- Pregnancy
- Hypothalamic malfunction:
  Emotional stress (endorphins?)
  Amenorrhoea
  Athletica (extreme exercise)
  Dieting, poor nutrition, weight loss, low body fat
  Anorexia
  Idiopathic (drugs, toxins, medications?)
- Pituitary gland malfunction:
  Hyperprolactinemia
  Tumour
  Surgery
  Trauma
  Empty sella syndrome
  Sheehan's syndrome
  Cushing's disease
- Hormonal feedback problems affecting pituitary gland:
  Hepatorenal disease
  Adrenal disease
  Cushing's syndrome
  Congenital adrenal hyperplasia
  Polycystic ovary
  Hypo/hyperthyroidism
  Obesity (excess oestrogen)
- Ovarian abnormalities:
  Ovarian cysts
  Endometriosis
  Infection
- Premature ovarian failure
- Incidental fertility findings:
  Asherman's syndrome (adhesions in the uterus)
  Cervical stenosis (cervix closed from surgery)
- Idiopathic (no identifiable cause).

Practical Evaluation of Hormonal Status

- The patients with a disorder of reproductive function serve as their own bioassay.
- The history and physical examination are most important in evaluating any patient with reproductive dysfunction.
- Evaluating the female patient with normal pubertal development as a reference is often useful in determining the cause of the reproductive dysfunction.
- Laboratory tests are used to confirm what is suspected on the basis of the initial evaluation.
- Immunoassays of WHO recommended standards are recommended for proper clinical correlation.
- Measurements of basal FSH, LH, PRL and TSH are warranted in all amenorrhoeic patients once pregnancy has been excluded.
- Radiographic studies of the sella turcica are indicated in amenorrhoeic women with low levels of circulating LH and FSH, whether prolactin is elevated or not. High sensitive immunoassays are required to ascertain the lower end values.
- Individuals with hypothlamic or pituitary tumours and those with presumptive hypopituitarism should undergo dynamic testing of pituitary function.
- Individuals with hirsutism should have serious aetiologic factor eliminated for appropriate laboratory testing.

ALGORITHM FOR EVALUATING AMENORRHOEA (Figs 17.10 to 17.15)

IMMUNOASSAYS FOR LH, FSH AND PRL

- **Sensitivity:** The LH and FSH levels can drop to very low concentrations as low as 1 mIU/ ml. Hence, assays have to be with very high sensitivity.

Sensitivity is of diagnostic importance in hypogonadism particularly when it is very essential to differentiate between the low and normal values of LH and FSH.

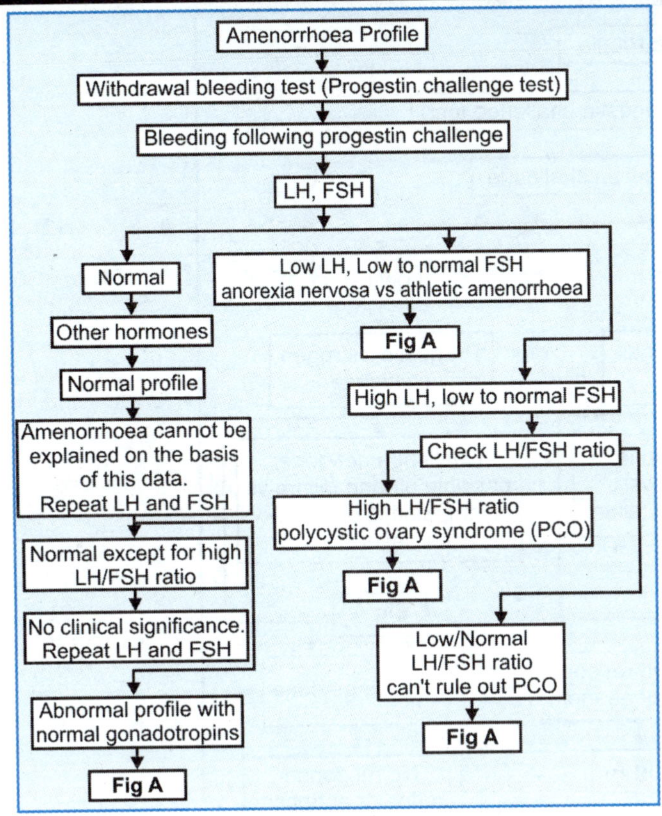

Fig. 17.10

Detection Limits of Various Immunoassays

- 2nd Gen Elisa 2.0 mIU/ml
- RIA 0.2 mIU/ml
- Chemiluminisence 0.2 mIU/ml
- 3rd Gen RIAC Elisa 0.02mIU/ml

Conditions in which LH/FSH levels can go below 2.0 mIU/ ml

- **Hypopituitarism (refer case history no. 1)**
  LH < 1.5 mIU/ml
  FSH < 1.0 mIU/ml
- **Pituitary tumour + Hypopituitarism (refer to case history no.2)**

— LH < 2.0 mIU/ml
— FSH < 1.5 mIU/ml

- **Non-functional pituitary tumour (refer to case history no.3)**

— LH < 1.2 mIU/ml
— FSH < 1.0 mIU/ml

- **Hypogonadism (refer to case history no.4)**

— LH < 1.5 mIU/ml
— FSH < 1.5 mIU/ml

- **Streptavidin-biotin assay system:** The strength and speed of the binding between avidin and biotin is used to provide amplification of signal and as the basis of generic signal generation reagents.

As compared to low sensitivity assays, streptavidin-biotin based assay systems offer an increase in signal ratio as well as improvement in rate of change of the measured signal which in turn offers the immunoassay users greater accuracy from the test system in question (Fig. 17.17).

Calibrator Matrix: Calibrators should ideally be prepared by using a base material identical to that in the test samples. For clinical applications, human serum is the preferred base matrix (Fig. 17.18).

WHO Std. Reference: The World Health Organization's International Laboratory for Biological Standards is now providing qualified investigators with an International Reference Preparation of Human Pituitary Gonadotrophins (LH and FSH) for Immunoassay (coded WHO 1st IRP 68/40 and WHO 2nd IRP 78/549). Data compared with these standard preparations can be reported in terms of International Units. These units differ from those obtained with use of the 2nd IRP-hMG).

Thus, the importance of knowing the "standard preparation" that is used and the "normal range" for any given laboratory is obvious. Also important is that commercially available assays may use different standards, and some of the kits do not even state what reference preparation is provided.

Cross Reaction: LH, FSH and PRL are pituitary hormones and are structurally similar to other pituitary hormones. Therefore, the tendency to cross react is very high when it comes to the estimation of these assays. For example, the tendency of PRL to cross react with GH is very high. Similarly, LH cross-reacts to a very high degree with hCG because of similar alpha chains. Hence, LH estimates are invalid in pregnant women or persons with hCG-secreting tumours. Immunoassays should be highly specific with minimal cross reaction.

Monoclonal Capture: Monoclonal captures are better compared to traditional polyclonal capture as it is more specific.

Assays having polyclonal capture antibodies give rise to different results. Monoclonal antibodies, which react against one highly specific antigenic determinant of a given hormone (epitype

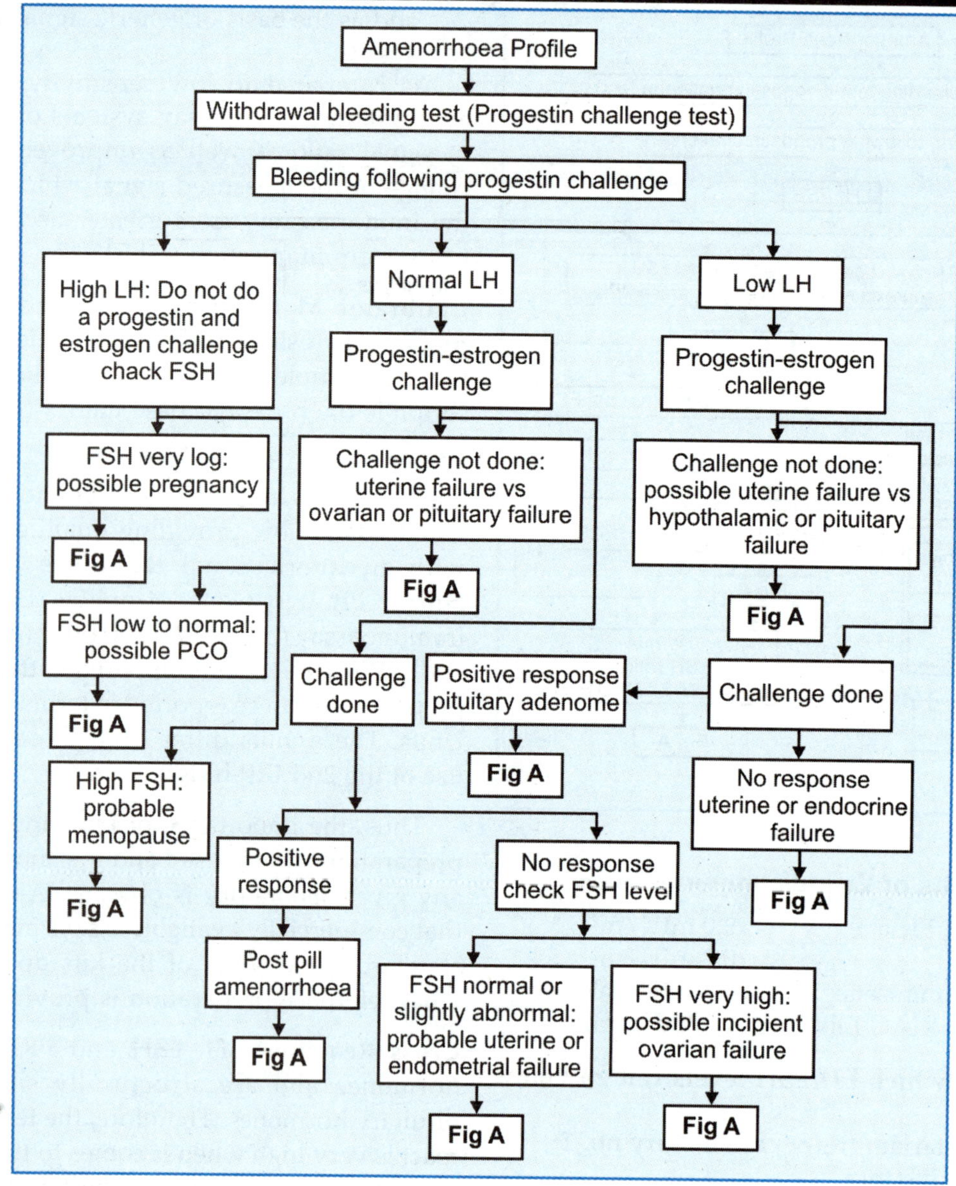

Fig. 17.11

characterisation), can help alleviate interlaboratory differences in results (Fig. 17.19).

Normal Ranges

	LH:mIU/ml	*FSHmIU/ml*	*PRL: (ng/ml)*
Women :			1.2 – 15.5
Follicular phase	0.8 – 10.5	3.0 – 12.0	
Mid-cycle	18.4 – 61.2	8.0 – 22.0	
Luteal phase	0.8 – 10.5	2.0 – 12.0	
Postmenopausal	8.2 – 40.8	35.0 – 151.0	1.5 – 18.5
Men	0.7 - 7.4	1.0 – 14.0	1.8 – 17

Sample Collection and Storage

LH and FSH: Plasma, serum or urine can be used for LH and FSH measurements. Both hormones are stable for 8 days at room temperature and for 2 weeks at 4°C; for longer periods, the specimen should be stored frozen at or below –20°C. Because of episodic, circadian and cyclic variations in the secretion of gonadotrophins, a meaningful clinical evaluation of these hormones may require determinations in pooled blood specimens, multiple serial blood specimens, or timed urine specimens.

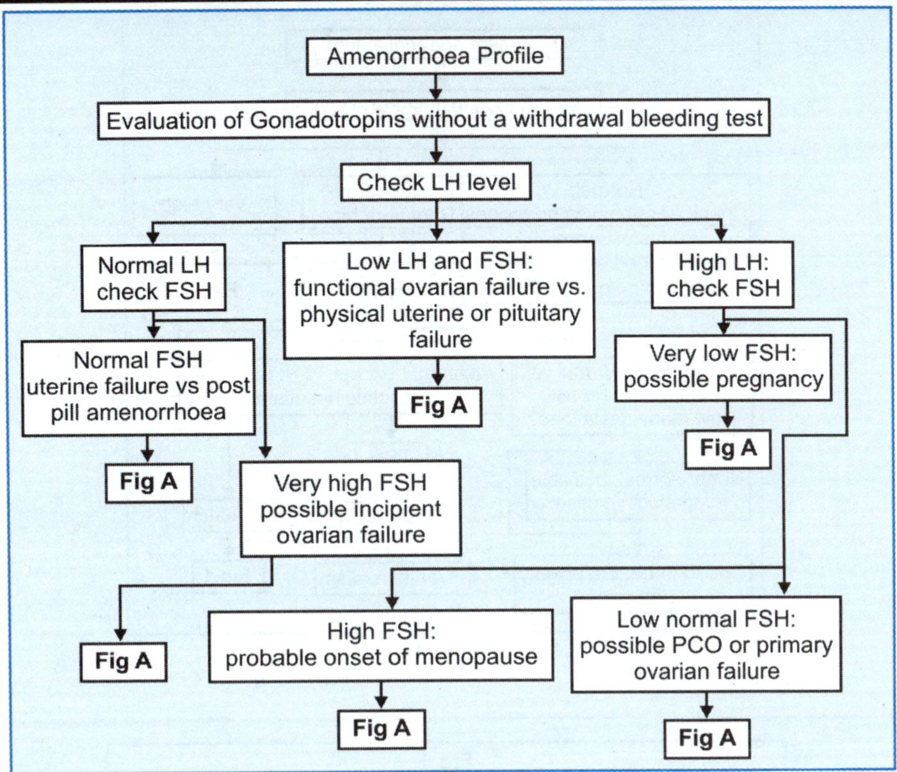

Fig. 17.12

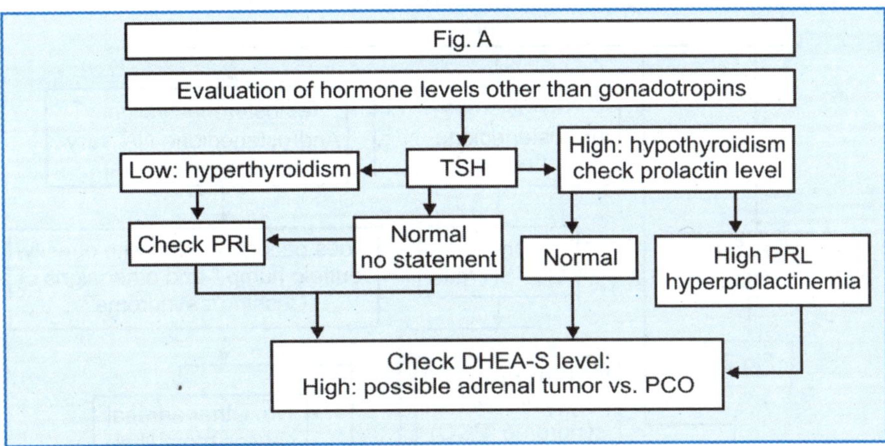

Fig. 17.13

Prolactin: Serum is the specimen of choice for PRL assays and can be stored at 4°C for 24 hours. Freezing is preferred for maintaining long-term stability. Specimens should be collected 3 to 4 hours after the patient has awakened, since PRL level rise rapidly during sleep and peak in early morning hours. Emotional stress, exercise, ambulation, and protein ingestion also elevate PRL levels. As PRL is secreted episodically, multiple sampling techniques may be advantageous (e.g., pooling equal volumes of sera from specimens drawn at 6 to 18 min intervals) (Fig. 17.20).

The ranges will differ from laboratory to laboratory and depend on the reference preparation used for the standards.

The dotted line represents the clinically important lower range.

The range of values is plotted on a logarythmic scale. Measured values differ significantly, depending on the laboratory and immunoassay system employed.

The dotted line signifies the upper limit of the normal range in many laboratories.

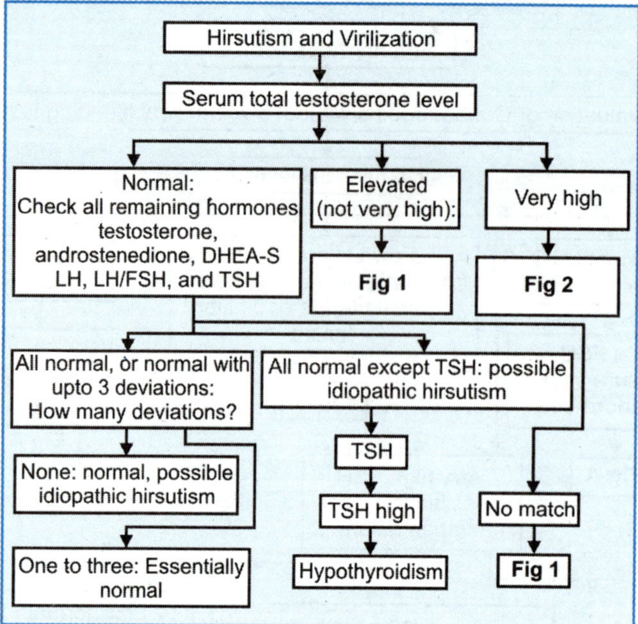

Fig. 17.14

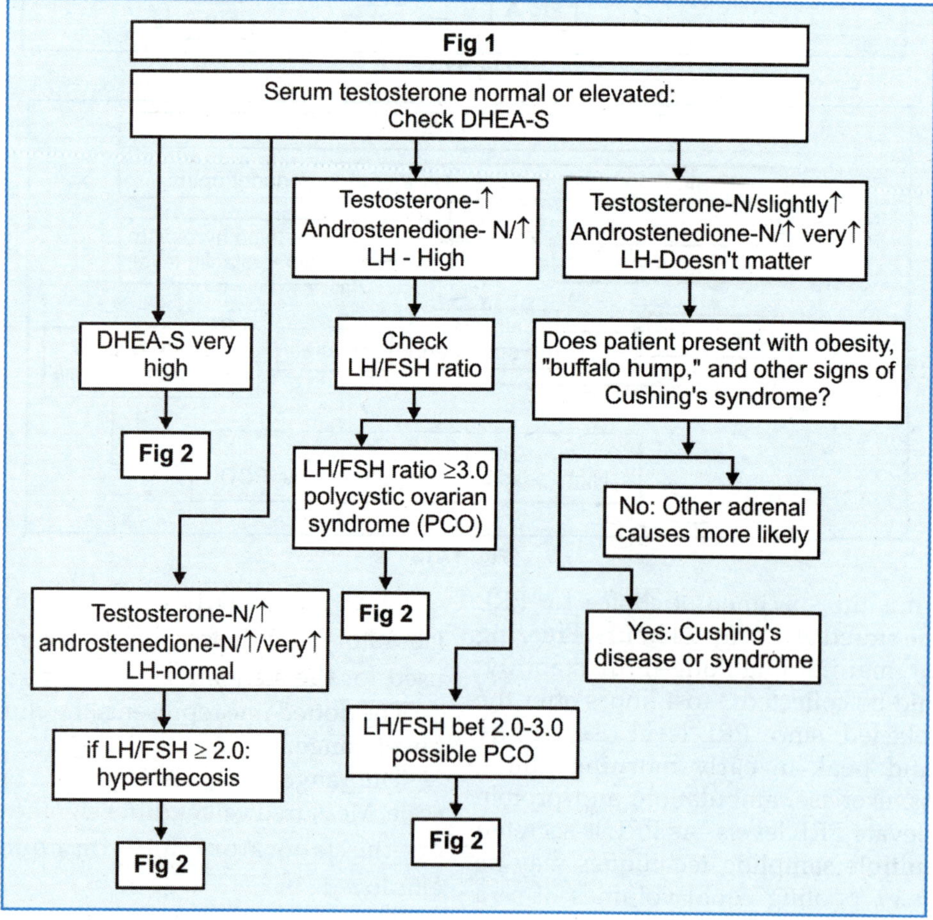

Fig. 17.15

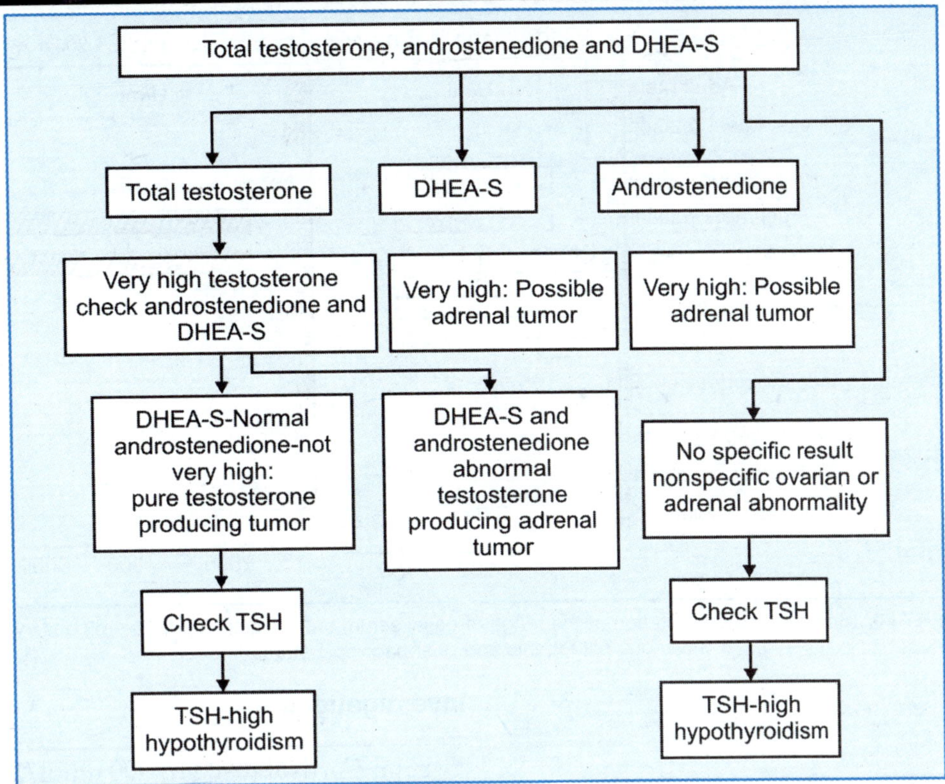

Fig. 17.16

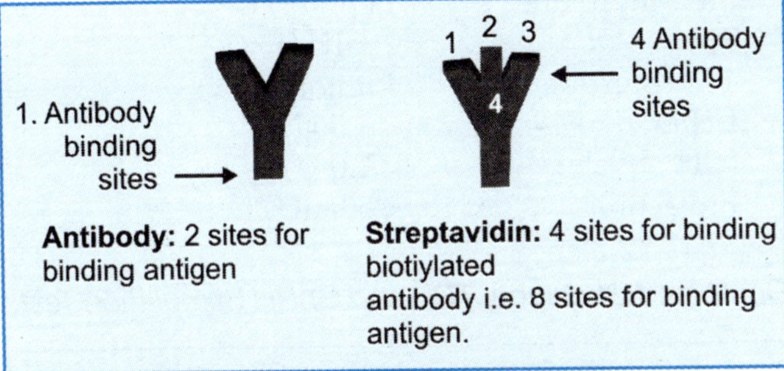

Fig. 17.17: Streptavidin-biotin assay system

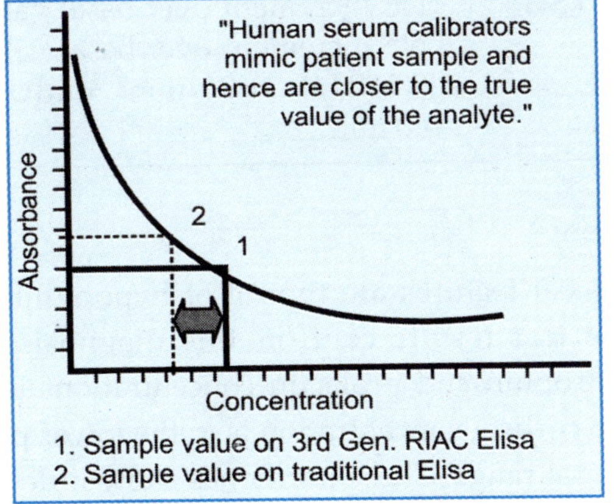

Fig. 17.18: Difference between ELISA generations

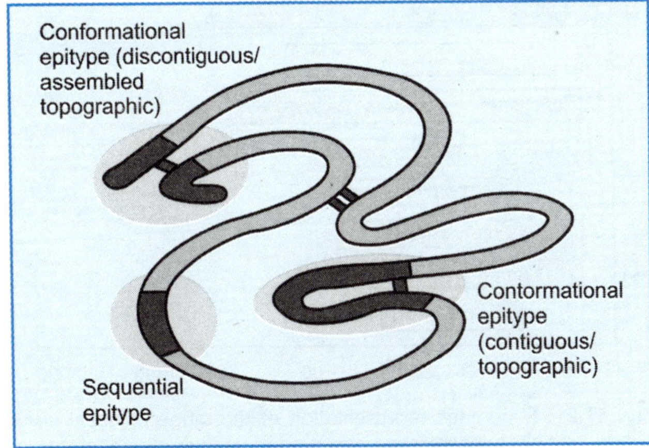

Fig. 17.19: Epitype Characterization

The arrow signifies the clinically important lower range (Fig. 17.21).

CASE HISTORIES

CASE HISTORY-1

A 50-year-old man tripped and fell as he was running for a bus. He hit his head against the kerb and was

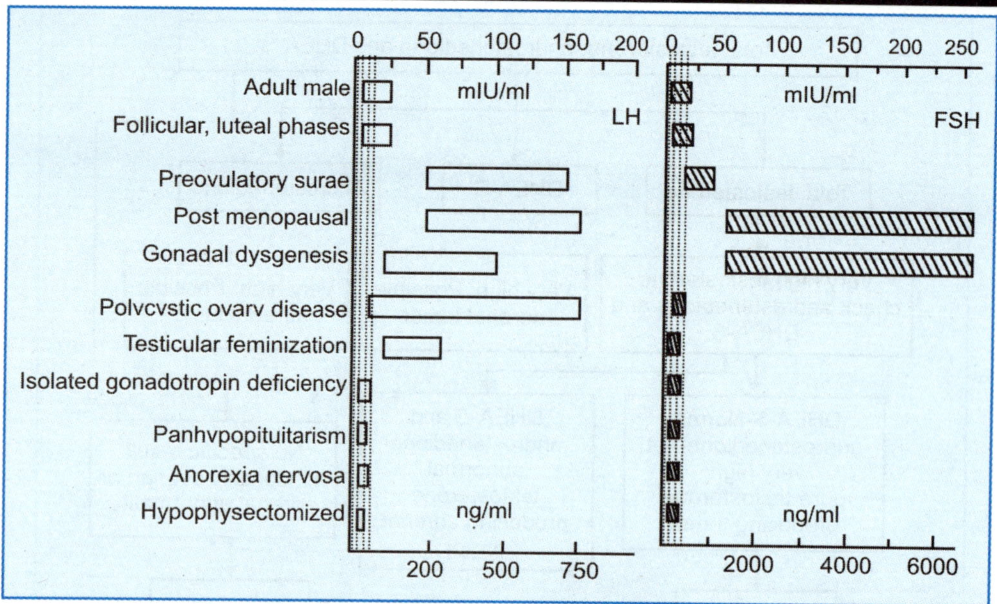

Fig. 17.20: Schematic representation of the range of basal serum the prolactin levels (ug/ml) observed in various pathogenic and pharmacologic states

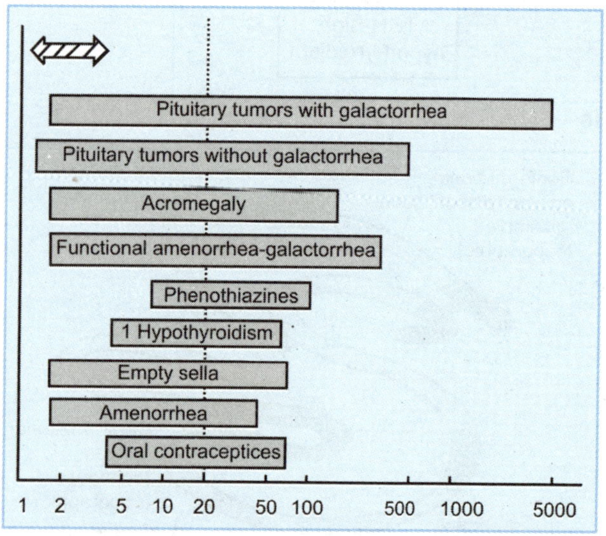

Fig. 17.21: Schematic representation of the range of basal serum gonadotrophin concentration observed in various clinical states

knocked out for a few seconds. An ambulance was called and he was taken to the local hospital.

There was no sign of physical injury on examination but a skull radiograph showed enlargement of the pituitary fossa. The casualty officer questioned the patient further. Over the preceding 12 months, he had lost his libido and found it necessary to shave less frequently than before; he had also noticed some loss of axillary and pubic hair. He frequently felt dizzy when getting out of bed in the morning and despite spending a lot of time in the sun he had not acquired his usual summer tan.

Investigations

Serum: Cortisol (0900 h)	300 nmol/L
GH	< 2 mIU/L
Free thyroxine	12 pmol/L
TSH	2 mIU/L
Testosterone	4 nmol/L
LH	< 1.5 U/L
FSH	< 1.0 U/L
Prolactin	< 50 mU/L

Combined Glucagon, TRH and GnRH Stimulation Test:

Serum: Cortisol (maximum)	350 nmol/L at 180 min
LH, FSH	No increment over basal values
GH	No increment over basal values
TSH	5 mIU/L at 20 min; 3 mIU/L at 60 min

Comment

The clinical features are typical of hypopituitarism and the test results confirm this diagnosis. GH, gonadotrophin and prolactin concentrations are all low; the cortisol concentration is in the lower part of the normal range. These hormones show little or no response to appropriate stimuli. The low testo-styerone is secondary to the lack of gonadotrophins.

The serum free thyroxine is near the lower end of the normal range; if these were related to incipient thyroid failure, a higher TSH concentration would be expected. There is a TSH response to TRH, but even this is towards the lower limit of normal.

Cortisol replacement therapy was started immediately and testosterone and thyroxine were also given. Within a few hours, the patient became polyuric and signs of water depletion developed. The serum sodium concentration, which was low on admission (128 nmol/L), rose to 149 nmol/L. Diabetes insipidus, due to impaired release of vasopressin, can be masked by simultaneous cortisol deficiency and revealed when replacement therapy is started, as in this case.

The patient was given synthetic vasopressin which controlled his polyuria. He subsequently underwent surgery and a chromophobe adenoma was successfully removed. On follow-up, there was no evidence of recovery of pituitary function and he continued to remain on therapy.

CASE HISTORY-2

A 40-year-old man consulted his general practitioner because he had become impotent. He had also been embarrassed by excessive sweating in the absence of exertion. His wife thought that his facial features had become coarser, and he had recently had to buy a larger pair of shoes than normal because his old ones had become uncomfortable. The GP found mild hypertension and a trace of glycosuria and referred him to an endocrine clinic with a presumptive diagnosis of acromegaly.

Investigations

Combined Pituitary Function Test

Time (min)	Blood glucose (mmol/L)	Serum cortisol (nmol/L)	Serum LH (U/L)	Serum FSH (U/L)	Serum TSH (mU/L)
0	7.6	400	2.0	1.5	0.8
15	3.4				
20		2.2	1.7	9.7	
30	2.0	700			
45	2.1				
60	3.3	680	2.1	1.5	4.3
90	4.0	600			
120	4.5	550			

Oral Glucose Tolerance Test

Blood glucose	(initial)	8.5 mmol/L
	(2 h)	11.5 mmol/L
serum GH	(initial)	22 mU/L
	(minimum)	20 mU/L
Serum:	Prolactin (at 0 min)	800 mU/L
	Testosterone	11 nmol/L

Visual fields: Partial bitemporal hemianopia

Skull radiograph: Enlarged pituitary fossa with erosion of anterior clinoid processes

Pituitary CT scan: Pituitary tumour with supracellar extension

Comment

The clinical diagnosis is confirmed by the high basal GH level which is not suppressed by glucose. The glucose tolerance test gives a diabetic result; abnormal glucose tolerance is seen in about 25 per cent of cases of acromegaly, but clinical diabetes mellitus is present in only about 10 per cent.

The basal prolactin concentrations is increased. Gonadotrophins are low and do not increase in response to GnRH. The serum testosterone concentration is at the low end of the normal range due to inadequate testicular stimulation by LH. The cortisol and TSH responses are normal.

The presence of a tumour is confirmed by the radiographic appearances; the optic chiasm lies immediately above the pituitary and compression of it can cause either visual field defects, characteristically a bitemporal hemi- or quadrantanopia, or threaten complete visual failure.

CASE HISTORY-3

A 42-year-old woman, who had been diagnosed as an insulin-dependent diabetic in childhood, complained of frequent episodes of hypoglycaemia, which had continued to occur in spite of reduction of her insulin dosage. She had also developed amenorrhoea. Her diabetes had previously been well controlled, with only occasional episodes of hypoglycaemia and HbA_{1c} in the range of 6.5-7.0 per cent. A review of her history showed that her insulin requirement had fallen from 48 to 28 U over the previous 12 months.

Investigations

HbA_{1c}	6.5 per cent
Serum LH	1.2 U/L
Serum FSH	1.0 U/L

Comment

Occasional hypoglycaemic episodes are common in patients with IDDM, and there may be obvious reasons for them, e.g. a missed meal or an increase in physical activity of counter regulatory hormones. In this instance, the development of amenorrhoea with low gonadotrophin concentrations suggested that the patient might have developed pituitary failure, with decreased production of GH and ACTH causing increased sensitivity to insulin. This was confirmed by formal pituitary function testing and shown to be due to a non-functioning pituitary tumour.

CASE HISTORY-4

A 20-year-old man presented with impotence. On examination, he was eunuchoid; there was only sparse pubic hair, the genitalia were infantile, muscular development was poor and his span exceeded his height with a sole-pubic symphysis distance greater than symphysis to crown.

Investigations

Serum	Testosterone	3 nmol/L
	LH	<1.5 U/L
	FSH	<1.5 U/L

Clomiphene test (3 ng/kg body weight clomiphene citrate daily for seven days)

Serum	*LH*	*<1.5 U/L*
	FSH	<1.5 U/L

Gonadotrophin-releasing hormone (GnRH) test (100 μg GnRH i.v.)

Time (min)	*FSH (U/L)*	*LH (U/L)*
0	<1.5	<1.5
20	2.0	2.0
60	2.5	3.0

(after 100 μg GnRH subcutaneously daily for two weeks)

0	3.5	4.5
20	8.4	21.5
60	4.5	8.0

Comment

The age onset of normal puberty may sometimes be delayed until 18 years of age and hypogonadism should be diagnosed with caution in patients who are younger than this. The low testosterone and gonadotrophins in this case suggest a lesion at the level of either the pituitary or the hypothalamus. This is confirmed by the failure of response to clomiphene. This drug competes with gonadal steroids for hypothalamic receptors; and in normal men, results in an increase in gonadotrophin secretion and thus testosterone secretion. Patients with pituitary lesions may have clinical or biochemical evidence of other pituitary abnormalities (none was present in this case).

The GnRH test is sometimes used in an attempt to distinguish between pituitary and hypothalamic causes of hypogonadism; but in practice it is of limited value. In pituitary disease, it might be expected that that the LH and FSH responses to GnRH would be diminished or absent, but they can be normal. In hypothalamic disease, the response can be delayed (greater at 60 min than 20 min, cf. TRH test), normal, or delayed. The pituitary can become insensitive to exogenous GnRH in hypothalamic disease and repeated injections of the hormone may correct this. When the GnRH test was repeated after GnRH priming, this patient's response was normal, indicating a hypothalamic, rather than a pituitary defect. He was later found to be anosmic (lacking a sense of smell). The association between anosmia and hypogonadotrophic hypogonadism is called Kallmann's syndrome. The eunuchoid habitus is a direct consequence of testosterone deficiency; this promotes epiphyseal fusion; and when its secretion is inadequate, there is continued growth of long bones which become disproportionate to the axial skeleton.

CASE HISTORY-5

A young woman consulted her doctor because she was embarrassed by excessive hair on her upper lip, lower abdomen and thighs. She was moderately obese. Her periods had always been irregular.

Investigations

Serum:	*Testosterone*	*3.5 nmol/L*
	LH (early follicular)	14 U/L
	FSH (early follicular)	3 U/L

Ultrasound examination of the ovaries: Multiple cysts present, bilaterally.

Comment

These findings are characteristic of the polycystic ovary syndrome; testosterone concentration is slightly elevated, and LH is high in relation to FSH. The clinical features of this condition include hirsutism, acne, menstrual disturbances and obesity, but there is a considerable variation on their prevalence and severity. Neither are the typical hormonal changes always present. The pathogenesis of the condition is uncertain. The normal ovaries synthesise androgens (principally testosterone and androstenedione), but their secretion is increased in PCOS. Conversions of androgens to oestrogens in liver and adipose tissue inhibit secretion of FSH (preventing ovulation) and stimulate that of LH (further stimulating androgen secretion). Hyperinsulinaemia is frequently present and may be fundamental to the increased ovarian androgen secretion.

CASE HISTORY-6

A couple in their late twenties were infertile in spite of regular intercourse over a two-year period. Each partner had a child by previous marriages. The woman's periods had recently become irregular. A semen sample contained a normal count of motile sperm. Physical examination revealed no abnormality. The woman was on steroid replacement for adrenal failure, which had been diagnosed in her late teens.

Investigations (woman)

Serum:	*Prolactin*	*300 mIU/L*
	LH	12 U/L
	FSH	25 U/L

Comment

This is secondary infertility. The elevated FSH concentration (due to decreased negative feedback by oestrogens) indicates incipient ovarian failure. The FSH is a more sensitive test for this than LH; although in established ovarian failure (after the menopause), the plasma concentrations of LH and FSH are both very high. The adrenal failure in the woman had shown to be due to autoimmune disease, and there is a recognized association between autoimmune adrenal and ovarian failure (Schmidt's syndrome). Two months later, she had not had her period, and measurement of plasma LH concentration gave a value of > 100 U/L. It is possible for hCG to cross react in assays for LH. A pregnancy test was positive. Ovarian failure develops gradually and occasional ovulation may still occur in the early stages.

CASE HISTORY-7

A 45-year-old man presented with weight loss, lassitude and weakness. His skin was noticeably bronzed, although it was winter and he had not been out of the country. On examination, he was found to have hepatosplenomegaly, rather sparse body hair and small testes. On further questioning, he admitted that he had lost his libido and become impotent.

Investigations

Urine		Positive for glucose
Blood glucose (fasting)		10 mmol/L
Serum:	Iron	70 μmol/L
	Iron-binding capacity	67 μmol/L
	Ferritin	5000 μg/L
	Testosterone	9 nmol/L
	LH	2 U/L

Comment

Skin pigmentation is virtually always present in idiopathic haemochromatosis, though it develops insidiously and may go unnoticed by the patient. It is a result of increased melanin deposition (and iron in advanced cases). Deposition of the iron in the pancreas causes islet cell destruction and diabetes. Parenchymal iron deposition in the liver leads to cirrhosis which may be complicated by hepatoma formation; the liver disease is often exacerbated by excessive alcohol ingestion. Both primary and secondary hypogonadism can occur; in this case, the luteinising hormone level suggests that the hypogonadism is secondary to pituitary damage. The joints are often involved and deposition of iron in the myocardium can cause arrthythmias and cardiac failure.

The total iron-binding capacity is normal in this case but may be decreased as a result of the impaired ability of the liver to synthesise transferrin. It is, however, fully saturated with iron with the result that the plasma iron concentration is always elevated. Plasma ferritin concentration is massively elevated; values of several thousand μg/L are typical of idiopathic haemochromatosis (mean normal 100 μg/L in males). The diagnosis of haemochromatosis can be confirmed by demonstration of the massive excess of parenchymal iron in a sample of the liver obtained by percutaneous biopsy.

The families of patients with haemochromatosis should be screened to detect homozygotes for the defective gene, who are at risk of developing the condition can be given prophylactic treatment. Treatment of homozygotes before the onset of overt disease has been shown to prevent the development of cirrhosis and reduce the (otherwise considerable) risk of hepatocellular carcinoma. The HLA typing and iron studies can be used for screening. Heterozygotes are not at risk; the results of iron studies in them may be normal but some can be detected by HLA typing.

THYROID FUNCTION TESTS

Introduction

When a patient is referred by a clinician for thyroid function tests, he may be symptomatic or asymptomatic.

Symptomatic patients present vague symptoms and complain that they just do not feel like themselves—may be they are a little tired, are experiencing hot or cold spells, or feel that their heartbeat is too fast or too slow. These symptoms could mean that the patient is suffering from thyroid disease or these could be symptoms related to nonthyroidal diseases.

At the same time, the asymptomatic patient may be suffering from thyroid illness and may be in need of immediate diagnosis and therapy. In such conditions, it is very crucial for the physician to accurately diagnose and treat the patient or monitor treatment.

It is here that the Clinical Laboratory plays an important role. The physician is totally dependent on the interpretation of the Pathologist. It is based on the Pathologist's interpretation that the physician can successfully diagnose and treat the patient.

Thyroid assays in general are extremely sensitive assays as they involve measurement of hormones in microgram and nanogram quantities. Also, the thyroid function and thyroid hormones interact as part of a multiple gland feedback loop, and hence are often interpreted together to detect disease and understand its aetiology.

In the past five years, important changes have taken place in the strategy of thyroid function testing. previously, thyroid tests were dominated by T3 (Total T3), T4 (Total T4) and TSH tests. People believed that if total T3 and total T4 are low, then TSH has to be high and vice versa. Here, they are considered *only* the feedback mechanism between the pituitary hormone TSH and thyroid gland hormones total T3 and total T4. What they failed to consider here is that there are other factors which affect total T3 and total T4 levels. Moreover, total T3 and total T4 being in bound form (bound to TBG) and are not the physiologically active hormones participating in metabolic functions; but it is the free hormones, free T3 and free T4, which are physiologically active.

Throughout the world, there is a trend for TSH and free T4 tests to replace the conventional total T3, total T4, TSH tests for screening thyroid functions with conventional thyroid screening strategy total T3, total T4 and TSH. When laboratory results are correlated with clinical findings, the relations may be either concordant or discordant.

Laboratarians often face the problem of physicians complaining that the reports do not match with the clinical history of the patient for eg. 'abnormal' total T4 in absence of thyroid disease. Here the laboratorian only correlates total T3, total T4 and TSH values; and as a result, in such situations, clinicians are in a dilemma and often doubt the methodology used.

If the laboratory results are discordant, a distinction needs to be made between a previously unsuspected diagnosis, subclinical disease, anomalous assay results, and a discrepancy caused by specific or nonspecific assay interference.

Tests for Thyroid Function

Laboratory tests of thyroid function are required to assist in the screening, diagnosis and monitoring of thyroid disease. Most laboratories offer a standard 'profile' of T3/T4/TSH. Measurement of plasma total T4 concentration was formerly widely used as test of thyroid function, but has a major disadvantage in that it is dependent on binding proteins concentration as well as thyroid activity. For example, a slightly elevated plasma total T4 concentration, compatible with mild hyperthyroidism, can occur with normal thyroid function if there is an increase in plasma-binding protein concentration. With the introduction of more reliable assays for free T4 (FT4), there is now little if any justification for laboratories continuing to measure total T4 as a test of thyroid function.

Plasma total T3 concentration is almost always raised in hyperthyroidism (usually to a proportionately greater extent than total T4, hence it is the more sensitive test for this condition) but may be normal in hypothyroidism. However, total T3 concentrations, like those of total T4, are dependent on the concentration of binding proteins in plasma and their measurement is being superseded by measurements of free T3 (FT3).

Binding Proteins

For both, the Clinician and Pathologist, protein binding can provide a major obstacle to the laboratory assessment of thyroid status.

It is a known fact that both T3 and T4, when they are released into the blood, are extensively bound to plasma proteins. There are two types of plasma proteins which are present in large concentration in blood: TBG—which has a very high affinity for T3 & T4 and TBPA—which has low affinity but high capacity for binding. Therefore, maximum T4 is bound to TBG and very little to TBPA. The precise physiological function of TBG is unknown. It has been suggested that the extensive binding of thyroid hormones to TBG provides a buffer, which maintains the free hormone levels constant in the face of any tendency to change. The binding may also reduce the amount of thyroid hormones lost through the kidneys.

Total thyroid hormone concentration is dependent upon the concentration of binding proteins present in the blood. If these were to increase, the temporary fall in free hormone concentration caused by increased protein binding would stimulate TSH release and this would restore the free hormone concentrations to normal. Conversely, if the protein concentrations were to fall, the reverse would occur. In either situation, there would be a change in the concentrations of the total hormones, but the free hormone concentrations would remain normal. Thus, measurement of total hormone concentrations can give misleading information.

This is a matter of considerable practical importance since changes in the concentrations of the binding proteins occur in many circumstances. Further, certain drugs, for example, salicylates and phenytoin, will displace thyroid hormones from their binding proteins, thus reducing the total, but not the free hormone concentrations, once a new steady state is attained. If an attempt is made to assess thyroid status in a patient who is not in a steady state, the results may be bizarre and misleading.

Only small amounts of T4 and T3 are excreted by the kidneys due to the extensive protein binding. The major route of thyroid hormone degradation is by deiodination and metabolism in tissues, but they are also conjugated in the liver and excreted in bile (Fig. 17.22).

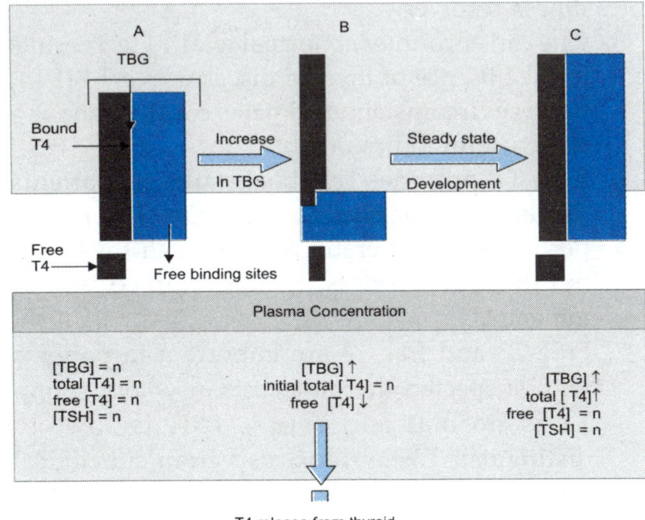

Fig. 17.22: Effect of an increase in TBG concentration on plasma T4 levels

a. In the initial steady state, TBG is one-third saturated with T4.
b. TBG levels increase causing more T4 to be bound, thus reducing the free T4 concentration. This stimulates TSH secretion which leads to an increase in the release of T4 from the thyroid.
c. The new T4 is re-distributed between the bound and the free states leading to a new steady state with the same free T4 level but an increased total T4.

Importance of Free T4 and Free T3

1. In pregnancy, the normal range for FT4 in euthyroid women decreases as the pregnancy progresses. There is an increase in TBG, due to the increased oestrogen levels, and in total T4, but these are disproportionate, causing the level of free T4 to fall. Thyroid status, as assessed clinically, does not change.
2. Free T3 is a sensitive test for hyperthyroidism. In hyperthyroid patients, both FT3 and FT4 are usually elevated (FT3 to a proportionately greater extent) but there are exceptions to this.
3. In a small number of patients with hyperthyroidism the FT3 concentration is elevated but the FT4 is not (though it is usually high-normal)—a condition called 'T3 thyrotoxicosis'.
4. Occasionally, FT4 is elevated but not FT3. This is usually due to concomitant nonthyroidal illness resulting in decreased conversion of T4 to T3, and FT3 concentration increases when this illness resolves.
5. One can encounter abnormal total T4 test results in the absence of thyroid disease. Free T4 (FT4) in these circumstances remains constant and is a more useful indicator.
6. Free T4 provides reliable results in patients displaying abnormalities in serum T4 binding particularly if alterations are caused by severe nonthyroidal illness or hereditary dysalbuminemias.
7. Free T3 and free T4 are important in patients with suspected thyrotoxicosis in whom serum T4 is normal and serum TSH is low, to distinguish T3 thyrotoxicosis from subclinical thyrotoxicosis.
8. In the estimation of the serum FT3 : FT4 ratio, a high ratio(>0.024 on a molar basis or >20 calculated as ng/mg) that persists during antithyroid drug treatment may indicate that patients with hyperthyroid Graves' disease are unlikely to achieve remission. This ratio usually is lower in patients with iodide-induced thyrotoxicosis or thyrotoxicosis caused by thyroiditis than in those with thyrotoxicosis caused by Graves' disease.
9. To detect early recurrence of thyrotoxicosis after cessation of antithyroid therapy.
10. To establish the extent of active hormone excess during high-dose replacement or suppressive therapy with T4 or when an intentional T4 overdose has been taken.
11. For diagnosis of amiodarone-induced thyrotoxicosis, which should not be based on T4 excess because of the occurrence of euthyroid hyperthyroxinemia in many amiodarone-treated patients.

Alterations in the Concentrations or Affinity of Thyroid Hormone-Binding-Proteins (Fig. 17.23).

Increases in

a. TBG concentration (or affinity):
   1. Genetic (inherited) determination
   2. Nonthyroidal illness (HIV infection, infectious and chronic active hepatitis, oestrogen-producing tumours acute intermittent porphyria)
   3. Physiology (pregnancy, newborn)
   4. Drug use (oral contraceptives, oestrogens, tamoxifen, methadone)
b. Prealbumin concentration
c. Albumin binding (familial dysalbuminaemic hyperthroxinaemia)
d. T4 binding by antibodies (autoimmune thyroid disease, hepatocellular carcinoma)

Decreases in

a. TBG concentration:
   1. Genetic (inherited) determination
   2. Nonthyroidal illness (major illness or surgical stress, nephrotic syndrome)
   3. Drug use (androgens, anabolic steroids, large doses or glucocorticoids)
b. TBG-binding capacity (drugs bound to TBG such as salicylates and phenytoin)
c. Prealbumin concentration

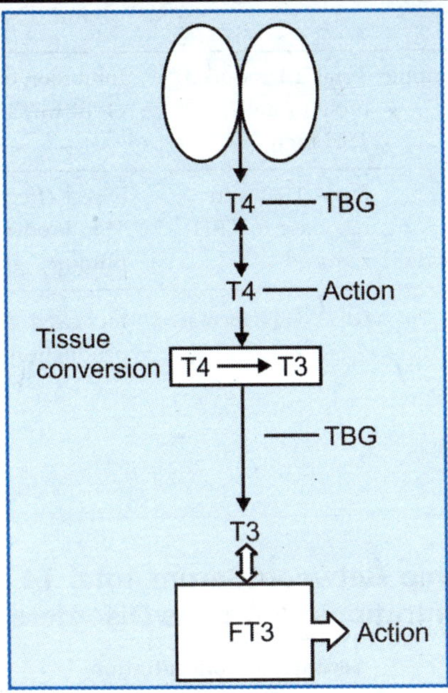

Fig. 17.23: Thyroid hormones and TBG

The TSH-Free T4 Relationship

If a sensitive serum TSH assay is used together with a valid serum free T4 estimate, a sensitive and specific assessment of thyroid status can usually be made from the general relation between the two hormones.

The following figure emphasises the distinction between primary target gland failure (high serum TSH, low free T4 : A), failure of TSH secretion (both low: B), autonomous or abnormally stimulated target gland function (high serum free T4, low TSH: C), and primary excess of TSH or thyroid hormone resistance (both high: D) Fig. 17.24.

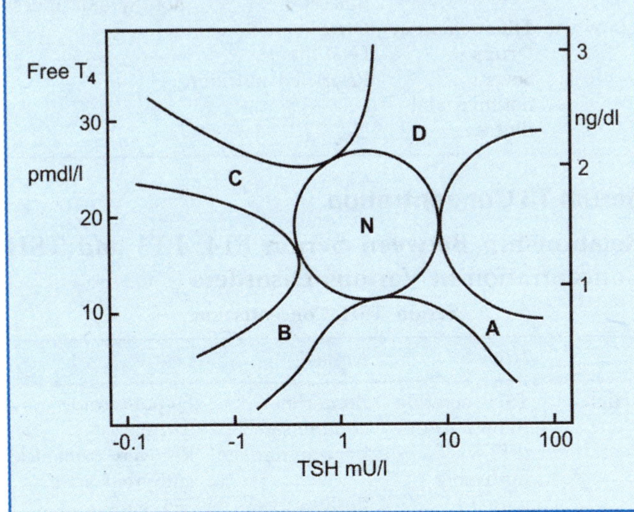

Fig. 17.24: TSH-FT4 relationship

The relationship between serum TSH and free T4 concentrations in normal subjects (N) and patients with various abnormalities of thyroid function: A, primary hypothyroidism; B, central (secondary) hypothyroidism; C, thyrotoxicosis (excluding TSH-induced thyrotoxicosis). Results in area D are uncommon but suggest a possible methodologic artefact, an unrecognised binding abnormality, generalised thyroid hormone resistance, or TSH-induced thyrotoxicosis. Findings that fall in the undefined areas suggest that an additional factor may be modifying the feedback relationship or that samples have been taken in nonsteady-state conditions. Serum free T4 is shown on a linear scale, whereas the scale for serum TSH is logarithmic.

Problems in the Interpretation of Thyroid Function Tests

It is difficult to guarantee reliable thyroid function results in patients with nonthyroidal illness. Abnormal results may occur in patients with infections, malignancy, myocardial infarction, following surgery, etc., who do not have thyroid disease.

Typically, during the acute phase of an illness, free T3 (FT3) concentration and less often, free T4 (FT4) concentration is decreased. The TSH is usually normal but may be undetectable in the severely ill. During recovery, TSH may rise transiently into the hypothyroid range as free hormone concentrations return to normal. In chronic illness, for example, chronic renal failure, free hormone concentrations are decreased (to an extent that may reflect the severity of the underlying disease); TSH is usually normal, but it is occasionally decreased.

The occurrence of abnormalities of thyroid function tests in patients with nonthyroidal illness has been termed the 'Sick Euthyroid Syndrome'. Causes include decreased peripheral conversion of T4 to T3; changes in the concentration of binding; increased plasma concentrations of free fatty acids, which displace thyroid hormones from their binding sites, and nonthyroidal influences on the hypothalamic-pituitary-thyroid axis, for example, by cortisol, which can inhibit TSH secretion.

Furthermore, many drugs can influence the results of tests of thyroid function. Many times, the levels of FT3, FT4 and TSH do not correlate.

Common Causes of TSH/FT4/FT3 Discrepancies

- Over replacement of thyroid hormone (TSH low, free T4 normal)
- Recent dose adjustment (TSH high, free T4 normal)
- Patient taking T3 (TSH low, free T4 normal)
- Patient noncompliant with hormone replacement (TSH high, free T4 normal)
- Nonthyroidal illness
- Drugs affecting thyroid hormones: Glucocorticoids, dopamine
- Thyroid hormone resistance (TSH high, free T4 high, patient euthyroid)
- TSH-secreting tumour (TSH high, free T4 high, patient hyperthyroid)
- During antithyroid drug therapy, there can be patients who have persistent serum T3 excess, despite normal or low serum T4 values.

Effects of Drugs on Thyroid Function

- Altered hypothalamic or pituitary function
- Altered biosynthesis or release of thyroid hormones
- Displacement of T4 and T3 from binding proteins
- Reduced peripheral conversions of T4 to T3
- Inhibition of peripheral hormone activity

Drugs that Affect Results of Thyroid Function Tests

Drugs	*Effect*	*Cause*
Salicylates, Phenylbutzone, Dphenylhydantoin	Total T4 and T3 reduced, Free T4 normal	Inhibition of serum protein binding
Propylthiouracil, Methimazole, Lithium, Iodides	Total T4 and T3 reduced	Inhibition of TSH production or release
Propylthiouracil	Total T3 reduced both T4 and	Inhibition of conversion of T4 to T3
Propranolol	Total T3 reduced, T4 normal, TSH normal	Inhibition of conversion of T4 to T3
Drugs	*Effect*	*Cause*
Glucocorticoids	Total T3 reduced, T4 and TSH low or normal	Inhibition of conversion of T4 to T3

Contd...

Contd...

Oral radiographic dyes	Total T3 reduced, both T4 and TSH high	Inhibition of conversion of T4 to T3
Dopamine, L-dopa, Glucocorticoids	Basal TSH and response to TRH reduced	Direct effect to inhibit TSH Production in pituitary gland
Amiodarone, TRH, Bensamide (transient), Metopramide, Sulpiride	Basal TSH increased	Increased TSH production

Relationship Between Serum Total T4 and Total T3 Concentrations in Various Disorders

Serum T3 Concentration

	Low	*Normal*	*High*
High	Iodide deficiency T3 treatment	T3-thyrotoxicosis T3-binding autoantibodies	Thyrotoxicosis of any cause Excess T4 ingestion Thyroid hormone resistance
	Antithyroid drug therapy	TBG excess	
Normal	Iodine deficiency		T4 treatment Euthyroid hyperthyroxinemia
	T3 treatment		Thyrotoxicosis with acute or moderate
	Hypothyroidism		T4 binding autoantibodies
	Severe hypothyroidism	Acute and chronic nonthyroidal illness	Thyrotoxicosis with severe nonthyroidal illness
Low	TBG deficiency Drugs Severe nonthyroidal illness	Drugs Fetal life Restricted nutrition	

Serum T3 Concentration

Relationship Between Serum FT4, FT3 and TSH Concentration in Various Disorders

Serum TSH Concentration

	High	*Normal*	*Low*
High	TSH-secreting tumour (rare) (FT3 = ↑) Euthyroid with T4	Borderline/ compensated hypothyroidism Euthyroid	Hypothyroid (primary) Recovery from sick euthyroid state Sick euthyroid

Contd...

Contd...

Normal	Autoantibodies (uncommon)		(FT3 = $\downarrow$) Hypopitutarism (other pituitary hormones = $\downarrow$)
	Hyperthy-roidism	T3 thyrotoxicosis	Hypopituitarism (other pituitary hormones = $\downarrow$)
Low		(FT3 = $\uparrow$) Sub-clinical (FT3 = N/ $\downarrow$)	hormones = $\downarrow$) Sick euthyroid (severe) (FT3 = $\downarrow$)

Free Thyroxine Measurements in Common Conditions Affecting Thyroid-Binding Proteins

Clinical conditions	Free T4 Levels
Near Normal Concentration of Serum-Binding Proteins	
Hypothyroidism	Low
Hyperthyroidism	High
Hyperoestrogenism	Low
Abnormal Concentration of Serum-Binding Proteins	
TBG excess	Normal
TBG deficiency	High
Dysalbuminaemia	Normal
Hypoalbuminaemia	Normal
T4 autoantibody	Normal
Low total T4 non-thyroidal illness	Normal or High
High total T4 Non-thyroidal illness	Normal or High

Free T4 and Free T3 in Various Disease Conditions

1. *Hyperthyroidism*
   - Hyperthyroidism produces a primary increase in Free T4, whereas oestrogens and idiopathic or genetic conditions may produce a primary increase in TBP. In both cases [T4 and TBP] increase, but in the former, the patient is ill and requires treatment; in the latter, the patient is euthyroid. Likewise, a low serum [T4 & TBP] any be due to a primary decrease in [FT4] or to a primary decrease in [TBP]. It is, therefore, clinically important to differentiate between changes in [T4 & TBP] that are due to primary changes in [FT4] (e.g. hyper-or hypothyroidism) and those that are due to primary changes in [TBP].
   - Serum TSH level is low in all forms of hyperthyroidism except in rare cases in which hyperthyroidism is mediated by TSH itself. When TSH level is low, free T4 concentration should be measured and will be elevated in most cases of hyperthyroidism. Finding a low TSH level and an elevated free T4 level is usually sufficient to establish the diagnosis of hyperthyroidism. If TSH level is low but free T4 level is normal, a T3 measurement should be performed, since serum T3 concentration is often elevated earlier in the course of hyperthyroidism and to a greater degree that is T4 concentration. Because only the free fraction of T3 is active, the estimation of free T3 is helpful in adjusting the total T3 for variations in binding proteins. It should be remembered that numerous medications as well as both acute and chronic illness may cause a transient lowering of T3 concentration as well as a reduction in TSH level.
   - In Grave's disease or toxic adenomas, serum total T3 and free T3 levels are typically elevated to a greater degree than total T4 and free T4.
   - T3 toxicosis—encountered in about 5 per cent of hyperthyroid population—total T3 and free T3 values increase.
   - Serum total T4 and free T4 are disproportionately elevated to a greater degree than total T3 and Free T3 values in most patients with toxic multinodular goitre.
   - Monitoring total T3 and free T3 values may also be of importance in evaluating both the severity and the response therapy in patients being treated for thyroid storm or crisis in that the antithyroid drug therapies are focused on reducing both thyroid gland T3 secretion and peripheral tissue T3 production from T4.
2. *Nonthyroidal Illness*
   - In nonthyroidal illness (NTI) and altered states of nutrition there are two categories:
     Low T3 state: Decrease in total T3 and free T3 while maintaining normal total T4 and free T4. Observed in mild or moderate NTIs or states of caloric deprivation (< 400 cal)
     Low T3-T4 state: Total T4 also decreased, a case of severe NTI.

- Free T4 levels remain within or near the normal range of values as serum total T4 levels decline.
- Decreased total T3 or normal free T4 or increased free T4 results from acquired defect in serum T4-binding proteins which accompany NTI.
- Also common are increases in the levels of the free fraction of T4 and T3 which are caused by decrease in serum concentrations of thyroid hormone-binding proteins, changes in binding properties induced by circulating inhibitors and drugs, or both. Low levels of total T4 may be seen in nonthyroidal illnesses, but total T4 concentrations in these patients are usually normal or above normal as determined using reference methods.
- Thus in nonthyroidal illnesses, abnormal thyroid test results are not necessarily indicative of thyroid disease but may demonstrate adaptations to the catabolic state, many of these changes revert to normal when the patient recovers.
- Several test abnormalities may be seen in nonthyroidal illnesses in euthyroid patients (the 'euthyroid sick syndrome'). The most common abnormalities are a reduction in the serum total T3 concentration and an elevation in the serum level of rT3. Also common are increases in the levels of the free fraction of T4 and T3 which are caused by decrease in serum concentrations of thyroid hormone-binding proteins, changes in binding properties induced by circulating inhibitors and drugs, or both. Low levels of total T4 may be seen in nonthyroidal illnesses, but total T4 concentrations in these patients are usually normal or above normal as determined using reference methods.

3. *Hypothyroidism*
   - If total T4 (or free T4) level is normal, hypothyroidism is most unlikely: however, a low T4 concentration is often seen in the euthyroid sick.

Assay Choice Application

For definitive diagnosis, assessment of both serum TSH and free T4 is required, but a more limited approach can be used for initial case finding and follow-up. In the interests of cost effectiveness, evaluation of thyroid status may often begin with an assay for either serum TSH or free T4, followed by further algorithm-based assessment if the initial result is abnormal. As an initial test, serum total T4 measurements give an unacceptable rate of abnormal results, due to the frequency of abnormalities in serum thyroid hormone-binding proteins.

Four distinct clinical situations in which evaluation of thyroid function is done can be considered: testing of unselected populations for case finding or screening, testing of untreated patients who have clinical features that suggest thyroid disease, assessment of the response to treatment for thyroid dysfunction, and evaluation of patients in whom associated illness or drug therapy are likely to complicate clinical and laboratory assessment or whose initial results are atypical or unclear.

Screening and Case Finding

About 2 per cent to 7 per cent of women over age 40 years may have slightly elevated serum TSH concentrations. The case for routine assessment of thyroid status is strongest in elderly women who have any symptoms that could be consistent with hypothyroidism. Among hospitalised patients, the large majority of abnormal results are due to nonthyroidal illness or medications.

Most persons found to have either high or low serum TSH values in screening or case-finding studies have subclinical disease. That is, they have no clinical manifestations of thyroid dysfunction and normal serum free T4 and T3 concentrations.

Regardless of which initial test is used, assessment of thyoid status has a high priority in patients at increased risk of having thyroid dysfunction, as for example in those with goitre, those treated previously for thyrotoxicosis or receiving lithium or amiodarone, and patients with associated autoimmune disease or connective tissue diseases or a history of neck or whole body irradiation.

Untreated Patients

In untreated ambulatory patients, a normal serum TSH concentration has high negative predictive value in ruling out thyroid disease. If serum TSH is abnormal, serum free T4 is given. Diagnostic strategies have been evaluated in which serum T4 measurements are done routinely only if the serum TSH is abnormal, unless pituitary disease is suspected.

Long-term assessment of this approach will need to balance cost savings against potentially serious adverse outcomes; for example, if thyrotoxicosis is missed because of normal serum TSH values, or central hypothyroidism is missed on the basis of normal serum TSH values.

The following groups of patients will be incompletely or incorrectly assessed if either serum TSH or free TSH or free T4 alone is measured.

- Patients with subclinical hypothyroidism (high serum TSH, normal free T4) in whom replacement therapy may be beneficial.
- Those with subclinical thyrotoxicosis (low serum TSH, normal free T4) in whom treatment with an antithyroid drug or thyroid ablation may be beneficial.
- Those being treated for thyrotoxicosis, in whom suppression of TSH secretion may persist for weeks or months after normalisation of serum T4 and T3 of drug.
- Those with central (secondary or hypothyrotropic) hypothyroidism (low serum free T4 low or normal TSH), who should be evaluated for adrenal insufficiency before T4 therapy is initiated.
- Those with binding abnormalities such as familial dysalbuminaemic hyperthyroxinaemia (FDH) or T4 or T4 binding autoantibodies in whom some serum free T4 estimates are invalid.
- Those with thyroid hormone resistance with high serum T4 and T3 concentrations and normal or high serum TSH concentrations, who are often not recognised until after inappropriate treatment has been given.
- Those with thyrotoxicosis caused by excess TSH secretion caused by a pituitary tumour or selective pituitary resistance to thyroid hormone.

Notwithstanding the widespread acceptance of serum TSH as a single initial test, some still advocate an estimate of free T4 as the best initial test for suspected thyrotoxicosis.

Assessment of the Response to Treatment

In the testing of ambulatory patients with known thyroid disease, the use of serum TSH alone can also be considered. In a study of ambulatory patients attending a thyroid clinic, hyperthyroid patients taking T4 for either replacement or suppression, seldom needed a serum free T4 measurement of the serum TSH was greater than 0.05 mU/L; although at lower values, the magnitude of hyperthyroxinaemia did influence management. In contrast, in patients with newly diagnosed thyrotoxicosis, measurements of serum free T4 or free T3, or both, were necessary in addition to serum TSH not only to establish the degree of hormone excess but also to evaluate the response to treatment. This study included a few new cases of hypothyroidism, in whom serum T4 measurement also would be required to establish the degree of hormone deficiency. In patients with thyroiditis and pituitary-hypothalamic disease, combined assessment was required.

In evaluating patients receiving T4 therapy, some have suggested that hormone measurements add little to a clinical assessment made by experts, but there is justification for periodic serum TSH assessment to avoid subtle tissue effects of thyroid hormone excess of deficiency. A serum TSH value in the low-normal range is, probably, the best single indicator of appropriate dosage and is certainly of more use than a serum free T4 value alone, which may be increased slightly depending on the time interval between dose and sampling. In some situations (e.g. patients with ischaemic heart disease and hypothyroidism), the appropriate dose of T4 should be based on clinical judgement rather than laboratory findings.

Difficult Diagnostic Situations

The prevalence of abnormal serum T4 or TSH values in patients with acute medical or psychiatric illness is high, but there is controversy as to the value of thyroid function testing in these situations, because most of the abnormalities do not indicate the presence of thyroid disease in acutely ill patients because of the potential importance of intercurrent thyroid disease and the difficulty in assessing clinical features of thyroid dysfunction, others suggest that testing should not be done without some clinical indication.

In patients hospitalised for acute illness one or more of the assumptions outlined above may not be justified; for example, when there are wide fluctuations from the steady state. Serum TSH values frequently are subnormal in the absence of thyrotoxicosis and serum free T4 estimates are subject to multiple interfering influences, depending often on the particular method. Dual assessment clearly is necessary to identify the serum free T4 TSH combinations that indicate true thyroid dysfunction.

When a patient has both thyroid dysfunction and a severe nonthyroidal illness, assessment becomes especially difficult because the effects of the illness, medications, or changes in nutrition can alter the expected changes in serum free T4 or TSH. Only clinical re-evaluation and repeated sampling may resolve the dilemma.

Thyroid Diagnosis and Treatment

There are three general principles upon which the physician should focus when evaluating thyroid function in a patient. These principles are:

- The thyroid gland is the principal site of thyroid dysfunction
- Autoimmune thyroid disease is the most common aetiology producing the dysfunction
- Thyroid status is best determined by a combined measurement employing a serum free thyroxine (FT4) estimate and thyrotrophin (TSH).

For both hypothyroidism and hyperthyroidism, TSH and an estimate of free T4 (FT4) are recommended.

T3 or free T3 may be needed to confirm hyperthyroidism if free T4 is within limits. Anti-thyroid antibodies, preferably antithyroid peroxidase (anti-TPO), may establish an autoimmune mechanism.

Recommendations for Thyroid Testing

Hyperthyroid	
Symptomatic	Free T4, TSH
Post-therapy	Free T4 (Free T3)
hypothyroid	
Symptomatic	TSH, Free T4 (anti-TPO)
Subclinical	TSH-first (T4, anti-TPO)
Monitor replacement	TSH
Hypopituitary	TSH and Free T4
Acutely Ill	None without suspicion
Pregnant	
Diagnosis	TSH, Free T4
Hypo, treated	TSH
Elderly	
Healthy	None
Ill	None
Women > 60 years	TSH
High risk*	TSH
Healthy adults	None without suspicion

*Ambigious symptoms, concurrent illness associated with thyroid disease, drugs associated with thyroid dysfunction.

Diagnostic Approach to Anomalous Serum T3, T4, and TSH Values

- Clinical re-evaluation, with particular attention to long-term features suggestive of thyroid disease and to the medication history.
- Measurement of serum TSH by a third-generation method to identify conclusively the degree of TSH suppression.
- Measurement of the serum T3 concentration with appropriate binding correction (free T3)
- An authentic estimate of serum free T4 (particularly in euthyroid hyperthyroxinaemia).
- Follow-up to establish whether the abnormality is transient or persistent.
- Search for evidence of unusual binding abnormalities or hormone resistance in the propositus and family members.

Typical Reference Ranges for Serum Thyroid Hormones and TSH in Humans*

Hormone	*Reference ranges*	*Variations unrelated to thyroid disease*
Total T3	69-202 ng/dl	Binding protein changes, binding competitors, age-related changes, nutrition, illness, surgery, drugs
Free T3	1.4-4.2 pg/ ml	Methodologic factors and influences on total T3
Total T4	4.4-11.6 μg/dl	Binding protein changes, binding competitors
Free T4	0.8-2.0 ng/dl	Methodologic factors, pregnancy
TSH	0.28-6.82 μIU/ ml	Diurnal variation, pulse secretion, age-related changes, drugs

*These ranges should be determined for the particular methods used in each laboratory. The neonatal period is excluded. Higher values in childhood.

CASE HISTORIES

CASE HISTORY 1

Knowing that thyroid disease is common in the elderly, a house physician requested thyroid function tests on an elderly women admitted to hospital with severe cellulite of the leg secondary to an infected in growing toe nail.

Investigations

Serum:	TSH	0.05 mU/L
	fT4	8.0 pmol/L
	fT3	2.0 pmol/L

Thyroid Levels in Different Disease Conditions

Disease	*T3*	*T4*	*TSH*	*FT3*	*FT4*	*T-Uptake*	*Tg*	*Anti-TPO*	*TRH*	*TBG*
Primary Hypothyroidism	↓	↓	↑	↓	↓	↓			R	
Hyperthyroidism	↑	↑	↓	↑	↑	↑	↑			
Pituitary insuffiency, tertiary hypothroidism		↓	↓		↓	↓			R*	
T3, thyrotoxicosis				↑	↓				R	
Subacute thyroiditis		↑	↓		↑	↑[a], ↓[b]	↑			
Nontoxic nodular goiter					↑		↑			
Graves disease				↑	↑			↑		
Hashimoto thyroiditis				↑		↑[d], ↓[e]		↑		
Lymphadenoid goiter								↑		
Iatrogenic hyperthyroidoidism					↑					
Myxedema			↑		↓					
Estrogen therapy, oral contraceptives, pregnancy		↑	↓[c]			↓				↑
Androgen therapy, steroid, hypoproteinemia (nephrosis, cirrhosis)		↓				↑				
Hypothyroidism treated with thyroxine					↓					
Hypothyroidism treated with hypoproteinemia thyroidism					↑					
Anti-thyroid drug for thyrotoxicosis		↓,N	↓			↓				
Benign adenoma							↑			
Untreated and metastatic carcinoma of thyroid							↑			
Acute psychiatric illness, acute medical illness, hepatic disease, malnutrition, addisons disease, acromegaly					↓					

a–recovery stage, b- active stage, c- 1st trimester, d- early, e-late, R- respose, R*- delayed response

Comment

The TSH, fT4, fT3 are all low results, which at first glance might suggest thyroid failure secondary to hypopituitarism. However, a TSH this low would be unusual except in severe hypopituitarism. The TSH secretion tends to be affected late in progressive pituitary disease. A random serum cortisol concentration was 950 nmol/L, indicating normal response of the hypothalamic-pituitary-adrenal axis to stress, and it was concluded that the thyroid function results were due to the sick euthyroid syndrome. The infection was treated successfully and thyroid function tests were repeated prior to discharge: serum TSH concentration was 6 mU/L, fT4 was 12 pmol/L and fT3, 4.7 pmol/L.

CASE HISTORY 2

A 24-year-old physiotherapist consulted her general practitioner because excessive moistness of her skin was causing embarrassment at work. She was also concerned that her eyes seemed to have become more prominent and that she had lost weight, although her appetite was unchanged. On examination, her doctor observed that her pulse was 92 per minute at rest and that she had slightly enlarged thyroid gland.

Investigations

Serum	TSH	<0.1 mU/L
	fT4	34 pmol/L
	fT3	12 pmol/L

An isotopic scan of the thyroid showed an enlarged gland with uniformly increased uptake. Autoantibodies to thyroid peroxidase and thyroglobulin were present in the serum in high titre.

Comment

The high fT3 and fT4 concentrations with low TSI I are diagnostic of thyrotoxicosis, and the presence of autoantibodies and scan appearances are characteristic of Grave's disease. Although the clinical features are typical of thyrotoxicosis, they are often less in milder cases and in the elderly. They may suggest an anxiety state. Some clinical features are specified to Grave's disease and can have a course independent of the hyperthyroidism. Grave's disease (ophthalmic Graves disease) yet be suppressed even though fT3 may not be elevated, and such patients eventually become biochemically and clinically thyrotoxic. The combination of low TSH with a normal (usually high-normal) fT3 (subclinical or borderline hyperthyroidism) can occur early in the course of Grave's disease and other conditions causing thyrotoxicosis.

CASE HISTORY 3

Shortly before her final examinations, a medical student experienced sleep disturbance, tachycardia with palpitation and noticed that her hands were warm and sweaty. Her doctor was sure that her symptoms were due to anxiety, but was persuaded to take a blood sample for thyroid function tests.

Investigations

Serum	T4	165 nmol/L
	T3	2.9 nmol/L
	Free T4	24 pmol/L

These results were considered to be equivocal and a TRH test was performed.

Serum TSH	0 min	1.2 mU/L
	20 min	5.4 mU/L
	60 min	3.1 mU/L

Comment

This patient was investigated before the introduction of presently available TSH assays, and exemplifies the problems posed by the effect of changes in binding protein concentration on measurements of total thyroid hormone concentration.

The total T4 is elevated and the T3 is at the upper limit of normal, the free T4 is near the upper limit of normal. Mild thyrotoxicosis could bot be excluded on the basis of these results. However, the TSH response to TRH is normal. Indicating that the patient is euthyroid. It trancontraceptive pill and the resulting increase in serum TBG would explain the abnormal total hormone concentrations.

In retrospect, the normal TSH response to TRH would have been predicted from the normal basal TSH concentration, which itself suggests that the patient is euthyroid.

CASE HISTORY 4

A senior civil servant was persuaded to seek medical advice because of his increasingly bizarre behaviour. He has slowed up mentally, become indecisive and he no longer has the energy to play. Whereas in the past he had annoyed his colleagues by opening windows even on cold day, he now no longer objected to them remaining closed. His appearance has changed, his skin appearing sallow and his hair coarse and lacking luster.

His general practitioner suspected hypothyroidism and elicited a history of recent constipation in addition to the other typical features. Bradycardia was present and when the peripheral reflexes were tested, slow quadriceps relaxation was noted. There was no goitre.

Investigations

Serum : TSH	>100 mU/L

Comment

The very high serum TSH concentration reflecting the lack of negative feedback from circulating thyroid hormone confirms the clinical diagnosis of hypothyroidism. Under such circumstances, measurement of fT4 is unnecessary for diagnosis, although as discussed on p.140, most laboratories routinely measure TSH and fT4 on all samples submitted for thyroid function tests, fT4 also provides an additional index against which to assess the response to treatment.

CASE HISTORY 5

A 55 year old businesswoman underwent the medical screening programme provided by her company.

Various tests were performed, including assessment of thyroid function.

Investigations

Serum	TSH	8 ml/L
	FT4	12 pmol/L

Comment

Serum TSH concentration is slightly elevated, and ft4, through within the reference range, is near the lower end, compatible with early or borderline hypothyroidism. Thyroid failure can be an insidious condition and sufficient function of the failing thyroid may be maintained by increased secretion of TSH in the early stages. Measurement of fT4 concentration, though useful for subsequent comparison, may not be of practical help in management. The decision made on clinical grounds, although the detection of thyroid autoantibodies in serum lends weight to the diagnosis of thyroid disease. Because the clinical features of hypothyroidism can be so nonspecific, patients may only appreciate, retrospectively, that they started. Often, the most prudent course is to follow-up the patient clinically, and repeat the tests after 3-6 months. In this case, thyroxine replacement was given initially; but six months later, serum TSH concentration had increased to 29mU/L and fT4 was 9 pmol/L. After thyroxine replacement had been started, the patient commented that she now realised that she had been feeling run down for some time beforehand.

CALCITONIN

Calcitonin is produced by the parafollicular cells of the thyroid. The main effect in man is to inhibit bone resorption, it lowers serum calcium and phosphorus. Hypocalcaemia decreases calcitonin secretion; hypercalcaemia increases calcitonin secretion. A syndrome of calcitonin excess—medullary carcinoma of the thyroid—is recognised in man. Little effect on calcium homeostasis is observed. However, the finding of elevated levels of the hormone is useful in the early detection of tumours.

Clinical Relevance

a. Increased levels are associated with:
   1. Medullary thyroid cancers
   2. C cell hyperplasia
   3. Chronic renal failure
   4. Pernicious anaemia
   5. Zollinger-Ellison syndrome
   6. Cancers of lung, breast and pancreas

b. In a small proportion of patients who do have medullary cancer, the fasting level of calcitonin is normal. In these instances, a provocative test using calcium or pentagastrin should be followed by an abnormally large increase in calcitonin levels.

Procedure

1. A pentagastin injection is administered. Blood samples are drawn before the injection and 1½ and 5 minutes after injection.
2. Another method is to infuse calcium (15 mg/kg) over a 4-hour period and collect blood samples before infusion and again at 3 to 4 hours.

Interfering Factors

Levels are normally increased in
- Pregnancy at term
- Newborns.

PARATHYROID

The production of parathormone varies inversely with the plasma levels of ionised calcium, which is ordinarily maintained within normal limits.

Actions

Parathormone acts by controlling metabolic reactions which:
1. Increase calcium and phosphorus reabsorption from bones,
2. Increase calcium reabsorption and phosphate excretion in the renal tubule,

3. Increase absorption of calcium from the gastrointestinal tract and,
4. Decrease calcium secretion in the lactating breast (secondary hyperparathyroidism may follow renal insufficiency).

Clinical Disorders

A. *Deficiency:* Tetany (acute deficiency), hypoparathyroidism (chronic deficiency), often with epileptiform seizures.
B. *Excess:* Hyperparathyroidism with symptoms of hypercalcaemia, renal calculi, bone resorption, sometimes peptic ulcer, hypertension, pancreatitis.

Methods of Evaluation

The X-ray of the bones of the hands, teeth, and skull, intravenous urography, serum calcium (repeated), serum phosphorus, urine calcium, serum alkaline phosphatase, bone biopsy, calcium and phosphorus tolerance, reabsorption and excretion tests. Test response of elevated calcium level to cortisone administration. Reduced blood magnesium levels (1.5-1.8 mg per cent) are frequent in hypoparathyroidism. Serum protein should be determined, as half of serum calcium is protein bound (while withdrawing blood, no tourniquet or pressure should be applied). Some of the important tests are mentioned below.

Serum Calcium

A finding of serum calcium levels above 11 mg per cent repeatedly suggests hyperparathyroidism. Hypercalcaemia also occurs in multiple myeloma, sarcoidosis, milk alkali syndrome, vitamin-D intoxication, acute osteoporosis, Addison's disease, after electroshock therapy, in the presence of metastatic malignant disease with or without bone involvement, and in thyrotoxicosis.

On a diet containing about 100 mg of calcium per day, the normal person excretes 125 ± 50 mg of calcium per 24 hours. If milk or cheese is not present in the diet, the urine normally forms a slight cloud when Sulkowitch reagent is added. In hyperparathyroidism, which may be intermittent, hypercalcaemia is usually associated with a daily urinary excretion of calcium greater than 200 mg. Hypercalcaemia due to this cause is usually unaffected by corticosteroids (hydrocortisone 100 mg/day, or prednisone 20 mg/day, for 1 week), which decrease hypercalcaemia in sarcoidosis, infantile hypercalcaemia, metastatic malignancy, the usual case of vitamin-D intoxication, and miliary tuberculosis. Bone biopsy and tracer studies are diagnostic.

Tubular Reabsorption of Phosphate (TRP)

This test may indicate hyperparathyroidism in patients with good renal function and a daily phosphate intake of 800 mg or more. False positives may occur with uraemia and in some cases of renal tubular disease, sarcoidosis and osteomalacia.

Method: A constant diet containing moderate amounts of calcium and phosphate is given for 3 days. Fasting blood is drawn in the morning when a timed 4-hour urine specimen is collected.

Urine phosphate (UP) and creatinine (UC) (in mg excreted/minute) and serum phosphate (SP) and creatinine (SC) (in mg/100 ml) are determined. Calculate TRP as:

$$\text{TRP (in per cent)} = 100 \times 1 - \frac{UP \times SC}{UC \times SP}$$

Interpretation: TRP is about 78 per cent on a normal diet, higher on a low-phosphate diet (430 mg/day for 3 days). In hyperparathyroidism, the TRP is 74 per cent or less after a normal diet, 85 per cent or less on a low-phosphate diet.

Calcium Infusion Test

Method: On a constant diet, 3 consecutive 24-hour urines are collected and measured for phosphate. On the second day, a 4-hour infusion of 1 litre of normal saline solution containing calcium gluconate-glucoheptonate (in a quantity enough to provide 15 mg of calcium per kg ideal body weight) is given.

Interpretation: A normal response consists of a marked reduction of urinary phosphate on the day of calcium infusion and a rebound increase on the third day. In hyperparathyroidism, minor alteration in urinary phosphate excretion is observed. Changes in urinary cyclic AMP parallel phosphate changes.

Ellsworth-Howard Test

This test distinguishes hypoparathyroidism from pseudohypoparathyroidism in which the level of parathyroid hormone is adequate, but the renal tubules are unresponsive. Anaphylactoid reactions to parathyroid extract may occur. Be sure the extract used is phosphuretic in humans and renal function is adequate.

Method: The fasting patient is given 2 ml (200 units) of parathyroid extract IV. The urinary phosphorus content is determined hourly for 3 hours prior to and for 3-5 hours following the injection.

Interpretation: Following the injection of parathyroid extract in normals, there is a 5-fold to 6-fold increase in urine phosphorus excretion. In hypoparathyroidism, following the injection of parathyroid extract, there is a 10-fold or greater increase in urine phosphorus excretion; with pseudohypoparathyroidism, there is utmost a 2-fold increase and urinary cyclic AMP does not increase in proportion.

Serum Parathyroid Hormone

Radioimmunoassay methods have been developed and results can be obtained. The relationship of parathyroid hormone assay to serum or ionised calcium levels are the best discriminators of parathyroid activity.

Parathyroid Hormone Assay; Parathyrin; Parathormone (PTH-C Terminal)

Normal values	*SI units*	
Serum 11-54 pg/ml laboratory specific:		
Cord	≤3 pg/ ml	≤3 ng/L
2-20 years	9-52 pg/ ml	9-52 ng/L
Adults	10-65 pg/ ml	10-65 ng/L
Plasma	1.0-5.0 pmol/L	
Mid-molecule and C terminal: Also check laboratory specific norms.		
Serum		
1-16 years	51-217 pg/ ml	51-217 ng/L
Adults	50-330 pg/ ml	50-330 ng/L
Plasma	<50 μLEq/ ml	<50 mLEq/L
N-terminal: Also check laboratory specific norms.		
Serum		
2-13 years	14-12 pg/ ml	14-21 ng/L
Adult	8-24 pg/ ml	8-24 ng/L
Plasma	<6.1 pmol/L	

The PTH is a polypeptide hormone produced in the parathyroid gland, and is one of the major factors in the regulation of calcium concentration in extracellular fluid. Three molecular forms of PTH exist:

1. Intact, also called native or glandular hormone
2. Multiple, N-terminal fragments and
3. C-terminal fragments.

Test Significance

Investigation is of importance in distinguishing nonparathyroid from parathyroid causes of hypercalcaemia. A decrease in the level of ionised calcium is the primary stimulus for PTH secretions, while a rise in calcium inhibits secretions. This relationship is lost in hyperparathyroidism, and PTH will be inappropriately high in relation to calcium. The C assays tend to have higher values and are more widely accepted as better indication of hyperparathyroidism. Creatinine is usually determined with all PTH assays to determine kidney function.

Clinical Relevance

1. Increased PTH values are seen in:
   a. Chronic renal failure. This is a cause of secondary hyperparathyroidism.
   b. Pseudohyperparathyroidism. There is a primary defect in renal tubular responsiveness to PTH (slight increase).
   c. Vitamin D deficiency (moderate)
   d. Malabsorption (moderate)
   e. Rickets (moderate)
   f. Osteomalacia (moderate)
2. Decreased PTH values occur in nonparathyroid hypercalcaemia, as in:
   a. Use of thiazide diuretics
   b. Milk alkali syndrome
   c. Vitamin A and D intoxication
   d. Haematologic malignancies (some of them)
   f. Sarcoidosis
   g. Graves' disease
   h. Permanent postoperative hypoparathyroidism
3. Increased PTH-N values occur in:
   a. Pseudohypoparathyroidism
   b. Secondary hyperparathyroidism
   c. Primary hyperparathyroidism
4. Decreased PTH-N values are seen in:
   a. Hypoparathyroidism
   b. Neoplasms
   c. Nonparathyroid hypercalcaemia
5. Increased PTH-C values are seen in:
   a. Pseudohypoparathyroidism
   b. Secondary hyperparathyroidism
   c. Primary hyperparathyroidism
   d. Neoplasms
6. Decreased PTH-C values occur in:
   a. Hypoparathyroidism
   b. Nonparathyroid hypercalcaemia

Interfering Factors

A. Fasting sample should be obtained:
   1. Elevated blood lipids interfere with results
   2. Milk ingestion will lower PTH levels

ADRENAL CORTEX

The adrenal cortex produces four major groups of hormones: (i) *glucocorticoids* (cortisol, cortisone), (ii) *androgens* (androstenedione, dehydroepiandrosterone), (iii) *Mineralocorticoids* (aldosterone, deoxycorticosterone, corticosterone), and (iv) *oestrogens* and *progesterone.*

Adrenal corticosteroid production is controlled by a number of factors originating in the hypothalamic-pituitary system. The ACTH is the major tropic substance of the system. Aldosterone is under minimal control of ACTH, and its secretion is mainly influenced by volume receptors, angiotensin II and potassium concentration. The plasma cortisol, in turn, regulates ACTH secretion. The direct feedback mechanism does not seem operative for aldosterone secretion.

Cortisol-binding globulin (CBG) avidly binds cortisol and corticosterone and is the main carrier protein at normal concentrations. Oestrogens increase CBG are inactive but are in equilibrium with free unbound steroid.

Actions

The mineralocorticoids increase reabsorption of sodium and chloride, increased excretion of potassium, and allow an exchange of intracellular potassium with extracellular sodium. Aldosterone is most effective in this regard. The glucocorticoids affect protein, carbohydrate, and fat metabolism, raising blood glucose, increasing gluconeogenesis and protein catabolism (with resulting osteoporosis), metabolising hepatic fat depots, decreasing tubular reabsorption of urates, increasing uropepsin secretion, and lysing eosinophils and lymphocytes.

Clinical Disorders of Adrenal Steroids

a. *Deficiency*
   1. Acute: Addisonian crisis, Waterhouse-Friderichsen syndrome
   2. Chronic: Addison's disease
b. *Excess*
   1. Principal glucocorticoids: Cushing's syndrome.
   2. Principal androgen excess: Adrenogenital syndrome in females, macrogenitosomia in males.
   3. Aldosterone excess: Primary hyperaldosteronism.

Methods of Evaluation of Glucocorticoids and Androgens

Evaluation of adrenocortical function may depend upon: (i) physical examination, noting particularly pigmentation of the skin and mucous membranes, pubic and axillary hair growth, blood pressure and the presence of oedema, (ii) determination of serum sodium, potassium, chloride, CO_2, urea and protein, (iii) X-ray studies of the bones for osteoporosis and of the adrenal region, with or without retroperitoneal pneumography and tomography, (iv) determination of blood and urine levels of 17-ketosteroids, 17-hydroxycorticosteroids, aldosterone and specific excretory products such as androsterone and etiocholanolone, pregnanetriol, and pregnenetriolone, (v) specific function tests such as the water loading test and the response of hormone excretion levels to stimulation by exogenous ACTH, inhibition of ACTH production by corticosteroids, or inhibition of 11-β hydroxylation by metyrapone; and (vi) in the absence of interfering factors, the number of circulating eosinophils, normally between 100 and 300/ml, varying inversely with adrenocortical activity.

Urinary 17-Hydroxycorticosteroids, 17-Ketosteroid Excretion, Ketogenic Steroids, or Free Cortisol

The basal 24-hour urine excretion of 17-hydroxycorticosteroids is the most frequently used test in assessing adrenocortical activity. Paraldehyde, quinine, colchicine, iodides, sulphamerazine, and chlorpromazine interfere with the Porter-Silber steroid determination. The 17, hydroxycorticosteroids are metabolites of cortisol and cortisone. Urinary 17-ketosteroids are metabolites of: (i) adrenocortical steroids such as cortisol, (ii) adrenal androgens, and (iii) gonadal androgens.

The test, hence, reflects the activity of the adrenal cortex and the gonads in the male and the adrenal cortex in the female. There is a diurnal variation in excretion of 17-hydroxycorticosteroids and 17-ketosteroids of adrenal origin. The contribution of testosterone metabolites to the ketosteroids in the urine is minimal.

The 17-ketosteroid levels determined by the Zimmermann reaction are greatly reduced by probenecid and meprobamate administration. These drugs should be stopped for several days before urine collection.

The patient should not be receiving androgens or cortisol when specimens are collected. Testosterone propionate is excreted in the urine and is measured as 17-ketosteroids, methyltestosterone does not appear in the urine.

Method: A 24-hour urine specimen is collected in a jug containing 5 ml of 2 per cent thymol glacial acetic acid.

Interpretation: High levels of excretion of both 17-hydroxycorticosteroids, 17-ketosteroids, ketogenic steroids, and urinary-free cortisol are found in adrenocortical carcinoma and adrenocortical hyperplasia, and of 17-ketosteroids and pregnanetriol in the adrenogenital syndrome. Low levels of excretion are found in hypopituitarism. Addison's disease, myxoedema, and occasionally in anorexia nervosa.

ALDOSTERONE

Aldosterone, Serum and Urine

Normal values

Average-Sodium diet	Serum	SI units	
Peripheral blood			
Supine	3-10 ng/dl	0.14-1.9 nmol/L	
Upright			
Adult Female pregnant	18-100 ng/dl	0.5-2.8 nmol/L	
Nonpregnant	5-30 ng/dl	0.14-0.8 nmol/L	
Adult male	6-22 ng/dl	0.17-0.61 nmol/L	
Adrenal vein			
Child			
1 week-12 mo	1-60 ng/dl	0.03-4.43 nmol/L	
Age 1-3	5-60 ng/dl	0.14-1.7 nmol/L	
Age 3-11	5-70 ng/dl	0.14-1.9 nmol/L	
Age 11-15	<5-50 ng/dl	<0.14-1.4 nmol/L	
Urinary aldosterone			
Norm urine	2-26 mg/24 h	5.6-73 nmol/day	
Urinary sodium	Plasma Renin	μg/day	nmol/day
<30 nmol/day	5-24 Al/ ml/h	35-80	97-220
20-50 nmol/day	2-7 Al/ ml/h	13-33	36-91
50-100 nmol/day	1-5 Al/ ml/h	5-24	14-66
100-150 nmol/day	0.5-4 Al/ ml/h	3-19	8-53
150-200 nmol/day		1-16	3-44
200-250 nmol/day		1-13	3-36

This cholesterol-derived hormone is the most potent of the mineralocorticoids. Its foremost physiologic effect is that of regulating the transport of ions across cell membranes, especially those of renal tubules. This hormone causes the retention of sodium and chloride and the elimination of potassium and hydrogen. The second is the maintenance of blood pressure. Minute quantities will depress the urinary and salivary sodium to potassium ratio primarily because of diminished sodium excretion.

The three main factors that apparently affect aldosterone levels include the renin-angiotensin system, the plasma-potassium concentration and ACTH. The renin-angiotensin system appears to be the major mechanism that controls extracellular fluid by regulation of aldosterone secretion. Potassium loading results in increased aldosterone levels, whereas a potassium-deficient diet in the presence of aldosterone excess will result in a lowered aldosterone level. Increased concentrations of potassium in the blood plasma directly stimulate adrenal production of the hormone. The ACTH may affect aldosterone production in conditions of acute stress, burns, haemorrhage, and other pathologic conditions. Under physiologic conditions, ACTH seems to have little effect on aldosterone production.

Method

1. A 24-hour urine specimen is obtained.
2. Urine should ideally be refrigerated during collection.
3. Venous blood specimen is added to a heparinised or EDTA vial. Separate the cells from plasma immediately. Specimen should be obtained in the morning after the patient has been upright for at least 2 hours.
4. Specify and record the source of the specimen (e.g. peripheral venous, etc).

Diuretic agents, progestational agents, oestrogens, and liquorice should be discontinued 2 weeks prior to test. The patient's diet for 2 weeks before the test should be normal and include 3 gm of sodium per day.

Test Significance

This test is useful in detecting primary or secondary aldosteronism. Patients with primary aldosteronism characteristically have hypertension, muscular pains and cramps, weakness, tetany, paralyses and polyuria.

Clinical Relevance

1. Elevated levels occur in primary aldosteronism as in:
   a. Aldosterone producing adenoma
   b. Adrenal cortical hyperplasia
   c. Glucucorticoid remediable hyperaldosteronism
2. Elevated levels also occur in secondary aldosteronism when aldosterone output is elevated due to external stimuli or because of greater activity in the renin-angiotensin system as in:
   a. Salt depletion
   b. Potassium loading
   c. Large doses of ACTH
   d. Cardiac failure
   e. Hepatic cirrhosis with ascites
   f. Nephrotic syndrome
   g. Bartter's syndrome
   h. Postsurgical syndrome
   i. Hypovolaemia and haemorrhage.

Interfering Factors

Values are increased in pregnancy and by posture.

CLINICAL DISORDERS OF MINERALOCORTICOIDS

Primary Hyperaldosteronism

Primary hyperaldosteronism is usually due to adrenocortical adenoma. The principal manifestations of excess aldosterone secretion are hypertension and hypokalaemia. Urinary aldosterone levels are high and plasma-renin activity is reduced or absent.

The most effective screening method is to determine whether hypertension is due to hyperaldosteronism or not in the serum potassium measurement. The disease must be suspected if more than 50 mEq of potassium are excreted in 24 hours and the serum potassium level is below 3 mEq/L. The patient should be on a high salt intake (2 gm of salt with each meal for 4 days before electrolyte measurements and ECG are done). The electrocardiographic changes are those of prolonged hypertension and hypokalaemia.

The patient with hyperaldosteronism frequently complains of severe headache. Potassium depletion causes weakness, paresthesis, flaccid paralysis, polyuria, and nocturia. Transient correction of hypokalaemia by administration of spironolactone, 400 mg daily in divided doses for 3 days, is presumptive evidence of primary hyperaldosteronism. A diabetic glucose tolerance curve is present in about half of cases.

Isothenuria which does not respond to vasopressin is also due to potassium depletion.

Sodium retention causes hypernatremia and dilutional anaemia due to increased plasma volume (low haematocrit). Autonomic dysfunction is manifested by a postural fall in blood pressure without changes in pulse rate.

Desoxycorticosterone acetate, 20 mg IM daily in divided doses for 3 days, causes no change in aldosterone production if an aldosterone-producing tumour is present. The measurement of plasma aldosterone can be used. Care must be taken because of its increased response to posture, activity, and salt restriction. The plasma aldosterone does not normally increase 2-to 3-fold after 4 hours upright in patients with adenoma. While 83 per cent of patients with the syndrome of primary aldosteronism have a solitary adenoma, the hypertension seen in patients with hyperplasia in the remaining 17 per cent usually does not respond to subtotal or total adrenalectomy.

Secondary Hyperaldosteronism

Excessive secretion of aldosterone is seen in oedematous states, such as cirrhosis with ascites, nephrosis, congestive heart failure, and toxemia of pregnancy; in nonoedematous states, such as malignant hypertension; in unilateral renal arterial narrowing, and after diuretic therapy. Useful differential diagnostic aids are: (i) low serum concentration, (ii) blood volume, usually reduced in hypertensive patients, and (iii) normal or elevated plasma-renin activity.

Islolated Hypoaldosteronism

Hyperkalaemia unexplained by diminished renal function can be the presenting finding in patients with reduced aldosterone levels. All other adrenal steroids are normal, and the defect resides in the defective release or production of renin.

ADRENAL MEDULLA

The adrenal medullary hormones are catecholamines: (i) epinephrine and (ii) norepinephrine, the parent compound from which epinephrine is formed by addition of a methyl group.

Catecholamines, Plasma

Normal values

		SI units
Fractionation		
Standing		
Epinephrine	0-140 pg/ ml	0-762 pmol/L
Norepinephrine	200-1700 pg/ ml	1088-9256 pmol/L
Dopamine	0-30 pg/ ml	0-163 pmol/L
Supine		
Epinephrine	0-110 pg/ ml	0-599 pmol/L
Norepinephrine	70-750 pg/ ml	381-4083 pmol/L
Dopamine	0-30 pg/ ml	0-163 pmol/L
Fractionation Free		
Total	150-650 pg/ ml	886-3843 pmol/L

Catecholamines, Urine

Normal values

		SI units
Random urine		
Total catecholamines	0-18 μg/dl	0-103 nmol/dl
Daytime specimen		
Total catecholamines	1.4-7.3 μg/h	8-43 nmol/h
24-hour urine		
Total catecholamines	0-135 $\mu g/M^2/D^2$	0-796 $nmol/m^2/D^2$
Panic level	>200 $\mu g/M^2/D^2$	>1180 $nmol/m^2/D^2$
Epinephrine		
Adult	0-15 μg	0-82 nmol/D
Children		
Age 1-4	0-6 μg/D	0-33 nmol/D
Age 4-10	0-10 μg/D	0-55 nmol/D
Age 10-15	0.5-20 μg/D	2.7-110 nmol/D
Epinephrine panic level	> 50 μg/D	> 295 nmol/D
Norepinephrine		
Adult	0-100 μg/D	0-590 nmol/D
Children		
Age 1-4	0-29 μg/D	0-170 nmol/D
Age 4-10	8-65 μg/D	47-380 nmol/D
Age 10-15	15-80 μg/D	89-470 nmol/D
Dopamine		
Age 4 years to adult	65-400 μg/D	384-2364 nmol/D
Age 4 years or less	40-260 μg/D	236-1535 nmol/D

Actions

Epinephrine is sympathomimetic, increases cardiac output and rate, systolic blood pressure, blood glucose, hepatic glycogenolysis, basal metabolic rate, sweating, and causes mydriasis and skin-vessel constriction. By contrast, norepinephrine causes bradycardia, peripheral vasoconstriction, and rise in diastolic blood pressure, and has much less prominent metabolic effects.

Clinical Disorders

A. *Deficiency:* Hypotension. Idiopathic spontaneous hypoglycaemia (failure of epinephrine response to hypoglycaemia).
B. *Excess:* Paroxysmal or persistent hypertension, headaches, sweating, tachycardia, elevated blood glucose.

Method of Evaluation

Chemical assay of epinephrine or norepinephrine in blood or urine, provocative and blocking tests for pheochromocytoma; glucose tolerance test; X-rays of suprarenal area.

Adrenal medullary hyperactivity, as in phaeochromocytoma, produces symptoms and signs, including hypertension, through the release of large amounts of epinephrine and norepinephrine into the bloodstream. The most satisfactory single diagnostic procedure is the discovery of plasma levels of norepinephrine in excess of 0.5 μg/L. Jaundice, azotaemia, and tetracycline administration also cause high levels.

When phaeochromocytoma is suspected and hypertension is intermittent, or the basal blood pressure is less than 170/110, a provocative test with histamine may cause a characteristic rise in the blood pressure and in the urine and plasma catecholamines. Higher levels of basal blood pressure are best investigated by the phentolamine test.

The levels of urinary catecholamines and their metabolites (such as Vanillylmandelic acid—VMA normetanephrine and metanephrine) are greatly increased (10-100 times) in the presence of phaeochromocytoma. The usual 24-hour excretion of epinephrine is up to 50 mg, of the metabolite, VMA, 2.5 μg/mg creatinine and less than 1.3 mg/24 hours for 1 ml metanephrine. The inigestion of tea, coffee, bananas, vanilla, salicylates, phenobarbital, fruit, morphine, iproniazid, and methocarbamol will invalidate the VMA measurement. Tetracyclines, vasopressors, and methyldopa can influence catechol determination. Monoamine oxidase inhibitors may cause a rise in metanephrine and a low VMA. The pressor amine output at rest is about half that during normal daily activity. If the urine contains increased amounts of epinephrine (40 per cent of cases), the tumour is almost always in one of the adrenal areas or the organ of Zuckerkandl. If urine contains increased amounts of norepinephrine (60 per cent of cases), the tumour may still be expected to be in or near one of the adrenal areas in two-third of cases; and in the remaining one-third, all possible sites must be considered.

In both, provocative and blocking tests, control blood pressure must be taken and the pressure must restabilise after venipuncture before the drug is given. Hypotensive drugs, e.g. rauwolfia, chlorothiazide, or sedatives, will confuse the results if given within 24 hours before testing. No diagnosis of phaeochromocytoma should be based on these tests alone.

Histamine Provocative Test

Keep phentolamine ready for a case where there is a severe blood pressure rise in a hypertensive patient.

Method: A cold pressure test is first performed by placing the patient's forearm in a water-ice bath for 1 minute after basal blood pressure reading has been taken, and then recording post-immersion blood pressure readings at 30-second intervals for 3 minutes or until the basal state is reachieved. At this time, 0.01-0.05 mg of histamine phosphate in 0.5 ml of isotonic saline is injected rapidly IV, and the readings are again followed to a basal level at 30-second intervals.

Interpretation: Normal subjects experience flushing, headache, and slight blood pressure fall. An elevation in blood pressure significantly greater than the cold pressure response within 2 minutes of the injection, or an increase in the basal levels of plasma catecholamines following histamine stimulation, may indicate phaeochromocytoma.

Phentolamine Blocking Test

This test is used for diagnosis of phaeo-chromocytoma in the hypertensive phase. Barbiturates interfere with the test.

Method: When the resting patient has achieved a basal blood pressure level, 5 mg of phentolamine are given rapidly IV and the blood pressure is determined at 30-second intervals. Maximum effect appears in 2 minutes and lasts for 3-5 minutes. If phaeochromocytoma is strongly suspected, a dose of 1 mg should be administered to avoid profound and prolonged hypotension.

Interpretation: In normal individuals, phentolamine causes a slight transient fall in blood pressure. In the presence of phaeochromocytoma with hypertension, a fall in systolic blood pressure of more than 35 mm Hg and a fall in diastolic blood pressure of more than 25 mm Hg appearing in 2 minutes and lasting for at least 2½ minutes is characteristic.

TESTES

From Leydig cells, the testis elaborates testosterone, androstenedione, and dehydroepiandrosterone (also from adrenal cortex). Luteinizing hormone from the pituitary stimulates the formation of tetosterone, which is inactivated and conjugated in the liver and excreted as glucuronide. Testosterone production rates in men are 2-8 mg/day; in women, 0.5-2.5 mg/day.

ACTIONS

Testosterone maintains sex organs and controls development of male sex characteristics, inhibits pituitary LH, promotes long-bone growth without closure of epiphyses, and has many anabolic effects (e.g. retention of sodium, chloride, water, decrease in gluconeogenesis). It is required for spermatogenesis. However, it cannot be taken exogenously for this purpose since it would suppress FSH and thus prevent this process.

CLINICAL DISORDERS

A. *Deficiency:* Before puberty, enunchoidism or cryptorchism. After puberty, asthenia, loss of beard and potency, atrophy of sex organs, hot flashes, nervousness, depression and osteoporosis. Partial deficiency syndromes may occur (e.g. Klinefelter, Del Castillo)
B. *Excess:* Masculinization as with adrenocortical tumors, Leydig cell tumors, testicular teratomas and seminomas. Administered excess may depress spermatogenesis which "rebounds" to supranormal level after withdrawal.

METHODS OF EVALUATION

A. *Physical examination:* Noting pubic and temporal hair, prostate, and testes. The study of male hypogonadism or sperm deficiencies involves testicular biopsy, examination of the semen and spermatozoa count, and such urinary hormone determinations as indication of androgen production (17-ketosteroid excretion) or inhibition or lack of the pituitary gonadotropins (FSH determination). The absence of hyaluronidase from semen may indicate an obstructive lesion of the ducts leading from the testes, where the enzyme is produced. Urinary testosterone and plasma testosterone measurements are very helpful. Plasma testosterone levels in adult men are 0.4-1 mg%. In castrates, the concentration is 0.015 mg%; in women, 0.05 mg%; in children 0.015 mg%.

B. *Gonadotropin Stimulation test:* Hypogonadism originating in the testis is accompanied by high excretory and serum levels of LH and FSH, whereas both are low when the defect is in the pituitary. Evidences of hypogonadism will disappear and 17-ketosteroid excretion will rise in a patient with hypopituitarism when gonadotropins are administered. This treatment is ineffective when the defect originates in the gonad.
The patient should not be receiving endocrine therapy at the time of testing.
Chorionic gonadotropin is given intramuscularly in a daily dose of 2000 IU for 3 weeks. The patient is watched for abatement of evidences of hypogonadism: in men, sperm count, testicular biopsy, 17-ketosteroids, testosterone, secondary sex characteristics, in women, vaginal smear for estrogenic effects, secondary sex characteristics.

Disappearance of the evidences of hypogonadism indicates hypogonadism secondary to pituitary failure.

TESTOSTERONE, FREE, BLOOD

Normal values

	pg/ml	*SI Units pmol/L*	*Percentage of Total Testosterone*
Males values			
Adults	50-210	174-729	1.0-2.7
Children			
Cord blood	5-22	17.4-76.3	2.0-4.4
Newborn	1.5-31.0	5.2-107.5	0.9-1.7
4 weeks-3 months	3.3-8.0	11.5-62.5	0.4-0.8
3-5 months	0.7-14.0	2.4-48.6	0.4-1.1
5-7 months	0.4-4.8	1.4-16.6	0.4-1.0
6-9 years	0.1-3.2	0.3-11.1	0.9-1.7

Contd...

Contd...

10-11 years	0.6-5.7	2.1-19.8	1.0-1.9
12-14 years	1.4-156	4.9-541	1.3-3.0
15-17 years	80-159	278-552	1.8-2.7
Female values			
Adults	1.0-8.5	3.5-29.5	0.5-1.8
Children			
Cord blood	4.0-16.0	13.9-55.5	2.0-3.9
Newborn	0.5-2.5	1.7-8.7	0.8-1.5
4 weeks-3 months	0.1-1.3	0.3-4.5	0.4-1.1
3-5 months	0.3-1.1	1.0-3.8	0.5-1.0
5-7 months	0.2-0.6	0.7-2.1	0.5-0.8
6-9 years	0.1-0.9	0.3-3.1	0.9-1.4
10-11 years	1.0-5.2	3.5-18.0	1.0-1.9
12-14 years	1.0-5.2	3.5-18.0	1.0-1.9
15-17 years	1.0-5.2	3.5-18.0	1.0-1.9

Increased Androgen resistance, hirsutism, polycystic ovary syndrome, tumor (virilizing). See also Testosterone, Total, Blood.

Decreased Hypogonadism, $P\text{-}450_{c17}$ enzyme deficiency. See also Testosterone, Total, Blood.

Description

Free testosterone is that portion of circulating testosterone that is not bound to the sex hormone-binding globulin (SHBG) plasma protein. This test is used to differentiate true abnormal testosterone levels from those caused by abnormally low or high amounts of circulating SHBG. (See also Testosterone, Total, Blood).

TESTOSTERONE, TOTAL, BLOOD

Normal values

	Male		*Female*	
	ng/dl	*SI Units nmol/L*	*ng/dl*	*SI Units mmol/L*
Adult	300-1200	10.4-41.6	30-95	1.0-3.3
Prepubertal values				
Cord blood	13-55	0.45-1.91	5-45	0.17-1.56
Premature infant	37-198	1.28-6.87	5-22	0.17-0.76
Newborn	75-400	2.6-13.9	20-64	0.69-2.22
1-5 months	1-177	0.03-6.14	1-5	0.03-0.17
6-11 months	2-7	0.07-0.24	2-5	0.07-0.17
12 months-5 years	2-25	0.07-0.87	2-10	0.07-0.35
6-9 years	3-30	0.10-1.04	2-20	0.07-0.69
Pubertal values				
Tanner stage				
1	2-23	0.07-0.80	2-10	0.07-0.35
2	5-70	0.17-23	5-30	0.17-1.04
3.	15-280	0.52-9.72	10-30	0.35-1.04
4.	105-545	3.64-18.91	15-40	0.52-1.39
5.	265-800	9.19-27.76	10-40	0.35-1.39

Increased Adrenal hyperplasia, adrenal tumor, arrhenoblastoma, central nervous system lesions, hirsutism (idiopathic), hyperthyroidism, ovairan tumor (virilizing), testicular feminization, testicular tumor, virilizing luteoma, and virilization. In women, idiopathic hirsutism, cystic acne, polycystic ovary syndrome, adrenogenic alopecia, abnormal menstruation, anovulation, adrenogenital syndrome with virilization, ovarian tumor, and Stein-Leventhal syndrome with virilization. Drugs include anticonvulsants, barbiturates, cimetidine, clomiphene, estrogens, gonadotropin (males), and oral contraceptives.

Decreased Anemia, cirrhosis, crypto-orchidism, Down syndrome, gynecomastia, hypogondism (male), hypopituitarism, impotence, Klinefelter's syndrome, male climacteric, obesity, and orchidectomy. Drugs include androgens, cyproterone, dexamethasone, diethylistilbestrol, digoxin (males), digitalis, estrogens (males), ethanol, glucose, glucocorticoids, gonadotropin-releasing hormone analogues, halothane, ketoconazole, metoprolol, metyrapone, phenothiazines, spironolactone, and tetracyline.

Description

Testosterone is the dominant androgen found in the adrenal glands, brain, ovary, pituitary, skin, kidney, and testes. It circulates both freely, and bound to plasma proteins (sex hormone-binding globulin [SHBG]). Testosterone promotes the growth and development of the male sexual organs, and increases body mass and hair replacement. This test measures total testosterone levels in clients with normal SHBG levels.

Interfering Factors

In adult males, an inverse correlation of free testosterone with age occurs. The upper limit of normal range generally decreases from the age of 20 to 60 years. The lower range of free normal does not change significantly with age.

TESTOSTERONE DIRECT IMMUNOENZYMATIC DETERMINATION OF TESTOSTERONE ON SERUM OR PLASMA: (Courtesy: Lilac Medicare)

1. PRINCIPLE

Testosterone (antigen) in the sample competes with horseradish peroxidase testosterone (enzyme-labelled antigen) for binding onto the limited number of antitestosterone (antibody) sites on the microplates (solid phase).

After incubation, the bound/free separation is performed by a simple solid-phase washing.

The enzyme substrate (H_2O_2) and the chromogen (TMB) are added. After an appropriate time has elapsed for maximum colour development, the enzyme reaction is stopped and the absorbance is determined.

Testosterone concentration in the sample is calculated based on a series of standard.

The colour intensity is inversely proportional to the testosterone concentration in the sample.

2. REAGENT, MATERIAL AND INSTRUMENTATION

2.1 Reagent and Material Supplied in the Kit

1. Standard (S_0-S_1-S_2-S_3-S_4) 1.0 ml/0.5 ml. Before use, mix for 5 min with rotating mixer.
   The standards have the following concentration of testosterone:

	S_0	S_1	S_2	S_3	S_4
ng/ml	0	0.2	1.0	4.0	16.0

2. Marker 11 ml /5.5 ml. Ready to use. Testosterone-HRP conjugate. Before use mix gently for 5 minutes with rotating mixer.
3. Microwell plate 8 × 12 strips. Anti-testosterone IgG adsorbed on microplate.
4. TMB-substrate 12 ml H_2O_2 TMB 0.25 g/L (avoid any skin contact).
5. Stop solution 12 ml HCl 1N (avoid any skin contact).

2.2 Notes

- Store all reagents between +2 and + 8°C in the dark.
- Open the bag with the microplate only when it is at room temperature and close immediately after use.
- Do not remove the adhesive sheets on the unutilised strips:

2.3 Reagents Necessary which are not supplied with the Kit

- Distilled water.

2.4 Auxiliary Materials and Instrumentation

- Disposable glass tubes
- Automatic dispenser
- Microplates reader

3. PREPARATION OF THE SAMPLE

The determination of testosterone can be performed in plasma as well as in serum of patients who have observed fast. Store reagent at –20°C if the determination is not performed on the same day of the sample collection.

3.1 Precaution

- Do not use heavily haemolysed samples.
- Maximum precision is required for reconstitution and dispensation of the reagents.
- This method allows the determination of testosterone from 0.2 ng/ml to 16.0 ng/ml.
- The clinical significance of the determination of testosterone can be invalidated if the patient was treated with cortisone or natural or synthetic steroids.

4. PROCEDURE

As it is necessary to perform the determination in duplicate, prepare two wells for each of the five points of the standard curve (S_0-S_4) and for each sample, one for blank.

Pipette

	Standard	*Sample*	*Blank*
Sample	....	25 ul	....
Standards S_0-S_4	25 ul	....	....
Marker	100 ul	100 ul	....
Mix well			
Incubate at 37°C for 1 hour			
Remove the contents from each well; wash the wells with 300 μl of distilled water. Repeat the washing procedure by draining the water completely.			
TMB-substrate	100 ul	100 ul	100 ul
Incubate at room temperature (20-25°C) for 15 minutes in the dark			
Stop solution	100 ul	100 ul	100 ul
Read the absorbance (E) at 450 nm against Blank			

5. STANDARD CURVE-CALCULATION OF RESULTS

5.1 Mean Absorbance and Relative Percentage

Calculate the mean of the absorbances (Em) corresponding to the single points of the standard curve and of each sample. Express data as the per centage of the mean absorbance of B_0. (EmS_0) with the following formula:

$$(B/B_0) \text{ per cent} = \frac{Em}{(Em\ S_0)} \times 100$$

5.2 Standard Curve

Plot the values of the standards expressed as (B/B_0) per cent on the enclosed logit-log paper.

Extrapolate the line passing through the points.

5.3 Calculation of Results

Interpolate the values of the samples expressed as (B/B_0) per cent on the standard curve to obtain the corresponding values of the concentrations expressed in ng/ml.

ESTRIOL

Direct Immunoenzymatic Determination of Unconjugated Oestriol of Serum Plasma (Courtesy: Lilac Medicare)

1. PRINCIPLE

"Unconjugated" estriol (antigen) in the sample competes with horseradish peroxidase oestriol (enzyme-labelled antigen) for binding onto the limited number of antioestriol (antibody) sites on the microplates (solid phase).

After incubation, the bound/free separation is performed by a simple solid-phase washing.

The enzyme substrate (H_2O_2) and the chromogen (TMB) are added. After an appropriate time has elapsed for maximum coluor development, the enzyme reaction is stopped and the absorbance is determined.

Estriol concentration in the sample is calculated based on a series of standard.

The colour intensity is inversely proportional to the oestriol concentration in the sample.

2. REAGENT, MATERIAL AND INSTRUMENTATION

2.1 Reagent and Material supplied in the Kit

*S_1-S_2-S_3-S_4

Oestriol Standards 1 × 1 ml having the following concentration of oestriol:

	S_1	S_2	S_3	S_4
ng/ml	0.1	1.0	4.0	12.0

1. Incubation buffer : 1 × 28 ml
   Phosphate buffer 50 mM pH 7.4; BSA 1 gr/L
2. Marker 200x conc. 1 × 0.5 ml/vial Estriol-HRP conjugate
3. Microplate:12./8 microwell strips Anti-Estriol IgG adsorbed on microplate
4. TMB-Substrat: 1 × 11 ml/vial TMB 0.25 g/L (avoid any skin contact)
5. Stop Solution 1 × 11 ml/vial 1 N HCl: Avoid contact with eyes and skin

2.2 Notes

- Store all reagents between +2 and + 8°C in the dark.
- Open the bag with the microplate only when it is at room temperature.and close immediately after use.
- Do not remove the adhesive sheets on the unutilized strips.

2.3 Reagents Necessary which are not Supplied with the Kit

- Distilled water

2.4 Auxiliary Materials and Instrumentation

- Automatic dispenser.
- Microplates reader.

2.5 Preparation of Reagents

Standard (S_1,S_2,S_3,S_4) (freeze-dried) Reconstitute each bottle with 1 mL of distilled water. Let stand until completely dissolved and mix gently. Before use, mix for 10 min with rotating mixer.

Diluted Marker (Prepare immediately before use) Add 10 µl stock solution (reagent 2) to 2.0 mL of Incubation Buffer (reagent 1). Mix gently.

3. PREPARATION OF THE SAMPLE

The determination of oestriol can be performed in plasma as well as in serum.

Store reagent at –20°C if the determination is not performed on the same day of the sample collection.

3.1 Precaution

- Do not use heavily haemolysed samples.
- Maximum precision is required for reconstitution and dispensation of the reagents.
- This method allows the determination of Estriol from 0.1 ng/mL to 12.0 ng/mL. For concentration of Estriol over 12 ng/mL dilute the serum (1+3) with saline solution, considering the diluting factor when calculating the results.
- The clinical significance of Estriol determination can be invalidated if the patient was treated with natural or synthetic steroids.

4. Procedure

As it is necessary to perform the determination in duplicate, prepare two wells for each of the four points of the standard curve (S_1-S_4), two for B_0 and for each sample, one for blank.

Pipette:

	B_0	Standard	Sample	Blank
Reagent 1	20 µl	......	......	......
Sample	......	......	20 µl	......
Standards S_1 -S_4	......	20 µl	......	......
Diluted marker	200 µl	200 µl	200 µl	......
Incubate at 37°C for 1 hour				
Remove the contents from each well; wash the wells with 300 nl of distilled water.Repeat the washing procedure by draining the water completely.				
Pipette				
	B_0	Standard	Sample	Blank
TMB-substrate	100 µl	100 µl	100 µl	100 µl
Incubate at 20-25°C for 15 minutes in the dark				
Pipette				
	B_0	Standard	Sample	Blank
Stop sol.	50 µl	50	50 µl	50 µl
Read the absorbance (E) at 450 nm against blank				

5. STANDARD CURVE-CALCULATION OF RESULTS

5.1 Mean Absorbance and Relative Percentage

Calculate the mean of the absorbances (Em) corresponding to the single points to the standard curve (S_1-S_4), and of each sample. Express data as the per centage of the mean absorbance of B_0 (EmB_0) with the following formula:

$$(B/B_0) \text{ per cent} = \frac{Em}{(EmB_0)} \times 100$$

5.2 Standard Curve

Plot the values of the standards (S_1-S_4) expressed as (B/B_0) per cent on the enclosed logit-log paper.

Extrapolate the line passing through the points.

5.3 Calculation of Results

Interpolate the values of the samples expressed as (B/B_0) per cent on the standard curve to obtain the corresponding values of the concentrations expressed in ng/mL.

6. REFERENCE VALUES

Estriol Serum	
	Normal Values in ng/ml
Weeks of pregnancy	
14	0.2-3.0
15	0.2-3.5
16	0.3-4.2
17	0.4-5.2
18	0.4-5.8
19	0.4-6.2
20	0.4-6.8
22	0.4-9.1
24	0.4-9.1
26	1.9-9.5
28	2.2-10.1
30	2.0-10.8
32	2.5-11.3
34	2.2-12.7
36	2.5-25.0
37	3.6-25.3
38	6.6-29.7
39	6.7-25.3
40	7.2-22.9
41	8.8-31.5

Estriol Values are Increased in

Feminising tumours, true precocious puberty, liver cirrhosis and multiple pregnancy. Drugs include oxytocin.

Estriol Values are Decreased in

Anencephaly, abortion, anemia, choriocarcinoma, diabetes mellitus, erythroblastosis, fetalis, fetal adrenal aplasia, fetal Down syndrome, fetal growth retardation, fetal encephalopathy, gynaecomastia, hepatic disease, haemoglobinopathy, hydatidiform mole, intrauterine death, menopause, postmaturity, pre-eclampsia, and Rh-immunisation, drugs include betamethasone, cascara, corticosteroids (large doses), dexamethasone, diuretics, glutethimide, oestrogens, mandelamine, meprobamate, penicillins, phenazopyridine, phenophthalein, probenecid and senna.

17-β-ESTRADIOL

Direct Immunoenzymatic Determination of 17-β-Estradiol in Serum, Plasma (Courtesy: Lilac Medicare)

Principle

The 17-β-oestradiol (antigen) in the sample competes with horseradish peroxidase 17-β-estradiol (enzyme-labelled-antigen) for binding onto the limited number of anti-17-β-estradiol (antibody) sites on the microplates (solid phase).

After incubation, the bound/free separation is performed by a simple solid-phase washing. The enzyme substrate (H_2O_2) and the chiromogen (TMB) are added. After an appropriate time has elapsed for maximum colour development, the enzyme reaction is stopped and the absorbance is determined.

The 17-β-estradiol concentration in the sample is calculated based on a series of standard.

The colour intensity is inversely proportional to the 17-β-estradiol concentration in the sample.

2. REAGENTS, MATERIAL AND INSTRUMENTATION

2.1 Reagents and Material Supplied in the Kit

S_1-S_2-S_3-S_4 : 1 × 1.0 ml/vial/1 × 0.5 ml/vial 17-β-Estradiol Standards having the following

Concentrations pg/ml	S1	S2	S3	S4
	10	60	400	1500

Stable until the expiration date reported on the kit.

1. Incubation buffer 2 × 12 ml/vial/phosphate buffer 50 mM pH 7.4; BSA 1 gr/L
2. Marker : 1 × 0.5 ml/vial/100 x conc. 17-β-estradiol-HRP conjugate
3. Microplate : 12 × 8 microwell strips Anti-17β-Estradiol IgG-adsorbed on microwells.

4. TMB-substrate: 1 × 12 ml/vial H_2O_2 TMB 0.25 g/L (avoid any skin contact)
5. Stop solution 1 × 12 ml/vial 1n HCl avoid contact with eyes and skin
6. Competitive solution : 2 × 2.5 ml/vial

2.2 Notes

- Store all reagents between + 2 to 8°C in the dark.
- Open the bag with the microwells only when it is at room temperature and close immediately after use. Do not remove the adhesive sheet from the unutilised strips.

2.3 Reagents Necessary which are not Supplied with the Kit

Distilled water

2.4 Auxiliary Materials and Instrumentation

Automatic dispenser.
Microplates reader

2.5 Preparation of Reagents

Diluted Marker (Prepare immediately before use) Add 10 μl stock solution (reagent 2) to 1.0 mL of Incubation Buffer (reagent 1). Mix gently.

3. PREPARATION OF THE SAMPLE

The determination of 17-β estradiol can be performed in plasma as well as in serum of patients who have observed fast.

Store reagent at –20°C if the determination is not performed on the same day of the sample collection.

3.1 Precaution

- Do not use heavily haemolysed samples
- Maximum precision is required for reconstitution and dispensation of the reagents.
- This method allows the determination of 170-β-estradiol from 20 pg/mL to 3000 pg/mL
- The clinical significance of the determination 170-β-estradiol can be invalidated if the patient was treated with cortisone or natural or synthetic steroids.

Procedure

As it is necessary to perform the determination in duplicate, prepare two wells for B_0.two for each of the four points of the standard curve (S_1-S_4), two for each sample, one for blank.

Dispense

	B_0	Standard	Sample	Blank
Incubation buffer	100 μl	.....	.....	.....
Sample	.....	.....	50 μl	.....
Competitive Sol	.....	.....	50 μl	.....
Standards S_1-S_4	.....	100 μl	.....	.....
Diluted marker	100 μl	100 μl	100 μl	.....
Incubate at +37°C for 1 hour				
Remove the contents from each well. Wash the wells with 300 nL of distilled water. Repeat the washing procedure draining the water completely. «				
Dispense				
	B_0	Standard	Sample	Blank
TMB-substrate	100 μl	100 μl	100 μl	100 μl
Incubate at room temperature (20-25°C) for *15 minutes* in the dark.				
Dispense				
	B_0	Standard	Sample	Blank
Stop solution	100 μl	100 μl	100 μl	100 μl
Read the absorbance (E) at 450 ran against blank.				

5. STANDARD CURVE-CALCULATION OF RESULTS

5.1 Mean Absorbance and Relative Percentage

Calculate the mean of the absorbances (Em) corresponding to the single points to the standard curve and of each sample. Express data as the per centage of the mean absorbance of B_0 (EmB_0) with the following formula:

$$(B/B_0) \text{ per cent} = \frac{Em}{(EmB_0)} \times 100$$

5.2 Standard Curve

Plot the values of the standards expressed as (B/B_0) per cent on the enclosed logit-log paper.
Extrapolate the line passing through the points.

5.3 Calculation of Results

Interpolate the values of the samples expressed as (B/B_0) per cent on the standard curve to obtain the corresponding values of the concentrations expressed in pg/mL.

Note

The standard concentrations are 2 times lower than the values reported in the logit-log paper because the quantity of standards dispensed is double than the samples.

6. REFERENCE VALUES

The serum or plasma 17-β-estradiol values are comprised in the following intervals:

Woman	Follicular phase	30-120 pg/mL
	Ovulatory peak	150-400 pg/mL
	Luteinic phase	70-200 pg/mL
	Manopause	< 60 pg/mL
Man		< 40 pg/mL
Children		< 60 pg/mL

The measurement of oestradiol is important for the evaluation of normal sexual development (menarche), causes of infertility (anovulation, amenorrhea, dysmenorrhoea), and menopause, normal oestradiol levels are lowest at menses and into the early follicular phase and then rise in the late follicular phase to a peak just before the LH surge, initiating ovulation. If conception occurs, estradiol levels continue to rise. At menopause, estradiol levels remain low.

Estradiol is Increased in

Adrenal tumours, cirrhosis, gynaecomastia in males, hyperthyroidism, Klinefelter's syndrome, liver tumours, ovarian neoplasm, polycystic ovary syndrome.

Estradiol is Decreased in

Amenorrhoea, anorexia nervosa, hypopituitarism, infertility, menopause, osteoporosis, ovarian hypofunction, pituitary disease, and polycytic ovary syndrome.

DHEA-S (DEHYDROEPIANDROSTERONE SULFATE)

Direct Immunoenzymatic Determination of Dehydroepiandrosterone Sulfate of Serum Plasma
Courtesy: Lilac Medicare

1. PRINCIPLE

Dehydroepiandrosterone sulfate (antigen) in the sample competes with horseradish peroxidase dehydroepiandrosterone sulfate (enzyme-labelled antigen) for binding onto the limited number of antidehydroepiandrosterone sulfate (antibody) sites on the microplates (solid phase).

After incubation, the bound/free separation is performed by a simple solid-phase washing.

The enzyme substrate (H_2O_2) and the chromogen (TMB) are added. After an appropriate time has elapsed for maximum colour development, the enzyme reaction is stopped and the absorbance is determined.

Dehydroepiandrosterone sulfate concentration in the sample is calculated based on a series of standard. The colour intensity is inversely proportional to the dehydroepiandrosterone sulfate concentration in the sample.

2. REAGENT, MATERIAL AND INSTRUMENTATION

2.1 Reagent and Material Supplied in the Kit

1. Microplate: 12 × 8 microwells strips microwells strips
   Antidehydroepiandrosterone sulfate IgG adsorbed on microwells
2. Dehydroepiandrosterone sulfate standards: Ixl ml/vial/1 × 0.5 ml/vial having the following concentration:

	S_1	S_2	S_3	S_4
ng/ml	1	3	12	40

   Stable until the expiration date reported on the kit
3. Incubation buffer: 1 × 28 ml/vial/Phosphate buffer 50 mM pH 7.4; BSA 1 g/L
4. Marker: 1 × 0.5 ml/vial/Dehydroepiandrosterone sulfate-HRP conjugate 100x conc.
5. TMB Substrate: 1 × 11 ml/vial/H_2O_2-TMB 0.25 g/L (avoid any skin contact)
6. Stop solution: 1 × 11 ml/vial/Sulphuric acid 0.15 mol/1:Avoid any skin contact.

2.2 Notes

Store all reagents between +2 and + 8°C in the dark. Open the bag with the microplate only when it is at room temperature.and close immediately after use.

Do not remove the adhesive sheet on the unused strips.

2.3 Reagents Necessary which are not Supplied with the Kit

- Distilled water
- 0.9 per cent saline solution

2.4 Auxiliary Materials and Instrumentation

- Disposable glass tubes
- Automatic dispenser
- Microplates reader

2.5 Preparation of Reagents

1. **Diluted Marker** (Prepare immediately before use)

Add 10 μl stock solution to 1.0 mL of incubation buffer. Mix gently.

3. PREPARATION OF THE SAMPLE

The determination of dehydroepiandrosterone sulfate can be performed in plasma as well as in serum of patients who have observed fast.

Store sera at –20°C if the determination is not performed on the same day of the sample collection.

Sample Dilution

Immediately before use, prepare a tube for each sample and pipette

Saline solution	mL	2
Sample	μL	10
Mix well		

3.1 Precaution

- Do not use heavily haemolysed samples.
- Maximum precision is required for dispensation of the reagents.
- This method allows the determination of dehydroepiandrosterone sulfate from 0.2 μg/mL to 8 μg/mL.

— The clinical significance of the determination of dehydroepiandrosterone sulfate can be invalidated if the patient was treated with cortisone or natural or synthetic steroids.

4. PROCEDURE

As it is necessary to perform the determination in duplicate, prepare two wells for each of the four points of the standard curve (S_1-S_4), two for B_0 and for each sample, one for blank.

Pipette

	B_0	Standard	Sample	Blank
Saline solution	50 μl	....	....	....
Diluted sample	....	....	50 μl	
Standards S_i-S_4	....	50 μl	....	....
Diluted marker	150 μl	150 μl	150 μl	....
Incubate at 37°C for *15 minutes*				

Remove the contents from each well; wash the wells with 300 ul of distilled water. Repeat the washing procedure by draining the water completely.

Pipette

	B_0	Standard	Sample	Blank
TMB-Substrate	100 μl	100 μl	100 μl	100 μl

Incubate at room temperature (20-25°C) for 15 minutes in the dark.

Pipette

	B_0	Standard	Sample	Blank
Stop solution	100 μl	100 μl	100 μl	100 μl

Read the absorbance (E) at 450 nm against blank.

5. STANDARD CURVE-CALCULATION OF RESULTS

5.1 Mean Absorbance and Relative Percentage

Calculate the mean of the absorbances (Em) corresponding to the single points to the standard curve and of each sample. Express data as the per centage of the mean absorbance of B_0 (EmB_0) with the following formula:

$$(B/B_0) \text{ per cent} = \frac{Em}{(Em\ B_0)} \times 100$$

5.2 Standard Curve

Plot the values of the standards expressed as (B/B_0) per cent on the enclosed logit-log paper.

Extrapolate the line passing through the points.

Note: The standard concentrations are 200 times lower than the values reported in the logit log paper because they are not diluted while the samples are diluted 1/200.

5.3 Calculation of Results

Interpolate the values of the samples expressed as (B/B_0) per cent on the standard curve to obtain the corresponding values of the concentrations expressed in μg/mL.

6. Reference Values

The serum or plasma dehydroepiandrosterone sulfate values are comprised in the following intervals:

	Women μg/mL	Man μg/mL
Newborns	0.9 - 1.8	0.9 - 1.8
Before puberty	0.25 -1.0	0.25-1.0
Adults	0.9 - 3.6	0.9 - 3.6
After menopause	< 0.25 - 1.0	
Pregnancy	0.25 -1.8	

Values are Increased in

Adrenal cortex adenoma and carcinoma, Cushing's disease, ectopic ACTH-producing tumours, female acne and hirsutism, oligomenorrhoea in female athletes, polycystic ovarian syndrome, Stein Levinthal syndrome, and virilising congenital hyperplasia.

Values are Decreased in

Primary and secondary adrenal insufficiency. Low levels in amniotic fluid indicate anencephaly in the foetus.

Δ4-ANDROSTENEDIONE

Direct Immunoenzymatic Determination of Δ 4-Androstenedione of Serum, Plasma (Curtesy: Lilac Medicare)

1. PRINCIPLE

Androstenedione (antigen) in the sample competes with horseradish peroxidase androstenedione (enzyme-labelled antigen) for binding onto the limited number of antiandrostenedione (antibody) sites on the microplates (solid phase).

After incubation, the bound/free separation is performed by a simple solid-phase washing. The enzyme substrate (H_2O_2) and the chromogen (TMB) are added. After an appropriate time has elapsed for maximum colour development, the enzyme reaction is stopped and the absorbance are determinated.

Androstenedione concentration in the sample is calculated based on a series of standard. The colour intensity is inversely proportional to the androstenedione concentration in the sample.

2. REAGENT, MATERIAL AND INSTRUMENTATION

2.1 Reagent and Material supplied in the Kit

* S_0 S_1,-S_2-S_3-S_4, S_5 (1 bottle each)
Androstenedione Standards

1. Incubation buffer: 1 × 28 ml
   Phosphate buffer 50 mM pH 7.4; BSA 1 g/L
2. Marker 1 × 0.5 ml 100x conc Androstenedione-HRP conjugate
3. Microplate : 12 × 8 microwells
   Antiandrostenedione IgG adsorbed on microplate
4. TMB-Substrate : 1 × 11 ml
   H_2O_2-TMB 0.25 g/L (avoid any skin contact)
5. Stop solution : 1 × 11 ml
   Sulphuric acid 0.15 mol/L (corrosive: avoid any skin contact)

2.2 Notes

- Store all reagents between +2 and + 8C°in the dark.
- Open the bag of reagent 3 (antibody) only when it is at room temperature and close immediately after use.
- Do not remove the adhesive sheet from the strips unutilized.

2.3 Reagents Necessary which are not Supplied with the Kit

- Distilled water

2.4 Auxiliary Materials and Instrumentation

- Automatic dispenser
- Microplates reader

2.5 Preparation of Reagents

Standard (S0, S1, S2, S3, S4, S5) (freeze-dried) Reconstitute each bottle with 1 mL of distilled water. Let stand until completely dissolved and mix gently. Before use, mix for 10 min with rotating mixer. The standard reconstituted in this way has the following concentration of androstenedione:

	S_0	S_1	S_2	S_3	S_4	S_5
ng/ml	0	0.1	0.4	1.2	4.0	10.0

Stable two weeks when stored at +4°C: Six months when stored at –20°C.

Diluted Marker (Prepare immediately before use) Add 10 μl stock solution (reagent 2) to 1.0 mL of incubation buffer (reagent 1). Mix gently.

3. PREPARATION OF THE SAMPLE

The determination of androstenedione can be performed in plasma as well as in serum of patients who have observed fast.

Store reagent at –20°C if the determination is not performed on the same day of the sample collected.

3.1 Precaution

- Do not use heavily haemolysed samples.
- Maximum precision is required for reconstitution and dispensation of the reagents.
- This method allows the determination of androstenedione from 0.1 ng/mL to 10 ng/mL.
- The clinical significance of androstenedione determination can be invalidated if the patient was treated with cortisone or natural or synthetic steroids.

4. Procedure

As it is necessary to perform the determination in duplicate, prepare two wells for each of the six points of the standard curve (S_0-S_5), two for each sample, one for blank.

Pipette

	Standard	*Sample*	*Blank*
Sample	.....	50 μl	.....
Standards S_0, -S_5	50 μl	.....	.....
Diluted marker	150 μl	150 μl	.....

Incubate at +37°C for 1 hour

Remove the contents from each well. Wash the wells with 300 uL of distilled water. Repeat the washing procedure by draining the water completely.

Pipette

	Standard	*Sample*	*Blank*
TMB-Substrate	100 μl 100 μl	1	00 μl

Incubate at; room temperature (20-25°C) for 15 minutes in the dark

Pipette

	Standard	*Sample*	*Blank*
Stop solution	100 μl	100 μl	100 μl

Read the absorbance (E) at 450 nm against blank.

5. STANDARD CURVE-CALCULATION OF RESULTS

5.1 Mean Absorbance and Relative Percentage

Calculate the mean of the absorbances (Em) corresponding to the single points to the standard curve and of each sample. Express data as the per centage of the mean absorbance of B_0 (EmS_0) with the following formula:

$$(B/B_0) \text{ per cent} = \frac{\text{Em}}{(\text{Em } S_0)} \times 100$$

5.2 Standard Curve

Plot the values of the standards expressed as (B/B_0) per cent on the enclosed logit-log paper.

Extrapolate the line passing through the points.

5.3 Calculation of Results

Interpolate the values of the samples expressed as (B/B_0) per cent on the standard curve to obtain the corresponding values of the concentrations expressed in ng/mL.

6. REFERENCE VALUES

The serum or plasma androstenedione values are comprised in the following intervals:

Women	Follicular phase	0.75 - 2.16 ng/mL
	Luteinic phase	0.94 - 2.33 ng/mL
Men		0.60-1.85 ng/mL

PROGESTERONE

Direct Immunoenzymatic Determination of Progesterone in Serum, Plasma (Courtesy: Lilac Medicare)

1. PRINCIPLE

Progesterone (antigen) in the sample competes with horseradish peroxidase progesterone (enzyme-labelled antigen) for binding onto the limited number of antiprogesterone (antibody) sites on the microplates (solid phase).

After incubation, the bound/free separation is performed by a simple solid-phase washing.

The enzyme substrate (H_2O_2) and the chromogen (TMB) are added. After an appropriate time has elapsed for maximum colour development, the enzyme reaction is stopped and the absorbances are determined.

Progesterone concentration in the sample is calculated based on a series of standards.

The colour intensity is inversely proportional to the progesterone concentration of the sample.

2. REAGENTS, MATERIAL AND INSTRUMENTATION

2.1 Reagents and Material Supplied in the Kit

Standard (S_0, S_1, S_2, S_3, S_4, S_5) (1 bottle each). Progesterone standards) having the following concentration of progesterone:

	S_0	S_1	S_2	S_3	S_4	S5
ng/ml	0	0.4	1.0	3.0	8.0	20.0

Incubation buffer: 1 × 28 ml/Phosphate buffer 50 mM pH 7.4; BSA 1 g/L;ANSAl mm/L

Marker 0.5 ml/vial 100x conc. Progesterone-HRP conjugate Microplate : 12 × 8 microwells. Anti Progesterone IgG adsorbed on microplate

TMB-Substrate 11 ml/vial H_2O_2-TMB 0.25 g/L (avoid any skin contact) Stop Solution 11 ml/vial Sulphuric acid 0.15 mol/l (Corrosive: Avoid contact any skin contact).

2.2 Notes

Store all reagents between +2 and + 8C° in the dark. Open the bag of the microwells only when it is at room temperature and close immediately after use. Do not remove the adhesive sheets on the strips unutilized.

2.3 Reagents Necessary which are not Supplied with the Kit

- Distilled water

2.4 Auxiliary Materials and Instrumentation

- Automatic dispenser
- Microplates reader

12.5 Preparation of Reagents

Diluted Marker (Prepare immediately before use) Add 10 μl stock solution (reagent 2) to 1.0 mL of incubation buffer (reagent 1). Mix gently.

3. PREPARATION OF THE SAMPLE

The determination of progesterone can be performed in plasma as well as in serum.

Store reagent at –20°C if the determination is not performed on the same day of the sample connection.

3.1 Precaution

- Do not use heavily haemolysed samples.
- Maximum precision is required for reconstitution and dispensation of the reagents.
- This method allows the determination of Progesterone from 0.4 ng/mL to 20.0 ng/mL.
- For higher values, for example, in pregnancy, dilute the sample; consider the diluting factor when calculating the result
- The clinical significance of the progesterone determination can be invalidated if the patient was treated with cortisone or natural or synthetic steroids.

4. Procedure

As it is necessary to perform the determination in duplicate, prepare two wells for each of the six points of the standard curve (S_0-S_5), and for each sample, one for blank.

Pipette

	Standard	*Sample*	*Blank*
Sample	....	20 μl	....
Standards S_0-S_5	20 μl	....	....
Diluted marker	200 μl	200 μl	....
Incubate at 37°C) for 1 hours			
Remove the contents from each well; wash the wells with 300 μL of distilled water. Repeat the washing procedure draining the water completely.			
Pipette			
	Standard	*Sample*	*Blank*
TMB-Substrate	100 μl	100 μl	100 μl
Incubate at room temperature (20-25°C) for 15 minutes in the dark.			
Pipette			
	Standard	*Sample*	*Blank*
Stop solution	100 μl	100 μl	100 μl
Read the absorbance (E) at 450 nm against blank.			

5. STANDARD CURVE: CALCULATION OF RESULTS

5.1 Mean Absorbance and Relative Percentage

Calculate the mean of the absorbances (Em) corresponding to the single points to the standard curve and of each sample. Express data as the per centage of the mean absorbance of B_0 (EmS_0) with the following formula:

$$(B/B_0) \text{ per cent} = \frac{Em}{(EmS_0)} \times 100$$

5.2 Standard Curve

Plot the values of the standards expressed as (B/B_0) per cent on the enclosed logit-log paper.

Extrapolate the line passing through the points.

5.3 Calculation of Results

Interpolate the values of the samples expressed as (B/B_0) per cent on the standard curve to obtain the corresponding values of the concentrations expressed in ng/mL.

Normal Values (Units- ng/ml)

Males		0.4-0.9
Females		
Follicular phase		0.40-1.7
Midluteal		4.9-18.8
Postmenopausal		Up to-1.0
On oral contraceptive pills		0.34-0.92
Pregnant Females		
18-21 wk	53-76	
22-25 wk	60-86	
26-29 wk	71-133	
30-33 wk	86-142	
34-37 wk	104-175	
38-41 wk	117-187	

Measurement of serum progesterone have also been used to check the effectiveness of ovulation induction, to monitor progesterone replacement therapy and to detect and evaluate patients at risk for abortion during the early weeks of pregnancy, progesterone levels are increased in luteal phase of menstrual cycle, luteal cysts of ovary, ovarian tumours (e.g. arrhenoblastoma) and adrenal tumours. While decreased levels of progesterone are seen in conditions of amenorrhoea, threatened abortion and fetal death, toxaemia of pregnancy and gonadal agenesis.

Values are Increased in

Adrenal hyperplasia (congenital males), corpus luteum cyst, lipid ovarian tumours, molar pregnancy, ovarian chorionepitheloima, ovarian neoplasms, placental tissue (retained postparturition), precocious puberty and theca lutein cysts. Drugs include adrenocortical hormones, oestrogens and progesterones.

Values are Decreased in

Adrenogenital syndrome, amenorrhoea, anovular menstruation, fetal abnormality or death, luteal deficiency, menstrual abnormalities, ovarian failure, panhypopituitarism, placental failure or insufficiency, pre-eclampsia, Stein-Levinthal syndrome, threatened abortion, toxaemia of pregnancy, Turner's syndrome, and primary/secondary hypogonadism. Drugs include ampicillin and ethinyl estradiol.

17αOH PROGESTERONE

Direct Immunoenzymatic Determination of 17α OH Progesterone of Serum, Plasma (Courtesy: Lilac Medicare)

1. PRINCIPLE

The 17αOH progesterone (antigen) in the sample competes with horseradish peroxidase 17αOH progesterone (enzyme-labelled antigen) for binding onto the limited number of anti 17αOH progesterone (antibody) sites on the microplates (solid phase).

After incubation, the bound/free separation is performed by a simple solid-phase washing.

The enzyme substrate (H_2O_2) and the chromogen (TMB) are added. After an appropriate time has elapsed for maximum colour development, the enzyme reaction is stopped and the absorbances are determined.

The 17αOH progesterone concentration in the sample is calculated based on a series of standard. The colour intensity is inversely proportional to the 17αOH progesterone concentration in the sample.

2. REAGENT, MATERIAL AND INSTRUMENTATION

2.1 Reagent and Material Supplied in the Kit

* S_1-S_2-S_3-S_4 (1 bottle each) 1 × 1 ml

17αOH progesterone standards having the following concentrations

	S	S_2	S_3	S_4
ng/ml	0.2	0.4	1.6	6.4

Stable until the expiration date reported on the kit.

1. **Incubation Buffer:** 1 × 28 ml
   Phosphate buffer 50 mM pH 7.4; BSA 1 gr/L
2. **Marker:** 1 × 0.5 ml 100 × conc
   17α OH Progesterone-HRP conjugate
3. **Microplate:** 12 × 8 microwells
   Anti-17αOH Progesterone IgG adsorbed on microplate
4. **TMB-Substrate:** 1 × 11 ml
   H_2O_2-TMB 0.25 g/L (avoid any skin contact)
5. **Stop solution:** 1 × 11 ml
   Sulphuric acid 0.15 mol/L (corrosive avoid any skin contact)

2.2 Notes

- Store all reagents between +2 and + 8C° in the dark.
- Open the bag of reagent 3 (Antibody) only when it is at room temperature.and close immediately after use.
- Do not remove the adhesive sheets on the strips unutilized.

2.3 Reagents Necessary which are not Supplied with the Kit

- Distilled water

2.4 Auxiliary Materials and Instrumentation

- Automatic dispenser
- Microplates reader

2.5 Preparation of Reagents

Diluted Marker: (Prepare immediately before use) Add 10 μl stock solution (reagent 2) to 1.0 mL of incubation buffer (reagent 1). Mix gently.

3. PREPARATION OF THE SAMPLE

3.1 Precaution

- Do not use heavily haemolysed samples.
- Maximum precision is required for reconstitution and dispensation of the reagents.
- This method allows the determination of 17αOH progesterone from 0.2 ng/mL to 6.4 ng/mL.
- The clinical significance of the determination of 17αOH progesterone can be invalidated if the patient was treated with cortisone or natural or synthetic steroids.

4. PROCEDURE

As it is necessary to perform the determination in duplicate, prepare two wells for each of the four points of the standard curve (S_1-S_4), two for B_0 and for each sample, one for blank.

Pipette

	Bo	*Standard*	*Sample*	*Blank*
Reagent 1	50 μl	....	....	....
Sample	....	....	50 μl	....
Standards S_1, -S_4	....	50 μl	....	....
Diluted Marker	150 μl	150 μl	150 μl	....

Incubate at 37°C for/1 hours

Remove the contents from each well; wash the wells with 300 ul of distilled water. Repeat the washing procedure by draining the water completely.

Pipette

	B_0	*Standard*	*Sample*	*Blank*
TMB-Substrate	100 μl	100 μl	100 μl	100 μl

Incubate at room temperature (20-25°C) for 15 minutes in the dark.

Pipette

	B_0	*Standard*	*Sample*	*Blank*
Stop solution	100 μl	100 μl	100 μl	100 μl

Read the absorbance (E) at 450 nm against blank.

5. STANDARD CURVE: CALCULATION OF RESULTS

5.1 Mean Absorbance and Relative Percentage

Calculate the mean of the absorbances (Em) corresponding to the single points to the standard curve and of each sample. Express data as the per centage of the mean absorbance of B_0 (EmB_0) with the following formula:

$$(B/B_0) \text{ per cent} = \frac{Em}{(Em\ B_0)} \times 100$$

5.2 Standard Curve

Plot the values of the standards expressed as (B/B_0) per cent on the enclosed logit-log paper.

Extrapolate the line passing through the points.

5.3 Calculation of Results

Interpolate the values of the samples expressed as (B/B_0) per cent on the standard curve to obtain the corresponding values of the concentrations expressed in ng/mL.

6. REFERENCE VALUES

The serum or plasma 17αOH progesterone values are comprised in the following intervals:

Woman	follicular phase	0.2 - 1.2 ng/mL
	luteinic phase	1.0 - 4.5 ng/mL
	menopause	0.2 - 0.8 ng/mL
Men		0.2 - 2.3 ng/mL
Children		0.2 - 0.9 ng/mL

It is measurement is of value in the diagnosis and measurement of congenital adrenal hyperplasia, hirsutism and infertility. Circulation 17 alpha hydroxy progesterone normally exhibits a diurnal variation similar to that of cortisol, with higher values in the morning. Serum measurement has been used in the differential diagnosis of hirsutism and infertility where 21 hydrolase deficiency is suspected. Since late-onset congenital adrenal hyperplasia can sometimes mimic the polycystic ovary syndrome, untreated congenital adrenal hyplasia in newborn is usually associated with markedly elevated 17 alpha hydroxy progesterone levels ranging from 10 to 400 times the upper limit of the normal.

CORTISOL

Direct Immunoenzymatic Determination of Cortisol in Serum, Plasma (Courtesy: Lilac Medicare)

1. PRINCIPLE

Cortisol (antigen) in the sample competes with horseradish peroxidase cortisol (enzyme-labelled antigen) for binding onto the limited number of anti cortisol (antibody) sites on the microplates (solid phase).

After incubation, the bound/free separation is performed by a simple solid-phase washing.

The enzyme substrate (H_2O_2) and the chromogen (TMB) are added. After an appropriate time has elapsed for maximum colour development, the enzyme reaction is stopped and the absorbances are determined.

Cortisol concentration in the sample is calculated based on a series of standard.

The colour intensity is inversely proportional to the cortisol concentration in the sample

2. REAGENTS, MATERIAL AND INSTRUMENTATION

2.1 Reagents and Material Supplied in the Kit

S_0-S_1-S_2-S_3-S_4 : 1 × 1.0 ml/via

Cortisol standards having the following concentration:

	S_0	S_1	S_2	S_3	S_4
ng/ml	0,0	10	50	150	500

Stable until the expiration date of the kit

Incubation buffer: 1 × 28 ml/vial

Phosphate buffer 50 mM pH 7.4; BSA 1 g/L, ANSA 0.5 g/L

Marker: 1 × 0.4 ml/vial 100 × conc.

Cortisol-HRP conjugate

Microplate: 12 × 8 microwells strips

Anti-Cortisol-IgG adsorbed on microplate

TMB-Substrate: 1 × 11 ml/vial Ready to use

H_2O_2-TMB 0.25 g/L (avoid any skin contact)

Stop solution: 1 × 11 ml/vial Sulphuric acid 0.15 mol/1 Warning: Avoid contact with eyes and skin.

2.2 Notes

- Store all reagents between + 2 and + 8°Cin the dark.
- Open the bag with the microplate only when it is at room temperature and close immediately after use.
- Do not remove the adhesive sheets on the strips unutilized.

2.3 Reagents Necessary which are not Supplied with the Kit

- Distilled water
- 0.9 per cent saline solution

2.4 Auxiliary Materials and Instrumentation

- Disposable glass tubes
- Automatic dispenser
- Microplates reader

2.5 Preparation of reagents

Diluted Marker. (Prepare immediately before use) Add 10 μl stock solution (reagent 2) to 1.0 mL of incubation buffer (reagent 1). Mix gently.

3. PREPARATION OF THE SAMPLE

The determination of cortisol can be performed in plasma as well as in serum.

Store reagent at –20°C if the determination is not performed on the same day of the sample connection.

3.1 Precaution

- Do not use heavily haemolysed samples.
- Maximum precision is required for reconstitution and dispensation of the reagents.
- This method allows the determination of cortisol from 10 ng/mL to 500 ng/mL.
- The clinical significance of the cortisol determination can be invalidated if the patient was treated with corticosteroids or natural or synthetic steroids.

4. PROCEDURE

As it is necessary to perform the determination in duplicate, prepare two wells for each of the four points of the standard curve (S_0-S_4), two for B_0 and for each sample, one for blank.

Pipette

	Standard	*Sample*	*Blank*
Sample	...	10 μl	....
Standards S_0-S_4	10 μl	....	....
Diluted marker	200 μl	200 μl	....

Cover the plate and incubate at 37°C for 1 hour. Remove the contents from each well; wash the wells with 300 ul of distilled water. Repeat the washing procedure draining the water completely.

Pipette

	Standard	*Sample*	*Blank*
TMB-Substrate	100 μl	100 μl	100 μl

Incubate at room temperature (20-25°C) for 15 minutes in the dark.

Pipette

	Standard	*Sample*	*Blank*
Stop solution	100 μl	100 μl	100 μl

Read the absorbance (E) at 450 nm against blank.

5. STANDARD CURVE-CALCULATION OF RESULTS

5.1 Mean Absorbance and Relative Percentage

Calculate the mean of the absorbances (Em) corresponding to the single points to the standard curve and of each sample. Express data as the per centage of the mean absorbance of S_0 (EmS_0) with the following formula:

$$(B/B_0) \text{ per cent} = \frac{\text{Em}}{(\text{Em So})} \times 100$$

5.2 Standard Curve

Plot the values of the standards expressed as (B/B_0) per cent on the enclosed logit-log paper. Extrapolate the line passing through the points.

5.3 Calculation of Results

Interpolate the values of the samples expressed as (B/B_0) per cent on the standard curve to obtain the corresponding values of the concentrations expressed in ng/mL.

CORTISOL

Plasma Cortisol

Unconjugated cortisol (free and protein-bound) concentration vary diurnally. At 8 am, the average concentration in plasma in 12 mg% (range 7-20 mg%). Diurnal variation is striking. In normal humans observing customary day night activity, the highest levels occur at about 8 am and the lowest level shortly after midnight cortisol plasma or serum norms. Peak occur at about 0800 (8 am) and troughts occur in late afternoon.

Normal Values

Cortisol Interpretation Normal Values in ng/ml	
Age/time	
Adult:	60-230
8-10 am	30-130
4-6 pm	< 50 per cent of am value
Child:	
8-10 am	180-230
4-6 pm	60-120
8 pm	< 50 per cent of am value
Patient treated with ACTH	280-600
Patient treated with dexamethasone	0-50

Cortisol Levels are Increased in

Burns, Cushing's disease, Cushing's syndrome, eclampsia, exercise, hepatic disease (severe), hyperpituitarism, hypertension, hyperthyroidism, infectious disease, obesity, acute pancreatitis, pregnancy, severe renal disease, shock, shock (severe heat, cold, trauma, psychological), surgery, and virilism. Drugs include corticotrophin, oestrogens, oral contraceptives, and vasopressin.

Cortisol Levels are Decreased in

Addison's disease, adrenal insufficiency adenogenital syndrome, chromophobe adenoma, cranipharyngioma, hypoglycaemia, hypophysectomy, hypotituitarism, hypothyroidism, liver disease, postpartum pituitary necrosis, and Waterhouse-Friderichsen syndrome. Drugs include dexamethasone, dexamethasone acetate, and dexamethasone sodium phosphate.

Interfering Factors

1. Pregnancy will cause an increased value
2. There is no normal diurnal variation in patients under stress
3. Drugs such as spironolactone and oral contraceptives will give falsely elevated results.

CORTISOL SUPPRESSION (DEXAMETHASONE SUPPRESSION)

Normal values

8 am : 7-20 μg/dl

4 pm : 2-10 μg/dl

Morning following administration of dexamethasone: 5 μg/dl.

Test Significance

This is screening test for Cushing's syndrome and depends on the fact that ACTH production will be suppressed in normal persons after a low dose of dexamethasone, whereas it is not in Cushing's syndrome.

Method

1. Venous blood sample is obtained at 8 am, 4 pm and again at 8 am the next day after dexamethasone has been administered.
2. At 4 pm, dexamethasone tablets are given orally. The dosage varies according to weight.

All medications should be discontinued for 24 to 48 hours before the study. Especially important are aldactone, oestrogens, contraceptive pills, cortisol, tetracyclines, stilbestrol and dilantin.

Clinical Relevance

No diurnal variation or suppression will occur in:

1. Cushing's syndrome
2. Conditions causing extreme stress
3. Failure to take dexamethasone
4. If dilantin has been administered.

CORTISOL STIMULATION (CORTROSYN STIMULATION)

Normal values

Rise : > 7 mg/dl

Peak : > 20 mg/dl

Test Significance

This is a good test to detect adrenal insufficiency. Cortrosyn is a synthetic subunit of ACTH that exhibits full corticosteroid-stimulating effect of ACTH in normal persons. Failure to respond is an indication of adrenal insufficiency.

Method

1. A fasting venous sample is obtained
2. Cortrosyn is administered intramuscularly
3. Additional blood samples are obtained 30 and 60 minutes after administration of cortrosyn.

Clinical Relevance

Absent or diminished response occurs in:

1. Adrenal insufficiency
2. Hypopituitarism
3. Prolonged steroid administration.

Tests for Adrenocortical Insufficiency

WATER EXCRETION TEST (SOFFER)

Method: The patient fasts overnight. In the morning he empties his bladder and drinks 1500 ml of water (about 20 ml/kg body weight) over a period of 15-45 minutes. A 5-hour urine specimen collected from the beginning of the test is measured. During the 5-hour period, the patient reclines or sits except while voiding. The test may be repeated 2 hours after the oral administration of 50 mg of cortisone.

Interpretation

Normal individuals excrete 1200 ml or more of urine over the 5-hour collection period. Patients with Addison's disease may excrete less than 800 ml of urine. False-positive results may be obtained if the rate of absorption of water from the gastrointestinal tract or its elimination by the kidney is decreased, e.g. in patients with nephritis, cirrhosis, celiac disease, or cardiac failure.

Patients with adrenal insufficiency (primary, or secondary to hypopituitarism) show substantial increase in diuresis when retested following cortisone.

Corticotrophin (ACTH) Response test (Thorn test)

If responsive adrenocortical tissue is present, the administration of potent corticotrophin results in an increased secretion of adrenocortical steroids, and increase in plasma cortisol, producing eosinopenia and increased urinary excretion of 17-ketosteroids and 17-hydroxycorticosteroids. If ACTH has been absent because of pituitary insufficiency, its daily administration leads to a stepwise increase in adrenocortical response over a period of 2-3 days.

Adrenal response to corticotrophin is retarded in myxoedema as well as in hypopituitarism. Allergic eosinophilia may mask a fall in eosinophils. The patient should be free of the effects of large doses of androgens, cortisone, and corticotrophin before urinary steroids are measured.

Method

1. The 4-hour corticotrophin test may be used for screening. The eosinophil count or plasma cortisol is measured before 25 USP units of corticotrophin are administered in a 4-hour infusion. Four hours later, another eosinophil count is done or plasma cortisol measured.
2. Eight-hour intravenous corticotrophin test. 2-5 USP units of corticotrophin in 500 ml of normal saline are administered IV as a continuous 8-hour infusion. An eosinophil count or plasma cortisol level is determined at the beginning and at the end of the 8-hour period. 24-hour urine collections are made on a control day prior to the test and on the day of corticotrophin administration. Urinary excretion levels of 17-ketosteroids, 17-hydroxycorticosteroids, ketogenic steroids, or urinary-free cortisol on each specimen are compared with the control value.
3. As an alternative to the intravenous test, 40-80 USP units of corticotrophin gel (repository corticotrophin injection) or corticotrophin zinc may be given intramuscularly twice daily over the testing period. Corticotrophin gel should not be used in suspected adrenal insufficiency.
4. The patient with Addison's disease may be protected from an untoward reaction to ACTH by the administration of 0.1-0.25 mg of fludrocortisone, urinary steroid levels are not significantly altered.
5. A synthetic 24 amino acid ACTH compound has made possible a rapid intramuscular test. 0.25 mg IM will take more than double normal plasma cortisol in less than 1 hour.

Interpretation

The 4-hour corticotrophin screening test normally decreases circulating eosinophils by more than half. In test (2) or (3) above, normal subjects respond with an 80-100 per cent fall in eosinophil levels, a 2-fold to 5-fold increase in 17-hydroxycorticosteroids, and 2-fold increase in 17-ketosteroid excretion levels. Plasma cortisol increases by 3 or 4 times.

When Cushing's syndrome is present due to adrenocortical hyperplasia, 17-hydroxycorticosteroid excretion levels may reach 75-100 mg/24 hours. The response is usually absent in the presence of the usually more autonomous adrenal carcinoma. The ACTH stimulation of patients with the adrenogenital syndrome produces an excessive response in 17-ketosteroid levels, not noted in cases of idiopathic hirsutism.

In Addison's disease, the 4-hour corticotrophin test elicits a fall of less than 50 per cent in circulating eosinophils. In the 8-hour IV corticotrophin test and the corticotrophin gelatin solution alternate, the addisonian patient shows little or no change in circulating eosinophils or urinary or plasma hormone levels. In order to rule out adrenal insufficiency unequivocally, at least 3 days of method (2) are recommended. The synthetic ACTH method is of value in identifying a normal adrenal response. If no response is observed, method (2) should be applied.

Patients with hypopituitarism and ACTH insufficiency show varying responses depending upon the degree of adrenocortical involution. Repetition of the test on 3-5 consecutive days shows a gradual rise in 17-ketosteroid and 17-hydroxycorticosteroid output and an increasing eosinopenia. Plasma cortisol usually shows an increase of 3-4 times in 4-hours.

All tests other than the IV administration of corticotrophin are subject to occasional false-negative responses due to extravascular inactivation of corticotrophin.

ADRENOCORTICAL INHIBITION TEST

1. *Test with dexamethasone:* Tests to determine the suppressibility of ACTH by glucocorticoids may be done using dexamethasone. Dexamethasone has little effect on sodium or potassium balance and does not interfere with corticosteroid determination.
   Method: 24-hour urine specimens are collected for analysis on 3 successive days. After the first specimen is obtained, 0.5 mg dexamethasone is given every 6 hours by mouth for 2 days. Excretion level is measured on each 24-hour urine specimen. In normal individuals, the repeated administration of the 0.5 mg dose reduces by 50 per cent the basal excretion of 17-hydroxycorticosteroids, urinary cortisol, and plasma cortisol per 24 hours by the end of the second day. If suppression is not obtained, the test is repeated with a dose of 2 mg every 6 hours for 2 days.
   Interpretation: The increased corticosteroid levels which occur in patients with adrenocortical hyperplasia is usually suppressed only by the larger (2 mg) doses, whereas the corticosteroid levels in patients with autonomous adrenocortical neoplasms may not be suppressed even with higher doses.
2. *Rapid dexamethasone test:* 1 mg of dexamethasone at midnight will reduce normal plasma levels to less than 5 mg per cent by 8.00 am. This will effectively rule out adrenal overactivity.
3. *Tests with metyrapone* (an endogenous ACTH test): Inhibition of 11 β-hydroxylase by metyrapone results in reduced blood levels of cortisol and loss of cortisol inhibition by ACTH. The ability of the pituitary to respond to this stimulus by release of ACTH may be measured by noting the increment in 17-ketosteroids, 17-hydroxycorticosteroids, or the metabolite of 11-deoxycortisol (compound-S) produced by the adrenal and excreted in the urine. Compound-S is formed by the adrenal cortex after inhibition of cortisol (hydrocortisone) formation. The rise in urinary 17-hydroxycorticosteroids is a result of increased amounts of this metabolite.

Method

1. *IV-Metyrapone,* 30 mg/kg body weight in 1 liter of normal saline is given IV for 4 hours, starting between 8.00 and 10.00 am. The same method is followed on another day, except that 25 USP units of ACTH are added to metyrapone infusion to compare the functional capacity of maximally stimulated adrenals with the response evoked by the endogenous ACTH released after administration of metyrapone alone.
2. *Oral:* A basal 24-hour urine 17-hydroxycorticosteroid measurement is obtained. 0.75 gm of metyrapone are given every 4 hours for 6 doses. A second 24-hour urine for 17-hydroxycorticosteroid levels is obtained the day following the drug administration.
   Interpretation: Normal subjects may double their basal 24-hour 17-hydroxycorticosteroid excretion after metyrapone, and ACTH adds nothing to this response. Hypopituitary patients show no increase in excretion with metyrapone, but their response to exogenous ACTH is adequate. Addisonian patients respond to neither stimulus. I/V metyrapone causes a vigorous response in patients with adrenal hyperplasia, but adrenal tumors fail to respond. Chlorpromazine blocks metyrapone responses.
   Direct measurements of the metabolite of compound-S and its plasma level are also available, and the direct measurement of their increase provides a more direct assessment of ACTH release.

TOTAL TRIIODOTHYRONINE (T3)

Intended Use: The Quantitative Determination of Total Triiodothyronine Concentration in Human Serum or Plasma by a Microplate Enzyme Immunoassay (Courtesy: Lilac Medicare)

SUMMARY AND EXPLANATION OF THE TEST

Measurement of serum tri-iodothyronine concentration is generally regarded as a valuable tool in the diagnosis of thyroid dysfunction. This importance has provided the impetus for the significant improvement in assay methodology that has occurred in the last two decades.

The advent of monospecific antiserum and the discovery of blocking agents to the T3-binding serum proteins has enabled the development of procedurally simple radioimmunoassays.

This microplate enzyme immunoassay methodology provides the technician with optimum sensitivity while requiring a few technical manipulations. In this method, serum reference, patient specimen, or control is first added to a microplate well. Enzyme-T3 conjugate is added, then the reactants are mixed. A competition reaction results between the enzyme conjugate and the native triiodothyronine for a limited number of antibody combining sites immobilised on the well.

After the completion of the required incubation period, the antibody-bound enzyme-triiodothyronine conjugate is separated from the unbound enzyme-triiodothyronine conjugate by aspiration or decantation. The activity of the enzyme present on the surface of the well is quantitated by reaction with a suitable substrate to produce color.

The employment of several serum references of known triiodothyronine concentration permits construction of a graph of activity and concentration. From comparison to the dose response curve, an unknown specimen's activity can be correlated with triiodothyronine concentration.

PRINCIPLE

Competitive Enzyme Immunoassay

The essential reagents required for a solid phase enzyme immunoassay include immobilized antibody, enzyme-antigen conjugate and native antigen.

Upon mixing immobilized antibody, enzyme-antigen conjugate and a serum containing the native antigen, a competition reaction results between the native antigen and the enzyme-antigen conjugate for a limited number of insolubulized binding sites. The interaction is illustrated by the following equation:

Abcw = Monospecific immobilised antibody (constant quantity)
Ag = Native antigen (variable quantity)
^{Enz}Ag = Enzyme-antigen conjugate (constant quantity)
AgAb cw = Antigen-antibody complex
^{Enz}Ag Abcw = Enzyme-antigen conjugate-antibody complex
k_a = Rate Constant of association
k_{-a} = Rate Constant of disassociation
$K = k_a / k_{-a}$ = Equilibrium constant

After equilibrium is attained, the antibody-bound fraction is separate from unbound antigen by decantation or aspiration. The enzym activity in the antibody-bound fraction is inversely proportional to the native antigen concentration. By utilising several different serurm references of known antigen concentration, a dose response curve can be generated from which the antigen concentration of an unknown can be ascertained.

REAGENTS FOR 96-Well MICROPLATE

A. Human Serum References-1.0 ml/vial

Six (6) vials of serum reference for triiodothyronine; concentrations of 0 (A), 50 (B), 100 (C), 250 (D), 500 (E) an 750 (F) ng/dl. Store at 2-8°C. A preservative has been added.

B. Enzyme-antigen Conjugate-10 ml/vial

One (1) vial of triiodothyronine-horseradish peroxidase (HRP conjugate in a bovine albumin-stabilizing matrix. A preservative has been added. Store at 2-8°C.

C. Enzyme-antigen Conjugate Buffer-11 ml

One (1) bottle containing buffer, red dye, preservative, and binding protein inhibitors. Store at 2-8°C.

D. Antibody-Coated Microplate-96 Wells

One 96-well microplate coated with sheep anti-T3 serum and packaged in an aluminum bag with a drying agent. Store at 2-8°C.

E. Wash Solution Concentrate-20 ml

One (1) vial Containing a surfactant in phosphate buffered saline A preservative has been added. Store at 2-30°C.

F. Substrate A-7.0 ml/vial

One (1) bottle containing tetramethyl benzidine (TMB) in buffer Store at 2-8°C.

G. Substrate B-7.0 ml/vial

One (1) bottle containing hydrogen peroxide (H_2O2> in buffer Store at 2-8°C.

H. Stop Solution-6.0 ml/vial

One (1) bottle of stop solution containing a strong acid (1N HCL Store at 2-30°C.

PRECAUTIONS

For *in vitro* Diagnostic Use Not for Internal or External Use in Humans or Animals

All products that contain human serum have been found to be nonreactive for Hepatitis B Surface Antigen, HIV 1-2 and HCV Antibodies by FDA required tests. Since no known test can offer complete assurance that infectious agents are absent, all human serum products should be handled as potentially hazardous and capable of transmitting disease. Good laboratory procedures for handling blood products can be found in the Center for Disease Control/ National Institute of Health, "Biosafety in Microbiological and Biomedical Laboratories," 2nd Edition, 1988, HHS Publication No. (CDC) 88-8395.

SPECIMEN COLLECTION AND PREPARATION

Collect sample(s) by venipuncture in ten (10) ml silicone evacuated tube(s) or evacuated tube(s) containing EDTA or heparin. The usual precautions in the collection of venipuncture samples should be observed. Separate the red blood cells by centrifugation, use serum or plasma for the total T4 procedure. Specimen(s) may be refrigerated at 2-8°C for a maximum period of 48 hours. If the specimen(s) cannot be assayed within 48 hours, the sample(s) may be stored at temperatures of –20°C for up to 30 days. When assayed in duplicate, 0.10 ml of the specimen is required.

The crossreactivity of the triiodothyronine antibody to selected substances was evaluated by adding the interfering substance to a serum matrix at various concentrations. The crossreactivity was calculated by deriving a ratio between dose of interfering substance to dose of triiodothyronine needed to displace the same amount of tracer.

Substance	*Crossreactivity*	*Concentration*
l-Triiodothyronine	1.0000	
l-Thyroxine	< 0.0002	10 μg/ml
Iodothyrosine	< 0.0001	10 μg/ml
Diiodothyrosine	< 0.0001	10 μg/ml
Diiodothyronine	< 0.0001	10 μg/ml
Phenylbutazone	< 0.0001	10 μg/ml
Sodium salicylate	< 0.0001	10 μg/ml

MATERIALS

Provided

1. Six (6) vials of triiodothyronine human serum References.
2. One (1) vial of triiodothyronine-enzyme conjugate concentrate.
3. One (1) vial of triiodothyronine-enzyme conjugate buffer.
4. One 96-well antibody-coated microplate.
5. One (1) bottle of wash buffer concentrate.
6. One (1) bottle of substrate A.
7. One (1) bottle of substrates B.
8. One (1) bottle of stop solution.
9. Instructions.

Required but not Provided

1. Pipette capable of delivering 50 μl volumes with a precision of better than 1.5 per cent.
2. Dispenser(s) for repetitive deliveries of 0.100 ml and 0.300 ml volumes with a precision of better than 1.5 per cent.
3. Adjustable volume (20-200 μl) and (200-1,000 μl) dispenser(s) for conjugate and substrate dilutions.
4. Microplate washer or a squeeze bottle (optional).
5. Microplate reader with 450 nm wavelength absorbance capability.
6. Test tubes for dilution of enzyme conjugate and substrates A and B.
7. Absorbent Paper for blotting the microplate wells.
8. Plastic wrap or microplate cover for incubation steps.
9. Vacuum aspirator (optional) for wash steps.
10. Timer
11. Quality control materials.

REAGENT PREPARATION

1. Working R eagent 1-T3-enzyme Conjugate Solution

Dilute the triiodothyronine-enzyme conjugate 1:11 with enzyme-antigen conjugate buffer in a suitable container. For example, dilute 160 μl of conjugate with 1.6 ml of buffer for 16 wells (a slight excess of solution is made). This reagent should be used within twenty-four hours for maximum performance of the assay. Store at 2-8°C.

General Formula

Amount of buffer required = Number of wells × 0.1

Quantity of enzyme conjugate necessary = # of wells × 0.01

i.e. = 16 × 0.1 = 1.6 ml for enzyme conjugate buffer

16 × 0.01 = 0.16 ml (160 μl) for T3-enzyme conjugate

2. Wash Buffer

Dilute contents of wash concentrate to 1000 ml with distilled or deionized water in a suitable storage container. Store at room temperature until expiration date printed on concentrate label.

3. Working Substrate Solution-Prepare Immediately Before Use

Determine the amount of reagent needed and prepare by mixing equal portions of Substrate A and Substrate B in a suitable container. For example, add 1 ml of A and 1 ml of B per two (2) eight well strips (a slight excess of solution is made). Use within one (1) hour of preparation for maximum performance of the assay.

TEST PROCEDURE

Before proceeding with the assay, bring all reagents, serum references and controls to room temperature (20-30°C).

1. Format the microplates' wells for each serum reference, control and patient specimen to be assayed in duplicate.
2. Pipette 0.050 ml (50 μl) of the appropriate serum reference, control or specimen into the assigned well.
3. Add 0.100 ml (100 μl) of Working reagent 1, triiodothyronine-enzyme conjugate solution, to all wells (see reagent preparation section).
4. Swirl the microplate gently for 20 to 30 seconds to mix and cover.
5. Incubate 60 minutes at room temperature.
6. Discard the contents of the microplate by decantation or aspiration. If decanting, blot the plate dry with absorbent paper.
7. Add 500 μl of wash buffer (see reagent preparation section), decant (tap and blot) or aspirate. Repeat two (2) additional times for a total of three (3) washes. An automatic or manual plate washer can be used. Follow the manufacturer's instruction for proper usage. If a squeeze bottle is employed, fill each well by depressing the container (avoiding air bubbles) to dispense the wash. Decant the wash and repeat two (2) additional times.
8. Add 0.100 ml (100 μl) of working substrate solution to all wells (see reagent preparation section). Always add reagents in the same order to minimize reaction time differences between wells.
9. Incubate at room temperature for fifteen (15) minutes.
10. Add 0.050 ml (50 μl) of stop solution to each well and gently mix for 15 to 20 seconds. Always add reagents in the same order to minimize reaction time differences between wells.
11. Read the absorbance in each well at 450 nm in a microplate reader. The results should be read within thirty (30) minutes of adding the stop solution.

Note: For re-assaying specimens with concentrations greater than 750 ng/dl, pipette 25 μl of the specimen and 25 μl of the 0 serum reference into the sample well (this maintains a uniform protein concentration). Multiply the readout value by 2 to obtain the triiodothyronine concentration.

QUALITY CONTROL

Each laboratory should assay controls at levels in the hypothyroid, euthyroid and hyperthyroid range for monitoring assay performance. These controls should be treated as unknowns and values determined in every test procedure performed. Quality control charts should be maintained to follow the performance of the supplied reagents. Pertinent statistical methods should be employed to ascertain trends. The individual laboratory should set acceptable assay performance limits. Other parameters that should be monitored include the 80, 50 and 20 per cent intercepts of the dose response curve for run-to-run reproducibility. In addition, maximum absorbance should be consistent with past experience. Significant deviation from established performance can indicate unnoticed change in experimental conditions or degradation of kit reagents. Fresh reagents should be used to determine the reason for the variations.

RESULTS

A dose response curve is used to ascertain the concentration of triiodothyronine in unknown specimens.

1. Record the absorbance obtained from the printout of the microplate reader as outlined in Example 1.
2. Plot the absorbance for each duplicate serum reference versus the corresponding T3 concen-

tration in ng/dl on linear graph paper (do not average the duplicates of the serum references before plotting).

3. Draw the best-fit curve through the plotted points.
4. To determine the concentration of T3 for an unknown, locate the average absorbance of the duplicates for each unknown on the vertical axis (y-axis) of the graph, find the intersecting point on the curve, and read the concentration (in ng/dl) from the horizontal axis (x-axis) of the graph (the duplicates of the unknown may be averaged as indicated). In the following example, the average absorbance 1.208 (intersects the dose response curve at (106 ng/dl) T3 concentration (See Figure 17.25).

Example

Well	*Serum references*	*Absorbance*
1	0 ng/dl	2.192
2	0 ng/dl	2.331
3	50 ng/dl	1.732
4	50 ng/dl	1.779
5	100 ng/dl	1.230
6	100 ng/dl	1.239
7	250 ng/dl	0.576
8	250 ng/dl	0.587
9	500 ng/dl	0.286
10	500 ng/dl	0.273
11	750 ng/dl	0.176
12	750 ng/dl	0.171

Well	Unknown ID	OD	Avg. OD	Value
13	Unknown #1	1.213		
14	Unknown #1	1.202	1.208	106 ng/dl

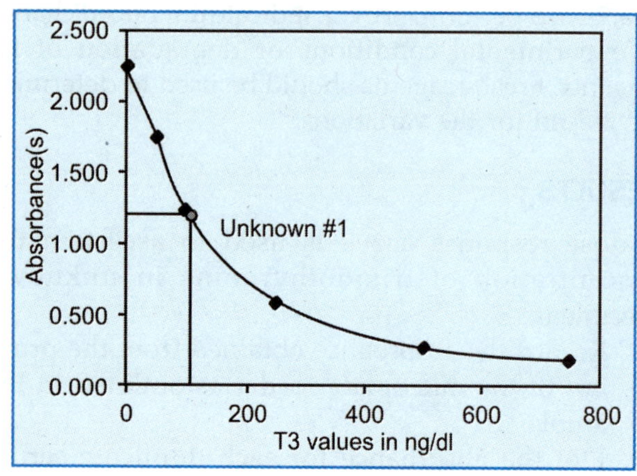

Fig. 17.25 T3 values in ng/dl

*The data presented in Example and Figure 17.25 are for illustration only and should not be used in lieu of a dose response curve prepared with each assay.

QC Parameters

Maximum absorbance (O calibrator) = 1.5-2.75.

LIMITATIONS OF PROCEDURE

A. Assay Performance

Serum references and controls should not exhibit cloudiness with time. Discard if cloudiness is observed.

Sample(s), which are contaminated microbiologically, should not be used in the assay. Highly lipaemeic or haemolysed specimen(s) should similarly not be used.

It is important that the time of reaction in each well is held constant for reproducible results. Pipetting of samples should not extend beyond ten (10) minutes to avoid assay drift. If more than one (1) plate is used, it is recommended to repeat the dose response curve.

Addition of the substrate solution initiates a kinetic reaction, which is terminated by the addition of the stop solution. Therefore, the addition of the substrate and the stopping solution should be added in the same sequence to eliminate any time deviation during reaction.

Plate readers measure vertically. Do not touch the bottom of the wells.

Failure to remove adhering solution adequately in the aspiration or decantation wash step(s) may result in poor replication and spurious results.

Unused microwell strips should be reinserted into the aluminum foil bag and resealed with the ziploc.

B. Interpretation

If computer-controlled data reduction is used to interpret the results of the test, it is imperative that the predicted values for the calibrators fall within 10 per cent of the assigned concentrations.

Total serum triiodothyronine concentration is dependent upon a multiplicity of factors: thyroid gland function and its regulation, thyroxine binding globulin (TBG) concentration, and the binding of triiodothyronine to TBG. Thus, total triiodothyronine concentration alone is not sufficient to assess clinical status.

A decrease in total triiodothyronine values is found with protein-wasting diseases, certain liver diseases and administration of testosterone, diphenylhydantoin or salicylates. A table of interfering drugs and conditions which affect total triiodothyronine values has been compiled by the Journal of the American Association of Clinical Chemists.

Expected Ranges of Values

A study of euthyroid adult population was undertaken to determine expected values for the T3 EIA Test System. The mean (R) values standard deviations (SD) and expected ranges (±2 SD) are presented below. The total number of samples was 105.

Expected values for the T3 EIA Test System

	(in ng/dl)
Mean(X)	135.5
Standard Deviation (SD)	33.4
Expected Ranges (±2 SD)	69-202

It is important to keep in mind that establishment of a range of values which can be expected to be found by a given method for a population of "normal"-persons is dependent upon a multiplicity of factors: the specificity of the method, the population tested and the precision of the method in the hands of the analyst. For these reasons, each laboratory should depend upon the range of expected values established by the manufacturer only until an in-house range can be determined by the analysts using the method with a population indigenous to the area in which the laboratory is located.

Interpretation of Total T3 in ng/ml

Age	
Adults	0.60-2.3
Children	
Cord blood	0.15-0.75
First 72 hours	0.32-2.16
7-14 days	AVG-2.5
2-14 weeks	1.60-2.40
4-16 weeks	1.17-2.09
16-52 weeks	1.10-2.80
1-5 years	1.05-2.69
5-10 years	0.94-2.41
10-15 years	0.83-2.31

FREE TRIIODOTHYRONINE (FT3) (Courtesy: Lilac Medicare)

Intended Use: The Quantitative Determination of Free Triiodothyronine Concentration in Human Serum by a Microplate Enzyme Immunoassay. Levels of fT3 are thought to reflect the amount of T3 available to the cells and may, therefore, determine the clinical metabolic status of T3.

Summary and Explanation of the Test

Triiodothyronine, a thyroid hormone, circulates in blood almost completely bound (> 99.5 per cent) to carrier proteins. The main transport protein is thyroxine-binding globulin (TBG). However, only the free (unbound) portion of triiodothyronine is believed to be responsible for the biological action. Further, the concentrations of the carrier proteins are altered in many clinical conditions, such as pregnancy. In normal thyroid function as the concentrations of the carrier proteins alters, the total triiodothyronine level changes so that the free triiodothyronine concentration remains constant. Thus, measurements of free triiodothyronine concentrations correlate more reliably with clinical status than total triiodothyronine levels.

For example, the increase in total triiodothyronine levels associated with pregnancy, oral contraceptives and oestrogen therapy result in higher total T3 levels, while the free T3 concentration remains basically unchanged.

This microplate enzyme immunoassay methodology provides the technician with optimum sensitivity while requiring a few technical manipulations in a direct determination of free T3. In this method, serum reference, patient specimen, or control is first added to a microplate well. Enzyme-T3 conjugate (analog method) is added, then the reactants are mixed. A competition reaction results between the enzyme conjugate and the free triiodothyronine for a limited number of antibody combining sites immobilized on the well.

After the completion of the required incubation period, the antibody-bound enzyme-triiodothyronine conjugate is separated from the unbound enzyme-triiodothyronine conjugate by aspiration or decantation. The activity of the enzyme present on the surface of the well is quantitated by reaction with a suitable substrate to produce color.

The employment of several serum references of known free triiodothyronine concentration permits construction of a graph of activity and concentration. From comparison to the dose response curve, an unknown specimen's activity can be correlated with free triiodothyronine concentration.

PRINCIPLE

Competitive Enzyme Immunoassay-Analog Method for Free T3

The essential reagents required for a solid phase enzyme immunoassay include immobilised T3 antibody, enzyme-T3 conjugate and native free T3 antigen. The enzyme-T3 conjugate should have no measurable binding to serum proteins, especially TBG and albumin. The method achieves this goal.

Upon mixing immobilised antibody, enzyme-T3 conjugate and a serum containing the native free T3 antigen, a competition reaction results between the native free T3 and the enzyme-T3 conjugate for a limited number of insolubulized binding sites. The interaction is illustrated by the following equation:

$$^{Enz}Ag + Ag + Ab\,cw \underset{k_{-a}}{\overset{k_a}{\rightleftharpoons}} AgAbcw + {}^{Enz}AgAb_c\,w$$

Abcw	= Monospecific immobilised antibody (constant quantity)
Ag	= Native free antigen (variable quantity)
^{Enz}Ag	= Enzyme-T3 antigen conjugate (constant quantity)
$AgAbc_w$	= Antigen-antibody complex
$^{Enz}Ag\,Ab_{cw}$	= Enzyme-antigen conjugate-antibody complex
k_a	= Rate constant of association
$k\text{-}_a$	= Rate constant of disassociation
$K = k_a/k_{-a}$	= Equilibrium constant

After equilibrium is attained, the antibody-bound fraction is separated from unbound antigen by decantation or aspiration. The enzyme activity in the antibody-bound fraction is inversely proportional to the native free antigen concentration. By utilising several different serum references of known antigen concentration, a dose response curve can be generated from which the antigen concentration of an unknown can be ascertained.

REAGENT FOR 96-WELL MICROPLATE

A. Human Serum References-1.0 ml/vial

Six (6) vials of serum reference for free triiodothyronine at approximate* concentrations of 0 (A), 0.4 (B), 1.2 (C), 4.5 (D), 8.0 (E) and 18.0 (F) pg/ml. Store at 2-8°C. A preservative has been added. *Exact levels are given on the labels on a lot specific basis. For SI units: 1 pg/ ml × 1.536 = pmol/L

B. Enzyme-antigen Conjugate-1.0 ml/vial

One (1) vial of triiodothyronine-horseradish peroxidase (HRP) conjugate in a bovine albumin-stabilizing matrix. A preservative has been added. Store at 2-8°C.

C. Enzyme-antigen Conjugate Buffer-11 ml

One (1) bottle reagent containing buffer, blue dye, and preservative. Store at 2-8°C.

D. Antibody-Coated Microplate-96 Wells

One 96-well microplate coated with sheep anti-triiodothyronine serum and packaged in an aluminum bag with a drying agent. Store at 2-8°C.

E. Wash Solution Concentrate-20 ml

One (1) vial containing a surfactant in phosphate buffered saline. A preservative has been added. Store at 2-30°C.

F. Substrate A -7.0 ml/vial

One (1) bottle containing tetramethylbenzidine (TMB) in buffer. Store at 2-8°C.

G. Substrate B-7.0 ml/vial

One (1) bottle containing hydrogen peroxide (hbCb) in buffer. Store at 2-8°C.

H. Stop Solution-6.0 ml/vial

One (1) bottle containing a strong acid (1N HCl). Store at 2-30°C.

Note 1: Do not use reagents beyond the kit expiration date.

Note 2: Opened reagents are stable for sixty (60) days when stored at 2-8°C.

Precautions

For In Vitro Diagnostic Use

Not for Internal or External Use in Humans or Animals

All products that contain human serum have been found to be nonreactive for Hepatitis B Surface Antigen, HIV 1 and 2 and HCV Antibodies by FDA required tests. Since no known test can offer complete assurance that infectious agents are absent, all human serum products should be handled as potentially hazardous and capable of transmitting disease. Good laboratory procedures for handling blood products can be found in the Center for Disease Control/ National Institute of Health, "Biosafety in Microbiological and Biomedical Laboratories," 2nd Edition, 1988, HHS Publication No. (CDC) 88-8395.

Specimen Collection and Preparation

Collect sample(s) by venipuncture in ten (10) ml silicone evacuated tube(s). The usual precautions in the collection of venipuncture samples should be observed. Separate the red blood cells by centrifugation, use serum for the free T3 procedure. Specimen(s) may be refrigerated at 2-8°C for a maximum period of 48 hours. If the specimen(s) cannot be assayed within 48 hours, the sample(s) may be stored at temperatures of –20°C for up to 30 days. When assayed in duplicate, 0.10 ml of the specimen is required.

The crossreactivity of the triiodothyronine antibody to selected substances was evaluated by adding the interfering substance to a serum matrix at various concentrations. The crossreactivity was calculated by deriving a ratio between dose of interfering substance to dose of triiodothyronine needed to displace the same amount of tracer.

Substance	*Crossreactivity*	*Concentration*
l-Triiodothyronine	1.0000	
l-Thyroxine	< 0.0002	10 μg/ ml
Iodothyrosine	< 0.0001	10 μg/ ml
Diiodothyrosine	< 0.0001	10 μg/ ml
Diiodothyronine	< 0.0001	10 μg/ ml
Phenylbutazone	< 0.0001	10 μg/ ml
Sodium Salicylate	< 0.0001	10 μg/ ml

MATERIALS

Provided

1. Six (6) vials of free triiodothyronine human serum references.
2. One (1) vial of T3-enzyme conjugate concentrate.
3. One (1) vial of Free T3/T4 conjugate buffer.
4. One 96-well antibody coated microplate.
5. One (1) bottle of wash buffer concentrate.
6. One (1) bottle of substrate A.
7. One (1) bottle of substrate B.
8. One (1) bottle of stop solution.
9. Instructions.

Required but Not Provided

1. Pipette capable of delivering 50 μl volumes with a precision of better than 1.5 per cent.
2. Dispenser(s) for repetitive deliveries of 0.100 ml and 0.300 ml volumes with a precision of better than 1.5 per cent.
3. Adjustable volume (20-200 μl) and (200-1000 μl) dispenser(s) for conjugate and substrate dilutions.
4. Microplate washer or a squeeze bottle (optional).
5. Microplate reader with 450 nm wavelength absorbance capability.
6. Test tubes for dilution of enzyme conjugate and substrates A and B.
7. Absorbent paper for blotting the microplate wells.
8. Plastic wrap or microplate cover for incubation steps.
9. Vacuum aspirator (optional) for wash steps.
10. Timer.
11. Quality control materials.

REAGENT PREPARATION

1. Working Reagent 1-Triiodothyronine-enzyme Conjugate Solution

Dilute the triiodothyronine-enzyme conjugate 1:11 with triiodothyronine-enzyme conjugate buffer in a suitable container. For example, dilute 160 μl of conjugate with 1.6 ml of buffer for 16 wells (a slight excess of solution is made). This reagent should be used within twenty-four hours for maximum performance of the assay. Store at 2-8°C.

General Formula

Amount of Buffer required = Number of wells × 0.1

Quantity of enzyme conjugate necessary = # of wells × 0.01 i.e. = 16 x 0.1 = 1.6 ml for TS conjugate buffer 16 × 0.01 = 0.16 ml (160 μl) for T3 enzyme conjugate.

2. Wash Buffer

Dilute contents of wash concentrate to 1000 ml with distilled or deionised water in a suitable storage container. Store at room temperature until expiration date printed on concentrate label.

3. Working Substrate Solution-Prepare Immediately before Use

Determine the amount of reagent needed and prepare by mixing equal portions of substrate A and substrate B in a suitable container. For example, add 1 ml of A and 1 ml of B per two (2) eight well strips (A slight excess of solution is made). Use within one (1) day of preparation for maximum performance of the assay.

Test Procedure

Before proceeding with the assay, bring all reagents, serum references and controls to room temperature (20-30°C).

1. Format the microplates' wells for each serum reference, control and patient specimen to be assayed in duplicate.
2. Pipette 0.050 ml (50 μl) of the appropriate serum reference, control or specimen into the assigned well.
3. Add 0.100 ml (100 μl) of working reagent 1, triiodothyronine-enzyme conjugate solution, to all wells (see reagent preparation section).
4. Swirl the microplate gently for 20 to 30 seconds to mix and cover.
5. Incubate 60 minutes at room temperature.
6. Discard the contents of the microplate by decantation or aspiration. If decanting, blot the plate dry with absorbent paper.
7. Add 300 μl of wash buffer (see reagent preparation section), decant (tap and blot) or aspirate. Repeat two (2) additional times for a total of three (3) washes. An automatic or manual plate washer can be used. Follow the manufacturer's instruction for proper usage. If a squeeze bottle is employed, fill each well by depressing the container (avoiding air bubbles) to dispense the wash. Decant the wash and repeat two (2) additional times.
8. Add 0.100 ml (100 μl) of working substrate solution to all wells (see reagent preparation section). Always add reagents in the same order to minimise reaction time differences between wells.
9. Incubate at room temperature for fifteen (15) minutes.
10. Add 0.050 ml (50 μl) of stop solution to each well and gently mix for 15 to 20 seconds. Always add reagents in the same order to minimise reaction time differences between wells.
11. Read the absorbance in each well at 450 nm in a microplate reader. The results should be read within thirty (30) minutes of adding the stop solution.

Quality Control

Each laboratory should assay controls at levels in the hypothyroid, euthyroid and hyperthyroid range for monitoring assay performance. These controls should be treated as unknowns and values determined in every test procedure performed. Quality control charts should be maintained to follow the performance of the supplied reagents. Pertinent statistical methods should be employed to ascertain trends. The individual laboratory should set acceptable assay performance limits. Other parameters that should be monitored include the 80, 50 and 20 per cent intercepts of the standard curve for run-to-run reproducibility. In addition, maximum absorbance should be consistent with past experience. Significant deviation from established performance can indicate unnoticed change in experimental conditions or degradation of kit reagents. Fresh reagents should be used to determine the reason for the variations.

Results

A dose response curve is used to ascertain the concentration of free triiodothyronine in unknown specimens.

1. Record the absorbance obtained from the printout of the microplate reader as outlined in Example 2.
2. Plot the absorbance for each duplicate serum reference versus the corresponding FT3 concentration in Pg/ml on linear graph paper do not average the duplicates of the serum references before plotting.
3. Draw the best-fit curve through the plotted points.
4. To determine the concentration of fT3 for an unknown, locate the average absorbance of the duplicates for each unknown on the vertical axis of the graph, find the intersecting point on the curve, and read the concentration (in pg/ml) from the horizontal axis of the graph (the duplicates of the unknown may be averaged as indicated). In the following example, the average absorbance 1.799 (intersects the standard curve at (1.2 pg/ml) fT3 concentration.

Example 2

Well	Serum	Reference	Absorbance
1	0.0	pg/ml	2.639
2	0.0	pg/ml	2.615
3	0.4	pg/ml	2.330
4	0.4	pg/ml	2.259
5	1.2	pg/ml	1.835
6	1.2	pg/ml	1.753
7	4.5	pg/ml	0.939
8	4.5	pg/ml	0.975
9	8.0	pg/ml	0.537
10	8.0	pg/ml	0.569
11	18.0	pg/ml	0.301
12	18.0	pg/ml	0.287

Well	Unknown ID	OD	Avg OD	Value
13	Unknown # 1	1.876		
14	Unknown # 1	1.721	1.799	1.2 pg/ml

The data presented in Example 2 are for illustration only and should not be used in lieu of a standard curve prepared with each assay.

QC Parameters

Maximum Absorbance (O calibrator) = 1.5-2.7

LIMITATIONS OF PROCEDURE

A. Assay Performance

Sample(s), which are contaminated microbiologically, should not be used in the assay. Highly lipaemeic or haemolysed specimen(s) should similarly not be used.

It is important that the time of reaction in each well is held constant for reproducible results. Pipetting of samples should not extend beyond ten (10) minutes to avoid assay drift. If more than one (1) plate is used, it is recommended to repeat the dose response curve.

Addition of the substrate solution initiates a kinetic reaction, which is terminated by the addition of the stop solution. Therefore, the addition of the substrate and the stopping solution should be added in the same sequence to eliminate any time deviation during reaction.

Plate readers measure vertically. Do not touch the bottom of the wells.

Failure to remove adhering solution adequately in the aspiration or decantation wash step(s) may result in poor replication and spurious results.

B. Interpretation

Corresponding fT3 concentration in pg/ml on linear graph paper Do. If computer-controlled data reduction is used to calculate the results of the test, it is imperative that the predicted values for the calibrators fall within 10 per cent of the assigned concentrations.

Several drugs are known to effect the binding of triiodothyronine to the thyroid hormone carrier proteins or its metabolism to T3 and complicate the interpretation of free T3 results.

Circulating autoantibodies to T3 and hormone-binding inhibitors may interfere.

Heparin has been reported to have *in vivo* and *in vitro* effects on free T3 concentration. Therefore, do not obtain samples in which this anticoagulant has been used.

In severe nonthyroidal illness (NTI), the assessment of thyroid status becomes very difficult. TSH measurements are recommended to identify thyroid dysfunction.

Familial dysalbuminemic conditions may yield erroneous results on direct free T3 assays.

"Not Intended for Newborn Screening"

Expected Ranges of Values

A study of euthyroid adult population was undertaken to determine expected values for the fT3 EIA Test System. The mean (R) values, standard deviations (SD) and expected ranges (±2 SD) are presented.

Expected Values for the Free T3 EIA Test System (in pg/ ml)

	Adult (110 specimens)	*Pregnancy (75 specimens)*
Mean (X)	2.8	3.0
Standard deviation (SD)	0.7	0.6
Expected ranges (±2 SD)	1.4-4.2	1.8-4.2

It is important to keep in mind that establishment of a range of values which can be expected to be found by a given method for a population of "normal" persons is dependent upon a multiplicity of factors; the specificity of the method, the population tested and the precision of the method in the hands of the analyst. For these reasons, each laboratory should depend upon the range of expected values established by the manufacturer only until an in-house range can be determined by the analysts using the method with a population indigenous to the area in which the laboratory is located.

UPTAKE (Courtesy: Lilac Medicare)

Intended Use: The Measurement of the Total Amount of Binding Sites Available for the Thyroid Hormones in Human Serum or Plasma by a Microplate Enzyme Immunoassay

Summary and Explanation of the Test

The thyroid gland under the regulatory control of thyrotrophin hormone secretes thyroxine (T4) and triiodothyronine (T3) into the general circulation. The released hormones do not circulate as free molecules but are almost entirely (99.9 per cent) bound to specific serum proteins.

Three protein fractions with varying affinities and capacities for interaction with T3 and T4 have been identified by reverse flow paper electrophoresis. Thyroxine-binding globulin (TBG) carries 65-75 per cent of the total circulating concentration. Thyroxine binding prealbumin (TBPA) has an intermediate avidity for thyroxine (carries approximately 15-25 per cent) but little if any avidity for triiodothyronine. Albumin with a low affinity but high capacity carries 10 per cent of thyroxine and 30 per cent of the available triiodothyronine.

Since the metabolic processes are regulated entirely by the concentration of the free thyroid hormones, which are inversely related to the levels of the binding proteins, an assessment of the binding capacity of human serum was developed in 1957 by Hamolsky. In this early method, radioactive T3 was added to a specimen of whole blood. After an incubation period, the mixture was centrifuged and the red cells washed. The radioactivity uptake of the red cells was inversely related to the binding capacity of the serum. Although this method had severe limitations, it proved to be a valuable diagnostic tool.

Further technical improvements in the assay methodology of the T-uptake test resulted as various separation agents such as coated charcoal, ion-exchange resins, denatured albumin, silicates, antibodies and organic polymers were employed in place of the red cells.

This microplate enzyme immunoassay methodology provides the technician with optimum sensitivity while requiring few technical manip μlations. In this method, serum reference, patient specimen, or control is first added to a microplate well. Enzyme-T4 conjugate and thyroxine (T4) are added, then the reactants are mixed. The endogenous binding proteins of the sample react with the thyroxine, but not with the enzyme conjugate. This leads to a higher binding of the enzyme conjugate to the antibody combining sites immobilised on the well as the binding capacity of the specimen increases.

After the completion of the required incubation period, the antibody-bound enzyme-thyroxine conjugate is separated from the unbound-enzyme-thyroxine conjugate by aspiration or decantation. The activity of the enzyme present on the surface of the well is quantitated by reaction with a suitable substrate to produce colour.

The employment of several serum references of known unsaturated thyroid hormone binding capacity permits construction of a graph of absorbance and concentration. From comparison to the dose response curve, an unknown specimen's absorbance can be correlated with thyroid hormone-binding capacity.

PRINCIPLE

Competitive Enzyme Immunoassay

The required components for assessing the binding capacity of human serum are enzyme-thyroxine conjugates, thyroxine-binding protein (P), and immobilised thyroxine antibody (Ab).

Upon mixing the enzyme-conjugate and thyroxine with the specimen, a binding reaction results between the patient's binding proteins and the added thyroxine but not with the enzyme conjugate. This interaction is represented below:

$T4 + P \rightarrow T4\text{-}P$ (1)

T4 = Thyroxine added (constant quantity)

P = Specific binding proteins (varying quantity)

The added thyroxine (T4) not consumed in reaction 1 then competes with the enzyme-antigen conjugate for a limited number of insolubulised binding sites. The interaction is illustrated by the following equation:

$$EnzT_4 + T_{4r} + Ab\ c.w \underset{k_{-a}}{\overset{k_a}{\rightleftharpoons}} T4\ Ab\ cw + {}^{Enz}T4Ab_{cw}\ (2)$$

Ab_{cw}	= Monospecific Immobilized T4 antibody (constant quantity)
$T4_r$	= Added thyroxine unreacted in reaction (1) (variable quantity)
Enz	= Enzyme-antigen conjugate (constant quantity)
$T4Ab_{cw}$	= Thyroxine-antibody complex
${}^{Enz}T4\ Ab_{cw}$	= Enzyme-thyroxine conjugate-antibody complex
k_a	= Rate constant of association 100
k_{-a}	= Rate constant of disassociation
$K = k_a / k_{-a}$	= Equilibrium constant

After equilibrium is attained, the antibody-bound fraction is separated from unbound enzyme-antigen by decantation or aspiration. The enzyme activity in the antibody-bound fraction is directly proportional to the binding capacity of the specimen. Thus, in hypothyroidism, the binding proteins are relatively unsaturated (due to the low level of thyroid hormones) resulting in higher consumption of the added thyroxine than a euthyroid specimen. This leads to higher binding of the enzyme-thyroxine conjugate caused by the reduced concentration of the available thyroxine. In hyperthyroidism, the reverse is true. The binding proteins are relatively saturated with thyroxine (due to the high level of thyroid hormone) resulting in lower consumption of the added thyroxine. The remaining thyroxine is relatively much higher than a euthyroid specimen resulting in lower enzyme-thyroxine antibody binding due to the increased competition of the thyroxine for the limited antibody sites.

REAGENT FOR 96-WELL MICROPLATE

A. Human Serum References -1.0 ml/vial

Four (4) vials of serum reference of unsaturated thyroid hormone binding capacity at approximate* levels of 15.0 (A), 26.5 (B), 35.5 (C), and 46.0 (D) per cent. Store at 2-8°C. A preservative has been added.

*Exact levels are given on the labels on a lot specific basis.

B. Enzyme-antigen Conjugate -1.0 ml/vial

One (1) vial of thyroxine-horseradish peroxidase (HRP) conjugate and thyroxine in a bovine albumin-stabilising matrix. A preservative has been added. Store at 2-8°C.

C. Enzyme-antigen Conjugate Buffer-11 ml

One (1) bottle reagent containing buffer, orange dye and preservative. Store at 2-8°C.

D. Antibody-Coated Microplate-96 wells

One 96-well microplate coated with sheep anti-thyroxine serum and packaged in an aluminum bag with a drying agent. Store at 2-8°C.

E. Wash Solution Concentrate-20 ml

One (1) vial containing a surfactant in phosphate buffered saline. A preservative has been added. Store at 2-30°C.

F. Substrate A-7.0 ml/vial

One (1) bottle containing tetramethyl benzidine (TMB) in buffer. Store at 2-8°C.

G. Substrate B-7.0 ml/vial

One (1) bottle containing hydrogen peroxide (H_2O_2) in buffer. Store at 2-8°C.

H. Stop Solution-6.0 ml/vial

One (1) bottle containing a strong acid (1N HCl). Store at 2-30°C.

Note 1: Do not use reagents beyond the kit expiration date.

Note 2: Opened reagents are stable for sixty (60) days when stored at 2-8°C.

Precautions

For In Vitro Diagnostic

Use Not for Internal or External Use in Humans or Animals

All products that contain human serum have been found to be nonreactive for Hepatitis B Surface Antigen, HIV 1 and 2 and HCV Antibodies by FDA required tests. Since no known test can offer complete assurance that infectious agents are absent, all human serum products should be handled as potentially hazardous and capable of transmitting disease. Good laboratory procedures for handling blood products can be found in the Center for Disease Control/ National Institute of Health, "Biosafety in Microbiological and Biomedical Laboratories," 2nd Edition, 1988, HHS Publication No. (CDC) 88-8395.

Specimen Collection and Preparation

Collect sample(s) by venipuncture in ten (10) ml silicone evacuated tube(s) or evacuated tube(s) containing EDTA or heparin. The usual precautions in the collection of venipuncture samples should be observed. Separate the red blood cells by centrifugation, use serum or plasma for the T-uptake procedure. Specimen(s) may be refrigerated at 2-8°C for a maximum period of 48 hours. If the specimen(s) cannot be assayed within 48 hours, the sample(s) may be stored at temperatures of –20°C for up to 30 days. When assayed in duplicate, 0.05 ml of the specimen is required.

The crossreactivity of the thyroxine antibody to selected substances was evaluated by adding the interfering substance to a serum matrix at various concentrations. The crossreactivity was calculated by deriving a ratio between dose of interfering substance to dose of thyroxine needed to displace the same amount of tracer.

Substance	*Cross Reactivity*	*Concentration*
I -Thyroxine	1.0000	
d-Thyroxine	0.9800	10 μg/dl
d-Triiodothyronine	0.0150	100 μg/dl
I-Triiodothyronine	0.0300	100 μg/dl
lodothyrosine	0.0001	100 μg/ml
Diiodothyrosine	0.0001	100 μg/ml
Diiodothyronine	0.0001	100 μg/ml

MATERIALS

Provided

1. Four (4) vials of T-uptake human serum references.
2. One (1) vial of thyroxine-enzyme conjugate concentrate.
3. One (1) vial of T-uptake conjugate buffer.
4. One 96-well antibody coated microplate.
5. One (1) bottle of Wash buffer concentrate.
6. One (1) bottle of substrate A.
7. One (1) bottle of substrate B.
8. One (1) bottle of stop solution.
9. Instructions.

Required but Not Provided

1. Pipette capable of delivering 25 μl volumes with a precision of better than 1.5 per cent.
2. Dispenser(s) for repetitive deliveries of 0.100 ml and 0.300 ml volumes with a precision of better than 1.5 per cent.
3. Adjustable volume (20-200 μl) and (200-1000 μl) dispenser(s) for conjugate and substrate dilutions
4. Microplate washer or a squeeze bottle (optional).
5. Microplate reader with 450 nm wavelength absorbance capability.
6. Test tubes for dilution of enzyme conjugate and substrates A and B.
7. Absorbent paper for blotting the microplate wells.
8. Plastic wrap or microplate cover for incubation steps.
9. Vacuum aspirator (optional) for wash steps.
10. Timer.
11. Quality control materials.

REAGENT PREPARATION

1. Working Reagent 1-T4-Enzyme Solution-Prepare Monthly

Dilute the thyroxine-enzyme conjugate 1:11 with thyroxine-enzyme conjugate buffer in a suitable container. For example, dilute 160 μl of conjugate with 1.6 ml of buffer for 16 wells (a slight excess of solution is made). This reagent should be used within thirty (30) days for maximum performance of the assay. Store at 2-8°C. General Formula:

Amount of buffer required = Number of wells × 0.1

Quantity of enzyme conjugate necessary = # of wells × 0.01 i.e. = 16 × 0.1 = 1.6 ml for T4 conjugate buffer 16 × 0.01 = 0.16 ml (160 μl) for T4 enzyme conjugate.

2. Wash Buffer

Dilute contents of wash concentrate to 1000 ml with distilled or deionised water in a suitable storage container. Store at room temperature until expiration date printed on concentrate label.

3. Working Substrate Solution-Prepare Daily

Determine the amount of reagent needed and prepare by mixing equal portions of substrate A and substrate B in a suitable container. For example, add 1 ml of A and 1 ml of B per two (2) eight well strips (a slight excess of solution is made). Use within twenty (24)) hours of preparation for maximum performance of the assay.

Test Procedure

Before proceeding with the assay, bring all reagents, serum references and controls to room temperature (20-30°C).

1. Format the microplates' wells for each serum reference, control and patient specimen to be assayed in duplicate.
2. Pipette 0.025 ml (25 μl) of the appropriate serum reference, control or specimen into the assigned well.
3. Add 0.100 ml (100 μl) of working reagent 1, T4-enzyme solution to all wells.
4. Swirl the microplate gently for 20 to 30 seconds to mix and cover.
5. Incubate 60 minutes at room temperature.
6. Discard the contents of the microplate by decantation or aspiration. If decanting, blot the plate dry with absorbent paper.
7. Add 300 μl of wash buffer (see reagent preparation section), decant (tap and blot) or aspirate. Repeat two (2) additional times for a total of three (3) washes. An automatic or manual plate washer can be used. Follow the manufacturer's instruction for proper usage. If a squeeze bottle is employed, fill each well by depressing the container (avoiding air bubbles) to dispense the wash. Decant the wash and repeat two (2) additional times.
8. Add 0.100 ml (100 μl) of working substrate solution to all wells (see reagent preparation section). Always add reagents in the same order to minimise reaction time differences between wells.
9. Incubate at room temperature for fifteen (15) minutes.
10. Add 0.050 ml (50 μl) of stop solution to each well and gently mix for 15 to 20 seconds. Always add reagents in the same order to minimise reaction time differences between wells.
11. Read the absorbance in each well at 450 nm in a microplate reader. The results should be read within thirty (30) minutes of adding the stop solution.

Quality Control

Each laboratory should assay controls at levels in the hypothyroid, euthyroid and hyperthyroid range for monitoring assay performance. These controls should be treated as unknowns and values determined in every test procedure performed. Quality control charts should be maintained to follow the performance of the supplied reagents. Pertinent statistical methods should be employed to ascertain trends. The individual laboratory should set acceptable assay performance limits. In addition, maximum absorbance should be consistent with past experience. Significant deviation from established performance can indicate unnoticed change in experimental conditions or degradation of kit reagents. Fresh reagents should be used to determine the reason for the variations.

QC Parameters

Maximum absorbance (O calibrator) = 1.5-2.8.

Results

A dose response curve is used to ascertain the unsaturated thyroid-binding capacity in unknown specimens.

1. Record the absorbance obtained from the printout of the microplate reader as outlined in Example given below.
2. Plot the absorbance for each duplicate serum references versus the corresponding T-uptake in% on linear graphs paper donot average the duplicates of the serum references befor plotting.
3. Connect the points with lines.
4. To determine the per cent T-uptake for an unknown, locate the average absorbance of the duplicates for each unknown on the vertical axis of the graph, find the intersecting point on the reference response, and read the per cent T-uptake (per cent U) from the horizontal axis of the graph (the duplicates of the unknown may be averaged as indicated). In the following example, the average absorbance 1.698 (intersects the reference curve at (27.3 per cent U) (see 17.26).

Example 1

Well	*Serum references*	*Absorbance*
1	15.0 per cent U	2.605
2	15.0 per cent U	2.638
3	26.5 per cent U	1.802
4	26.5 per cent U	1.719
5	35.5 per cent U	1.082
6	35.5 per cent U	1.030
7	46.0 per cent U	0.582
8	46.0 per cent U	0.547

Well	**Unknown ID**	**OD**	**Avg OD**	**Value**
9	Unknown#1	1.701		
10	Unknown#1	1.695	1.698	27.3 % U

The T-uptake can also be expressed as a T-uptake ratio. Divide the per cent U by 30 per cent to convert into a T-uptake ratio.

Example 2

27.3 per cent U/Example 23.0 per cent = 0.910.

*The data presented in Example 3 and Figure 17.26. are for illustration only and should not be used in lieu of a standard curve prepared with each assay

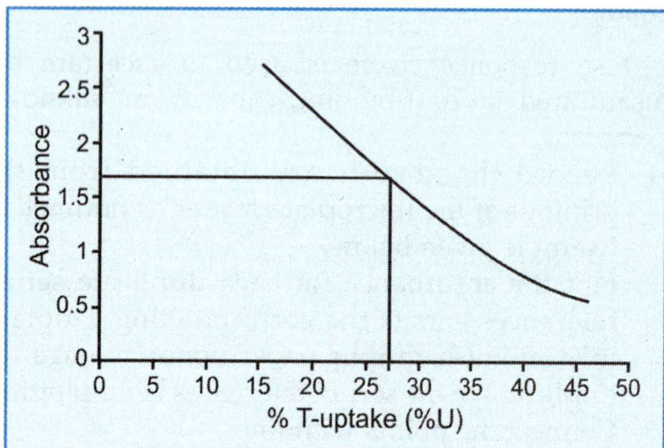

Fig. 17.26: Estimation of T-uptake

LIMITATIONS OF PROCEDURE

A. Assay Performance

It is important that the time of reaction in each well is held constant for reproducible results. Pipetting of samples should not extend beyond ten (10) minutes to avoid assay drift. If more than one (1) plate is used, it is recommended to repeat the dose response curve.

Addition of the substrate solution initiates a kinetic reaction, which is terminated by the addition of the stop solution. Therefore, the addition of the substrate and the stopping solution should be added in the same sequence to eliminate any time deviation during reaction.

Plate readers measure vertically. Do not touch the bottom of the wells. Failure to remove adhering solution adequately in the aspiration or decantation wash step(s) may result in poor replication and spurious results.

B. Interpretation

The T-uptake test is dependent upon a multiplicity of factors: thyroid gland and its regulation, thyroxine binding globulin (TBG) concentration, and the binding of the thyroid hormones to TBG. Thus, the T-Uptake Test alone is not sufficient to assess clinical status.

The free thyroxine index (FTI), which is the product of the T-uptake ratio and the total thyroxine concentration, has gained wide clinical acceptance as a more accurate assessment of thyroid status. The FTI value compensates for any condition or drug, such as pregnancy or oestrogens, which alters the TBG and the T4 levels but does not change the thyrometabolic status. A table of interfering drugs and conditions which .affect the T-Uptake Test has been compiled by the Journal of the American Association of Clinical Chemists.

Expected Ranges of Values

A study of a euthyroid adult population (85 specimens) was undertaken to determine expected values for the T-uptake and are presented.

Expected Values for the T-uptake EIA test system

Thyroid Status	per cent T-Uptake	T- Ratio
Euthyroid	25-35	0.83-1.17
Hypothyroid or TBG (Excess binding)	less than 25	less than 0.83
Hyperthyroid or TBG (Reduced binding)	greater than 35	greater than 1.17

It is important to keep in mind that establishment of a range of values which can be expected to be found by a given method for a population of "normal" persons is dependent upon a multiplicity of factors: the specificity of the method, the population tested and the precision of the method in the hands of the analyst. For these reasons, each laboratory should depend upon the range of expected values established by the manufacturer only until an in-house range can be determined by the analysts using the method with a population indigenous to the area in which the laboratory is located.

TOTAL THYROXINE (T4) (Courtesy: Lilac Medicare)

Intended Use: The Quantitative Determination of Total Thyroxine Concentration in Human Serum or Plasma by a Microplate Enzyme Immunoassay

Summary and Explanation of the Test

Measurement of serum thyroxine concentration is generally regarded as an important *in vitro* diagnostic test for assessing thyroid function. This importance has provided the impetus for the significant improvement in assay methodology that has occurred in the last three decades. This procedural evolution can be traced from the empirical protein-bound iodine (FBI) test to the theoretically sophisticated radioimmunoassay.

This microplate enzyme immunoassay methodology provides the technician with optimum sensitivity while requiring a few technical manipulations. In this method, serum reference, patient specimen, or control is first added to a microplate well. Enzyme-T4 conjugate is added, then the reactants are mixed. A competition reaction results between the enzyme conjugate and the native thyroxine for a limited number of antibody-combining sites immobilised on the well.

After the completion of the required incubation period, the antibody-bound enzyme-thyroxine conjugate is separated from the unbound enzyme-thyroxine conjugate by aspiration or decantation. The activity of the enzyme present on the surface of the well is quantitated by reaction with a suitable substrate to produce color.

The employment of several serum references of known thyroxine concentration permits construction of a graph of activity and concentration. From comparison to the dose response curve, an unknown specimen's activity can be correlated with thyroxine concentration.

PRINCIPLE

Competitive Enzyme Immunoassay

The essential reagents required for a solid phase enzyme immunoassay include immobilized antibody, enzyme-antigen conjugate and native antigen.

Upon mixing immobilized antibody, enzyme-antigen conjugate and a serum containing the native antigen, a competition reaction results between the native ar.tigen and the enzyme-antigen conjugate for a limited number of insolubulized binding sites. The interaction is illustrated by the following equation:

$$Enz_{Ag} + Ag + Ab\ c.w. \underset{k\text{-}a}{\overset{ka}{\rightleftharpoons}} AgAb\ c.w. + Enz\ Ag\ Abc.w$$

Ab_{cw} = Monospecific immobilized antibody (constant quantity)

Ag = Native antigen (variable quantity)

^{Enz}Ag = Enzyme-antigen conjugate (constant quantity)

$AgAbc_{w}$ = Antigen-antibody complex

$^{Enz}Ag\ Abcw$ = Enzyme-antigen conjugate -antibody complex

k_{a} = Rate constant of association

k_{-a} = Rate constant of disassociation

$K = k_{a}/k_{-a}$ = Equilibrium constant

After equilibrium is attained, the antibody-bound fraction is separated from unbound antigen by decantation or aspiration. The enzyme activity in the antibody-bound fraction is inversely proportional to the native antigen concentration. By utilizing several different serum references of known antigen concentration, a dose response curve can be generated from which the antigen concentration of an unknown can be ascertained.

REAGENTS FOR 96-WELL MICROPLATE

A. Human Serum References-1.0 ml/vial

Six (6) vials of serum reference for thyroxine at concentrations of 0 (A), 2.0 (B), 5.0 (C), 10.0 (D), 15.0 (E) and 25.0 (F) µg/dl. Store at 2-8°C. A preservative has been added.

B. Enzyme-antigen Conjugate-1.0 ml/vial

One (1) vial of thyroxine-horseradish peroxidase (HRP) conjugate in a bovine albumin-stabilizing matrix. A preservative has been added. Store at 2-8°C.

C. Enzyme-antigen Conjugate Buffer-11 ml

One (1) bottle reagent containing buffer, red dye, preservative, and binding protein inhibitors. Store at 2-8°C.

D. Antibody-Coated Microplate-96 Wells

One 96-well microplate coated with sheep anti-thyroxine serum and packaged in an aluminum bag with a drying agent. Store at 2-8°C.

E. Wash Solution Concentrate-20 ml

One (1) vial containing a surfactant in phosphate buffered saline. A preservative has been added. Store at 2-30°C.

F. Substrate A ~7.0 ml/vial

One (1) bottle containing tetramethylbenzidine (TM8) in buffer. Store at 2-8°C.

G. Substrate B-7.0 ml/vial

One (1) bottle containing hydrogen peroxide (HaOz) in buffer. Store at 2-8°C.

H. Stop Solution-6.0 ml/vial

One (1) bottle containing a strong acid (1N HCl). Store at 2-30°C.

Note 1: Do not use reagents beyond the kit expiration date.

Note 2: Opened reagents are stable for sixty (60) days when stored at 2-8°C.

Precautions

For In Vitro Diagnostic Use

Not for Internal or External Use in Humans or Animals

All products that contain human serum have been found to be nonreactive for Hepatitis B Surface Antigen, HIV 1 and 2 and HCV Antibodies by FDA required tests. Since no known test can offer complete assurance that infectious agents are absent, all human serum products should be handled as potentially hazardous and capable of transmitting disease. Good laboratory procedures for handling blood products can be found in the Center for Disease Control/ National Institute of Health, "Biosafety in Microbiological and Biomedical Laboratories," 2nd Edition, 1988, HHS Publication No. (CDC) 88-8395.

Specimen Collection and Preparation

Collect sample(s) by venipuncture in ten (10) ml silicone evacuated tube(s) or evacuated tube(s) containing EDTA or heparin. The usual precautions in the collection of venipuncture samples should be observed. Separate the red blood cells by centrifugation, use serum or plasma for the total T4 procedure. Specimen(s) may be refrigerated at 2-8°C for a maximum period of 48 hours. If the specimen(s) can not be assayed within 48 hours, the sample(s) may be stored at temperatures of -20°C for up to 30 days. When assayed in duplicate, 0.05 ml of the specimen is required.

The cross-reactivity of the thyroxine antibody to selected substances was evaluated by adding the interfering substance to a serum matrix at various concentrations. The cross-reactivity was calculated by deriving a ratio between dose of interfering substance to dose of thyroxine needed to displace the same amount of tracer.

Substance	*Cross Reactivity*	*Concentration*
I -Thyroxine	1.0000	
d-Thyroxine	0.9800	10 μg/dl
d-Triiodothyronine	0.0150	100 μg/dl
I-Triiodothyronine	0.0300	100 μg/dl
Iodothyrosine	0.0001	100 μg/ml
Diiodothyrosine	0.0001	100 μg/ml
Diiodothyronine	0.0001	100 μg/ml

MATERIALS

Provided

1. Six (6) vials of thyroxine human serum references.
2. One (1) vial of thyroxine-enzyme conjugate concentrate.
3. One (1) vial of thyroxine-enzyme conjugate buffer.
4. One 96-well antibody coated microplate.
5. One (1) bottle of wash buffer concentrate.
6. One (1) bottle of substrate A.
7. One (1) bottle of substrate B.
8. One (1) bottle of stop solution.
9. Instructions.

Required but Not Provided

1. Pipette capable of delivering 25 μl volumes with a precision of better than 1.5 per cent.
2. Dispenser(s) for repetitive deliveries of 0.100 ml and 0.300 ml volumes with a precision of better than 1.5 per cent.
3. Adjustable volume (20-200 μl) and (200-1000 μl) dispenser(s) for conjugate and substrate dilutions.
4. Microplate washer or a squeeze bottle (optional).
5. Microplate reader with 450 nm wavelength absorbance capability.
6. Test tubes for dilution of enzyme conjugate and substrates A and B.
7. Absorbent paper for blotting the microplate wells.
8. Plastic wrap or microplate cover for incubation steps.
9. Vacuum aspirator (optional) for wash steps.
10. Timer
11. Quality control materials.

REAGENT PREPARATION

1. Working Reagent 1-Thyroxine-enzyme Conjugate Solution

Dilute the thyroxine-enzyme conjugate 1:11 with thyroxine-enzyme conjugate buffer in a suitable container. For example, dilute 160 μl of conjugate with 1.6 ml of buffer for 16 wells (a slight excess of solution is made). This reagent should be used within twenty-four hours for maximum performance of the assay. Store at 2-8°C. General Formula:

Amount of buffer required = Number of wells × 0.1

Quantity of enzyme conjugate necessary = # of wells × 0.01

i.e. = 16 × 0.1 = 1.6 ml for T4 conjugate buffer

16 × 0.01 = 0.16 ml (160 μl) for T4 enzyme conjugate

2. Wash Buffer

Dilute contents of wash concentrate to 1000 ml with distilled or deionized water in a suitable storage container. Store at room temperature until expiration date printed on concentrate label.

3. Working Substrate Solution-Prepare immediately before use

Determine the amount of reagent needed and prepare by mixing equal portions of substrate A and substrate B in a suitable container. For example, add 1 ml of A and 1 ml of B per two (2) eight well strips (a slight excess of solution is made). Use within one (1) hour of preparation for maximum performance of the assay.

Test Procedure

Before proceeding with the assay, bring all reagents, serum references and controls to room temperature (20-30°C).

1. Format the microplates' wells for each serum reference, control and patient specimen to be assayed in duplicate.
2. Pipette 0.025 ml (25 μl) of the appropriate serum reference, control or specimen into the assigned well.
3. Add 0.100 ml (100 μl) of working reagent l, Thyroxine-enzyme conjugate solution, to all wells (see reagent preparation section).
4. Swirl the microplate gently for 20-30 seconds to mix and cover.
5. Incubate 60 minutes at room temperature.
6. Discard the contents of the microplate by decantation or aspiration. If decanting, blot the plate dry with absorbent paper.
7. Add 300 μl of wash buffer (see reagent preparation section), decant (tap and blot) or aspirate. Repeat two (2) additional times for a total of three (3) washes. An automatic or manual plate washer can be used. Follow the manufacturer's instruction for proper usage. If calculated, a squeeze bottle is employed, fill each well by depressing the container (avoiding air bubbles) to dispense the wash. Decant the wash and repeat two (2) additional times.
8. Add 0.100 ml (100 μl) of working substrate solution to all wells (see reagent preparation section). Always add reagents in the same order to minimize reaction time differences between wells.
9. Incubate at room temperature for fifteen (15) minutes.
10. Add 0.050 ml (50 μl) of stop solution to each well and gently mix for 15-20 seconds. Always add reagents in the same order to minimize reaction time differences between wells.
11. Read the absorbance in each well at 450 nm in a microplate reader. The results should be read within thirty (30) minutes of adding the stop solution.

Note: For reassaying specimens with concentrations greater than 25 μg/dl, pipe the 12.5 μl of the specimen and 12.5 μl of the 0 serum reference into the sample well (this maintains a uniform protein concentration). multiply the readout value by 2 to obtain the thyroxine concentration.

Quality Control

Each laboratory should assay controls at levels in the hypothyroid, euthyroid and hyperthyroid range for monitoring assay performance. These controls should be treated as unknowns and values determined in every test procedure performed. Quality control charts should be maintained to follow the performance of the supplied reagents. Pertinent statistical methods should be employed to ascertain trends. The individual laboratory should set acceptable assay performance limits. Other parameters that should be monitored include the 80, 50 and 20 per cent intercepts of the standard curve for run-to-run reproducibility. In addition, maximum absorbance should be consistent with past experience. Significant deviation from established performance can indicate unnoticed change in experimental conditions or degradation of kit reagents. Fresh reagents should be used to determine the reason for the variations.

Results

A dose response curve is used to ascertain the concentration of thyroxine in unknown specimens.

1. Record the absorbance obtained from the printout of the microplate reader as outlined in Example 4.
2. Plot the absorbance for each duplicate serum reference versus the corresponding T4 concentration in μg/dl on linear graph paper (do not average the duplicates of the serum references before plotting).
3. Draw the best-fit curve through the plotted points.
4. To determine the concentration of T4 for an unknown, locate the average absorbance of the duplicates for each unknown on the vertical axis of the graph, find the intersecting point on the curve, and read the concentration (in μg/dl) from the horizontal axis of the graph (the duplicates of the unknown may be averaged as indicated). In the following example, the average absorbance 1.123 (intersects the standard curve at 8.1 μg/dl) T4 concentration (See Figure 17.27).

Example 4

Well	*Serum references*	*Absorbance*
1	0.0 μg/dl	2.374
2	0.0 μg/dl	2.358
3	2.0 μg/dl	1.843
4	2.0 μg/dl	1.897
5	5.0 μg/dl	1.409
6	5.0 μg/dl	1.393
7	10.0 μg/dl	0.952
8	10.0 μg/dl	1.012
9	15.0 μg/dl	0.757
10	15.0 μg/dl	0.752
11	25.0 μg/dl	0.474
12	25.0 μg/dl	0.502

Well	Unknown ID	OD	Avg. OD	Value
13	Unknown #1	1.105		
14	Unknown #1	1.142	1.123	8.1 μg/dl

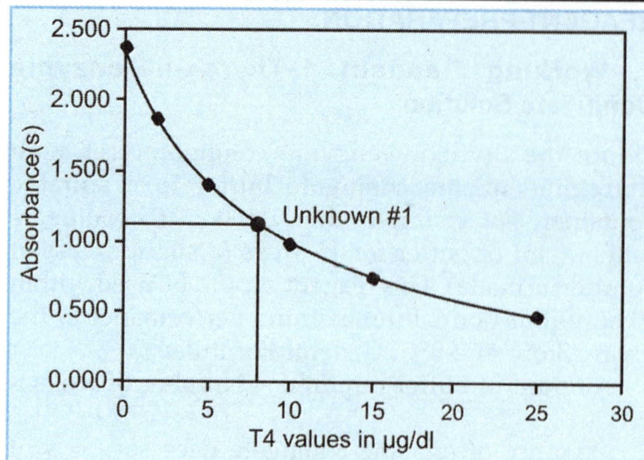

Fig. 17.27: Estimation of T_4

*The data presented in Example 4 and Figure 17.27 are for illustration only and should not be used in lieu of a standard curve prepared with each assay.

QC Parameters

Maximum absorbance (O calibrator) = 1.5- 2.7

LIMITATIONS OF PROCEDURE

A. Assay Performance

Serum references and controls should not exhibit cloudiness with time. Discard if cloudiness is observed.

Sample(s), which are contaminated microbiologically, should not be used in the assay. Highly lipaemeic or haemolysed specimen(s) should similarly not be used.

It is important that the time of reaction in each well is held constant for reproducible results. Pipetting of samples should not extend beyond ten (10) minutes to avoid assay drift. If more than one (1) plate is used, it is recommended to repeat the dose response curve.

Addition of the substrate solution initiates a kinetic reaction, which is terminated by the addition of the stop solution. Therefore, the addition of the substrate and the stopping solution should be added in the same sequence to eliminate any time deviation during reaction.

Plate readers measure vertically. Do not touch the bottom of the wells.

Failure to remove adhering solution adequately in the aspiration or, decantation wash step(s) may result in poor replication and spurious results.

Unused microwell strips should be re-inserted into the aluminum foil bag and re-sealed with the ziploc.

B. Interpretation

If computer controlled data reduction is used to interpret the results of the test, it is imperative that the predicted values for the calibrators fall within 10 per cent of the assigned concentrations.

Total serum thyroxine concentration is dependent upon a multiplicity of factors: thyroid gland function and its regulation, thyroxine-binding globulin (TBG) concentration, and the binding of thyroxine to TBG. Thus, total thyroxine concentration alone is not sufficient to assess clinical status.

Total serum thyroxine values may be elevated under conditions such as pregnancy or administration of oral contraceptives. A T3 uptake test may be performed to estimate the relative TBG concentration in order to determine if the elevated T4 is caused by TBG variation.

A decrease in total thyroxine values is found with protein-wasting diseases, certain liver diseases and administration of testosterone, diphenylhydantoin or salicylates. A table of interfering drugs and conditions which affect total thyroxine values has been compiled by the Journal of the American Association of Clinical Chemists.

"Not Intended for Newborn Screening".

Expected Range of Values

A study of euthyroid adult population was undertaken to determine expected values for the T4 EIA test system. The mean (R) values, standard deviations (SD) and expected ranges (±2 SD) are presented below.

Expected Values for the T4 EIA Test System (in μg/dl)

	Male (42 specimens)	*Female* (58 specimens)*
Mean (X)	7.6	8.2
Standard Deviation (SD)	1.6	1.7
Expected Ranges	(±2 SD) 4.4-10.8	4.8-11.6

*Normal patients with high TBG levels were not excluded except if pregnant.

It is important to keep in mind that establishment of a range of values which can be expected to be found by a given method for a population of "normal" persons is dependent upon a multiplicity of factors: the specificity of the method, the population tested and the precision of the method in the hands of the analyst. For these reasons, each laboratory should depend upon the range of expected values established by the manufacturer only until an in-house range can be determined by the analysts using the method with a population indigenous to the area in which the laboratory is located.

Normal Values (µg/dl)

Age	
Adults	5.0-12.0
Pregnant > 14 weeks	9.1-14.0
Elderly (> 60 years)	
Female	5.5-10.5
Male	5.0-10.0
Children	
Cord blood	
First 72 hours	7.4-13.0
7-14 days	11.8-22.6
4-16 weeks	9.8-16.6
4-12 months	7.2-14.4
1-5 years	7.8-16.5
5-10 years	7.3-15.0
	6.4-13.3
10-15 years	5.6-11.7
Panic levels	
Thyroid storm possible	> 20.0
Myxoedema possible	< 2.0

FREE THYROXINE (FT4) (Courtesy: Lilac Medicare)

Intended Use: The Quantitative Determination of Free Thyroxine Concentration in Human Serum or Plasma by a Microplate Enzyme Immunoassay. Levels of fT4 are thought to reflect the amount of T4 available to the cells and may, therefore, determine the clinical metabolic status of T4.

Summary and Explanation of the Test

Thyroxine, the principal thyroid hormone, circulates in blood almost completely bound to carrier proteins. The main carrier is thyroxine-binding globulin (TBG). However, only the free (unbound) portion of thyroxine is responsible for the biological action. Further, the concentrations of the carrier proteins are altered in many clinical conditions, such as pregnancy. In normal thyroid function as the concentrations of the carrier proteins alter, the total thyroxine level changes so that the free thyroxine concentration remains constant. Thus, measurements of free thyroxine concentrations correlate better with clinical status than total thyroxine levels.

For example, the increase in total thyroxine associated with pregnancy, oral contraceptives and oestrogen therapy occasionally result in total T4 levels over the limits of normal while the free thyroxine concentration remains in the normal reference range. Masking of abnormal thyroid function can also occur in both hyper- and hypothyroid conditions by alterations in the TBG concentration. The total T4 can be elevated or lowered by TBG changes such that the normal reference levels result. Again, the free thyroxine concentration typically uncovers the patient's actual clinical status.

This microplate enzyme immunoassay methodology provides the technician with optimum sensitivity while requiring a few technical manipulations. In this method, serum reference, patient specimen, or control is first added to a microplate well. Enzyme-T4 conjugate (analog method) is added, then the reactants are mixed. A competition reaction results between the enzyme conjugate and the free thyroxine for a limited number of antibody-combining sites immobilised on the well.

After the completion of the required incubation period, the antibody-bound enzyme-thyroxine conjugate is separated from the unbound enzyme-thyroxine conjugate by aspiration or decantation. The activity of the enzyme present on the surface of the well is quantitated by reaction with a suitable substrate to produce color.

The employment of several serum references of known free thyroxine concentration permits construction of a graph of activity and concentration. From comparison to the dose response curve, an unknown specimen's activity can be correlated with free thyroxine concentration.

PRINCIPLE

Competitive Enzyme Immunoassay-Analog Method for Free T4

The essential reagents required for a solid phase enzyme immunoassay include immobilised antibody, enzyme-antigen conjugate and native antigen.

Upon mixing immobilised antibody, enzyme-antigen conjugate and a serum containing the native free antigen, a competition reaction results between the native free antigen and the enzyme-antigen conjugate for a limited number of insolubulized binding sites. The interaction is illustrated by the following equation:

$$^{Enz}Ag + Ag + Abcw \underset{k_{-a}}{\overset{k_a}{\rightleftharpoons}} AgAbcw + {}^{Enz}AgAbcw$$

Abcw	= Monospecific immobilized antibody (constant quantity)
Ag	= Native antigen (variable quantity)
^{Enz}Ag	= Enzyme-antigen conjugate (constant quantity)
AgAbcw	= Antigen-antibody complex
^{Enz}Ag Abcw	= Enzyme-antigen conjugate -antibody complex
k_a	= Rate constant of association
k_{-a}	= Rate constant of disassociation
$K = k_a/k_{-a}$	= Equilibrium constant

After equilibrium is attained, the antibody-bound fraction is separated from unbound antigen by decantation or aspiration. The enzyme activity in the antibody-bound fraction is inversely proportional to the native free antigen concentration. By utilising several different serum references of known antigen concentration, a dose response curve can be generated from which the antigen concentration of an unknown can be ascertained.

REAGENTS FOR 96-WELL MICROPLATE

A. Human Serum References-1.0 ml/vial

Six (6) vials of serum reference for thyroxine at approximate* concentrations of 0 (A), 0.3 (B), 0.95 (C), 2.1 (D), 3.6 (E) and 7.0 (F) ng/dl. Store at 2-8°C. A preservative has been added.

*Exact levels are given on the labels on a lot specific basis.

B. Enzyme-antigen Conjugate-1.0 ml/vial

One (1) vial of thyroxine-horseradish peroxidase (HRP) conjugate in a bovine albumin-stabilising matrix. A preservative has been added. Store at 2-8°C.

C. Enzyme-antigen Conjugate Buffer-11 ml

One (1) bottle reagent containing buffer, blue dye, and preservative. Store at 2-8°C.

D. Antibody-Coated Microplate-96 wells

One 96-well microplate coated with sheep anti-thyroxine serum and packaged in an aluminum bag with a drying agent. Store at 2-8°C.

E. Wash Solution Concentrate-20 ml

One (1) vial containing a surfactant in phosphate buffered saline. A preservative has been added. Store at 2-30°C.

F. Substrate A-7.0 ml/vial

One (1) bottle containing tetramethylbenzidine (TMB) in buffer. Store at 2-8°C.

G. Substrate B-7.0 ml/vial

One (1) bottle containing hydrogen peroxide (H_2O_2) in buffer. Store at 2-8°C.

H. Stop Solution-6.0 ml/vial

One (1) bottle containing a strong acid (1N HCl). Store at 2-30°C.

Note 1: Do not use reagents beyond the kit expiration date.

Note 2: Opened reagents are stable for sixty (60) days when stored at 2-8°C.

Precautions

For In Vitro Diagnostic Use

Not for Internal or External Use in Humans or Animals

All products that contain human serum have been found to be nonreactive for Hepatitis B Surface Antigen, HIV 1 and 2 and HCV Antibodies by FDA required tests. Since no known test can offer complete assurance that infectious agents are absent, all human serum products should be handled as potentially hazardous and capable of transmitting disease. Good laboratory procedures for handling blood products can be found in the Center for Disease Control/ National Institute of Health, "Biosafety in Microbiological and Biomedical Laboratories," 2nd Edition, 1988, HHS Publication No. (CDC) 88-8395.

Specimen Collection and Preparation

Collect sample(s) by venipuncture in ten (10) ml silicone evacuated tube(s) or evacuated tube(s) containing EDTA or heparin. The usual precautions in the collection of venipuncture samples should be observed. Separate the red blood cells by centrifugation, use serum or plasma for the total T4 procedure. Specimen(s) may be refrigerated at 2-8°C for a maximum period of 48 hours. If the specimen(s) cannot be assayed within 48 hours, the sample(s) may be stored at temperatures of –20°C for up to 30 days. When assayed in duplicate, 0.05 ml of the specimen is required.

The crossreactivity of the thyroxine antibody to selected substances was evaluated by adding the interfering substance to a serum matrix at various concentrations. The crossreactivity was calculated by deriving a ratio between dose of interfering substance to dose of thyroxine needed to displace the same amount of tracer.

Substance	*Crossreactivity*	*Concentration*
I-Thyroxine		1.0000
d-Thyroxine	0.9800	10 μg/dl
d-Triiodothyronine	0.0150	100 μg/dl
I-Triiodothyronine	0.0300	100 μg/dl
Iodothyrosine	0.0001	100 μg/ ml
Diiodothyrosine	0.0001	100 μg/ ml
Diiodothyronine	0.0001	100 μg/ ml

MATERIALS

Provided

1. Six (6) vials of free thyroxine human serum references.
2. One (1) vial of thyroxine-enzyme conjugate concentrate.
3. One (1) vial of thyroxine-enzyme conjugate buffer.
4. One 96-well antibody coated microplate.
5. One (1) bottle of wash buffer concentrate.
6. One (1) bottle of substrate A.
7. One (1) bottle of substrate B.
8. One (1) bottle of stop solution.
9. Instructions.

Required but Not Provided

1. Pipette capable of delivering 50 μl volumes with a precision of better than 1.5 per cent.
2. Dispenser(s) for repetitive deliveries of 0.100 ml and 0.300 ml volumes with a precision of better than 1.5 per cent.
3. Adjustable volume (20-200 μl) and (200-1000 μl) dispenser(s) for conjugate and substrate dilutions.
4. Microplate washer or a squeeze bottle (optional).
5. Microplate reader with 450 nm wavelength absorbance capability.

6. Test tubes for dilution of enzyme conjugate and substrates A and B.
7. Absorbent paper for blotting the microplate wells.
8. Plastic wrap or microplate cover for incubation steps.
9. Vacuum aspirator (optional) for wash steps.
10. Timer.
11. Quality control materials.

REAGENT PREPARATION

1. Working Reagent 1-Thyroxine-enzyme

Conjugate Solution

Dilute the thyroxine-enzyme conjugate 1:11 with thyroxine-enzyme conjugate buffer in a suitable container. For example, dilute 160pl of conjugate with 1.6 ml of buffer for 160 wells (a slight excess of solution is made). This reagent should be used within twenty-four hours for maximum performance of the assay. Store at 2-8°C. General Formula:

Amount of buffer required = Number of wells × 0.1

Quantity of Enzyme conjugate necessary = # of wells × 0.01

i.e. = 16 × 0.1 = 1.6 ml for T4 conjugate buffer

16 × 0.01 = 0.16 ml (160 μl) for T4 enzyme conjugate

2. Wash Buffer

Dilute contents of wash concentrate to 1000 ml with distilled or deionized water in a suitable storage container. Store at room temperature until expiration date printed on concentrate label.

3. Working Substrate Solution-Prepare immediately before use

Determine the amount of reagent needed and prepare by mixing equal portions of substrate A and substrate B in a suitable container. For example, add 1 ml of A and 1 ml of B per two (2) eight well strips (a slight excess of solution is made). Use within one (1) hour of preparation for maximum performance of the assay.

Test Procedure

Before proceeding with the assay, bring all reagents, serum references and controls to room temperature (20-30°C).

1. Format the microplates' wells for each serum reference, control and patient specimen to be assayed in duplicate.
2. Pipette 0.050 ml (50 μl) of the appropriate serum reference, control or specimen into the assigned well.
3. Add 0.100 ml (100 μl) of working reagent, Thyroxine-enzyme conjugate solution, to all wells (see reagent preparation section).
4. Swirl the microplate gently for 20-30 seconds to mix and cover.
5. Incubate 60 minutes at room temperature.
6. Discard the contents of the microplate by decantation or aspiration. If decanting, blot the plate dry with absorbent paper.
7. Add 300 μl of wash buffer (see reagent preparation section), decant (tap and blot) or aspirate. Repeat two (2) additional times for a total of three (3) washes. An automatic or manual plate washer can be used. Follow the manufacturer's instruction for proper usage, if a squeeze bottle is employed, fill each well by depressing the container (avoiding air bubbles) to dispense the wash. Decant the wash and repeat two (2) additional times.
8. Add 0.100 ml (100 μl) of working substrate solution to all wells (see reagent preparation section). Always add reagents in the same order to minimise reaction time differences between wells.
9. Incubate at room temperature for fifteen (15) minutes.
10. Add 0.050 ml (50 μl) of stop solution to each well and gently mix for 15-20 seconds. Always add reagents in the same order to minimise reaction time differences between wells.
11. Read the absorbance in each well at 450 nm in a microplate reader. The results should be read within thirty (30) minutes of adding the stop solution.

Quality Control

Each laboratory should assay controls at levels in the hypothyroid, euthyroid and hyperthyroid range for monitoring assay performance. These controls should be treated as unknowns and values determined in every test procedure performed. Quality control charts should be maintained to follow the performance of the supplied reagents. Pertinent statistical methods should be employed to ascertain trends. The individual laboratory should set acceptable assay performance limits. Other parameters that should be monitored include the 80, 50 and 20 per cent intercepts of the standard curve for run-to-run reproducibility. In addition, maximum absorbance should be consistent with past experience. Significant deviation from established performance can indicate unnoticed change in experimental conditions or degradation of kit reagents. Fresh reagents should be used to determine the reason for the variations.

Results

A dose response curve is used to ascertain the concentration of thyroxine in unknown specimens.

1. Record the absorbance obtained from the print-out of the microplate reader as outlined in Example 5.
2. Plot the absorbance for each duplicate serum reference versus the corresponding FT_4 concentration in ng/dl on linear group paper donot average the duplicates of the serum references before plotting.
3. Draw the best-fit curve through the plotted points.
4. To determine the concentration of T4 for an unknown, locate the average absorbance of the duplicates for each unknown on the vertical axis of the graph, find the intersecting point on the curve, and read the concentration (in ng/dl) from the horizontal axis of the graph (the duplicates of the unknown may be averaged as indicated). In the following example, the average absorbance 1.123 (intersects the standard curve at 8.1 ng/dl) T4 concentration (See Figure 17.28).

Example 5

Well	Serum references	Absorbance
1	0.0 ng/dl	2.462
2	0.0 ng/dl	2.531
3	0.3 ng/dl	2.330
4	0.3 ng/dl	2.255
5	0.95 ng/dl	1.915
6	0.95 ng/dl	1.892
7	2.1 ng/dl	1.328
8	2.1 ng/dl	1.262
9	3.6 ng/dl	0.834
10	3.6 ng/dl	0.804
11	7.0 ng/dl	0.399
12	7.0 ng/dl	0.421

Well	Unknown ID	OD	Avg. OD	Value
13	Unknown#1	1.783		
14	Unknown#1	1.676	1.730	1.3 ng/dl

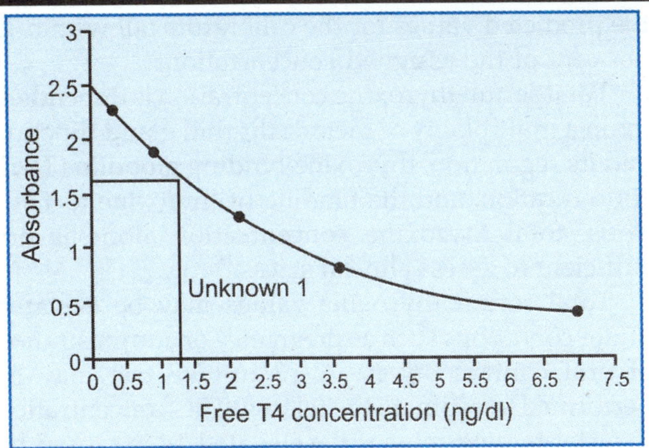

Fig. 17.28: Estimation of FT4

The data presented in Example 5 and Figure 17.28 are for illustration only and should not be used in lieu of a standard curve prepared with each assay.

QC Parameters

Maximum absorbance (O callibrator) = 1.5-2.7

LIMITATIONS OF PROCEDURE

A. Assay Performance

Serum references and controls may exhibit cloudiness with time. This occurrence does not affect the accuracy or performance of the test. Use until exhausted or until expiration date on the label.

It is important that the time of reaction in each well is held constant for reproducible results. Pipetting of samples should not extend beyond ten (10) minutes to avoid assay drift. If more than one (1) plate is used, it is recommended to repeat the dose response curve.

Addition of the substrate solution initiates a kinetic reaction, which is terminated by the addition of the stop solution. Therefore, the addition of the substrate and the stopping solution should be added in the same sequence to eliminate any time deviation during reaction.

Plate readers measure vertically. Do not touch the bottom of the wells.

Failure to remove adhering solution adequately in the aspiration or decantation wash step(s) may result in poor replication and spurious results.

B. Interpretation

If computer controlled data reduction is used to interpret the results of the test, it is imperative that the predicted values for the calibrators fall within 10 per cent of the assigned concentrations.

Total serum thyroxine concentration is dependent upon a multiplicity of factors: thyroid gland function and its regulation, thyroxine-binding globulin (TBG) concentration, and the binding of thyroxine to TBG. Thus, total thyroxine concentration alone is not sufficient to assess clinical status.

Total serum thyroxine values may be elevated under conditions such as pregnancy or administration of oral contraceptives. A T3 uptake test may be performed to estimate the relative TBG concentration in order to determine if the elevated T4 is caused by TBG variation.

A decrease in total thyroxine values is found with protein-wasting diseases, certain liver diseases and administration of testosterone, diphenylhydantoin or salicylates. A table of interfering drugs and conditions which affect total thyroxine values has been compiled by the Journal of the American Association of Clinical Chemists.

"Not Intended for Newborn Screening"

Expected Range of Values

A study of euthyroid adult population was undertaken to determine expected values for the free T4 EIA test system. The mean (R) values, standard deviations (SD) and expected ranges (±2 SD) are presented below.

Expected values for the free T4 EIA test system (in ng/dl)

Adult (110 specimens)	*Pregnancy* (30 specimens)	
Mean (X)	1.4	1.5
Standard Deviation (SD)	0.6	0.7
Expected Ranges (±2S. D.)	0.8-2.0	0.8-2.2

It is important to keep in mind that establishment of a range of values which can be expected to be found by a given method for a population of "normal" persons is dependent upon a multiplicity of factors: the specificity of the method, the population tested and the precision of the method in the hands of the analyst. For these reasons, each laboratory should depend upon the range of expected values established by the manufacturer only until an in-house range can be determined by the analysts using the method with a population indigenous to the area in which the laboratory is located.

THYROTROPIN (TSH) Courtesy: Lilac Medicare

Intended Use: The Quantitative Determination of Thyrotrophin Concentration in Human Serum by a Microplate Immunoenzymometric Assay

Summary and Explanation of the Test

Measurement of the serum concentration of thyrotrophin (TSH), a glycoprotein with a molecular weight of 28,000 daltons and secreted from the anterior pituitary, is generally regarded as the most sensitive indicator available for the diagnosis of primary and secondary (pituitary) hypothyroidism (1,2). Increase in serum concentrations of TSH, which is primarily responsible for the synthesis and release of thyroid hormones, is an early and sensitive indicator of decrease thyroid reserve and in conjunction with decreased thyroxine (T4) concentrations is diagnostic of primary hypothyroidism. The expected increase in TSH concentrations demonstrates the classical negative feedback system between the pituitary and thyroid glands. That is, primary thyroid gland failure reduces secretion of the thyroid hormones, which in turn stimulates the release of TSH from the pituitary.

Additionally, TSH measurements are equally useful in differentiating secondary and tertiary (hypothalamic) hypothyroidism from the primary thyroid disease. TSH release from the pituitary is regulated by thyrotrophin-releasing hormone (TRH), which is secreted by the hypothalamus, and by direct action of T4 and triiodothyronine (T3), the thyroid hormones, at the pituitary, increase levels of T3 and T4 reduces the response of the pituitary to the stimulatory effects of TRH. In secondary and tertiary hypothyroidism, concentrations of T4 are usually low and TSH levels are generally low or normal. Either pituitary TSH deficiency (secondary hypothyroidism) or insufficiency of stimulation of the pituitary by TRH tertiary hypothyroidism causes this. The TRH stimulation test differentiates these conditions. In secondary hypothyroidism, TSH response to TRH is blunted while a normal or delayed response is obtained in tertiary hypothyroidism.

Further, the advent of immunoenzymometric assays has provided the laboratory with sufficient sensitivity to enable the differentiating of hyperthyroidism from euthyroid population and extending the usefulness of TSH measurements. This method is a third-generation assay, which provides the means for discrimination in the hyperthyroid-euthyroid range. The functional sensitivity (<20 per cent between assay CV) of the one hour procedure is 0.195 μIU/ml while the two hour procedure has a functional sensitivity of 0.095 μIU/ml.

In this method, TSH calibrator, patient specimen or control is first added to a streptavidin-coated well. Biotinylated monoclonal and enzyme-labelled antibodies are added and the reactants mixed. Reaction between the various TSH antibodies and native TSH forms a sandwich complex that binds with the streptavidin coated to the well.

After the completion of the required incubation period, the antibody-bound enzyme-thyrotrophin conjugate is separated from the unbound enzyme-thyrotrophin conjugate by aspiration or decantation. The activity of the enzyme present on the surface of the well is quantitated by reaction with a suitable substrate to produce color.

The employment of several serum references of known thyrotrophin levels permits construction of a dose response curve of activity and concentration. From comparison to the dose response curve, an unknown specimen's activity can be correlated with thyrotrophin concentration.

PRINCIPLE

Immunoenzymometric Assay

The essential reagents required for an immunoenzymometric assay include high affinity and specificity antibodies (enzyme and immobilised), with different and distinct epitope recognition, in excess, and native antigen. In this procedure, the immobilisation takes place during the assay at the surface of a microplate well through the interaction of streptavidin coated on the well and exogenously added biotinylated monoclonal anti-TSH antibody.

Upon mixing monoclonal biotinylated antibody, the enzyme-labeled antibody and a serum containing the native antigen, reaction results between the native antigen and the antibodies, without competition or steric hindrance, to form a soluble sandwich complex. The interaction is illustrated by the following equation:

$$^{Enz}Ab_{(p)} + AgisH + {}^{Bln}Ab_{(m)} \underset{k\text{-}a}{\overset{k_a}{\rightleftharpoons}} {}^{Enz}Ab_{(p)}AgTSH\text{-}{}^{B/n}Ab_{(m)}$$

$^{Btn}Ab_{(m)}$ = Biotinylated monoclonal antibody (excess quantity)

AgrsH = Native antigen (variable quantity)

$^{Enz}Ab_{(p)}$ = Enzyme labeled polyclonal antibody (excess quantity)

$^{En2}Ab_{(p)}\text{-}Ag_TsH\text{-}{}^{Btn}Ab_{(m)}$ = Antigen-antibodies sandwich complex

k_a = Rate constant of association

$k\text{-}_a$ = Rate constant of dissociation

Simultaneously, the complex is deposited to the well through the high affinity reaction of streptavidin and biotinylated antibody. This interaction is illustrated below:

$^{Enz}Ab_(p)\text{-}Ag_TsH\text{-}{}^{Btn}Ab(m)$ + Streptavidin c.w.→ immobilised complex

Streptavidin cw = Streptavidin immobolised on well

Immobilised complex = Sandwich complex bound to the solid surface.

After equilibrium is attained, the antibody-bound fraction is separated from unbound antigen by decantation or aspiration. The enzyme activity in the antibody-bound fraction is directly proportional to the native antigen concentration. By utilising several different serum references of known antigen values, a dose response curve can be generated from which the antigen concentration of an unknown can be ascertained.

REAGENTS FOR 96-WELL MICROPLATE

A. Thyrotrophin Calibrators-1.0 ml/vial

Seven (7) vials of references for TSH antigen at levels of 0(A), 0.5(B), 2.5(C), 5.0(D), 10(E), 20(F) and 40(G) μIU/ml. Store at 2-8°C. A preservative has been added.

Note: The calibrators, human serum based, were calibrated using a reference preparation, which was assayed against the WHO 2nd IRP 80/558.

B. Enzyme-Polyclonal Conjugate and Biotinylated Monoclonal Antibody—11 ml/vial

One (1) vial containing enzyme-labeled affinity purified goat antibody, biotinylated monoclonal mouse IgG in buffer, dye, and preservative. Store at 2-8°C.

C. Streptavidin-Coated Microplate-96 Wells

One 96-well microplate coated with Streptavidin and packaged in an aluminum bag with a drying agent. Store at 2-8°C.

D. Wash Solution Concentrate-20 ml

One (1) vial containing a surfactant in phosphate buffered saline. A preservative has been added. Store at 2-30°C.

E. Substrate A—7.0 ml/vial

One (1) bottle containing tetramethylbenzidine (TMB) in buffer. Store at 2-8°C.

F. Substrate B-7.0 ml/vial

One (1) bottle containing hydrogen peroxide (H_2O_2) in buffer. Store at 2-8°C.

G. Stop Solution-6.0 ml/vial

One (1) bottle containing a strong acid (1N HCl). Store at 2-30°C.

Note 1: Do not use reagents beyond the kit expiration date.

Note 2: Opened reagents are stable for sixty (60) days when stored at 2-8°C.

FOR IN VITRO DIAGNOSTIC USE NOT FOR INTERNAL OR EXTERNAL USE IN HUMANS OR ANIMALS

Precautions

All products that contain human serum have been found to be nonreactive for Hepatitis B Surface Antigen, HIV 1 and 2 and HCV Antibodies by FDA required tests. Since no known test can offer complete assurance that infectious agents are absent, all human serum products should be handled as potentially hazardous and capable of transmitting disease. Good laboratory procedures for handling blood products can be found in the Center for Disease Control/ National Institute of Health, "Biosafety in Microbiological and Biomedical Laboratories," 2nd Edition, 1988, HHS.

Specimen Collection and Preparation

The specimens shall be blood serum in type and the usual precautions in the collection of venipuncture samples should be observed. For accurate comparison to established normal values, a fasting morning serum sample should be obtained. The blood should be collected in a plain red-top venipuncture tube without additives or gel barrier. Allow the blood to clot. Centrifuge the specimen to separate the serum from the cells.

Samples may be refrigerated at 2-8°C for a maximum period of five (5) days. If the specimen(s) cannot be assayed within this time, the sample(s) may be stored at temperatures of –20°C for up to 30 days. Avoid repetitive freezing and thawing. When assayed in duplicate, 0.100 ml of the specimen is required.

MATERIALS

Provided

1. Seven (7) vials of thyrotrophin serum calibrators.
2. One (1) vial of biotinylated and enzyme labeled antibody reagent.
3. One 96-well Streptavidin-coated microplate.
4. One (1) bottle of wash buffer concentrate.
5. One (1) bottle of substrate A.
6. One (1) bottle of substrate B.
7. One (1) bottle of stop solution.
8. Instructions.

Required but Not Provided

1. Pipette(s) capable of delivering 50 μl and 100 μl volumes with a precision of better than 1.5 per cent.
2. Dispensers for repetitive deliveries of 0.100 ml and 0.300 ml volumes with a precision of better than 1.5 per cent (optional).
3. Microplate washer or a squeeze bottle (optional).
4. Microplate reader with 450 nm wavelength absorbance capability.
5. Adjustable volume (200-1000 μl) dispenser for reagent dilution.
6. Container(s) for mixing of reagents (see below).
7. Absorbent paper for blotting the microplate wells.
8. Plastic wrap or microplate cover for incubation steps.
9. Vacuum aspirator (optional) for wash steps.
10. Timer.
11. Storage container for storage of wash buffer.
12. Distilled or deionized water.
13. Quality control materials.

REAGENT PREPARATION

1. Working Reagent 1-Wash Buffer

Dilute contents of wash concentrate to 1000 ml with distilled or deionized water in a suitable storage container. Store at room temperature.

2. Working Reagent 2-Substrate Solution-Prepare before Use

Determine the amount of reagent needed and prepare by mixing equal portions of substrate A and substrate B in a suitable container. For example, add 1 ml of A and 1 ml of B per two (2) eight well strips (a slight excess of solution is made). Use within one (1) hour of preparation for maximum performance of the assay.

Test Procedure

Before proceeding with the assay, bring all reagents, serum references and controls to room temperature (20-30°C).

1. Format the microplates' wells for each serum reference, control and patient specimen to be assayed in duplicate. Replace any unused microwell strips back into the aluminum bag, seal and store a 2-8°C.
2. Pipette 0.050 ml (50 µl) of the appropriate serum reference, control or specimen into the assigned well.
3. Add 0.100 ml (100 µl) of the biotinylated/enzyme-labeled antibodies to each well. It is very important to dispense all reagents close to the bottom of the coated well.
4. Swirl the microplate gently for 20-30 seconds to mix and cover.
5. Incubate 60 minutes at room temperature.
6. Discard the contents of the microplate by decollation or aspiration decanting, tap and blot the plate dry with absorbent paper.
7. Add 300 µl of wash buffer (see reagent preparation section), decant (tap and blot) or aspirate. Repeat two (2) additional times for a total of three (3) washes. An automatic or manual plate washer can be used. Follow the manufacturer's instruction for proper usage. If a squeeze bottle is employed, fill each well by depressing the container (avoiding air bubbles) to dispense the wash. Decant the wash and repeat two (2) additional times.
8. Add 0.100 ml (100 µl) of working substrate solution to all wells (see reagent preparation section). Always add reagents in the same order to minimise reaction time differences between wells.
9. Incubate at room temperature for fifteen (15) minutes.
10. Add 0.050 ml (50 µl) of stop solution to each well and mix gently for 15-20 seconds. Always add reagents in the same order to minimize reaction time differences between wells.
11. Read the absorbance in each well at 450 nm in a microplate reader. The results should be read within thirty (30) minutes of adding the stop solution.

For better low-end sensitivity (< 0.5 µIU/ml). Incubate 120 minutes at room temperature. The 40 µIU/ml calibrator should be excluded since absorbance over 3.0 units will be experienced. Follow the remaining steps.

Quality Control

Each laboratory should assay controls at levels in the hypothyroid, euthyroid and hyperthyroid range for monitoring assay performance. These controls should be treated as unknowns and values determined in every test procedure performed. Quality control charts should be maintained to follow the performance of the supplied reagents. Pertinent statistical methods should be employed to ascertain trends. The individual laboratory should set acceptable assay performance limits. Other parameters that should be monitored include the 80, 50 and 20 per cent intercepts of the dose response curve for run-to-run reproducibility. In addition, maximum absorbance should be consistent with past experience. Significant deviation from established performance can indicate unnoticed change in experimental conditions or degradation of kit reagents. Fresh reagents should be used to determine the reason for the variations.

Results

A dose response curve is used to ascertain the concentration of thyrotrophin in unknown specimens.

1. Record the absorbance obtained from the printout of the microplate reader as outlined in Example 6 (an example of the 120-minute incubation is presented in italic type).
2. Plot the absorbance for each duplicate serum reference versus the corresponding TSH concentration in µIU/ml on linear graph paper (do not average the duplicates of the serum references before plotting).
3. Draw the best-fit curve through the plotted points.

4. To determine the concentration of TSH for an unknown, locate the average absorbance of the duplicates for each unknown on the vertical axis of the graph, find the intersecting point on the curve, and read the concentration (in μIU/ml) from the horizontal axis of the graph (the duplicates of the unknown may be averaged as indicated). In the following example, the average absorbance (1.019) intersects the dose response curve at (15.3 μIU/ml) TSH concentration (See Figure 17.29).

Note: Computer data reduction software designed for IEMA assays may also be used for the data reduction.

Example 6

Incubation Time

Well	*Serum References*	*60 Minute Absorbance*	*120 Minute Absorbance*
1	0.0 μIU/ml	0.011	0.008
2	0.0 μIU/ml	0.009	0.009
3	0.5 μIU/ml	0.034	0.065
4	0.5 μIU/ml	0.033	0.065
5	2.5 μIU/ml	0.177	0.375
6	2.5 μIU/ml	0.175	0.375
7	5.0 μIU/ml	0.377	0.758
8	5.0 μl/ml	0.366	0.734
9	10.0 μl/ml	0.743	1.448
10	10.0 μIU/ml	0.748	1.412
11	20.0 μIU/ml	1.452	2.679
12	20.0 μIU/ml	1.431	2.498
13	40.0 μIU/ml	2.633	
14	40.0 μIU/ml	2.530	

Well	**Unknown ID**	**OD**	**Avg OD**	**Value**
15	Unknown #1	1.028		
16	Unknown #1	1.011	1.019	15.3 μIU/ ml

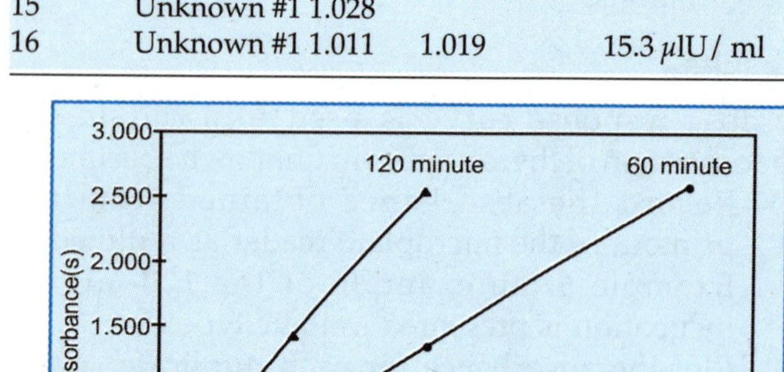

Fig. 17.29: Estimation of TSH in μIU/ml

The data presented in Example 6 is for illustration only and should not be used in lieu of a dose response curve prepared with each assay.

QC Parameters

Maximum absorbance (40 μIU/ml) =1.8-2.7

LIMITATIONS OF PROCEDURE

A. Assay Performance

It is important that the time of reaction in each well is held constant for reproducible results. Pipetting of samples should not extend beyond ten (10) minutes to avoid assay drift. If more than one (1) plate is used, it is recommended to repeat the dose response curve.

Sample(s), which are contaminated microbiologically, should not be used in the assay. Highly lipaemeic or haemolysed specimen(s) should similarly not be used.

Addition of the substrate solution initiates a kinetic reaction, which is terminated by the addition of the stop solution. Therefore, the addition of the substrate and the stopping solution should be added in the same sequence to eliminate any time deviation during reaction. Plate readers measure vertically. Do not touch the bottom of the wells.

Failure to remove adhering solution adequately in the aspiration or decantation wash step(s) may result in poor replication and spurious results.

Patient specimens with TSH concentrations above 40 μIU/ml may be diluted with the zero calibrator and re-assayed. The sample's concentration is obtained by multiplying the result by the dilution factor. Each component in one assay should be of the same lot number and stored under identical conditions.

Unused microwell strips should be re-inserted into the aluminum foil bag and re-sealed with the ziploc.

B. Interpretation

If computer controlled data reduction is used to interpret the results of the test, it is imperative that the predicted values for the calibrators fall within 10 per cent of the assigned concentrations.

Serum thyrotrophin concentration is dependent upon a multiplicity of factors: hypothalamus gland function, thyroid gland function, and the responsiveness of pituitary to TRH. Thus, thyrotrophin concentration alone is not sufficient to assess clinical status.

Serum thyrotrophin values may be elevated by pharmacological intervention. Domperiodone, amiodazon, iodide, phenobarbital, and phenytoin have been reported to increase TSH levels.

A decrease in thyrotrophin values has been reported with the administration of propranolol, methimazol, dopamine and d-thyroxine.

Genetic variations or degradation of intact TSH into subunits may affect the binding characteristics of the antibodies and influence the final result. Such samples normally exhibit different results among various assay systems due to the reactivity of the antibodies involved.

"Not Intended for Newborn Screening".

Expected Ranges of Values

A study of euthyroid adult population was undertaken to determine expected values for the TSH IEMA microplate test system. The number and determined range are given in below. A nonparametric method (95 per cent per centile estimate) was used.

Expected values for the TSH IEMA test system

	(in μIU/ ml)
Number	139
Low normal range	0.39
High normal range	6.16
70 per cent confidence intervals for 2.5 per centile	
Low range	0.28-0.53
High range	5.60-6.82

It is important to keep in mind that establishment of a range of values which can be expected to be found by a given method for a population of "normal'-persons is dependent upon a multiplicity of factors: the specificity of the method, the population tested and the precision of the method in the hands of the analyst. For these reasons, each laboratory should depend upon the range of expected values established by the manufacturer only until an in-house range can be determined by the analysts using the method with a population indigenous to the area in which the laboratory is located.

Normal Values (μIU/ ml)

Age	
Adults/infants/children	0.3-6.2
Adults > age 80 years	Up to 10.0
Newborn by day 3	< 20.0
Newborn by day 10	< 10.0
Newborn by day 14	< 6.2

For understanding thyroid hormone levels vis-a-vis ultrasensitive TSH assay, refer to Fig. 17.30.

THYROGLOBULIN ANTIBODIES (Courtesy: Lilac Medicare)

Intended Use: The Quantitative Determination of Thyroglobulin (Tg) Autoantibodies in Human Serum or Plasma by a Microplate Enzyme Immunoassay. Measurements of Tg autoantibodies may aid in the diagnosis of certain thyroid diseases such as Hashimoto's and Graves' as well as nontoxic goiter.

Summary and Explanation of the Test

Antibodies to thyroglobulin have been shown to be characteristically present from patients with thyroiditis and primary thyrotoxicosis. This has lead to the clinical measurement becoming a valuable tool in the diagnosis of thyroid dysfunction.

Passive haemaglutination (PHA) methods have been employed in the past for measurements of antibodies to Tg. PHA tests do not have the sensitivity of enzyme immunoassay and are limited by subjective interpretation. This procedure, with the enhanced sensitivity of EIA, permits the detectability of subclinical levels of antibodies to Tg. In addition, the results are quantitated by a spectrophotometer, which eliminates subjective interpretation.

Monobind's microplate enzyme immunoassay methodology provides the technician with optimum sensitivity while requiring a few technical manipulations. In this method, serum reference, diluted patient specimen, or control is first added to a microplate well. Biotinylated thyroglobulin (Tg) is added, then the reactants are mixed. Reaction results between the autoantibodies to Tg and the biotinylated Tg to form an immune complex, which is deposited to the surface of streptavidin-coated wells through the high affinity reaction of biotin and streptavidin.

After the completion of the required incubation period, aspiration or decantation separates the

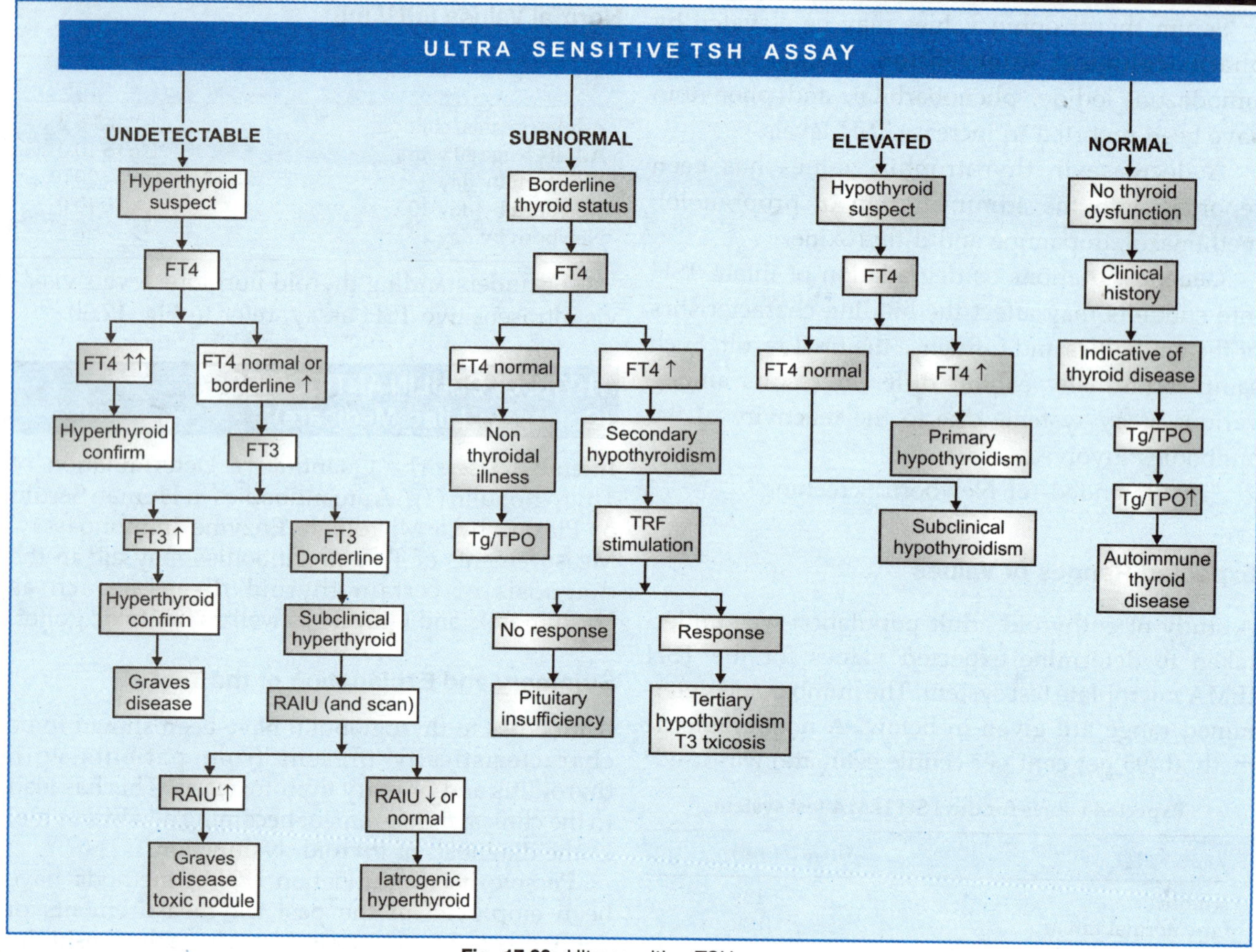

Fig. 17.30: Ultrasensitive TSH assay

reactants that are not attached to the wells. An enzyme anti-human IgG conjugate is then added to permit quantitation of reaction through interaction with human IgG of the immune complex. After washing, the enzyme activity is determined by reaction with substrate to produce color.

The employment of several serum references of known antibody activity permits construction of a graph of enzyme and antibody activities. From comparison to the dose response curve, an unknown specimen's enzyme activity can be correlated with autoimmune antibody level.

PRINCIPLE

A Sequential ELISA Method

The reagents required for the sequential ELISA assay include immobilised antigen, circulating autoantibody and enzyme-linked species specific antibody. In this procedure, the immobilisation takes place during the assay at the surface of a microplate well through the interaction of streptavidin coated on the well and exogenously added biotinylated thyroglobulin antigen.

Upon mixing biotinylated antigen and a serum containing the autoantibody, reaction results between the antigen and the antibody to form an immunocomplex. The interaction is illustrated by the following equation:

$$\text{h-Ab}_{(X\text{-}Tg)} + {}^{Btn}Ag_{(Tg)} \underset{k_{-a}}{\overset{k_a}{\rightleftharpoons}} \text{h-Ab}_{(x\text{-}Tg)}\text{-}{}^{Btn}Ag_{(Tg)}$$

${}^{Btn}Ag_{(Tg)}$ = Biotinylated antigen (constant quantity)

$\text{h-Ab}_{(x\text{-}Tg)}$ = Human auto-antibody (variable quantity)

$Ab_{(x\text{-}Tg)}\text{-}{}^{Btn}Ag_{(T8)}$ = Immune complex (variable quantity)

k_a = Rate constant of association

k_{-a} = Rate constant of disassociation

Simultaneously, the complex is deposited to the well through the high affinity reaction of streptavidin and biotinylated antigen. This interaction is illustrated below:

$h\text{-}Ab_{(x\text{-}Tg)}$ - ${}^{Btn}Ag_{(Tg)}$ + Streptavidin cw→ immobilised complex (IC)

Streptavidin cw = Streptavidin immobolised on well

Immobilised complex = sandwich complex bound to the solid surface

After the incubation time, the well is washed to separate the unbound components by aspiration and/or decantation. The enzyme-linked species specific antibody (anti-h-IgG) is then added to the microwells. This conjugate binds to the immune complex that formed:

IC (h-LgG) + Ab(x-h-LgG)→ Ab(x-h-LgG)-IC (h-IgG)

IC (h-IgG) = Immobilised immune complex (variable quantity)

^{ENZ}Ab(x-h-Igc) = Enzyme-antibody conjugate (constant quantity)

^{ENZ}Ab(x-h-IgG)-IC (h-IgG) = Antigen-antibody complex (variable quantity)

The anti-h-IgG enzyme conjugate that binds to the immune complex in a second incubation is separated from unreacted material by a wash step. The enzyme activity in this fraction is directly proportional to the antibody concentration in the specimen. By utilising several different serum references of known antibody activity, a reference curve can be generated from which the antibody activity of an unknown can be ascertained.

REAGENTS FOR 96-WELL MICROPLATE

A. Anti-Thyroglobulin Calibrators-1.0 ml/vial

Six (6) vials of references for anti-Tg at levels of 0(A), 50(8), 125(C), 500(D), 1000(E), and 2000(F) lU/ml. Store at 2-8°C. A preservative has been added.

Note: The calibrators, human serum based, were calibrated using a reference preparation, which was assayed against the Medical Research Council (MRC) Research Standard A 65/93 for antithyroglobulin activity.

B. Thyroglobulin Biotin Conjugate-11 ml/vial

One (1) vial of biotinylated thyroglobulin in a buffering matrix. A preservative has been added. Store at 2-8°C.

C. Enzyme-antigen Conjugate-11 ml/vial

One (1) vial of anti-human IgG-horseradish peroxidase (HRP) conjugate in a buffering matrix. A preservative has been added. Store at 2-8°C.

D. Streptavidin-Coated Microplate—96 Wells

One 96-well microplate coated with Streptavidin and packaged in an aluminum bag with a drying agent. Store at 2-8°C.

E. Serum Diluent Concentrate-20 ml

One (1) vial of serum diluent containing buffer salts and a dye. Store at 2-8°C (see note below).

F. Wash Solution Concentrate-20 ml Icon

One (1) vial containing a surfactant in phosphate buffered saline. A preservative has been added. Store at 2-8°C.

G. Substrate A ~7.0 ml/vial

One (1) bottle containing tetramethylbenzidine (TMB) in buffer. Store at 2-8°C.

H. Substrate B-7.0 ml/vial

One (1) bottle containing hydrogen peroxide (H_2O_2) in buffer. Store at 2-8°C.

I. Stop Solution-6.0 ml/vial

One (1) bottle of stop solution containing a strong acid (1N HCl). Store at 2-8°C.

Note 1: Do not use reagents beyond the kit expiration date.

Note 2: Opened reagents are stable for sixty (60) days when stored at 2-8°C.

Note 3: The serum diluent concentrate can cloud or show precipitation when stored at 2-8°C. This is normal as the reagent supplied is highly concentrated. Please warm to room temperature to solubilise any precipitant before dilution.

PRECAUTIONS

For In Vitro Diagnostic Use Not for Internal or External Use in Humans or Animals

All Monobind products that contain human serum have been found to be nonreactive for Hepatitis B Surface Antigen, HIV 1 and 2, and HCV Antibodies by FDA required tests. Since no known test can offer complete assurance that infectious agents are absent, all human serum products should be handled as potentially hazardous and capable of transmitting disease. Good laboratory procedures for handling blood products can be found in the Center for Disease Control/National Institute of Health, "Biosafety in Microbiological and Biomedical Laboratories," 2nd Edition, 1988, HHS Publication No. (CDC) 88-8395.

Specimen Collection and Preparation

Collect sample(s) by venipuncture in ten (10) ml silicone evacuated tube(s) or evacuated tube(s) containing EDTA or heparin. The usual precautions in the collection of venipuncture samples should be observed. Separate the red blood cells by centrifugation, use serum or plasma for the anti-Tg procedure. Specimen(s) may be refrigerated at 2-8°C for a maximum period of 48 hours. If the specimen(s) cannot be assayed within 48 hours, the sample(s) may be stored at temperatures of –20°C for up to 30 days. When assayed in duplicate, 0.100 ml of the diluted specimen is required.

MATERIALS

Provided

1. Six (6) vials of serum reference for antithyroglobulin.
2. One (1) vial of thyroglobulin biotin conjugate.
3. One (1) vial of enzyme-anti-h-IgG conjugate.
4. One 96-well streptavidin-coated microplate.
5. One (1) bottle of serum diluent concentrate.
6. One (1) bottle of wash buffer concentrate
7. One (1) bottle of substrate A.
8. One (1) bottle of substrate B.
9. One (1) bottle of stop solution.
10. Instructions.

Required but Not Provided

1. Pipett(s) capable of delivering 10 μl and 50 μl volumes with a precision of <1.5 per cent.
2. Dispenser(s) for repetitive deliveries of 0.100 ml, 0.300 ml and 1.0 ml volumes with a precision of better than 1.5 per cent.
3. Microplate washer (optional) or squeeze bottle to wash plates.
4. Microplate reader with 450 nm wavelength absorbance capability.
5. Test tubes for dilution of patient samples and substrates A and B.
6. Absorbent paper for blotting the microplate wells.
7. Plastic wrap or microplate cover for incubation steps.
8. Vacuum aspirator (optional) for wash steps.
9. Timer.

REAGENT PREPARATION

1. Serum Diluent

Dilute the serum diluent concentrate to 200 ml in a suitable container with distilled or deionized water. Store at 2-8°C.

2. Wash Buffer

Dilute contents of wash concentrate to 1000 ml with distilled or deionized water in a suitable storage container. Store at room temperature until expiration date printed on concentrate label.

3. Patient Sample Dilution (1/100)

Dispense 0.010 ml (10 μl) of each patient specimen into 1 ml of serum diluent. Cover and vortex or mix thoroughly by inversion. Store at 2-8°C for up to forty-eight (48) hours.

4. Working Substrate Solution-Prepare Immediately before Use

Determine the amount of reagent needed and prepare by mixing equal portions of substrate A and substrate B in a suitable container. For example, add 1 ml of A and 1 ml of B per two (2) eight well strips (a) slight excess of solution is made). Use within one (1) hour of preparation for maximum performance of the assay.

Test Procedure

Before *proceeding with the assay, bring all reagents, serum references and controls to room temperature (20-30°C).*

1. Format the microplates wells for each serum reference, control and patient specimen to be assayed in duplicate.
2. Pipette 0.050 ml (50 μl) of the appropriate serum reference.
3. Add 0.100 ml (100 μl) of Tg biotinylated conjugate solution.

4. Swirl the microplate gently for 20-30 seconds to mix and cover.
5. Incubate 60 minutes at room temperature.
6. Discard the contents of the microplate by decantation or aspiration. If decanting, blot the plate dry with absorbent paper.
7. Add 300 μl of wash buffer (see reagent preparation section), decant (blot and tap) or aspirate. Repeat two (2) additional times for a total of three (3) washes. An automatic or manual plate washer can be used. Follow the manufacturer's instruction for proper usage. If a squeeze bottle is employed, fill each well by depressing the container (avoiding air bubbles) to dispense the wash. Decant the wash and repeat two (2) additional times.
8. Add 0.100 ml (100 μl) of enzyme anti-h-IgG conjugate solution to all wells. Always add reagents in the same order to minimise reaction time differences between wells.
9. Swirl the microplate gently, cover and incubate for thirty (30) minutes at room temperature.
10. Repeat steps (6 and 7) as explained above.
11. Add 0.100 ml (100 μl) of working substrate solution to all wells (see reagent preparation section). Always add reagents in the same order to minimise reaction time differences between wells.
12. Incubate at room temperature for fifteen (15) minutes.
13. Add 0.050 ml (50 μl) of stop solution to each well and mix gently for 15-20 seconds. Always add reagents in the same order to minimise reaction time differences between wells.
14. Read the absorbance in each well at 450 nm in a microplate reader. The results should be read within thirty (30) minutes of adding the stop solution.

Note: For re-assaying specimens with concentrations greater than 2000 ID/ml, dilute the sample an additional 1:10 or 1:50 using the original diluted material. Multiply by the dilution factor to obtain the concentration of the specimen.

Quality Control

Each laboratory should assay and establish reference intervals for clinically relevant controls to monitor assay performance. These controls should be treated as unknowns and values determined in every test procedure performed. Quality control charts should be maintained to follow the performance of the supplied reagents. Pertinent statistical methods should be employed to ascertain trends. The individual laboratory should set acceptable assay performance limits. Other parameters that should be monitored include the 80, 50 and 20 per cent intercepts of the dose response curve for run-to-run reproducibility. In addition, maximum absorbance should be consistent with past experience. Significant deviation from established performance can indicate unnoticed change in experimental conditions or degradation of kit reagents. Fresh reagents should be used to determine the reason for the variations.

Results

A reference curve is used to ascertain the concentration of anti-Tg in unknown specimens.

1. Record the absorbance obtained from the printout of the microplate reader as outlined in Example 7.
2. Plot the absorbance for each duplicate serum reference versus the corresponding anti-Tg activity in IU/ml on linear graph paper (do not average the duplicates of the serum references before plotting).
3. Draw the best-fit curve through the plotted points.
4. To determine the level of Anti-Tg activity for an unknown, locate the average absorbance of the duplicates for each unknown on the vertical axis of the graph, find the intersecting point on the curve, and read the concentration (in ID/ml) from the horizontal axis of the graph (the duplicates of the unknown may be averaged as indicated). In the following example, the average absorbance 1.387 (intersects the dose response curve) at 790 ID/ml anti-Tg concentration (See Figure 17.31). *

Example 7

Well	Calibrator	Absorbance
1	0 ID/ml	0.022
2	0 IU/ml	0.028
3	50 IU/ml	0.135
4	50 IU/ml	0.131
5	125 IU/ml	0.280
6	125 IU/ml	0.261
7	500 IU/ml	0.962
8	500 IU/ml	0.936
9	1000 IU/ml	1.709
10	1000 IU/ml	1.698
11	2000 IU/ml	2.739
12	2000 IU/ml	2.667

Well	Unknown ID	OD	Avg OD	Value
13	Unknown #1	1.390		
14	Unknown #1	1.383	1.387	790 IU/ ml

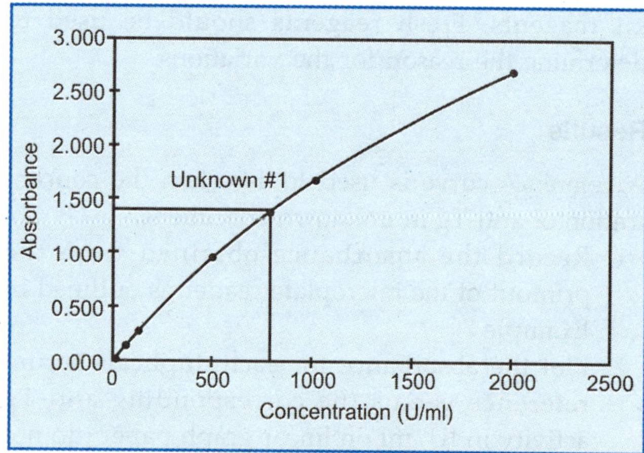

Fig. 17.31: Estimation of antithyroglobulin in u/ml

*The data presented in Example 7 and Fig 17.31 are for illustration only and should not be used in lieu of a standard curve prepared with each assay.

QC Parameters

Maximum Absorbance (2000 IU/ml calibrator) =1.8-2.8. Anti-Tg concentration at 80 per cent maximum absorbance = 1460 + 250 IU/ml

Anti-Tg Concentration at 50 per cent maximum absorbance = 765 ± 125 IU/ml Anti-Tg Concentration at 20 per cent maximum absorbance = 275 ± 50 IU/ ml.

LIMITATIONS OF PROCEDURE

A. Assay Performance

It is important that the time of reaction in each well is held constant for reproducible results. Pipetting of samples should not extend beyond ten (10) minutes to avoid assay drift. If more than one (1) plate is used, it is recommended to repeat the dose response curve.

Addition of the substrate solution initiates a kinetic reaction, which is terminated by the addition of the stop solution. Therefore, the addition of the substrate and the stopping solution should be performed in the same sequence to eliminate any time deviation during reaction.

Plate readers measure vertically. Do not touch the bottom of the wells.

Failure to remove adhering solution adequately in the aspiration or decantation wash step(s) may result in poor replication and spurious results.

Very high concentration of anti-Tg in patient specimens can contaminate samples immediately following these extreme levels. Bad duplicates are indicative of cross contamination. Repeat any sample, which follows any patient specimen with over 3.0 units of absorbance.

Samples, which are contaminated microbiologically, should not be used.

B. Interpretation

If computer-controlled data reduction is used to interpret the results of the test, it is imperative that the predicted values for the calibrators fall within 10 per cent of the assigned concentrations.

The presence of autoantibodies to Tg is confirmed when the serum level exceeds 125 IU/ml. The clinical significance of the result, coupled with antithyroid peroxidase activity, should be used in evaluating the thyroid condition. However, clinical inferences should not be solely based on this test but rather as an adjunct to the clinical manifestations of the patient and other relevant tests.

The cost benefits should be considered in the use of thyroglobulin antibodies testing when performed in concent with antithyroid peroxidase (TPO). The widespread practice of performing both tests has been questioned.

Expected Range of Values

A study of normal population was undertaken to determine expected values for the anti-Tg microplate test system. The number (n), mean (x) and standard deviation are given below. Values in excess of 125 IU/ml are considered positive for the presence of anti-Tg autoantibodies.

Expected values for the anti-Tg ELISA test system

	(in IU/ml)
Number (n)	100
Mean (x)	74.3
Standard deviation (*)	25.2
Upper 95 per cent (+2*) level	124.7

It is important to keep in mind that establishment of a range of values which can be expected to be found by a given method for a population of "normal"persons is dependent upon a multiplicity of factors: the specificity of the method, the population tested and the precision of the method in the hands of the analyst. For these reasons, each laboratory should depend upon the range of expected values established by the manufacturer only until an in-house range can be determined by the analysts using the method with a population indigenous to the area in which the laboratory is located.

THYROID PEROXIDASE ANTIBODIES (Courtesy; Lilac Medicare)

Intended Use: The Quantitative Determination of Thyroid Peroxidase (TPO) Autoantibodies in Human Serum or Plasma by a Microplate Enzyme Immunoassay. Measurements of TPO autoantibodies may aid in the diagnosis of certain thyroid diseases such as Hashimoto's and Graves' as well as nontoxic goitre.

Summary and Explanation of the Test

Antibodies to thyroid peroxidase have been shown to be characteristically present from patients with Hashimoto's thyroiditis (95 per cent), idiopathic myxoedema (90 per cent) and Graves' disease (80 per cent). In fact, 72 per cent of patients positive for anti-TPO exhibit some degree of thyroid dysfunction. This has lead to the clinical measurement becoming a valuable tool in the diagnosis of thyroid dysfunction.

Measurements of antibodies to TPO have been done, in the past, by passive haemaglutination (PHA). PHA tests do not have the sensitivity of enzyme immunoassay and are limited by subjective interpretation. This procedure, with the enhanced sensitivity of EIA, permits the detectability of subclinical levels of antibodies to TPO. In addition, the results are quantitated by a spectrophotometer, which eliminates subjective interpretation.

Monobind's microplate enzyme immunoassay methodology provides the technician with optimum sensitivity, while requiring a few technical manipulations. In this method, serum reference, diluted patient specimen, or control is first added to a microplate well. Biotinylated thyroid peroxidase Antigen (TPO) is added, then the reactants are mixed. Reaction results between the autoantibodies to TPO and the biotinylated TPO to form an immune complex, which is deposited to the surface of streptavidin-coated wells through the high affinity reaction of biotin and streptavidin.

After the completion of the required incubation period, aspiration or decantation separates the reactants that are not attached to the wells. An enzyme anti-human IgG conjugate is then added to permit quantitation of reaction through interacting with human IgG of the immune complex. After washing, the enzyme activity is determined by reaction with substrate to produce color.

The employment of several serum references of known antibody activity permits construction of a graph of enzyme and antibody activities. From comparison to the dose response curve, an unknown specimen's enzyme activity can be correlated with autoimmune antibody level.

PRINCIPLE

A Sequential ELISA Method

The reagents required for the sequential ELISA assay include immobilised antigen, circulating autoantibody and enzyme-linked species specific antibody. In this procedure, the immobilisation takes place during the assay at the surface of a microplate well through the interaction of streptavidin-coated on the well and exogenous added biotinylated thyroid peroxidase antigen.

Upon mixing biotinylated antigen and a serum containing the autoantibody, reaction results between the antigen and the antibody to form an immunocomplex. The interaction is illustrated by the following equation:

$$\text{h-Ab}_{(\text{a-TPO})} + {}^{\text{Bln}}\text{Ag}_{(\text{TPO})} \underset{\text{k-a}}{\xrightarrow{\text{ka}}} \text{h-Ab}\,(\text{x-}_{\text{T}}\text{po})\text{-}^{\text{Btn}}\text{Agn}_{(\text{TPO})}$$

${}^{\text{Btn}}\text{Ag}_{(\text{TPO})}$ = Biotinylated antigen (constant quantity)

$\text{h-Ab}_{(\text{a-TPO})}$ = Human auto-antibody (variable quantity)

$\text{Ab}_{(\text{a-TPO})}\text{-}^{\text{Btn}}\text{Ag}_{(\text{TPO})}$ = Immune complex (variable quantity)

k_a = Rate constant of association

k_a = Rate constant of disassociation

Simultaneously, the complex is deposited to the well through the high affinity reaction of streptavidin and biotinylated antigen. This interaction is illustrated below:

h-Ab(x-TPoi -^{Btn}Ag(Tpo) + Streptavidin cw→ immobilised complex (IC)

Streptavidin cw = Streptavidin immobolized on well

Immobilised complex = Sandwich complex bound to the solid surface

After the incubation time, the well is washed to separate the unbound components by aspiration and/or decantation. The enzyme-linked species specific antibody (anti-h-IgG) is then added to the microwells. This conjugate binds to the immune complex that formed.

$$IC_{(h\text{-}IgG)} + {}^{ENZ}Ab_{(x\text{-}h\text{-}IgG)} \rightarrow Ab_{(x\text{-}h\text{-}IgG)}\text{-}IC\ (h\text{-}IgG)$$

IC (hIgG)	= Immobilised immune complex (variable quantity)
^{ENZ}Ab(x-h-IgG)	= Enzyme-antibody conjugate (constant quantity)
^{ENZ}Ab(x-h-IgG)- I-C (h-IgG)	= Antigen-antibody complex (variable quantity)

The anti-h-IgG enzyme conjugate that binds to the immune complex in a second incubation is separated from unreacted material by a wash step. The enzyme activity in this fraction is directly proportional to the antibody concentration in the specimen. By utilising several different serum references of known antibody activity, a reference curve can be generated from which the antibody activity of an unknown can be ascertained.

REAGENTS FOR 96-WELL MICROPLATE

A. Anti-TPO Calibrators-1.0 ml/vial

Six (6) vials of references for anti-TPO at levels of 0(A), 25(B), 50(C), 100(D), 250(E) and 500(F) ID/ml. Store at 2-8°C. A preservative has been added.

Note: The calibrators, human serum based, were calibrated using a reference preparation, which was assayed against the Medical Research Council (MRC) International Standard 66/287 for thyroid microsome.

Thyroid Peroxidase Biotin Conjugate-11 ml/vial-Icon One (1) vial of biotinylated thyroid perxidase (TPO). The widespread practice of performing both tests has been questioned.

B. Thyroid Peroxidase Biotin Conjugate-11 ml/vial

One (1) vial of biotinylated thyroid peroxidase in a buffering matrix. A preservative has been added. Store at 2-8°C.

C. Enzyme-antigen Conjugate-11 ml/vial

One (1) vial of anti-human IgG-horseradish peroxidase (HRP) conjugate in a buffering matrix. A preservative has been added. Store at 2-8°C.

D. Streptavidin-Coated Microplate-96 Wells

One 96-well microplate coated with Streptavidin and packaged in an aluminum bag with a drying agent. Store at 2-8°C.

E. Serum Diluent Concentrate—20 ml

One (1) vial of serum diluent containing buffer salts and a dye. Store at 2-8°C (See note 3).

F. Wash Solution Concentrate-20 ml

One (1) vial containing a surfactant in phosphate buffered saline. A preservative has been added. Store at 2-8°C.

G. Substrate A-7.0 ml/vial

One (1) bottle containing tetramethylbenzidine (TMB) in buffer. Store at 2-8°C.

H. Substrate B-7.0 ml/vial

One (1) bottle containing hydrogen peroxide (H_2O_2) in buffer. Store at 2-8°C.

I. Stop Solution-6.0 ml/vial

One (1) bottle containing a strong acid (1N HCl). Store at 2-8°C.

Note 1: Do not use reagents beyond the kit expiration date.

Note 2: Opened reagents are stable for sixty (60) days when stored at 2-8°C.

Note 3: The serum diluent concentrate can cloud or show precipitation when stored at 2-8°C. This is normal as the reagent supplied is highly concentrated. Please warm to room temperature to solubilise any precipitant before dilution.

Precautions

For In Vitro Diagnostic Use

Not for Internal or External Use in Humans or Animals

All products that contain human serum have been found to be nonreactive for Hepatitis B Surface Antigen, HIV 1 and 2 and HCV Antibodies by FDA required tests. Since no known test can offer complete assurance that infectious agents are absent, all human serum products should be handled as potentially hazardous and capable of transmitting disease. Good laboratory procedures for handling blood products can be found in the Center for Disease Control/ National Institute of Health, "Biosafety in Microbiological and Biomedical Laboratories," 2nd Edition, 1988, HHS Publication No. (CDC) 88-8395.

Specimen Collection and Preparation

Collect sample(s) by venipuncture in ten (10) ml silicone evacuated tube(s) or evacuated tube(s) containing EDTA or heparin. The usual precautions in the collection of venipuncture samples should be observed. Separate the red blood cells by centrifugation, use serum or plasma for the anti-TPO procedure. Specimen(s) may be refrigerated at 2-8°C for a maximum period of 48 hours. If the specimen(s) cannot be assayed within 48 hours, the sample(s) may be stored at temperatures of –20°C for up to 30 days. When assayed in duplicate, 0.05 ml of the diluted specimen is required.

MATERIALS

Provided

1. Six (6) vials of serum reference for anti-thyroid peroxidase.
2. One (1) vial of thyroid peroxidase biotin conjugate.
3. One (1) vial of enzyme-anti-h-IgG conjugate.
4. One 96-well streptavidin-coated microplate.
5. One(1) vial of serum diluent concentrate
6. One (1) bottle of wash buffer concentrate.
7. One (1) bottle of substrate A.
8. One (1) bottle of substrate B.
9. One (1) bottle of stop solution.
10. Instructions.

Required but Not Provided

1. Pipette(s) capable of delivering 10 μl and 25 μl volumes with a precision of <1.5 per cent.
2. Dispenser(s) for repetitive deliveries of 0.100 ml, 0.300 ml and 1.0 ml volumes with a precision of better than 1.5 per cent.
3. Microplate washer (optional) or squeeze bottle to wash plates.
4. Microplate reader with 450 nm wavelength absorbance capability.
5. Test tubes for dilution of patient samples and substrate A and B.
6. Absorbent paper for blotting the microplate wells.
7. Plastic wrap or microplate cover for incubation steps.
8. Vacuum aspirator for wash steps (optional).
9. Timer.

REAGENT PREPARATION

1. Serum Diluent

Dilute the serum diluent concentrate to 200 ml in a suitable container with distilled or deionized water. Store at 2-8°C.

2. Wash Buffer

Dilute contents of wash concentrate to 1000 ml with distilled or deionized water in a suitable storage container. Store at room temperature until expiration date printed on concentrate label.

3. Patient Sample Dilution (1/100)

Dispense 0.010 ml (10 μl) of each patient specimen into 1 ml of serum diluent. Cover and vortex or mix thoroughly by inversion. Store at 2-8°C for up to forty-eight (48) hours.

4. Working Substrate Solution-Prepare Immediately before use

Determine the amount of reagent needed and prepare by mixing equal portions of substrate A and substrate B in a suitable container. For example, add 1 ml of A and 1 ml of B per two (2) eight well strips (a slight excess of solution is made). Use within one (1) hour of preparation for maximum performance of the assay.

Test Procedure

Before proceeding with the assay, bring all reagents, serum references and controls to room temperature (20-30°C).

1. Format the microplates' wells for each serum reference, control and patient specimen to be assayed in duplicate.
2. Pipette 0.025 ml (25 μl) of the appropriate serum reference, control or diluted patient specimen into the assigned well.
3. Add 0.100 ml (100 μl) of TPO biotinylated conjugate solution.
4. Swirl the microplate gently for 20-30 seconds to mix and cover.
5. Incubate 60 minutes at room temperature.
6. Discard the contents of the microplate by decantation or aspiration. If decanting, blot the plate dry with absorbent paper.
7. Add 300 μl of wash buffer (see reagent preparation section), decant (blot) or aspirate. Repeat two (2) additional times for a total of three (3) washes. An automatic or manual plate washer can be used. Follow the manufacturer's instruction for proper usage. If a squeeze bottle is employed, fill each well by depressing the container (avoiding air bubbles) to dispense the wash. Decant the wash and repeat two (2) additional times.
8. Add 0.100 ml (100 μl) of enzyme anti-h-IgG conjugate solution to all wells. Always add reagents in the same order to minimise reaction time differences between wells.
9. Swirl the microplate gently, cover and incubate for thirty (30) minutes at room temperature.
10. Repeat steps (6 and 7) as explained above.
11. Add 0.100 ml (100 μl) of working substrate solution to all wells (see reagent preparation section). Always add reagents in the same order to minimise reaction time differences between wells.
12. Incubate at room temperature for fifteen (15) minutes.
13. Add 0.050 ml (50 μl) of stop solution to each well and mix gently for 15-20 seconds. Always add reagents in the same order to minimise reaction time differences between wells.
14. Read the absorbance in each well at 450 nm in a microplate reader. The results should be read within thirty (30) minutes of adding the stop solution.

Note: For re-assaying specimens with concentrations greater than 500 IU/ml, dilute the sample an additional 1:10 or 1:100 using the original diluted material. Multiply by the dilution factor to obtain the concentration of the specimen.

Quality Control

Each laboratory should assay and establish reference intervals for clinically relevant controls to monitor assay performance. These controls should be treated as unknowns and values determined in every test procedure performed. Quality control charts should be maintained to follow the performance of the supplied reagents. Pertinent statistical methods should be employed to ascertain trends. The individual laboratory should set acceptable assay performance limits. Other parameters that should be monitored include the 80, 50 and 20 per cent intercepts of the standard curve for run-to-run reproducibility. In addition, maximum absorbance should be consistent with past experience. Significant deviation from established performance can indicate unnoticed change in experimental conditions or degradation of kit reagents. Fresh reagents should be used to determine the reason for the variations.

Results

A reference curve is used to ascertain the concentration of anti-TPO in unknown specimens.

1. Record the absorbance obtained from the printout of the microplate reader as outlined in Example 8.
2. Plot the absorbance for each duplicate serum reference versus the corresponding anti-TPO activity in ID/ml on linear graph paper (do not average the duplicates of the serum references before plotting).
3. Draw the best-fit curve through the plotted points.
4. To determine the level of anti-TPO activity for an unknown, locate the average absorbance of the duplicates for each unknown on the vertical axis of the graph, find the intersecting point on the curve, and read the concentration (in ID/ml) from the horizontal axis of the graph (the duplicates of the unknown may be averaged as indicated). In the following example, the aver-

age absorbance 1.15 (intersects the dose response curve) at 200 IU/ ml anti-TPO concentration (See Figure 17.32).*

Example 8

Well	Calibrator	Absorbance
1	0 IU/ml	0.068
2	0 IU/ml	0.069
3	25IU/ml	0.209
4	25 IU/ml	0.215
5	50 IU/ml	0.380
6	50 IU/ml	0.367
7	100 IU/ml	0.691
8	100 ID/ml	0.680
9	250 IU/ml	1.400
10	250 ID/ml	1.366
11	500 IU/ml	2.312
12	500 IU/ml	2.203

Well	Unknown ID	OD	Avg. OD	Value
13	Unknown #1	1.125		
14	Unknown#1	1.175	1.150	200 IU/ml

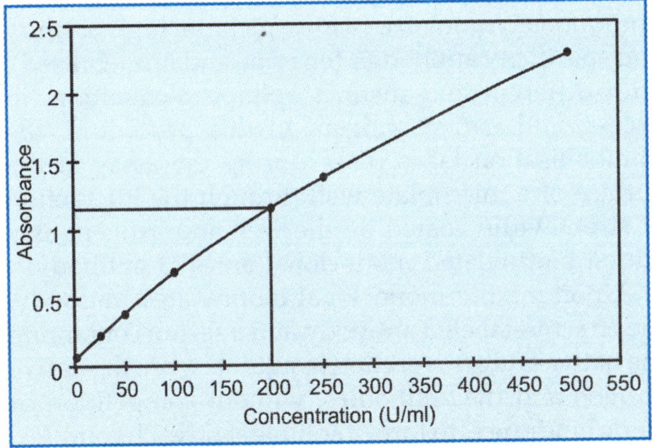

Fig. 17.32: Estimation of anti TPO in U/ml

*The data presented in Example 8 and Figure 17.32 are for illustration only and should not be used in lieu of a standard curve prepared with each assay.

QC Parameters

Maximum absorbance (500 IU/ ml calibrator) = 15-2.7 Anti-TPO Concentration at 80 per cent maximum absorbance = 370 ± 50 IU/ml. Anti-TPO concentration at 50 per cent maximum absorbance = 210 ± 35 IU/ ml. Anti-TPO concentration at 20 per cent maximum absorbance = 65 + 25 IU/ml.

LIMITATIONS OF PROCEDURE

A. Assay Performance

It is important that the time of reaction in each well is held constant for reproducible results. Pipetting of samples should not extend beyond ten (10) minutes to avoid assay drift. If more than one (1) plate is used, it is recommended to repeat the dose response curve.

Addition of the substrate solution initiates a kinetic reaction, which is terminated by the addition of the stop solution. Therefore, the addition of the substrate and the stopping solution should be added in the same sequence to eliminate anytime deviation during reaction.

Plate readers measure vertically. Do not touch the bottom of the wells.

Failure to remove adhering solution adequately in the aspiration or decantation wash step(s) may result in poor replication and spurious results.

Very high concentration of anti-TPO in patient specimens can contaminate samples immediately following these extreme levels. Bad duplicates are indicative of cross contamination. Repeat any sample, which follows any patient specimen with over 3.0 units of absorbance.

Samples, which are contaminated microbiologically, should not be used.

B. Interpretation

If computer-controlled data reduction is used to interpret the results of the test, it is imperative that the predicted values for the calibrators fall within 10 per cent of the assigned concentrations.

The presence of autoantibodies to TPO is confirmed when the serum level exceeds 40 ID/ml. The clinical significance of the result, coupled with antithyroglobulin activity, should be used in evaluating the thyroid condition. However, clinical inferences should not be solely based on this test but rather as an adjunct to the clinical manifestations of the patient and other relevant tests.

Expected Range of Values

A study of normal population was undertaken to determine expected values for the Anti-TPO microplate test system. The number (n), mean (x) and standard deviation are given below. Values in excess of 40 IU/ ml are considered positive for the presence of anti-TPO autoantibodies.

Expected values for the anti-TPO ELISA test system

	(in IU/ ml)
Number (n)	100
Mean (x)	17.6
Standard deviation (r)	10.8
Upper 95 per cent (+2a) level	39.2

It is important to keep in mind that establishment of a range of values which can be expected to be found by a given method for a population of "normal" persons is dependent upon a multiplicity of factors: the specificity of the method, the population tested and the precision of the method in the hands of the analyst. For these reasons, each laboratory should depend upon the range of expected values established by the manufacturer only until an in-house range can be determined by the analysts using the method with a population indigenous to the area in which the laboratory is located.

LUTEINISING HORMONE (LH) Courtesy: Lilac Medicare

Intended Use: The Quantitative Determination of Luteinising Hormone Concentration in Human Serum by a Microplate Immunoenzymometric Assay

Summary and Explanation of the Test

Luteinising hormone (LH) is a glycoprotein consisting of two subunits with a molecular mass of 30,000 daltons. The cc-subunit is similar to other pituitary hormones [follicle-stimulating hormone (FSH) thyroid-stimulating hormone (TSH) and chorionic gonadotrophin hCG)], while the β-subunit is unique. The β-subunit confers the biological activity to the molecule. The α-subunit consists of 89 amino acid residues, while the p-subunit contains 129 amino acids. The carbohydrate content is between 15 and 30 percent.

The clinical usefulness of the measurement of luteinising hormone (LH) in ascertaining the homeostasis of fertility regulation via the hypothalamic-pituitary-gonadal axis has been well established. In addition, the advent of *in vitro* fertilisation (IVF) technology to overcome infertility associated problems has provided the impetus for rapid improvement in LH assay methodology from the technically demanding bioassay to the procedurally simple and rapid immunoenzymometric assays.

In this method, LH calibrator, patient specimen or control is first added to a streptavidin-coated well. Biotinylated monoclonal and enzyme-labelled antibodies (directed against distinct and different epitopes of LH) are added and the reactants mixed. Reaction between the various LH antibodies and native LH forms a sandwich complex that binds with the streptavidin-coated to the well.

After the completion of the required incubation period, the enzyme-luteinising hormone antibody bound conjugate is separated from the unbound enzyme-luteinising hormone conjugate by aspiration or decantation. The activity of the enzyme present on the surface of the well is quantitated by reaction with a suitable substrate to produce color.

The employment of several serum references of known luteinising hormone levels permits construction of a dose response curve of activity and concentration. From comparison to the dose response curve, an unknown specimen's activity can be correlated with luteinising hormone concentration.

PRINCIPLE

Immunoenzymometric Assay

The essential reagents required for an immunoenzymometric assay include high affinity and specificity antibodies (enzyme and immobilised), with different and distinct epitope recognition, in excess, and native antigen. In this procedure, the immobilisation takes place during the assay at the surface of a microplate well through the interaction of streptavidin coated on the well and exogenously added biotinylated monoclonal anti-LH antibody.

Upon mixing monoclonal biotinylated antibody, the enzyme-labeled antibody and a serum containing the native antigen, reaction results between the native antigen and the antibodies, without competition or steric hindrance, to form a soluble sandwich complex. The interaction is illustrated by the following equation:

$$^{Enz}Ab_{(p)} + Ag_{LH} + {^{Btn}Ab_{(m)}} \underset{k_{-a}}{\overset{k_a}{\rightarrow}} {^{Enz}AB_{(p)}}\text{-}Ag_{LH}\text{-}{^{Btn}Ab_{(m)}}$$

$^{Btn}Ab_{(m)}$ = Biotinylated monoclonal antibody (excess quantity)

Ag_{LH} = Native antigen (variable quantity)

$^{Enz}Ab_{(p)}$ = Enzyme-labeled polyclonal antibody (excess quantity)

$^{Enz}Ab_{(p)}–Ag_{LH}–{^{Btn}Ab_{(m)}}$ = Antigen-antibodies sandwich complex

k_a = Rate constant of association

$k\text{-}_a$ = Rate constant of dissociation

Simultaneously, the complex is deposited to the well through the high affinity reaction of streptavidin and biotinylated antibody. This interaction is illustrated below:

$^{Enz}Ab_{(p)}$-AgLH-$^{Btn}Ab_{(m)}$ + Streptavidin$_{cw}$→ immobilised complex

Streptovidin$_{cw}$ = Streptavidin immobolised on well

Immobilised complex = Sandwich complex bound to the solid surface

After equilibrium is attained, the antibody-bound fraction is separated from unbound antigen by decantation or aspiration. The enzyme activity in the antibody-bound fraction is directly proportional to the native antigen concentration. By utilising several different serum references of known antigen values, a dose response curve can be generated from which the antigen concentration of an unknown can be ascertained.

REAGENTS FOR 96-WELL MICROPLATE

A. Luteinising Hormone Calibrators—1.0 ml/vial

Six (6) vials of references for LH Antigen at levels of 0(A), 5(B), 25(C), 50(D), 100(E) and 200(F) mlU/ml. Store at 2-B°C. A preservative has been added.

Note: The calibrators, human serum based, were calibrated using a reference preparation, which was assayed against the WHO IRP (68/40).

B. Enzyme-Polyclonal Conjugate and Biotinylated Monoclonal Antibody—11 ml/vial

One (1) vial containing enzyme-labeled affinity purified goat antibody, biotinylated monoclonal mouse IgG in buffer, dye, and preservative. Store at 2-8°C.

C. Streptavidin-Coated Microplate - 96 Wells

One 96-well microplate coated with streptavidin and packaged in an aluminum bag with a drying agent. Store at 2-8°C.

D. Wash Solution Concentrate - 20 ml

One (1) vial containing a surfactant in phosphate buffered saline. A preservative has been added. Store at 2-30°C.

E. Substrate A -7.0 ml/vial

One (1) bottle containing tetramethylbenzidine (TMB) in buffer. Store at 2-8°C.

F. Substrate B - 7.0 ml/vial

One (1) bottle containing hydrogen peroxide (H_2O_2) in buffer. Store at 2-8°C.

G. Stop Solution - 6.0 ml/vial

One (1) bottle containing a strong acid (1N HCl). Store at 2-30°C.

Note 1: Do not use reagents beyond the kit expiration date.

Note 2: Opened reagents are stable for sixty (60) days when stored at 2-8°C.

For In Vitro Diagnostic Use Not for Internal or External Use in Humans or Animals

Precautions

All products that contain human serum have been found to be nonreactive for Hepatitis B Surface Antigen, HIV 1 and 2 and HCV Antibodies by FDA required tests. Since no known test can offer complete assurance that infectious agents are absent, all human serum products should be handled as potentially hazardous and capable of transmitting disease. Good laboratory procedures for handling blood products can be found in the Center for Disease Control/ National Institute of Health, "Biosafety in Microbiological and Biomedical Laboratories," 2nd Edition, 1988, HHS.

Specimen Collection and Preparation

The specimens shall be blood serum in type and the usual precautions in the collection of venipuncture samples should be observed. For accurate comparison to established normal values, a fasting morning serum sample should be obtained. The blood should be collected in a plain redcap venipuncture tube without additives or gel barrier. Allow the blood to clot. Centrifuge the specimen to separate the serum from the cells.

Samples may be refrigerated at 2-8°C for a maximum period of five (5) days. If the specimen(s) cannot be assayed within this time, the sample(s) may be stored at temperatures of –20°C for up to 30 days. Avoid repetitive freezing and thawing. When assayed in duplicate, 0.100 ml of the specimen is required.

MATERIALS

Provided

1. Six (6) vials of luteinising hormone serum calibrators.
2. One (1) vial of combined biotinylated monoclonal antibody and enzyme-labeled polyclonal reagent.
3. One 96-well streptavidin-coated microplate.
4. One (1) bottle of wash buffer concentrate.
5. One (1) bottle of substrate A.
6. One (1) bottle of substrate B.
7. One (1) bottle of stop solution.
8. Instructions.

Required but Not Provided

1. Pipette(s) capable of delivering 50 µl and 100 µl volumes with a precision of better than 1.5 per cent
2. Dispenser(s) for repetitive deliveries of 0.100 ml and 0.300 ml volumes with a precision of better than 1.5 per cent (optional)
3. Microplate washer or a squeeze bottle (optional)
4. Microplate reader with 450 nm wavelength absorbance capability
5. Container(s) for mixing of reagents (see below)
6. Absorbent paper for blotting the microplate wells
7. Plastic wrap or microplate cover for incubation steps
8. Vacuum aspirator (optional) for wash steps
9. Timer
10. Storage container for storage of wash buffer
11. Distilled or deionized water.

REAGENT PREPARATION

1. Working Reagent 1 - Wash Buffer

Dilute contents of wash concentrate to 1000 ml with distilled or deionized water in a suitable storage container. Store at room temperature.

2. Working Reagent 2-Substrate Solution - Prepare before Use

Determine the amount of reagent needed and prepare by mixing equal portions of substrate A and substrate B in a suitable container. For example, add 1 ml of A and 1 ml of B per two (2) eight well strips (a slight excess of solution is made). Use within one (1) hour of preparation for maximum performance of the assay.

Test Procedure

Before proceeding with the assay, bring all reagents, serum references and controls to room temperature.

1. Format the microplates' wells for each serum reference, control and patient specimen to be assayed in duplicate. Replace any unused microwell strips back into the aluminum bag, seal and store at 2-8°C.
2. Pipette 0.050 ml (50 µl) of the appropriate serum reference, control or specimen into the assigned well.
3. Add 0.100 ml (100 µl) of the biotinylated/enzyme-labeled antibodies to each well. It is very important to dispense all reagents close to the bottom of the coated well.
4. Swirl the microplate gently for 20-30 seconds to mix and cover.
5. Incubate 60 minutes at room temperature.
6. Discard the contents of the microplate by decantation or aspiration. If decanting, tap and blot the plate dry with absorbent paper.
7. Add 300 µl of wash buffer (see reagent preparation section), decant (tap and blot) or aspirate. Repeat two (2) additional times for a total of three (3) washes. An automatic or manual plate washer can be used. Follow the manufacturer's instruction for proper usage. If a squeeze bottle is employed, fill each well by depressing the container (avoiding air bubbles) to dispense the wash. Decant the wash and repeat two (2) additional times.
8. Add 0.100 ml (100ul) of working substrate solution to all wells (see reagent preparation section). Always add reagents in the same order to minimise reaction time differences between wells.
9. Incubate at room temperature for fifteen (15) minutes.
10. Add 0.050 ml (50 µl) of stop solution to each well. Always add reagents in the same order to minimise reaction time differences between wells.
11. Read the absorbance in each well at 450 nm in a microplate reader. The results should be read within thirty (30) minutes of adding the stop solution.

Quality Control

Each laboratory should assay controls at levels in the low, normal and elevated range for monitoring assay performance. These controls should be treated as unknowns and values determined in every test procedure performed. Quality control charts should be maintained to follow the performance of the supplied reagents. Pertinent statistical methods should be employed to ascertain trends. The individual laboratory should set acceptable assay performance limits. Other parameters that should be monitored include the 80, 50 and 20 per cent intercepts of the dose response curve for run-to-run reproducibility. In addition, maximum absorbance should be consistent with past experience. Significant deviation from established performance can indicate unnoticed change in experimental conditions or degradation of kit reagents. Fresh reagents should be used to determine the reason for the variations.

Results

A dose response curve is used to ascertain the concentration of luteinising hormone in unknown specimens.

1. Record the absorbance obtained from the printout of the microplate reader as outlined in Example 9.
2. Plot the absorbance for each duplicate serum reference versus the corresponding LH concentration in mlU/ml on linear graph paper (do not average the duplicates of the serum references before plotting).
3. Draw the best-fit curve through the plotted points.
4. To determine the concentration of LH for an unknown, locate the average absorbance of the duplicates for each unknown on the vertical axis of the graph, find the intersecting point on the curve, and read the concentration (in mill/ml) from the horizontal axis of the graph (the duplicates of the unknown may be averaged as indicated). In the following example, the average absorbance (0.578) intersects the dose response curve at (43 mlU/ml) LH concentration (See Figure 17.33).

Note: Computer data reduction software designed for IEMA assays may also be used for the data reduction.

Example 9

Well	*Serum References*	*Absorbance*
1	0.0 mlU/ml	0.012
2	0.0 mlU/ml	0.012
3	5.0 mlU/ml	0.065
4	5.0 mlU/ml	0.070
5	25.0 mlU/ml	0.322
6	25.0 mlU/ml	0.350
7	50.0 mlU/ml	0.687
8	50.0 mlU/ml	0.710
9	100.0 mlU/ml	1.325
10	100.0 rnlU/ml	1.351
11	200.0 mlU/ml	2.495
12	200.0 mlU/ml	2.403

Well	**Unknown ID**	**OD**	**Avg. OD**	**Value**
13	Unknown #1	0.575		
14	Unknown #1	0.580	0.578	43m IU/ml

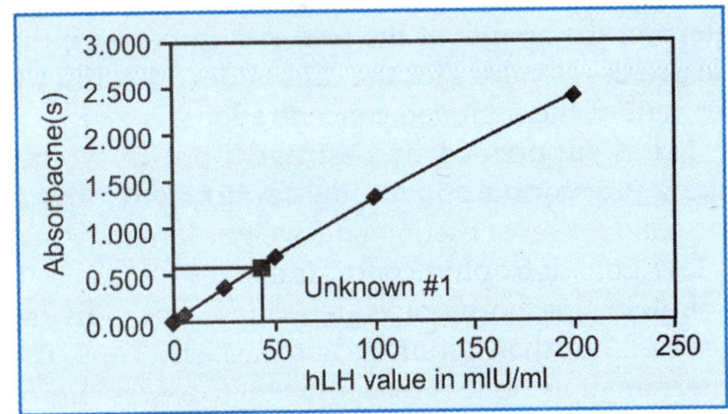

Fig. 17.33: Estimation of LH in mIU/ml

*The data presented in Example 9 and Figure 17.33 are for illustration only and should not be used in lieu of a dose response curve prepared with each assay.

LIMITATIONS OF PROCEDURE

A. Assay Performance

It is important that the time of reaction in each well is held constant for reproducible results. Pipetting of samples should not extend beyond ten (10) minutes to avoid assay drift. If more than one (1) plate is used, it is recommended to repeat the dose response curve.

Addition of the substrate solution initiates a kinetic reaction, which is terminated by the addition of the stop solution. Therefore, the addition of the substrate and the stopping solution should be added in the same sequence to eliminate any time deviation during reaction.

Plate readers measure vertically. Do not touch the bottom of the wells.

Failure to remove adhering solution adequately in the aspiration or decantation wash step(s) may result in poor replication and spurious results.

Sample(s), which are contaminated microbiologically, should not be used in the assay. Highly lipaemeic or haemolysed specimen(s) should similarly not be used.

Each component in one assay should be of the same lot number and stored under identical conditions.

B. Interpretation

If computer-controlled data reduction is used to interpret the results of the test, it is imperative that the predicted values for the calibrators fall within 10 per cent of the assigned concentrations.

LH is suppressed by oestrogen; but in women taking oral contraceptives, the level may be low or normal. Excessive dieting and weight loss may lead to low gonadotrophin concentrations.

Luteinising hormone is dependent upon diverse factors other than pituitary homeostasis. Thus, the-determination alone is not sufficient to assess clinical status.

Expected Range of Values

A study of an apparent normal adult population was undertaken to determine expected values for the LH IEMA microplate test system. The expected values are presented below.

Expected values for the LH IEMA test system (in mlU/ml (IRP 68/40}

Women	Follicular phase	0.8-10.5
	Midcycle	18.4-61.2
	Luteal phase	0.8-10.5
	Postmenopausal	8.2-40.8
Men		0.7-7.4

It is important to keep in mind that establishment of a range of values which can be expected to be found by a given method for a population of "normal" persons is dependent upon a multiplicity of factors: the specificity of the method, the population tested and the precision of the method in the hands of the analyst. For these reasons, each laboratory should depend upon the range of expected values established by the manufacturer only until an in-house range can be determined by the analysts using the method with a population indigenous to the area in which the laboratory is located.

Usage: To evaluate infertility in women and men (high serum values are related to gonadal dysfunction, and low values of LH are related to dysfunction or failure of the hypothalamus or pituitary galnd) to evaluate hormonal therapy for inducing ovulation and to evaluate endocrine problems related to precocious puberty in children.

Values are Increased in

Amenorrhoea, endocrine, problems related to precocious puberty in children, hyperpituitarism, Klinefelter's syndrome, liver disease, menopause, menstruation, ovarian or testicular failure (primary gonadal dysfunction) Stein-Levinthal syndrome (polycystic ovarian disease), tumour, (pituitary, testicular), and Turner's syndrome (ovarian dysgenesis). Drugs includeanticonvulsants, clomiphene, naloxone, and spironolactone.

Values are Decreased in

Adrenal hyperplasia or tumour, amenorrhoea, (pituitary failure, secondary gonadal insufficiency), anorexia nervosa, anovulation, hypophysectomy, hypopituitarism, hypothalamic disorder, malnutrition, pituitary disorder, and testicular failure (related to pituitary failure). Drugs include digoxin, oestrogen compounds, oral contraceptives, phenothiazines, progesterone, stanozlol, and testosterone administration.

FOLLICLE STIMULATING HORMONE (FSH)

Courtesy: Lilac Medicare

Intended Use: The Quantitative Determination of FSH Concentration in Human Serum and Plasma by a Microplate Immunoenzymometric assay (ELISA). Measurements of FSH are used in the diagnosis of pituitary gland and gonadotrophin disorders.

Summary and Explanation of the Test

Follicle-stimulating hormone (FSH) is a glycoprotein consisting of two subunits with an approximate molecular mass of 35,500 daltons. The α-subunit is similar to other pituitary hormones [luteinizing stimulating hormone (LH), thyroid-stimulating hormone (TSH) and chorionic gonadotrophin (CG)] while the β-subunit is unique. The β-subunit confers the biological activity to the molecule. Stimulation by gonadotrophin-releasing hormone (GnRH) causes release of FSH as well as LH, from the pituitary and is transported by the blood to their sites of action, the testes or ovary.

In men, FSH acts on the Sertoli cells of the testis, stimulating the synthesis of inhibin, which appears to specifically inhibit further FSH secretion, and androgen-binding protein. Thus, it indirectly supports spermatogenesis.

In women, FSH acts on the granulosa cells of the ovary, stimulating steroidogenesis. All ovulatory menstrual cycles have a characteristic pattern of FSH, as well as LH, secretion. The menstrual cycle is divided into a follicular phase and a luteal phase by the midcycle surge of the gonadotrophins (LH and FSH). As the follicular phase progresses, FSH concentration decreases. Near the time ovulation occurs, about midcycle, FSH peaks (lesser in magnitude than LH) to its highest level.

The clinical usefulness of the measurement of follicle-stimulating hormone (FSH) in ascertaining the homeostasis of fertility regulation via the hypothalamic-pituitary-gonadal axis has been well established.

In this method, FSH calibrator, patient specimen or control is first added to a streptavidin-coated well. Biotinylated monoclonal and enzyme-labeled antibodies (directed against distinct and different epitopes of FSH) are added and the reactants mixed. Reaction between the various FSH antibodies and native FSH forms a sandwich complex that binds with the streptavidin coated to the well.

After the completion of the required incubation period, the enzyme-follicle-stimulating hormone antibody-bound conjugate is separated from the unbound enzyme-follicle-stimulating hormone conjugate by aspiration or decantation. The activity of the enzyme present on the surface of the well is quantitated by reaction with a suitable substrate to produce color.

The employment of several serum references of known follicle-stimulating hormone levels permits construction of a dose response curve of activity and concentration. From comparison to the dose response curve, an unknown specimen's activity can be correlated with follicle-stimulating hormone concentration.

PRINCIPLE

Immunoenzymometric Assay

The essential reagents required for an immunoenzymometric assay include high affinity and specificity antibodies (enzyme and immobilised), with different and distinct epitope recognition, in excess, and native antigen. In this procedure, the immobilisation takes place during the assay at the surface of a microplate well through the interaction of streptavidin coated on the well and exogenously added biotinylated monoclonal anti-FSH antibody.

Upon mixing monoclonal biotinylated antibody, the enzyme-labeled antibody and a serum containing the native antigen, reaction results between the native antigen and the antibodies, without competition or steric hindrance, to form a soluble sandwich complex. The interaction is illustrated by the following equation:

$$^{Enz}Ab_{(p)} + Ag_{FSH} + {}^{Btn}Ab_{(m)} \underset{k_{-a}}{\overset{k_a}{\rightleftharpoons}} {}^{En}zAb_{(p)}\text{-}Ag_{FSH}\text{-}{}^{Btn}Ab_{(m)}$$

$^{Btn}Ab(m)$ = Biotinylated monoclonal antibody (excess quantity)

Ag_{FSH} = Native antigen (variable quantity)

$^{Enz}Ab(p)$ = Enzyme labeled polyclonal antibody (excess quantity)

$^{Enz}Ab(p)\text{-}Ag_{FSH}\text{-}{}^{Btn}Ab_{(m)}$ = Antigen-antibodies sandwich complex

k_a = Rate constant of association

k_a = Rate constant of dissociation

Simultaneously, the complex is deposited to the well through the high affinity reaction of streptavidin and biotinylated antibody. This interaction is illustrated below:

$^{Enz}Ab(p)\text{-}AgFSH\text{-}{}^{Btn}Ab_{(m)}$ + Streptavidinc w. => Immobilised complex

Streptavidin c.w. = Streptavidin immobolised on well

Immobilised complex = Sandwich complex bound to the solid surface

After equilibrium is attained, the antibody-bound fraction is separated from unbound antigen by decantation or aspiration. The enzyme activity in the antibody-bound fraction is directly proportional to the native antigen concentration. By utilising several different serum references of known antigen values, a dose response curve can be generated from which the antigen concentration of an unknown can be ascertained.

REAGENTS FOR 96-WELL MICROPLATE

A. FSH Calibrators -1.0 ml/vial

Six (6) vials of references for FSH Antigen at levels of 0(A), 5(B), 10(C), 25(D), 50(E) and 100(F) mIU/ml. Store at 2-8°C. A preservative has been added.

Note: The calibrators, human serum based, were calibrated using a reference preparation, which was assayed against the WHO 2nd IRP (78/549).

B. Enzyme-Polyclonal Conjugate and Biotinylated Monoclonal antibody—11 ml/vial

One (1) vial-containing enzyme-labeled affinity purified goat antibody, biotinylated monoclonal mouse IgG in buffer, dye, and preservative. Store at 2-8°C.

C. Streptavidin-Coated Microplate-96 Wells

One 96-well microplate coated with Streptavidin and packaged in an aluminum bag with a drying agent. Store at 2-8°C.

D. Wash Solution Concentrate - 20 ml

One (1) vial containing a surfactant in phosphate buffered saline. A preservative has been added. Store at 2-30°C.

E. Substrate A ~7.0 ml/vial

One (1) bottle containing tetramethylbenzidine (TMB) in buffer. Store at 2-8°C.

F. Substrate B - 7.0 ml/vial

One (1) bottle containing hydrogen peroxide (H_2O_2) in buffer. Store at 2-8°C.

G. Stop Solution ~ 6.0 ml/vial

One (1) bottle containing a strong acid (1N HCl). Store at 2-30°C.

Note 1: Do not use reagents beyond the kit expiration date.

Note 2: Opened reagents are stable for sixty (60) days when stored at 2-8°C.

For In Vitro Diagnostic Use Not for Internal or External Use in Humans or Animals

Precautions

All products that contain human serum have been found to be nonreactive for Hepatitis B Surface Antigen, HIV 12 and HCV Antibodies by FDA required tests. Since no known test can offer complete assurance that infectious agents are absent, all human serum products should be handled as potentially hazardous and capable of transmitting disease. Good laboratory procedures for handling blood products can be found in the Center for Disease Control/ National Institute of Health, "Biosafety in Microbiological and Biomedical Laboratories," 2nd Edition, 1988, HHS

Specimen Collection and Preparation

The specimens shall be blood serum in type and the usual precautions in the collection of venipuncture samples should be observed. For accurate comparison to established normal values, a fasting morning serum sample should be obtained. The blood should be collected in a plain redcap venipuncture tube without additives or gel barrier. Allow the blood to clot. Centrifuge the specimen to separate the serum from the cells.

Samples may be refrigerated at 2-8°C for a maximum period of five (5) days. If the specimen(s) cannot be assayed within this time, the sample(s) may be stored at temperatures of –20°C for up to 30 days. Avoid repetitive freezing and thawing. When assayed in duplicate, 0.100 ml of the specimen is required.

MATERIALS

Provided

1. Six (6) vials of follicle-stimulating hormone serum calibrators
2. One (1) vial of combined biotinylated monoclonal antibody and enzyme-labeled polyclonal reagent
3. One 96-well streptavidin-coated microplate
4. One (1) bottle of wash buffer concentrate

5. One (1) bottle of substrate A
6. One (1) bottle of substrate B
7. One (1) bottle of stop solution
8. Instructions

Required but Not Provided

1. Pipette(s) capable of delivering 50 μl and 100 μl volumes with a precision of better than 1.5 per cent.
2. Dispenser(s) for repetitive deliveries of 0.100 ml and 0.300 ml volumes with a precision of better than 1.5 per cent (optional).
3. Microplate washer or a squeeze bottle (optional)
4. Microplate reader with 450 nm wavelength absorbance capability
5. Container(s) for mixing of reagents (see below).
6. Absorbent paper for blotting the microplate wells.
7. Plastic wrap or microplate cover for incubation steps.
8. Vacuum aspirator (optional) for wash steps.
9. Timer
10. Storage container for storage of wash buffer
11. Distilled or deionized water
12. Quality control materials

REAGENT PREPARATION

1. Working Reagent 1 - Wash buffer

Dilute contents of wash concentrate to 1000 ml with distilled or deionized water in a suitable storage container. Store at room temperature (20-30°C).

2. Working Reagent 2-Substrate Solution-Prepare before Use

Determine the amount of reagent needed and prepare by mixing equal portions of substrate A and substrate B in a suitable container. For example, add 1 ml of A and 1 ml of B per two (2) eight well strips (a slight excess of solution is made). Use within one (1) hour of preparation for maximum performance of the assay.

Test Procedure

Before proceeding with the assay, bring all reagents, serum references and controls to room temperature (20-30°C).

1. Format the microplates' wells for each serum reference, control and patient specimen to be assayed in duplicate. Replace any unused microwell strips back into the aluminum bag, seal and store at 2-8°C.
2. Pipette 0.050 ml (50 μl) of the appropriate serum reference, control or specimen into the assigned well.
3. Add 0.100 ml (100 μl) of the biotinylated/enzyme-labeled antibodies to each well. It is very important to dispense all reagents close to the bottom of the coated well.
4. Swirl the microplate gently for 20-30 seconds to mix and cover.
5. Incubate 60 minutes at room temperature.
6. Discard the contents of the microplate by decantation or aspiration. If decanting, tap and blot the plate dry with absorbent paper.
7. Add 300 μl of wash buffer (see reagent preparation section), decant (tap and blot) or aspirate. Repeat two (2) additional times for a total of three (3) washes. An automatic or manual plate washer can be used. Follow the manufacturer's instruction for proper usage. If a squeeze bottle is employed, fill each well by depressing the contsainer (avoiding air bubbles) to dispense the wash. Decant the wash and repeat two (2) additional times.
8. Add 0.100 ml (100 ul) of substrate solution to all wells (see reagent preparation section). Always add reagents in the same order to minimise reaction time differences between wells.
9. Incubate at room temperature for fifteen (15) minutes.
10. Add 0.050 ml (50 ul) of stop solution to each well and swirl the microplate gently for 15-20 seconds to mix. Always add reagents in the same order to minimise reaction time differences between wells.
11. Read the absorbance in each well at 450 nm in a microplate reader. The results should be read within thirty (30) minutes of adding the stop solution.

Note: For assaying specimens with concentration greater than 100 mlU/ ml, pipette 25 μl of the specimen and 25 μl of the 0 serum calibrator into the sample well (this maintains a uniform protein environment). Multiply the result by 2 to obtain the FSH concentration of the specimen.

Quality Control

Each laboratory should assay controls at levels in the low, normal and elevated range for monitoring assay performance. These controls should be treated as unknowns and values determined in every test procedure performed. Quality control charts should be maintained to follow the performance of the supplied reagents. Pertinent statistical methods should be employed to ascertain trends. The individual laboratory should set acceptable assay performance limits. Other parameters that should be monitored include the 80, 50 and 20 per cent intercepts of the dose response curve for run-to-run reproducibility. In addition, maximum absorbance should be consistent with past experience. Significant deviation from established performance can indicate unnoticed change in experimental conditions or degradation of kit reagents. Fresh reagents should be used to determine the reason for the variations.

Results

A dose response curve is used to ascertain the concentration of follicle-stimulating hormone in unknown specimens.

1. Record the absorbance obtained from the printout of the microplate reader as outlined in Example 10.
2. Plot the absorbance for each duplicate serum reference versus the corresponding FSH concentration in mlU/ml on linear graph paper (do not average the duplicates of the serum references before plotting).
3. Draw the best-fit curve through the plotted points.
4 To determine the concentration of FSH for an unknown, locate the average absorbance of the duplicates for each unknown on the vertical axis of the graph, find the intersecting point on the curve, and read the concentration (in mlU/ml) from the horizontal axis of the graph (the duplicates of the unknown may be averaged as indicated). In the following example, the average absorbance (1.186) intersects the dose response curve at (42.2 mlU/ml) FSH concentration (See Figure 17.34).

Note: Computer data reduction software designed for ELISA assays may also be used for the data reduction.

Example 10

Well	*Serum References*	*Absorbance*
1	0.0 mlU/ml	0.018
2	0.0 mlU/ml	0.019
3	5.0 mlU/ml	0.171
4	5.0 mlU/ml	0.165
5	10.0 mlU/ml	0.296
6	10.0 mlU/ml	0.288
7	25.0 mlU/ml	0.745
8	25.0 mlU/ml	0.703
9	50.0 mlU/ml	1.424
10	50.0 mlU/ml	1.365
11	100.0 mlU/ml	2.459
12	100.0 mlU/ml	2.406

Well	**Unknown ID**	**OD**	**Avg. OD**	**Value**
13	Unknown #1	1.206		
14	Unknown #	1 1.165	1.186	42.2 mlU/ml

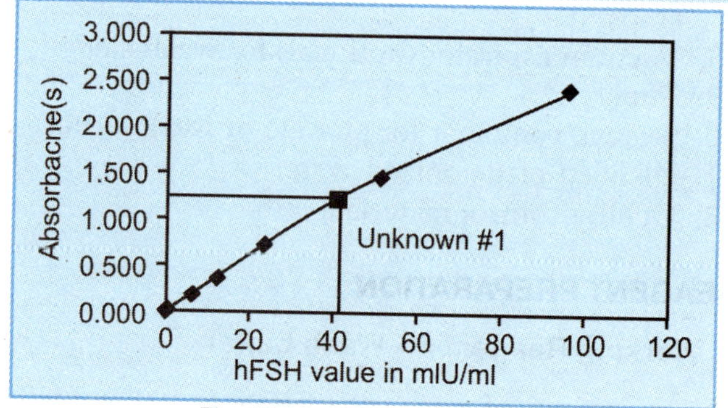

Fig. 17.34: FSH concentration

The data presented in Example 10 and Figure 17.34 are for illustration only and should not be used in lieu of a dose response curve prepared with each assay.

LIMITATIONS OF PROCEDURE

A. Assay Performance

It is important that the time of reaction in each well is held constant for reproducible results. Pipetting of samples should not extend beyond ten (10) minutes to avoid assay drift. If more than one (1) plate is used, it is recommended to repeat the dose response curve.

Addition of the substrate solution initiates a kinetic reaction, which is terminated by the addition of the stop solution. Therefore, the addition of the substrate and the stopping solution should be in the same sequence to eliminate any time deviation during reaction.

Plate readers measure vertically. Do not touch the bottom of the wells.

Failure to remove adhering solution adequately in the aspiration or decantation wash step(s) may result in poor replication and spurious results.

Sample(s), which are contaminated microbiologically, should not be used in the assay. Highly lipaemic or haemolysed specimen(s) should similarly not be used.

Each component in one assay should be of the same lot number and stored under identical conditions.

B. Interpretation

If computer-controlled data reduction is used to interpret the results of the test, it is imperative that the predicted values for the calibrators fall within 10 per cent of the assigned concentrations.

The FSH is suppressed by oestrogen, but in women taking oral contraceptives, the level may be low or normal. Excessive dieting and weight loss may lead to low gonadotrophin concentrations.

Follicle-stimulating hormone is dependent upon diverse factors other than pituitary homeostasis. Thus, the determination alone is not sufficient to assess clinical status.

Normal Values in MIU/ml

Sex / phase	
Males	1.0-14.0
Females:	
Follicular phase	3.0-12.0
Midcycle	8.0-22.0
Luteal phase	2.0-12.0
On oral contraceptives	Up to 3.0
Postmenopausal	35.0-151.0

Values are Increased in

Acromegaly (early), amenorrhoea (primary), anorchism, castration, gonadal failure, hyperpituitarism, hypogonadism, hypothalamic tumour, hysterectomy, Klinefelter's ovarian failure, pituitary tumours, precocious puberty, premature menopause, seminiferous tubule failure, seminoma, Stein-Levinthal syndrome (polycystic ovary syndrome), testicular agenesis, testicular destruction (due to radiation or mumps orchitis), testicular failure, testicular feminsation syndrome (complete), and Turner's syndrome (primary hypogonadism).

Values are Decreased in

Adrenal hyperplasia, amenorrhoea (secondary), anorexia nervosa, anovulatory menstrual cycle, delayed puberty, hypogonadotropism, hypophysectomy, hypothalamic dysfunction, neoplasm (adrenal, ovarian, testicular), panhypopituitarism, and prepubertal child. Drugs include chlorpromazine, oestrogens, oral contraceptives, progesterone, and testosterone.

PROLACTIN HORMONE (PRL)
Courtesy: Lilac Medicare

Intended Use: The Quantitative Determination of Prolactin Hormone Concentration in Human Serum by a Microplate Immunoenzymometric Assay

Summary and Explanation of the Test

Prolactin hormone (PRL), secreted from the lactotrophs of the anterior pituitary, is a protein consisting of a single polypeptide chain containing approximately 200 amino acids. The primary biological action of the hormone is on the mammary gland where it is involved in the growth of the gland and in the induction and maintenance of milk production. There is evidence to suggest that prolactin may be involved in steroidogenesis in the gonad, acting synergistically with luteinising hormone (LH). High levels of prolactin appear to inhibit steroidogenesis as well as inhibiting LH and follicle-stimulating hormone (FSH) synthesis at the pituitary gland.

The clinical usefulness of the measurement of prolactin hormone (PRL) in ascertaining the diagnosis of hyperprolactinaemia; and for the subsequent monitoring, the effectiveness of the treatment has been well-established.

In this method, PRL calibrator, patient specimen or control is first added to a streptavidin-coated well. Biotinylated monoclonal and enzyme-labeled antibodies (directed against distinct and different epitopes of PRL) are added and the reactants mixed. Reaction between the various PRL antibodies and native PRL forms a sandwich complex that binds with the streptavidin coated to the well.

After the completion of the required incubation period, the enzyme-prolactin hormone antibody-bound conjugate is separated from the unbound enzyme-prolactin hormone conjugate by aspiration or decantation. The activity of the enzyme present on the surface of the well is quantitated by reaction with a suitable substrate to produce color.

The employment of several serum references of known prolactin hormone levels permits the construction of a dose response curve of activity and concentration. From comparison to the dose response curve, an unknown specimen's activity can be correlated with prolactin hormone concentration.

PRINCIPLE

Immunoenzymometric Assay

The essential reagents required for an immunoenzymometric assay include high affinity and specificity antibodies (enzyme and immobilised), with different and distinct epitope recognition, in excess, and native antigen. In this procedure, the immobilisation takes place during the assay at the surface of a microplate well through the interaction of streptavidin coated on the well and exogenously added biotinylated monoclonal anti-PRL antibody.

Upon mixing monoclonal biotinylated antibody, the enzyme-labeled antibody and a serum containing the native antigen, reaction results between the native antigen and the antibodies, without competition or steric hindrance, to form a soluble sandwich complex. The interaction is illustrated by the following equation:

$$^{Enz}Ab_{(p)} + A_{gp}R_L + {}^{Btn}Ab_{(m)} \underset{k\text{-}a}{\overset{k_a}{\rightleftharpoons}} {}^{Enz}Ab(p)\text{-}Ag_{PRL}\text{-}{}^{Btn}Ab_{(m)}$$

$^{Btn}Ab_{(m)}$ = Biotinylated monoclonal antibody (excess quantity)

Ag_{PRL} = Native antigen (variable quantity)

$^{Enz}Ab_{(p)}$ = Enzyme labeled polyclonal antibody (excess quantity)

$^{Enz}Ab_{(p)}$-AgpRL-$^{Btn}Ab_{(m)}$ = Antigen-antibodies sandwich complex

k_a = Rate constant of association

k_- = Rate constant of dissociation

Simultaneously, the complex is deposited to the well through the high affinity reaction of streptavidin and biotinylated antibody. This interaction is illustrated below:

$^{Enz}Ab_{(p)}$-Ag_{PRL}-$^{Btn}Ab_{(m)}$ + Streptavidin cw => immobilised complex

Streptavidin cw = Streptavidin immobilised on well

Immobilised complex = Sandwich complex bound to the solid surface

After equilibrium is attained, the antibody-bound fraction is separated from unbound antigen by decantation or aspiration. The enzyme activity in the antibody-bound fraction is directly proportional to the native antigen concentration. By utilising several different serum references of known antigen values, a dose response curve can be generated from which the antigen concentration of an unknown can be ascertained.

REAGENTS FOR 96-WELL MICROPLATE

A. Prolactin Hormone Calibrators -1.0 ml/vial

Six (6) vials of references for PRL Antigen in human serum at levels of 0(A), 5(B), 10(C), 25(D), 50(E) and 100(F) ng/ml. Store at 2-8°C. A preservative has been added.

B. Enzyme-Poiyclonal Conjugate and Biotinylated Monoclonal antibody—11 ml/vial

One (1) vial containing enzyme labeled affinity purified rabbit antibody, biotinylated monoclonal mouse IgG in buffer, dye, and preservative. Store at 2-8°C.

C. Streptavidin Coated Microplate - 96 wells

One 96-weli microplate coated with streptavidin and packaged in an aluminum bag with a drying agent. Store at 2-8°C.

D. Wash Solution Concentrate - 20 ml

One (1) vial containing a surfactant in phosphate buffered saline. A preservative has been added. Store at 2-8°C.

E. Substrate A ~7.0 ml/vial

One (1) bottle containing tetramethylbenzidine (TMB) in buffer. Store at 2-8°C.

F. Substrate B - 7.0 ml/vial

One (1) bottle containing hydrogen peroxide (H_2O_2) in buffer. Store at 2-8°C.

G. Stop Solution— 6.0 ml/vial

One (1) bottle containing a strong acid (1N HCl). Store at 2-8°C.

Note 1: Do not use reagents beyond the kit expiration date.

Note 2: Opened reagents are stable for sixty (60) days when stored at 2-8°C.

For In Vitro Diagnostic Use Not for Internal or External Use in Humans or Animals

Precautions

All products that contain human serum have been found to be nonreactive for Hepatitis B Surface Antigen, HIV 1 and 2 and HCV Antibodies by FDA required tests. Since no known test can offer complete assurance that infectious agents are absent, all human serum products should be handled as potentially hazardous and capable of transmitting disease. Good laboratory procedures for handling blood products can be found in the Center for Disease Control/ National Institute of Health, "Biosafety in Microbiological and Biomedical Laboratories," 2nd Edition, 1988, HHS.

Specimen Collection and Preparation

The specimens shall be blood serum in type and the usual precautions in the collection of venipuncture samples should be observed. For accurate comparison to established normal values, a fasting morning serum sample should be obtained. The blood should be collected in a plain red-top venipuncture tube without additives or gel barrier. Allow the blood to clot. Centrifuge the specimen to separate the serum from the cells.

Samples may be refrigerated at 2-8°C for a maximum period of five (5) days. If the specimen(s) cannot be assayed within this time, the sample(s) may be stored at temperatures of –20°C for up to 30 days. Avoid repetitive freezing and thawing. When assayed in duplicate, 0.100 ml of the specimen is required.

MATERIALS

Provided

1. Six (6) vials of prolactin hormone human serum calibrators.
2. One (1) vial of combined biotinylated monoclonal antibody and enzyme labeled polyclonal reagent.
3. One 96-well streptavidin coated microplate.
4. One (1) bottle of wash buffer concentrate.
5. One (1) bottle of substrate A.
6. One (1) bottle of substrate B.
7. One (1) bottle of stop solution.
8. Instructions.

Required but Not Provided

1. Pipette(s) capable of delivering 50 μl and 100 pl volumes with a precision of better than 1.5 per cent.
2. Dispenser(s) for repetitive deliveries of 0.100 ml and 0.300 ml volumes with a precision of better than 1.5 per cent (optional).
3. Microplate washer or a squeeze bottle (optional).
4. Microplate reader with 450 nm wavelength absorbance capability.
5. Container(s) for mixing of reagents (see below).
6. Absorbent paper for blotting the microplate wells.
7. Plastic wrap or microplate cover for incubation steps.
8. Vacuum aspirator (optional) for wash steps.
9. Timer.
10. Storage container for storage of wash buffer.,
11. Distilled or deionized water.
12. Quality control materials.

REAGENT PREPARATION

1. Working Reagent 1—Wash Buffer

Dilute contents of wash concentrate to 1000 ml with distilled or deionized water in a suitable storage container. Store at room temperature.

2. Working Reagent 2—Substrate Solution - Prepare before use

Determine the amount of reagent needed and prepare by mixing equal portions of substrate A and substrate B in a suitable container. For example, add 1 ml of A and 1 ml of B per two (2) eight well strips (A–. slight excess of solution is made). Use within one (1) hour of preparation for maximum performance of the assay.

Test Procedure

Before proceeding with the assay, bring all reagents, serum references and controls to room temperature (20-30°C).

1. Format the microplates' wells for each serum reference, control and patient specimen to be assayed in duplicate. Replace any unused microwell strips back into the aluminum bag, seal and store at 2-8°C.
2. Pipette 0.050 ml (50 μl) of the appropriate serum reference, control or specimen into the assigned well.
3. Add 0.100 ml (100 μl) of the biotinylated/enzyme-labeled antibodies to each well. It is very important to dispense all reagents close to the bottom of the coated well.
4. Swirl the microplate gently for 20-30 seconds to mix and cover.
5. Incubate 60 minutes at room temperature.
6. Discard the contents of the microplate by decantation or aspiration. If decanting, tap and blot the plate dry with absorbent paper.
7. Add 300 μl of wash buffer (see reagent preparation section), decant (tap and blot) or aspirate. Repeat two (2) additional times for a total of three (3) washes. An automatic or manual plate washer can be used. Follow the manufacturer's instruction for proper usage. If a squeeze bottle is employed, fill each well by depressing the container (avoiding air bubbles) to dispense the wash. Decant the wash and repeat two (2) additional times.
8. Add 0.100 ml (100 μl) of working substrate solution to all wells (see reagent preparation section). Always add reagents in the same order to minimise reaction time differences between wells.
9. Incubate at room temperature for fifteen (15) minutes.
10. Add 0.050 ml (50 μl) of stop solution to each well and swirl the microplate gently for 15-20 seconds to mix. Always add reagents in the same order to minimize reaction time differences between wells.
11. Read the absorbance in each well at 450 nm in a microplate reader. The results should be read within thirty (30) minutes of adding the stop solution.

Note: For assaying specimens with concentration greater than 100 ng/ml, pipett 25 μl of the sample and 25 μl of the 0 serum calibrator into the assigned well (this maintains a uniform protein environment). Multiply the result by 2 to obtain the prolactin concentration of the specimen.

Quality Control

Each laboratory should assay controls at levels in the low, normal and elevated range for monitoring assay performance. These controls should be treated as unknowns and values determined in every test procedure performed. Quality control charts should be maintained to follow the performance of the supplied reagents. Pertinent statistical methods should be employed to ascertain trends. The individual laboratory should set acceptable assay performance limits. Other parameters that should be monitored include the 80, 50 and 20 per cent intercepts of the dose response curve for run-to-run reproducibility. In addition, maximum absorbance should be consistent with past experience. Significant deviation from established performance can indicate unnoticed change in experimental conditions or degradation of kit reagents. Fresh reagents should be used to determine the reason for the variations.

Results

A dose response curve is used to ascertain the concentration of prolactin (PRL) hormone levels in unknown specimens.

1. Record the absorbance obtained from the print-out of the microplate reader as outlined in Example 11.
2. Plot the absorbance for each duplicate serum reference versus the corresponding PRL concentration in ng/ml on linear graph paper (do not average the duplicates of the serum references before plotting).
3. Draw the best-fit curve through the plotted points.
4. To determine the concentration of PRL for an unknown, locate the average absorbance of the duplicates for each unknown on the vertical axis of the graph, find the intersecting point on the curve, and read the concentration (in ng/ml) from the horizontal axis of the graph (the duplicates of the unknown may be averaged as indicated). In the following example, the average absorbance (0.891) intersects the dose response curve at (26.8 ng/ml) PRL concentration (See Figure 17.35).

Note: Computer data reduction software designed for IEMA assays may also be used for the data reduction.

Example 11

Well	Serum References	Absorbance
1	0.0 ng/ml	0.017
2	0.0 ng/ml	0.017
3	5.0 ng/ml	O.T84
4	5.0 ng/ml	0.174
5	10.0 ng/ml	0.366
6	10.0 ng/ml	0.365
7	25.0 ng/ml	0.841
8	25.0 ng/ml	0.851
9	50.0 ng/ml	1.480
10	50.0 ng/ml	1.460
11	100.0 ng/ml	2.290
12	100.0 ng/ml	2.295

Well	Unknown ID	OD	Avg. OD	Value
13	Unknown #	1 0.895		
14	Unknown #	1 0.888	0.891	26.8 ngml

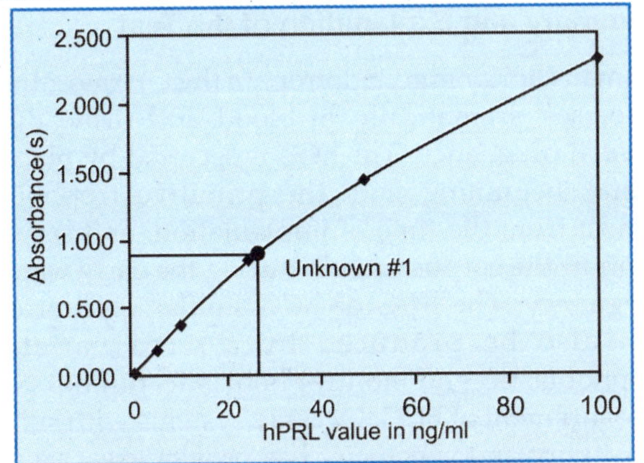

Fig. 17.35: Estimation of PRL in ng/ml

The data presented in Example 11 and Figure 17. 35 are for illustration only and should not be used in lieu of a dose response curve prepared with each assay.

LIMITATIONS OF PROCEDURE

A. Assay Performance

It is important that the time of reaction in each well is held constant for reproducible results. Pipetting of samples should not extend beyond ten (10) minutes to avoid assay drift. If more than one (1) plate is used, it is recommended to repeat the dose response curve.

Addition of the substrate solution initiates a kinetic reaction, which is terminated by the addition of the stop solution. Therefore, the addition of the substrate and the stopping solution should be added in the same sequence to eliminate any time deviation during reaction.

Plate readers measure vertically. Do not touch the bottom of the wells.

Failure to remove adhering solution adequately in the aspiration or decantation wash step(s) may result in poor replication and spurious results.

Sample(s) that are contaminated microbiologically should not be used in the assay. Highly lipaemic or haemolysed specimen(s) should similarly not be used.

Each component in one assay should be of the same lot number and stored under identical conditions.

B. Interpretation

If computer-controlled data reduction is used to interpret the results of the test, it is imperative that the predicted values for the calibrators fall within 10 per cent of the assigned concentrations.

Patient specimens with abnormally high prolactin levels can cause a hook effect, that is, paradoxical low absorbance results. If this is suspected, dilute the specimen 1/100 with 0 calibrator, reassay (multiply the result by 100). However, values as high as 3000 ng/ml have been found to absorb greater than the absorbance of the highest calibrator.

Patients receiving preparations of mouse monoclonal antibodies for diagnosis or therapy may contain human antimouse antibodies (HAMA) and may show either falsely elevated or depressed values when assayed.

Pregnancy, lactation, and the administration of oral contraceptives can cause an increase in the level of prolactin.

Drugs such as morphine, reserpine and the psychotropic drugs increase prolactin secretion.

Since prolactin hormone concentration is dependent upon diverse factors other than pituitary homeostasis, the determination alone is not: sufficient to assess clinical status.

Expected Range of Values

A study of an apparent normal adult population was undertaken to determine expected values for the PRL IEMA microplate test system. The expected values (95 per cent confidence intervals) are presented below.

Expected Values for the PRL IEMA Test System (in ng/ml)

Women (Number = 60)	1.2-15.5
Postmenopausal (Number = 10)	1.5-18.5
Men (Number = 50)	1.8-17.0

It is important to keep in mind that establishment of a range of values which can be expected to be found by a given method for a population of "normal" persons is dependent upon a multiplicity of factors: the specificity of the method, the population tested and the precision of the method in the hands of the analyst. For these reasons, each laboratory should depend upon the range of expected values established by the manufacturer only until an in-house range can be determined by the analysts using the method with a population indigenous to the area in which the laboratory is located.

Normal range of HPRL in ng/ml)

Age/sex/phase	
Newborn	> 250
Adult male	< 20
Adult female, nonlactating	< 25
Follicular phase	< 28
Luteal phase	5-40
Postmenopausal	< 12
Pregnancy	
Trimester 1	< 80
Trimester 2	< 160
Trimester 3	< 400
Pituitary tumour	> 100

HPRL Levels are Increased in

Acromegaly, Addison's disease, amenorrhoea, anorexia nervosa, breast stimulation, bronchogenic carcinoma, Chiari-Frommel syndrome, coitus, Del Castillo's syndrome, ectopic tumours, endometriosis, exercise.

Forbes-Albright syndrome, galactorrhoea, hyper-estrogen states, Hyperpituitarism, hypothalamic disorders, hypothyroidism (primary), hysterectomy, idiopathic causes (e.g., early micro-adenoma that are undetectable by radiology), impotence, lactation, Nelson's syndrome, neurogenic causes, pituitary tumours, polycystic ovaries, pregnancy. Chronic renal failure, sleep and stress, drugs include amitryptiline, amoxapine, amphetamines, benzamides, chlorpr-thixine, desipramine, doxepin, droperidol, oestrogens, haloperidol, imipramine, isoniazid, maprotiline, meprobamate, methyldopa, metoclopra-mide, nortriptyline, opiates, oral contraceptives, phenothiazines, procainamide hydrochloride, protriptyline, reserpine, thioridazine, thiothixene, thyrotrophin, triavli, and trimipramine maleate.

HPRL Levels are Decreased in

Gynaecomastia, hirsutism, osteoporosis, and pituitary necrosis/infarction. Drugs include apomorphine hydrochloride, clonidine, bromocripine mesylate, dihydroergotamine, mesylate, dopamine, ergonovine maleate, ergotamine tartarate, ergoloid mesylate, lergotrile, levodopa, and lisuride hydrogen maleate.

CHORIONIC GONADOTROPHIN (HCG)

Intended Use: The Quantitative Determination of Chorionic Gonadotrophin Concentration in Human Serum by a Microplate Immunoenzymometric Assay.

Summary and Explanation of the Test

Human chorionic gonadotrophin (hCG) concentration increases dramatically in blood and urine during normal pregnancy. The hCG is secreted by placental tissue, beginning with the primitive trophoblast, almost from the time of implantation, and serves to support the corpus luteum during the early weeks of pregnancy. The hCG or hCG similar glycoproteins can also be produced by a wide variety of trophoblastic and nontrophoblastic tumours. The measurement of hCG, by assay systems with suitable sensitivity and specificity has proven great value in the detection of pregnancy and the diagnosis of early pregnancy disorders.

According to the literature, hCG is detectable as early as 10 days after ovulation, reaching 100 mlU/ml by the first missed period. At the time for the next ovulation, the hCG level is 200 mlU/ml (approximately 28 days after conception). A peak of 50,000 or even 100,000 mlU/ml is attained by the third month, then a gradual decline is observed.

In this method, hCG calibrator, patient specimen or control is first added to a streptavidin-coated well. Biotinylated monoclonal and enzyme-labeled antibodies (directed against distinct and different epitopes of hCG) are added and the reactants mixed. Reaction between the various hCG antibodies and native hCG forms a sandwich complex that binds with the streptavidin coated to the well.

After the completion of the required incubation period, the enzyme-chorionic gonadotrophin antibody bound conjugate is separated from the unbound enzyme-chorionic gonadotrophin conjugate by aspiration or decantation. The activity of the enzyme present on the surface of the well is quantitated by reaction with a suitable substrate to produce color.

The employment of several serum references of known chorionic gonadotrophin levels permits construction of a dose response curve of activity and concentration. From comparison to the dose response curve, an unknown specimen's activity can be correlated with chorionic gonadotrophin concentration.

PRINCIPLE

Immunoenzymometric Assay

The essential reagents required for an immunoenzymometric assay include high affinity and specificity antibodies (enzyme and immobilised), with different and distinct epitope recognition, in excess, and native antigen. In this procedure, the immobilisation takes place during the assay at the surface of a microplate well through the interaction of streptavidin coated on the well and exogenously added biotinylated monoclonal anti-hCG antibody.

Upon mixing monoclonal biotinylated antibody, the enzyme-labeled antibody and a serum containing the native antigen, reaction results between the native antigen and the antibodies, without competition or steric hindrance, to form a soluble sandwich complex. The interaction is illustrated by the following equation:

$$^{Enz}Ab_{(p)} + Ag_{hC}G + {}^{Btn}Ab_{(m)} \underset{k_{-a}}{\overset{kg}{\longrightarrow}} {}^{Enz}Ab_{(p)}\text{-}Ag_{h}cG - {}^{Btn}Ab_{(m)}$$

$^{Btn}Ab_{(m)}$ = Biotinylated monoclonal antibody (excess quantity)

Ag_{hCG} = Native antigen (variable quantity)

$^{Enz}Ab_{(p)}$ = Enzyme labeled polyclonal antibody (excess quantity)

$^{Enz}Ab_{(p)}\text{-}AghCG\text{-}{}^{Bln}Ab_{(m)}$ = Antigen-antibodies sandwich complex

k_a = Rate constant of association

k-a = Rate constant of dissociation

Simultaneously, the complex is deposited to the well through the high affinity reaction of streptavidin and biotinylated antibody. This interaction is illustrated:

$$^{Enz}Ab_{(p)}\text{-}AghCG\text{-}{}^{Btn}Ab_{(m)} + \text{Streptavidin cw} \Rightarrow \text{immobilised complex}$$

Streptavidin cw = Streptavidin immobolised on well

Immobilised complex = Sandwich complex bound to the solid surface

After equilibrium is attained, the antibody-bound fraction is separated from unbound antigen by decantation or aspiration. The enzyme activity in the antibody-bound fraction is directly proportional to the native antigen concentration. By utilising several different serum references of known antigen values, a dose response curve can be generated from which the antigen concentration of an unknown can be ascertained.

REAGENTS FOR 96-WELL MICROPLATE

A. Chorionic Gonadotrophin Calibrators -1.0 ml/vial

Six (6) vials of references for hCG Antigen at levels of 0(A), 5(B), 25(C), 50(D), 100(E) and 250(F) mill/ml. Store at 2-8°C. A preservative has been added.

Note: The calibrators, human serum based, were calibrated using a reference preparation, which was assayed against the WHO 3rdIS (75/537).

B. Enzyme-Polyclonal Conjugate and Biotinylated Monoclonal Antibody—11 ml/vial

One (1) vial containing enzyme-labeled affinity purified goat antibody, biotinylated monoclonal mouse IgG in buffer, dye and preservative. Store at 2-8°C.

C. Streptavidin-Coated Microplate— 96 Wells

One 96-well microplate coated with streptavidin and packaged in an aluminum bag with a drying agent. Store at 2-8°C.

D. Wash Solution Concentrate - 20 ml

One (1) vial containing a surfactant in phosphate buffered saline. A preservative has been added. Store at 2-30°C.

E. Substrate A ~7.0 ml/vial

One (1) bottle containing tetramethylbenzidine (TMB) in buffer. Store at 2-8°C.

F. Substrate B— 7.0 ml/vial

One (1) bottle containing hydrogen peroxide (H_2O_2) in buffer. Store at 2-8°C.

G. Stop Solution - 6.0 ml/vial

One (1) bottle containing a strong acid (1N HCl). Store at 2-30°C.

Note 1: Do not use reagents beyond the kit expiration date.

Note 2: Opened reagents are stable for sixty (60) days when stored at 2-8°C.

For In Vitro Diagnostic Use Not for Internal or External Use in Humans or Animals

Precautions

All products that contain human serum have been found to be nonreactive for Hepatitis B Surface Antigen, HIV 1 and 2 and HCV Antibodies by FDA required tests. Since no known test can offer complete assurance that infectious agents are absent, all human serum products should be handled as potentially hazardous and capable of transmitting disease. Good laboratory procedures for handling blood products can be found in the Center for Disease Control/ National Institute of Health, "Biosafety in Microbiological and Biomedical Laboratories," 2nd Edition, 1988, HHS.

Specimen Collection and Preparation

The specimens shall be blood serum in type and the usual precautions in the collection of venipuncture samples should be observed. For accurate comparison to established normal values, a fasting morning serum sample should be obtained. The blood should be collected in a plain redtop venipuncture tube without additives or gel barrier. Allow the blood to clot. Centrifuge the specimen to separate the serum from the cells.

Samples may be refrigerated at 2-8°C for a maximum period of five (5) days. If the specimen(s) cannot be assayed within this time, the sample(s) may be stored at temperature of –20°C for up to 30 days. Avoid repetitive freezing and thawing. When assayed in duplicate, 0.050 ml of the specimen is required.

MATERIALS

Provided

1. Six (6) vials of chorionic gonadotrophin serum calibrators.
2. One (1) vial of combined biotinylated monoclonal antibody and enzyme labeled polyclonal reagent.
3. One 96-well streptavidin-coated microplate.
4. One (1) bottle of wash buffer concentrate.
5. One (1) bottle of substrate A.
6. One (1) bottle of substrate B.
7. One (1) bottle of stop solution.
8. Instructions.

Required but Not Provided:

1. Pipette(s) capable of delivering 25 μl and 100 μl volumes with a precision of better than 1.5 per cent.
2. Dispenser(s) for repetitive deliveries of 0.100 ml and 0.300 ml volumes with a precision of better than 1.5 per cent (optional).
3. Microplate washer or a squeeze bottle (optional).
4. Microplate reader with 450 nm wavelength absorbance capability.
5. Container(s) for mixing of reagents (see below).
6. Absorbent paper for blotting the microplate wells.
7. Plastic wrap or microplate cover for incubation steps.
8. Vacuum aspirator (optional) for wash steps.
9. Timer.
10. Storage container for storage of wash buffer.
11. Distilled or deionized water.

REAGENT PREPARATION

1. Working Reagent 1— Wash Buffer

Dilute contents of Wash concentrate to 1000 ml with distilled or deionized "~ water in a suitable storage container. Store at room temperature.

2. Working Reagent 2—Substrate Solution - Prepare before Use

Determine the amount of reagent needed and prepare by mixing equal portions of substrate A and substrate B in a suitable container. For example, add 1 ml of A and 1 ml of B per two (2) eight well strips (a slight excess of solution is made). Use within one (1) hour of preparation for maximum performance of the assay.

Test Procedure

Before proceeding with the assay, bring all reagents, serum references and controls to room temperature.

1. Format the microplates' wells for each serum reference, control and patient specimen to be assayed in duplicate. Replace any unused microwell strips back into the aluminum bag, seal and store at 2-8°C.
2. Pipette 0.025 ml (25 μl) of the appropriate serum reference, control or specimen into the assigned well.
3. Add 0.100 ml (100 μ1) of the biotinylated/enzyme-labeled antibodies to each well. It is very important to dispense all reagents close to the bottom of the coated well.
4. Swirl the microplate gently for 20-30 seconds to mix and cover.
5. Incubate 60 minutes at room temperature.
6. Discard the contents of the microplate by decantation or aspiration. If decanting, tap and blot the plate dry with absorbent paper.
7. Add 300 μl of wash buffer (see reagent preparation section), decant (tap and blot) or aspirate. Repeat two (2) additional times for a total of three (3) washes. An automatic or manual plate washer can be used. Follow the manufacturer's instruction for proper usage. If a squeeze bottle is employed, fill each well by depressing the container (avoiding air bubbles) to dispense the wash. Decant the wash and repeat two (2) additional times.
8. Add 0.100 ml (100 μl) of working substrate solution to all wells (see reagent preparation section). Always add reagents in the same order to minimise reaction time differences between wells.
9. Incubate at room temperature for fifteen (15) minutes.
10. Add 0.050 ml (50 μl) of stop solution to each well and mix gently for 15-20 seconds. Always add reagents in the same order to minimise reaction time differences between wells.
11. Read the absorbance in each well at 450 nm in a microplate reader. The results should be read within thirty (30) minutes of adding the stop solution.

Quality Control

Each laboratory should assay controls at levels in the low, normal and elevated range for monitoring assay performance. These controls should be treated as unknowns and values determined in every test procedure performed. Quality control charts should be maintained to follow the performance of the supplied reagents. Pertinent statistical methods should be employed to ascertain trends. The individual laboratory should set acceptable assay performance limits. Other parameters that should be monitored include the 80, 50 and 20 per cent intercepts of the dose response curve for run-to-run reproducibility. In addition, maximum absorbance should be consistent with past experience. Significant deviation from established performance can indicate unnoticed change in experimental conditions or degradation of kit reagents. Fresh reagents should be used to determine the reason for the variations.

Results

A dose response curve is used to ascertain the concentration of chorionic gonadotrophin in unknown specimens.

1. Record the absorbance obtained from the printout of the microplate reader as outlined in Example 12.
2. Plot the absorbance for each duplicate serum reference versus the corresponding hCG concentration in mlU/ml on linear graph paper (do not average the duplicates of the serum references before plotting).
3. Draw the best-fit curve through the plotted points.
4. To determine the concentration of hCG for an unknown, locate the average absorbance of the duplicates for each unknown on the vertical axis of the graph, find the intersecting point on the curve, and read the concentration (in mlU/ml) from the horizontal axis of the graph (the duplicates of the unknown may be averaged as indicated). In the following example, the average absorbance (1.949) intersects the dose response curve at (169 mlU/ml) hCG concentration (See Figure 17.36).

Note: Computer data reduction software designed for IEMA assays may also be use'd for the data reduction.

Example 12

Well	*Serum references*	*Absorbance*
1	0.0 mlU/ml	0.012
2	0.0 mlU/ml	0.012
3	5.0 mlU/ml	0.077
4	5.0 mlU/ml	0.074
5	25.0 mlU/ml	0.407
6	25.0 mlU/ml	0.410
7	50.0 mlU/ml	0.817
8	50.0 mlU/ml	0.785
9	100.0 mlU/ml	1.431
10	100.0 mlU/ml	1.438
11	250.0 mlU/ml	2.611
12	250.0 mlU/ml	2.603

Well	Unknown ID	OD	Avg. OD	Value
13	Unknown #1	1.918		
14	Unknown #1	1.981	1.949	169 mlU/ ml

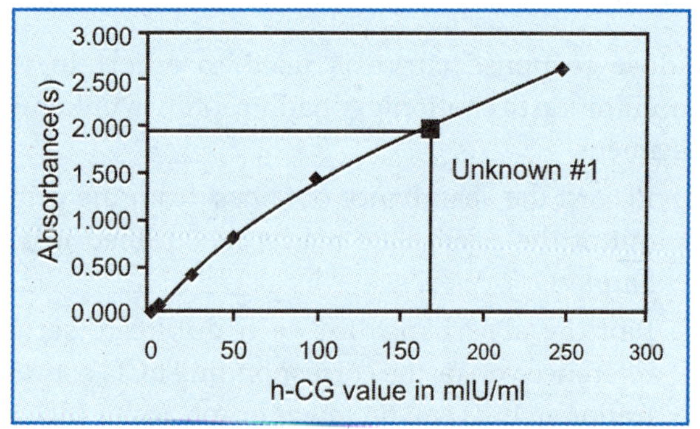

Fig. 17.36: Estimation of hCG in mIU/ml

*The data presented in Example 1 and Fig.17.36 are for illustration only and should not be used in lieu of a dose response curve prepared with each assay.

QC Parameters

Maximum absorbance (250 mlU/ml) = 1.8-2.7.

hCG concentration at 80 per cent maximum absorbance = 155 ± 25 mlU/ml.

hCG concentration at 50 per cent maximum absorbance = 82 + 185 mlU/ml.

hCG concentration at 20 per cent maximum absorbance = 31 ± 102 mlU/ml.

LIMITATIONS OF PROCEDURE

A. Assay Performance

It is important that the time of reaction in each well is held constant for reproducible results. Pipetting of samples should not extend beyond ten (10) minutes to avoid assay drift. If more than one (1) plate is used, it is recommended to repeat the dose response curve.

Addition of the substrate solution initiates a kinetic reaction, which is terminated by the addition of the stop solution. Therefore, the addition of the substrate and the stopping solution should be added in the same sequence to eliminate any time deviation during reaction.

Plate readers measure vertically. Do not touch the bottom of the wells.

Failure to remove adhering solution adequately in the aspiration or decantation wash step(s) may result in poor replication and spurious results.

Sample(s), which are contaminated microbiologically, should not be used in the assay. Highly lipaemeic or haemolysed specimen(s) should similarly not be used.

Patient specimens with hCG concentrations above 200 mlU/ml may be diluted with normal male serum (hCG < 1 mlU/ml) and re-assayed. The sample's concentration is obtained by multiplying the result by the dilution factor.

Each component in one assay should be of the same lot number and stored under identical conditions.

B. Interpretation

If computer-controlled data reduction is used to interpret the results of the test, it is imperative that the predicted values for the calibrators fall within 10 per cent of the assigned concentrations.

False-positive results may occur in the presence of a wide variety of trophoblastic and non-trophoblastic tumours that secrete hCG. Therefore, the possibility of an hCG secreting neoplasia should be eliminated prior to diagnosing pregnancy.

Also, false-positive results may be seen when assaying specimens from individuals taking the drugs Pergonal* and Clomid**. Additionally, Pergonal will often be followed with an injection of hCG.

Spontaneous microabortions and ectopic pregnancies will tend to have values which are lower than expected during a normal pregnancy, while somewhat higher values are often seen in multiple pregnancies.

Following therapeutic abortion, detectable hCG may persist for as long as three to four weeks. The disappearance rate of hCG, after spontaneous abortion, will vary depending upon the quantity of viable residual trophoblast.

*Pergonal is a registered trademark of Serono Laboratories, Inc.

**Clomid is a registered trademark of Merriell-National Laboratories.

Expected Range of Values

A study of an apparent normal adult population was undertaken to determine expected values for the hCG IEMA microplate test system. The mean (X) values, standard deviations (S.D.) and expected ranges (±2 SD) are presented below.

Expected Values for the hCG IEMA test system (in mIU/ml (3rd IS 75/537)

Number	25
Mean (X)	2.9
Standard Deviation (SD)	1.4
Expected Ranges (±2 SD)	0.1-5.7

Normal Values

Males	< 5.0
Females:	
Non pregnant	< 20.0
< 1 week gestation	Up to 50.0
2 weeks gestation	50-500
3 weeks gestation	100-10,000
4 weeks gestation	1000-30,000
5 weeks gestation	3,500-115,000
6-8 weeks gestation	12,000-270,000
12 weeks gestation	15,000-220,000

Values are Increased in

Choriocarcinoma, eclampsia, ectopic pregnancy, erythroblastosi foetalis, germ cell tumours, gynaecomastia, hydatidiform mole, insulinoma, neoplasms (colon, lung, pancreas, stomach), ovarian cancer, pregnancy, seminoma, and testicular cancers and possibly bladder cancer.

Values are Decreased in Abortion and Ectopic Pregnancy

The hCG testing may help differentiate actual pregnancy from an ectopic pregnancy in conjunction with an ultrasound.

Avoid medications such as anticonvulsants, antiparkinsonism agents, hypnotics, tranquilizers which may cause a false-positive result.

Factors that Affect Results

— False-positive results may be due to incorrect handling of the test sample, excessive production of luteinising hormone (LH) of the pituitary gland, absence of gonadal hormones in menopausal women or hCG producing tumours.

— False-negative results may be due to the test being performed too early in pregnancy.

Other Data

Although not usually present in healthy males or nonpregnancy females, elevated levels of hCG may be detected in patients with certain malignant tumours.

INSULIN Courtesy: Lilac Medicare

Intended Use: Monobind Insulin Microplate Elisa test is intended to be used for the quantitative determination of insulin levels in human serum. The test is for *in vitro* diagnostic use only.

Summary and Explanation of the Test

Human insulin is a peptide produced in the beta cells of the pancreas and is responsible for the metabolism and storage of carbohydrates. As a result of biofeedback, the insulin levels increase with intake of sugars and decline when sugar content is low for absorption. In the diabetic population the mechanism of insulin production is impaired because of genetic predispositions (Type 1) or because of lifestyle and/ or hereditary factors (Type II). In such cases, either the insulin production has to be boosted by medication or it has to be supplemented by oral or intravenous methods. The quantitative determination of insulin can help in dose selection the patient has to be subjected to.

On the other hand, the circulatory insulin can be found at much higher levels like in patients with pancreatic tumours. These tumours secrete abnormally high levels of insulin and thus cause hypoglycaemia. Accordingly, fasting hypoglycaemia associated with inappropriately high concentrations of insulin strongly suggests an islet-cell tumour (insulinoma). To distinguish insulinomas from factitious hypoglycaemia due to insulin administration, serum C-peptide values are recommended. These insulinomas can be localized by provocative intravenous doses of tolbutamide and calcium.

PRINCIPLE

Immunoenzymometric Assay

The essential reagents required for an immunoenzymometric assay include high affinity and specificity antibodies (enzyme conjugated and immobilised), with different and distinct epitope recognition, in excess, and native antigen. In this procedure, the immobilisation takes place during the assay at the surface of a microplate well through the interaction of streptavidin coated on the well and exogenously added biotinylated monoclonal anti-Insulin antibody.

Upon mixing monoclonal biotinylated antibody, the enzyme-labeled antibody and a serum containing the native antigen, reaction results between the native antigen and the antibodies, without competition or steric hindrance, to form a soluble sandwich complex. The interaction is illustrated by the following equation:

$$^{EnZ}Ab(p) + {}^{Btn}Agins + {}^{Ptn}Ab_{(m)} \underset{k_{-a}}{\overset{k_a}{\rightleftharpoons}} {}^{EnZ}Ab_{(p)}Ag_{TSH}-{}^{Btn}Ab_{(m)}$$

$^{Btn}Ag_{INS}$ = Biotinylated monoclonal antibody (excels quantity)

Ag_{INS} = Native antigen (variable quantity)

$^{EnZ}Ab_{(p)}$ = Enzyme labeled monoclonal antibody (excess quantity)

$Ab_{(p)}$-Ag_{INS}-$^{Btn}Ab_{(m)}$ = Antigen-antibodies sandwich complex

k_a = Rate constant of association

k_{-a} = Rate constant of dissociation

Simultaneously, the complex is deposited to the well through the high affinity reaction of streptavidin and biotinylated antibody. This interaction is illustrated below

$^{ENZ}Ab_{(p)}$-AgI_{NS}-$^{Btn}Ab_{(m)}$ + $Streptavidin_{cw}$ => immobilised complex

Streptavidin cw = Streptavidin immobolized on well

Immobilised complex = Sandwich complex bound to the solid surface

After equilibrium is attained, the antibody-bound fraction is separated from unbound antigen by decantation or aspiration. The enzyme activity in the antibody-bound fraction is directly proportional to the native antigen concentration. By utilising several different serum references of known antigen values, a dose response curve can be generated from which the antigen concentration of an unknown can be ascertained.

For In Vitro Diagnostic Use Not for Internal or External Use in Humans or Animals

Precautions

All products that contain human serum have been found to be nonreactive for Hepatitis B Surface antigen, HIV 1 and 2 and HCV antibodies by FDA required tests. Since no known test can offer complete assurance that infectious agents are absent, all human serum products should be handled as potentially hazardous and capable of transmitting disease. Good laboratory procedures for handling blood products can be found in the Center for Disease Control/ National Institute of Health, "Biosafety in Microbiological and Biomedical Laboratories," 2nd Edition, 1988, HHS.

Specimen Collection and Preparation

The specimens shall be blood serum in type and the usual precautions in the collection of venipuncture samples should be observed. For accurate comparison to established normal values, a fasting morning serum sample should be obtained. The blood should be collected in a plain red-top venipuncture tube without additives or gel barrier. Allow the blood to clot. Centrifuge the specimen to separate the serum from the cells.

Samples may be refrigerated at 2-8°C for a maximum* period of five (5) days. If the specimen(s) cannot be assayed within this time, the sample(s) may be stored at temperatures of –20°C for up to 30 days. Avoid repetitive freezing and thawing. When assayed in duplicate, 0.100 ml of the specimen is required.

REAGENTS AND MATERIALS PROVIDED

1. Insulin Calibrators - 2.0 ml/vial (Dried)

Six (6) vials of references for insulin antigen at levels of 0(A), 5(B), 25(C), 50(D), 100(E), and 300(F) mlU/

ml. Reconstitute each vial with 2 ml of distilled or deionized water. The reconstituted calibrators are stable for sixty (60) days at 2-8°C. A preservative has beer, added.

Note: The calibrators, human serum based, were calibrated using a reference preparation, which was assayed against the WHO 1st IRP 66/304.

2. Enzyme-Insulin Antibody Conjugate and Biotinylated Monoclonal Antibody —13 ml/vial

One (1) vial containing enzyme-labeled affinity purified monoclonal mouse antibody, biotinylated monoclonal mouse IgG in buffer, dye, and preservative. Store at 2-8°C.

3. Streptavidin-Coated Microplate—96 Wells

One 96-well microplate coated with Streptavidin and packaged in an aluminum bag with a drying agent. Store at 2-8°C.

4. Wash Solution Concentrate—20 ml

One (1) vial containing a surfactant in phosphate buffered saline. A preservative has been added. Store at 2 to 30°C.

5. Substrate A —7.0 ml/vial

One (1) bottle containing tetramethylbenzidine (TMB) in buffer. Store at 2-8°C.

6. Substrate B — 7.0 ml/vial

One (1) bottle containing hydrogen peroxide (H_2O_2) in buffer. Store at 2-8°C.

7. Stop Solution—8.0 ml/vial

One (1) bottle containing a strong acid (1N HCl). Store at 2 to 30°C.

8. Instructions

Required but Not Provided

1. Pipettete(s) capable of delivering 50 μl and 100 μl volumes with a precision of better than 1.5 per cent.
2. Dispenser(s) for repetitive deliveries of 0.100 ml and 0.300 ml volumes with a precision of better than 1.5 per cent (optional).
3. Microplate washer or a squeeze bottle (optional).
4. Microplate reader with 450 nm and 620 nm wavelength absorbance capability (The 620 nm filter is optional)
5. Adjustable volume (200-1000 μl) dispenser.
6. Container(s) for mixing of reagents (see below).
7. Absorbent paper for blotting the microplate wells.
8. Plastic wrap or microplate cover for incubation steps.
9. Vacuum aspirator (optional) for wash steps.
10. Timer
11. Storage container for storage of wash buffer.
12. Distilled or deionized water.
13. Quality control materials.

REAGENT PREPARATION AND STORAGE

1. Wash Buffer

Dilute contents of wash concentrate to 1000 ml with distilled or deionized water in a suitable storage container. Store at room temperature for sixty days. It is essential that all the contents of the wash buffer concentrate dissolve. Crystal formation in the wash concentrate can be eliminated by briefly (approx. 5 minutes) heating in a water bath at 37°C or storing the wash concentrate at room temperature.

2. Working Substrate Solution

Mix substrate A and substrate B by pouring the contents of substrate B into the vial of substrate A. Use within sixty days of preparation

Note 1: Do not use reagents beyond the kit expiration date.

Note 2: Opened reagents are stable for sixty (60) days when stored at 2-8°C.

Note 3: If the substrate solution turns blue, discard the reagent.

Test Procedure

Before proceeding with the assay, bring all reagents, serum references and controls to room temperature (20-25°C).

1. Format the microplates' wells for calibrator, control and patient specimen to be assayed in duplicate. Replace any unused microwell strips back into the aluminum bag, seal and store at 2-8°C.
2. Pipettete 0.050 ml (50 μl) of the appropriate calibrators, controls and samples into the assigned wells.

3. Add 0.100 ml (100 μl) of the biotinylated/enzyme-labeled antibodies to each well. It is very important to dispense all reagents close to the bottom of the microwell.
4. Swirl the microplate gently for 20-30 seconds to mix. Cover with a plastic wrap.
5. Incubate for 120 minutes at room temperature (22-25°C).
6. Discard the contents of the microplate by decantation or aspiration. If decanting, tap and blot the plate dry with absorbent paper.
7. Add 300 μl of wash buffer (see reagent preparation section), decant (tap and blot) or aspirate. Repeat two (2) additional times for a total of three (3) washes. An automatic or manual plate washer can be used. Follow the manufacturer's instruction for proper usage. If a squeeze bottle is used, fill each well to the top by squeezing the container. Avoiding air bubbles. Decant the wash and repeat two (2) additional times.
8. Add 0.100 ml (100 μl) of working substrate solution to all wells (see reagent preparation section). Always add reagents in the same order to minimize reaction time differences between wells.
9. Incubate at room temperature for fifteen (15) minutes.
10. Add 0.050 ml (50 μl) of stop solution to each well and mix gently for 15-20 seconds. Always add reagents in the same order to minimize reaction time differences between wells.
11. Read the absorbance in each well at 450 nm (using a reference wavelength of 620-630 nm to minimize well imperfections) in a microplate reader. The results should be read within thirty (30) minutes of adding the stop solution.

Quality Control

Each laboratory should assay controls at levels in the low, normal and elevated ranges for monitoring assay performance. These controls should be treated as unknowns and values determined in every test procedure performed. Quality control trends should be maintained to monitor batch-to-batch consistency.

Calculation Control

1. Record the absorbance obtained from the printout of the microplate reader as outlined in Example 13
2. Average the absorbance of each duplicate. Plot the mean absorbance for each duplicate calibrator versus the corresponding insulin concentration in μIU/ml on linear graph paper.
3. Draw a dose *response curve (DRC)* using the best-fit through the plotted points.
4. Interpolate the concentration of the controls and the unknowns from the DRC.

Example 13

Sample	*Well*		*Mean*	*Value*
IU	*Number*	*Abs (A)*	*Abs (B)*	*(μl U/ml)*
Cal A	A1	0.011	10	0
	B1	0.009		
Cal B	C1	0.063	0.062	5
	D1	0.061		
Cal C	E1	0.269	0.266	25
	F1	0.262		
Cal D	G1	0.507	0.482	50
	H1	0.456		
Cal E	A2	0.942	0.933	100
	B2	0.923		
Cal F	C2	2.492	2.394	300
	D2	2.296		
Ctrl 1	E2	0.067	0.065	5.2
	F2	0.063		
Ctrl 2	G2	0.249	0.274	22.3
	H2	0.245		
Patient 1	A3	0.24	0.242	22
	B3	0.244		

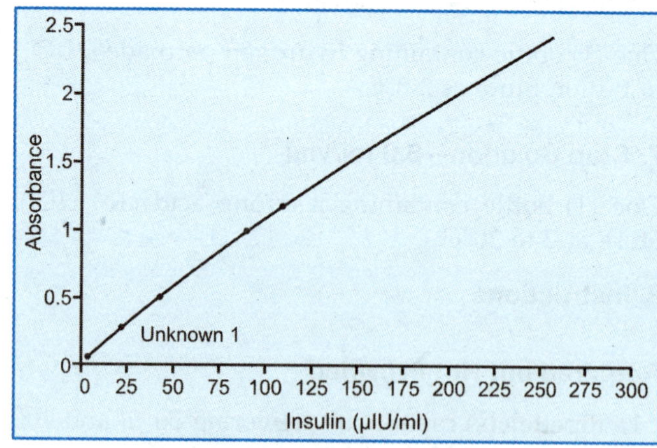

Fig. 17.37: Estimation insulin (μIU/ml)

*The data presented in Example 13 and Figure 17.37 are for illustration only and should not be used in lieu of a dose response curve prepared with each assay.

Quality Control

In order for the assay results to be considered valid, the following criteria should be met:

1. The absorbance (OD) of calibrators 0 μl IU/ml should be < 0.1.
2. The absorbance (OD) of calibrators 300 μl IU/ml should be > 1.2.
3. Four out of six quality control pools should be within the established ranges.

Limitations of Procedure

1. It is important that the time of reaction in each well is held constant for reproducible results.
2. Pipeting of samples should not extend beyond ten (10) minutes to avoid assay drift.
3. If more than one (1) plate is used, it is recommended to repeat the dose response curve.
4. Addition of the substrate solution initiates a kinetic reaction, which is terminated by the addition of the stop solution. Therefore, the addition of the substrate and the stopping solution should be added in the same sequence to eliminate any time deviation during reaction.
5. Plate readers measure vertically. Do not touch the bottom of the wells.
6. Failure to remove adhering solution adequately in the aspiration or decantation wash step(s) may result in poor replication and spurious results.
7. Highly lipaemeic, haemolysed or grossly contaminated specimen(s) should not be used.
8. Patient samples with insulin concentrations above 300 μlU/ml may be diluted with the zero calibrator and re-assayed. Multiply the value obtained by the dilution factor to obtain the corrected value.
9. Use components from the same lot. No intermixing of reagents from different batches.

Expected Values

Insulin values are consistently higher in plasma than in serum; thus, serum is preferred. Compared with fasting values in nonobese nondiabetic individuals, insulin levels are higher in obese nondiabetic subjects and lower in trained athletes. Although proinsulin cross reacts with most competitive insulin assays, there is virtually less than 0.01 per cent cross reaction found with proinsulin using the Monobind Insulin Microwell Elisa.

Each laboratory is advised to establish its own ranges for normal and abnormal populations. These ranges are always dependent upon locale, population, laboratory, technique and specificity of the method.

Based on the clinical data gathered by Monobind in concordance with the published literature the following ranges have been assigned. These ranges should be used as guidelines only

Children < 12 yr	< 10 μlU/ml
Adult (Normal)	0.7 - 9.0 μlU/ml
Diabetic (Type II)	0.7 - 25 μlU/ml

C-PEPTIDE (Courtesy: Lilac Medicare)

Intended Use: The Quantitative Determination of Circulating C-Peptide Concentrations in Human Serum by a Microplate Immunoenzymometric Assay

Summary and Explanation of the Test

Diabetes is one of the leading causes of disability and death in the US. It affects an estimated 16 million Americans, about one third of them do not even know they have the disease. The causes of diabetes are not precisely known, but both genetic and environmental factors play a significant role. The disease is marked by deficiencies in the body's ability to produce and properly use insulin. The most common forms of diabetes are type 1, in which the body's ability to produce insulin is destroyed, and type 2, in which the body is resistant to insulin even though some amount of insulin may be produced.

In vitro determination of insulin and C-peptide levels help in the differential diagnosis of liver disease, acromegaly, Cushing's syndrome, familial glucose intolerance, insulinoma, renal failure, ingestion of accidental oral hypoglycaemic drugs or insulin-induced factitious hypoglycaemia. Both insulin and C-peptide are produced by enzymatic cleavage of proinsulin. Proinsulin is stored in the secretory granules of pancreatic p-cells and is split into a 31 amino acid connecting peptide (C-peptide; MW 3600) and insulin (MW 6000). C-peptide is devoid of any biological activity but appears to be necessary to maintain the structural integrity of insulin. Although insulin and C-peptide are secreted into portal circulation in equimolar concentrations, fasting levels of C-peptide are 5-10 fold higher than those of insulin owing to the longer half-life of C-peptide. The liver does not extract C-peptide however, it is removed from the circulation by degradation in the kidneys with a fraction passing out unchanged in urine. Hence urine C-peptide levels correlate well with fasting C-peptide levels in serum. The glucagon stimulated C-peptide determination is often used for differential diagnosis of insulin-dependent from noninsulin-dependent diabetic patients.

PRINCIPLE

Immunoenzymometric Assay

The essential reagents required for an immunoenzymometric assay include high affinity and specificity antibodies (enzyme conjugated and immobilised), with different-and distinct epitope recognition, in excess, and native antigen. In this procedure, the immobilisation takes place during, the assay at the surface of a microplate well through the interaction of streptavidin coated on the well and exogenously added biotinylated monoclonal anti-insulin antibody.

Upon mixing monoclonal biotinylated antibody, the enzyme-labeled antibody and a serum containing the native antigen, reaction results between the native antigen and the antibodies, without competition or steric hindrance, to form a soluble sandwich complex. The interaction is illustrated by the following equation

$$^{Enz}Ab_{(m)} + Agc_{-Pep} + {}^{Btn}Ab_{(m)} \quad {}^{Enz}Ab_{(m)}\text{-}Ag_{TSH}\text{-}{}^{Btn}Ab_{(m)}$$

$^{Btn}Ab_{(m)}$ = Biotinylated monoclonal antibody (excess quantity)

$^{ENZ}Ab_{(m)}$ = Enzyme labeled monoclonal antibody (excess quantity)

$^{ENZ}Ab_{(m)}\text{-}Agc\text{-}_{PEP}\text{-}{}^{Btn}Ab_{(m)}$ = Antigen-antibodies complex

k_a = Rate constant of association

k_a = Rate constant of dissociation

Simultaneously, the complex is deposited to the well through the high affinity reaction of streptavidin and biotinylated antibody. This interaction is illustrated below

$^{Enz}Ab_{(m)}\text{-}Agc\text{-}_{PEP-}{}^{Btn}Ab_{(m)}$ + Streptavidin cw →Immobilised complex

Streptavidin cw = Streptavidin immobolised on well

Immobilised complex = Sandwich complex bound to the solid surface

After equilibrium is attained, the antibody-bound fraction is separated from unbound antigen by decantation or aspiration. The enzyme activity in the antibody-bound fraction is directly proportional to the native antigen concentration. By utilising several different serum references of known antigen values, a dose response curve can be generated from which the antigen concentration of an unknown can be ascertained.

PRECAUTIONS

For In Vitro Diagnostic Use Not for Internal or External Use in Humans or Animals

All products that contain human serum have been found to be nonreactive for Hepatitis B Surface antigen, HIV 1 and 2 and HCV antibodies by FDA required tests. Since no known test can offer complete assurance that infectious agents are absent, all human serum products should be handled as potentially hazardous and capable of transmitting disease. Good laboratory procedures for handling blood products can be found in the Center for Disease Control/ National Institute of Health, "Biosafety in Microbiological and Biomedical Laboratories," 2nd Edition, 1988, HHS.

Specimen Collection and Preparation

The specimens shall be blood serum in type and the usual precautions in the collection of venipuncture samples should be observed. For accurate comparison to established normal values, a fasting morning serum sample should be obtained. The blood should be collected in a plain red-top venipuncture tube without additives. Allow the blood to clot. Centrifuge the specimen to separate the serum from the cells.

Samples may be refrigerated at 2-8°C for a maximum period of two (2) days. If the specimen(s) cannot be assayed within this time, the sample(s) may be stored at temperatures of –20°C for up to 30 days. Avoid repetitive freezing and thawing. When assayed in duplicate, 0.100 ml of the specimen is required.

Reagents and Materials Provided

1. **C-Peptide Calibrators - 2.0 ml/vial (Lyophilized):** Six (6) vials of references for C-peptide antigen at levels of 0(A). 0.2(B), 1.0(C),

2.0(D), 5.0(E), and 10.0(F) ng/ml. Reconstitute each vial with 2.0 ml of distilled or deionised water.

The reconstituted calibrators are stable for 7 days at 2-8°C. In order to store for a longer period of time aliquot the reconstituted calibrators in cryo vials and store at –10°C. Do not freeze thaw more than once. A preservative has been added.

Note: The calibrators, human serum based, were calibrated using a reference preparation, which was assayed against the WHO 1st IRR 84/510.

2. **Anti-C-Peptide-HRP and Biotinylated monoclonal antibodies — 13 ml/vial**
   One (1) vial containing enzyme-labeled affinity purified monoclonal mouse antibody, biotinylated monoclonal mouse IgG in buffer, dye, and preservative. Store at 2-8°C.
3. **Streptavidin Microplate - 96 wells**
   One 96-well microplate coated with Streptavidin and packaged in an aluminum bag with a drying agent. Store at 2-8°C.
4. **Wash Solution Concentrate - 20 ml**
   One (1) vial containing a surfactant in buffered saline. A preservative has been added. Store at 2 to 30°C.
5. **Substrate A -7.0 ml/vial**
   One (1) bottle containing tetramethyl benzidine (TMB) in buffer. Store at 2-8°C.
6. **Substrate: B - 7.0 ml/vial**
   One (1) bottle containing hydrogen peroxide (H_2O_2) in buffer. Store at 2-8°C.
7. **Stop solution-8.0 ml/vial**
   One (1) bottle containing a strong acid (1N HCI). Store at 2 to 30°C.
8. Instructions.

Required but Not Provided

1. Pipettete(s) capable of delivering 50 μl and 100 μl volumes with a precision of better than 1.5 per cent.
2. Dispenser(s) for repetitive deliveries of 0.100 ml and 0.300 ml volumes with a precision of better than 1.5 per cent (optional).
3. Microplate washer or a squeeze bottle (optional).
4. Microplate reader with 450 nm and 620 nm wavelength absorbance capability (The 620 nm filter is optional)
5. Adjustable volume (200-1000 μl) repeat dispenser.
6. Container(s) for mixing of reagents (see below).
7. Absorbent paper for blotting the microplate wells.
8. Plastic wrap or microplate cover for incubation steps.
9. Vacuum aspirator (optional) for wash steps.
10. Timer
11. Storage container for storage of wash buffer
12. Distilled or deionized water
13. Quality control materials.

REAGENT PREPARATION

1. Wash Buffer

Dilute contents of wash concentrate to 1000 ml with distilled or deionized water in a suitable storage container. Store at room temperature 20-27°C for up to 60 days.

2. Working Substrate Solution

Pour the contents of the vial labeled Solution 'A' into the vial labeled Solution 'B'. Mix and store at 2-8°C. Use within 60 days. Or for longer periods of usage, determine the amount of reagent needed and prepare by mixing equal portions of substrate A and substrate B in a suitable container. For example, add 1 ml of A and 1 ml of B per two (2) eight well strips (a slight excess of solution is made). Discard the unused portion.

Note: Do not use the working substrate if it looks blue.

Test Procedure

Before proceeding with the assay, bring all reagents, serum references and controls to room temperature (20 -25°C).

1. Format the microplates' wells for calibrator, control and patient specimen to be assayed in duplicate. Replace any unused microwell strips back into the aluminum bag, seal and store at 2-8°C.
2. Pipette 0.050 ml (50 μl) of the appropriate calibrators, controls and samples into the assigned wells.
3. Add 0.100 ml (100 μl) of the biotinylated/enzyme-labeled antibodies to each well. It is very important to dispense all reagents close to the bottom of the microwell.

4. Swirl the microplate gently for 20-30 seconds to mix. Cover with a plastic wrap.
5. Incubate for 120 minutes at room temperature (20-25°C).
6. Discard the contents of the microplate by decantation or aspiration. If decanting, tap and blot the plate dry with absorbent paper.
7. Add 300 μl of wash buffer (see reagent preparation section), decant (tap and blot) or aspirate. Repeat two (2) additional times for a total of three (3) washes. An automatic or manual plate washer can be used. Follow the manufacturer's instruction for proper usage. If a squeeze bottle is used, fill each well to the top by squeezing the container. Avoiding air bubbles. Decant the wash and repeat two (2) additional times.
8. Add 0.100 ml (100 μl) of working substrate solution to all wells *(see reagent preparation section).*
9. Incubate at room temperature for fifteen (15) minutes.
10. Add 0.050 ml (50 μl) of stop solution to each well and mix gently for 15-20 seconds. Read the absorbance in each well at 450 nm (using a reference wavelength of 620-630 nm to minimise well imperfections) in a microplate reader. The results should be read within thirty (30) minutes of adding the stop solution.

Note: Always add reagents in the same order to minimise reaction time differences between wells.

Quality Control

Each laboratory should assay controls at levels in the low, normal and elevated ranges for monitoring assay performance. These controls should be treated as unknowns and values determined in every test procedure performed. Quality control trends should be maintained to monitor batch-to-batch consistency.

Calculation of Results

1. Record the absorbance obtained from the printout of the microplate reader as outlined in Example 14.
2. Average the absorbance of each duplicate. Plot the mean absorbance for each duplicate calibrator versus the corresponding C-peptide concentration in ng/ml on linear graph paper.
3. Draw a dose response curve (DRC) using the best-fit through the plotted points.
4. Interpolate the concentration of the controls and the unknowns from the DRC.

Example 14

Sample IU	*Well Number*	*Abs (A)*	*Mean Abs (B)*	*Value (μl U/ml)*
Cal A	A1	0.022	0.022	0
	B1	0.023		
Cal B	C1	0.097	0.103	0.2
	D1	0.421		
Cal C	E1	0.439	0.429	1
	F1	0.889		
Cal D	G1	0.91	0.901	2
	H1	1.976		
Cal E	A2	1.966	1.971	5
	B2	2.717		
Cal F	C2	2.57	2.643	10
	D2	0.429		
Ctrl 1	E2	0.437	0.433	1.03
	F2	1.861		
Ctrl 2	G2	1.913	1.887	4.64
	H2	0.388		
Patient 1	A3	0.421	1.502	3.38
	B3			

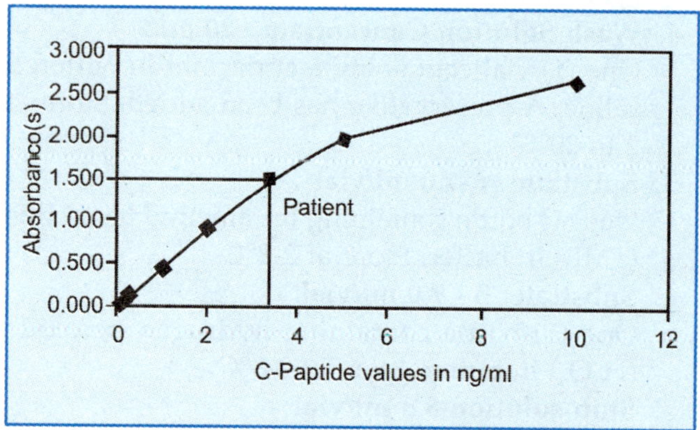

Fig. 17.38: Estimation of C-peptide in ng/ml

*The data presented in Example 14 and Figure 17.38 are for illustration only and should not be used in lieu of a dose response curve prepared with each assay.

Quality Control

In order for the assay results to be considered valid, the following criteria should be met:

1. The absorbance (OD) of calibrators 0 ng/ml should be < 0.1.
2. The absorbance (OD) of calibrators 10 ng/ml should be > 1.2.
3. Four out of six quality control pools should be within the established ranges.

Limitations of Procedure

1. It is important that the time of reaction in each well is held constant for reproducible results.
2. Pipeting of samples should not extend beyond ten (10) minutes to avoid assay drift.
3. If more than one (1) plate is used, it is recommended to repeat the dose response curve.
4. Addition of the substrate solution initiates a kinetic reaction, which is terminated by the addition of the stop solution. Therefore, the addition of the substrate and the stopping solution should be added in the same sequence to eliminate any time deviation during reaction.
5. Plate readers measure vertically. Do not touch the bottom of the wells.
6. Failure to remove adhering solution adequately in the aspiration or decantation wash step(s) may result in poor replication and spurious results.
7. Highly lipaemic, haemolysed or grossly contaminated specimen(s) should not be used.
8. Patient samples with C-peptide concentrations above 10 ng/ml may be diluted with the zero calibrator and re-assayed. Multiply the value obtained by the dilution factor to obtain the corrected value.
9. Use components from the same lot. No intermixing of reagents from different batches.

Expected Values

C-peptide values are consistently higher in plasma than in serum; thus, serum is preferred. Compared with fasting values in nonobese nondiabetic individuals, C-peptide levels are higher in obese nondiabetic subjects and lower in trained athletes.

Each laboratory is advised to establish its own ranges for normal and abnormal populations. These ranges are always dependent upon locale, population, laboratory, technique and specificity of the method.

Based on the clinical data gathered by Monobind in concordance with the published literature, the following range has been assigned. Thus range should be used as guideline only.

Adult (Normal) 0.7 - 1.9 ng/ml

ANTI-INSULIN (Courtesy: Lilac Medicare)

Immunometric Enzyme Immunoassay for the Quantitative Determination of Autoantibodies to Bovine, Porcine and recombinant human Insulin in Serum or Plasma

Warnings and Precautions

All reagents of this test kit are strictly intended for *in vitro* use only.

Please adhere strictly to the sequence of pipeting steps provided in this protocol. Observe the guidelines for performing quality control in medical laboratories by assaying controls and/or pooled sera.

All reagents should be stored refrigerated at 2-8°C in their original container.

Do not interchange kit components from different lots. The expiration dates stated on the labels of the shipping container and all vials have to be observed. Do not use kit components beyond their expiration dates.

Allow all kit components and specimen to reach room temperature prior to use and mix well.

During handling of all kit reagents, controls and serum samples, observe the existing legal regulations. The following precautions should be taken while handling potentially infectious materials:

- do not eat, drink or smoke in areas where -specimens or kit reagents are handled
- do not pipette by mouth
- wear disposable gloves while handling specimens or kit reagents and wash hands thoroughly afterwards.

The test kit contains components of human origin which, when tested by FDA-licensed methods, were found negative for hepatitis B surface antigen and for HIV antibody. No known test can guarantee, however, that products derived from human blood will not be infectious. Handle, therefore, all reagents and human blood derivatives, like plasma or serum samples, as if capable of transmitting infection.

Avoid contact with the TMB (3, 3', 5, 5'-tetramethyl benzidine). If TMB comes into contact with skin, wash thoroughly with water and soap.

The stop solution contains hydrochloric acid. If it comes into contact with skin, wash thoroughly with water and seek medical attention.

Avoid contact between the buffered peroxide solution and easily oxidised materials; extreme temperatures may initiate spontaneous combustion.

Material Supplied

Package size 96 determination.

Divisible microplate consisting of 12 modules of 8 wells each, 1 coated with a mixture of highly purified preparations of bovine, porcine and recombinant human insulin.

Anti-insulin calibrators in la PBS/BSA matrix containing 0; 6.3; 12.5; 25; 50 and 100 U/ ml (A-F)	1 Set 6 vials 1 ml each
Anti-Insulin controls in a PBS/feSA matrix (positive and negative), for the respective concentrations see the enclosed package insert	1 Set 2 vials 1 ml each
sample buffer, yellow, concentrate	1 vial 20 ml
Enzyme conjugate solution (light red), containing polyclonal rabbit anti-h-lgG-IgG, labelled with horseradish peroxidase	1 vial 15 ml
TMB substrate solution, containing 3,3,'5,5'-tetramethyl-benzidine in buffered peroxide solution ready to use	1 vial 15 ml
Stop solution (1 M hydrochloric acid)	1 vial 15 ml
Buffered wash solution, concentrate	1 vial 20 ml

Controls

A set of two controls is provided with the kit.

Technical Data

Sample material	Serum or plasma
Required sample size	10 μl of sample to be diluted 1 100 with sample buffer
100 μl prediluted sample per single determination	
Total incubation time	60 minutes at room temperature (18-28°C)
Calibration range	6.3 -100 U/ml
Sensitivity	0.5 U/ml
Storage	refrigerated at 2-8°C
Shelf-life	9 months after manufacturing or until the expiration date printed on the labels
Package size	96 tests

Principle of the Procedure

Anti-insulin is an indirect solid phase enzyme immunometric assay (ELISA). It is designed for the quantitative measurement of IgG class autoantibodies directed against insulin. The assay is based on microplates coated with a mixture of highly purified preparations of bovine, porcine and recombinant human insulin. The assay is useful in the primary diagnosis of Type I Diabetes, as well as for screening purposes to detect developing insulin autoantibodies in patients under insulin therapy.

The microplate can be divided into 12 modules of 8 wells each or can be used completely for 96 determinations.

Reaction Phases

During this procedure, the binding of present autoantibodies, as well as the formation of the sandwich complexes and enzymatic colour reaction take place during three different reaction phases.

Phase 1

Calibrators, controls and prediluted patient samples are pipetted into the wells of the microplate. Any present antibodies bind to the inner surface of the wells. After a 30-minute incubation, the microplate is washed with wash buffer for removing non-reactive serum components.

Phase 2

An anti-human-IgG horseradish peroxidase conjugate solution is pipetted into the wells of the microplate to recognise the autoantibodies bound to the immobilised antigens. After a 15-minute incubation, any excessive enzyme conjugate, which is not specifically bound, is washed away with wash buffer.

Phase 3

A chromogenic substrate solution containing TMB (3, 3'5, 5'-teramethyl-benzidine) is dispensed into the wells. During 15 minutes of incubation, the colour of the solutions change into blue. Colour development is stopped by adding 1 M hydrochloric acid as stop solution. The solutions' colour change into yellow.

The amount of colour is directly proportional to the concentration of IgG present in the original sample. The optical density for each calibrator may be graphically plotted against the concentration of IgG and unknowns extrapolated from the curve.

To read the optical density, a microplate reader with a 450 nm filter is required. Bichromatic measurement with a 600-650 nm reference is recommended.

Clinical Relevance

Type 1 Diabetes is mainly characterised by limited or fully missing secretion of the hormone insulin. Morphological studies demonstrated a destruction of the beta cells of the so-called Langerhans' Islet Cells in Type 1 diabetics. Numerous researchers described the appearance of antibodies directed against the islet cells and insulin as the causal reason for the onset of the disease.

Anti-insulin antibodies are found in 37 per cent of patients with newly detected Type I Diabetes, in 4 per cent of their relatives of the first degree and in up to 1-5 per cent of healthy controls. A positive correlation between the appearance of anti-insulin and anti-islet cell antibodies has been reported.

Anti-insulin autoantibodies may be detected several months and in some cases years before the onset of the fully clinical manifestation of the diseases. Occasionally also autoantibodies to pro-insulin may appear.

These "true" anti-insulin autoantibodies directed against endogenous insulin have to be distinguished from those autoantibodies which are developed in insulin-dependent diabetics undergoing therapy with insulin preparations of animal origin. In fact, the latter have to be referred to side effects. These side effects may occur as local reactions of the skin by development of insulin-specific autoantibodies. These autoantibodies are causing the formation of an insulin depot and they may simulate a resistance against the hormonal treatment with animal insulin.

Additionally, other immunological phenomena have been reported for Type I diabetics. A lot of other autoantibody specificities have been detected in those patients too, but these antibodies must not cause additional autoimmune phenomenon.

Figure 17.39 shows the incidence (in per cent) of various autoantibodies occurring in Type 1 diabetics compared to healthy controls

Autoantibody specificity	type 1 diabetics (%)	healthy controls (%)
Anti-islet cell antibodies	32	1
Antibodies against islet cell surface antigens	approx. 50	2
Anti-insulin antibodies	up to 70	0
Anti-thyroid peroxidase ab's (Anti-TPO)	18	6
Anti-single-stranded DNA ab's (Anti-ssDNA)	85	9

Indications

- Anti-insulin antibodies in Type I diabetics
- Development of anti-insulin antibodies under insulin therapy.

Normal Values

In a normal range study with serum samples from healthy blood donors, the following ranges have been established with the anti-insulin test

Anti-insulin	[U/ml]
Normal	< 5
Borderline	5-10
Elevated	> 10

Positive results should be verified concerning the entire clinical status of the patient. Also, every decision for therapy should be taken individually.

It is recommended that each laboratory establishes its own normal and pathological ranges. The reference ranges below should be regarded as guidelines only.

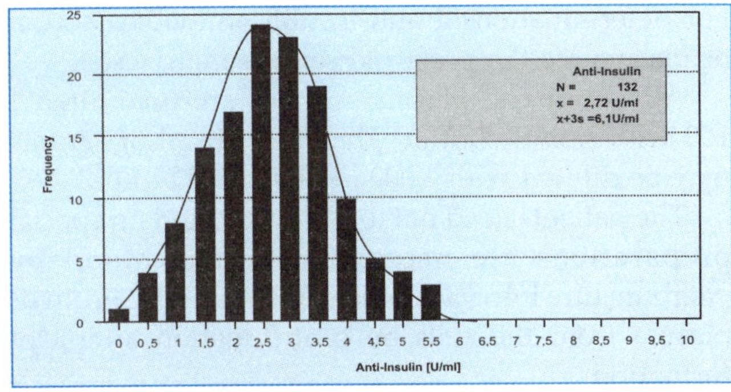

Fig. 17.39: Anti-Insulin [U/ ml] frequency distribution of Anti-Insulin antibodies in healthy blood donors

Specificity

The microplate is coated with a mixture of highly purified preparations of bovine, porcine and recombinant human insulin. Therefore, the anti-insulin test kit recognises only IgG-class autoantibodies specific for these insulins. No crossreactivities have been observed.

Calibration

Since no international reference preparation for anti-insulin autoantibodies is available, the assay system is calibrated in relative arbitrary units.

IMMUNOASSAY PROCEDURE

Materials Required

Equipment

- Microplate reader capable for endpoint measurements at 450 nm
- Vortex mixer
- Pipettes of 10 µl, 100 µl and 1000 µl

Preparation of Reagents

- Distilled water
- Graduated cylinder for 100 and 1,000 ml
- Plastic container for storage of the wash solution

Optional

- Multichannel dispenser
- Or Repeatable pipette for 100 µl
- Data reduction software

Specimen Collection and Preparation

For determination of anti-insulin antibodies serum or plasma are the preferred sample matrixes.

All serum and plasma samples are prediluted 1 100 with sample buffer. Therefore, 10 µl of sample may be diluted with 1,000 µl of sample buffer.

The patients need not to be fasting, and no special preparations are necessary. Collect blood by venipuncture into vacutainers and separate serum or plasma from the cells by centrifugation after clot formation.

Samples may be stored refrigerated at 2-8°C for at least 5 days. For longer storage of up to six months, samples should be stored frozen at –20°C. To avoid repeated thawing and freezing, the samples should be aliquoted.

Neither bilirubin nor haemolysis have significant effect on the procedure.

Preparation and Storage of Reagents

All components of this test kit are supplied in a liquid format and ready to use, except the sample buffer and wash buffer. When stored, refrigerated at 2-8°C, the components are stable for at least 30 days after opening or until the expiration date printed on the labels.

Remaining modules of the microplate should be stored refrigerated at 2-8°C protected from moisture; stored together with desiccant and carefully sealed in the plastic bag.

Preparation of Sample Buffer

Dilute the contents of each vial of the sample buffer concentrate (5x) with distilled water to a final volume of 100 ml prior to use. Store refrigerated stable at 2-8°C for at least 30 days after preparation or until the expiration date printed on the label.

Preparation of Buffered Wash Solution

Dilute the contents of each vial of the buffered wash solution concentrate (50x) with distilled water to a final volume of 1000 ml prior to use. Store refrigerated stable at 2-8°C for at least 30 days after preparation or until the expiration date printed on the label.

Notes on Technique

Control sera or pools should routinely be assayed as unknowns to check performance of the reagents and the assay.

Pipetting and Sample Handling

Use a disposable-tip micropipette to dispense sera and plasma samples. Pipette directly to the bottom of the wells. To avoid carryover contamination, change the tip between samples.

Patient samples expected to contain high concentrations should be additionally diluted with sample buffer before. Additional dilutions must be considered during calculation.

Immunoassay Procedure

Do not interchange components of different lots.

All components should be at room temperature before use.

Dilute all patient samples 1:100 with sample buffer before assay. Therefore, combine 10 µl of sample with 1,000 µl of sample buffer in a polystyrene tube. Mix well. Calibrators and controls are ready to use and need not to be diluted.

1. Prepare a sufficient number of microplate modules to accommodate calibrators, controls and prediluted patient samples in duplicates.

	1	2	3	4	5	6	7	8	9	10	11	12
a	SA	SE	P1	P..								
b	SA	SE	P1	P..								
c	SB	SF	P2									
d	SB	SF	P2									
e	SC	C1	P3									
f	SC	C1	P3									
g	SD	C2	P..									
h	SD	C2	P..									

2. Pipette 100 μl of calibrators, controls and prediluted patient samples into the wells.
3. Incubate for 30 minutes at room temperature (18-28°C).
4. Discard the contents of the microwells and wash 3 times with 300 μl of wash solution.
5. Dispense 100 μl of enzyme conjugate solution into each well.
6. Incubate for 15 minutes at room temperature.
7. Discard the contents of the microwells and wash 3 times with 300 μl of wash solution.
8. Dispense 100 μl of 1 MB substrate solution into each well.
9. Incubate for 15 minutes at room temperature.
10. Add 100 μl of stop solution to each well of the modules and let it stand for 5 minutes.
11. Read the optical density at 450 nm and calculate the results. Bichromatic measurement with a reference at 600-690 nm is recommended.

The developed colour is stable for at least 30 minutes. Read optical densities during this time.

Calculation of Results

For the anti-insulin test a 4-parameter-fit with lin-log coordinates for optical density and concentration is recommended. Smoothed Spline approximation and log-log coordinates are also suitable.

Recommended Lin-Log Plot

First, calculate the averaged optical densities for each calibrator well. Use lin-log graph paper and plot the averaged optical density of each calibrator versus the concentration. Draw the best fitting curve approximating the path of all calibrator points. The calibrator points may also be connected with straight line segments. The concentration of unknowns may then be estimated from the calibration curve by interpolation.

Calculation Example

The data given below show typical results for anti-insulin. These data are intended for illustration only and should not be used to calculate results from another run.

Calibrators

No	Position	OP 1	OP 2	Mean	Cone. 1	Cone. 2	Mean	decl. Cone.	CV per cent
STA	A1/B1	0.036	0.032	0.034	0.1	0.1	0.1	0.0	8
STB	C1/D1	0.354	0.345	0.349	6.3	6.1	6.2	6.3	2
STC	E1/F1	0.621	0.602	0.611	12.9	12.4	12.7	12.5	2
STD	G1/H1	0.984	1.005	0.994	25	25	25	25	1
STE	A2/B2	1.503	1.500	1.502	50	50	50	50	0
STF	C2/D2	2.057	2.035	2.046	102	99	100	100	1

ASSAY CHARACTERISTICS

Sensitivity

The lower detection limit for anti-insulin has been determined at 0.5 U/ml.

Chapter 18

Diabetes Mellitus Laboratory Diagnosis

DIABETES MELLITUS

Diabetes mellitus is a chronic metabolic disorder with vascular components that is characterised by disturbances in carbohydrate, lipid and protein metabolism. So, hyperglycaemia and glycosuria reflect the major metabolic lesion in carbohydrate metabolism, with secondary metabolic disturbances in proteins (gluconeogenesis) and lipids (ketosis and hypercholesterolaemia).

With hyperglycaemia, renal glycosuria occurs with an osmotic diuresis (polyuria) ultimately leads to dehydration and associated polydipsia (increased thirst). Glycogenolysis and gluconeogenesis (protein depletion) are augmented to generate glucose that contributes to or sustains hyperglycaemia. Muscle glycogen cannot contribute glucose directly to the blood because of the absence of glucose-6-phosphatase. A failure of glucose to penetrate adipose tissue cells mobilises fat and produces a rise in the free fatty acid and triglycerides in the liver. A diabetic fatty liver may result from the absence of lipoprotein synthesis when protein synthesis is compromised by accelerated gluconeogenesis (negative nitrogen balance). When glucose oxidation is impaired, fatty acids form the major source of energy and generate an excess of acetyl coenzyme. A that cannot be oxidised to water and carbon dioxide or be disposed of in other metabolic routes. The condensation of two carbon fragments of acetyl coenzyme A results in formation of ketone bodies, ketonaemia and ketonuria. The three ketone bodies are acetone, β hydroxybutyric acid and acetoacetic acid. Ketoacidosis is the hallmark of potentially fatal complications of diabetes mellitus.

Classification and Causes of Diabetes

Primary
- Maturity-onset (adult) type
- Growth-onset (juvenile) type
- Hyperpituitarism
  - pituitary basophilism
  - acromegaly
- Hyperadrenalism
  - cortical: Cushing's syndrome, aldosteronism
  - medullary: phaeochromocytoma.
- Hyperthyroidism
- Iatrogenic
  - corticosteroids and ACTH
  - growth hormone
  - thyroid extract and triiodothyronine.

Destruction of pancreatic islets:
- Surgical removal of pancreas
- Haemochromatosis
- Fibrocystic disease of pancreas
- Neoplasm.

Miscellaneous
- Diuretics and derivatives (thiazide therapy)
- Stress reactions, surgery and pregnancy
- Starvation and low carbohydrate intake.

The course of the disease can be divided into four stages:

1. Prediabetes,
2. Suspected diabetes,
3. Chemical or latent diabetes,
4. Overt diabetes.

The period from birth until the first evidence of the disease characterises prediabetes. In suspected diabetes, the patient displays an abnormal glucose tolerance test (GTT) or even diabetic symptoms after stressful influences (e.g. obesity, pregnancy, trauma, infections), but usually is normal in all respects. In chemical or latent diabetes, there are no signs or symptoms of disease but an abnormal GTT or fasting hyperglycaemia are evident when the patient is not under stress. With overt diabetes, symptoms of polyuria, polydipsia and weight loss (and possibly ketoacidosis) are often associated with fasting hyperglycaemia and glycosuria. For diagnosis of diabetes in individuals with marked glucose intolerance, the provocative tests should not be performed (as in an insulin requiring diabetic). In patients who have neither glycosuria nor fasting hyperglycaemia—in these individuals provocative tests may be needed to demonstrate impaired glucose tolerance. Glycosuria associated with ketonuria is almost always pathognomonic of diabetes mellitus.

SCREENING TESTS

These include urine and blood glucose estimations.

Urine Glucose (Methods mentioned elsewhere)

While evaluating glycosuria, it should be remembered that venous "true glucose" must exceed 180 mg% of blood before any glucose will spill over into urine (renal threshold). In diabetic nephropathy, the renal threshold may be elevated considerably (very little filtration apparatus left, i.e. glomeruli) even in the presence of hyperglycaemia. Also, the renal threshold increases with age, and in some elderly patients no glycosuria will be present with serum levels of 200 mg% of glucose.

Fasting Blood Sugar

For this, plasma is the blood fraction of choice. Fasting plasma glucose values in excess of 120 mg% (true glucose) are considered indicative of diabetes mellitus; values between 110-120 mg% are equivocal and should be confirmed with a GTT. The 2-hour postprandial (PP) test should be done instead of fasting glucose levels. Emotional hyperglycaemia from secretion of epinephrine as well as cerebral lesions (skull fractures, tumours, vascular accident, and encephalitis) and carbon monoxide poisoning, often provoke hyperglycaemia and glycosuria, must be considered in the evaluation of blood glucose measurements.

Two-hour Postprandial Blood Glucose

After an overnight fast (12 hours), the patient is given a breakfast of 100 gm of carbohydrate or a 100 gm glucose load. Previous to the test, the patient should have been on an adequate carbohydrate diet (300 gm daily) and all medications that influence glucose tolerance should have been discontinued three days prior to the test. Two hours later (2 hours PP or pc, postcibum) a single blood sample is withdrawn for analysis. A value within normal limits makes the diagnosis of diabetes mellitus unlikely, plasma glucose values in the range of 110-120 mg% are suspicious and in excess of 120 mg% (true glucose), diagnosis is most likely and should be confirmed by GTT.

The limitations of a single 2-hour PP glucose value include the following:

1. Slow absorption, which may delay the peak.
2. Rapid absorption with early hyperglycaemia, rapid fall in concentration of blood glucose (due to insulin release), and then a second hyperglycaemic peak due to the effects of counter regulatory responses (epinephrine, glucagon, growth hormone), and
3. Errors in timing specimen collection.

Criteria for the Diagnosis of Diabetes Mellitus and Impaired Glucose Homeostasis

Diabetes mellitus—positive findings from any two of the following tests on different days:

Symptoms of diabetes mellitus* plus casual† plasma glucose concentration > = 200 mg per dL (11.1 mmol per L)

or

FPG > = 126 mg per dL (7.0 mmol per L)

or

2 hrPPG > 200 mg per dL (11.1 mmol per L) after a 75-g glucose load

Impaired glucose homeostasis

Impaired fasting glucose: FPG from 110 to <126 (6.1 to 7.0 mmol per L)

Impaired glucose tolerance: 2hrPPG from 140 to <200 (7.75 to <11.1 mmol per L)

Normal

FPG < 110 mg per dL (6.1 mmol per L)

2hrPPG < 140 mg per dL (7.75 mmol per L)

†--Casual is defined as any time of day without regard to time since last meal.

*--Symptoms include polyuria, polydipsia or unexplained weight loss.

FPG=fasting plasma glucose; 2hrPPG=two-hour postprandial glucose.

DIAGNOSTIC TESTS

Oral Glucose Tolerance Test (OGTT)

This is performed to establish a diagnosis in:

1. Patients with transient or sustained glycosuria who have no clinical symptoms of diabetes (polyuria) and with normal fasting and post-prandial blood glucose levels,
2. Patients with symptoms of diabetes but with no glycosuria and normal fasting level,
3. Persons with a strong family history of diabetes but with no overt diabetes,
4. Patients whose glycosuria is associated with pregnancy, thyrotoxicosis, liver disease, and/or infections,
5. Women who have characteristically large babies (>9 lbs) or individuals who were large babies and,
6. Patients with neuropathies and retinopathies of undetermined origin.

The patient should ingest a daily diet of at least 300 gm of carbohydrate for 3 days prior to the test. Therefore, on an acutely ill-hospitalised patient, this test should not be conducted. As far as possible it should be performed on an ambulatory patient. Preferably, the test should be performed in the morning. Various malignancies, fever, cachexia, liver dysfunction and renal failure may be associated with mild to moderate degrees of abnormal GTT. There is an age-related factor that decreases glucose tolerance and hence makes the interpretation of OGTT in elderly subjects difficult. Timing of glucose administration and blood sampling must be accurate.

Patient Preparation

1. Instruct the patient about the purpose and procedure of the test:
   a. Stress a normal diet with high carbohydrate (150-300 gm) for 3 days preceding the test.
   b. Fasting is required for at least 10 hours before the test and not more than 16 hours.
   c. Water is permitted and encouraged.
2. Determine the patient's weight and record it.
3. Collect urine and blood samples and test for glucose, recording exact time of collection. Have the patient empty his or her bladder for each specimen:
   a. No liquids other than water can be taken. Have the patient empty his or her bladder for each urine sample.
   b. No food is to be taken during the test period.
   c. No alcohol to be consumed the previous evening.
   d. Encourage the patient to stay in bed or rest quietly during the test period. Weakness or feeling faint may occur during test, and exercise also changes, glucose results.
   e. No smoking is allowed during the test.
   f. Coffee and unusual physical exercise should be avoided for at least 8 hours before the test.

Carbohydrate meal (or glucose) to be given in 25% (w/v) solution according to the age.

Age	*Dose*
0-18 months	2.5 gm/kg
1½-3 years	2.0 gm/kg
8-12 years	1.75 gm/kg
> 12 years	1.25 gm/kg

Preferably, the samples of urine and whole blood be taken at fasting, 30 minutes, 1, 1½, 2, 3, and 4 hours after ingestion of the carbohydrate meal. If nausea and vomiting occur during the test, the interpretation becomes difficult.

Interpretation

Three popular methods for evaluating GTT for diabetes mellitus are:

1. *Wilkerson point system*

Time	*mg% plasma*	*Points*
Fasting	130 or more	1
1 hr	195 or more	½
2 hr	140 or more	½
3 hr	130 or more	1

Two or more points are judged diagnostic of diabetes mellitus (DM)

2. *The Fajans-Conn criteria*

Time	*mg% plasma*
Fasting	
1 hr	195 or more
1½ hr	165 or more
2 hr	140 or more

A diagnosis of DM in otherwise healthy and ambulatory individuals under age 50 is made if the above criteria are met.

3. *The university group diabetes mellitus programme*

The fasting 1 hr, 2 hr and 3 hr blood glucose levels are adjusted for plasma glucose as above, and the subject is judged diabetic if the sum of values obtained equals 500 or more.

Abnormally, high values in the first hour with a rapid fall to normal values or a flat curve with no appreciable rise usually reflect primary alterations in intestinal absorption of glucose. The former is characteristic of hyperthyroidism and the latter of hypothyroidism or malabsorptive states. A very flat rise in blood glucose followed by a prolonged and pronounced hypoglycaemic phase may be observed in primary (islet cell adenoma or hyperplasia) and secondary hyperinsulinism (hypoadrenocorticism). In the elderly, especially in females, interpretation of OGTT must be made in light of what is an age-dependent carbohydrate intolerance.

Interfering Factors

1. Smoking will increase glucose level.
2. Inadequate diet (such as a weight reducing diet) before testing can diminish carbohydrate tolerance and suggest a false diabetes.
3. Levels tend to increase normally in older people, the maximum can reach 200 mg/dl
4. Prolonged administration of oral contraceptives will give significantly higher glucose levels in the second hour or in later blood samples.
5. Bedrest over a lengthy period of time will influence glucose tolerance. For this reason, the test should be performed on ambulatory patients, not on patients whose condition requires bedrest.
6. Infectious diseases and surgery will affect tolerance. Two weeks of recovery should be permitted before the test.
7. Drugs that impair glucose tolerance:
   - Insulin
   - Oral hypoglycaemics
   - Salicylates in larger doses
   - Oral contraceptives
   - Thiazide diuretics
   - Corticosteroids
   - Oestrogen
   - Ferrous ascorbinate
   - Nicotinic acid
   - Phenothiazines
   - Lithium
   - Metapyrone.

Discontinue these drugs for 3 days prior to test.

This test is contraindicated in patients who have had a recent history of surgery, myocardial infarction, a labour and delivery for these conditions can cause erroneous results. Record and report any reactions that may occur during the test. Weakness, faintness, and sweating may occur between the second and third hours. If this occurs, a blood sample for sugar is drawn and the test is discontinued. Test should be postponed in the event of unexpected illness such as fever or gastritis or if there has been ingestion of food within 8 hours. If the fasting blood sugar is over 200 mg/dl, the GTT is usually not done. If it is done, the patient should be monitored very carefully for severe reaction or even coma.

I/V GTT

In patients with gastrointestinal disorders an intravenous GTT may be done. These patients may be suffering from sprue or malabsorption syndrome or may be post-gastrectomy patients. A sterile glucose solution is given I/V (20% w/v) over a 30-minute period in an amount of 0.5 gm/kg of ideal body weight. Similar blood collection intervals, including a fasting specimen, are followed, and a curve is plotted for evaluation (F, 1/2, 1, 1½, 2, 2½ and 3 hours). In a normal individual, the fasting specimen of blood contains a normal amount of glucose, the concentration of any single specimen does not exceed 250 mg%, and by 1 hour 30 minutes to 2 hours, the blood glucose level approximately comes to the fasting level (this test, however, is a less sensitive indicator of mild abnormalities of carbohydrate tolerance than the standard OGTT).

RAPID I/V GTT

Here a rapid I/V (50% w/v) GTT (0.5 gm glucose/kg ideal body weight) to a maximum dose of 25 gm may be given over a 3-4 minute period. Blood samples are obtained at intervals of 10 minutes for at least 2 hours. Under these conditions, disappearance of glucose from blood follows an exponential curve and a glucose disappearance constant can be calculated. In normal subjects glucose disappearance usually exceeds 1.5% of the administered dose per minute, values below 1% are compatible with diabetes mellitus.

CORTISONE GLUCOSE TOLERANCE TEST

This may reveal prediabetic patients, especially in relatives of known diabetics. Cortisone promotes intolerance in a latent or mild diabetic. After performance of an initial GTT a standard dose of cortisone (50 mg) for adults is given parenterally 8½ hours and again 2 hours before a regular GTT. A positive test shows a blood glucose concentration of 140 mg% or higher with 2 hour specimen. Follow-up studies are necessary for such individuals.

PARENTERAL ADMINISTRATION OF GLUCAGON OR EPINEPHRINE

Will cause a slight elevation of blood glucose concentration from glycogenolysis in normal subjects—this is much greater and more sustained in diabetics. It is also a measure of glycogen storage and release, so it may be used to study patients suspected of having a glycogen storage disease.

I/V TOLBUTAMIDE TEST

Oral hypoglycaemic agent administration results in secretion of insulin from pancreas. This principle is taken advantage of to indicate (active) insulin reserve in patients. Sodium tolbutamide (1 gm) is given I/V in 20 ml of saline over 2 minutes to a (12 hr) fasting subject. A fasting preinjection blood specimen and postinjection samples at 2, 5, 10, 20, 30, 60, 120, and 180 minutes are collected for glucose estimation. Juvenile diabetics (insulinopenic) reveal virtually no response, while adult (maturity-onset) diabetics show a delayed increase in blood glucose concentrations. Patients with an insulin-secreting tumour (islet cell adenoma or hyperplasia) reveal a profound depression of blood glucose values which persists below 50 mg% at 2 hours, this is associated with maximum insulin values as early as 15 minutes. Appropriate medical precautionary measures must be readily available (sterile glucose injection) and used promptly with any stress tolerance test whenever a patient's condition warrants intervention and cessation of test.

I/V INSULIN TOLERANCE TEST

Here insulin 0.1 unit/kg of ideal body weight is administered I/V in a fasting state, blood specimens are collected at appropriate intervals over a 2-hour period for glucose analyses. Within 30 minutes the blood glucose concentration falls to about 50 or 60% of the fasting level and returns to normal fasting levels between 1 hour 30 minutes, and 2 hours. A failure to observe such a depression in blood glucose concentration may imply insulin resistance. This may be occasionally seen in adult type diabetes, as well as in acromegaly and Cushing's syndrome. In panhypopituitarism and adrenocortical insufficiency (Addison's disease) a more profound and sustained decrease in blood glucose may be observed, hence caution should be exercised in patients suspected of having these disorders.

GLYCOSYLATED HAEMOGLOBIN (HBA_{1C}); GLYCO-HAEMOGLOBIN (G-HB); DIABETIC CONTROL INDEX

Normal values (kits available commercially)

Normal Values

	Percentage of Total Hb
Total of HbA_1a, HbA_1b, and HbA_1c	5.5-8.8
Diabetes under control	7.5-11.4
Diabetes less well controlled	11.5-15
Diabetes out of control	>15
Ketoacidosis	14.3-20
High-performance liquid chromatography	
Hb A_1a	1.8
Hb A_1b	0.8
Hb A_1c	3.5-6.0

Increased Diabetes mellitus, glycosuria, and hyperglycaemia.

Decreased See, below, Factors that affect results.

Description

Glycosylated-haemoglobin is blood glucose bound to haemoglobin (Hb) and includes from Hb A_1a, Hb A_1b, and Hb A_1c. Hb A_1c is formed as haemoglobin, is gradually glycosylated throughout the 120-day red blood cell lifespan, and forms the largest portion of the three glycosylated Hb fractions. The amount of glycosylated haemoglobin found and stored in erythrocytes depends on the amount of glucose available. Hb A_1c is a reflection of how well blood glucose levels have been controlled for up to the prior 4 months. Hyperglycaemia in diabetics if usually a cause of an increase in Hb A_1c.

Factors that Affect Results

a. Reject haemolysed specimens.
b. Falsely increased values may be due to foetal-maternal transfusion, haemodialysis, hereditary persistence of foetal haemoglobin, neonates, and pregnancy.
c. Falsely decreased values may be due to anaemia (haemolytic, pernicious, sickle cell); chronic loss of blood ; effects of splenectomy; renal failure (chronic); and thalassaemias.

Other Data

a. Glycosylated haemoglobin cannot be used to monitor control of diabetic clients with chronic renal failure, as levels are significantly lower due to shortened erthyrocyte survival.

Approximately 8.5% of total haemoglobin: HbA_1

Glycohaemoglobin is one of the types of minor haemoglobins found in every individual. Haemoglobin A, undergoes change or glycosylation to haemoglobin A_{1a}, A_{1b}, A_{1c} by a slow, nonenzyme process within the RBCs during their circulating life-span of 120 days. Simply putting it, glycohaemoglobin is blood glucose bound to haemoglobin. The RBC, as it circulates, combines, some of the glucose from the bloodstream with its own content of haemoglobin to form glycohaemoglobin in a one-way reaction. The amount of glycosylated haemoglobin found and stored by the RBC depends on the amount of glucose available to it over the RBCs 120 days lifespan. In diabetics with hyperglycaemia, the increase in G-Hb is usually caused by an increase in HbA_{1c}. The glucose concentration will increase when hyperglycaemia caused by insulin deficiency develops. This glycosylation is irreversible.

Test Significance

This test is an index of long-term glucose control. GHb monitoring reflects the average blood sugar level for the 2- to 3-month period before the test. The more glucose the RBC is exposed to, the higher the percentage of GHb. The test provides vital information about the success of treatment of diabetes such as the adequacy of dietary or insulin therapy, allows determination of duration of hyperglycaemia in new cases of juvenile onset diabetes with acute ketoacidosis, provides a sensitive estimate of glucose imbalance in mild cases of diabetes, and is an evaluation of effectiveness of old and new forms of therapy such as oral hypoglycaemic agents, single or multiple insulin injections, and B-cell transplantation. Test results are not affected by time of day, meal intake, exercise, just administered diabetic drugs, emotional stress, patient cooperation or accuracy.

The estimation of GHb is of greater importance for specific groups of patients. These groups include diabetic children, diabetics in whom the renal threshold for glucose is abnormal, unstable insulin-dependent diabetics in whom blood sugars vary markedly from day to day, patients who do not test urine regularly for glucose, and people who, before their scheduled appointments, will change their usual habits, dietary or otherwise, so that their metabolic control appears better than it actually is.

Clinical Relevance

1. Values are increased in poorly controlled and newly diagnosed diabetes. In these instances, HbA_{1c} levels comprise 8% to 12% of the total haemoglobin.
2. With optimal insulin control, the HbA_{1c} levels return toward normal.
3. A diabetic patient who has only recently come under good control may still have a high concentration of glycosylated haemoglobin. This level will only gradually decline as newly formed RBCs with nearly normal GHb replace older RBCs with high concentrations of GHb.

Interfering Factors

1. Spurious results should be expected in every case of haemoglobinopathy distinguishable from haemoglobin A by electrophoresis.
2. Decreased value in pregnancy and sickle cell anaemia, increased value in thalassaemia.

Confusion in interpretation of results may occur because there are two tests for determining glycosilated haemoglobin. The most specific test measures Hb_{A1}, which includes haemoglobin A_{1a}, A_{1b} and A_{1c}. There are different expected values for each test. Keep in mind that HbA, is always 2% to 4% higher than HbA_{1c}.

GLYCOSYLATED HEMOGLOBIN KIT (Ion Exchange Resin method) For the quantitative determination of Glycohemoglobin in Blood (For in vitro Diagnostic use only)

Summary

Glycosylated hemoglobin (GHb) is formed continuously by the adduction of glucose by co-valent bonding to the amino-terminal valine of the hemoglobin beta chain progressively and irreversibly over a period of time and is stable till the life of the RBC. This process is slow, nonenzymatic and is dependent on the average blood Glucose concentration over a period of time.

A single glucose determination reflects the glucose level at the time. GHb on the other hand reflects the mean glucose level over an extended period of time. Thus GHb reflects the metabolic control of glucose level over a period of time unaffected by diet, insulin, other drugs, or exercise on the day of testing. GHb is now widely recognised as an important test for the diagnosis of diabetes mellitus and is a reliable indicator of the efficacy of therapy.

Principle

Glycosylated hemoglobin (GHb) has been defined operationally as the fast fraction hemoglobins HbA1 (Hb A1a, A1b, A1c) which elute first during column chromatography. The nonglycosylated hemoglobin, which consists of the bulk of hemoglobin, has been designated HbAo.

A haemolysed preparation of whole blood is mixed continuously for 5 minutes with a weakly binding cation-exchange resin. The labile fraction is eliminated during the hemolysate preparation and during the binding. During this mixing, HbAo binds to the ion exchange resin leaving GHb free in the supernatant. After the mixing period, a filter separator is used to remove the resin from the supernatant. The percent glycosylated hemoglobin is determined by measuring absorbances of the glycosylated hemoglobin (GHb) fraction and the total hemoglobin (THb) fraction. The ratio of the absorbances of the Glycosylated hemoglobin and the Total hemoglobin fraction of the Control and the Sample is used to calculate the percent Glycosylated hemoglobin of the sample.

Normal Reference Values

Normal	:	4.5 - 8.0 %
Good control	:	8.0 - 9.0 %
Fair control	:	9.0 - 10.0 %
Poor control	:	> 10.0 %

It is recommended that each laboratory establish its own normal range representing its patient population.

Contents	10 Tests	25 Tests
Ion Exchange Resin (Predispensed Tubes)	10 × 3 ml	25 × 3 ml
Lysing Reagent	5 ml	12.5 ml
Control (10% GHb)	1 × 1 ml	1 × 1 ml
Resin Separators	10 Nos.	25 Nos.

Storage/Stability

Contents stable at 2-8°C till the expiry mentioned on the label. Do not freeze. The Resin separators can be removed on opening the kit and stored at R.T.

Reagent Preparation

The ion exchange resin tubes and the lysing reagent are ready to use.

Reconstitute the control with 1 ml of distilled water. Allow to stand for 10 min. with occasional mixing. The reconstituted control is stable for at least 7 days when stored at 2-8°C tightly sealed, and at least 4 weeks when stored at -20°C. Do not thaw and refreeze.

Sample Material

Whole blood. Preferably fresh and collected in EDTA. GHb in whole blood is reported to be stable for one week at 2-8°C.

Procedure

Wavelength/Filter : 415 nm (Hg 405 nm)
Temperature : R.T.
Light path : 1 cm

A. Haemolysate Preparation
1. Dispense 0.5 ml lysing reagent into tubes labeled as control (C) and test (T).
2. Add 0.1 ml of the reconstituted control and well-mixed blood sample into the appropriately labeled tubes. Mix until complete lysis is evident.
3. Allow to stand for 5 minutes.

B. Glycosylated hemoglobin (GHb) Separation
1. Remove cap from the Ion-exchange resin tubes and label as control and test.
2. Add 0.1 ml of the hemolysate from Step A into the appropriately labeled Ion exchange resin tubes.
3. Insert a resin separator into each tube so that the rubber sleeve is approximately 1 cm above the liquid level of the resin suspension.
4. Mix the tubes on a rocker, rotator or a vortex mixer continuously for 5 minutes.
5. Allow the resin to settle, then push the resin separator into the tubes until the resin is firmly packed.
6. Pour or aspirate each supernatant directly into a cuvette and measure each absorbance against distilled water.

C. Total hemoglobin (THb) fraction
1. Dispense 5.0 ml of distilled water into tubes labeled as Control and Test.
2. Add to it 0.02 ml of hemolysate from Step A into the appropriately labeled tube. Mix well.
3. Read each absorbance against distilled water.

Calculations

$$\text{Ratio of Control (RC)} = \frac{\text{Abs. Control GHb}}{\text{Abs. Control THb}}$$

$$\text{Ratio of Test (RT)} = \frac{\text{Abs. Test GHb}}{\text{Abs. Test THb}}$$

$$\text{GHb in \%} = \frac{\text{Ratio of Test (RT)}}{\text{Ratio of Control (RC)}} \times 10 \text{ (Value of Control)}$$

Linearity

The glycosylated hemoglobin procedure shows linearity for GHb levels in the range of 4.0% - 20.0%.

Notes

Blood samples with hemoglobin greater than 18 g/dl should be diluted 1 + 1 with normal saline before the assay.

Samples from patients with Hemoglobinopathies, decreased red cell survival times, gross lipemia may show incorrect results.

Do not use Ion Exchange Resin tubes in case of turbidity or visible discolouration.

Diabetics with metabolic imbalance may have extremely high levels of the labile aldimine form. In such cases the incubation time during hemolysate preparation may be increased to 15 minutes to ensure elimination of this instable fraction.

INSULIN

Normal values

		SI Units
Adult		
Fasting level	<17 μU/ml	42-243 pmol/L or 1.00 mg/L
Newborn	3-20 μU/ml	21-139 pmol/L
Infant	<13 μU/ml	≤89 pmol/L
Prepubertal child	<13 μU/ml	≤89 pmol/L
Panic levels	>30 μU/ml	>290 pmol/L
Last trimester, amniotic fluid	11.3 μU/ml	78 pmol/L

Insulin is a hormone produced in pancreas by the beta cells of the islets of Langerhans, regulates the metabolism of carbohydrates along with liver,

Table for the conversion of Glycosylated Hemoglobin A1 (GHbA1)
to Gylcosylated Hemoglobin A1c (HbA1c) and to the Mean Blood Glucose level (MBG)

GHbA1	HbA1c	MBG	GHbA1	HbA1c	MBG	GHbA1	HbA1c	MBG	GHbA1	HbA1c	MBG
5.0	3.46	—	9.0	6.81	141	13.0	10.16	252	17.0	13.51	—
5.1	3.54	—	9.1	6.89	144	13.1	10.25	255	17.1	13.60	—
5.2	3.63	—	9.2	6.98	146	13.2	10.33	258	17.2	13.68	—
5.3	3.71	—	9.3	7.06	149	13.3	10.41	261	17.3	13.68	—
5.4	3.79	—	9.4	7.15	152	13.4	10.50	264	17.4	13.85	—
5.5	3.88	—	9.5	7.23	155	13.5	10.58	266	17.5	13.93	—
5.6	3.96	—	9.6	7.31	158	13.6	10.66	269	17.6	14.02	—
5.7	4.04	—	9.7	7.40	160	13.7	10.75	272	17.7	14.10	—
5.8	4.13	—	9.8	7.48	163	13.8	10.83	275	17.8	14.18	—
5.9	4.21	—	9.9	7.56	166	13.9	10.92	278	17.9	14.27	—
6.0	4.30	57	10.0	7.65	169	14.0	11.00	280	18.0	14.35	—
6.1	4.38	60	10.1	7.73	171	14.1	11.08	—	18.1	14.44	—
6.2	4.46	63	10.2	7.82	174	4.2	11.17	—	18.2	14.52	—
6.3	4.55	65	10.3	7.90	177	14.3	11.25	—	18.3	14.60	—
6.4	4.63	68	10.4	7.98	180	14.4	11.34	—	18.4	14.69	—
6.5	4.71	71	10.5	8.07	183	14.5	11.42	—	18.5	14.77	—
6.6	4.80	74	10.6	8.15	185	14.6	11.50	—	18.6	14.85	—
6.7	4.88	77	10.7	8.23	188	14.7	11.59	—	18.7	14.94	—
6.8	4.97	79	10.8	8.32	191	14.8	11.67	—	18.8	15.02	—
6.9	5.05	82	10.9	8.40	194	14.9	11.75	—	18.9	15.11	—
7.0	5.13	85	11.0	8.49	197	15.0	11.84	—	19.0	15.19	—
7.1	5.22	88	11.1	8.57	199	15.1	11.92	—	19.1	15.27	—
7.2	5.30	91	11.2	8.65	202	15.2	12.01	—	19.2	15.36	—
7.3	5.39	93	11.3	8.74	205	15.3	12.09	—	19.3	15.44	—
7.4	5.47	96	11.4	8.82	208	15.4	12.17	—	19.4	15.53	—
7.5	5.55	99	11.5	8.91	211	15.5	12.26	—	19.5	15.61	—
7.6	5.64	102	11.6	8.99	213	15.6	12.34	—	19.6	15.69	—
7.7	5.72	104	11.7	9.07	216	15.7	12.42	—	19.7	15.78	—
7.8	5.80	107	11.8	9.16	219	15.8	12.51	—	19.8	15.86	—
7.9	5.89	110	11.9	9.24	222	15.9	12.59	—	19.9	15.94	—
8.0	5.97	113	12.0	9.32	224	16.0	12.68	—	20.0	16.03	—
8.1	6.06	116	12.1	9.41	227	16.1	12.76	—			
8.2	6.14	118	12.2	9.49	230	16.2	12.84	—			
8.3	6.22	121	12.3	9.58	233	16.3	12.93	—			
8.4	6.31	124	12.4	9.66	236	16.4	13.01	—			
8.5	6.39	127	12.5	9.74	238	16.5	13.09	—			
8.6	6.47	130	12.6	9.83	241	16.6	13.18	—			
8.7	6.56	132	12.7	9.91	244	16.7	13.26	—			
8.8	6.64	135	12.8	9.99	247	16.8	13.35	—			
8.9	6.73	138	12.9	10.08	250	16.9	13.43	—			

MBG in mg/dl = 33.3 x HbA1c value - 86
These values are linear in the range of 6.5 - 13% of HbA1c values

adipose, muscle, and other target cells and is responsible for maintaining a constant level of blood glucose. The rate of insulin secretion is determined primarily by the level of blood glucose perfusing the pancreas and is affected by hormonal status, the autonomic nervous system, and nutritional status.

Test Significance

This measurement of the insulin secretory response to glucose may be of value in establishing the diagnosis of insulinoma and in the evaluation of abnormal carbohydrate and lipid metabolism. Insulin levels are also helpful in supporting the diagnosis of diabetes in persons with borderline abnormalities of the GTT. This determination is invaluable in the investigation of fasting hypoglycaemic patients and may be useful in the differentiation of islet cell neoplasms. Insulin levels may be ordered along with GTT.

Clinical Relevance

Increased values are associated with:

A. Insulinoma: diagnosis of insulinoma is based on
   1. Association of insulinoma with hypoglycaemia
   2. Persistent hypoglycaemia along with hyperinsulinaemia between 2 and 3 hours after injection of tolbutamide.
   3. Failure of C-peptide suppression when plasma glucose is 40 mg/dl or less. After 100 gm of glucose, normal insulin will rise less than 2 μU/ml to 25 to 231 in half hour, 18 to 276 in one hour, 16 to 166 in 2 hours, 4 to 38 in 3 hours. The results may be too variable to be of diagnostic importance.

B. Acromegaly

C. Cushing's syndrome.

Interfering Factors

Falsely increased values are associated with food intake, obesity, and use of oral contraceptives.

C-PEPTIDE

Normal values

		SI Units
Qualitative	Negative	
Quantitative		
Adult	68-8200 ng/ml or 20 mg/dl or < 8 μg/ml	68-8200 μg/L
Cord blood	10-350 ng/ml	10-350 μg/L

C-peptide is formed during the conversion of proinsulin to insulin in the beta cells of the pancreas. It is secreted into the bloodstream in almost equal concentration with insulin. Normally, a strong correlation exists between levels of insulin and C-peptide, except possibly in obese subjects and in the presence of islet cell tumours.

Test Significance

C-peptide level measurement provides a reliable indication of beta and secretory function and insulin secretions. This determination has its most useful application in the evaluation of endogenous secretion of insulin when the presence of circulatory insulin antibodies interferes with the direct assay of insulin. This situation is most likely to occur in diabetics who have been treated with bovine pork insulin. The test is also useful in evaluating hypoglycaemic states in identifying surreptitious injection of insulin, and in confirmation of remission of diabetes mellitus. Furthermore, monitoring following pancreatectomy for removal of cancer can provide a means of detecting the presence of residual tissue.

Clinical Relevance

1. *Increased values* are associated with endogenous hyperinsulinism in insulin-dependent diabetic persons when a high level of insulin is also present.
2. *Decreased levels* are associated with persons who have been surreptitiously injecting insulin and who have both hypoglycaemia and high insulin levels.
3. Normal levels are found in persons who have had a remision of diabetes mellitus.

GLUCAGON

Normal values

1. 50-200 pg/ml plasma
2. Glucagon response in normal people after a standard test meal of carbohydrates, fat and protein is a gradual increase from 92 plus or minus 12 pg/ml to a peak of 125 plus or minus 13 pg/ml.
3. In a glucose tolerance test, glucagon levels will significantly decline from fasting levels during the hyperglycaemic first hour in normal people.

Glucagon is a peptide hormone produced by alpha cells of the islets of Langerhans in the pancreas. In the liver, this hormone promotes glucose production. This action of glucagon is opposed to that of insulin. The normal coordinated release patterns of this hormone provide a sensitive control mechanism for glucose production and storage. For example, low glucose levels result in release, whereas conditions of hyperglycaemia reduce circulating glucagon levels to approximately 50% of the amount in the fasting state.

Kidneys play an important role in the metabolism of glucagon.

Abnormally high levels of glucagon recede once insulin therapy begins to control diabetes, and levels slowly revert to normal in persons on maintenance doses of insulin. Also, in contrast to the normal glucagon, secretion in diabetics does not decrease following ingestion of a carbohydrate meal. However, an arginine infusion causes greatly increased glucagon secretion in normal persons.

Test Significance

This measurement has clinical significance in two ways. Glucagon deficiency reflects a general loss of pancreatic tissue. Compelling evidence for glucagon deficiency is the failure of glucagon levels to rise during arginine infusion. Hyperglucagonaemia occurs in diabetics, acute pancreatitis, and in situations where catecholamine secretion is greatly augmented as in phaeochromocytoma and in the presence of infection.

Clinical Relevance

1. Increased levels are associated with:
   a. Acute pancreatitis
   b. Diabetes mellitus. Persons with severe diabetic ketoacidosis are reported to have levels five times normal fasting levels despite marked hyperglycaemia.
   c. Glucagonoma
   d. Uraemia
   e. Infections
   f. Phaeochromocytoma
2. Reduced levels are associated with:
   a. Inflammatory disease with loss of pancreatic tissue
   b. Neoplastic replacement of pancreas
   c. Surgical removal of pancreas

Interfering Factors

Increased levels occur in vigorous exercise and in trauma.

Other Important Tests in Diabetics

Urine — ketone bodies (present in diabetic ketoacidosis).

Serum — cholesterol (raised)
— triglycerides (raised)
} Can be assessed chemically or by serum electrophoresis

— ketones (raised in presence of ketonuria).

HYPOGLYCAEMIA

By definition means blood glucose levels less than 50 mg%.

Causes of Hypoglycaemia

Spontaneous (fasting) Hypoglycaemia

1. Excessive insulin
   - Insulinoma or insulin-secreting carcinoma
   - Erythroblastosis foetalis.
2. Non-endocrine tumour–retroperitoneal fibroma.
3. Glycogen storage disease of the liver.
4. Malnutrition or malabsorption.
5. Adrenocortical or pituitary failure.
6. Liver necrosis.
7. Hereditary galactosaemia.
8. Reye's syndrome and other forms of ketotic hypoglycaemia in children.

Induced Hypoglycaemia

1. Excessive insulin:
   - Overtreated insulin.
   - Leucine (includes some islet cell tumours).
   - Sulphonylureas.
   - Functional:
     - Prediabetic
     - Postgastrectomy.
     - Haemodialysis with hypertonic glucose.
     - Idiopathic.
2. Reduced gluconeogenesis
   - Ethanol.
   - Hypoglycin.
   - Hereditary fructose intolerance.
   - Failure of glucagon secretion.
3. Persistent increase of peripheral glucose uptake.
   - Failure of catecholamine secretion.
   - Propranolol blockade of catecholamine effect.
4. Cause uncertain
   - Pentamidine.

RAPID DIAGNOSTICS

1. Urine sugar: See urinalysis chapter for dipstick tests.
2. Blood sugar: Various instant blood glucose meters are available.

CHAPTER 19

Liver Function Tests

Liver function tests can be classified as:

a. Tests of excretion by the liver
b. Evaluation of synthesis in liver
c. Evaluation of enzyme activity

Liver function tests are most often employed to determine: (i) the presence of liver disease, (ii) the type of liver disease, and (iii) the extent and progression of liver disease.

TESTS OF EXCRETION BY THE LIVER

Bile Pigment

Serum bilirubin concentration depends on the rate of removal of bilirubin from destruction of haemoglobin.

Types of bilirubin

In the plasma, bilirubin is present as 'indirect' reacting bilirubin, which is not water-soluble; and 'direct'-reacting esterified bilirubin (bilirubin glucuronide), which is water soluble. In the van den Bergh reaction, the water soluble ester reacts readily with diazo reagent (*'direct reaction'*), the addition of alcohol renders the unesterified bilirubin soluble so that diazotisation may occur (*'indirect reaction'*). Jaundice: is a term used in clinical medicine to describe a visible yellow discolouration of the skin and sclera.

CLASSIFICATION OF THE CAUSES OF JAUNDICE

UNCONJUGATED BILIRUBIN

Prehepatic (haemolytic retention jaundice)

1. *Excessive red cell haemolysis*
   a. *Familial:* e.g. spherocytosis, enzyme defects in red cell.

Bilirubin--Urobilinogen Cycle (Solid arrows = conjugated bilirubin; dotted arrows = urobilinogen)

NORMAL

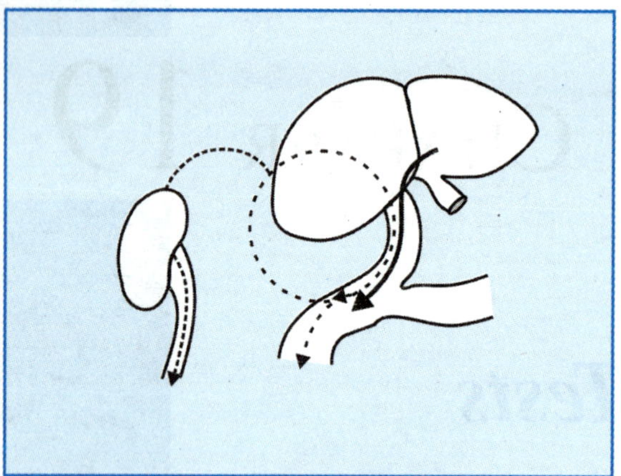

Fig. 19.1: Urine urobilinogen 0-4 mg/24 hrs; Bilirubin absent
Fecal urobilinogen 40-280 mg/24 hrs.

HEPATITIS

Bilirubin--Urobilinogen Cycle
(Solid arrows = Conjugated bilirubin; dotted arrows = urobilinogen)

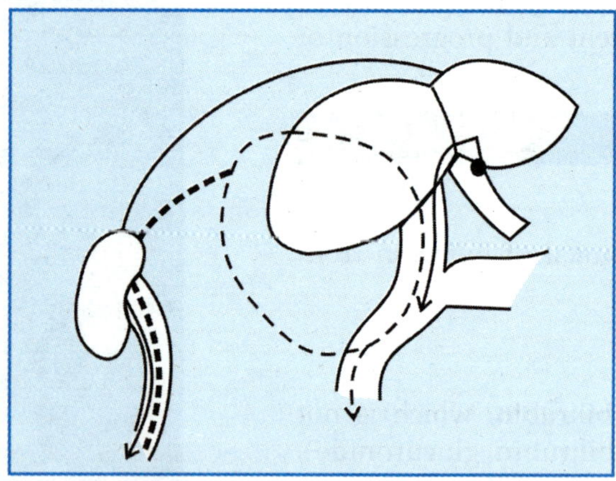

Fig. 19.3: Urine urobilinogen increased; bilirubin present
Bilirubin excretion decreased
Fecal urobilinogen decreased

b. *Acquired*
   Traumatic, e.g. haematomas
   Toxic, e.g. phenylhydrazine
   Infective, e.g. malaria
   Neoplastic, e.g. Hodgkin's disease.

2. Excessive "shunt" production.

Hemolytic jaundice

Bilirubin formation increased

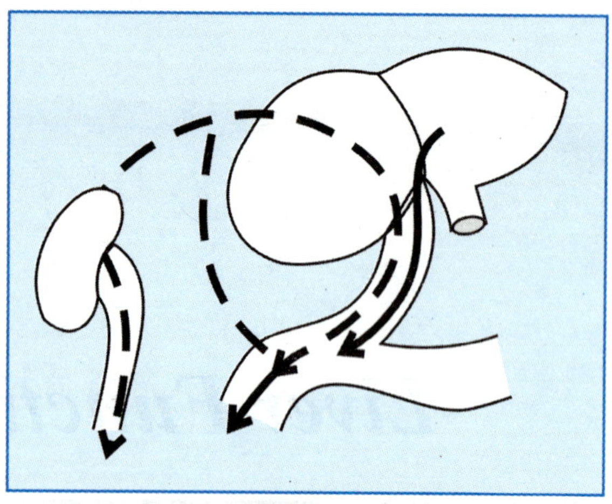

Fig. 19.2: Urine urobilinogen increased; bilirubin absent
Fecal urobilinogen increased

OBSTRUCTION

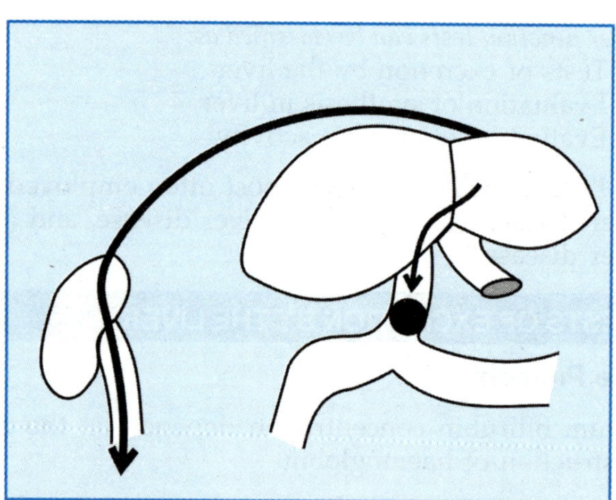

Bilirubin present-->

Fig.19.4:

	Urine urobilinogen	Fecal urobilinogen
COMPLETE Tumor Stricture Severe hepatitis (rarely)	Absent	Trace to Absent
INTERMITTENT Stone	Fluctuates	Fluctuates

Hepatic

1. Nonhemolytic retention jaundice (defect of transport into cell or microsomes).
   a. *Familial:*
      UDP glucuronyl transferase deficiency (Types I and II) Gilbert's disease

Crigler-Najjar syndrome

b. *Acquired or uncertain inheritance*
Neonatal jaundice, e.g. physiological breast milk, or serum factor.

Conjugated Bilirubin

Intrahepatic Cholestasis (regurgitation jaundice)

A. *Hepatocellular injury*
- *Toxic,* e.g. carbon tetrachloride necrosis
- *Infective,* e.g. viral hepatitis
- *Neoplastic,* e.g. primary or secondary carcinoma of liver
- *Cirrhosis,* e.g. familial or acquired.

B. *Bile duct injury*
- *Familial,* e.g. Dubin-Johnson syndrome. Rotor syndrome, recurrent familial cholestasis.
- *Toxic,* e.g. drugs (phenothiazines, steroids).
- *Inflammatory,* e.g. sclerosing cholangitis.
- *Neoplastic,* e.g. cholangiocarcinoma
- *Others,* e.g. primary biliary cirrhosis, pregnancy, intrahepatic atresias

C. *Posthepatic* (extrahepatic cholestasis): Various causes are:
1. *Intramural:* e.g. Stones, parasites.
2. *Mural:*
   - *Congenital,* e.g. extrahepatic biliary atresia
   - *Inflammatory,* e.g. acute cholangitis
   - *Neoplastic,* e.g. cholangiocarcinoma, carcinoma of ampulla of Vater.
3. *Extramural:*
   - *Inflammatory,* e.g. acute pancreatitis
   - *Neoplastic,* e.g. carcinoma of pancreas, lymphoma.
   - ***Hyperbilirubinemia***—various causes have been discussed, rise in conjugated or unconjugated bilirubin in blood / serum has been indicated.
   - ***Urine urobilinogen***—urobilinogen is normally formed from bilirubin by bacterial action in the bowel. Normally all urobilinogen absorbed from the gut is excreted by the liver, only up to 4 mg appearing in urine in 24 hours.

     Urine urobilinogen increased (> 4 mg / 24 hours);

A. Impaired liver function or partial duct obstruction.

B. 'Overloading' of the liver as a result of increased urobilinogen production following hemolytic disease.

Urine urobilinogen absent: If biliary duct obstruction is complete, no bilirubin enters the gut, no urobilinogen is formed, and none is found in the urine or feces.

Faecal Urobilinogen

If the hepatobiliary system is functioning, faecal urobilinogen varies directly with rate of red cell haemolysis.

Faecal urobilinogen increased occurs when blood destruction is increased and when biliary obstruction is relieved.

In the case of haemolysis, the daily excretion is related to the existing total body haemoglobin mass. If there is a reduced total body haemoglobin mass, accelerated rates of haemolysis may only yield an amount of urobilinogen that would be within normal limits for an individual with normal haemoglobin mass.

Faecal urobilinogen absent occurs with exclusion of bilirubin from the gut in complete biliary tract obstruction and in extreme cases of hepatocellular disease. Absence of urobilinogen in feces is important in indicating biliary tract obstruction, persistent absence is a strong indication of malignant obstructive disease. Decreased fecal urobilinogen excretion may occur when antibiotics which alter intestinal flora are used (tetracyclines, streptomycin, etc).

Bromsulphalein (Sulphobromophthalein) Excretion Test

Sulphobromophthalein sodium (Bromsulphalein, BSP, is a dye which is bound avidly by albumin, the complex is picked up by the liver cell, and the BSP is transported into the microsomes, conjugated and excreted in the bile, in a manner analogous to bilirubin.

BSP is given intravenously and its amount present in the blood after 30, 45 or 60 minutes indicate hepatic function. The greater the liver function loss, greater the amount BSP present in blood (This test is of no significant value in differential diagnosis). BSP retention in blood conjugated / unconjugated runs parallel to bilirubin related disorders. In the presence of fevers, administration of anabolic steroids, Telepaque, Dubin-Johnson syndrome and in Gilbert's disease, BSP retention is increased. In the latter two disorders the uptake by liver cells is normal (so normal retention at 45 minutes) but after getting conjugated it regurgitates back into blood (so BSP retention is marked at 3 hours period).

Method

1. Lipemic/jaundiced sera may cause interference. In any case one should not perform the test in the presence of acute liver/gallbladder disease.
2. Know the patient's weight, inject 5 mg BSP/kg body weight intravenously, over a period of 60 seconds. Having injected set the time to 45 minutes.
3. After 45 minutes withdraw 8-10 ml blood from the other arm, let it clot, remove serum after centrifuging.
4. Take 2 test tubes marked test and blank

Test	*Blank*
1.0 ml serum +4.0 ml N/10 NaOH mix by gentle inversion	1.0 ml serum +4.0 ml N/10 HCl mix by gentle inversion.

   The full reddish colour develops in the alkaline solution, and the dye is colourless in acid solution.
5. Read the absorbance of test at 575 nm (or 590 nm) setting the zero with the blank.
6. Refer the absorbance reading to the calibration curve to obtain the percentage of the dye dose remaining in the blood after the 45 minute interval. Report as percentage of dye retention after-minutes," giving the dose used. Normal retention is upto 4% (average 2.8%).

Calibration: Into a 1 litre volumetric flask pipette very accurately 2.0 ml of 5% BSP. Dilute to the mark with distilled water and mix well. Into 4 clean test tubes pipette accurately the following amounts of the diluted dye: 0.25, 0.50, 0.75, and 1.0 ml. Make each to 1.0 ml with distilled water. To each tube add exactly 4.0 ml of N/10 NaOH. Mix by inversion and read the absorbance at 575/590 nm. These standards correspond to values of 25, 50, 75 and 100% retention in the test. Plotted on graph paper, the readings should fall on a straight line passing through the origin.

Conditions Associated with Increased BSP Retention

Hepatobiliary System

- Jaundice from any cause except Gilbert's syndrome
- Viral hepatitis
- Toxic hepatitis
- Fatty liver
- Cirrhosis
- Bile duct obstruction
- Metastatic carcinoma
- Lymphomatous or leukemic infiltration
- Granulomatous inflammation
- Amyloidosis
- Dubin-Johnson syndrome.

Extrahepatic Conditions

- Congestive heart failure
- Fever above 39°C
- Oral contraceptive use
- Prolonged fasting or malnutrition
- Contrast media used for gallbladder examination.

Artefacts

- Obesity
  Spuriously high retention because excessive weight results in excessive dose
- Hypoalbuminemia
  Spuriously low retention because binding is reduced
- Ascites
  Spuriously low retention because the dye enters the ascitic fluid
- Proteinuria
  Spuriously low retention because albumin bound dye enters urine.

EVALUATION OF SYNTHESIS IN LIVER

Serum Proteins (albumin especially)

Since serum albumin and a small fraction of globulin are synthesized in liver, serum proteins are affected both quantitatively and qualitatively in liver disease. In any disease causing hepatocellular damage, the concentration of serum albumin decreases. In many liver disorders, serum globulins may rise to such a level so as to maintain normal or increased total protein concentration even when there is severe albumin depletion.

The changing levels of serum albumin thus provide valuable indices of severity, progress, and prognosis in hepatic disease. Decreased albumin and elevated globulins in serum indicate hepatocellular origin of jaundice or liver disease. In obstructive jaundice, serum protein changes occur late, after secondary hepatocellular damage has occurred. Cholangitis and biliary cirrhosis, however, result in liver damage which may not be accompanied by protein alteration. Furthermore, serum protein changes many return to normal before convalescence from hepatitis is complete. However, liver disease is not the only cause of serum protein alterations.

Chemical methods and electrophoretic methods are available for serum proteins estimation. Electrophoresis is most precise and specific way of assessing serum proteins. The flocculation and turbidity methods crudely estimate globulins and hence are not specific and obsolete in today's context.

Prothrombin Concentration

Deficiency of prothrombin may occur as a result of

1. Inadequate absorption of bile from the intestinal tract, or
2. Inability of a damaged liver to convert vitamin-K to prothrombin.

A normal prothrombin concentration does not rule out abnormal liver function.

Low Prothrombin in Presence of Jaundice

When a low prothrombin level is found in a jaundice patient, give 2-4 mg vitamin K, I/V or I/M, and measure prothrombin concentration later.

1. Return to normalcy of prothrombin concentration (85-100% of normal) indicates that the capacity of liver cells to synthesize prothrombin is good.
2. A poor response implies hepatocellular disease, either primary or following prolonged obstructive disease.

Low Prothrombin in the Absence of Jaundice

In the absence of jaundice, a low prothrombin level usually indicates serious liver damage, and no response to large doses (60-70 mg) of parenteral water-soluble vitamin K confirms it. This is true if jaundice is also present.

Cholesterol and its Esters

Decrease of Both Substances

Associated with extensive destruction of liver parenchyma is reduction in serum levels of cholesterol and cholesterol esters, extremely low concentration implies a poor prognosis. Persistently low cholesterol ester concentration or ester/total cholesterol ratio indicates continuing hepatocellular damage, a rise in cholesterol ester is considered as a good sign and heralds improvement.

Increase of Total but Decrease of Esters

Accompanying biliary obstruction is usually a rise in total cholesterol, but the cholesterol ester concentration is often unaffected. The determination of cholesterol ester, however, is not a fruitful exercise clinically.

DETOXIFICATION

The liver removes noxious materials or renders them harmless by conjugation of toxic substances with amino acids, glucuronate and inorganic radicals (e.g. sulphate), by oxidation or reduction, by excretion, etc.

Serum Protein changes in Selected Diseases

Disease	*Albumin*	*Globulin*	*ß Globulin*	*γ Globulin*
Acute hepatitis	N or Sl ↓	N or Sl ↑	Sl ↑	↑ (IgG and M)
Laennec's cirrhosis	↓↓	N	Sl ↑	↑↑ (IgM and A)
Chronic active hepatitis	↓↓	N	↑	↑↑ (IgG)
Biliary cirrhosis	↓	↑	↑↑	↑ (IgM)
Extrahepatic biliary obstruction	N	N or Sl ↑	↑	N

N=normal Sl=slightly, ↑ =moderately elevated, ↓ = moderately depressed, ↓↓ =severely depressed, ↑↑ =markedly elevated

Hippuric Acid Test

This test depends upon conjugation by liver of sodium benzoate with glycine to produce hippuric acid, which is excreted in the urine. It is preferrable to give sodium benzoate-1.77 gm-I/V (instead of orally in which case the absorption may be irregular), one hour later at least 0.7 gm of hippuric acid should be excreted in the urine. Consideration of low values is permissible only if impaired renal function is ruled out for retention of hippuric acid.

EVALUATION OF ENZYME ACTIVITY

Serum Transaminases

Liver and muscle are rich in enzymes of Krebs cycle. Among such enzymes is a group responsible for transfer of NH_2 groups from amino acids to keto acids, thus, providing for metabolism of amino acids. Destruction of muscle or of liver cells releases the enzymes, with consequent rise in their values in plasma. In obstructive jaundice and more so in acute hepatitis, the serum levels of SGOT and SGPT rise to very high levels (300-1500 units, normal being 5-40 units), as does LDH concentration (normal concentration, 200-450 units). Chronic hepatitis may produce moderate elevations of serum transaminases. Liver cell destruction incident to neoplastic disease metastatic to the liver produces moderate elevation of transaminases concentration in the serum.

In many cases, there seems to be a correlation between the differences in the degree of elevation of SGOT and SGPT and the cause of jaundice. Rise of SGPT is greater than elevation of SGOT in extrahepatic obstruction, acute hepatitis and toxic hepatitis, the reverse is true in cirrhosis of liver, intrahepatic neoplasm, and haemolytic jaundice.

Serum Alkaline Phosphatase

The concentration of this enzyme often increases in the plasma of an icteric patient. It is normally present in the liver and excreted in the bile so that elevation of serum alkaline phosphatase may be a manifestation of retention; this is a convenient explanation for the observation that serum alkaline phosphatase concentration increases in obstructive jaundice. In acute and chronic hepatocellular disease, serum alkaline phosphatase is raised, but not to the extent typical of obstructive jaundice. In hemolytic jaundice, normal levels are the rule. In some cases of metastatic carcinoma of liver, serum alkaline phosphatase may rise in the absence of jaundice. It should be kept in mind that phosphatase levels may be normal early in obstructive disease and with relief of obstruction. Pregnancy and such diseases as Paget's disease of bone, hyperparathyroidism, and rickets/osteomalacia, are also associated with elevated serum alkaline phosphatase concentration and these must be ruled out.

SUGGESTED LIVER FUNCTION TESTS

A. *Jaundice absent*: Urine bilirubin, urine urobilinogen, serum bilirubin, BSP excretion, transaminases.
B. *Jaundice present*: As mentioned above (except BSP excretion), plus alkaline phosphatase, prothrombin response, serum proteins.
C. *Possible metastatic cancer*: Alkaline phosphatase, transaminases, and bilirubin. If alkaline phosphatase and transaminases are high in the presence of normal bilirubin and normal or mildly increased BSP retention, one should suspect metastatic cancer in the liver.

Rapid Diagnostics

Bilirubin Tester (Manufactured by Wako Pure Chemicals). The bilirubin assay is based on the spectrophotometric method of White et al, using the absorbance of bilirubin at 455 nm. The system performs automatic correction for haemoglobin in the sample. Its features are:

1. The amount of blood required for the assay can be obtained in a single capillary tube and as little as one drop (0.05 ml) of serum is sufficient.
2. No reagents or diluent solutions are required.
3. Errors due to oxyhaemoglobin in the sample are corrected automatically.
4. There is no chance of contaminating the sample because the capillary tube used for sample collection is utilised as the cell.
5. The measured value of total bilirubin content is presented digitally and hence reading errors are eliminated.
6. The last digit of the read out represents tenths of a milligram per deciliter.

LIVER BATTERY (PROFILE), SERUM

Normal Values are Dependent Upon Methods Used

Normal Value

		SI units
Alanine Aminotransferase (ALT or SGPT)		
Adult female	4-35 U/L	
Adult male	7-46 U/L	
Children		
<12 months	≤54 U/L	
Age 1-2 years	3-37 U/L	
Age 2-8 years	3-30 U/L	
Age 8-16 years	3-38 U/L	
Alkaline Phosphatase (ALP)		
Adults		
Age 20-60 years		
Bodansky	2-4 U/dl	10.7-21.5 IU/L
King-Armstrong	4-13 U/dl	25.0-92.3 IU/L
Bessey-Lowery-Brock	0.8-2.3 U/dl	13.3-38-3 IU/L
Elderly	Slightly Higher	
Newborn	1-4 times adult values	
Children	Values remain high until epiphyses close.	
Female		
Age 2-10 years	100-350 U/L	
Age 10-13 years	110-400 U/L	
Males		
Age 2-13 years	100-350 U/L	
Age 13-15 years	125-500 U/L	
Aspartate Aminotransferase		
Adult females		
≤Age 60 years	8-20 U/L	8-20 U/L
>Age 60 years	10-20 U/L	10-20 U/L
Adult males		
≤Age 60	8-20 U/L	8-20 U/L
>Age 60	11-26 U/L	11-26 U/L
Children		
Newborn	16-72 U/L	16-72 U/L
Infant	15-60 U/L	15-60 U/L
Age 1 year	16-35 U/L	16-35 U/L
Age 5 years	19-28 U/L	19-28 U/L
Bilirubin		
1 month-adult	<1.5 mg/dl	1.7-20.5 μmol/L
Premature infant		
Cord	<2.8 mg/dl	<48 μmol/L
24 hours	1-6 mg/dl	17-103 μmol/L
48 hours	6-8 mg/dl	103-137 μmol/L
3-5 days	10-12 mg/dl	171-205 μmol/L
Full-term infant		
Cord	<2.8 mg/dl	<48 μmol/L
24 hours	2-6 mg/dl	34-103 μmol/L
48 hours	6-7 mg/dl	103-120 μmol/L
3-5 days	4-6 mg/dl	68-103 μmol/L

Gamma-Glutamyl Transferase/Transpeptidase (GGT/GGTP)

Adult female	4-25 U
	9-31 mU/ml
	3.5-13 IU/L
	3-33 U/L> 37°C
Adult males	7-40 U
	12-38 mU/ml
	4-23 mU/ml
	9-69 U/L>37°C
Children	
Cord blood	190-270 U/L >37°C
Premature infant	<140 U/L >37°C
1-3 days	56-233 U/L >37°C
4-21 days	0-130 U/L >37°C
3-12 weeks	4-120 U/L >37°C
3-6 months, female	5-35 U/L >37°C
3-6 months, male	5-5 U/L >37°C
>6 months, female	15-85 IU/L
>6 months, male	5-55 IU/L
1-15 years	0-23 U/L >37°C

Hepatitis B Profile

Negative

Lactate Dehydrogenase (LD/LDH)

Wroblewski method 30°C	150-450 U/L	72-217 IU/L
Adults		
<Age 60	45-90 U/L	45-90 U/L
>Age 60	55-102 U/L	55-102 U/L
Children		
Newborn	160-500 U/L	160-500 U/L
Neonate	300-1500 U/L	300-1500 U/L
Infant	100-250 U/L	100-250 U/L
Child	60-170 U/L	60-170 U/L

Leucine Aminopeptidase (LAP)

12-33 IU/dl	<50 IU/L

5′Nucleotidase (5′NT or 5′N)

2-15 IU/L
0-17 U/L
0-1.6 U
0.3-3.2 Bodansky units

Protein Electrophoresis

Normals are dependent on laboratory procedure. Percentage values are for the Agarose method and represent the percentage of total protein:

Adult (Agarose method)		
Total protein		5.90-8.00
Albumin	58-74%	0.58-0.74
Alpha$_1$, globulin	2.0-3.5%	0.02-0.04
Alpha$_2$ globulin	5.4-10.6%	0.05-0.11
Beta globulin	7.0-14.0%	0.07-0.14
Gamma globulin	8.0-18.0%	0.08-0.18
Adult		
Total protein	6.0-8.0 gm/dl	60-80gm/L
Albumin	3.3-5.0 gm/dl	35-50gm/L
Alpha$_1$ globulin	0.1-0.4 gm/dl	1-4gm/L

Alpha$_2$ globulin	0.5-1 gm/dl	5-10gm/L
Beta globulin	0.7-1.2 gm/dl	7-12 gm/L
Gamma globulin	0.8-1.6 gm/dl	8-16 gm/L
Premature infant		
Total protein	4.4-6.3 gm/dl	44-63 gm/L
Albumin	3.0-4.2 gm/dl	30-42gm/L
Alpha$_1$ globulin	0.11-0.5 gm/dl	1.1-5 gm/L
Alpha$_2$ globulin	0.3-0.7 gm/dl	3-7 gm/L
Beta globulin	0.3-1.2 gm/dl	3-12 gm/L
Gamma globulin	0.3-1.4 gm/dl	3-14 gm/L
Newborn		
Total protein	4.6-7.4 gm/dl	46-74 gm/L
Albumin	3.5-5.4 gm/dl	35-54 gm/L
Alpha$_1$ globulin	0.1-0.3 gm/dl	1-3 gm/L
Alpha$_2$ globulin	0.3-0.5 gm/dl	3-5 gm/L
Beta globulin	0.2-0.6 gm/dl	2-6 gm/L
Gamma globulin	0.2-1.2 gm/dl	2-12 gm/L
Infant		
Total protein	6.0-6.7 gm/dl	60-67 gm/L
Albumin	4.4-5.4 gm/dl	44-54 gm/L
Alpha$_1$ globulin	0.2-0.4 gm/dl	2-4 gm/L
Alpha$_2$ globulin	0.5-0.8 gm/dl	5-8 gm/L
Beta globulin	0.5-0.9 gm/dl	5-9 gm/L
Gamma globulin	0.3-0.8 gm/dl	3-8 gm/L
Child		
Total protein	6.2-8.0 gm/dl	62-80 gm/L
Albumin	4.0-5.8 gm/dl	40-58 gm/L
Alpha$_1$ globulin	0.1-0.4 gm/dl	1-4 gm/L
Alpha$_2$ globulin	0.4-1.0 gm/dl	4-10 gm/L
Beta globulin	0.5-1.0 gm/dl	5-10 gm/L
Gamma globulin	0.3-1.0 gm/dl	3-10 gm/L

Contd...

Contd...

Prothrombin time	
Adult	10-15 seconds
Newborn	<17 seconds
Child	11-14 seconds

Usage: Work-up for liver disease, bilary disease, hepatoma, liver metastatic chronic active hepatitis, cirrhosis, including biliary cirrhosis, hepatic complications associated with medications or TPN.

Increased: See individual test listings.

Decreased: See individual test listings.

Description

Liver battery includes testing for several blood levels that reflect hepatic function. In general, a liver battery includes the following: *Alanine, Aminotransferase, Serum; Alkaline Phosphafase, Serum; Aspartate Aminotransferase, Serum; Bilirubin. Gamma-Glutamyl Transpeptidase, Blood; Hepatitis B Surface Antigen, Blood; Lactate Dehydrogenase. Blood: Leucine Aminopeptidase, Blood; 5′ Nucleotidase. Blood: Protein, Electrophoresis, Serum; Prothrombin time, Blood.* See individual test listings for specific descriptions.

CHAPTER 20

Clinical Chemistry

COLORIMETRY

Colorimetry is the science that deals with the measurement of the capacity of a chemical, coloured system to absorb light. Since it makes specific quantitative measurements, it is very useful and widely used in laboratories in the form of **colorimeter or spectrophotometer.** To understand colorimetry, it is essential to have some knowledge and understanding of what is meant by **Light, Colour and Beer's Law.**

- **Light** is a form of energy (radiant energy)
- It moves in space in the form of waves like the electromagnetic waves.
- The peak of the wave is called the **CREST.**
- The lowest point of the wave is called the **Trough.**
- The distance between two identical points on a wave cycle is called the **wavelength.**
- The unit of measure for wavelength is **nanometer (nm).**
- Wavelengths are also expressed as **lamda (λ).**

The colours are the wavelength we see. It is the wavelength that determines the colour of the light. The human eye can only see the wavelengths of energy between about 400 and 750 nm. This is called the **visible spectrum.**

The total light spectrum can be divided into 3 distinct regions—the ultraviolet region, the visible region and the infrared region. The wavelengths of the various regions and colours are shown below.

UV								Infrared

Light whose wavelength is 400 nm is violet. Light with wavelength less than 400 nm is not visible to the human eye and is known as ultraviolet. Light with wavelengths of more than 700 is not visible and is known as infrared light. The visible spectrum occurs between the wavelengths of 400 nm and 700 nm. Here we have the colours of violet, blue, green, yellow, orange and red or the "rainbow". Thus, while light is seen colourless, it is composed of all colours of the visible spectrum.

The colour of a substance will depend on the wavelength absorbed by the substance and which are transmitted to the observer's eye.

Beer's Law: When a coloured solution is illuminated with monochromatic light, its absorbance is directional proportional to the concentration of the colored solution when the light path is constant.

Absorbance α Concentration
(when light path length is constant)

Lambert's Law: When a coloured solution is illuminated with light, it's absorbance is directly proportional to the light path when concentration of the solution is constant.

Absorbance α Length,
(when concentration is constant).

If we combine both we get the Beer Lambert's Law; "When a coloured solution illuminated with monochromatic light, it's absorbance is proportional to the concentration of the colored solution and the length of the light path."

Absorbance (A) α Concentration (C) X Length (L)

$$A = \epsilon CL$$

Where ϵ is the molar absorption coefficient.

In all the colorimetric determinations, a reference standard of known concentration is used and its color intensity is compared with color intensity of the test sample,

$$A_t = \epsilon C_t L$$

$$A_s = \epsilon C_s L \text{ (t = test, s = standard)}$$

Since the same cuvette is used for the test and standard, L is constant.

$$A_t = C_t$$
$$A_s = C_s$$

If concentration of the standard, i.e. C_s is known then $C_t = \frac{A_t \times C_s}{A_s}$

Calculation of Absorbance (A):

Usually *colorimeters measure transmittance* rather than absorbance. *Transmittance and Absorbance has an inverse relationship.*

T is the ratio of intensity of emergent light (Ie) to the intensity of incident light (Io)

$$T = Ie / Io$$
$$A = -\log T\,\%$$
$$A = 1 / \text{Log } T\,\% \text{ or } A = -\log T\,\%$$
$$A = -\log T\,\%$$
$$= \log 1/T\,\%$$
$$= \log 100 - \log T = 2.0 - \log T$$

In *clinical chemistry* there are two ways of expressing the amount of light absorbed by a solution. These are

- **Amount transmission (%T)** Per cent transmission is the amount of light, which passes through a coloured solution compared to the amount of light, which passes through a blank or colourless solution. As the concentration of the coloured solution increases the amount of light absorbed increases while the %T decreases.
- **Optical density (OD)** The OD may be calculated from the % T and is the units preferred in clinical chemistries, the reason OD is usually preferred is that there is a *direct relationship* between the *concentration of a solution* and the OD, i.e. as the concentration of a solution increases, the absorbance or OD also increases.

By taking the unknown, we can use the derived formula from Beer's Law to find the concentration of the unknown, which is:

$$\frac{\text{Concentration unknown}}{\text{Concentration standard}} = \frac{\text{OD unknown}}{\text{OD standard}}$$

$$\text{i.e. Concentration of unknown} = \frac{\text{OD unknown}}{\text{OD standard}} \times \text{concentration of standard}$$

PHOTOMETER

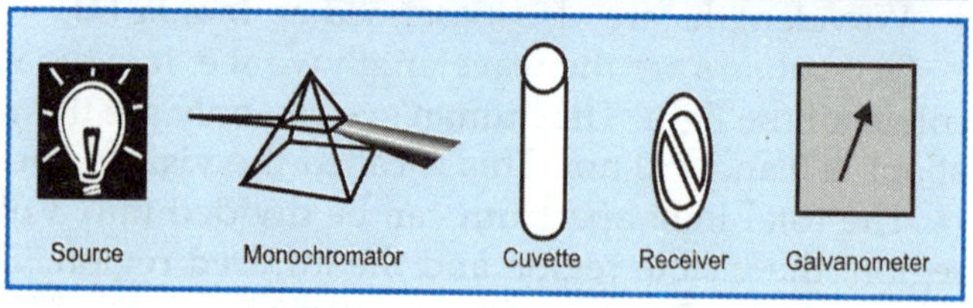

Source Monochromator Cuvette Receiver Galvanometer

The basic components of a photometer are as shown above. They are:

- **Light source**
- **Filter or monochromator**
- **Cuvette**
- **Photodiode cell** (receiving light signals)
- **Galvanometer**

A. Light source

A tungsten filament lamp is usually used as source for light (radiant energy). Its intensity varies upon the type of photometers. A uniform voltage supply is very important for a stable source of light. Ageing of the lamp or accumulation if dirt can result in range in absorbance reading.

B. Wavelength selectors

In most instruments **filters** are used for this purpose. The filter chosen is usually complementary to the colour of the solution to be measured (see table below).

Colour of solution	Usual filter
Blue	yellow
Bluish-green	Red
Purple	Green
Red	Bluish-green
Yellow	Blue
Yellowish-green	Violet

Filters are made of glass or dyed gelatine between glass plates and have a limited transmission band at which they transmit maximally. To understand the use of **light filters** consider a bluish-green solution which absorbs light in the red part of the spectrum. Such a solution when illuminated by white light absorbs red colour wavelengths and emits bluish-green light together with a small amount of red. The greater the concentration of the solution the smaller the amount of red light transmitted. The most sensitive readings of the galvanometer will therefore be obtained by allowing only the transmitted red light to activate the photoelectric cell. The red filter achieves this by stopping the transmission of bluish-green light and allowing only the red light to pass through the solution.

In the more expensive type of equipment, a **diffraction grating** or a **prism** is used to obtain the required wavelength.

In **diffraction grating** the white light is dispersed into a continuous spectrum. By turning a wavelength adjustment, the grating is rotated and different parts of the spectrum are allowed to fall onto the photocell.

In **glass prism** spectrophotometers, light is focused onto the prism. Light passes through and forms an extended spectrum. On adjusting the exit slit (wavelength adjustment) light can pass through the cuvette, and illuminate the photocell.

C. Cuvettes and flow-through cells

These are used to hold coloured solutions and must be scrupulously clean, with no dirty finger marks or spillage of fluid on the outside of the optical side. Spillage of fluid or dirty finger marks will absorb light and interfere in the measurement of the colour. Scratches on the glass must be avoided and if badly scratched it must be discarded.

In order to speed up laboratory work, a more recent development in colorimetry is the introduction of **follow-through cells.** These cells enable colorimetric readings to be speeded up considerably, since the cells or cuvettes can be drained without being removed from the colorimeters.

D. Photoelectric cell

A photoelectric cell consists of photoelectric elements; light falling on these elements generates an electric current which deflects a galvanometer needle, the deflection being proportional to the light intensity.

E. Galvanometer

The galvanometer measures the output of the photosensitive element, and in good instruments a very sensitive is used.

Requirements of Colorimetric Analysis

When colorimetric determinations are made, it is essential to ensure that the colour being measured is only due to the substance under investigation and is not due to any of the reagents used. It is, therefore, essential to include the following solutions.

1. **Test solution:** This contains the unknown concentration of the substance together with the reagents used in the test.
2. **Standard solution:** This is usually identical to the test solution, except that it contains a known amount of the substance being determined and is approximately equal in concentration to that expected in the test.
3. **Blank solution:** This solution is identical to both the test and standard solution and it is carried through the complete test procedure and contains all the reagents used, but without any test or standard substance. Any colour given by the reagents used in the analysis can be detected and eliminated.

In order to be sure that the absorbance is due solely to the substance under test, the reading given by the 'blank' solution must be considered with the reading obtained from the 'test' and 'standard' solutions. The photoelectric absorptiometer is set to read zero absorbance with distilled water. The Blank, Test and Standard absorbance readings are recorded, rechecking the zero absorbance between each reading. The blank reading is then subtracted from the test and standard reading as follows:

$$\frac{\text{Test} - \text{Blank}}{\text{Standard} - \text{Blank}} \times \text{concentration of standard}$$

This procedure will usually ensure that only the substance under investigation is being measured. Satisfactory results are only obtained with absorbance ranging from 0.2 to 0.8, so that if possible the determination should be modified in order that the lower and upper limits of deflection fall within this range.

Sources of error in photometry

Errors in photometry can be attributed to three sources

1. Inherent properties of the solution being measured
2. Instrument
3. Operator

Inherent Properties of the Solution

The factors, which may be included in this group, influence the absorption of light by the solution and can be the cause of deviations from Beer's Law.

a. **Chemical Nature of the Solvent and Solution**
   Deviations from Beer's Law may occur either as a result of a shift in the shape of a given portion of the absorption curve as the concentration changes or because of the absence of a linear relationship between optical density and concentration. A shift in the shape of a portion of the absorption curve can indicate a chemical transformation of a portion of the coloured component being analyzed into a second component of a different colour. The production of a second coloured component may also occur due to an impurity in the solvent in which the original coloured component is dissolved. For example, iodine dissolved in carbon tetrachloride is deep purple but dissolved in alcohol is brown. The presence of only 1 % alcohol as an impurity in carbon tetrachloride is sufficient to change the colour and hence, the shape of the absorption curve of iodine in carbon tetrachloride. Thus, the absolute purity of the solvent is very important in spectrophotometric work. This is particularly true for analysis carried out in the ultraviolet region. The breakdown of a linear relationship between optical density and concentration can be due to the dissociation of a colourless substance to give coloured ions, or vice versa.

b. **Exposure to Light**
   Certain compounds tend to bleach or discolour or get coloured when exposed to light. Such photochemical reactions are likely to occur when the test sample is stored in a warm, brightly-lighted room. This may occur while the sample is in the photometer, if the intensity of illumination is too high, but in most instruments the intensity is below the danger level. Methods in which photochemical reactions are likely to occur usually mention the precautions to be taken against light exposure. For example, the reconstituted glucose reagent kit is recommended to be stored in a dark bottle, because on exposure to light a photochemical reaction takes place and the reagent gets oxidised and develops a pink colour.

c. **Colour Instability**
   In some colorimetric reactions, the colour may be stable for only a short period of time. It is then necessary to time the reaction carefully so that the readings of all samples and standards are made during the time that the colour remains constant. Instability of colour may be due to temperature or absorption by the walls of the container where these factors have an influence, they must be kept constant for test samples and standards.

d. **Foreign Matter and Air Bubbles**
   Solutions in the cuvettes must be free of lint or other foreign matter, and air bubbles. A scrupulous cleaning of the cuvettes and other glassware used in the analysis should help to eliminate foreign matter from the solution. For example, in a flow through cuvette of most semi-automated analysers an air bubble trapped in it, will lead to a decrease in optical density of the solution.

e. **Errors of weighing and dilution:**
Simple errors of weighing and dilution in preparing reagents, sample and standards can affect photometric results appreciably. A good analytical balance and reliable volumetric glassware should be used. For example, while reconstituting a control serum care should be taken while dispensing the volume of distilled water to the control sera bulb. An error in dilution will result in change in the concentration of the constituents.

Instrument

Instruments are capable of considerable precision of measurement. The instrumental precision is of a higher order than that normally resulting from the development of colour in the test solutions. Inherent errors of the solution as mentioned above actually cause greater deviation than do instrumental errors.

a. **Light Source**
Unless a double-cell photometer is being used, the consistancy and reproducibility of the light source is important. Fluctuations in voltage should be overcome by the use of a voltage stabilizer in line-operated instruments. Lamps should be allowed to warm up for at least 5 minutes before steady output can be expected.

b. **Stray light**
Stray light from windows or overhead lighting striking the instrument can cause error since invisible particles suspended in solutions can reflect these rays. The covering of the cuvette compartment with a light-tight cover (as usually provided with the instrument) before taking readings will reduce this error.

c. **Slit Width**
In the prism spectrophotometer, the purity of the monochromatic band depends on the width of the entrance and exit slits. The use of a narrow slit width will produce more accurate results.

d. **Moisture**
Moisture can be the cause of fluctuating readings in spectrophotometric operation. In instruments employing desicant, it is advisable to change to freshly dried silica gel at regular intervals. This is particularly important in an environment of high humidity.

e. **Linearity of Photocell Response**
Reliable results depend upon the current output of the photocell being proportional to the light striking the photocell. This relationship can be disturbed if the photocell is not adequately protected from moisture and from overheating. Some instruments are fitted with heat absorbing filters in the optical system and provided with thermal insulation of the light source.

f. **Cuvettes**
An important source of error and one which requires constant checking is the cuvette. It is necessary that cuvettes be optically matched so that readings will not be influenced by their individual variation when a series is used for making measurements. When it is necessary to re-use cuvettes that have not had adequate time to dry after cleaning, a rinse with alcohol and ether or acetone may be used to speed up the drying process. If cuvettes are dirty, etched, scratched or marked with fingerprints, erroneous readings will result.

g. **Wavelength Calibration**
A wavelength scale which is off calibration can be a source of error in spectrophotometers.

Operator Errors

Errors of the operator can be minimized by the practice of good technique in the laboratory preparation of the solutions and in the operation of the instrument. The operator should be guided in the latter instance by the instructions provided by the manufacturer. An awareness, of the sources of error in the preceding categories should tend to reduce these errors.

CLINICAL CHEMISTRY

Specimen Collection and Processing

With the exception of glucose, triglycerides and inorganic phosphorus, most blood chemical constituents reveal no significant change after a standard breakfast, so it is not essential for the patient to be in an absolute fasting state prior to blood specimen collection. However, lipemia (lactescence), caused by transient rise in triglycerides as chylomicrons following a meal containing fat may cause interference with a large number of chemical determinations because of turbidity. Therefore, blood is always collected from a patient in the post-absorptive state. This can be accomplished with an overnight fast (12-14 hours, especially for lipids), although a four to six hour fast will usually suffice.

Venipuncture should be performed for obtaining blood. Disposable needles eliminate the hazard of serum hepatitis transmission. Heparin is the most ideal anticoagulant for plasma determination. The cost is quite prohibitive so others EDTA, and trisodium citrate can be used without significant alteration in reading and results. For glucose, oxalate-fluoride mixture is used. Fluoride impairs glycolysis of the blood cells. Prompt separation of plasma/serum is essential to yield a proper specimen for most chemical estimations. Always collect a little more blood than required so as not to fall short of it subsequently. For 1 ml of serum about 2.5 ml of blood should be withdrawn. Labelling and identification is important.

Pipettes: For dispensing test materials or reagents, etc., exact quantities are needed. For volumes till 0.1 ml Borosil's pipettes can be used. Otherwise autopipettes for micro to macro sampling can be used. Dispensing exact amounts of test samples/reagents is the first step to accurate clinical chemistry.

Proper Specimen Collection

If the commercially available kits are being used, follow the manufacturers guidelines and collect the requisite amount of blood.

Specimen Collection

Chemistry (plain tube)

Amylase	Lipase
Alcohol	Lithium
Bilirubin	LATS and TSH
Barbiturate	Triglyceride
Salicylate	Electrolytes
BSP	BUN
Calcium	Uric acid
Cholesterol	
Copper	
Creatinine	
CPK	
SGOT	
SGPT	
Urea	
T_4	
Iron and iron binding capacity	
LDH	

Chemistry (Heparin)
pH
Ammonia
RBC Potassium
Renin
Plasma testosterone
Cholinesterase
Plasma cortisol
Methemoglobin
Plasma haemoglobin

Chemistry
Oxalate, fluoride tube
Glucose
Glucose tolerance test

Haematology (EDTA)
Complete Blood counts
WBC, RBC, Hb, PCV,
MCV, MCH, MCHC
Differential count
Absolute eosinophil count

Haematology (EDTA)
Hb electrophoresis
G_6PD screening
Reticulocyte count
ESR

Haematology (plain tube)
Haptoglobin,
LE preparation
Serum viscosity

Haematology (Sodium citrate)
PTTK
Prothrombin time
Thrombin time
Fibrinogen titer
Fibrinogen level

Blood bank (plain tube)
Crossmatch
Typing
Coombs' test
Antibody identification

Serology (plain tube)
α_1 antitrypsin
Antinuclear antibody
Antistreptolysin-O
Antithyroid antibodies

Ceruloplasmin
C-Reactive protein
Cold agglutinins
Paul Bunnel test
Immunoglobulins
Leptospira agglutination test
VDRL
Australia antigen
Sickling test
Platelet count

Processing

Ideally all measurements should be performed within 1 hour after collection. Tests where proteins are first precipitated with tungstic acid, trichloroacetic acid or barium sulphate—samples for these tests can be stored in a refrigerator at 4-6°C if the interval before the analysis exceeds 30 minutes. In medical chemistry, plasma can be used for virtually all measurements (ideal anticoagulant being heparin), although a few require serum (serum enzymes and protein electrophoresis), while whole blood can for all practical purposes be eliminated. Whenever a delay of more than 1 hour is anticipated, refrigerate the sample at 4ºC. For extracting serum–let the blood clot at room temperature (takes about 20-30 minutes), loosen the clot at the top by a stick. Centrifuge blood for 10 minutes at 3,000 rpm, serum can be removed with the use of a pasteur pipette. Label and store the serum in a refrigerator at 4-6ºC until analyzed or freeze at–20ºC if the analysis is to be delayed by more than 4 hours.

Centrifuge

While centrifuging the principle of balance must always be observed. Tubes of equal weight, shape, and size should be placed in opposing positions in the centrifuge head (using water filled tubes whenever necessary). Tubes should be supported by appropriately shaped rubber cushions in the carrier of the centrifuge head. The speed of the centrifuge should be slowly accelerated.

Difficulties

1. All tubes should be chemically clean, i.e. free of actual or potential organic and/or inorganic constituents that may alter the result of a chemical analysis. They need not be sterile.
2. Haemolysis: It should always be avoided as release of RBC contents (e.g. LDH, acid phosphatase and potassium) or through colour change (especially for photometric measurements using shorter wavelengths of the visible spectrum 400-500 nm) results may be falsely high. Haemoglobin interferes with specific chemical reactions (e.g. diazotization inhibition in bilirubin estimation).

Blood Collection, Precautions and Errors

1. Excessive venous stasis by prolonged application of tourniquet should be avoided. This would also raise concentration of certain constituents of blood hormones, calcium, K^+, Lactic acid, etc).
2. The syringe, needle and the tube should be moisture free.
3. Blood should be withdrawn by needle of gauge less than 21.
4. Expelling blood through the needle into the container should be avoided.
5. Do not shake blood in container to mix with anticoagulants. Mix by gentle repetitive inversion—about 6 to 8 times.
6. Clotted specimens should not be disturbed for 20-30 minutes.
7. Prolonged contact of serum or plasma with blood cells should be avoided to minimize glycolysis and/or shift of constituents from cells to serum or plasma.
8. If the patient is already on an I/V drip, withdraw blood from the other arm.
9. Refrigeration of freshly collected blood specimen before clotting has occurred or freezing of whole blood before separation should be avoided.
10. Lactescence: Milky or lipemic plasma and serum are frequently obtained with blood samples collected 1 to 2 hours after a fatty meal or patients with hyperlipoproteinemia. It is associated with blood neutral fat levels. This interferes with certain photometric measurements, e.g. uric acid and enzymes. It also produces false elevations when serum is used in final test mixture but not in the reagent blanks.
11. *Concentration changes*: Changes in drawn blood samples from the original constituent concentrations occur through dilution or evaporation.

12. *Composition changes*: The major sources of composition alteration in blood specimens are bacterial and enzymatic effect, loss of volatile blood constituents by diffusion or evaporation and interchange of substance between the liquid and cellular components of blood. Protection from light is essential for certain constituents (e.g. bilirubin).
13. *Bacterial changes*: These include ammonia formation from urea and can be minimized by
    a. Sterile handling of the blood samples wherever possible
    b. Prompt separation of cells from plasma or serum
    c. Storage of the specimen at 4-6°C until analysed or freezing at –20°C (minus 20°C) when possible.
14. *Enzymatic changes*: Glycolysis is minimized by the same measures as bacterial changes, except that sterility has no effect unless an enzymatic method is employed.

Clinical Chemistry and Drug Interference (See Appendix II)

Drug interference can occur in two ways

1. *Pharmacologic interference*: whereupon some action of the drug or its metabolite can cause an alteration *(in vivo)* in the concentration of the substance being measured by the test, or
2. *Chemical interference*: in which some physical or chemical property of the drug can alter the analysis directly.

CONTROL SERA

Before one proceeds for knowing the unknown, one must have some known standards with which to compare and obtain the results of the unknown. Most kits do provide a standard solution of the substance to be measured but the following are outstanding and are extremely useful for preparation of calibration curves.

NORMAL VALUES DIFFER WITH DIFFERENT KITS AND MANUFACTURES. ALWAYS CONSULT THE PRODUCT INSERT FOR EXACT METHOD FOR A PARTICULAR KIT, FOLLOW THE MANUFACTURES INSTRUCTIONS STRICTLY.

Kits of all tests mentioned in this and the next chapter can be obtained from **CORAL CLINICAL SYSTEMS, GOA.**

BLOOD UREA NITROGEN (BUN)

Courtesy: Tulip Group of Companies

Normal Values

		SI Units
Young adult <40	5-18 mg/dl	1.8-6.5 mmol/L
Adult	5-20 mg/dl	1.8-7.1 mmol/L
Elderly >60	8-21 mg/dl	2.9-7.5 mmol/L
Mild azotemia	20-50 mg/dl	7.1-17.7 mmol/L
Children		
Cord blood	21-40 mg/dl	7.5-14.3 mmol/L
Premature infant, first 7 days	3-25 mg/dl	1.1-7.9 mmol/L
Full-term Newborn	4 18 mg/dl	1.4-6.4 mmol/L
Infant	5-18 mg/dl	1.8-6.4 mmol/L
Child	5-18 mg/dl	1.8-6.4 mmol/L
Panic level	>100 mg/dl	>35.7 mmol/L

Control Sera from Boehringer

Product	*Standardises*
1. Precibil	Bilirubin
2. Preciflo (for Technicon systems)	23, chemical parameters
3. Precilip (normal range)	26, chemical parameters
4. Precilip EL (elevated range)	6 parameters (mainly lipids)
5. Precinorm E (normal range)	16 enzyme parameters
6. Precipath E (elevated range)	16 enzymic parameters
7. Precinorm S (normal range)	5 chemical parameters
8. Precipath S (elevated range)	15 chemical parameters
9. Precinorm U (normal range) Suitable for both automated and manual	38 chemical and enzymic parameters. procedures
10. Precipath U (abnormal range)	-do-
11. Precinorm protein (normal range)	For IgG, IgM and transferrin values
12. Special control serum for HDL cholesterol.	

(For all the above mentioned controls the exact assay values are provided by the manufacturers)

UREA (DAM METHOD)

For the determination of Urea in serum, plasma and urine. (for in vitro diagnostic use only)

Summary

Urea is the end product of the protein metabolism. It is synthesised in the liver from the ammonia produced by the catabolism of amino acids. It is transported by the blood to the kidneys from where it is excreted. Increased levels are found in renal diseases, urinary obstructions, shock, congestive heart failure and burns. Decreased levels are found in liver failure and pregnancy.

Principle

Urea in an acidic medium condenses with Diacetyl monoxime at 100°C to form a red coloured complex. Intensity of the colour formed is directly proportional to the amount of urea present in the sample.

$$\text{Urea} + \text{Diacetyl monoxime} \xrightarrow{100°C} \text{Red Coloured Complex}$$

Normal reference values

Serum, Plasma : 14 - 40 mg/dl
Urine : upto 20 g/Litre

It is recommended that each laboratory establish its own normal range representing its patient population.

Contents	25 Tests	50 Tests
L1: Urea Reagent	75 ml	150 ml
L2: Acid Reagent	75 ml	150 ml
L3 : DAM Reagent	75 ml	150 ml
S: Urea Standard (40 mg/dl)	5 ml	5 ml

Storage/stability

All reagents are stable at RT till the expiry mentioned on the labels.

Reagent Preparation

Reagents are ready to use. Do not pipette with mouth.

Sample material

Serum, plasma or urine. Urine should be of 24 hours collection. Dilute the urine specimen 1:20 with distilled/deionised water before the assay. Urea is reported to be stable in serum for 5 days at 2-8°C.

Procedure

Wavelength/filter : 520 nm (Hg 546 nm) / Green
Temperature : 100°C
Light path : 1 cm

Pipette into clean dry test tubes labeled as Blank (B), Standard (S), and Test (T):

Addition Sequence	B (ml)	S (ml)	T (ml)
Urea Reagent (L1)	1.0	1.0	1.0
Acid Reagent (L2)	1.0	1.0	1.0
DAM Reagent (L3)	1.0	1.0	1.0
Distilled water	0.01	—	—
Urea Standard (S)	—	0.01	—
Sample	—	—	0.01

Mix well and keep the test tubes in boiling water (100°C) for 10 minutes. Cool under running tap water and measure the absorbance of the Standard (Abs S), and Test Sample (Abs T) against the Blank.

Calculations

$$\text{Urea in mg/dl} = \frac{\text{Abs T}}{\text{Abs S}} \times 40$$

$$\text{Urine Urea in g/Litre} = \frac{\text{Abs T}}{\text{Abs S}} \times 8$$

Urea Nitrogen in mg/dl = Urea in mg/dl × 0.467

Linearity

The procedure is linear upto 70 mg/dl. If values exceed this limit, dilute the sample with distilled water and repeat the assay, Calculate the value using the proper dilution factor.

Note

The presence of ammonia does not interfere in this test.

System Parameters			
Reaction	End point	Interval	:
Wavelength	: 520 nm	Sample vol	: 0.01 ml
Zero Setting	: Reagent blank	Reagent vol	: 3.00 ml
Incub Temp	: 100°C	Standard	: 40 mg/dl
Incub time	: 10 min.	Factor	:
Delay time	:	React slope	: Increasing
Read time	: —	Linearity	: 70 mg/dl
No of read	: —	Units	: mg/dl

UREA (MOD. BERTHELOT METHOD) (COURTESY: TULIP GROUP OF COMPANIES)

For the determination of Urea in serum, plasma and urine. (for in vitro diagnostic use only)

Summary

Urea is the end product of protein metabolism. It is synthesised in the liver from the ammonia produced by the catabolism of amino acids. It is transported by the blood to the kidneys from where it is excreted. Increased levels are found in renal diseases, urinary obstructions, shock, congestive heart failure and burns. Decreased levels are found in liver failure and pregnancy.

Principle

Urease hydrolyses urea to ammonia and CO_2. The ammonia formed further reacts with a phenolic chromogen and hypochlorite to form a green coloured complex. Intensity of the colour formed is directly proportional to the amount of urea present in the sample.

$$\text{Urea} + H_2O \xrightarrow{\text{Urease}} \text{Ammonia} + CO_2$$

Ammonia + Phenolic chromogen + Hypochlorite ⟶ Green coloured complex

Normal reference values

Serum/Plasma : 14-40 mg/dl
Urine : Upto 20 g/L

It is recommended that each laboratory establish its own normal range representing its patient population.

Contents	75 assays	3 × 75 assays
L1: Buffer Reagent	75 ml	3 × 75 ml
L2: Enzyme Reagent	7.5 ml	3 × 7.5 ml
L3: Chromogen Reagent	15 ml	45ml
S: Urea Standard (40 mg/dl)	5 ml	5 ml

Storage/stability

Contents are stable at 2-8°C till the expiry mentioned on the labels.

Reagent Preparation

Reagents are ready to use for the given procedure.

Working Enzyme Reagent: For the flexibility and convenience in performing large assay series, a working enzyme reagent may be made by pouring 1 bottle of L2 (Enzyme Reagent) into 1 bottle of L1 (Buffer Reagent). For smaller series combine 10 parts of L1 (Buffer Reagent) and 1 part of L2 (Enzyme Reagent). Use 1 ml of the working reagent per assay instead of 1 ml of L1 and 0.1 ml of L2 as given in the procedure. The working enzyme reagent is stable for at least 4 weeks when stored at 2-8°C.

Working Chromogen Reagent: For larger volume cuvettes, dilute 1 part of L3 (Chromogen Reagent) with 4 parts of fresh ammonia free distilled/deionised water. Use 1 ml of working chromogen instead of 0.2 ml in the assay. The working chromogen reagent is stable for atleast 8 weeks when stored at 2-8°C in a tightly stoppered plastic bottle.

Sample Material

Serum, plasma, Urine. Dilute urine 1 + 49 with distilled water before the assay (results × 50). Urea is reported to be stable in the serum for 5 days when stored 2-8°C.

Procedure

Wavelength/filter : 570 nm (Hg 578 nm)/yellow
Temperature : 37°C / RT
Light path : 1 cm

Pipette into clean dry test tubes labelled as Blank (B), Standard (S), and Test (T) :

Addition	B	S	T
Sequence	(ml)	(ml)	(ml)
Buffer Reagent (L1)	1.0	1.0	1.0
Enzyme Reagent (L2)	0.1	0.1	0.1
Distilled water	0.01	—	—
Urea Standard (S)		0.01	—
Sample	—	—	0.01
Mix well and incubate for 5 min. at 37°C or 10 min. at RT (25°C)			
Chromogen Reagent (L3)	0.2	0.2	0.2

Mix well and incubate for 5 min. at 37°C or 10 min. at RT (25°C). Measure the absorbance of the Standard (Abs S), and Test Sample (Abs T) against the Blank, within 60 Min.

Calculations

$$\text{Urea in mg/dl} = \frac{\text{Abs T}}{\text{Abs S}} \times 40$$

Urea Nitrogen in mg/dl = Urea in mg/dl x 0.467

Linearity

This procedure is linear upto 250 mg/dl. Using the working chromogen reagent (1 ml) the linearity is increased to 400 mg/dl. If values exceed this limit, dilute the serum with normal saline (NaCI 0.9%) and repeat the assay. Calculate the value using the proper dilution factor.

Note

Any contamination by ammonia or ammonium salts lead to erroneous results, hence plasma should not be collected with Fluoride or Heparin Ammonium salts. The working enzyme reagent is not stable at elevated temperatures and should be stored back at 2-8°C immediately after use. The chromogen reagent contains chlorine. The bottle should be opened only when required and closed tightly after use to prevent the loss of active chlorine.

System Parameters			
Reaction	: End point	No of read	:
Wavelength	: 570 nm	Interval	:
Zero setting	: Reagent blank	Sample Vol	: 0.01 ml
Incub. temp	: 37°C/RT	Reagent Vol	: 1.30 ml
Incub. time	: 5 min + 5 min or 10 min +10 min	Standard Factor	: 40 mg/dl
		React slope	: Increasing
Delay time	:	Linearity	: 250 mg/dl
Read time	:	Units	: mg/dl

UREA (GLDH Kinetic method) (Courtesy: Tulip Group of Companies)

For the determination of Urea in serum or plasma. (for in vitro diagnostic use only)

Summary

Urea is the end product of protein metabolism. It is synthesised in the liver from the ammonia produced by the catabolism of amino acids. It is transported by the blood to the kidneys from where it is excreted. Increased levels are found in renal diseases, urinary obstructions, shock, congestive heart failure and burns. Decreased levels are found in liver failure and pregnancy.

Principle

Urease hydrolyzes urea to ammonia and CO_2. The ammonia formed further combines with a Ketoglutarate and NADH to form Glutamate and NAD. The rate of oxidation of NADH to NAD is measured as a decrease in absorbance in a fixed time which is proportional to the urea concentration in the sample.

$$\text{Urea} + H_2O + 2\,H^+ \xrightarrow{\text{Urease}} 2\,NH_4 + CO_2$$

$$2\,NH_4^+ + 2\,\alpha\text{Ketoglutarate} + 2NADH \xrightarrow{\text{GLDH}} 2\ \text{L-glutamate} + 2\,NAD^+ + 2H_2O$$

Normal reference values

Serum/plasma : 14-40 mg/dl
Urine : Upto 20 g/l

It is recommended that each laboratory establish its own normal range representing its patient population.

Contents	75ml	2 ×75 ml
L1: Enzyme Reagent	60 ml	2 × 60 ml
L2: Starter Reagent	15 ml	2 × 15 ml
S: Urea Standard (40mg/dl)	5 ml	5 ml

Storage/stability

Contents are stable at 2-8°C till the expiry mentioned on the labels.

Reagent Preparation

Reagents are ready to use.

Working reagent: For sample start assays a single reagent is required. Pour the contents of 1 bottle of L2 (Starter Reagent) into 1 bottle of L1 (Enzyme Reagent).

This working reagent is stable for at least 10 days when stored at 2-8°C. Alternatively for flexibility as much of working reagent may be made as and when desired by mixing together 4 parts of L1 (Enzyme Reagent) and 1 part of L2 (Starter Reagent). Alternatively 0.8 ml of L1 and 0.2 ml of L2 may also be used instead of 1 ml of the working reagent directly during the assay.

Sample Material

Serum, plasma, Urine. Dilute urine 1+ 49 with distilled water before the assay (results × 50). Urea is reported to be stable in the serum for 5 days when stored at 2-8°C.

Procedure

Wavelength/filter : 340 nm
Temperature : 37°C / 30°C / 25°C
Light path : 1 cm

Substrate Start Assay

Pipette into a clean dry test tube labelled Standard (S) or Test (T):

Addition	(S)/(T)
Sequence	37°C / 30°C / 25°C
Enzyme Reagent (L1)	0.8 ml
Urea Standard/Serum/Diluted urine	0.01 ml
Incubate at the assay temperature for 1 minute and add	
Starter Reagent (L2)	0.2 ml

Mix well and read the initial absorbance A for the Standard and Test after exactly 30 seconds. Read another absorbance A_2 of the Standard and Test exactly 60 seconds later. Calculate the change in absorbance ΔA for both the Standard and Test.

Sample Start Assay

Pipette into a clean dry test tube labelled Standard (S) or Test (T):

Addition Sequence	(S)/(T) 37°C / 30°C / 25°C
Working reagent Bring to assay temperature and add	1.0 ml
Urea standard/serum/diluted urine	0.01 ml

Mix well and read the initial absorbance A_1 for the Standard and Test after exactly 30 seconds. Read another absorbance A_2 of the Standard and test exactly 60 seconds later. Calculate the change in absorbance ΔA for both the Standard and Test.

For Standard $\Delta AS = A_2S - A_1S$

For Test $\Delta AT = A_2T - A_1T$

Calculations

$$\text{Urea in mg/dl} = \frac{\Delta A\ T}{\Delta A\ S} \times 40$$

Linearity

This procedure is linear upto 250 mg/dl. If values exceed this limit, dilute the serum with normal saline (NaCI 0.9%) and repeat the assay. Calculate the value using the proper dilution factor.

Note

Plasma should not be collected with Fluoride or Heparin salts as contamination by ammonia or ammonium salts lead to erroneous results.

System Parameters			
Reaction	: Fixed Time Kin.	Interval	: 60 sec.
Wavelength	: 340 nm	Sample vol	: 0.01 ml
Zero Setting	: Distilled Water	Reagent Vol	: 1.00ml
Incub temp	: 30°C / 37°C	Standard	: 40 mg/dl
Incub time	—	Factor	:
Delay time	: 30 sec.	React slope	: Decreasing
Read time	: 60 sec.	Linearity	: 250 mg/dl
No of read	: 2	Units	: mg/dl

NORMAL VALUES (GENERAL REFERENCE)

Adults: BUN is 8-18 mg%, Urea = 15-40 mg%

Adults over 60 years : may have a little higher values normally. Low values may be found during pregnancy and in full-term infants, whereas premature infants may have slightly higher values than the adult range.

CLINICAL RELEVANCE

COMMON CAUSES OF UREMIA

Prerenal

- Reduced blood flow to kidney
  Shock, blood loss, dehydration
- Increased protein catabolism
  Crush injuries, burns, fever, haemorrhage into soft tissue or body cavities, haemolysis

Renal

- Acute renal failure
  Glomerulonephritis, malignant hypertension, nephrotoxic drugs or metals, renal cortical necrosis
- Chronic renal disease
  Glomerulonephritis, pyelonephritis, diabetes mellitus, arteriosclerosis, renal tubular disease, collagen-vascular diseases.

Post-renal:

- Ureteral destruction by stones, tumor, inflammation, surgical trauma, obstruction of bladder neck or urethra by prostate, stones, tumor, inflammation.

DECREASED BUN IS ASSOCIATED WITH

a. Liver failure
b. Negative nitrogen balance as may occur in malnutrition, excessive use of IV fluids and physiologic hydremia of pregnancy.
c. Impaired absorption as in celiac disease.
d. Occasionally in nephrotic syndrome
e. Overhydration.

Interfering Factors

1. A combination of a low protein and a high carbohydrate diet cause a decreased BUN level.
2. The BUN is normally lower in children and women because they have a smaller muscle mass than adult men.
3. Increased BUN values occur in late pregnancy and infancy because of increased use of protein.
4. Older people may have an increased BUN when their kidneys are not able to concentrate urine adequately.
5. Decreased BUN values may normally occur earlier in pregnancy because of physiologic hydremia.
6. Many drugs can cause increased BUN levels.
7. Drugs that may cause decreased BUN levels include
   - Dextrose infusions
   - Phenothiazines
   - Thymol

Comments

1. Ammonium oxalate should not be used as an anticoagulant. Plasma can be used if it is obtained from EDTA, citrate, potassium oxalate or heparin.
2. If the serum sample is very lipemic, prepare a special blank tube by adding the phenol colour reagent to the urease before adding the serum. Set the zero absorbance for the particular sample with this blank.
3. For urgent test–the incubation time can be reduced to 5 minutes if the water bath temperature is raised to 55-56°C.
4. Plasma or serum preserved with fluoride cannot be used as this inactivates the enzyme. Urea is stable in frozen serum for months.
5. Make sure that there is no contamination by ammonia or heavy metal ions.
6. For a small laboratory, commercially available multi/monostep kits can be used.

PLASMA OR SERUM CREATININE (Courtesy: Tulip Group of Companies)

Normal Values

		SI Units
Jaffe, manual method	0.8-1.5 mg/dl	70-133 μmol/day
Jaffe, kinetic or enzymatic method		
Adult		
Female	0.5-1.1 mg/dl	44-97 μmol/L
Males	0.6-1.2 mg/dl	53-106 μmol/L
Eldery	May be lower	May be lower
Children		
Cord blood	0.6-1.2 mg/dl	53-106 μmol/L
Newborn	0.8-1.4 mg/dl	71-124 μmol/L
Infant	0.7-1.7 mg/dl	62-150 μmol/L
Age 1 female	≤0.5 mg/dl	≤44 μmol/L
Age 1 male	≤0.6 mg/dl	≤53 μmol/L
Age 2-3 female	≤0.6 mg/dl	≤53 μmol/L
Age 2-3 male	≤0.7 mg/dl	≤62 μmol/L
Age 4-7 female	≤0.7 mg/dl	≤62 μmol/L
Age 4-7 male	≤0.8 mg/dl	≤71 μmol/L
Age 8-10 female	≤0.8 mg/dl	≤71 μmol/L
Age 8-10 male	≤0.9 mg/dl	≤80 μmol/L
Age 11-12 female	≤0.9 mg/dl	≤80 μmol/L
Age 11-12 male	≤1.0 mg/dl	≤88 μmol/L
Age 13-17 female	≤1.1 mg/dl	≤97 μmol/L
Age 13-17 male	≤1.2 mg/dl	≤106 μmol/L
Age 18-20 female	≤1.2 mg/dl	≤106 μmol/L
Age 18-20 male	≤1.3 mg/dl	≤115 μmol/L

CREATININE (Alkaline Picrate method) (Courtesy: Tulip Group of Companies)

For the determination of Creatinine in serum and urine. (for *in vitro* diagnostic use only)

Summary

Creatinine is the catabolic product of creatinine phosphate which is used by the skeletal muscle. The daily production depends on muscular mass and it is excreted out of the body entirely by the kidneys. Elevated levels are found in renal dysfunction, reduced renal blood flow (shock, dehydration, congestive heart failure) diabetes acromegaly. Decreased levels are found in muscular dystrophy.

Principle

Picric acid in an alkaline medium reacts with creatinine to form a orange coloured complex with the alkaline picrate. Intensity of the colour formed is directly proportional to the amount of creatinine present in the sample.

Creatinine + Alkaline picrate→Orange coloured complex

Reference values

	Serum	Urine, 24hrs. collection
Males	: 0.6 - 1.2 mg%	1.1-3.0 gm
Females	: 0.5 - 1.1 mg%	1.0-1.8 gm

It is recommended that each laboratory establish its own normal range representing its patient population.

Contents	15 Tests	35 Tests
L1: Picric Acid Reagent	60 ml	140 ml
L2: Buffer Reagent	5 ml	12 ml
S: Creatinine Standard (2 mg/dl)	5 ml	5 ml

Storage/stability

All reagents are stable at RT till the expiry mentioned on the labels.

Reagent Preparation

Reagents are ready to use. Do not pipette with mouth.

Sample Material

Serum or Urine

Creatinine is stable in serum for 1 day at 2-8°C

Urine of 24 hours collection is preferred. Dilute the specimen 1:50 with distilled/deionised water before the assay.

Procedure

Wavelength/filter 520 nm (Hg 546 nm)/Green
Temperature RT
Light path 1 cm

Deproteinization of specimen

Pipette into a clean dry test tube
Picric acid reagent (L1) 2.0 ml
Sample 0.2 ml

Mix well and centrifuge at 2500 - 3000 rpm for 10 min. to obtain a clear supernatant

Colour development

Pipette into clean dry test tubes labelled as Blank (B), Standard (S), and Test (T):

Addition Sequence	B (ml)	S (ml)	T (ml)
Supernatant	-	-	1.1
Picric Acid Reagent (L1)	1.0	1.0	
Distilled water	0.1		
Creatinine Standard (S)	-	0.1	
Buffer Reagent (L2)	0.1	0.1	0.1

Mix well and keep the test tubes at RT for exactly 20 minutes. Measure the absorbance of the standard (Abs S), and test sample (Abs T) against the blank.

Calculations

$$\text{Creatinine in mg\%} = \frac{\text{Abs T}}{\text{Abs S}} \times 2.0$$

$$\text{Urine Creatinine in gm/Lit.} = \frac{\text{Abs T}}{\text{Abs S}} \times 1.0$$

Urine Creatinine gm/24Hrs = Urine Creatinine in gm/L × Vol. of urine in 24 mrs.

Linearity

The procedure is linear upto 8 mg% of creatinine.

If values exceed this limit, dilute the sample with distilled water and repeat the assay. Calculate the value using the proper dilution factor.

Note

Maintain the reaction time of 20 min. as closely as possible since a longer incubation causes an increase in the values due to the reaction of pseudo-chromogens. The determination is not specific and may be affected by the presence of large quantities of reducing substances in the sample. The reaction is temperature sensitive and all the tubes should be maintained at a uniform temperature.

System Parameters			
Reaction	: End point	Interval	:
Wavelength	: 520 nm	Sample Vol	: 0.20 ml
Zero setting	: Reagent blank	Reagent	: Vol. 1.10 ml
Incub temp	: RT	Standard	: 2 mg/dl
Incub time	: 20 min.	Factor	:
Delay time	: —	React slope	: Increasing
Read time	: —	Linearity	: 8 mg/dl
No of read	: —	Units	: mg/dl

CREATININE (Mod Jaffa's Kinetic method) (Courtesy: Tulip Group of Companies)

For the determination of Creatinine in serum and urine. (for in vitro diagnostic use only)

Summary

Creatinine is the catabolic product of creatinine phosphate which is used by the skeletal muscle. The daily production depends on muscular mass and it is excreted out of the body entirely by the kidneys. Elevated levels are found in renal dysfunction, reduced renal blood flow (shock, dehydration, congestive heart failure) diabetes acromegaly. Decreased levels are found in muscular dystrophy.

Principle

Picric acid in an alkaline medium reacts with creatinine to form a orange coloured complex with the alkaline picrate. Intensity of the colour formed during the fixed time is directly proportional to the amount of creatinine present in the sample.

Creatinine + Alkaline Picrate→Orange coloured complex.

Reference values

	Serum	Urine in 24 hrs. collection
Males	: 0.6 - 1.2 mg%	1.1-3.0 gm
Females	: 0.5 - 1.1 mg%	1.0-1.8 gm

It is recommended that each laboratory establish its own normal range representing its patient population.

Contents	2 × 35 ml	2 × 75 ml
L1: Picric Acid Reagent	35 ml	75 ml
L2: Buffer Reagent	35 ml	75 ml
S: Creatinine Standard (2 mg/dl)	5 ml	5 ml

Storage/stability

All reagents are stable at RT till the expiry mentioned on the label.

Reagent Preparation

Reagents are ready to use. Do not pipette with mouth.

Working reagent: For larger assay series a working reagent may be prepared by mixing equal volumes of Picric Acid Reagent and Buffer Reagent. The Working reagent is stable at RT (25-30°C) for at least one week.

Sample Material

Serum or Urine

Creatinine is stable in serum for 1 day at 2-8°C

Urine of 24 hours collection is preferred. Dilute the specimen 1:50 with distilled/deionised water before the assay.

Procedure

Wavelength/filter	: 520 nm (Hg 492 nm)/Green
Temperature	: 30°C/37°C
Light path	: 1 cm

Pipette into a clean dry test tube labelled Standard (S) or Test (T):

Addition Sequence	(S)/(T) 30°C/37°C
Picric Acid Reagent (L1)	0.5 ml
Buffer reagent (L2)	0.5 ml
Bring reagents to the assay temperature and add	
Creatinine Standard (S)/Sample/Diluted Urine	0.1 ml

Mix well and read the initial absorbance A_1 for the standard and Test after exactly 30 seconds. Read another absorbance A_2 of the Standard and Test exactly 60 seconds later. Calculate the change in absorbance ΔA for both the Standard and Test.

For Standard	$\Delta A S$	=	A_2S	-	A_1S
For Test	ΔAT	=	A_2T	-	A_1T

Calculations

$$\text{Creatinine in mg/dl} = \frac{\Delta AT}{\Delta AS} \times 2.0$$

$$\text{Urine Creatinine in g/L} = \frac{\Delta AT}{\Delta AS} \times 1.0$$

Urine Creatinine g/24Hrs.= Urine Creatinine in g/L × Vol. of urine in 24 Hrs.

Linearity

The procedure is linear upto 20 mg/dl of Creatinine. If values exceed this limit, dilute the sample with distilled water and repeat the assay. Calculate the value using the proper dilution factor.

Note

The Buffer Reagent may turn milky or show white precipitates at cold temperatures. This is not a deterioration of the reagent. Dissolve/clear the same by warming the reagent to 37°C with gentle swirling before use. The determination is not specific and may be affected by the presence of large quantities of reducing substances.

As the test is temperature sensitive it is essential to maintain the indicated reaction timings and temperatures meticulously during the test procedure.

System Parameters			
Reaction	: Fixed Time Kin	Interval	: 60 sec.
Wavelength	: 520 nm	Sample vol	: 0.10 ml
Zero Setting	: Distilled Water	Reagent vol	: 1.00 ml
Incub temp	: 30°C/37°C	Standard	: 2 mg/dl
Incub time	: -	Factor	: -
Delay time	: 30 sec.	React slope	: Increasing
Read time	: 60 sec.	Linearity	: 20 mg/dl
No of read.	: 2	Units	: mg/dl

CLINICAL RELEVANCE

Causes of raised serum creatinine levels

All renal causes of uremia are usually associated with raised serum creatinine values. Elevated BUN levels in a patient with normal creatinine usually signal a nonrenal cause for the uremia. With severe, permanent renal damage, urea levels continue to climb, but creatinine values tend to plateau. At very high creatinine levels, some is excreted across the alimentary tract.

Decreased Creatinine levels occur in

Muscular dystrophy

Interfering Factors

1. High levels of ascorbic acid can give a falsely increased level.
2. Drugs influencing kidney function (diuretics and dextran), chloral hydrate, marijuana, aceto-hexamide, guanethidine, furosemide, chloram-phenicol, and sulphonamides can cause a change in blood creatinine.
3. A diet high is roast meat will cause increased levels.
4. Many drugs may cause a change in the blood creatinine. Refer to Appendix II.

   A normal blood serum creatinine does not always indicate unimpaired renal function. A normal value cannot be used as standard for a patient who is known to have existing renal disease.

SERUM BILIRUBIN

Normal Values

		SI Units
Total bilurubin		
1 month-adult	<1.5 mg/dl	1.7-20.5 μmol/L
Premature infant		
Cord	<2.8 mg/dl	<48 μmol/L
24 hours	1-6 mg/dl	17-103 μmol/L
48 hours	6-8 mg/dl	103-137 μmol/L
3-5 days	10-12 mg/dl	171-205 μmol/L
Full-term infant		
Cord	<2.8 mg/dl	<48 μmol/L
24 hours	2-6 mg/dl	34-103 μmol/L
48 hours	6-7 mg/dl	103-120 μmol/L
3-5 days	4-6 mg/dl	68-103 μmol/L
Direct bilirubin	0.0-0.3 mg/dl	1.7-5.1 μmol/L
Indirect bilirubin	0.1-1.0 mg/dl	1.7-17.1 μmol/L

BILIRUBIN (Mod Jendrassik and Grof's method) (Courtesy: Tulip Group of Companies)

For the determination of Direct and Total Bilirubin in serum. (for in vitro diagnostic use only)

Summary

Bilirubin is mainly formed from the heme portion of aged or damaged RBCs. It then combines with albumin to form a complex which is not water soluble. This is referred to as indirect or unconjugated Bilirubin. In the liver this Bilirubin complex is combined with glucuronic acid into a water soluble conjugate. This is referred to as conjugated or direct Bilirubin. Elevated levels of bilirubin are found in liver diseases (Hepatitis, cirrhosis), excessive hemolysis/destruction of RBC (hemolytic jaundice) obstruction of the biliary tract (obstructive jaundice) and in drug induced reactions. The differentiation between the direct and indirect bilirubin is important in diagnosing the cause of hyperbilirubinemia.

Principle

Bilirubin reacts with diazotised sulphanilic acid to form a coloured azobilirubin compound. The unconjugated bilirubin couples with the sulphanilic acid in the presence of a caffein- benzoate accelerator. The intensity of the colour formed is directly proportional to the amount of bilirubin present in the sample.

Bilirubin + Diazotized Sulphanilic acid→ Azobilirubin Compound

Normal reference values

Serum	(Direct)	:	upto 0.2 mg/dl
	(Total)	:	upto 1.0 mg/dl

It is recommended that each laboratory establish its own normal range representing its patient population.

Contents	30 tests	75 tests
L1: Direct Bilirubin Reagent	75 ml	150 ml
L2: Direct Nitrite Reagent	4 ml	4 ml
L1: Total Bilirubin Reagent	75 ml	150 ml
L2: Total Nitrite Reagent	4 ml	4 ml
S: Artificial Standard (10 mg/dl)	10 ml	10 ml

Storage/Stability

All reagents are stable at RT till the expiry mentioned on the label.

Reagent Preparation

Reagents are ready to use. Do not pipette with mouth.

Sample material

Serum. Bilirubin is reported to be stable in the sample for 4 days at 2-8°C protected from light as it is photosensitive.

Procedure

Wavelength/filter : 546 nm/yellow-Green
Temperature : RT
Light path : 1 cm

Direct Bilirubin Assay

Pipette into clean dry test tubes labelled as Blank (B), and Test (T):

Addition Sequence	B (ml)	T (ml)
Direct Bilirubin Reagent (L1)	1.0	1.0
Direct Nitrite Reagent (L2)	-	0.05
Sample	0.1	0.1

Mix well and incubate at RT for exactly 5 min. Measure the absorbance of the Test Samples (Abs T) immediately against their respective Blanks.

Total Bilirubin Assay

Pipette into clean dry test tubes labelled as Blank (B), and Test (T) :

Addition Sequence	B (ml)	T (ml)
Total Bilirubin Reagent (L1)	1.0	1.0
Total Nitrite Reagent (L2)	-	0.05
Sample	0.1	0.1

Mix well and incubate at RT for 10 min. Measure the absorbance of the Test Samples (Abs T) immediately against their respective Blanks.

Calculations

Total or Direct Bilirubin in mg/dl = Abs T × 13

Linearity

This procedure is linear upto 20 mg/dl. If values exceed this limit, dilute the sample with distilled water and repeat the assay. Calculate the value using the proper dilution factor.

Note

In case the exact wavelength is not available the artificial standard (S) may be used. Measure the absorbance of the artificial standard against distilled water with the appropriate filter and keep the same for future calculations by dividing the Abs T with the Abs. of the Std. x 10. Discard the Artificial Standard after use.

In case of neonates where the sample quantity is a limitation, and the samples have high bilirubin (above 3 mg/dl), only 0.05 ml/0.02 ml of the sample may be used for bilirubin estimation. The calculation factor in this case would be 24.9/60.5 respectively instead of 13. In case of using the standard the value of the same would be 19.1/46.5 mg/dl respectively instead of 10 mg/dl.

System Parameters			
Reaction	: End point	Interval	:
Wavelength	: 546 nm	Sample Vol	: 0.10 ml
Zero Setting	: Sample Blank	Reagent Vol	: 1.05 ml
Incub temp	: RT	Standard	:
Incub time	: 5 min/10 min.	Factor	: 13
Delay time	: —	React slope	: Increasing
Read time	: —	Linearity	: 20 mg/dl
No. of read	: —	Units	: mg/dl

CAUSES OF HYPERBILIRUBINEMIA

Unconjugated (Indirect) Hyperbilirubinemia

I. Overproduction of bilirubin
   A. Hemolytic disorders.

1. Congenital (e.g. hemoglobinopathies)
2. Acquired (e.g. Coombs' positive anaemia)
3. Liver disease (e.g. hepatitis and cirrhosis).

B. Shunt hyperbilirubinemia

II. Defective uptake and storage of bilirubin

A. Idiopathic unconjugated hyperbilirubinaemia.
1. Hereditary–Gilbert's syndrome.
2. Acquired
— Post-viral hepatitis.
— Post-portacaval shunt

B. Decreased availability of cytoplasmic binding proteins (Y and Z) in newborn and premature infants.

C. Drugs (e.g. flavispidic acid).

III. Defective glucuronyl transferase activity.

A. Deficiency.
1. In newborn and premature infants.
2. Crigler-Najjar syndrome.

B. Inhibition
1. Abnormal steroids in breast milk or maternal plasma (Lucey-Driscoll type).
2. Drugs (e.g. Novobiocin).

CONJUGATED (DIRECT) HYPERBILIRUBINEMIA

Defective excretion of conjugated bilirubin

A. Hereditary
1. Dubin-Johnson syndrome.
2. Rotor syndrome.

B. Obstructive
1. Intrahepatic cholestasis.
   a. Cirrhosis (occasionally)
   b. Hepatitis (often)
   c. Alcoholic liver disease (occasionally)
   d. Drugs (e.g. chlorpromazine and methyltestosterone).
   e. Primary biliary cirrhosis
2. Extrahepatic obstruction.
   a. Gall stones
   b. Carcinoma of the bile duct, pancreas, ampulla of Vater.
   c. Bile duct stricture.
   d. Biliary atresia.

Interfering Factors

1. A 1 hour exposure of the specimen to sunlight or high intensity artificial light at room temperature will reduce the bilirubin content.
2. Contrast media 24 hours before measurement may cause an altered reaction.
3. A high fat meal may cause decreased bilirubin levels by interfering with the clinical reactions.
4. Air bubbles and shaking of the specimen may cause decreased levels.
5. Foods (carrots, etc.) and drugs increase the yellowish hue in the serum.
6. Refer to the Appendix II for a listing of the many drugs that may interfere with testing for bilirubin.
7. Hemolysed blood will falsely elevate bilirubin level.

Comments

1. In severe obstructive jaundice with formation of biliverdin, low results for the degree of jaundice will be obtained since biliverdin does not react with the diazo reagent and cannot be determined.
2. An unusual source of otherwise unexplained elevated serum bilirubin has been described following 48 hours fasting. A normal bilirubin value from 0.68 mg% may rise to the abnormal range at 1.87 mg%.

ICTERUS INDEX

The icterus index is a measure of the degree of icterus (yellowish-green colour) in a plasma or serum specimen in cases of jaundice. This is just a screening test for hyperbilirubinemia. Substances other than bilirubin in the serum (carotene, xanthophyll, haemoglobin, etc.) may contribute to the icterus index, therefore, limiting its clinical utility. The test is now considered to be obsolete.

Reagents

A. Potassium dichromate solution
1. Stock solution (1%)
   Dissolve 1 gram of potassium dichromate in 70 ml of water placed in a 100 ml volumetric flask. Add 2 drops of sulphuric acid and dilute to 100 ml mark with distilled water. Store in a glass-stoppered brown/amber coloured bottle.
2. Working standard solution (0.1%)
   Pipette 10 ml of the stock solution into a 100 ml volumetric flask and dilute to 100 ml mark with distilled water.

B. Saline (0.9% NaCl) isotonic.

Method

A. Dilute the serum specimen ten times with saline (1 ml of serum mixed with 9 ml of saline) in a test tube and mix.
B. Transfer the diluted serum into a cuvette and read absorbance at 420 to 460 nm. If too dark, dilute further and multiply the final reading with the dilution factor utilised here.
C. Determine the icterus index from the calibration curve. Multiply the result by dilution factor. If the serum is diluted ten times, the dilution factor is 10.

Calibration Curve

A. Prepare three concentrations of the standard by diluting appropriate quantities of the stock solution of potassium dichromate in three 100 ml volumetric flasks
   1. Five ml stock mixed with 95 ml of water (1:20). This corresponds to 5 units.
   2. Twenty five ml of stock solution made to 100 ml with water (1:4 dilution). This corresponds to 25 units.
   3. Fifty ml of stock solution made to 100 ml with water (1:2 dilution). This corresponds to 50 units.
B. Read the absorbance of each working standard solution corresponding to 5, 25 and 50 units at 420 to 460 nm using water as blank.
C. Tabulate the results with the units of icterus index and the corresponding absorbance values.
D. Plot a calibration curve and use this for the determination of icterus index.

TOTAL PROTEIN

TOTAL PROTEIN (Biuret method)
Courtesy: Tulip Group of Companies

For the determination of Total Proteins in serum and plasma (for in vitro diagnostic use only)

Summary

Proteins are constituents of muscle, enzymes, hormones and several other key functional and structural entities in the body. They are involved in the maintenance of the normal distribution of water between blood and the tissues. Consisting mainly of albumin and globulin the fractions vary independently and widely in diseases. Increased levels are found mainly in dehydration. Decreased levels are found mainly in malnutrition, impaired synthesis, protein losses as in haemorrhage or excessive protein catabolism.

Principle

Proteins, in an alkaline medium, bind with the cupric ions present in the biuret reagent to form a blue-violet coloured complex. The intensity of the colour formed is directly proportional to the amount of proteins present in the sample.

Proteins + $Cu^{++} \rightarrow$ Blue violet coloured complex

Normal reference values

Serum and Plasma : 6.0 - 8.0 g/dl

It is recommended that each laboratory establish its own normal range representing its patient population.

Contents	150 ml	2 × 150 ml
Carton 1		
L1: Biuret reagent	150 ml	2 × 150 ml
Carton 2		
S: Protein Standard (8 g/dl)	5 ml	5 ml

Storage/stability

Carton 1: Biuret Reagent is stable at RT till the expiry mentioned on the label.

Carton 2: Protein Standard is stable at 2-8°C till the expiry mentioned on the label.

Reagent preparation

Reagents are ready to use. Protect from bright light.

Sample material

Serum or plasma. Proteins are reported to be stable in the sample for 6 days at 2 - 8°C.

Procedure

Wavelength/filter : 550 nm (Hg 546 nm)/yellow - Green
Temperature : RT/37°C
Light path : 1 cm

Pipette into clean dry test tubes labeled as Blank (B), Standard (S), and Test (T)

Addition Sequence	B (ml)	S (ml)	T (ml)
Biuret reagent (L1)	1.0	1.0	1.0
Distilled water	0.02		
Protein Standard (S)	-	0.02	
Sample	-	-	0.02

Mix well and incubate at 37°C for 10 min. or at RT for 30 min. Measure the absorbance of the standard (Abs S), and test sample (Abs T) against the blank, within 60 min.

Calculations

$$\text{Total Proteins in g/dl} = \frac{\text{Abs T}}{\text{Abs S}} = \times 8$$

Linearity

This procedure is linear upto 15 g/dl. If values exceed this limit, dilute the sample with distilled water and repeat the assay. Calculate the value using the proper dilution factor.

Note

Do not use if the reagent shows turbidity or black precipitates.

System Parameters			
Reaction	: End point	Interval	:
Wavelength	: 550 nm	Sample vol	: 0.02 ml
Zero setting	: Reagent blank	Reagent vol	: 1.00 ml
Incub temp.	: 37°C/RT	Standard	: 8 g/dl
Incub time	: 10 mm./30 min	Factor	:
Delay time	:	React slope	: Increasing
Read time	:	Linearity	: 15 g/dl
No of read	:	Units	: g/dl

SERUM ALBUMIN

DETERMINATION OF SERUM ALBUMIN (BCG method) (Courtesy: Tulip Group of Companies)

For the determination of Albumin in serum or plasma. (for in vitro diagnostic use only)

Summary

Albumin consists of approximately 60% of the total proteins in the body, the other major part being globulin. It is synthesized in the liver and maintains the osmotic pressure in blood. Albumin also helps in the transportation of drugs, hormones and enzymes. Elevated levels are rarely seen and are usually associated with dehydration. Decreased levels are seen in liver diseases (Hepatitis, Cirrhosis). Malnutrition, kidney disorders, increased fluid loss during extensive burns and decreased absorption in gastrointestinal diseases.

Principle

Albumin binds with the dye Bromocresol Green in a buffered medium to form a green coloured complex. The intensity of the colour formed is directly proportional to the amount of albumin present in the sample.

Albumin + Bromocresol Green→Green Albumin BCG Complex.

Normal reference values

Serum, Plasma (Albumin)	:	3.7 - 5.3 g/dl
Globulin	:	2.3 - 3.6 g/dl
A/G Ratio	:	1.0 -2.3

It is recommended that each laboratory establish its own normal range representing its patient population.

Contents	150 ml	2 × 150 ml
Carton 1 L1: BCG Reagent	150 ml	2 × 150 ml
Carton 2 S: Albumin Standard (4 g/dl)	5 ml	5 ml

Storage/stability

Carton 1 : BCG Reagent is stable at RT till the expiry mentioned on the label.

Carton 2 : Albumin Standard is stable at 2-8°C till the expiry mentioned on the label.

Reagent Preparation

Reagents are ready to use. Protect from bright light.

Sample material

Serum, EDTA plasma. Albumin is reported to be stable in the sample for 6 days at 2-8°C.

Procedure

Wavelength/filter	: 630 nm (Hg 623 nm)/Red
Temperature	: RT
Light path	: 1 cm

Pipette into clean dry test tubes labelled as Blank (B), Standard (S), and Test (T) :

Addition Sequence	B (ml)	S (ml)	T (ml)
BCG reagent (L1)	1.0	1.0	1.0
Distilled water	0.01	-	-
Albumin Standard (S)	-	0.01	-
Sample	-	-	0.01

Mix well and incubate at RT for 5 min. Measure absorbance of the Standard (Abs S), and Test Sample (Abs T) against the Blank.

Calculations

$$\text{Albumin in g/dl} = \frac{\text{Abs T}}{\text{Abs S}} \times 4$$

$$\text{Globulin in g/dl} = \underset{\text{(in g/dl)}}{\text{(Total Proteins)}} - \underset{\text{(in g/dl)}}{\text{(Albumin)}}$$

$$\text{A/G Ratio} = \frac{\text{Albumin in g/dl}}{\text{Globulin in g/dl}}$$

Linearity

The procedure is linear upto 7 g/dl. If values exceed this limit, dilute the sample with distilled water and repeat the assay. Calculate the value using the proper dilution factor.

Note

Gross haemolysis, ampicillin and heparin interfere with the results. Elevated bilirubin and lipemic samples may have a slight effect on accuracy. For grossly lipemic samples run a sample blank by adding 0.02 ml sample in 2 ml distilled water. Read the absorbance against D.W. and substract the blank absorbance from the test absorbance.

System Parameters

Reaction	: End point	Interval	:
Wavelength	: 630 nm	Sample vol	: 0.01 ml
Zero setting	: Reagent blank	Reagent vol	: 1.00 ml
Incub temp.	: RT	Standard	: 4 g/dl
Incub time	: 5 min	Factor	:
Delay time	: —	React slope	: Increasing
Read time	: —	Linearity	: 7 g/dl
No of read	: —	Units	: g/dl

NORMAL VALUES

Total Proteins

		SI Units
Adults	6.0-8.0 gm/dl	60-80 gm/L
Children		
Premature	4.3-7.6 gm/dl	43-76 gm/L
Newborn	4.6-7.4 gm/dl	46-74 gm/L
Infant	6.0-6.7 gm/dl	60-67 gm/L
Child	6.2-8.0 gm/dl	62-80 gm/L

Specimen Collection and storage

1. Serum is the specimen of choice.
2. Avoid excessive haemolysis since every 100 mg/dl of haemoglobin corresponds to about 100 mg/dl of albumin.
3. Albumin in serum is reported stable for one week at room temperature (18-30°C) and approximately one month when stored in the refrigerator (2-8°C) and protected against evaporation.

CLINICAL RELEVANCE

Causes of Hypoalbuminemia

Reduced Synthesis

- Malnutrition
- Malabsorption syndromes
- Chronic inflammatory diseases
- Acute hepatitis (lasting 14 days or more)
- Chronic liver disease
- Genetic abnormalities

Increased Loss

- Nephrotic syndrome
- Massive burns
- Protein-losing enteropathy

Increased Catabolism

- Massive burns
- Widespread malignancy

Multifactorial

- Cirrhosis
- Congestive heart failure
- Pregnancy

Increased albumin levels are generally not observed (When albumin concentration decreases there is a relative increase in globulins. However, there is a definite rise in globulins in mono/polyclonal gammopathies).

Disorders Associated with Polyclonal Gammopathies

Chronic Liver Disease

- Nutritional cirrhosis
- Primary biliary cirrhosis
- Chronic active hepatitis
- Viral hepatitis

Collagen Diseases

- Rheumatoid arthritis
- Systemic lupus erythematosus
- Sjögren's syndrome
- Felty's syndrome
- Polymyositis
- Scleroderma

Chronic Infections

- Tuberculosis
- Osteomyelitis
- Deep fungi
- Syphilis
- Bronchitis

Miscellaneous

- Metastatic carcinoma
- Cystic fibrosis
- Recovery from trauma

Causes of Monoclonal Gammopathies

- Multiple myeloma
- Waldenstrom's macroglobulinemia
- Benign idiopathic monoclonal gammopathy
- Heavy chain diseases
- Collagen disorders, autoimmune diseases
- Certain lymphomas
- Cirrhosis liver
- Neoplasms of colon, prostate, breast, female genital tract, stomach and lungs
- Myeloproliferative disorders-CML, polycythemia, myclofibrosis, erythrimic myelosis, erythroleukemia, other acute leukemias
- Aberrations in lipid metabolism
- Diabetes mellitus.

Interfering Factors

1. Low levels of albumin occur normally in all trimester's of pregnancy.
2. Bromsulphalein may cause a false elevation. Therefore, a serum protein test should not be done within 48 hours following a BSP test.
3. See appendix for complete listing of drugs that interfere with total protein levels.

SERUM CHOLESTEROL

CHOLESTEROL (CHOD/PAP method)
Courtesy: Tulip Group of Companies

For the determination of Cholesterol in serum or plasma. (for in vitro diagnostic use only)

Summary

Cholesterol is the main lipid found in blood, bile and brain tissues. It is the main lipid associated with arteriosclerotic vascular diseases. It is required for the formation of steroids and cellular membranes. The liver metabolizes the cholesterol and it is transported in the blood stream by lipoproteins. Increased levels are found in hypercholesterolaemia, hyperlipidaemia, hypothyroidism, uncontrolled diabetes, nephrotic syndrome, and cirrhosis. Decreased levels are found in malabsorption, malnutrition, hyperthyroidism, anaemias and liver diseases.

Principle

Cholesterol esterase hydrolyses esterified cholesterols to free cholesterol. The free cholesterol is oxidised to form hydrogen peroxide which further reacts with phenol and 4-aminoantipyrine by the catalytic action of peroxidase to form a red coloured quinoneimine dye complex. Intensity of the colour formed is directly proportional to the amount of cholesterol present in the sample.

$$\text{Cholesterol esters} + H_2O \xrightarrow{\text{Cholesterol esterase}} \text{Cholesterol} + \text{Fatty acids}$$

$$\text{Cholesterol} + O_2 \xrightarrow{\text{Cholesterol Oxidase}} \text{Cholestenone} + H_2O_2$$

$$H_2O_2 + 4\ \text{Aminoantipyrine} + \text{Phenol} \xrightarrow{\text{Peroxidase}} \text{Red Quinoneimine dye} + H_2O$$

Normal reference values

Serum/plasma	(Suspicious)	: 220 mg/dl and above
	(Elevated)	: 260 mg/dl and above

It is recommended that each laboratory establish its own normal range representing its patient population.

Contents	2 × 75 ml	2 × 150 ml
L1: Enzyme Reagent 1	2 × 60 ml	2 × 120 ml
L2: Enzyme Reagent 2	2 ×15 ml	2 × 30 ml
S: Cholesterol Standard (200 mg/dl)	5 ml	5 ml

Storage/stability

Contents are stable at 2-8°C till the expiry mentioned on the labels.

Reagent Preparation

Reagents are ready to use.

Working reagent: Pour the contents of 1 bottle of L2 (Enzyme Reagent 2) into 1 bottle of L1 (Enzyme Reagent 1).This working reagent is stable for at least 8 weeks when stored at 2-8°C. Upon storage the working reagent may develop a slight pink colour however, this does not affect the performance of the reagent. Alternatively for flexibility as much of working reagent may be made as and when desired by mixing together 4 parts of L1 (Enzyme Reagent 1) and 1 part of L2 (Enzyme Reagent 2). Alternatively 0.8 ml of L1 and 0.2 ml of L2 may also be used instead of 1 ml of the working reagent directly during the assay.

Sample material

Serum, EDTA plasma. Cholesterol is reported to be stable in the sample for 7 days when stored at 2-8°C. The sample should preferably be of 12 to 14 hours fasting.

Procedure

Wavelength/filter : 505 nm (Hg 546 nm)/Green
Temperature : 37°C /RT
Light path : 1 cm

Pipette into clean dry test tubes labelled as blank (B), standard (S), and test (T):

Addition Sequence	B (ml)	S (ml)	T (ml)
Working reagent	1.0	1.0	1.0
Distilled water	0.01	-	-
Cholesterol Standard (S)	-	0.01	
Sample	-	-	0.01

Mix well and incubate at 37°C for 5 min. or at RT (25°C) for 15 min. Measure the absorbance of the Standard (Abs S), and Test Sample (Abs T) against the Blank, within 60 Min.

Calculations

$$\text{Cholesterol in mg/dl} = \frac{\text{Abs T}}{\text{Abs S}} \times 200$$

Linearity

This procedure is linear upto 750 mg/dl. If the value exceeds this limit, dilute the serum with normal saline (NaCI 0.9%) and repeat the assay. Calculate the value using the proper dilution factor.

Note

Anticoagulants such as fluorides and oxalates result in false low values. The test is not influenced by Hb values upto 20 mg/dl and bilirubin upto 10 mg/dl.

System Parameters			
Reaction	: End point	Interval	: ...
Wavelength	: 505 nm	Sample vol	: 0.01 ml
Zero Setting	: Reagent blank	Reagent vol	: 1.00 ml
Incub temp	: 37°C / RT	Standard	: 200 mg/dl
Incub time	: 5 min./15 min.	Factor	:
Delay time	: —	React slope	: Increasing
Read time	: —	Linearity	: 750 mg/dl
No of read	: —	Units	: mg/dl

Normal Values

	Male		*Female*	
Age	*mg/l*	*SI Units mmol/L*	*mg/dl*	*SI Units mmol/L*
Total Cholesterol				
Adult				
20-24	124-218	3.21-5.64	122-216	3.16-5.59
25-29	133-244	3.44-6.32	128-222	3.32-5.75
30-34	138-254	3.57-6.58	130-230	3.37-5.96
35-39	146-270	3.78-6.99	140-242	3.63-6.27
40-44	151-268	3.91-6.94	147-252	3.81-6.53
45-49	158-276	4.09-7.15	152-265	3.94-6.86
50-54	158-277	4.09-7.17	162-285	4.20-7.38
55-59	156-276	4.04-7.15	172-300	4.45-7.77
60-64	159-276	4.12-7.15	172-297	4.45-7.69
65-69	158-274	4.09-7.10	171-303	4.43-7.85
>70	144-265	3.73-6.86	173-280	4.48-7.25
Child				
Cord blood	44-103	1.14-2.66	50-108	1.29-2.79
<4	114-203	2.95-5.25	112-200	2.90-5.18
5-9	121-203	3.13-5.25	126-205	3.26-5.30
10-14	119-202	3.08-5.23	124-201	3.21-5.20
15-19	113-197	2.93-5.10	119-200	3.08-5.18
High-density Lipoprotein Cholesterol (HDL)				
Adult				
20-24	30-63	0.78-1.63	33-79	0.85-2.04
25-29	31-63	0.80-1.63	37-83	0.96-2.15
30-34	28-63	0.72-1.63	36-77	0.93-1.99

Contd...

Contd...

35-39	29-62	0.75-1.60	34-82	0.88-2.12
40-44	27-67	0.70-1.73	34-88	0.88-2.28
45-49	30-64	0.78-1.66	34-87	0.88-2.25
50-54	28-63	0.72-1.63	37-92	0.96-2.38
55-59	28-71	0.72-1.84	37-91	0.96-2.35
60-64	30-74	0.78-1.91	38-92	0.98-2.38
65-69	30-75	0.78-1.94	35-96	0.91-2.48
> 70	31-75	0.80-1.94	33-92	0.85-2.38
Child				
Cord blood	6-53	0.16-1.37	13-56	0.34-1.45
5-9	38-75	0.98-1.94	36-73	0.93-1.89
10-14	37-74	0.96-1.91	37-70	0.96-1.81
15-19	30-63	0.78-1.63	35-74	0.91-1.91
Low-Density lipoprotein Cholesterol (LDL)				
Adult				
20-24	66-147	1.71-3.81	57-159	1.48-4.12
25-29	70-165	1.81-4.27	71-164	1.84-4.25
30-34	78-185	2.02-4.79	70-156	1.81-4.04
35-39	81-189	2.10-4.90	75-172	1.94-4.45
40-44	87-186	2.25-4.92	74-174	1.92-4.51
45-49	97-202	2.51-5.23	79-186	2.05-4.82
50-54	89-197	2.31-5.10	88-201	2.28-5.21
55-59	88-203	2.28-5.26	89-210	2.31-5.44
60-64	83-210	2.15-5.44	100-224	2.59-5.80
65-69	98-210	2.54-5.44	92-221	2.38-5.72
>70	88-186	2.28-4.82	96-206	2.49-5.34
Child				
Cord blood	20-56	0.52-1.45	21-58	0.54-1.50
5-9	63-129	1.63-3.34	68-140	1.76-3.63
10-14	64-133	1.66-3.44	68-136	1.76-3.52
15-19	62-130	1.61-3.37	59-137	1.53-3.55

		SI Units
Cholesterol Esters	60-75% of total or <210 mg/dl	0.60—0.75 <5.43 mmol/L
Free cholesterol	<50 mg/dl	<1.29 mmol/L
LDL:HDL ratio	<3	<3

Clinical Relevance

1. Increased levels of cholesterol
   a. Levels above 250 mg/dl are considered elevated and call for a triglyceride test.
   b. Conditions related to elevated cholesterol
      1. Cardiovascular disease and atherosclerosis
      2. Type II, familial hypercholesterolemia
      3. Obstructive jaundice (also an increase in bilirubin)
      4. Hypothyroidism (decreased in hyperthyroidism)
      5. Nephrosis
      6. Xanthomatosis
      7. Uncontrolled diabetes
      8. Nephrotic syndrome
      9. Obesity
   c. Free versus esterified cholesterol.
      There is a markedly abnormal ratio of free to esterified cholesterol in disease of the liver biliary tract, infectious disease, and extreme cholesterolemia.
2. Decreased levels of cholesterol
   a. Conditions where cholesterol is not absorbed from the gastrointestinal tract
      1. Malabsorption
      2. Liver disease
      3. Hyperthyroidism
      4. Anaemia
      5. Sepsis
      6. Stress
      7. Drug therapy such as antibiotics
   b. Other disorders related to decreased cholesterol levels
      1. Pernicious anaemia
      2. Hemolytic jaundice
      3. Hyperthyroidism
      4. Severe infections
      5. Terminal stages of debilitating diseases such as cancer
      6. Hypolipoproteinemias
   c. Esterol fraction decreases in liver diseases, liver cell injury, malabsorption syndrome, and malnutrition.
3. Increased levels of cholesterol esters are associated with familial deficiency of LCAT.
4. Decreased levels of cholesterol are associated with liver disease. This is because persons with liver diseases may have impaired formation of LCAT with a resulting deficiency of the enzyme.
5. Cholesterol ester storage disease causes accumulation of cholesterol esters in the tissues, but it has no effect on the percentage of esterified cholesterol in the blood.
6. The higher the cholesterol phospholipid ratio, the greater the possible risk of developing atherosclerosis.

Interfering Factors

1. Cholesterol is normally slightly elevated in pregnancy.

2. Estrogen decreases plasma cholesterol and oophorectomy increases it.
3. Many drugs may cause a change in the blood cholesterol (see Appendix II for complete listing).

Patient Preparation

1. Advise patient about fasting for a night for 12 hours before the test.
2. Water is permitted.
3. Before fasting, the patient should be on a normal diet for 7 days before testing.
4. No alcohol should be consumed 24 hours before testing.
5. Lipid lowering drugs such as estrogen, oral contraceptives, and salicylates should be withheld.

HDL CHOLESTEROL

HDL CHOLESTEROL KIT (PEG/CHOD-PAP method) Courtesy: Tulip Group of Companies

For the determination of HDL Cholesterol in serum or plasma. (For In vitro Diagnostic Use Only)

Summary

Lipoproteins are the proteins which mainly transport fats in the blood stream. They can be grouped into chylomicrons, very low density lipoproteins (VLDL), low density lipoproteins (LDL) and high density lipoproteins (HDL). Chylomicrons and VLDL transport mainly triglycerides, though VLDLs also transport some amount of cholesterol. LDL carries cholesterol to the peripheral tissues where it can be deposited and increase the risk of arteriosclerotic heart and peripherial vascular disease. Hence, high levels of LDL are atherogenic. HDL transports cholesterol from the peripherial tissues to the liver for excretion, hence, HDL has a protective effect. The measurement of total and HDL cholesterol and triglycerides provide valuable information for the risk assessment of coronary heart diseases.

Principle

When the serum is reacted with the Polyethylene Glycol contained in the precipitating reagent, all the VLDL and LDL are precipitated. The HDL remains in the supernatant and is then assayed as a sample for cholesterol using the Cholesterol (CHOD/PAP) reagent.

Normal reference values

		Prognostically favourable	Standard Risk Level	Risk Indicator
HDL Chol. (mg/dl)	males	> 55	35 - 55	< 35
	females	> 65	45 - 65	< 45
LDL Chol. (mg/dl)	males females	<150	150-190	>190
Total Chol.	males	> 3.8	3.8 - 5.9	< 5.9
HDL Chol.	females	> 3.1	3.1 - 4.6	< 4.6

It is recommended that each laboratory establish its own normal range representing its patient population.

Contents	75 ml
L1 : Enzyme Reagent 1	60 ml
L2 : Enzyme Reagent 2	15 ml
L3 : Pricipitating Reagent	2.5 ml
S : HDL Cholesterol Standard (25 mg/dl)	5 ml

Storage/stability

Contents are stable at 2-8°C till the expiry mentioned on the labels.

Reagent Preparation

Reagents are ready to use.

Working reagent : Pour the contents of 1 bottle of L2 (Enzyme Reagent 2) into 1 bottle of L1 (Enzyme Reagent 1). This working reagent is stable for at least 8 weeks when stored at 2-8°C. Upon storage the working reagent may develop a slight pink colour however this does not affect the performance of the reagent.

Alternatively for flexibility as much of working reagent may be made as and when desired by mixing together 4 parts of L1 (Enzyme Reagent 1) and 1 part of L2 (Enzyme Reagent 2). Alternatively 0.8 ml of L1 and 0.2 ml of L2 may also be used instead of 1 ml of the working reagent directly during the assay.

Sample material

Serum, EDTA plasma. Cholesterol & HDL Cholesterol are reported to be stable in serum for 7 days when stored at 2-8°C.The sample should preferably be of 12 to 14 hours fasting.

Procedure

Wavelength/filter : 505 nm (Hg 546 nm)/Green
Temperature : 37°C/RT.
Light path : 1 cm

Precipitation of VLDL & LDL :

Pipette into a clean dry test tube :
Precipitating Reagent (L3) } 0.1 ml
Sample } 0.1 ml
Mix well and incubate at RT for 5 min. Centrifuge at 2500-3000 rpm to obtain a clear supernatant.

Cholesterol Assay

Pipette into clean dry test tubes labelled as Blank (B), Standard (S), and Test (T) :

Addition Sequence	B (ml)	S (ml)	T (ml)
Working reagent	1.0	1.0	1.0
Distilled water	0.05	-	-
HDL Standard (S)	-	0.05	-
Supernatant *	-	-	0.05

Mix well and incubate at 37°C for 5 min. or at RT (25°C) for 15 min. Measure the absorbance of the Standard (Abs.S), and Test Sample (Abs.T) against the Blank, within 60 Min.

* If only Total Cholesterol is to be determined use only 0.01 ml of DW/Chol. Std./Sample directly in the cholesterol assay.

Calculations

$$\text{HDL Cholesterol in mg/dl} = \frac{\text{Abs.T}}{\text{Abs.S}} \times 25 \times 2$$

(Where 2 is the dilution factor due to the deprotenization step)

Calculation of LDL Cholesterol (mg/dl)

(Freidewald's Formula)

$$= \text{Total cholesterol} - \left(\frac{\text{Triglycerides}}{5}\right) - \text{HDL Cholesterol}$$

Freidewald's Formula is reliable provided that:

1. No chylomicrons are present i.e. it is a fasting sample.
2. Triglyceride values are below 400 mg/dl.
3. Type III hyperlipoproteinemia is absent.

Linearity

This procedure is linear upto 150 mg/dl of HDL Cholesterol. If values exceed this limit, dilute the serum with normal saline (NaCl 0.9%) and repeat the assay. Calculate the value using the proper dilution factor.

Note

The supernatant should be clear. If it is hazy or cloudy, the sample should be diluted 1 + 1 with normal saline (NaCl 0.9%) and the precipitation step should be repeated. (Results × 2)

Anticoagulants such as fluoride, oxalates and haemolysed serums should not be used.

System Parameters			
Reaction	: End Point	**Interval**	: —
Wavelength	: 505 nm	**Sample Vol.**	: 0.05 ml
Zero Setting	: Reagent Blank	**Reagent Vol.**	: 1.00 ml
Incub. Temp.	: 37°C/RT	**Standard**	: 25 mg/dl x 2
Incub. Time	: 5 min./15 min.	**Factor**	: —
Delay Time	: —	**React. Slope**	: Increasing
Read Time	: —	**Linearity**	: 150 mg/dl
No. of read.	: —	**Units**	: mg/dl

RISK FACTOR

Coronary heart disease (CHD) risk factor can be calculated using total lipid profile, as suggested by Castelli *et al*. The risk factor gives a most accurate and definite assessment of heart disease risk.

The factors are calculated by the ratio of total cholesterol to HDL—cholesterol and by the ratio of LDL—cholesterol (Low density lipoproteins—cholesterol) to HDL—cholesterol.

Risk	*Ratio: Total/ HDL–Cholesterol*		*Ratio: LDL/ HDL–Cholesterol*	
	Men	*Women*	*Men*	*Women*
½ Average	3.43	3.27	1.00	1.47
Average	4.97	4.44	3.55	3.22
2 × Average	9.55	7.05	6.25	5.03
3 × Average	23.99	11.04	7.99	6.14

HDL CHOLESTEROL PPT SET (PEG Precipitation Method) (Courtesy: Tulip group of Companies)

For the determination of HDL Cholesterol in serum or plasma. (for in vitro diagnostic use only)

Summary

Lipoproteins are the proteins which mainly transport fats in the blood stream. They can be grouped into chyiomicrons, very low density lipoproteins VLDL, low density lipoproteins (LDL) and high density lipoproteins (HDL). Chyiomicrons and VLDL transport mainly triglycerides, though VLDLs also transport some amount of cholesterol. LDL carries cholesterol to the peripheral tissues where it can be deposited and increase the risk of arteriosclerotic heart and peripheral vascular disease. Hence, high levels of LDL are atherogenic. HDL transports cholesterol from the peripheral tissues to the liver for excretion, hence HDL has a protective effect. The measurement of total and HDL cholesterol and triglycerides provide valuable information for the risk assessment of coronary heart diseases.

Principle

When the serum is reacted with the Polyethylene Glycol contained in the precipitating reagent, all the VLDL and LDL are precipitated. The HDL remains in the supernatant and is then assayed as a sample for cholesterol using the Cholesterol (CHOD/PAP) reagent.

Normal reference values

		Prognostically favourable	*Standard Risk Level*	*Risk Indicator*
HDL Chol (mg/dl)	males	> 55	35-55	< 35
	females	> 65	45-65	< 45
LDL Chol.	males females	< 150	150-190	>190
Total Chol	males	> 3.8	3.8 - 5.9	< 5.9
HDL Chol	females	> 3.1	3.1 - 4.6	< 4.6

It is recommended that each laboratory establish its own normal range representing its patient population.

Contents	**10 ml**
L1: Precipitating Reagent	10 ml
S: HDL Cholesterol Standard (25 mg/dl)	5 ml

Storage/stability

Contents are stable at 2-8°C till the expiry mentioned on the labels.

Reagent Preparation

Reagents are ready to use.

After the precipitation step Cholesterol reagent is required additionally for conducting the Cholesterol assay.

Sample material

Serum, EDTA plasma. HDL Cholesterol is reported to be stable in serum for 7 days when stored at 2-8°C. The sample should preferably be of 12 to 14 hours fasting.

Procedure

Precipitation of VLDL and LDL:

Pipette into a clean dry test tube

Precipitating Reagent (L1)	0.1 ml
Sample	0.1 ml

Mix well and incubate at RT for 5 min. Centrifuge at 2500-3000 rpm to obtain a clear supernatant.

Procedure for the cholesterol assay

Wavelength/filter	: 505 nm (Hg 546 nm)/Green
Temperature	:37°C/RT
Light path	: 1 cm

Pipette into clean dry test tubes labeled as blank (B), standard (S), and test (T):

Addition Sequence	**B** (ml)	**S** (ml)	**T** (ml)
Working reagent	1.0	1.0	1.0
Distilled water	0.05	-	-
HDL Standard (S)	-	0.05	-
Supernatant	-	-	0.05

Mix well and incubate at 37°C for 5 mm. or at RT (25°C) for 15 min. Measure the absorbance of the standard (Abs S), and test Sample (Abs T) against the blank, within 60 Min.

Calculations

$$\text{HDL Cholesterol in mg/dl} = \frac{\text{Abs T}}{\text{Abs S}} \times 25 \times 2$$

(Where 2 is the dilution factor due to the deprotenization step)

Calculation of LDL Cholesterol (mg/dl):

(Freidewald's Formula)

$$=(\text{Total cholesterol})-\left(\frac{\text{Triglycerides 1}}{5}\right)-(\text{HDL cholesterol})$$

Freidewald's Formula is reliable provided that:
1. No chylomicrons are present, i.e, it is a fasting sample.
2. Triglyceride values are below 400 mg/dl.
3. Type III hyperlipoproteinemia is absent.

Linearity

This procedure is linear upto 150 mg/dl of HDL Cholesterol. If values exceed this limit, dilute the serum with normal saline (NaCl 0.9%) and repeat the assay. Calculate the value using the proper dilution factor.

Note

The supernatant should be clear. If it is hazy or cloudy, the sample should be diluted 1 + 1 with normal saline (NaCI 0.9%) and the precipitation step should be repeated. (Results × 2)

Anticoagulants such as fluoride, oxalates and haemolysed serums should not be used.

System Parameters

Reaction	: End point	Interval	:
Wavelength	: 505 nm	Sample vol	: 0.05 ml
Zero Setting	: Reagent blank	Reagent vol	: 1.00 ml
Incub temp	: 37°C / RT	Standard	: 25 mg/dl x 2
Incub time	: 5 min/15 min	Factor	
Delay time	: —	React slope	: Increasing
Read time	: —	Linearity	: 150 mg/dl
No of read	: —	Units	: mg/dl

CLINICAL RELEVANCE

1. Increased values are associated with a chronic liver disorder.
2. Decreased values are associated with
   a. Increased risk of coronary heart disease when HDL—Cholesterol is less than 45 mg/dl in men and less men 55 mg/dl in women.
   b. Inheritance and chronic physical inactivity (25-35 mg/dl). Long level distance runners have higher levels of HDL.
3. Levels can be either high or low in primary biliary cirrhosis, chronic hepatitis, or alcoholism.

Interfering Factors

1. Decreased HDL is associated with smokers.
2. Increased HDL is associated with moderate intake of alcohol.
3. Iodine contrast substances interfere with test results.
4. Recent weight gains or losses can interfere with the test results.

Patient Preparation

1. Overnight fasting is required. Water is permitted.
2. If possible, all medication should be withheld for 24 to 48 hours before testing—confer with attending physician regarding this.
3. Ask patient if there has been any drastic change in weight in last few weeks before testing.

Patient Aftercare

Person with decreased HDL can be counselled to take measures to increase levels by losing weight, cutting down on calories consumption, eating less red meat, and taking lecithin supplements. Moderate alcohol consumption is believed by some to be a factor in increased HDL.

CHOLESTEROL: LDL AND VLDL

Very low density lipoproteins (VLDL) and low-density lipoproteins (LDL).

Normal Values

VLDL cholesterol: 25%-50%
LDL cholesterol: 62-185 mg/dl

VLDL is a major carrier of triglyceride (60-70% triglyceride, 10-15% cholesterol). Degradation of VLDL leads to a major source of LDL. Circulating fatty acids are vitalised by the liver to form triglycerides that are packaged with apoprotein and cholesterol and exported into the blood as very low density lipoproteins.

LDLs are the cholesterol rich remnants of the lipid transport vehicle, VLDL. Since LDL has a longer half-life (3-4 days) than its precursor, VLDL, LDL is more prevalent in the blood. It is finally catabolised in the liver and possibly in nonhepatic cells as well.

LDL-CHOLESTEROL FULLY ENZYMATIC, COLORIMETRIC TEST, Courtesy: Randox

Principle

Low-density lipoproteins (LDL) are precipitated by heparin at their isoelectric point (pH 5.04). After centrifugation the high-density lipoproteins (HDL) and the very low-density lipoproteins (VLDL) remain in the supernatant. These can then be determined by enzymatic methods.

LDL-cholesterol = Total cholesterol-cholesterol in the supernatent.

Sample

Serum

Reagents

Contents Initial Concentration of Solution

1. Precipitation Reagent
   Heparin 50,000 IU/1
   Sodium citrate 0.064 mol/l, pH 5.04

Preparation of Reagents

1. Precipitation Reagent
   Ready for use
   Stable up to expiry date when stored at +2 to +8°C.
2. Reagent solution for Cholesterol Determination (see fore-going pages).

Procedure

Wavelength 500 nm.Hg 546
Cuvette 1 cm light path
Temperature +20 to +25°C, 37°C
Pipette into centrifuge tube
Serum 100 µl
Precipitation reagent (1) 1000 µ1
Mix well, have to stand for 10 min at + 15 to + 25°C and centrifuge for 15 min at approx. 4000 rpm. Determine the cholesterol concentration of the supernatant within 1 hour after centrifugation.

Pipette into test tubes:

	Reagent Blank	*Standard*	*Sample*
Distilled water	50 µl		
Standard		50 µl	
Supernatant			50 µl
Reagent (2) (Cholesterol reagent)	1000 µl	1000 µl	1000 µl

Mix well, incubate for 10 min at +20 to +25°C or for 5 min at 37°C and measure the absorbance of the sample (A_{sample}) against the reagent blank.

Calculation

Using a Standard

Conc. of cholesterol in the supernatant:

$$\frac{A_{sample}}{A_{standard}} \times \text{conc. of std.}$$

Calculation of the LDL-cholesterol

LDL-cholesterol = Total chol.-chol. in the supernatant.

Using a Factor

Cholesterol concentration of the supernatant = A_{sample} x F

Factor (F) is given in Table below:

	mmol/L	*mg/dl*
Hg 546	49.63	1920
500 nm	32.70	1265

Calculation the LDL-Cholesterol

LDL—Cholesterol = total cholesterol— cholesterol in the supernatant

Clinical Interpretation

	mg/dl	*mmol/L*
No treatment required	<150	3.9
Suspect range	150-190	3.9-4.9
Treatment required	>190	>4.9

Note

Low-density lipoproteins and the very rare atherogenic Lp(a) are precipitated qualitatively. There is a slight coprecipitation of the VLDL but as the cholesterol content of these is low, the LDL cholesterol values are not increased significantly and the estimation of cardiovascular risk is not affected.

Test Significance

This test is specifically done to determine the risk of coronary heart disease. The low-density lipoproteins are closely correlated with an increased incidence of atherosclerosis and coronary heart disease. One on the other hand, a decreased incidence of coronary heart disease is seen in persons with high levels of HDL.

The VLDL cholesterol concentration is expressed as percent of total cholesterol.

SERUM TRIGLYCERIDES

Normal Values

		SI Units
Adult females		
Age 20-29	10-100 mg/dl	0.11-1.13 mmol/L
Age 30-39	10-110 mg/dl	0.11-1.24 mmol/L
Age 40-49	10-122 mg/dl	0.11-1.38 mmol/L
Age 50-59	10-134 mg/dl	0.11-1.51 mmol/L
Age >59	10-147 mg/dl	0.11-1.66 mmol/L
Adult males		
Age 20-29	10-157 mg/dl	0.11-1.77 mmol/L
Age 30-39	10-182 mg/dl	0.11-2.05 mmol/L
Age 40-49	10-193 mg/dl	0.11-2.18 mmol/L
Age 50-59	10-197 mg/dl	0.11-2.22 mmol/L
Age >59	10-199 mg/dl	0.11-2.24 mmol/L
Children		
Female, age 1-19	10-121 mg/dl	0.11-1.36 mmol/L
Male, age 1-19	10-103 mg/dl	0.11-1.16 mmol/L

Note: Plasma values are lower by about 3%.

Classification of Triglyceride Levels

Borderline high	200-400 mg/dl	2.3 mmol/L
High	400-1000 mg/dl	4.5-11.3 mmol/L
Very high	>1000 mg/dl	>11.3 mmol/L

TRIGLYCERIDES (GPO/PAP method) Courtesy: Tulip Group of Companies

For the determination of Triglycerides in serum or plasma. (for in vitro diagnostic use only).

Summary

Triglycerides are a form of fatty acid esters. They are produced in the liver by binding glycerol and other fatty acids. They are transported by VLDL and LDL and act as a storage source for energy. Increased levels are found in hyperlipidemias, diabetes, nephrotic syndrome, hypothyroidism. Increased levels are risk factor for arteriosclerotic coronary disease and peripheral vascular disease. Decreased levels are found in malnutrition and hyperthyroidism.

Principle

Lipoprotein lipase hydrolyses triglycerides to glycerol and free fatty acids. The glycerol formed with ATP in the presence of glycerol kinase forms glycerol 3 phosphate which is oxidised by the enzyme glycerol phosphate oxidase to form hydrogen peroxide. The hydrogen peroxide further reacts with phenolic compound and 4-aminoantipyrine by the catalytic action of peroxidase to form a red coloured quinoneimine dye complex. Intensity of the colour formed is directly proportional to the amount of triglycerides present in the sample.

$$\text{Triglycerides} \xrightarrow{\textit{Lipoprotein Lipase}} \text{Glycerol} + \text{Free fatty acids}$$

$$\text{Glycerol} + \text{ATP} \xrightarrow{\textit{Glycerol Kinase}} \text{Glycerol 3 Phosphate} + \text{ADP}$$

$$\text{Glycerol 3 Phosphate} + O_2 \xrightarrow{\textit{Glycerol 3 PO}} \text{Dihydroxyacetone phos} + H_2O_2$$

$$H_2O_2 + \text{4 Aminoantipyrine} + \text{Phenol} \xrightarrow{\textit{Peroxidase}} \text{Red Quinoneimine dye} + H_2O$$

Normal reference values

Serum/Plasma	(Suspicious)	: 150 mg/dl and above
	(Elevated)	: 200 mg/dl and above

It is recommended that each laboratory establish its own normal range representing its patient population.

Contents	25 ml	2 × 75 ml
L1: Enzyme Reagent 1	20 ml	2 × 60 ml
L2: Enzyme Reagent 2	5 ml	2 × 15 ml
S: Triglycerides Standard (200 mg/dl)	5 ml	5 ml

Storage/stability

Contents are stable at 2-8°C till the expiry mentioned on the labels.

Reagent Preparation

Reagents are ready to use.

Working reagent: Pour the contents of 1 bottle of L2 (Enzyme Reagent 2) into 1 bottle of L1 (Enzyme Reagent 1). This working reagent is stable for at least 8 weeks when stored at 2-8°C. Upon storage the working reagent may develop a slight pink colour however, this does not affect the performance of the reagent. Alternatively for flexibility as much of working reagent may be made as and when desired by mixing together 4 parts of L1 (Enzyme Reagent 1) and 1 part of L2 (Enzyme Reagent 2). Alternatively 0.8 ml of L1 and 0.2 ml of L2 may also be used instead of 1 ml of the working reagent directly during the assay.

Sample Material

Serum, plasma. Triglycerides is reported to be stable in the sample for 5 days when stored at 2-8°C.

Procedure

Wavelength/filter : 505 nm (Hg 546 nm)/Green
Temperature : 37°C/RT
Light path : 1 cm

Pipette into clean dry test tubes labeled as Blank (B), Standard (S), and Test (T):

Addition Sequence	B (ml)	S (ml)	T (ml)
Working reagent	1.0	1.0	1.0
Distilled water	0.01		
Triglycerides Standard (S	-	0.01	
Sample	-	-	0.01

Mix well and incubate at 37°C for 5 min. or at RT (25°C) for 15 min. Measure the absorbance of the Standard (Abs. S), and Test Sample (Abs. T) against the blank, within 60 Min.

Calculations

$$\text{Triglycerides in mg/dl} = \frac{\text{Abs T}}{\text{Abs S}} \times 200$$

Linearity

This procedure is linear upto 1000 mg/dl. If values exceed this limit, dilute the serum with normal saline (NaCI 0.9%) and repeat the assay.

Note

Fasting samples of 12 to 14 hrs. are preferred. Fatty meals and alcohol may cause elevated results. Patient should not drink alcohol for 24 hrs. before the test.

System Parameters			
Reaction	: End point	**Interval**	: —
Wavelength	: 505 nm	**Sample vol**	: 0.01 ml
Zero Setting	: Reagent blank	**Reagent vol**	: 1.00 ml
Incub temp	: 37°C/RT	**Standard**	: 200 mg/dl
Incub time	: 5 mm/15 min	**Factor**	:
Delay time	: —	**React slope**	: Increasing
Read time	: —	**Linearity**	: 1000 mg/dl
No of read	: —	**Units**	mg/dl

CLINICAL IMPLICATIONS

1. *Increased triglyceride levels* are believed to be a factor in increased risk for atherosclerosis
   A. Increased levels occur in
      1. Types I, IIb, III, IV, and V hyperlipoproteinemias
      2. Liver disease
      3. Nephrotic syndrome
      4. Hypothyroidism
      5. Poorly controlled diabetes
      6. Pancreatitis
      7. Glycogen storage disease
      8. Myocardial infarction (increases may last one year)
      9. Metabolic disorders related to endocrinopathies.
   B. Many of the clinical conditions that cause an increase in cholesterol levels also cause increase in triglycerides
      1. Nephrotic syndrome
      2. Pancreatic dysfunction
      3. Toxemia
      4. Hypothyroidism
2. *Decreased levels* occur in malnutrition and congenital alpha-beta lipoproteinemia.

BLOOD GLUCOSE

GLUCOSE (GOD/POD method)
Courtesy: Tulip Group of Companies

For the determination of Glucose in serum, plasma, and CSF. (for in vitro diagnostic use only)

Summary

Glucose is the major carbohydrate present in blood. Its oxidation in the cells is the source of energy for the body. Increased levels of glucose are found in diabetes mellitus, hyperparathryroidism, pancreatitis, renal failure. Decreased levels are found in Insulinoma, hypothyroidism, hypopituitarism and extensive liver disease.

Principle

Glucose is oxidised to gluconic acid and hydrogen peroxide in the presence of glucoseoxidase. Hydrogen peroxide further reacts with phenol and 4- aminoantipyrine by the catalytic action of peroxidase to form a red coloured quinoneimine dye complex.

Intensity of the colour formed is directly proportional to the amount of glucose present in the sample.

$$\text{Glucose} + O_2 + H_2O \xrightarrow{\text{Glucose Oxidase}} \text{Gluconate} + H_2O_2$$

$$H_2O_2 + 4\ \text{Aminoantipyrine} + \text{Phenol} \xrightarrow{\text{Peroxidase}} \text{Red Quinoneimine dye} + H_2O$$

Normal reference values

Serum/Plasma (Fasting) : 70-110 mg/dl
(2 hrs. PP) : upto 150 mg/dl
CSF : 50-80 mg/dl

It is recommended that each laboratory establish its own normal range representing its patient population.

Contents	2 × 150 ml	1000 ml
L1: Glucose Reagent	2 × 150 ml	1000 ml
S: Glucose Standard (100 mg/dl)	5 ml	5 ml

Storage/stability

Contents are stable at 2-8°C till the expiry mentioned on the labels. Upon storage the Glucose reagent may develop a slight pink colour. This does not affect the performance of the test.

Reagent Preparation

Reagents are ready to use.

Sample material

Serum, plasma, CSF. Glucose is reported to be stable in the sample for 7 days when stored at 2-8°C.

Procedure

Wavelength/filter : 505 nm (Hg 546 nm)/Green
Temperature : 37°C/RT
Light path : 1 cm

Pipette into clean dry test tubes labelled as Blank (B), Standard (S), and Test (T):

Addition Sequence	B (ml)	S (ml)	T (ml)
Glucose Reagent (L1)	1.0	1.0	1.0
Distilled water	0.01		
Glucose Standard (S)	-	0.01	
Sample	-	-	0.01

Mix well and incubate at 37°C for 10 min. or at RT (25°C) for 30 min. Measure the absorbance of the Standard (Abs S), and Test Sample (Abs T) against the Blank, within 60 Min.

Calculations

$$\text{Total Glucose in mg/dl} = \frac{\text{Abs T}}{\text{Abs S}} \times 100$$

Linearity

This procedure is linear upto 500 mg/dl. If values exceed this limit, dilute the serum with normal saline (NaCI 0.9%) and repeat the assay. Calculate the value using the proper dilution factor.

Note

To avoid glycolysis the serum should be separated from the clot as soon as possible, and plasma should be collected in an EDTA + fluoride bulb (0.5 mg + 1 mg per ml of blood).

System Parameters			
Reaction	: End point	Interval	:
Wavelength	: 505 nm	Sample vol	: 0.01 ml
Zero Setting	: Reagent blank	Reagent vol	: 1.00 ml
Incub temp	: 37°C/RT	Standard	: 100 mg/dl
Incub time	: 10 min./ 30 min.	Factor	:
Delay time	: —	React slope	: Increasing
Read time	: —	Linearity	: 500 mg/dl
No. of read	: —	Units	: mg/dl

BODY FLUID, GLUCOSE, SPECIMEN

Normal Values

		SI Units
Cerebrospinal fluid Lags behind blood glucose levels by 2-4 hours. Fasting to 4 hours postpradially 50-80% of serum glucose.		
Adult	40-80 mg/dl	2.2-4.4 mmol/L
Premature infant	24-63 mg/dl	1.3-3.5 mmol/L
Full-term infant	34-119 mg/dl	1.9-6.6 mmol/L
Child	35-75 mg/dl	1.9-4.1 mmol/L
Peritoneal fluid	70-100 mg/dl	3.8-5.5 mmol/L
Pleural fluid	Same as blood glucose level, with a time lag of 2-4 hours or no less than 40 mg/dl (2.2 mmol/L) below blood glucose	
Fasting blood	60-110 mg/dl	3.3-6.1 mmol/L
Synovial fluid	No more than 10 mg/dl (0.6 mmol/L SI units) lower than good glucose level.	

CAUSES OF ABNORMAL GLUCOSE LEVELS

Persistent Hyperglycemia

- Diabetes mellitus
- Adrenal cortical hyperactivity (Cushing's syndrome)
- Acromegaly
- Obesity

Transient Hyperglycemia

- Pheochromocytoma
- Severe liver disease
- Acute stress reaction (physical or emotional)
- Shock
- Convulsions

Persistent Hypoglycemia

- Insulinoma
- Adrenal cortical insufficiency
- Hypopituitarism
- Galactosemia
- Ectopic insulin production from tumors

Transient Hypoglycemia

- Acute alcohol ingestion
- Drugs: Salicylates, anti-tuberculosis agents
- Severe liver disease
- Several glycogen storage diseases
- "Functional" hypoglycemia
- Hereditary fructose intolerance.

URIC ACID

URIC ACID (Uricase/PAP method)
Courtesy: Tulip Group of Companies

For the determination of Uric Acid in serum or plasma. (for *in vitro* diagnostic use only)

Summary

Uric acid is the end product of purine metabolism. Uric acid is excreted to a large degree by the kidneys and to a smaller degree in the intestinal tract by microbial degradation. Increased levels are found in Gout, arthritis, impaired renal functions and starvation. Decreased levels are found in Wilson's disease, Fanconis syndrome and yellow atrophy of the liver.

Principle

Uricase converts uric acid to allantoin and hydrogen peroxide. The hydrogen peroxide formed further reacts with a phenolic compound and 4 aminoantipyrine by the catalytic action of peroxidase to form a red coloured quinoneimine dye complex. Intensity of the colour formed is directly proportional to the amount of uric acid present in the sample.

$$\text{Uric acid} + H_2O \xrightarrow{\text{Uricase}} \text{Allantoin} + H_2O_2$$

$$H_2O_2 + 4\ \text{Aminoantipyrine} + \text{Phenolic Compound} \xrightarrow{\text{Peroxidase}} \text{Red Quinoneimine dye} + H_2O$$

Normal reference values

Serum/Plasma (Males) : 3.4 - 7.0 mg/dl
(Females) : 2.5 - 6.0 mg/dl

It is recommended that each laboratory establish its own normal range representing its patient population.

Contents	25 ml	75 ml
L1: Buffer Reagent	20 ml	60 ml
L2: Enzyme Reagent	5 ml	15 ml
S: Uric Acid Standard (8 mg/dl)	5 ml	5 ml

Storage/stability

Contents are stable at 2-8°C till the expiry mentioned on the labels.

Reagent Preparation

Reagents are ready to use.

Working reagent: Pour the contents of 1 bottle of L2 (Enzyme Reagent) into 1 bottle of L1 (Buffer Reagent). This working reagent is stable for at least 4 weeks when stored at 2-8°C. Upon storage the working reagent may develop a slight pink colour however, this does not affect the performance of the reagent. Alternatively for flexibility as much of working reagent may be made as and when desired by mixing together 4 parts of L1 (Enzyme Reagent 1) and 1 part of L2 (Enzyme Reagent 2). Alternatively 0.8 ml of L1 and 0.2 ml of L2 may also be used instead of 1 ml of the working reagent directly during the assay.

Sample Material

Serum, plasma. Uric Acid is reported to be stable in the sample for 3 to 5 days when stored at 2-8°C.

Procedure

Wavelength/filter : 520 nm (Hg 546 nm) / yellow Green
Temperature : 37°C/RT
Light path : 1 cm

Pipette into clean dry test tubes labeled as Blank (B), Standard (S), and Test (T) :

Addition Sequence	B (ml)	S (ml)	T (ml)
Working reagent	1.0	1.0	1.0
Distilled water	0.02		
Uric Acid Standard (S)	-	0.02	-
Sample	-	-	0.02

Mix well and incubate at 37°C for 5 min. or at RT (25°C) for 15 min. Measure the absorbance of the Standard (Abs S), and Test Sample (Abs T) against the Blank, within 30 Min.

Calculations

$$\text{Uric Acid in mg/dl} = \frac{\text{Abs T}}{\text{Abs S}} \times 8$$

Linearity

This procedure is linear upto 20 mg/dl. If values exceed this limit, dilute the serum with normal saline (NaCl 0.9%) and repeat the assay. Calculate the value using the proper dilution factor.

System Parameters			
Reaction	: End point	**Interval**	:
Wavelength	: 520 nm	**Sample vol**	: 0.02 ml
Zero Setting	: Reagent blank	**Reagent vol**	: 1.00 ml
Incub temp	: 37°C / RT	**Standard**	: 8 mg/dl
Incub time	: 5 min./15 min.	**Factor**	:
Delay time	: —	**React slope**	: Increasing
Read time	: —	**Linearity**	: 20 mg/dl
No of read	: —	**Units**	: mg/dl

Normal Values

		SI Units
Adult females	2.5-6.0 mg/dl	143-357 µmol/L
Adult males	3.4-7.0 mg/dl	202-416 µmol/L
Children	2.5-5.5 mg/dl	119-327 µmol/L
Panic level	>12 mg/dl	>714 µmol/L

CLINICAL RELEVANCE

Factors Affecting Serum Uric Acid levels

Increased Production, Raised Serum Levels

- Idiopathic mechanisms associated with primary gout.
- Excessive dietary purines (organ meats, legumes, anchovies, etc.)
- Cytolytic treatment of malignancies, especially leukemias and lymphomas
- Polycythemia
- Myeloid metaplasia
- Psoriasis
- Sickle cell anaemia.

Decreased Excretion, Raised Serum Levels

- Alcohol ingestion
- Thiazide diuretics
- Lactic acidosis
- Aspirin doses < 2 gm/day
- Ketoacidosis especially diabetes or starvation.
- Renal failure due to any cause.

Increased Excretion, Lowered Serum Levels

- Probenecid, sulphinpyrazone, aspirin doses above 4 gm/day
- Corticosteroids and ACTH
- Coumarin anticoagulants.
- Estrogens.

Decreased Production, Lowered Serum Levels

- Allopurinol

CALCIUM

CALCIUM (OCPC method) Courtesy: Tulip Group of Companies

For the determination of Calcium in serum or plasma. (for in vitro diagnostic use only)

Summary

Calcium, in the body, is found mainly in the bones (approximately 99%). In serum calcium exists equally in a free ionised form and in a bound form (with albumin). Hence a decrease in Albumin causes lower Calcium levels and vice versa. The levels of Calcium in serum depend on the parathyroid hormone. Increased Calcium levels are found in bone tumours, hyperparathyroidism. Decreased levels are found in hypoparathyroidism, renal failure, rickets, Vitamin D deficiency and pancreatitis.

Principle

Calcium in an alkaline medium combines with o-Cresolphthalein Complexone to form a purple coloured complex. Intensity of the colour formed is directly proportional to the amount of calcium present in the sample.

Calcium + OCPC ⟶ Purple coloured complex

Normal reference values

Serum/Plasma : 8.7 - 11.0 mg/dl (general)

It is recommended that each laboratory establish its own normal range representing its patient population.

Contents	2 × 35 ml	2 × 75 ml
L1: Buffer Reagent	35 ml	75 ml
L2: Colour Reagent	35 ml	75 ml
S: Calcium Standard (10 mg/dl)	5 ml	5 ml

Storage/stability

Contents are stable at 2-8°C till the expiry mentioned on the labels.

Reagent Preparation

Reagents are ready to use. Protect from bright light.

Working Reagent: For convenience a single working reagent may be prepared by mixing equal parts of the Buffer Reagent and Colour Reagent. This combined reagent is stable for 7 days at 2-8°C.

Sample material

Serum/Heparinized plasma. Calcium is reported to be stable in serum for 7 days at 2-8°C.

Procedure

Wavelength/filter : 570 nm (Hg 578 nm)/yellow
Temperature : RT
Light path : 1 cm

Pipette into clean dry test tubes labelled as Blank (B), Standard (S), and Test (T):

Addition Sequence	B (ml)	S (ml)	T (ml)
Buffer Reagent (L1)	0.5	0.5	0.5
Colour Reagent (L2)	0.5	0.5	0.5
Distilled water	0.02	-	-
Calcium Standard (S)	-	0.02	-
Sample	-	-	0.02

Mix well and incubate at RT (25°C) for 5 min. Measure the absorbance of the Standard (Abs S), and Test Sample (Abs T) against the Blank, within 60 Min.

Calculations

$$\text{Calcium in mg/dl} = \frac{\text{Abs T}}{\text{Abs S}} \times 10$$

Linearity

This procedure is linear upto 18 mg/dl. If values exceed this limit, dilute the sample with distilled water and repeat the assay. Calculate the value using the proper dilution

Note

As calcium is a very widely distributed ion, care should be taken to avoid any contamination. All glassware being used for the test should first be rinsed with 1% or 0.1 N HCI and then with good quality deionised water before use.

It is suggested that after the rinsing of the tubes with HCI the reagent be pipetted in their respective tubes and the tubes be rinsed with the reagent. The reagent then should be pooled together in the 'blank' tube and repipetted out into the 'standard' and 'test' test tubes. This will ensure that any remaining contamination will be carried over equally in all the tubes. For flow cell cuvettes it is suggested that some reagent be aspirated before the blank to take away any contamination in the flow through tubing or cuvette which may cause a higher than the actual blank of the reagent.

Chelating agents such as EDTA, present even in traces, prevent the formation of the colour complex, hence necessary care should be taken during the assay.

System Parameters			
Reaction	: End point	**Interval**	:
-Wavelength	: 570 nm	**Sample vol**	: 0.02 ml
Zero Setting	: Reagent blank	**Reagent vol**	: 1.00 ml
Incub temp	: RT	**Standard**	: 10 mg/dl
Incub time	: 5 min	**Factor**	:
Delay time	: —	**React slope**	: Increasing
Read time	: —	**Linearity**	: 18 mg/dl
No of read	: —	**Units**	: mg/dl

CALCIUM (Arsenazo III method)
Courtesy: Tulip Group of Companies

For the determination of Calcium in serum or plasma. (for in vitro diagnostic use only).

Summary

Calcium, in the body, is found mainly in the bones (approximately 99%). In serum calcium exists equally in a free ionised form and in a bound form (with albumin). Hence a decrease in Albumin causes lower Calcium levels and vice versa. The levels of Calcium in serum depend on the parathyroid hormone. Increased Calcium levels are found in bone tumours, hyperparathyroidism. Decreased levels are found in hypoparathyroidism, renal failure, rickets, Vitamin D deficiency and pancreatitis.

Principle

Calcium combines specifically with Arsenazo III at a neutral pH to form a blue purple coloured complex. Intensity of the colour formed is directly proportional to the amount of calcium present in the sample.

Calcium + Arsenazo III ⟶ Blue Purple coloured complex

Normal reference values

Serum/Plasma : 8.7 - 11.0 mg/dl

It is recommended that each laboratory establish its own normal range representing its patient population.

Contents	75 ml	3 × 75 ml
L1: Calcium Reagent	75 ml	3 × 75 ml
S: Calcium Standard (10 mg/dl)	5 ml	5 ml

Storage/stability

Contents are stable at 2-8°C till the expiry mentioned on the labels.

Reagent Preparation

Reagents are ready to use. Protect from bright light.

Sample material

Serum/heparinized plasma. Calcium is reported to be stable in serum for 7 days at 2-8°C.

Procedure

Wavelength/filter : 650 nm (Hg 623 nm)/Red
Temperature : RT
Light path : 1 cm

Pipette into clean dry test tubes labelled as Blank (B), Standard (S), and Test (T):

Addition Sequence	B (ml)	S (ml)	T (ml)
Calcium Reagent (L1)	1.0	1.0	1.0
Distilled water	0.01		
Calcium Standard (S)	-	0.01	
Sample	-	-	0.01

Mix well and incubate at RT (25°C) for 5 min. Measure the absorbance of the Standard (Abs S), and Test Sample (Abs T) against the Blank, within 60 Min.

Calculations

$$\text{Calcium in mg/dl} = \frac{\text{Abs T}}{\text{Abs S}} \times 10$$

Linearity

This procedure is linear upto 15 mg/dl. If values exceed this limit, dilute the sample with distilled water and repeat the assay. Calculate the value using the proper dilution factor.

Note

As calcium is a very widely distributed ion, care should be taken to avoid any contamination. All glassware being used for the test should first be rinsed with 1% or 0.1 N HCI and then with good quality deionised water before use.

It is suggested that after the rinsing of the tubes with HCI the reagent be pipetted in their respective tubes and the tubes be rinsed with the reagent. The reagent then should be pooled together in the 'blank' tube and repipetted out into the 'standard' and 'test' test tubes. This will ensure that any remaining contamination will be carried over equally in all the tubes. For flow cell cuvettes it is suggested that some reagent be aspirated before the blank to take away any contamination in the flow through tubing or cuvette which may cause a higer than the actual blank of the reagent.

Chelating agents such as EDTA, present even in traces, prevent the formation of the colour complex, hence necessary care should be taken during the assay.

System Parameters			
Reaction	: End point	**Interval**	:
Wavelength	: 650 nm	**Sample vol**	: 0.01 ml
Zero Setting	: Reagent blank	**Reagent vol**	: 1.00 ml
Incub temp	: RT	**Standard**	: 10 mg/dl
Incub time	: 5 min	**Factor**	:
Delay time	: —	**React slope**	: Increasing
Read time	: —	**Linearity**	: 15 mg/dl
No of read	: —	**Units**	: mg/dl

NORMAL VALUES

Adults		
18-60 years	8.6-10.0 mg/dl	2.15-2.50 mmol/L
60-90 years	8.8-10.2 mg/dl	2.20-2.55 mmol/L
>90 years	8.2-9.6 mg/dl	2.05-2.40 mmol/L
Children		
Cord blood	8.2-11.2 mg/dl	2.05-2.80 mmol/L
Premature infant	6.2-11.0 mg/dl	1.55-2.75 mmol/L
<10 days	7.6-10.4 mg/dl	1.90-2.60 mmol/L
10 days-2 years	9.0-11.0 mg/dl	2.25-2.75 mmol/L
2-12 years	8.8-10.8 mg/dl	2.20-2.70 mmol/L
12-18 years	8.4-10.2 mg/dl	2.10-2.55 mmol/L
Panic levels		
Tetany	<7 mg/dl	<1.75 mmol/L
Coma	>12 mg/dl	>2.99 mmol/L
Possible death	<6 mg/dl	<1.50 mmol/L

Specimen Collection and Storage

1. Fresh, unhemolysed serum is the preferred specimen.
2. Heparinised plasma may also be used.
3. Anticoagulants other than heparin should not be used.
4. Remove serum from clot as soon as possible since red cells can absorb calcium.
5. Older serum specimens containing visible precipitate should not be used.
6. Serum calcium is stable for 24 hours at room temperature, one week at 2-8°C, and up to five months frozen (-15 to -25°C.)and protected from evaporation. Specimens should not be thawed and refrozen.

CLINICAL RELEVANCE

Normal levels of total calcium combined with other findings

1. Normal calcium levels with overall normal findings in other tests indicate that there are no problems with calcium metabolism.
2. Normal calcium and abnormal phosphorus indicate impaired calcium absorption due to alteration of parathyroid hormone activity or secretion. In rickets, the calcium level may be normal or slightly lowered and the phosphorus level is depressed.
3. Normal calcium and elevated BUN indicates
   a. Possible secondary hyperparathyroidism. Initially lowered serum calcium results from uremia and acidosis. The lower calcium level stimulates the parathyroid to release parathyroid hormone, which acts on bone to release more calcium.
   b. Possible primary hyperparathyroidism. Excessive amounts of parathormone cause elevation in calcium levels, but secondary kidney disease would cause retention of phosphate and concomitant lower calcium.
4. Normal calcium and decreased serum albumin. This is indicative of hypercalcemia, since there should be a decrease in calcium when there is a decrease in albumin because of the 50% of serum calcium that is protein-bound.

Hypercalcemia (increased total calcium). Hypercalcemia is associated with many disorders, but its greatest clinical importance rests in its association with cancer, including multiple myeloma, parathyroid tumours, nonendocrine tumours producing a parathormone-like substance, and cancers metastasizing to the bone. Increased calcium levels are caused by or associated with.

1. Hyperparathyroidism due to
   a. Parathyroid adenoma associated with hypophosphatemia
   b. Hyperplasia of parathyroid glands associated with hypophosphatemia
2. Cancer
   a. Metastatic cancers involving bone cancers of lung, breast, thyroid, kidney, and testes may metastasize to bone
   b. Hodgkin's disease other lymphomas
   c. Multiple myeloma in which there is extensive bone destruction

   d. Lung and renal cancers may produce parathormone resulting in symptoms of hypercalcemia
   e. Sarcoidosis due to increased IgG or IgA
   f. Leukemia
3. Addison's disease
4. Hyperthyroidism
5. Paget's disease of bone (also accompanied by high levels of alkaline phosphatase)
6. Prolonged immobilisation
7. Bone fractures combined with bed rest
8. Excessive intake of vitamin D
9. Prolonged use of diuretics, thiazides
10. Respiratory alkalosis
11. Milk alkali syndrome (history of peptic ulcer could indicate excessive intake of milk and antacids)

Hypocalcemia (decreased total calcium levels) Commonly caused by/associated with

1. Pseudohypocalcemia (hyperproteinemia). Actually, what looks like hypocalcemia is really a reflection of diminished albumin (as revealed by a serum protein electrophoresis). It is the reduced protein that is responsible for the low calcium, since 50% of the calcium total is protein-bound. (Excessive use of IV fluids will decrease albumin levels and thus, decrease the amount of calcium).
2. Hypoparathyrodism (primary is very rare) may be due to accidental removal of parathyroid glands during a thyroidectomy, irradiation, hypomagnesemia, GI disorders, renal wasting.
3. Hyperphosphatemia
   Due to renal failure, laxatives, cytotoxic drugs
4. Malabsorption
   Due to sprue, celiac disease, pancreatic dysfunction (fatty acids combine with calcium and are precipitated and excreted in the faeces).
5. Acute pancreatitis
6. Alkalosis (calcium ions become bound to protein)
7. Osteomalacia
8. Diarrhea
9. Rickets

Increased ionised calcium

1. Primary hyperparathyroidism
2. Ectopic parathyroid hormone producing tumours
3. Excess intake of vitamin D
4. Various malignancies

Decreased ionised calcium

Primary hypoparathyroidism is associated with low ionised calcium level and low total calcium level

Be Careful

1. Thiazide diuretics may lead to impairment of urinary calcium excretions and consequent hypercalcemia.
2. Patients with renal insufficiency who are undergoing dialysis, a calcium-ion exchange resin is sometimes used for hyperkalemia. The use of this resin may lead to increased calcium levels.
3. Increased intake of magnesium and phosphates and the excessive use of laxatives may lower the blood calcium level. This occurs because of the increased intestinal loss of calcium produced by these elements.
4. When decreased calcium levels are due to magnesium deficiency, as in poor absorption from the bowel, the administration of magnesium will correct the calcium deficiency.
5. If a patient is known to have or suspected of having a pH abnormality, a concurrent pH should be requested with ionised calcium.

Interfering Factors

See Appendix II for the list of drugs that may alter blood calcium level.

PHOSPHORUS

PHOSPHORUS (Molybdate UV method)
Courtesy: Tulip Group of Companies

For the determination of Inorganic Phosphorus in serum, plasma and urine. (for in vitro diagnostic use only)

Summary

Phosphorus is mainly combined with calcium and is found in the bones. Approximately 15% exists as inorganic phosphorus or phosphate esters. It is involved in the carbohydrate metabolism and is a component of many other substances. Increased levels are found in hypoparathyroidism, renal failure, bone metastatis and liver diseases. Decreased levels are found in hyperparathyroidism, rickets and Vitamin D deficiency.

Principle

Phosphate ions in an acidic medium react with ammonium molybdate to form a phosphomolybdate complex. This complex has an absorbance in the ultraviolet range and is measured at 340 nm. Intensity of the complex formed is directly proportional to the amount of inorganic phosphorus present in the sample.

Phosphorus + Ammonium Molybdate ⟶ Phosphomolybdate complex

Normal reference values

Serum	(Adults)	: 2.5 - 5.0 mg/dl
	(Children)	: 4.0 - 6.5 mg/dl
Urine		: 0.3-1.0 g/24 hours

It is recommended that each laboratory establish its own normal range representing its patient population.

Contents	75 ml	2 × 75 ml
L1: Acid Reagent	60 ml	2 × 60 ml
L2: Molybdate Reagent	15 ml	2 × 15 ml
S: Phosphorus Standard (5mg/dl)	5 ml	5 ml

Storage/stability

Reagents are stable at RT (25-30°C) till the expiry mentioned on the labels

Reagent Preparation

Reagents are ready to use.

Working reagent: Pour the contents of 1 bottle of L2 (molybdate reagent) into 1 bottle of L1 (Acid Reagent). This working reagent is stable for at least 6 months when stored at 2-8°C. Upon storage the working reagent may develop a slight blue colour, however this does not affect the performance of the reagent.

Alternatively for flexibility as much of working reagent may be made as and when desired by mixing together 4 parts of L1 (acid reagent) and 1 part of L2 (molybdate reagent 2). Alternatively 0.8 ml of L1 and 0.2 ml of L2 may also be used instead of 1 ml of the working reagent directly during the assay.

Sample Material

Serum heparinized/EDTA Plasma or urine. Acidify the urine with a few drops of conc. Hydrochloric acid and dilute 1+19 before the assay, (results × 20).

Inorganic phosphorus is reported to be stable in serum for 7 days at 2-8°C.

Procedure

Wavelength/filter	: 340 nm (Hg 365 nm)
Temperature	: RT
Light path	: 1 cm

Pipette into clean dry test tubes labeled as Blank (B), Standard (S), and Test (T):

Addition Sequence	B (ml)	S (ml)	T (ml)
Working reagent	1.0	1.0	1.0
Distilled water	0.01		
Phosphorus Standard (S)	-	0.01	
Sample	-	-	0.01

Mix well and incubate at RT for 5 min. Measure the absorbance of the Standard (Abs S), and Test Sample (Abs T) against the Blank, within 60 Min.

Calculations

$$\text{Phosphorus in mg/dl} = \frac{\text{Abs T}}{\text{Abs S}} \times 5$$

Linearity

This procedure is linear upto 20 mg/dl. If values exceed this limit, dilute the sample with distilled water and repeat the assay. Calculate the value using the proper dilution factor.

Note

Hemolysis interferes with the test.

Use clean glassware washed with N/10 HCI as detergents may contain phosphate ions.

System Parameters			
Reaction	: UV End point	**Interval**	:
Wavelength	: 340 nm	**Sample vol**	: 0.01 ml
Zero Setting	: Reagent blank	**Reagent vol**	: 1.00 ml
Incub temp	: RT	**Standard**	: 5 mg/dl
Incub time	: 5 min	**Factor**	:
Delay time	: —	**React slope**	: Increasing
Read time	: —	**Linearity**	: 20 mg/dl
No of read	: —	**Units**	: mg/dl

PHOSPHORUS (Mod Gomorri's method)
Courtesy: Tulip Group of Companies

For the determination of Inorganic Phosphorus in serum, plasma and urine. (for in vitro diagnostic use only)

Summary

Phosphorus is mainly combined with calcium and is found in the bones. Approximately 15% exists as inorganic phosphorus or phosphate esters. It is involved in the carbohydrate metabolism and is a component of many other substances. Increased levels are found in hypoparathyroidism, renal failure, bone metastasis and liver diseases. Decreased levels are found in hyperparathyroidism, rickets and Vitamin D deficiency.

Principle

Phosphate ions in an acidic medium react with ammonium molybdate to form a phosphomolybdate complex. This complex reacts with Metol and is reduced to a molybdinum blue complex. Intensity of the molybdinum blue complex formed is directly proportional to the amount of inorganic phosphorus present in the sample.

Phosphorus + Ammonium Molybdate→Phosphomolybdate complex

Phosphomolybdate complex + Metol→MolybdinumBlue Complex

Normal reference values

Serum (Adults) : 2.5 - 5.0 mg/dl
(Children): 4.0 - 6.5 mg/dl

Urine : 0.3- 1.0g/24 hours

It is recommended that each laboratory establish its own normal range representing its patient population.

Contents	10 Tests	25 Tests
L1: Acid Reagent	30 ml	75 ml
L2: Molybdate Reagent	30 ml	75 ml
L3: Colour Reagent	30 ml	75 ml
S: Phosphorus Standard (5 mg/dl)	5 ml	5 ml

Storage/stability

Reagents are stable at RT (25-30°C) till the expiry mentioned on the labels.

Reagent Preparation

Reagents are ready to use.

Sample material

Serum, heparinized/EDTA Plasma or urine. Acidify the urine with a few drops of cone. Hydrochloric acid and dilute 1+19 before the assay, (results x 20). Inorganic phosphorus is reported to be stable in serum for 7 days at 2-8°C.

Procedure

Wavelength/filter : 650 nm (Hg 623 nm)/Red
Temperature : RT
Light path : 1 cm

Pipette into clean dry test tubes labeled as Blank (B), Standard (S), and Test (T):

Addition Sequence	B (ml)	S (ml)	T (ml)
Acid Reagent	1.0	1.0	1.0
Molybdate Reagent	1.0	1.0	1.0
Distilled water	0.1		
Phosphorus Standard (S)	-	0.1	
Sample	-	-	0.1
Colour Reagent	1.0	1.0	1.0

Mix well and incubate at RT for 5 min. Measure the absorbance of the Standard (Abs S), and Test Sample (Abs T) against the Blank, within 30 Min.

Calculations

$$\text{Phosphorus in mg/dl} = \frac{\text{Abs T}}{\text{Abs S}} \times \text{L5}$$

Linearity

This procedure is linear upto 15 mg/dl. If values exceed this limit, dilute the sample with distilled water and repeat the assay. Multiply the value obtained with an appropriate dilution factor.

Notes

Hemolysis interferes with the test.

Use clean glassware washed with N/10 HCI as many detergents contain phosphate ions.

The addition sequence of the reagents and the sample is important and should not be changed.

System Parameters			
Reaction	: End point	**Interval**	:
Wavelength	: 650 nm	**Sample vol**	: 0.1 ml
Zero Setting	: Reagent blank	**Reagent vol**	: 3.00 ml
Incub temp	: RT	**Standard**	: 5 mg/dl
Incub time	: 5 min	**Factor**	:
Delay time	: —	**React slope**	: Increasing
Read time	: —	**Linearity**	: 15 mg/dl
No. of read	: —	**Units**	: mg/dl

NORMAL VALUES

		SI Units
Adults <age 60	2.7-4.5 mg/dl	0.87-1.45 mmol/L
Females >age 60	2.8-4.1 mg/dl	0.90-1.30 mmol/L
Males>age 60	2.3-3.7 mg/dl	0.74-1.20 mmol/L
Cord blood	3.7-8.1 mg/dl	1.20-2.62 mmol/L
Premature infant	5.4-10.9 mg/dl	1.74-3.52 mmol/L
Newborn	4.5-9 mg/dl	1.45-2.91 mmol/L
Infant (10 days-24 months)	4.5-6.7 mg/dl	1.45-2.16 mmol/L
Child (24 months-12 years)	4.5-5.5 mg/dl	1.45-1.78 mmol/L

CLINICAL RELEVANCE

Hyperphosphatemia (increased phosphorus levels)

The most common causes of elevated blood phosphate levels are found in association with kidney dysfunction and uremia. This is because phosphate is so closely regulated by the kidneys.

Increased phosphorus levels are associated with

a. Renal insufficiency and severe nephritis accompanied by elevated BUN and creatinine.
b. Hypoparathyroidism (accompanied by elevated phosphorus, decreased calcium, and normal renal function).
c. Hypocalcemia
d. Excessive intake of alkali (possible history of peptic ulcer)
e. Excessive intake of vitamin D
f. Fractures in the healing stage
g. Bone tumours
h. Addison's disease
i. Acromegaly

Hypophosphatemia (Decreased phosphorus levels)

Decreased phosphorus levels may be associated with

a. Hyperparathyroidism (accompanied by increased calcium, no renal disease)
b. Rickets (childhood), Osteomalacia (adults)
c. Diabetic coma because of increased carbohydrate metabolism
d. Hyperinsulinism
e. Continuous administration of intravenous glucose in a non-diabetic patient.

Interfering Factors

1. Normally high in children
2. Falsely increased by haemolysis of blood
3. Drugs causing possible elevation
   a. Diphenylhydantoin (phenytoin)
   b. Heparin
   c. Pituitrin
   d. Vitamin-D
   e. Methicillin
   f. Tetracyclines
   g. Alkaline antacids
   h. Lipomol
4. The use of laxatives or enemas containing large amounts of sodium phosphate will cause increased phosphorus levels.
5. Drugs causing possible decreases
   a. Aluminum hydroxide
   b. Epinephrine (adrenaline)
   c. Insulin
   d. Mannitol
   e. Mithramycin
   f. Parathyroid injection.

CHLORIDE

CHLORIDE (Thiocyanate Method)
Courtesy: Tulip Group of Companies

Chloride is a major extracellular anion and maintains the cation/anion balance between intra and extra cellular fluids, mostly as a salt with sodium. Increased levels are usually found in dehydration, kidney dysfunction, and anaemia. Decreased levels are found in extensive burns, vomiting, diarrhoea, intestinal obstructions, and salt losing nephritis.

Principle

Chloride ions combine with free mercurie ions and release thiocyanate from mercuric thiocyanate. The thiocyanate released combines with the ferric ions to form a red brown ferric thiocyanate complex. Intensity of the colour formed is directly proportional to the amount of chloride present in the sample.

$$2\,Cl^- + Hg\,(SCN)_2 \longrightarrow HgCl_2 + 2\,(SCN)^-$$

$$3\,(SCN) + Fe^{3+} \longrightarrow Fe(SCN)_3$$

Normal reference values

Serum/Plasma Chloride	: 96-106 mmol/l
Urine Chloride	: 170 - 250 mmol/24 hours
CSF Chloride	: 120 -135 mmol/l

It is recommended that each laboratory establish its own normal range representing its patient population.

Chloride Kit

L1 :Chloride reagent	75 ml
S : Chloride standard (100 mmol/1)	5 ml

Storage/stability

All reagents are stable at RT till the expiry mentioned.

Reagent Preparation

Reagents are ready to use.

For Chloride: Serum, plasma, urine, and CSF. Dilute urine samples 1+1 with distilled water before the assay. Chloride is reported to be stable in serum for 7 days at 2-8°C.

Procedure

Wavelength/filter	:505 nm (Hg 546/ Green)
Temperature	:RT
Light path	:1 cm

Chloride Assay

Pipette into clean dry test tubes labeled as Blank (B), Standard (S), and Test (T)

Addition Sequence	B (ml)	S (ml)	T (ml)
Chloride Reagent (L1)	1.0	1.0	1.0
Deionised water	0.01	–	–
Chloride Standard (S)	–	0.01	
Sample	–	–	0.01

Mix well and incubate at RT for 2 min. Measure the absorbance of the Standard (Abs S), and Test Sample (Abs T) against Blank, within 60 min.

Linearity

The Chloride assay is linear between 70-140 mmol/L. If values exceed this limit, dilute the sample with deionised water (free from $Na^+/K^+/Cl^-$ ions) and repeat the assay. Calculate the value using the proper dilution factor.

Notes

Bring all reagents to RT before use.

Turbid or icteric samples may produce falsely elevated results.

The procedure for chloride measures total halides such as bromides, iodides, and fluorides in addition to chlorides hence, their contamination should be avoided. Since the test is temperature sensitive so a constant temperature should be maintained during incubation and reading.

System Parameters, Cl^-			
Reaction	: End point	**Interval**	:
Wavelength	: 505 nm	**Sample vol**	: 0.01 ml
Zero Setting	: Reagent blank	**Reagent vol**	: 1.00 ml
Incub temp	: RT	**Standard**	: 100 mmol/1
Incub time	: 2 min	**Factor**	:
Delay time	: —	**React slope**	: Increasing
Read time	: —	**Linearity**	: 70-140 mmol/1
No. of read	: —	**Units**	: mmol/1

Calculation

$$\text{Chloride in mmol/L} = \frac{\text{Abs. T}}{\text{Abs. S}} \times 100$$

Normal Values

		SI Units
Children and adults	97-106 mEq/L	97-107 mmol/L
Premature infants	95-110 mEq/L	95-110 mmol/L
Full-term infants	96-106 mEq/L	96-106 mmol/L
Panic levels	<80 mEq/L	<80 mmol/L
	>115 mEq/L	>115 mmol/L

CLINICAL RELEVANCE

1. Whenever the serum level is much lower than 100 mEq/L, the urinary excretion of chloride falls to a very low level.
2. The reason why decreased chloride levels often occur in acute infections is not clear.
3. Chloride measurements are of limited value in renal diseases for the reason that plasma chloride can be maintained near normal limits even when a considerable degree of renal failure is present.
4. Increased chloride levels occur in
   a. Cushing's syndrome
   b. Dehydration
   c. Hyperventilation
   d. Eclampsia
   e. Anaemia

f. Cardiac decompensation
g. Some renal disorders.

5. Decreased chloride levels occur in
   a. Severe vomiting
   b. Severe diarrhoea
   c. Ulcerative colitis
   d. Pyloric obstruction
   e. Severe burns
   f. Heat exhaustion
   g. Diabetic acidosis
   h. Addison's disease
   i. Fever
   j. Acute infections such as pneumonia
   k. Use of drugs such as mercurial and chlorothiazide diuretics.

Interfering Factors

1. The plasma chloride concentration of infants is usually higher than that of children and adults.
2. Many drugs may cause a change in chloride levels. See appendix II for a detailed listing.

Be Careful

1. In intravenous therapy, if the solution contains 100 mEq/L, there is ample chloride present for the correction of urine metabolic acidosis.
2. If an electrolyte disorder is suspected, daily weight and accurate intake and output should be recorded.

SERUM IRON AND TIBC

IRON AND TIBC (Ferrozine method)
Courtesy: Tulip Group of Companies

For the determination of Iron and Total Iron Binding Capacity in serum. (Laboratory Reagent for Professional Use Only)

Summary

Iron found in blood is mainly present in the haemoglobin of the RBCs. It's role in the body is mainly in the transportation of oxygen and cellular oxidation. Iron is absorbed in the small intestine, and bound to a globulin in the plasma, called transferrin.and transported to the bone marrow for the formation of haemoglobin. Increased serum levels are found in haemolytic anaemias, hepatitis, lead and iron poisoning. Decreased serum levels are found in anaemias caused by iron deficency due to insufficient intake or absorption of iron, chronic blood loss, late pregnancy and cancer. Increase in TIBC is found in Iron defecient anaemias and pregnancy. Decrease in TIBC is found in hypoproteinaemia, haemolytic/pernicious/sicklecell anaemias, inflammatory diseases and cirrhosis.

Principle

Iron, bound to Transferrin, is released in an acidic medium and the Ferric ions are reduced to Ferrous ions. The Fe (II) ions react with Ferrozine to form a violet coloured complex. Intensity of the complex formed is directly proportional to the amount of Iron present in the sample. For TIBC, the serum is treated with excess of Fe (II) to saturate the iron binding sites on transferrin. The excess Fe (II) is adsorbed and precipitated and the Iron content in the supernatant is measured to give the TIBC.

$$Fe(III) \xrightarrow{\text{Acidic Medium}} Fe(II)$$

$$Fe\,(II) + \text{Ferrozine} \longrightarrow \text{Violet Coloured Complex}$$

Normal reference values

Serum Iron	(Males)	: 60-160 µg/dl
	(Females)	: 35-145 µg/dl
	(Neonates)	: 150-220 µg/dl
TIBC		: 250-400 µg/dl
UBIC		: 160-360 µg/dl

It is recommended that each laboratory establish its own normal range representing its patient population.

Contents	35 ml	75 ml
Iron Reagents		
L1: Iron Butter Reagent	35 ml	75 ml
L2: Iron Colour Reagent	2 ml	4 ml
S: Iron Standard (100 µg/dl)	2 ml	2 ml
TIBC Reagents		
L1: TIBC Saturating Reagent	10 ml	20 ml
L2: TIBC Precipitating Reagent	1 gm	2 gm

Storage/stability

Contents are stable at 2-8°C till the expiry mentioned on the labels.

Reagent Preparation

Reagents are ready to use.

Sample material

Serum, free from haemolysis. Iron is reported to be stable in serum for 7 days at 2-8°C.

Procedure

Wavelength/filter : 570 nm (Hg 578 nm)/yellow
Temperature : RT
Light path : 1 cm

Iron assay

Pipette into clean dry test tubes labeled as Blank (B), Standard (S), Sample Blank (SB) and Test (T):

Addition Sequence	B (ml)	S (ml)	SB (ml)	T (ml)
Iron Buffer Reagent (L1)	1.0	1.0	1.05	1.0
Distilled water	0.2	-	-	-
Iron Standard (S)	-	0.2	-	-
Sample	-	-	0.2	0.2
Iron Colour Reagent (L2)	0.05	0.05	-	0.05

Mix well and incubate at RT for 5 min. Measure the absorbances of the blank (Abs.B), standard (Abs S), sample blank (Abs SB) and test sample (Abs T) against DW

TIBC assay

Pipette into a clean dry test tube

Serum	0.5 ml
TIBC Saturating Reagent (L1)	1.0 ml
Mix well and allow to stand at RT for 10 min. and add	
TIBC Precipitating Reagent (L2)	Approx 50 mg

Mix well and allow to stand at RT for 10 min. Centrifuge at 2500-3000 rpm for 10 min. to obtain a clear supernatant. Determine the Iron content in the supernatant as above mentioned iron assay.

Calculations

$$\text{Iron in } \mu g/dl = \frac{\text{Abs T- (Abs. SB + Abs.B)}}{\text{Abs. S - Abs. B}} \times 100$$

$$\text{TIBC in } \mu g/dl = \frac{\text{Abs T - (Abs. SB + Abs.B)}}{\text{Abs. S - Abs. B}} \times 300$$

UBIC in µg/dl = TIBC in µg/dl - Iron in µg/dl

Linearity

This procedure is linear upto 1000 µg/dl. If values exceed this limit, dilute the sample with distilled water and repeat the assay. Calculate the value using the proper dilution factor.

Notes

Haemolysis interferes with the test as the haemoglobin present in the RBCs have a very high iron content.

All glassware being used for the test should first be rinsed with 1 % or 0.1 N HCI and then with good quality deionised water before use.

System Parameters			
Reaction	: End point + SB	**Interval**	:
Wavelength	: 578 nm	**Sample vol**	: 0.2 ml
Zero Setting	: Deionised water	**Reagent vol**	: 1.05 ml
Incub temp	: RT	**Standard**	: 100 ng/dl
Incub time	: 5 min	**Factor**	:
Delay time	: —	**React slope**	: Increasing
Read time	: —	**Linearity**	: 1000 µg/dl
No of read	: —	**Units**	: µg/dl

CLINICAL RELEVANCE

1. TIBC is raised in
   a. Inadequate dietary iron
   b. Iron deficiency anaemia due to haemorrhage
   c. Acute hepatitis
   d. Polycythaemia
   e. Oral contraceptive use
2. Decreased levels of TIBC are caused by
   a. Pernicious anaemia
   b. Thalassemia
   c. Sickle cell anaemia
   d. Chronic infection
   e. Cancer
   f. Hepatic disease
   g. Uremia
   h. Rheumatoid arthritis.

Interfering Factors

1. Transferrin is elevated in
   a. Children 2 ½ to 10 years of age
   b. Pregnant women during the third trimester
2. Drugs that may cause increased TIBC are
   a. Chloramphenicol
   b. Fluorides.

TRACE ELEMENTS

The term trace elements refers to inorganic substances which occur in concentration <0.01% of the body mass, i.e. in amounts $<10^{-6}$ g/g of body weight. They are divided into essential and nonessential trace elements. In humans, Cr, Co, Cu, Fe, I, Mn, Mo, Ni, Se, Zn belong to the former category; Al, Ag, As, Au, Ba, Bi, Cs, Cd, Pb, Ti, and V belong to the group of nonessential trace elements. The latter also include elements without physiological functions as well as toxic heavy metals. Magnesium, in a strict sense, is not a trace element but is customarily considered to be one. In this issue three trace elements are considered.

ZINC

Oxidation state +2,
Atomic number 30,
Atomic symbol Zn,
Atomic weight 65.38,
Electron configuration-8-18-2.

ZINC (Colorimetric Method)
Courtesy: Tulip Group of Companies

For the determination of Zinc in serum and urine (laboratory reagent for professional use only).

Summary

Zinc is important in man for growth and sexual development. It is present in various organs and is a component of many enzymes. Zinc found in serum is totally bound to protein with over 60% being bound to albumin. Increased levels are found in patients associated with gastrointestinal disorders accompanied with nausea, vomiting, high fever and a metallic taste. Decreased levels are found in cirrhosis lung carcinomas, sickle cell anaemia, acute myocardial infarction, renal failure, corticosteroid and oral contraceptive therapy.

Principle

Zinc in an alkaline medium reacts with nitro-PAPS to form a purple coloured complex. Intensity of the complex formed is directly proportional to the amount of zinc present in the sample.

$$\text{Zinc} + \text{Nitro-PAPS} \xrightarrow[\text{Medium}]{\text{Alkaline}} \text{Purple coloured complex}$$

Normal reference values

Serum : 60-120 µg/dl
Urine : 100-1000 µg/24 hrs.

It is recommended that each laboratory establish its own normal range representing its patient population.

Contents	25 ml	75 ml
L1: Buffer Reagent	20 ml	60 ml
L2: Colour Reagent	5 ml	15
S: Zinc Standard (200 µg/dl)	2 ml	2 ml

Storage/stability

Contents are stable at 2-8°C till the expiry mentioned on the labels.

Reagent Preparation

Reagents are ready to use.

Working reagent : Pour the contents of 1 bottle of L2 (Enzyme Reagent 2) into 1 bottle of L1 (Enzyme Reagent 1). This working reagent is stable for at least 2 weeks when stored at 2-8°C.

Alternatively for flexibility as much of working reagent may be made as and when desired by mixing together 4 parts of L1 (enzyme reagent 1) and 1 part of L2 (enzyme reagent 2). Alternatively 0.8 ml of L1 and 0.2 ml of L2 may also be used instead of 1 ml of the working reagent directly during the assay.

Sample material

Serum (Free from hemolysis) or urine.

Zinc is reported to be stable in serum for 7 days at 2-8°C.

Procedure

Wavelength/filter : 570 nm (Hg 578 nm)/yellow
Temperature : RT
Light path : 1 cm

Pipette into clean dry test tubes labeled as Blank (B), Standard (S), and Test (T):

Addition Sequence	B (ml)	S (ml)	T (ml)
Working Reagent	1.0	1.0	1.0
Distilled water	0.05		
Zinc Standard (S)	-	0.05	
Sample	-	-	0.05

Mix well and incubate at RT (25°C) for 5 min. Measure the absorbance of the Standard (Abs S), and Test Sample (Abs T) against the Blank, within 20 Min.

Calculations

$$\text{Zinc in } \mu g/dl = \frac{\text{Abs T}}{\text{Abs S}} \times 200$$

Linearity

This procedure is linear upto 700 µg/dl. If values exceed this limit, dilute the sample with distilled water and repeat the assay. Calculate the value using the proper dilution factor.

Notes

Chelating agents such as EDTA, Oxalate and Citrate, present even in traces, prevent the formation of the colour complex, hence necessary care should be taken during the assay.

Highly lipemic samples could interfere and should be cleared by centrifugation of filtration before use.

For a Seminal fluid assay, centrifuge the sample for 10 min at 3000 RPM. Dilute the supernatant 1+ 99 with normal saline before use.

System Parameters			
Reaction	: End point	**Interval**	:
Wavelength	: 578 nm	**Sample vol**	: 0.05 ml
Zero Setting	: Reagent blank	**Reagent vol**	: 1.00 ml
Incub temp	: RT	**Standard**	: 200 µg/dl
Incub time	: 5 min	**Factor**	:
Delay time	: —	**React slope**	: Increasing
Read time	: —	**Linearity**	: 700 µg/dl
No. of read	: —	**Units**	: µg/dl

NORMAL VALUES

Serum : 60-120µg/dl or 9.18-18.4 µmol/L
Urine : 100-1000 µg/24hrs.

Less than 60 µg/dl is considered as deficiency state.

Toxic level symptoms

Cough, chest discomfort, tachycardia, hypertension, gastrointestinal discomfort, nausea, vomiting, diarrhoea, metallic taste in the mouth. Treatment includes removal of intake and peritoneal dialysis.

Deficiency Symptoms

May progress from decreased weight, low sperm count, and impaired wound healing to alopecia, hypogonadism, ataxia, tremors, and impaired resistance to infection. Treatment includes dietary replenishment, medication or hyperalimentation.

Values are increased in

Anaemia, arteriosclerosis, coronary heart disease, dietary intake of acidic food or beverages from galvanised containers, industrial exposure to zinc (welding), and primary osteosarcoma of bone. Drugs include cisplatin, corticosteroids, estrogens, interferon, oral contraceptives (containing estrogen), phenytoin, and thiazides.

Values are decreased in

Acrodermatitis enteropathica, alopecia, alcoholism, anaemia (haemolytic), celiac sprue, cirrhosis, diarrhoea, gallbladder disease, hepatic metastases, hypoalbuminaemia, hypogonadal dwarfism, acute infections, leukaemias, lymphomas, malabsorption, myocardial infarction, dietary deficiency, pregnancy (especially third trimester), receiving parenteral nutrition, chronic renal failure, acute stress, thalassaemia major, enteric fever, and pulmonary tuberculosis. Drugs include antimetabolites, chlorthalidone, cisplatin, diuretics, estrogens, histidine, and penicillamine.

COPPER

Oxidation state + 1+ 2,
Atomic number 29,
Atomic symbol Cu,
Atomic weight 63.546,
Electron configuration-8-18-1.

COPPER (Colorimetric Method)
Courtesy: Tulip Group of Companies

For the determination of Copper in serum. (Laboratory reagent for professional use only)

Summary

Copper is widely distributed in the various organs of the body. The highest concentration is found in the liver followed by the brain and kidneys. It plays an important part in the iron metabolism by converting the ferrous ions to a ferric state. Over 90% of the copper in plasma is bound to the protein ceruloplasmin. Increased levels are found in chronic/ malignant diseases, e.g. leukaemia, cirrhosis, various infections and in patients on oral contraceptives and oestrogens. Decreased levels are found in Wilson's disease, decreased synthesis of ceruloplasmin, malabsorption, malnutrition, and nephrotic syndrome.

Principle

Copper, released from ceruloplasmin, in an acidic medium, reacts with Di-Br-PAESA to form a coloured complex. Intensity of the complex formed is directly proportional to the amount of Copper present in the sample.

$$\text{Copper} + \text{Di-Br-PAESA} \xrightarrow[\text{Medium}]{\text{Acidic}} \text{Coloured complex}$$

Normal reference values

Serum (Males)	: 80-140 µg/dl
(Females)	: 80-155 µg/dl
(Newborns)	: 12 - 67 µg/dl
(Children upto 10 yrs)	: 30 - 150 µg/dl

It is recommended that each laboratory establish its own normal range representing.

Contents	25 ml	75 ml
L1: Buffer Reagent	12.5 ml	37.5 ml
L2: Colour Reagent	12.5 ml	37.5 ml
S: Copper Standard (200 µg/dl)	2 ml	2 ml

Storage/stability

Contents are stable at 2-8°C till the expiry mentioned on the labels.

Reagent Preparation

Reagents are ready to use. Protect from bright light.

The cold Buffer (L1) when retrieved from 2-8°C may have a particulate suspension. The suspension clears up once the Buffer attains a temperature over 25°C.

Working reagent

For larger assay series a working reagent may be prepared by mixing equal volumes of L1 (Buffer Reagent) and L2 (Colour Reagent). The Working reagent is stable at 2-8°C for at least 3 weeks. Keep tightly closed.

Sample material

Serum, free from hemolysis. Copper is reported to be stable in the sample for 6 days when stored at 2-8°C.

Procedure

Wavelength/filter	: 580 nm (Hg 578 nm)/yellow
Temperature	: RT
Light path	: 1 cm

Pipette into clean dry test tubes labeled as Blank (B), Standard (S), and Test (T) :

Addition Sequence	B (ml)	S (ml)	T (ml)
Buffer Reagent (L1)	0.5	0.5	0.5
Colour Reagent (L2)	0.5	0.5	0.5
Distilled water	0.05		
Copper Standard (S)	-	0.05	
Sample	-	-	0.05

Mix well and incubate at RT (25°C) for 10 min. Measure the absorbance of the Standard (Abs S), and Test Sample (Abs T) against the Blank, within 30 Min.

Calculations

$$\text{Copper in µg/dl} = \frac{\text{Abs T}}{\text{Abs S}} \times 200$$

Linearity

This procedure is linear upto 500 µg/dl. If the value exceeds this limit, dilute the serum with normal saline (NaCl 0.9%) and repeat the assay. Calculate the value using the proper dilution factor.

Notes

Chelating agents such as EDTA, Oxalate and Citrate, present even in traces, prevent the formation of the colour complex, hence necessary care should be taken during the assay.

Highly lipemic samples could interfere and should be cleared by centrifugation or filtration before use.

The assay can be run at 600 nm, however the absorbances would be approx. 30% lower as compared to 570 nm.

System Parameters			
Reaction	: End point	**Interval**	:
Wavelength	: 578 nm	**Sample vol**	: 0.05 ml
Zero Setting	: Reagent blank	**Reagent vol**	: 1.00 ml
Incub temp	: RT	**Standard**	: 200 µg/dl
Incub time	: 10 min.	**Factor**	:
Delay time	: —	**React slope**	: Increasing
Read time	: —	**Linearity**	: 500 µg/dl
No of read	: —	**Units**	: µg/dl

Toxic level symptoms

Jaundice, hepatic injury, headache, vomiting, and may lead to haemolytic shock.

Deficiency symptoms

Impaired erythrocyte production and survival time and lowered catabolism by copper-containing enzymes

Values are Increased in

Alzheimer's disease, anaemia (aplastic, pernicious, megaloblastic anaemia of pregnancy; iron deficiency), cirrohosis (billiary), elevated CRP, glomerulonephritis, haemochromatosis, Hodgkin's disease, hyperestrogenemia, hypothyroidism, hyperthyroidism, infections, leukaemia, lymphoma, Lofgren syndrome, myocardial infarction, pellagra, pregnancy (especially third trimester), rheumatic fever, rheumatoid arthritis, sarcoidosis, and systemic lupus erythematosus. Drugs include carbamazepine, estrogens and oral contraceptives, henobarbital, and phenytoin sodium.

COPPER URINE

Normal Values

All ages	0-60 µg/24 hours
Wilson's disease	> 100µg/24 hours

Values are increased in

Alzheimer's disease, aminoaciduria, cirrhosis (billiary, Indian childhood), hepatitis (chronic active), hyperceruloplasminemia, nephritic syndrome, pellagra, proteinuria, and Wilson's disease.

Values are decreased in

Burns, hypoproteinaemia, kwashiorkor, malabsorption, Menkes' hair syndrome, nephrosis, and Wilson's disease.

MAGNESIUM

Oxidation +2,
Atomic number 12,
Atomic symbol Mg,
Atomic weight 24.305,
Electron configuration 2-8-2

MAGNESIUM (Calmagite Method)
Courtesy: Tulip Group of Companies

For the determination of Magnesium in serum, urine and CSF (Laboratory Reagent for Professional Use Only).

Summary

Magnesium, along with potassium, is a major intracellular cation. It is an activator of various enzymes. It is also involved in amino acid activation and protein synthesis. Increased levels are found in dehydration, addison's disease and uremia. Decreased levels are found in malabsorption, during treatment of diabetic coma, chronic renal disease, chronic alcoholism, pancreatitis and hyperthyroidism.

Principle

Magnesium combines with Calmagite in an alkaline medium to form a red coloured complex. Interference of calcium and proteins is eliminated by the addition of specific chelating agents and detergents. Intensity of the colour formed is directly proportional to the amount of magnesium present in the sample.

$$\text{Magnesium} + \text{Calmagite} \xrightarrow[\text{Medium}]{\text{Alkaline}} \text{Red coloured complex}$$

Normal reference values

Serum (Children)	: 1.5 - 2.0 mEq/L
(Adults)	: 1.3 - 2.5 mEq/L
CSF	: 2.0 - 3.0 mEq/L
Urine	: 6.0 - 8.5 mEq/24 hrs

It is recommended that each laboratory establish its own normal range representing its patient population.

Note : 2 mEq/L = 1 mmol/L = 2.44 mg/dl

Contents	25 ml	75 ml
L1: Buffer Reagent	12.5 ml	37.5 ml
L2: Colour Reagent	12.5 ml	37.5 ml
S: Magnesium Standard (2.0 mEq/L)	2 ml	2 ml

Storage/stability

Contents are stable at 2-8°C till the expiry mentioned on the labels.

Reagent Preparation

Reagents are ready to use. Protect from bright light.

Working reagent: For larger assay series a working reagent may be prepared by mixing equal volumes of L1 (Buffer Reagent) and L2 (Colour Reagent). The Working reagent is stable at 2-8°C for at least one month. Keep tightly closed.

Sample material

Serum (Free from haemolysis), Urine and CSF.

24 hr. collected urine should be acidified to a pH of 2-3 by the addition of approx. 10 to 15 ml of HCI and diluted 1+ 3 with D.Water before use. Multiply results by 4. Magnesium is reported to be stable in serum/plasma for 7 days at 2-8°C.

Procedure

Wavelength/filter : 510 nm (Hg 546 nm)/green
Temperature : RT
Light path : 1 cm

Pipette into clean dry test tubes labeled as Blank (B), Standard (S), and Test (T):

Addition Sequence	B (ml)	S (ml)	T (ml)
Buffer Reagent (L1)	0.5	0.5	0.5
Colour Reagent (L2)	0.5	0.5	0.5
Distilled water	0.01		
Magnesium Standard (S)	-	0.01	
Sample	-	-	0.01

Mix well and incubate at RT (25°C) for 5 min. Measure the absorbance of the Standard (Abs S), and Test Sample (Abs T) against the Blank, within 30 Min.

Calculations

$$\text{Magnesium in mEq/L} = \frac{\text{AbS.T}}{\text{Abs S}} \times 2$$

Linearity

This procedure is linear upto 10 mEq/L. If values exceed this limit, dilute the sample with distilled water and repeat the assay. Calculate the value using an appropriate dilution factor.

Notes

All glassware being used for the test should first be rinsed with 1% or 0.1 N HCI and then with good quality deionised water before use.

Chelating agents such as EDTA, Oxalate and Citrate, present even in traces, prevent the formation of the colour complex, hence necessary care should be taken during the assay.

RBCs have double the magnesium content compared to serum, and hence hemolysed samples should not be used.

System Parameters			
Reaction	: End point	Interval	:
Wavelength	: 510 nm	Sample vol	: 0.01 ml
Zero Setting	: Reagent blank	Reagent vol	: 1.00 ml
Incub temp	: RT	Standard	: 2.0 mEq/L
Incub time	: 5 min	Factor	:
Delay time	: —	React slope	: Increasing
Read time	: —	Linearity	: 10 mEq/L
No. of read	: —	Units	: mEq/L

NORMAL VALUES

Serum (children)	1.5-2.0 mEq/L
(adults)	1.3-2.5 mEq/L
CSF	2.0-3.0 mEq/L
Urine	6.0-8.5 mE1/24 hours
Panic level (serum)	> 3.0 mEq/L or < 0.5 mEq/L
Toxic level (serum)	>12 mEq/L

Toxic Level Symptoms

Lethargy, drowsiness, flushing, nausea, vomiting, slurred speech, hypotension, weak or absent deep tendon reflexes, ECG changes (prolonged PR and QT intervals, widened QRS, bradycardia), respiratory depression. (Treatment includes stop magnesium intake, promote excretion, give calcium salts, haemodialysis).

Deficiency Symptoms

Muscle tremors, twitching, tetany, hypocalcemia, hyperactive deep tendon reflexes, ECG changes (prolonged PR and QT intervals, broad flat T-waves, premature ventricular contractions, ventricular tachycardia, fibrillation), anorexia, nausea, vomiting, lethargy, insomnia.

Values are increased in

Addison's disease adrenalectomy, ataxia, dehydration (severe), diabetes (uncontrolled diabetes, diabetic acidosis before treatment, controlled diabetes in older patients), dysarrhythmias, hypercalcemia, hypothyroidism, hypophosphatemia, renal lithiasis, leukemias (lymphocytic and myelocytic), renal insufficiency and failure. Drugs include antacids containing magnesium, calcium containing medications, cathartics, ethacrynic acid, laxatives (epsom salt and magnesium citrate), loop diuretics, and thyroid medications.

Values are decreased in

Acute tubular necrosis (diuretic phase), alcholism (chronic), Bartter's syndrome, bowel resection complications, convulsions, diabetic ketoacidosis, diarrhoea (chronic), dysarrythmias, excessive lactation, excessive sweating, hepatitis, hepatic cirrhosis, hepatic insufficiency, hungry bone syndrome, hypokalaemia, hypercalcaemia, hyperthyroidism, hypoparathyroidism, hypocalcaemia, IV solutions without magnesium, ketoacidosis, kwashiorkor (severe malnutrition), laxative abuse, magnesium deficiency tetany syndrome, pancreatitis (acute and chronic), phosphate depletion, postobstructive diuresis, postoperartively, primary hyperaldostreronism, prolonged gastric drainage, reduced magnesium intake, reduced magnesium absorption (specific magnesium malabsorption, generalised malabsorption syndrome, excessive bowel resection, diffuse bowel disease or injury), renal tubular acidosis, stress states with catecholamine excess, tetany, toxaemia of pregnancy, ulcerative colitis, volume expansion (extracellular fluid). Drugs include alcohol, amphotericin B, some antibiotics (neomycin, aminoglycosides), calcium gluconate, corticosteroids, cyclosporine, diuretics (e.g. mercurial, ethacrynic acid), glucose, insulin, mannitol, and urea.

MAGNESIUM URINE

Values are increased in: Alcoholism, Bartter's syndrome, hypermagnesaemia, and nephrolithiasis. Drugs include aldosterone, cisplastin, corticosteroids, diuretics (ethacrynic acid), and thiazide.

Values are decreased: Renal disease, magnesium deficit, osteoporosis, and syndrome of inappropriate antidiuretic hormone secretion (SIADHS).

AUTOMATION IN CLINICAL CHEMISTRY

INSTRUMENTATION

Till very recently the only machine one could find in a pathologist's biochemistry laboratory was the centrifuge. That added by a simple colorimeter, a microscope, some chemicals and test tubes were typical exhibits in a laboratory. This picture is changing very rapidly. New instruments are entering the laboratory. With the advancements made in the field of computer sciences more and more automation is entrusted to instrumentation.

Automation, in general is expected to bring in convenience, speed and reliability without compromising accuracy. Let us see how these aspects are served by clinical chemistry analysers for analysing blood samples. Analysers system consists of two parts: (i) chemical reagents which are mixed with blood samples whereby the particular substance to be estimated is reacted with the specific reagent and (ii) optoelectronic analyser to process/monitor/estimate the above reaction and thereby establish the exact amount of the substance.

PRESENT STATUS

For convenience there are three broad categories of automatic analysers presently available:

1. Random access auto analyser
2. Batch analyser
3. Semiauto analyser.

Category (1) is very popular in most of the advanced countries. In India, such machines are found only in very large hospitals and in big towns, their price is approximately Rs.15 lacs and more. Batch analysers are available at a range of Rs. 4 to 9 lacs, whereas semiauto analysers are in the range of around 2.5 lacs. There are a large number of semiautomatic analyser installations in India and newer models are coming in the market regularly.

Semiautomatic analysers offer a big leap in a laboratory's capability. It forms a major breakthrough, since it offers enhancement of speed and convenience. Let us first see what should normally be the expectations of a laboratory from an analyser and how would a semiautomatic analyser answer them.

BENEFITS OF A SEMIAUTOMATIC ANALYSER

Economy

As compared with a colorimeter the analyser is a considerably more expensive instrument. The first and foremost expectation from it therefore, is that it should justify the higher investment.

Semiautomatic analysers work on in general 1.0 ml of reagent volume per test. There are some which work on as low a volume as 0.5 ml. The colorimeter requires 5.0 ml of reagent though some are now available for use with 2.5 ml or 3 ml. The main pay back comes from the savings on recurring costs of reagents.

Other benefits such as savings on time costs (employing less number of persons) glassware work space, etc. are also available, but the amount of savings on reagents costs form the major part of economy of operation.

Wide Spectrum of Tests

All tests based on the principle of colorimetry can be performed on analysers. The analysers have high quality filters or a spectrophotometer for selection of wavelengths. More important, kinetic and end point mode chemistries can be performed on analysers. An ultraviolet wavelength of 340 nm is available and the combination 340 nm and kinetic and end point mode opens out a very wide range of chemistries. A particular chemistry may possibly be done at a different wavelength on a colorimeter, but analyser will make available a quicker and accurate method of latest technology.

Entire range of organ functions like cardiac, hepatic and renal profiles can be performed by analysers.

Speed

A typical workload in a laboratory is expected to be finished in a couple of hours. Samples collected during the morning hours are analysed in the afternoon. Before the evening, results are compiled and patient reports prepared to be delivered in the evening. A medium size laboratory can meet its work load through a semiautomatic analyser (about 100 tests per day). As the number of tests per day increases, a batch analyser or large random access analyser is called for.

Accuracy and Reliability

The chances of manual errors are reduced in analysers because of automatic settings of wavelength, temperature, factors and other variable parameters which have to be set up on machines. Pipetting errors are also eliminated by use of automatic micro pipettes. The analysers are computer-based instruments and have self-monitoring features. They monitor the progress of chemical reactions and indicate any abnormality. Manual steps at various stages are reduced and the results obtained are accurate and reliable.

Convenience

The convenience achieved through the use of the analyser is manifold. Three main features are: (i) elimination of manual calculations, (ii) digital display and print out of results, (iii) emergency requests can be handled with speed and accuracy. For example, a colorimeter based test for SGOT/SGPT would take 1½ to 2 hours whereas on an analyser the results are available within minutes.

Non-dependence on Technicians

An analyser is easy to operate as most of the steps are automatic. A technician requires only a few days to learn operations of the machine. Besides, in absence of the technician it is not very difficult for the senior person/doctor to handle the workload in case of a small/medium laboratory.

Business Growth

With an automatic analyser installed in the laboratory, physicians as well as patients develop a great amount of confidence in the results. This added by wider range of tests make the business of the laboratory grow fast.

WHICH LAB NEEDS AUTOMATION?

Given above are some of the expectations that can be fulfilled by an analyser. The importance given to a particular factor would depend on the choice of an individual lab. Even if the analyser is purchased primarily for any one of the above mentioned reasons, all of the remaining purposes are served.

Earlier, the main criterion used to be speed, keeping in mind the requirement of finishing the lab workload in 2 to 3 hours. The ideas have changed. There are laboratories which have purchased it for handling the 'night' (emergency) workload—by keeping the laboratories open all 24 hours. There are laboratories which have started with the purchase of a semi-automatic analyser and established themselves in the group of reputable laboratories in the towns in a span of one year. There are quality conscious buyers wanting to give adequate confidence to their referring physicians and patients. There are nursing homes who have started laboratories with an analyser not limiting the facilities only to their in-house and OPD patients but making them available to any patient.

In short, presently there is no predictable trend of particular laboratories buying analysers. It is quite understandable looking to the varied purposes an analyser can serve. Any laboratory is fully justified in its purchase of an analyser unit.

SELECTION OF A MODEL

While selecting a particular model the primary objective of the laboratory for purchase has to be well-defined. It could be anyone or a combination of the above mentioned points. A particular model may have an advantage in one area (say economy), whereas another will be a better choice for some other features (say, an elaborate display or print out). Quicker pay back of the analyser's investment is the next point that one must consider. This should be looked at from different angles. One model may be available at a price, say, Rs.20,000 less but if its recurrent costs on reagents, etc. are comparatively more that would not turn out to be the best alternative. The cost analysis should be done for a period of 5 years minimum.

After-sales service forms an important part for all instrumentation systems. The company selling it should be of repute and should have a network of field service engineers. Failure rate is normally more in a country with tropical weather conditions. As far as possible the system should be proven to be working reliably in various places and be tropicalized. A modular system can be of advantage.

The selling company should also have a good reagent support. It is better to have the total system from one company. This makes sure that the company personnel also understand the exact application of the unit rather than only the engineering aspects.

ANALYSER CLASSIFICATION

Broad based classification of analysers can fall under the following three categories.

Semiauto Analysers

Serum sample-reagent mixture is done manually outside the unit and fed manually. The unit performs/monitors/evaluates the chemical reaction and gives the result on display and/or printer. The setting of the unit is normally automatic as regards wavelength, temperature, etc.

Batch Analysers

Serum sample-reagent mixing is normally automatic and the mix is fed automatically to the analyser. The analyser performs the same function as a semiauto analyser unit. Here a batch of a particular chemistry test (say, glucose, urea) can be set up and performed automatically. One reagent is stored on the machine at a time.

Random Access Auto Analyser

On the machine more than one reagent is stored. Patient samples are kept on the machine. The computer is programmed to carry out selected tests on individual samples. Any particular sample and reagent can be selected, mixed, incubated and monitored as per the programme. The patient report is fully compiled by the unit and printed out.

CLIN CHECK PLUS (Courtesy: Tulip Group of Companies)

The clin check plus is a clinical chemistry/biochemistry analyser, designed for a precise and fast execution of almost all-clinical chemistry analysis. Automatic selection of filters and temperature controller is all managed by the microprocessor. The CCP is a fully open machine with 40 locations. Following arrays can be performed on the machine:

EP/KIN/FXT/MSD AND ABS MODE

Excellent features; with only 4 operating keys; very simple to handle; reads OD up to 2.0 A; In-built incubation (2 positions); RS 232 port makes compatible with PC Communication; which can also handle Data from machine to PC. It's a lightweight and sturdy machine with less breakdown and low maintenance cost.

The machine is ideally suited for growing or nascent laboratories. CCP picture.

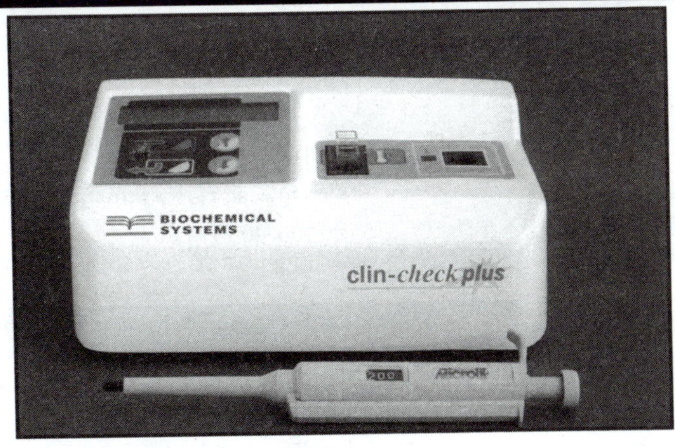

CCP picture

Features

- User Friendly, Fully Open System with 40 programmable locations.
- Only 4 operating keys- very simple to handle.
- Reads OD up to 2.0A- large working range.
- Two inbuilt incubator positions.
- RS 232 software support for external serial port printer.
- Data handling software available.
- Lightweight, only 3.8 kg.
- Service support by instruments division, Tulip diagnostics Pvt Ltd.

Technical features CCP

Photometric Systems:	
Light Source	2 W long-life tungsten incandescent lamp
Spectral field	340 to 700 nm
Filter change	automatic
Filters	340, 405, 505, 546, 630 nm; 8 m pass-band
Detector	solid state device
Thermostating	
Heating element	semiconductor
Temperature	37°C
Temperature Accuracy	± 0.2 ° C
Stabilisation Period	10-20 Min.
Thermostatic Unit	Two Places for Square or Cylindrical Cuvettes
Measuring System	
Reset:	Automatic
Measuring Range	0 to +2000 OD
Photometric Linearity	± 2% from 0 to 1700 OD
Photometric Accuracy	± 2% from 0 to 1700 OD
Precision	± 2 digit
Drift	Lower than 0.005 OD per hour
Reagent Volume	1ml minimum.
Measure Method	End point, Kinetics, Fixed-Time, Differential
Data Display and Programming:	
Keyboard	With 4 Function Keys
Display	32 Characters, Liquid Crystals, Alpha-Numeric
Serial Output	RS-232 Standard
Power Supply	220 V, 50 Hz., 117V, 60Hz., 40 VA
Size	cm. 27.5 × 21 × 9
Weight	3.8 Kg.

SCREEN MASTER 3000 (Courtesy: Tulip Group of Companies)

A typical clinical chemistry semi-auto analyser with unmatched features designed for Indian laboratories. Quality at par and performance as per international standards which can perform. EP/KIN/FXT/MSD with ABS mode.

The machine uses both flow cell (18 µl) and cuvettes (semi-micro cuvettes) also ensuring less carry over effect and less breakdown period of the machine. It covers the entire range of spectrum for measurements, (340-700 nm). Automatic selection of filters and is managed by microprocessors with in-built 10 position incubator which is regulated by Peltier heat pumps.

Its very simple to handle and is user friendly as its operation and programming of machine is done by keyboard and set of instruction displayed on the display. All results are interpreted by units and also Graphs are available for KIN/MSD. Also has dynamic display (real time display of OD) for KIN and also Reagent blank OD (save)-ensures minimum consumption of reagents. Any errors or malfunction in the machine is denoted on the display or printout.

The machine is capable of storing 500 results in memory and is able to retrieve also for later use. Also has inbuilt 20 column Thermal printer (optional). A Built in QC program which validates the overall performance of system. Gives Mean, SD, CV and Levy-Jennings chart. Computer compatibility with RS 232 port, which also supports data handling software.

Features

- User Friendly, Fully Open System with 90 programmable locations.

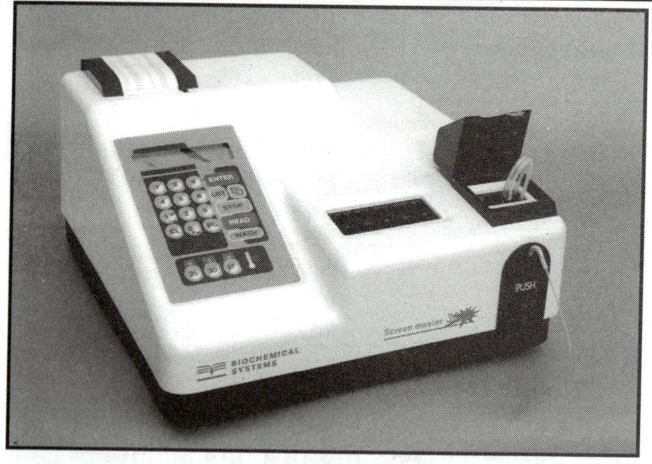

Biochemical systems

- 18 µl Flowcell minimizes reagent consumption and avoids carry over.
- Reads OD up to 2.5 A-large working range.
- Built in 24-column graphic thermal printer.
- 10 position incubator at 25°, 30°, 37°C.
- Incubated flowcell resting chamber.
- Stores 500 test results in memory.
- Built in Software for QC program with mean, SD, CV and Levy Jennings chart.

Technical Features of Screenmaster 3000

Operating modes	Absorbance, end point, fixed-time, kinetic and multi-standard and tests.
For Flow Cell	
Flowcell volume	18 µl
Typical working volume	500 µl
Minimum working volume	350 µl
Aspiration	Peristaltic pump with programmable intake volume
For Cuvette	
Wavelength range	340-700 nm
Filters	340-405-505-546-578-630 nm
Reagents volumes in cuvette	1 ml (min) for macro cuvette, 0.3 for micro cuvette
Measuring System	
Reset	Automatic
Measuring range	from -200 to + 2500 OD units
Photometric accuracy	±2% from 0 to 2000 OD units
Photometric linearity	±2% from 0 to 2000 OD units
Reproducibility	±1% digit
General	
Incubator	10 positions at 25/30/37°C + 0.2°C
Printer	built-in graphic printer with 20 columns
Power supply	220V, 50 Hz or 110V, 60 Hz
Dimensions	40 × 40 ×17 cm
Weight	13.0 Kg

MAP LAB PLUS

Unique and the only semi-auto analyser with True Elisa reader available in Indian market. Exclusively marketed and serviced by Tulip Diagnostics Pvt Ltd.

The machine is capable of performing routine biochemistry test as well as Elisa tests in a single machine, which can perform the following operations: EP / KIN / FXT /MSD / latex / QLT and ELISA.

Uses both cuvettes and flowcell for measurement ensures low carry over effect and less breakdown period of the machine.

Machine has 2 separate set of optical system (Lamps as well as Filters): 6 (biochemistry) and 4 (Elisa).

Covers entire range of spectrum for biochemistry (340-700 nm), and Also for ELISA: 405, 450, 492, 630.

Selection of filters is automatically managed by microprocessors. This minimizes errors in the selection of filters. Separate lamp source is used 20W and 2W. (biochemistry and ELISA). Also has 10 positions for In-built Incubator fixed at 37°C with the help of semiconductor (less power consumption).

In-built thermal printer with graphical printouts and results made interpretation much easier. The analytical results are directly displayed or printed with preset units as programmed.

Dynamic display (real time display of OD) in KIN gives extra check for chemistry being performed.

Especially 40 locations are available for MSD mode, which cover entire ElA conc.; EIA, QLT, latex, etc. can take 7 standards to plot a curve. With the help of special algorithm the machine can recalibrate the graph with the help of 2 stands. Partial calibration.

PC compatible with RS 232 ports; helps to communicate with machines, Data and PC. Also supports data handling software and also support data management software provided with machine for ELISA section only.

Machine has built in QC program which validates the overall performance of system. Gives mean, SD, CV and Levy Jennings chart.

Ideally suitable for any lab with workload of biochemistry plus ELISA (MSD).

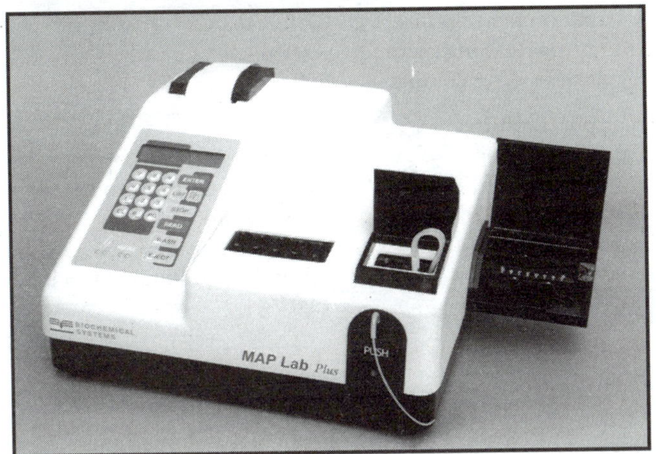

MLP

Features

- User friendly, fully open system with 90 programmable locations.
- Separate optical systems for clinical chemistry and ELISA.
- 18 µl flowcell minimizes reagent consumption and avoids carry over.
- Reads OD up to 3.2 A-large working range.
- Dynamic display for kinetics.
- Built in 24-column graphic thermal printer.
- 10 position Incubator.
- Incubated flowcell resting chamber.
- Built in QC with mean, SD, CV and Levy Jennings chart.
- RS 232 software support with DMS and DHS.
- Service support by instruments division, Tulip diagnostics Pvt Ltd.

Technical Features of Maplab Plus

Operating modes	Absorbance, end point, fixed-time, kinetic, multistandard and qualitative tests
For Flow Cell	
Flowcell volume	18 µl
Typical working volume	500 µl
Minimum working volume	350 µl
Aspiration	Peristaltic pump with programmable intake volume
For Cuvette	
Wavelength range	340-700 nm
Filters	340-405-505-546-578-630 nm
Reagents volumes in cuvette	1 ml (min) for macro cuvette, 0.3 for micro cuvette
For Micro well strip	
Wavelength range	405-700 nm
Filters	405-450-492-630 nm
Micro well strips type	All kind of 8-micro well strips
Measuring System	
Reset	Automatic
Measuring range	from -200 to + 3200 OD units
Photometric accuracy	± 2% from 0 to 2500 OD units
Photometric linearity	± 2% from 0 to 2500 OD units
Reproducibility	± 1% digit
General	
Incubator	10 positions at 37°C ± 0.2°C
Printer	built-in graphic printer with 20 columns
Power supply	220V, 50 Hz or 110V, 60 Hz
Dimensions	40 × 40 × 17 cm
Weight	13.5 Kg

FULLY

Innovative technology for user friendly meeting all requirement simplicity, reliability, accuracy and competitive. Today's laboratory environment demands an expert system with an economic advantage. The revolutionary design makes FULLY a compact and complete Clinical Chemistry Analyser. FULLY machine is uniquely designed to answer the real needs of laboratories low acquisition and operating costs, simple and flexible use minimum maintenance.

System Overview

- The special design of the reagent bottle has been developed in order to avoid reagent loss.
- 20 position reagent tray to maximize the number of tests per sample at a time.
- Flexibility to run both single and two reagent chemistries.
- Open system that enables the programming of an unlimited number of techniques.

Modern

- Common shape of reaction wells and cups is easily available in local market.

- Programmable washing cycle between samples and tests for minimizing carry over.
- Fully walk away system capable of running 54 samples at a time.
- Auto rerun with pre dilution.

Compact

- Proven and high technique will assure accurate measuring system and easy maintenance.
- 18 µl flow cell volume for economical running cost.
- Peltier controlled flow cell temperature.
- Washing and waste tanks level sensors.
- Auto level sensing.
- Built in high performance PC.

Software

- Discover the simplicity of operations with windows environment.
- Very user friendly, enables skilled laboratory staff to run FULLY within short time.
- Easy selection of menus by icons.
- Reagent positions are automatically determined by the workplan with volumes required once the sample and reagent have been programmed.
- Nine profiles of up to unlimited chemistries each to simplify your task of profile management.
- Continuous working status monitoring.
- QC program with Levey-Jennings plot.
- Intelligent error management.
- Multilanguage support.
- Network integration facilities.
- Built in thermal printer and additional output for external connection.

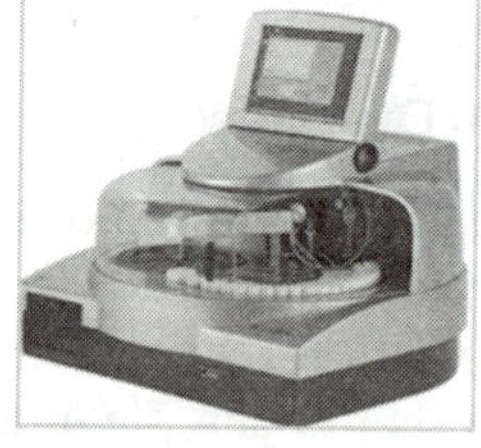

Fully

Technical Specifications of Fully

Measuring System

Operating modes	Absorbance, End-Point, Fixed Time, Kinetic, Multistandard
Throughput	Up to 120 tests/hour.
Light source	Halogen lamp 12V 20W
Spectral Range	320-690 nm
Filter Wavelength	340, 405, 492, 505, 546, 578, 630 nm, one free position
Measuring Range	from -0.200 to 2.500 OD
Flow Cell	18 µl
Incubation temperature	37°C ± 0.2°C
Minimum Reading volume	350 ml
Typical Reading volume	500 ml
Sample Handling	
Sample number	54 positions including samples, calibrators and controls/tray
Sample container	Cup (1.2 ml)
Sample volume	2-200 µl (l µ l steps)
Automatic dilution	Pre and post dilution ration: 1:2-1:20
Reagent Handling	
Reagent tray	20 bottles + 1 bottle for diluent
Reagent bottle	45 ml
Reagent volume	Reagent 1 volume range: 30 to 1000 µl (1 µl steps) Reagent 2 volume range: 0 to 1000 µl (1 µl steps)
Liquid detection	Sensor
Reagent warming	Pre-heated ARM
Reagent identification	Position ID
Tray exchange	Possible with reagent bottles
Reaction	
Number of wells	144 wells (12 wells × 12 strips)
Well volume	1ml
Well temperature	37°C ± 2°C
Diluter	
Syringe	1000 µl, 1 µl steps
Accuracy	± 1% at 5 µl
Computer	
Computer	Built-in
Computer description	Intel® Processor, 20 GB HD, 128 MB RAM
Operating system	Microsoft Windows® Display TFT 12", 800 × 600
Network adapter	Built-in
Printer	Built-in thermal printer, 120 mm
Output	RS232, LPT
Drive	CD ROM, Floppy disk 3.5" 1.44 M bytes
General	
Power Supply	AC115-230V 50-60Hz full range
Dimensions	720 (W) × 680 (D) × 750 (H) open or 530 (H) close mm
Weight	55 kg

CHAPTER 21

Enzymology

For most enzymic estimations, special care has to be taken regarding storage specifications of reagents/kits. During testing one has to be extremely cautious about temperature (incubation), pH, time settings, etc. otherwise reproducible results may not be obtained. All precautions listed in this chapter or those mentioned by manufacturers should be cautiously followed to every minutest detail.

SERUM/PLASMA

α AMYLASE

SERUM AND URINE (Direct Substrate Method) (Courtesy: Tulip Group of Companies)

For the determination of α Amylase activity in serum, plasma or urine (for *in vitro* diagnostic use only).

Summary

α Amylase is secreted by the pancreas into the duodenum where it aids the catabolism of carbohydrates to simple sugars. Damage to the pancreas or obstruction to the pancreatic duct causes the enzyme to enter the blood stream. Elevated levels are found in acute pancreatitis, perforated/penetrating peptic ulcers, paraotitis (mumps). Patients with chronic pancreatic disorders having pancreatic cell destruction do not have high levels as less amylase is produced by the pancreas.

Principle

α Amylase catalyses the hydrolysis of a 2-chloro-4 nitro phenol salt to chloro nitrophenol (CNP). The rate of hydrolysis is measured as an increase in absorbance due to the formation of chloro nitrophenol which is proportional to the α Amylase activity in the sample.

$$CNP - Gal - G2 + H_2O \xrightarrow{\alpha \text{ Amylase}} CNP + Gal - G2$$

Normal reference values

Serum : up to 90 U/L at 37°C
Urine : up to 490 U/L at 37°C

It is recommended that each laboratory establish its own normal range representing its patient population.

Contents	2 × 10 ml	2 × 30 ml
L1: Amylase reagent	2 × 10 ml	2 × 30 ml

Storage/stability

Contents are stable at 2-8°C till the expiry mentioned on the label.

Reagent Preparation

Reagents are ready to use. Do not pipette with mouth.

Sample material

Serum, heparinised plasma, urine.
α Amylase is reported to be stable in the sample for 5 days at 2-8°C. Separate serum from clot as soon as possible.

Procedure

Wavelength/filter : 405/(Hg405)/violet
Temperature : 37°C
Light path : 1 cm
For Serum as Sample:
Pipette into a clean dry test tube labelled as Test (T):

Addition Sequence	(T) 37°C
Amylase Reagent (L1)	1.0 ml
Sample	0.02 ml

Mix well and read the initial absorbance A_0 after 1 minute and repeat the absorbance reading after every 1, 2, and 3 minutes. Calculate the mean absorbance change per minute (ΔA/min)

For Urine as Sample

Pipette into a clean dry test tube labelled as Test (T):

Addition Sequence	(T) 37°C
Amylase Reagent (L1)	1.0 ml
Sample	0.01 ml

Mix well and read the initial absorbance A_0 after 1 minute and repeat the absorbance reading after every 1, 2, and 3 minutes. Calculate the mean absorbance change per minute (ΔA/min)

Calculations

αAmylase Activity in U/L (Serum) = ΔA/min × 3954
αAmylase Activity in U/L (Urine) = ΔA/min × 7830

Linearity

The procedure is linear upto 1000 U/L at 37°C. If the absorbance change (ΔA/min) exceeds 0.300, use only the value of the first two minutes to calculate the result, or dilute the sample 1 + 9 with normal saline (NaCI 0.9%) and repeat the assay (Results x 10).

Note

Anticoagulants like oxalate and EDTA bind Calcium which is needed for α Amylase activity and should not be used. Heparin may be used. Saliva and sweat contain α Amylase. Avoid contamination of reagent and sample during use.

For users to convert the values obtained by this method to the EPS substrate methods, multiply the results obtained by 2.45.

System Parameters			
Reaction	: Kinetic	**Interval**	: 60 sec.
Wavelength	: 405 nm	**Sample vol**	: 0.02 ml/0.01 ml
Zero setting	: Distilled water	**Reagent vol**	: 1.00 ml
Incub temp.	: 37°C	**Standard**	:
Incub time.	: —	**Factor**	: 3954/7830
Delay time	: 60 sec.	**Factor**	: Increasing
Read time	: 180 sec.	**Linearity**	: 1000 U/L
No. of read	: 4	**Units**	: U/L

Normal Values

Normal Values Urine	
Mayoclonic method	10-80 amylase U/hour
Somogyi method	26-950 U/24 hours
Beckman method	1-17 U/hour

Normal Values Serum		*SI Units*
Somogyi method	50-180 U/dl	92-330 U/L
Beckman method		20-125 U/L
Over age 70		20-160 U/L
Panic level	Three times the upper limit of normal	

CLINICAL RELEVANCE

Increased levels are found in

Pronounced elevation (5 or more times normal)
- Acute pancreatitis
- Pancreatic pseudocyst
- Morphine administration

Moderate elevation (3 to 5 times normal)
- Pancreatic carcinoma affecting head of pancreas (late manifestation)
- Mumps
- Salivary gland inflammation
- Perforated peptic ulcer (sometimes)
- Acute exacerbation of chronic pancreatitis
- Partial gastrectomy
- Obstruction of pancreatic duct
- Alcohol poisoning
- Acute cholecystitis
- Intestinal obstruction with strangulation
- Ruptured tubal ectopic
- Ruptured aortic aneurysm

Decreased Levels are found in

- Acute pancreatitis subsidence
- Hepatitis
- Cirrhosis of liver
- Toxemia of pregnancy
- Severe burns
- Severe thyrotoxicosis

LIPASE

Lipase, Serum

Normal Value

<200 U/L with triolein;<160 U/L with olive oil.

		SI Units
Adults	13-141 U/L	0.22-2.40 μKat/L
Age 20-60	31-186 U/L	0.53-3.16 μKat/L
Over age 60	<302 U/L	<5.13 μKat/L
Over age 90	26-267 U/L	0.44-4.54 μKat/L
Children	20-136 IU/L	
Infants	9-105 IU/L	

Increased: Cholecystitis, cirrhosis, duodenal ulcers, fat embolism, gallstone colic, pain (abdominal), pancreatic carcinoma, pancreatic cholera, pancreatic trauma, pancreatitis, peritonitis trauma, pancreatitis, peritonitis, renal disease with impaired output, and strangulated bowel. Drugs include bethanechol, heparin, and narocotic analgesics.

Description

Lipase is a pancreatic enzyme that changes fats and triglycerides into fatty acids and glycerol. The pancreas is the only body organ that demonstrates significant lipase activity. In acute pancreatitis, serum lipase begins to increase in 2-6 hours, peaks at 12-30 hours, and remains elevated, but slowly decreases for 2-4 days. Lipase rises and falls in tandem with amylase in acute pancreatitis, but is a more specific marker for this condition.

PHOSPHATASES

Phosphatases belong to the class of enzymes called hydrolases, and they are characterized, by their ability to hydrolyse a large variety of organic phosphate esters with the formation of an alcohol and a phosphate ion.

Phosphatases of diagnostic significance are of two kinds: alkaline phosphatase and acid phosphatase. These are differentiated by their reaction in alkaline and acidic medium. The pH for measuring the alkaline phosphatase activity is 10, and for acid phosphatase it is 5.0. Various substrates have been used from time to time, but the current use of p-nitrophenyl phosphate (PNPP) appears to be universal. The PNNP is not a natural substrate for the phosphatases. It is used because it gives a reasonably rapid rate of reaction and because it is analytically convenient to measure the product formed (p-nitrophenol). The liberated phenol is yellow in colour in alkaline medium and is colourless in acid medium. Continuous assay can be done for alkaline phosphatase by measuring the rate of formation of p-nitrophenol at pH 10. For this one will need a recording spectrophotometer. The manual two-point method is described here.

Units For Reporting Phosphatase Activity

Several units are used in expressing phosphatase activity—Bodansky unit, King-Armstrong unit, Bessey-Lowry-Brock unit and U/L (International unit). As the current trend is to express all enzyme activity by the International unit, one U/L signifies 1.0 mmole of chromogen from the substrate used per minute (and thus releases 1.0 mmole of chromogen from the substrate per minute) under the conditions of the assay.

Specimen

Serum is the preferred specimen but plasma (heparinized) can also be used. Other anticoagulants inhibit the activity of ALP. A blood specimen after overnight fasting is recommended, but a specimen collected at any other time can also be used. Separate the serum promptly and store in a refrigerator if immediate analysis is not possible. Red blood cells are high in acid phosphatase concentration and hence a haemolysed serum specimen is not acceptable for acid phosphatase determination of serum. In case of increased acid phosphatase activity due to haemolysis, check for "tartrate-inhibition". Acid phosphatase of red blood cells is not "tartrate-labile" and hence is not inhibited. Alkaline phosphatase (ALP) activity increases with storage, hence, as a general rule, it is best to analyse ALP specimens the same day they are drawn. Acid phosphatase (ACP) is best stored in acid medium, hence, maintain an acid pH with citric acid ("acid stabilizer"). Control sera must be treated in the same way after reconstitution. ACP is measured in vaginal washings in suspected rape cases and this must also be acidified.

ALKALINE PHOSPHATASE (ALP)

Clinical Significance

Increased alkaline phosphatase activity may be related to hepatobiliary and bone diseases. Very high alkaline phosphatase activity in serum is seen in patients with bone cancer, and marked increase also occur in obstructive jaundice and biliary cirrhosis. Moderate elevations have been noted in case of Hodgkin's disease, congestive heart failure, infective hepatitis and abdominal problems.

ALKALINE PHOSPHATASE, SERUM

Normal Values

Total Alkaline Phosphatase		*SI Units*
King-Armstrong Method		
Adult age 20-60	4.5-13 U/dl	32-92 U/L
Eldery	Slightly higher	
Newborn	5-15 U/dl	36-107 U/L
Premature newborn	1.5-2 times adult value	
Children: Values remain high until epiphyses close.		
1 month	10-30 U/dl	71-213 U/L
3 years	10-20 U/dl	71-142 U/L
10 years	15-30 U/dl	107-213 U/L
Bodansky Method		
Adults age 20-60	2-4 U/dl	10.7-21.5 U/L
Eldery	Slightly higher	
Children	5-14 U/dl	27-75 U/L
Bessey-Lowrey-Brock Method		
Adults age 20-60	0.8-2.3 U/dl	13.3-38.3 U/L
Eldery	Slightly higher	
Bowers and McComb Method		
Females		
Age 1-12	<350 U/L	<5.95 μKat/L
Puberty: Values may triple.		
Age >15	25-100 U/L	0.43-17.0 μKat/L
Males		
Age 1-12	<350 U/L	<5.95 μKat/L
Age 12-14	<500 U/L	<8.50 μKat/L
Puberty: Values may triple		
Age >20	25-100 U/L	0.43-1.70 μKat/L
Isoenzyme Normal Values		
Heat Inactivation Method	Percentage of Isoenzyme Inactivated After 16 Minutes at 55°C	Fraction of Isoenzyme Inactivated After 16 Minutes at 55°C
Liver isoenzyme	50-70	0.50-0.70
Bone isoenzyme	90-100	0.90-1.00
Intestinal isoenzyme	50-60	0.50-0.60
Placental isoenzyme		
Trimester 1 to 1 month postpartum 50% of total		

ALKALINE PHOSPHATASE (Mod. Kind and King's Method) (Courtesy: Tulip Group of Companies)

For the determination of Alkaline Phosphatase activity in serum. (for *in vitro* diagnostic use only)

Summary

Alkaline Phosphatase (ALP) is an enzyme of the Hydrolase class of enzymes and acts in an alkaline medium. It is found in high concentrations in the liver, biliary tract epithelium and in the bones. Normal levels are age dependent and increase during bone development. Increased levels are associated mainly with liver and bone disease. Moderate increases are seen in Hodgkin's disease and congestive heart failure.

Principle

ALP at an alkaline pH hydrolyses di sodium phenylphosphate to form phenol. The phenol formed reacts with 4-aminoantipyrine in the presence of potassium ferricyanide, as an oxidising agent, to form a red coloured complex. The intensity of the colour formed is directly proportional to the activity of ALP present in the sample.

di Na. Phenylphosphate + H_2O —ALP, pH 10.0→ Phenol + di Na. Hydrogen Phosphate

Phenol + 4-Aminoantipyrine —Alkaline Medium, $K_3Fe(CN)_6$→ Red Coloured Complex

Normal reference values

Total ALP activity : 3.0-13.0 KA units

It is recommended that each laboratory establish its own normal range representing its patient population.

Contents	15 Tests	30 Tests
L1: Buffer reagent	60 ml	120 ml
L2: Substrate reagent	6 ml	12 ml
L3: Colour reagent	60 ml	120 ml
S: Phenol standard (10 mg/dl)	5 ml	5 ml

Storage/stability

Contents are stable at 2-8°C till the expiry mentioned on the labels.

Reagent Preparation

All reagents are ready to use.

Sample Material

Serum free from hemolysis. ALP is reported to be stable in serum for 3 days at 2-8°C.

Procedure

Wavelength/filter : 510 nm (Hg 546 nm)/green
Temperature : 37°C
Light path : 1 cm
Assay:

Pipette into four clean dry test tubes labeled as Blank (B), **Standard** (S), (C), Test (T).

Addition	B	S	C	T
Sequence	ml	ml	ml	ml
Distilled water	1.05	1.00	1.0	1.0
Buffer reagent (L1)	1.0	1.0	1.0	1.0
Substrate reagent (L2)	0.10	0.10	0.10	0.10
Mix well and allow to stand at 37°C for 3 minutes and add.				
Sample	-	-	-	0.05
Phenol standard (S)	-	0.05	-	-
Mix well and allow to stand at 37°C for 15 minutes and add.				
Colour reagent (L3)	1.0	1.0	1.0	1.0
Sample	-	-	0.05	-

Mix well after each addition. Measure the absorbances of the blank (Abs. B), standard (Abs. S), control (Abs. C), and test (Abs. T) against distilled water.

Calculations

$$\text{Total ALP activity in KA units} = \frac{\text{Abs. T-Abs. C}}{\text{Abs. S-Abs. B}} \times 10$$

Linearity

If enzyme activity 60 KA. **Units** dilute the sample with distilled water and repeat the assay. Multiply the value with the proper dilution factor.

Note

In case or multiple samples to be assayed simultaneously, only one blank and standard can be run for the entire series, however for each sample a control and test assay has to be run additionally.

System Parameters			
Reaction	: End point abs	**Interval**	: —
Wavelength	: 510 nm	**Sample vol**	: 0.05 ml
Zero setting	: Distilled water	**Reagent vol**	: Calculate
Incub temp.	: 37°C	**Standard**	: Calculate
Incub time.	: 15 min	**Factor**	: —
Delay time	: —	**Reaction slope**	
Increasing			
Read time	: —	**Linearity**	: 60 KA units
No. of read	: —	**Units**	: KA units

ALKALINE PHOSPHATASE (DEA) (pNPP Kinetic Method) (Courtesy: Tulip Group of Companies)

For the determination of Alklaline Phosphatase activity in serum (For *in vitro* diagnostic use only)

Summary

Alkaline Phosphatase (ALP) is an enzyme of the Hydrolase class of enzymes and acts in an alkaline medium. It is found in high concentrations in the liver, biliary tract epithelium and in the bones. Normal levels are age dependent and increase during bone development. Increased levels are associated mainly with liver and bone disease. Moderate increases are seen in Hodgkin's disease and congestive heart failure.

Principle

ALP at an alkaline pH hydrolyses p-Nitrophenyl-phosphate to form p-Nitrophenol and Phosphate. The rate of 'formation of p-Nitrophenol is measured as an increase in absorbance which is proportional to the ALP activity in the sample.

$$\text{p-Nitrophenylphosphate} \xrightarrow{\text{ALP}} \text{p-Nitrophenol} + \text{Phosphate}$$

Normal reference values

Serum (Adults) : 80 - 290 U/L at 37°C
(Children) : 245 - 770 U/L at 37°C

It is recommended that each laboratory establish its own normal range representing its patient population.

Contents	10 × 3 ml	5 × 15 ml
L1 : Buffer Reagent	35 ml	80 ml
T1 : Substrate Reagent	10 Nos	5 Nos

Storage/stability

Contents are stable at 2-8°C till the expiry mentioned on the labels.

Reagent Preparation

Working reagent : Dissolve 1 substrate tablet in 3.2 ml (10 × 3 ml pack) or 15 ml (5 × 15 ml pack) of buffer reagent.

This working reagent is stable for at least 15 days when stored at 2-8°C.

The substrate is light and temperature sensitive. Take adequate care, especially after reconstitution.

Sample material

Serum. Free from hemolysis. ALP is reported to be stable in serum for 3 days at 2-8°C.

Procedure

Wavelength/filter : 405 nm
Temperature : 37°C/30°C/25°C
Light path : 1 cm

Pipette into a clean dry test tube labeled as Test (T):

Addition Sequence	(T) (ml)
Working Reagent	1.0
Incubate at the assay temperature for 1 minute and add	
Sample	0.02

Mix well and read the initial absorbance A_0 after minute and repeat the absorbance reading after every 1, 2, and 3 minutes. Calculate the mean absorbance change per minute (ΔA/min).

Calculations

ALP Activity in U/L=ΔA/min. × 2754.

Temperature Conversion Factors

Assay Temperature	Desired 25°C	Reporting 30°C	Temperature 37°C
25°C	1.00	1.22	1.64
30°C	0.82	1.00	1.33
37°C	0.61	0.75	1.00

Linearity

The procedure is linear upto 700 U/L at 37°C. If the absorbance change (ΔA/min) exceeds 0.250, use only the value of the first two minutes to calculate the result, or dilute the sample 1 + 9 with normal saline (NaCI 0.9%) and repeat the assay (Results × 10).

Note

Samples having a very high activity show a very high initial absorbance. If this is suspected then dilute the sample and repeat the assay.

System Parameters			
Reaction	: Kinetic	**Interval**	: 30
Wavelength	: 405 nm	**Sample vol**	: 0.02 ml
Zero setting	: Distilled water	**Reagent vol**	: 1.00 ml
Incub temp.	: 37°C	**Standard**	: —
Incub time.	: —	**Factor**	: 2754
Delay time	: 30 sec.	**Factor**	: Increasing
Read time	: 120 sec.	**Linearity**	: 700 U/L
No. of read	: 4	**Units**	: U/L

Clinical Relevance

Elevated Levels

1. Liver disease (correlates with abnormal liver function tests). An elevation of serum alkaline phosphatase is often associated with elevated SGOT/SGPT and raised bilirubin
   a. Marked increases
      1. Obstructive jaundice (gallstones obstructing major biliary ducts, accompanies elevated bilirubin).
      2. Space occupying lesions of the liver such as cancer and abscesses.
      3. Hepatocellular cirrhosis.
      4. Biliary cirrhosis.
   b. Moderate increases
      1. Hepatitis
      2. Cirrhosis of liver
2. Bone disease
   a. Marked increases
      1. Paget's disease
      2. Metastatic bone disease
      3. Osteitis deformans
   b. Moderate increases
      1. Osteomalacia (in osteoporosis, no increase in ALP)
      2. Rickets
3. Other diseases
   a. Hyperparathyroidism (accompanied by hypercalcemia)
   b. Infectious mononucleosis

Reduced Levels

1. Hypophosphatasia (markedly reduced)
2. Malnutrition
3. Hypothyroidism
4. Pernicious anaemia
5. Scurvy
6. Milk-alkali syndrome
7. Placental insufficiency.

Interfering Factors

1. Many drugs produce mild to moderate elevations of ALP, e.g.
   a. Phenothiazine tranquillisers
   b. Methyltestosterone
   c. Oral contraceptives
   d. Allopurinol
   e. Methyldopa
   f. Procainamide
   g. Tolbutamide
   h. Isoniazid
   i. PAS
   j. Erythromycin
   k. Oxacilin
   l. Ergoesterol
2. Young children, pregnant women in the third trimester, and all women have physiologically high levels of alkaline phosphatase.
3. The level is slightly increased in older people.
4. After IV administration of albumin there is sometimes a marked increase lasting for several days.
5. Drugs that may cause decreased levels
   a. Fluoride
   b. Oxalates
   c. Phosphates
   d. Propranolol
   e. Vitamin D.

ALKALINE PHOSPHATASE ISOENZYMES

Normal Values

AP-1, Alpha 2: Values are reported as weak, moderate, or strong

AP-2, Beta 1: Values are reported as weak, moderate, or strong

AP-3, Beta 2: Values are reported as weak, moderate, or strong

The isoenzymes of alkaline phoshphatase (ALP) are produced by various tissues. AP-1, Alpha 2 is heat labile and is produced in the liver and by proliferating blood vessels. AP-2, Beta 1 is heat stable and is produced by bone and placenta. The intestinal isoenzymes AP-3, Beta 2 is present in small quantities in Group O and B individuals AP-1 and 2 can be distinguished partially in the laboratory by heating and urea testing. Placental alkaline phosphatase is still more stable to heat than urea.

The test is conducted (when the total alkaline phosphatase is raised) to distinguish between bone and liver origin of alkaline phosphatase.

Clinical Relevance

1. Osteoblastic bone tumors, increase the bone alkaline phosphatase in the blood serum; less than 25% is thermostable in bone disease.
2. Liver diseases such as cancer and biliary obstruction increase the liver isoenzyme, more than 25% in thermostable in hepatic disease.

3. The intestinal isoenzyme may be increased in patients with cirrhosis.
4. The placental isoenzymes is increased in some patients with cancer (cancinopla-cental antigen) and normally in pregnancy.

ACID PHOSPHATASE

Clinical Significance

Request for the analysis of serum acid phosphatase is often done in male patients with suspected prostatic cancer. The increase of serum acid phosphatase activity in such patients is found to be inhibited by tartrate. Acid phosphatase is also present in very high concentrations in semen, a fact utilised in forensic medicine in the investigations of rape offences.

Normal Values

Method		*SI Units*
Bodansky	0.5-2 U/L	2.7-10.7 IU/L
King-Armstrong	0.1-5 U/L	0.2-8.8 IU/L
Bessey-Lowery-Brock	0.1-0.8 U/L	1.7-13.4 IU/L
Gutman	0.1-2 U/L	1.7-13.4 IU/L

Specimen

Serum is the most commonly used specimen; haemolysed serum specimens are contaminated with red cell acid phosphatase and should be rejected.

ACID PHOSPHATASE (Mod. King's Method) Courtesy: Tulip Group of Companies

For the determination of Acid Phosphatase activity in serum. (For *in vitro* diagnostic use only)

Summary

Acid phosphatase (ACP) is an enzyme of the Hydrolase class of enzymes and acts in an acidic medium. It is widely distributed and found in high concentrations in the liver, RBCs and the prostate. Increased levels of the prostatic fraction are associated with prostatic carcinomas. Increased levels of the non prostatic fraction are associated with liver diseases, hyperparathyroidism, and Paget's disease.

Principle

ACP at an acidic pH hydrolyses di Sodium Phenylphosphate to form phenol. The Phenol formed reacts with 4-Aminoantipyrine in the presence of Potassium Ferricyanide, as an oxidising agent, to form a red coloured complex. The intensity of the colour formed is directly proportional to the activity of ACP present in the sample. Tartrate inhibits prostatic ACP and the testing in its presence is done to find the non prostatic ACP. The difference between the activities of the total and non prostatic ACP gives the activity of the prostatic ACP.

$$\text{di Na. Phenyl Phosphate} + H_2O \xrightarrow[\text{pH } 5.0]{\text{ACP}} \text{Phenol} + \text{di Na. Hydrogen Phosphate}$$

$$\text{Phenol} + \text{4-Aminoantipyrine} \xrightarrow[K_3Fe(CN)_6]{\text{Alkaline Medium}} \text{Red Coloured Complex}$$

Normal reference values

Total ACP Activity : 1.0 - 4.0 KA Units
Prostatic ACP Activity : 0.0 - 0.8 KA Units

It is recommended that each laboratory establish its own normal range representing its patient population.

Contents	10 Tests	25 Tests
L1: Buffer Reagent	50 ml	125 ml
L2: Substrate Reagent	5 ml	12.5 ml
L3: Colour Reagent	50 ml	125 ml
L4: Tartrate Reagent	2 ml	2 ml
S : Phenol **Standard** (10 mg/dl)	5 ml	5 ml

Storage/stability

Contents are stable at 2-8°C till the expiry mentioned on the labels.

Reagent Preparation

All reagents are ready to use.

Sample material

Serum. Free from haemolysis.

ACP, especially the prostatic fraction, is unstable in a collected sample hence the serum should be separated from the clot, as soon as possible, and assayed. In case of a delay in testing the serum should be acidified to a pH of 5.0 with 0.02 ml Acetate Buffer (5M) for each ml of serum.

Procedure

Wavelength/filter : 510 nm (Hg 546 nm) / Green
Temperature : 37°C
Light path : 1 cm

Assay

Pipette into five clean dry test tubes labeled as Blank (B), **Standard** (S), Control (C), Test (T), and Tartrate Stable (TS).

Addition Sequence	B (ml)	S (ml)	C (ml)	T (ml)	TS (ml)
Distilled water	1.1	1.05	1.0	1.0	1.0
Buffer Reagent (L1)	1.0	1.0	1.0	1.0	1.0
Substrate Reagent (L2)	0.10	0.10	0.10	0.10	0.10
Mix well and allow to stand at 37°C for 3 minutes and add.					
Tartrate Reagent (L4)	-	-	-	-	0.02
Sample	-	-	-	0.1	0.1
Phenol **Standard** (S)	-	0.05			
Mix well and allow to stand at 37°C for 60 minutes and add.					
Colour Reagent (L3)	1.0	1.0	1.0	1.0	1.0
Sample	-	-	0.1	-	

Mix well after each addition. Measure the absorbances of the Blank (Abs.B), **Standard** (Abs.S), Control (Abs.C), Test (Abs.T), and Tartrate Stable (Abs.TS) against Distilled water.

Calculations

$$\text{Total ACP activity in K.A. Units} = \frac{\text{Abs. T - Abs. C}}{\text{Abs. S - Abs. B}} \times 5.0$$

$$\text{Prostatic ACP activity in KA units} = \frac{\text{Abs. T - Abs. TS}}{\text{Abs. S - Abs. B}} \times 5.0$$

Linearity

If Enzyme activity exceeds 40 KA.Units dilute the sample with distilled water\and repeat the assay. Multiply the value obtained with an appropriate dilution factor.

Notes

In case of multiple samples to be assayed **simultaneously,** only one Blank and Standard can be run for the entire series, however for each sample a Control, Test and Tartrate Stable assay has to be run additionally. It has been seen that in a collected sample ACP, especially the prostatic form, may loose around 50% of its activity in an hour at R.T.

System Parameters			
Reaction	: End Point Abs.	**Interval**	:
Wavelength	: 510 nm	**Sample vol**	: 0.10 ml
Zero setting	: Distilled water	**Reagent vol**	: 3.10 ml
Incub temp.	: 37°C	**Standard**	: Calculate
Incub time.	: 60 min	**Factor**	:
Delay time	: —	**Factor**	: Increasing
Read time	: —	**Linearity**	: 40 KA **Units**
No. of read	: —	**Units**	: KA **Units**

ACID PHOSPHATASE (α Naphthylphosphate Kinetic Method) (Courtesy: Tulip Group of Companies)

For the determination of Acid Phosphatase activity in serum (For *in vitro* diagnostic use only)

Summary

Acid Phosphatase (ACP) is an enzyme of the Hydrolase class of enzymes and acts in an acidic medium. It is widely distributed and found in high concentrations in the liver, RBCs and the prostate. Increased levels of the prostatic fraction are associated with prostatic carcinomas. Increased levels of the non prostatic fraction are associated with liver diseases, hyperparathyroidism, and Paget's disease.

Principle

ACP at an acidic pH hydrolyses α Naphthylphosphate to form α Naphthol and Inorganic Phosphate. The α Naphthol formed is coupled with Fast Red TR salt to form a diazo dye complex. The rate of formation of this complex is measured as an increase in absorbance which is proportional to the ACP activity in the sample. Tartrate inhibits prostatic ACP and the testing in it's presence is done to find the non prostatic ACP. The difference between the activities of the total and non prostatic ACP gives the activity of the prostatic ACP.

$$\alpha \text{ Naphthylphosphate} + H_2O \xrightarrow{\text{ACP}} \alpha \text{ Naphthol} + \text{Phosphate}$$
$$\alpha \text{ Naphthol} + \text{Fast Red TR Salt} \longrightarrow \text{Diazo dye complex}$$

Normal reference values

Serum (male) : upto 4.2 U/L at 30°C/upto 4.7 U/L at 37°C
(female) : upto 3.0 U/L at 30°C/upto 3.7 U/L at 37°C
Prostatic ACP : upto 1.5 U/L at 30°C/upto 1.6 U/L at 37°C

It is recommended that each laboratory establish its own normal range representing its patient population.

Contents	10 × 2 ml	30 × 2 ml
L1 : Buffer Reagent	25 ml	75 ml
T1 : Substrate Tablets	10 Nos	30 Nos
L2 : Tartrate Reagent	2 ml	2 ml
L3 : Acetate Buffer	2 ml	2 ml

Storage/stability

Contents are stable at 2-8°C till the expiry mentioned on the labels.

Reagent Preparation

Reagents L2 and L3 are ready to use.

The Buffer (L1) when retrieved from 2-8°C may appear turbid. However the turbidity clears up on attaining RT. In case the turbidity persists a little warning of the Buffer to 30°C/37°C may be required.

Working reagent: Dissolve 1 Substrate tablet (T1) in 2.2 ml of Buffer Reagent (L1). Allow the tablet to hydrate for around 5 min and then shake to dissolve. This working reagent is stable for at least 3 days when stored at 2-8°C. The working reagent may be used for the Total ACP assay or the non prostatic ACP assay as required.

Sample material

Serum. Free from haemolysis.

ACP, especially the prostatic fraction, is unstable in a collected sample hence the serum should be separated from the clot, as soon as possible, and assayed. In case of a delay in testing the serum should be acidified to a pH of 5.0 with 0.02 ml Acetate Buffer (5M) provided for each ml of serum.

Procedure

Wavelength/filter : 405 nm
Temperature : 30°C/37°C
Light path : 1 cm

Total ACP Assay

Pipette into a clean dry test tube labeled as Test (T) :

Addition Sequence	(T) (ml)
Working Reagent	1.0
Sample	0.1

Mix well and read the initial absorbance A_0 after 5 minutes and repeat the absorbance reading after every 1, 2, and 3 minutes. Calculate the mean absorbance change per minute (ΔA/min)

Non Prostatic ACP Assay : (Tartrate Inhibited)

Pipette into a clean dry test tube labelled as Test (T):

Addition Sequence	(T) (ml)
Working Reagent Tartrate Reagent	1.0 0.02
Incubate at the assay temperature for 1 minute and add	
Sample	0.1

Mix well and read the initial absorbance A_0 after 5 minutes and repeat the absorbance reading after every 1, 2, and 3 minutes. Calculate the mean absorbance change per minute (ΔA/min)

Calculations

ACP Activity in U/L = ΔA/min × 750
Prostatic ACP Activity in U/L = Total ACP-Non Prostatic ACP

Linearity

The procedure is linear upto 75 U/L at 37°C. If the absorbance change (ΔA/min) exceeds 0.100, dilute the sample 1 + 4 with normal saline (NaCI 0.9%) and repeat the assay (Results ×5).

Notes

Samples having a high activity show a very high initial absorbance. If this is suspected then dilute the sample and repeat the assay.

The working reagent should have an absorbance below 0.800 against distilled water at 405 nm. Discard the reagent if the absorbance is above 0.800. It has been seen that in a collected sample ACP, especially the prostatic form, may loose around 50% of its activity in an hour at RT.

System Parameters			
Reaction	: Kinetic	**Interval**	: 60
Wavelength	: 405 nm	**Sample vol**	: 0.1 ml
Zero setting	: Distilled water	**Reagent vol**	: 1.00 ml
Incub temp.	: 30°C/37°C	**Standard**	:
Incub time.	: —	**Factor**	: 750.0
Delay time	: 300 sec.	**Read scope**	: Increasing
Read time	: 180 sec	**Linearity**	: 75 U/L
No. of read	:	**Units**	: U/L

CLINICAL RELEVANCE

1. A significantly elevated value nearly always indicative of metastatic cancer of the prostate. If the tumour is successfully treated, this enzyme level will drop within 3 to 4 days after surgery or 3 to 4 weeks after estrogen adminstration.
2. Moderately increased values also occur in the absence of prostate disease in
   a. Paget's disease
   b. Gaucher's disease
   c. Hyperparathyroidism
   d. Multiple myeloma
   e. Any cancer that has metastasized to the bone
   f. Hepatitis
   g. Obstructive jaundice
   h. Acute renal impairment
   i. Sickle cell crisis/hemolytic anemia
   j. Excessive destruction of platelets
3. Levels are reported to be elevated in the bone marrow of patients with prostatic cancer metastatic to the bone.

Interfering Factors

1. Drugs that may cause increased levels include
   a. Androgen in females
   b. Clofibrate
2. Drugs that may cause decreased levels include
   a. Fluorides
   b. Oxalates
   c. Phosphates

Serum Alkaline Phosphatase and Acid Phosphatase

The following table gives the differences between the two:

Serum Alkaline Phosphatase	*Serum Acid Phosphatase*
1. Alkaline optimum (pH=10.0)	Acid optimum (pH=4.9)
2. Three isoenzymes known —from bone, liver and intestine	Two isoenzymes known
3. Inhibited by EDTA	Inhibited by oxalate and fluoride — Prostatic acid phosphatase is inhibited by tartrate
4. Tissue sources— Osteoblast of bone, liver cells, intestine, kidney and placenta	Bone, liver, spleen, kidney, prostate and red cells
5. Normal values 3-13 KA units	1-4 KA units

TRANSAMINASES

Transmination is a process in which an amino group is transferred from an amino acid to an alpha-ketoacid. It is an important step in the metabolism of amino acids. The enzymes responsible for transamination are called transaminase (now called, aminotransferases). Two diagnostically useful transaminases are glutamate oxalacetate transminase or GOT or aspartate, aminotransferase and glutamate pyruvate transaminase or GPT alanine amino transferase. These enzymes catalyse the following reactions:

$$\text{L-aspartate + Oxoglutarate (or ketoglutarate)} \xrightarrow{\text{GOT/AST}} \text{Oxalacetate+ Glutamate}$$

$$\text{L-alanine + Oxoglutarate (or ketoglutarate)} \xrightarrow{\text{GPT/ALT}} \text{Pyruvate + Glutamate}$$

Clinical Significance

Increased serum transaminase activity is seen in liver dysfunction. Greater activity of GOT (AST) over GPT (ALT) is typical of myocardial infarction.

Evaluation of Methods

The two methods applied in the analysis of transaminase activity are colorimetry and ultraviolet spectrophotometry. The latter procedure requires NADH, coenzyme. The colorimetric method is discussed below.

Specimen

The serum specimen submitted for the enzyme assay of SGOT and SGPT should be free from haemolysis.

Collect the serum by the usual procedure described earlier. Prompt analysis is recommended and if this is not possible, refrigerate the specimen.

SGOT (AST) (Reitman and Frankel's Method) Courtesy: Tulip Group of Companies

For the determination of SGOT (AST) activity in serum (For *in vitro* diagnostic use only)

Summary

SGOT is an enzyme found mainly in heart muscle, liver cells, skeletal muscle and kidneys. Injury to these tissues results in the release of the enzyme in blood stream. Elevated levels are found in myocardial infarction, Cardiac operations, Hepatitis, Cirrhosis, acute pancreatitis, acute renal diseases, primary muscle diseases. Decreased levels may be found in Pregnancy, Beri Beri and Diabetic ketoacidosis.

Principle

SGOT converts L-Aspartate and α Ketoglutarate to Oxaloacetate and Glutamate. The Oxaloacetate formed reacts with 2,4,Dinitrophenyl hydrazine to produce a hydrazone derivative, which in an alkaline medium produces a brown coloured complex whose intensity is measured. The reaction does not obey Beer's law and hence a calibration curve is plotted using a Pyruvate standard. The activity of SGOT (ASAT) is read off this calibration curve.

$$\text{L-Aspartate} + \alpha\text{Ketoglutarate} \xrightarrow[\text{pH 7.4}]{\text{SGOT}} \text{Oxaloacetate} + \text{L-Glutamate}$$

$$\text{Oxaloacetate} + \text{2,4,DNPH} \xrightarrow[\text{Medium}]{\text{Alkaline}} \text{2,4,Dinitrophenyl Hydrazone (Brown coloured complex)}$$

Normal reference values

Serum : 8-40 **Units**/ml

It is recommended that each laboratory establish its own normal range representing its patient population.

Contents	40 assays
L1 : Substrate reagent	25 ml
L2 : DNPH reagent	2 × 12.5 ml
L3 : NaOH reagent (4N)	25 ml
S : Pyruvate standard (2 mM)	5 ml

Storage/stability

Contents are stable at 2-8°C till the expiry mentioned on the labels. Sodium hydroxide can be stored at RT till the expiry mentioned.

Reagent Preparation

All reagents are ready to use except NaOH reagent (4N) which has to be diluted 1:10 with distilled/ deionised water.

Working NaOH reagent: Dilute the sodium hydroxide to 250 ml or for every 1.0 ml of NaOH reagent (4N) add 9.0 ml of distilled water. The working sodium hydroxide reagent is stable at RT till the expiry mentioned, in a plastic bottle.

Sample Material

Serum. Free from hemolysis SGOT (ASAT) is reported to be stable in serum for 3 days at 2-8°C.

Procedure

Wavelength/filter : 505 nm (Hg 546 nm)/green
Temperature : 37°C and RT
Light path : 1 cm

Plotting of the calibration curve.

Pipette into five clean dry test tubes labeled as 1, 2, 3, 4, and 5.

Addition sequence Enzyme activity (U/ml)	1 0 ml	2 24 ml	3 61 ml	4 114 ml	5 190 ml
Substrate reagent (L1)	0.50	0.45	0.40	0.35	0.30
Pyruvate standard (S)	-	0.05	0.10	0.15	0.20
Distilled water	0.10	0.10	0.10	0.10	0.10
DNPH reagent (L2)	0.50	0.50	0.50	0.50	0.50
Mix well and allow to stand at RT for 20 minutes					
Working NaOH reagent (L3)	5.00	5.00	5.00	5.00	5.00

Mix well and allow to stand at RT for 10 min. Measure the absorbances of the tubes 2-5 against tube 1 (blank). Plot a graph of the absorbances of tubes 2-5 on the 'Y' axis versus the corresponding enzyme activity on the 'X' axis.

Assay

Pipette into clean dry test tubes labeled as blank (B) and Test (T):

Addition Sequence	B ml	T ml
Substrate reagent (L1)	0.50	0.50
Incubate at 37°C for 3 minutes		
Sample	-	0.10
Mix well and incubate at 37°C for 60 minutes		
DNPH reagent (L2)	0.50	0.50
Mix well and allow to stand at RT for 20 minutes		
Distilled water	0.10	-
Working NaOH reagent (L3)	5.00	5.00

Mix well and allow to stand at RT for 10 min. Measure the absorbance of the test (T) against blank (Blank) and read the activity of the test from the calibration curve plotted earlier.

Note

One sample blank is sufficient for each assay series.

If enzyme activity exceeds 190 U/ml dilute the sample with distilled water and repeat the assay. Multiply the value with the proper dilution factor.

High concentration of aldehydes and ketones in the sample or icteric or lipemic, samples may cause slightly elevated results. It is recommended to run a sample blank for these samples using serum instead of distilled water in the blank. High levels of serum pyruvate may interfere with results.

System Parameters

Reaction	: End point	**Interval**	: —
Wavelength	: 505 nm	**Sample vol**	: 0.10 ml
Zero setting	: Reagent blank	**Reagent vol**	: 6.00 ml
Incub temp.	: 37°C	**Standard**	: Calib curve
Incub time.	: 80 min	**Factor**	: —
Delay time	: —	**React slope**	: Increasing
Read time	: —	**Linerity**	: 190 U/ml
No. of read	: —	**Units**	: U/ml

SGOT (AST) (Mod. IFCC Method) Courtesy: Tulip Group of Companies

For the determination of SGOT (ASAT) activity in serum (For *in vitro* diagnostic use only)

Summary

SGOT is an enzyme found mainly in heart muscle, liver cells, skeletal muscle and kidneys. Injury to these tissues results in the release of the enzyme in blood. Elevated levels are found in myocardial infarction, Cardiac operations, Hepatitis, Cirrhosis, acute pancreatitis, acute renal diseases, primary muscle diseases. Decreased levels may be found in Pregnancy, Beri Beri and Diabetic ketoacidosis.

Principle

SGOT (ASAT) catalyzes the transfer of amino group between L-Aspartate and α Ketoglutarate to form Oxaloacetate and Glutamate. The Oxaloacetate formed reacts with NADH in the presence of Malate Dehydrogenase to form NAD. The rate of oxidation of NADH to NAD is measured as a decrease in absorbance which is proportional to the SGOT (ASAT) activity in the sample.

$$\text{L-Aspartate} + \alpha\ \text{Ketoglutarate} \xrightarrow{\text{SGOT}} \text{Oxaloacetate} + \text{L-Glutamate}$$

$$\text{Oxaloacetate} + \text{NADH} + H^+ \xrightarrow{\text{MDH}} \text{Malate} + \text{NAD}^+$$

Normal reference values

Serum(males) : upto 37 U/L at 37°C

(females) : upto 31 U/L at 37°C

It is recommended that each laboratory establish its own normal range representing its patient population.

Contents	25 ml	75 ml
L1 : Enzyme Reagent	20 ml	60 ml
L2 : Starter Reagent	5 ml	15 ml

Storage/stability

Contents are stable at 2-8° C till the expiry mentioned on the labels.

Reagent Preparation

Reagents are ready to use.

Working reagent : For sample start assays a single reagent is required. Pour the contents of 1 bottle of L2 (Starter Reagent) into 1 bottle of L1 (Enzyme Reagent). This working reagent is stable for at least 3 weeks when stored at 2-8°C.

Alternatively for flexibility as much of working reagent may be made as and when desired by mixing together 4 parts of L1 (Enzyme Reagent) and 1 part of L2 (Starter Reagent). Alternatively 0.8 ml of L1 and 0.2 ml of L2 may also be used instead of 1 ml of the working reagent directly during the assay.

Sample material

Serum. Free from hemolysis. SGOT (ASAT) is reported to be stable in serum for 3 days at 2-8°C.

Procedure

Wavelength/filter : 340 nm
Temperature : 37°C/30°C/25°C
Light path : 1 cm

Substrate Start Assay

Pipette into a clean dry test tube labeled as Test (T):

Addition Sequence	(T) 25°C / 30°C	(T) 37°C
Enzyme Reagent (L1)	0.8 ml	0.8 ml
Sample	0.2 ml	0.1ml
Incubate at the assay temperature for 1 minute and add		
Starter Reagent (L2)	0.2 ml	0.2 ml

Mix well and read the initial absorbance A_0 and repeat the absorbance reading after every 1, 2, and 3 minutes. Calculate the mean absorbance change perminute (ΔA/min)

Sample Start Assay

Pipette into a clean dry test tube labeled as Test (T):

Addition Sequence	(T) 25°C / 30°C	(T) 37°C
Working Reagent	1.0 ml	1.0 ml
Incubate at the assay temperature for 1 minute and add		
Sample	0.2 ml	0.1 ml

Mix well and read the initial absorbance A_0 after 1 minute and repeat the absorbance reading after every 1, 2, and 3 minutes. Calculate the mean absorbance change per minute (ΔA /min).

Calculations

Substrate/sample start

SGOT (ASAT) Activity in U/L 25°C/30°C = ΔA /min × 952
SGOT (ASAT) Activity in U/L 37°C = ΔA /min × 1746

TEMPERATURE CONVERSION FACTORS

Assay Temperature	Desired Reporting Temperature 25°C	30°C	37°C
25°C	1.00	1.37	2.08
30°C	0.73	1.00	1.54
37°C	0.48	0.65	1.00

Linearity

The procedure is linear upto 500 U/L at 37°C. If the absorbance change (ΔA /min) exceeds 0.250, use only the value of the first two minutes to calculate the result, or dilute the sample 1+9 with normal saline (NaCI 0.9%) and repeat the assay (Resultsx10).

Note

Samples having a very high activity show a very low initial absorbance as most of the NADH is consumed prior to the start of measurement. If this is suspected then dilute the sample and repeat the assay.

The working reagent or the combined reagent should have an absorbance above 1.000 against distilled water at 340 nm. Discard the reagent if the absorbance is below 1.000

System parameters			
Reaction	: UV kinetic	**Interval**	: 60
Wavelength	: 340 nm	**Sample vol**	: 0.10 ml
Zero setting	: Distilled water	**Reagent vol**	: 1.00 ml
Incub temp.	: 37°C	**Standard**	: —
Incub time.	: —	**Factor**	: 1746
Delay time	: 60 sec	**Reac. slope**	: Decreasing
Read time	: 180 sec	**Linerity**	: 500 U/L
No. of read	: 4	**Units**	: U/L

SGPT (ALT) (Reitman and Frankel's Method) Courtesy: Tulip Group of Companies

For the determination of SGPT (ALAT) activity in serum (For *in vitro* diagnostic use only)

Summary

SGPT is found in a variety of tissues but is mainly found in the liver. Increased levels are found in hepatitis, cirrhosis, obstructive jaundice and other hepatic diseases. Slight elevation of the enzymes is also seen in myocardial infarction.

Principle

SGPT converts L-Alanine and α Ketoglutarate to Pyruvate and Glutamate. The Pyruvate formed reacts with 2,4,Dinitrophenyl hydrazine to produce a hydrazone derivative, which in an alkaline medium produces a brown coloured complex whose intensity is measured. The reaction does not obey Beer's law and hence a calibration curve is plotted using a Pyruvate standard. The activity of SGPT (ALAT) is read off this calibration curve.

$$\text{L-Alanine} + \alpha\text{Ketoglutarate} \xrightarrow[\text{pH 7.4}]{\text{SGPT}} \text{Pyruvate} + \text{L-Glutamate}$$

$$\text{Pyruvate} + \text{2,4,DNPH} \xrightarrow[\text{Medium}]{\textit{Alkaline}} \text{2,4,Dinitrophenyl Hydrazone (Brown coloured complex)}$$

Normal reference values

Serum =5-35 Units/ml

It is recommended that each laboratory establish its own normal range representing its patient population.

Contents	40 assays
L1 : Substrate Reagent	25 ml
L2 : DNPH Reagent	2 × 12.5 ml
L3 : NaOH Reagent (4N)	25 ml
S : Pyruvate **Standard** (2mM)	5 ml

Storage/stability

Contents are stable at 2-8°C till the expiry mentioned on the labels. Sodium Hydroxide can be stored at RT till the expiry mentioned.

Reagent Preparation

All reagents are ready to use except NaOH Reagent (4N) which has to be diluted 1:10 with distilled/deionised water.

Working NaOH reagent: Dilute the sodium hydroxide to 250 ml or for every 1.0 ml of NaOH reagent (4N) add 9.0 ml of water. The working sodium hydroxide reagent is stable at RT till the expiry mentioned, in a plastic bottle.

Sample material

Serum. Free from haemolysis. SGPT (ALAT) is reported to be stable in serum for 3 days at 2-8°C.

Procedure

Wavelength/filter : 505 nm (Hg 546 nm)/Green
Temperature : 37°C and RT
Light path : 1 cm

Plotting of the Calibration curve

Pipette into five clean dry test tubes labeled as 1, 2, 3, 4, and 5:

Addition sequence Enzyme Activity (U/ml)	1 0 (ml)	2 28 (ml)	3 57 (ml)	4 97 (ml)	5 150 (ml)
Substrate Reagent (L1)	0.50	0.45	0.40	0.35	0.30
Pyruvate Standard (S)	-	0.05	0.10	0.15	0.20
Distilled water	0.10	0.10	0.10	0.10	0.10
DNPH Reagent (L2)	0.50	0.50	0.50	0.50	0.50
Mix well and allow to stand at RT for 20 minutes.					
Working NaOH Reagent (L3)	5.00	5.00	5.00	5.00	5.00

Mix well and allow to stand at R.T. for 10 min Measure the absorbances of the tubes 2 - 5 against tube 1 (Blank). Plot a graph of the absorbances of tubes 2-5 on the Y axis versus the corresponding Enzyme activity on the 'X' axis.

Assay

Pipette into clean dry test tubes labeled as Blank (B) and Test (T).

Addition Sequence	(B) (ml)	(T) (ml)
Substrate Reagent (L1)	0.50	0.50
Incubate at 37°C for 3 minutes		
Sample	-	0.10
Mix well and incubate at 37°C for 30 minutes		
DNPH Reagent (L2)	0.50	0.50
Mix well and allow to stand at R.T. for 20 minutes.		
Distilled water	0.10	
Working NaOH reagent (L3)	5.00	5.00

Mix well and allow to stand at R.T. for 10 min Measure the absorbances of the Test (T) against Blank (Blank) and read the activity of the test from the calibration curve plotted earlier.

Note

One sample blank is sufficient for each assay series.

If enzymes activity exceeds 150 U/ml dilute the sample with distilled water and repeat the assay. Multiply the value with proper dilution factor.

High concentration of aldehydes and ketones in the sample or icteric or lipemic, samples may cause slightly elevated results. It is recommended to run a sample blank for these samples using serum instead of distilled water in the blank. High levels of serum pyruvate may interfere with the results.

System Parameters			
Reaction	: End point	**Interval**	: —
Wavelength	: 505 nm	**Sample vol**	: 0.10 ml
Zero setting	: Reagent blank	**Reagent vol**	: 6.00 ml
Incub temp.	: 37°C	**Standard**	: Calib curve
Incub time.	: 50 min	**Factor**	: —
Delay time	: —	**Reac. slope**	: Increasing
Read time	: —	**Linearity**	: 150 U/ml
No. of read	: —	**Units**	: U/ml

SGPT (ALT) (Mod. IFCC Method)
Courtesy: Tulip Group of Companies

For the determination of SGPT (ALAT) activity in serum (For *in vitro* diagnostic use only).

Summary

SGPT is found in a variety of tissues but is mainly found in the liver. Increased levels are found in hepatitis, cirrhosis, obstructive jaundice and other hepatic diseases. Slight elevation of the enzymes is also seen in myocardial infarction.

Principle

SGPT (ALAT) catalyzes the transfer of amino group between L-Alanine and α Ketoglutarate to form Pyruvate and Glutamate. The Pyruvate formed reacts with NADH in the presence of Lactate Dehydrogenase to form NAD. The rate of oxidation of NADH to NAD is measured as a decrease in absorbance which is proportional to the SGPT (ALAT) activity in the sample.

$$\text{L- Alanine} + \alpha\ \text{Ketoglutarate} \xrightarrow{\text{SGPT}} \text{Pyruvate} + \text{L-Glutamate}$$

$$\text{Pyruvate} + \text{NADH} + \text{H} \xrightarrow{\text{LDH}} \text{Lactate} + \text{NAD}^+$$

Normal reference values

Serum (males) : upto 40 U/L at 37°C
(females) : upto 31 U/L at 37°C

It is recommended that each laboratory establish its own normal range representing its patient population.

Contents	25 ml	75 ml
L1 : Enzyme Reagent	20 ml	60 ml
L2 : Starter Reagent	5 ml	15 ml

Storage/stability

Contents are stable at 2-8° C till the expiry mentioned on the labels.

Reagent Preparation

Reagents are ready to use.

Working reagent : For sample start assays a single reagent is required. Pour the contents of 1 bottle of L2 (Starter Reagent) into 1 bottle of L1 (Enzyme Reagent). This working reagent is stable for at least 3 weeks when stored at 2-8 degree C. Alternatively for flexibility as much of working reagent may be made as and when desired by mixing together 4 parts of L1 (Enzyme Reagent) and 1 part of L2 (Starter Reagent). Alternatively 0.8 ml of L1 and 0.2 ml of L2 may also be used instead of 1 ml of the working reagent directly during the assay.

Sample material

Serum. Free from hemolysis. SGPT (ALAT) is reported to be stable in serum for 3 days at 2-8° C.

Procedure

Wavelength/filter : 340 nm
Temperature : 37°C/30°C/25°C
Light path : 1 cm

Substrate Start Assay

Pipette into a clean dry test tube labeled as Test (T):

Addition Sequence	(T) 25°C / 30°C	(T) 37°C
Enzyme Reagent (L1) Sample	0.8 ml 0.2 ml	0.8 ml 0.1 ml
Incubate at the assay temperature for 1 minute and add		
Starter Reagent (L2)	0.2 ml	0.2 ml

Mix well and read the initial absorbance A_0 and repeat the absorbance reading after every 1,2, and 3 minutes. Calculate the mean absorbance change per minute (ΔA /min)

Sample Start Assay

Pipette into a clean dry test tube labeled as Test (T):

Addition Sequence	(T) 25°C / 30°C	(T) 37°C
Working Reagent	1.0 ml	1.0 ml
Incubate at the assay temperature for 1 minute and add		
Sample	0.2 ml	0.1 ml

Mix well and read the initial absorbance A_0 after 1 minute and repeat the absorbance reading after every 1, 2, and 3 minutes. Calculate the mean absorbance change per minute (ΔA/min)

Calculations

Substrate/Sample start

SGPT (ALAT) Activity in U/L 25°C/30°C = ΔA /min x 952

SGPT (ALAT) Activity in U/L 37°C = ΔA /min x 1746

TEMPERATURE CONVERSION FACTORS

Assay Temperature	Desired 25°C	Reporting 30°C	Temperature 37°C
25°C	1.00	1.32	1.82
30°C	0.76	1.00	1.38
37°C	0.55	0.72	1.00

Linearity

The procedure is linear upto 500 U/L at 37°C. If the absorbance change (ΔA/min) exceeds 0.250, use only the value of the first two minutes to calculate the result, or dilute the sample 1 + 9 with normal saline (NaCI 0.9%) and repeat the assay (Results ×10).

Note

Samples having a very high activity show a very low initial absorbance as most of the NADH is consumed prior to the start of measurement. If this is suspected then dilute the sample and repeat the assay.

The working reagent or the combined reagent should have an absorbance above 1.000 against distilled water at 340 mn. Discard the reagent if the absorbance is below 1.000.

System Parameters

Reaction	: UV Kinetic	**Interval**	: 60
Wavelength	: 340 nm	**Sample vol**	: 0.10 ml
Zero setting	: Distilled water	**Reagent vol**	: 1.00 ml
Incub temp.	: 37°C	**Standard**	:
Incub time.	: —	**Factor**	: 1746
Delay time	: 60 sec.	**Reac. slope**	: Decreasing
Read time	: 180 sec.	**Linearity**	: 500 U/L
No. of read	: 4	**Units**	: U/L

CLINICAL RELEVANCE OF SGPT ESTIMATION

A. *Increased levels are found in*
1. Hepatocellular disease (moderate to high increase)
2. Active cirrhosis (mild increase)
3. Metastatic liver tumour (mild increase)
4. Obstructive jaundice/biliary obstruction (mild to moderate increase)
5. Infection or toxic hepatitis (markedly increased)
6. Liver congestion (mild to moderate increase)
7. Pancreatitis (mild increase)
8. Hepatic injury in myocardial infarction complicated by shock
9. Infectious mononucleosis (moderate increase)
10. Chronic active hepatitis (moderate increase)
11. Reye's syndrome (moderate increase)
12. Laennec's cirrhosis (mild increase)
13. Alcoholic fatty liver (mild increase).

B. **SGOT/SGPT Comparison**
1. Although SGOT level is always increased in acute myocardial infarction, the SGPT level does not always increase proportionately.
2. SGPT is usually increased more than SGOT in acute extrahepatic biliary obstruction.

CLINICAL RELEVANCE OF SGOT ESTIMATION

A. *Increased levels occur in*
1. Myocardial infarction (MI)
   a. In MI, the SGOT level may be increased 4 to 10 times the normal values
   b. The SGOT level reaches a peak in 24 hours and returns to normal by the third or fourth day. Secondary rises in SGOT levels suggest extension or recurrence of MI
   c. The SGOT curve in MI parallels that of CPK
   d. Elevated levels do not always indicate MI in suspected patients. Severe arrhythmias and severe angina can also cause elevation.

2. *Liver disease*
   a. Level is alway enhanced in cirrhosis of the liver
   b. In liver disease the level may be 10 to 100 times the normal.
   c. Liver disorders associated with elevated SGOT levels
      1. Acute hepatitis
      2. Active cirrhosis
      3. Infectious mononucleosis with hepatitis
      4. Hepatic necrosis
      5. Metastatic or primary tumour of liver
3. *Other diseases associated with elevated SGOT levels*
   a. Acute pancreatitis
   b. Trauma and irradiation of skeletal muscle
   c. Acute haemolytic anaemia.
   d. Acute renal disease
   e. Severe tumours
   f. Cardiac catheterization and angiography
   g. Recent brain trauma with brain necrosis
   h. Crushing injuries
   i. Progressive muscular dystrophy
   j. Delirium tremens
   k. Pulmonary infarction
   l. Paricarditis
   m. Cerebrovascular accident

B. **Decreased** levels occur in
   1. Beriberi
   2. Uncontrolled diabetes mellitus with acidosis
   3. Occasional liver disease may cause a decrease instead of the expected increase.

C. **Interfering factors**
   1. Slight decreases occur during pregnancy when there is abnormal metabolism of pyridoxine
   2. Drugs that can cause elevated levels
      a. Aspirin
      b. Codeine
      c. Cortisone
      d. Cholinergics
      e. Theophylline
      f. Vitamin A
      g. Large doses of nicotinic acid
      h. Hydralazine
      i. Mepiridine
      j. Erythromycin
      k. Morphine
      l. Tolbutamide
      m. Guanethidine analogues
      n. Griseofulvin
   3. Salicylates may cause falsely decreased or increased SGOT levels

For diagnosis of myocardial infarction, the SGOT levels should be done on three consecutive days because the peak is reached in 24 hours and levels are back to normal in 3 to 4 days.

GAMMA-GLUTAMYL TRANSPEPTIDASE (GGTP) BLOOD

Normal Values

Adult females	4-25 U 9-31 mU/ml 3.5-13 IU/L 3-33 U/L at 37°C
Adult males	7-40 U 12-38 mU/ml 4-23 IU/L 9-69 U/L at 37°C
Children	
Cord blood	190-270 U/L at 37° C
Premature infants	< 140 U/L at 37 ° C
1-3 days	56-233U/L at 37 ° C
4-21 days	0-130U/L at 37 ° C
3-12 weeks	4-120U/L at 37 ° C
3-6 months, female	5-35U/L at 37 ° C
3-6 months, male	5-65U/L at 37 ° C
> 6 months, female	15-85 IU/L
> 6 months, male	5-55 IU/L
1-15 years	0-23 U/L at 37 ° C

GLUTAMYL TRANSFERASE (Carboxy Substrate Method)

For the determination of γ-Glutamyl Transferase activity in serum (For *in vitro* diagnostic use only)

Summary

γ-Glutamyl Transferase (GGT) is an enzyme found mainly in serum from hepatic origin, though the highest levels are in the kidneys. Elevated levels are found in hepatobiliary and pancreatic diseases, Chronic alcoholism, myocardial infarction with secondary liver damage, and diabetics.

Principle

GGT catalyzes the transfer of amino group between L-γ-Glutamyl-3-carboxy-4 nitroanilide and Glycylglycine to form L-γ-Glutamylglycylglycine and 5-amino-2-nitrobenzoate. The rate of formation of 5-amino-2-nitrobenzoate is measured as an increase in absorbance which is proportional to the GGT activity in the sample.

L-γ-Glutamyl-3-carboxy-4-nitroanilide + Glycylglycine —GGT→ L-γGlutamylglycyl-glycine + S-amino-2-nltrobenzoate

Normal reference values

Serum (Males) : 10-50 U/L at 37°C
(Females) : 7 - 35 U/L at 37°C

It is recommended that each laboratory establish its own normal range representing its patient population.

Contents	10 × 2 ml	35 × 2 ml
L1 : Buffer Reagent	25 ml	80 ml
T1 : Substrate Tablets	10 Nos.	35 Nos.

Storage/stability

Contents are table at 2-8° till the expiry mentioned on the labels.

Reagent Preparation

Working reagent: Dissolve 1 substrate tablet in 2.2 ml of buffer reagent. This working reagent is stable for at least 15 days when stored at 2-8°C.

Sample material

Serum. Free from haemolysis. GGT is reported to be stable in serum for 3 days at 2-8°C.

Procedure

Wavelength/filter : 405 nm
Temperature : 37°C / 30°C / 25°C
Light path : 1 cm

Peptite into a clean dry test tube labeled as test (T)

Addition Sequence	(T) (ml)
Working Reagent	1.0
Incubate at the assay temperature for 1 minute and add	
Sample	0.1

Mix well and read the initial absorbance A_0 after minute and repeat the absorbance reading after every 1, 2, and 3 minutes. Calculate the mean absorbance change per minute (ΔA/min)

Calculations

GGT Activity in U/L = ΔA/min × 1158

TEMPERATURE CONVERSION FACTORS

Assay Temperature	Desired Reporting Temperature 25°C	30°C	37°C
25°C	1.00	1.37	1.79
30°C	0.73	1.00	1.30
37°C	0.56	0.77	1.00

Linearity

The procedure is linear upto 700 U/L at 37°C. If the absorbance change (ΔA/min) exceeds 0.250, use only the value of the first two minutes to calculate the result, or dilute the the sample 1 + 9 with normal saline (NaCI 0.9%) and repeat the assay (Results × 10).

Note

Samples having a very high activity show a very high initial absorbance.If this is suspected then dilute the sample and repeat the assay.

System Parameters			
Reaction	: Kinetic	**Interval**	: 30
Wavelength	: 405 nm	**Sample vol**	: 0.10 ml
Zero setting	: Distilled water	**Reagent vol**	: 1.00 ml
Incub temp.	: 37°C	**Standard**	:
Incub time.	: —	**Factor**	: 1158
Delay time	: 30 sec.	**React. slope**	: **Increasing**
Read time	: 120 sec.	**Linearity**	: 700 U/L
No. of read	: 4	**Units**	: **U/L**

CLINICAL RELEVANCE

1. Increased GGTP levels are associated with:
   a. Cholecystitis
   b. Cholelithiasis
   c. Cancer metastasis to the liver
   d. Cirrhosis of the liver
   e. Acute pancreatitis
   f. Cancer of the bile duct
   g. Alcoholism
   h. Barbiturate use
   i. Lipoid nephrosis
   j. Obstruction of biliary tract
   k. Hepatotoxic drugs for treatment of cancer increase levels more than the cancer itself.

2. In myocardial infarction, GGTP is usually normal. However, if there is an increase, it occurs about the fourth day after myocardial infarction and probably implies liver damage secondary to cardiac insufficiency.
3. Values are not enhanced in:
   a. Bone disorders
   b. Pregnancy
   c. Skeletal muscle disease
   d. Neonatal hepatitis
   e. Renal failure

LACTIC DEHYDROGENASE

Lactic dehydrogenase (LDH) is a hydrogen transfer enzyme that catalyses the following reaction:

$$\text{Lactic acid + NAD} \underset{}{\overset{\text{LD}}{\rightleftharpoons}} \text{Pyruvic acid + NADH}$$

The reaction is reversible but the conditions for the reverse reaction are different than those for the forward (e.g. the pH for the forward reaction is 8.8 to 9.8 and for the reverse reaction is 7.4 to 7.8).

LD activity can be determined colorimetrically using 2, 4-dinitrophenyl-hydrazine (2, 4-DNPH) as the chromogen in alkaline medium. It is a discrete or two-point method. The alternative method of kinetic measurement or continuous monitoring enzyme assay is definitely superior to the colorimetric method.

LD activity is present in almost all the tissues of the body yet its increased activity in serum reflects several pathologic states. The five isoenzymes of LD (1 to 5) can be separated by electrophoresis. Increased activity of LD-1 is related to myocardial infarction while that of LD-5 is interpreted to be due to liver disorder. LD-1 and LD-5 can also be separated by thermal treatment. If serum is heated to 65°C for 30 minutes, the thermolabile LD-5 is destroyed. Thus the difference between the total LD activity of a non-heated serum specimen and the activity of the thermostable isoenzyme (LD-1) gives the measure of LD-5 activity.

Clinical Significance

Serum LD activity is related to myocardial infarction, liver diseases, pernicious anaemia, megaloblastic anaemia, renal diseases, malignant diseases, and progressive muscular dystrophy.

Normal Values

		SI Units
Wroblewski method 30° C	150-450 U/L	72-217 U/L
Adult		
< Age 60	45-90 U/L	45-90U/L
> Age 60	55-102 U/L	55-102 U/L
Newborn	160-500 U/L	160-500 U/L
Neonate	300-1500 U/L	300-1500 U/L
Infant	100-250 U/L	100-250 U/L
Child	60-170 U/L	60-170 U/L

LDH (P-L) (Mod. IFCC Method) Courtesy: Tulip Group of Companies

For the determination of LDH activity in serum (For *in vitro* diagnostic use only)

Summary

LDH is found in many body tissues particularly heart, liver, skeletal muscle, kidney and RBCs. LDH is found in the form of isoenzymes based on their electrophoretic mobility with each isoenzyme being primarily from different organs. Increased levels are found in myocardial infarction, pulmonary diseases, hepatic diseases, haemolytic anaemias, renal diseases and muscular dystrophy.

Principle

LDH catalyses the reduction of pyruvate with NADH to form NAD. The rate of oxidation of NADH to NAD is measured as a decrease in absorbance which is proportional to the LDH activity in the sample.

$$\text{Pyruvate + NADH + H}^+ \xrightarrow{\text{LDH}} \text{Lactate + NAD}^+$$

Normal reference values

Serum : 230 - 460 U/L at 37°C

It is recommended that each laboratory establish its own normal range representing its patient population.

Contents	25 ml	2x75 ml
L1 : Buffer Reagent	20 ml	2 x 60 ml
L2 : Starter Reagent	5 ml	2 x 15 ml

Storage/stability

Contents are stable at 2-8°C till the expiry mentioned.

Reagent Preparation

Reagents are ready to use.

Working reagent: For sample start assays a single reagent is required. Pour the contents of 1 bottle of L2 (Starter Reagent) into 1 bottle of L1 (Buffer Reagent). This working reagent is stable for at least 1 week when stored at 2-8°C. Alternatively for flexibility as much of working reagent may be made as and when desired by mixing together 4 parts of L1 (Buffer Reagent) and 1 part of L2 (Starter Reagent). Alternatively 0.8 ml of L1 and 0.2 ml of L2 may also be used instead of 1 ml of the working reagent directly during the assay.

Sample material

Serum. Free from hemolysis. Total LDH is reported to be stable in serum for 1-3 days at 2-8°C. **Freezing inactivates the liver isoenzyme.**

Procedure

Wavelength/filter : 340 nm
Temperature : 37°C/30°C/25°C
Light path : 1 cm

Substrate Start Assay

Pipette into a clean dry test tube labeled as Test (T):

Addition Sequence	(T) 25°C / 30°C	(T) 37°C
Buffer Reagent	0.8 ml	0.8
Sample	0.05 ml	0.02
Incubate at the assay temperature for 1 minute and add		
Starter Reagent	0.2 ml	0.2 ml

Mix well and read the initial absorbance A_0 and repeat the absorbance reading after every 1, 2, and 3 minutes. Calculate the mean absorbance change per minute (ΔA/min)

Sample Start Assay

Pipette into a clean dry test tube labeled as Test (T):

Addition Sequence	(T) 25°C/30°C	(T) 37°C
Working Reagent	1.0 ml	1.0 ml
Incubate at the assay temperature for 1 minute and add		
Sample	0.05 ml	0.02 ml

Mix well and read the initial absorbance after 1 minute and repeat the absorbance reading after every 1, 2, and 3 minutes. Calculate the mean absorbance change per minute (ΔA/min)

Calculations

Substrate/Sample Start

LDH Activity in U/L 25°C/30°C = ΔA/min x 3333
37°C = ΔA/min. × 8095

TEMPERATURE CONVERSION FACTORS

Assay Temperature	Desired Reporting Temperature 25°C	30°C	37°C
25°C	1.00	1.33	1.92
30°C	0.75	1.00	1.44
37°C	0.52	0.70	1.00

Linearity

The procedure is linear upto 2000 U/L at 37°C. If the absorbance change (ΔA/min) exceeds 0.250, use only the value of the first two minutes to calculate the result, or dilute the sample 1 + 9 with normal saline (NaCl 0.9%) and repeat the assay (results × 10).

Note

Samples having a high activity show a very low initial absorbance as most of the NADH is consumed prior to the start of measurement. If this is suspected then dilute the sample and repeat the assay.

The working reagent or the combined reagent should have an absorbance above 1.000 against distilled water at 340 nm. Discard the reagent if the absorbance is below 1.000.

RBCs have a very high LDH content and hence, haemoysed samples should not be used.

System Parameters			
Reaction	: U.V. Kinetic	Interval	: 60
Wavelength	: 340 nm	Sample vol	: 0.02 ml
Zero setting	: Distilled water	Reagent vol	: 1.00 ml
Incub temp.	: 37°C	Standard	:
Incub time	: —	Factor	: 8095
Delay time	: 60 sec.	React. slope	: Decreasing
Read time	: 180 sec.	Linearity	: 2000 U/L
No. of read	: 4	Units	: U/L

CLINICAL RELEVANCE

Myocardial infarction

The elevation of LDH that follows an MI is characterised by:

1. High levels within 12 to 24 hours of infarction (18 hour) and 2 to 10 times normal.
2. Elevation that may continue for 6 to 10 days (larger than SGOT or CK). For this reason, LDH determination may be useful in the late diagnosis of MI. Elevations return to normal in 8 to 14 days.

Pulmonary infarction

In pulmonary infarction, there is usually an increased LDH within 24 hours of the onset of pain. The pattern of normal SGOT and elevated LDH that levels 1 to 2 days after an episode of chest pain provides evidence for pulmonary infarction.

Conditions in general and according to degree of increase in levels.

1. Elevated levels of LDH are observed in a variety of conditions.
   a. Acute MI
   b. Acute leukaemia
   c. Haemolytic anaemias
   d. Hepatic disease
   e. Skeletal muscle necrosis
   f. Sprue
   g. Acute pulmonary infarction
   h. Malignant neoplasms, extensive cancer
   i. Acute renal infarction and chronic renal disease
   j. Shock with necrosis of minor organs
   k. Myxoedema
2. The greatest increase (2-40 times normal) is seen in
   a. Megaloblastic anaemia
   b. Extensive cancer (especially hepatic metastases)
   c. Shock and anoxia
3. Moderate increase (2-4 times normal) is seen in
   a. MI
   b. Pulmonary infarction
   c. Haemolytic anaemia
   d. Granulocytic or acute leukaemia
   e. Infectious mononucleosis
   f. Progressive muscular dystrophy
4. Slight increase occurs in
   a. Delirium tremens
   b. Hepatitis
   c. Obstructive jaundice/cholangitis
   d. Cirrhosis
   e. Nephrotic syndrome
   f. Hypothyroidism

Decreased LDH levels are associated with a good response to cancer therapy.

Elevated urine LDH levels occur in

1. Cancer of kidney or bladder
2. Glomerulonephritis
3. Malignant hypertension
4. Lupus nephritis
5. Acute tubular necrosis
6. Renal transplantation and haemograft rejection
7. Pyelonephritis (sometimes)

Interfering Factors

1. Strenuous exercise and the muscular exertion involved in childbirth will cause increased levels.
2. Skin diseases can cause falsely increased levels.
3. Haemolysis of RBCs due to freezing, heating, or shaking the blood sample will cause falsely increased levels.
4. Drugs that may elevate levels comprise.
   a. Codeine
   b. Clofibrate
   c. Meperidine
   d. Mithramycin
   e. Morphrine
   f. Procainamide
5. Oxalate is known to cause decreased levels

Electrophoresis of LDH Isoenzymes

Normal values

Isoenzyme	Organ related	Percentage of total LDH
Isoenzyme 1	Cardiac	(25% – 40%)
Isoenzyme 2	Cardiac	(35% – 46%)
Isoenzyme 3	Pulmonary	(17% – 32%)
Isoenzyme 4	Hepatic	(9% – 18%)
Isoenzyme 5	Hepatic	(6% – 17%)

Variation of 2 to 4% are considered physiologically normal (isoenzymes 1 to 5 are also present in human skeletal muscle).

Test Significance

Electrophoresis or separation of LDH identifies the five isoenzymes or fractions of LDH, each with its own characteristics physical and chemical properties. Fractionating the LDH activity multiplies its diagnostic relevance since LDH is found in many organs. The LDH isoenzymes are released into the blood stream when tissue necrosis occurs. However, a complete knowledge of the clinical history is necessary to properly interpret the resulting patterns. The isoenzymes are evaluated in terms of patterns established, not on the basis of the value of a single isoenzyme. The five isoenzyme fractions of LDH show different patterns in various disorders. Abnormalities in the pattern suggest which tissue has been damaged and help to diagnose myocardial infarction, pulmonary infarction, and liver disease. This test is sensitive enough to detect hepatic fraction in infectious hepatitis before clinical jaundice appears. It is in confirming the diagnosis of suspected MI that the separation of LDH isoenzymes finds its most frequent application, especially when a second infarct occurs shortly after the first. In these cases, the ECG is already abnormal, but the isoenzyme pattern will show increased LDH_1, indicating the release of more of the cardiac enzyme.

Clinical Relevance

Abnormal patterns reflect damaged tissue

1. LDH_1 and LDH_2 are increased in MI and in some hemolytic anaemias
2. LDH_3 is increased in pulmonary infarction and extensive pneumonia.
3. LDH_5 is increased in liver disease.
4. An increase in LDH_2, LDH_3, LDH_4 is common in malignant disease.
5. The LDH pattern will be essentially the same in MI, pernicious anaemia, and renal infarction. This is because RBC's and the kidney have an isoenzyme pattern simllar to that of heart muscle.
6. In most cancers, one to three of the bands (LDH_2, LDH_3, and LDH_4) are frequently increased. A notable exception is in seminomas and dysgermi-nomas when LDH_1, and LDH_2 are increased. Frequently, an increase in LDH_3 may be the first indication of the presence of cancer.

CK (NAC ACT) (Mod. IFCC Method)
Courtesy: Tulip Group of Companies

For the determination of CK activity in serum (For *in vitro* diagnostic use only).

Summary

CK is mainly found in all muscle and brain tissue. It plays an important role in the energy storing mechanism of the tissues. Increased levels are found in myocardial infarction, cerebrovascular diseases, muscular dystrophy, pulmonary infarction and, electrical shocks. Increased levels can also be caused by intra muscular injections, strenuous exercise and recent surgery. Early pregnancy may produce decreased levels.

Principle

Creatine Kinase catalyse the reaction between creatinine phosphate and ADP to form creatine and ATP. The ATP formed along with glucose is catalysed by Hexokinase to form Glucose 6 phosphate. The glucose 6 phosphate reduces NADP to NADPH in the presence of glucose 6 phosphate dehydrogenase. The rate of reduction of NADP to NADPH is measured as an increase in absorbance which is proportional to the CK activity in the sample.

$$\text{Creatine Phosphate} + \text{ADP} \xrightarrow{\text{Creatine Kinase}} \text{Creatine} + \text{ATP}$$

$$\text{Glucose} + \text{ATP} \xrightarrow{\text{Hexokinase}} \text{Glucose 6 phosphate} + \text{ADP}$$

$$\text{G-6-P} + \text{NADP} \xrightarrow{\text{G-6-PDH}} \text{Gluconate-6-P} + \text{NADPH} + \text{H}$$

Normal reference values

Serum (male) : 24 - 195 U/L at 37°C
(female) : 24-170 U/L at 37°C

It is recommended that each laboratory establish its own normal range representing its patient population.

Contents	2 × 10 ml	2 × 25 ml
L1 : Enzyme Reagent	2 × 8 ml	2 × 20 ml
L2 : Starter Reagent	2 × 2 ml	2 × 5 ml

Storage/stability

Contents are stable at 2-8°C till the expiry mentioned on the labels.

Reagent Preparation

Reagents are ready to use.

Working reagent: For sample start assays a single reagent is required. Pour the contents of 1 bottle of L2 (Starter Reagent) into 1 bottle of L1 (Enzyme Reagent). This working reagent is stable for at least

10 days when stored at 2 to 8°C. Alternatively for flexibility as much of working reagent may be made as and when desired by mixing together 4 parts of L1 (Enzyme Reagent) and 1 part of L2 (Starter Reagent). Alternatively 0.8 ml of L1 and 0.2 ml of L2 may also be used instead of 1 ml of the working reagent directly during the assay.

Sample material

Serum. Free from hemolysis. CK is reporter to be stable in serum for 3 days at 2 to 8°C.

Procedure

Wavelength/filter : 340 nm
Temperature : 37°C / 30°C / 25°C
Light path : 1 cm

Substrate Start Assay :

Pipette into a clean dry test tube labelled as Test (T):

Addition Sequence	(T) 25°C / 30°C /	(T) 37°C
Enzyme Reagent (L1)	0.8 ml	0.8 ml
Sample	0.05 ml	0.02 ml
Incubate at the assay temperature for 5 minutes and add		
Starter Reagent (L2)	0.2 ml	0.m

Mix well and read the initial absorbance A_0 and repeat the absorbance reading after every 1, 2, and 3 minutes. Calculate the mean absorbance change per minute (ΔA/min.)

Sample Start Assay

Pipette into a clean dry test tube labelled as Test (T):

Addition Sequence	(T) 25°C / 30°C/	(T) 37°C
Working Reagent	1.0 ml	1.0 ml
Incubate at the assay temperature for 1 minute and add		
Sample	0.05 ml	0.02 ml

Mix well and read the initial absorbance A_0 after 10 minutes and repeat the absorbance reading after every 1, 2, and 3 minutes. Calculate the mean absorbance change per minute (ΔA/min)

Calculations

Substrate/Sample start

CK Activity in U/L 25°C / 30°C $= \Delta A / \text{min} \times 3333$
37°C $= \Delta A / \text{min} \times 8095$

TEMPERATURE CONVERSION FACTORS

Assay Temperature	Desired Reporting Temperature 25°C	30°C	37°C
25°C	1.00	1.56	2.44
30°C	0.64	1.00	1.56
37°C	0.41	063	1.00

Linearity

The procedure is linear upto 2000 U/L at 37°C. If the absorbance change (ΔA/min) exceeds 0.250, use only the value of the first two minutes to calculate the result, or dilute the sample 1+ 9 with normal saline (NaCl 0.9%) and repeat the assay (Results × 10).

Note

Samples having a high activity show a very high initial absorbance as most of the NADP is converted prior to the start of measurement. If this is suspected then dilute the sample and repeat the assay.

The working reagent or the combined reagent should have an absorbance below 0.800 against distilled water at 340 nm. Discard the reagent if the absorbance is above 0.800.

System Parameters			
Reaction	: UV Kinetic	**Interval**	: 60
Wavelength	: 340 nm	**Sample vol**	: 0.02 ml
Zero setting	: Distilled water	**Reagent vol**	: 1.00 ml
Incub temp.	: 37°C	**Standard**	:
Incub time.	: -	**Factor**	: 8095
Delay time	: 60 sec.	**React. slope**	: Increasing
Read time	: 180 sec.	**Linearity**	: 2000 U/L
No. of read	: 4	**Units**	: U/L

CK MB (NAC ACT) (IMMUNOINHIBITION/MOD. IFCC METHOD) Courtesy: Tulip Group of Companies

For the determination of CK-MB activity in serum (For *in vitro* diagnostic use only)

Summary

CK is dimeric molecule composed of M and B submlts, which are immunologically distinct. It exists as three main iso enzymes CK - MM, CK - MB, and CK - BB. The CK - MM is found in the muscle while CK - MB is found mainly in the myocardial cells. The CK - BB is found mainly in the brain and lungs, and enters the blood stream only on injury to these organs like cerebrovascular accident or pulmonary infarction. Normally CK - MM is found in the blood. CK - MB levels increase significantly 4-6 hours following a myocardial infarction and peak at around 12 to 24 hours after the infarct. The levels return to normal, in case of no further myocardial damage, after 24 to 48 hours. Hence, the increased levels of CK - MB along with elevated levels of total CK is a good indicator of myocardial infarction. CK - MB levels usually do not rise in chest pain caused by angina, pulmonary embolism or congestive heart failure.

Principle

CK - M fractions of the CK - MM and the CK - MB in the sample are completely inhibited by an anti CK - M antibody present in the reagent. Then the activity of the CK - B fraction is measured by the CK (NAC act.) method, the CK - MB activity is obtained by multiplying the CK - B activity by two.

Normal reference values

Serum =upto 24 U/L at 37°C

Indication of myocardial infarction is based on the the following factors:

Total CK (male) : > 195 U/L at 37°C
(female) : > 170 U/L at 37°C
CK - MB : > 24 U/L at 37°C
CK - MB to Total CK : > 6% - 25%

It is recommended that each laboratory establish its own normal range representing its patient population.

Contents	2 × 10 ml	2 × 25 ml
L1 : Enzyme Reagent	2 × 8 ml	2 × 20 ml
L2 : Starter Reagent	2 × 2 ml	2 × 5 ml

Storage/stability

Contents are stable at 2-8° C till the expiry mentioned on the labels.

Reagent Preparation

Reagents are ready to use.

Working reagent: For sample start assays a single reagent is required. Pour the contents of 1 bottle of L2 (Starter Reagent) into 1 bottle of L1 (Enzyme Reagent). This working reagent is stable for at least 10 days when stored at 2-8°C. Alternatively for flexibility as much of working reagent may be made as and when desired by mixing together 4 parts of L1 (Enzyme Reagent) and 1 part of L2 (Starter Reagent). Alternatively 0.8 ml of L1 and 0.2 ml of L2 may also be used instead of 1 ml of the working reagent directly during the assay.

Sample material

Serum. Free from hemolysis.

Procedure

Wavelength/filter : 340 nm
Temperature : 37°C / 30°C / 25°C
Light path : 1 cm

Substrate Start Assay

Pipette into a clean dry test tube labelled as Test (T):

Addition Sequence	(T) 25°C / 30°C/37°C
Enzyme Reagent (L1)	0.8 ml
Sample	0.05 ml
Incubate at the assay temperature for 1 minute and add	
Starter Reagent (L2)	0.2 ml

Mix well and read the initial absorbance A_0 after 5 minutes and repeat the absorbance reading after every 1, 2, and 3 minutes. Calculate the mean absorbance change per minute (ΔA/min)

Substrate Start Assay

Pipette into a clean dry tube labelled as test (T)

Addition Sequence	25°C/30°C/37°C (T)
Working reagent	1.0 ml
Incubate at the assay temperature for 1 minute and add	
Sample	0.05 ml

Mix well and read the initial absorbance A_0 after 10 minutes and repeat the absorbance reading after every 1, 2 and 3 minutes. Calculate the mean absorbance change per minute (ΔA/min)

Calculations

Substrate/Sample start

CK - B activity in U/L 25°C / 30°C /37°C = ΔA/min x 3333
CK-MB activity in U/L 25°C / 30°C /37°C = ΔA /min x 6666

TEMPERATURE CONVERSION FACTORS

Assay Temperature	Desired Reporting Temperature 25°C	30°C	37°C
25°C	1.00	1.56	2.44
30°C	0.64	1.00	1.56
37°C	0.41	0.63	1.00

Linearity

This procedure linear upto 1000 U/ml. Inhibition of CK - MM is upto 1500 U/L at 37°C. If the total CK activity exceeds this limit dilute the sample 1 + 9 with normal saline (NaCl 0.9%) before estimating CK - MB (Results x 10).

Note

This method will also measure any CK - BB isoenzyme present in the sample. The amount of CK - BB is usually negligible in serum from normal individuals or in patients with myocardial infarction.

A macro form of BB has been observed and this will be measured as CK - B activity, if the CK - B activity exceedes 20% of the total CK activity the presence of macro BB should be suspected.

The working reagent or the combined reagent should have an absorbance below 0.800 against distilled water at 340 nm. Discard the reagent if the absorbance is above 0.800.

System Parameters

Reaction	: UV Kinetic	**Interval**	: 60 sec.
Wavelength	: 340 nm	**Sample vol**	: 0.05 ml
Zero setting	: Distilled water	**Reagent vol**	: 1.00ml
Incub temp.	: 37°C	**Standard**	:
Incub time.	: —	**Factor**	: 6666
Delay time	: 300 sec.	**React. slope**	: Increasing
Read time	: 180 sec.	**Linearity**	: 1000 U/L
No. of read	: 4	**Units**	: U/L

CREATINE KINASE (CK)

Clinical Relevance

The two enzymes CK and adenylate kinase (AK) play a decisive role in the synthesis of ATP, the immediate energy source of the muscle, the CNS and many proliferating tissues. Human creatinine kinase is synthesised by a number of different genes. The respective gene products are called CK-M (muscle), CK-B (brain) and CK-Mi (mitochondria). The total CK activity measurable in serum is composed of the activities of the cytoplasmic, dimeric isoenzymes (CK-MM, CK-MB, CK-BB) and their postsynthetically modified forms, and the activities of the macro creatinine kinase (macro CK).

C K Isoenzymes

Isoenzyme of total C K

CK-BB (brain) 0-3 (found mainly in brain, also in smooth muscle, thyroid, lungs and prostate)

CK-MB (heart) 0-6 (found mainly in myocardium, also in tongue, diaphragm and skeletal muscle)

CK-MM (muscle) 90 - 97 (found mainly in the skeletal muscle).

Approximate distribution of the CK isoenzymes in human organs

Tissue	U/g	CK-MM	CK-MB	CK-BB	CK-mito
Skeletal muscle	800-4000	++++	(+)	(+)	+
Myocardium	240-800	+ + +	++	(+)	+ +
Brain	≤550	-	-	+ + +	+ +
Bladder	≤135	-		++++	+
Blood	≤0.2	++++	(+)		
Colon	≤200	(+)	(+)	+ + + +	+
Umbilical cord blood	≤1.0	+ + + +	(+)	+	?
Prostate	≤135	-	-	+ + + +	?
Uterus	≤400	-	-	+ + + +	+
Vein wall	≤60	-	-	+ + + +	?

(+ + + +:>75%, + + +:50-75%, + +:25-50%, +:5-25%, (+):<5% at 37°C)

Normal Values (at 37°C)

CK

Adult males 24-195 U/L, Adult females 24-170 U/L

Children: Umbilical cord 175-402 U/L, Newborns; ≤5 days 195-700 U/L, < 6 months 41-330 U/L, > 6 months 24-229 U/L. (Conversion of U/L into μ, Kat/L: 1 μKat/L=60 U/L)

CK-MB: Normal value ≤ 24 U/L. CK-BB:, For adults < 2 U/L.

CK-MM: Reference values for total CK activity for adults can be used.

CK-mito: Normal value is < 2U/L

Clinical data, EGG findings and the results of CK determination complement each other with regard to clinical sensitivity and specificity. In spite of determination of CK-MB the differential diagnosis of myocardial infarction /skeletal damage presents problems in the following circumstances: extensive skeletal muscle damage and concomitant small infarction, chronic skeletal muscle disease and myocardial involvement or MI after coronary artery bypass grafting. In these cases determination of one of the cardiospecific troponins is necessary.

Diagnostic Alert

As adenylate kinase interferes with CK estimation and AK is found to a greater extent in the Indian population. It becomes imperative to use reagents that are capable of inhibiting AK so as not to over estimate CK. A report generated by employing inappropriate kits can initiate unnecessary therapy.

Total CK and CK-MB trends in acute myocardial infarction

	Total CK	*CK-MB*
Initial rise:	2-6 hours after onset of damage	4-8 hours after onset of damage.
Peak levels:	18-36 hours after onset of damage	18-24 hours after the onset of damage.
Return to basal levels:	3-6 days after onset of damage	3 days after onset of damage

6% Rule

The decision criterion is an increase in the total CK activity to > 240 U/L (37°C) within the diagnostic time window and a simultaneous increase in CK-MB activity. A CK-MB fraction more than 6% of the total CK activity is regarded as diagnostic for MI. A fraction < 6% indicates skeletal muscle damage. The clinical specificity of the 6% rule is high as the number of false positive results caused by presence of extracardiac CK-MB is small. However, following this rule, smaller MIs may be missed. False positive values can be caused by Adenylate Kinase, which occurs in large quantities in the liver and in blood cells.

Increased Total CK: Amyotrophic lateral sclerosis, anoxia, atresia (biliary), bowel injury, brain tumour, burns (thermal, electrical), cancer (breast, lung, oat cell, gastrointestinal, prostatic), carbon monoxide poisoning, cardiomyopathy (cobalt-beer), carrier state (for Duchenne's muscular dystrophy), cerebrovascular accident, CNS trauma, coma (hepatic), convulsions, coughing (severe), delirium tremens, dermatomyositis, eosinophilia-myalgia syndrome, exercise, head injury, haemodialysis, hypokalemia (severe), hypothermia, hypothyroidism, infarction (bowel, cerebral, myocardial, prostate), intoxication (alcohol, salicylate), intramuscular injection (recent), labour, leptospirosis, malignant hyperthermia, meningoencephalitis, muscle spasms, muscular dystrophy (Duchenne's, limb-girdle, fascioscapulohumeral), myocarditis, myoglobinuria, myopathy (from alcoholism), myotonic dystrophy, myxedema, necrosis of striated muscle, organ rejection (heart transplant), parturition, polymyositis, pregnancy, prostatic injury, psychosis (acute with agitation), pulmonary edema, pulmonary embolism, renal failure, renal insufficiency (chronic), Reye's syndrome, rhabdomyolysis, Rocky Mountain spotted fever, shock, skeletal muscle disorders, status epliepticus, striated muscle atrophy (acute), subarachnoid haemorrhage, surgery (bowel, cardiac, CNS, prostate), tachycardia, thyrotoxicosis, toxic shock syndrome (day 7), trauma (muscular), typhoid fever, and very muscular people.

Increased CK-BB : Anoxia, atresia (biliary), cancer (breast, gastrointestinal, oat cell, prostatic, widespread malignancies), cerebrovascular accident (haemorrhage, infarction), haemodialysis, hypothermia, intestinal necrosis, labour, malignant hyperthermia, renal failure, shock, surgery (CNS), and uraemia.

Increased CK-MB: Anoxia, burns (electrical, thermal), cancer (lung), carbon monoxide poisoning, cardiomyopathy (cobalt-beer), collagen vascular diseases, congestive heart failure (rare), coronary angiography (rare), coronary insufficiency (rare), hypothermia, hypothyroidism, malignant hyperthermias, muscular dystrophy (Duchenne's), myocardial infarction, myocarditis, myoglobinuria (severe), polymyositis, pulmonary embolism, renal insufficiency (chronic), Reye's syndrome, rhabdomyolysis, Rocky Mountain spotted fever, surgery (cardiac, valve replacement), SLE, and trauma (cardiac).

Increased CK-MM: Cardiac catheterisation (with myocardial damage), cardioversion, coronary arteriography (with myocardial damage), hypothyroidism, intramuscular injection, muscle trauma, myocardial infarction, psychosis (acute with agitation), Reye's syndrome, shock, surgery, and trauma (skeletal muscle).

Decreased Total CK : Addison's disease, anterior pituitary hyposecretion, connective tissue disease, hepatic disease (alcoholic), low muscle mass, metastatic neoplasia, and pregnancy (first half). Drugs include steroids.

Decreased CK-BB, CK-MB, CK-MM: Clinically insignificant/not applicable.

Interfering Factors

1. Strenuous exercise (up to 3 times normal) and surgical procedures that damage skeletal muscle may cause increased levels.
2. High doses of salicylates may cause increased levels
3. Athletes have a higher value because of greater muscle mass.
4. Multiple intramuscular injections may cause increased levels
5. Drugs that may cause increased levels include
   a. Amphotericin B
   b. Ampicillin IM
   c. Carbenicillin IM
   d. Chlorpromazine IM
   e. Clofibtrate.

ENZYMOLOGY IN RELATION TO HEART DISEASE

Introduction

Myocardial Infarction (MI) is the gross necrosis of the myocardium due to interruption of blood supply to the area. In over 90% of patients with acute MI, an acute thrombus, often associated with plaque rupture, occludes the arteries (usually it is already partially obstructed by an atherosclerotic plaque) that supply the damaged area. Altered platelet function induced by endothelial change in the atherosclerotic plaque presumably contributes to thrombogenesis. Spontaneous thrombolysis occurs in about two thirds of the patients so that, 24 hrs later, thrombotic occlusion is found in only about 30% of the patients.

MI is rarely caused by arterial embolization for example in mitral or aortic stenosis, infective endocarditis, and marantic endocarditis. MI has been reported in patients with coronary spasm and otherwise normal coronary arteries. Cocaine causes intense coronary arterial spasm, and users may present with cocaine-induced angina or MI. Autopsy studies and coronary angiography have shown that cocaine-induced coronary thrombosis may occur in normal coronary arteries or be superimposed on pre-existing atheroma. MI is predominantly a disease of the left ventricle (LV), but damage may extend into the right ventricle (RV) or the atria. RV infarction usually results from occlusion of the right coronary or a dominant left circumflex artery and is characterised by high RV filling pressure, often with severe tricuspid regurgitation and reduced cardiac output. Some degree of RV dysfunction occurs in about half of patients with an inferior-posterior infarction, producing haemodynamic abnormality in 10 to 15%. RV dysfunction should be considered in any patient with inferior-posterior infarction and elevated jugular venous pressure with hypotension or shock (Anatomy of human heart is given in Fig. 21.1).

The ability of the heart to continue functioning as a pump relates directly to the extent of myocardial damage. Patients who die of cardiogenic shock usually have an infarct, or a combination of scar and new infarct, of about 50% of LV mass. Anterior infarcts tend to be larger and have a worse prognosis than inferior-posterior infarcts. They are usually due to occlusion in the left coronary arterial tree, especially the anterior descending artery, whereas inferior-posterior infarcts reflect right coronary occlusion or occlusion of a dominant left circumflex artery. Transmural infarcts involve the whole thickness of myocardium from epicardium to endocardium and are usually characterised by abnormal Q waves on ECG. Nontransmural or subendocardial infarcts do not extend through the ventricular wall and cause only ST segment and T-wave abnormalities. Subendocardial infarcts usually involve the inner one third of the myocardium where wall tension is highest and myocardial blood flow is most vulnerable to circulatory changes. They may also follow prolonged hypotension. Because the transmural depth of necrosis cannot be precisely determined clinically, infarcts are better classified by ECG as Q wave and non-Q wave.

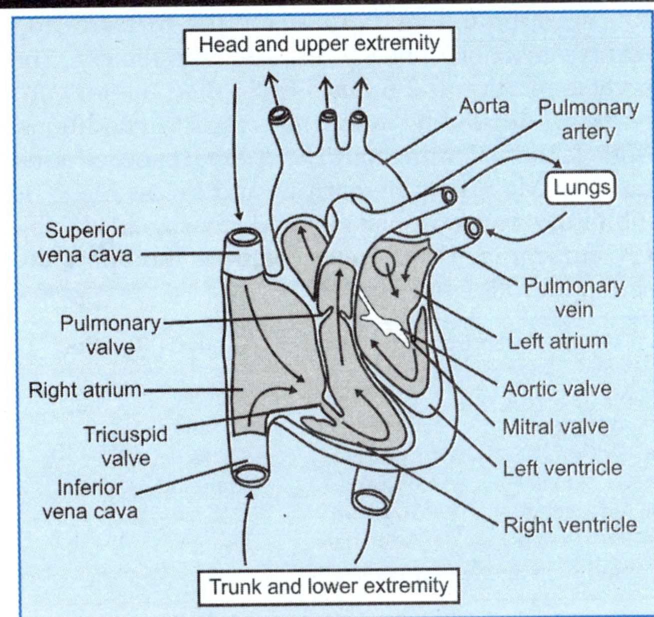

Fig. 21.1: The Human Heart

CLINICAL PRESENTATION

It is accepted that the term MI reflects a loss of cardiac myocytes (necrosis) caused by prolonged ischaemia. Ischaemia is the result of a perfusion-dependent imbalance between supply and demand. Ischaemia in a clinical setting can be identified from the patient's history and from the ECG. Possible ischaemic symptoms include chest, epigastric, arm, wrist or jaw discomfort with exertion or at rest. The discomfort associated with acute MI usually lasts at least 20 min, but may be shorter in duration. The discomfort may develop in the central or left chest and then radiate to the arm, jaw, back or shoulder. The discomfort is usually not sharp or highly localised and may be associated with dyspnoea, diaphoresis, nausea, vomiting or light-headedness. The discomfort can develop in the epigastrium, which is often confused with indigestion, arm, shoulder, wrist, jaw or back, without occurring in the chest, but such a pattern is atypical. The discomfort is not affected by moving the muscles of the region where the discomfort is localised, nor is it worsened by deep inspiration. The discomfort is not positional in nature. Symptoms can also include unexplained nausea and vomiting, persistent shortness of breath secondary to left ventricular failure and unexplained weakness, dizziness, lightheadedness or syncope, or a combination of these. These symptoms may be noted in association with chest discomfort or they may occur in the absence of chest symptoms. Although many patients have symptoms such as those just described, these complaints may go unrecognised or may be erroneously labeled as another disease entity, such as indigestion or a viral syndrome. Myocardial necrosis may also occur without symptoms.

DIAGNOSIS OF MI

Electrocardiogram (ECG)

An electrocardiogram is usually the first diagnostic test performed. Diagnostic specificity is approximately 100 percent, and a positive tracing, signalled by an elevated ST segment, essentially confirms a diagnosis of AMI. The diagnostic sensitivity, however, has been estimated to range from only 63-82%. ECG tracings are therefore, indeterminate in a substantial fraction of MI patients. One of the major advantages of ECG is that it allows assessment of most nonischaemic causes of acute chest pain, such as perimyocarditis, valvular heart disease (aortic stenosis), pulmonary embolism and aortopathies (aortic dissection).

This sensitivity limitation necessitates reliance on biochemical serum cardiac markers for triaging patients with indeterminate ECGs.

Imaging

Imaging techniques have been used to assist in:

- Ruling out or confirming the presence of acute infarction or ischaemia in the Emergency Departments.
- Identifying nonischemic conditions causing chest pain.
- Defining short- and long-term prognosis.
- Identifying mechanical complications of acute infarction.

The rationale of imaging using echocardiographic or nuclear techniques in patients suspected of having acute ischaemia is that ischaemia results in regional myocardial hypoperfusion, leading to a cascade of events that can include myocardial dysfunction and ultimately cell death. Some imaging methods are:

- Cross-sectional Echocardiography
- Radionuclide Angiography
- Myocardial Single Photon Emission Computed Tomographic (SPECT) perfusion imaging

Radionuclide techniques enable the physician to assess perfusion at the time of patient presentation; this can be performed with immediate tracer injection, because image acquisition can be delayed for 60 to

90 minutes. Quantitative analysis is an advantage of this technique. The accuracy of the studies is high when interpreted by skilled observers. These studies also provide simultaneous information on myocardial perfusion and function.

Biomarkers are more sensitive, more specific and less costly than imaging techniques for the diagnosis of myocardial necrosis. Injury involving >20% of myocardial wall thickness is required before a segmental wall motion abnormality can be detected by Echocardiography. In general, >10 g of myocardial tissue must be injured before a radionuclide perfusion defect can be resolved. Neither technique can distinguish ischaemia from infarction.

Thus the sensitivity limitation in ECG, requirement of expensive equipment and skilled personnel for imaging, necessitates reliance on biochemical serum cardiac markers for routine diagnosis and follow-up of MI.

Biochemical Markers of Myocardial Necrosis

Myocardial necrosis results in and can be recognised by the appearance in the blood of different markers released into the circulation due to the damaged myocytes: Creatine Kinase (CK), Myoglobin, cardiac Troponin T and Troponin I, Lactate dehydrogenase (LDH), SGOT as well as many others. Myocardial infarction is diagnosed when blood levels of sensitive and specific biomarkers are increased in the clinical setting of acute ischaemia. These biomarkers reflect myocardial damage but do not indicate its mechanism. Thus, an elevated value in the absence of clinical evidence of ischaemia should prompt a search for other causes of cardiac damage, such as myocarditis.

CK and its Isoenzymes—The Time-tested Biomarker

Creatine kinase (CK), also called as creatine phosphokinase (CPK), catalyses the reversible phosphorylation of creatine by ATP, as shown in the following equation (Fig. 21.2):

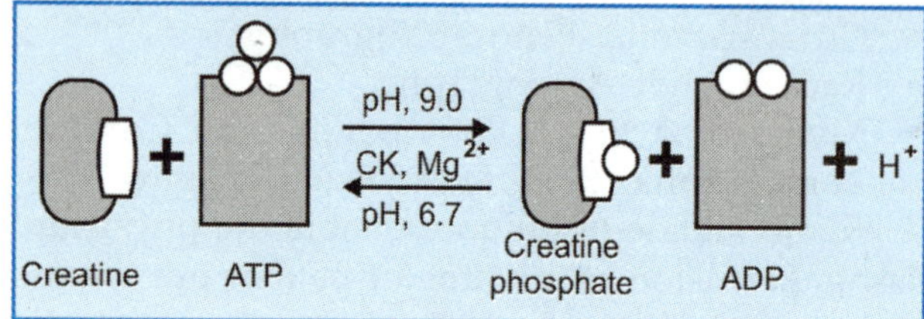

Fig. 21.2: Catalytic action of creatine kinase

The optimum pH values for the forward and reverse reactions are 9.0 and 6.7 respectively. The reverse reaction is 2-6 times faster than the forward reaction, depending upon the reaction conditions. Mg^{2+} is the activating ion. The optimal concentration range of Mg^{2+} is quite narrow, and excess Mg^{2+} is inhibitory. Several metal ions and other agents inhibit CK enzyme activity. Some common inhibitors are shown in following figure:

Some Common Inhibitors of CK Catalytic Reaction

• Mn^{2+}ions	• Excess ADP	• Iodide
• Zn^{24}ions	• Citrate	• Bromide
• Ca^{2+}ions	• Fluoride	• Chloride
• Cu^{2+}ions	• Nitrate	• Malonate
• Iodoacetate	• Sulphate	• L-thyroxine
• Sulfhydryl-binding reagents	• Adenylate Kinase enzyme	• Urate

Diagnostic Applications of CK and its Isoenzymes

- Suspected cardiac muscle disease in patients with clinical and ECG signs typical of myocardial infarction.
- In patients in whom an intervention is contraindicated.
- For evaluation of thrombolytic therapy.
- For risk stratifications in patients with angina.
- Myocarditis.
- Suspected skeletal muscle damage.
- Monitoring cardiac and skeletal muscle disease.

Special Findings

Serum CK is particularly valuable for the following reasons:

- Serial total CK has sensitivity close to 100% early in course of Myocardial Infarction (MI).
- It allows early diagnosis because increased levels appear within 3-6 hours after onset of MI and reaches its peak at 24-36 hours.
- It is more sensitive indicator than other enzymes because an increased CK level shows a larger amplitude of change (6-12 times normal).

Isoforms of CK

CK is a dimer composed of two subunits, each with a molecular weight of about 40000 Daltons. These subunits - B (brain) and M (muscle), are the products of the loci on chromosomes 14 and 19 respectively.

Only three different pairs of subunits exist - CK-BB, CK-MB and CK-MM. Although CK-MB is not an isoenzyme in the true sense but a hybrid moleclue consisting of one CK-M and one CK-B subunit, this term is, nevertheless, widely used.

There exists a fourth form of CK that differs from the others based on both immunologic and electrophoretic mobility. This isoenzyme, CK-Mt (or CK-Mi), is located between the inner and the outer membranes of mitochondria. Its structure is determined by a locus on chromosome 15. Unlike other subunits, no hybridisation (e.g CK-MB) between subunits of CK-Mt has been found.

CK activity may also be found in macromolecular form—macro CK. Macro-CK is sometimes found in hospitalised patients in small proportions. It exists in two forms MacroCK-Type 1 and MacroCK-Type 2. MacroCK-Type 1 is a complex of CK-BB+IgG or CK-MM+lgA. It is associated with gastrointestinal diseases, adenoma, carcinoma, myocardial/vascular diseases and other life-threatening conditions. It often occurs in women older than 50 yrs.

MacroCK-Type 2 is oligomeric mitochondrial CK. It is found predominantly in adults who are severely ill with malignancies/liver disease or in children with myocardial disease. Both the M and B subunits have a C-terminal lysine residue, but only the former can be hydrolysed by the action of carboxypeptidases normally present in blood. Based on this hydrolysis, several isoforms are possible with different nomenclatures (Fig. 21.3).

Biochemistry and Physiology

The two enzymes CK and Adenylate kinase (AK) play a decisive role in the synthesis of ATP, the immediate energy source of the muscle, the CMS and many proliferating tissues. CK is involved in providing energy for the muscle in two ways. In mitochondria, the site of energy production, CK-Mt catalyses the synthesis of Creatine phosphate (CrP) from ATP. The energy-rich CrP is carried in the CrP shuttle from the mitochondria to the cytoplasm where it is converted back into ATP by CK at the sites of energy consumption. Some of the intracellular CK is present in free form, some attached to the respective cell structure. After release of CK into the blood (post-injury/infarct/damage), the enzyme undergoes the so-called postsynthetic modifications producing the forms known as CK-variants. Variants with normal molecular masses of about 80 K ΔA occur when carboxypeptidase successively removes the C-terminal lysine of both M-chains. The tissue form CK-MM_3 becomes first CK-MM_2 and finally CK-MM_1. The analogous action on the tissue form CK-MB_2 results in CK-MB.

As described earlier, variants with higher molecular mass > 200kDA can occur when CK is bound by specific immunoglobulins (macro CK type 1) or when CK-Mt occurs in preferred oligomeric form (macro CK type 2).

The total CK activity measurable in serum is composed of the activities of the cytoplasmic dimeric isoenzymes CK-MM, CK-MB, CK-BB and their post-synthetically modified forms and of the activities of the macro CK. In healthy individuals the total activity consists mainly of CK-MM while the other CK isoenzymes and variants are only present in trace amounts or are undetectable. If the total activity of CK or of a particular isoenzyme is increased, the isoenzyme pattern can provide information on the underlying organ damage.

Tissue distribution of CK and its isoenzymes

Tissue	CK activity U/gm wet Weight	CK-MM %	CK-MB %	CK-BB %
Skeletal muscle	2500-3000	95-99	1-5	<0.1
Myocardium	500-700			
-Normal		90	5	
-Pathologically altered		70-80	20-30	
Brain	200-300			100
Gastrointestinal tract	120-150			100
Bladder	85			100
Uterus				
-Non Pregnant	165			100
-Pregnant	245		6	94
Placenta	250	19	1	80
Prostate gland	85			100
Lung	15	0-20		80-100

CK ACTIVITY—SKELETAL MUSCLE DISEASE

Serum CK activity is greatly elevated, at some time during the course of the disease in all types of muscular dystrophy like Duchenne Muscular Dystrophy (DMD) and Becker Muscular Dystrophy (BMD). Levels up to 50 times the upper limit of normal may be observed. In progressive muscular dystrophies like DMD/BMD, serum CK activity is the highest at 7-10 yrs of age and falls, as the patient

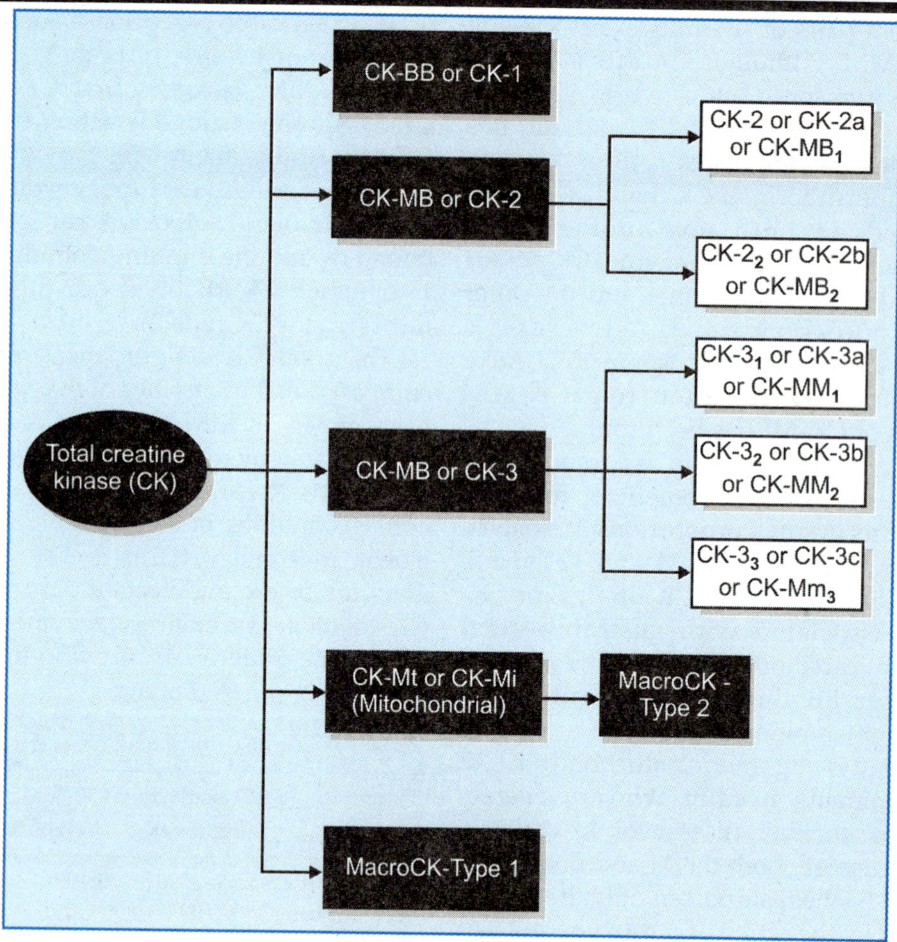

Fig. 21.3: Isoforms of creatine kinase

gets older. 50-80% of asymptomatic female carriers of DMD show a 3-6-fold rise in CK activity, but values may be normal if specimens are obtained after patients have experienced a period of physical inactivity. High to very high values of CK are noted in viral myositis, polymyositis, acute rhabdomyolysis and malignant hyperthermia. Hence, attention needs to be paid when interpreting the results with the clinical findings. Fructose-bisphosphate aldolase (FBPA) is also present in high concentrations in skeletal muscle and thus could be used to support the conclusions reached from the assay of CK. However, FBPA is also present in many other tissues, though not at such high concentrations. Particularly important in this respect is the high FBPA content of red blood cells. It is, therefore, essential that a sample of serum to be assayed for CK does not contain lysed red blood cells, i.e. the serum should be free from haemolysis.

Apparently, CK-MB replaces part of the CK-MM form in the muscles, resulting in impaired storage of Creatine Phospahte in the muscle. In dystrophies and myopathies, usually only CK-MM is present in serum; but if total CK activity is high, some CK-MB can also be detected (<6%) because diseased skeletal muscle may contain a significant proportion of this isoenzyme owing to the phenomenon of fetal reversion, in which fetal pattern of protein synthesis reappear.

In polymyositis, CK-MM isoform pattern correlates well with the course of the disease. Total CK activity can also be elevated by direct trauma to muscle, including IM injections and surgical interventions, hypo or hyperthermia seizures, neuroleptic malignant syndrome, sepsis, exposure to certain drugs and chronic endocrinopathies.

Activity of total CK and CK-MB as a result of ACUTE skeletal muscle damage

Disease	Assessment
Acute damage (general)	• Total CK can increase to well above 5000 U/L (37°C) in proportion to the damage • The CK-MB activity is < 3% of the total CK • CK-MB concentration shows the same behaviour
Physical activity **Work** **Sport**	• All strenuous exercises increases CK activity. • There is no limit which permits a distinction between a normal reaction and pathological muscle damage. • High activity is observed after some forms of exercise • (Like running downhill) and rhabdomyolysis • Excessive training (like marathon runners) leads to CK-MB activity > 3%
Diseases	Increased CK activity is observed in diseases like tetany, cramps, Parkinson's disease, cough attacks, status asthmaticus, psychosis and delirium tremens.
Intramuscular injections	• Depending upon the substance, volume, concentration and osmolality, IM injections increases CK activity and can interfere with diagnosis of infarction. • Some drugs chlorpromazine, diazepam and promethazine are known to cause muscle damage that causes a rise in CK activity.
Surgery, Trauma, arterial embolism	• Surgery or trauma (also burns, electrical injuries and pressure necroses) leads to an increase in CK activity embolism proportional to the severity of damage. • CK-MB increase after chest injuries is thought to indicate myocardial damage
Polymyositis viral myositis	In acute and sub acute myositis, the CK activity > 20000 U/L (37°C) • No dynamic changes in CK activity observed with pharmacological doses
Medications and drugs of abuse, chemicals	Drugs of intoxication (abuse) like amphetamines barbiturates, heroin, etc. • In extreme cases of rhabdomyolysis or malignant hyperthermia CK activities > 20000 U/L (37°C) are found
Contd...	
Chronic damage (general)	• CK is elevated depending upon the severity of the disease • CK-MB activity may be >10% of the total CK due to isoenzyme synthesis of the chronically stressed muscle. Thus an elevated CK-MB, in this case, is not due to myocardial involvement.
Muscular dystrophy-DMD and BMD	• Disease with X-Linked recessive inheritance and extreme CK activities > 25000 U/L (37°C), particularly in the initial phase. • The CK-MB activity is also increased. This does not confirm myocardial involvement. • In other type of dystrophies like limb-girdle type, ocular type, myotonic dystrophy, CK activities are sometimes within reference range and rarely > 2000 U/L (37 °C)
Myotonia congenita, Glycogenosis type V, myastenia, gravis, spinal muscular atrophieseference	These primary myopathies also have CK activities which are within the range or only slightly increased depending on the phase of the disease.
Polymyositis, dermatomyositis, ocular myositis.	The CK activities in the chronic forms of myositis are considerably lower than in the acute forms. Activities within the reference are also possible.
Secondary myopathies	Secondary increase in CK activity may be seen in endocrine diseases, intoxications, seizure disorders, paralysis, Lupus erythematosus, multiple sclerosis and taking certain drugs. The CK activity returns to the reference range with improvement in underlying conditions.
Medications and drugs of abuse.	• Pharmacological doses of anti-arrhythmic drugs, beta-blockers, potassium lowering drugs, Lithium, halothane, etc. lead to increased CK activity. • Prednisone and related steroids and chemotheraphy agents lead to lower CK activity.

CK activity—HEART DISEASE

Total CK activity shows an increase following Ml in which it is increased earlier than other enzymes, beginning at 4-6 hrs, peaking on an average at 24hrs and returning to normal within 2-3 days. The area under the peak and slope of the initial rise are proportional to the size of the infarct. False negatives are rare and are usually due to technical errors. False positives may occur, and for accurate diagnosis of Ml CK-MB activity should be measured. If the Total CK- activity is raised and CK-MB contributes more than 6% of the activity then Ml is considered highly probable.

After Ml the maximum CK activity rarely exceeds 7500U/L (37°C). Higher CK activities suggest concomitant skeletal muscle damage. Early reperfusion is marked by a particularly rapid rise and early peak of the CK-MB. A characteristic second peak of CK-MB indicates a second trauma or reinfarction.

As CK-MB also occurs in skeletal muscles, it is, therefore, not absolutely cardiospecific; a diagnostic strategy for careful preselection of patients based on clinical criteria is necessary. It is also necessary, that, the **ratio of total CK to CK-MB activities** be measured. This helps in differential diagnosis of Ml and skeletal muscle damage. If this is done, the clinical questions can be answered in most cases.

Activity of Total CK and CK-MB as a result of CARDIAC muscle damage

Disease	Assessment
Acute myocardial damage	• The CK increases in proportion to the damage; the CK -MB activity is more than 6% of the total CK. • Total CK activities > 7500U/L (37°C) indicate additional skeletal muscle trauma, e.g. as a result of resuscitation • CK-MB activities > 25% after immunoinhibition require determination of CK variants.
Myocarditis, Endocarditis and pericarditis	Elevated total CK and CK-MB Levels are typical in myocarditis; activity time curves resembling infarction are possible.
Angina pectoris	• No increases in CK-MB are observed in stable angina with immunoinhibition method; unstable angina can show small increases in CK-MB concentration, which are within the reference interval. • Uncomplicated cardiac catheterisation and coronary angiography do not lead to significant increase in CK-MB. • Resuscitation, defibrillation and chest trauma lead to increased CK activities, which correspond to the extent of skeletal muscle damage; if there is myocardial involvement the CK-MB increases.
Diagnostic and therapeutic interventions, trauma	• Surgical procedures involving the myocardium release CK-MB. • CK-MB activities > 50 U/L (37°C) after coronary artery bypass grafting suggest infarction. Valve replacement and transplantation lead to increases in CK and CK-MB • Stress tests (exercise, etc.) do not lead to pathological concentrations.
Tachycardia, heart failure and valve defects	These conditions do not usually lead to a significant increase in activity.

CLINICAL ENZYMOLOGY IN MI—A BRIEF ANALYSIS

Enzymological methods have been particularly useful in providing supporting evidence for myocardial infarction (Ml) and also monitoring the course of the infarct.

In Ml, a coronary artery becomes obstructed and this leads to irreversible damage and necrosis of the heart tissue. Enzymes are released from the necrotic tissue into the plasma; the three enzymes most commonly assayed are creatine kinase (CK), aspartate aminotransferase (SGOT) and lactate dehydrogenase (LDH). Each enzyme shows a different time course for release into the plasma and subsequent disappearance (Fig. 21.4). These differences depend upon the concentration of each present in the cardiac tissue, their rate of release and their subsequent rate of clearance or degradation. Their **half-life** in the plasma is:

- CK: »15 hrs
- SGOT: » 17 hrs
- LDH: »110 hrs

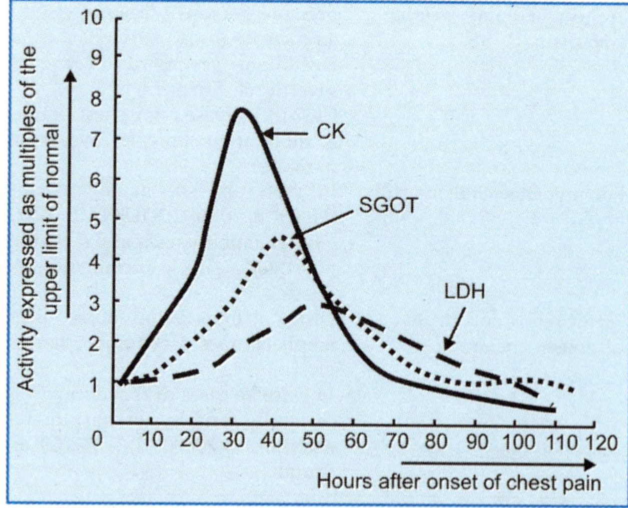

Fig. 21.4: Typical changes in CK, SGOT and LDH activities following MI

CK is the earliest to be detectable, rising 4-6 hrs after onset of pain, reaching a peak at 24-36 hrs and then rapidly declining. SGOT reaches a peak between 48 and 60 hrs and LDH between 48 and 72 hrs, the latter declines more slowly than the former. The prognosis and progress can be assessed by the increase in the activities of these enzymes. CK, which does not occur in the liver unlike SGOT and LDH, can therefore be used to differentiate heart disease from liver disease. Thus, CK can be used in the early detection and prognosis of myocardial infarction.

Comparison of sensitivity and specificity of various test in MI

Test	Sensitivity %	Specificity %
EGG	63-84	100
Increased SGOT	89 - 97	48 - 88
Increased LDH	87	88
LDH1 >LDH2 (on 3rd day after chest pain)	61-96	94-99
Increased Total CK	93 -100	57- 88
Increased CK-MB	94-100	93-100

Determination of CK and CK-MB activity alone is not suitable for assessment of the risk of Ml. It can be particularly useful in interpretation, if its estimation is accompanied by determination of the isoenzyme (CK-MB), serial tests (enzyme-time curves), or ECG under exercise testing. The CK-MB results can be interpreted on the basis of the 6% rule, a limit of 12U/L or preferably the dynamic activity time curve of an enzymogram.

The 6% Rule: The decision criterion is an increase in the total CK activity to > 100 U/L (25°C) within the diagnostic time window and a simultaneous increase in CK-MB activity. A CK-MB fraction more than 6% of the total activity is regarded as diagnostic for Ml. A fraction less than 6% indicates skeletal muscle damage. The clinical specificity of this rule is high as the number of false positive results caused by the presence of extracardiac CK-MB is small. This high clinical specificity is of course obtained at the expense of some loss of sensitivity in the detection of smaller infarctions.

The 12U/L limit: The decision criterion is—increased total CK activity during diagnostic time window and a simultaneous increase in CK-MB activity to > 10U/L (25°C)/15U/L (30°C)/24U/L (37°C). This is equivalent to 12U/L CK-B activity (25°C). This strategy is characterised by a higher clinical sensitivity, which also permits identification of small infarctions. This high diagnostic sensitivity is obtained at the expense of some loss of specificity if the prevalence of infarction is low.

Dynamic activity-time curves (cardioenzymogram): If an acute Ml is suspected serial determination of total CK and CK-MB activity are carried out so that the changes in the enzyme activities observed in this dynamic condition can be taken into account in the diagnosis and monitoring of treatment. This strategy is characterised by high levels of diagnostic sensitivity, specificity and flexibility as regards to medical and logistic requirements.

METHOD OF DETERMINATION—TOTAL CK

The methodology recommended by International Federation of Clinical Chemistry (IFCC) is a photometric rate assay. The reaction conditions are so robust that the measurements can be performed without problems at reaction temperatures of 37°C, 30°C or 25°C under optimal reaction conditions. The principle of the IFCC method can be depicted as per the equation given in Fig. 21.5.

METHOD OF DETERMINATION—CK ISOENZYMES

At present only determination of the isoenzyme CK-MB is of clinical significance.

Immunoinhibition method

This is currently the most economical, practical and widely used method in clinical laboratories worldwide. The theoretical basis for the clinical application of the Immunoinhibition method is the assumption that only CK-MM and CK-MB are released into the blood stream after muscle damage. The reagent used contain anti CK-M antibodies, which completely inhibit all CK-M activity, i.e., both M subunits in CK-MM and the single M subunit in CK-MB. The remaining non-CK-M activity corresponding to the CK-B activity of CK-MB is measured. Since, only CK-B activity of the dimeric CK-MB molecule is measured, multiplication by a factor of 2 gives the CK-MB activity in the specimen.

Isoenzyme electrophoresis method

The CK isoenzymes are separated on cellulose acetate strips or agarose gel and the activity bands then visualised fluormetrically using the total CK reagent. The fluorescence of the $NADPH_2$ formed in the reaction permits quantitative analysis.

This method is useful only to exactly differentiate between isoenzymes. It is labour intensive, complicated and hence expensive. Moreover, the interference due to AK makes the interpretation difficult. Not practical for routine use in a clinical laboratory.

Immunoassay for Determination of CK-MB Mass (Concentration)

Here CK-MB is determined with a combination of CK-B and CK-M specific antibodies or with CK-MB specific antibodies. The first generation assays use the double antibody technique with CK-M and CK-B specific antibodies. The second-generation assays use CK-MB specific monoclonal antibodies, in some cases, in combination with CK-M and CK-B specific antibodies. The assay format may be EIA, Fluorescent immunoassay, Luminiscent immunoassay, radio immunoassay, etc.

Interferences have been described in these assays too

- Apart from interference typical of immunoassays (like HAMA-human anti-mouse antibody), specific interference by high concentrations of CK-MM and CK-BB or by CK-B binding autoantibodies has been demonstrated.
- Lack of a universal standardisation has influenced the non-comparability of results.
- The data on reference ranges, decision limit and specific activities are therefore not uniform but vary from reagent-to-reagent.

CRITICAL DETERMINANTS OF CK AND CK-MB REAGENT SYSTEM DESIGN

Appropriate activator

During storage, CK is rapidly inactivated by the oxidation of the sulphydryl groups at the active site of the enzyme. The need to reactivate the enzyme has been demonstrated and the various sulphydryl reagents like cysteine, dithiothreitol, glutathione, 2- mercaptoethanol and N- acetylcysteine have been used as an activator in the reagent. But:

- Cysteine deteriorates rapidly in solution.
- Dithiothreitol causes turbidity by precipitation of albumin.
- Glutathione is unstable since it allows interference by glutathione reductase released from red cells in haemolysed specimens.
- 2-mercaptoethanol cause turbidity and its decomposition products inhibits CK.

N- acetylcysteine (NAC) suffers none of these shortcomings and is accepted to be the best thiol (sulphydryl) activator for maintenance and

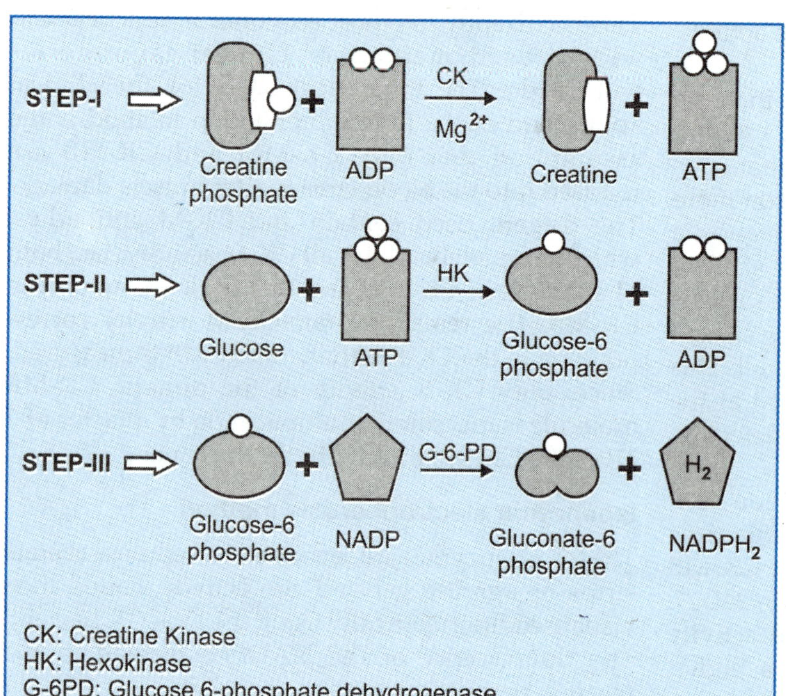

Fig. 21.5: The IFCC principle of photometric rate assay for CK
CK: Creatine Kinase
HK: Hexokinase
G-6PD: Glucose 6-phosphate dehydrogenase

reactivation of CK activity in serum. The optimum concentration of NAC is of utmost importance. A small imbalance in its concentration may cause free cysteine to be released. This may cause the reagent system to behave erroneously.

Adenylate Kinase (AK) Interference

AK is present in many tissues and cells including skeletal and cardiac muscle, liver, brain, and erythrocytes. The enzyme is also present in normal serum and may be markedly raised in haemolysed specimens. Adenylate kinase deficiency in the erythrocytes, a rare genetic disorder, is associated with haemolytic anaemia. AK catalyses the reaction as shown in figure 21.6.

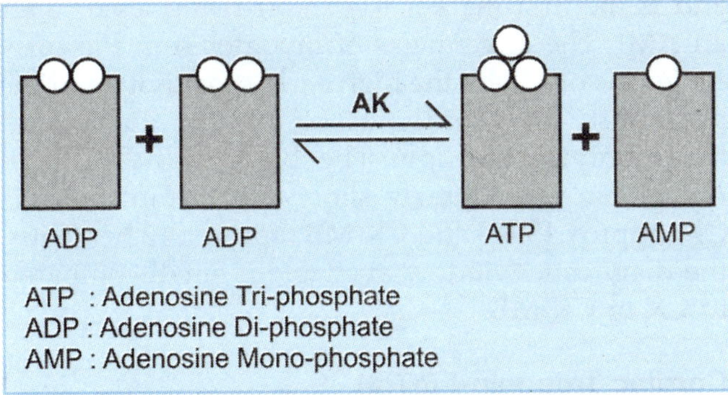

Fig. 21.6: Adenylate Kinase catalytic action

The ATP generated in this catalytic action of AK enters the reaction of the CK assay and leads to an apparent increase or false positive values of CK.

AK activity can be inhibited by adding:

- Fluoride
- AMP or
- Diadenosine pentaphosphate (DAPP)

Although Fluoride is an effective inhibitor, it may form insoluble magnesium fluoride with magnesium ion in CK assay. AMP alone can competitively inhibit product formation (2ADPF = ATP + AMP). Thus, to adequately inhibit AK from red cell and muscle and to ensure better results, an **optimised blend** of AMP and DAPP should be used. DAPP competitively inhibits the AK of muscle and erythrocytes while AMP inhibits AK derived from liver and kidney.

Fildes and Harris (1966) found electrophoretic variation in red cells and defined 3 phenotypes, designated AK1, AK2-1 and AK2. In India, in majority of the populations the AK1 gene occurs in high frequencies, approaching 90% and above. Thus, this demographic pattern also indicates that, in India, to get accurate results, a CK assay system should contain optimised blend of AK inhibitors.

Cation Inhibitor

CK is readily inhibited by polyvalent cations such as Ca^{2+}. This can be prevented by addition of EDTA. EDTA also helps in the protection of the thiol reagent from oxidation by metal ions.

Anti CK-M Antibody used in Immunoinhibition Method

The anti CK-M antibodies quantitatively inhibit all M subunits of the sample within the incubation time. These antibodies should have high specificity and corresponding affinity.

Since, the specificity of the antibody used as anti-CK-M reagent is of utmost importance, a brief discussion on antibody structure would be worthwhile.

The antibody molecule is made up of two identical heavy and two identical light chains held together by interchain disulphide bonds. These chains can be separated by reduction of the S-S bonds and acidifications. The exposed hinge region is extended in structure due to high proline content and therefore, vulnerable to proteolytic attack. The molecule is split by papain to yield two identical fragments, each with a single combining site for antigen, called F_{ab} fragment (Fragment antigen binding). A third fragment, known as F_c fragment, is also formed. The F_c fragment lacks the ability to bind to antigens. The F_{ab} fragment of the "Y-shaped" antibody carries the paratopes, the binding sites that bind to the epitopes on the CK-M antigen. In an intact antibody molecule F_{ab} is present along with the F_c fragment. Because the F_c fragment binds to complements, certain bacterial proteins (like staphylococcal Protein A) and other non-specific molecules such as heterophillic antibodies, the reagent for inhibition should preferably be devoid of the F_c fragment. Since, the F_{ab} fragment is specific with high antigen binding capacity, to achieve adequate inhibition of CK-M activity without interference, a reagent system should preferably use the purified F_{ab}fragment in the anti-CK-M reagent (Fig. 21.7).

Liquid Reagent System

In the CK/CK-MB assay, the calculations to arrive at the results involve a multiplication step with a

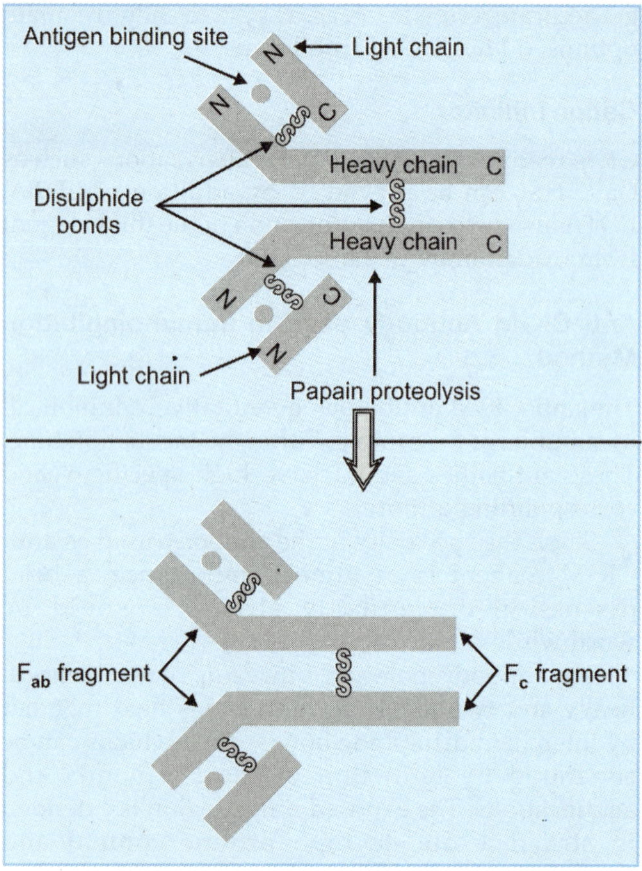

Fig. 21.7: Antibody model showing proteolytic fragments

relatively high value of factor-over 6000 for CK-MB and over 8000 for total CK. This means a small change in the optical density (OD) would result in a significant change in the final results of CK /CK-MB activities.

In a dry powder-based assay system, the reagent powder is reconstituted with deionised water or buffer to make the working reagent. This reconstituted reagent may contain suspended microparticles, though apparently, it may seem to be **optically clean.** These microparticles are heterogeneous molecular aggregates derived from the lyophilised reagent. During the course of photometric measurement, the passage of light through the solution cause "excitation" of these microparticles leading to erroneous OD readings. This error is compounded by multiplication with the high factor. Consequently, the final results of CK/CK-MB activities may show unexpected variation leading to erroneous/inadequate clinical decisions. This problem can be solved by filtration of the reconstituted reagent through a 0.22 micron sterile filter. But, in a routine clinical laboratory this may not be a practical option. Thus, the best option is to use ready-made liquid reagent system available with some manufacturers. These reagents are optically clean and do not cause the interference from suspended microparticles.

OTHER BIOMARKERS OF MI

Myoglobin

Myoglobin, a relatively small (17.8 kDa) heme protein that transports oxygen within muscle cells, constitutes about 2 percent of muscle protein in both skeletal and cardiac muscle. Thus, the marker is not cardiospecific. Because of its low molecular weight, myoglobin is rapidly released into the circulation and is the first marker to exhibit rising levels after an AMI. The advantages of myoglobin in the early diagnosis of MI are the high early sensitivity and the possibility of rapidly assessing the success of thrombolytic therapy. The biologic half-life of myoglobin is extremely short (10-20 min) vis-ávis CK (approx.15 hr) and CK-MB (approx. 12 hr). Thus, the diagnostic window available is small compared to CK or CK-MB.

Cardiac Troponin-I (cTnl)

- Troponin is a complex consisting of three single-chain polypeptides:
- Troponin-l, which prevents muscle contraction in the absence of calcium.
- Troponin-T, which connects the troponin complex to tropomyosin.
- Troponin-C, which binds calcium

Together with tropomyosin and under the influence of calcium, troponin regulates muscle contraction. The cardiac muscle-specific isoform cTnl (24 kDa) exhibits approximately 60 percent homology with the skeletal isoforms (sTnl), and has a unique 31 amino acid extension of the N-terminus. After myocardial infarction, elevated cTnl levels appear within 3 to 6 hours. Levels peak within 14 to 20 hours, and return to normal after 5 to 7 days. Cardiac Troponin-I is 100% cardiospecific. Unfortunately, the standardisation of cardiac troponin—I assays is problematic. Up to 20-fold variation of serum cTnl mass determinations may be observed for a given patient sample when measured by different assay systems. As a result, significant ambiguity often exists in the clinical interpretation of serum cTnl concentrations. Recent efforts have been directed toward the biochemical standardization of cTnl assays. However, the heterogeneous nature and biochemical complexity of the serum forms of cTnl and differences of the epitope recognition by the various methods have hindered the harmonisation of serum cTnl assays.

IMPORTANT TERMS

Angina pectoris

Angina pectoris is the medical term used to describe chest pain caused by poor blood flow to certain areas of the heart muscle. Often, the name is shortened to angina.

Angiography

It is a description of blood vessels and lyphatics. The relative inaccessibility of the blood vessels and lyphatics for physical examination requires investigation with other means, primarily radiologic examinations that include lung scintigraphy, conventional or digital subtraction pulmonary angiography (DSPA), pulmonary computed tomography angiography (PCTA), and pulmonary magnetic resonance angiography (PMRA).

Aortic stenosis

Aortic stenosis (AS) is the obstruction of blood flow across the aortic valve.

AS has several etiologies: congenital unicuspid or bicuspid valve, rheumatic fever, and degenerative calcific changes of the valve.

Arterial embolism

Embolism is the obstruction of a blood vessel by foreign substances or a blood clot. If the blood vessel concerned is an artery it is called arterial embolism. Obstruction in the pulmonary artery is called pulmonary embolism (PE). In PE the blood clot is in the lung. PE is usually caused by an embolus from thrombosis in lower extremities, pelvis, arms, or heart. When a clot forms in the legs or arms, it is referred to as a deep venous thrombosis (DVT).

Atheroma

Fatty degeneration or thickening of the walls of the larger arteries occurring in atherosclerosis.

Atria

A chamber or cavity communicating with another structure.

Defibrillation

Fibrillation is a small, local, involuntary, muscular contraction, due to spontaneous activation of single muscle cells or muscle fibres. Defibrillation is the termination of atrial or ventricular fibrillation, usually by electroshock.

Delirium Tremens

Delirium tremens (DTs) is a severe manifestation of alcohol withdrawal. Pearson first described it in 1813 as an acute psychosis following abstinence from alcohol. Although it only occurs in a relatively small number of patients who undergo alcohol withdrawal, it can be fatal. DT is a medical emergency that requires prompt recognition and treatment.

Diaphoresis

Profuse sweating.

Dyspnoea

Air hunger resulting in laboured or difficult breathing, sometimes accompanied by pain.

Endocarditis

Endocarditis refers to an infection of a heart valve. Although several different types of organisms can cause endocarditis, it is usually caused by a bacterial infection.

Endocardium

Serous lining membrane of inner surface and cavities of the heart. It is continuous with the intima or interior coat of arteries.

Epicardium

The inner or visceral layer of the pericardium, which forms a serous membrane forming the outermost layer of the wall of the heart.

Epigastrium

Region over the pit of the stomach.

Glycogenosis Type V

Also known as McArdle disease. It is caused by a deficiency of myophosphorylase (alpha-1,4-glucan orthophosphate glycosyl transferase), which normally initiates glycogen breakdown by removing 1,4-

glucosyl groups from the glycogen molecule with release of glucose- 1-phosphate.

Malignant Hyperthermia

Malignant hyperthermia (MH) is a genetic disease, which may result in rhabdomyolysis. In this disease, episodes of hyperthermia and rhabdomyolysis are triggered by exposure to volatile anaesthetics such as halothane, or succinylcholine, a depolarising muscle relaxant. MH appears to be an autosomal dominant condition.

Marantic Endocarditis

Endocarditis is the inflammation of the lining membrane of the heart. It is usually confined to the external lining of the valve, sometimes to the lining membrane of its chambers. May be due to invasion of microorganisms or an abnormal immunological reaction. Marantic endocarditis, also known as Nonbacterial Thrombotic Endocarditis (NBTE), is the endocarditis due to non-bacterial causes.

Muscular Dystrophy

Muscular dystrophy (MD) is a collective group of inherited noninflammatory but progressive muscle disorders without a central or peripheral nerve abnormality. The disease affects the muscles, with definite fiber degeneration but without evidence for morphologic aberrations. Dystrophin was found to be at the root of the disorder. Defects in the genetic code for this 427-kDa-muscle protein resulted in the various manifestations commonly associated with MD.

Myasthenia Gravis

Myasthenia gravis (MG) is an acquired autoimmune disorder characterised clinically by weakness of skeletal muscles and fatigability on exertion. Thomas Willis reported the first clinical description in 1672.

Myocarditis

Myocarditis is an inflammatory disease of the myocardium with a wide range of clinical presentation, from subtle to devastating. It usually manifests in an otherwise healthy person and can result in rapidly progressive (and often fatal) heart failure and arrhythmia.

Myocardium

The middle layer of the walls of the heart composed of cardiac muscle.

Myocytes

Muscular tissue cells.

Myositis

Inflammation of muscle tissue especially voluntary muscles.

Myotonia Congenita

A benign disease characterised by tonic spasms of the muscles induced by voluntary movements; usually congenital and transmitted from one generation to another.

Ocular Myositis

Inflammation of muscle tissues of the eye.

Parkinson's Disease

Parkinson disease (PD) is a progressive neurodegenerative disorder associated with a loss of dopaminergic nigrostriatal neurons. It is named after James Parkinson, the English physician who described the shaking palsy in 1817.

Pericarditis

Pericarditis is the inflammation of the lining of the heart. Pericarditis is a commonly found syndrome in the hospital setting, particularly in the coronary care unit. It most often affects men aged between 20 and 50 yr, usually following respiratory infections.

Polymyositis

Polymyositis (PM) is an inflammatory muscle disease of unknown etiology. PM, dermatomyositis (DM), and inclusion body myositis are the major members of a group of syndromes called the idiopathic inflammatory myopathies. In much of the literature, PM and DM are grouped as one disease.

Regurgitation

A backward flowing, as in the return of solids or fluids from stomach or the backward flow of blood through a defective heart valve.

Resuscitation

Restoration to life of one apparently dead. Also may be used for cardiopulmonary resuscitation (CPR). CPR is the re-establishing of heart and lung action by artificial ventilation and closed-chest cardiac massage, after cardiac arrest or apparent sudden death resulting from electric shock, drowning, respiratory arrest, and other causes.

Rhabdomyolysis

Rhabdomyolysis is the breakdown of muscle fibres with leakage of potentially toxic cellular contents into the systemic circulation. The final common pathway of rhabdomyolysis may be a disturbance in myocyte calcium homeostasis.

Spinal Muscular Atrophy

The spinal muscular atrophies (SMAs) are a clinically and genetically heterogeneous group of disorders. They are characterised by primary degeneration of the anterior horn cells of the spinal cord and often of the bulbar motor nuclei without evidence of primary peripheral nerve or long-tract involvement.

Status Asthmaticus

Status asthmaticus is a medical emergency in which asthma symptoms are refractory to initial bronchodilator therapy in the emergency department. Patients complain of chest tightness, rapidly progressive shortness of breath, dry cough, and wheezing. Typically, patients present a few days after the onset of a viral respiratory illness or following exposure to a potent allergen or irritant.

Syncope

Syncope (fainting) is a sudden fall of blood pressure resulting in loss of consciousness.

Tachycardia

Abnormally rapid heart rate.

Tetany

A syndrome manifested by sharp flexion of the wrist and ankle joints, muscle twitching, cramps and convulsions due to abnormal calcium metabolism and occurring in parathyroid hypofunction, vitamin D deficiency, alkalosis and as a result of alkaline salts.

Thrombogenesis

The formation of a blood clot.

Transmural

Across the wall of an organ or structure, as in transmural myocardial thrombosis, in which the tissue in the entire thickness of the portion of the cardiac wall is affected.

Triage

Triage is a French word that literally means, "to separate". Medical Triage refers to the classification of patients or casualties to determine priority of need and proper place of treatment.

Viral Myositis

Viral myositis is an acute, subacute, or chronic infection of skeletal muscle. Once considered a tropical disease, it is now seen in temperate climates as well, particularly with the emergence of HIV infection. In addition to HIV, other viruses, bacteria, mycobacteria, fungi, and parasites can cause myositis.

LIVER DISEASE (SERUM ENZYME PATTERNS) VALUES ARE X TIMES THE UPPER NORMAL LIMITS

Condition	*GOT*	*GPT*	*LDH*	*SAP*
Acute viral hepatitis	15-20	15-20	6-8	1-2
Obstructive jaundice (intra/extra hepatic)	3-4	3-4	1-2	3-6
Cirrhosis (portal)	2-3	2-3	1-2	1-2
Secondary deposits in liver without jaundice	1-2	1-2	1-3	1-3

GOT—glutamic-oxaloacetic transaminase

GPT—glutamic pyruvic transaminase (tends to be higher than GOT in acute liver disorders)
LDH—lactate dehydrogenase
SAP—(Serum) alkaline phosphatase
(In obstructive jaundice in addition to others, 5-nucleotidase rises 4-6 times the upper normal limit (UNL) and in tumour deposits in liver GGTP-

Gamma-lutamyl Transpeptidase rises 4-20 times the UNL.

AUTOMATION IN CLINICAL CHEMISTRY RANDOM ACCESS AUTO ANALYSER

These kind of completely automatic analysers are best suited for laboratories with moderate to heavy workload.

For a laboratory considering an automated clinical chemistry system, there are a number of criteria which are very important to the Indian/tropical environment:

1. Design
2. Support
3. Cost.

Design

System design is an important factor and one should answer questions as:

a. Does it have miles of tubing which can leak and which will need replacing?
b. Is the dispensing mediated by banks of syringes which can (and will) leak, and will need replacing?
c. Are the moving parts easily accessible?
d. Does the system need external drains?
e. Does the system need external water supplies?
f. Is the software open (can I change volumes, times etc)?
g. Is the system open (can I use any reagent I like)?
h. Is the system flexible (can I do drugs, drug abuse in urine-DAU, special proteins, and general developmental work etc.)?
i. Is the system truly walkaway?
j. Can the system be interlinked with other equipment?
k. Can the system work with a data management system?

Support

Is the system supported in India by an organisation with true accountability, professionalism, and infrastructure such that you can depend on getting help when you need it?

Cost

1. Capital cost of the equipment
2. Recurrent cost of reagents and consumables.

When looking at the cost of an instrument it is vital to compare "like" with "like". This means that it is important to develop an understanding of the design feature differences which can translate into very real benefits to the user. This means in turn that one should not just compare quoted prices on the assumption that one system is much like another, they are not.

To summarize, when choosing an analyser one should think very seriously about the suitability of the equipment to India. Issues of throughput, and unit price should not distract the buyer from fundamentals of good design because in the long run good design will save money.

MARS (Courtesy: Lilac Medicare)

MARS (Multi-Analyte Random Access System), manufactured by Infopia, Korea and marketed in India by Aster Biologicals, Mumbai (Clinical Chemistry Division of Lilac Medicare (P) Ltd), is a Fully Automated Random Access Clinical Chemistry Analyser. The revolutionary design makes MARS a compact and complete analyzer. The low running cost and wide routine chemistry test menu makes MARS a brilliant choice for laboratories having small to medium workload. The instrument can perform several testing methods like End-point, Fixed-time kinetic, Kinetic and Immuno-turbidimetry with multi point calibration facility in both monochromatic and bichromatic modes.

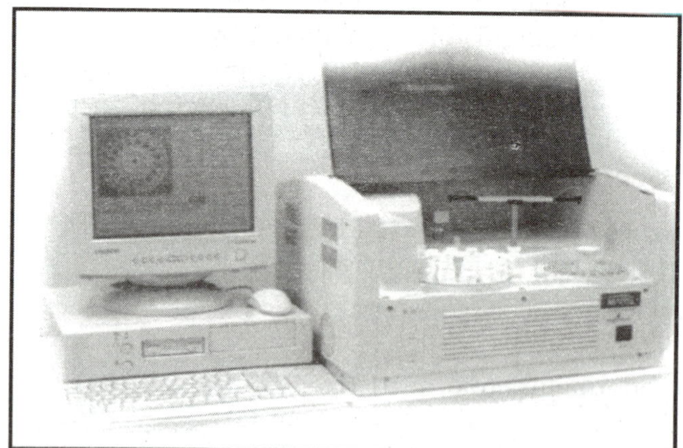

This state-of-the-art instrument has Open System Architecture. Clinical Chemistry reagents sourced from any manufacturers can be used on this system. MARS has a high throughput of up to 180 tests per hour. The fully automated sample/reagent pippeting, stirring mechanism and programmable on–board laundry system enables the system to achieve the desired throughput. Other significant features of MARS include: Dual probes (dedicated-sample and reagent probes) that avoids the carryover, 18-reagent positions with 36 reagents programming facility & 40+40 sample positions.

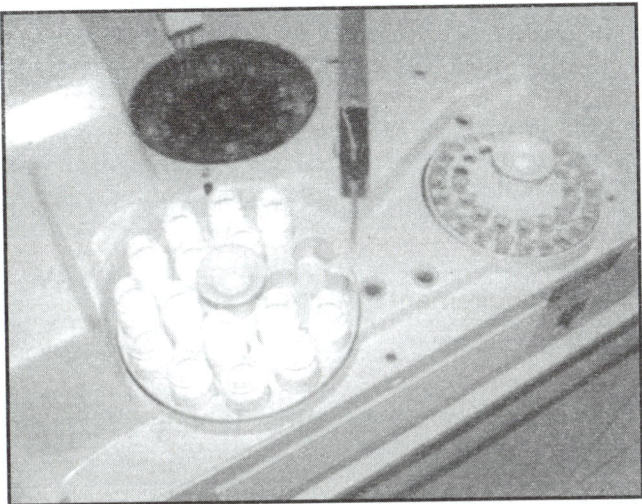

The functioning of dual probes is guided by two world class Hamilton syringes. MARS is equipped with level sensor detector and can aspirate sample from both, sample cups and primary tubes. Reaction takes place in the 48 semi disposable reaction polycarbonate cuvettes.

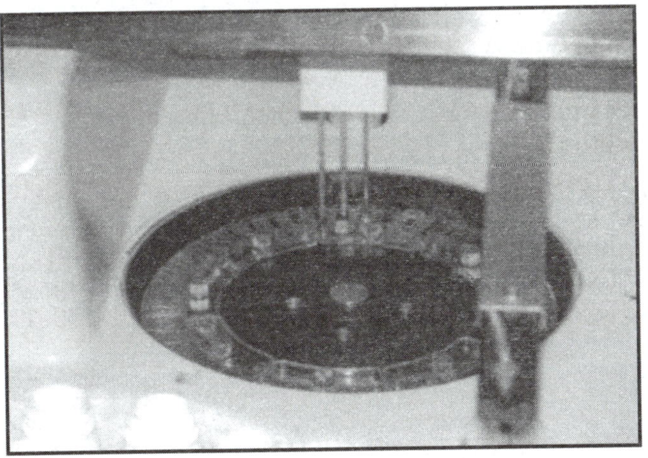

This system is designed on basis of the analytical method of the absorption of light using a diffraction Grating monochromator (spectrum photometer). The continuous grating allows free wavelenth selection from 320 nm to 720 nm in 1 nm increment enabling the operator to select the specific wavelength required for the analyte detection.

MARS proves to be a true economical instrument for the laboratory for its minimal volumes of sample & reagents. The sample volume ranges from 3-30 ml while reagent volume from 50-300 ml. To add to economical aspect the instrument requires no consumables for processing and maintenance. The commonly available distilled water is minimally used for priming and rinsing.

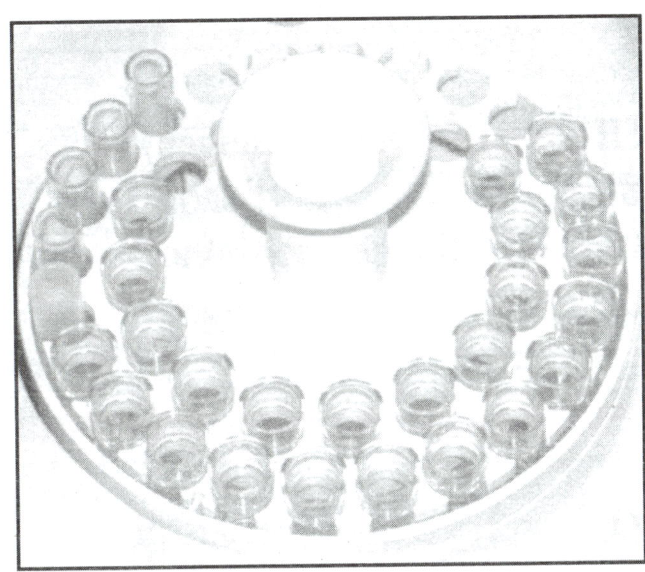

The system is driven by user-friendly software. The software has Graphic Mode Display of ongoing process and results. The Online QC with Levy Jenning chart happens to be one of the important features of the software. The step-by-step instructions on the display make the operation easy.

MARS- TECHNICAL SPECIFICATIONS

System

Model	: Table top, Compact Unit, Fully Automated clinical Chemistry Analyser
Type	: Multi Analyte, Random Access System
Throughput	: Up to 180 Tests/Hour

Sample

Sample Type	: Serum, Plasma, Urine & CSF

Capacity	: 40 samples, 80 Samples in double Sample Trays.
Sample Container	: Sample Cup (2 ml), Primary tube
Sample Volume	: 3-30 ml
Pre-dilution	: Available

Reagent

Reagent type	: R1/R2
Capacity	: 18 Reagents, 36 in Double Reagent Trays
Container Capacity	: 20 ml
Reagent Volume	: 50–300 ml

Pipetting System

Probes	: Two Independent Probes
Liquid Level Detection	: Available
Stirrer	: Integrated Stirrer
Dispensing	: Two Hamilton Syringes With Stepper Motor and Diaphragm Pump.
Probe Washing	: Internal and External

Photometry

Measuring Method	: End Point, Kinetic, Fixed Time & HIA
Light Source	: Halogen Lamp 12 Volts/20 Watts
Wavelength	: 320–720 nm, Free Wavelength Control
Reading	: Monochromatic and Bichromatic
Optics	: Grating monochromator
Absorbance	: - 0.000 To 3.000

Cuvette System

Number	: 48 Cuvettes
Material	: Polycarbonate
Capacity	: 1200 ml
Washing	: On Board Fully Automatic Absorption and Supply of Water Through Probes

Incubation

Reaction Temperature	: 37 ± 0.2°C/-0.2°C
Calculation Methods	: Linear 1 Point, K Factor, Linear 2 Point Linear N Point, Non Linear N^{th}

Water Requirement

Consumption	: Very Low, 1-2 Litre/Run
De-ioniser	: Not Required
Container Capacity	: 5 Litres (With In-built Filter)
Special Solutions	
Washing	: Distilled Water
Cleaning	: Distilled Water
Priming	: Distilled Water
Any Special Solution	: Not Required
Hidden Cost	: Nil

Waste

Container Capacity	: 5 Litres
On Line Waste Disposal	: Available
Computer Interface	: External, Standard : RS 232
Power Requirement	: AC 85-250 V, 50-60 Hz, 300 W
Environment (Non Condensing)	: 15-32°C, 5-70% Humidity
Dimensions	: 615 (W) X 483 (D) X 350 (H) mm, 45 Kg

CHAPTER 22

Blood Gases and Electrolytes

BLOOD GASES

Introduction

Reasons for obtaining blood gases:
1. Assessment of adequacy of oxygenation
2. Assessment of adequacy of ventilation
3. Assessment of acid-base status by measuring the respiratory and non-respiratory components

Reasons for using *arterial* blood rather than *venous* blood to measure blood gases.
1. Arterial blood is a good way to sample a mixture of blood that has come from various parts of the body.
   a. Venous blood in an extremity gives information mostly about that extremity. The metabolism in the extremity can differ from the metabolism in the body as a whole. This difference is accentuated.
      i. In shock, when the extremity is cold or under-perfused
      ii. With local exercise of extremity, as opening and closing the fist
      iii. In local infection of the extremity.
   b. Blood from a central venous catheter usually is an incomplete mix of venous blood from various parts of the body. For a sample of completely mixed blood, a sample would have to be obtained from the right ventricle or pulmonary artery, and even then information is not obtained about how well the lungs are oxygenating the blood.
2. Arterial blood gives the added information of how well the lungs are oxygenating the blood.
   a. If it is known that arterial O_2 concentration is normal (indicating that the lungs are functioning normally), but the mixed venous O_2 concentration is low, it can be inferred that the heart and circulation are failing.
   b. Oxygen measurements of central venous catheter blood can tell if the tissues are getting oxygenated, but they do not separate the contribution of the

heart from the lungs. If central venous catheter blood has a low O_2 concentration, it means either that:

i. The lungs have not oxygenated the arterial blood well so that venous blood has a low concentration or
ii. The heart is not circulating the blood well. In this case, the tissues of the body must take more than the usual amount of O_2 from each cardiac cycle because the blood is flowing slowly. This produces a low venous O_2 concentration.

Note: The site of arterial puncture must satisfy three requirements:
1. Available collateral blood flow
2. Superficial or easily accessible
3. Periarterial tissues (should be nonsensitive)

The radial artery satisfies the criteria tested above, although the brachial and femoral are also arteries of choice.

Procedure for Obtaining Arterial Blood Sample

1. Place the patient either in a sitting or supine position.
2. Elevate the wrist with a small pillow and ask the patient to extend fingers downward (this will flex the wrist and move the radial artery closer to the surface).
3. Palpate the artery and rotate the patient's hand back and forth until a good strong pulse is felt.
4. Swab the area liberally with an antiseptic agent such as betadine.
5. Optional: Anaesthetise the area with a small amount of 1% xylocaine (approximately ¼ ml or less). This allows a second attempt without undue pain if the first attempt is a failure.
6. Using a 20-or 21-gauge needle, make the puncture and then attach the preheparinised 12 ml syringe once the artery has been entered.
7. Pull the plunger on the syringe (being careful not to accidentally pull the needle out of the artery) and collect a 3 to 5 ml sample.
8. Withdraw needle and place a 4" × 4" absorbent bandage over the puncture site and maintain pressure with two fingers for a minimum of 2 minutes.
9. Meanwhile, any air-bubbles in the blood sample should be expelled as quickly as possible; the syringe should be capped and gently rotated to mix heparin with blood.
10. If the sample is not going to be analysed for 15-20 minutes, place it in an icewater container until it can be analysed.

Clinical Alert

1. Arterial gases will not indicate to what degree the patient is suffering from an abnormality. For this reason, the vital signs and mental function of the patient must be used as guides to determine adequacy of tissue oxygenation.
2. Arterial puncture site must have pressure applied and be watched carefully for bleeding.
3. Blood for gases (and electrolytes) must be drawn without trauma and be protected from room air at all times. Be aware that air bubbles in the syringe will also change gas values.

Blood Gas Symbols

Large capital letters are used as primary symbols for blood.

C = Concentration of gas in blood
S = Per cent saturation of haemoglobin with CO_2 or O_2
Q = Volume of blood
QT = Volume of blood per unit time
P = Gas pressure or partial pressure of a gas in a gas mixture or in blood.

To indicate whether blood is capillary, venous, arterial, lower case letters are used as subscripts:

v = Venous blood
a = Arterial blood
c = Capillary blood
s = Shunted blood

Combination of Symbols

PO_2 = Oxygen tension or partial pressure of oxygen.
PvO_2 = Venous oxygen tension or partial pressure of oxygen in venous blood.
PaO_2 = Arterial oxygen tension or partial pressure of oxygen in arterial blood.
PCO_2 = Partial pressure of carbon dioxide.
$PaCO_2$ = Partial pressure of carbon dioxide in arterial blood.

$PvCO_2$ = Partial pressure of carbon dioxide in venous blood
SO_2 = Oxygen saturation
SaO_2 = Per cent saturation of oxygen in arterial blood
SvO_2 = Per cent saturation of oxygen in venous blood
TCO_2 = Total carbon dioxide content

Blood Gases, Arterial (ABG), Blood

Normal Values

Must be corrected for body temperature.

		SI Units
pH		
Adults	7.35-7.45	7.35-7.45
Panic values	<7.2 and >7.6	<7.2 and >7.6
Children		
Birth-2 months	7.32-7.49	7.32-7.49
2 months-2 years	7.34-7.46	7.34-7.46
Over 2 years	7.35-7.45	7.35-7.45
$PaCO_2$	35-45 mmHg	4.7-6.0 kPa
Panic values	<20 mmHg	<2.7 kPa
PaO_2	75-100 mmHg	10.0-13.3 kPa
Panic values	<40 mmHg	<5.3 kPa
HCO_3	22-26 mEq/L	22-26 mmol/L
Panic values	<10 mEq/L	<10 mmol/L
O_2 Saturation	96-100%	0.96-1.00
Panic values	<60%	<0.60
Oxyhaemoglobin Dissociation Curve	No shift	

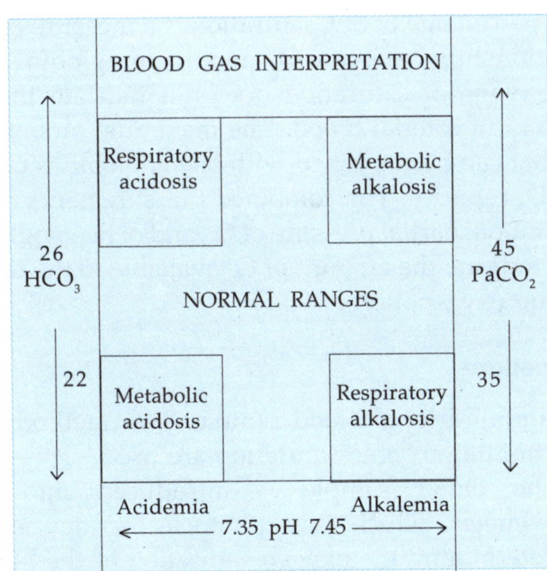

Blood Gases, Capillary, Blood

Normal Values

Must be corrected for body temperature.

		SI Units
pH		
Adults	7.35-7.45	7.35-7.45
Panic Values	<7.2 or >7.6	<7.2 or >7.6
Children (arterialized capillary sample)		
Birth-2 months	7.32-7.49	7.32-7.49
2 months-2 years	7.34-7.46	7.34-7.46
Over 2 years	7.35-7.45	7.35-7.45
PCO_2	26.4-41.2 mmHg	3.5-5.4 kPa
Panic values	<20 mmHg	<2.7 kPa
	>70 mmHg	
PO_2	75-100 mmHg	10.0-13.3 kPa
Panic values	<40 mmHg	<5.3 kPa
HCO_3	22-26 mEq/L	22-26 mmol/L
Panic values	<10 mEq/L	<10 mmol/L
O_2 Saturation	96-100%	0.96-1.00
Panic value	<60%	<0.60

Blood Gases, Venous, Blood

Normal Values

Must be corrected for body temperature.

		SI Units
pH	7.32-7.43	7.32-7.43
Panic value	<7.2 or >7.6	<7.2 or >7.6
PCO_2	38-50 mmHg	5.0-6.7 kPa
PO_2	20-49 mmHg	2.6-6.5 kPa
HCO_3	22-26 mEq/L	22-26 mmol/L
Panic value	<10 mEq/L	<10 mmol/L
	>40 mEq/L	>40 mEq/L
O_2 saturation	60-80%	0.60-0.80

PARTIAL PRESSURE OF CARBON DIOXIDE (PCO_2)

Normal Values

$PaCO_2$ (arterial blood) 35-45 torr
$PvCO_2$ (venous blood) 38-50 torr

Carried in blood in two ways: 10% carried in plasma, 90% carried in RBCs

Explanation of Test

This test is a measurement of the pressure or tension exerted by dissolved CO_2 in the blood and is proportional to the partial pressure of CO_2 in the alveolar air. The test is commonly used to detect a respiratory abnormality and to determine the alkalinity or acidity of the blood. In order to maintain CO_2 within normal limits, the rate and depth of respiration vary automatically with changes in metabolism. It is an index of alveolar ventilation and is the most physiologically reflective blood gas measurement. When taken as an arterial sample, it directly reflects how well air is exchanging with blood in the lungs.

CO_2 tension in the blood and cerebrospinal fluid (CSF) is the major chemical factor regulating alveolar ventilation. When the CO_2 of arterial blood rises from 40 torr to 45 torr, it causes a three-fold increase in alveolar ventilation. A CO_2 of 63 torr in arterial blood increases alveolar ventilation tenfold. When the CO_2 concentration of breathed air exceeds 5%, the lungs can no longer be ventilated fast enough to present a dangerous rise of CO_2 concentration in tissue fluids. Any further increase in CO_2 begins to depress the respiratory centre, causing a progressive decline in respiratory activity rather than an increase.

Procedure

1. Obtain an arterial blood sample
2. Do not expose sample to air
3. A small amount of blood is then introduced into a blood gas analyser and the CO_2 tension is measured with a silver-silver chloride electrode (Severinghaus electrode).

Clinical Implications

1. A rise in PCO_2 is usually associated with hypoventilation, a decrease, with hyperventilation. Reduction in PCO_2 through its effect on plasma bicarbonate concentration decreases renal bicarbonate reabsorption. For each mEq/L fall in HCO_3, the PCO_2 falls by 1 to 1.3 mm of Hg. Because HCO_3 and PCO_2 bear this close mathematical relationship, and this ratio in turn defends the hydrogen ion concentration, the outcome is that the steady state PCO_2 in simple metabolic acidosis is equal to the last two digits of the pH. Also, addition of 15 to the bicarbonate level also equals the last two digits of the pH. Failure of the PCO_2 to achieve predicted levels defines the presence of superimposed respiratory acidosis on alkalosis.
2. The causes of *decreased* PCO_2 include:
   - Hypoxia
   - Nervousness
   - Anxiety
   - Pulmonary emboli
   - Pregnancy
   - Other cause of hyperventilation
3. The causes of *increased* PCO_2 are:
   a. Obstructive lung disease
      - Chronic bronchitis
      - Emphysema

   b. Reduced function of respiratory centre
      - Over-reaction
      - Head trauma
      - Anaesthesia

   c. Other more rare causes of hypoventilation, such as pickwickian syndrome.

Clinical Alert

Increased PCO_2 may occur even with normal lungs if the respiratory centre is depressed. Always check laboratory reports for abnormal values. In interpreting laboratory reports remember that PCO_2 is a gas and is regulated by the lungs, not the kidneys.

OXYGEN SATURATION (SO_2)

Normal Values

Arterial blood saturation SaO_2 = 95% or higher mixed venous blood saturation SvO_2 = 75%.

Explanation of Test

This measurement is a ratio of the actual oxygen (O_2) content of the haemoglobin compared to the potential maximum O_2 carrying capacity of the haemoglobin. The percentage of SO_2 saturation is a measure of the relationship between O_2 and haemoglobin. The percentage of saturation does not indicate the O_2 content of arterial blood. The maximum amount of O_2 that can be combined with haemoglobin is called the O_2 capacity. The combined measurements of O_2 saturation, partial pressure of O_2, and of haemoglobin will indicate the amount of O_2 available to the tissue (tissue oxygenation).

Procedure

Obtain an arterial blood sample. Two methods for determining oxygen saturation are used.

1. The blood sample is introduced into the oximeter, which is a photoelectric device for determining the oxygen saturation of the blood. The value is measured directly with an oximeter (i.e., spectrometry).
2. Oxygen saturation is calculated from the oxygen content and oxygen capacity determinations.

$$\text{Percentage saturation} = \frac{100 \times O_2 \text{ content volume\%}}{O_2 \text{ capacity volume\%}}$$

That is

Percentage saturation =

$$\frac{100 \times \text{vol. of } O_2 \text{ actually combined with Hb}}{\text{vol of } O_2 \text{ with which Hb is capable of combination}}$$

The O_2 content of blood sample is measured before and after exposure to atmosphere.

OXYGEN (O_2) CONTENT

Normal Values

Aterial blood : 15%-22 vol%
Venous blood : 11%-16 vol%
(Vol% = volume percentage = ml/100 ml of blood)

Explanation of Test

The actual amount of oxygen (O_2) in the blood is termed the oxygen content. Blood can contain less O_2 than it is capable of carrying. About 98% of all O_2 delivered to the tissues is transported in chemical combination with haemoglobin. One gram of haemoglobin can carry or is capable of combining with 1.34 ml of O_2, whereas 100 ml of blood plasma can carry upto 0.3 ml of O_2. This measurement is determined mathematically by multiplying the number of grams of haemoglobin in 100 ml of blood by 1.34 times the partial pressure of oxygen in the blood.

Procedure

1. An arterial or venous blood sample is obtained
2. Mathematical formula
   O_2 content = $SaO_2 \times Hb \times 1.34 + PaO_2 \times 0.003$

Clinical Implications

Decreased arterial blood O_2 associated with increased arterial blood CO_2 can be due to:
1. Chronic obstructive lung disease
2. Patients with respiratory complications postoperatively
3. Flail chest
4. Kyphoscoliosis
5. Neuromuscular impairment
6. Obesity hypoventilation.

PARTIAL PRESSURE OF OXYGEN (PO_2)

Normal Values

PaO_2 80 torr or greater: arterial sample
PvO_2 30-40 torr : venous or peripheral blood sample.

Background

Oxygen (O_2) is carried in the blood in two forms dissolved and in combination with haemoglobin. Most of the O_2 in the blood is carried by haemoglobin. It is the partial pressure of a gas that determines the force it exerts in attempting to diffuse through the pulmonary membrane. The partial pressure reflects the amount of O_2 passing from the pulmonary alveoli into the blood and is directly influenced by the amount of O_2 being inhaled.

Explanation of Test

This is a measure of the pressure exerted by the amount of O_2 dissolved in the plasma. It is a test that measures the effectiveness of the lungs to oxygenate the blood. The severity of impairment of the ability of the lungs to diffuse O_2 across the alveolar membrane into the circulating blood is indicated by the level of partial pressure of oxygen (PO_2).

Procedure

1. An arterial blood sample is obtained.
2. A small amount of blood is then introduced into a blood gas analysing machine and the O_2 tension is measured with a polarographic electrode (Clark electrode).

Clinical Implications

1. Increased levels are associated with:
   a. Polycythaemia
   b. Hyperventilation in an arterial blood sample
2. Decreased levels are associated with:
   a. Anaemias
   b. Cardiac decompensation
   c. Insufficient atmospheric O_2
   d. Intracardiac shunts
   e. Chronic obstructive disease
   f. Restrictive pulmonary disease
   g. Hypoventilation due to neuromuscular disease
3. Decreased arterial PO_2 with normal or decreased arterial blood PCO_2 tension is associated with:
   a. Diffuse interstitial pulmonary infiltration
   b. Pulmonary oedema
   c. Pulmonary embolism
   d. Postoperative extracorporeal circulation.

CARBON DIOXIDE (CO_2) CONTENT OR TOTAL CARBON DIOXIDE (TCO_2)

Normal Values

24-30 mEq/litre

Background

In normal blood plasma, more than 95% of the total CO_2 content is contributed by bicarbonate (HCO_3), which is regulated by the kidneys. The other 5% of the CO_2 is contributed by the dissolved CO_2 gas and carbonic acid (H_2CO_3). Dissolved CO_2 gas, which is regulated by the lungs, therefore, contributes little to the total CO_2 content. Total CO_2 content gives little information about the lungs.

HCO_3^- in the extracellular spaces exists first as CO_2 then as H_2CO_3, and thereafter, much of it is changed to sodium bicarbonate ($NaHCO_2$) by the buffers of the plasma and red cells.

Explanation of Test

This test is a general measure of the alkalinity or acidity of the venous, arterial or capillary blood. This test measures CO_2 from:

1. Dissolved CO_2
2. Total H_2CO_3
3. HCO_3^-
4. Carbamino carbon dioxide
   Total $CO_2 = HCO_3^- + 0.03 \times PCO_2$

Procedure

1. A venous or arterial blood sample of 6 ml is collected in a heparinised syringe.
2. If the collected blood sample cannot be studied immediately, the syringe should be placed in an iced container.

Clinical Implications

1. Elevated CO_2 content levels occur in:
   a. Severe vomiting
   b. Emphysema
   c. Aldosteronism
   d. Use of mercurial diuretics
2. Decreased CO_2 content levels occur in:
   a. Severe diarrhoea
   b. Starvation
   c. Acute renal failure
   d. Salicylate toxicity
   e. Diabetic acidosis
   f. Use of chorothiazide diuretics

(**Note:** In diabetic acidosis the supply of ketoacids exceeds the demands of the cell. Blood plasma acids rise. Blood plasma HCO_3 decreases because it is used in neutralising these acids).

Clinical Alert

A double use of the CO_2 is one of the main reasons why understanding acid-base problems may be difficult. Use the terms CO_2 content and CO_2 gas to avoid confusion. Remember the following:

1. CO_2 content is mainly bicarbonate and a base. It is a solution and is regulated by kidneys.
2. CO_2 gas is mainly acid. It is regulated by the lungs.

Interfering Factors

1. Drugs that may cause increased or decreased levels include:
   a. Nitrofurantoin
   b. Salicylates
2. Drugs that may cause decreased levels include:
   a. Dimercaprol (BAL)
   b. Lipomul oil injection
   c. Methicillin.

BLOOD pH

Normal Values

Arterial blood : 7.35-7.45
Venous blood : 7.32-7.43

Background

The pH is the negative logarithm of the hydrogen ion concentration in the blood. The sources of hydrogen ions are: (i) volatile acids, which can vary between a liquid and a gaseous state, and (ii) non-volatile acids that cannot be volatilised and are fixed (e.g., dietary acids, lactic acids and ketoacids).

Explanation of Test

This is a measurement of the chemical balance in the body and is a ratio of acids to bases. A determination of the blood pH is one of the best ways to tell if the body is too acid or too alkaline. Low pH numbers (< 7.35) indicate an acid stage, and higher pH numbers

(> 7.45) indicate an alkaline state. This balance is extremely intricate and must be kept within the very slight margin of 7.35 to 7.45 pH (alkaline) in the extracellular fluid. pH limits compatible with life are 6.9 to 7.8.

The respiratory response to changes in blood pH is almost instantaneous. Acidosis (CO_2 retained; pH falls) stimulates ventilation; alkalosis (CO_2 blown off; pH rises) depresses ventilation. The respiratory centre in the medulla appears to respond to a pH intermediate between those of the blood and CSF (7.35-7.40).

Procedure

1. An arterial blood sample is obtained.
2. Two methods of determining the pH are used, the direct method and the indirect method:
   a. *Direct method:* A small amount of blood is introduced into a blood gas machine and the pH is measured.
   b. *Indirect method:* The Henderson-Hasselbatch equation is solved.

$$\text{pH} = \text{pk} + \log \frac{(H_2CO_3^-) \text{ major blood base}}{(H_2CO_3^-) \text{ major blood acid}}$$

Clinical Implications

1. Generally speaking, the pH is decreased in acidaemia because of increased formation of acids. pH is increased in alkalaemia because of a loss of acids.
2. When attempting to interpret an acid-base abnormality, one must:
   a. Check the pH to see if there is an alkalaemia or an acidaemia.
   b. Check PCO_2 to see if there is a respiratory abnormality.
   c. Check HCO_3^- or base excess to see if there is a metabolic abnormality.
3. Refer to table given later for a more complete explanation of the changes occurring in respiratory and metabolic acidaemia and respiratory and metabolic alkalaemia.
4. Metabolic acidaemia:
   a. Renal failure
   b. Ketoacidosis in starvation and diabetes
   c. Lactic acidosis
   d. Strenuous exercise
5. Metabolic alkalaemia:
   a. Deficient potassium
   b. Hypochloraemia
   c. Gastric suction or vomiting
   d. Massive administration of steroids
   e. Sodium bicarbonate administration
   f. Aspirin intoxication.
6. Respiratory alkalaemia:
   a. Acute pulmonary disease
   b. Myocardial infarction
   c. Chronic and acute heart failure
   d. Adult cystic fibrosis
   e. Third trimester of pregnancy
   f. Anxiety, neurosis, psychoses
   g. CNS disease
   h. Pain
   i. Anaemia
   j. Carbon monoxide poisoning
   k. Acute pulmonary embolus
   l. Shock
7. Respiratory acidaemia:
   a. Acute respiratory distress syndrome
   b. Ventilatory failure

Clinical Alert

Ventilation failure is a medical emergency. Aggressive and supportive measures must be taken immediately.

Observing the rate and depth of respiration may give a clue to blood pH:

1. Acidosis usually increases respirations.
2. Alkalosis usually decreases respirations.

Interfering Factors

1. Drugs that may cause increased levels include:
   - Potassium oxalate
   - Sodium bicarbonate
   - Sodium oxalate
2. Drugs that may cause decreased levels include:
   - Acetazolamide
   - Ammonium chloride
   - Ammonium oxalate
   - Calcium chloride
   - EDTA
   - Methyl alcohol
   - Paraldehyde
   - Salicylates
   - Sodium citrate.

BASE EXCESS/DEFICIT

Normal Values (± 3 mEq/litre)

Positive value indicates a base excess (i.e. a non-volatile acid deficit)

Negative value indicates a deficit (i.e., a non-volatile acid excess)

Explanation of Test

This determination is an attempt to quantify the patient's total base excess or deficit so that clinical treatment of acid-base disturbances (specifically those that are nonrespiratory in nature) can be initiated. It is also referred to as the whole blood buffer base and is the sum of the concentration of buffer anions (in mEq/litre) contained in whole blood. These buffer anions are the bicarbonate (HCO_3^-) ion in plasma and RBCs, and the haemoglobin, plasma proteins, and phosphates in plasma and RBCs.

Total quantity of buffer anions is 45 to 50 mEq per liter or about twice that of HCO_3^-, which is 24 to 28 mEq/litre. Thus, the quantity of HCO_3^- ions accounts for only about half of total buffering capacity of the blood. Therefore, the base excess/deficit measurement provides a more complete picture of the buffering taking place and is a critical index of nonrespiratory changes in acid-base balance versus respiratory changes.

Procedure

Calculation is made from the measurements of pH, $PaCO_2$, and haematocrit. These values are plated on a nomogram and the base excess/deficit is read.

Clinical Implications

1. Negative value (below 3 mEq/liter) reflects a nonrespiratory or metabolic disturbance. It indicates acid accumulation due to:
   a. Dietary intake of organic and inorganic acids.
   b. Lactic acid.
   c. Ketoacidosis
2. Positive value (above 3 mEq/litre) reflects a non-volatile acid deficit.

AUTOMATION IN BLOOD GAS ANALYSIS BLOOD GAS ANALYSERS (FROM AVL)

Automatic blood gas analysers have been in operation for over a decade now. However, most of them had a warming-up time of half-an-hour or so. That is each time power fails or when instrument is started on a fresh day or when an emergency strikes half-an-hour must elapse before readings can be obtained. AVL-995 blood bas analyser (Fig. 22.1) has shortened this warming-up time for an investigation that is requested mostly as an urgent one.

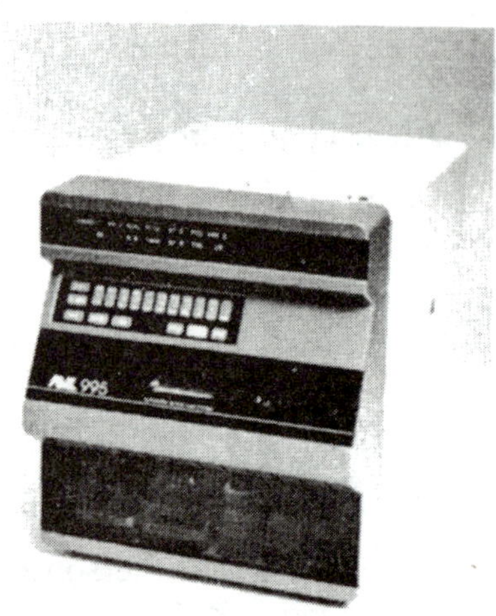

Fig. 22.1: AVL blood gas analyser

1. Very short warm-up time (only 5 minutes)
2. Power fail protection of calibration Data through EEPROMS.
3. Facility to calibrate individual electrodes separately. No need to go through the entire cycle of calibrating all the electrodes when not required.
4. Totally automatic sampling (micro-sample of 25 ml acceptable) calibration and cleaning cycles.
5. Automatic filling of humidifiers and reference electrodes along with automatic periodic cleaning of measuring chamber with special cleaning solution built in.
6. Built-in barometric pressure sensor.
7. Fully visible, illuminated and optically magnified measuring chamber for easy and quick detection and handling of clots and air bubbles.
8. Easy and quick maintenance of electrodes.
9. Built, in service log book (software).
10. Comprehensive self-test protocols for easy and quick troubleshooting by operating staff.
11. AVL-995 blood gas analyser is highly economical, as costs of consumables are minimal. Expensive callibrating gas mixtures are not needed (only CO_2 is used because of built-in gas mixing unit). A wash-solution locally prepared

Table 22.1: Four basic forms of acid-base imbalance and their compensatory mechanism

Form	*Cause*	*Occurrence*	*Compensatory mechanism*
1. Respiratory acidaemia	Primary increase in PCO_2 and decreased pH	*Depression of respiratory centres* a) Drug overdose b) Barbiturate toxicity c) Use of anaesthetics *Interference with mechanical function of thoracic cage* a) Deformity of thoracic cage b) Kyphoscoliosis *Airway obstruction* a) Extrathoracic tumours b) Asthma c) Bronchitis d) Emphysema *Circulatory disorders* a) Congestive heart failure b) Shock	Renal reabsorption of the bicarbonate ion. Examples: a) Uncompensated respiratory acidemia (acute ventilatory failure) *Values* pH = 7.26 ↓ PCO_2 = 56 ↑ Bicarbonate = 4 Normal b) Compensated respiratory acidaemia (chronic respiratory failure) *Values*: pH = 7.36 PCO_2= 63 Bicarbonate = 34
2. Respiratory alkalaemia	Primary decrease in PCO_2 and in increased pH	*Hyperventilation* —Hysteria *Lack of oxygen.* *Toxic stimulation of the respiratory centres* a) High fever b) Cerebral haemorrhage c) Excessive artificial respiration d) Salicylates	Glomerular filtration of the bicarbonate ion. Examples a) Uncompensated respiratory alkalaemia (acute alveolar hyperventilation) *Values*: pH = 7.52 ↑ PCO_2=28↓ Bicarbonate = 22 Normal b) Compensated respiratory alkalemia (Chronic alveolar hyperventilation) pH=7.43 PCO_2=24 Bicarbonate=15
3. Nonrespiratory acidaemia metabolic acidaemia	Increase in hydrogen ions with a secondary decrease in bicarbonate	*Acid addition* a) Renal failure b) Diabetic ketoacidosis c) Lactic acidosis d) Anaerobic metabolism *Hypoxia* *Base subtraction* a) Diarrhoea b) Renal tubular acidosis	Hyperventilation through stimulation of central chemoreceptors. Examples a) Uncompensated nonrespiratory acidaemia (acute) *Values*: pH = 7.20 ↓ PCO_2 = 38 ↓ Bicarbonate = 15 ↓ b) Compensated respiratory acidaemia (chronic) *Values*: pH = 7.35 PCO_2 = 25 Bicarbonate = 15
4. Nonrespiratory alkalaemia or metabolic alkalaemia	Increase in bicarbonate secondary to a decrease in hydrogen ions	*Acid subtraction* a) Loss of gastric juice b) Vomiting *Potassium or chloride depletion base addition* a) Excessive bicarbonate or lactate administration	Hypoventilation. Examples a) Uncompensated nonrespiratory alkalaemia (acute) *Values*: pH = 7.56 ↑ PCO_2 = 44 ↑ Bicarbonate = 38 ↑ b) Compensated respiratory alkalemia (chronic) *Values*: pH = 7.44 PCO_2 = 55 Bicarbonate = 38

Note

1. Although these four basic imbalances occur individually, more frequently a combination of two or more is observed. These disturbances may have an antagonistic or a synergistic effect upon each ones.
2. Compensation is most efficient is respiratory and non-respiratory acidemia.
3. The degree of hypoventilation is precisely related to the degree of hypobicarbonatemia. For each mEq/L fall in bicarbonate, PCO_2 falls by 1-1.3 torr. A close mathematical relationship prevails between bicarbonate and PCO_2. Their ratio (HCO_3 and PCO_2) defines the prevailing hydrogen ion concentration. For this reason, the steady state PCO_2 in simple metabolic acidosis is equal to the last two digits of the pH. Failure of the PCO_2 to reach predicted levels defines the presence of superimposed respiratory acidosis or alkalosis.

costs only half-a-rupee. Extremely small volumes of regents are consumed.

12. Results can be read-off of the LCD display or a hard copy obtained through the in-built thermal printer.

Measured Parameters

pH, PO_2, PCO_2, and barometric pressure.

Calculated Parameters

Base excess (BE), base excess (BE-ECF), buffer base (BB), actual bicarbonate (HCO_3-), total CO_2 (TCO_2), standard bicarbonate ($STHCO_3$), standard pH (STpH), oxygen saturation (O_2 Sat), oxygen content (O_2CT), H_2 ion concentration (CH^+), alveolar-arterial oxygen gradient ($AaDO_2$) and haemoglobin indicator (dBE/dTHb).

Another system AVL-995 Hb measures Hb in addition to all other parameters mentioned above. AVL-990 is further economically priced and comes without the thermal printer.

ELECTROLYTE ANALYSIS BY FLAMEPHOTOMETER

In this instrument the solution under test is passed under carefully controlled conditions as a very fine spray in the air supply to a burner. In the flame, the solution evaporates and the salt dissociates to give neutral atoms. Some of these though only a very small proportion, move into a higher energy state (their electrons move to the outer orbits). When the electrons of these atoms fall back to their original orbits, they release energy in the form of light. Which is used in flame photometry of this type and is called emission flame photometry. Light of characteristic wavelengths is emitted and passes through a suitable filtre, grating or prism on to a photocell, and the amount of current thus produced is measured. This varies with the concentration of sodium; for example, in the solution being tested. Using solutions of known sodium concentrations, a calibration curve can be made and this is used for reading the sodium content of the fluids examined.

Many gases have been used for the flame. These include acetylene, propane, butane and coal gas. Both the gas pressure and air pressure have to be carefully regulated so as to maintain a constant steady flame, which should be blue in colour and have no yellow streaks. The spray is formed by passing compressed air through an atomiser, into which the liquid which is being tested is drawn either by suction or gravity, and then enters the burner in its air supply. The pressure used is usually about 10 to 15 lb per square inch. The atomiser is a very important part of the apparatus. A steady fine spray of droplets of uniform size should be produced if there is to be a constant emission of light.

The light produced is first passed through a lens to focus it and then through suitable filters, a diffraction grating or prism before it falls on to the photocell. For determining sodium, an orange or yellow (589 nm) filter can be used. Potassium emits light at 404.4 and 766.5 nm. For the former, a violet; and for the latter a deep red filter should be used. Lithium (671 nm) needs a near red filter for its measurement.

The most satisfactory dilution to use should be established experimentally. For sodium, this may be 1 in 100, 1 in 200, even 1 in 500; for potassium, it is usually lower, often 1 in 50, but it is possible by varying the sensitivity to use the same dilution for both. Both sodium and potassium can interfere with each other, therefore, in standard solution both the elements are added.

Equipment: Systronics provides digital read-out flame photometer (Mediflame 127/128/129) that provides two parameters at a time.

FLAME PHOTOMETER 129 (FROM SYSTRONICS)

Microprocessor-Based Automation

Systronics flame photometer 129 is a microprocessor-based unit designed for medical applications (Fig. 22.2). The microprocessor provides automation in operation, measurements, and end-result presentation. The unit can do the estimation of sodium (Na), potassium (K), calcium (Ca) and lithium (Li) in single aspiration of a sample.

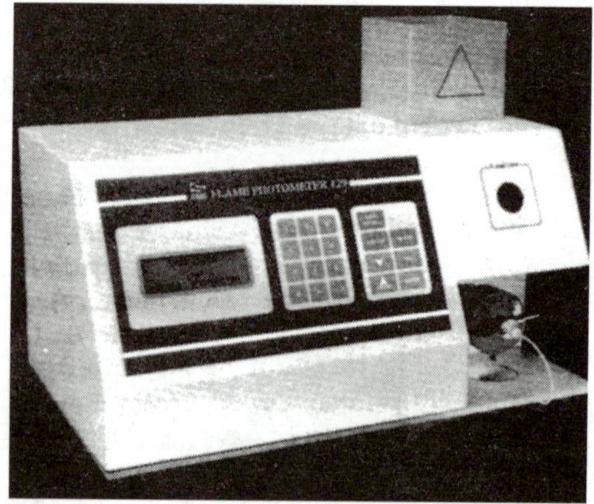

Fig. 22.2: Flame photometer

For user's convenience, the unit offers three measuring modes: (i) serum, (ii) urine, and (iii) bio-fluid, general. The last mode is helpful for analysing Biological samples other than serum and urine.

Frequently used measurement setups can be stored once (in a battery-back-up memory) and recalled whenever required with a stroke of a button. This eliminates the typical chores of instructions required to be given to a microprocessor-based instrument before it starts the operation. Facility for restandardisation with a single standard is available to minimise the effect of any unforeseen drift without going for the full recalibration.

A 4-line 20-character LCD readout provides easy user interface and presentation of results. A Centronics printer port is provided for Epson compatible dot matrix/inkjet and HP compatible laser printers. Printer is optional (Fig. 22.3).

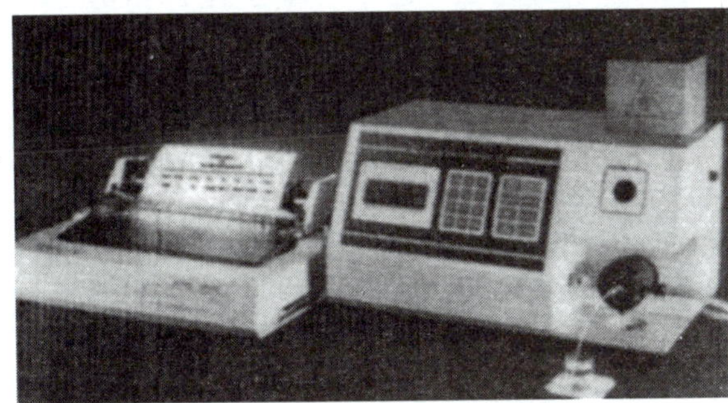

Fig. 22.3: Measurement results can be printed immediately or later on

Salient Features

- Specifically designed for medical applications.
- Up to four elements measured with single aspiration.
- Automatic filter selection (narrow band interference).
- Curve fittings for nonlinear range (up to 5 standards).
- Calibration stored in memory.
- Restandardisation cuts on full recalibration.
- Record kept of date and time of analysis.
- Saved set-ups cut operation steps.
- Measurement results can be recalled later on for display and printout (330 max).
- Measurement results can be printed (individual, full Batch, of the day, all in memory).
- 4-line, 20-character Alphanumeric LCD readout.
- Centronics printer port for Epson compatible dot matrix/inkjet and HP laser printers.
- RS-232 interface (optional).
- Compressor with built-in air filter and air regulator.

Easy Menu Driven Operation

Operating Mode
1. Serum
2. Urine
3. Bio-Fluids (GEN)

Specifically designed for medical use.

SET FLAME
Ignite Flame,
Aspirate DW,
Press ENTER

Step-by-step guidance for operation.

Adjust FUEL for
best FLAME stability
<0578.7)

Digital monitoring of flame stability.

RE-STANDARDISATION
Enter Std. Value
Na = 140

A restandardisation facility cuts on full recalibration

MEASUREMENT RECALL
Enter Date: 23/02
Enter Batch No.: 1
Enter Sample No.: 01

Measurement results can be recalled later on for display.

SETUP
1. DIRECTORY
2. CALL SETUP
3. EDIT SETUP

Saved setups drastically cut operation steps.

Technical Specifications

Range of Operation

Element	*Serum*	*Urine*	*BIP-Fluids*
Na	100-200 mEq/L 1: 100 dil	0-250 mEq/L 1: 100 dil	All the four elements up to
K	0-10 mEq/L 1: 100 dil	0-100 mEq/L 1: 100 dil	250 mEq/L with 1: 100 dil
Li	0-2 mEq/L 1: 10 dil		
Ca		0-10 mEq/L 1: 2 dil	

i. Curve fit software is provided for urine and bio-fluids.
ii. Curve fit accuracy: ± 2% f.s.
iii. Suitable dilution for concentrations higher than given in the above table.

- Filters (10 nm Typical): Na and K supplied; Li and Ca (optional)
- Reproducibility: ± 2% f.s.
- Minimum Sample: Approximately 3 ml per element (at Avg. time of 4 sec.)
- Averaging: 2 to 15 seconds, selectable
- Aspiration Time: (5 sec + Avg. time) per element + 4 sec.
- Operating air pressure: 0.45 kg/cm^2 (typical)
- Air compressor: With built-in air regulator and air filter to deliver stable and moisture/oil free air supply.
- Fuel Gas: LPG
- Power Supply: 230 Vac +/- 10%, 50 Hz.

System: The system consists of main unit with one each of NA and K narrow band filters, a compressor with built-in air regulator and air filter. Li and Ca filters and printer are optional (Fig. 22.4).

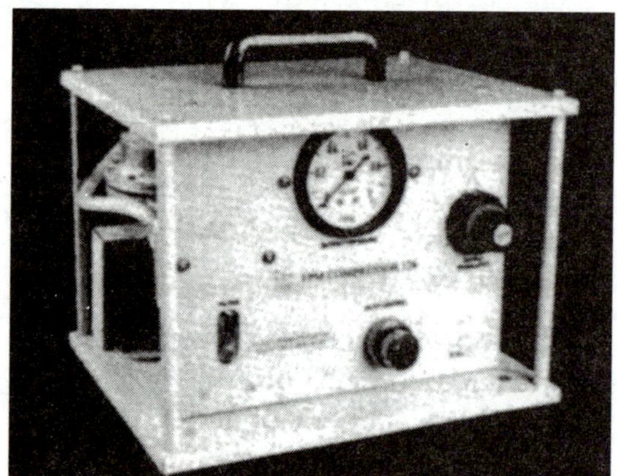

Fig. 22.4: Compressor with air filter and regulator

Standards: With flame photometers—obtaining standards is a persistent problem—it has been eradicated by the FLAMECAL standards provided by the Tulip Group of Companies.

Standard Solutions

Standards should be put through each time determinations are made. Prepare suitable solutions as follows:

a. Stock sodium solution, 1,000 mEq/L, 58.5 grams of sodium chloride per litre of solution.
b. Stock potassium, 100 mEq/L, 7.46 grams of potassium chloride per litre of solution.

A series of stock standard solutions can be prepared from these as follows:

For sodium:					
mEq. Na/L	120	130	140	150	160
ml stock solution A	60	65	70	75	80
ml stock solution B	25	25	25	25	25
	Made up to 500 ml with water				
For potassium:					
mEq. K/L	3	4	5	6	8
ml stock solution B	15	20	25	30	40
ml stock solution A	70	70	70	70	70
	Made up to 500 ml with water				

These solutions then be diluted in the same way as the serum to give standards for use in the instrument. When carrying out a series of determinations, insert an appropriate standard solution at frequent intervals to ensure that constancy of reading is obtained.

Normal Values

		SI Units
Potassium		
Adults	3.5-5.3 mEq/L	3.5-5.3 mmol/L
Premature infants	5.0-10.2 mEq/L	5.0-10.2 mmol/L
Cord blood	5.0-10.2 mEq/L	5.0-10.2 mmol/L
2 days	3.0-6.0 mEq/L	3.0-6.0 mmol/L
Full-term newborn		
Cord blood	5.6-12.0 mEq/L	5.6-12.0 mmol/L
Newborn	3.7-5.0 mEq/L	3.7-5.0 mmol/L
Infants	4.1-5.3 mEq/L	4.1-5.3 mmol/L
Children	3.4-4.7 mEq/L	3.4-4.7 mmol/L

Contd...

Contd...

Panic levels		
Adults	<2.5 mEq/L	<2.5 mmol/L
	or >6.6 mEq/L	or >6.6 mmol/L
Newborn	<2.5 mEq/L	<2.5 mmol/L
	or >8.1 mEq/L	or >8.1 mmol/L
Sodium		
Adults	136-145 mEq/L	136-145 mmol/L
Umbilical cord	116-166 mEq/L	116-166 mmol/L
Infants	139-146 mEq/L	139-146 mmol/L
Children	138-145 mEq/L	138-145 mmol/L

Alterations of Sodium and Extracellular Fluid (ECF)

Hyponatraemia (serum sodium concentration lower than normal)

Total-body sodium and ECF volume low:
- GIT fluid loss
- Burns
- "Third compartment" accumulation
- Salt losing renal disorders
- Diuretic overuse

Total body sodium and ECF volume normal:
- Acute water intoxication, usually iatrogenic
- Syndrome of inappropriate ADH secretion.
- Glucocorticoid deficiency.
- Severe whole body potassium depletion.

Total body sodium and ECF volume increased:
- Acute renal failure with superimposed water load.
- Congestive heart failure.
- Cirrhosis.
- Nephrotic syndrome.

Hypernatraemia (serum sodium concentration higher than normal)

Total body sodium normal, ECF volume low:
- Gastroenteritis
- Osmotic diuresis
- Pronounced sweating

Total body sodium increased proportionately more than increased ECF volume:
- Salt ingestion, deliberate or accidental.
- Inappropriate intravenous therapy.

Hyperosmolality, without sodium alterations:
- High blood ethanol
- Hyperglycemia
- Radiographic contrast media.

Abnormalities of Serum and Whole Body Potassium

Hyperkalaemia (serum potassium concentration more than normal)

Inappropriate cellular metabolism:
- Insulin deficiency
- Acidaemia
- Hypoaldosteronism
- Cell necrosis (burns, crush, haemolysis, anti-leukaemia therapy)

Decreased renal excretion:
- Acute renal failure
- Chronic interstitial nephritis
- Tubular unresponsiveness to aldosterone
- Hypoaldosteronism

Increased potassium intake:
- Inappropriate use of salt substitutes or K^+ replacement.
- Potassium salts of antibiotics.

Hypokalemia (serum potassium concentration lower than normal)

Inappropriate cellular metabolism
- Alkalaemia
- Familial periodic paralysis
- Very rapid generation of cells (leukaemia, treated megaloblastic anaemia)

Increased excretion:
- Vomiting and/or diarrhoea
- Diuretic overuse
- Hyperaldosteronism
- Renal tubular acidosis

Decreased potassium intake:
- Anorexia nervosa
- Diet deficient in vegetables, meat
- Clay eating (binds potassium and prevents absorption)

RAPID DIAGNOSTICS IN ELECTROLYTE ANALYSIS

Within a remarkably short period of only a few years, a variety of analysers have appeared in the market which use ion-selective electrodes (ISE) for quantitative measurements of biologically relevant cations and anions. The electrode (ISE) permits measurement of the activity of a specific ion under the presence of a given amount of other ions. The selective transport of a certain ion species from the solution into the membrane phase of the electrode allows a potential difference that can be calculated and the ion concentration can be deduced thereof.

Ion selective electrodes are available for H^+ (for pH measurement), Li^+ (Lithium), Na^+, K^+, Ca^{++} and Cl^-.

Easylyte Systems from Medica

Three models to choose from

Easylyte Sodium Potassium Analyser

Fast and efficient, the Easylyte provides clinically accurate Na^+/K^+ results at the lowest operating cost.

Customer Support

- Installation
- Troubleshooting
- Warranty service
- Order information

Ease of Operation

- Two button operation
- Automatic calibration
- No sample preparation
- No daily maintenance

Economy

- Low reagent cost
- Long electrode warranty
- Low supply costs
- Extended warranty plan

Print Outs

- Patient results
- Calibration values
- Result summaries daily/weekly/all
- Quality control data

Easylyte Lithium (Sodium, Potassium, Lithium Analyser)

Economy

- Long electrode life
- Low purchase price
- Low reagent cost
- Automatic standby mode

Easy Operation

- Yes/No prompted operation
- Automatic calibration
- Minimal sample contact
- All reagents in single pack

Easy Maintenance

- Modular electrodes
- All components accessable
- Diagnostic software
- No flame or gas

Reliability

- QC programme computes statistics
- Abnormal values flagged
- ISE technology
- Software monitored performance

Easylyte Plus (Sodium, Potassium and Chloride Analyser)

It delivers fast, accurate and economical tests of sodium, potassium and chloride levels in whole blood, serum, plasma or urine—emphasising extreme safety for the operator, who never touches the specimen or reagents. It is also extremely compact, occupying counter space about the size of a notebook. And EasyLyte PLUS is one of the least expensive electrolyte analysers you can buy.

Chapter 23

Serology/Immunology

TECHNOLOGIES

RAPID IMMUNOCHROMATOGRAPHIC TECHNIQUES

Perspective on Membrane-based Rapid Diagnostic Tests and Detection of hCG Using these Tests

The need for a rapid, reliable, simple, sensitive *in vitro* diagnostic assay for use at point-of-care, have lead to the commercialisation of *in vitro* Rapid Diagnostic Tests based on the principle of immunochromatography.

Rapid Diagnostic Tests are membrane-based immunoassays that allow visual detection of an analyte in liquid specimens. In clinical assays, specimens such as urine, whole blood, serum or plasma, saliva and other body fluids may be employed.

What are the Principles of Membrane-based Rapid Diagnostic Tests?

Currently available Rapid Diagnostic Tests comprise of a base membrane such as nitrocellulose. A detector reagent (antigen/antibody-indicator complex) specific to the analyte, impregnated at one end of the membrane. A capture reagent is coated on the membrane at the test region.

When the specimen is added to the sample pad, it rapidly flows through the conjugate pad. Analyte if present in the specimen, binds to the detector reagent. As the specimen passes over the test band to which the capture reagent is coated, the analyte-detector reagent complex is immobilised. A coloured band proportional to the amount of analyte present in the sample, develops. The excess unbound detector reagent moves further up the membrane and is immobilised at the control band.

What are the Components of Membrane-based Rapid Diagnostic Tests and how are they Constructed?

Rapid Diagnostic Tests consists of (Fig. 23.1)

1. Sample pad

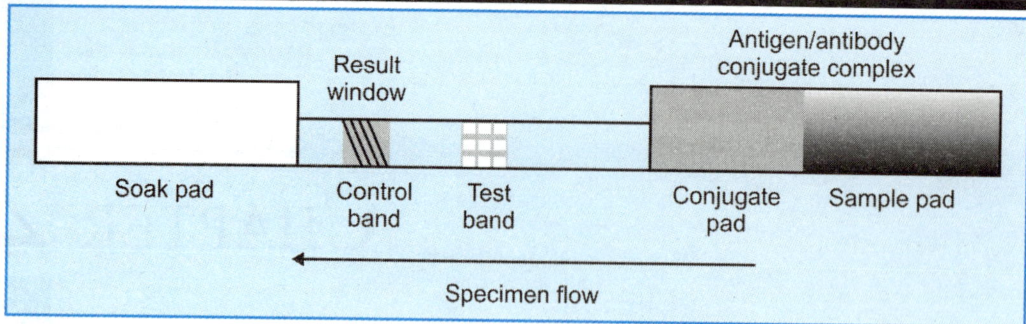

Fig. 23.1: Construction of Rapid Diagnostic Tests

2. Detector reagent/conjugate: Antigen/antibody-indicator complex specific to the analyte, impregnated in the conjugate pad but remains unbound
3. Test band: Coated on nitrocellulose membrane; specific to the analyte
4. Control band: Usually antidetector antibodies coated on the membrane, served to validate the test results
5. Soak pad

Currently, immunochromatography tests are available in two formats; "Lateral flow" and "Transverse flow or flow through". The lateral flow formats are available in device or dipstick format. The lateral flow formats are commonly employed where rapid detection of pregnancy, drug abuse, infectious disease or parasitology is required, and serve as qualitative screening assay at laboratories, physician's office or at homes due to their simplicity and ease of performance. The flow through format is less common as the assay requires greater operator involvement. However, some of these assays enable semiquantitative estimation of the analyte by visual comparison with an in-built reference.

Regardless of the format used, the desired specificity, sensitivity and assay performance depends upon reliable formulation and proper assay assembly.

What are the Limitations and Effects of Various Components on the Performance of Membrane Rapid Diagnostic Tests?

This section highlights the role of various components of Rapid Diagnostic Tests and their effect on attaining the desired performance characteristics.

How does the Nitrocellulose Membrane affect the Sensitivity of Rapid Diagnostic Tests?

Rapid Diagnostic Tests are fabricated on a solid support membrane, usually made of nitrocellulose. Membranes employed in Rapid Diagnostic Tests are porous. Depending upon the porosity, some membranes are better suited for applications with certain specimens than others. This is because, the pore size of the membrane has significant effect on the capture reagent binding properties and the lateral flow rate. The combined effects of these two phenomena in turn determine the sensitivity and performance of the test assay.

Pore Size and Capture Reagent Binding Properties

It has been observed that as the pore size decreased the effective surface area available for binding of capture reagent increases. Greater effective surface area available for binding, results in optimal coating of the capture reagent, which is essential for attaining the desired sensitivity of the assay.

Pore Size and Lateral Flow Rate

It has been observed that as the pore size increases, the lateral flow rate increases. However, slower flow rate increases the effective concentration (concentration required for interaction) of the analyte, since a slower flow rate allows the analyte and the capture reagent to be in close proximity for a longer times. As it is well known, immunological reactions are time-dependent and prolonged exposure of the analyte with the capture reagent allows better interaction and thus, results in increased sensitivity. The flow rate is important when the analyte is present in low concentrations, such as borderline samples.

The relationship between lateral flow rate and effective analyte concentration is: effective analyte concentration

$$\alpha \frac{1}{(\text{flow rate})^2}$$

Thus, it is important to optimise the membranes such that Rapid Diagnostic Tests can achieve rapid results which are also reliable and accurate.

Why are Colloidal Gold Sol Particles commonly employed in the Detector Reagent in Membrane-based Rapid Diagnostic Tests?

Interpretation of results in Rapid Diagnostic Tests depends upon the development of a signal at the stipulated time. A signal is generated when capture reagent—analyte-detector reagent complex is formed. The detector reagent/conjugate consists of an antibody or antigen bound to the indicator. The indicator imparts colour to the signal, enabling visual interpretation of results.

Coloured latex particles, colloidal gold sol particles, dyes, enzymes and carbon particles are some of the indicator used in immunochromatographic assays. However, stability, protein-binding properties, and particles' size are critical factors that determine their use in immunochromatographic assays. The most popular indicators used in immunochromatographic assays is the colloidal gold sol particle.

Colloidal Gold Sol Particles as Indicator

Homogeneous colloidal gold sol particles are inert and can couple with antibody/antigen, which is stable in dry as well as in liquid forms. All the above-mentioned parameters are determined by the particles' shape and size of colloidal gold.

Effect of Shape of Colloidal Gold Sol Particles on Stability

Colloidal gold sol particles have a net negative charge called "zeta potential". This zeta potential maintains the minimal distance between two particles resulting in long term stability. Ideally, colloidal gold sol particles should be spherical in shape, since this shape allows uniform distribution of zeta potential at the surface. In case of nonhomogeneous particles, the zeta potential is not uniformly distributed, thus the particles may come together to form aggregates. These aggregates may permanently get impregnated into the conjugate pad, or during the test assay may deposit on the nitrocellulose membrane leading to discrepant results. Such nonhomogeneous colloidal gold is usually blue/black in colour.

Effect of Shape of Colloidal Gold Sol Particles on Sensitivity

Spherical, homogeneous colloidal gold sol particles also allow uniform coating of the detector reagent at their surface. Whereas nonhomogeneous colloidal gold sol particles do not allow uniform coating of detector reagent, resulting in decreased assay sensitivity and specificity.

Effect of Size on Colour of Colloidal Gold Sol Particles

It has been observed that as the colloidal gold sol particles increase in size, the colour turns from light pink to cherry red to red-purple to blue-black to grey-black. Darker coloured particles are preferred in Rapid Diagnostic Tests since darker colours allow easy interpretations of results. However, as the colloidal gold sol particles increase in size, these particles are less stable and aggregate together. Secondly, due to the steric hindrance, the larger colloidal gold sol particles tend to dwarf the coated antigen/antibody making interaction with the analyte difficult (Fig. 23.2).

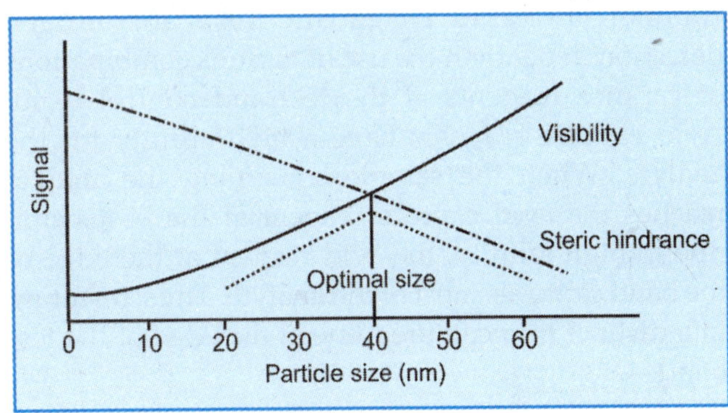

Fig.23.2: Graph of particle's size v/s signal colour of colloidal gold sol

Ideally, the colloidal gold sol used in immunochromatographic assay is ~40 nm in size and imparts a cherry red colour, which enables optimal visualisation of results against a clear white background and is stable in dry and liquid forms. However, purple coloured colloidal gold sol particles if properly stabilised, can also be used in Rapid Diagnostic Tests.

Why are Variations in Band Appearance Commonly Observed in Membrane-based Rapid Diagnostic Tests Employed for Antigen Detection?

The sensitivity/specificity of Rapid Diagnostic Tests primarily depends upon the detector and capture reagent pair. Ideally, the detector reagent should be specific to one epitope of the analyte and the capture reagent specific to another epitope of the same analyte, thereby enabling two-site sandwich immunoassay. To illustrate the same, please refer to Fig. 23.3.

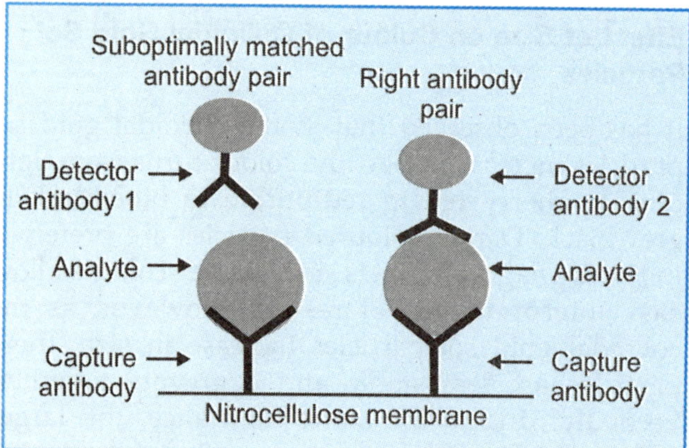

Fig. 23.3: Two-site sandwich immunoassay

For higher analyte sensitivity, manufacturers of commercial Rapid Diagnostic Tests for antigen detection depend on the use of various combinations of capture reagents at the test and control band. Avid capture reagents have a high affinity for the analyte. When the sample containing the analyte reaches the avid capture reagent at the best band, due to high affinity, the avid reagent at the edge of the band captures most of the analyte. Thus, resulting in a distinct thin coloured line at the edge of the test band.

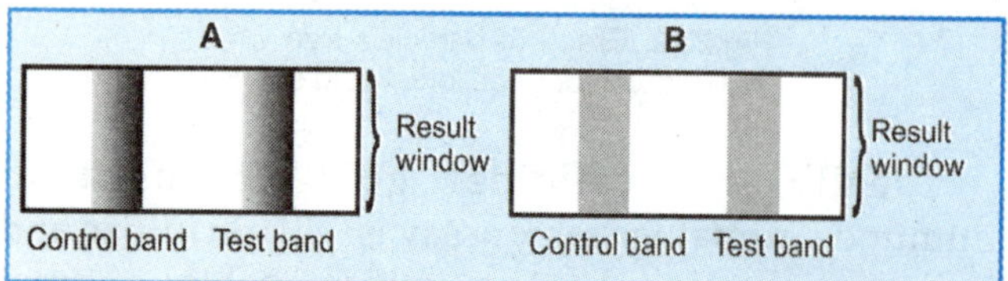

Figs 23.4A and B : A. Band appearance due to avid antibodies. B. Band appearance due to less avid antibodies

On the other hand, use of less avid capture reagent (lesser affinity for the analyte) results in capture of the analyte uniformly across the test or control band. Thus, broader bands are generated by less avid antibodies.

Variations in band appearance in different assays is due to use of varying avidity of the antibodies at the test/control band.

What is the Role of Sample Pad in Membrane-based Rapid Diagnostic Tests?

Rapid Diagnostic Tests enable detection of the analyte in several specimens such as urine, whole blood, serum or plasma. However, the pH, viscosity, ionic concentraction, turbidity, and total protein content may vary from specimen to specimen. Variations in these factors can cause alterations in the colloidal gold particles or the capture reagent leading to nonspecific results. For example, highly turbid specimens can cause invalid results since the particles from the specimen may block the membrane preventing sample flow. Urine specimen becomes acidic on storage due to bacterial growth. Due to a shift in the pH, the colloidal gold particles come together to form aggregates which may interfere in the performance of the test.

Rapid Diagnostic Tests incorporating serum as specimen may give false-positive results due to the presence of heterophillic antibodies. These antibodies have multispecificity and bind the capture reagent to the detector reagent leading to false positive results. Use for Rapid Diagnostic Tests incorporating heterophillic blocking reagents (HBR) is recommended to avoid this intereference.

A sample pad with a bed volume of minimum retention capacity facilitates transfer of the entire specimen dispensed. This not only ensures minimal wastage of specimen but also the excess specimen can be used to wash away unbound conjugate from the test region for better visualisation of results.

Thus, use of sample pad that allows incorporation of buffer salts, stabilisers and HBR, to a large extent eliminates variation in pH, ionic concentration and interference of heterophillic antibodies.

What is the Role of Soak Pad in Membrane-based Rapid Diagnostic Test?

Use of a soak pad with high bed volume is preferred in Rapid Diagnostic Tests because the total volume of specimen that enters the test assay can be increased. This increased volume can be used to dislodge the conjugate as well as wash away the unbound/unreacted conjugate from the test region contributing to clearer background and better visualisation of results.

Why do "Faint Ghost Bands" Appear at the Test Region if the Device is left out on the Worktable?

A common phenomenon observed in the device format is appearance of faint ghost bands at the test region after some time. After completion of the test, if the device is exposed to warm ambient temperatures, evaporation occurs from the result window. Due to evaportion, the excess sample along with unreacted/unbound conjugate from the soak pad flows back to reaction area. This unreacted or unbound conjugate may then get deposited on the test band resulting in appearance of a "Faint Ghost Band" after some time (Fig. 23.5).

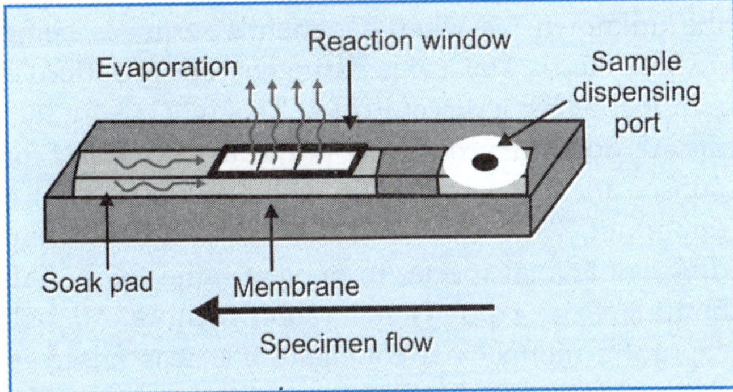

Fig. 23.5: Appearance of "Faint Ghost Band"

Results must be recorded at the end of the recommended reaction time for correct interpretation

How do we Interpret "Broken Bands" at the Test/Control Region?

To prevent evaporation of the specimen from the test window, the membrane of the device is laminated with the help of a thin transparent tape. Sometimes, during the process of lamination, air pockets may be formed between the membrane and the tape. These air pockets prevent uniform sample flow, which may result in appearance of broken bands at the test/control region.

However, appearance of even a broken band at the test region indicates positive results.

In the following section, we shall discuss the role of hCG as a marker for diagnosing pregnancy and certain conditions that may give discrepant results.

Excess Sample Volume Dispensed

Adding excess sample in no way improves the performance of the test. The excess sample added, cannot be absorbed by the sample pad and thus flows out through the sides of the device. Sometimes, the excess sample may flow out along with the conjugate. The amount of the conjugate left in the device is insufficient to perform the assay, leading to invalid results. Secondly, once the specimen flows through the device, the soak pad cannot retain the excess volume of the sample, which then may flow out through the sides of the device or may also flow back to the membrane along with unreacted/ unbound conjugate. This unreacted/unbound conjugate may then deposit onto the membrane resulting in apparently discrepant results.

ENZYME IMMUNOASSAY

Introduction

An immunoassay can be defined as a qualitative or quantitative assay, which relies on the reaction between an antigen and its specific antibody. The antigen being bound is called "ligand" and the antibody is the "binder" of the ligand. Enzyme labelled conjugates were introduced first in 1966 for localisation of antigens in tissues, as an alternative for fluorescent conjugates. In 1971, enzyme-labelled antigens and antibodies were developed as serological reagents for assay of antibodies and antigens. Their versatility, sensitivity, simplicity, economy and absence of radiation hazard have made EIAs the most widely used procedure in clinical serology. The availability of test kits and facility of automation have added to their popularity.

The enzyme-linked immunosorbent assay (ELISA), [(Enzyme immunoassay (EIA) or solid-phase immuosorbent assay (SPIA)] is a sensitive laboratory method used to detect the presence of antigens (Ag) or antibodies (Ab) of interest in a wide variety biological sample.

Many variations in the methodology of the ELISA have evolved since its development in the 1960s, but the basic concept is still the immunological detection and quantitation of single or multiple Ag or Ab in a patient sample (usually serum).

CLASSIFICATION OF ELISA

ELISA can be classified in different ways (see Fig. 23.13):

1. Direct ELISA

Direct ELISA is the most basic of ELISA configurations. It is used to detect an Ag after it has been attached to the solid phase (e.g. a membrane or dipstick). An Ab conjugated with a label (e.g. HRPO, AP, FITC) is then incubated with the captured antigen. After washing off excess conjugate and incubating with a substrate and chromogen, the presence of an expected colour indicates a specific Ab-Ag interaction. The conjugate could be a commercial preparation specific for the Ag of interest, or an in-house conjugated monoclonal or polyclonal Ab, or even patient serum (Fig. 23.6).

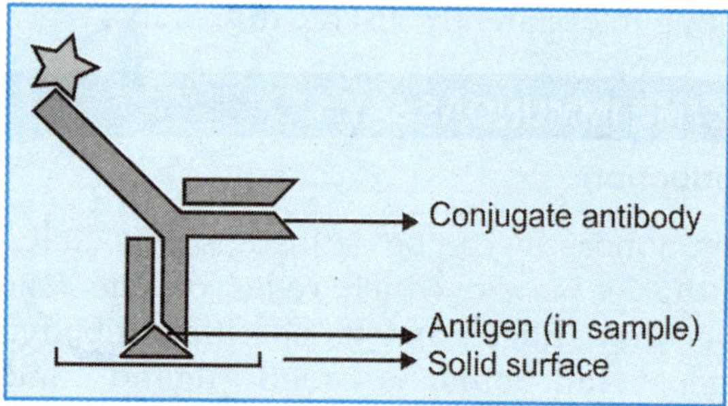

Fig. 23.6: Direct ELISA

2. Indirect ELISA

This is extensively used for the detection and/or titration of specific antibodies from serum samples. The specificity of the assay is directed by the antigen on the solid phase, which may be highly purified and characterized. The first, or **primary** Ab is incubated with the Ag, and then the excess is washed off. A second or **secondary** Ab conjugate is then incubated with the samples. The excess is again removed by washing. For colour to develop, a primary Ab that is specific for the Ag must have been present in the sample (e.g. human serum, CSF or saliva). This indicates a positive reaction. It is important, during assay optimisation, to ensure that the secondary Ab does not bind nonspecifically to the Ag preparation or impurities within it, nor to the solid phase (Fig. 23.7).

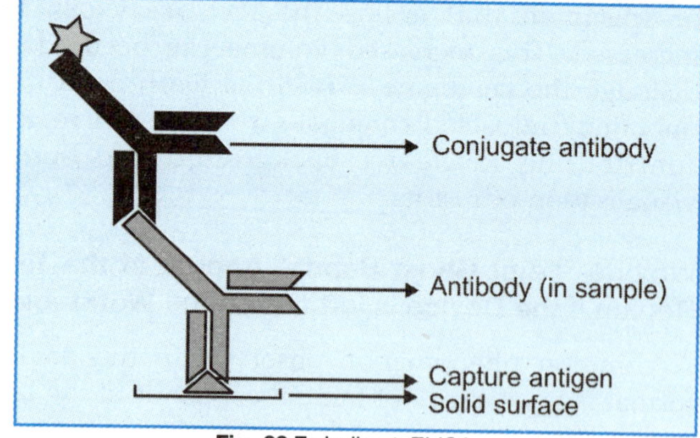

Fig. 23.7: Indirect ELISA

3. Capture ELISA

a. Antigen Capture

In this, more specific approach, a capturing Ab is adsorbed onto the solid phase. The capture antibody may be the reagent to be tested (e.g. the titre of a patients immune response to a known Ag). However, the Ab may be a standard reagent and the antigen the unknown (as when a patient's serum is being investigated). The same stringent optimisation is required as for indirect ELISA. This will ensure that the Ab does not cross-react in the absence of Ag, or nonspecifically binds to the solid phase. It is also important, when detecting the Ag, to use Ab from different animal species to prevent same-species Ab binding (e.g. a polyclonal rabbit capture Ab will capture a monoclonal conjugate if it was raised in rabbits. This will produce a positive result in the absence of Ag) (Fig. 23.8).

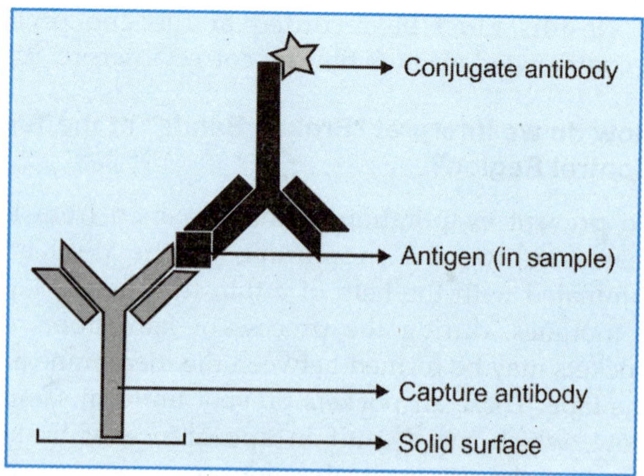

Fig. 23.8: Antigen capture

b. Antibody Capture

In this approach, a capturing Ab is adsorbed onto the solid phase. The Ab is designed to capture a class of human Ab (e.g. IgG, IgA or IgM). Next, the sample is applied, containing the Ab under investigation. After washing, an Ag specific for the Ab is added and finally an anti-Ag conjugate provides the signal (Fig. 23.9).

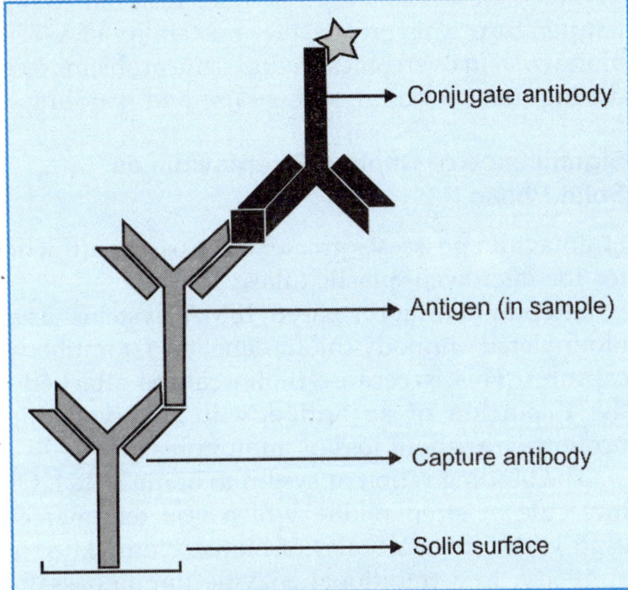

Fig. 23.9: Antibody capture

Another approach is to coat antigen on the solid surface. The antibody (from the sample) binds with it. After washing an anti-antibody (antibody against antibody) conjugated with enzyme is added.

4. Competitive ELISA

This implies that two reactants are trying to bind to a third. Proper competition assays involve the simultaneous addition of two competitors. It can be of various types.

a. Direct Antibody Competition

In this, the solid phase is coated with antigen. The labelled and unlabelled antibodies both compete for the limited binding sites for the antigen (Fig. 23.10).

b. Direct Antigen Competition

This is same as above except that the solid phase is coated with antibody, while labelled and unlabelled antigens (from the patient sample) compete for the antibody.

In a competitive ELISA, the amount of colour developed is inversely proportional to the amount of Ag-specific patient Ig present. Careful standardisation is required to interpret the results.

<u>Analytes tested by competitive ELISA</u>

- Thyroid hormones T3, T4, FT3, FT4
- Steroid hormones:
  - Androgens, Testosterone, Androstenedione, DHEA-S
  - Estrogens Estradiol (E2), Estriol (E3)
  - Progesterones Progesterone, 17-OH Progesterone
- Cortisol
- Hepatitis Markers: HAV, HBc Antibody

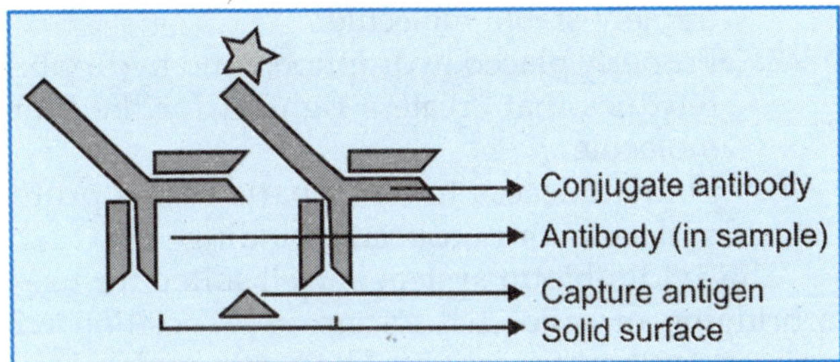

Fig. 23.10: Competitive ELISA-direct antibody competition

5. Streptavidin-Biotin ELISA

This is also a type of sandwich ELISA. In this, the solid phase is coated with streptavidin instead of antigen or antibody.

Avidin, found in hen egg white, is a fascinating protein because of its high binding affinity for the vitamin Biotin (vitamin H). In fact, avidin and a related protein, streptavidin (found in the bacteria *Streptomyces avidinii*), exhibit the highest known affinity in nature between a protein and a ligand (Ka.1015 M/L). The rate constant for the avidin/biotin association reaction is also fast (K=7 × 10^7 M-1s-1).

Because of its extraordinary binding capacity, biotin is used to develop modern ultrasensitive quantitative enzyme immunoassays. The tetrameric avidin/streptavidin system (crosslinking with biotinylated molecules) has been used for developing third generation ultrasensitive quantitative endocrine and other related immunoassays.

The active form of avidin is a tetramer composed of four glycosylated subunit (mol. wt = 62,400). The avidin tetramer has the capacity to bind up to four biotin molecules through noncovalent linkages. Each avidin monomer consists of 128 residues arranged in an orthogonal eight-stranded "B barrel". Biotin binds with the barrel towards one end only.

Avidin-Biotin relation of Ag-Ab binding

Every antibody has two antigen binding sites (F_{ab}), the structure and shape of the particular antigen-binding site of an antibody (also termed as Paratope) and its corresponding antigen (more specifically Epitope) is such that they tightly fit (high attraction force and minimum repulsive force between participating molecules) to each other. Similarly, biotin gets tightly fit into the avidin molecule because of the following structural characteristics of avidin:

1. Strong hydrogen bonding between the monomers of avidin makes streptavidin an extremely stable molecule.
2. Properly placed hydrophobic and hydrophilic residues that create a tight fit for the biotin molecule.
3. Limited access to other parts of the protein molecule for nonspecific binding.

The avidin-biotin system is well suited for use as a bridging or sandwich system in association with antigen-antibody reactions. The biotin molecule can be easily coupled to either antigens or antibodies, and avidin can be conjugated to enzymes and other immunological markers.

Advantages of Streptavidin

Streptavidin is used in preference to avidin because of the following reasons:

- It has a neutral isoelectric point and it does not contain carbohydrates.
- Streptavidin is more inert in assay systems.
- It reportedly exhibits less nonspecific binding than avidin; and hence, offer, greater specificity.

Streptavidin-biotin based IEMA systems are a better choice for Indian laboratories because of the following.

Stability: The binding of avidin and biotin is not disturbed by extremes of salt, pH or temperature.

Specificity and Sensitivity: Avidin has a very high binding affinity for biotin and so the system avidin-biotin is highly specific; moreover, the rate constant for the avidin-biotin association is also fast; and as a result, assay protocols become rapid and simple.

Speed of the Reaction: The solid phase is coated with avidin and the capture antibody is biotinylated, this minimises the need for the other coating methods and facilitates the use of antibodies with high affinities, reducing overall assay incubation time.

Temperature Stability and Other Problems: Non-bound avidin is very thermostable for the folded-unfolded transition, Tm=85 degree Celsius (pH 7-9). When biotin is found, the protein acquires greater thermostability (Tm=132 degree celsius).

Thus, the avidin-biotin is more resistant to high temperature. This greater thermostability of avidin-biotin system overcomes/reduces the problems faced during transportation, storage use and handling.

Significance of Coating Streptavidin as Solid Phase

Streptavidin possesses greater electrostatic attraction for the microwell/plastic tubes.

Streptavidin-biotin based IEMA systems use a biotinylated antibody (biotin-labelled 1st antibody/ capture). This is because biotin can be attached to the F_c portion of an antibody in relatively high proportion without loss of immunoreactivity.

The binding ration of avidin to biotin is 1: 4. One molecule of streptavidin, which is a tetramer can bind with four molecules of biotin/biotinylated 1st antibody. In a traditional enzyme immunoassay, a limited space is normally available for coating the capture/1st antibody in the bottom of the microwell/ plastic tube. Ideally, if one can increase the number of capture/1st antibodies coated on the microwell. The assay sensitivity goes up because more number of antigen-binding sites becomes available in case of low concentration of analytes (antigens) present in the sample.

Streptavidin biotin based systems coat streptavidin on the microwell/plastic tubes instead of directly coating the capture/1st antibody. Capitalising the tetrameric valency of streptavidin binds with four molecules of biotinylated capture/ 1st antibody thus providing an excess of binding sites to the system, which ensures four-fold higher sensitivity of the IEMA system (Fig. 23.11).

Analytes tested by Streptavidin-Biotin ELISA

Pituitary hormones: TSH, FSH, LH, PRL
Tumor Markers: PSA, CEA, AFP, CA 125, CA 15.3, CA 242, hCG
Antibody estimation: Anti-thyroglobulin, anti-thyroid peroxidase (TPO), anti-*H. pylori*

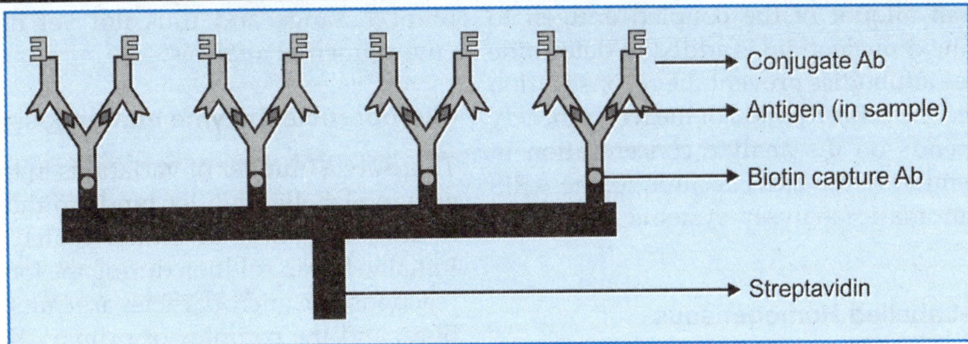

Fig. 23.11: Streptavidin-biotin ELISA

6. Immunocapture ELISA

This is also a type of sandwich ELISA and is commonly known as µ-capture/IgM-capture ELISA. It is mainly used for the identification of IgM class of antibodies. In this, there is an "immunocomplex" (antigen complexed with conjugate) is used. The microwell is coated with anti-human IgM, which is IgG in nature, which is specific against the µ-chain of IgM class antibody (from the patient sample). After binding the conjugate, it is added followed by substrate (Fig. 23.12).

<u>Analytes tested by Immunocapture ELISA</u>

Infectious serology IgM panels:
ToRCH infections: Toxo, Rubella, CMV, HSV
Hepatitis markers: HAV IgM, HBc IgM, HDV IgM

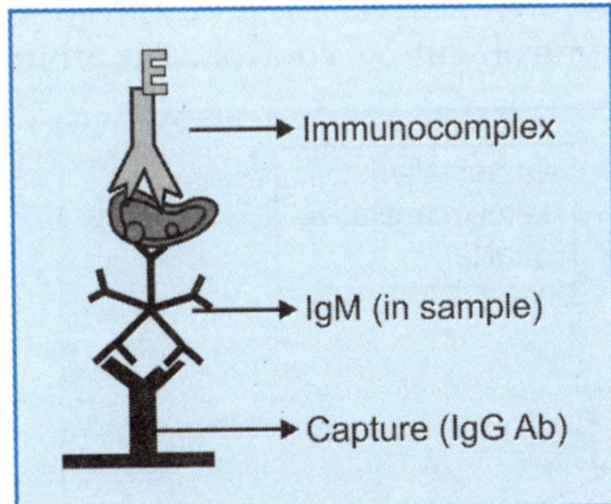

Fig. 23.12: Immunocapture ELISA

7. Interference Corrected ELISA

It is also one type of sandwich ELISA and is used for infectious diseases immunoassays. This ELISA is best for overcoming all the false positives and false negatives, which affect the correct result. For ToRCH (Toxo, Rubella, CMV, HSV) IgM assays, many factors can give false positives and false negatives. This leads to wrong reporting and wrong diagnosis. "Interference correction" is a principle by which one can remove all these factors. A few manufacturers have this feature. For ToRCH assays, it is always suggested to use interference corrected ELISA kits.

<u>Based on separation steps, ELISA can be classified as</u>

Homogeneous ELISA

Do not require separation of free and bound label. Bound label selectively separates or label is inactive when bound.

Latex Particle Agglutination Immunoassay (LPAIA)

A large number of latex agglutination immunoassays have been adopted from clinical chemistry. These assays are based on the visualisation of antigen-antibody complexes by the attachment of latex particles or gold colloids. Entities of this type with dimensions in the nanometer or micrometer range can be quantified by turbidimetry, nephelometry, light scattering techniques, and particle counters.

Enzyme-Multiplied Immunoassay Technique (EMIT)

In the EMIT, the analyte is covalently bound to the enzyme in spatial proximity to the active site; and consequently, the formation of the antibody-antigen complex inactivates the enzyme; addition of hapten results in a reduction of this inactivation. Over a limited range, the enzyme activity is approximately proportionate to analyte concentration. This method has been widely employed for therapeutic drug monitoring.

Apoenzyme Reconstitution Immunoassay System (ARIS)

If, however, the antigen is covalently bound to the prosthetic group of an enzyme such as glucose oxidase and an aliquot of the coupled antigen to flavin – adenine dinucleotide) is added to determine an analyte, free antibodies prevent the reconstitution of the enzyme. The concentration of the free antibody naturally depends on the analyte concentration in the sample. Similar to the EMIT technique, the ARIS is used in automatic analyser systems in clinical chemistry.

Fluorophore-Labelled Homogeneous Immunoassay (FLHIA)

At first glance, fluorescent labelling appears to have a much higher detection strength compared to colourimetric detection, but this is not the case. First, the affinity constant generally limits the detection strength of a process. Second, fluorophores are exposed to many influences, such as quenching by impurities, or even adsorption of the fluorophore molecule. However, the fact that the detection can be repeated is advantageous, whereas a chemical reaction is irreversible.

Homogeneous Fluorescence Polarisation Immunoassay (FPIA)

Direct observation of the formation of a hapten-(fluorescent labelled) antibody complex is also possible in polarised light. The presence of free hapten reduces the antibody-tracer complex concentration, and the degree of polarisation is lowered. The detection strength of this test is in the µmol/L range and thus not yet high enough for environmental analysis.

Microparticle Enzyme Immunoassay (MEIA)

There are a number of variations in this method. The enzyme-labelled binder binds to the analyte, which in turn is bound to binder-coated microparticles. Initially, free in solution during the foregoing chemical reactions, the microparticles are immobilised on glass fibre, and the complex of primary binder (capture), ligand (analyte) and labelled binder (conjugate) is exposed to substrate, producing a coloured product.

Heterogeneous ELISA

This requires separation of free and bound label. Most ELISAs described above, fall into this category.

Based on the functional results ELISA can be classified as shown in Fig. 23.13.

Quantitative ELISA

In this type the concentration of the analyte is measured and expressed in standardized units (ng/dl for T3, ng/ml for PSA). Standards are run and graph is plotted against which the concentration of the analyte is estimated, e.g. T3, T4, TSH, FSH, LH, etc.

Semi-quantitative ELISA

In this type, the controls are used (positive control, negative control, cut-off control). An arbitrary unit

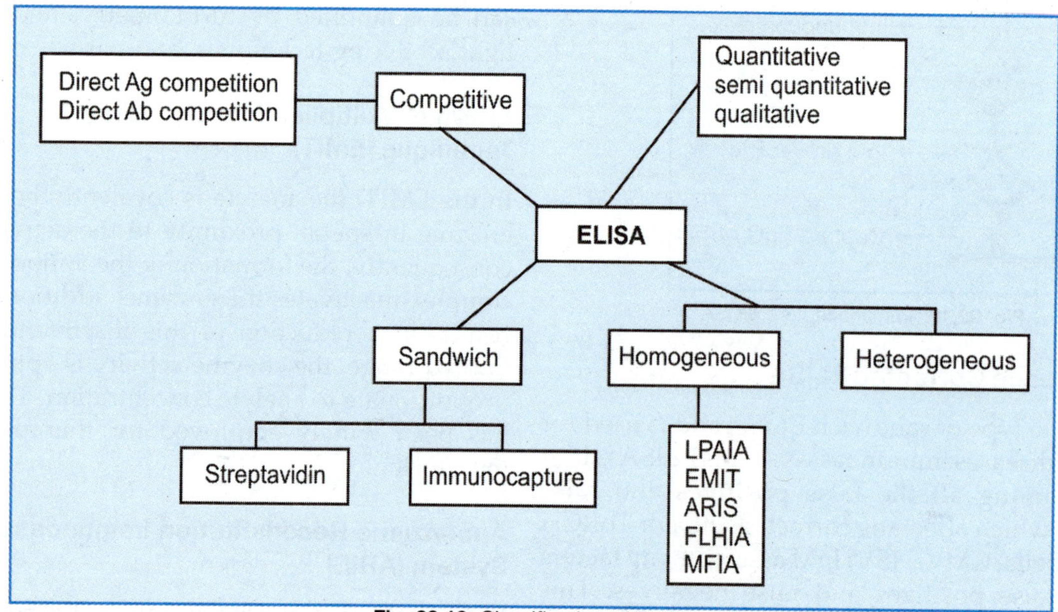

Fig. 23.13: Classification of ELISA

is given to express the concentration (EU/ml). Graph may or may not be used, e.g. ToRCH, ANA, etc.

Qualitative ELISA

In this type, the controls are used and is formula based. No graphs are required, e.g. HIV, HBsAg, etc.

ELISA: PRACTICAL ASPECTS

The different components of ELISA are packed together. This is commonly known as "Kit". The components are as follows.

Solid surface: It can be a microwell, coated tube or bead. This can be compared to a plate on which the reaction takes place. The microwell can be breakable or unbreakable. The coated tubes may be of polystyrene or polypropylene in nature. The solid phase may be coated with antigen, antibody or streptavidin. The choice of solid phase influences the measurement of optical density. In the case of Microwell, it is measured with an ELISA reader; and in coated tube it is measured by an analyser.

The process of fixing onto the solid phase is called "adsorption" and is commonly called coating. Most proteins adsorb to plastic surfaces, probably, as a result of hydrophobic interactions between nonpolar protein structures and plastic matrix. There may be nonspecific binding of unwanted proteins in available free sites. This can be avoided by adding "immunologically inert" proteins so as to block the free sites. These blocking agents may be added during the coating process.

Calibrators/Controls They are references against which the value of the analyte in the sample is estimated. An important fact is that immunoassays do not actually measure the analyte. They can only provide a quantitative estimate of concentration by direct comparison with standard/calibrator material.

The Features of an Ideal Calibrator are:

- A prerequisite for standardisation is that the standard/calibrator and analyte are identical.
- The calibrator should contain the analyte in a form identical to that found in the sample.
- Calibrators should ideally be prepared by using a base material identical to that in the test sample.
- For clinical applications, human serum is the preferred base matrix.

References

The matrix of a calibrator needs to behave in a similar way to the sample matrix.

For assay of hormones that are bound to serum protein, it is hard to use any other matrix other than human serum.

A prerequisite for standardisation is that the standard/calibrator and analyte are identical. In other words, the calibrator should contain the analyte in the form identical to that found in the sample.

Conjugate: It is the binder in the immunoassay system. The analyte in the sample may compete (in case of competitive ELISA) or bind with (in sandwich ELISA) the conjugate. It is either an antigen or antibody tagged with an enzyme (depending upon what it is being detected). The conjugate should have certain characteristics:

- The enzyme must be capable of binding to an antigen or antibody (the enzyme will react with the substrate to give colour).
- Should be stable at typical assay temperature.
- Should be stable when stored at 2 to 8°C.
- It must undergo only low-grade inactivation of reagent and enzyme.
- Long-term stability without loss of immunological and enzymatic activities.

Most commonly used enzymes in immunoassays are: Alkaline phosphatase, horseradish peroxidase, acetylcholinesterase, carbonic anhydrase, glucose oxidase, glucamylase, glucose-6 phosphate dehydrogenase, lysozyme, malate dehydrogenase.

Substrate: The confirmation of an antigen-antibody reaction is done by a suitable indicator. In ELISA this is done by the substrate. The substrate reacts with the enzyme (in the conjugate) to give a coloured end product. The intensity of the coloured product is directly/inversely proportional to the antigen-antibody reaction (in turn to the presence/absence or concentration of the analyte in the sample). The coloured end product may be soluble which is measured colourimetrically. This is mainly used in quantitative immunoassays. The end product may also be insoluble which is measured visually. It is suitable for dot blot assays. The end product remains as a permanent record. (e.g. Western blot strips, Rapid test cartridges, etc.). The substrate should have the following features:

- It should be able to produce intense coloured end product.

- Fast reaction rate or rate of conversion of substrate to end product.
- Ability to produce a broad range of coloured end product in a given time depending upon the amount of conjugate (analyte) it has reacted with.

The commonly used substrates are: TMB (tetramethyl benzidine), OPD (o-phenlyenediamine), DAB [diaminobenzidine (with enzyme HRP)] and BCIP (5-bromo4-chloro 3-indolyl phosphate), [NBT (Nitroblue tetrazolium)] (with enzyme alkaline phosphatase).

The factors affecting the performance of substrate are: temperature, pH, buffer composition, etc.

Stop Solution: The enzyme substrate reaction needs to be stopped to measure the optical density of the end product. The stop solution acts by destroying the enzyme component. The commonly used stop solutions are 1N HCl, 4N H_2SO_4, NaOH.

STEPS IN ELISA

There are multiple steps involved in an ELISA procedure. They can be grouped as follows.

Dilution: This is the first step. The reagents like conjugate, controls, sample diluent, wash buffer, stop solution, substrate, etc. are mixed in required proportions. In some cases, sample may also be diluted in given ratios before adding them in the well. Proper calculation of dilution ratios should be made. It is advisable to prepare slight excess of the quantity required to avoid pipetting errors. In some cases, the dilution itself will have excess volumes to offset the pipetting errors.

Addition: This is the pipetting step. It is done by either manual or electronic dispensing systems. The tips used must be compatible with the pipette. Multichannel pipettes can be used for addition of common reagents like conjugates, substrates, stop solution, etc. The advantage of electronic dispensing system is that errors are minimised. During pipetting some bubbles may be formed in the well. They should be burst using a pin. Different pins should be used for breaking different wells, as usage of same pin may lead to carry over.

Incubation: It is time period during which antigen combines with antibody or enzyme reacts with substrate. There are two types of incubation–stationary and rotatory incubation. In stationary—incubation, mixing takes place through diffusion of reagents. Because stationary incubation relies on diffusion of molecules, the role of temperature becomes extremely critical. To ensure complete reaction, longer incubation time is recommended. Rotatory incubation ensures complete mixing of reagents. This leads to increased contact between analyte and the capture/adsorbed reactant. Rotation gives additional kinetic energy to the system and hence, the reaction is less dependent on temperature.

Wash: It is actually a dilution process to optimally dilute the original solution without stripping off the bound/capture protein. It is one of the critical steps in ELISA. The optimal dilution step requires 3-5 cycles. Less than 3 cycles will leave behind residual proteins in the wells. The volume of wash solution dispensed per well should be high enough to cover the entire surface coated with antigen/antibody. The entire well must be filled during the wash cycle. Enough care is needed to prevent well-to-well overflowing of wash solution. During washing, more specifically in aspiration step, it is recommended to leave a small amount of wash buffer in the wells. This creates a film on the well and thus, prevents denaturation due to drying effect. The liquid used to wash wells is usually buffered (PBS) in order to maintain isotonicity, since most Ag-Ab reactions are optimal under such conditions. Tap water is not recommended, since tap water varies greatly in composition (pH, molarity, and so on).

Estimation: The estimation of colour can be done either visually (for rapid tests, Western blots, etc.) or using an ELISA reader. It is an instrument to measure the optical density and give the interpretation according to the program. The instrument can be programmed to do calculation and print the results. In case of coated tubes, the measurement is done by an analyser (Fig. 23.14).

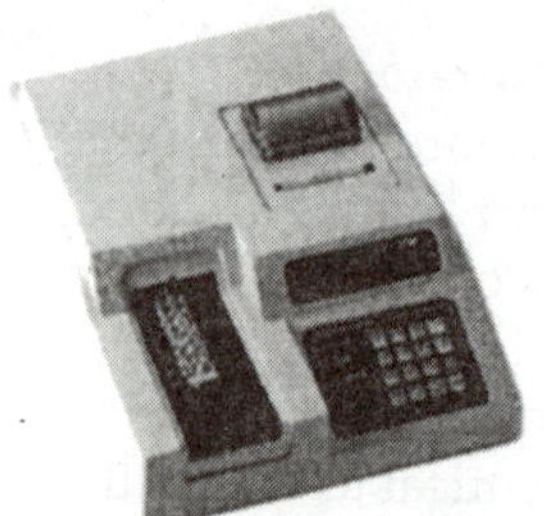

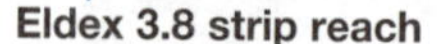

Eldex 3.8 strip reach

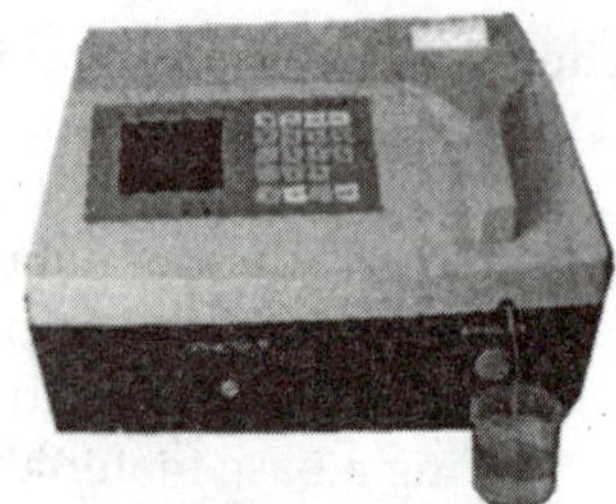

AE 600 semi-auto analyser

Fig. 23.14: Analysers (Courtesy: Lilac Medicare)

INTERFERENCES IN IMMUNOASSAYS

Despite advances in the design of immunoassays, the problems of unwanted interference have yet to be completely overcome. An ideal immunoassay should have the following attributes:

- The immunochemical reaction behaviour should be identical and uniform for both the reference (standard/calibrator) preparation and the analyte in the sample.
- The immunochemical reaction of the reagent is uniform from batch to batch.
- The immunochemical method is well standardised to ensure that the size of measurement signal is caused only by the antigen-antibody reaction.
- For macromolecules, the results declared in arbitrary units (IU—International Units), the conversion to (SI) units is not constant and depends on many factors.

Definition of Interference: Interference may be defined as "the effect of a substance present in an analytical system which causes a deviation of the measured value from the true value, usually expressed as concentration or activity".

The IFCC (International Federation of Clinical Chemistry) offers the following definition: "Analytical interference is the systematic error of measurement caused by a sample component, which does not, by itself, produce a signal in the measuring system."

Assay interference can be "analyte dependent or analyte independent" and can increase or decrease the measured result.

Increase (positive interference) is due to lack of specificity.

Decrease (negative interference) is due to lack of sensitivity.

Assay interference can be of different types:

- Preanalytical errors
- Analytical errors
- Postanalytical errors (see Fig. 23.15)

PREANALYTICAL VARIABLES

All factors associated with the procedures before the actual performance of the test are known as preanalytical errors. They can be as follows:

Patient based: Such as incorrect sampling times and environmental factors such as smoking, etc. may change analyte concentration and consequently interpretation.

Specimen based: There are many factors that constitute this.

Blood collection procedure and time of collection. Certain hormones are affected by the time of collection.

Nature of the sample: For all immunoassays, serum is the matrix of choice. Samples collected in to tubes containing sodium fluoride may be unsuitable for some enzymatic immunoassay methods; preservation with sodium fluoride may affect results. Impurities in tracers interfere with direct dialysis methods for free hormones.

Hemolysis and Hyperbilirubinaemia

Lipaemia may cause interference with assays for fat-soluble compounds such as steroids.

Stability and storage of reagents and samples are as follows:

Assay based: Certain procedures before the test is performed like:

- Bringing the kit to the room temperature
- Checking the incubator temperature
- Checking the room temperature
- Formatting and arranging the workbench
- Planning for assays to be performed
- Proper dilution calculation
- Maintaining the fridge temperature
- Dilution of samples with distilled water instead of zero calibrator.

Manufacturing error:

- Batch problem
- Packing error
- Assay protocol error
- Labelling error
- Wrong pack insert.

ANALYTICAL VARIABLES

These form the major part of all errors that affects the results in immunoassays. Mostly, these are overlooked and so attention is not paid to rectify them. These will lead to erroneous results. They are mainly the procedural errors. They are mostly confined to the different steps—addition, washing, incubation, dilution, pipetting, reading the protocol suggested by the manufacturer is not followed. Some of the errors are as follows.

Washing Errors

- High pressure washing
- Carry over during washing
- Drying of wells
- Splashing during washing
- Non removal of all wash solution from wells or tubes
- Not following soak time (if present) during washing
- Using a syringe to wash
- Leaving bubbles in the well after washing
- Not tapping the well after washing
- Use of contaminated wash buffer
- Wells/tubes falling off while washing.

Pipetting error

- Reuse of pipette tips
- Pipette tip blocked
- Pipette/dispenser not primed
- Pipette barrel contaminated
- Using tips to break bubbles
- Using same tips to break bubbles.

Equipment error

- Incubators not maintained at right temperature
- Heating not uniform throughout
- Washer probes blocked, contaminated
- Refrigerator not maintaining right temperature
- Defrost water falling on kits
- Use of dry incubators instead of water bath
- Instrument filters not checked periodically.

Procedural errors

- Interchange of reagent lots
- Wells not covered during incubation
- Not blanking when required
- Not running all calibrators to plot a graph
- Reuse of pipette tips
- Bubbles in wells
- Use of contaminated or uncleaned tubes to prepare reagents
- Using kits/reagents beyond expiry
- Using negative wells again
- Not mixing after adding stop solution.

POSTANALYTICAL VARIABLES

The errors that occur after the performance of the test are called as postanalytical errors. These are like:

- Calculation mistakes.
- Choosing a wrong graph scale.
- Comparison of result with inappropriate reference interval.
- Not correlating the results with clinical history.
- Transcription error when report is prepared.

Use of Wrong Reference Values

The reference ranges (normal ranges) of various parameters are different. Manufacturers specify the reference ranges. The units for reference ranges may differ. One should only compare with reference intervals given in the pack insert or should establish their own reference interval.

Comparison with results of different reference intervals will create confusion. Many laboratories make the mistake of comparing results with other labs without knowing the assay conditions and other factors that affect ELISA.

Use of Wrong Units

The units given by manufacturers may be different. For example, T3 ng/dl is different from ng/ml. A kit having a sensitivity of 0.4 ng/dl is more sensitive than 0.4 ng/ml (it is 40 ng/dl).

One should always make note of the units. Reports from different laboratories may differ in this aspect and create confusion.

The errors may be of any kind, but the outcome is that the result is incorrect and hence a wrong report is given. To overcome this, one should follow all the steps and adhere to the protocol strictly.

ELISA TROUBLESHOOTING

ELISA is a technique of multiple steps. The steps must be followed strictly to achieve good results. Errors at any levels will affect the final result. Complete understanding of the process is necessary for troubleshooting.

PRACTICAL TIPS ON ELISA

Normal Washing

In washing plate manually, the most important factor is that each well receives the washing solution so that, no air bubbles are trapped in the well or a thumb is not placed over corner wells.

Strip/Plate Washers

Various washing cycles can be programmed. Careful maintenance is essential, since they are prone to machine errors, such as having a particular nozzle being blocked.

Washing Tips

- Follow procedure for preparation of wash buffer.
- Check washer alignment daily as part of routine instrument start-up procedures.
- Ensure that the plate is levelled.
- Make certain well is completely filled, when washing, to ensure residual conjugate is removed.
- Examine that the plate is levelled.
- Make certain well is completely filled, when washing, to ensure residual conjugate is removed.
- Examine the fill volume (a slight dome should be observed at the top of the well).
- When washing does not allow wells to overflow.
- Reduce pressure in wash system.
- Check washers before use to determine they are working properly. Perform routine maintenance.
- Be certain to wash the specified number of times.
- Allow approximately 20 seconds between the addition of wash solution and subsequent aspiration.
- Examine the wells for complete aspiration of contents.
- Upon completion of wash cycle, blot to remove residual fluid.

Pipetting Tips

- Calibrate pipettes regularly according to manufacturer's instructions.
- Avoid touching sidewall of well with tips.
- Avoid splashing of sample and reagents.
- Avoid blowing out tip contents.
- Use a new tip for each sample/control/reagent addition.
- New tips should be used on the multichannel pipettes for each reagent to be added.
- Reverse pipette when using the multichannel pipette to add conjugate and substrate solution.
- Forward pipette when using the multichannel pipettes to add stop solution.
- Check pipette tips are long enough to provide air space between top of tip and pipette barrel.
- Check pipette barrel for residual fluid or dried material, remove if present.
- Ensure pipettes tips are fitted tightly.
- Service pipettes periodically by the manufacturers or authorised person.
- Do not open the pipette without proper tools.

Microplates

- Bring microplate pouches to room temperature before opening.
- Level microwells evenly in microplate frame as the individual breakaway wells have very flexible plate frames leading to bowing of wells and yield poor washes.
- Place plates in dark immediately after addition of substrate solution, provided the substrate is sensitive to light.
- Grasp holder on grip marks when tapping to avoid strips slipping from holder.
- Rotate strips 180°C and re-insert or use correct holder if strips do not fit in holder.
- Seal unused wells in pouches along with the desiccant.
- Date the pouches when first opened.
- Clean bottom surface of plates with wash buffer to remove fingerprints.
- Make sure microwells are at level during washing, reagent addition and plate/strip reading.
- Wipe the bottom of the plate with a lint-free cloth/towel before reading.
- Do not allow microwells to become dry once the assay has begun.

Substrate Preparation

- Use freshly prepared substrate A and substrate B.
- Do not hold substrate solution longer than 1 hour.
- Follow procedure of working substrate solution.
- The temperature of solution is important because it affects rate of colour reaction.
- Do not add fresh substrate to reagent bottle containing old substrate.
- Clean old substrate solution bottle with H_2SO_4 and thoroughly rinse with distilled water.

Conjugates

- Store at recommended temperature.

- Never store exclusively diluted conjugate for use at some later time.
- Always make up the working dilution of conjugate just before you need it.
- Never leave conjugates on the bench for excessive time.

General tips

- Plan the assay properly.
- Ensure all necessary items are chosen before starting the assay.
- Maintain a logbook on calibration and results data.
- While performing the assay, do not divert attention.

MATRIX EFFECTS

A fundamental problem with the analysis of components in biological materials is the effect of the extremely complex and variable mixture of proteins, carbohydrates, lipids, and small molecules and salts constituting the sample. The effect of these compounds on analytical techniques is termed as matrix effect.

It can be defined as "the sum of the effects of all the components, qualitative or quantitative, in a system with the exception of the analyte to be measured".

1. The Effect of Reagents

Assay buffers: The ionic strength and pH of buffers are vitally important, particularly in the case of monoclonal antibodies with pI values of 5-9. The use of binding displacers (blockers) may change the binding characteristics of antibodies, particularly those of low affinity. Detergents used in the buffers may contain peroxides, which inhibit antigen-antibody reaction.

Immunoassay labels: Labels have a profound effect on assays. The structure of most molecules, especially haptens, may be dramatically changed by labelling, e.g., by attachment of a radioactive iodine atom to a steroid. Labelling antibodies with enzymes is less of a problem because of their large size.

Separation of the antibody-bound and free fractions: The proportion of free analyte in the bound fraction and vice versa is known as the "misclassification error". Antibody bound fraction may be efficiently separated from the free analyte using solid-phase systems in which the antibody is covalently linked to an inert support e.g. the reaction tube, a polystyrene bead, a cellulose or nylon.

2. Effect of Proteins

Interfering proteins of general relevance include the following.

Albumin: It may interfere as a result of its comparatively huge concentration and its ability to bind as well as to release large quantities of ligands.

Rheumatoid factors: These are autoantibodies usually IgM class, and directed against the Fc portion of IgG. They are not specific to rheumatoid arthritis and are found in other autoimmune diseases, including systemic lupus erythematosus, scleroderma and chronic active hepatitis.

Complement: These proteins bind to the Fc fragment of immunoglobulins, blocking the analyte specific binding sites.

Lysozyme: Strongly associates with proteins having low isoelectric points (pI). Immunoglobulins have a pI of around 5 and lysozyme may form a bridge between the solid-phase IgG and the signal antibody.

Endogeneous hormone-binding proteins—These are present in varying concentrations in all serum and plasma samples and may markedly influence assay performance. For example, **HBG** (sex hormone binding globulin) interferes in immunoassay of testosterone and estradiol **TBG**, (thyroxine binding globulin) and **NEFA** (non-esterified fatty acid) interfere with the estimation of free T4.

Abnormal forms of endogeneous binding proteins: These are present in the plasma of some patients. They are present in familial dysalbuminaemic hyperthyroxinaemia (FDH) in which albumin molecules bind to thyroxine (T4). Individuals with FDH can be diagnosed as thyrotoxic, in spite of being normal.

Heterophilic antibodies: They may arise as a consequence of intimate contact, either intentional or unintentional, with animals. The most familiar effect of heterophilic antibodies is observed in two-site sandwich reagent-excess assays, in which a 'bridge' is formed between the two antibodies forming the sandwich. Assays that are affected by heterophilic antibodies include CEA, CA 125, hCG, TSH, T3, T4, free T4, prolactin, HBsAg and Digoxin.

MECHANICAL INTERFERENCE

Fibrinogen from incompletely clotted samples interferes with sampling procedures on automated immunoassay instruments and may produce spurious results. Paraproteinaemia causes interferences in many assays by increasing the viscosity of the sample. They may also nonspecifically bind either analytes or reagents that may affect the result.

NONSPECIFIC INTERFERENCE

Nonspecific interference may arise from excessive concentrations of other constituents of plasma. Free fatty acids affect some assays for free T4 by displacement of T4 from endogeneous binding proteins.

HOOK EFFECT

The "Hook Effect" is characterised by the production of artefactually low results from samples that have extraordinarily high concentrations of antigen (analyte), far exceeding the concentration of the upper standard in the assay concerned.

The hook effect is most commonly found in single-step immunometric assays, a popular format, chosen for its specificity and speed, particularly with high-throughput immunoassay analysers. The assays most affected are those that have analyte concentration that may range over several orders of magnitude. For example, alpha fetoprotein (AFP), CA-125, hCG, PSA, TSH, prolactin and ferritin are most affected by hook effect.

Reduction of Hook Effect

The incidence of hook effect can be reduced (but not eliminated) by careful assay design—incorporating a wash step prior to addition of the second antibody, thereby avoiding simultaneous saturation of both antibodies.

Despite attempts to eliminate or reduce the hook effect by careful assay design, the only reliable method of routinely eliminating the effect is to test the samples that are likely to be affected by hook effect in undiluted and also at a suitable dilution. Such samples should be diluted using either the assay diluent or serum from a normal subject until a stable quantitative response is achieved.

EDGE EFFECT

Sometimes with ELISA performed in a microwell plate unexpectedly higher (or lower) optical densities (OD) are measured in the peripheral wells than in the central wells. This phenomenon is called "edge effect". The most probable causes of this effect are illumination or temperature differences between the peripheral and the central wells.

Light may cause edge effect if the substrate is photosensitive (i.e. converted by light exposure) like the H_2O_2/OPD substrate in the peroxidase system. Thus, if strong light is coming from one side (e.g. sunlight from a window) during the substrate reaction, the peripheral wells closest to the light source may give elevated OD values. Temperature difference, however, is the most common cause of edge effect.

Incubation at 37°C instead of room temperature is often used for shortening incubation time, which is not correct. Also, a common mistake is to use reactant liquids straight from a refrigerator and then incubate in a 37°C incubator (or at room temperature). Temperature changes of these magnitudes may, especially with short incubation times, destroy the assay homogeneity in microwell plates. The peripheral wells will normally be heated up first because of their position closest to the lower edge of the plate, which is in direct contact with the warm incubator shelf, which may result in higher OD values in these wells, other things being equal. The edge effect may be more pronounced if plates are stacked during incubation, especially in plates in the middle of the stack because their central wells are shielded from the warmer surroundings by the plates above and beneath.

To avoid the above-mentioned problems, the following precautions should be taken:

- Incubations should take place in subdued light or in the dark (if protocol requires).
- Reactant liquids (and plates) should be adjusted to the temperature intended for incubation.
- Plates should be sealed with adhesive tape or placed in a 100% relative humidity environment during incubation.

ASSAY SPECIFICITY

It is one of the most important requirements of immunoassays. Interference occurs in all situations in which the antibody is not absolutely specific for the analyte. Consequently, assessment of specificity is a vital step in the optimisation of every new immunoassay. Poor specificity results in interference from compounds of similar molecular structure or which carry similar immunoreactive epitopes. In determining the overall specificity of an assay, a major factor is the crossreactivity of the antibody.

Some of the major specificity problem areas are related to measurement of steroids and structurally related compounds. All commonly used testosterone assays, cross react in varying degrees with 5 α-dihydrotesterone, and all cortisol assays cross react with prednisolone.

Assessment of the specificity of immunometric assays is complex and quite different from that used for single-site assays. In most assays, two different antibodies are employed, each having unique specificity for a different epitope on the antigen. It is usual practice to employ at least one monoclonal antibody, which can be selected by epitope mapping to react only with predetermined sites on the antigen molecule. Use of two monoclonal antibodies can introduce extreme specificity.

ASSAY SENSITIVITY

The ability of a kit to detect very low concentrations of an analyte (in quantitative ELISA) is mainly understood by the sensitivity of the kit. Many manufacturers mention the sensitivity and specificity after the result interpretation. This is overlooked commonly. One should observe this carefully. Higher sensitivity is a desirable property in any kit. Some doubts have been expressed regarding the value of ultrasensitive assays, which detect very minute amounts of analyte, which may be below the clinically or diagnostically significant values.

Most diagnostic kits are not exhausted overnight. Repeated usage and storage exposes the kit to multiple thermal shocks. This affects the performance of the kit over a period of time due to lowering of sensitivity. This shift in sensitivity affects the ultra-

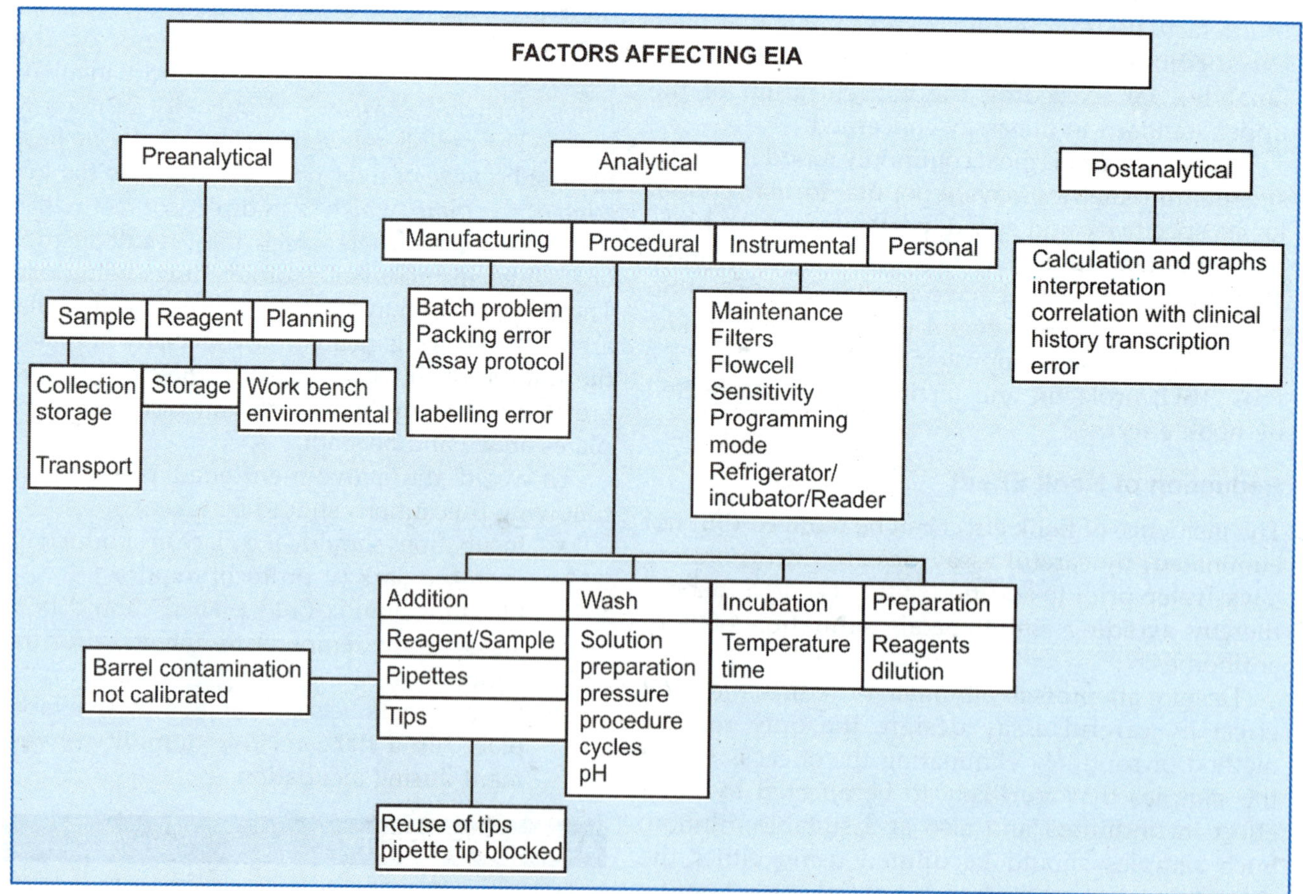

Fig. 23.15 Factors Affecting EIA

sensitive kits lesser than those with less sensitivity.

A good example of ultra sensitive kit is "Third Generation TSH kits" which are very useful in the diagnosis of hypothyroidism.

As compared to low sensitive kits, ultrasensitive kits are more robust, more accurate that improve the reliability of results and provide confidence to the clinicians on the laboratory results.

CHEMILUMINESCENCE: THE TECHNOLOGY

Introduction

"Chemiluminescence" is defined as the production of electromagnetic (ultraviolet, visible or near-infrared) radiation as a result of a chemical reaction. One of the reaction products is in an excited state and emits light on returning to its ground state.

The generation of signal and its estimation varies from technology to technology. In RIA (Radio Immunoassay) the radioactive signal is measured in gamma counter. In ELISA, the enzyme and substrate react to produce colour, which is measured using an ELISA reader. Fluorescence immunoassays involve a similar principle where enzyme and substrate react to produce a fluorophor, which is measured fluorometrically. In case of chemiluminescence immunoassays, the light is produced which is measured.

Measurement of light from a chemical reaction is highly useful because the concentration of unknown can be inferred from the rate at which light is emitted. The rate of light output is directly related to the amount of light emitted. This type of luminescence is frequently compared with fluorescence, which also involves emission of light as a result of relaxation of excited states. Since chemiluminescence does not involve initial absorption of light, measurement of chemiluminescence emission are made against a lower background noise that is not possible with conventional fluorescence, thus potentially allowing greater sensitivities of detection in chemiluminescent technology. This lack of inherent background and the ability to easily measure very low and very high light intensities with simple instrumentation provide a large potential dynamic range of measurement. Linear measurement over a dynamic range of 10^6 or 10^7 using purified compounds and standards has become possible with developments in the technology.

Light, as we see it, consists of billions of tiny packets of energy called photons, which are measured in the detection process. There are different factors that affect the emission and measurement of light.

- The efficiency of light emission from a chemiluminescent molecule is expressed as the chemiluminescence quantum yield, ÖCL, which describes the number of moles of photons emitted per mole of reactant
- The signal
- The quantity of signal required to produce the emission
- The duration of emission
- Instrumentation employed for the quantification of emission

COMPONENTS OF CHEMILUMINESCENT SYSTEM

The Signal

The signal (or substrate) used for generation of light should have optimum stability. There are many signal reagent available—luminol, 1,2 Dioxetanes, Acridinium ester, ruthenium salts, etc. Luminol is preferred of all these because of its stability and its advantage of being enhanced by iodophenol and phenothiazine.

Signal Quantity

The light emission in a chemiluminescent reaction is influenced by the quantity of signal used for generation of light. The manufacturing capabilities are limited globally and hence a prohibitive cost in procuring the signal for use in commercial scale. This limits the volume of signal for generation and also the sensitivity (lesser quantum of light produced, compromising the assay sensitivity).

The solution for this impediment can be achieved by increasing the quantity of signal generated in the reaction process. This is best done by using enhancers, which increase the intensity of signal produced. In 1985, Kircka and co-workers discovered that iodophenol compounds are strong enhancers that intensify luminol chemiluminescence about 1000 times, while also prolonging the duration of chemiluminescence.

Since the appearance of enhanced chemiluminescence, where enzymes like iodophenol, phenothiazine, etc. are employed to improve the light output of reactions, enzyme-sensitive chemiluminescent compounds have been the basis of several new clinical laboratory tests. These compounds increase the duration and quantum of signal produced by the reaction. Both peroxidase (HRP) - and phosphatase-sensitive chemiluminescent tags are commercially available. More tests employing these compounds can be expected to reach the clinical laboratory soon. Also, the recent introduction of enzyme-sensitive chemiluminescent tags with amplified light output has resulted in clinical tests with much-improved sensitivity.

This process of enhancement improves the performance of chemiluminescence immunoassay kits.

Signal Duration

Equally important is the fact that the light produced by the reaction process be measured within a specific time. The chemiluminescent reactions can be of two types depending on the duration of light produced.

Flash: In this, the addition of signal causes the immediate emission of light, typically over milliseconds or seconds. The instrumentations generating this type use a module for injecting the signal into the reaction system (injector module). These systems have moderate efficiencies. These systems have the benefit of a traditional chemiluminescent systems by increased sensitivity and dynamic range, but with its inherent inadequacies like homogenisation effect, difficult for photon counting and impossibility of repeat measurements in a reaction. Particularly the repeat measurement is important because, it gives more confidence in reporting. This is not possible by these systems and one has to repeat the entire test for second measurement.

Glow: The emission of light builds and reaches a maximum. The emission is stable for a longer period of time making re-measurement possible. Glow type systems are excellent for quantitative systems such as immunoassays and detection of proteins. In the case of glow reactions, procedure development is relatively simple and the timing of reagent addition and reagent/sample mixing are not critical as in flash reactions.

Instrumentation

The instrumentations perform the function of quantification of emission and read out design. There are many ways of doing this depending on the level of sensitivity and sophistication required. The instrument employs a photomultiplier tube (PMT) for this purpose. These devices can be used in either a current measuring or photon-counting mode. Photon-counting systems are the latest development in chemiluminescence technology and provide greater sensitivity and long-term stability than the traditional current measuring chemiluminescent systems. Different types of PMTs exhibit different sensitivities to different wavelengths and it is, therefore, important to select the PMT with maximum spectral response for maximum sensitivity. There are a very few good manufacturers of PMT present globally.

The instrumentations are available from simple one, which can count photon emissions from a single tube to fully automated systems capable of counting microplates by photon-counting mode. These often carry the software on board to be able to perform data reduction of standards and samples. The PMT count every single electron generated by secondary emission from the system in the form of a pulse and gives the output.

These pulse chemiluminescent systems are better than other chemiluminescent systems.

Comparison with Other Technologies

The detection of antigen-antibody binding can be done by many ways. Methods like RIA, ELISA, and fluorescence immunoassay have been used widely. Of this, ELISA is adopted commonly for many parameters.

Drawbacks of Other Technologies

Radio Immunoassay

- Low sensitivity
- Disposal issues, health hazard pertaining to radioactivity
- Older technology.

Enzyme Immunoassay

- Limitation of photometric measuring range.
- Low sensitivity in 2nd generation assays.
- Smaller dynamic range and linearity.

Fluorescence Immunoassay

- Compromised sensitivity
- Background fluorescence
- Protein quenching
- Sensitivity to temperature, pH
- Interference from haemoglobin, bilirubin.

References

"Interference from light scattering, background fluorescence and quenching can reduce the potential sensitivity of fluorescence immunoassay by factors between 100 and 1000.

"Fluorescent EIAs are identical to other EIAs. There may be substances in the system that emit fluorescent light. These substances increase the background signal which may interfere with the assay's sensitivity" (Fig. 23.16).

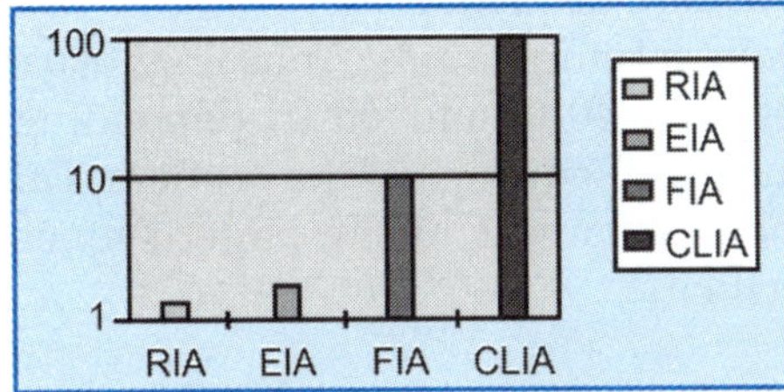

Fig. 23.16: Relative sensitivity

Advantages of Chemiluminescence Technology

1. **Linearity:** In chemiluminescence, since the individual photons are counted, there is very high linearity. Very high values can be obtained without dilution.
2. **Stability:** The signal generated in chemiluminescence is stable for long time making it better than other technologies.
3. **Sensitivity:** The lower detection limit is more in chemiluminescene than other technology.
4. **Convenience:** There is no second incubation in chemiluminescence since there is no substrate incubation step.
5. **Cost:** Since less signal quantity is used in "Enhanced pulse chemiluminescence" systems, the reagent and instrumentation cost are less than the closed chemiluminescent systems.

Overall, enchanced pulse chemiluminescence is favoured for the following reasons:

- No excitation source is required
- Chemiluminescent substrates have a shelf-life of about a year, whereas those of fluorescence (which contain a fluorescein molecule) will last only about a week.
- The level of detection is also lower with that of chemiluminescence—femtogram level has been well documented.
- Fluorescence due to its limited availability is very expensive. Chemiluminescence is much more affordable.
- Extraordinary sensitivity; a wide dynamic range; inexpensive instrumentation; and the emergence of novel luminescent assays make this technique very popular.
- Superior sensitivity and low background distinguish chemiluminescence from other analytical methods.
- Chemiluminescence is up to 100,000 times more sensitive than absorption spectroscopy and is at least 1,000 times more sensitive than fluorometry.
- The background light component is much lower in chemiluminescence than in other analytical techniques such as spectrophotometry and fluorometry.
- Wide dynamic range and low instrument cost are also distinct advantages of chemiluminescence. Samples can be measured across decades of concentration without dilution or modification of the sample cell.

Enhanced pulse chemiluminescence immunoassays are available in two formats.

1. Impulse 9.0—An open semi automated chemiluminescent immunoassay system (Fig. 23.17).

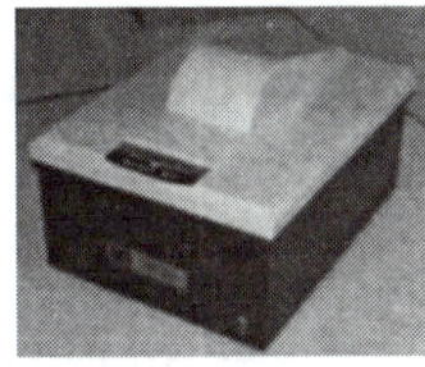

Fig. 23.17: Impulse 9.0 enhanced pulse chemilunescence system. Courtesy: Lilac Medicare

Advantages

- First of its kind in the category of chemiluminescent instruments in India.
- Wide range of assay menu.
- No protein quenching problem as in fluorescence.
- Better sensitivity out of all available immunoassay technologies.
- Simple operation, performs single tests.
- Robust instrument design. Ideal for distant locations for engineer free operations.

2. Alpha Prime LS—fully automated walkaway chemiluminescent immunoassay system (fig. 23.18).

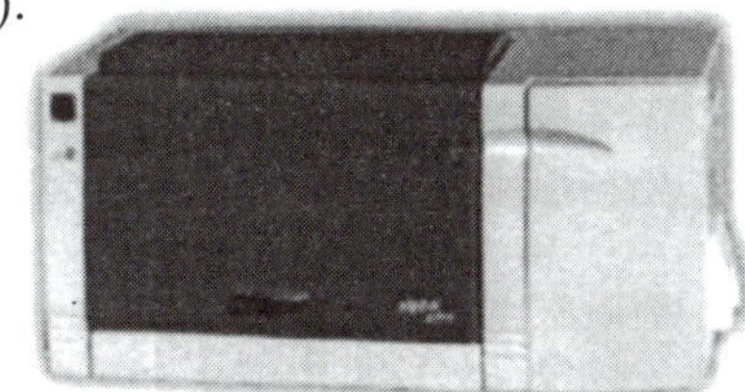

Fig. 23.18: Alpha prime LS. Courtesy: Lilac Medicare

Advantages

- Fully automated multiparametric immunoassay system.
- Can run up to 384 samples at a time.
- Can perform 18 different parameters simultaneously.
- Can operate in CLIA and EIA technology also (for infectious and autoimmune diseases parameters).

POLYMERASE CHAIN REACTION

PCR stands for the Polymerase Chain Reaction and was developed in 1987 by Kary Mullis and associates. It is capable of producing enormous amplification (i.e. identical copies) of a short DNA sequence from a single molecule of starter DNA. It is used to amplify a specific DNA (**target**) sequence lying between known positions (**flanks**) on a double-stranded (ds) DNA molecule.

The amplification process is mediated by oligonucleotide primers that, typically, are 20-30 nucleotides long. The primers are single-stranded (ss) DNA that have sequences complementary to the flanking regions of the target sequence. Primers anneal to the flanking regions by complementary-base pairing (G≡C and A=T) using hydrogen bonding.

The amplified product is known as an amplicon.

Generally, PCR amplifies smallish DNA targets 100-1000 base pairs (bp) long. (It is technically difficult to amplify targets >5000 bp long.)

PCR has many applications in research, medicine and forensic science.

One PCR cycle consists of three steps:

- Denaturation
- Annealing
- Extension

Denaturation by Heat

Heat (usually >90°C) separates double-stranded DNA into two single strands, referred to as "denaturation". Since the hydrogen bonds linking the bases to one another are weak, they break at high temperatures, whereas the bonds between deoxyribose and phosphates, which are stronger covalent bonds, remain intact.

Annealing Primer Binding to Target

Primers are short, synthetic sequences of single-stranded DNA typically consisting of 20-30 bases, with a biotin-labelled 5' end to aid in detection. They are specific for the target region of the organism. Two primers are included in the PCR, one for each of the complementary single DNA strands that was produced during denaturation. The beginning of the DNA target sequence of interest is marked by the primers that anneal (bind) to the complementary sequence.

Annealing Temperature: Annealing usually takes place between 40°C and 65°C, depending on the length and base sequence of the primers. This allows the primers to anneal to the target sequence with high specificity.

Extension

Once the primers anneal to the complementary DNA sequences, the temperature is raised to approximately 72°C and the enzyme Taq DNA polymerase is used to replicate the DNA strands. Taq DNA polymerase is a recombinant thermostable DNA polymerase from the organism *Thermus aquaticus* and, unlike normal polymerase enzymes is active at high temperatures.

Taq DNA polymerase, begins the synthesis process at the region marked by the primers. It synthesises new double-stranded DNA molecules, both identical to the original double-stranded target DNA region, by facilitating the binding and joining of the complementary nucleotides that are free in solution (dNTPs). Extension always begins at the 3' end of the primer making a double strand out of each of the two single strands. Taq DNA polymerase synthesises exclusively in the 5' to 3' direction. Therefore, free nucleotides in the solution are only added to the 3' end of the primers constructing the complementary strand of the targeted DNA sequence.

Following primer extension, the mixture is heated (again at 90-95°C) to denature the molecules and separate the strands and the cycle repeated.

Each new strand then acts as a template for the next cycle of synthesis. Thus amplification proceeds at an exponential (logarithmic) rate, i.e. amount of DNA produced doubles at each cycle. 30-35 cycles of amplification can yield around 1 µg DNA of 2000 bp length from 10^{-6} µg original template DNA. This is a million-fold amplification.

Initially, the 3 different stages at 3 different temperatures were carried out in separate water baths but nowadays, a thermal cycler is used (a machine that automatically changes the temperature at the correct time for each of the stages and can be programmed to carry out a set number of cycles).

A typical thermal cycle might be as follows:

Heat denaturation at 94°C for 20 seconds

Primer annealing at 55°C for 20 seconds

Primer extension at 72°C for 30 seconds

Total time for one cycle = approx. 4 minutes.

1. **DNA is denatured.** Primers attach to each strand. A new DNA strand is synthesised behind primers on each template strand.
2. **Another round:** DNA is denatured, primers are attached, and the number of DNA strands are doubled.
3. **Another round:** DNA is denatured, primers are attached, and the number of DNA strands are doubled.
4. **Another round:** DNA is denatured, primers are attached, and the number of DNA strands are doubled.
5. **Continued rounds** of amplification swiftly produce large numbers of identical fragments. Each fragment contains the DNA region of interest.

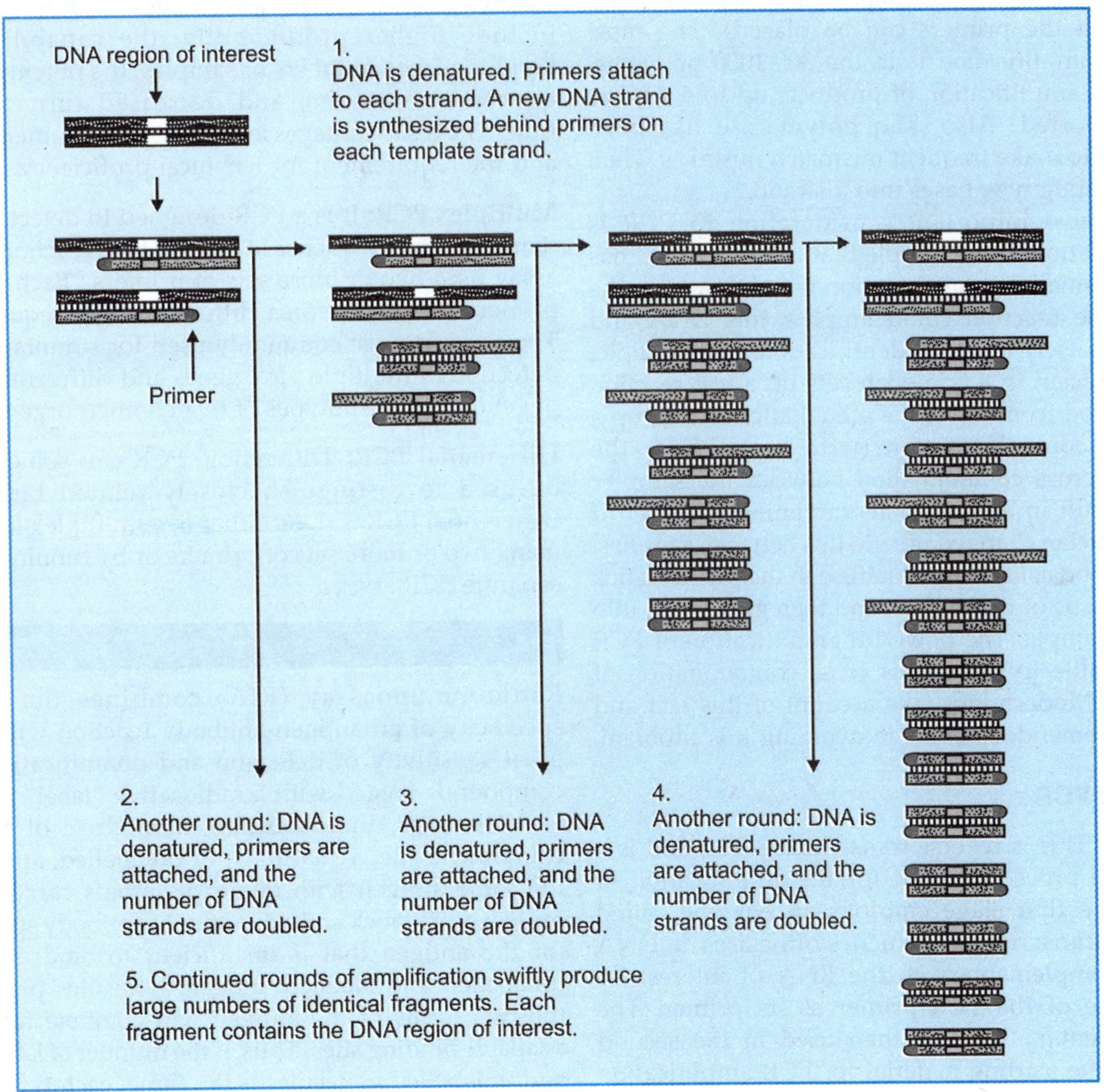

Fig. 23.19: Polymerase chain reaction

Limitations/Difficulties

While a very powerful technique, PCR can also be very tricky. The polymerase reaction is very sensitive to the levels of divalent cations (especially Mg^{2+}) and nucleotides, and the conditions for each particular application must be worked out. Primer design is extremely important for effective amplification. The primers for the reaction must be very specific for the template to be amplified. Crossreactivity with non-target DNA sequences results in nonspecific amplification of DNA. Also, the primers must not be capable of annealing to themselves or each other, as this will result in the very efficient amplification of short nonsense DNAs. The reaction is limited in the size of the DNAs to be amplified (i.e., the distance apart that the primers can be placed). The most efficient amplification is in the 300-1000 bp range, however, amplification of products up to 4 Kb has been reported. Also, Taq polymerase has been reported to make frequent mismatch mistakes when incorporating new bases into a strand.

The most important consideration in PCR is contamination. If the sample that is being tested has even the smallest contamination with DNA from the target, the reaction could amplify this DNA and report a falsely positive identification. For example, if a technician in a crime lab sets up a test reaction (with blood from the crime scene) after setting up a positive control reaction (with blood from the suspect) cross contamination between the samples could result in an erroneous incrimination, even if the technician changed pipette tips between samples. A few blood cells could volatilise in the pipette, stick to the plastic of the pipette, and then get ejected into the test sample. The powerful amplification of PCR may be able to detect this cross contamination of samples. Modern labs take account of this fact and devote tremendous effort to avoiding this problem.

Types of PCR

RT-PCR: This is reverse transcriptase-PCR and is a two-stage procedure used for the amplification of RNA. The first stage employs an enzyme called reverse transcriptase, which synthesises a DNA strand complementary to the RNA of interest by using one of the PCR primer as its primer. The complementary DNA is then used in the second stage as the starting material for PCR amplification by a conventional thermostable DNA polymerase.

Nested PCR: It is a PCR done in two steps, a primary PCR reaction and a nested reaction. The primary (or first) reaction uses a set of primers to generate a product that serves as the template for the nested (or second) reaction. The nested reaction uses a set of PCR primers specific for a region within the amplified product from the first reaction. Therefore, the nested reaction often serves as a confirmation for the specificity of the PCR products amplified in the primary reaction.

Real-Time PCR: Combines PCR amplification and detection into a single step. The basic principle of real-time quantitative PCR is the detection of target sequences using a fluorogenic 5′ nuclease assay (often called 'TaqMan'). The advantages of this system include high reproducibility, the capability of handling large numbers of samples, the potential for quantitative results, and decreased turnaround time. The disadvantages include high instrument cost and the requirement for technical proficiency.

Multiplex PCR: It is a PCR designed to detect more than one target sequence in a single PCR reaction. The assay uses two or more sets of primers. Each set of primers is specific for a different target sequence. The assay is most commonly used for simultaneous detection of multiple viral genes and differentiation of genotypes or subtypes of related microorganisms.

Differential PCR: Differential PCR can sometimes be used to distinguish closely related targets. Differential PCR is done either in a multiplex format using two or more sets of primers or by running two separate PCR assays.

RIA

Radioimmunoassay (RIA) combines the high specificity of an antigen-antibody reaction with the great sensitivity of detection and quantification of compounds tagged with a radioactive "label" atom.

If there is, in a solution, a mixture of three components, i.e. a "natural", or unlabelled, antigen, the same antigen with one of its atoms carrying a radioactivity label, and a quantity of antibody specific for the antigen that is insufficient to bind all the unlabelled and labelled antigen molecules present, the two forms of the antigen will compete for the available binding sites. Thus, if the number of labelled and unlabelled molecules is the same, each type has an equal chance of finding a free binding site, half the available antibody-binding sites will carry labelled antigen and half will carry unlabelled antigen. If the number of unlabelled antigen molecules is greater than the number of labelled ones, a large number of antibody-binding sites will become occupied by unlabelled antigen molecules. Thus, the larger the number of unlabelled antigen molecues in the mixture, the smaller the fraction of the original quantity of labelled antigen that will become bound by antibody. Since the firmly bound combination of antigen and antibody can be separated from the remaining components of the original mixture and its radioactivity determined and compared with that of the original labelled antigen addition; and since the relative amounts of bound and free labelled antigen will depend upon the number of unlabelled antigen molecules originally present, a calibration curve can be made by adding known amounts of unlabelled antigen to the system of labelled antigen and antibody, separating and determining the ratio of radioactivity of bound to original labelled antigen, and plotting this ratio against the known amounts of added unlabelled antigen. If a sample containing an unknown amount of natural (unlabelled) antigen is then mixed with the same amounts of labelled antigen and antibody as in the calibration curve mixture, the antigen-antibody complex separated and the ratio of its radioactivity determined when compared with that of the original amount of labelled antigen, this ratio, usually expressed as a percentage, when referred to the calibration curve, will give the amount of unlabelled (natural) antigen in the sample.

The unique combination of specificity and sensitivity of the RIA principle makes it particularly suitable for the assay of substances such as insulin, growth hormone, thyroxine, testosterone, progesterone, angiotensin, aldosterone, and drugs such as digoxin in serum or plasma at the level of nanogram per ml.

The procedures involved in RIA differ in the radioactive element used as the label, in the method used to separate the antigen-antibody combination from the unbound antigen, and in the standardisation. The majority of current methods use ^{125}I (radioactive iodine) or ^{3}H (tritium, the radioactive isotope of hydrogen) as the labels. For separation of antigen-antibody combination, charcoal coated with dextran is used. The dextran acts as a molecular sieve that passes only unbound antigen molecules for retention by the charcoal, the antigen-antibody combinations are too large to cross the dextran coating. After centrifuging, the relatively dense charcoal grains with their adsorbed antigen molecules will be packed at the bottom of the tube, and the supernatant containing the antigen-antibody combinations can be separated. Measurement of the ratio of radioactivities of the two components completes the assay. A more sophisticated method of precipitating the antigen-antibody combination is to add a second antibody prepared to react with the protein of the first antibody, usually a gamma globulin. The resultant complex can then be separated either by centrifugation or cellulose acetate filters. Standardisation can be done as described in the description of general principles above.

The RIA technique promises to provide reliable data by relatively simple methods about biological substances that present considerable analytical problems when more orthodox procedures are used. In practice, of course, RIA has its own sources of error. These include:

- Lability of compound analysed.
- Antibody cross reaction with related antigens.
- Interfering substances in the sample, e.g. urea and bilirubin.
- Poor pipetting technique (good pipetting technique is critical, because of the very small volumes).
- Contamination of equipment from extraneous radioactive materials.
- Change in the antigen's chemical or immunological identity owing to the process of adding radioactive label to the antigen.

The RIA methods measure the amounts of particular molecular structures, not their biological activity.

Measurement of Radioactivity

The radioactive atoms used as labels produce different types of emitted radiation. ^{125} emits short-wavelength, high-energy gamma rays; ^{3}H (tritium) produces beta-type radiation, which is actually high-speed particles, positively or negatively charged electrons. Gamma rays are detected by a so-called scintillation counter, which consists of a large sodium iodide crystal that contains thallium as an activator. The crystal is in close contact with a photomultiplier tube; and when an emitted quantum of gamma radiation strikes a sodium iodide molecule in the crystal lattice, it produces a photon of light energy.

This light is picked up and amplified by the assopifeted photomultiplier tube and converted to a pulse of electrical energy. The number of pulses is proportional to the quantity of radioactive material in the sample, the power or energy of the pulse is determined by the energy of the original gamma ray. The scintillation counter incorporates "discriminators," which pass through only those pulses whose energy levels correspond to those of the gamma radiation emitted from the particular radioactive atom whose detection is required. Finally, the scintillation counter uses a sealer to count the number of pulses arriving in a preset time or to determine the time required for a preset number of pulses to occur. To detect beta particles, which have less energy than gamma radiation is used.

The preparation of serology reagents and antisera is much too complex and beyond the scope of this book. It is, therefore, advised that ready-made kits available commercially be used. Basic principles are mentioned. Product insert must, however, be read and followed strictly.

TEST FOR SYPHILIS

VDRL TEST

CONVENTIONAL VDRL TEST

Serological testing, for the diagnosis of syphilis, traditionally has been based on the detection of "Reagin" by the use of antigen, prepared from normal tissues, most commonly beef heart. VDRL slide test can be used both qualitatively and quantitatively for the detection of "Reagin" in serum.

Principle

A phospholipid viz. cardiolipin, derived from beef heart muscle together with cholesterol and lecithin, is used as an antigen. After mixing the antigen with patient's serum, the reaction is accelerated by rotatory agitation either on a mechanical shaker or by hand. The antigen reacts with reagin and forms floccules. These floccules can be observed with naked eye, hand lens or under a low power objective of a microscope when the reaction is weak.

Equipment Required

1. VDRL Test Slide: A 2" × 3" glass slide with 12 paraffin or ceramic rings of approximately 14 mm inside diameter.
2. Hypodermic needles without bevels (18, 19 gauge).
3. Syringe (1-2 ml).
4. Thirty ml flat or concave inner bottomed glass stoppered, narrow mouth bottle, approximately thirty-five mm in diameter (bottles with convex inner bottom surface are unsatisfactory).

Precautions

1. Use clean and dry glassware.
2. Allow all reagents and samples to reach room temperature before starting the test.
3. Carry out the test at room temperature (preferably between 23 and 29°C).

Sample

Serum (0.05 ml is required for qualitative test and 0.1 ml is needed for quantitative test.

Preparation of Patient's Serum (Inactivation)

Heat clear serum sample in a water bath at 56°C for 30 minutes. Examine all serum samples after removing from the water bath and those found to contain particulate debris should be recentrifuged. Serum samples to be tested more than 4 hours after inactivation should be reheated at 56°C and allowed to cool to room temperature.

Reagents Usually Supplied

- Reagent 1 VDRL Antigen
- Reagent 2 Buffered Saline Diluent
- Reagent 3 Positive Control Serum
- Reagent 4 Negative Control Serum

Preparation of Working Solutions

Working Antigen Suspension

a. Pipette 0.4 ml of Buffered Saline Diluent into a glass stoppered bottle (with concave or flat inner bottom) and make the reagent completely cover the inner bottom as a thin layer.
b. Add 0.5 ml of VDRL Antigen from the lower half of a 1.0 ml pipette, which is graduated to the tip, directly to the Buffered Saline Diluent while continuously but gently rotating the bottle. Add the antigen drop by drop but rapidly, allowing 6 seconds for completing the

addition of 0.5 ml of the antigen. The pipette tip should remain in the upper third of the bottle and rotation should not be vigorous enough to splash Buffered Saline Diluent on to the pipette. The proper speed of rotation is obtained when the centre of the bottle circumscribes a 5 cm diameter circle approximately three times a second.

c. The last drop of the antigen should be blown from the pipette tip so that the pipette tip does not touch the surface of the contents of the bottle.
d. Continue rotation of the bottle for 10 more seconds.
e. Now add 4.1 ml of Buffered Saline Diluent to the bottle. Close the bottle with the stopper and shake it for approximately 10 seconds. The working antigen suspension is now ready for preliminary testing.

Note

There is some indication that maturation of the antigen increases the sensitiveness and this is almost complete within 15 to 30 minutes after preparing Working Antigen suspension. This may then be used within 24 hours.

Under condition of high temperature and low humidity, the Working Antigen should be stored in a refrigerator, but should be brought to room temperature before use. Mix the working antigen suspension gently each time it is used. Do not mix it by forcing it back and forth through the syringe and needle as this may lead to breakdown of antigen particles which results in loss of activity.

Preliminary Testing of the Working Antigen Suspension

1. Each time the Working Antigen Suspension is prepared, it has to be tested with negative and positive control sera by means of slide qualitative test method described under Procedure, using the controls in place of test sera.
2. The Working Antigen Suspension should give expected typically reactive and nonreactive results respectively. Also, the size and number of antigen particles per microscopic field in the nonreactive serum should be optimum. If the antigen particles in nonreactive serum appear too large, the fault will usually be in the preparation of the Working Antigen Suspension although other factors are sometimes responsible.
3. The antigen control (suspension in saline) should be smooth in appearance with antigen particles well dispersed.
4. Do not use Working Antigen Suspension if it does not give satisfactory performance in the preliminary testing.

Storage and Stability

The VDRL Antigen and Buffered Saline Diluent are to be stored exclusively in a cool and dark place at room temperature (preferably at 23-29°C); and at these conditions, the reagents are stable till the expiry date mentioned.

The control sera are stable at 2 to 8°C till the expiry date mentioned.

Working Antigen Suspension prepared for any day must NOT under any circumstances be kept and used for the subsequent days.

Procedure

Qualitative Test

1. Pipette 0.05 ml of patient's inactivated serum into the concavity of the VDRL slide.
2. Pipette 0.05 ml each of positive and negative control sera into other two concavities of the VDRL slide.
3. Add one drop (1/75 ml) of the *Working Antigen Suspension* to each of the above concavities, with a calibrated 23-gauge needle without bevel.
4. Rotate the slide for 4 minutes with hand on a flat surface (this movement should circumscribe roughly about 5 cm diameter circle 120 times per minute) or on a VDRL rotator.
5. Read the tests immediately under a low power objective of a microscope.

Quantitative Test

For quantitative test with sera reacting strongly in qualitative test, the following procedure should be followed:

1. Prepare different dilutions of test serum, in test tubes, in the range of 1:2, 1:4, 1:8, 1:16, 1:32 or more with normal saline.
2. Transfer 0.05 ml of each of the above diluted sera into separate concavities of the VDRL slide.
3. With the help of a 23-gauge needle and syringe, add one drop (1/75 ml) of Working Antigen Suspension to each of the above concavities.
4. Rotate the slide for 4 minutes with hand on a flat surface (this movement should circumscribe roughly about 5 cm diameter circle 120 times per minute) or on a VDRL rotator.
5. Read the test immediately under a low power objective of a microscope.

Note

The results of controls should be satisfactory for validating the results of tests.

Interpretation of Test Results

The antigen particles are seen as small fusiform needles which remain more or less evenly dispersed in case of a nonreactive serum and aggregate into clumps with reactive serum. The conclusions can be drawn from the observations as follows:

	Observation	*Conclusion*
(i)	No clumps or very slight roughness	Nonreactive
(ii)	Small clumps	Weakly reactive
(iii)	Medium/Large clumps	Reactive

Notes

1. Zonal reactions occasionally occur in serological tests. In such cases, a strongly reactive serum may show a weak or atypical reaction when undiluted serum is tested (prozone phenomenon). A completely negative reaction with very strongly reactive sera is extremely rare.
2. A reactive or weakly reactive test result indicates the presence of reagin, which almost invariably is formed in *Treponema* infection, but which may be produced by a variety of other conditions. In actual practice, a reactive result in the presence of clinical symptoms is considered as a confirmatory evidence of syphilitic infection. However, in the absence of clinical findings, test reactivity can represent any of the following: (a) Latent syphilis, (b) A biological false-positive reaction, either temporary or chronic or (c) A technical or clinical error.

Limitation of the Test

1. Acute or chronic infections such as malaria, leprosy, infectious mononucleosis and upper respiratory diseases as well as collagen and immunologic diseases such as rheumatoid arthritis and lupus erythematosus can produce false-positive reagin tests.
2. Other less well-known conditions include tissue regeneration, pregnancy, heroin addiction and the use of certain drugs for hypertension.
3. Reliable test results require strict attention to details of technique, including proper identification of specimens, accurate measurement, temperature control, correct timing and observation of principles of quality control.

MODIFIED VDRL REAGENT (TREPOLIPIN®, Courtesy: Tulip Group of Companies)

Summary

Syphilis is a sexually transmitted (venereal) disease caused by the spirochaete *Treponema* pallidum. After infection, the host forms *Treponema* antibodies to *Treponema pallidum*; in addition, the host also forms non-*Treponema* antilipoidal antibodies in response to the lipoidal material released from the damaged host cell. These antibodies are traditionally referred to as 'REAGINS'. Cardiolipin, a phospholipid, reacts with the 'Reagins' to give a non-*Treponema* flocculation reaction. Non-*Treponema* tests such as TREPOLIPIN® are of great value when used for screening and follow-up of therapy.

Reagent

1. TREPOLIPIN® reagent A ready to use stabilised emulsion of cardiolipin, lecithin and cholesterol.
2. Positive control, reactive with TREPOLIPIN® reagent.
3. Negative control, nonreactive with TREPOLIPIN® reagent.

The TREPOLIPIN® detects antilipoidal antibodies in serum, plasma and cerebrospinal fluid (CSF). As against the conventional VDRL reagents, test samples do not require heat inactivation.

Each batch of reagents undergoes rigorous quality control at various stages of manufacture for its specificity, sensitivity and performance.

Reagent Storage and Stability

1. Store the reagent at 2 to 8°C. Do not freeze.
2. The shelf-life of reagent is as per the expiry date mentioned on the reagent vial label. Avoid exposure to elevated temperature and air as the reagent is highly sensitive to denaturation and drying.

Principle

When serum, plasma or cerebrospinal fluid (CSF) containing antilipoidal antibodies is reacted with TREPOLIPIN® reagent, a flocculation reaction is produced.

Flocculation is a positive test result and indicates presence of antilipoidal antibodies in the sample. No flocculation is a negative test result and indicates absence of antilipoidal antibodies in the sample.

Note

1. *In vitro* diagnostic reagent for laboratory and professional use only. Not for medicinal use.
2. Reagent contains sodium azide 0.1% as preservative. Avoid contact with skin and mucosa. On disposal, flush with large quantities of water.
3. The antigen suspension should be gently but thoroughly mixed by swirling before testing to homogenise the reagent and improve test readability.
4. Performance of the reagent must be verified with positive and negative controls and it is recommended that controls be run with each test series.
5. Accessories provided with the kit only must be used for optimum results.

Sample Collection and Storage

1. No special preparation of the patient is required prior to sample collection by approved techniques. Do not use haemolysed samples.
2. Fresh serum, plasma or CSF should be used for testing.
3. Haematogeneous CSF should not be used for testing. For cloudy samples, centrifuge and use the clear supernatant for testing.

Material Provided with the Kit

1. Stabilised cardiolipin suspension.
2. Reagent dropper assembly for dispensing the antigen suspension.
3. Positive control, reactive with reagent.
4. Negative control, nonreactive with reagent.

Additional Material Required

Conventional VDRL cavity slide (glass), microscope (with magnification of 100 x), Pasteur pipettes, mechanical rotor (180 rpm), isotonic saline.

Note: For TREPOLIPIN® 5 × 5 ml kit. Known reactive and nonreactive samples would be required additionally.

Test Procedure

Bring reagent and samples to room temperature before testing.

1. Thoroughly mix the TREPOLIPIN® reagent suspension by gentle agitation before testing.
2. With cerebrospinal fluid, the test specimen volume is 0.01 ml.
3. For use with cerebrospinal fluid, each drop of TREPOLIPIN® reagent should be diluted with 0.02 ml of good isotonic saline before testing.

Qualitative Method

1. Pipette 0.05 ml of serum or plasma to the VDRL slide cavity.
2. Dispense one drop of TREPOLIPIN® reagent to the surface of the test sample in the same cavity using the reagent dropper provided.
3. Rotate the slide continuously at 180 rpm for four minutes, observing for flocculation.
4. Read the results macroscopically or microscopically at four minutes.
5. All positive test results may be further tested by the quantitative test procedure.

Quantitative Method

1. Pipette 0.1 ml of isotonic saline into seven test tubes.

2. Pipette 0.1 ml of the test sample into the first test tube.
3. Transfer 0.1 ml of the diluted test sample from the first tube to the second tube.
4. Continue the serial dilution of the test sample till dilutions of 1:2, 1:4, 1:8, 1:16, 1:32, 1:64, 1:128 are achieved.
5. Transfer 0.05 ml each dilution of the test sample from tubes 1 to 7 to a conventional VDRL slide.
6. Dispense one drop of TREPOLIPIN® reagent to each dilution of the sample on the VDRL slide.
7. Rotate the slide continuously at 180 rpm for four minutes.
8. Observe for flocculation macroscopically or microscopically at four minutes.

INTERPRETATION OF RESULTS

Qualitative Method

Flocculation is a positive test result and indicates presence of antilipoidal antibodies in the test sample.

No flocculation is a negative test result and indicates absence of antilipoidal antibodies in the test sample. The strength of flocculation may vary, depending upon the degree of positivity of the test sample.

Quantitative Method

The antilipoidal antibody titre is the highest dilution of the test sample giving a positive test result (flocculation).

Remarks

1. Quantitative procedure must be performed to determine the response to treatment and detect reinfection.
2. False-positive reactions occur not infrequently and have been attributed to a variety of acute and chronic conditions.
3. In the absence of supporting clinical, historical or epidemiological evidence reactive results must be confirmed with more specific *Treponema* tests.
4. It is recommended that results of the test should be correlated with clinical findings to arrive at the final diagnosis.
5. Microscopic evaluation of test results requires well-trained and experienced professional. It is recommended that a few known negatives should be run with each batch of the tests so as to familiarise and differentiate effectively the appearance of nonreactive samples from the reactive ones.

TOLUIDINE RED UNHEATED SERUM TEST FOR RAPID SERODIAGNOSIS OF SYPHILIS (REDGEN, Courtesy: Tulip Group of Companies)

Summary

Syphilis is a sexually transmitted (venereal) disease caused by the spirochaete *Treponema pallidum*. After infection, the host forms *Treponema* antibodies to *Treponema pallidum*; in addition, the host also forms non-*Treponema* antilipoidal antibodies in response to the lipoidal material released from the damaged host cell. These antibodies are traditionally referred to as 'Reagin'.

Toluidine Red Unheated Serum Test (TRUST) is a macroscopic non-*Treponema* flocculation test for the detection and quantitation of antilipoidal antibodies. Non-*Treponema* tests like REDGEN are of great value when used for screening and follow-up of therapy.

Reagent

1. REDGEN reagent: A participate suspension containing a red micronised dye coated with lipid complexes.
2. Positive control, reactive with the REDGEN latex reagent.
3. Negative control, non reactive with the REDGEN latex reagent.

REDGEN detects antilipoidal antibodies in serum or plasma. As against the conventional VDRL reagents, test samples do not require heat inactivation.

Each batch of reagents undergoes rigorous quality control at various stages of manufacture for its specificity, sensitivity and performance.

Reagent Storage and Stability

1. Store the reagent at 2 to 8°C. Do not freeze.
2. The shelf-life of the reagent is as per the expiry date mentioned on the reagent vial label.

Avoid exposure to elevated temperature and air as the reagent is highly sensitive to denaturation and drying.

Principle

During the test procedure, the specimen, serum or plasma is mixed with REDGEN reagent and allowed to react for eight minutes. If antilipoidal antibodies are present in the specimen, they will react with REDGEN reagent forming visible red floccules against the white background of the reaction card. If antilipoidal antibodies are not present in the specimen, there will be no flocculation, resulting in an even pink mat on the reaction circle.

Note

1. *In vitro* diagnostic reagent for laboratory or professional use only. Not for medicinal use.
2. The reagent contains thiomersal 0.1% as preservative. Avoid contact with skin and mucosa. On disposal, flush with large quantities of water.
3. The REDGEN reagent suspension should be gently but thoroughly mixed before testing to disperse the dye particles uniformly and improve test readability.
4. Performance of the reagent must be verified with positive and negative controls and it is recommended that controls be run with each test series.
5. Accessories provided with the kit should be used for optimum results.

Sample Collection and Storage

1. No special preparation of the patient is required prior to sample collection by approved techniques. Haemolysed or lipaemic samples are not suitable for testing. In case of oxalated blood samples, it is advisable to avoid excess of oxalate as it may interfere with the test results.
2. Fresh serum or plasma should be used for testing.
3. Samples not tested immediately may be stored at 2 to 8°C for up to 48 hours.
4. Hazy samples should be centrifuged. Use the clear supenatant for testing.

Material Provided with the Kit

The TRUST antigen, positive control reactive with the reagent, negative control nonreactive with the reagent, disposable slides with eight reaction circles, disposable sample/control dispensing pipettes, mixing sticks, rubber teats, reagent dropper for dispensing the REDGEN reagent suspension.

Additional Material Required

Stopwatch, high intensity light source, isotonic saline, pipettetes, test tubes, mechanical rotor at 180 rpm circumscribing a circle 2 cm in diameter on a horizontal plane.

Test Procedure

Bring all reagents and samples to room temperature before testing.

Thoroughly mix the REDGEN reagent suspension by gentle agitation before testing.

Qualitative Method

1. Place one drop of the test sample, positive and negative controls onto separate reaction circles of the disposable slide using a sample dispensing pipette.
2. Add one drop of well mixed REDGEN reagent next to the test sample or controls by using the reagent dropper provided with the kit. Do not let the dropper tip touch the liquid on slide.
3. Using a mixing stick, mix the test sample and REDGEN reagent thoroughly, spreading uniformly over the entire reaction circle.
4. Immediately start a stopwatch. Rotate the slide gently and continuously either manually or on a mechanical rotor at 180 rpm.
5. Observe for flocculation macroscopically at 8 minutes.

Quantitative Method

1. Using isotonic saline, prepare serial dilutions of the test sample positive in the qualitative method 1:2, 1:4, 1:8, 1:16, 1:32, 1:64, 1:128 and so on.
2. Perform the qualitative test procedure using each dilution as a specimen.
3. The titre is reported as reciprocal of the highest dilution which shows a positive test result.

INTERPRETATION OF TEST RESULTS

Qualitative Method

1. Large and medium RED coloured floccules against white background: Reactive
2. Small RED coloured floccules against white background: Weakly reactive
3. No floccules, smooth pink background : Nonreactive

Flocculation is a positive test result and indicates presence of antilipoidal antibodies in the test sample. No flocculation is a negative test result and indicates absence of antilipoidal antibodies in the test sample.

Quantitative Method

The titre of antilipoidal antibodies is the highest dilution of test sample giving a positive test result.

Remarks

1. Quantitative procedure must be performed to determine response to treatment and detect reinfection.
2. False-positive reactions occur not infrequently and have been attributed to a variety of acute and chronic conditions.
3. In the absence of supporting clinical, historical or epidemiological evidence, reactive result must be confirmed with more specific *Treponema* tests.
4. It is strongly recommended that results of the test should be correlated with clinical findings to arrive at the final diagnosis.
5. Dispose all used and contaminated material as per Standard Biohazard Safety Guidelines.
6. The reagent dropper provided for dispensing the REDGEN antigen should be thoroughly cleaned with distilled water and air dried after use, to ensure that it does not contaminate the reagent during subsequent use.
7. Very slight roughness should be interpreted as a negative test result.

LATEX SLIDE TEST FOR VDRL (SYPHFINAL, MFD: Tulip Group of Companies)

Summary

Syphilis is a sexually transmitted disease caused by *Treponema pallidum*, a bacterium classified under the category of Spirochaetes. After infection, the host in response to *Treponema pallidum* forms *Treponema* antibodies.

In addition to *Treponema* antibodies, the host also forms non-*Treponema* antilipoidal antibodies in response to the lipoidal material released from the host cell during infection. This antibody is traditionally referred to as reagin.

Cardiolipin, a phospholipid derived from the beef heart, reacts with antilipoidal antibodies and this antigenic property of cardiolipin is used in non-*Treponema* tests such as the VDRL, modified VDRL, USR tests and Syphfinal. Non-*Treponema* tests are of great value when used for screening and follow-up of therapy.

Reagent

Syphfinal reagent is a ready-to-use, uniform suspension of polystyrene latex particles coated with cardiolipin, suspended in a suitable buffer of proprietary composition.

Though Syphfinal reagent, in performance, corresponds to the other USRs, it accords better readability to the test results, thereby giving better confidence in reporting results. As against the conventional VDRL tests, the samples do not require heat inactivation.

Each batch of reagent undergoes rigorous quality control at various stages of its manufacture for its sensitivity, specificity and performance.

Reagent Storage and Stability

Store the reagent at 2-8°C. Do not freeze. The shelf life of the reagent is as per the expiry date mentioned on the reagent vial labels. Avoid exposure to elevated temperatures, air and direct sunlight as the reagents are highly sensitive to denaturation, drying and microbial contamination.

Principle

Syphfinal, latex VDRL reagent, is based on the principle of agglutination. The test specimen, serum or plasma is mixed with Syphfinal latex VDRL reagent and allowed to react for six minutes. If antilipoidal antibodies are present in the specimen, they will react with the latex reagent forming a visible agglutination. If antilipoidal antibodies are not present in the specimen, then no agglutination is observed.

Note

1. *In vitro* diagnostic reagent for laboratory and professional use only. Not for medicinal use.
2. The reagent contains sodium azide 0.1% as preservative. Avoid contact with skin and mucosa. On disposal, flush with large quantities of water.
3. All reagents derived from human source are tested for HBsAg and anti-HIV antibodies and found to be nonreactive. However, handle the material as if infectious.
4. Syphfinal latex VDRL reagent should be gently but thoroughly mixed before testing to disperse the latex particles uniformly and improve test readability.
5. Performance of the reagents must be verified with positive and negative controls provided with the kit and it is recommended that controls be run with each test series.

Sample Collection and Storage

No special preparation of the patient is required prior to sample collection by approved techniques. Do not use haemolysed samples. Fresh serum or plasma should be used for testing. Samples not tested immediately may be stored at 2 to 8°C for up to 48 hours. Hazy samples should be centrifuged. Use clear supernatant for testing.

Material Provided with the Kit

Latex VDRL reagent, positive control reactive with the reagent, negative control nonreactive with the reagent, disposable slides with eight reaction circles, disposable sample/control dispensing pipettes, mixing sticks, rubber teats.

Additional Material Required

Stopwatch, high intensity direct light source, isotonic saline, pipettes, test tubes.

Test Procedure

Bring all reagents and samples to room temperature before testing.

Qualitative Method

1. Pipette one drop of test sample onto one of the reaction circles of the disposable slide using a sample dispensing pipette. The disposable slides and the sample dispensing pipettes are provided with the kit.
2. Repeat the procedure with positive and negative controls.
3. Add one drop of well-mixed Syphfinal latex reagent to the test sample, positive control and negative control respectively. Do not let the dropper tip touch the liquid on the slide.
4. Using a mixing stick, mix the test sample and Syphfinal reagent thoroughly spreading uniformly over the entire reaction circle.
5. Immediately start a stopwatch. Rotate the slide gently and continuously, observing for agglutination macroscopically at six minutes.

Quantitative Method

1. Using isotonic saline prepare serial dilutions of the test sample, e.g. 1:2, 1:4, 1:8, 1:16, 1:32, 1:64, 1:128, etc.
2. Perform qualitative test procedure using each dilution as test specimen.
3. The titre is reported as the reciprocal of the highest dilution which shows a positive test result.

INTERPRETATION OF TEST RESULT

Qualitative Method

Agglutination is a positive test result and indicates the presence of antilipoidal antibodies in the test sample. No agglutination is a negative test result indicating the absence of detectable levels of antilipoidal antibodies in the test specimen.

Quantitative Method

The titre of antilipoidal antibodies is the highest dilution of the test sample giving a positive test result (i.e. agglutination).

Performance Characteristics

Twenty five known VDRL positive samples and 217 known negative samples were evaluated with Syphfinal latex VDRL reagent in parallel with modified VDRL test and RPR tests by both qualitative and quantitative techniques. Syphfinal was found to correlate 100% with modified VDRL test and the

RPR tests by the qualitative technique. Syphfinal was found to correlate 96% with modified VDRL and 100% with RPR tests by the quantitative technique.

Remarks

1. Quantitative procedure must be performed to determine the response to treatment and detect reinfection.
2. False-positive reactions occur not infrequently and have been attributed to a variety of acute and chronic conditions.
3. In the absence of supporting clinical, historical or epidemiological evidence, reactive results must be confirmed with more specific *Treponema* tests.
4. It is recommended that the results of the test should be correlated with the clinical findings to arrive at the final diagnosis.
5. Dispose all used and contaminated materials as per Standard Biohazard Safety Guidelines.

RAPID PLASMA REAGIN (RPR) CARD TEST/ CARBON ANTIGEN FOR SYPHILIS TESTING (CARBOGEN), Courtesy: Tulip Group of Companies

Summary

Syphilis is a sexually transmitted (venereal) disease caused by the spirochaete *Treponema pallidum*. After infection, the host forms *Treponema* antibodies to *Treponema pallidum*; in addition, the host also forms non-*Treponema* antilipoidal antibodies in response to the lipoidal material released from the damaged host cell. These antibodies are traditionally referred to as 'Reagins'.

The Rapid Plasma Reagin (RPR)/Carbon Antigen test is a macroscopic non-*Treponema* flocculation test for the detection and quantitation of antilipoidal antibodies. Non-*Treponema* tests like CARBOGEN are of great value when used for screening and follow-up of therapy.

Reagent

1. CARBOGEN reagent: A particulate carbon suspension coated with lipid complexes.
2. Positive control, reactive with the CARBOGEN reagent.
3. Negative control, nonreactive with the CARBOGEN reagent.

The CARBOGEN detects antilipoidal antibodies in serum or plasma. As against the conventional VDRL reagents, test samples do not require heat inactivation.

Each batch of reagent undergoes rigorous quality control at various stages of manufacture for its specificity, sensitivity and performance.

Reagent Storage and Stability

Store the reagent at 2 to 8°C. Do not freeze. The shelf-life of the reagent is as per the expiry date mentioned on the reagent vial label. Avoid exposure to elevated temperatures and air as the reagent is highly sensitive to denaturation and drying.

Principle

During the test procedure, the specimen, serum or plasma is mixed with CARBOGEN reagent and allowed to react for eight minutes. If antilipoidal antibodies are present in the specimen, they will react with CARBOGEN reagent forming visible black floccules. If antilipoidal antibodies are not present in the specimen, there will be no flocculation.

Note

1. *In vitro* diagnostic reagent for laboratory or professional use only. Not for medicinal use.
2. The reagent contains sodium azide 0.1% as preservative. Avoid contact with skin and mucosa. On disposal, flush with large quantities of water.
3. CARBOGEN RPR/Carbon antigen should be gently but thoroughly mixed before testing to disperse the carbon particles uniformly and improve test readability.
4. Performance of the reagent must be verified with positive and negative controls and it is recommended that controls be run with each test series.
5. Accessories provided with the kit only must be used for optimum results.

Sample Collection and Storage

1. No special preparation of the patient is required prior to sample collection by approved techniques. Haemolysed or lipaemic samples are not suitable for testing.
2. Fresh serum or plasma should be used for testing.

3. Samples not tested immediately may be stored at 2 to 8°C for up to 48 hours.
4. Hazy samples should be centrifuged. Use the clear supernatant for testing.

Material Provided with the RPR Kit

1. Carbon antigen.
2. Positive control, reactive with the reagent.
3. Negative control, nonreactive with the reagent.
4. Disposable slides with eight reaction circles.
5. Disposable sample/control dispensing pipettes.
6. Mixing sticks.
7. Rubber teats.
8. Reagent dropper for dispensing the carbon antigen.

Additional Material Required

Stop watch, high intensity light source, isotonic saline, pipettes, test tubes, mechanical rotor at 180 rpm. circumscribing a circle 2 cm in diameter on a horizontal plane.

Note: For CARBOGEN Carbon Antigen: Item Nos. 2 to 7 listed above under RPR kit, would be required additionally.

Test Procedure

Bring reagent and samples to room temperature before testing.

Thoroughly mix the CARBOGEN reagent suspension by gentle agitation before testing.

Qualitative Method

1. Place one drop of the test specimen, positive and negative controls onto separate reaction circles of the disposable slide using a sample dispensing pipette.
2. Add one drop of well-mixed CARBOGEN reagent next to the test specimen, positive control and negative control by using the reagent dropper provided with the kit. Do not let the dropper tip touch the liquid on the slide.
3. Using a mixing stick, mix the test specimen and the CARBOGEN reagent thoroughly spreading uniformly over the entire reaction circle.
4. Immediately start a stopwatch. Rotate the slide gently and continuously either manually or on a mechanical rotor at 180 rpm.
5. Observe for flocculation macroscopically at 8 minutes.

Quantitative Method

1. Using isotonic saline, prepare serial dilutions of the test specimen positive in the qualitative method 1:2, 1:4, 1:8, 1:16, 1:32, 1:64, 1:128 and so on.
2. Perform the qualitative test procedure using each dilution as a test specimen.
3. The titre is reported as the reciprocal of the highest dilution which shows a positive test result.

INTERPRETATION OF TEST RESULTS

Qualitative Method

1. Large and medium black floccules against white background : Reactive
2. Small black floccules against white background: Weakly reactive
3. No floccules, even grey background: Nonreactive

Flocculation is a positive test result and indicates presence of antilipoidal antibodies in the test specimen.

No flocculation is a negative test result and indicates absence of antilipoidal antibodies in the test specimen.

Quantitative Method

The titre of antilipoidal antibodies is the highest dilution of the test specimen giving a positive test result.

Remarks

1. Quantitative procedure must be performed to determine response to treatment and detect reinfection.
2. False-positive reactions occur not infrequently and have been attributed to a variety of acute and chronic conditions.
3. In absence of supporting clinical, historical or epidemiological evidence, reactive result must be confirmed with more specific *Treponema* tests.

4. It is strongly recommended that results of the test should be correlated with clinical findings to arrive at the final diagnosis.
5. Dispose all used and contaminated material as per Standard Biohazard Safety Guidelines.
6. The reagent dropper provided for dispensing the carbon antigen should be thoroughly cleaned with distilled water and air dried after use, to ensure that it does not contaminate the reagent during subsequent use.
7. Very slight roughness should be interpreted as a negative test result.

ONE-STEP TEST FOR SYPHILIS: DIPSTICK (Syphicheck®, Mfd: Tulip Group of Companies)

Introduction

Syphicheck is a one-step; rapid, self-performing, qualitative, two-site double antigen sandwich immunoassay for the detection of syphilis.

Summary

Syphilis is a sexually transmitted (venereal) disease caused by the spirochaete *Treponema pallidum.* The disease can also be transmitted congenitally thereby attaining its importance in antenatal screening. After infection, the host forms non-*Treponema* antilipoidal antibodies (reagins) to the lipoidal material released from the damaged host cells as well as *Treponema* specific antibodies. Serological tests for non-*Treponema* antibodies such as VDRL, RPR, TRUST, etc. are useful as screening tests. Tests for *Treponema* specific antibodies such as TPHA, FTA-ABS, rapid *Treponema* antibody tests are gaining importance as screening as well as confirmatory tests because they detect the presence of antibodies specific to *Treponema pallidum.*

Syphicheck qualitatively detects the presence of IgM and IgG class of *Treponema* specific antibodies during syphilis in serum or plasma specimen within 15 minutes.

Principle

Syphicheck utilises the principle of immunochromatography, a unique two-site immunoassay on a membrane. As the test sample flows through the membrane assembly of the dipstick, the recombinant *Treponema* antigen-colloidal gold conjugate forms a complex with *Treponema* specific antibodies in the sample. This complex moves further on the membrane to the test region where it is immobilised by the recombinant *Treponema pallidum* antigen coated on the membrane leading to the formation of a pink to deep purple coloured band at the test region which confirms a positive test result. Absence of this coloured band in test region indicates a negative test result. The unreacted conjugate and the unbound complex if any move further on the membrane and are subsequently immobilised by the anti-rabbit antibodies coated on the membrane at the control region, forming a pink to deep purple coloured band. The control band serves to validate the test results.

Reagents and Materials Supplied

Each individual pouch contains:

1. **Dipstick:** Membrane assembly predispensed with recombinant *Treponema pallidum* antigen-colloidal gold conjugate, recombinant *Treponema pallidum* antigen and anti-rabbit antiserum coated at the respective regions.
2. **Desiccant pouch**

Additional Material Required

12 × 75 mm test tubes

Storage and Stability

The sealed pouches in the test kit may be stored between 4 and 30°C for the duration of shelf-life as indicated on the pouch.

Note

1. For *in vitro* diagnostic use only. Not for medicinal use
2. Do not use beyond expiry date.
3. Read the instructions carefully before performing the test.
4. Handle all specimens as potentially infectious.
5. Follow standard biosafety guidelines for handling and disposal of potentially infective material.

Specimen Collection and Preparation

No special preparation of patient is necessary prior to specimen collection by approved techniques. Though fresh serum/plasma is preferable, serum/plasma specimens may be stored at 2 to 8°C for up to 24 hours, in case of delay in testing. Do not use haemolysed or contaminated specimens. Turbid specimens should be centrifuged or allowed to settle and only the clear supernatant should be used for testing.

Testing Procedure and Interpretation of Results

Bring kit components, specimen to room temperature prior to testing.

1. Collect serum/plasma in a clean test tube (approximately 0.5-1 ml may be required). Ensure that only sufficient quantity of the specimen is collected to allow submerging the red area on the dipstick (about 1 cm high).
2. Bring the sealed pouch to room temperature, open the pouch and remove the dipstick. Once opened, the dipstick must be used immediately.
3. Dip the dipstick in serum/plasma specimen submerging only the red area.
4. The dipstick should be left submerged for the entire duration of the test ensuring only the red area is submerged in the specimen.
5. At the end of 15 minutes read the results as follows:

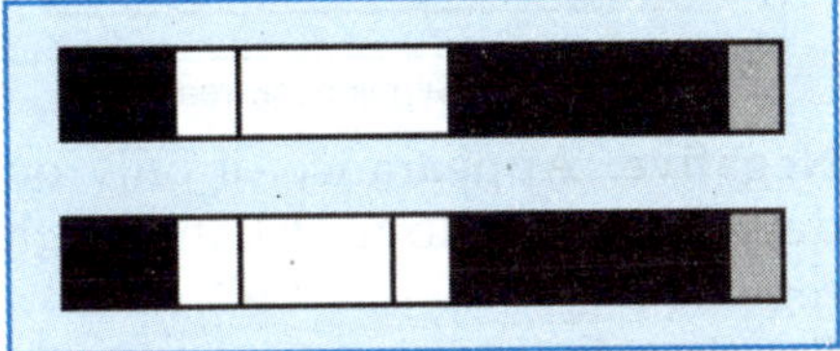

Fig. 23.20: Syphicheck reading

   Negative: Only one pink to deep purple coloured band appears on the dipstick
   Positive: Two distinct pink to deep purple coloured bands appear on the dipstick
6. The test should be considered invalid if neither the test band nor the control band appears. Repeat the test with a new dipstick.
7. Although depending on the concentration of *Treponema* antibodies in the specimen, positive results may appear as early as 2 minutes, negative results must be confirmed only at the end of 15 minutes.

Performance Characteristics

1. Syphicheck detects the presence of *Treponema* antibodies; thus, a positive result indicates a past or present infection. Positive results should be evaluated in correlation with the clinical condition before arriving at a final diagnosis.
2. Low levels of antibodies to *Treponema pallidum* such as those present at a very early primary stage of infection can give a negative result. But a negative result does not exclude the possibility of exposure to or infection with *Treponema pallidum.* Retesting is indicated after two weeks if clinically syphilis is still suspected.
3. In order to assess the clinical response to treatment, it is advisable to use a reagin test such as VDRL, RPR.
4. Syphicheck detects *Treponema* antibodies in serum/plasma; other body fluids may not give accurate results.
5. In immunocompromised patients the test results must be interpreted with caution.

ONE-STEP TEST FOR SYPHILIS (DEVICE) SYPHICHECK, Courtesy: Tulip Group of Companies

Introduction

Syphicheck is a one-step; rapid, self-performing, qualitative, two-site double antigen sandwich immunoassay for the detection of syphilis.

Summary

Syphilis is a sexually transmitted (venereal) disease caused by the spirochaete *Treponema pallidum.* The disease can also be transmitted congenitally thereby attaining its importance in antenatal screening. After infection the host forms non-*Treponema* antilipoidal antibodies (reagins) to the lipoidal material released from the damaged host cells as well as *Treponema* specific antibodies. Serological tests for non-*Treponema* antibodies such as VDRL, RPR, TRUST, etc. are useful as screening tests. Tests for *Treponema* specific antibodies such as TPHA, FTA-ABS, rapid *Treponema* antibody tests are gaining importance as screening as well as confirmatory tests because they detect the presence of antibodies specific to *Treponema pallidum.*

Syphicheck qualitatively detects the presence of IgM and IgG class of *Treponema* specific antibodies during syphilis in serum or plasma specimen within 15 minutes.

Principle

Syphicheck utilises the principle of immunochromatography, a unique two-site immunoassay on a membrane. As the test sample flows through the membrane assembly of the test device, the recombinant *Treponema* antigen-colloidal gold conjugate forms a complex with *Treponema* specific antibodies in the sample. This complex moves further on the membrane to the test region where it is immobilised by the recombinant *Treponema pallidum* antigen coated on the membrane leading to the formation of a pink to deep purple coloured band at the test region 'T' which confirms a positive test result. Absence of this coloured band in test region 'T' indicates a negative test result. The unreacted conjugate and the unbound complex if any move further on the membrane and are subsequently immobilised by the anti-rabbit antibodies coated on the control region 'C' of the membrane assembly, forming a pink to deep purple coloured band. The control band serves to validate the test results.

Reagents and Materials Supplied

Each individual pouch contains:

1. Test device: Membrane assembly predispensed with recombinant *Treponema pallidum* antigen-colloidal gold conjugate, recombinant *Treponema pallidum* antigen and anti-rabbit antiserum coated at the respective regions.
2. Disposable plastic dropper
3. Desiccant pouch

Storage and Stability

The sealed pouches in the test kit may be stored between 4 and 30°C for the duration of shelf-life as indicated on the pouch.

Note

1. For *in vitro* diagnostic use only. Not for Medicinal use
2. Do not use beyond expiry date
3. Read the instructions carefully before performing the test
4. Handle all specimens as potentially infectious
5. Follow standard biosafety guidelines for handling and disposal of potentially infective material.

Specimen Collection and Preparation

No special preparation of patient is necessary prior to specimen collection by approved techniques. Though fresh serum/plasma is preferable, serum/plasma specimens may be stored at 2 to 8° C for up to 24 hours, in case of delay in testing. Do not use haemolysed or contaminated specimens. Turbid specimens should be centrifuged or allowed to settle and only the clear supernatant should be used for testing.

Testing Procedure and Interpretation of Results

Bring kit components, specimen to room temperature prior to testing.

1. Bring the sealed pouch to room temperature, open the pouch and remove the device. Once opened, the device must be used immediately.
2. Dispense two drops of serum/plasma specimen into the sample well 'S' using the dropper provided.
3. At the end of 15 minutes, read the results as follows:

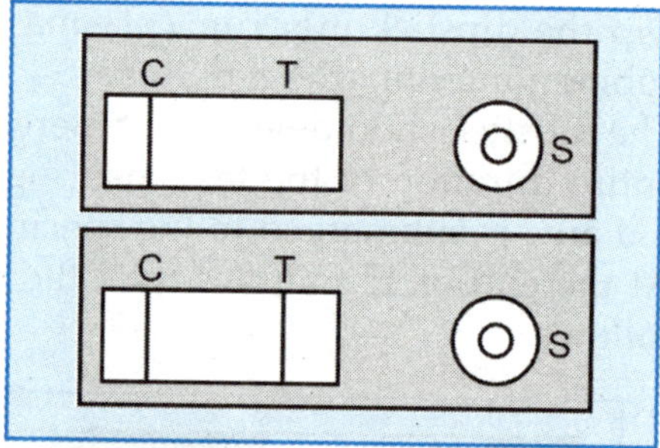

Fig. 23.21: Syphicheck reading

   Negative: Appearance of only one pink to deep purple coloured band at the control region 'C'.

   Positive: In addition to the control band, a distinct pink to deep purple coloured band also appears on the test region 'T'.
4. The test should be considered invalid if neither the test band nor the control band appear. Repeat the test with a new device.
5. Although, depending on the concentration of *Treponema* antibodies in the specimen, positive results may appear as early as 2 minutes, negative results must be confirmed only at the end of 15 minutes.

Remarks

1. Syphicheck detects the presence of *Treponema* antibodies; thus, a positive result indicates a past or present infection. Positive results should be evaluated in correlation with the clinical condition before arriving at a final diagnosis.
2. Low levels of antibodies to *Treponema pallidum* such as those present at a very early primary stage of infection can give a negative result.

But a negative result does not exclude the possibility of exposure to or infection with *Treponema pallidum*. Retesting is indicated after two weeks if clinically syphilis is still suspected.

3. In order to assess the clinical response to treatment, it is advisable to use a reagin test such as VDRL, RPR.
4. Syphicheck detects *Treponema* antibodies in serum/plasma; other body fluids may not give accurate results.
5. In immunocompromised patients the test results must be interpreted with caution.

WIDAL ANTIGEN SET/ANTIGENS FOR TUBE TESTS (TYPHOCHEK) Courtesy: Tulip Group of Companies

Summary

Enteric fever occurs when pathogenic microorganisms like *S. typhi, S. paratyphi A, S. paratyphi B* infect the human body. During the course of disease, the body responds to this antigenic stimulus by producing antibodies whose titre rises slowly in early stages, to a maxima and then slowly falls till it is undetectable. Antibodies to *Salmonella* organisms may be detected in the patient serum from the second week after onset of infection. Information regarding the titres and whether or not they are rising or falling can be obtained by performing serological tests using Typhochek antigen suspensions.

Reagent

Typhochek contains ready-to-use coloured, smooth antigen suspensions of the bacilli; *S. typhi 'O'*, *S. typhi 'H'*, *S. paratyphi 'AO'*, *S. paratyphi 'BO'*, *S. paratyphi 'AH'*, *S. paratyphi 'BH'*.

Typhochek reagents are versatile and standardised for use in a standard tube test procedure for the detection of *S. typhi* and *S. paratyphi* antibodies in the patient's serum.

Each batch of reagents undergoes rigorous quality control at various stages of manufacture for its specificity and performance.

Reagent Storage and Stability

1. Store the reagents at 2 to 8°C. Do not freeze.
2. The shelf-life of reagents is as per the expiry date mentioned on the reagent bottle labels.

Principle

When the coloured, smooth suspension of attenuated Typhochek antigen suspensions are incubated with patient serum, anti-*Salmonella* antibodies present in the patient's serum react with the antigen suspensions to produce an agglutination. Agglutination is a positive test result, indicating presence of *Salmonella* antibodies in the patient's serum. No agglutination is a negative test result indicating absence of *Salmonella* antibodies in the patient's serum.

Note

1. *In vitro* diagnostic reagent for laboratory and professional use only. Not for medicinal use.
2. The *S. typhi 'O'* reagent contains phenol 0.5%, *S. typhi 'H'*, *S. paratyphi 'AH'*, *S. paratyphi 'BH'* reagents contain formal dehyde 0.3% and *S. paratyphi 'AO'*, *S. paratyphi 'BO'* reagents contain ethanol 0.7% as preservatives. Avoid contact with skin and mucosa. On disposal, flush with large quantities of water.

Sample Collection and Storage

1. No special preparation of the patient is required prior to sample collection by approved techniques. Do not use haemolysed samples.
2. Clean and dry glassware free from detergents must be used for sample collection.
3. Do not heat/inactivate the serum.
4. Though freshly collected serum is preferable, store samples at 2 to 8°C in case of delay in testing, for up to 72 hours.

MATERIAL PROVIDED WITH THE KIT

Reagent Pack

Typhochek 4 × 50 ml set contains item Nos. 1, 2, 5 and 6 mentioned below.

1. Typhochek *S. typhi 'O'* Antigen suspension
2. Typhochek *S. typhi 'H'* Antigen suspension
3. Typhochek *S. paratyphi 'AO'* Antigen suspension
4. Typhochek *S. paratyphi 'BO'* Antigen suspension
5. Typhochek *S. paratyphi 'AH'* Antigen suspension
6. Typhochek *S. paratyphi 'BH'* Antigen suspension

Note: Item Nos. 1 to 6 each is available as individual reagent packs.

Additional Material Required

Timer, Kahn tubes/test tubes, pipettes (0.1 ml, 1 ml), isotonic saline, incubator (37°C), test tube rack.

Procedure

a. Bring reagents to room temperature before testing.
b. Shake and mix antigens well before dispensing.
c. Carefully label test tubes for sample and reagent identity when more than one antigens is used during test procedure.

a. Standard Tube Test Method

1. Take appropriate number of sets (as required; one set for each antigen suspension) of 8 Kahn tubes/test tubes and label them 1 to 8.
2. Pipette into tube No. 1 of all sets 0.9 ml of isotonic saline.
3. To each of the remaining tubes (2 to 8 of each set), add 0.5 ml of isotonic saline.
4. To tube No. 1 of all sets, add 0.1 ml of serum sample to be tested and mix well.
5. Transfer 0.5 ml of the diluted serum sample from tube No. 1 to tube No.2 and mix well.
6. Transfer 0.5 ml of the diluted serum sample from tube No. 2 to tube No. 3 and mix well. Continue this serial dilution till tube No. 7 in each set.
7. Discard 0.5 ml of the diluted serum from tube No. 7 of each set.
8. Tube No. 8 in all the sets serves as a saline control.
9. To all the tubes of the respective sets, add 0.5 ml of the respective Typhochek antigen suspensions and mix well.
10. This will give final dilutions in tube 1 to 7 as 1:20, 1:40, 1:80, 1:160, 1:320, 1:640, 1:1280.
11. Cover and incubate at 37°C overnight (approximately 18 hours).
12. Dislodge the sedimented button gently and observe for agglutination macroscopically.

Interpretation of Results

The titre of the patient serum using Typhochek antigen suspensions is the highest dilution of the serum sample that gives a visible agglutination.

Remarks

1. TAB vaccinated patients may show a high titre of antibodies to each of the antigens.
2. 'O' being a somatic antigen brings about a coarse, compact, granular agglutination, whereas 'H' being a flagellar antigen brings about larger, loose, flocculant agglutination.
3. Apart from the pattern of sedimented antigens, in the tube test method a decrease in opacity as compared to the saline control must also be considered while judging the degree of agglutination.
4. While the 'O' antigen is species specific, the 'H' antigen is specific to the serotype.
5. Turbid and contaminated sera should not be used for testing.
6. Generally, antibody titres of 180 or more are considered clinically and diagnostically significant. However, the significant titre may vary from population to population and needs to be established for each area.
7. It is recommended that results of the tests should be correlated with clinical findings to arrive at the final diagnosis.
8. Since techniques and standardisation vary from lab to lab one tube difference in tube titres can be expected.
9. Do not interchange reagent caps.

WIDAL ANTIGEN SET/ANTIGENS FOR SLIDE AND TUBE TESTS (TYDAL) Courtesy: Tulip Group of Companies

Summary

Enteric fever occurs when pathogenic microorganisms like *S. typhi, S. paratyphi A, S. paratyphi B* infect the human body. During the course of disease, the body responds to this antigenic stimulus by producing antibodies whose titre rises slowly in early stages, to a maxima and then slowly falls till it is undetectable. Antibodies to *Salmonella* organisms may be detected in the patient serum from the second week after onset of infection. Information regarding the titres and whether or not they are rising or falling can be obtained by performing serological tests using TYDAL antigen suspensions. Usually, tube titres of 180 and above are taken as diagnostically significant, however, for endemic areas, higher cut-offs may need to be established.

Reagent

The TYDAL contains ready-to-use concentrated, vitally stained, smooth antigen suspensions of the bacilli; *S typhi 'O'*, *S typhi 'H'*, *S paratyphi 'AO'*, *S. paratyphi 'BO'*, *S paratyphi 'AH'*, *S paratyphi 'BH'* and/or polyspecific positive control reactive with these antigens. Each batch of reagents undergoes rigorous quality control at various stages of manufacture for its specificity and performance.

Reagent Storage and Stability

1. Store the reagents at 2 to 8°C. Do not freeze.
2. The shelf-life of reagents is as per the expiry date mentioned on the reagent vial labels.

Principle

When the coloured, smooth, attenuated TYDAL antigen suspensions are mixed/incubated with patient serum, anti-*Salmonella* antibodies present in the patient serum react with the antigen suspensions to give agglutination. Agglutination is a positive test result, indicating presence of anti-*Salmonella* antibodies in the patient serum. No agglutination is a negative test result indicating absence of anti-*Salmonella* antibodies.

Note

1. *In vitro* diagnostic reagent for laboratory and professional use only. Not for medicinal use.
2. The *S typhi 'O'* reagent contains phenol 0.5%, *S. typhi 'H'*, *S. paratyphi 'AH'*, *S. paratyphi 'BH'* reagents contain formal dehyde 0.3% and *S paratyphi 'AO'* , *S paratyphi 'BO'* reagents contain ethanol 0.7% as preservatives. Avoid contact with skin and mucosa. On disposal flush with large quantities of water.
3. Only a clean and dry glass slide must be used. Clean the glass slide with distilled water and wipe dry.
4. Accessories provided with the kit only must be used for optimum results, (applicable only for TYDAL 4 × 5 ml set and 4 × 10 ml set).

Sample Collection and Storage

1. No special preparation of the patient is required prior to sample collection by approved techniques. Do not use haemolysed samples.
2. Clean and dry glassware free from detergents must be used for sample collection.
3. Do not heat inactivate the serum.
4. Though freshly collected serum is preferable, store samples at 2 to 8°C in case of delay in testing, for upto 72 hour.

MATERIAL PROVIDED WITH THE KIT

Reagent Pack

The TYDAL 4 × 5 ml set and TYDAL 4 x 10 ml set contain item Nos 1, 2, 5, 6, 7 and 8 mentioned below. TYDAL 2 × 5 ml set contains item Nos. 1, 2 and 7 mentioned below:

1. *S. typhi 'O'* Antigen suspension
2. *S. typhi 'H'* Antigen suspension
3. *S. paratyphi 'AO'* Antigen suspension
4. *S. paratyphi 'BO'* Antigen suspension
5. *S. paratyphi 'AH'* Antigen suspension
6. *S. paratyphi 'BH'* Antigen suspension
7. Polyspecific positive control (Goat)
8. Glass slide with six reaction circles, mixing sticks, disposable sample dispensing pipettes with rubber teats.

Note: Item Nos. 1 to 6 each is available as individual reagent packs.

Additional Material Required

Slide test method Stop watch, variable micropipettes.
Note: Item No 8 from reagent pack is additionally required for TYDAL 2 × 5 ml set. Item No. 7 and 8 from reagent pack are additionally required for individual reagent packs of TYDAL 'O', TYDAL 'H', TYDAL 'AO', TYDAL 'BO', TYDAL 'AH', TYDAL 'BH' antigens.

Quantitative Method

Timer, Kahn tubes/test tubes, pipettes (0.1 ml, 1 ml), isotonic saline, incubator (37°C), test tube racks.

Procedure

a. Bring reagents to room temperature before testing.
b. Shake and mix antigens well before dispensing.

Slide Screen Method

1. Place one drop of positive control onto a reaction circle of the glass slide.

2. Place one drop of isotonic saline onto the next reaction circle of the glass slide.
3. Place one drop of patient serum to be tested onto each of the required number of reaction circles.
4. Add one drop of appropriate TYDAL antigen suspensions to the reaction circles containing positive control and isotonic saline.
5. Add one drop of appropriate TYDAL antigen suspensions to the reaction circles containing the patient serum.
6. Mix contents of each circle uniformly over the entire circle with separate mixing sticks.
7. Rock the slide gently back and forth, and observe for agglutination macroscopically at one minute.

Slide Semiquantitative Method

1. Using a pipette, place 80 µl, 40 µl, 20 µl, 10 µl, and 5 µl of patient serum to be tested on 5 different reaction circles on the glass slide. The corresponding titres obtained will be 1:20, 1:40, 1:80. 1:160, and 1:320 respectively.
2. Follow step No. 5 to 7 of slide screen method.

Note: This method is recommended for obtaining quick approximate titres only.

Quantitative Method

Tube Test Procedure

1. Take appropriate number of sets (as required; one set for each antigen suspension) of 8 Kahn tubes/test tubes and label them 1 to 8.
2. Pipette into tube No. 1 of all sets 1.9 ml of isotonic saline.
3. To each of the remaining tubes (2 to 8), add 1 ml of isotonic saline.
4. To tube No. 1 of all sets add 0.1 ml of serum sample to be tested and mix well.
5. Transfer 1 ml of the diluted serum sample from tube No. 1 to tube No. 2 and mix well.
6. Transfer 1 ml of the diluted serum sample from tube No. 2 to tube No. 3 and mix well. Continue this serial dilution till tube No. 7 in each set.
7. Discard 1.0 ml of the diluted serum from tube No. 7 of each set.
8. Now the dilutions of the serum sample achieved from tube No. 1 to 7 respectively in each set is as follows 1:20, 1:40, 1:80. 1:160, 1:320, 1:640, 1:1280. Tube No. 8 in all the sets serves as a saline control.
9. To all the tubes (1 to 8) of each set, add one drop of the respective well mixed TYDAL antigen suspensions from the reagent vials and mix well.
10 Cover and incubate at 37°C overnight (approximately 18 hours).
11. Dislodge the sedimented button gently and observe for agglutination.

Interpretation of Results

Slide Screen Method

Agglutination is a positive test result and indicates presence of the corresponding antibody in the patient serum.

No agglutination is a negative test result and indicates absence of the corresponding antibody in the patient serum.

Slide Semiquantitative Method

Agglutination is a positive test result. The titre of the patient serum corresponds to the visible agglutination in the test circle with the smallest amount of serum sample.

Quantitative Method

The titre of the patient serum using TYDAL antigen suspensions is the highest dilution of the serum sample that gives a visible agglutination.

Remarks

1. Positive results obtained in the slide test should be confirmed with the tube test to establish whether the titres are diagnostically significant or not.
2. TAB vaccinated patients may show a high titre of antibodies to each of the antigens.
3. 'O' being a somatic antigen brings about a coarse, compact, granular agglutination whereas 'H' being a flagellar antigen brings about larger, loose, flocculant agglutination.
4. While the 'O' antigen is species specific, the 'H' antigen is specific to the serotype.
5. Turbid and contaminated sera should not be used for testing.

6. Generally antibody titres of 1:80 or more are considered clinically and diagnostically significant. However, the significant titre may vary from population to population and needs to be established for each area.
7. It is recommended that results of the tests should be correlated with clinical findings to arrive at the final diagnosis.
8. Since techniques and standardisation vary from lab to lab one tube difference in tube titres can be expected.
9. The performance of the reagents should be validated occasionally using know positive control. Good physiological saline may be used as a negative control.

REDUCED WIDAL ANTIGEN SET: O AND H FOR TUBE TESTS (VITAL WIDAL) Courtesy: Tulip Group of Companies

Summary

In enteric fever, specific agglutinins are usually detectable in patient's blood after six days of fever. During the course of disease, the body responds to this antigenic stimulation by producing antibodies whose titre rises slowly in early stages to a maxima and then slowly falls till it is undetectable. Antibodies to *Salmonella* organisms may be detected in the patient's serum from second week after the onset of infection. Information regarding the titres and whether or not they are rising or falling can be obtained by performing serological tests using Vital Widal antigen suspensions.

Reagent

Vital Widal contains ready-to-use coloured, smooth antigen suspensions of the bacilli; *S. typhi O* and *S. typhi H* along with a polyspecific positive control reactive with these antigens. Vital Widal reagents are versatile and standardised for use in a modified tube test procedure for the detection of *S. typhi* antibodies in the patient's serum.

Each batch of reagents undergoes rigorous quality control at various stages of manufacture for its specificity and performance.

Reagent Storage and Stability

1. Store the reagent at 2 to 8°C. Do not freeze.
2. The shelf-life of the reagent is as per the expiry date mentioned on the reagent bottle labels.

Principle

When the coloured, smooth suspension of attenuated Vital Widal antigen suspensions are incubated with the patient's serum, anti-*Salmonella* antibodies if present in the patient's serum react with the antigen suspension to produce an agglutination. Agglutination is a positive test result, indicating presence of *Salmonella* antibodies in the patient's sample. No agglutination is a negative test result indicating absence of *Salmonella* antibodies in the patient's sample.

Note

In vitro diagnostic reagent for laboratory and professional use only. Not for medicinal use.

The reagent contains 0.5% Phenol/0.3% Formal dehyde as preservative. Avoid contact with skin and mucosa. On disposal, flush with large quantities of water.

Sample Collection and Storage

1. No special preparation of the patient is required prior to sample collection by approved techniques. Do not use haemolysed samples.
2. Clean and dry glassware free from detergents must be used for sample collection.
3. Do not heat/inactivate the serum.
4. Though freshly collected serum is preferable, store samples at 2 to 8°C in case of delay in testing.

Material Provided with the Kit

- Antigen suspension, *S. typhi 'O'*
- Antigen suspension, *S. typhi 'H'*
- Polyspecific positive control (goat)
- Colour coded vial top squeeze droppers

Additional Material Required

1. Test tubes/Kahn Tubes (preferably)
2. Pipettes 0.1 ml, 1.0 ml
3. Incubator (37°C)
4. Pasteur pipettes
5. Isotonic saline

1. Procedure

a. Tear off aluminium seals from the antigen vials. Fit on to each antigen vial, vial top squeeze dropper.
b. Bring all reagents to room temperature before testing.
c. Shake antigens well before dispensing.
d. Carefully label test tubes for sample and reagent identity.
e. Ensure squeeze dropper tips are wiped dry with clean tissues, before recapping

Tube Test Method

1. Take two sets of 8 Kahn tubes and test tubes and label them as 1 to 8 for O and H antibody detection.
2. Pipette into tube No 1 of all sets 1.9 ml of isotonic saline.
3. To each of the remaining tubes (2 to 8 each set), add 1.0 ml of isotonic saline.
4. To the tube No. 1 of all sets, add 0.1 ml of serum sample to be tested and mix well.
5. Transfer 1.0 ml of the diluted serum from the tube No. 1 to tube No. 2 and mix well.
6. Transfer 1.0 ml of the diluted serum from the tube No. 2 to tube No. 3 and mix well. Continue this serial dilution till tube No. 7.
7. Discard 1.0 ml of the diluted serum from tube No. 7.
8. This will give final dilutions in tubes 1 to 7 as 1:20, 1:40, 1:80, 1:160, 1:320, 1:640, 1:1280.
9. Tube No. 8 serves as saline control.
10. To all the tubes (1 to 8) of each set add one drop of well mixed Vital Widal suspension of the respective specificity. Mix well.
11. Incubate at 37°C overnight (approximately 18 ± 2 hours).
12. Dislodge the sedimented button gently and observe for agglutination macroscopically.

Interpretation of Results

The titre of the patient serum using Vital Widal is the highest dilution of serum that gives a visible agglutination. Generally antibodies having titres of 1:80 or more are considered diagnostically significant.

Apart from the pattern of sedimented antigens, in the tube test method a decrease in opacity as compared to the saline control must also be considered while judging the degree of agglutination.

Remarks

1. Serum from individuals vaccinated with TAB may also show moderately elevated titres of 'H' agglutinin.
2. 'O' being a somatic antigen, brings about coarse, compact and granular agglutination, whereas 'H' being a flagellar antigen, brings about larger, loose, flocculant agglutination.
3. 'H' antigen, being species specific, is more reliable in determining the type of infection.
4. Turbid and contaminated serum should not be used for testing.
5. It is recommended that results of the tests should be correlated with clinical findings to arrive at the final diagnosis.
6. Do not interchange vial top squeeze dropper cap.

POSITIVE CONTROL FOR WIDAL TEST

Summary

Enteric fever occurs when pathogenic microorganisms like *S. typhi, S. paratyphi A, S. paratyphi B, S. paratyphi C* infect the human body During the course of disease, the body responds to this antigenic stimulus by producing antibodies. Antibodies to *Salmonella* organisms may be detected in the patient serum from the second week after onset of infection. Information regarding the titres and whether or not they are rising or falling can be obtained by performing serological tests using Widal antigen suspensions. The performance of the Widal antigen suspensions can be validated with the help of Positive Control for Widal test.

Reagent

The Widal Positive Control contains ready-to-use standardised goat antiserum with polyspecific antibodies having specific reactivity towards *S. typhi 'O' and 'H'* antigens, S, *paratyphi 'AH'* and *'BH'* antigens, S *paratyphi 'AO'* and *'BO'* antigens and *S. paratyphi 'CO'* and *'CH'* antigens and is useful in the validation of the performance of Widal reagents.

Reagent Storage and Stability

1. Store the reagent at 2 to 8°C. Do not freeze.
2. The shelf-life of the reagent is as per the expiry date mentioned on the reagent bottle label.

Each batch of reagent undergoes rigorous quality control at various stages of manufacture for its specificity, sensitivity and performance.

Principle

The positive control is mixed with the Widal antigen suspensions to be tested and allowed to react. Specific reactivity of *Salmonella* antigens if present in the antigen suspensions will produce an agglutination reaction. No agglutination indicates the deterioration of the performance of the antigen suspensions.

Note

1. *In vitro* diagnostic reagent for laboratory and professional use only. Not for medicinal use.
2. The reagent contains sodium azide 0.1% as preservative. Avoid contact with skin and mucosa. On disposal flush with large quantities of water.

Additional Material Required

Stopwatch, isotonic saline, glass slide with clear/white background, appropriate pipettes/micropipettes, mixing sticks and a high intensity direct light source.

Procedure

a. Bring reagent to room temperature before testing.
b. Shake and mix the positive control for Widal test well before dispensing.

Slide test Method

1. Place one drop of positive control onto the reaction circle of the glass slide.
2. Place 50 µl of saline onto the next reaction circle of the glass slide.
3. Add one drop of test reagent (*Salmonella* antigen suspensions) in each of the above circles.
4. Mix contents of each circle uniformly over the entire circle with separate mixing sticks.
5. Gently rock the slide back and forth, observe for agglutination macroscopically at one minute against a white background.

Interpretation of Results Slide Test Method

Agglutination is a positive test result and indicates that the test reagent (*Salmonella* antigen suspension) are performing satisfactorily.

No agglutination is a negative test result and indicates the deterioration of the test reagent (*Salmonella* antigen suspension).

SLIDE AND TUBE TEST FOR DETECTION OF ANTIBODIES TO BRUCELLA ABORTUS/ MELITENSIS BRUCEL A/M®, Courtesy: Tulip Group of Companies

Summary

Human brucellosis (diurnal, or undulant fever) is a common febrile illness caused by infection with bacteria of some of the *Brucella* species (*abortus*, melitensis). This undulant fever is associated with symptoms, which are often variable and nonspecific with chills, fever, sweats and anorexia. On exposure, the body responds to this antigenic stimulation by producing specific antibodies whose titres rise slowly at early stages and then increases. Specific antibodies to the *Brucella* species are detectable a few weeks after exposure and are of considerable importance in the diagnosis of brucellosis. Information regarding the titre of antibodies can be obtained by using specific Tulip Brucel antigen suspensions.

Reagent

The Brucel-A/Brucel-M reagents contain ready-to-use standardised, attenuated, stained, smooth specific antigen suspensions of *Brucella* having specific reactivity towards antibodies to *Brucella abortus* (Brucel-A), and *Brucella melitensis* (Brucel-M).

Reagent Storage and Stability

Store the reagent at 2 to 8°C. Do not freeze.

The shelf-life of the reagents is as per the expiry date mentioned on the reagent vial labels.

Each batch of reagents undergoes rigorous quality control at various stages of manufacture for its specificity, sensitivity, and performance.

Principle

The smooth, attenuated, stained Bruce antigen suspensions are mixed with the patient's serum. Specific antibodies to *Brucella* antigens if present in the patient serum will react with the antigen suspension to produce an agglutination reaction. No agglutination indicates the absence of specific antibodies to *Brucella* antigens.

Note

1. *In vitro* diagnostic reagent for laboratory and professional use only. Not for medicinal use.
2. The reagent contains thimerosal 0.01% as preservative. Avoid contact with skin and mucosa. On disposal, flush with large quantities of water.

Sample Collection and Storage

1. No special preparation of patient is required prior to sample collection by approved techniques. Do not use haemolysed serum samples.
2. Clean and dry glassware free from detergents must be used for sample collection.
3. Do not heat/inactivate the serum.
4. Though freshly collected serum is preferred, samples can be stored at 2 to 8°C, for 24 hours or frozen for 8 days should a delay in testing occur.

Materials Provided with the Kit
Stained Brucel-A/Brucel-M antigen suspensions.
Additional Material Required
Slide test method

Stop watch, positive control, isotonic saline, and glass slide with clear/white background, appropriate pipettes/micropipettes, mixing sticks and a high intensity direct light source.

Quantitative Method

Timer, test tubes (12 mm × 75 mm), test tube rack, appropriate pipettes/micropipettes, isotonic saline/ 0.25% phenol saline, incubator (37°C).

PROCEDURE

Bring all reagents to room temperature.

Shake and mix the *Bruce* antigen suspensions well before dispensing.

The procedure for Brucel-A and Brucel-M is identical.

Slide Test Method

Qualitative Method

1. Place one drop of positive control (available as Brucel Positive Control, CAT. No. BPS005) onto the reaction circle of glass slide.
2. Place 80 µl of saline onto the next reaction circle of the glass slide.
3. Place 80 µl of patient serum to be tested onto the next reaction circle.
4. Add one drop of the appropriate Brucel antigen suspensions in each of the above circles. (containing positive control, saline, and the patient serum to be tested.)
5. Mix contents of each circle uniformly over the entire circle with separate mixing sticks.
6. Gently rock the slide back and forth, observe for agglutination macroscopically, at one minute against white background.

Semiquantitative Method

1. Using a pipette place 80 µl, 40 µl, 20 µl, 10 µl, and 5 µl of patient serum to be tested on 5 different circles on the glass slide. The corresponding titres obtained will be 1:20, 1:40, 1:80, 1:160, and 1:320 respectively.
2. Place one drop of appropriate Brucel antigen suspension to each circle.
3. Mix contents of each circle uniformly over the entire circle with separate mixing sticks.
4. Gently rock the slide back and forth, observe for agglutination macroscopically at one minute against a white background.

Tube Test Method

1. Take 8 test tubes and label them 1 to 8.
2. Pipette 1.9 ml of isotonic saline or preferably 0.25% phenol saline to tube No. 1.
3. To each of the remaining tubes (2-7), add 1.0 ml of isotonic saline or preferably 0.25% phenol saline.
4. To the tube No. 1, add 0.1 ml of serum sample to be tested. Mix well.
5. Transfer 1.0 ml of the diluted serum from tube No. 1 to tube No. 2 and mix well.
6. Transfer 1.0 ml of the diluted serum from tube No. 2 to tube No. 3 and mix well. Continue this serial dilution till tube No. 7.
7. Discard 1.0 ml of the diluted serum from tube No. 7.
8. Pipette 1.0 ml of isotonic saline in tube No. 8, which serves as a negative control.
9. To all the tubes add 1 drop of appropriate Brucel antigen suspensions and mix well.
10. Cover the tubes and incubate at 37°C for 24 hours.
11. Observe for agglutination macroscopically in each tube of the dilution series.

INTERPRETATION OF RESULTS

Slide Test Method

Qualitative Method

Agglutination is a positive test result and indicates the presence of specific antibodies to *Brucella* in the patient serum.

No agglutination is a negative test result and indicates absence of specific antibodies to *Brucella* in the patient serum.

Semiquatitative Method

Agglutination is a positive test result. The titre of patient serum corresponds to the visible agglutination in the test circle with the minimum amount of serum sample.

Tube Test Method

The titre of patient serum is the reciprocal of the last dilution of the serum sample that gives a granular agglutination.

In negative reaction, the appearance of the suspension remains unchanged, which shows a typical swirl when the tube is flicked.

Remarks

1. Turbid and contaminated serum should not be used for testing.
2. In the semi quantitative test the reactions obtained are roughly equivalent to those which would occur in a tube test.
3. Agglutinins are found in high proportion of normal individuals and titres less than 180 are of doubtful significance. A rising titre is more significant than a single high titre.
4. False-positive reactions may occur in sera of patients infected with *Pasteurella tularensis* or vaccinated with *Vibrio cholerae.*
5. False positive results are likely if the test is read more than one minute after mixing on slide test.
6. It is recommended that results of the tests should be correlated with the clinical findings to arrive at the final diagnosis.
7. Prozoning may sometimes be encountered in serum containing very high titres on slide test.
8. Since techniques and standardisation vary from laboratory to laboratory one tube difference in titres can be expected.

SLIDE SCREENING TEST FOR *BRUCELLA* Antibodies (Brucel-RB) Courtesy: Tulip Group of Companies

Summary

Human brucellosis (diurnal, or undulant fever) is a common febrile illness caused by infection with bacteria of some of the *Brucella* species *(abortus, melitensis).* This undulant fever is associated with symptoms, which are often variable and nonspecific with chills, fever, sweats and anorexia. Specific antibodies to the *Brucella* species are detectable a few weeks after exposure and are of considerable importance in the diagnosis of brucellosis.

Reagent

The BRUCEL-RB reagent contains smooth, killed buffered suspensions of *Brucella abortus* strain 99, coloured with rose bengal, standardised against the 2nd International preparation, having specific reactivity towards antibodies to *Brucella.*

Reagent Storage and Stability

1. Store the reagent at 2 to 8°C. Do not freeze.
2. The shelf-life of the reagents is as per the expiry date mentioned on the reagent vial labels.

Each batch of reagents undergoes rigorous quality control at various stages of manufacture for its specificity, sensitivity, and performance.

Principle

The smooth, coloured, killed BRUCEL-RB antigen suspension is mixed with the patient serum. Specific antibodies to *Brucella* antigens if present in titres $\geq$ 120, in the patient serum will react with the antigen suspension to produce an agglutination reaction. No agglutination indicates the absence of detectable levels of specific antibodies to *Brucella.*

Note

1. *In vitro* diagnostic reagent for laboratory and professional use only. Not for medicinal use.

2. The reagent contains 0.01% thimerosal as preservative. Avoid contact with skin and mucosa. On disposal, flush with large quantities of water.

Sample Collection and Storage

1. No special preparation of patient is required prior to sample collection by approved techniques. Do not use haemolysed serum samples.
2. Clean and dry glassware free from detergents must be used for sample collection.
3. Do not heat/inactivate the serum.
4. Though freshly collected serum is preferred, samples can be stored at 2 to 8°C, for 24 hours, or frozen for 8 days should a delay in testing occur.

Material Provided with the Kit

BRUCEL-RB *Brucella* rose bengal coloured antigens.

Additional Material Required

Stop watch, positive control, isotonic saline, glass slide with clear/white background, appropriate pipettes/micropipettes, mixing sticks and a high intensity direct light source.

PROCEDURE

Bring all reagents to room temperature.

Shake and mix the BRUCEL-RB antigen suspension well before dispensing.

Slide Test Method

Qualitative Method

1. Place one drop of positive control (available as Brucellosis Positive Control, CAT. No. BPS005) onto the reaction circle of glass slide.
2. Place 80 µl of saline onto the next reaction circle of the glass slide.
3. Place 80 µl of patient serum to be tested onto the next reaction circle.
4. Add one drop of well mixed BRUCEL-RB antigen suspension in each of the above circles containing positive control, isotonic saline and the patient serum to be tested.
5. Mix contents of each circle uniformly over the entire circle with separate mixing sticks.
6. Gently rock the slide back and forth, observe for agglutination macroscopically, at one minute against a white background.

Semiquantitative Method

1. Using a pipette, place 80 µl, 40 µl, 20 µl, 10 µl, and 5 µl of patient serum to be tested on 5 different circles on the glass slide. The corresponding titres obtained will be 1 20, 1 40, 1 80, 1:160, and 1 320 respectively.
2. Place one drop of BRUCEL-RB antigen suspension to each circle.
3. Mix contents of each circle uniformly over the entire circle with separate mixing sticks.
4. Gently rock the slide back and forth, observe for agglutination macroscopically at one minute against a white background.

INTERPRETATION OF RESULTS

Qualitative Method

Agglutination is a positive test result and indicates the presence of antibodies to *Brucella* in titres $\geq$ 1:20 in the patient serum.

No agglutination is a negative test result and indicates absence of antibodies to *Brucella* in titres 1:20 in the patient serum.

Semiqualitative Method

Agglutination is a positive test result. The titre of patient serum corresponds to the visible agglutination in the test circle with the minimum amount of serum sample.

Remarks

1. Turbid and contaminated serum should not be used for testing.
2. Agglutinins are found in high proportion of normal individuals and titres less than 1:80 are of doubtful significance. A rising titre is more significant than a single high titre.
3. False-positive reactions may occur in sera of patients infected with *Pasteurella tularensis* or vaccinated with *Vibrio cholerae*.
4. False-positive results are likely if the test is read more than one minute after mixing on the slide.
5. It is recommended that results of the test should be correlated with the clinical findings to arrive at the final diagnosis.
6. Prozoning may sometimes be encountered in serum containing very high titres on slide test.

7. Since techniques and standardisation vary from laboratory to laboratory a difference of titre corresponding to next or previous titre can be expected.

BRUCELLOSIS POSITIVE CONTROL
Courtesy: Tulip Group of Companies

Summary

Human brucellosis (diurnal, or undulant fever) is a common febrile illness caused by infection with bacteria of some of the *Brucella* species *(abortus, melitensis).* This undulant fever is associated with symptoms, which are often variable and nonspecific with chills, fever, sweats and anorexia. On exposure, the body responds to this antigenic stimulation by producing specific antibodies whose titres rise slowly at early stages and then increases. Specific antibodies to the *Brucella* species are detectable a few weeks after exposure and are of considerable importance in the diagnosis of Brucellosis. Information regarding the titre of antibodies can be obtained by using specific Brucel antigen suspensions.

The performance of the Brucel-A/Brucel-M antigen suspensions can be validated with the help of BRUCELLOSIS Positive Control.

Reagent

The Brucellosis Positive Control contains ready-to-use standardised goat antiserum with polyspecific antibodies having specific reactivity towards *Brucella abortus* and *Brucella melitensis* antigens and is useful in the validation of the performance of Brucel-A/Brucel-M reagents.

Reagent Storage and Stability

Store the reagent at 2 to 8°C. Do not freeze.

The shelf-life of the reagent is as per the expiry date mentioned on the reagent bottle label.

Each batch of reagents undergoes rigorous quality control at various stages of manufacture for its specificity, sensitivity, and performance.

Principle

The Brucellosis Positive Control is mixed with the *Brucella* antigen suspensions to be tested and allowed to react. Specific reactivity of *Brucella* antigens if present in the antigen suspensions will produce an agglutination reaction. No agglutination indicates the deterioration of the performance of the antigen suspensions.

Note

1. *In vitro* diagnostic reagent for laboratory and professional use only. Not for medicinal use.
2. The reagent contains thimerosal 0.01% as preservative. Avoid contact with skin and mucosa. On disposal, flush with large quantities of water.

Additional Material Required

Stopwatch, isotonic saline, glass slide with clear/white background, appropriate pipettes/micropipettes, mixing sticks and a high intensity direct light source.

Procedure

Bring all reagents to room temperature. Shake and mix the Brucellosis Positive Control well before dispensing.

Slide Test Method

1. Place one drop of Brucellosis Positive Control onto the reaction circle of glass slide.
2. Place 80 µl of saline onto the next reaction circle of the glass slide.
3. Add one drop of test reagent *(Brucella* antigen suspensions) in each of the above circles.
4. Mix contents of each circle uniformly over the entire circle with separate mixing sticks.
5. Gently rock the slide back and forth, observe for agglutination macroscopically at one minute against a white background.

INTERPRETATION OF RESULTS

Slide Test Method

Agglutination is a positive test result and indicates that the *Brucella* antigen reagents are performing satisfactorily. No agglutination is a negative test result and indicates the deterioration of *Brucella* antigen reagents.

RAPID TEST FOR IgM AND IgG ANTIBODIES TO DENGUE VIRUS:DENGUE FEVER (Denguecheck-WB) (Device) (Courtesy: Tulip Group of Companies

Introduction

Dengucheck-WB is a rapid immunochromatographic test for the simultaneous detection of IgM and IgG antibodies to Dengue virus in human serum/plasma/whole blood. The test can be used as a screening test for Dengue viral infection and as an aid for differential diagnosis of the self-limiting primary Dengue infections and the potentially fatal secondary Dengue infections in conjunction with other criteria.

Summary

Dengue fever virus (serotypes 1-4) belong to the family of *Flaviviridae*, which is widely distributed in the epidemic and endemic areas throughout tropical and subtropical regions of the world. Dengue virus infection is considered significant in terms of morbidity, mortality and economic cost associated with it, an estimated 100 million cases of dengue fever occurring throughout the world yearly. Dengue virus is transmitted in nature principally by the day-biting *Aedes aegypti* and *Aedes albopictus* mosquitoes. The mosquito vector is highly domesticated and an urban species. Dengue presents typically as a fever of sudden onset with headache, retro-orbital pain, pain in the back and limbs (break-bone fever), lymphadenopathy and maculopapular rash. Patients diagnosed with dengue infection in endemic areas generally have secondary infection, whereas patients in nonendemic areas are usually diagnosed with primary infection. Specific antibody response to Dengue virus enables serodiagnosis and differentiation between primary and secondary dengue infections and detection of potentially life-threatening conditions such as DHF and DSS.

Dengucheck-WB is a new generation rapid immunochromatographic test using highly specific and purified immunodominant, Recombinant Dengue 'Env.' antigens. It is a simple test for the differential diagnosis of Dengue virus infection.

Principle

Dengucheck-WB utilszes the principle of immunochromatography, a unique two-site, self-performing immunoassay on a membrane. Specific human IgM and human IgG antibody-binding proteins are immobilised on the nitrocellulose membrane as two individual test bands (IgM and IgG) in the test window "T" of the test device at region "M" and region "G" respectively. The IgM band in the test window "T" is closer to the sample well and the IgG band is close to the control window "C". As the test sample flows through the membrane assembly within the test device, the coloured-Dengue specific recombinant antigen-colloidal gold conjugate complexes with specific antibodies (IgM and IgG) to Dengue virus, if present in the sample. This complex moves further on the membrane to the test region where it is immobilised by the specific human IgM antibody and/or human IgG antibody binding proteins coated on the membrane leading to formation of a coloured band which confirms a positive test result. Absence of these coloured bands in the test window "T" indicates a negative test result. A built-in control band in the control window "C" appears when the test has been performed correctly, regardless of the presence or absence of anti-Dengue virus antibodies in the specimen and serves to validate the test performance.

Reagents and Materials Supplied

Each kit contains:

A. Individual pouches, each containing:
   1. Dengucheck-WB (Device) Membrane test assembly predispensed with recombinant Dengue virus specific antigen colloidal gold conjugate, streptavidin gold conjugate, anti-human IgM at test region 'M' Protein A at the test region 'G' and Biotin at the control region 'C'.
   2. Desiccant pouch
   3. 5 µl sample loop

B. Sample running buffer

C. Package insert

Storage and Stability

The sealed pouches in the test kit and the kit components may be stored between 4 and 30°C for the duration of the shelf-life as indicated on the pouch.

Optional Material Required: 5 µl precision micropipettes.

Note

1. For *in vitro* diagnostic use only. Not for Medicinal Use.
2. Do not use beyond expiry date.
3. Read the instructions carefully before performing the test.
4. Handle all specimen as potentially infectious
5. Follow standard biosafety guidelines for handling and disposal of potentially infective material.

Specimen Collection and Preparation

1. No special preparation of the patient is necessary prior to specimen collection by approved techniques.
2. Though fresh serum/plasma is preferable, specimen may be stored at 2-8° C for up to 24 hours, in case of delay in testing.
3. Whole blood samples collected with a suitable anticoagulant such as EDTA or Heparin or Oxalate can also be used.
4. Do not use turbid, lipaemic, icteric and haemolysed specimen.
5. Repeated freezing, thawing of the specimen should be avoided.
6. Specimen containing precipitates or particulate matter must be centrifuged and the clear supernatant only should be used for testing.

Testing Procedure and Interpretation of Results

1. Bring the kit components to room temperature before testing.
2. Open the pouch and retrieve the test device. Once opened, the device must be used immediately.
3. Label the test device with patient identity.
4. Add 5 µl of serum/plasma/whole blood, with the micropipette into the sample port 'A', or using the 5 µl sample loop provided with the-kit, dip the loop into the sample and then blot into the sample port 'A'. Ensure that the loop does not retrieve clots or debris from the sample.
5. Add five drops of sample running buffer in the reagent port 'B'.
6. Exactly at the end of 15 minutes, read the test results.

INTERPRETATION OF RESULTS

Negative Test Result

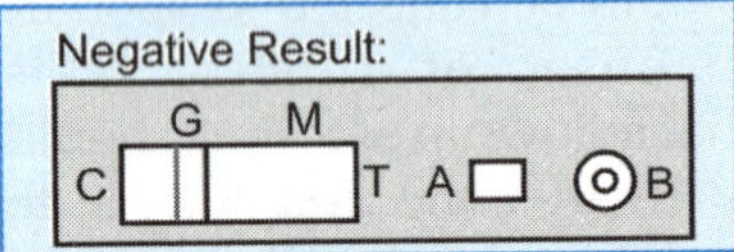

Negative results

The presence of only the single red/purple coloured band in the control window "C" indicates the absence of specific antibodies against dengue virus or that the amount of antibodies is below the detection limit of the test.

Positive Test Result

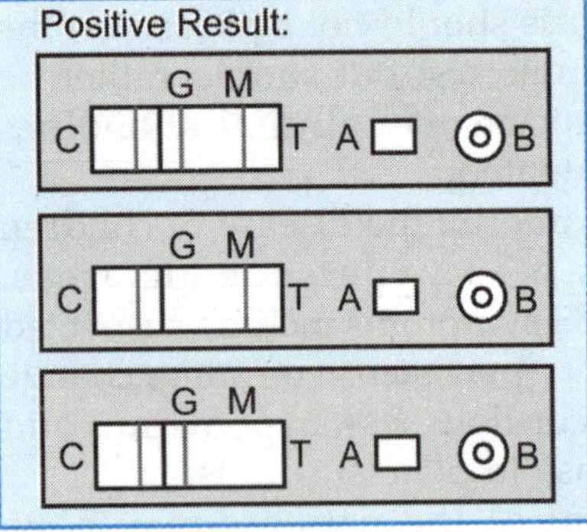

Positive result reading

1. In addition to the band in the control window 'C', appearance of two red/purple coloured bands in the test window at region 'M' and region 'G' indicates the presence of Dengue virus specific IgM and IgG antibodies (acute secondary infection).
2. In addition to the control band in the control window 'C', appearance of a red/purple coloured band in the test window at region 'M' indicates the presence of Dengue virus specific IgM antibodies (acute primary infection).
3. In addition to the control band in the control window 'C', the appearance of a red/purple coloured band in the test window at region

'G' indicates the presence of Dengue virus specific IgG antibodies (acute secondary infection).

Invalid Result: If, after 15 minutes, no band is visible either in the test or control window, the result is considered invalid. The test should be react with a new device.

Remarks

1. Do not use test kit beyond expiration date.
2. While sample should be collected as soon as possible after onset of illness, it is recommended that follow-up of testing should be done on day 10 after the first sample to allow seroconversion, especially when the test is negative and Dengue virus infection is clinically suspected.
3. Though *Dengucheck*-WB does provide evidence to distinguish the past (secondary) infection from current (primary) ongoing infection, a negative result does not preclude the possibility of infection with Dengue virus.
4. As with all diagnostic tests, a definitive clinical diagnosis should not be based on the results of a single test but should rather be made by a clinician after all clinical findings have been evaluated.
5. The DHF is primarily the disease of children under 15 years in hyperendemic areas. Impending DSS symptoms include suspected abdominal pain, persistent vomiting, change in the level of conciousness, hypothermia and sudden decrease in platelet counts.
6. Eighty percent of the patients may have detectable levels of IgM antibody by day 5 of illness and 99% by day 10.
7. IgM levels rise quickly and peak by two weeks after onset of symptoms and then fall to become undetectable over 2 to 3 months. IgG antibodies rise quickly and peak at about two weeks postinfection and then decline slowly over 3 to 6 months.

TEST FOR INFECTIOUS MONONUCLEOSIS (IMMUTEX®), Courtesy: Tulip Group of Companies

Summary

Infectious mononucleosis is a self-limited prolonged illness strongly associated with Epstein-Barr Virus. Though specific treatment is rarely required since the disease is usually asymptomatic, potential complications, such as inflammation of the liver, enlargement of the spleen, pericarditis, myocarditis and encephalitis as well as haemolytic anaemia associated with this disease, require physician's attention.

In individuals with suppressed or abnormal immunodeficiency disorders, cancer or those with recent organ transplant, infectious mononucleosis occurs with severe complications.

Studies have cited the presence of heterophile antibodies during the course of infection with infectious mononucleosis.

Reagent

Immutex is a ready-to-use, uniform suspension of stabilised, specially treated horse erythrocytes highly specific for heterophile antibodies associated with infectious mononucleosis. The reagent does not react with normal Forssman antibodies.

Each batch of reagent undergoes rigorous quality control at various stages of manufacture for its specificity, sensitivity and performance.

Reagent Storage and Stability

Store the reagents at 2 to 8°C. Do not freeze. The shelf-life of the reagents is as per the expiry date mentioned on the reagent vial labels.

Principle

Immutex is a rapid slide haemagglutination test for the detection of heterophile antibodies. Immutex IM reagent will agglutinate when mixed with serum containing heterophile antibodies. No agglutination indicates absence of heterophile antibodies.

Note

1. *In vitro* diagnostic reagent for laboratory and professional use only. Not for medicinal use.
2. All the components derived from human source have been tested for HBsAg and Anti-HIV antibodies and found to be nonreactive. However, handle the material as if infectious.
3. The reagents contain thimerosal 0.01% as preservative. Avoid contact with skin or mucosa. On disposal, flush with large quantities of water.

4. The reagent can be damaged due to microbial contamination or on exposure to extreme temperatures. It is recommended that the performance of reagents should be verified with known positive and negative controls provided with the kit.
5. Ensure resuspension of the stabilised erythrocyte reagent before use to improve test readability by gently inverting the vial.
6. Do not interchange vial droppers.
7. Only a clean and dry glass slide must be used. Clean the slide with distilled water and wipe dry.

Sample Collection and Preparation

No special preparation of the patient is necessary prior to specimen collection by approved techniques. Though fresh serum is preferable, serum specimens stored at 2 to 8°C for up to 24 hours, can also be used in case of delay in testing. Do not use haemolysed or contaminated specimens. Turbid specimens should be centrifuged or allowed to settle and only the clear supernatant should be used for testing.

Materials Provided with the Kit

Reagent

Immutex IM reagent, Positive Control, Negative Control.

Accessories

Glass slide with six reaction circles, sample dispensing pipettes, mixing sticks and rubber teats.

Additional Material Required

A high intensity direct light source, stopwatch.

TEST PROCEDURE

Bring all reagents and samples to room temperature before use.

Qualitative Method

1. Gently mix the Immutex IM reagent to resuspend the stabilised horse erythrocyte reagent.
2. Place one drop of the sample to be tested onto one of the reaction circles of the glass slide using a sample dispensing pipette provided with the kit.
3. Place one drop of the positive and negative control onto separate reaction circles of the glass slide.
4. Add one drop of Immutex IM reagent to the test specimen on the slide. Do not let the dropper tip touch the liquid on the slide.
5. Add one drop of Immutex IM reagent to each of the controls.
6. Mix with separate mixing sticks, spreading the mixture uniformly over the entire reaction circle.
7. Immediately start the stopwatch. Rock the slide gently, back and forth, for 2 minutes.
8. Leave the slide undisturbed on the work table for a further 1 minute.
9. Pick up the slide at the end of 1 minute and observe for agglutination by rocking the slide gently back and forth.

INTERPRETATION OF RESULTS

Agglutination is a positive test result and indicates presence of heterophile antibodies in the test specimen. No agglutination is a negative test result and indicates absence of heterophile antibodies in the test specimen.

Remarks

1. Markedly lipaemic, haemolysed and contaminated serum sample could produce nonspecific results.
2. Use of plasma rather than serum can lead to false-positive results.
3. Heterophile antibodies may be found in disease other than infectious mononucleosis. Low titres have been detected in cytomegalic inclusion disease and toxoplasmosis.
4. Do not read the results beyond indicated testing time limit.
5. As with all diagnostic tests, the result of the test should be correlated with clinical findings to arrive at the final diagnosis.
6. The reagent performance should be validated by occasionally running the positive and negative controls provided with the kit.

RAPID TEST FOR IgM ANTIBODIES TO *LEPTOSPIRA:* LEPTOSPIROSIS (LEPTOCHEK WB) *(*DEVICE), Courtesy: Tulip Group of Companies

Introduction

Leptocheck-WB is a rapid, self-performing, qualitative, sandwich immunoassay for the detection of *Leptospira* specific IgM antibodies in human serum/ plasma or whole blood specimen. It is useful for the serodiagnosis of current or recent leptospirosis. The broadly reactive genus specific antigen employed in the test allows the detection of *Leptospira* infections caused by a wide range of strains of different serovars.

Summary

Leptospira are actively motile, delicate spirochaetes possessing a large number of closely wound spirals and characteristic hooked ends. There are several species of *Leptospira* and they may be saprophytic or parasitic. They can be distinguished only under dark ground illumination in the living state or by electron microscopy. *Leptospirosis* is a zoonotic disease of worldwide prevalence. Humans are infected when the water contaminated by the urine of carrier animals enters the body through cuts or abrasions on the skin or through intact mucosa of the mouth, nose or conjunctiva. Clinical symptoms include fever, chills, headache, conjunctivitis, myalgia and Gl-related symptoms, kidney infection is a common sequelae.

Diagnosis may be made by demonstration of *Leptospira* microscopically in blood or urine, by isolating them in culture or by inoculation of guinea pigs, or by serological tests.

Leptocheck-WB, qualitatively detects the presence of IgM class of *Leptospira* specific antibodies in human serum/plasma or whole blood specimen.

PRINCIPLE

Leptocheck-WB utilises the principle of immuno-chromatography, a unique two-site immunoassay on a membrane. As the test sample flows through the membrane assembly of the test device, the anti-human IgM-colloidal gold conjugate forms a complex with IgM antibodies in the sample. This complex moves further on the membrane to the test window 'T' where it is immobilised by the broadly reactive *Leptospira* genus specific antigens coated on the membrane, leading to the formation of a red to deep purple coloured band at the test region 'T' which confirms a positive test result. Absence of this coloured band in test region 'T' indicates a negative test result. The unreacted conjugate and the unbound complex if any move further on the membrane and are subsequently immobilised by the anti-rabbit antibodies coated on the control window 'C' of the membrane assembly, forming a red to deep purple coloured band. The control band serves to validate the test results.

Reagents and Material Supplied

Each kit contains:

A. Individual pouches, each containing:
   1. Test Device Membrane test assembly predispensed with Anti Human IgM-colloidal gold conjugate, *Leptospira* genus specific antigens at test window 'T' and anti-rabbit antiserum predispensed at the control window 'C'.
   2. Desiccant pouch
   3. 5 µl sample loops

B. Sample running buffer

C. Package insert

Storage and Stability

The sealed pouches in the test kit and the kit components may be stored between 4 and 30°C for the duration of the shelf-life as indicated on the pouch.

Optional Material Required: 10 µl precision micropipettes.

Note

1. For *in vitro* diagnostic use only. Not for Medicinal Use.
2. Do not use beyond expiry date.
3. Read the instructions carefully before performing the test.
4. Handle all specimens as potentially infectious.
5. Follow standard biosafety guidelines for handling and disposal of potentially infective material.

Specimen Collection and Preparation

1. Blood samples collected with a suitable anti-coagulant such as EDTA or Heparin or Oxalate can also be used.

2. No prior preparation of the patient is required before sample collection by approved techniques.
3. Fresh serum/plasma is preferable. Anticoagulated whole blood can also be used as specimen. Serum/plasma may be stored at 2 to 8°C up to 24 hours in case of delay in testing. For long-term storage, freeze the specimen at –20°C for 3 months or –70°C for longer periods. Whole blood should be used immediately and should not be frozen.
4. Repeated freezing and thawing of the specimen should be avoided.
5. Do not use haemolysed, clotted, contaminated, viscous/turbid specimen.
6. Specimen containing precipitates or particulate matter must be centrifuged and the clear supernatant only used for testing.
7. For each sample, a new sample loop should be used.

Testing Procedure and Interpretation of Results

1. Bring the kit components to room temperature before testing.
2. Open the pouch and retrieve the test device. Once opened, the device must be used immediately.
3. Label the test device with the patient's identity.
4. Add 10 µl of serum/plasma or whole blood with a micropipette into the sample port "A", OR using the 5 µl sample loop provided with the kit. Dip the loop into the sample and then blot into the sample port 'A'. Repeat this step twice for each sample. Ensure that the loop does not retrieve clots or debris from the sample.
5. Add 5 drops of sample running buffer to the reagent port 'B'.
6. At the end of 15 minutes read the results as follows.

Negative Test Result

Only one coloured band appears in the control window 'C'.

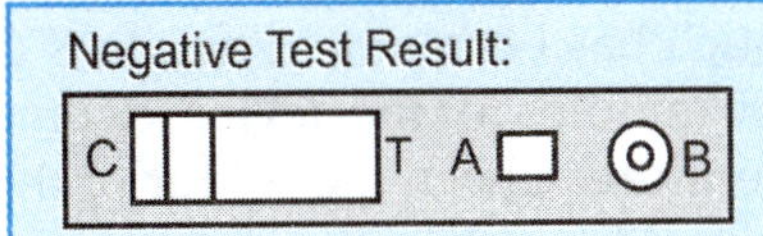

Negative result

Positive Test Result

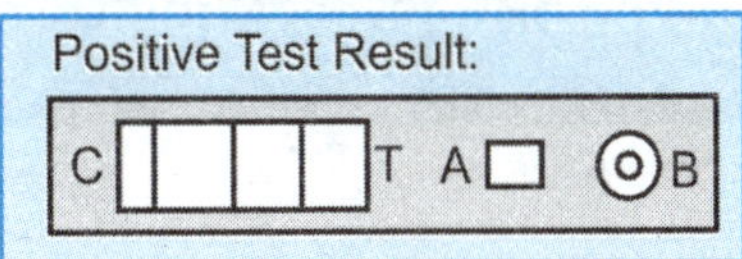

Positive result

In addition to the band in control window 'C', another red/purple band appears in the test window 'T' indicating the presence of specific IgM antibodies to *Leptospira*.

- The test should be considered invalid if neither the control band 'C' nor the test band 'T' appears. Repeat the test with a new device.

Performance Characteristics

Leptocheck-WB was evaluated at the Royal Tropical Institute, Amsterdam in parallel with other licensed tests for the serodiagnosis of *leptospirosis*. The 47 sera evaluated were from diverse serogroups of *Leptospira*. Leptocheck-WB had a performance comparable to the other tests.

Remarks

1. The intensity of the test line depends upon the stage of the disease and the titres of the antibodies in the test specimen.
2. As specific antibodies reach detectable levels about one week after the onset of disease, a sample collected very early may yield a negative test result.
3. If the test is negative and if leptospirosis is still suspected, the test should be repeated with the second sample collected at a later date in conjunction with clinical re-examination.
4. In endemic areas, faint bands may appear occasionally due to borderline IgM titres present as a result of previous exposures.
5. It is recommended that the positive results obtained must be reconfirmed using a confirmatory test such as the MAT (microscopic agglutination test).
6. High titres of RF and heterophile antibodies may interfere with the test; in such cases, the results must be interpreted with caution.
7. The results must be correlated with clinical findings to arrive at the diagnosis.
8. Do not use the test kit beyond expiration date.

RAPID TEST FOR *P. FALCIPARUM* MALARIA (PARACHECK Pf) (DEVICE), Courtesy: Tulip Group of Companies

Introduction

Paracheck Pf is a rapid self-performing, qualitative, two-site sandwich immunoassay for the determination of *P. falciparum* specific histidine-rich protein-2 (Pf HRP-2) in whole blood samples.

Summary

Four species of the *Plasmodium* parasites are responsible for malaria infections in human viz *P. falciparum, P. vivax, P. ovale* and *P. malariae.* Of these, *P. falciparum* is the most prevalent and severe species that is responsible for most of the morbidity and mortality worldwide. Early detection of *P. falciparum* malaria is of paramount importance due to incidence of cerebral malaria and drug resistance associated with it. The Pf HRP-2 is a water-soluble protein that is released from parasitised erythrocytes of infected individuals and is specific to the *P. falciparum* species.

Paracheck Pf detects the presence of Pf HRP-2 in whole blood specimen and is a sensitive and specific test for the detection of *P. falciparum* malaria.

Principle

Paracheck Pf is a rapid test for the detection of *P. falciparum* malaria that utilises the principle of immunochromatography. As the test sample flows through the membrane assembly of the device after addition of the clearing buffer, the coloured anti Pf HRP-2 colloidal gold conjugate (monoclonal) antisera complexes the Pf HRP-2 in the lysed sample. This complex moves further on the membrane to the test region where it is immobilised by the anti-Pf HRP-2 (monoclonal) antisera coated on the membrane leading to formation of a pink coloured band which confirms a positive test result. Absence of this coloured band in the test region indicates a negative test result. The unreacted conjugate and unbound complex if any, move further on the membrane and are subsequently immobilised by antimouse antibodies coated on the membrane at the control region, forming a pink band. This control band serves to validate the test performance.

Reagents and Materials Supplied

Paracheck Pf Kit contains

1. Individually pouched devices: Membrane assembly predispensed with anti Pf HRP-2 colloidal gold conjugated antisera, anti-Pf HRP-2 antisera and antimouse antisera at the respective regions and sample applicator pipette.
2. Clearing buffer in a dropper bottle.

Optional Material Required

Calibrated micropipette capable of delivering 5 µl sample accurately.

Storage and Stability

The test kit may be stored between 4 and 30°C till the duration of the shelf-life as indicated on the pouch/carton. Do not freeze.

Note

Read the instructions carefully before performing the test.

- For *in vitro* diagnostic use only. Not for Medicinal Use.
- Do not use beyond expiry date.
- Do not intermix reagents from different lots.
- Handle all specimens as potentially infectious.
- Follow standard biosafety guidelines for handling and disposal of potentially infective material.

Specimen Collection and Preparation

Fresh anticoagulated whole blood should be used as test sample and EDTA or Heparin or Oxalate can be used as suitable anticoagulant. The specimen should be collected in a clean glass or plastic container. If immediate testing is not possible, then specimen may be stored at 2-8°C for up to 72 hours before testing. Clotted or contaminated blood samples should not be used for performing the test. Fresh blood from finger prick/puncture may also be used as a test specimen.

Test Procedure

1. Bring the Paracheck Pf kit components to room temperature before testing.
2. In case the pouch has been stored at 2 to 8°C allow at least 30 minutes for the device to come to room temperature. Check the colour of the desiccant. It should be blue. If it has turned

colourless or faint blue, discard the device and use another device.

3. Open the pouch and remove the device. Once opened, the device must be used immediately.
4. Evenly mix the anticoagulated blood sample by gentle swirling. Touch the sample applicator pipette to the surface of the blood in the sample container. Blot the blood so collected onto the sample pad in the sample well 'A' (this delivers approximately 5 µl of the whole blood specimen).

   Or

   In case finger prick blood is being used, touch the sample applicator pipette to the blood on the finger prick and immediately blot the specimen onto the sample pad in the sample well 'A' (care should be taken that the blood sample has not clotted and the transfer to the sample pad is immediate).

   Or

   Alternatively, 5 µl of the anticoagulated or the finger prick specimen may be delivered to the sample pad in the sample well 'A' using a micropipette.

   Note: Ensure the blood from the sample applicator pipette has been completely taken up by the sample pad.
5. Dispense six drops (300 µl) of the clearing buffer into well 'B' by holding the plastic dropper bottle vertically.
6. At the end of 15 minutes, read the results as follows

   Negative: for *P. falciparum* malaria: Only one pink coloured band appears in the control window 'C'.

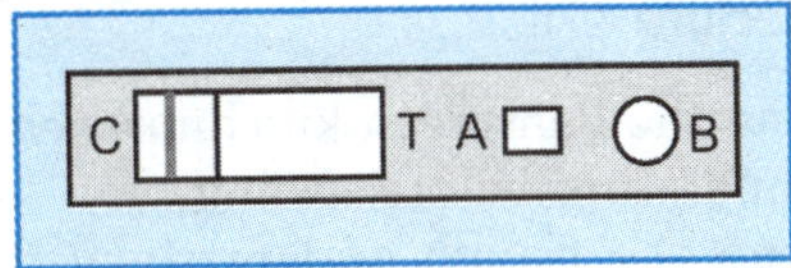

Negative result

   Positive: for *P. falciparum* malaria: In addition to the control band, a distinct pink coloured band also appears in the test window 'T'.

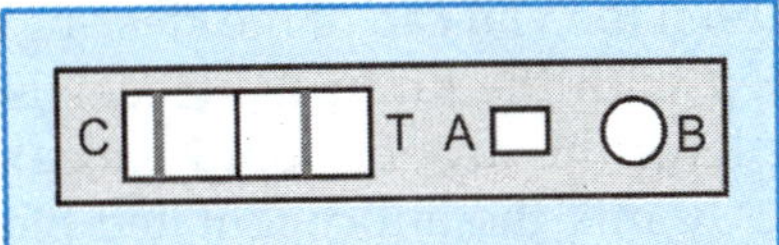

Positive result

7. The test results should not be interpreted after 15 minutes.
8. The test should be considered invalid if no bands appear on the device. Repeat the test with a new device ensuring that the test procedure has been followed accurately.

Limitations of the Test

1. Since the Pf HRP-2 persists for up to a fortnight even after successful therapy, a positive test result does not indicate a failed therapeutic response.
2. In case the test needs to be used to monitor success of therapy, testing is advised only from 15 days after the completion of therapy.
3. As with all diagnostic tests, the results must always be correlated with clinical findings.

RAPID TEST FOR MALARIA (Parascreen) Pan/Pf (Device), Courtesy: Tulip Group of Companies

Introduction

Parascreen is a rapid self-performing, qualitative, two-site sandwich immunoassay, utilising whole blood for the detection of *P. falciparum* specific histidine-rich protein-2 (Pf HRP-2) and pan specific pLDH. The test may also be used for differentiation of *P. falciparum* and other malarial species and for the follow-up of antimalarial therapy, in whole blood samples.

Summary

Four species of the *Plasmodium* parasites are responsible for malaria infections in human viz. *P. falciparum, P. vivax, P. ovale* and *P. malariae*. Of these, *P. falciparum* and *P. vivax* are the most prevalent. Early detection and differentiation of malaria is of paramount importance due to incidence of cerebral malaria and drug resistance associated with falciparum malaria and due to the morbidity associated with the other malarial forms.

Parascreen detects the presence of pan malaria specific pLDH released from the parasitised blood cells, for the detection of all malarial parasites. Whereas for the detection of *P. falciparum* malaria.

Parascreen utilises the detection of *P. faiciparum* specific histidine-rich protein-2 (Pf HRP-2), which is a water-soluble protein that is released from parasitised erythrocytes of infected individuals.

In the absence of *P.faiciparum* specific Pf HRP-2, the presence of the pan malaria specific band points to the presence of other malarial species viz.; *P.vivax, P.ovale* or *P.malariae.* Speciation is done and results inferred in the context of prevalence rates of the malarial species prevalent in the particular region.

Since pLDH is a product of viable parasities, the pan band may also be used to monitor success of antimalarial therapy.

Principle

Parascreen utilises the principle of immunochromatography. As the test sample flows through the membrane assembly of the device after addition of the clearing buffer, the coloured monoclonal anti-HRP-2 specific/anti-pan specific colloidal gold conjugate antibodies complexes the proteins in the lysed sample. This complex moves further on the membrane to the test region where it is immobilised by the monoclonal anti Pf. HRP-2/anti-pan specific antibody coated on the membrane leading to formation of pink-purple coloured band/s which confirm(s) a positive test result. While both the bands will appear at the test region in falciparum positive samples, only one band would appear in nonfalciparum malaria positive samples. Absence of this coloured band/s in the test region indicates a negative test result.

The unreacted conjugate along with the rabbit globulin-colloidal gold conjugate and unbound complex if any, move further on the membrane and are subsequently immobilised by anti-rabbit antibodies coated on the membrane at the control region, forming a pink-purple band. This control band serves to validate the test performance.

Reagents and Material Supplied

Parascreen kit contains:

A. Individual pouches, each containing:
   1. Test Device Membrane assembly predispensed with monoclonal anti-HRP-2 colloidal gold conjugate, monoclonal anti-pan specific pLDH colloidal gold conjugate, rabbit globulin-colloidal gold conjugate and monoclonal anti-Pf. HRP-2 antibody, monoclonal anti-pan specific pLDH antibody and anti-rabbit antibody at the respective regions.
   2. Desiccant pouch.
   3. 5 µl sample loop.

B. Clearing buffer in a dropper bottle.

C. Package insert.

Optional Material Required

Calibrated micropipettes capable of delivering 5 µl sample accurately.

Storage and Stability

The test kit may be stored between 4-30°C till the duration of the shelf-life as indicated on the pouch/carton. Do not freeze.

Note

Read the instructions carefully before performing the test For *in vitro* diagnostic use only. Not for Medicinal Use. Do not use beyond expiry date. Do not intermix reagents from different lots. Handle all specimens as potentially infectious. Follow standard biosafety guidelines for handling and disposal of potentially infective material.

Specimen Collection and Preparation

Fresh anti-coagulated whole blood should be used as a test sample and EDTA or Heparin or Oxalate can be used as suitable anticoagulant. The specimen should be collected in a clean glass or plastic container. If immediate testing is not possible, then the specimen may be stored at 2 to 8°C for up to 72 hours before testing. Clotted or contaminated blood samples should not be used for performing the test. Fresh blood from finger prick/puncture may also be used as a test specimen.

Test Procedure

1. Bring the Panscreen kit components to room temperature before testing.
2. Open the pouch and retrieve the device, sample loop and desiccant. Check the colour of the desiccant. It should be blue. If it has turned colourless or pink, discard the device and use another device. *Once opened, the device must be used immediately.*
3. Tighten the vial cap of the clearing buffer provided with the kit in the clockwise direction to pierce the dropper bottle nozzle.
4. Evenly mix the anticoagulated blood sample by gentle swirling. Dip the sample loop into the sample. Ensuring that a loop full of blood

is retrieved, blot the blood so collected on to the sample pad in the sample port 'A' (this delivers approximately 5 µl of the whole blood specimen).

Or

In case finger prick blood is being used, touch the sample loop to the blood on the finger prick. Ensuring that a loop full of blood is retrieved, immediately blot the specimen onto the sample pad in the sample port 'A' (care should be taken that the blood sample has not clotted and the transfer to the sample pad is immediate).

Or

Alternatively, 5 µl of the anticoagulated or finger prick specimen may be delivered to the sample pad in the sample port 'A' using a micropipette.

Note: Ensure the blood from the sample applicator pipette has been completely taken up by the sample pad.

5. Dispense four drops of the clearing buffer into port 'B', by holding the plastic dropper bottle vertically.
6. At the end of 15 minutes, read the results as follows

Negative for Malaria

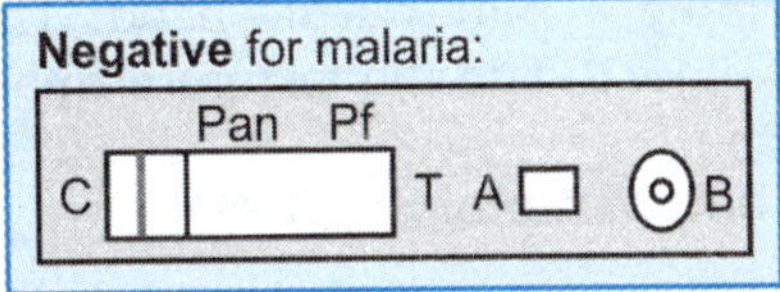

- Only one pink-purple band appears in the control window 'C'.

Positive for Malaria

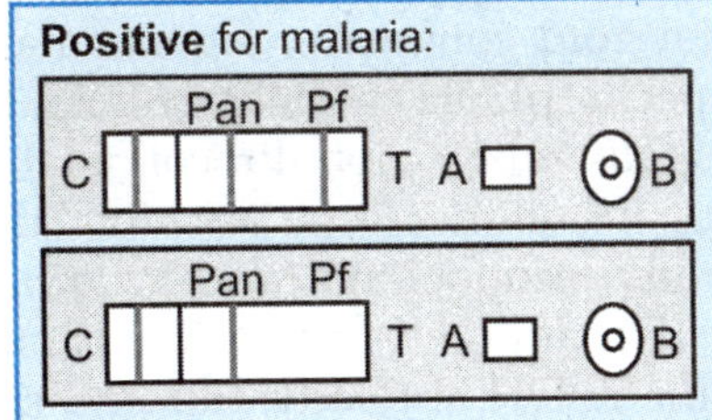

- *P. falciparum* or mixed infection: In addition to the control band, two pink-purple bands appear at regions 'Pf' and 'Pan' in the test window 'T'.
- Other species (non falciparum) In addition to the control band, one pink-purple band appears only at region 'Pan' in the test window 'T'.

7. The test result should not be interpreted after 15 minutes.
8. The test should be considered invalid if no bands appear on the device. Repeat the test with a new device ensuring that the test procedure has been followed accurately.

Limitations of the Test

1. As with all diagnostic tests, the test result must always be correlated with clinical findings.
2. The results of test are to be interpreted within the epidemiological, clinical and therapeutic context. When it seems indicated, the parasitological techniques of reference should be considered (microscopic examination of the thick smear and thin blood films).
3. Any modification to the above procedure and/or use of other reagents will invalidate the test procedure.
4. The device and buffer of different lots must not be mixed and used.
5. In case of mixed infection (*P falciparum* with other malarial species), both, 'Pf' and 'Pan' malaria band will be positive. Hence, differentiation of infection due to *P. vivax, P. ovale* or *P. malariae* cannot be done.
6. While monitoring therapy, using the 'Pan' band, if the reaction of the test remains positive with the same intensity after 5-10 days, post-treatment, the possibility of a resistant strain of malaria has to be considered.
7. Usually, the 'Pan' band turns negative after successful antimalarial therapy. However, since treatment duration and medication used affect the clearance of parasites, the test should be repeated after 5-10 days of start of treatment.
8. In *P. falciparum* malaria infection, HRP-2 is not secreted in the gametogony stage. Hence, in "Carriers", the HRP-2 band may be absent.
9. The HRP-2 levels, post-treatment, persists up to 15 days, the 'Pan' band can be used to monitor success of therapy, in *P falciparum* malaria cases.
10. In a few cases, where the HRP-2 band is positive and the 'Pan' malaria band is negative,

it may indicate a case of post-treatment malaria. However, such a reaction pattern may also be obtained in a few cases of untreated malaria. Retesting after 2 days is advised, in such cases.

RAPID TEST FOR MALARIA PAN/PV/PF (PARAMAX-3) (DEVICE), Courtesy: Tulip Group of Companies

Introduction

Paramax-3 is a rapid self-performing, qualitative, two-site sandwich immunoassay utilising whole blood for the detection of *P. falciparum* specific histidine-rich protein-2 (Pf HRP-2), *P.* vivax specific pLDH and pan malaria specific pLDH. The test can be used for the specific detection of *P. falciparum* and *P. vivax* malaria, differentiation of other malarial species and for the follow-up of antimalarial therapy.

Summary

Four species of the *Plasmodium* parasites are responsible for malaria infections in human viz. *P. falciparum, P. vivax, P. ovale* and *P. malariae.* Of these, *P. falciparum* and *P. vivax* are the most prevalent. Early detection and differentiation of malaria is of utmost importance due to incidence of cerebral malaria and drug resistance associated with falciparum malaria and due to the morbidity associated with the other malarial forms. As the course of treatment is dependent on the species, differentiation between *P. falciparum* and *P. vivax* is of utmost importance for better patient management and speedy recovery.

In Paramax-3 the detection system for *P. falciparum* malaria is based on the detection of *P. falciparum* specific histidine-rich protein-2 (Pf HRP-2) which is a water-soluble protein that is released from parasitised erythrocytes of infected individuals. The detection system of *P. vivax* is based on the presence of *P. vivax* specific pLDH. Further the detection of other malarial infections such as *P. ovale* and *P. malariae* is achieved through the pan malaria specific pLDH. Since pLDH is a product of viable parasites, the pan band may also be used to monitor course of effective antimalarial therapy.

Paramax-3 detects the presence of *P. falciparum* specific Pf HRP-2, *P.vivax* specific pLDH and pan specific pLDH in whole blood specimen and is a sensitive and specific test for the detection of all malaria species, differentiation for *P. falciparum* and *P. vivax* and monitoring successful antimalarial therapy.

Principle

Paramax-3 utilises the principle of immunochromatography. As the test sample flows through the membrane assembly of the device after addition of the clearing buffer, the coloured colloidal gold conjugates of anti-HRP-2 antibody, anti-*P. vivax* specific pLDH antibody and anti-pan specific pLDH antibody complexes the HRP-2/corresponding pLDH in the lysed sample. This complex moves further on the membrane to the test region where it is immobilised by the monoclonal anti-Pf. HRP-2 antibody and/or monoclonal anti-*P. vivax* specific pLDH antibody and/or monoclonal pan specific pLDH antibody coated on the membrane leading to formation of a pink-purple coloured band in the respective regions which confirms a positive test result. Absence of a coloured band in the test region indicates a negative test result for the corresponding antigen. The unreacted conjugate along with the rabbit globulin colloidal gold conjugate and unbound complex if any, move further on the membrane and are subsequently immobilised by anti-rabbit antibodies coated on the membrane at the control region, forming a pink-purple band. This control band serves to validate the test performance.

Reagents and Material Supplied

Paramax-3 kit contains:

A. Individual pouches, each containing:
   1. Test Device Membrane assembly predispensed with monoclonal anti-HRP-2 antibody-colloidal gold conjugate, monoclonal anti-*P.vivax* specific pLDH antibody-colloidal gold conjugate, monoclonal anti-pan specific pLDH antibody-colloidal gold conjugate, rabbit globulin colloidal gold conjugate, monoclonal anti-Pf. HRP-2 antibody, monoclonal anti-*P. vivax* specific pLDH antibody, monoclonal anti-pan specific pLDH antibody and anti-rabbit antibody at the respective regions.
   2. Desiccant pouch.
   3. 5 μl sample loop.

B. Clearing buffer in a dropper bottle.

C. Package insert.

Optional Material Required

Calibrated micropipettes capable of delivering 5 µl sample accurately.

Storage and Stability

The test kit may be stored between 4-30°C till the duration of the shelf-life as indicated on the pouch/ carton. Do not freeze.

Note

Read the instructions carefully before performing the test. For *in vitro* diagnostic use only. Not for Medicinal Use. Do not use beyond expiry date. Do not intermix reagents from different lots. Handle all specimens as potentially infectious. Follow standard biosafety guidelines for handling and disposal of potentially infective material.

Specimen Collection and Preparation

Fresh anticoagulated whole blood should be used as a test sample and EDTA or Heparin or Oxalate can be used as suitable anticoagulant. The specimen should be collected in a clean glass or plastic container. If immediate testing is not possible, then the specimen may be stored at 2 to 8°C for up to 72 hours before testing. Clotted or contaminated blood samples should not be used for performing the test. Fresh blood from finger prick/puncture may also be used as a test specimen.

Test Procedure

1. Bring the Paramax-3 kit components to room temperature before testing.
2. Open the pouch and retrieve the device, sample loop and desiccant. Check the colour of the desiccant. It should be blue. If it has turned colourless or pink, discard the device and use another device. *Once opened, the device must be used immediately.*
3. Tighten the vial cap of the clearing buffer provided with the kit in the clockwise direction to pierce the dropper bottle nozzle.
4. Evenly mix the anticoagulated blood sample by gentle swirling. Dip the sample loop into the sample. Ensuring that a loop full of blood is retrieved, blot the blood so collected onto the sample pad in the sample port 'A' (this delivers approximately 5 µl of the whole blood specimen).
   Or
   In case finger prick blood is being used, touch the sample loop to the blood on the finger prick. Ensuring that a loop full of blood is retrieved, immediately blot the specimen on to the sample pad in the sample port 'A'. (Care should be taken that the blood sample has not clotted and the transfer to the sample pad is immediate).
   Or
   Alternatively, 5 µl of the anti coagulated or finger prick specimen may be delivered to the sample pad in the sample port 'A' using a micro pipette.
   Note: Ensure that the blood from the sample loop has been completely taken up by the sample pad.
5. Dispense four drops of the clearing buffer into port 'B', by holding the plastic dropper bottle vertically.
6. At the end of 15 minutes, read the results as follows.

Negative for Malaria

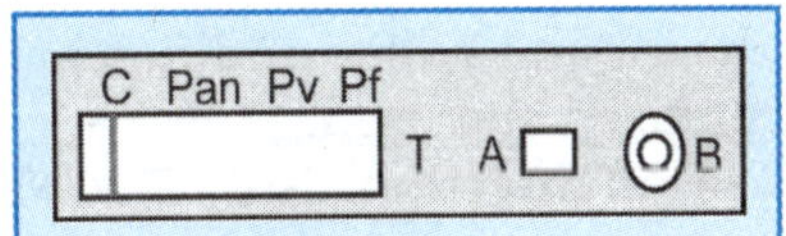

- Only one pink-purple band appears at the control region 'C'.

Positive for Malaria

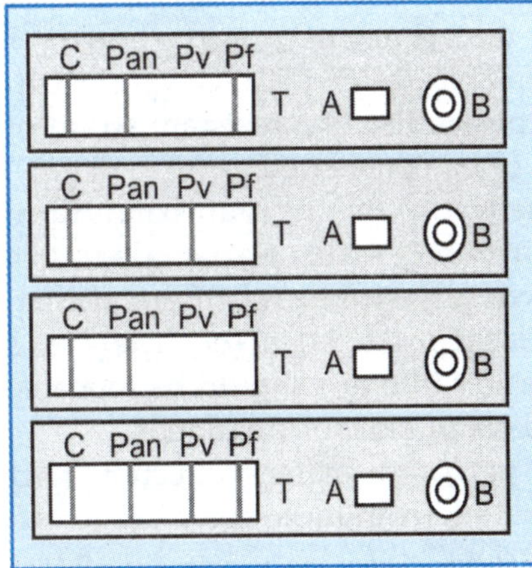

- *P. falciparum* malaria: In addition to the control band, a pink-purple band appears at the 'Pf' and 'Pan' regions respectively.
- *P. vivax* malaria: In addition to the control band, a pink-purple band appears at 'Pv' and 'Pan' regions respectively.
- Other species: In addition to the control band, one pink-purple band appears only at 'Pan' region.

- Mixed infection: In addition to the control band, a pink-purple band appears at 'Pf', 'Pv' and 'Pan' regions respectively.

7. The test should be considered invalid if no bands appear on the device. Repeat the test with a new device ensuring that the test procedure has been followed accurately.

Limitation of the Test

1. As with all diagnostic tests, the test result must always be correlated with clinical findings.
2. The results of test are to be interpreted within the epidemiological, clinical and therapeutic context. When it seems indicated, the parasitological techniques of reference should be considered (microscopic examination of the thick smear and thin blood films).
3. Any modification to the above procedure and/or use of other reagents will invalidate the test procedure.
4. The device and buffer of different lots must not be mixed and used.
5. In case of infection due to *P.vivax or P. falciparum*, or due to mixed infection by these species, the 'Pan' malaria band will also be positive. Hence, differentiation of infection due to *P. ovale* or *P.malariae* cannot be done.
6. While monitoring therapy, if the reaction of the test remains positive with the same intensity after 5 to 10 days, post-treatment, the possibility of a resistant strain of malaria has to be considered.
7. Usually, the 'Pv' and 'Pan' bands turn negative after successful anti-malarial therapy. However, since treatment duration and medication used affect the clearance of parasites, the test should be repeated after 5-10 days of start of treatment.
8. In *P. falciparum* malaria infection, HRP-2 is not secreted in gametogony stage. Hence, in "Carriers", the HRP-2 band may be absent.
9. The HRP-2 levels, post-treatment, persist up to 15 days, the 'Pan' band can be used to monitor success of therapy, in *P. falciparum* malaria cases.
10. In a few cases, where the HRP-2 band is positive and the 'Pan' malaria band is negative, it may indicate a case of post-treatment malaria. However, such a reaction pattern may also be obtained in a few cases of untreated malaria. Retesting after 2 days is advised, in such cases.

SLIDE TEST FOR C-REACTIVE PROTEIN (Rhelax CRP), Courtesy: Tulip Group of Companies

Summary

The C-reactive protein (CRP) is a serum protein which is synthesised in the liver. Its rate of synthesis and secretion increases within hours of an acute injury or the onset of inflammation and may reach as high as 20 times the normal levels. Elevated serum concentration of CRP is an unequivocal evidence of an active tissue damage process; and CRP measurement, thus provides a simple screening test for organic disorders. Apart from indicating inflammatory disorders, CRP measurement helps in differential diagnosis, in the management of neonatal septicaemia and meningitis where standard microbiological investigations are difficult.

Its use in postoperative surveillance is of great importance. CRP levels invariably rise after major surgery but fall to normal within 7-10 days. Absence of this fall is indicative of possible septic or inflammatory postoperative complications. Serum CRP measurement also provides useful information in patients with myocardial infarction there being an excellent correlation between peak levels of CRP and creatine phosphokinase (CPK).

Reagent

1. RHELAX CRP reagent: A uniform suspension of polystyrene latex particles coated with anti-CRP antibodies. The reagent is standardised to detect CRP concentrations greater than 0.6 mg/dl.
2. Positive control, reactive with RHELAX CRP reagent.
3. Negative control, non-reactive with RHELAX CRP reagent.

Each batch of reagents undergoes rigorous quality control at various stages of manufacture for its specificity, sensitivity and performance.

Reagent Storage and Stability

1. Store the reagent at 2 to 8°C. Do not freeze.
2. The shelf-life of reagent is as per the expiry date mentioned on the reagent vial label.

Principle

The RHELAX CRP slide test for detection of CRP is based on the principle of agglutination. The test specimen (serum) is mixed with RHELAX CRP latex reagent and allowed to react. If CRP concentration is greater than 0.6 mg/dl, a visible agglutination is observed. If CRP concentration is less than 0.6 mg/dl, then no agglutination is observed.

Note

1. *In vitro* diagnostic reagent for laboratory and professional use only. Not for medicinal use.
2. All the reagents derived from human source have been tested for HBsAg and anti-HIV antibodies and are found to be nonreactive.
3. The Reagent contains sodium azide 0.1% as preservative. Avoid contact with skin and mucosa. On disposal, flush with large quantities of water.
4. The reagent can be damaged due to microbial contamination or on exposure to extreme temperatures. It is recommended that the performance of the reagent be verified with the positive and negative controls provided with the kit.
5. Shake the latex reagent well before use to disperse the latex particles uniformly and improve test readability.
6. Only a clean and dry glass slide must be used. Clean the slide with distilled water and wipe dry.
7. Accessories provided with the kit only must be used for optimum results.

Specimen Collection and Preparation

No special preparation of the patient is required prior to specimen collection by approved techniques.

Only serum should be used for testing. Should a delay in testing occur, store the sample at 2 to 8°C. Samples can be stored for up to a week. Do not use hemolysed serum.

Material Provided with the Kit

Reagent

The RHELAX CRP latex reagent, positive control, negative control.

Accessories

Glass slide with six reaction circles, sample dispensing pipettes, mixing sticks, rubber teat.

Additional Material Required

Stopwatch, test tubes, a high intensity direct light source, isotonic saline.

Test Procedure

Bring reagent and samples to room temperature before testing.

Qualitative Method

1. Pipette one drop of the test specimen (serum) on the glass slide using a disposable pipette provided with the kit.
2. Add one drop of RHELAX CRP latex reagent to the drop of test specimen on the slide. Do not let the dropper tip touch the liquid on the slide.
3. Using a mixing stick, mix the test specimen and the RHELAX CRP latex reagent uniformly over the entire circle.
4. Immediately start a stopwatch. Rock the slide gently back and forth, observing for agglutination macroscopically at two minutes.

Semiquantitative Method

1. Using isotonic saline, prepare serial dilutions of the test specimen positive in the qualitative method 1:2, 1:4, 1:8, 1:16 and so on.
2. Pipette each dilution of the test specimen onto separate reaction circles.
3. Add one drop of RHELAX CRP latex reagent to the drop of test specimen on the slide. Do not let the dropper tip touch the liquid on the slide.
4. Using a mixing stick, mix the test specimen and the latex reagent uniformly over the entire circle.
5. Immediately start a stopwatch. Rock the slide gently, back and forth, observing for agglutination macroscopically at two minutes.

Interpretation of Test Results Qualitative Method

Agglutination is a positive test result and indicates the presence of detectable levels of CRP in the test specimen. No agglutination is a negative test result and indicates the absence of detectable levels of CRP in the test specimen.

Semiquantitative Method

Agglutination in the highest serum dilution corresponds to the amount of CRP in mg/dl present in the test specimen.

Concentration of CRP can be calculated as follows:

CRP (mg/dl) = S × D

where S = Sensitivity of the reagent, i.e. 0.6 mg/dl.

D = Highest dilution of serum showing agglutination.

Remarks

1. Markedly lipaemic, haemolysed and contaminated serum samples could produce nonspecific results.
2. Use of plasma rather than serum can lead to false-positive results.
3. The CRP is found to be present after the first trimester of pregnancy and persists until delivery.
4. The CRP levels increase in women who are on oral contraceptives.
5. The CRP response is not affected by the commonly used anti-inflammatory or immunosuppresive drugs, including steroids, unless the disease activity is affected and it covers an exceptionally broad incremental range upto 3000 times.
6. Do not read results beyond indicated testing time limits.
7. Since CRP production is a non-specific response to tissue injury, it is recommended that results of the test should be correlated with clinical findings to arrive at the final diagnosis.
8. In cases where an increase in CRP levels is suspected, but the screening test shows a negative result, semiquantitation should be done to rule out prozone effect.

SLIDE TEST FOR ANTI STREPTOLYSIN O (Rhelax ASO), Courtesy: Tulip Group of Companies

Summary

Streptococcus belongs to the family of Lactobacillaceae and the majority are facultative anaerobes. The facultative anaerobic streptococci are divided into two categories:

a. those which produce soluble haemolysin and
b. those which do not produce soluble haemolysin

The first group of streptococci are called (3-haemolytic streptococci which can be further subdivided into group (a), group (b), group (c) and group (d). It includes most of the species associated with primary streptococcal infections in humans. The group (a) (3-haemolytic streptococci produce various exotoxins such as streptolysin O and streptolysin S that can act as antigens. The affected individuals produce specific antibodies against streptolysin O, namely anti streptolysin O (ASO). Determination of these antibodies is very useful for the diagnosis of streptococcal infections and their relative effects such as rheumatic fever and acute glomerulonephritis. An elevated ASO titre of more than 200 IU/ml may indicate an acute streptococcal infection.

Reagent

1. RHELAX ASO reagent: A uniform suspension of polystyrene latex particles coated with streptolysin O.
2. Positive control, reactive with RHELAX ASO reagent.
3. Negative control, nonreactive with RHELAX ASO reagent.

The RHELAX ASO reagent system is standardised to detect antibodies to streptolysin O in concentrations ranging from 200 to 4000 IU/ml.

Each batch of reagents undergoes rigorous quality control at various stages of manufacture for its specificity, sensitivity and performance.

Reagent Storage and Stability

1. Store the reagent at 2 to 8°C. Do not freeze.
2. The shelf-life of reagent is as per the expiry date mentioned on the reagent vial labels.

Principle

The RHELAX ASO slide test for detection of antibodies to streptolysin O is based on the principle of agglutination. The test specimen (serum) is mixed with RHELAX ASO latex reagent and allowed to react. If antibodies to streptolysin O are present in concentrations more than 200 IU/ml, but less than 4000 IU/ml, then a visible agglutination is observed.

If antibodies to streptolysin O are not present or are in concentrations less than 200 IU/ml, then no agglutination will be observed.

Note

1. *In vitro* diagnostic reagent for laboratory and professional use only. Not for medicinal use.
2. All the reagents derived from human source have been tested for HBsAg and anti-HIV antibodies and are found to be non-reactive. However, handle the material as if infectious.
3. The reagent contains sodium azide 0.1% as preservative. Avoid contact with skin and mucosa. On disposal, flush with large quantities of water.
4. The reagent can be damaged due to microbial contamination or on exposure to extreme temperatures. It is recommended that the performance of the reagent be verified with the positive and negative controls provided with the kit.
5. Shake the RHELAX ASO latex reagent well before use to disperse the latex particles uniformly and improve test readability.
6. Only a clean and dry glass slide must be used. Clean the slide with distilled water and wipe dry.
7. Accessories provided with the kit only must be used for optimum results.

Specimen Collection and Preparation

No special preparation of the patient is required prior to specimen collection by approved techniques.

Only serum should be used for testing. Should a delay in testing occur, store the sample at 2 to 8°C. Samples can be stored for up to a week. Do not use haemolysed serum.

Material Provided with the Kit

Reagent

RHELAX ASO latex reagent, positive control, negative control.

Accessories

Glass slide with six reaction circles, sample dispensing pipettes, mixing sticks, rubber teat.

Additional Material Required

Stopwatch, high intensity direct light source, isotonic saline, pipettetes, test tubes.

Test Procedure

Bring reagent and samples to room temperature before testing.

Qualitative Method

1. Pipettete one drop of test sample onto the glass slide using a disposable pipette provided with the kit.
2. Add one drop of RHELAX ASO latex reagent to the drop of test sample on the slide.
3. Using a mixing stick, mix the serum and the RHELAX ASO latex reagent uniformly over the entire circle. Do not let the dropper tip touch the liquid on the slide.
4. Immediately start a stopwatch. Rock the slide gently, back and forth, observing for agglutination macroscopically at two minutes.

Semiquantitative Method

1. Using isotonic saline, prepare serial dilutions of the serum sample positive in the qualitative method 1:2, 1:4, 1:8, 1:16 and so on.
2. Pipette the diluted specimens onto the slide. Start with the 1:2 diluted test specimen.
3. Add a drop of RHELAX ASO reagent to it and mix well. Spread the mixture uniformly over the entire circle.
4. Immediately start a stopwatch. Rock the slide gently, back and forth, observing for agglutination macroscopically at two minutes. Proceed similarly with each dilution as test specimen.

INTERPRETATION OF TEST RESULTS

Qualitative Method

Agglutination is a positive test result and indicates the presence of detectable levels of antistreptolysin O in the test specimen.

No agglutination is a negative test result and indicates the absence of detectable levels of antistreptolysin O in the test specimen.

Semiquantitative Method

Agglutination in the highest serum dilution corresponds to the amount of ASO in IU/ml present in the test specimen. The concentration of ASO can be calculated as follows:

ASO (IU/ml) = S × D

where S = Sensitivity of the reagent, i.e. 200 IU/ml.

D = Highest dilution of serum showing agglutination.

Remarks

1. Markedly lipaemic, haemolysed and contaminated serum samples could produce non-specific results.
2. Serum samples having markedly higher protein content may produce nonspecific reagent aggregation.
3. Use of plasma rather than serum can lead to false-positive results.
4. Do not read results beyond two minutes.
5. It is recommended that all positive test results should be further tested with methods enabling quantitation of ASO titres.
6. It is recommended that results of the tests should be correlated with clinical findings to arrive at the final diagnosis.

SLIDE TEST FOR RHEUMATOID FACTORS (Rhelax RF), Courtesy: Tulip Group of Companies

Summary

Sometimes autoantibodies are produced by the human body against self-antigens. The precise role that this aberrant immunity plays in the pathogenesis of certain rheumatic diseases is unknown. However, the presence of these autoantibodies serve as credible marker of the disease.

In rheumatoid arthritis, diagnostically useful autoantibodies termed as "Rheumatoid factors (RF) can be detected which are immunoglobulins of the classes IgM, IgG, IgA and IgE. Practically, IgM class RF with specificity to human IgG (Fc) is the most useful prognostic marker of RF. The clinical significance of RF determinations consists in differentiation between rheumatoid arthritis, in which RFs of modified IgM class have been demonstrated in the serum of approximately 80 percent of the cases examined and rheumatic fever, in which RFs are almost always absent. The agglutination test is most frequently used because of its greater sensitivity and simplicity. The RHELAX RF is a latex agglutination slide test for detection of rheumatoid factors of the IgM class.

Reagent

1. RHELAX RF reagent: A uniform suspension of polystyrene latex particles coated with suitably modified Fc fraction of IgG. The reagent is standardised to detect 10 IU/ml of RF or more.
2. Positive control, reactive with the RHELAX RF reagent.
3. Negative control, nonreactive with the RHELAX RF reagent.

Each batch of reagents undergoes rigorous quality control at various stages of manufacture for its specificity, sensitivity and performance.

Reagent Storage and Stability

1. Store the reagents at 2 to 8°C. Do not freeze.
2. The shelf-life of the reagent is as per the expiry date mentioned on the reagent vial label.

Principle

The RHELAX RF slide test for detection of rheumatoid factors is based on the principle of agglutination. The test specimen is mixed with RHELAX RF latex reagent and allowed to react. If RF is present within detectable levels, then a visible agglutination is observed. If RF is absent below detectable levels, then no agglutination is observed.

Note

1. *In vitro* diagnostic reagent for laboratory and professional use only. Not for medicinal use.
2. All the reagents derived from human source have been tested for HBsAg and anti-HIV antibodies and are found to be nonreactive. However, handle the material as if infectious.
3. The reagent contains sodium azide 0.1% as preservative. Avoid contact with skin and mucosa. On disposal, flush with large quantities of water.
4. The reagent can be damaged due to microbial contamination or on exposure to extreme

temperatures. It is recommended that the performance of the reagent be verified with the positive and negative controls provided with the kit.

5. Shake the RHELAX RF latex reagent well before use to disperse the latex particles uniformly and improve test readability.
6. Only a clean and dry glass slide must be used. Clean the slide with distilled water and wipe dry.
7. Accessories provided with the kit only must be used for optimum results.

Specimen Collection and Preparation

No special preparation of the patient is required prior to specimen collection by approved techniques,

Only serum should be used for testing. Should a delay in testing occur, store the sample at 2 to 8°C. Samples can be stored for up to a week. Do not use haemolysed serum.

Material Provided with the Kit

Reagent

Rhelax RF latex reagent, positive control, negative control.

Accessories

Glass slide with six reaction circles, sample dispensing pipettes, mixing sticks, rubber teat.

Additonal Material Required

Stopwatch, test tubes, high intensity direct light source, isotonic saline.

Test Procedure

Bring reagent and samples to room temperature before use.

Qualitative Method

1. Pipette one drop of serum onto the glass slide using the disposable pipette provided with the kit.
2. Add one drop of RHELAX RF latex reagent to the drop of serum on the slide. Do not let the dropper tip touch the liquid on the slide.
3. Using a mixing stick, mix the serum and the RHELAX RF latex reagent uniformly over the entire circle.
4. Immediately start a stopwatch. Rock the slide gently, back and forth, observing for agglutination macroscopically at two minutes.

Semiquantitative Method

1. Using isotonic saline, prepare serial dilutions of the serum sample positive in the qualitative method 1:2, 1:4, 1:8, 1:16, 1:32, 1:64 and so on.
2. Pipette each dilution of the serum sample onto separate reaction circles.
3. Add one drop of RHELAX RF latex reagent to each drop of the diluted serum sample on the slide. Do not let the dropper tip touch the liquid on the slide.
4. Using a mixing stick, mix the sample and the latex reagent uniformly over the entire circle.
5. Immediately start a stopwatch. Rock the slide gently, back and forth, observing for agglutination macroscopically at two minutes.

INTERPRETATION OF TEST RESULTS

Qualitative Method

Agglutination is a positive test result and indicates the presence of rheumatoid factors in the test specimen. No agglutination is a negative test result and indicates the absence of rheumatoid factors in the test specimen.

Semiquantitative Method

Agglutination in the highest serum dilution corresponds to the approximate amount of rheumatoid factors in IU/ml present in the test specimen.

To calculate the RF in lU/ml, use the following formula:

RF (IU/rnl) = S x D

Where S = Sensitivity of the reagent, i.e. 10 IU/ml.

D = Highest dilution of serum showing agglutination.

Remarks

1. Markedly lipaemic, haemolysed and contaminated serum samples could produce nonspecific results.
2. Use of plasma rather than serum can lead to false-positive results.

3. Do not read results beyond two minutes.
4. Rheumatoid factors are not exclusively found in rheumatoid arthritis but sometimes in syphilis, systemic lupus erythematosus, hepatitis, hypergammaglobulinaemia also.
5. It is recommended that results of the test should be correlated with clinical findings to arrive at the final diagnosis.
6. The RHELAX RF reagent is free from prozone effect at RF levels between 10 IU/ml to 2300 IU/ml of RF concentration.
7. The RHELAX RF reagent is sensitive to the presence of IgM RF with heterogeneous specificity.

Serological diagnosis rheumatic disorders with latex agglutination tests RF, CRP, ASL

Spectrum			*Probable diagnosis*	*Further test indicated*
Latex agglutination tests				
CRP	ASL	RF		
–	+	–	Rheumatic fever	Anti-streptolysin titre determination
+	+	–	Acute rheumatic fever	ADNase B, AHy, ANADase
–	–	+	Chronic polyarthritis (CP)	Quantitative RF determination
+	–	+	Inflammation in acute attack	Quantitative RF determination
+	–	–	Acute inflammatory (CP) (early stage)	Quantitative RF determination
–	–	+	Lupus erythematosus (LE), Polyarteritis nodosa, Dermatomyositis, Polymyositis, scleroderma	ANA (antinuclear Ab) Anti-ds-DNA against native double filament
–	–	–	Seronegative chronic polyarthritis (e.g., juvenile arthritis)	ANA/HLA B-27
(+)	–	–	Bechcet's disease	HLA B 27
			Collagen/MCTD (mixed connective tissue disease)	ANA, Anti-ds-DNA
			Reiter disease	HLA B 27, Yersinia antibody detection
			Psoriasis	-
			LE	ANA
			Pseudo-LE (drug induced)	AMA (antimitochondrial antibody)
+	–	–	Inflammatory-degenerative rheumatic disorders	—
			Gout (acute attack)	Uric acid
			Reactive arthritis (after infection)	Gonococcal detection, virus serology (e.g., Rubella infection)
+	–	+	By chronic appearance of age and other inflammatory conditions	Quantitative RF

– = Negative, + = Positive, (+) = Weakly positive

SLIDE TEST FOR ANTI DEOXYRIBONUCLEOPROTEIN (Rhelax SLE) Courtesy: Tulip Group of Companies

Summary

The presence of autoantibodies to nuclear proteins is a common finding in Systemic Lupus Erythematosus (SLE) and other collagen diseases.

Anti-DNP is present in high titres in the serum of majority of SLE patients with active disease but is present occasionally in remission states. Although anti-DNP is found exclusively in SLE, only low titres may be detected in diseases such as chronic hepatitis, periarteritis nodosa, dermatomyositis, scleroderma and drug hypersensitivity.

Reagent

The Rhelax SLE reagent is a ready-to-use uniform suspension of polystyrene latex particles coated with deoxyribonucleoprotein (DNP). Each batch of reagents undergoes rigorous quality control at various stages of manufacture for its specificity, sensitivity and performance.

Reagent Storage and Stability

Store the reagent at 2 to 8°C. Do not freeze. The shelf-life of the reagent is as per the expiry date mentioned on the reagent vial label.

Principle

Latex particles coated with DNP will agglutinate when mixed with serum containing anti-DNP. No agglutination indicates absence of anti-DNP in the serum.

Note

1. In vitro diagnostic reagent for laboratory and professional use only. Not for medicinal use.
2. All the components derived from human source have been tested for HBsAg and anti-HIV antibody and are found to be non-reactive. However, handle the material as if infectious.
3. The reagents contain sodium azide 0.1% as preservative. Avoid contact with skin and mucosa. On disposal, flush with large quantities of water.
4. The reagent can be damaged due to microbial contamination or exposure to extreme temperatures. It is recommended that the

performance of the reagent be verified with the positive and negative controls provided with the kit.

5. Shake the latex reagent well before use to disperse the latex particles uniformly and to improve test readability.
6. Only a clean and dry glass slide must be used. Clean the slide with distilled water and wipe dry.

Sample Collection and Preparation

No special preparation of the patient is required prior to sample collection by approved techniques. Use fresh clear serum samples. In case of delay in testing, store the serum samples at 2 to 8°C for up to 72 hours. For longer storage, freeze the serum. However, repeated freezing and thawing of samples should be avoided.

Material Provided with the Kit

Reagent Pack

Rhelax SLE latex reagent, positive control, negative control.

Accessories Pack

Glass slide with six reaction circles, mixing sticks, rubber teats, sample dispensing pipettes.

Additional Material Required

Test tube (10 × 75 mm), Pipettes, isotonic saline, stopwatch, direct light source.

TEST PROCEDURE

Bring all reagents and samples to room temperature before use.

Qualitative Method

1. Place one drop of sample to be tested onto one of the reaction circles of the glass slide using a sample dispensing pipette provided with the kit.
2. Place one drop of positive and negative control onto separate reaction circles of the glass slide.
3. Gently shake the latex reagent and add one drop to each sample and control taken on the slide.
4. Mix with separate mixing sticks, spreading the mixture uniformly over the entire reaction circle.
5. Immediately start a stopwatch. Rock the slide gently, back and forth, observing for agglutination macroscopically at three minutes.

Semiquantitative Method

1. Using isotonic saline prepare serial dilutions of the serum sample 1:2, 1:4, 1:8, 1:16, 1:32 and soon.
2. Place each dilution of the serum sample onto separate reaction circles of the slide.
3. Add one drop of well-mixed latex reagent to each dilution of the sample on the slide.
4. Mix with separate mixing sticks, spreading the mixture uniformly over the entire reaction circle.
5. Immediately start a stopwatch. Rock the slide gently, back and forth, observing for agglutination macroscopically at three minutes.

INTERPRETATION OF RESULTS

Qualitative Method

Agglutination is a positive test result and indicates presence of anti-DNP in the test specimen.

No agglutination is a negative test result and indicates absence of anti-DNP in the test specimen.

Semiquantitative Method

The titre of the serum is the reciprocal of the highest dilution which gives agglutination.

Remarks

1. Markedly lipaemic, haemolysed and contaminated serum samples could produce nonspecific results.
2. Use of plasma rather than serum can lead to false-positive results.
3. Anti-DNP may be found in diseases other than SLE. Low titres have been detected in rheumatoid arthritis, chronic hepatitis, periarteritis nodosa, dermatomyositis, scleroderma, atypical pneumonia, tuberculosis and lymphoma.

AUTOIMMUNE DISORDERS AND ANA

Introduction

If we have had mumps as children, we know that we are not susceptible to a second episode of mumps. We say we are immune to mumps. Here we have acquired immunity through natural exposure to the disease. If we are vaccinated or immunised, we acquire our immunity through an artificial means.

In other words, we acquire immunity, either through natural exposure to the disease or through artificial means, such as vaccination.

If immunity is going to benefit us, it has to be directed against something foreign, something outside the body. This implies that there is some mechanism by which the body can distinguish what is itself from what is not itself—we now say the immune response shows self, non-self discrimination.

A number of key discoveries were made—which turned that doctrine of self, non-self distinction on its head. It was found that there are a number of instances in which the immune response is directed to something in the body of the host itself. This is what we call Autoimmunity. Autoimmunity is nothing more than the immune response directed to the body of the patient himself or herself. When this produces a disease in a person, it is called autoimmune disease.

This LPAP contains information about autoimmunity and autoimmune diseases. Since autoimmune diseases are complex, the information presented here is restricted to basics and moves to greater depths when it comes to the diagnosis of the disease.

How does the Immune System Work?

The immune system defends the body from attack by invaders recognised as foreign. It is an extraordinarily complex system that relies on an elaborate and dynamic communications network that exists among the many different kinds of immune system cells that patrol the body. At the heart of the system is the ability to recognise and respond to substances called *antigens* whether they are infectious agents or part of the body (self-antigens) (Fig. 23.22).

- Our immune response is of two kinds
- Cell mediated immune response
- Humoral immune response

Cell-mediated immune response is mounted by the immune system with the help of T cells (T lymphocytes) and macrophages, where they attack the antigen directly.

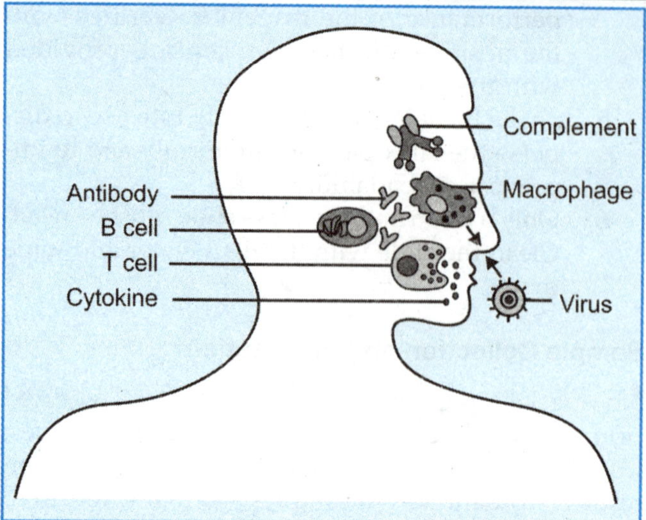

Fig. 23.22: Cells and molecules of the immune system protect the nose from attack by a virus

The humoral response is the result of the collaboration between macrophages, T cells and B cells (B lymphocytes), wherein the macrophages activate the T cells, and the T cells activate the B cells to start producing antibodies to bring about the destruction of the antigen.

Thus, the overall performance of the immune mechanisms depends mainly on the degree of reactivity of the T cell population, whether it is the cell-mediated immunity or the humoral immune response.

Components of the Immune System

Macrophages and Neutrophils: *Housekeeper and frontline defender.*

Macrophages and neutrophils circulate in the blood and survey the body for foreign substances. When they find foreign antigens, such as bacteria, they engulf and destroy them (Fig. 23.23).

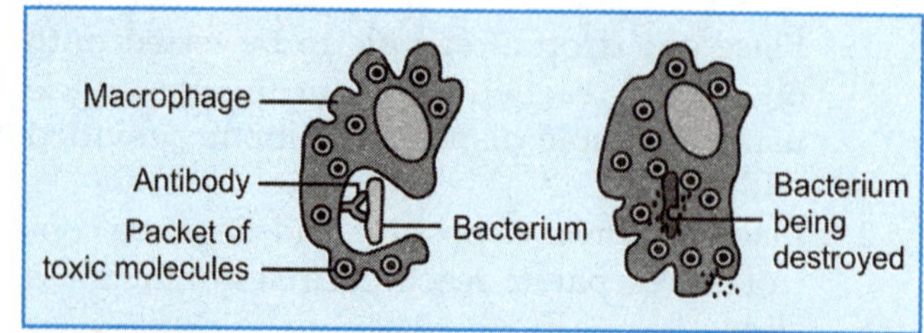

Fig. 23.23: A macrophage engulfing a bacterium and releasing packets of toxic molecules (reactive oxygen intermediates) that break down and destroy the bacterium

If production of these toxic molecules continues unchecked, not only are the foreign antigens destroyed, but tissues surrounding the macrophages and neutrophils are also destroyed. For example, in individuals with the autoimmune disease called Wegener's granulomatosis, overactive macrophages and neutrophils that invade blood vessels produce many toxic molecules and contribute to the damage of the blood vessels. In rheumatoid arthritis, reactive oxygen intermediate molecules and other toxic molecules are made by overproductive macrophages and neutrophils invading the joints. The toxic molecules contribute to inflammation, which is observed as warmth and swelling, and participate in damage to the joint.

T-Cells: T cells are critical immune system cells that help to destroy infected cells and coordinate the overall immune response. The T cell has a molecule on its surface called the *T-cell receptor*. This receptor interacts with molecules called *MHC (major histocompatibility complex)*. The MHC molecules are on the surfaces of most other cells of the body and help T cells recognise antigen fragments (Fig. 23.24).

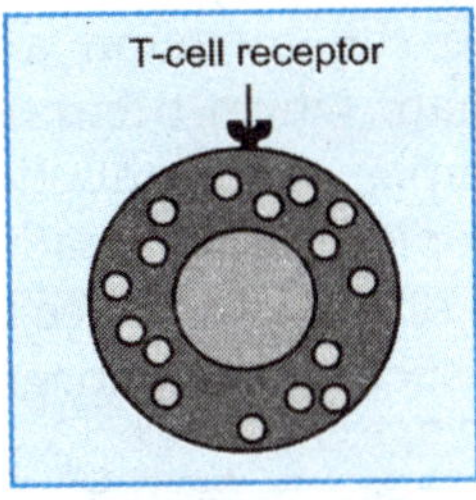

Fig. 23.24: T-cell receptor

Helper T-Cell: *Commander-in-chief of the immune system*

It identifies the enemy and rushes to the spleen and lymph nodes where it stimulates the production of other cells to fight the infection.

Killer T Cell: *Recruited and activated by helper T cells*

It specialises in killing cells of the body that have been invaded by foreign organisms as well as that have turned cancerous.

Suppressor T Cell: *Keeping in control*

A third type of T cell, it is able to slow down or stop the activities of B cells and other T cells playing a vital role in calling off the attack after an infection has been conquered.

B Cell: *Biologic arms factory*

B cells are another critical type of immune system cell. They participate in the removal of foreign antigens from the body by using a surface molecule to bind the antigen or by making specific antibodies that can search out and destroy specific foreign antigens. However, the B cell can only make antibodies when it receives the appropriate command signal from a T cell. Once the T cell signals the B cell with a type of cytokine that acts as a messenger molecule, the B cell is able to produce a unique antibody that targets a particular antigen (Fig. 23.25).

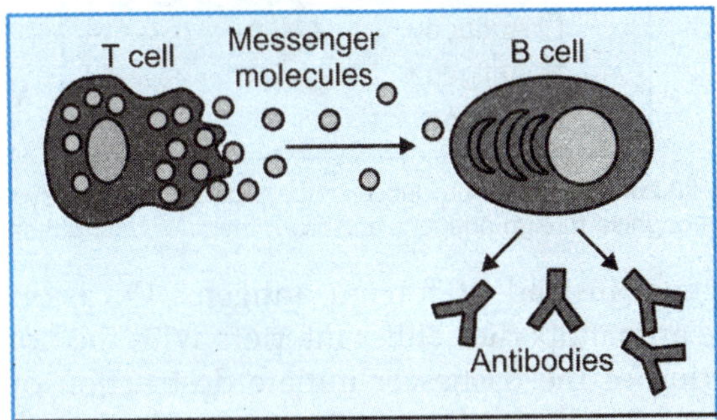

Fig. 23.25: A T cell sends messenger molecules, e.g. cytokines, to the B cell, which allow the B cell to start making antibodies

Antibody: *Ammunition of the immune system*

Engineered to target a specific invader, this Y-shaped protein molecule is rushed to the infection site where it either neutralizes the enemy or tags it for attack by other cells or chemicals.

The antibodies that B cells produce are basic templates with a special region that is highly specific to target a given antigen.

Different antibodies are destined for different purposes. Some coat the foreign invaders to make them attractive to the circulating scavenger cells, phagocytes, that will engulf an unwelcome microbe.

When some antibodies combine with antigens, they activate a cascade of nine proteins, known as complement, that have been circulating in inactive form in the blood. Complement forms a partnership with antibodies, once they have reacted with antigen, to help destroy foreign invaders and remove them from the body. Still other types of antibodies block viruses from entering cells (Fig. 23.26).

Autoantibodies

In some autoimmune diseases, B cells mistakenly make antibodies against tissues of the body (self-

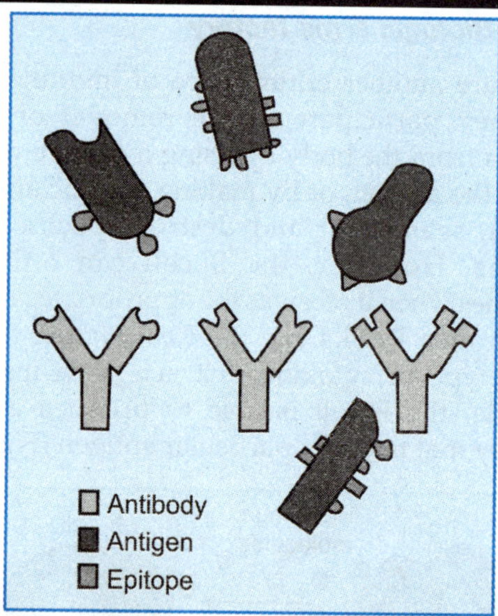

Fig. 23.26: Antibodies produced by cells of the immune system recognise foreign antigens and mark them for destruction

antigens) instead of foreign antigens. Occasionally, these autoantibodies either interfere with the normal function of the tissues or initiate destruction of the tissues. People with myasthenia gravis experience muscle weakness because autoantibodies attack a part of the nerve that stimulates muscle movement. In the skin disease pemphigus vulgaris, autoantibodies are misdirected against cells in the skin. The accumulation of antibodies in the skin activates other molecules and cells to break down, resulting in skin blisters.

Memory Cell: *Watchdogs of the immune system*

Generated during an initial infection this defense may circulate in the blood or lymph for years, enabling the body to respond more quickly to subsequent infections.

Antigen Presenting Cells

When a virus infects a cell, an MHC molecule binds to a piece of a virus (antigen) and displays the antigen on the cell's surface. Cells that have the capability of displaying antigen with MHC are called antigen-presenting cells. Each MHC molecule that displays an antigen is recognised by a matching or compatible T-cell receptor. Thus, an *antigen-presenting cell* is able to communicate with a T cell about what may be occurring inside the cell (Fig. 23.27).

Cytokines and Chemokines: Couriers of the immune system

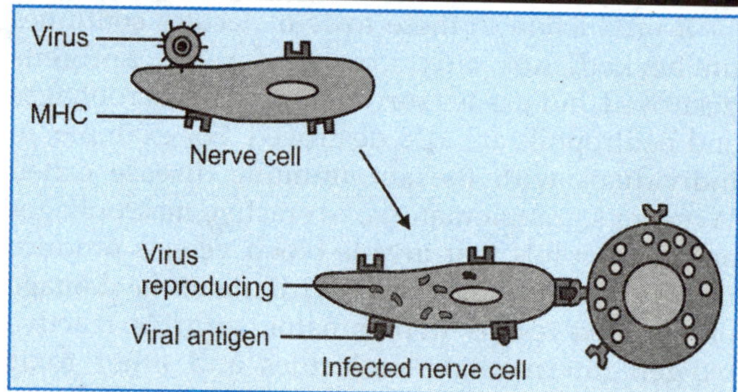

Fig. 23.27: A virus attacking a nerve cell. Lower right: a T cell with a T-cell receptor recognising a piece of a virus (antigen) on the MHC of the infected never cell

These are proteins by which immune cells communicate with each other.

Cytokines are proteins that may cause surrounding immune system cells to become activated, grow, or die. They also may influence nonimmune system tissues. For example, some cytokines may contribute to the thickening of the skin that occurs in people with scleroderma.

Chemokines are small cytokine molecules that attract cells of the immune system. Overproduction of chemokines contributes to the invasion and inflammation of the target organ, which occurs in autoimmune diseases. For example, overproduction of chemokines in the joints of people with rheumatoid arthritis may result in invasion of the joint space by destructive immune system cells such as macrophages, neutrophils, and T cells (Fig. 23.28).

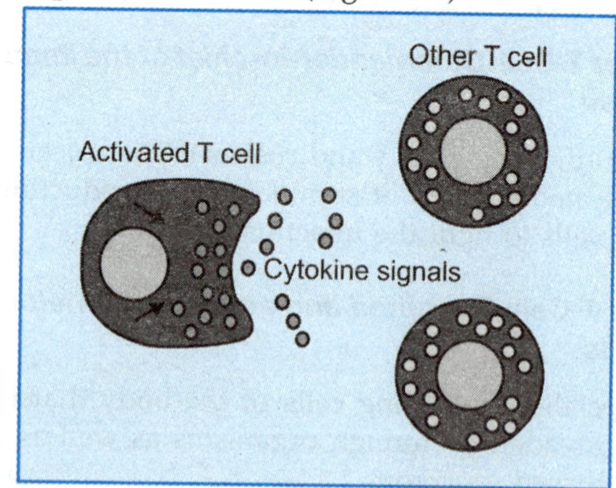

Fig. 23.28: After the antigen-presenting cell and T cell interact through the MHC, T-cell receptor and co-stimulatory and molecules, the T cell becomes activated, sending cytokine signals to other cells

Immune Complexes and the Complement System

When many antibodies are bound to antigens in the bloodstream, they form a large lattice network called an *immune complex*. Immune complexes are harmful when they accumulate and initiate inflammation within small blood vessels that nourish tissues. Immune complexes, immune cells, and inflammatory molecules can block blood flow and ultimately destroy organs such as the kidney. This can occur in people with systemic lupus erythematosus (SLE) (Fig. 23.29).

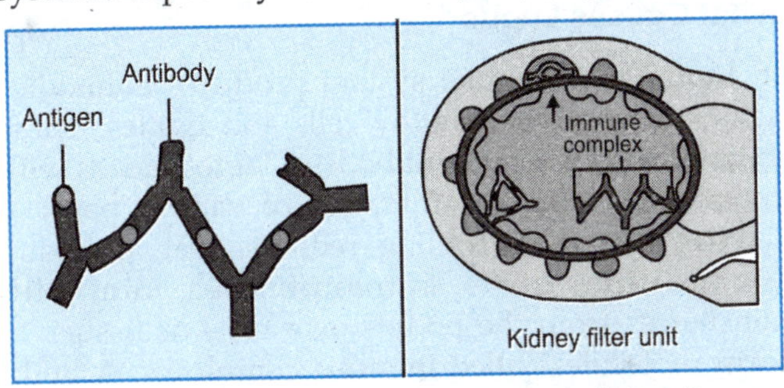

Fig. 23.29 : If immune complexes accumulate in the kidney, they may promote movement of other inflammatory cells and molecules into the kidney

What Happens During an Immune Response

The forces multiply: Once activated, helper T cells begin to multiply. They then stimulate the multiplication of those few killer T cells and B cells that are insensitive to the invading antigens. As the number of B cells increase, helper T cells signal them to start producing antibodies.

Conquering the infection: Meanwhile some of the antigens (e.g. virus) has entered cells of the body, the only place they are able to replicate. Killer T cells will surface these cells by chemically puncturing their membranes letting the contents spill out thus disrupting the antigen. Antibodies then neutralise the antigens by binding directly to their surfaces preventing them from attacking other cells. Additionally, they precipitate chemical reactions that actually destroy infected cells.

Calling a Truce: As the invasion by the antigen is contained, suppressor T cells halt the entire range of immune responses preventing them from spiraling out of control. Memory T and B cells are left in the blood and lymphatic system ready to move quickly should the same antigen once again invade the body.

Classification of Autoimmune Disorders

Autoimmune disorders can be broadly classified as organ specific and nonorgan specific-systemic (since they are spread all over the body system).

In case of organ specific diseases, the auto antibodies are directed against the tissue cells of the concerned organ; whereas in systemic autoimmune disease, the autoantibodies are directed to the cellular core or parts of the core, of the tissues and the body cell nucleus.

Organ specific autoimmune diseases are mostly isolated in one organ and, therefore, the damage is also localised to the organ concerned. In systemic autoimmune diseases the damage of tissue is spread all over the body. However, main effects are subsequently felt at the kidney, skin and joints. The clinical symptoms are various and show a disseminated (diffused) picture.

The damage in autoimmune diseases is the consequence of precipitation of immune complexes on the concerned parts of the body.

Factors Influencing Autoimmunity

Sex: Autoimmune disorders appear more in women than men (9:1). Certain female hormones affect (influence) the autoantibody formation.

Genetics: It is a confirmed fact that autoantibodies are genetically transmittable and autoimmune diseases within families are very often seen. The HLA (human leukocyte antigens) association of many autoimmune disorders is another evidence of the genetic transmission of autoimmune disorders. Autoimmune diseases can be detected in persons of every age but many autoantibodies (such as RF, ANA, Anti-Tg Abs) are found more commonly in aged individuals than in young individuals.

Pregnancy: During pregnancy, some autoimmune disorders may surface. Clinical manifestations of SLE (or polyarthritis) are more common during pregnancy. Though pregnancy may be a cause of an autoimmune disorder but only when the pregnant female has previously acquired these genes from the parents. Such manifestations are normally not during the first but subsequent pregnancies.

Drugs: Drugs do cause the production of autoimmune Abs, especially procainmide and hydrazine which are used for the treatment of heart and they support the production of anti-SS DNA and anti-histone antibodies.

Environment: The SLE patients are very sensitive to radiation by sunlight, especially body parts like hands and face which are exposed. UV radiation accelerates the deterioration of disease status in SLE. In future cases of active SLE will probably increase due to worldwide increase in UV levels (deterioration of ozone layer).

SYSTEMIC LUPUS ERYTHEMATOSUS-SLE (LUPUS)

Lupus is a type of autoimmune disease. Lupus can affect many parts of the body, including the joints, skin, kidneys, heart, lungs, blood vessels, and brain. Although people with the disease may have many different symptoms, some of the most common ones include extreme fatigue, painful or swollen joints (arthritis), unexplained fever, skin rashes, and kidney problems. Lupus is also known as a rheumatic disease. The rheumatic diseases are a group of disorders that cause aches, pain, and stiffness in the joints, muscles, and bones.

At present, there is no cure for lupus. However, the symptoms of lupus can be controlled with appropriate treatment, and most people with the disease can lead active, healthy lives. Lupus is characterised by periods of illness, called flares, and periods of wellness, or remission. Understanding how to prevent flares and how to treat them when they do occur help people with lupus maintain better health. Intense research is underway and scientists are continuing to make great strides in understanding the disease, which ultimately may lead to a cure.

- Although "lupus" is used as a broad term, there actually are several kinds of lupus:
- Systemic lupus erythematosus (SLE) is the form of the disease that most people are referring to when they say "lupus." The word "systemic" means the disease can affect many parts of the body. The symptoms of SLE may be mild or serious. Although SLE usually first affects people between the ages of 15 and 45 years, it can occur in childhood or later in life as well.
- Discoid lupus erythematosus is a type of lupus that primarily affects the skin. A red, raised rash may appear on the face, scalp, or elsewhere. The raised areas may become thick and scaly. The rash may last for days or years and may recur. A small percentage of people with discoid lupus later develop SLE.
- Drug-induced lupus refers to a form of lupus caused by medication.
- Neonatal lupus can affect some newborn babies of women with SLE or certain other immune system disorders. Babies with neonatal lupus may have a serious heart defect. Neonatal lupus is very rare, and most infants of mothers with SLE are entirely healthy.

What Causes Lupus

In lupus, the immune system produces antibodies against the body's healthy cells and tissues. These antibodies, called autoantibodies ("auto" means self), contribute to the inflammation of various parts of the body, causing swelling, redness, heat, and pain. In addition, some autoantibodies join with substances from the body's own cells or tissues to form molecules called immune complexes. A build up of these immune complexes in the body also contributes to inflammation and tissue injury in people with lupus.

Symptoms of Lupus

Each person's experience with lupus is different. Symptoms can range from mild to severe and may come and go over time. Common symptoms of lupus include extreme fatigue, painful or swollen joints, unexplained fever, and skin rashes. A characteristic skin rash may appear across the nose and cheeks—the so-called butterfly or malar rash. Other rashes occur elsewhere on the face and ears, upper arms, shoulders, chest, and hands.

Other symptoms of lupus include chest pain, hair loss, sensitivity to the sun, anaemia (a decrease in red blood cells), and pale or purple fingers and toes from cold and stress. Some people also experience headaches, dizziness, depression, or seizures. New symptoms may continue to appear years after the initial diagnosis, and different symptoms can occur at different times.

Common Symptoms of Lupus

- Painful or swollen joints and muscle pain
- Unexplained fever
- Extreme fatigue
- Red rash or colour change on the face
- Chest pain upon deep breathing
- Unusual loss of hair
- Pale or purple fingers or toes from cold or stress (Raynaud's phenomenon)

- Sensitivity to the sun
- Swelling (oedema) in legs or around eyes
- Swollen glands

In some people with lupus, only one system of the body such as the skin or joints is affected. Other people experience symptoms in many parts of their body. Just how seriously a body system is affected also varies from person to person. Most commonly, joints and muscles are affected, causing arthritis and muscle pain. Skin rashes also are quite common. The following systems in the body also can be affected by lupus, kidneys, central nervous system, blood vessels, blood, lungs, and heart.

Diagnosing Lupus

Diagnosing lupus can be difficult. It may take months or even years for doctors to piece together the symptoms to accurately diagnose this complex disease. Making a correct diagnosis of lupus requires knowledge and awareness on the part of the doctor and good communication on the part of the patient. This information, along with a physical examination and the results of laboratory tests, helps the doctor consider other diseases that may mimic lupus, or determine if the patient truly has the disease.

No single test can determine whether a person has lupus, but several laboratory tests may help the doctor to make a diagnosis. The most useful tests are blood tests that identify certain autoantibodies often present in people with lupus.

Some tests are used less frequently but may be helpful if the cause of a person's symptoms remains unclear. The doctor may order a biopsy of the skin or kidneys if those body systems are affected. Some doctors may order a syphilis test because some lupus antibodies in the blood may cause the test to be falsely positive. A positive test does not mean that a patient has syphilis. Again, all these tests merely serve as tools to give the doctor clues and information in making a diagnosis. The doctor will look at the entire picture—medical history, symptoms, and test results—to determine if a person has lupus.

Other laboratory tests are used to monitor the progress of the disease once it has been diagnosed. A complete blood count (CBC), urinalysis, blood chemistries, and erythrocyte sedimentation rate (ESR) test can provide valuable information (the ESR is a measure of inflammation in the body). It tests how quickly red blood cells drop to the bottom of a tube of unclotted blood.) Another common test measures the blood level of a group of proteins called complement. People with lupus often have low complement levels, especially during flares of the disease.

Treating Lupus

Several types of drugs are used to treat lupus. The treatment the doctor chooses is based on the patient's individual symptoms and needs. For people with joint pain, fever, and swelling, drugs that decrease inflammation, referred to as nonsteroidal anti-inflammatory drugs (NSAIDs), are often used.

Antimalarials are another type of drug commonly used to treat lupus. The mainstay of lupus treatment involves the use of corticosteroid hormones. Corticosteroids are related to cortisol, which is a natural anti-inflammatory hormone. They work by rapidly suppressing inflammation. For patients who cannot take corticosteroids, a type of immuno-suppressive drug called methotrexate may be used to help control the disease.

SCLERODERMA

Scleroderma is a chronic disease of the connective tissues (skin, ligaments, cartilage and bone), which results from an overproduction of the protein collagen. The terms "sclero" or "sclerosis" refer to the process of hardening, particularly due to excessive growth of fibrous tissue. "Derma" refers to the skin. Scleroderma causes a hardening of the skin and other tissues or organs. Because connective tissue is found throughout the body, scleroderma also can affect internal organs.

The disease is very individualised and can range from mild to lifethreatening. When the skin is affected, symptoms are visible. When internal organs and structures are affected but the skin is not, the disease may not be apparent. Nonetheless, involvement of internal organs and tissues signals a more severe form of scleroderma.

Causes

The precise cause of scleroderma is not known. It is considered an "autoimmune disease," which means that the body's immune system reacts against itself, causing an overproduction of collagen. Some people appear to have a genetic predisposition to developing the disease, but it is not directly inherited. Environment also may play a causal role. Despite the body's uncontrolled production of collagen, scleroderma is not malignant (cancerous). Nearly 80 percent of people with scleroderma are female.

Symptoms of Scleroderma

Symptoms vary widely between individuals, but may include:

- Thickening of the skin
- Swelling of the hands and feet
- Pain and stiffness in the joints
- Aching of the muscles, joints and bones
- Problems with the digestive system
- Sjögren's syndrome (dry mucous membranes)
- Oral, facial and dental problems
- Complications of the heart, lungs, kidneys and other internal organs.
- High blood pressure
- General weakness and fatigue
- Weight loss.

There are several classifications of scleroderma, based on the areas affected and the degree of severity.

1. Localised (or "limited") scleroderma:
   - Usually confined to a few areas of skin, such as the fingers or face
   - Progresses slowly, with good prognosis
   - Rarely advances to the systemic form of the disease
   - More common in children.
2. Systemic (or "diffused") sclerosis:
   - Internal organs and tissues are affected (oesophagus, gastrointestinal tract, lungs, heart, kidneys)
   - Blood vessels, muscles and joints may be affected
   - Thickening of skin on the arms, legs, face, abdomen and back
   - May begin with tissue inflammation, but progresses quickly to hardening
   - Can be degenerative and lifethreatening as hardening from scar tissue limits the functioning of internal organs.
3. CREST, a milder form of systemic sclerosis. People may exhibit some or all of these "CREST" symptoms
   - *Calcinosis*: Painful calcium deposits in the skin. They appear as white spots, often on elbows, knees and fingers.
   - *Raynaud's phenomenon*: Spasm of tiny arteries in response to cold or stress. Hinders blood flow to the finger, toes, ears and tongue.
   - *Oesophageal dysfunction*: Difficulty swallowing because of scarring in the esophagus. This may cause acid reflux and heartburn
   - *Sclerodactyly*: Thickening and tightening of skin on the fingers and toes. This can limit motion.
   - Telangiectasis tiny red spots on the hands, palms, forearms, face and lips. These are caused by dilated capillaries.

Diagnosis

Diagnosis can be difficult, particularly in the early stages of the disease because many of the symptoms of scleroderma are common to other connective tissue diseases such as rheumatoid arthritis or lupus. The diagnostic process begins with a comprehensive physical examination. In addition, it may include:

- Blood tests to identify various antibodies [antinuclear antibodies (ANAs), anti-centromere antibody, or anti-Scl-70 antibody].
- Nail-fold capillary test, which takes a skin sample from beneath the fingernail and studies it under the microscope. The test can detect abnormal capillary function, which is an early sign of scleroderma
- Various tests to identify any internal disease (chest X-ray, upper and lower GI endoscopy, electrocardiogram).

Treatment

Although scleroderma cannot be cured, many of its symptoms can be managed in most cases. Early treatment is critical, particularly during the first three years after skin symptoms appear. Organ inflammation and scarring usually occur within this critical three-year period. After that time, the risk of organ involvement lessens.

Treatment focuses on the most troublesome symptoms. It may include:

- Medications to reduce inflammations, such as colchicines
- Lotions and creams to soften and moisturise skin, including over-the-counter and prescribed moisturisers

- Medications to control high blood pressure and prevent kidney failure. Treatment of Raynaud's symptoms
- Antacids for oesophageal heartburn
- Immunosuppressant drugs to suppress the body's overactive immune system
- Localised laser therapy to remove telangiectasis (red spots on skin).

SJÖGREN'S SYNDROME

Sjögren's syndrome is a slowly progressive inflammatory disorder involving the exocrine glands. Mikulicz and others recognised the findings of keratoconjunctivitis and xerostomia as an entity in the late 1800s. In 1933, Sjögren recognised the association of this symptom complex with polyarthritis. Subsequent studies showed that Sjögren's syndrome may be a primary disorder or may be secondary to other autoimmune disorders, including systemic lupus erythematosus (SLE), rheumatoid arthritis, scleroderma, biliary cirrhosis, and others.

Pathophysiology: The characteristic abnormality found on the lacrimal or salivary gland biopsy is the lymphocytic infiltration in the glandular lobules. The predominant cells are memory $CD4^+$ T cells, suggesting a central role in the pathogenesis of this disorder. Activated B cells are also found in the lesions, which may be responsible for the production of the autoantibodies to autoantigens Ro (SS-A) and LA (SS-B). Anti-Ro (SS-A) is found in 40-45% and anti-LA (SS-B) in 50% of patients with Sjögren syndrome. Because these autoantibodies are also observed in other autoimmune disorders, including SLE, further diagnostic tools must be used for the correct diagnosis.

A higher incidence of Sjögren's syndrome exists in family members of these patients. The association of Sjögren's syndrome with human leukocyte antigen (HLA)–B8, HLA-Dw3, HLA-DR3, and with the DQA1*0501 allele supports the notion of genetic susceptibility.

Symptoms

- Sicca syndrome
- Keratoconjunctivitis: Dry eyes with reduced tear production with gritty or sandy sensation under the lids; red eyes; photosensitivity
- Xerostomia: Decreased saliva production leading to difficulties with chewing, swallowing, and even speech; abnormality in taste and smell; dental caries; mucosal burning sensation; sensitivity to spicy and acidic foods and beverages; increased risk for oral candidiasis; hoarseness of voice
- Musculoskeletal symptoms
- Arthralgia, morning stiffness, nonerosive arthritis
- Myalgia, muscle weakness
- Cutaneous findings
- Raynaud's phenomenon
- Nonthrombocytopenic purpura, especially of lower extremities
- Nasal, vaginal, and cutaneous dryness
- Gastrointestinal symptoms
- Dysphagia, nausea, epigastric pain
- Achalasia (in children)
- Achlorhydria, chronic atrophic gastritis
- Primary biliary cirrhosis
- Pulmonary findings
- Dyspnea due to mild interstitial disease
- Dry cough
- Renal findings—interstitial nephritis
- Other symptoms—fatigue, depression

Physical

- Parotid gland enlargement
- Corneal ulceration, vascularisation
- Vasculitic lesions—purpura
- Lymphadenopathy
- Autoimmune thyroiditis
- Neuromuscular manifestations
- Arthritis
- Oral cavity
- Mild erythema and thinning of the mucosa
- Erythema, fissuring, coating, and depapillation of the dorsal tongue
- Traumatic erosions and ulcers, angular cheilitis, and chapped lips
- Frothy, ropey, and thickened saliva

Lab Studies

- CBC count with differential: Mild anaemia and leukopenia are present.
- Erythrocyte sedimentation rate (ESR): Elevated ESR is observed in 80 to 90% of patients; however, C-reactive protein (CRP) usually is within the reference range.
- Immunoglobulin levels: Hypergammaglobulinaemia, up to several grams of immunoglobulin G (IgG), is observed in 80% of patients.

- Autoantibodies
- Antinuclear antibody (ANA) and rheumatoid factor (RF)—usually elevated
- Anti-Ro (SS-A), anti-La (SS-B)
- Other autoantibodies to thyroglobulin, thyroid microsomal, mitochondrial, smooth muscle, and salivary duct

Treatment

Cholinergic agonists: Stimulate salivary secretion.

Immunosuppressive agents: Used to treat extraglandular disease (i.e., interstitial pneumonitis, glomerulonephritis, vasculitis, pseudolymphoma, malignancy).

Nonsteroidal anti-inflammatory drugs (NSAIDs): Use of NSAIDs similar to those used for juvenile arthritis may be used to treat polyarthritis associated with Sjögren's syndrome.

Disease-modifying antirheumatic drugs (DMARDs): Used for polyarthritis not controlled with NSAIDs. Methotrexate (MTX) has been shown to be effective in managing polyarthritis. Other DMARDs (e.g., hydroxychloroquine, sulphasalazine, D-penicillamine) may be synergistic when coadministered with methotrexate.

MIXED CONNECTIVE TISSUE DISEASE (MCTD)

Mixed connective tissue disease (MCTD) is an autoimmune disease that encompasses symptoms of other rheumatoid autoimmune diseases. Symptoms of scleroderma, polymyositis and systemic lupus erythematosus are most common. However, people with MCTD also may have symptoms of rheumatoid arthritis and dermatomyositis. Because it comprises symptoms of several diseases, MCTD is sometimes called "overlap syndrome" or "undifferentiated mixed connective tissue disease." (Some medical experts consider MCTD and undifferentiated MCTD as different forms of the same disease. For purposes of this overview, they will be considered the same).

Mixed connective tissue disease affects the body's connective tissues. Made up of collagen and elastin, connective tissues are found throughout the body in the joints, ligaments, cartilage, muscles, skin and organs.

Causes

Mixed connective tissue disease is up to 15 times more common among women than men. Some theorise that this high prevalence in women is related to hormones.

The exact cause of MCTD is not known. The disorder is characterized by immune system abnormalities. Lab tests show that most patients diagnosed with MCTD have a pattern of high levels of antinuclear antibodies as well as antibodies to ribonucleoprotein (anti-RNP).

Symptoms

Typically, symptoms of MCTD mimic symptoms of other rheumatoid diseases, and can vary from person to person. Early symptoms can be subtle and are sometimes disregarded until the disease progresses. Initial symptoms often include:

- Raynaud's phenomenon in response to cold (blood vessel spasm followed by numbness and whiteness in fingers and toes).
- Swollen fingers or hands.
- Rashes (including butterfly rash on the nose, similar to rash caused by lupus).
- Red patches over the knuckles.
- Purplish discolouration of the eyelids.
- Alopecia (hair loss).
- Telangiectasia (dilation of blood vessels), causing lesions on the hands and face.
- Irritable bowel and other digestive problems.
- Allergies.
- Fatigue.
- Sleep disturbances.
- Sore throat.

Symptoms of MCTD can progress gradually or rapidly. In some people, MCTD remains mild for years, then will flare up and create a medical crisis. As the disease progresses, more body systems are affected. More advanced symptoms may include:

- Arthritis (usually nondeforming, but erosive deformities like those caused by rheumatoid arthritis can develop).
- Muscle weakness.
- Pain in the joints or muscles.
- Abnormalities of the oesophagus.
- Frequent infections in the gums, stomach and lungs.
- Pleuritis (inflammation of membranes surrounding the lungs), which may cause shortness of breath or more serious problems.

- Kidney disease.
- Heart disease.
- Trigeminal sensory neuropathy.

Diagnosis

Initial laboratory evaluation should include the following:

- Complete blood count with platelets and reticulocyte count: Leukopaenia, thrombocytopaenia, or haemolytic anaemia is a common finding. If the patient has a combination of these findings, carefully consider the possibility of leukaemia.
- Complete chemistry panel to evaluate electrolytes, liver, and kidney function.
- Unsuspected autoimmune hepatitis may be found based on elevated LFTs.
- Nephritic patients may have elevated creatinine and abnormal electrolytes.
- Patients with nephrosis may have low albumin and high cholesterol.
- Urine analysis
- Patients with MCTD and nephritis may have protein, RBCs, WBCs, or casts on evaluation of urine.
- Patients with nephrotic syndrome have high urinary protein.
- Muscle enzymes: Myositis may be found by measurement of creatine kinase, aldolase, aspartate aminotransferase, alanine aminotransferase, and lactic dehydrogenase.
- Acute phase reactants: Measurement of acute phase reactants can include erythrocyte sedimentation rate or C-reactive protein.

Diagnostic laboratory studies include the following:

- Antinuclear antibody: This test is usually positive in very high titres.
- Anti–double-stranded DNA: This test is usually negative but is occasionally positive in individuals with MCTD.
- Autoantibody panel including antibodies against RNP, Smith, Ro(SSA), La(SSB), Scl-70, phospholipids, cardiolipin and histone, total haemolytic complement, C3, C4, quantitative immunoglobulins, and thyroid studies.
- Other than anti-RNP and anti-Sm, these lab tests may be either positive or negative depending on the characteristics of the individual patient's disease.
- By definition, anti-RNP should be positive, and anti-Sm should be negative.
- Antibodies against purified proteins of Sm and RNP should be identified, i.e. antibodies should be against specific epitopes of Sm (Sm-B/B', Sm-D, Sm-E, Sm-F, Sm-G) and RNP (RNP-70 or U1 RNP, RNP-A, RNP-C).

Treatment

Treatment focuses on the individual's specific symptoms, and on suppressing inflammations caused by the immune system. Treatment methods may include:

- Nonsteroidal anti-inflammatory drugs (NSAIDs).
- Aspirin, acetaminophen.
- Immunosuppressant medications.
- Corticosteroids.
- Cytoxic medications.
- Heart medications.
- Antidiarrhoea medications.

POLYMYOSITIS AND DERMATOMYOSITIS

Polymyositis (PM) is an inflammatory disease of striated muscle. When polymyositis is associated with typical skin changes, it is called dermatomyositis. Autoantibodies are directed against tRNA synthetases. Antibodies are typically to Jo-1 (histidyl tRNA synthetase).

ANTINUCLEAR ANTIBODIES

There are many different types of antinuclear antibodies which are directed towards various antigenic epitopes found in two different nuclear structures; chromatin and snRNPs.

1. *Chromatin:*
   - Consists of DNA and histones
   - Histones are small basic proteins which bind tightly to DNA
   - There are 2 autoantibodies to DNA
   - There are 5 autoantibodies to histones
2. *Small nuclear ribonucleoproteins (snRNPs):*
   - There are four forms of RNA; messenger, transfer, ribosomal, and a heterogeneous group of small RNA molecules
   - When specific proteins bind to the different forms of RNA, the complex is called a ribonucleoprotein (RNP)
   - RNPs are also called 'extractable nuclear antigens' (ENAs) because they are soluble in aqueous buffers

- There are at least 4 autoantibodies to snRNPs; anti-Sm, anti-U1RNP, Anti-Ro, and Anti-La
- Autoantibodies to one or more snRNPs are common in SLE.

Autoantibodies to DNA

- Natural DNA (nDNA)
- Also called double-stranded (dsDNA)
- Anti-dsDNA antibodies are directed against the glycoprotein "backbone" of the helical, DNA molecule.
- Autoantibodies to NDNA are virtually pathognomonic of SLE
- Specific for SLE (i.e., rarely associated with other rheumatic diseases)
- Present in high titres in children with active nephritis.
- Anti-dsDNA antibodies are indicative of poor prognosis and have been implicated in lupus glomerulonephritis.

Single-Stranded DNA (ssDNA)

- Also called denatured DNA
- Anti-ssDNA antibodies are directed against the purine/pyrimadine base pairs located within the DNA helix (epitopes not available for binding in the stable, helical DNA molecule).
- Is present in 50% of children with SLE
- Nonspecific for SLE (i.e., found in a variety of rheumatic diseases and infections)
- Of little diagnostic significance

Autoantibodies to Histones

- There are at least 5 different histones H1, H2A, H2B, H3, H4
- Less specific for natural SLE as autoantibodies to histones are also found in drug-induced SLE (i.e., procainamide, hydralazine)
- In those with SLE, the strongest responses are directed against the histones H1 and H2B
- Patients with autoantibodies to DNA usually have auto- antibodies to Histones

Autoantibodies to snRNPs

1. *Anti-Sm antibodies:*
   - Sm (Smith)
   - These autoantibodies are specific for SLE
   - Presence is related to CNS disease
   - The Sm antigen is comprised of 5 small Uridine-rich nuclear RNAs and a number of polypeptides (B/B′, D, E, F, and G). Autoantibodies may be directed against specific epitopes.
   - For diagnostic purposes it is important to identify antibodies against all epitopes.
2. *Anti-U1RNP antibodies:*
   - The RNP antigen represents a portion of a polypeptide associated with U1 RNA (70 KD protein)
   - These autoantibodies are less specific for SLE
   - Found in low titres in children with SLE
   - Found in high titres in patients with mixed connective tissue disease
   - Antibodies against RNP isotypes–RNP-70, RNP-A, RNP-C help confirm MCTD.
3. *Anti-Ro antibodies:*
   - Aso called SS-A (Sjögren's syndrome A antigen)
   - These autoantibodies are less specific for SLE
   - Found in about 25% of cases of SLE and associated with renal and pulmonary manifestations of SLE
   - Most often found in Sjögren's syndrome
   - Found in neonatal lupus syndrome and associated with complete congenital heart block
   - Found in subacute cutaneous lupus
   - Found in 5-15% of normal individuals
   - Found as two isotypes: Ro-60 and Ro-52.
   - Ro-60 has a stronger association with SLE while Ro-52 has a stronger association with Sjögren's syndrome.
4. *Anti-La antibodies:*
   - Also called SS-B (Sjögren's syndrome B antigen)
   - These autoantibodies are less specific for SLE
   - Most often found in Sjögren's syndrome
   - Found in neonatal lupus syndrome
   - Found at low levels in 5% of normal individuals
   - Anti-La antibodies are almost always found in association with anti-Ro antibodies.

Anti-Scl Antibodies

- Also called scleroderma antibodies.
- Two isotypes may be identified Scl-70 and Scl-100 (PM-Scl-100)
- Antibodies to Scl-70 is useful in subtyping and prognostic judgement with systemic sclerosis or with early scleroderma associated symptoms.
- Antibodies to PM-Scl-100 is diagnostic of polymyositis or dermatomyositis.

Anti-Jo-1 Antibodies

- Suspicion of polymyositis or dermatomyositis.
- Fibrolysing alveolitis.
- Antisynthetase syndrome.

Antibodies to Poly-Nucleosomes and Mono-Nucleosomes

- Suspicion of SLE, scleroderma, MCTD.
- It is an earlier marker than anti-dsDNA.

Centromere B

- Suspicion of systemic sclerosis.
- Subtyping and prognostic judgement with systemic sclerosis or with early scleroderma associated symptoms, e.g. Raynaud's phenomenon.

Other Autoantibodies

1. *Lupus anticoagulant:*
   - This autoantibody binds to a phospholipids which results in the inhibition of the prothrombin-activator complex (Xa, V, calcium, phospholipids) which interferes with the conversion of prothrombin to thrombin in the common coagulation pathway
   - This results in the haemorrhagic disorder seen in some patients with SLE (i.e., menorrhagia)
   - Associated with an increased PT and PTT
2. *Anticardiolipin antibody:*
   - Also called anti-phospholipid antibody
   - These are autoantibodies which cross-react with negatively charged phospholipids
   - Are present in 50-100% of children with SLE
   - May be related to the CNS manifestations of SLE
   - May be responsible for the clinical manifestations of recurrent venous and arterial thromboses, livedo reticularis, emboli, stroke, chorea, hypertension, thrombocytopenia, spontaneous abortions, and foetal loss
3. *Rheumatoid factor (Rf):*
   - Autoantibodies to IgM
   - Found in 10-30% of children with SLE
   - High Rf titres are found in children with mixed connective tissue disease

DIAGNOSTIC METHODS FOR DETECTING ANTINUCLEAR ANTIBODIES

ANA Immunoflourescence (FANA)

It is called the immunofluorescent antinuclear antibody test (ANA or FANA). Provides a high degree of sensitivity for the detection of antinuclear antibodies (ANA).

The patient's blood is mixed with rat or mouse liver cells or HEp-2 cells, exposed to fluorescein-tagged anti-IgG antibodies, and then examined under a microscope. The preparations are assessed in two ways.

1. ANA Titre

This tells how many times the patient's plasma had to be diluted to get a sample free of the fluorescein-tagged anti-IgG antibodies.

2. ANA Pattern

This looks at the distribution of fluorescein-tagged anti-IgG antibodies on the cells. There are four patterns.

Peripheral (Rim or Shaggy): Most specific pattern for SLE. Is found almost exclusively in patients with SLE and suggests the presence of antibodies to natural (double-stranded) DNA.

Speckled: Less specific for SLE. Is found in patients with SLE and mixed connective tissue disease. Associated with Anti-U1RNP Antibodies.

Homogeneous (Smooth): Less specific for SLE. Is found in patients with a variety of connective tissue diseases and in those taking certain drugs (anti-arrhythmics, anticonvulsants, antihypertensives).

Nucleolar: Is found in patients with scleroderma.

Disadvantages

Fluorescent staining patterns (i.e. homogeneous, speckled, nucleolar, cytoplasmic) are reported in conjunction with positive sera. These patterns may or may not be related to the presence of specific autoantibodies (for example, anti-dsDNA antibodies are frequently associated with peripheral staining patterns; however, pheripheral staining does not necessarily indicate the presence of anti-dsDNA antibodies, nor do anti-dsDNA always result in a pheripheral pattern). FANA also provides total anti-nuclear antibody semiquantisation in doubling dilutions (titre) with an expected error of +/– one dilution. Although considered the "gold standard" for ANA testing, the labour intensive, subjective interpretation of FANA and high level of positivity in normal individuals (<30%) present method associated limitations.

First and Second Generation EIA

These tests are more objective and attempt to overcome the drawbacks of FANA. These tests offer quantification of the antibodies.

The antigens are coated on a microplate (microwell) and antinuclear antibodies, if present bind to these antigens. The end result (colour) is measured spectrophotometrically.

They provide screening tests, profile tests and individual assays.

The Units are Internationally Approved or Arbitrary (based on the manufacturer).

Disadvantages

Commercial kits are not available to detect all the antigenic epitopes. Hence cannot correlate with IFA results. For example:

Anti-nucleolar pattern: Diagnosed scleroderma. Although there are commercial kits available for the detection of anti-Scl-70 (DNA topoisomerase 1), several other antigens are implicated in antinucleolar patterns associated with scleroderma (i.e. anti-Pm/Scl -100, RNP-C, etc) for which assays are generally unavailable. The presence of a nucleolar pattern on FANA is then an indicator of more severe (systemic) sclerosis.

Anti-Sm and Anti-RNP: The difficulty in measuring anti-Sm and anti-RNP independently lies in the fact that Sm-RNP are parts of the same molecule. Although anti-Sm is stable, anti-(U1) RNP is heat labile and, therefore, unstable as an independent entity. Therefore, all tests designed to detect anti-RNP are actually detecting anti-RNP/Sm (total).

Some second generation EIAs offer an independent anti-Sm assay and a total anti-RNP(Sm) assay. A positive anti-RNP result is interpreted as positive for anti-RNP and/or anti-Sm.

The Sm and RNP have various epitopes Sm-B/B′, Sm-D, Sm-E, Sm-F, Sm-G and RNP-70, RNP-A, RNP-C. Autoantibodies may be present against each epitope. These EIAs could not identify each epitope, they were designed to identify Sm/RNP as a whole or only Sm as whole.

Third Generation EIAs

Offers a simple, objective and highly sensitive method for detection of antinuclear antibodies. Complete antigen representation (including all epitopes), antigen stability and quality as well as method of adhesion to the microtitre well, define the clinical utility of these assays. These assays help overcome the overlap syndrome and offer a clear diagnosis. Characterise 20 ANAs and hence a better solution to autoimmune disorders.

ANA TESTING (MFD: Orgentec, Courtesy: Lilac Medicare)

Warnings and Precautions

All reagents of this test kit are strictly intended for *in vitro* use only.

Please adhere strictly to the sequence of pipetting steps provided in this protocol. Observe the guideline for performing quality control in medical laboratories by assaying controls and/or pooled sera.

All reagents should be stored refrigerated at 2 to 8°C in their original container.

Do not interchange kit components from different lots. The expiration dates stated on the labels of the shipping container and all vials have to be observed. Do not use kit components beyond their expiration dates.

Allow all kit components and specimen to reach room temperature prior to use and mix well.

During handling of all kit reagents, controls and serum samples, observe the existing legal regulations.

The following precautions should be taken handling potentially infectious materials:

- — do not eat, drink or smoke in areas where specimens or kit reagents are handled
- — do not pipette by mouth
- — wear disposable gloves while handling specimens or kit reagents and wash hands thoroughly afterwards.

The test kit contains components of human origin which, when tested by FDA-licensed methods, were found negative for hepatitis B surface antigen and for HIV antibody. No known test can guarantee, however, that products derived from human blood will not be infectious. Handle, therefore, all reagent and human blood derivatives, like plasma or serum samples, as if capable of transmitting infection.

Avoid contact with the TMB (3,3′,5,5′-Tetramethyl-benzidine). If TMB comes into contact with skin, wash thorughly with water and soap.

The stop solution contains hydrochloric acid. If it comes into contact with skin, wash thorougly with water and seek medical attention.

Avoid contact between the buffered peroxide solution and easily oxidised materials; extreme temperatures may initiate spontaneous combustion.

Material Supplied

- Package size 96 determinations
- Divisible microplate consisting of 12 modules of 8 wells each, 1 coated with highly purified SSA-52 (Ro 52), SSA-60 (Ro 60), SSB (La), RNP/Sm, RNP-70 Kd, RNA-A, RNP-C, Sm-BB, Sm-D, Sm-E, Sm-F, SM-G, Scl-70, Jo-1, dsDNA, ssDNA, poly-nucleosomes, mononucleosomes, histone-complex, histone-H1, histone H2A, histone H2B, histone H3, histone H4, PM-Scl-100, centromere B.
- Anti-ANA controls in a serum/buffer matrix 3 vials 1.5 ml each
- Negative control (NC), cut-off control (CC), positive control (PC) 1 vial, 20 ml
- Sample buffer, yellow concentrate
- Enzyme conjugate solution, (light red) containing polyclonal rabbit anti-h-IgG; labelled with horseradish peroxidase 1 vial, 15 ml
- TMB substrate solution 1 vial, 15 ml
- Stop solution (1 M hydrochloric acid) 1 vial, 15 ml
- Buffered wash solution, concentrate 1 vial, 20 ml

Technical Data

- Sample material: Serum or plasma
- Required sample size 10 µl of sample to be diluted 1:100 with sample buffer 100 µl prediluted sample per single determination
- Total incubation time 60 minutes at room temperature (18-28°C)
- Storage refrigerated at 2 to 8°C
- Shelf-life: 12 months after manufacturing or until the expiration date printed on the labels
- Package size 96 tests

Principle of the Procedure

The ANA detect ELISA is an indirect solid-phase enzyme immunometric assay (ELISA). It is designed for the qualitative screening on IgG class autoantibodies directed against the antigen SSA-52 (Ro 52), SSA-60 (Ro 60), SSB (La), RNP/Sm, RNP-70 Kd, RNP-A, RNP-C, Sm-BB; SM-D, Sm-E, Sm-F, Sm-G, Scl-70, Jo-1, dsDNA, ssDNA, polynucleosomes, mononucleosomes, histone-complex, histone-H1, histone-H2A, histone-H2B, histone-H3, histone-H4, PM-Scl-100, centromere B. The antigens were coated in microplates, which can be divided into 12 modules of 8 wells each or can be used complete for 96 determinations.

Reaction Phase

The binding of present autoantibodies, the formation of the sandwich complexes and the enzymatic colour reaction take place during three different reaction phases.

Phase 1

Controls and prediluted patient samples are pipetted into the wells of the microplate. Any present anti bodies bind to the immobilised antigens. After a 30 minute incubation, the microplate is washed with wash buffer for removing nonreactive serum components.

Phase 2

An anti-human-IgG horseradish peroxidase conjugate solution is pipetted into the wells of the microplate to recognise the autoantibodies bound to the immobilised antigen. After a 15-minute incubation any excessive enzyme conjugate, which is not specifically bound is washed away with wash buffer.

Phase 3

A chromogenic substrate solution containing TMB (3,3′,5,5′-Tetramethy-benzidine) is dispensed into the wells. During 15 minutes of incubation, the colour of the solution changes into blue. Colour development is stopped by adding 1 M hydrochloric acid as stop solution. The solution's colour changes into yellow. The amount of colour is directly proportional to the concentration of IgG present in the original sample.

To read the optical density, a microplate reader with a 450 nm filter is required. Bichromatic measurement with a 600-690 nm reference is recommended.

Specificity

The microplate is coated with highly purified SSA-52 (Ro 52), SSA-60 (Ro 60), SSB (La), RNP/Sm, RNP-70 Kd, RNP-A, RNP-C, Sm-BB; Sm-D, Sm-E, Sm-F, Sm-G, Scl-70, Jo-1, dsDNA, ssDNA, polynucleosomes, mononucleosome, histone-complex, histone-H1, histone-H2A, histone-H2B, histone-H3, histone-H4, PM-Scl-100, centromere B. The ANA detect ELISA test is specific only for autoantibodies directed to these antigens. No crossreactivities have been observed.

Calibration

The assay is calibrated against the internationally recognised reference sera from CDC, Atlanta, USA. And against the WHO reference preparation for human anti-dsDNA Wo/80.

Clinical Relevance

The serological detection of antinuclear antibodies (ANA) in patients with suspected autoimmune disorders is a common practice in every immunological lab.

Inflammatory connective tissue diseases are characterised by idiopathic genesis along with disturbances in terms of cellular and humoral immunity, systemic organ failure, and a chronic course of disease. Additionally, connective tissue diseases exhibit overlapping symptomatic features thus making a right diagnosis extremely difficult.

Systemic lupus erythematosus (SLR), Sjögren's syndrome, progressive systemic scleroderma along with CREST syndrome, Sharp's syndrome (mixed connective tissue disease) and myositis belong to the inflammatory rheumatic diseases.

Considering the diversity of mixed connective tissue diseases, such disorders exhibit a common serological characteristic, the presence of antinuclear antibodies. These antibodies are directed against parts of the cell nucleus and the cytoplasm. For the most part the presence of a particular ANA in a patient serum can be assigned to a special inflammatory disease.

When an autoimmune disorder is suspected, the first diagnostic step is the performance of a screening test on antinuclear antibodies. Common practice is indirect immunofluorescence on HEp-2 cells. The second step in the ANA algorithm is the isolated detection of the particular antibodies specificities (e.g. with ANA-combi, ORG 539). In between an additional screening test can be performed.

The wells of the ORGen Tec ANA detect ELISA are coated with a large number of autoantigens in order to allow a screening on the most important antinuclear antibodies SS-52 (Ro 52), SSA-60 (Ro 60), SSB (La), RNP/Sm, RNP-70 Kd, RNP-A, RNP-C, Sm-BB, Sm-D, Sm-E, Sm-F, Sm-G, Scl-70, Jo-1, dsDNA, ssDNA, polynucleosomes, mononucleosomes, histone-complex, histone-H1, histone-H2A, histone-H2B, histone-H3, histone-H4, PM-Scl-100, Centromere B. Thus, the ANA detect ELISA kit allows a sensitive screening on one or more autoantibodies possibly being present in patient serum.

IMMUNOASSAY PROCEDURE

Materials Required

Equipment

- Microplate reader capable for endpoint measurement at 450 nm
- Vortex mixer
- Pipettes for 10 µl, 100 µl, 1000 µl

Preparation of reagents

- distilled water
- graduated cylinder for 100 and 1000 ml
- plastic container for storage of the wash solution

Optional

— multichanel dispenser
— or repeatable pipette for 100 µl
— data reduction software

Specimen Collection and Preparation

For determination of anti-ANA antibodies, serum or plasma are the preferred sample matrixes. All serum and plasma samples are prediluted 1:100 with sample buffer. Therefore, 10 µl of sample may be diluted with 1000 µl of sample buffer.

The patients need to be fasting, and no special preparations are necessary. Collect body by venipunture into vacutainers and separate serum or plasma from the cells by centrifugation after clot formation.

Sample may be stored, refrigerated at 2 to 8°C for at least 5 days. For longer storage of up to six months, sample should be stored frozen at –20°C. To avoid repeated thawing and freezing the samples should be aliquoted.

No interference has been observed with haemolytic, lipemic or billirubin containing sera. Nor have any interfering effects been noticed with the use of anticoagulants.

Preparation and Storage of Reagents

All components of this test kit are supplied in a liquid format and ready to use, except the sample buffer and wash buffer. When stored refrigerated at 2 to 8°C the diluted components are stable for at least 30 days after opening or until the expiration date printed on the labels.

Remaining modules of the microplate should be stored refrigerated at 2 to 8°C protected from moisture; store together with desiccant and carefully sealed in the plastic bag.

Preparation of Sample Buffer

Dilute the contents of each vial of the sample buffer concentrate (5x) with distilled water to a final volume of 100 ml prior to use. Store refrigerated stable at 2 to 8°C for at least 30 days after preparation or until the expiration date printed on the label.

Preparation of Buffered Wash Solution

Dilute the contents of each vial of the buffered wash solution concentrate (50x) with distilled water to a final volume of 1000 ml prior to use. Store refrigerated stable 2 to 8°C for at least 30 days after preparation or until the expiration date printed on the label.

Notes on Technique

Control sera or pools should routinely be assayed as unknowns to check performance of the reagents and the assay.

For all controls, the respective concentrations are provided on the labels of each vial. Using these concentrations, a calibration curve may be calculated to read off the patient results semiquantitatively.

Pipetting and Sample Handling

Use a disposable-tip micropipette to dispense sera and plasma samples. Pipette directly to the bottom of the wells. To avoid carryover contamination, change the tip between samples. Patient samples expected to contain high concentrations should be additionally diluted with sample buffer before. Additional dilutions must be considered during calculation.

Immunoassay Procedure

- Do not interchange components of different lots.
- All components should be at room temperature before use.
- Dilute all patient samples 1:100 with sample buffer before assay
- Therefore combine 10 µl of sample with 1000 µl of sample buffer in a polystyrene tube.
- Mix well. controls are ready to use and need not to be diluted
  1. Prepare a sufficient number of microplate modules to accommodate controls and prediluted patient samples.

	1	2	3	4	5	6
A	CC	P..				
B	NC	P..				
C	PC					
D	P1					
E	P2					
F	P3					
G	P4					
H	P5					

P1, P2...Patient samples 1, 2....
CC : Cut off control

NC : Negative control
PC : Positive Control

2. Pipette 100 µl of controls and prediluted patient samples into the wells.
3. Incubate for 30 minutes at room temperature (20-28°C).
4. Discard the contents of the microwells and wash 3 times with 300 µl of wash solutions.
5. Dispense 100 µl of enzyme conjugate into each well.
6. Incubate for 15 minutes at room temperature.
7. Discard the contents of the microwells and wash 3 times with 300 µl of wash solution.
8. Dispense 100 µl of TMB substrate solution into each well.
9. Incubate for 15 minutes at room temperature
10. Add 100 µl of stop solution to each well of the modules and let it stand for 5 minutes.
11. Read the optical density at 450 nm and calculate the results. Bi-chromatic measurement with a reference at 600-690 nm is recommended.

    This developed colour is stable for at least 30 minutes. Read optical densites during this time.

CALCULATION OF RESULTS

Semiquantitative Results

For detailed semiquantification of the results, each patient OD value can be expressed by the "index value". The index value is calculated by dividing the sample OD by the cut-off OD:

$$\text{Index value} = \frac{OD_{sample}}{OD_{cut\text{-}off}}$$

ANA Detect ELISA
(Index Value)

Negative	< 1.0
Borderline	1.0-1.2
Positive	≥ 1.2

The calculation of index values is not influenced by variations of the sample-OD and/or cut-off-OD. Index values are recommended for long-term validations (i.e. internal quality control samples).

Qualitative Results

Evaluation of the ANA detect ELISA test is easily carried out by direct comparison of the optical density of each patient sample with the optical density of the cut-off control.

Patient samples exhibiting optical densities higher than the optical density of the cut-off control are considered to be positive.

Negative	OD patient <	OD cut-off
Positive	OD Patient ≥	OD cut-off

Calculation Example

The table shows typical results for ANA detect ELISA. These data are intended for illustration only and should not be used to calculate results from another run.

Sample No	*Sample OD*	*OD cut-off*	*Index value*	*Interpretation*
1	0.107	0.435	0.25	Negative
2.	0.435	0.435	1.00	Borderline
3.	1.294	0.435	2.97	Positive
4.	2.496	0.43	5.74	Positive

Due to additive effects of each of the coated antigens, sera with positive results in the ANA detect ELISA test may be determined as negative using the ANA combi or the quantitative Anti-ANA tests.

Further differentiation and typing should be carried out by using the ANA combi test or the quantitative anti-ANA test kits.

Incubation Scheme

1. Pipette 100 µl control or diluted patient sample
   ↘Incubate for 30 minutes at room temperature ↘
   Discard the contents of the wells and wash 3 times with 300 µl wash solution
2. Pipette 100 µl enzyme conjugate
   ↘Incubate for 15 minutes at room temperature ↘
   Discard the contents of the wells and wash 3 times with 300 µl wash solution.
3. Pipette 100 µl substrate solution
   ↘Incubate for 15 minutes at room temperature
4. And 100 µl stop solution
   ↘Leave untouched for 5 minutes
   ↘Read at 450 nm

ANA: Description

The ANA are antibodies the body produces against its own DNA and nuclear material that cause tissue damage and characterise autoimmune diseases. Highest titres occur in SLE.

ANA/ANF is positive in

Deramatomyositis, hepatitis (chronic active), mixed connective tissue disease, myasthenia gravis, polymyositis, pulmonary fibrosis (idiopathic) Raynaud's syndrome, rheumatoid arthritis, scleroderma, some healthy older adults, systemic lupus erythematosus (SLE), Sjögren's syndrome. Drugs include beta-adrenergic blockers, carbamazepine, lowastatin, methyldopa, nitrofurantion sodium, penicillamine, and tocainide.

Drugs that may cause false positive results due to drug-induced syndrome resembling SLE include:

acetazolamide, aminosalicylic acid, carbidopa, chlorothiazide, chlorpromazine, clofibrate, diphenylhydantoin, ethosuximide, gold salt, griseofulvan microsize, griseofulvan ultramicrosize, hydralazine hydrochloride, hydroxytryptophan, isoniazid, mephenytoin, methylined methylodopate hydrochloride, methythiouricil, methysergide maleate, contraceptives, penicilin, phenylbutazone, phenytoin, primil procainamide hydrochloride, propylthiouricil, quinidine glucone quinidine polygalacturonate, quinidine sulphate, resprine, strepton sulphate, sulphadimethoxine, sulphonamides, tetracyclines, thiouracil trimethadione.

ANTI-dsDNA (MFD: Orgentec, Courtesy: Lilac Medicare)

Immunometric enzyme immunoassay for the quantitative determination of autoantibodies to doubl-stranded DNA (recombinant)

Warnings and Precautions

All reagents of this test kit are strictly intended for *in vitro* use only.

Please adhere strictly to the sequence of pipetting steps provided in the protocol. Observe the guidelines for performing quality control in medical laboratories by assaying control and/or pooled sera.

All reagents should be stored, refrigerated at 2 to 8°C in their original container.

Do not interchange kit components from different lots. The expiration dates stated on the labels of the shipping container and all vials have to be observed. Do not use kit components beyond their expiration dates.

Allow all kit components and specimen to reach room temperature prior to use and mix well.

During handling of all kit reagents, controls and serum samples, observe the existing legal regulations. The following precautions should be taken handling potentially infectious materials:

- do not eat, drink or smoke in areas where specimens or kit reagents are handled
- do not pipette by mouth
- wear disposable gloves while handling specimens or kit reagents and wash hands thoroughly afterwards.

The test kit contains components of human origin which, when tested by FDA-licensed methods, were found negative for hepatitis B surface antigen and for HIV antibody. No known test can guarantee, however, that products derived from human blood will not be infectious. Handle, therefore, all reagents and human blood derivatives, like plasma or serum samples, as if capable of transmitting infection.

Avoid contact with TMB (3,3′, 5,5′-Tetramethylbenzidine). If TMB comes into contact with skin, wash thoroughly with water and soap.

The stop solution contains hydrochloric acid. If it comes into contact with skin, wash thoroughly with water and seek medical attention.

Avoid contact between the buffered peroxide solution and easily oxidised materials; extreme temperature may initiate spontaneous combustion.

Materials Supplied

Package size	96 determinations
Divisible microplate consisting of 12 modules of 8 wells coated with recombinant double-stranded DNA (dsDNA)	1
Anti-dsDNA calibrators in a serum/buffer matrix containing 0:12.5; 25; 50; 100 and 200 IU/ml	6 vials, 1.5 ml each
Anti-dsDNA controls in a serum/buffer matrix (positive and negative), for the respective concentrations see the enclosed package insert	1 set, 2 vials, 1.5 ml each
Anti-dsDNA sample buffer, yellow, concentrate	1 vial, 20 ml
Enzyme conjugate solution (light red), containing polyclonal rabbit anti-h-IgG-IgG, labelled with horseradish peroxidase	1 vial, 15 ml

TMB substrate solution	1 vial, 15 ml
Stop solution (1 M hydrochloric acid)	1 vial, 15 ml
Buffered wash solution, concentrate	1 vial, 20 ml

Controls

A set of two controls is provided with the kit.

Technical Data

Sample material	:	Serum of plasma
Required sample volume	:	10 µl of sample to be diluted 1:100 with sample buffer 100 µl prediluted sample per single determination
Total incubation time	:	60 minutes at room temperature (20-28°C)
Calibration range	:	12.5-200 IU/ml
Sensitivity	:	1 IU/ml
Storage	:	Refrigerated at 2 to 8°C
Shelf-life	:	12 months after manufacturing or until the expiration date printed on the labels
Package size	:	96 tests

Principle of the Procedure

Anti-dsDNA is an indirect solid-phase enzyme immunometric assay (ELISA). It is designed for the quantitative measurement of IgG class autoantibodies directed against double-stranded DNA. The assay is based on microplates coated with recombinant double-stranded DNA. The microplate can be divided into 12 modules of 8 wells each or can be used complete for 96 determinations.

Reaction Phases

During this procedure the binding or present autoantibodies, as well as the formation of the sandwich complexed and enzymatic colour reaction take place during three different reaction phases.

Phase 1

Controls and prediluted patient samples are pipetted into the wells of the microplate. Any present antibodies bind to the immobilised antigens. After a 30-minute incubation, the microplate is washed with wash buffer for removing nonreactive serum components.

Phase 2

An anti-human-IgG horseradish peroxidase conjugate solution is pipetted into the wells of the microplate to recognise the autoantibodies bound to the immobilised antigens. After a 15-minutes incubation, any excessive enzyme conjugate, which is not specifically bound is washed away with wash buffer.

Phase 3

A chromogenic substrate solution containing TMB (3,3′, 5,5′-Terametheyl-benzidine) is dispensed into the wells. During 15 minutes of incubation, the colour of the solutions changes into blue. Colour development is stopped by adding 1 M hydrochloric acid as stop solution. The solution colour changes into yellow.

The amount of colour is directly proportional to the concentration of IgG present in the original sample. The optical density (OD) of the controls serve as reference for the determination of the cut-off OD. Patient results may be classified in terms of negative, positive or strong positive. Alternatively, the concentrations of the controls may be used to calculate a calibration curve from semiquantitative results.

To read the optical density, a microplate reader with a 450 nm filter is required. Bichromatic measurement with a 600-690 nm reference is recommended.

Clinical Relevance

Autoimmune diseases are characterised by the occurrence of antibodies against own antigenic structures, the so-called autoantibodies. Presence of autoantibodies to native deoxyribonucleic acids (n-DNA, dsDNA, double-stranded DNA) is typical for the clinical picture of systemic lupus erythematosus (SLE).

Antibodies against dsDNA belong to the group of antinuclear antibodies (ANA), which are directed against various structures of the nucleus of the cell. They appear in a variety of rheumatoid diseases. Besides the ANA antibodies, another group of autoantibodies is of interest, which are directed against the so-called extractable nuclear antigens (ENA). The ARA criteria of the American Rheumatism Association Provide an extensive diagnostic scheme for the diagnosis of SLE. In case that at least 4 of the eleven ARA criteria are fulfilled, SLE is highly predictive.

Antibodies to dsDNA are found during the active phases of SLE, where the serum concentration exhibits positive correlation to the severity of the disease. An ongoing therapy may be monitored by the aid of autoantibody determination. Diagnostic sensitivity of the anti-dsDNA determination in cases of SLE is approximately 91% combined with a diagnostic specificity of nearly 96 percent.

Antibodies against DNA can be differentiated into two groups:

1. Antibodies, that bind only to native double-stranded DNA (dsDNA).
2. Antibodies recognising single-stranded DNA (ssDNA) too.

Measurement of antinuclear antibodies (ANA, or antinuclear factor (ANF) by indirect immunofluorescence test (IFT) is widely accepted as screening method in suspected SLE. Since in some stages of the diseases or during therapy, IFT sometimes gives false results, a more specific test system is needed. Negative IFT for antinuclear antibodies does not exclude the presence of anti-dsDNA antibodies, since the antigenic structures may be masked by other structures. Furthermore, the ANA titres determined by IF test show only week correlation to the severity of the disease.

Most antibodies against dsDNA are directed against the phosphate units of DNA. Thus, these autoantibodies also bind to DNA single strains. For quantitation of anti-dsDNA, it has to be proven, that the antigen preparation exhibits no contamination with single-stranded DNA.

Autoantibodies against single-stranded DNA are mainly directed against its basic compound, which in the native DNA is masked inside the helical structure. In serum of SLE patients anti-ssDNA antibodies are found with a frequency of up to 87 percent during acute phases and 43 percent during inactive phases.

The SLE-like diseases are caused by some drugs. For differential diagnosis of drug-induced LE, the determination of anti-ssDNA is a valuable diagnostic tool. In drug-induced LE anti-ssDNA is elevated in more than 50 percent of all cases. Furthermore, elevated anti-ssDNA serum concentrations have been reported in mononucleosis, hepatitis and various forms of leukaemia.

Table below gives the frequency of anti-dsDNA and anti-ssDNA in various diseases.

	Frequency (%)	
Disorders	*dsDNA-Ab*	*ssDNA-Ab*
Systemic lupus erythematosus (active)	60-90	78-87
Systemic lupus erythematosus (inactive)	60	43
Discoid lupus erythematodes	25	20
Drug-induced lupus	3	52
Collagenosis with negative ANA-test	5	27
Sharp-syndrome (MCTD)	22	
Sclerodermia		27
Sjögren's syndrome	25	
Juvenile rheumatoid arthritis	4	35-50
Polymyositis/dermatomyositis	21	
Myasthenia gravis	12	
Thyreotoxicosis	20	
Infectious mononucleosis		40
Autoimmune, chronic aggressive hepatitis		58
Acute myelotic leukaemia		89
Acute lymphatic leukaemia		83
Chronic myelotic leukaemia		60
Healthy	0-5	4

Determination of autoantibodies to double-stranded DNA (anti-dsDNA) and single-stranded DNA (anti-ssDNA) is mainly induced in:

— Systemic lupus erythematosus
— Drug-induced LE and
— Other systemic autoimmune diseases.

Normal Values

In a normal range study, with serum samples from healthy blood donors, the following ranges have been established with the anti-dsDNA test:

	anti-dsDNA [IU/ml]
Cut-off	20

Positive results should be verified concerning the entire clinical status of the patient. Also, every decission for therapy should be taken individually.

It is recommended that each laboratory establishes its own normal and pathological ranges. The values below should be regarded as guidelines only.

Specificity

The solid phase is coated with recombinant double-stranded DNA (dsDNA). Due to a newly developed coating process, the antigenic structure is conserved; and during coating; no sequences of single-stranded DNA occur. Therefore, the anti-dsDNA test kit recognises only autoantibodies specific for double-stranded DNA.

Calibration

The quantitative test system for anti-dsDNA autoantibodies is calibrated against the WHO reference preparation for human anti-dsDNA Wo/80 finding a concentration of 200 IU/ml when reconstituted in 0.5 ml.

Materials Required

Equipment

- Microplate reader capable for endpoint measurement at 450 nm
- Vortex mixer
- Pipettes for 10 µl, 100 µl and 1000 µl

Preparation of Reagents

- Distilled water
- Graduated cylinder for 100 and 1000 ml
- Plastic container for storage of the wash solution

Optional

- multichanel dispenser
- or repeatable pipette for 100 µl
- data reduction software

Specimen Collection and Preparation

For determination of anti-dsDNA antibodies serum or plasma are the preferred sample matrices. All serum and plasma samples are prediluted 1:100 with sample buffer. Therefore, 10 µl of sample may be diluted with 1000 µl of sample buffer.

The patients need not be fasting, and no special preparations are necessary. Collect blood by venipunture into vacutainers and separate serum or plasma from the cells by centrifugation after clot formation.

Samples may be stored, refrigerated at 2 to 8°C for at least 5 days. For longer storage of up to six months, samples should be stored frozen at 20°C. To avoid repeated thawing and freezing, the samples should be aliquoted.

Neither bilirubin nor haemolysis have significant effect on the procedure.

Preparation and Storage of Reagents

All components of this test kit are supplied in a liquid format and ready to use, except the sample buffer and wash buffer. When stored refrigerated at 2 to 8°C the components are stable for at least 30 days after opening or until the expiration date printed on the labels.

Remaining modules of the microplate should be stored refrigerated at 2 to 8°C protected from moisture; store together with desiccant and carefully sealed in the plastic bag.

Preparation of Sample Buffer

Dilute the contents of each vial of the sample buffer concentrate (5x) with distilled water to a final volume of 100 ml prior to use. Store refrigerated stable at 2 to 8° C for at least 30 days after preparation or until the expiration date printed on the label.

Preparation of Buffered Wash Solution

Dilute the contents of each vial of the buffered wash solution concentrate (50x) with distilled water to a final volume of 1000 ml prior to use. Store refrigerated stable at 2 to 8°C for at least 30 days after preparation or until the expiration date printed on the label.

Notes on Technique

Control sera or pools should routinely be assayed as unknowns to check performance of the reagents and the assay.

For all controls, the respective concentrations are provided on the labels of each vial. Using these concentrations, a calibration curve may be calculated to read off the patient results semiquantitatively.

Pipetting and Sample Handling

Use a disposable-tip micropipette to dispense sera and plasma samples. Pipette directly to the bottom of the wells. To avoid carryover contamination, change the tip between samples. Patient samples expected to contain high concentration should be additionally diluted with sample buffer before. Additional dilutions must be considered during calculation.

Assay Characteristics

Sensitivity

The lower detection limit for anti-dsDNA has been determined at 1.0 IU/ml.

Parallelism

In dilution experiments sera with high antibody concentrations were diluted with sample buffer and assayed in the anti-dsDNA kit. The assay shows linearity over the full measuring range.

Precision

Statistics were calculated for each of the three samples from the results of 24 determinations in a single run for intraassay precision. Run-to-run precision was calculated from the results of 5 different runs with 6 determinations each:

Intraassay			Interassay		
Sample No	*Mean (IU/ml)*	*CV (%)*	*Sample No*	*Mean (IU/ml)*	*CV (%)*
1	26	4.5	1	29	14.4
2	61	3.1	2	68	7.3
3	114	6.4	3	138	5.2

Immunoassay Procedure

Do not interchange components of different lots.

All components should be at room temperature before use.

Dilute all patient samples 1:100 with sample buffer before assay. Therefore, combine 10 µl of sample with 1000 µl of sample buffer in a polystyrene tube. Mix well. Calibrators and controls are ready to use and need not to be diluted.

1. Prepare a sufficient number of microplate modules to accommodate calibrates controls and prediluted patient samples in duplicates.

	1	2	3	4	5	6
A	SA	SE	P1	P5		
B	SA	SE	P1	P5		
C	SB	SF	P2	P..		
D	SB	SF	P2	P..		
E	SC	C1	P3			
F	SC	C1	P3			
G	SD	C2	P4			
H	SD	C2	P4			

SA-SF Standards A to F
P1, P2, Patient sample 1, 2...
C1 Positive control
C2 Negative control

2. Pipette 100 µl of calibrators, controls and prediluted patient samples into the wells.
3. Incubate for 30 minutes at room temperature (20-28°C).
4. Discard the contents of the microwells and wash 3 times with 300 µl of wash solution..
5. Dispense 100 µl of enzyme conjugate solution into each well.
6. Incubate for 15 minutes at room temperature.
7. Discard the contents of the microwells and wash 3 times with 300 µl of wash solution.
8. Dispense 100 µl of TMB substrate solution into each well.
9. Incubate for 15 minutes at room temperature protected from light.
10. Add 100 µl of stop solution to each well of the modules and leave untouched for 5 minutes.
11. Read the optical density at 450 nm and calculate the results. Bichromatic measurement with reference at 600-650 nm is recommended.

The developed colour is stable for at least 30 minutes. Read optical densities during this time.

Calculation of Results

For the anti-dsDNA tests a 4-parameter-fit with lin-log coordinates for optical density and concentration is recommmended. Smoothed spine approximation and log-log coordinates are also suitable.

Recommended Lin-Log Plot

First calculate the averaged optical densities for each calibrator well. Use lin-log graph paper and plot the averaged optical density of each calibrator versus the concentration. Draw the best fitting curve approximating the path of all calibrator points. The calibrator points may also be connected with straight line segments. The concentration of unknowns may then be estimated from the calibration curve by interpolation.

Calculation Example

The figures below show typical results for anti-dsDNA. These data are intended for illustration only and should not be used to calculate results from another run.

No	*Position*	*OD 1*	*OD 20*	*Mean*	*Conc 1*	*Conc 2*	*Mean*	*decl Conc*	*CV%*
ST1	A1/A2	0.023	0.021	0.022	0.0	0.0	0.0	0.0	9
ST2	B1/B2	0.174	0.174	0.174	13	13	13	12	0
ST3	C1/C2	0.0336	0.335	0.336	25	25	25	25	0
ST4	D1/D2	0.643	0.658	0.651	49	50	50	50	2
ST5	E1/E2	1.172	1.173	1.173	101	101	101	100	0
ST6	F1/F2	1.809	1.788	1.799	201	197	199	200	1

Incubation Scheme

1. Pipette 100 µl calibrator, control or diluted patient sample
   ↘Incubate for 30 minutes at room temperature↘
   Discard the contents of the wells and wash 3 times with 300 µl wash solution
2. Pipette 100 µl enzyme conjugate
   ↘Incubate for 15 minutes at room temperature↘
   Discard the contents of the wells and wash 3 times with 300 µl wash solution
3. Pipette 100 µl substarte solution
   ↘Incubate for 15 minutes at room temperature
4. Add 100 µl stop solution
   ↘Leave untouched for 5 minutes
   ↘Read at 450 nm

Anti-dsDNA Ab Interpretaton

Anti dsDNA Ab IU level	*Interpretation*
Less than 25	Negative
25-30	Borderline
30-60	Low positive
60-200	Positive
> 200	Strong positive

Anti-dsDNA antibodies are characteristically seen in systemic lupus erythematosus.

ANACOMBI (ANA PROFILE TESTING) IMMUNOMETRIC ENZYME IMMUNOASSAY FOR THE QUALITATIVE DETERMINATION OF ANA-AUTOANTIBODIES (MFD: Orgentec, Courtesy: Lilac Medicare)

Warnings and Precautions

All reagents of this test kit are strictly intended for *in vitro* use only.

Please adhere strictly to the sequence of pipetting steps provided in this protocol. Observe the guidelines for performing quality control in medical laboratories by assaying controls and/or pooled sera.

All reagents should be stored, refrigerated at 2 to 8°C in their original container.

Do not interchange kit components from different lots. The expiration dates stated on the labels of the shipping container and all vials have to be observed. Do not use kit components beyond their expiration dates.

Allow all kit components and specimen to reach room temperature prior to use and mix well.

During handling of all kit reagents, controls and serum samples, observe the existing legal regulations. The following precautions should be taken while handling potentially infectious materials:

— do not eat, drink or smoke in areas where specimens or kit reagents are handled
— do not pipette by mouth
— wear disposable gloves while handling specimens or kit reagents and wash hands thoroughly afterwards.

The test kit contains components of human origin which, when tested by FDA licensed methods, were found negative for hepatitis B surface antigen and for HIV antibody. No known test can guarantee, however, that products derived from human blood will not be infectious. Handle, therefore, all reagents and human blood derivatives, like plasma or serum samples, as if capable of transmitting infection.

Avoid contact with the TMB (3,3′, 5,5′-Tetramethyl-benzidine). If TMB comes into contact with skin, wash thoroughly with water and soap.

The stop solution contains hydrochloric acid. If it comes into contact with skin, wash thoroughly with water and seek medical attention.

Avoid contact between the buffered peroxide solution and easily oxidised materials; extreme temperatures may initiate spontaneous combustion.

Materials Supplied

Package size	96 determinations
Divisible microplate consisting of 12 modules of 8 wells each coated with highly purified antigens: RNP-70, RNP/Sm, Sm, SS-A, SS-B, Scl-70, Centromer B, Jo-1	1
ANA controls in a PBS/BSA matrix: negative control (NC), calibrator control (CC)	2 vials, 3 ml each
Sample buffer, yellow, concentrate	1 vial, 20 ml
Enzyme conjugate solution, (light red) containing polyclonal rabbit anti-h-IgG-IgG; labelled with horseradish peroxidase	1 vial, 15 ml
TMB substrate solution	1 vial, 15 ml
Stop solution (1 M hydrochloric acid)	1 vial, 15 ml
Buffered wash solution, concentrate	1 vial, 20 ml

Technical Data

Sample material	Serum or plasma
Required sample size	10 µl of sample to be diluted 1:100 with sample buffer 800 µl prediluted sample per profile
Total incubation time	60 minutes at room temperature (20-28°C)
Storage	Refrigerated at 2 to 8°C
Shelf-life	12 months after manufacturing or unitl the expiration date printed on the labels
Package size	12 profiles

Principle of the Procedure

The ANAcombi is an indirect solid-phase enzyme immunometric assay (ELISA). It is designed for the qualitative determination ANA autoantibodies directed against RNP-70, RNP/sm, Sm, SS-A, SS-B, Scl-70, Centromer B and Jo-1. The assay system recognises IgG class autoantibodies. The wells of the microplate were coated with RNP-70, RNP/Sm, Sm, SS-A, SS-B, Scl-70, centromer B and Jo-1 in row A to H, respectively. The microplate can be divided into 12 modules of 8 wells each.

Reaction Phases

During this procedure, the binding of present autoantibodies, as well as the formation of the sandwich complexes and enzymatic colour reaction take place during three different reaction phases

Phase 1

Controls and prediluted patient samples should be pipetted into the wells of the microplate. Any present antibodies bind to the antibodies antigens. After a 60-minutes incubation, the microplate is washed with wash buffer for removing nonreactive serum components.

Phase 2

An anti-human IgG horseradish peroxidase conjugate solution to pipetted into the wells of the microplate to recognise the autoantibodies bound to the immobilised antigens. After a 15-minute incubation, any excess enzyme conjugate, which is not specifically bound is washed away with wash buffer.

Phase 3

A chromogenic substrate solution containing TMB (3,3′, 5,5′-Tetramethyl-benzidine) is dispensed into the wells. During 15-minutes of incubation, the colour of the solutions change into blue. Colour development is stopped by adding 1 M hydrochloric acid as stop solution. The solutions colour change into yellow.

The amount of colour is directly proportional to the concentration of IgG present in the original sample. The optical density of the controls serve as reference for the determination of the cut-off OD. Patient results may be classified in terms of negative or positive.

To read the optical, density a microplate reader with a 450 nm filter is required. Bichromatic measurement with a 600-690 nm reference is recommended.

Clinical Relevance

The serological detection of antinuclear antibodies (ANA) in patients with suspected autoimmune disorders is common practice in every immunological lab.

Inflammatory connective tissue diseases are characterised by idiopathic genesis along with disturbances in terms of cellular and humoral immunity, systemic organ failure, and a chronic course of disease. Additionally, connective tissue diseases exhibit overlapping symptomatic features, thus making a right diagnosis extremely difficult.

Systemic lupus erythematosus (SLE), Sjögren's syndrome, progressive systemic scleroderma along with CREST syndrome, Sharp's syndrome (mixed connective tissue disease) and myositis belong to the inflammatory rheumatic diseases.

Considering the diversitivity of mixed connective tissue diseases such disorders exhibit a common serological characteristic the presence of antinuclear antibodies. Those antibodies are directed against parts of the cell nucleus and the cytoplasm. For the most part, the presence of a particular ANA in a patient serum can be assigned to a special inflammatory disease.

When an autoimmune disorder is suspected the first diagnostic step is the performance of a screening test on antinuclear antibodies. Common practice is indirect immunofluorescence on HEp-2 cells. The second step in the ANA algorithm is the isolated detection of the particular antibodies specilfities (e.g. with ANAcombi, ORG 530). In between, an additional screening test can be performed.

The wells of the ORGenTec ANAscreen ELISA are coated with a mixture of eight autoantigens in order to allow a screening on the most important antinuclear antibodies anti RNP 70 (also called Anti-RNP-68), Anti-Sm, Anti-RNP-Sm (= Anti-U1-snRNP), Anti-SS-A, Anti-SS-B, Anti-Scl-70, Anti-Centromer B and Anti-Jo-1). Thus the ANAscreen kit allows a sensitive screening on one or more autoantibodies possibly being present in a patient serum.

Specificity

The microplate is coated with the antigens RNP-70, RNP/Sm, Sm, SS-A, SS-B, Scl-70, centromer B and Jo-1, respectively. All antigen preparations, native and recombinant, are highly purified by affinity chromatography. The ANAcombi test is specific only for autoantibodies directed to these antigens. No cross reactivities have been observed.

Calibration

The assay system is calibrated against the internationally recognised reference sera from CDC, Atlanta, USA, since no other international standards are available.

Materials Required

Equipment

- Microplate reader capable for endpoint measurement at 450 nm
- Vortex mixer
- Pipettes for 10 µl, 100 µl and 1000 µl

Preparation of Reagents

- Distilled water
- Graduated cylinder for 100 and 1000 ml
- Plastic container for storage of the wash solution

Optional

- Multichannel Dispenser or
- Repeatable pipette for 100 µl
- Data reduction software

Specimen Collection and Preparation

For determination of ANA antibodies serum or plasma are the preferred sample matrices.

All serum and plasma samples are prediluted 1:100 with sample buffer. Therefore, 10 µl of sample may be diluted with 1000 µl of sample buffer.

The patients need not to be fasting, and no special preparations are necessary. Collect blood by venipuncture into vacutainers and separate serum or plasma from the cells by centrifugation after clot formation.

Samples may be stored refrigerated at 2 to 8°C for at least 5 days. For longer storage of up to six months samples should be stored frozen at –20°C. To avoid repeated thawing and freezing, the samples should be aliquoted.

Neither bilirubin nor haemolysis have significant effect on the procedure.

Preparation and Storage of Reagents

All components of this test kit are supplied in a liquid format and ready to use, except the sample buffer and wash buffer. When stored refrigerated at 2 to 8°C the components are stable for at least 30 days after opening or until the expiration date printed on the labels.

Remaining modules of the microplate should be stored refrigerated at 2 to 8°C protected from moisture; store together with desiccant and carefully sealed in the plastic bag.

Preparation of Sample Buffer

Dilute the contents of each vial of the sample buffer concentrate (5x) with distilled water to a final volume of 100 ml prior to use. Store regfrigerated stable at 2 to 8° C for at least 30 days after preparation or until the expiration date printed on the label.

Preparation of Buffered Wash Solution

Dilute the contents of each vial of the buffered wash solution concentrate (50x) with diluted water to a final volume of 1000 ml prior to use. Store refrigerated: stable at 2-8ºC for at least 30 days after preparation or until the expiration date printed on the label.

NOTES ON TECHNIQUE

Control sera or pools should routinely be assayed as unknowkns to check performance of the reagents and the assay.

For all controls, the respective concentrations are provided on the labels of each vial. Using these concentrations a calibration curve may be calculated to read off the patient results semi-quantitatively.

Pipetting and Sample Handling

Use a disposable-tip micropipette to dispense sera and plasma samples. Pipette directly to the bottom of the wells. To avoid carryover contamination change the tip between samples.

Patient samples expected to contain high concentration should be additionally diluted with sample buffer before. Additional dilutions must be considered during calculation.

Immunoassay Procedure

Do not interchange components of different lots.

All components should be at room temperature before use.

Dilute all patient samples 1:100 with sample buffer before assay. Therefore, combine 10 µl of sample with 1000 µl of sample buffer in a polystyrene tube. Mix well. Calibrators and controls are ready to use and need not to be diluted.

1. Prepare a sufficient number of microplate modules to accommodate controls and prediluted patient samples in duplicates.

	1	2	3	4	5	6
RNP/70	A	CC	NC	P1	P2	P..
RNP/Sm	B	CC	NC	P1	P2	P..
Sm	C	CC	NC	P1	P2	P..
SS-A	D	CC	NC	P1	P2	P..
SS-B	E	CC	NC	P1	P2	P..
Scl-70	F	CC	NC	P1	P2	P..
Centromer B	G	CC	NC	P1	P2	P..
Jo-1	H	CC	NC	P1	P2	P..

CC Calibrator
NC negative control
P1, P2 patient samples

2. Pipette 100 µl of controls and prediluted patient samples into the wells.
3. Incubate for 30 minutes at room temperature (20-28°C).
4. Discard the contents of the microwells and wash 3 times with 300 µl of wash solution.
5. Dispense 100 µl of enzyme conjugate solution into each well.
6. Incubate for 15 minutes at room temperature.
7. Discard the contents of the microwells and wash 3 times with 300 µl of wash solution.
8. Dispense 100 µl of TMB substrate solution into each well.
9. Incubate for 15 minutes at room temperature protected from light.
10. Add 100 µl of stop solution to each well of the modules and leave untouched for 5 minutes.
11. Read the optical density at 450 nm and calculate the results. Bichromatic measurement with reference at 600-650 nm is recommended.

The developed colour is stable for at least 30 minutes. Read optical densities during this time.

Calculation of Results

OD Quotient Calculation

For each patient sample 8 index values should be calculated according to the following equation:

$$\text{Index value} = \frac{OD_{Sample}}{OD_{Cut\text{-}off}}$$

A sample is positive for one ANA parameter if its index-value is ≥ 1.2

	ANAcombi (Index value)
Negative	< 1.0
Borderline	1.0-1.2
Positive	≥ 1.2

Alternative Calculation

Evaluation of the ANAcombi test is carried out by comparison of the optical densities of the patient sample with the optical density of the calibrator control.

For each antigen, the OD cut-off value should be calculated according to the following equation:

$$OD_{Cut\text{-}off} = OD_{Calibrator\ control} \times \text{specific factor}$$

A sample is positive for one ANA parameter if OD sample is > OD cut-off

	ANAcombi (OD-sample)
Negative	< OD Cut-off
Positive	≥ OD Cut-off

For detailed quantitative analyses we recommend to use the individual ANA-ELISA test systems.

Calculation Example

The chart below shows typical results for ANAcombi. These data are intended for illustration only and should not be used to calculate results from another run.

Sample No.	Anti	Row	OD Calibrator	Factor	OD Cut-off	OD Sample	Result
1	RNP-70	A	0.48	1.10	0.53	0.083	Negative
1	RNP/Sm	B	0.50	1.00	0.50	0.420	Negative
1	Sm	C	0.40	1.25	0.50	0.138	Negative
1	SS-A	D	0.42	0.85	0.36	0.133	Negative
1	SS-B	E	0.53	0.75	0.39	0.505	Positive
1	Scl-70	F	0.57	1.00	0.57	0.820	Positive
1	Centromer B	G	0.49	0.80	0.39	0.212	Negative
1	Jo-1	H	0.50	0.80	0.40	0.189	Negative

Incubation Scheme

1. Pipette 100 µl control or 8 × 100 µl patient sample
   - Incubate for 30 minutes at room temperature
     - Discard the contents of the wells and wash 3 times with 300 µl wash solution
2. Pipette 100 µl enzyme conjugate
   - Incubate for 15 minutes at room temperature
     - Discard the contents of the wells and wash 3 times with 300 µl wash solution
3. Pipette 100 µl substrate solution
   - Incubate for 15 minutes at room temperature
4. Add 100µl stop solution
   - Leave untouched for 5 minutes
     - Read at 450 nm

ANA PROFILE

ANA Profile Positivities

	ANA	dsDNA	DNP	Sm	RNP	SS-A	SS-B	Scl-70	Jo-1	RAF
Positivity in%										
Rheumatoid arth	30-60	5	5			5	2			72 to 85
SLE	95-10060		70	25	32	20	20			20
MCTD	95-100									20
Sjögren's syndrome	N					70	70			75
Diffuse sclerod	95							33		33
CREST	95							20		33
Polymyositis		95						10	30	33

Sm, RNP, SS-A, SS-B, Scl-70 and Jo-1 are collectively called extractable nuclear antigens or ENAs

SS-A/Ro Interpretation

Antibodies to SS-A/Ro have been detected in approximately 25-30% of patients with Sjögren's syndrome. In addition, anti-SS-A/Ro antibodies have been associated with homozygous compliment C2 and C4 deficiencies, subacute cutaneous lupus eryhtomatosus (SCLE), and neonatal lupus.

SS-B/La Interpretation

Antibodies to SS-B/La are nearly always found in association with antibodies to SS-A/Ro and occur in 15% of SLE patients. Anti-SS-B/La are also detected in approximately 50-60 % of Sjögren's syndrome patients and are considered a serological marker for that disease. The SS-B/La antigen is a 43-50 kD phosphorylated polypeptide that binds a large number of small RNA polymerase III transcripts and also small RNAs produced by some viruses, such as the Epstien-Barr virus, adenovirus and vesicular stomatitis virus. Evidence suggests that the SS-B/La particle is either a termination factor for RNA polymerase III or is involved in post-termination processing events. Anti-SS-B/La antibodies have also been detected in patients with systemic sclerosis, neonatal lupus, false negative immunofluorescence ANA, and are also found in normal individuals.

Sm Interpretation

Antibodies to Sm, a non-histone nuclear antigen, was first detected in a patient with SLE. These antibodies have been identified in the sera of approximately 25-40% of patients with SLE. Anti-Sm is both a diagnostic marker and a reliable measure of disease activity in SLE. Anti-Sm is considered to be a highly specific marker for SLE since it has not been detected in the normal sera or in the sera of patients with rheumatoid arthritis, Sjögren's syndrome (SS), progressive systemic sclerosis, mixed connective tissue disease, or drug induced lupus.

SmRNP Interpretation

Antibodies to RNP, A nonhistone nuclear antigen, occurs in many of the connective tissue diseases including SLE, MCTD, SS, PSS, RA, and polymyositis. High titres of anti-RNP antibodies are usually considered diagnostic of MCTD. Sm and RNP antigens are composed of small nuclear RNA (U-RNA) complexed with proteins which are extractable with physiologic saline.

Scl-70 Interpretation

Antibodies to Scl-70, are also known as topoisomerase I, are found almost.

Exclusively in patients with scleroderma. The Scl-70 antigen is a basic chromosomal nonhistone protein with a molecular weight of 70 kD. Anti-Scl-70 antibodies are highly specific for scleroderma and are found in 20-28% of patients with the disease. Anti-Scl-70 antibodies have also been found in patients with the crest variant of scleroderma, and with primary Raynaud's phenomenon.

Jo-1 Interpretation

Antibodies to Jo-1, also known as histidyl-tRNA synthetase, are commonly found in a subgroup of connective tissue disease patients with polymyositis and dermatomyositis. The Jo-1 antigen is a 50 kD molecular weight nuclear polypeptide that is the protein moiety of histidyl-tRNA synthetase. Anti-Jo-1 antibodies are present in 18-36% patients with polymyositis. Anti-Jo-1 antibodies have also been found in patients with interstitial lung disease.

ANTINEUTROPHIL CYTOPLASMIC ANTIBODIES ANCA PROFILE ANCAcombi MFD: Orgenetec, Courtesy: Lilac Medicare

Immunometric Enzyme Immunoassay for the Qualitative Determination of ANCA-Autoantibodies

Warnings and Precautions

All reagents of this test kit are strictly intended for *in vitro* use only.

Please adhere strictly to the sequence of pipetting steps provided in this protocol. Observe the guidelines for performing quality control in medical laboratories by assaying controls and/or pooled sera.

All reagents should be stored refrigerated at 2 to 8°C in their original container.

Do not interchange kit components from different lots. The expiration dates stated on the labels of the shipping container and all vials have to be observed. Do not use kit components beyond their expiration dates.

Allow all kit components and specimen to reach room temperature prior to use and mix well.

During handling of all kit reagents, controls and serum samples observe the existing legal regulations. The following precautions should be taken while handling potentially infectious materials:

— do not eat, drink or smoke in areas where specimens or kit reagents are handled
— do not pipette by mouth
— wear disposable gloves while handling specimens or kit reagents and wash hands thoroughly afterwards.

The test kit contains components of human origin which, when tested by FDA-licensed methods, were found negative for hepatitis B surface antigen and for HIV antibody. No known test can guarantee, however, that products derived from human blood will not be infectious. Handle, therefore, all reagents and human blood derivatives, like plasma or serum samples, as if capable of transmitting infection.

Avoid contact with the TMB (3,3′, 5,5′-Tetramethyl-benzidine). If TMB comes into contact with skin, wash thoroughly with water and soap.

The stop solution contains hydrochloric acid. If it comes into contact with skin, wash thorougly with water and seek medical attention.

Avoid contact between the buffered peroxide solution and easily oxidised materials; extreme temperatures may initiate spontaneous combustion.

Materials Supplied

Package size	96 determination
divisible microplate consisting	
of 12 modules of 8 wells,	1
coated with highly purified	
antigens: PR3, MPO, BPI, Elastase,	
Cathepsin G, Lysozyme and	
Lactoferrin	
ANCA controls in	
a PBS/BSA matrix	1 set
Negative control (A)	3 vials
Cut-off control (B)	1.5 ml each
Positive control (C)	
Sample buffer, yellow	1 vial
concentrate	20 ml
Enzyme conjugate solution 1 vial	
(light red) containing polyclonal rabbit	
anti-h-IgG-IgG	12 ml
labelled with horseradish	
peroxidase	
TMB substrate solution	1 vial
	12 ml
Stop solution	1 vial
(1 M hydrochloric acid)	12 ml
Buffered wash solution,	1 vial
concentrate	20 ml

Controls

A set of 3 controls is provided with the kit.

Technical Data

Sample material	Serum or plasma
Required sample size	10 µl of sample to be diluted 1:100 with sample buffer 100 µl prediluted sample per single determination
Total incubation time	60 minutes at room temperature (18-28°C)
Storage	Refrigerated at 2 to 8°C
Shelf-life	9 months after manufacturing or until the expiration date printed on the labels
Package size	96 tests

Principle of the Procedure

The ANCAcombi is an indirect solid-phase enzyme immunometric assay (ELISA). It is designed for the qualitative determination of anti-neutrophil cytoplasmic antibodies (ANCA) directed against PR3, MPO, BPI, elastase, cathepsin G, lysozyme and lactoferrin. The assay system recognises IgG class autoantibodies.

The wells of the microplate were coated with mixed antigen, PR3, MPO, BPI, elastase, cathepsin G, lysozyme and lactoferrin in row A to H, respectively. The microplate can be divided into 12 modules of 8 wells each or can be used completely for 96 determinations.

During the procedure the binding of present autoantibodies, as well as the formation of the sandwich complexes and enzymatic colour reaction take place during three different reaction phases.

Phase 1

Controls and prediluted patient samples are pipetted into the wells of the microplate. Any present antibodies bind to the immobilised antigens. After a 30-minutes incubation the microplate is washed with wash buffer for removing nonreactive serum components.

Phase 2

An anti-human-IgG horseradish peroxidase conjugate solution is pipetted into the wells of the microplate to recognise the autoantibodies bound to the immobilised antigens. After a 15-minute incubation, any excess enzyme conjugate, which is not specifically bound, is washed away with wash buffer.

Phase 3

A chromogenic substrate solution containing TMB (3,3′,5,5′-Tetramethyl-benzidine) is dispensed into the wells. During 15 minutes of incubation, the colour of the solutions changes into blue. Colour development is stopped by adding 1 M hydrochloric acid as stop solution. The solutions colour changes into yellow.

The amount of colour is directly proportional to the concentration of IgG present in the original sample. The optical density of the controls serve as reference for the determination of the cut-off OD. Patient results may be classified in terms of negative or positve.

To read the optical density a microplate reader with a 450 nm filter is required. Bichromatic measurement with a 600-690 nm reference is recommended.

Clinical Relevance

The acronym ANCA (Antineutrophil Cytoplasmic Autoantibodies) is defined by an accumulation of autoantibodies with specificity against different granulocytic, monozytic and probably endothelial cytoplasmic antigens.

Autoantibodies against endocellular components of neutrophile granulocyte (PMN) are known for a longer period. At first, in 1964 they have been described as granulocyte specific factor directed against anti nuclear components (GS-ANA). Under the term ANCA, they were first reported in 1982 in a few patients who has necrotising glomerulonephritis without immune deposits, but the relevance was still unclear. The next report of ANCA was in 1984 were these autoantibodies has been observed in four patients with systemic vasculitis and three of whom has also necrotising glomerulonephritis. In 1985, a collaborative study in the Netherlands and Denmark described these factors, showing a high sensitivity for active Wegener's granulomatosis, as APCA (Anti Cytoplasmic Antibodies) and they suggested that APCA could be used as a marker for disease activity. In 1988, further investigations substantiated the associaton of ANCA with Wegener's granulomatosis and polyarthritis nodosa, and also noted that ANCA occur in patients with pauci-immune (idiopathic) necrotising and crescentic glomerulonephritis who have no evidence for extrarenal disease. Proteinase 3 (PR3), showing a central accentuated pattern (cANCA) has been described as major antigen for Wegener's granulomatosis. A new pattern, showing a high specificity for the microscopic polyangitis, with perinuclear fluorescence (pANCA) was also observed in 1988. At first, only myeloperoxidase (MPO) was described as antigen. In the last years, newer investigations discovered and characterized a couple of new pANCA antigens: Elastase, Cathepsin G, Lysozyme and Lactoferrin.

In the meantime, PR3 and MPO are well defined as reliable serological markers for a definite group of primary systemic vasculitides (PSV), which were also named ANCA-associated vasculitides (AAV). The occurrence of AAV is clearly higher than supposed. The incidence is 1.5 per 1000 and in the group of older persons nearly 5 per 1000. The clinical appearance of the AAV is characterised trough manifestations in lung, kidney and respiratory tract.

Up to now, ANCA screening has been done with immunofluorescence techniques, but often there have been difficulties in the evaluation and in clinical findings. Therefore, the results have to be scrutinised with counter examinations on other cells or in other test system like ELISA. Moreover, it was not possible to differentiate the single cANCA and pANCA antigens.

Proteinase 3

The major antigen for the cANCA reactivity is the neutral serin protease 3 (synonyms p29, AGP7, Wegener autoantigen), which belongs to the trypsin/chymotrypsin family. In 1988, several groups showed that the antigen is a protein with a molecular weight of 29 kDa. PR3 was already described in 1973 by Ohlsson and Olsson under the name neutrophile collagenase. In the meantime it seems certain, that autoantibodies against PR3 are highly specific as serological marker for the diagnosis of Wegener's granulomatosis (specificity initial phase 50%, generalisation phase > 90%). Moreover there is a correlation between the concentration of the autoantibodies and the disease activity.

Myeloperoxidase

Myeloperoxidase was first isolated by Anger in 1941, who gave it the name "verdoperoxidase", because of its green colour and ability to catalyse peroxidase reactions. It is MPO that gives pus its greenish tone. In nearly 60% of the pANCA findings MPO is the major antigen. The occurrence of autoantibodies against MPO is classified as relevant marker for the rapid progressive nephritis Moreover these antibodies occur in 70-90% in all patients with serious kidney injury. Over and about they have also been detected at the Churg-Strauss syndrome (CSS), microscopic polyangitis (MPA) and other vasculitis diseases. The concentration of the autoantibodies correlates well with the disease acitivity of MPA. The MPA is also characterised by clinical manifestations of lung, kidney and respiratory tract, but these manifestations are, in contrast to WG, not granulomatous, However, these antibodies have, in contrast to the high specificity of PR3 antibodies for WG, a minor specificity of 60% in the diagnosis of MPA. The absence of autoantibodies against MPO and PR3, by simultaneous detection of ANA can be used as a tool for differential diagnosis between AAV and SLE-induced vasculitis.

BPI

Bactericidal permeability-increasing protein, BPI is a membrane-located protein of 55 kDa molecular weight and is classed as an ANCA-antigen of polymorph-nuclear granulocytes and monocytes that bind endotoxin. Its autoantibodies are now classified as cANCA. Due to BPI's high affinity to lipopolysaccharides its antimicrobial effect against gram-negative bacteria is significant. The BPI's splitted and thus inactivated by using elastase or other serine protease. Autoantibodies against BPI are above all detected in chronically infectious intestinal diseases such as Morbus Crohn or colitis ulcerosa. In contrast to anti-MPO and anti-PR3 autoantibodies, those against BPI seem not to have any association with vasculitis.

Elastase

Elastase is a serine protease with a sequence homology of 54% to that of proteinase 3. It occurs mainly in polymorphonuclear neutrophilic granulocytes (PMN), in macrophages and endothelial cells. The dismantling of proteoglycans by neutrophiles is mainly due to elastase proteolytic activity. Furthermore, elastase participates decisively in tissue destruction connected with emphysemas and rheumatoid arthritis. Autoantibodies against this antigen are generally associated with inflammatory rheumatic disorders, e.g. rheumatoid arthritis and vasculitis.

Cathepsin G

The cathepsins belong to a group of intracellular proteases mainly found in lysosomes, especially of the spleen, the liver and the kidney. Cathepsin G is a serine protease and a further pANCA antigen. It participates to a great part in the destruction of osteid tissue as of its hydrolytic properties. The autoantibodies against cathepsin G occur mainly in collagenosis and other related inflammatory rheumatic diseases, e.g. SLE, Sjögren syndrome and Felty's syndrome.

Lysozyme

In 1922, lysozyme (LZ) was accidentally discovered by Alexander Flemming. The LZ is a glykosidase consisting of 129 amino acid residues with a molecular weight of 14, 6 kDa, which decomposes the glycosidic bond between C-1 MNAc and C-4 of GlcNAc. Lysozyme is localised in the azurophilic as well as in the specific granules of neutrophiles and in extracellular liquid compartments like tears and salivary, where it spreads out its antimicrobial activities against invading bacteria. The LZ belongs also to the pANCA and autoantibodies against lysozyme occur in higher frequency in rheumatoid vasculitis and inflammatory bowel disease like colitis ulcerosa.

Lactoferrin

Lactoferrin (LF) is an iron-binding protein, with a molecular weight of 77-93 kDa, which occurs in high concentrations in secretions at mucosa surfaces, in tears and in milk. The LF also resides in the specific granules of polymorphonuclear (PMN) neutrophil leukocytes and becomes exocytosed upon PMN activation. During active inflammatory disease, raised serum levels of LF can be measured. The physiological antimicrobial effect of lactoferrin depends on its iron-binding capacity, because most of the bacteria require iron for their own physiological pathways. The LF inhibits myelopoiesis, prevents complement activation and prevents the formation of hydroxyl radicals. It is quite possible that LF has several important roles, like secretory IgA, as a nonspecific antiphlogistic defence factor at mucosal surfaces. The LF belongs to the pANCA, depending on the redistribution from the granules toward the nuclei, upon ethanol fixation. Autoantibodies against lactoferrin occur in higher frequency in patients with rheumatoid vasculitis (RV), colitis ulcerosa (CU) and primary sclerosing cholangitis (PSC).

Specificity

The microplate is coated with the antigens PR3, MPO, BPI, elastase, cathepsin G, lysozyme and lactoferrin, respectively. All antigen preparations are highly purified by affinity chromatography. The ANCAcombi test is specific only for autoantibodies directed to these antigens. No crossreactivities have been observed.

Calibration

Since no international reference preparations for ANCA autoantibodies are available, the assay system is calibrated arbitrarily.

IMMUNOASSAY PROCEDURE

Materials Required

Equipment

- Microplate reader capable for endpoint measurements at 450 nm
- Vortex mixer
- Pipettes for 10 µl, 100 µl and 1000 µl

Preparation of reagents

- Distilled water
- Graduated cylinder for 100 and 1,000 ml
- Plastic container for storage of the wash solution

Optional

- Multichannel dispenser
- Repeatable pipette for 100 µl
- Data reduction software

Specimen Collection and Preparation

For determination of ANCA antibodies, serum or plasma are the preferred sample matrices.

All serum and plasma samples are prediluted 1:100 with sample buffer. Therefore, 10 µl of sample may be diluted with 1,000 µl of sample buffer.

The patients need not to be fasting, and no special preparations are necessary. Collect blood by venipuncture into vacutainers and separate serum or plasma from the cells by centrifugation after clot formation.

Samples may be stored refrigerated at 2 to 8°C for at least 5 days. For longer storage of up to six months, samples should be stored frozen at –20°C. To avoid repeated thawing and freezing, the samples should be aliquoted.

Neither bilirubin nor haemolysis have significant effect on the procedure.

Preparation and Storage or Reagents

All components of this kit are supplied in a liquid format and ready to use, except the sample buffer and wash buffer. When stored refrigerated at 2 to 8°C the components are stable for at least 30 days after opening or until the expiration date printed on the labels.

Remaining modules of the microplate should be stored refrigerated at 2 to 8°C protected from moisture; store together with desiccant and carefully sealed in the plastic bag.

Preparation of Sample Buffer

Dilute the contents of each vial of the sample buffer concentrate (5x) with distilled water to a final volume of 100 ml prior to use. Store refrigerated stable at 2 to 8°C for at least 30 days after preparation or until the expiration date printed on the label.

Preparation of Buffered Wash Solution

Dilute the contents of each vial of the buffered wash solution concentrate (50x) with distilled water to a final volume of 1000 ml prior to use. Store refrigerated stable at 2 to 8°C for at least 30 days after preparation or until the expiration date printed on the label.

Notes on Technique

Control sera or pools should routinely be assayed as unknown to check peformance of the reagents and the assay.

The positive control (C) provided with the kit contains antibodies against each antigen. It can, therefore, be used to check the performance of each antigen separately.

Pipetting and Sample Handling

Use a disposable-tip micropipette to dispense serum and plasma samples. Pipette directly to the bottom of the wells. To avoid carryover contamination, change the tip between samples.

Patient samples expected to contain high concentrations should be additionally diluted with sample buffer before. Additional dilutions must be considered during calculation.

Immunoassay Procedure

Do not interchange components of different lots. All components should be at room temperature before use.

Dilute all patient samples 1:100 with sample buffer before assay. Therefore, combine 10 μl of sample with 1,000 μl of sample buffer in a polystyrene tube. Mix well. Controls are ready to use and need not to be diluted.

1. Prepare a sufficient number of microplate modules to accommodate controls and prediluted patient samples.

			1	2	3	4	5	6
Mixed antigen	⇒	a	A	B	C			
PR3	⇒	b	P1	P2	P3	P..		
MPO	⇒	c	P1	P2	P3	P..		
BPI	⇒	d	P1	P2	P3	P..		
Elastase	⇒	e	P1	P2	P3	P..		
Cathepsin G	⇒	f	P1	P2	P3	P..		
Lysozyme	⇒	g	P1	P2	P3	P..		
Lactoferrin	⇒	h	P1	P2	P3	P..		

2. Pipette 100 μl of calibrators, controls and prediluted patient samples into the wells.
3. Incubate of 30 minutes at room temperature (20-28°C).
4. Discard the contents of the microwells and wash 3 times with 300 μl of wash solution.
5. Dispense 100 μl of enzyme conjugate solution into each well.
6. Incubate for 15 minutes at room temperature.
7. Discard the contents of the microwells and wash 3 times with 300 μl of wash solution.
8. Dispense 100 μl of TMB substrate solution into each well.
9. Incubate for 15 minutes at room temperature.
10. Add 100 μl of stop solution to each well of the modules and let it stand for 5 minutes.
11. Read the optical density at 450 nm and calculate the results. Bichromatic measurement with a reference at 600-690 nm is recommended.

The developed colour is stable for at least 30 minutes. Read optical densities during this time.

Calculation of Results

Evaluation of the ANCAcombi test is carried out by comparison of the optical densities of the patient sample with the optical density of the cut-off control. Previously, each patient's OD must be corrected by a specific factor (please refere to the certificate).

For each patient sample 7 OD-Quotients should be calculated according to the following equation:

$$\text{OD-Quotient} = \frac{OD_{sample} \times \text{Factor}}{OD_{\text{Cut-off control B}}}$$

A sample is positive for one ANCA parameter if its OD-Quotient is ≥ 1.0

	ANCAcombi (OD-Quotient)
Negative	< 1.0
Positive	≥ 1.0

For detailed quantitative analyses we recommend to use the individual ANCA-ELISAs.

Calculation Example

The chart below shows typical results for ANCAcombi. These data are intended for illustration only and should not be used to calculate results from another run.

Sample No	*Anti*	*Row*	*OD_{sample}*	*Factor*	*$OD_{Cut\text{-}off}$*	*OD-Quotient*	*Result*
1	PR3	B	0.083	1.10		0.22	Negative
1	MPO	C	0.920	1.00		2.19	Positive
1	BPI	D	0.138	1.25		0.41	Negative
1	Elastase	E	0.133	0.85	0.420	0.27	Negative
1	Cath. G	F	0.505	0.75		0.90	Negative
1	Lysozyme	G	0.420	1.00	1.00	0.21	Negative
1	Lactoferrin	H	0.112	0.80		5.61	Negative
2	PR3	B	2.143	1.10		5.61	High pos.
2	MPO	C	0.240	1.00	0.420	0.57	Negative
2	BPI	D	0.079	1.25		0.24	Negative

Incubation Scheme

ANCAcombi

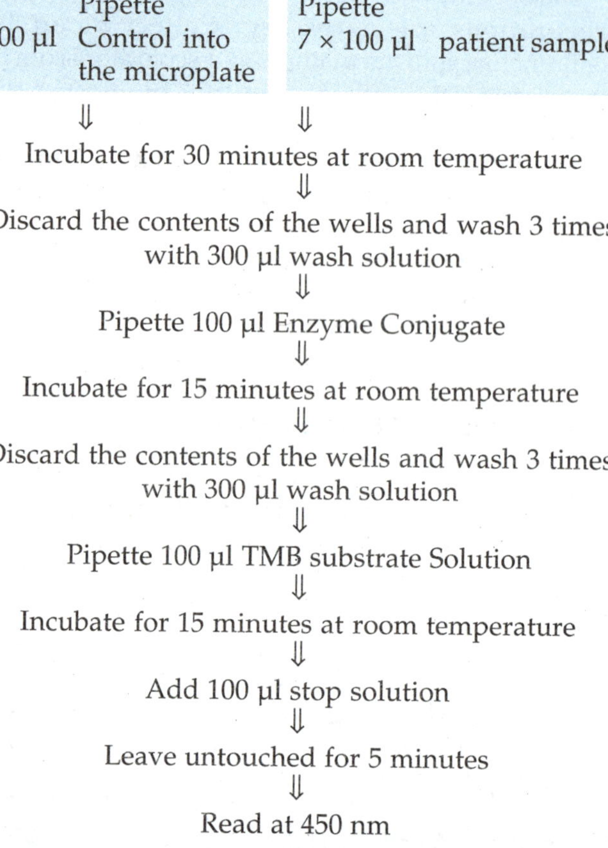

ANTIPHOSPHOLIPID SYNDROME

Introduction

Most people tend to think of infertility as the inability to become pregnant. It really is, however, the inability to have a baby. Thus, couples with recurrent pregnancy losses also have a fertility problem even though the woman is able to conceive.

There is now increasing evidence that abnormalities in the immune system affect a woman's ability to carry a pregnancy to term and deliver a healthy baby. Our immune system is designed to fight off foreign invaders such as viruses and bacteria. In many people (women are more commonly affected than men) the immune system becomes activated in an abnormal way and antibodies are formed against the person's own tissues. Our body then literally begins to attack itself. There are many diseases where this is occurring and we call these diseases "autoimmune". Common examples of autoimmune diseases include diabetes, lupus, rheumatic fever, rheumatoid arthritis, etc.

Many years ago, it was recognised that women with systemic lupus frequently aborted pregnancies in the first trimester. It was discovered that these women had, in their blood, a substance that affected the tests that used to measure the ability of the blood to clot. This substance prolonged certain coagulation tests. Women who had the substance in the bloodstream, when tested, behaved as if they were taking an anticoagulant such as heparin. This substance, but because it was found initially in women who had lupus, was named "the lupus anticoagulant".

It is critically important to understand that the lupus anticoagulant (LAC) is not an anticoagulant itself. It simply affects certain coagulation studies and, therefore, gives the appearance of being an anticoagulant. In fact, it is undoubtedly a substance that promotes the formation of blood clots. Lupus anticoagulant is also an autoimmune antibody.

Over the years other antibodies have been found that behave similarly to the lupus anticoagulant. These are called antiphospholipid antibodies. This led to the term antiphospholipid syndrome (APLS), because it included a series of symptoms as follows:

a. Repeated clotting in veins (for example - a pulmonary embolus) or arteries (examples include a stoke, a blood clot in an arm or a leg, or a coronary).
b. Recurrent pregnancy loss, usually in mid to late pregnancy as opposed to early pregnancy.

The above symptoms are specifically characteristic of APLS. However, there are a lot of other symptoms that are also associated with APLS. Such symptoms include skin changes and low platelets.

(*A syndrome is a collection of events which constitute a specific illness*).

History of APLS

In the 1900s, certain people had false-positive test results for syphilis. This data was a curiosity without clinical importance at the time, but rediscovered in the 1940s.

By the 1950s, it was realised that this false positive syphilis test had something to do with lupus. Today, although known as a clue to diagnosis, a false positive syphilis test is not sufficient for a diagnosis of lupus or APLS.

In the 1950s and 1960s, it was realised that the antiphospholipid antibodies had something to do with blood clots.

In 1983, Hughes, Gharavi, and Harris developed a simple test for the antibodies called an ELISA. Clinical descriptions of various things that occurred when people had this antibody were also noted.

In 1985, descriptions of what happened in pregnancy for people with this antibody were also noted.

Up until 1989, it was thought that APLS was a subset of lupus. However, enough cases were seen in which people had APLS without having lupus. It was decided that it should be categorised as a separate illness. Several names have been used to describe it. The most common name is PAPS (primary antiphospholipid syndrome). It is also sometimes called Hughes' syndrome. The term secondary antiphospholipid syndrome is used for people who had APLS and lupus.

In 1990, the β2-glycoprotein 1 was discovered. The importance of this protein will be reviewed later.

What is a Phospholipid?

A phospholipid is a type of fat. It contains phosphate and lipids (which means fat).

The six phospholipids that are important are:

1. Cardiolipin
2. Phosphatidyl serine
3. Phosphatidyl ethanolamine
4. Phosphatidic acid
5. Phosphatidyl inositol
6. Glycerol

All cells in the body have membranes that are made of phospholipids. These membranes hold the cell together. Bacteria and viruses also have phospholipids. They occur everywhere in nature.

The illustration (Fig. 23.30) shows that the cell has a membrane, and contains a nucleus which also has a membrane. Phospholipids make up the membrane and, as seen in the illustration, they are set opposed to one another on the outside and inside of the membrane. There is a difference between the phospholipids on the outside and inside. This will be an important issue.

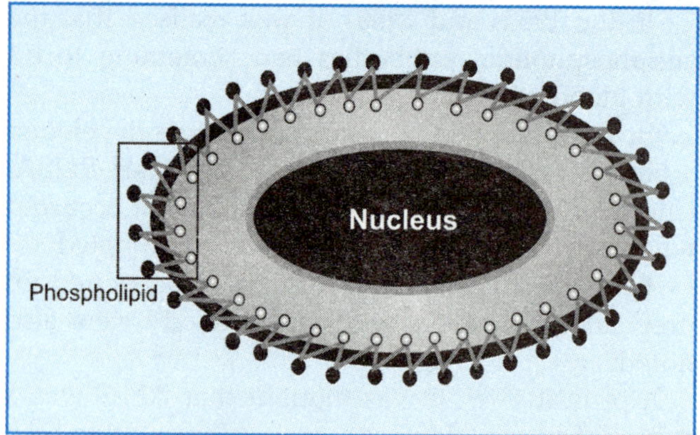

Fig. 23.30: Phospholipids on a cell membrane

What are Antiphospholipid Antibodies (APLs)?

Under normal circumstances, antibodies are proteins (immunoglobulins) made by our immune system to fight substances recognised as foreign by our body. Some examples of foreign substances are bacteria and viruses. Sometimes, the body's own cells are recognised as foreign. These antibodies are then called autoantibodies which lead to autoimmune disease.

In antiphospholipid antibody syndrome the body recognises phospholipids as foreign and produces antibodies against them. There are different types of antiphospholipid antibodies—IgG, IgM and IgA types. Secondly these antibodies may be against any of the phospholipids. Of these anticardiolipin and antiphosphatidyl serine are more important.

β2-Gycoprotein and its Relationship to APLS?

β2-glycoprotein 1 is bound to internal phospholipids that have flipped to the outside of the cell. Under certain circumstances, such as when a cell is injured, infected or because of some drugs, the inside phospholipids will flip to the outside. The β2-glycoprotein 1 then binds to these phospholipids (Fig. 23.31).

People with infections, such as syphilis, will make antibody directed against the phospholipids surrounding the cell. But, people with APLS make antibodies directed against the β2-glycoprotein 1, which binds to the phospholipid.

Mechanism of Action of APLs

How do antiphospholipid antibodies cause clotting disorders?

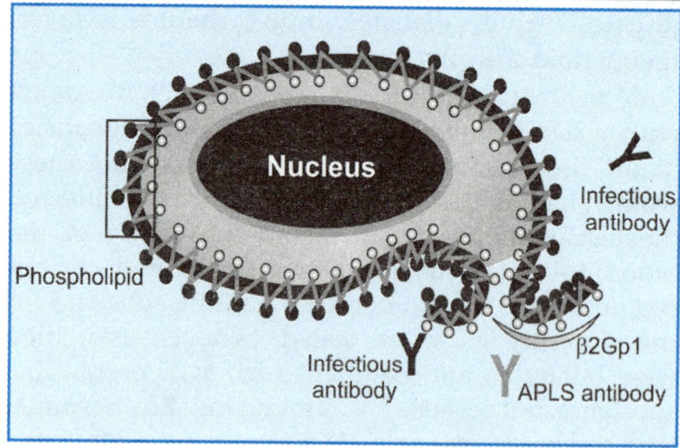

Fig. 23.31: Illustration 2: antiphospholipid antibodies and infectious antibodies

Our circulatory system has a self-sealing mechanism known as blood clotting to prevent life-threatening injury. Bleeding is rapidly stopped by a process known as haemostasis that involves the following processes.

Vascular injury leads to the margination of platelets to the site of vessel injury. The platelets adhere to the damaged endothelial cells via von Willebrand factor (small amounts of fibrinogen assist in creating this platelet plug). The platelets are then stimulated to degranulate and express receptors for factors V and VIII as well as leukocytes. At this same time, blood is exposed to tissue factor and the clotting pathways are initiated. The necessary cofactors (V and VIII) bind to receptors on platelet surfaces and allow for efficient propagation of the cascade. This eventually leads to the formation of fibrin. Since fibrin strands are formed in the vicinity of platelets, the two can easily come together and form a clot. Leukocyte receptors on the platelets bind PMNs and monocytes. PMNs initiate inflammatory reactions, and monocytes produce tissue factor to help in generating the thrombus and allowing for the first steps in wound healing (Fig. 23.32).

Blood clotting has to be initiated only when required as in the case of injuries. Under normal circumstances (when there is no injury), the blood has to be kept in a free flowing state. Therefore, all the clotting factors have to be controlled. Similarly, the aggregation of platelets also has to be controlled. This is achieved by two ways. In the coagulation cascade, the two major cofactors Factor V and Factor VIII are converted to Va and VIIIa to initiate the clotting process. Under normal conditions, Factor

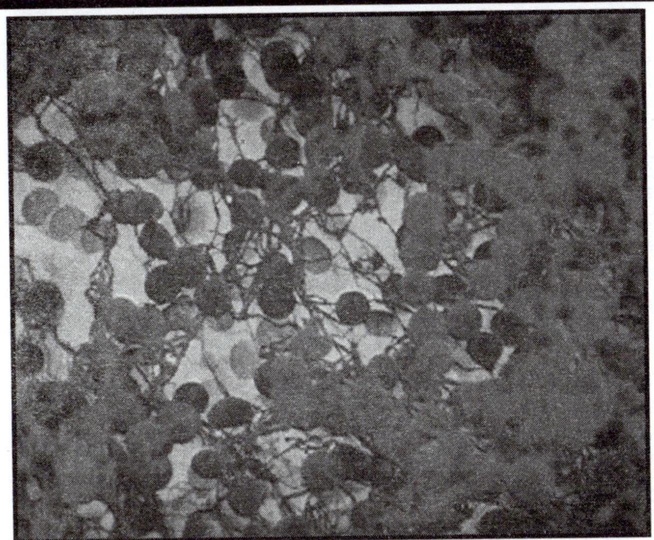

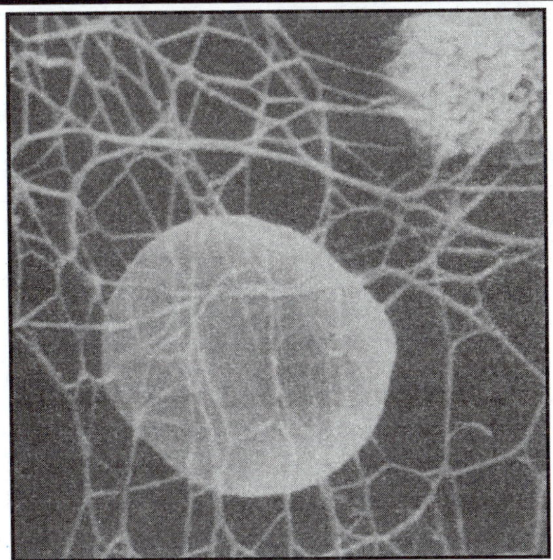

Fig. 23.32: Blood clotting and fibrin network

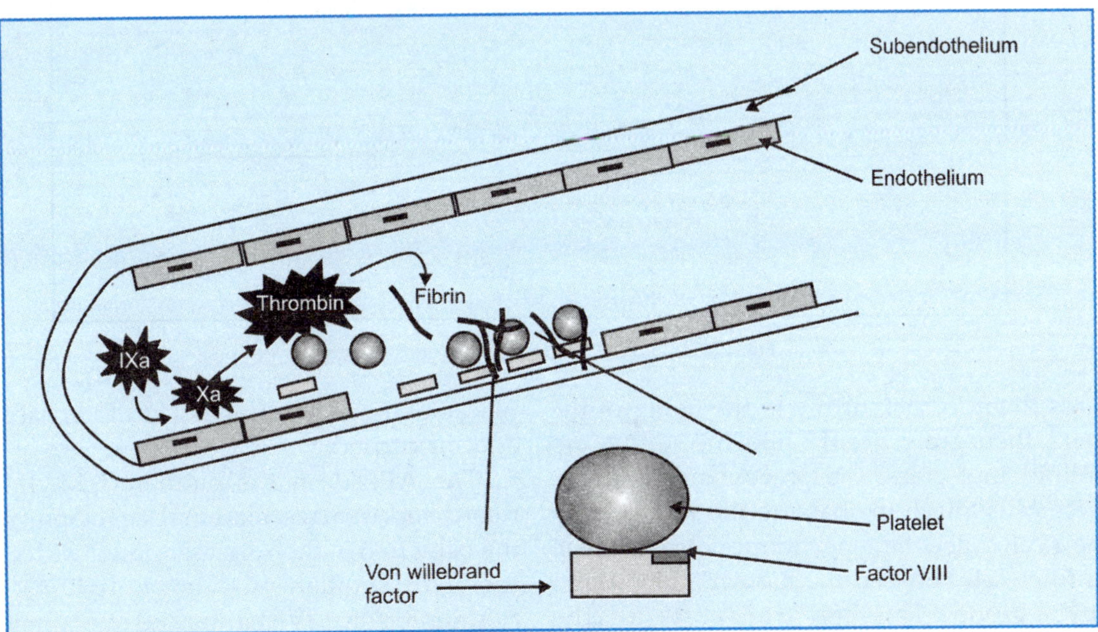

Fig. 23.33: Clotting process

Va and VIIIa are inactivated to Vai and VIIIai, so that clotting process is inhibited. This is achieved through protein C (PC to APC) (Fig. 23.33).

Antiphospholipid antibodies impair the normal functioning of protein C and as a result Factors Va and VIIIa are not inactivated. This leads to formation of clots even when they are not required.

Similarly, binding of antiphospholipid antibodies to platelets causes them to aggregate and clump together when it is not required.

The Illustration (Fig. 23.34) describes the blood clotting process in humans, which is divided into two pathways: intrinsic and extrinsic pathways. The inactivation of Va and VIIIa by protein C is described in the yellow box. Inhibition of PC by antiphospholipid antibodies is described in red.

Antiphospholipid Antibodies and Pregnancy

The six phospholipid molecules are components of every cell membrane. In the placenta they function in cytotrophoblast to syncytiotrophoblast formation. The cytotrophoblast, are the first cells of the placenta that attach the pregnancy to the uterus. The glue

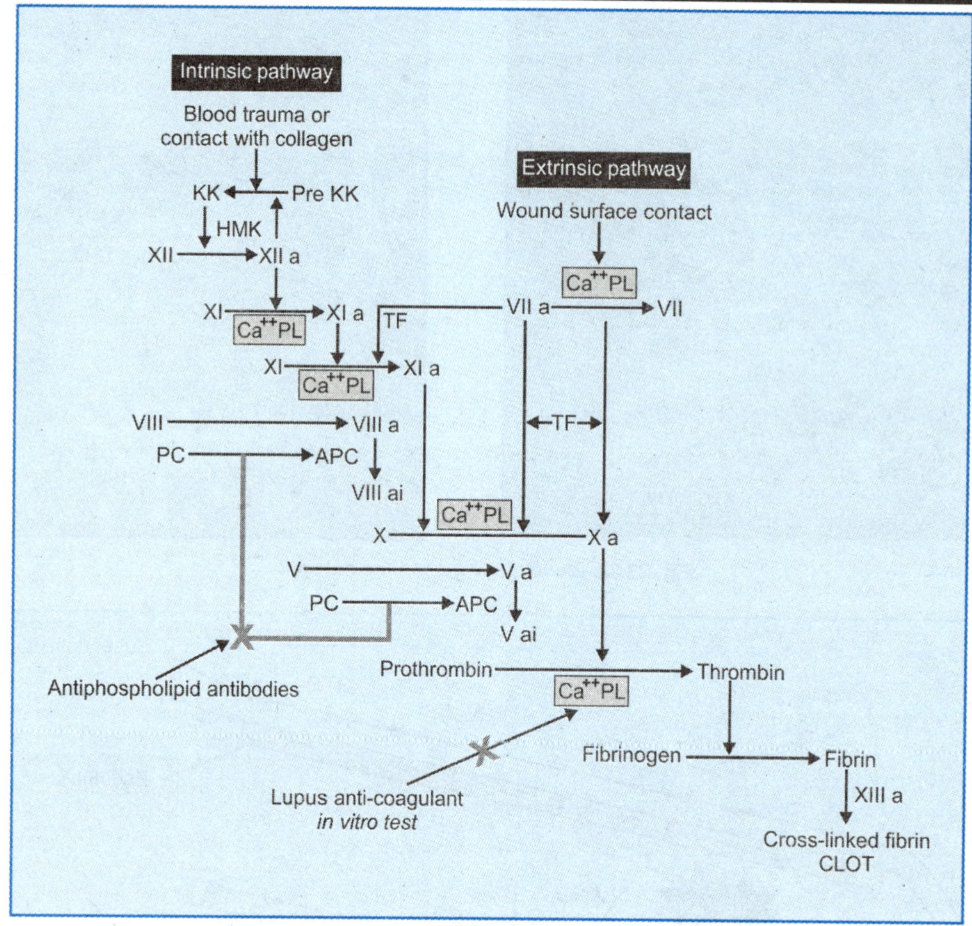

Fig. 23.34: Intrinsic pathway and extrinsic pathway

that causes them to stick firmly to the lining of the uterus and then grow deeply into the uterus are phospholipid molecules. Every woman has them. Once these cells attach the baby to the uterus, they form a new cell called the syncytiotrophoblast, which is like a filter cell between the mother's blood and the baby's blood. This cell transports all the nourishment to the baby and removes the waste from the baby's blood so that the mother can eliminate it for her baby.

In the blood the phospholipids are present on platelets. When the antibodies attach to the phospholipids, the tendency of the platelets to clump together is increased. This is one of the initial steps in clot formation. The woman's blood clots too fast, cutting off support to the baby; the cell is retarded in its development and the baby can "whither on the vine" and die. These antibodies also cause the embryo to attach too weakly to the uterus. This abnormality can be seen by doing immune pathology of the placental tissue paraffin blocks of the baby that died and miscarried.

The APLAs in the mother (IgM, IgG or IgA) retard and damage placental development, causing the baby to die; they are associated with a history of recurrent spontaneous abortion (RSA), endometriosis, infertility, IVF failure and implantation failure. APLAs are very common in women with blood clots, autoimmune diseases and inherited thrombophilia. Their incidence and titres increase with each successive pregnancy loss when compared to controls. In addition to pregnancy loss, several obstetrical complications are associated with APLAs, such as pre-eclampsia, foetal growth retardation in the second or early third trimester, abnormal fetal heart-rate tracing, abruption of the placenta, bleeding during pregnancy, subchorionic haemorrhages and preterm delivery. It has also been found that women who are HLA DQ A1, and who gestate a foetus of the same phenotype, are at the risk to develop APLAs to phospholipid molecules and lose their pregnancy despite of optimal therapy.

Each pregnancy that is lost makes the problem worse. A woman effectively vaccinates herself against a successful pregnancy. Many doctors are responsible for this because they tell the couple that nothing is wrong and simply try again. When a baby dies something is wrong; this is a common problem in many women with miscarriages, infertility, IVF failure and implantation failure. It is important to know that it is not necessary to lose one baby after another just to qualify for testing and treatment.

The most specific clinical features or problems that a woman experiences are:

1. Thrombotic events.
2. Blood clots (venous or arterial).
3. Autoimmune thrombocytopenia (low platelet count).
4. Anaemia (low red blood cell count).

The problems that are experienced with the pregnancies are:

1. Intrauterine foetal death.
2. Intrauterine growth retardation.
3. Low amniotic fluid volume.
4. Subchorionic haemorrhages.
5. Toxaemia of pregnancy.
6. Unexplained stillborn babies.

Other Clinical Features Associated with Antiphospholipid Antibodies

In some patients the only manifestation of the syndrome is recurrent miscarriage. In others, it is headaches or speech or visual/neurological disturbance. Both these aspects are discussed separately.

Deep Vein Thrombosis

The most dramatic sign that the disease is present is thrombosis, for example, deep vein thrombosis (DVT), in the leg or arm. This may be a 'one off', or be recurrent, or complicated by a lung clot (pulmonary embolus). In some women, it happens soon after the start of the oral contraceptive pill. Some of the most severe 'pill-associated' blood clots have been seen in individuals with antiphospholipid antibodies, clearly an important medical issue.

"Internal" veins may also clot, affecting organs such as the eye, the kidney, liver and so on—a diagnosis which will impinge on almost every speciality.

Arteries can also Clot

By definition, artery blockage is more serious than in the veins. Clinically, apart from the small artery disease in the brain, discussed later, major artery thrombosis seems to be less common than venous.

Blotchy Skin

A variety of other clinical features are seen in patients with primary APLS (Hughes' syndrome). A peculiar blotchiness (blue knees, purplish vein colouration on the back of the wrists, etc.) of the skin, called livedo reticularis is prominent in some patients.

In a small percentage of patients, the platelet numbers are affected and rarely, platelet counts may fall to dangerously low numbers. Thus, patients who have been diagnosed as having low platelet counts, thrombocytopenia, should be checked for primary APLS.

Headaches and Migraines

In quite a few patients, headaches, frequently with migraine features, e.g. flashing lights, speech disturbances, are important symptoms.

Interestingly, in many patients the headaches predate the clotting problem by many years. For example, a 25-year-old woman with recurrent miscarriages due to primary APLS gave a history of troublesome teenage migraine, possibly suggesting that the antibodies had been there for at least a decade before.

Memory Loss

For reasons not completely understood, the brain appears particularly sensitive to the clotting effects of antiphospholipid antibodies. The brain only has a limited number of ways of complaining at any disturbances in its supply of blood. The patient may develop transient memory loss, or slight speech disturbance, suggestive of a mini-stroke.

In others, the effect may be more insidious, with a gradually failing ability to put words, sentences, lists and so on, together.

The onset can be very dramatic. For example, in one patient, a woman who was her local village darts champion, the first sign of the problem was an inability to recognise and hit the "20". In another, a successful sculptress, there was difficulty in recognising three-dimensional shapes. In another, a

29 year old labourer, the first frightening sign occurred when standing on the station when "my speech became drunk my friends didn't know what I was saying."

Transient loss of blood supply to the brain (transient ischaemic attacks or TIAs) are capable of causing an infinitesimal variety of symptoms like epilepsy or fits.

One of the most interesting aspects of the syndrome is to see epilepsy, present in a patient for several years, apparently improve or even stop once proper anticoagulation treatment is started.

Who should be Tested for Antiphospholipid Antibodies?

Women who have had a history of recurrent pregnancy losses should be tested for antiphospholipid antibodies in addition to other routine tests. A history of unexplained poor foetal growth and/or the early onset of severe pre-eclampsia (toxaemia, also known as high blood pressure in pregnancy) or an unexplained placental abruption are indications for testing. A history of thrombosis (clots in the blood vessels), stroke, heart attack, thrombocytopenia (low platelet count), presence of other autoimmune disorders such as lupus, an abnormal VDRL, or PTT blood tests would suggest the need for testing.

LABORATORY DIAGNOSIS FOR APLS

1. Venereal Disease Research Laboratory (VDRL)

This was the first test to detect an antiphospholipid antibody. Reviews of patients with biologic false-positive test for syphilis, however, did not identify an increased risk of thrombosis or foetal loss. Therefore, this test is not diagnostic and the biologic false-positive test for syphilis is not even considered a strong associate of antiphospholipid syndrome.

2. Coagulation-based Tests

Antiphospholipid antibodies (APLA) react with phospholipid. The phospholipids provide a surface for the coagulation reaction to take place on. The basis of all these tests is that if there are antibodies on the phospholipid, it will prolong the coagulation reactions and the test time.

2a. Lupus Anticoagulant (LA)

The lupus anticoagulant is an immunoglobulin, either IgG or IgM, that prolongs clotting time *in vitro* because they agglutinate phospholipids present in the plasma thereby preventing their participation as cofactors in coagulation steps. Its *in vitro* action appears to be the inhibition of the conversion of prothrombin to thrombin.

The lupus anticoagulant test is a clotting test that measures how long it tales for blood to clot in a test tube. Blood is put in a test tube containing phospholipids. If the patients blood contains the antibody to these phospholipids, it will bind to the phospholipids in the test tube, and the blood will not clot.

No lupus anticoagulant test is 100% sensitive. Therefore, the following criteria are required for a positive lupus anticoagulant test:

1. Prolonged partial thromboplastin time, Russel Viper Venom time, or Kaolin clotting time;
2. Failure to correct the test by mixing patient plasma with normal plasma (suggesting a clotting inhibitor is present);
3. Normalisation of the test with freeze-thawed platelets, or phospholipids.

2b. APTT

Only sensitive to 30% of APLA. One can increase sensitivity by using different reagents.

2c. Dilute Rusell Viper Venom Time (dRVVT)

This test is very sensitive to any interference with phospholipid and is very sensitive to APLA. It is performed by initiating the coagulation cascade with Russell Viper Venom.

2d. Kaolin Clotting Time

This test uses no added phospholipid and is the most sensitive test to APLA.

2e. Platelet Neutralisation Test

This test takes a reaction that is prolonged by plasma which does not correct with a 50:50 mix and adds extracts of platelet. The platelet phospholipid "soak up" the antiphospholipid antibody and corrects the aPTT. If it corrects to normal, this is very specific for APLA.

2f. Hexagonal Phospholipid Neutralisation

Based on the same principle as the platelet test except using hexagonal phospholipid which are more specific for antiphospholipid antibodies.

3. Anticardiolipin Test (aCl)

Realising that cardiolipin was the major antigenic component of the false-positive test for syphilis, an immunoassay was created directed against this phospholipid. Of the many phospholipids, cardiolipin serves as a representative antigen in the system and antibodies against cardiolipin are used to screen for APLS. Anticardiolipin antibody is one of the few autoantibodies that have assays which allows the identification and quantification of specific isotypes (IgG, IgM and IgA). The IgG isotype was the major predictor of thrombosis and pregnancy loss while the IgM class was associated, especially with haemolytic anaemia in addition to thrombosis. Besides the identification of different isotypes, the antibody titre seems an useful predictor of pathogenicity (even though it is still not clear that quantity of antibody is the best or the only one). The higher-titre of IgG anticardiolipin antibody (>40 GPL) correlates strongly with thrombosis and foetal loss. Most patients with antiphospholipid syndrome have medium to high IgG anticardiolipin antibody levels with or without other isotypes.

4. Antiphosphatidyl Serine Test (aPS)

Other than cardiolipin, phosphatidyl serine seems to be the most antigenic. Phosphatidyl serine is normally on the interior surface of the platelet and endothelial cell membranes. When the cell is activated, phosphatidyl serine is redistributed to the cell surface and participates in clot formation. Cellular damage may result in inappropriate phosphatidyl serine expression on the cell surface giving rise to antibody formation. Therefore, antibodies against phosphatidyl serine are a more physiologically relevant antibody group.

Unlike cardiolipin, phosphatidyl serine is a more physiologically relevant phospholipid due to its presence in cell membranes of endothelial cells and platelets and its role in the coagulation cascade. The detection of antiphosphatidyl serine antibodies has been recommended for the serological diagnosis of antiphospholipid syndrome. Patients with positive results to both cardiolipin and phosphatidyl serine are more likely to have clinical complications than those who are positive for only one antibody.

APPROACH TO THE PATIENTS SUSPECTED OF HAVING APLAs

Relationship of LA, aCL and aPS

Unfortunately, there is no one test that can screen a patient for APLA. One must do the whole panel on patients suspected with APLA. This would include both lupus anticoagulant and ELISA testing for aCL and aPS. Since cardiolipin is only a representative of phospholipids an accurate test should include all the phospholipids for confirmation. The laboratory diagnosis of antiphospholipid antibody syndrome is positive when either the lupus anticoagulant or anticardiolipin/antiphosphatidyl serine/other phospholipid antibody is positive or when both tests are positive.

Up to 5% of apparently normal people have detectable aPL, especially low levels of aCL, but far fewer have LA or medium-or-high positive aCL. In contrast, most patients with APLS have LA, medium-to-high positive IgG aCL, or both. A few patients with APLS will be positive for LA and negative for aCL or vice versa. Thus, both LA and aCL should be ordered when considering the diagnosis of APLS.

Low-positive IgG aCL results and IgM aCL without the presence of LA or IgG aCL are of questionable significance. Physicians must exercise careful clinical judgement in the interpretation of low-positive IgG aCL or isolated IgM aCL results (Fig. 23.35).

Differential Diagnosis

The differential diagnosis will vary depending on the clinical manifestations. In cases in which thrombosis is the main presentation, other procoagulation states—such as protein C, protein S or antithrombin III deficiency, malignancy, oral contraceptives, nephrotic syndrome, polycythaemia, thrombocitosis, dysfibrinogaemia, paroxysmal nocturnal haemoglobinuria, homocystinuria—should be in mind and excluded. In the case of pregnancy loss, other mechanisms may be responsible for the foetal loss. These include foetal chromossomal abnormalities, anatomic anomalies of the maternal reproductive tract and others such as endocrine, infectious, autoimmune, drug-induced disorders.

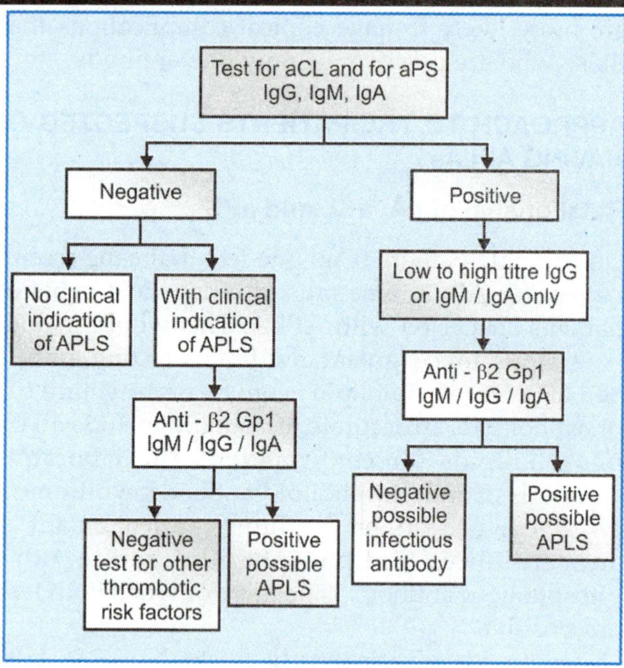

Fig. 23.35: Algorithm for APLS

Commercial Kits Used for Antiphospholipid Antibodies

The APLAs are measured using an ELISA system. There are different commercial kits in the market for measurement of these antibodies that vary greatly in their sensitivity and specificity.

The international standards for testing APLAs recommend a specific test system that reports results in GPL and MPL, units that are directly traceable to the standards of the Phospholipid Standardisation Laboratory at the University of Louisville.

The kit should contain β2-glycoprotein which is a serum cofactor necessary for the binding of antiphospholipid antibodies in the patient's serum to the phospholipid coating the test system wells. Both IgG and IgM antibodies should be measured.

Antiphospholipid antibodies are β-2 GPI dependent and β-2 GPI independent. For assured clinical correlation, it is mandatory that one should test for β-2 GPI dependent (IgG-2) antiphospholipid antibodies. β-2 GPI-independent antibodies are the antibodies produced during infections (syphilis) and this may cause false-positive results if detected.

Specimen Requirement for Antiphospholipid Testing

Lupus anticoagulant: 3 ml frozen citrated plasma. *Plasma must be* platelet free. *Double spin or filter* the *specimen to ensure that all platelets have been removed. Any remaining platelets in* the *specimen may contribute enough phospholipid to result in a false-negative test for LA.*

Antiphospholipid antibodies 1 ml frozen serum.

Hexagonal phase lupus anticoagulant 1 ml frozen plasma platelet free as above for LA.

TREATMENT

What is the Treatment for a Person who has Antiphospholipid Antibodies?

If a person has the lupus anticoagulant or anticardiolipin antibody, but has never had a thrombotic complication, treatment is not currently recommended. If a patient has had a thrombotic complication and has these antibodies, treatment may depend on where the clot (thrombosis) occurred. In general, treatment consists of "thinning" the blood to prevent future clots, using either aspirin or warfarin (Coumadin). The length of time that this treatment is necessary is unclear. Many physicians recommend long-term or even life-long treatment to prevent future episodes of thrombosis.

If a woman has Antiphospholipid Antibodies and is Pregnant, how is it Treated?

If the woman has antiphospholipid antibodies and is pregnant for the first time, or has had normal pregnancies in the past, no treatment may be advised. However, if the woman has had miscarriages in the past, several different treatment regimens are available, including aspirin, prednisone, and/or subcutaneous shots of a blood thinner called heparin. Pregnancies in women with antiphospholipid antibodies are considered to be "high-risk pregnancies."

Some women are helped by combinations of aspirin, prednisone, and/or subcutaneous heparin, whereas other women continue to have miscarriages even when they are taking these medications. Subcutaneous heparin is less likely than prednisone to cause diabetes and an increase in blood pressure during pregnancy. Other treatments, including plasmapheresis or intravenous gammaglobulin, may be considered in individual cases.

It is necessary for the obstetrician or gynaecologist to work closely with the rheumatologist or other physician who evaluates a woman with miscarriages for antiphospholipid antibodies. Miscarriages, especially early in pregnancy, are not rare. Women who have had multiple miscarriages should be checked to see if they have antiphospholipid antibodies as part of an overall obstetric evaluation for causes of miscarriage.

Asymptomatic patients with antiphospholipid Ab: Reduce risk factors for vascular disease

Those with high titres: Avoid oral contraceptive.

Lifestyle change maintain ideal weight, cholesterol level and physical activity.

Control blood pressure, avoid smoking.

ANTI-CARDIOLIPIN IgM/IgG WITH HUMAN β2-GLYCOPROTEIN I AS COFACTOR MFD: Orgentec, Courtesy: Lilac Medicare

Immunometric Enzyme Immunoassay for the Quantitative Determination of Anticardiolipin Antibodies of IgG and IgM class.

Warnings and Precautions

All reagents of this test kit are strictly intended for *in vitro* use only.

Please adhere strictly to the sequence of pipetting steps provided in this protocol. Observe the guidelines for performing quality control in medical laboratories by assaying controls and/or pooled sera.

All reagents should be stored refrigerated at 2 to 8°C in their original container.

Do not interchange kit components from different lots. The expiration dates stated on the labels of the shipping container and all vials have to be observed. Do not use kit components beyond their expiration dates.

Allow all kit components and specimen to reach room temperature prior to use and mix well.

During handling of all kit reagents, controls and serum samples observe the existing legal regulations. The following precautions should be taken while handling potentially infectious materials.

- do not eat, drink or smoke in areas where specimens or kit reagents are handled
- do not pipette by mouth
- wear disposable gloves while handling specimens or kit reagents and wash hands thoroughly afterwards.

The test kit contains components of human origin which, when tested by FDA-licensed methods, were found negative for hepatitis B surface antigen and for HIV antibody. No known test can guarantee, however, that products derived from human blood will not be infectious. Handle, therefore, all reagents and human blood derivatives, like plasma or serum samples, as if capable of transmitting infection.

Avoid contact with the TMB (3,3',5,5'-Tetramethylbenzidine). If TMB comes into contact with skin, wash thoroughly with water and soap.

The stop solution contains hydrochloric acid. If it comes into contact with skin, wash thoroughly with water and seek medical attention.

Avoid contact between the buffered peroxide solution and easily oxidised materials; extreme temperatures may initiate spontaneous combustion.

Material Supplied

Package size	96 determination
Divisible microplate consisting of	
12 modules of 8 wells each,	1
coated with highly purified	
Cardiolipin and saturated with	
highly purified human	
β_2-Glycoprotein I	
Combined calibrators with	
IgG and IgM class anticardiolipin	1 set
antibodies in a PBS/BSA	
matrix containing:	6 vials
IgG 0; 7.5; 15; 30; 60;	
120 GPL U/ml and	1, 5 ml each
IgM 0; 5; 10; 20; 40;	
80 MPL U/ml	
Anticardiolipin controls in a	
PBS/BSA matrix	1 Set
(positive and negative), for	
the respective:	2 vials
concentrations see the enclosed	
package insert	1 ml each
Cardiolipin sample buffer	
(yellow), concentrate	1 vial, 20 ml
containing BSA in PBS buffer	
Enzyme conjugate solution	
(light red), containing polyclonal	1 vial
rabbit anti-h-lgG-IgG, labelled	
with horseradish peroxidase	15 ml
in a PBS/BSA matrix	
enzyme conjugate solution	
(light red), containing polyclonal	1 vial
rabbit anti-h-lgM-IgG, labelled	
with horseradish peroxidase	15 ml
in a PBS/BSA matrix	

TMB substrate solution	1 vial, 15 ml
Stop solution	1 vial
(1 M hydrochloric acid)	15 ml
buffered wash solution,	1 vial
Concentrate	20 ml

Controls

A set of two controls is provided with the kit.

Technical Data

Sample material	Serum or plasma
Required sample size	10 µl of sample to be diluted 1:100 with sample buffer 100 µl prediluted sample per single determination
Total incubation time	60 minutes at room temperature (20-28°C)
Calibration range	7.5-120 GPL U/ml 5-80 MPL U/ml
Sensitivity	1 GPL U/ml resp. 0.5 MP U/ml
Storage	refrigerated at 2 to 8°C
Shelf-life	9 months after manufacturing or until the expiration date printed on the labels
Package size	96 tests

Principle of the Procedure

The anticardiolipin IgG/IgM is an indirect solid-phase enzyme immunometric assay (ELISA). It is designed for the quantitative measurement of IgG or IgM class autoantibodies directed against cardiolipin. The microplate is coated with highly purified cardiolipin and saturated with highly purified human β_2-Glycoprotein I (β_2GPI). The β_2-Glycoprotein I is known as a co-factor for the binding of anticardiolipin antibodies. This new coating procedure guarantees reproducible results independent of endogeneous β_2GPI.

The microplate can be divided into 12 modules of 8 wells each or can be used completely for 96 determinations. Each well can be separated from the module ("break-away").

The binding of present autoantibodies, formation of the sandwich complexes and enzymatic colour reaction take place during three different reaction phases.

Phase 1

Calibrators, controls and prediluted patient samples will be pipetted into the wells of the microplate. Any present antibodies bind to the inner surface of the wells. After a 30-minute incubation, the microplate is washed with wash buffer for removing non-reactive serum components.

Phase 2

An anti-human-IgG (or anti-human-IgM) horseradish peroxidase conjugate solution is pipetted into the wells of the microplate to recognise IgG class auto-antibodies (or IgM class autoantibodies) bound to the immobilised antigens. After a 15-minute incubation, any excess enzyme conjugate, which is not specifically bound is washed away with wash buffer.

Phase 3

A chromogenic substrate solution containing TMB (3,3',5,5'-Teramethyl-benzidine) is dispensed into the wells. During 15-minute of incubation the colour of the solutions changes into blue. Colour development is stopped by adding 1 M hydrochloric acid as stop solution. The solutions colour change into yellow.

The amount of colour is directly proportional to the concentration of IgG resp. IgM antibodies present in the original sample.

To read the optical density, a microplate reader with a 450 nm filter is required. Bichromatic measurement with a 600-690 nm reference is recommended.

Clinical Relevance

Cardiolipin (diphosphotidylglycerine) belongs to the group of negatively charged phospholipids. Antibodies to these phospholipids are described to be often—but not necessarily—identical to the lupus anticoagulants (LA), a class of antibodies responsible for a prolonged clotting process.

Autoantibodies to cardiolipin are described for various autoimmune diseases. The presence of anticardiolipin antibodies in systemic lupus erythematosus (SLE) can be related to the development of thrombosis and thrombocytopenia; in gynaecology, they are supposed to cause intrauterine death or recurrent abortion. Furthermore, anticardiolipin antibodies have been found in some nonthrombotic neurological disorders like cerebrovascular insufficiency, cerebral ischaemia or chorea and in myocardial infarction.

Anticardiolipin autoantibodies are found in the immunoglobulin classes IgG, IgM and/or IgA. The determination of IgM antibodies is a valuable indicator in the diagnosis of beginning autoimmune diseases, whereas IgG antibodies will be found in progressive stages of manifested autoimmune disorders. Anti-Cardiolipin IgG antibodies show a good correlation to the clinical status of the patient in thrombosis, thrombocytopenia, foetal loss and some neurological disorders. Anticardiolipin IgA antibodies are often associated with IgG antibodies. The determination of IgA antibodies seems to have a greater validity in thrombosis and foetal loss.

Major diseases associated with anticardiolipin antibodies are deep vein thrombosis and other thrombotic disorders. Anticardiolipin antibodies will be found in the sera of approximately 60 percent of the SLE patients. The presence of these antibodies is a high-risk factor for the development of thrombo-embolism and thrombocytopenia.

In gynaecology, anticardiolipin antibodies seems to be a good indicator in the prognosis of recurrent abortion or intrauterine death. Furthermore, routine determination of anticardiolipin antibodies in risky pregnancies of women with SLE or thrombosis is recommended. Quantitative measurements of anticardiolipin antibodies, especially IgG, is an important parameter with high specificity in therapy-monitoring.

The presence of anticardiolipin antibodies is also described in neurological diseases. Therefore, cerebral thrombosis may cause ischaemia. Non-thrombotic diseases of the central nervous system, like chorea or epilepsy, are also associated with anticardiolipin antibodies.

The anticardiolipin antibody test shows no correlation to the VDRL antibody test (Reagins Test) in the diagnosis of syphilis. Also, no cross-reactivities with anti-DNA antibodies are observed, because both types of antibodies belong to separate antibody populations.

Recent studies have shown that anticardiolipin antibodies require a plasma/serum co-factor for binding to cardiolipin. The co-factor has been identified as β_2-glycoprotein I (β_2GPI) also called apolipoprotein H, a 50 kDa β_2-globulin which occurs in plasma at a level of 200 ug/ml. The β_2GPI is associated *in vivo* with lipoproteins, anionic phospholipids, platelets and mitochondria. It has been found that β_2GPI inhibits the intrinsic coagulation pathway and the ADP-mediated platelet aggregation. Therefore, it is suggested that β_2GPI plays a role in the regulation of blood coagulation.

The presence of β_2GPI is absolutely required for the binding of anticardiolipin antibodies to cardiolipin. Recent studies have shown that anticardiolipin antibodies either recognise cardiolipin on its own or the complex of cardiolipin and β_2GPI.[18]

For ELISA-tests, sufficient concentrations of β_2GPI could be achieved either by addition of ABS/FCS or by coating with purified β_2GPI. The latter version provides constant quality and quantity for maintaining reproducible results.

Indication for determination of anti-cardiolipin antibodies:

- — SLE
- — Thrombosis
- — Thrombocytopenia
- — Cerebral ischaemia
- — Chorea
- — Epilepsy
- — Recurrent abortion
- — Intrauterine death

Normal Values

In a normal range study with serum samples from healthy blood donors, the following ranges have been established with the anticardiolipin tests

	anticardiolipin-Ab	
	IgG (GPL U/ml)	IgM (MPL U/ml)
Normal	< 10	< 7
Elevated	> 10	>7

Positive results should be verified concerning the entire clinical status of the patient. Also every, decision for therapy should be taken individually.

It is recommended that each laboratory establishes its own normal and pathological ranges of serum anticardiolipin. The values below should be regarded as guidelines only.

Specificity

The microplate is coated with highly purified cardiolipin and highly purified human β_2-Glycoprotein I. Special coating processes, developed by the manufacturer guarantee for the native immunogenic structure of cardiolipin after immobilisation on the solid phase. The anticardiolipin test kits are specific only for autoantibodies directed against cardiolipin or to the complex of cardiolipin and β_2-glycoprotein I.

No crossreactivity was observed to anti-DNA antibodies and those types of antibodies occurring in syphilis.

Calibration

The assay system is calibrated against the internationally recognised reference sera from EN Harris, Louisville, since no other international standards are available.

IMMUNOASSAY PROCEDURE

Materials Required

Equipment

- Microplate reader capable for endpoint measurements at 450 nm
- Vortex mixer
- Pipettes for 10 µl, 100 µl and 1000 µl

Preparation of reagents

- Distilled water
- Graduated cylinder for 100 and 1,000 ml
- Plastic container for storage of the wash solution

Optional

- Multichanel dispenser
- Repeatable pipette for 100 µl
- Data reduction software

Specimen Collection and Preparation

For determination of anticardiolipin, serum or plasma are the preferred sample matrices.

All serum and plasma samples are prediluted 1:100 with sample buffer. Therefore, 10 µl of sample may be diluted with 1,000 µl of sample buffer.

The patients need not to be fasting, and no special preparations are necessary. Collect blood by venipuncture into vacutainers and separate serum or plasma from the cells by centrifugation after clot formation.

Samples may be stored refrigerated at 2 to 8°C. for at least 5 days. For longer storage of up to six months, samples should be stored frozen at –20°C. To avoid repeated thawing and freezing, the samples should be aliquoted.

Neither bilirubin nor haemolysis have significant effect on the procedure.

Preparation and Collection of Reagents

All components of this test kit are supplied in a liquid format and ready to use, except the sample buffer and wash buffer. When stored refrigerated at 2 to 8°C. the components are stable for at least 30 days after opening or until the expiration date printed on the labels.

Remaining modules of the microplate should be stored refrigerated at 2 to 8°C. protected from moisture; store together with desiccant and carefully sealed in the plastic bag.

Preparation of Sample Buffer

Dilute the contents of each vial of the sample buffer concentrate (5x) with distilled water to a final volume of 100 ml prior to use. Store refrigerated stable at 2 to 8°C for at least 30 days after preparation or until the expiration date printed on the label.

Preparation of Buffered Wash Solution

Dilute the contents of each vial of the buffered wash solution concentrate (50 x) with distilled water to a final volume of 1000 ml prior to use. Store refrigerated stable at 2 to 8°C. for at least 30 days after preparation or until the expiration date printed on the label.

Notes on Technique

Control sera or pools should routinely be assayed as unknowns to check performance of the reagents and the assay.

Pipetting and Sample Handling

Use a disposable-tip micropipette to dispense sera and plasma samples. Pipette directly to the bottom of the wells. To avoid carryover contamination, change the tip between samples.

Patient samples expected to contain high concentrations should be additionally diluted with sample buffer before. Additional dilutions must be considered during calculation.

Immunoassay Procedure

Do not interchange components of different lots. All components should be at room temperature before use.

Dilute all patient samples 1:100 with sample buffer before assay. Therefore, combine 10 µl of sample with 1,000 µl of sample buffer in a polystyrene tube. Mix well. Calibrators and controls are ready to use and need not to be diluted.

1. Prepare a sufficient number of microplate modules to accommodate calibrators, controls and prediluted patient samples in duplicates.

	1	2	3	4	5	6	7
a	SA	SE	P1	P..			
b	SA	SE	P1	P..			
c	SB	SF	P2				
d	SB	SF	P2				
e	SC	C1	P3				
f	SC	C1	P3				
g	SD	C2	P4				
h	SD	C2	P4				

2. For the determination of one class of autoantibodies, pipette 100 µl of calibrators, controls and prediluted patient samples into the wells. For determination of both IgG and IgM autoantibodies, calibrators, controls and patient samples have to be pipetted in two attempts.
3. Incubate for 30 minutes at room temperature (20-28°C).
4. Discard the contents of the microwells and wash 3 times with 300 µl of wash solution.
5. Dispense 100 µl of enzyme conjugate solution (anti-h-lgG-IgG or anti-h-lgM-IgG) into each well.
6. Incubate for 15 minutes at room temperature.
7. Discard the contents of the microwells and wash 3 times with 300 µl of wash solution.
8. Dispense 100 µl of 1 MB substrate solution into each well.
9. Incubate for 15 minutes at room temperature.
10. Add 100 µl of stop solution to each well of the modules and let it stand for 5 minutes.
11. Read the optical density at 450 nm and calculate the results. Bichromatic measurement with a reference at 600-690 nm is recommended.

The developed colour is stable for at least 30 minutes. Read optical densities during this time.

Calculation of Results

For anticardiolipin IgG and IgM, α 4-parameter-fit with lin-log coordinates for optical density and concentration is the data reduction method of choice. Smoothed Spline Approximation and log-log coordinates are also suitable.

Recommended Lin-Log Plot

First calculate the averaged optical densities for each calibrator well. Use lin-log graph paper and plot the averaged optical density of each calibrator versus the concentration. Draw the best fitting curve approximating the path of all calibrator points. The calibrator points may also be connected with straight line segments. The concentration of unknowns may then be estimated from the calibration curve by interpolation.

Calculation Example

The figures and graph below show typical results for anticardiolipin IgG. These data are intended for illustration only and should not be used to calculate results from another run.

Calibrators									
No	Position	OD 1	OD 2	Mean	Conc. 1	Conc. 2	Mean	decl Conc.	CV%
STA	A1/B1	0.050	0.050	0.050	0.1	0.1	0.1	0.0	0
STB	C1/D1	0.322	0.300	0.311	7.8	7.0	7.4	7.5	7
STC	E1/F1	0.520	0.519	0.520	15.2	15.2	15.2	15.0	0
STD	G1/H1	0.803	0.824	0.814	29.2	30.5	29.9	30.0	3
STE	A2/b2	1.226	1.191	1.209	61.6	58.2	59.9	60.0	3
STF	C2/D2	1.640	1.637	1.638	120.5	119.9	120.2	120.0	0

ASSAY CHARACTERISTICS

Sensitivity

The lower detection limit for anticardiolipin IgG was determined at 1.0 GPL U/ ml. Anticardiolipin IgM yielded a sensitivity of 0.5 MPL U/ml.

Parallelism

In dilution experiments sera with high IgG-and IgM-antibody concentrations were diluted with sample buffer and assayed in the anticardiolipin kit.

Anticardiolipin	*Sample*	*Dilution*	*Observed (U/ml)*	*Expected (U/ml)*	*O/E*
IgG	1	1.200	126.7		
		1.400	63.7	63.4	100%
		1.800	32.9	31.7	104%
		1.1600	14.1	15.8	89%
		1.3200	7.2	7.9	91%
IgG	2	1.100	112.3		
		1.200	56.1	56.2	100%
		1.400	25.0	28.1	89%
		1.800	12.0	14.0	86%
		1.1600	6.0	7.0	86%
IgM	3	1.100	55.0		
		1.200	27.0	27.5	98%
		1.400	13.0	13.8	94%
		1.800	6.4	6.9	93%
IgM	4	1.200	46.5		
		1.400	23.2	23.3	100%
		1.800	10.9	11.6	94%
		1.1600	5.2	5.8	90%
		1.3200	2.8	2.9	97%

Precision

Statistics for coefficients of variation (CV) were calculated for each of three samples from the results of 24 determinations in a single run for intra assay precision. Run-to-run precision was calculated from the results of 5 different runs with 6 determinations each.

Anticardiolipin (IgG)			**Anticardiolipin (IgM)**		
Intraassay			**Intra assay**		
Sample No	Mean x (GPL U/ml)	CV (%)	Sample No	Mean x (MPL U/ml)	CV (%)
1	29.1	5.4	1	8.4	3.7
2	62.5	5.8	2	40.1	4.5
3	109.4	4.1	3	58.6	5.3
Interassay			**Interassay**		
Sample No	Mean x (GPL U/ml)	CV (%)	Sample No	Mean x (MPL U/ml)	CV (%)
1	32.9	3.8	1	10.3	3.4
2	70.9	2.5	24	7.0	3.3
3	118.3	2.7	3	79.1	2.5

Incubation Scheme

Anticardiolipin (IgG/IgM)

100 µl Pipette Calibrator into the microplate | 100 µl Control or patient sample

⇓ ⇓

Incubate for 30 minutes at room temperature

⇓

Discard the contents of the wells and wash 3 times with 300 µl wash solution

⇓

Pipette 100 µl enzyme conjugate solution

⇓

Incubate for 15 minutes at room temperature

⇓

Discard the contents of the well and wash 3 times with 300 µl wash solution

⇓

Pipette 100 µl TMB substrate solution

⇓

Incubate for 15 minutes at room temperature

⇓

Add 100 µl stop solution

⇓

Leave untouched for 5 minutes

⇓

Read at 450 nm

ANTICARDIOLIPIN IgA WITH HUMAN β2-GLYCOPROTEIN I AS COFACTOR Mfd: Orgentec, Courtesy: Lilac Medicare

Immunometric Enzyme Immunoassay for the Quantitative Determination of Anticardiolipin Antibodies of IgA Class

Warnings and Precautions

All reagents of this test kit are strictly intended for *in vitro* use only.

Please adhere strictly to the sequence of pipetting steps provided in this protocol. Observe the guidelines for performing quality control in medical laboratories by assaying controls and/or pooled sera.

All reagents should be stored refrigerated at 2 to 8°C in their original container.

Do not interchange kit components from different lots. The expiration dates stated on the labels of the shipping container and all vials have to be observed.

Do not use kit components beyond their expiration dates.

Allow all kit components and specimen to reach room temperature prior to use and mix well.

During handling of all kit reagents, controls and serum samples observe the existing legal regulations. The following precautions should be taken while handling potentially infectious materials:

— do not eat, drink or smoke in areas where specimens or kit reagents are handled
— do not pipette by mouth
— wear disposable gloves while handling specimens or kit reagents and wash hands thoroughly afterwards.

The test kit contains components of human origin which, when tested by FDA-licensed methods, were found negative for hepatitis B surface antigen and for HIV antibody. No known test can guarantee, however, that products derived from human blood will not be infectious. Handle, therefore, all reagents and human blood derivatives, like plasma or serum samples, as if capable of transmitting infection.

Avoid contact with the TMB (3,3', 5,5'-Tetramethyl-benzidine). If TMB comes into contact with skin wash thoroughly with water and soap.

The stop solution contains hydrochloric acid. If it comes into contact with skin, wash thoroughly with water and seek medical attention.

Avoid contact between the buffered peroxide solution and easily oxidised materials; extreme temperatures may initiate spontaneous combustion.

Material Supplied

Package size	96 determinations
Divisible microplate consisting of 12 modules of 8 wells each, coated with highly purified cardiolipin and saturated with highly purified human β_2-glycoprotein I	1
Calibrators with anti-Cardiolipin antibodies of IgA class in a PBS/BSA matrix containing: 0; 7.5; 15; 30; 60; 120 APL U/ml	1 set 6 vials 1,5 ml each
Anticardiolipin controls in a PBS/BSA matrix (positive and negative), for the respective concentrations see the enclosed package insert	1 set 2 vials 1 ml each
Cardiolipin sample buffer (yellow), concentrate containing BSA in PBS buffer	1 vial, 20 ml
Enzyme conjugate solution (light red) containing polyclonal rabbit anti-h-IgA-IgG, labelled with horseradish peroxidase in a PBS/BSA matrix	1 vial 15 ml
1 MB substrate solution	1 vial, 15 ml
Stop solution (1 M hydrochloric acid)	1 vial 15 ml
Buffered wash solution, concentrate	1 vial 20 ml

Controls

A set of two controls is provided with the kit.

Technical Data

Sample material:	Serum or plasma
Required sample size:	10 µl of sample to be diluted 1:100 with sample buffer 100 µl prediluted sample per single determination
Total incubation time:	60 minutes at room temperature (18-28°C)
Calibration range:	7.5 -120 APL U/ml
Sensitivity:	1 APL U/ml
Storage:	refrigerated at 2 to 8°C
Shelf-life:	9 months after manufacturing or until the expiration date printed on the labels
Package size:	96 tests

Principle of the Procedure

The anticardiolipin IgA is an indirect solid-phase enzyme immunometric assay (ELISA). It is designed for the quantitative measurement of IgA class autoantibodies directed against cardiolipin. The microplate is coated with highly purified cardiolipin and saturated with highly purified human β_2-glycoprotein I (β_2GPI). β_2-Glycoprotein I is known as a co-factor for the binding of anticardiolipin antibodies. This new coating procedure guarantees reproducible results independent of endogeneous β_2GPI.

The microplate can be divided into 12 modules of 8 wells each or can be used completely for 96 determinations. Each well can be separated from the module ("break-away").

The binding of present autoantibodies, formation of the sandwich complexes and enzymatic colour reaction take place during three different reaction phases.

Phase 1

Calibrators, controls and prediluted patient samples are pipetted into the wells of the microplate. Any present antibodies bind to the inner surface of the wells. After a 30-minute incubation, the microplate is washed with wash buffer for removing non-reactive serum components.

Phase 2

An anti-human-IgA horseradish peroxidase conjugate solution is pipetted into the wells of the microplate to recognise IgA class autoantibodies bound to the immobilised antigens. After a 15-minute incubation, any excess enzyme conjugate, which is not specifically bound, is washed away with wash buffer.

Phase 3

A chromogenic substrate solution containing TMB (3,3',5,5'-Terametһyl-benzidine) is dispensed into the wells. During 15 minutes of incubation, the colour of the solutions changes into blue. Colour development is stopped by adding 1 M hydrochloric acid as stop solution. The solutions colour, changes into yellow.

The amount of colour is directly proportional to the concentration of IgA class antibodies present in the original sample.

To read the optical density, a microplate reader with a 450 nm filter is required. Bichromatic measurement with a 600-690 nm reference is recommended.

Clinical Relevance

Cardiolipin (Diphosphatidyl glycerin) belongs to the group of negatively charged phospholipids. Antibodies to these phospholipids are described to be often—but not necessarily—identical to the lupus anticoagulants (LA), a class of antibodies responsible for a prolonged clotting process.

Autoantibodies to cardiolipin are described for various autoimmune diseases. The presence of anticardiolipin antibodies in systemic lupus erythematosus (SLE) can be related to the development of thrombosis and thrombocytopenia; in gynaecology, they are supposed to cause intrauterine death or recurrent abortion. Furthermore, anticardiolipin antibodies have been found in some nonthrombotic neurological disorders like cerebrovascular insufficiency, cerebral ischaemia or chorea and in myocardial infarction.

Anticardiolipin autoantibodies are found in the immunoglobulin classes IgG, IgM and/or IgA. The determination of IgM antibodies is a valuable indicator in the diagnosis of beginning autoimmune diseases, whereas IgG antibodies will be found in progressive stages of manifested autoimmune disorders. Anticardiolipin IgG antibodies show a good correlation to the clinical status of the patient in thrombosis, thrombocytopenia, foetal loss and some neurological disorders. Anticardiolipin IgA antibodies are often associated with IgG antibodies. The determination of IgA antibodies seems to have a greater validity in thrombosis and foetal loss.

Major diseases associated with anticardiolipin antibodies are deep vein thrombosis and other thrombotic disorders. Anticardiolipin antibodies will be found in the sera of approximately 60 percent of the SLE patients. The presence of these antibodies is a high risk factor for the development of thrombo-embolism and thrombocytopenia.

In gynaecology, anticardiolipin antibodies seems to be a good indicator in the prognosis of recurrent abortion or intrauterine death. Furthermore, routine determination of anticardiolipin antibodies in risky pregnancies of women with SLE or thrombosis is recommended. Quantitative measurements of anticardiolipin antibodies, especially IgG, is an important parameter with high specificity in therapy-monitoring.

The presence of anticardiolipin antibodies is also described in neurological diseases. Therefore, cerebral thrombosis may cause ischemia. Non-thrombotic diseases of the central nervous system, like chorea or epilepsy, are also associated with anticardiolipin antibodies.

The anticardiolipin antibody test shows no correlation to the VDRL antibody test (Reagins Test) in the diagnosis of syphilis. Also, no cross reactivities with anti-DNA antibodies are observed, because both types of antibodies belong to separate antibody populations.

Recent studies have shown that anticardiolipin antibodies require a plasma/serum cofactor for binding to cardiolipin. The cofactor has been identified as β_2-glycoprotein I (β_2GPI) also called apolipoprotein H, a 50 kDa (β_2-globulin which occurs in plasma at a level of 200 ug/ml. β_2GPi is associated *in vivo* with lipoproteins, anionic phospholipids, platelets and mitochondria. It has been found that β_2GPI inhibits the intrinsic coagulation pathway and the ADP-mediated platelet aggregation. Therefore, it is suggested that β_2GPI plays a role in the regulation of blood coagulation.

The presence of β_2GPI is absolutely required for the binding of anticardiolipin antibodies to cardiolipin. Recent studies have shown that anticardiolipin antibodies either recognise cardiolipin on its own or the complex of cardiolipin and li_2GPI.

For ELISA-tests sufficient concentrations of β_2GPI could be achieved either by addition of ABS/FCS or by coating with purified β_2GPI. The latter version provides constant quality and quantity for maintaining reproducible results.

Indication for determination of anticardiolipin antibodies.

— SLE
— Thrombosis
— Thrombocytopenia
— Cerebral Ischaemia
— Chorea
— Epilepsy
— Recurrent abortion
— Intrauterine death

Specificity

The microplate is coated with highly purified cardiolipin and highly purified human β_2-glycoprotein I. Special coating processes, developed by the manufacturer guarantee for the native immunogenic structure of cardiolipin after immobilisation on the solid phase. The anticardiolipin test kits are specific only for autoantibodies directed against cardiolipin or to the complex of cardiolipin and β_2-glycoprotein I.

No crossreactivity was observed to anti-DNA antibodies and those types of antibodies occurring in syphilis.

Normal Values

In a normal range study with serum samples from healthy blood donors the following ranges have been established with the anticardiolipin IgA test:

	anticardiolipin-Ab (APL U/ml)
Normal:	< 10
Elevated:	> 10

Positive results should be verified concerning the entire clinical status of the patient. Also, every decision for therapy should be taken individually.

It is recommended that each laboratory establishes its own normal and pathological ranges of serum anticardiolipin. The values below should be regarded as guidelines only.

Calibration

The assay system is calibrated against the internationally recognised reference sera from EN Harris, Louisville, since no other international standards are available.

IMMUNOASSAY PROCEDURE

Material Required

Equipment

- Microplate reader capable for endpoint measurements at 450 nm
- Vortex mixer
- Pipettes for 10 µl, 100 µl and 1000 µl

Preparation of reagents

- Distilled water
- Graduated cylinder for 100 and 1,000 ml
- Plastic container for storage of the wash solution

Optional

- Multichannel dispenser
- Repeatable pipette for 100 µl
- Data reduction software

Specimen Collection and Preparation

For determination of anticardiolipin serum or plasma are the preferred sample matrices.

All serum and plasma samples are prediluted 1:100 with sample buffer. Therefore, 10 µl of sample may be diluted with 1,000 µl of sample buffer.

The patients need not to be fasting, and no special preparations are necessary. Collect blood by venipuncture into vacutainers and separate serum or plasma from the cells by centrifugation after clot formation.

Samples may be stored refrigerated at 2 to 8°C for at least 5 days. For longer storage of up to six months, samples should be stored frozen at –20°C. To avoid repeated thawing and freesing the samples should be aliquoted.

Neither bilirubin nor haemolysis have significant effect on the procedure.

Preparation and Storage of Reagents

All components of this test kit are supplied in a liquid format and ready to use, except the sample buffer and wash buffer. When stored refrigerated at 2 to 8°C the components are stable for at least 30 days after opening or until the expiration date printed on the labels.

Remaining modules of the microplate should be stored refrigerated at 2 to 8°C protected from moisture; store together with desiccant and carefully sealed in the plastic bag.

Preparation of Sample Buffer

Dilute the contents of each vial of the sample buffer concentrate (5x) with distilled water to a final volume of 100 ml prior to use. Store refrigerated: stable at 2 to 8°C for at least 30 days after preparation or until the expiration date printed on the label.

Preparation of Buffered Wash Solution

Dilute the contents of each vial of the buffered wash solution concentrate (50x) with distilled water to a final volume of 1000 ml prior to use. Store refrigerated: stable at 2 to 8°C for at least 30 days after preparation or until the expiration date printed on the label.

Notes on Technique

Control sera or pools should routinely be assayed as unknowns to check performance of the reagents and the assay.

Pipetting and Sample Handling

Use a disposable-tip micropipette to dispense sera and plasma samples. Pipette directly to the bottom of the wells. To avoid carryover contamination change the tip between samples.

Patient samples expected to contain high concentrations should be additionally diluted with sample buffer before. Additional dilutions must be considered during calculation.

Immunoassay Procedure

Do not interchange components of different lots.

All components should be at room temperature before use.

Dilute all patient samples 1:100 with sample buffer before assay. Therefore, combine 10 µl of sample with 1,000 µl of sample buffer in a polystyrene tube. Mix well. Calibrators and controls are ready to use and need not to be diluted.

1. Prepare a sufficient number of microplate modules to accommodate calibrators, controls and prediluted patient samples in duplicates.

	1	2	3	4	5	6	7
a	SA	SE	P1	P..			
b	SA	SE	P1	P..			
c	SB	SF	P2				
d	SB	SF	P2				
e	SC	C1	P3				
f	SC	C1	P3				
g	SD	C2	P4				
h	SD	C2	P4				

2. Pipette 100 µl of calibrators, controls and prediluted patient samples into the wells.
3. Incubate for 30 minutes at room temperature (20-28°C).
4. Discard the contents of the microwells and wash 3 times with 300 µl of wash solution.
5. Dispense 100 µl of enzyme conjugate solution (anti-h-lgG-IgG or anti-h-lgM-IgG) into each well.
6. Incubate for 15 minutes at room temperature.
7. Discard the contents of the microwells and wash 3 times with 300 µl of wash solution.
8. Dispense 100 µl of 1 MB substrate solution into each well.
9. Incubate for 15 minutes at room temperature.
10. Add 100 µl of stop solution to each well of the modules and let it stand for 5 minutes.
11. Read the optical density at 450 nm and calculate the results. Bichromatic measurement with a reference at 600-690 nm is recommended.

The developed colour is stable for at least 30 minutes. Read optical densities during this time.

Calculation of Results

For anticardiolipin IgA, α 4-parameter-fit with lin-log coordinates for optical density and concentration is the data reduction method of choice. Smoothed spline approximation and log-log coordinates are also suitable.

Recommended Lin-Log Plot

First calculate the averaged optical densities for each calibrator well. Use lin-log graph paper and plot the averaged optical density of each calibrator versus the concentration. Draw the best fitting curve approximating the path of all calibrator points. The calibrator points may also be connected with straight line segments. The concentration of unknowns may then be estimated from the calibration curve by interpolation.

Calculation Example

The Table below shows typical results for anticardiolipin IgA. These data are intended for illustration only and should not be used to calculate results from another run.

Calibrators									
No	Position	OD 1	OD 2	Mean	Conc. 1	Conc. 2	Mean	decl. Conc.	CV %
STA	A 1/B 1	0.038	0.039	0.038	0.0	0.1	0.1	0.0	2
STB	C 1/D 1	0.223	0.223	0.223	7.5	7.5	7.5	7.5	0
STC	E 1/F1	0.428	0.430	0.429	15.2	15.3	15.3	15.0	0
STD	G 1/H 1	0.786	0.771	0.779	29.7	29.0	29.4	30.0	1
STE	A 2/b2	1.411	1.389	1.400	61.6	60.2	60.9	60.0	1
STF	C2/D2	2.144	2.109	2.127	121.3	117.5	119.4	120.0	1

Assay Characteristics

Sensitivity

The lower detection limit for anticardiolipin IgA was determined at 1.0 APL U/ml.

Parallelism

In dilution experiments sera with high IgA-antibody concentrations were diluted with sample buffer and assayed in the anticardiolipin kit.

Anticardiolipin	*Sample*	*Dilution*	*Observed (APLU /ml)*	*Expected (APLU /ml)*	*O/E*
IgA	1	1:200	120.2		
		1:400	59.9	60.1	100%
		1:800	28.7	30.1	95%
		1:1600	14.4	15.0	96%
		1:3200	7.3	7.5	97%
IgA	2	1:100	112.3		
		1:200	55.7	56.2	99%
		1:400	26.1	28.1	93%
		1:800	12.6	14.0	90%
		1:1600	I 6.2	I 7.0	89%

Precision

Statistics for coefficients of variation (CV) were calculated for each of three samples from the results of 24 determinations in a single run for intraassay precision. Run-to-run precision was calculated from the results of 5 different runs with 6 determinations each:

Intraassay			*Interassay*		
Sample No	*Mean x(APL U/ml)*	*CV (%)*	*Sample No*	*Mean x (APL U/ml)*	*CV (%)*
1 11.9	5.9	1	97	3.3	
2 40.0	4.0	2	37.6	3.9	
3 82.7	4.1	3	97.9	3.3	

Incubation Scheme

Anticardiolipin IgA

100 µl	Pipette control into the microplate	7 × 100 µl	Pipette patient sample

⇓ ⇓

Incubate for 30 minutes at room temperature

⇓

Discard the contents of the wells and wash 3 times with 300 µl wash solution

⇓

Pipette 100 µl enzyme conjugate

⇓

Incubate for 15 minutes at room temperature

⇓

Discard the contents of the well and wash 3 times with 300 µl wash solution

⇓

Pipette 100 µl TMB substrate solution

⇓

Incubate for 15 minutes at room temperature

⇓

Add 100 µl stop solution

⇓

Leave untouched for 5 minutes

⇓

Read at 450 nm

ANTIPHOSPHOLIPID SCREEN (IgG/IgM) WITH HUMAN β2-GLYCOPROTEIN I AS COFACTOR Mfd: Orgentec. Courtesy: Lilac Medicare

Immunometric Enzyme Immunoassay for the Quantitative Determination of the sum of Autoantibodies against Cardiolipin, Phosphatidyl Serine, Phosphatidyl Inositol and Phosphatidic Acid (IgG and/or IgM class).

Warnings and Precautions

All reagents of this test kit are strictly intended for in vitro use only.

Please adhere strictly to the sequence of pipetting steps provided in this protocol. Observe the guidelines for performing quality control in medical laboratories by assaying controls and/or pooled sera.

All reagents should be stored refrigerated at 2-8°C in their original container.

Do not interchange kit components from different lots. The expiration dates stated on the labels of the shipping container and all vials have to be observed. Do not use kit components beyond their expiration dates.

Allow all kit components and specimen to reach room temperature prior to use and mix well.

During handling of all kit reagents, controls and serum samples observe the existing legal regulations. The following precautions should be taken while handling potentially infectious materials:

- do not eat, drink or smoke in areas where specimens or kit reagents are handled
- do not pipette by mouth
- wear disposable gloves while handling specimens or kit reagents and wash hands thoroughly afterwards.

The test kit contains components of human origin which, when tested by FDA-licensed methods, were found negative for hepatitis B surface antigen and for HIV antibody. No known test can guarantee, however, that products derived from human blood will not be infectious. Handle, therefore, all reagents and human blood derivatives, like plasma or serum samples, as if capable of transmitting infection.

Avoid contact with the TMB (3,3',5,5'-Tetramethylbenzidine). If TMB comes into contact with skin, wash thoroughly with water and soap.

The stop solution contains hydrochloric acid. If it comes into contact with skin, wash thoroughly with water and seek medical attention.

Avoid contact between the buffered peroxide solution and easily oxidised materials; extreme temperatures may initiate spontaneous combustion.

Material Supplied

Package size	96 determinations
Divisible microplate consisting of 12 modules of 8 wells each, coated with a mixture of highly purified phospholipids: Cardiolipin, Phosphatidyl Serine, Phosphatidyl Inositol, Phosphatidic Acid and saturated with highly purified human β_2-Glycoprotein I	1
Combined calibrators with IgG and IgM class anti-Phospholipid antibodies in a PBS/BSA matrix containing: IgG: 0; 6.3; 12.5; 25; 50; 100 GPL U/ml and IgM: 0; 6.3; 12.5; 25; 50; 100 MPL U/ml	1 set 6 vials 1 ml each
Antiphospholipid controls in a PBS/BSA matrix (positive and negative), for the respective concentrations see the enclosed package insert	1 set 2 vials 1 ml each
Sample buffer (yellow), concentrate containing BSA in PBS buffer	1 vial 20 ml
Enzyme conjugate solution (light red), containing polyclonal rabbit anti-h-IgG-IgG, labelled with horseradish peroxidase in a PBS/BSA matrix	1 vial 15 ml
enzyme conjugate solution (light red), containing polyclonal rabbit anti-h-IgM-IgG, labelled with horseradish peroxidase in a PBS/BSA matrix	1 vial 15 ml
TMB substrate solution	1 vial, 15 ml
Stop solution (1 M hydrochloric acid)	1 vial 15ml
Buffered wash solution, concentrate	1 vial 20 ml

Controls

A set of two controls is provided with the kit.

Technical Data

Sample material:	Serum or plasma
Required sample size:	10 µl of sample to be diluted 1:100 with sample buffer 100 µl prediluted sample per single determination
Total incubation time:	60 minutes at room temperature (18-28°C)
Calibration range:	IgG and IgM: 6.3-100 U/ml
Sensitivity:	IgG and IgM: 0.5 U/ml
Storage:	Refrigerated at 2-8°C
Shelf-life:	9 months after manufacturing or until the expiration date printed on the labels
Package size:	96 tests

Principle of the Procedure

Antiphospholipid screen (IgG/IgM) is an indirect solid-phase enzyme immunometric assay (ELISA). It is designed for the quantitative measurement of IgG or IgM class autoantibodies directed against phospholipids. The microplate is coated with a mixture of highly purified negatively charged phospholipids: cardiolipin, phosphatidyl serine, phosphatidyl inositol and phosphatidic acid. antiphospholipid autoantibodies require (β_2-Glycoprotein I as a cofactor for binding. The microplate is therefore saturated with highly purified human β_2-glycoprotein I.

The microplates can be divided into 12 modules of 8 wells each or can be used completely for 96 determinations. Each well can be separated from the module ("break-away").

The binding of present autoantibodies, formation of the sandwich complexes and enzymatic colour reaction take place during three different reaction phases.

Phase 1

Calibrators, controls and prediluted patient samples are pipetted into the wells of the microplate. Any present antibodies bind to the inner surface of the wells. After a 30-minute incubation, the microplate is washed with wash buffer for removing non-reactive serum components.

Phase 2

An anti-human-IgG (or anti-human-IgM) horseradish peroxidase conjugate solution is pipetted into the wells of the microplate to recognise IgG class autoantibodies (or IgM class autoantibodies) bound to the immobilised antigens. After a 15-minute incubation, any excess enzyme conjugate, which is not specifically bound, is washed away with wash buffer.

Phase 3

A chromogenic substrate solution containing TMB (3,3',5,5'-Tetramethyl-benzidine) is dispensed into the wells. During 15 minutes of incubation, the colour of the solutions changes into blue. Colour development is stopped by adding 1 M hydrochloric acid as stop solution. The solutions colour changes into yellow.

The amount of colour is directly proportional to the concentration of IgG resp. IgM antibodies present in the original sample.

To read the optical density, a microplate reader with a 450 nm filter is required. Bichromatic measurement with a 600-690 nm reference is recommended.

Clinical Relevance

The first study of antiphospholipid antibodies began in 1906, when Wasserman introduced a serological test for syphilis. In 1942, the active component was found to be a phospholipid, which was designated cardiolipin. In the 1950s it became clear that a number of people had positive tests for syphilis without any evidence of the disease. This phenomenon was referred to as the biological false-positive serological test for syphilis. A high prevalence of autoimmune disorders, including systemic lupus erythematosus (SLE) and Sjögren syndrome occurred in this group of patients.

The presence of circulating anticoagulants in patients with SLE was first documented in 1952 and was associated with increased risk of paradoxical thrombosis in 1963. The term lupus anticoagulant (LA), first used in 1972, is clearly a misnomer, because LA is more frequently encountered in patients without lupus and is associated with thrombosis rather than abnormal bleeding.

During the last years it became clear that the optimal binding of antiphospholipid antibodies is depending on a cofactor termed β_2-glycoprotein (apolipoprotein H) (β_2GPI). β_2GPI is a 50 kDa β_2-globulin occurring in plasma at a level of 200 ug/ml. It has been found that β_2-glycoprotein I inhibits the intrinsic coagulation pathway and, therefore, it is involved in the regulation of blood coagulation. β_2GPI is associated *in vivo* with negatively charged substances, e.g. anionic phospholipids, heparin and lipoproteins. The phospholipid-binding region is located on its fifth domain.

Under the acronym "aPL" (antiphospholipid antibodies) antibodies against negatively charged phospholipids, such as CL (cardiolipin), LA (lupus anticoagulant), PS (phosphatidyl serine), PI (phosphatidyl inositol) and PA (phosphatidic acid) are summarised. Of these, cardiolipin is the phospholipid most commonly used as antigen to test for aPL by ELISA. Some antisera which bind cardiolipin-coated ELISA plates can also bind to plates coated with other negatively charged phospholipids, such as phosphatidyl serine (PS), phosphatidyl inositol and phosphatidic acid (PA).

Some investigators have suggested that the use of PS in place of cardiolipin in ELISA tests enables more specific diagnosis. These antigens are less commonly used and their additional use can improve the clinical sensitivity in patient samples with suspected APS (antiphospholipid syndrome), but they cannot replace the measurement of autoantibodies against cardiolipin.

Normal Values

In a normal range study with serum samples from healthy blood donors the following ranges have been established with the antiphospholipid screen test:

	antiphospholipid-Ab	
	IgG (GPL U/ml)	IgM (MPL U/ml)
Normal:	< 10	< 10
Elevated:	≥ 10	≥ 10

Positive results should be verified concerning the entire clinical status of the patient. Also, every decision for therapy should be taken individually.

It is recommended that each laboratory establishes its own normal and pathological ranges of antiphospholipid antibodies.

Specificity

The microplate is coated with a mixture of highly purified cardiolipin, phosphatidyl serine, phosphatidyl inositol, phosphatidic acid and highly purified human (β_2-Glycoprotein I. special coating processes, developed by the manufacturer guarantee for the native immunogenic structure of the phospholipids after immobilisation on the solid phase. The antiphospholipid screen test kit is specific for autoantibodies directed against phospholipids or the complex of negatively charged phospholipids and β_2-Glycoprotein I.

No crossreactivity was observed to anti-DNA antibodies and those types of antibodies occurring in syphilis.

Calibration

The assay system is calibrated against the internationally recognised reference sera from EN Harris, Louisville, since no other international standards are available.

IMMUNOASSAY PROCEDURE

Materials Required

Equipment

- Microplate reader capable for endpoint measurements at 450 nm
- Vortex mixer
- Pipettes for 10 µl, 100 µl and 1000 µl.

Preparation of reagents

- Distilled water
- Graduated cylinder for 100 and 1,000 ml
- Plastic container for storage of the wash solution.

Optional:

- Multichannel dispenser
- Repeatable pipette for 100 µl
- Data reduction software.

Specimen Collection and Preparation

For determination of antiphospholipid antibodies serum or plasma are the preferred sample matrixes.

All serum and plasma samples are prediluted 1:100 with sample buffer. Therefore 10 ul of sample may be diluted with 1,000 µl of sample buffer.

The patients need not to be fasting, and no special preparations are necessary. Collect blood by venipuncture into vacutainers and separate serum or plasma from the cells by centrifugation after clot formation.

Samples may be stored refrigerated at 2-8°C for at least 5 days. For longer storage of up to six months samples should be stored frozen at -20°C. To avoid repeated thawing and freezing, the samples should be aliquoted.

Neither bilirubin nor haemolysis have significant effect on the procedure.

Preparation and Storage of Reagents

All components of this test kit are supplied in a liquid format and ready to use, except the sample buffer and wash buffer. When stored refrigerated at 2-8°C, the components are stable for at least 30 days after opening or until the expiration date printed on the labels.

Remaining modules of the microplate should be stored refrigerated at 2-8°C protected from moisture; store together with desiccant and carefully sealed in the plastic bag.

Preparation of Sample Buffer

Dilute the contents of each vial of the sample buffer concentrate (5x) with destilled water to a final volume of 100 ml prior to use. Store refrigerated: stable at 2-8°C for at least 30 days after preparation or until the expiration date printed on the label.

Preparation of Buffered Wash Solution

Dilute the contents of each vial of the buffered wash solution concentrate (50x) with distilled water to a final volume of 1000 ml prior to use. Store refrigerated: stable at 2-8°C for at least 30 days after preparation or until the expiration date printed on the label.

Notes on Technique

Control sera or pools should routinely be assayed as unknowns to check performance of the reagents and the assay.

Pipetting and Sample Handling

Use a disposable-tip micropipette to dispense sera and plasma samples. Pipette directly to the bottom of the wells. To avoid carryover contamination, change the tip between samples.

Patient samples expected to contain high concentrations should be additionally diluted with sample buffer before. Additional dilutions must be considered during calculation.

Immunoassay Procedure

Do not interchange components of different lots.

All components should be at room temperature before use.

Dilute all patient samples 1:100 with sample buffer before assay. Therefore combine 10 µl of sample with 1,000 µl of sample buffer in a polystyrene tube. Mix well. Calibrators and controls are ready to use and need not to be diluted.

1. Prepare a sufficient number of microplate modules to accommodate calibrators, controls and prediluted patient samples in duplicates.

	1	2	3	4 5 6 7 8 9 10 11 12
a	SA	SE	P1	P..
b	SA	SE	P1	P..
c	SB	SF	P2	
d	SB	SF	P2	
e	SC	C1	P3	
f	SC	C1	P3	
g	SD	C2	P4	
h	SD	C2	P4	

2. For the determination of one class of autoantibodies pipette 100 µl of calibrators, controls and prediluted patient samples into the wells. For determination of both IgG and IgM autoantibodies calibrators, controls and patient samples have to be pipetted in two attempts.
3. Incubate for 30 minutes at room temperature (20-28°C).
4. Discard the contents of the microwells and wash 3 times with 300 µl of wash solution.
5. Dispense 100 µl of enzyme conjugate solution (anti-h-IgG-IgG or anti-h-IgM-IgG) into each well.
6. Incubate for 15 minutes at room temperature.
7. Discard the contents of the microwells and wash 3 times with 300 µl of wash solution.
8. Dispense 100 µl of TMB substrate solution into each well.
9. Incubate for 15 minutes at room temperature.

10. Add 100 µl of stop solution to each well of the modules and let it stand for 5 minutes.
11. Read the optical density at 450 nm and calculate the results. Bichromatic measurement with a reference at 600-690 nm is recommended.

The developed colour is stable for at least 30 minutes. Read optical densities during this time.

Calculation of Results

For antiphospholipid screen IgG and IgM a 4-parameter-fit with lin-log coordinates for optical density and concentration is the data reduction method of choice. Smoothed spline approximation and log-log coordinates are also suitable.

Recommended Lin-Log Plot

First calculate the averaged optical densities for each calibrator well. Use lin-log graph paper and plot the averaged optical density of each calibrator versus the concentration. Draw the best fitting curve approximating the path of all calibrator points. The calibrator points may also be connected with straight line segments. The concentration of unknowns may then be estimated from the calibration curve by interpolation.

Calculation Example

The table below shows typical results for anti-Phospholipid Screen IgG and IgM. These data are intended for illustration only and should not be used to calculate results from another run.

Calibrators

anti-PL	No	Position	OD 1	OD 2	Mean	Conc. 1	Conc. 2	Mean	decl. Conc.	CV%
IgG	STA	A 1/B 1	0.051	0.049	0.050	0.3	0.1	0.2	0.0	3
IgG	STB	C 1/D 1	0.163	0.160	0.161	6.4	6.3	6.3	6.3	1
IgG	STC	E 1/F 1	0.310	0.273	0.291	12.8	11.2	12.0	12.5	9
IgG	STD	G 1/H 1	0.603	0.630	0.616	25	26	26	25	3
IgG	STE	A 2/B 2	1.122	1.054	1.088	51	47	49	50	4
IgG	STF	C 2/D 2	1.742	1.787	1.765	98	103	101	100	2
IgM	STA	A 7/B 7	0.022	0.021	0.022	0.2	0.1	0.2	0.0	3
IgM	STB	C 7/D 7	0.211	0.205	0.208	6.1	6.0	6.1	6.3	2
IgM	STC	E 7/F 7	0.465	0.462	0.464	13.0	12.9	13.0	12.5	0
IgM	STD	G 7/H 7	0.788	0.879	0.833	23	26	24	25	8
IgM	STE	A 8/B 8	1.411	1.382	1.397	52	50	51	50	1
IgM	STF	C 8/D 8	1.868	1.852	1.860	101	98	99	100	1

HEPATITIS MARKERS

AUSTRALIA ANTIGEN HBSAG (VIRUTEX HBsAG)
Courtesy: Tulip Group of Companies

Slide Test for Hepatitis B Surface Antigen

Summary

Blood containing hepatitis B virus (HBV) is potentially infectious. In most cases detectable levels of hepatitis B surface antigen (HBsAg) circulate in the bloodstream of an infected person, two to three weeks prior to the appearance of clinical symptoms. These levels are especially elevated in the symptomatic phase, thereafter the levels slowly decline. Detection of HBV using HBsAg as a marker to screen blood donors is essential to reduce the risk of transmission of hepatitis B by blood transfusion.

Reagent

1. Virutex HBsAg reagent A uniform suspension of polystyrene latex particles coated with IgG class of monoclonal Anti-HBsAg antibodies.
2. Positive control, reactive with the Virutex latex reagent.
3. Negative control, nonreactive with the Virutex latex reagent.

Virutex HBsAg reagent conforms to the sensitivity requirements of a "Third generation" test. Each batch of reagent undergoes rigorous quality control at various stages of manufacture for its specificity, sensitivity and performance.

Reagent Storage and Stability

1. Store the reagent at 2 to 8°C. Do not freeze.
2. The shelf life of reagent is as per the expiry date mentioned on the reagent vial label.

Principle

Latex particles coated with anti-HBsAg antibodies will agglutinate when mixed with serum or plasma containing hepatitis B surface antigen within the detectable levels. Agglutination is absent when the hepatitis B surface antigen is absent or not within the detectable levels.

Note

1. *In vitro* diagnostic reagent for laboratory and professional use only. Not for medicinal use.

2. All the reagents derived from human source have been tested for HBsAg and anti-HIV antibody and are found to be nonreactive. However, handle the material as if infectious.
3. Reagent contains sodium azide 0.1% as preservative. Avoid contact with skin and mucosa. On disposal, flush with large quantities of water.
4. The reagents can be damaged due to microbial contamination or exposure to elevated temperatures. It is recommended that the performance of the reagents be verified by testing with the negative or positive controls provided with the kit.
5. Shake the latex antigen vial gently before use to disperse the latex particles uniformly and improve the test readability.
6. Use only a thoroughly clean and dry glass slide. Clean the slide with distilled water and wipe dry before use.
7. Accessories provided with the kit only must be used for optimum results.

Sample Collection and Storage

No special preparation of the patient is required prior to sample collection by approved techniques. Do not use haemolysed samples. Though plasma may be used, fresh serum is preferable. In case of delay in testing, store the samples at 2 to 8°C for up to 24 hours.

Material Provided with the Kit

Reagent Pack

Latex reagent coated with anti-HBsAg antibody, positive control reactive with the latex reagent, negative control nonreactive with the latex reagent.

Accessories Pack

Glass slide with six reaction circles, mixing sticks, rubber teats, sample dispensing pipettes.

Additional Material Required

Test tubes (10 × 75 mm), pipettes, isotonic saline, stopwatch, direct light source.

Procedure

Bring reagent and samples to room temperature before testing.

1. Pipette one drop of sample to be tested onto one of the reaction circles of the glass slide using a sample dispensing pipette, provided with the kit.
2. Prepare a 1: 40 dilution (0.05 ml serum +1.95 ml isotonic saline) of samples to be tested in isotonic saline.
3. Pipette one drop of the diluted sample on the next reaction circle of the glass slide.

3a. In steps 1 and 3 above, carefully aspirate the sample into the dispensing pipette avoiding sample entering the rubber teat and subsequent cross contamination.

4. Place one drop of positive and negative control onto the remaining reaction circles of the slide (do not dilute controls).
5. Shake the latex reagent vial gently to uniformly disperse the reagent suspension. Add one drop of the latex reagent to each of the samples and controls on the slide.
6. Mix with separate mixing sticks, spreading the mixture uniformly over the entire reaction circle.
7. Immediately start a stopwatch. Rock the slide gently back and forth, observing for agglutination macroscopically at five minutes.

Interpretation of Results

1. No agglutination with diluted and neat samples is a negative test result: HBsAg absent
2. Agglutination with neat sample but no agglutination with diluted sample is a positive test result: HBsAg present (weak positive)
3. Agglutination with both neat and diluted samples is a positive test result: HBsAg present (moderate positive)
4. Agglutination with diluted sample but no agglutination with neat sample is a positive test result: HBsAg present (strong positive)

Remarks

1. The positive control has been inactivated at 60°C for 10 hours and is not expected to be infectious.
2. Presence of autoantibodies such as RF and heterophile antibodies may interfere with the test giving a false-positive result. Probability of such an occurrence is low (less than 1% of all samples).

3. Since Virutex is only a quick screening test, for confirmation of the results, a confirmatory test should be used.
4. Positive and negative controls should be run with each series of tests and the results compared with unknown specimens to distinguish possible granularity from agglutination.
5. It is recommended that results of the tests should be correlated with clinical findings to arrive at the final diagnosis.
6. The reusable glass slide should be first immersed in sodium hypochlorite 5% solution and then rinsed with tap water and then distilled water. Wipe thoroughly dry before use.
7. As the biggest risk to laboratory personnel is from uncharacterised random samples, it is strongly recommended that as a safety measure hand gloves should be worn during the entire test procedure.
8. Samples that are contaminated, haemolysed, lipaemic or highly icteric may give nonspecific reactions.

ONE STEP TEST FOR HBsAG VIRUCHECK® DIPSTICK, Courtesy: Tulip Group of Companies

Introduction

Virucheck, one-step test for AHBsAg is a rapid, self-performing, qualitative, two-site, sandwich immunoassay for the detection of hepatitis B surface antigen, a marker for hepatitis B infections, in serum/plasma specimen.

Summary

Blood containing hepatitis B virus (HBV) is potentially infectious. Hepatitis B surface antigen (HBsAg), earlier known as Australia antigen, is among the first serological markers that circulate in the blood of infected persons even two to three weeks prior to the appearance of clinical symptoms. The levels of HBsAg are especially elevated during the symptomatic phase and decline thereafter.

Detection of HBV using HBsAg as the marker to screen blood donors is essential to reduce the risk of transmission of hepatitis B by blood transfusion. The HBsAg detection is also useful for screening high risk groups for HBV and for differential diagnosis of hepatitis infection.

Virucheck, one-step test for HBsAg detects the presence of HBsAg in serum/plasma specimens, qualitatively, at concentrations as low as 0.8 ng/ml.

Principle

Virucheck, one-step test for HBsAg utilizes the principle of Immunochromatography, a unique two-site immunoassay on a membrane. As the test sample flows through the membrane assembly of the dipstick, the coloured anti-HBsAg-colloidal gold conjugate complexes with HBsAg in the sample. The complex moves further on the membrane to the test region where it is immobilised by the anti-HbsAg antiserum coated on the membrane leading to formation of a pink coloured band which confirms a positive test result. Absence of this coloured band in the test region indicates a negative test result. The unreacted conjugate and unbound complex if any move further on the membrane and are subsequently immobilised by the antimouse antiserum coated on the membrane at the control region, forming a pink band. This control band serves to validate the test results.

Reagents and Materials Supplied

Each individual pouch contains:

1. Dipstick: Membrane assembly predispensed with anti-HBsAg antiserum-colloidal gold conjugate and anti-HBsAg antiserum and anti-mouse antiserum coated at the respective regions.
2. Desiccant pouch.

Storage and Stability

The sealed pouches in the test kit may be stored between 4-30°C for the duration of the shelf-life as indicated on the pouch.

Note

1. For *in vitro* diagnostic use only. Not for Medicinal Use.
2. Do not use beyond expiry date.
3. Read the instructions carefully before performing the test.
4. Handle all specimens as potentially infectious.
5. Follow standard biosafety guidelines for handling and disposal of potentially infective material.

Specimen Collection and Preparation

No special preparation of the patient is necessary prior to specimen collection by approved techniques. Though fresh serum/plasma is preferable, serum/

plasma specimen may be stored at 2 to 8°C for up to 24 hours, in case of delay in testing. Do not use haemolysed, turbid or contaminated samples. Turbid samples must be centrifuged and clear supernatant must be used for testing.

Test Procedure

1. Collect serum/plasma specimen in clean test tubes. Ensure that only sufficient quantity of the specimen is collected to allow submerging the red area of the dipstick (about 1 cm high).
2. Bring the sealed pouch to room temperature, open the pouch and remove the dipstick. Once opened, the dipstick must be used immediately.
3. Dip the dipstick in the serum/plasma specimen submerging only the red area.
4. At the end of 14 minutes, read results as follows

   Negative: Only one pink coloured band appears on the dipstick.

   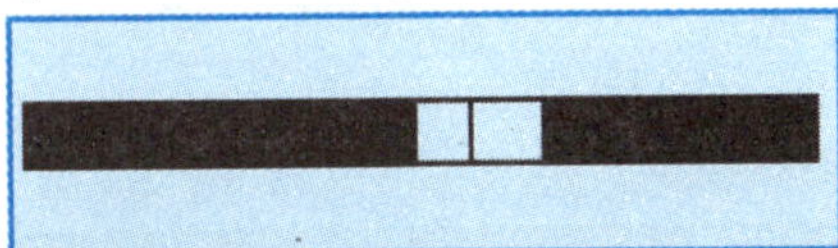

   Positive: Two distinct pink coloured bands appear on the dipstick.

   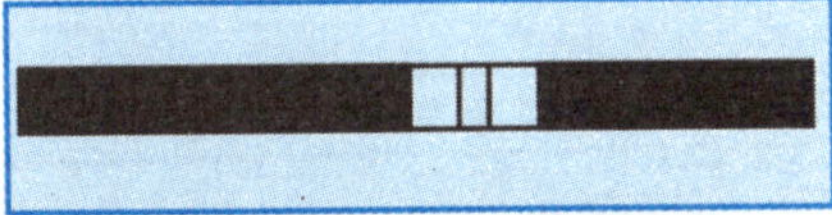

5. The test should be considered invalid if no band appears. Repeat the test with a new dipstick.
6. Although, depending on the concentration of HBsAg in the specimen, positive results may start appearing as early as 2 minutes, negative results must be confirmed only at the end of fifteen minutes.
7. In case of a doubtful result at 15 minutes, the test may be extended up to 30 minutes to get a clear background.

Limitations of the Test

1. Presence of elevated levels of other antigens such as RF and cross reacting autoantibodies such as antibodies to HLA DR4 may yield false-positive results. This may occur in less than 1% of the specimens. For confirmation of results, a confirmatory test must be used.
2. This test detects the presence of HBsAg in the specimen and hence should not be used as the sole criterion for the diagnosis of hepatitis infection.
3. As with all diagnostic tests, the results must be correlated with clinical findings.

ONE-STEP TEST FOR HBsAG VIRUCHECK® DEVICE, Courtesy: Tulip Group of Companies

Introduction

Virucheck one-step test for rapid, self-performing, qualitative, two-site, sandwich, immunoassay for the detection of hepatitis B surface antigen, a marker for hepatitis B infections, in serum/plasma specimen.

Virucheck one-step test for HBsAg detects the presence of HBsAg in serum/plasma specimens, qualitatively, at concentrations as low as 0.8 ng/ml.

Principle

Virucheck one-step test for HBsAg utilises the principle of immunochromatography, a unique two-site immunoassay on a membrane. As the test sample flows through the membrane assembly within the test device, the coloured anti-HBsAg colloidal gold conjugate complexes with HBsAg in the sample. This complex moves further on the membrane to the test region where it is immobilised by the anti-HBsAg antiserum coated on the membrane leading to formation of a pink coloured band which confirms a positive test result. Absence of this coloured band in the test region indicates a negative test result. The unreacted conjugate and unbound complex if any move further on the membrane and are subsequently immobilised by the antimouse antiserum coated on the membrane at the control region, forming a pink band. This control band serves to validate the test results.

Regents and Materials Supplied

Each individual pouch contains:

1. Test device: Contains membrane assembly predispensed with anti-HBsAg antiserum-colloidal gold conjugate and anti-HBsAg antiserum and antimouse antiserum coated at the respective regions.
2. Disposable plastic dropper.

Storage and Stability

The sealed pouches in the test kit may be stored between 4-30°C for the duration of the shelf-life as indicated on the pouch.

Note

1. For *in vitro* diagnostic use only. *Not for medicinal use.*
2. Do not use beyond expiry date.
3. Read the instruction carefully before performing the test.
4. Handle all specimens as potentially infectious.
5. Follow standard biosafety guidelines for handling and disposal of potentially infective material.

Specimen Collection and Preparation

No special preparation of the patient is necessary prior to collection by approved techniques. Though fresh serum/plasma is preferable, serum/plasma specimen may be stored at 2 to 8°C for up to 24 hours, in case of delay in testing. Do not use haemolysed, turbid or contaminated samples. Turbid samples must be centrifuged and clear supernatant must be used for testing.

Testing Procedure and Interpretation of Results

1. Bring the sealed pouch to room temperature, open the pouch and remove the device. Once opened, the device must be used immediately.
2. Dispense two drops of serum/plasma specimen into the sample well 'S' using the dropper provided. Refrigerated specimens must be brought to room temperature prior to testing.
3. At the end of fifteen minutes, read the results as follows (Fig. 23.36):

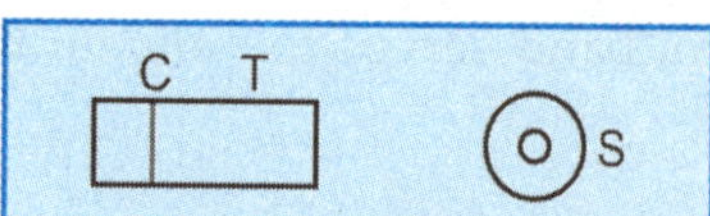

Negative: Only one coloured band appears on the control region 'C'.

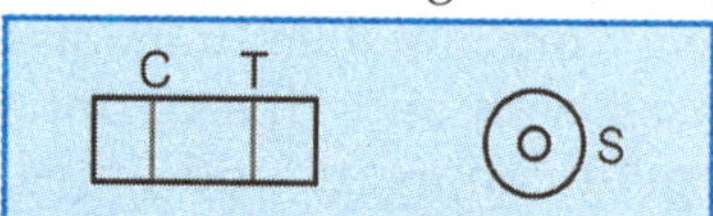

Positive: In addition to the control band, a distinct coloured band also appears on the test region 'T'.

4. The test should be considered invalid if neither the test band nor the control band appear. Repeat the test with a new device.
5. Although, depending on the concentration of HBsAg in the specimen, positive results may start appearing as early as 2 minutes, negative results must be confirmed only at the end of fifteen minutes.
6. In case of doubtful result at 15 minutes, the test may extended up to 30 minutes to get a clear background.

Limitation of the Test

1. Presence of elevated levels of other antigens such as RF and cross reacting autoantibodies such as antibodies to HLA DR4 may yield false-positive results. This may occur in less than 1% of the specimens. For confirmation of results, a confirmatory test must be used.
2. This test detects the presence of HBsAg in the specimen and hence should not be used as the sole criterion for the diagnoses of hepatitis infection.
3. As with all diagnostic test, the results must be correlated with clinical findings.

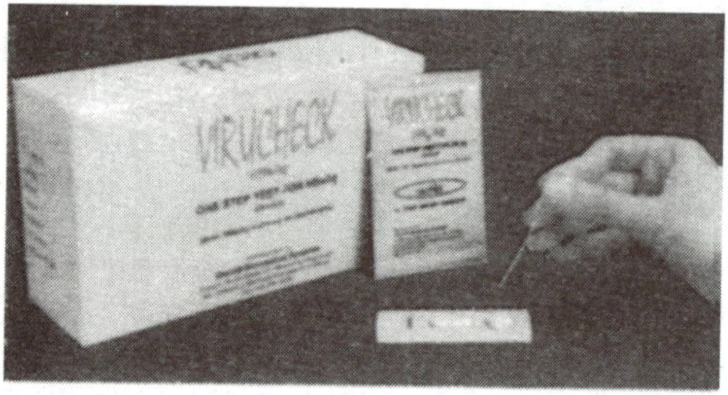

15 minutes

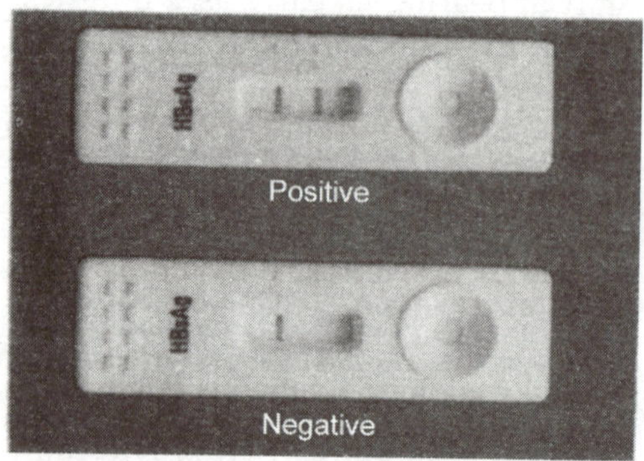

Fig. 23.36: Virucheck result reading

HCV FLAVICHECK® DEVICE, Courtesy: Tulip Group of Companies

One-Step Immunochromatographic Test for HCV Antibodies

Introduction

Flavicheck-HCV is a rapid self-performing, third generation, qualitative one-step, two-site sandwich immunoassay for the detection of antibodies specific to the hepatitis C virus in human serum and plasma. The test employs recombinant proteins derived from the core, NS3, NS4, and NS5 regions of the HCV genome. Combination of these proteins in a double antigen sandwich system not only affords antibody detection to greater number of HCV-encoded epitopes but also earlier detection of seroconversion following HCV infection.

Summary

Hepatitis C virus (HCV) is a single-stranded RNA virus of the Flaviviridae family. The HCV is now known to be the causative agent for most, if not all non-A, non-B hepatitis (NANBH). Antibodies to the hepatitis C encoded antigens are prevalent in the sera of HCV infected individuals. Detection of these antibodies indicates exposure to the hepatitis C virus.

Principle

Flavicheck-HCV utilises the principle of lateral flow immunochromatography, a unique two site double antigen sandwich immunoassay on a membrane. As the test specimen flows through the membrane assembly of the test device, the coloured HCV specific recombinant antigen-colloidal gold conjugate complexes with HCV antibodies in the sample. This complex moves further on the membrane to the test region 'T where it is immobilised by the HCV specific recombinant antigens coated on the membrane leading to formation of a coloured band which confirms a positive test result. Absence of this coloured band in the test region indicates a negative test result. The unreacted conjugate and unbound complex, if any, move further on the membrane and are subsequently immobilised by the antirabbit antibodies coated on the membrane at the control region 'C', forming a coloured band. This control band serves to validate the reagent and assay performance.

Reagents and Materials Supplied

Kit Components

1. Flavicheck-HCV membrane test assembly (device) comprises of HCV specific recombinant antigen-colloidal gold conjugate co-dispensed with rabbit IgG colloidal gold conjugate; pre-dispensed with HCV specific recombinant antigen at region T', and antirabbit antiserum predispensed at the region 'C', along with a plastic sample dropper and desiccant.
2. Package insert

Storage and Stability

The test kit should be stored between 4-30°C for the duration of the shelf-life of the kit as indicated on the pouch/kit label.

Note

1. *In vitro* diagnostic test. Not for medicinal use.
2. Do not use beyond expiry date.
3. Read the package insert carefully before performing the test.
4. Handle all specimen as potentially infectious.
5. Follow standard biosafety guidelines for personal protection, handling and disposal of potentially infectious material.

Specimen Collection and Preparation

1. No prior preparation of the patient is required before sample collection by approved techniques.
2. Fresh serum/plasma is preferable. Serum/plasma may be stored at 2 to 8°C up to 24 hours in case of delay in testing. For long-term storage, freeze the specimen at –20°C for 3 months or –70°C for longer periods.
3. Repeated freezing and thawing of the specimen should be avoided.
4. Do not use haemolysed, clotted, contaminated, viscous/turbid specimen.
5. Specimen containing precipitates or particulate matter must be centrifuged and the clear supernatant only used foresting.
6. Do not heat inactivate the sample.

Test Procedure and Interpretation of Results

1. Let the sealed pouches attain room temperature (25-30°C).
2. Tear open the sealed pouches and retrieve the appropriate number of test devices as required. Label the test devices appropriately. Once opened, the devices must be used immediately. The addition of sample must be done at the centre of the sample port holding the sample dropper in a vertical position. Ensure the drops are free falling. Use a new sample dropper for each specimen to avoid cross contamination.
3. Dispense two drops of specimen in to the sample port (S) using the dropper provided.
4. At the end of 15 minutes, read the results as follows:

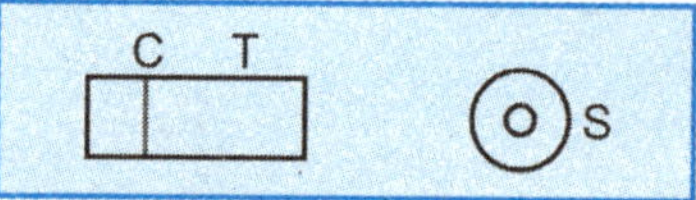

Negative test result: Appearance of only one coloured band at the control region'C'.

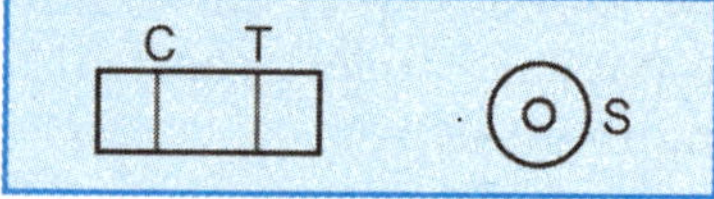

Positive test result: Appearance of a coloured band at the test region 'T'in addition to the band at control region 'C'.

6. The test should be considered invalid if neither the test nor the control bands appear. Repeat the test with a new device.
7. Based on the concentration of antibodies to HCV in the specimen a positive result may start appearing as early as two minutes, however, negative results must be confirmed only at the end of fifteen minutes.
8. In case of doubtful results at fifteen minutes, the test may be extended up to a maximum of 30 minutes if required.

Remarks

1. Though Flavicheck-HCV is a sensitive and reliable screening test, it should not be used as a sole criterion for diagnosis of HCV infection.
2. All positive specimen should be further tested using appropriate supplemental confirmatory tests. Test samples that are positive by a third generation double antigen sandwich-based assays may be reactive with very early seroconversion samples, which are negative/intermediate with blot-based assays. Such samples should be reconfirmed with the RNA-PCR-based method or must be followed up for seroconversion at a later date.
3. As with all diagnostic tests, results must be correlated with clinical findings to arrive at the final diagnosis.
4. Absence of antibodies to HCV does not indicate that an individual is absolutely free of HCV infection as the collection of sample and its timing vis-a-vis seroconversion will influence the test outcome.
5. Do not compare the intensity of test lines and the control lines to judge the concentration of antibodies in the test specimen.
6. Since various tests for HCV differ in their performance characteristics and antigenic composition, their reactivity patterns may differ.
7. Testing of pooled samples is not recommended.

ELISA-BASED TESTS
HAV AB, Courtesy: Lilac Medicare

Enzyme Immunoassay for the Determination of Antibodies to Hepatitis A Virus or HAV Ab—for *in vitro* Diagnostic Use Only.

Introduction

Hepatitis A virus (HAV) is a nonenveloped icosahedral RNA virus with a linear single-strand genome, encoding for only one known serotype. HAV has four major, structural polypeptides and it localises exclusively in the cytoplasm of human hepatocites. The route of infection is predominantly oral-faecal with an incubation period of 2-7 weeks during which HAV can be detected in stools. The HAV infection does not originate any chronic hepatitis and complications are uncommon. The infection stimulates a strong immunological response in the patient with elevated titres first of IgM and then of IgG, whose final presence lasts for years after infection. The determination of both IgM and IgG can distinguish the infective nature of the illness, the classification of the virus and phase of the infection cycle, as well.

Principle of the Assay

Anti-HAV antibodies, if present in the sample, compete with a virus-specific polyclonal IgG, labelled with peroxidase (HRP), for a fixed amount of HAV, affinity purified, coated on the microplate, in a simultaneous incubation of sample and tracer. The concentration of the bound enzyme on the solid phase is inversely proportional to the amount of anti-HAV antibodies in the sample and it is detected by acting on the chromogen/substrate mixture in the second incubation. The concentration of HAV-specific antibodies in the sample is determined by means of a cut-off value that allows for a semiquantitative detection of anti-HAV antibodies.

Content of the Kit and Reagents Preparation

1. **Microtitre strips:** 1 microtitre plate. 12 × 8-wells strips 6 × 8-wells coated with affinity purified HAV antigens. The plate is contained in a sealed bag with dessicant. Bring the plate to room temperature before use, to prevent any moisture formation inside the bag.
2. **Enzyme conjugate:** 1 vial of 0.5 ml 1 × 0.25 ml. Proteic buffer solution containing anti-HAV polyclonal antibody, conjugated with HRP, 20 × concentrated. It contains proteic stabilisers, 0.2 mg/ml gentamicin sulphate, 0.1% Kathon GC and 0.01% Cialit as preservatives.
3. **Conjugate diluent:** 1 vial of 10 ml 1 × 5 ml. Proteic buffer solution for the dilution of the concentrated tracer. It contains 0.2 mg/ml gentamicin sulphate, 0.1% Kathon GC and 0.01% Cialit as preservatives.
4. **Washing solution:** 1 vial of 50 ml 25 × concentrated solution to be diluted up to 1250 ml with bidistilled water. Contains PBS/Tween. Once diluted, the wash solution is stable for 1 month at 4-8°C or 1 week at room temperature.
5. **Chromogen:** 1 vial of 8 ml 1 × 4 ml. The solution contains tetramethyl-benzidine (TMB) with activators and stabilisers, diluted in phosphate/citrate buffer.
   Warning: Store protected from light!
6. **Substrate:** 1 vial of 8 ml 1 × 4 ml. The solution contains urea peroxide diluted in phosphate/citrate buffer.
7. **Stop solution:** 1 vial of 12 ml. It contains a solution of 1N HCl.
   Warning: Avoid contact with eyes or skin.
8. **Negative control:** 1 vial of 1 ml 1 × 0.5 ml. Human serum base, not reactive for anti-HAV IgG antibodies. It contains 0.2 µg/ml gentamicin sulphate, 0.1% Kathon GC and 0.01% Cialit as preservatives.
9. **Positive control:** 1 vial of 1ml 1 × 0.5 ml. Human serum base, reactive for anti-HAV IgG antibodies. It contains 0.2 mg/ml gentamicin sulphate, 0.1% Kathon GC and 0.01% Cialit as preservatives.
10. **Cardboard sealers:** 2 cardboard sealers to be used to cover the plate during the incubations.

Conditions and Notices

1. All the reagents contained in the kit are for *in vitro* diagnostic use only.
2. Do not use the kit or reagents after the expiry date stated on the labels. Do not mix reagents from different lots.
3. Procedures should be performed carefully, in order to obtain reliable results and clinical interpretations.
4. Bring all reagents to room temperature at least 60 minutes before the analysis.
5. Avoid contaminating reagents when taking them from the vials. We recommend to use automatic pipettes with disposable tips. When dispensing reagents, do not touch with tips the wall of wells in order to avoid cross contaminations.
6. For the washing step, use only the washing solution provided in the kit and follow carefully the indications reported at point "washing instruction". It is recommended anyway to use a good quality microplate washer.
7. Avoid the substrate/chromogen to come in contact with oxidising agents or metallic surfaces; avoid intense light exposure during incubation or reagent preparation. When preparing chromogen/substrate, we recommend the use of plastic disposable sterile containers.
8. Samples and materials potentially infected have to be handled with care as they could transmit the infection. All objects come in direct contact with samples and all residuals

of the assay should be treated or eliminated as potentially infected. Best procedures for inactivation are treatments with autoclave at 121°C for 30 minutes or with sodium hypochlorite at a final concentration of 2.5% for 24 hours. This last method can be used for treating the liquid washes that have to be neutralised before with sodium hydroxide.

9. Avoid any contact with skin and mucosas, especially with the blocking reagent.
10. In any case, use protective talk-free gloves.

Storage and Stability of the Kit

1. The kit has to be stored at 2 to 8°C and used before the expiry date stated on the label.
2. Unused strips have to be placed in the bag containing the dessicant and firmly sealed before restore at 2 to 8°C. After opening, strips are stable until the dessicant turns pink.
3. The diluted washing solution can be stored for one week at room temperature or 3 weeks at + 2 to 8°C.
4. The chromogen/substrate solution is stable for 4 hours at room temperature, protected from light.
5. The dissolved conjugate is stable for 1 week at 2 to 8°C, when stored in disposable sterile container.
6. All other liquid reagents are stable when stored at 2 to 8°C, provided that they are handled carefully to avoid any environment contamination.

Materials not Provided in the Kit

1. Semiautomatic pipettes of 50, 100 and 1000 µl.
2. Vortex mixer and absorbent paper.
3. Ultrapure water (bidistilled).
4. Chronometer.
5. Photometric reader of microplates or microstrips, linear up to at least 2 OD and supplied with filters of 450 nm and 620-630 nm.
6. Incubator set at + 37°C.
7. Automatic microplates washing device or manual apparatus capable of aspirating and dispensing volumes of 300 µl.

Samples

Either fresh sera or plasma can be used. If not used immediately, they can be stored at 2 to 8°C for 1 week; in case of longer storage, freeze at –20°C. Samples should be without particles or microbial contaminations; in case, centrifuge at 2000 g for 20 minutes or filtrate with a 0.2 µ filter. Highly lipaemic or haemolised samples can give uncorrect analytical results.

Reagents Preparation

1. Washing solution: Dilute 1:25 with bidistilled water and mix carefully before use. Stable one week at room temperature.
2. Conjugate: Dilute 1:20 the concentrated conjugate with the conjugate diluent. Mix carefully on vortex. The reagent is stable for 1 week when stored at 2 to 8°C in a sterile container.
3. Chromogen/substrate: About 5 minutes before use, prepare in disposable plastic container, according to needs, the substrate/chromogen solution by mixing the chromogen with the substrate in equal volumes. The reagent is not stable and must be used immediately.

Washing Instruction

A good washing procedure is essential to obtain correct and precise analytical results. We, therefore, recommend to use a good quality ELISA microplate washer, maintained at a good level of washing mechanical performances. Generally, 4-5 automatic washing cycles of 0.3 ml/well are sufficient to avoid false-positive reactions and remove high background. Anyhow we recommend to calibrate the washing system on the kit itself so to match the declared analytical performances. In case, of manual washing, we suggest to perform 5 washing cycles, dispensing and aspirating 0.3 ml/well per cycle leaving a soak time of 30 sec between each cycle. In any case, the liquid washed out from the plates must be inactivated with a sodium hypochlorite solution at a final concentration of 2.5%, before being thrown away or autoclaved, as it must be considered as potentially infected.

Assay Procedure

1. At least one hour before use, bring all reagents, controls and samples to room temperature (18-30°C), mixing them carefully on vortex.
2. Do not mix reagents from different lots.

3. We recommend to distribute the controls and the samples in duplicate.
4. Distribution and incubation times must be the same for all wells in the same analysis.
5. Avoid long interruptions between each step of the assay procedure.
6. It is suggested to eliminate the excess of washing solution from the microplate after washing by blotting it gently on an absorbent paper pad.
7. The colour developed in the last incubation is stable for a maximum of one hour in the dark.
8. We recommend to read the plate with an ELISA automatic reader able to substract the background at 620-630 nm and to read the absorbance of samples and controls at 450 nm. The "blanking" of the instrument is to be carried out in the blank reagent well (well A1).

HAV antigens coated microplate

Reagents	*A1 Blank*	*Negative Control*	*Positive Control*	*Sample*
Negative control	-	50 µl	-	-
Positive control	-	-	50 µl	-
Sample	-	-	-	50 µl
Diluted conjugate	-	50 µl	50 µl	50 µl
Cover strips with adhesive film.				
Incubate 120 min. at + 37°C.				
Peel out the adhesive film and the reaction solution from all wells.				
Wash 4-5 times with 300 µl of diluted washing solution, carefully aspirating off the remaining liquid.				
Reagents Chromogen/ Substrate Mixed:1	100 µl	100 µl	100 µl	100 µl
Cover strips with a new adhesive film				
Incubate 20 min. at room temperature protected from light.				
Stop solution	100 µl	100 µl	100 µl	100 µl
Read the absorbance of each well against A1 blanking-well at 450 nm and 620-630 nm				

Validity of the Assay

The assay is considered valid if:

1. The OD 450 nm of the A1 blank well is < 0.100.
2. After blanking on A1, the OD 450 nm mean value of the negative control or NC is > 1.000.
3. After blanking on A1, the OD 450 nm mean value of the positive control or PC is < 0.200.

In case data above do not match the correct values, before repeating the test check carefully the expiration date of the kit, the performances of the instruments used for the assay and the procedure of distribution of controls and samples.

Calculation of Results

If the test turns out to be valid, calculate the cut-off value through the following formula:

Cut-off = (NC + PC)/2

Samples with an OD 450 nm value equal or higher than the cut off are classified as negative for anti-HAV Ab. Samples with an OD 450 nm value lower than the cut off are classified as positive for anti-HAV Ab (content of antibodies higher than 10 WHO IU/lt).

Example of Calculation

Negative control mean OD 450 nm	1.800
Positive control mean OD 450 nm	0.200
Cut-off = (NC + PC)/2 =	1.000
Sample # 1 OD 450 nm = 1.680	Negative
Sample # 2 OD 450 nm = 0.158	Positive

Assay Performances

Sensibility: The sensitivity of the assay has been calculated by means of the international standard for HAV Ab supplied by WHO.

The test shows a sensitivity at the cut-off of about 10 WHO IU/Lt.

Specificity: It has been calculated on panels of negative and positive samples, preclassified with an FDA approved kit present on the market. The assay shows a specificity > 99% on plasma and sera.

Reproducibility: It has been calculated on the negative and positive controls run in replicates in different days. CV's between 6-15% have been obtained depending on their OD 450 nm value.

Note: 1 PE IU/lt = 1.3 WHO IU/lt

HAV IgM, Courtesy: Lilac Medicare

Enzyme "Capture" Immunoassay for the Qualitative Determination of IgM Class Antibodies to Hepatitis

A Virus or HAV IgM For *in vitro* Diagnostic Use Only

Introduction

Hepatitis A virus (HAV) is a nonenveloped icosahedral RNA virus with a linear single-strand genome, encoding for only one known serotype. The HAV has four major, structural polypeptides and it localises exclusively in the cytoplasm of human hepatocytes. The route of infection is predominantly oral-foecal with an incubation period of 2-7 weeks during which HAV can be detected in stools. The HAV infection does not originate any chronic hepatitis and complications are uncommon. The infection stimulates a strong immunological response in the patient with elevated titres first of IgM and then of IgG, whose final presence lasts for years after infection. The determination of both IgM and IgG can distinguish the infective nature of the illness the classification of the virus and phase of the infection cycle, as well.

Principle of the Assay

Microplates are coated with a monoclonal anti-IgM antibody that in the first step captures specifically this class of antibodies. After washing out all the other components of the sample, bound anti-HAV specific IgM are detected by the addition of a preformed immunocomplex, made of HAV and an antigen specific IgG antibody, labelled with peroxidase (HRP). The captured enzyme, acting on the substrate/chromogen mixture, generates an optical signal that is proportional to the presence of anti-HAV IgM in the sample.

Content of the Kit and Reagents Preparation

1. **Microtitre strips:** 1 microtitre plate 12 × 8-wells strips 6 × 8-wells strips 3 × 8-wells strips coated with anti-human IgM monoclonal antibody. The plate is contained in a sealed bag with dessicant. Bring the plate to room temperature before use, to prevent any moisture formation inside the bag.
2. **Enzyme Conjugate:** 1 vial of 0.8 ml 1 × 0.4 ml 1 × 0.2 ml 20 × concentrated solution containing an IgG antibody specific to HAV labelled with HRP, in presence of 0.2 mg/ml gentamicin sulphate, 0.1% Kathon GC and 0.01% Cialit as preservatives.
3. **HAV Antigen:** 1 vial of 8 ml, 4 ml, 2 ml. The vial contains a 2x concentrated solution of inactivated HAV dissolved in a proteic buffered solution with 0.2 mg/ml gentamicin sulphate and 0.1% Kathon GC as preservatives.
4. **Antigen/conjugate Diluent:** 1 vial of 8 ml, 4 ml, 2 ml. Proteic buffer solution for the dilution of the concentrated enzyme. It contains proteic stabilisers.0.2 mg/ml gentamicin sulphate and 0.1% Kathon GC as preservatives.
5. **Washing Solution:** 1 vial of 50 ml 25x concentrated solution to be diluted up to 1250 ml with bidistilled water. It contains PBS/Tween. The diluted solution, when stored at room temperature, is stable for at least 1 week.
6. **Chromogen:** 1 vial of 8 ml: 4 ml, 2 ml. The solution contains tetramethyl benzidine (TMB) with activators and stabilisers, diluted in phosphate/citrate buffer.
   Warning: Store protected from light!
7. **Substrate:** 1 vial of 8 ml, 4 ml, 2 ml. The solution contains urea peroxide diluted in phosphate/citrate buffer.
8. **Stop solution:** 1 vial of 12 ml It contains 1 NHCI.
   Warning: Avoid contact with eyes or skin.
9. **Negative control:** 1 vial of 2 ml 1 ml, 0.5 ml. Human serum base not reactive for anti-HAV IgM antibodies, prediluted and ready for use. It contains 0.09% sodium azide and 0.1% Kathon GC as preservatives.
10. **Positive control:** 1 vial of 2 ml 1 ml, 0.5 ml. Human serum base reactive for anti-HAV IgM antibodies, prediluted and ready to use. It contains 0.09% sodium azide and 0.1% Kathon GC as preservatives.
11. **Sample dilute ml:** 2 vials of 50 ml each, 1 × 50 ml, 1 × 25 ml. Protein solution for samples preparation; it contains a detergent, proteic stabilisers, 0.09% sodium azide and 0.1% Kathon GC as preservatives.
12. **Cardboard sealers:** Cardboard sealers to be used to cover the plate during the incubations.

Note: All the materials of human origin have been tested as negative for HBsAg HLV and HCV with FDA approved kits.

Conditions and Notices

1. All the reagents contained in the kit are for *in vitro* diagnostic use only.

2. Do not use the kit or reagents after the expiry date stated on the labels. Do not mix reagents from different lots.
3. Procedures should be performed carefully in order to obtain reliable results and clinical interpretations.
4. Bring all reagents to room temperature at least 60 minutes before the analysis.
5. Avoid contaminating reagents when taking them from the vials. We recommend to use automatic pipettes with disposable tips. When dispensing reagents, do not touch with tips the wall of wells in order to avoid cross contaminations.
6. For the washing step, use only the washing solution provided in the kit and follow carefully the indications reported at point 'washing instruction'. It is recommended anyway to use a good quality microplate washer.
7. Avoid the substrate/chromogen to come in contact with oxidising agents or metallic surfaces, avoid intense light exposure during incubation or reagent preparation. When preparing chromogen/substrate, we recommend the use of plastic disposable sterile containers.
8. Samples and materials potentially infected have to be handled with care as they could transmit the infection. All objects come in direct contact with samples and all residuals of the assay should be treated or eliminated as potentially infected. Best procedures for in activation are treatments with autoclave at 121°C for; 30 minutes or with sodium hypochlorite at a final concentration of 2.5% for 24 hours. This last method can be used for treating the liquid washes that have to be neutralised before with sodium hydroxide.
9. Avoid any contact with skin and mucosas, specially with the blocking reagent.
10. In any case, use protective talk-free gloves.

Storage and Stability of the Kit

1. The HAV IgM kit has to be stored at 2 to 8°C and used before the expiry date stated on the label.
2. Unused strips have to be placed in the bag containing the dessicant and firmly sealed before re-store at 2 to 8°C. After opening, strips are stable until the dessicant turns pink.
3. The diluted washing solution can be stored for one week at room temperature or 3 weeks at + 2 to 8°C.
4. The chromogen/substrate solution is stable for 4 hours at room temperature, protected from light.
5. The diluted immunocomplex is not stable. Dilute only the volume needed for the test.
6. All other liquid reagents are stable when stored at 2 to 8°C, provided that they are handled carefully to avoid any environment contamination.

Materials not Provided in the Kit

1. Semi-automatic pipettes of 10,200 and 1000 µl.
2. Vortex mixer and absorbent paper
3. Ultrapure water (bidistilled)
4. Chronometer
5. Photometric reader of microplates or microstrips, linear up to at least 2 OD and supplied with filters of 450 nm and 620-630 nm.
6. Incubator set at + 37°C.
7. Automatic microplates washing device or manual apparatus capable of aspirating and dispensing volumes of 300 µl.

Samples

Either fresh sera or plasma can be used. If not used immediately, they can be stored at 2 to 8°C for 1 week in case of longer storage, freeze at –20°C. Samples should be without particles or microbial contaminations in case, centrifuge at 2000 g for 20 minutes or filtrate with a 0.2 µl filter. Highly lipaemic or haemolysed samples can give uncorrect analytical results.

Reagents Preparation

1. **Washing solution: Dilute** 1:25 with bidistilled water and mix carefully before use.
2. **Immunocomplex:** It is recommended to prepare a volume of immunocomplex necessary only to run the programmed analysis, as the immunocomplex is not stable upon prolonged storage.
   About 10-20 min before its use, dilute the HAV Antigen with an identical volume of antigen/conjugates diluent. Then use this to dilute 20x the concentrated enzyme. Carefully mix on vortex before use.

3. **Chromogen/substrate:** 5 min before use, prepare in disposable plastic container, according to needs, the substrate/chromogen solution by mixing the chromogen with the substrate in equal volumes.

Washing Instruction

A good washing procedure is essential to obtain correct and precise analytical results. We, therefore, recommend to use a good quality ELISA microplate washer, maintained at a good level of washing mechanical performances. Generally, 4-5 automatic washing cycles of 0.3 ml/well are sufficient to avoid false-positive reactions and remove high background eventually adding a soak time between each washing cycle (see manual washing). Anyhow, we recommend to calibrate the washing system on the kit itself so to match the declared analytical performances

In case, of manual washing, we suggest to carry out 5 cycles, dispensing and aspirating 300 µl/well and leaving a soak time of 30 sec between each cycle.

In any case, the liquid washed out from the plates must be inactivated with a sodium hypochlorite solution at a final concentration of 2.5%, before being thrown away or autoclaved, as it must be considered as potentially infected.

Assay Procedure

1. At least one hour before use, bring all reagents, calibration set and samples to room temperature (18-30°C), mixing them carefully on vortex.
2. Do not mix reagents from different lots.
3. We recommend to distribute the calibration set and the samples in duplicate.
4. Distribution and incubation times must be the same for all wells in the same analysis.
5. Avoid long interruptions between each step of the assay procedure.
6. It is suggested to eliminate the excess of washing solution from the microplate after washing by blotting it gently on an absorbent paper pad.
7. The colour developed in the last incubation is stable for a maximum of one hour in the dark.
8. We recommend to read the plate with an ELISA automatic reader able to substract the background at 620-630 nm and to read the absorbance of samples and standards at 450 nm. The "blanking" of the instrument is to be carried out in the blank reagent well (well A1).

Assay Scheme

1. Dilute the sample 1:20 with the sample diluent (e.g. 5 µl sample + 1000 µl diluent). Controls are ready-to-use. Do not dilute. Mix carefully on vortex before dispensing.
2. Follow this scheme:

Monoclonal antibody coated wells

Reagents	*A1 Blank*	*Controls*	*Sample*
Controls	–	100 µl	–
Sample	–	–	100 µl
Cover strips with adhesive film			
Incubate 60 min at + 37°C			
Peel out the adhesive film and aspirate the reaction solution from all wells.			
Wash 4-5 times with 300 µl of diluted washing solution, carefully aspirating off the remaining liquid.			
Immunocomplex	-	100 µl	100 µl
Cover strips with adhesive fiim			
Incubate 60 min at + 37°C			
Peel out the adhesive film and aspirate the reaction solution from all wells.			
Wash 4-5 times with 300 µl of diluted washing solution, carefully aspirating off the remaining liquid.			
Reagents Chromogen/ Susbstrate Mixed 1:1	100 µl	100 µl	100 µl
Cover strips with a new adhesive film			
Incubate 20 min. at room temperature, protected from light			
Stop solution	100 µl	100 µl	100 µl
Read the absorbance of each well against A1 blanking-well at 450 nm and 620-630 nm			

Validity of the Assay

The assay is to be considered valid if :

1. The OD 450 nm of the blanking well is lower than 0.100. Higher values indicate a chromogen/substrate contamination. In such a case, repeat the assay carefully checking the reagent.
2. After subtracting the blank, the OD 450 nm or the negative control is lower than 0.200. Higher values indicate an uncorrect washing procedure. In such a case, check the efficiency of the washing device.

3. The value of the positive control is higher than 0.500 OD 450 nm. Lower values indicate kit or calibrator decay. In such a case, check expiry date of the kit before repeating the assay.

Calculation of Results

Calculate the mean OD 450 nm values for the negative control (NC) and the positive control (PC); then verify the validity of the assay. The cut-off value of the assay is calculated according to the following formula:

Cut-off = NC + 0.15

Calculate the mean OD 450 nm value of the samples. Samples with an OD 450 nm value lower than the cut-off are considered not reactive for anti-HAV IgM antibody. Samples with an OD 450 nm value higher than the cut-off are considered positive for anti-HAV IgM antibody.

Example of Calculation

Negative control mean OD 450 nm (NC) 0.080
Positive control mean OD 450 nm (PC) 1.120
Cut-off = NC + 0.250
Sample #1 OD 450 nm = 0.095 negative
Sample #2 OD 450 nm = 0.565 positive

Assay Performance

Sensibility: The sensitivity of the assay has been calculated on a panel of seroconversion and of positive samples by comparing with an FDA-approved kit present in the market.

The test shows a sensitivity > 98%.

Specificity: It has been calculated on panels of negative and positive samples, preclassified with an FDA-approved kit present on the market. The assay shows a specificity > 98% on plasma and sera.

Reproducibility: It has been calculated on the negative and positive controls tested in replicates in different days. CVs between 4-12% have been obtained depending on their OD 450 nm value.

HBc Ab, Courtesy: Lilac Medicare

One-step "competitive" Enzyme Immunoassay for the Determination of antibodies to Hepatitis B core Antigen or HBcAb.

—For *"in vitro"* diagnostic use only

Introduction

Hepatitis B core Antigen (or HBcAg) is the major component of the core particles of hepatitis B virus (or HBV). Particles have a size of 27 nm and contain a circular double-stranded DNA molecule, a specific DNA-polymerase and HbeAg; HBcAg is composed of a single polypeptide of about 17 kD that is released upon disaggregation of the core particles; the antigen contains at least one immunological determinant.

Upon primary infection, anti-HBcAg antibodies are one of the first markers of HBV hepatitis appearing in the serum of the patient, together or slightly later than HBsAg, the viral surface antigen.

Anti-HBcAg antibodies are produced usually at high titres and their presence is detectable even years after infection. Isolated HBcAb, in absence of other HBV markers, have been observed in blood units, suggesting the use of this test for screening HBV, in addition of HBsAg.

The determination of HBcAb has become important for the classification of the viral agent, together with the detection of the other markers of HBV infection, in sera and plasma.

Principle of the Assay

Anti-HbcAg IgG and IgM antibodies, if present in the sample, compete with a virus-specific monoclonal IgG, labelled with peroxidase (HRP), for a fixed amount of recombinant HBcAg, in a one-step incubation.

The concentration of the bound enzyme on the solid phase becomes inversely proportional to the amount of anti-HBcAg antibodies in the sample and its activity is detected by adding the chromogen/ substrate.

The concentration of HBcAg specific antibodies in the sample is determined by means of a cut-off value that allows for the semiquantitative detection of anti-HBcAg antibodies.

Test Conditions and Notices

1. All the reagents contained in the kit are for *"in vitro"* diagnostic use only.
2. Do not use the kit or reagents after the expiry date stated on labels. Do not mix reagents of different lots.
3. Procedures should be performed carefully in order to obtain reliable results and clinical interpretations.

4. Bring all the reagents to room temperature for at least 60 min, before the test is started.
5. Avoid any contamination of reagents when taking them out of vials. We recommend to use automatic pipettes and disposable tips. When dispensing reagents, do not touch the wall of microplate wells with tips, in order to avoid any cross-contamination.
6. In the washing procedure, use only the washing solution provided with the kit and follow carefully the indications reported in the "Washing instruction" section.
7. Ensure that the substrate/chromogen mixture does not come in contact with oxidising agents or metallic surfaces; avoid any intense light exposure during the incubation step or the reagent preparation. When preparing the substrate/chromogen mixture for the analysis, use only plastic, disposable, clean or sterile containers.
8. Samples and materials potentially infective have to be handled with care as they could transmit infection.
   All objects come in direct contact with samples and all residuals of the assay should be treated or wasted as potentially infective. Best procedures for inactivation are treatments with autoclave at 121°C for 30 min or with sodium hypochlorite at a final concentration of 2.5% for 24 hr. This last method can be used for the treatment of the liquid waste after that it has been neutralised with NaOH.
9. Avoid any contact of liquids with skin and mucosas.
   Use always protective talk-free gloves, glasses and laboratory coats, according to the safety regulations.

Content of the Kit

a. **Strips Microplate:** 12 × 8 and 6 × 8 wells strips coated with purified recombinant HBcAg. The plate is contained in a sealed bag with dessicant. Bring the plate to room temperature before use, to prevent any moisture formation inside the bag.
b. **Enzyme conjugate: 1 vial of 0.8 ml of 0.4 ml** Proteic buffer solution containing anti-HBcAg monoclonal IgG, labelled with HRP, 20 x concentrated. It contains proteic stabilizers, 0.2 mg/ml gentamicin sulphate and 0.1% Kathon GC as preservatives.
c. **Conjugate Diluent: 1 vial of 16 ml, of B ml** Proteic buffer solution for the dilution of the concentrated conjugate. It contains proteic stabilisers, 0.2 mg/ml gentamicine sulphate and 0.1% Kathon GC as preservatives.
d. **Washing solution: 1 vial of 50 ml** 25x concentrated solution to be diluted up to 1250 ml with EIA grade water, it contains a phosphate buffer, Tween 20 and Kathon GC as preservative. The diluted solution, when stored at room temperature, is stable for at least 1 week.
e. **Chromogen: 1 vial of 8 ml, of 4 ml** The solution contains tetramethylbenzidine (TMB) with activators and stabilizers, diluted in a phosphate/citrate buffer. Warning: Store protected from light.
f. **Substrate: 1 vial of 8 ml, of 4 ml** The solution contains stabilised hydrogen peroxide diluted in a phosphate/citrate buffer.
g. **Stop solution: 1 vial of 12 ml** It contains a solution of 1 N HCI. Warning avoid contact with eyes and skin.
h. **Negative control: 1 vial of 1 ml, of 0.5 ml** Human serum base not reactive for HBcAb. It contains 0.2 mg/ml gentamicine sulphate and 0.1% Kathon GC as preservatives.
i. **Cut-off Control: 1 vial of 1 ml, of 0.5 ml** Human serum base reactive for HBcAb at a concentration of 1 PEI U/ml. It contains 0.2 mg/ml gentamicine sulphate and 0.1% Kathon GC as preservatives.
j. **Positive control: 1 vial of 1 ml, of 0.5 ml** Human serum base strongly reactive for HBcAb. It contains 0.2 mg/ml gentamicine sulphate and 0.1% Kathon GC as preservatives.
m. **Cardboard Sealers: 2** Plastic transparent sealers to cover plates when incubating at + 37°C.

Note: All the materials of human origin have been tested and found negative for HBsAg, HCV Ab and HIV Ab with FDA-approved kits.

Storage and Stability

1. The kit has to be stored at 2 to 8°C and used before the expiration date declared on the external label.
2. Unused strips have to be returned into their bag containing the dessicant and firmly sealed with tape before storing them back at 2 to 8°C

After the bag has been opened the first time, strips are stable till the dessicant turns pink.

3. The diluted washing solution is stable at room temperature for 1 week or for 3 weeks at 2 to 8°C.
4. The chromogen/substrate mixture is stable for 4 hr at rt when stored protected from light.
5. The diluted conjugate is stable for 1 week at 2 to 8°C, when stored in a sterile disposable container.
6. All the other liquid reagents are stable at 2 to 8°C when handled carefully to avoid contaminations.

Materials not Provided

1. Micropipettes of 50,100 and 1000 µl
2. Vortex mixer and adsorbent papers
3. ELISA grade water for dilutions
4. Timer
5. Photometric ELISA reader linear up to at least 2 OD and supplied with filters of 450 nm and 620-630 nm
6. Incubator set at + 37°C
7. Automatic microplate washer or manual apparatus capable to deliver 300 µl and aspirate.

Samples

Either fresh sera or plasma can be used for the assay.

If not used immediately, they can be stored at 2 to 8°C for 1 week. In case of longer storage freeze them at –30°C.

Samples should be clear and not contaminated by microrganisms.

If necessary, remove contaminating particles by centrifugation at 2000 g × 20 min at rt or by filtration on 0.22 µl filters.

Highly lipaemic, icteric or haemolised samples should not be used as they can give false results in the assay.

Preparation of Reagents

a. **Washing Solution:** The concentrated solution has to be diluted 25x in ELISA grade water before use.
b. **Conjugate:** Dilute the concentrated conjugate 20x with the conjugate diluent and mix gently on vortex. Prepare only the volume necessary to the test.
c. **Chromogen/substrate:** About 5 minutes before use, prepare this reagent in a disposable plastic container by mixing 1 volume of chromogen with 1 volume of substrate. Prepare only the volume necessary to the test.

Washing Instructions

A good washing procedure is essential to obtain correct and precise analytical data.

We, therefore, recommend to use a good quality ELISA microplate washer, maintained at the best level of washing performances. Generally, 4-5 automatic washing cycles of 300/well are sufficient to avoid false-positive reactions and high background.

Anyhow, we recommend to calibrate the washing system on the kit itself so to match the declared analytical performances eventually adding a soak time between each washing cycle (see manual washing). In case of manual washing, we suggest to perform 5 washing cycles, dispensing and aspirating 0.3 ml/well per cycle and leaving a soak time of 30 sec between each cycle. In any case, the liquid aspirated out the strips must be treated with a sodium hypochloride solution at a final concentration of 2.5% for 24 hr, before liquids are wasted in an appropriate way.

Assay Procedure

Important Notes

- At least 1 hr before use, bring all the components of the kit to rt and mix the liquid reagents carefully on vortex.
- Do not mix reagents of different lots.
- We recommend to distribute the controls in duplicate. Distribution and incubation times should be the same for all the wells. Avoid long interruptions among the different steps of the assay.
- It is suggested to eliminate the excess of washing solution from wells by blotting them gently on a paper adsorbent pad.
- The colour developed in the last incubation is stable for maximum 1 hr in the dark. We recommend to read the microplate at 450 nm (reading filter) and subtract the blank at 620-630 nm (blanking filter). Use well A1 to carry out blanking operations.

1. Dispense controls and samples according to the following scheme

Position	Calibrator/sample
A1	Blanking well
B1 + C1	50 µl of negative control
D1 + E1	50 µl of cut-off control
F1	50 µl of positive control
G1...H12	50 µl of samples

Then add 50 µl of diluted conjugate in all the wells, except A1 used for blanking. Incubate the microplate sealed for 120 min at + 37°C.

2. Peel out the plate sealer and wash the microplate according to instructions.
3. Add 100 µl of the chromogen/substrate mixture, prepared as described, to all the wells, A1 included. Incubate the microplate for 20 min at rt, protected from light.
4. Stop the enzymatic reaction by adding 100 µl stop solution to all the wells, A1 included. Read the microplate at 450 nm and 620-630 nm blanking the instrument on A1 well.

Validity of the Assay

The assay is considered valid if:

1. The OD 450 nm of the A1 blank well is < 0.100.
2. After blanking on A1 the OD 450 nm mean value of the negative control or NC is > 1.000.
3. After blanking, the OD 450 nm mean value of the positive control or PC is < 0.200.
4. After blanking, the OD 450 nm mean value of the cut-off control is lower than 1/3rd the OD 450 nm value of the negative control.

In case data above do not match the correct values, before repeating the test check carefully the expiration date of the kit, the performances of the instruments used for the assay and the procedure of distribution of controls and samples.

Calculation of Results

If the test turns out to be valid, calculate the cut-off value through the following formula mean OD 450 nm cut-off control = cut-off

Samples with an OD 450 nm value equal or higher than the cut-off are classified as negative for HBcAb.

Samples with an OD 450 nm value lower than the cut-off are classified as positive for HBcAb (content of antibodies higher than 1 PEI U/ml).

Example of Calculation

Negative control mean OD 450 nm	1.800
Positive control mean OD 450 nm	0.050
Cut-off control mean OD 450 nm	0.400
Cut-off =	0.400
Sample # 1 OD 450 nm =	1.680 negative
Sample #2 OD 450 nm =	0.158 positive

Assay Performances

1. **Sensibility:** The sensitivity of the assay has been calculated by means of the international standard for HBcAb supplied by Paul Erlich Institute. The test shows a sensitivity at the cut-off of about 1 PEI U/ml.
2. **Specificity:** It has been calculated on panels of negative and positive samples, preclassified with an FDA-approved kit present on the market. The assay shows a specificity >99% on plasma and sera.
3. **Reproducibility:** It has been calculated on the negative and positive controls tested in replicates in different days. CVs between 6-15% have been obtained depending on their OD 450 nm value.

HBc IgM, Courtesy: Lilac Medicare

Enzyme Immunoassay for the Determination of IgM Class Antibodies to Hepatitis B "core" Antigen —For *in vitro* diagnostic use only

Introduction

Hepatitis B core antigen (HBcAg) is the major component of the core particles of hepatitis B virus (HBV), particles of 27 nm that contain a circular double-stranded DNA molecule, a specific DNA-polymerase activity and HBeAg. The HBcAg is composed of a single structural polypeptide of about 17000 daltons, that is released upon disaggregation of the core particles and that contains at least one immunological determinant. Upon primary infection, anti-HBcAg IgM are one of the first markers of HBV hepatitis appearing in the serum of the patient, together with HBsAg, the viral surface antigen. Anti-HBcAg IgM titres, very high during the acute phase, decrease along the illness as IgG appears, down to undetectable levels in convalescent sera. In chronic hepatitis, however, spikes of anti-HBcAg IgM synthesis are present, confirming reactivation of HBV in hepatocytes and giving origin to permanent IgM low titres. The determination of HBc IgM has become very important for the fast classification of the virus, of the phase of the illness and for the monitoring of patients under treatment with interferon.

Principle of the Assay

Microplates are coated with a monoclonal anti-IgM antibody that in the first step captures specifically this class of antibodies. After washing out all the other components of the sample, bound anti-HBcAg specific IgM are detected by the addition of a preformed immunocomplex, made of a recombinant HBcAg and a specific monoclonal antibody, labelled with peroxidase (HRP). The captured enzyme, acting on the substrate/chromogen mixture, generates an optical signal that is proportional to the presence of anti-HBcAg IgM in the sample. The HBc IgM may be determined quantitatively by means of a standard curve, calibrated against the PEI, reference preparation.

Content of the Kit and Reagents Preparation

1. **Microtitre strips:** 1 microtitre plate 12 × 8 wells strips coated with anti-human IgM monoclonal antibody. The plate is contained in a sealed bag with dessicant. Bring the plate to room temperature before use, to prevent any moisture formation inside the bag.
2. **Enzyme conjugate:** 1 vial of 1.1 ml 20x concentration buffered solution of an anti-HBcAg monoclonal antibody labelled with HRP. It contains proteic stabilisers with 0.2 mg/ml gentamicin sulphate and 0.3% Kathon GC as preservatives.
3. **Conjugate diluent:** 1 vial of 22 ml. Proteic buffer solution for the dilution of the concentrated conjugate. It contains 0.2 mg/ml gentamicin sulphate and 0.3% Kathon GC.
4. **Antigen: 1 vial of 1.1 ml:** 20x concentrated buffered solution of Sec-HBcAg. It contains proteic stabilisers with 0.2 mg/ml gentamicin sulphate and 0.3% Kathon GC as preservatives.
5. **Washing solution:** 1 vial of 50 ml 25 x concentrated solution to be diluted up to 1250 ml with bidistilled water. lt contains a Imidazole buffer, Tween 20 and Kathon GC as preservative. The diluted solution, when stored at room temperature, is stable for at least one week.
6. **Chromogen:** 1 vial of 8 ml. The solution contains tetramethylbenzidine (TMB) with activators and stabilizers, diluted in phosphate/citrate buffer.
   Warning: Store protected from light.
7. **Substrate:** 1 vial of 8 ml. The solution contains urea peroxide diluted in phosphate/citrate buffer.
8. **Stop solution:** 1 vial of 12 ml. It contains 1 N HCI.
   Warning: Avoid contact with eyes and skin.
9. **Negative control:** 1 vial of 2 ml. Human serum base not reactive for HBc IgM; it contains 0.09% Na-azide and 0.1% Kathon GC as preservatives. The control is prediluted and ready to use.
10. **Positive control:** 1 vial of 2 ml. Human serum base positive for HBcIgM; it contains 0.09% Na-azide and 0.1% Kathon GC as preservatives. The control is prediluted and ready to use.
    Warning: Handle as potentially infective.
11. **Sample diluent:** 2 vials of 50 ml each. Proteic solution for samples preparation; it contains a detergent, proteic stabilisers, 0.09% sodium azide and 0.1% Kathon GC as preservatives.
12. **Cardboard sealers:** 2 cardboard sealers to be used to cover the plate during the incubations.
13. **Calibration curve:** 6 vials of 2.0 ml each. The calibration set contains the following ready-to-use standards 0-5-10-20-50-100 PEI lU/ml. Standards are calibrated in units and prediluted in the sample diluent. Vials contain sodium azide and Kathon GC as preservatives. Do not dilute again.
    Warming: Handle as potentially infective.

Conditions and Notices

1. All the reagents contained in the kit are for *in vitro* diagnostic use only.
2. Do not use the kit or reagents after the expiry date stated on the labels. Do not mix reagents from different lots.
3. Procedures should be performed carefully in order to obtain reliable results and clinical interpretations.
4. Bring all reagents to room temperature at least 60 minutes before the analysis.

5. Avoid contaminating reagents when taking them from the vials. We recommend to use automatic pipettes with disposable tips. When dispensing reagents, do not touch with tips the wall of wells in order to avoid cross contaminations.
6. For the washing step, use only the washing solution provided in the kit and follow carefully the indications reported at point "washing instruction." It is recommended- anyway to use a good quality microplate washer.
7. Avoid the substrate/chromogen to come in contact with oxidising agents or metallic surfaces, avoid intense light exposure during incubation or reagent preparation. When preparing chromogen/substrate, we recommend the use of plastic disposable sterile containers.
8. Samples and materials potentially infected have to be handled with care as they could transmit the infection. All objects come in direct contact with samples and all residuals of the assay should be treated or eliminated as potentially infected. Best procedures for inactivation are treatments with autoclave at 121°C for 30 minutes or with sodium hypochlorite at a final concentration of 2.5% for 24 hours. This last method can be used for treating the liquid washes that have to be neutralised before with sodium hydroxide.
9. Avoid any contact with skin and mucosas, specially with the blocking reagent.
10. In any case, use protective talk-free gloves.

Storage and Stability of the Kit

1. The kit has to be stored at 2 to 8°C and used before the expiry date stated on the label.
2. Unused strips have to be placed in the bag containing the dessicant and firmly sealed before re-store at 2 to 8°C.
3. The diluted washing solution can be stored for one week at room temperature or 3 weeks at + 2 to 8°C.
4. The chromogen/substrate solution is stable for 4 hours at room temperature, protected from light.
5. The diluted enzyme is not stable. Dilute only the volume needed for the test.
6. All other liquid reagents are stable when stored at 2 to 8°C, provided that they are handled carefully to avoid any environment contamination.

Materials not Provided in the Kit

1. Semiautomatic pipettes of 10, 200 and 1000 µl.
2. Vortex mixer and absorbent paper.
3. Ultrapure water (bidistilled).
4. Chronometer.
5. Photometric reader of microplates or microstrips, linear up to at least 2 OD and supplied with filters of 450 nm and 620-630 nm.
6. Incubator set at + 37°C.
7. Automatic microplates washing device or manual apparatus capable of aspirating and dispensing volumes of 300 µl.

Samples

Either fresh sera or plasma can be used. If not used immediately, they can be stored at 2 to 8°C for 1 week in case of longer storage, freeze at –20°C. Samples should be without particles or microbial contaminations in case, centrifuge at 2000 g for 20 minutes or nitrate with a 0.22 µ filter. Highly lipaemic or haemolised samples can give uncorrect analytical results.

Reagents Preparation

1. **Washing solution:** Dilute 1: 25 with bidistilled water and mix carefully before use.
2. **Immunocomplex:** Dilute 1:20 concentrated conjugate with its diluent. 10-15 min before use add 1/20 volume of concentrated antigen into it. Mix carefully the solution on vortex.
3. **Chromogen/substrate:** About 5 minutes before use, prepare in disposable plastic container, according to needs, the substrate/chromogen solution by mixing the chromogen with the substrate in equal volumes.

Washing Instruction

A good washing procedure is essential to obtain correct and precise analytical results. We, therefore, recommend to use a good quality ELISA microplate washer, maintained at a good level of washing mechanical performances. Generally, 4-5 automatic washing cycles of 0.3 ml/well are sufficient to avoid false-positive reactions and remove high background.

Anyhow, we recommend to calibrate the washing system on the kit itself so to match the declared analytical performances, if necessary adding a soak time of 30 sec (see manual washing). In case of manual washing, we suggest to perform 5 washing cycles, dispensing and aspirating 0.3 ml/well per cycle and leaving a soak time of 30 sec between each cycle. In any case, the liquid washed out from the plates must be inactivated with a sodium hypochlorite solution at a final concentration of 2.5%, before being thrown away or autoclaved, as it must be considered as potentially infected.

Assay Procedure

1. At least one hour before use, bring all reagents, calibration set and samples to room temperature (18-30°C), mixing them carefully on vortex.
2. Do not mix reagents from different lots.
3. We recommend to distribute the calibration set and the samples in duplicate.
4. Distribution and incubation times must be the same for all wells in the same analysis.
5. Avoid long interruptions between each step of the assay procedure.
6. It is suggested to eliminate the excess of washing solution from the microplate after washing by blotting it gently on an absorbent paper pad.
7. The colour developed in the last incubation is stable for a maximum of one hour in the dark.
8. We recommend to read the plate with an ELISA automatic reader able to subtract the background at 620-630 nm and to read the absorbance of samples and standards at 450 nm. The "blanking" of the instrument is to be carried out in the blank reagent well (well A1).

Assay Scheme

1. Dilute the sample 1:201 with the sample diluent (e.g. 5 µl sample + 1000 µl diluent). Controls are ready-to-use. Do not dilute. Mix carefully on vortex before dispensing. Dispense the controls or the standard curve in proper wells in duplicate.
2. Follow this scheme monoclonal antibody coated wells

Reagents	*A1 Blank*	*Calibrators*	*Sample*
Calibrators	-	**100 ul**	-
Sample	-	-	**100ul**
Cover strips with adhesive film and Incubate 60 min. at + 37°C.			
Peel out the adhesive film and aspirate the reaction solution from all wells.			
Wash 4-5 times with 300ul of diluted washing solution, carefully aspirating off the remaining liquid			
Immunocomplex	-	**100ul**	**100ul**
Cover strips with adhesive film			
Incubate 60 min. at + 37°C			
Peel out the adhesive film and aspirate the reaction solution from all wells			
Wash 4-5 times with 300ul of diluted washing solution, carefully aspirating off -the remaining liquid			
Reagents Chromogen/ Substrate Mixed 1:1	100ul	100ul	100ul
Cover strips with a new adhesive film			
Incubate 20 min at room temperature, protected from light			
Stop solution	**100 µl**	**100 µl**	**100 µl**
Read the absorbance of each well against A1 blanking-well at 450 nm and 620-630 nm			

Validity of the Assay

The assay is to be considered valid if:

1. The OD 450 nm of the blanking well is lower than 0.100. Higher values indicate a chromogen/substrate contamination. In such a case, repeat the assay carefully checking the reagent.
2. After subtracting the blank, the OD 450 nm of the negative control or the 0 PEI IU/ml is lower than 0.200. Higher values indicate an uncorrect washing procedure. In such a case, check the efficiency of the washing device.
3. The OD 450 nm of the 5 PEI IU/ml standard is higher than the OD 450 nm of the 0 PEI IU/ml standard + 0.100.
4. The value of the positive control or the 100 PEI IU/ml standard is higher than 1.200 OD 450 nm. Lower values indicate kit or calibrator decay. In such a case, check expiry date of the kit before repeating the assay.

Calculation of Results

Check for the validity of the assay and then calculate the cut-off value with the following formulation

Negative control mean OD 450 nm + 0.200 = cut-off

Samples with an OD 450 nm value lower than the cut-off are considered negative for HbcIgM.

Samples with an OD 450 nm value higher than the cut-off are considered positive.

We recommend to elaborate the standard curve with the 4 parameters (lin-lin) curve fitting system and calculate the concentration of anti-HbcAg IgM antibodies in the sample. Values are expressed in units per ml (PEI IU/ml). Samples with an OD 450 nm lower than the 5 PEI IU/ml standard value have to be considered not reactive to HBc IgM. Samples with HBc IgM concentrations between 5 and 10 PEI IU/ml have to be considered in the grey-zone.

In the follow-up of chronic hepatitis, however, values higher than 5 PEI IU/ml are considered positive for HbcIgM. Values between 10 and 100 PEI IU/ml are to be considered by literature as representative of chronic hepatitis when anti-HbcAg IgG antibodies are present, or representative of primary acute hepatitis in resolution phase if IgG antibodies are missing or are present at low titre.

Values with a concentration higher than 100 PEI IU/ml are considered by literature as representative of acute hepatitis.

Assay Performances

1. **Sensibility:** The sensitivity of the assay has been calculated on a panel of seroconversion and of positive samples by comparing with a FDA-approved kit present in the market. The test shows a sensitivity better than 5 PEI IU/ ml.
2. **Specificity:** It has been calculated on panels of negative samples, preclassified with an FDA-approved kit present on the market. The assay shows a specificity > 98% on plasma and sera.
3. **Reproducibility:** It has been calculated on the negative and positive controls tested in replicates in different days. CVs between 4-12% have been obtained depending on their OD 450 nm value.

Example of Calculation

Negative control mean OD 450 nm	0.050
Positive control mean OD 450 nm	1.200
Cut-off = NC + 0.200 =	0.250
Sample # 1 OD 450 nm =	0.080 negative
Sample #2 OD 450 nm =	1.200 positive

Example of standard curve

0	IU/ml	0.050	OD 450 nm
5	IU/ml	0.250	OD 450 nm
10	IU/ml	0.900	OD 450 nm
20	IU/ml	1.600	OD 450 nm
50	IU/ml	2.000	OD 450 nm
100	IU/ml	2.500	OD 450 nm

HBeAb, Courtesy: Lilac Medicare

Competitive Enzyme Immunoassay for the Determination of Hepatitis B "envelope" Antibodies or HbeAb —For *in vitro* diagnostic use only

Introduction

Hepatitis B "e" antigen (HBeAg) is known to be intimately associated with hepatitis B virus (HBV) replication and the presence of infective Dane particles in the blood.

Recently, it has been found that the "e" antigen is a product of proteolytic degradation of hepatitis B core antigen (HBcAg) occurring in hepatocytes, whose expression is under the control of the precore region of HBV genome.

If HBeAg is considered a specific marker of infectivity, the presence of anti-HBeAg antibody in blood is recognized to be a clinical sign of recovery from infection to convalescence. The determination of these two analytes in samples from HBV patients has become important for the classification of the phase of the illness and as a prognostic value in the follow-up of infected patients.

Principle of the Assay

Anti-HBeAg antibodies, if present in the sample, compete with a recombinant HBeAg preparation for a fixed amount of an anti-HBeAg antibody, coated on the microplate wells.

The competitive assay is carried out in two incubations, the first with the sample and recHBeAg, and the second with a enzyme conjugate, composed of two anti-HBeAg monoclonal antibodies, labeled with peroxidase (HRP).

The concentration of the bound enzyme on the solid phase becomes inversely proportional to the amount of anti-HBeAg antibodies in the sample and its activity is detected by adding the chromogen/ substrate in the third incubation.

The concentration of HBeAg specific antibodies in the sample is determined by means of a cut-off value that allows for the semiquantitative detection of anti-HBeAg antibodies.

Content of the Kit and Reagents Preparation

1. **Microtitre strips:** 1 microtitre plate. 12 × 8-wells-strips, 6 × 8 wells, 3 × 8 wells coated with purified anti-HBeAg antibody. The plate is contained in a sealed bag with dessicant. Bring the plate to room temperature before using it, so to prevent any moisture formation inside the bag.
2. **Enzyme conjugate:** 1 vial of 1.75 ml 1 × 0.8 ml 1 × 0.4 ml. Solution containing specific monoclonal antibody conjugated with HRP, 20x concentrated. It contains proteic stabilizers, 0.2 mg/ml gentamicin sulphate and 0.1% Kathon GC as preservatives.
3. **Conjugate diluent:** 1 vial of 35 ml 1× 16 ml 1 × 8 ml. Proteic buffer solution for the dilution of the concentrated tracer. It contains proteic stabilisers ,0.2 mg/ml gentamicin sulphate and 0.1% Kathon GC as preservatives.
4. **Washing solution:** 1 vial of 50 ml 25 x concentrated solution to be diluted up to 1250 ml with bidistilled water. Contains PBS/Tween.
5. **Chromogen:** 1 vial of 16 ml × 8 ml 1 × 4 ml. The solution contains tetramethyl benzidine (TMB) with activators and stabilisers, diluted in phosphate/citrate buffer Warning Store protected from light.
6. **Substrate:** 1 vial of 16 ml 1 × 8 ml × 4 ml. The ready-to-use solution contains urea peroxide diluted in phosphate/citrate buffer.
7. **Stop solution:** 1 vial of 12 ml. It contains 1N HCL. Warning avoid contact with eyes and skin.
8. **Neutraliser:** 1 vial of 1.1 ml 1 × 0.5 ml 1 × 0.25 ml. 20 x concentrated proteic solution containing non infective recombinant HBeAg; it contains 0.09% sodium azide and 0.1% Katnon as preservatives.
9. **Neutraliser diluent:** 1 vial of 22 ml 1 × 10 ml 1 × 5 ml. Solution for the dilution of the neutraliser; it contains 0.09% sodium azide and 0.1% Kathon GC as preservatives.
10. **Negative control:** 1 vial of 2 ml 1 × 1 ml 1 × 0.5 ml. Serum base non-reactive to HBeAb and containing 0.09% sodium azide as preservative.
11. **Positive control:**1 vial of 2 ml 1 × 1 ml 1 × 0.5 ml. Serum base active to HBeAb, with 0.09% sodium azide as preservative.
12. **Cardboard sealers:** cardboard sealers to be used for protecting the plate during the incubations.

Conditions and Notices

1. All the reagents contained in the kit are for *in vitro* diagnostic use only.
2. Do not use the kit or reagents after the expiry date stated on the labels. Do not mix reagents from different lots.
3. Procedure should be performed carefully in order to obtain reliable results and interpretations.
4. Bring all reagents to room temperature at least 60 minutes before the analysis.
5. Avoid contaminating reagents when taking them from the vials. We recommend to use automatic pipettes with disposable tips when dispensing reagents. Do not touch with tips the wall of wells in order to avoid cross-contaminations.
6. For the washing step, use only the washing solution provided in the kit and follow carefully the indications reported at point "washing instruction". It is recommended anyway to use a good quality microplate washer.
7. Avoid the substrate/chromogen to come in contact with oxidising agents or metallic surfaces; avoid intense light exposure during incubation or reagent preparation. When preparing chromogen/substrate, we recommend the use of plastic disposable sterile containers.
8. Samples and materials potentially infected have to be handled with care as they could transmit the infection. All objects come in direct contact with samples and all residuals of the assay should be treated or eliminated as potentially infected. Best procedures for inactivation are treatments in autoclave at 121°C for 30 minutes or with sodium

hypochlorite at a final concentration of 2.5% for 24 hours. This last method can be used for treating the liquid washes that have to be neutralised before with sodium hydroxide.

9. Avoid, contact with skin and mucosas, specially with the blocking reagent.
10. In any case, use protective talc-free gloves.

Storage and Stability of the Kit

1. The HBeAb kit must be stored at 2 to 8°C and used before the expiry date stated on the label.
2. Unused strips have to be placed in the bag containing dessicant and firmly sealed before re-store at 2 to 8°C. After opening, strips are stable until the dessicant turns pink.
3. The diluted washing solution can be stored for one week at room temperature or for 3 weeks at + 2 to 8°C.
4. The chromogen/substrate solution is stable for 4 hours at room temperature, protected from light.
5. The diluted conjugate is stable for 1 week at 2 to 8°C when stored in a sterile disposable container.
6. All the other liquid reagents are stable when stored at 2 to 8°C provided that they are handled carefully to avoid any environment contamination.

Materials not Provided in the Kit

1. Semiautomatic pipettes of 100, 200 and 1000 µl.
2. Vortex mixer and absorbent paper
3. Bidistilled water.
4. Chronometer.
5. Photometric reader of microplates or microstrips, linear up to at least 2 OD and provided with filters of 450 nm and 620-630 nm.
6. Incubator set +37°C.
7. Microplates automatic washing device or manual apparatus capable of aspirating and dispensing volumes of 300 µl.

Samples

Either fresh sera or plasma can be used. If not used immediately, they can be stored at 2 to 8°C for 1 week in case of longer storage, freeze at –20°C. Samples should be without microbial contaminations. In case, centrifuge at 2000 g for 20 minutes or filtrate with a 0.2 µ filter. Highly lipaemic or haemolysed samples can give uncorrect analytical results. Samples containing high titres of rheumatoid factor and anti-mouse heterophylous antibodies could give false-positive results.

Reagents Preparation

1. **Washing solution:** Dilute 1:25 with bidistilled water and mix carefully before use.
2. **Conjugate:** Dilute the conjugate 1:20 with corresponding diluent. Mix carefully on vortex. The diluted conjugate is not stable; prepare only the quantity necessary to the assay.
3. **Neutraliser:** Dilute 1:20 with the corresponding diluent. Mix carefully on vortex. The diluted neutraliser is not stable prepare only the quantity necessary to the assay.
4. **Chromogen/substrate:** Prepare in disposable plastic container according to needs, the substrate/chromogen solution by mixing the chromogen with the sustrate in equal volumes.

Washing Instruction

A good washing procedure is essential to obtain correct and precise analytical results. We, therefore, recommend to use a good quality ELISA microplate washer, maintained at a good level of washing mechanical performance. Generally, 4-5 automatic washing cycles of 0.3 ml/each well are sufficient to avoid false-positive reactions and remove high background. Anyhow, we recommend to calibrate the washing system on the kit itself so to match the declared analytical performances. In case of manual washing, we suggest to perform 5 washing cycles, dispensing and aspirating 0.3 ml/well per cycle. In any case, the liquid from the plates must be inactivated with a sodium hypochlorite solution at a final concentration of 2.5%, before being thrown away or autoclaved, as it must be considered as potentially infective.

Assay Procedure

1. At least one hour before use, bring all reagents, controls and samples to room temperature (18-30°C), mixing them carefully on vortex.
2. Do not mix reagents from different lots.

3. For the test, we recommend to distribute the controls in duplicate.
4. Distribution and incubation times must be the same for all wells in the same analysis.
5. Avoid long interruptions between each step of the assay procedure.
6. It is suggested to eliminate the excess of washing solution from the microplate after washing by blotting it gently on an absorbent paper pad.
7. The colour developed in the last incubation is stable for a maximum of one hour in the dark.
8. We recommend to read the plate with an ELISA automatic reader able to subtract the background at 620-630 nm and to read the absorbance of samples and controls at 450 nm. The "blanking" of the instrument is to be carried out in the blank reagent well (well A1).

Assay Scheme

Follow this scheme:

Reagents	*A1 Blank*	*Negative Control*	*Positive Control*	*Sample*
Negative control	-	100 µl	-	-
Positive control	-	-	100 µl	-
Sample	-	-	-	100 µl
Diluted Neutrallzer	-	100 µl	100 µl	100 µl
Cover strips with adhesive film				
Incubate 120 mm. at + 37°C, Peel out the adhesive film and aspirate the reaction solution from all wells. Wash 4-5 times with 300 of diluted washing solution, carefully aspirating off the remaining liquid				
Diluted conjugate	200µl	200µl	200µl	200µl
Cover strips with adhesive film ***Incubate 60 mm at + 37°C*** Peel out the adhesive film and aspirate the reaction solution from all wells, Wash 4-5 times with 300ul of diluted washing solution, carefully aspirating off the remaining liquid				
Reagent Chromogen/ substrate mixed 1:1	200 µl	200 µl	200 µl	200 µl
Cover strips with a new adhesive film				
Incubate 20 min. at room temperature, protected from light.				
Stop solution	100 µl	100 µl	100 µl	100 µl
Read the absorbance of each well against At blanking-well at 450 nm and 620-630 nm.				

Validity of the Assay

The assay is to be considered valid if:

1. The OD 450 nm of the blanking well is lower than 0.100. Higher values indicate a chromogen/substrate contamination. In such a case, repeat the assay carefully checking the reagent.
2. After subtracting the blank, the mean OD value for the negative control is higher than 1.000. Lower values indicate an uncorrect washing procedure. In such a case, check the efficiency of the washing device.
3. The OD 450 nm ratio between of the negative control and the positive control is higher than 2.
4. The OD 450 nm of the positive control is lower than CO.

Calculation of Results

If the test turns out to be valid, calculate the cut-off value through the following formula:
mean OD 450 nm positive control = cut-off

Samples with an OD 450 nm value equal or higher than the cutoff are classified as negative for HBeAb. Samples with an OD 450 nm value lower than the cut-off are classified as positive for HBeAb (content of antibodies higher than 0.3 PEI U/ml).

Characteristics of the Assay

Sensitivity: The sensitivity of the assay has been calculated by means of the international standard for HbeAb supplied by Paul Erlich Institute. The test shows a sensitivity at the cut-off of about 0.3 PEI U/ml.

Specificity: It has been calculated on panels of negative and positive samples preclassified with an FDA-approved kit present on the market. The assay shows a specificity > 99% on plasma and sera.

Reproducibility: It has been calculated on the Negative and positive controls tested in replicates in different days. CVs between 4-15% have been obtained depending on their OD 450 nm value.

Example of Calculation

Mean OD 450 nm negative control	1.800
Mean OD 450 nm positive control	0.050
Cut-off =	0.450
Sample 1 OD 450 nm 1.897	negative
Sample 2 OD 450 nm 0.090	positive

HBeAG, Courtesy: Lilac Medicare

Enzyme immunoassay for the Determination of Hepatitis B "e" Antigen or HbeAg
— For *in vitro* diagnostic use only

Introduction

Hepatitis B "e" antigen (HBeAg) is known to be intimately associated with hepatitis B virus (HBV) replication and the presence of infective Dane particles in the blood. Recently, it has been found that the "e" antigen is a product of proteolytic degradation of hepatitis B core antigen (HBcAg) occurring in hepatocytes, whose expression is under the control of the precore region of HBV genome. If HBeAg is considered a specific marker of infectivity, the presence of anti-HBeAg antibody in blood is recognised to be a clinical sign of recovery from the infection. The determination of these two analytes in samples from HBV patients has become important for the classification of the phase of the illness and as a prognostic value in the follow-up of the infection cycle.

Principle of the Assay

Microplates are coated with a monoclonal antibody specific for HBeAg. In the antigen test (HBeAg), the "e" antigen if present in the sample binds to the solid phase and it is detected in a second incubation by another specific monoclonal antibody, labelled with peroxidase (HRP). The bound enzyme generates a signal that is proportional to the amount of antigen in the sample. Results are calculated by means of a cut-off that allows for the discrimination between negative and positive individuals.

Content of the Kit and Reagents Preparation

1. **Microtitre strips:** 1 microtitre plate 12 × 8-wells-strips/6 × 8 wells strips/3 × 8 wells strips coated with specific anti-HBeAg monoclonal antibody. The plate is contained in a sealed bag with dessicant. Bring the plate to room temperature before using it, so to prevent any moisture formation inside the bag.
2. **Enzyme Conjugate:** 1 vial of 1.1 ml 1 × 0.5 ml 1 × 5 ml Proteic buffer solution containing specific monoclonal antibody conjugated with HRP, 20x concentrate. It contains proteic stabilisers and 0.2 mg/ml gentamicin sulphate as preservative.
3. **Conjugate dilutent:** 1 vial of 22 ml /1 × 10 ml /1 × 5 ml. Proteic buffer solution for the dilution of the concentrated tracer. It contains proteic stabilisers and 0.2 mg/ml gentamicin sulphate as preservatives.
4. **Washing solution:** 1 vial of 50 ml 25x concentrated solution to be diluted up to 1250 ml with bidistilled water. Contains PBS/Tween.
5. **Chromogen:** 1 vial of 8 ml/1 × 4 ml /1×2 ml. The solution contains tetramethyibenzidine (TMB) with activators and stabilisers, diluted in phosphate/citrate buffer.
   Warning: Store protected from light.
6. **Substrate:** 1 vial of 8 ml/1 × 4 ml/1 × 2 ml. The solution contains urea peroxide diluted in phosphate/citrate buffer.
7. **Stop solution:**1 vial of 12 ml. It contains 1N HCI.
   Warning: Avoid contact with eyes and skin.
8. **Negative control:** 1 vial of 2 ml 1 × 1 ml /1 × 0.5 ml. Serum base, non-reactive to HBeAg and containing 0.09% sodium azide as preservative.
9. **Positive control:** 1 vial of 2 ml /1 × 1 ml /1 × 0.5 ml. Serum base reactive to recombinant and not infective HBeAg, with 0.09 % sodium azide as preservative.
10. **Cardboard sealers:** Cardboard sealers to be used for protecting the plate during the incubations.

Conditions and Notices

1. All the reagents contained in the kit are for *in vitro* diagnostic use only.
2. Do not use the kit or reagents after the expiry date stated on the labels. Do not mix reagents from different lots.
3. Procedure should be performed carefully in order to obtain reliable results and interpretations.
4. Bring at reagents to room temperature at least 60 minutes before the analysis.
5. Avoid contaminating reagents when taking them from the vials. We recommend to use automatic pipettes with disposable tips. When dispensing reagents, do not touch with tips the wall of wells, in order to avoid cross contaminations.
6. For the washing step, use only the washing solution provided in the kit and follow carefully the indications reported at point "washing instruction". It is recommended anyway to use a good quality microplate washer.

7. Avoid the substrate/chromogen to come in contact with oxidising agents or metallic surfaces. Avoid intense light exposure during incubation or reagent preparation. When preparing chromogen/substrate, we recommend the use of plastic disposable sterile containers.
8. Samples and materials potentially infected have to be handled with care as they could transmit the infection. All objects come in direct contact with samples and all residuals of the assay should be treated or eliminated as potentially infected. Best procedures for inactivation are treatments in autoclave at 121°C for 30 minutes or with sodium hypochlorite at a final concentration of 2.5% for 24 hours. This last method can be used for treating the liquid washes that have to be neutralised before with sodium hydroxide.
9. Avoid contact with skin and mucosas, especially with the blocking reagent.
10. In any case, use protective talc-free gloves.

Storage and Stability of the Kit

1. The HBeAg kit must be stored at 2 to 8°C and used before the expiry date stated on the label.
2. Unused strips have to be placed in the bag containing dessicant and firmly sealed before re-store at 2 to 8°C. After opening, strips are stable until the dessicant turns pink.
3. The diluted washing solution can be stored for one week at room temperature or 3 weeks at + 2 to 8°C.
4. The chromogen/substrate solution is stable for 4 hours at room temperature, protected from light.
5. The diluted conjugate is not stable. We recommend to dilute only the quantity necessary to the test.
6. All other liquid reagents are stable when stored at 2 to 8°C, provided that they are handled carefully to avoid any environment contamination.

Materials not Provided in the Kit

1. Semiautomatic pipettes of 100, 200 and 1000 µl
2. Vortex mixer and absorbent paper
3. Bidistilled water
4. Chronometer
5. Photometric reader of microplates or microstrips, linear up to at least 2 OD and provided with filters of 450 nm and 620-630 nm.
6. Incubator set +37°C.
7. Microplates automatic washing device or manual apparatus capable of aspirating and dispensing volumes of 300 µl.

Samples

Either fresh sera or plasma can be used. If not used immediately, they can be stored at 2 to 8°C for 1 week in case of longer storage, freeze at –20°C. Samples should be without microbial contaminations, in case, centrifuge at 2000 g for 20 minutes or filtrate with a 0.2 µ filter. Highly lipaemic or haemolysed samples can give uncorrect analytical results. Samples containing high titres of rheumatoid factor and anti-mouse heterophylous antibodies could give false-positive results.

Reagents Preparation

1. **Washing solution:** Dilute 1: 25 with bidistilied water and mix carefully before use.
2. **Conjugate:** Dilute the conjugate 1 20 with corresponding diluent; mix carefully on vortex.
3. **Chromogen/substrate:** Prepare in disposable plastic container, according to needs, the substrate/chromogen solution by mixing the chromogen with the substrate in equal volumes.

Washing Instruction

A good washing procedure is essential to obtain correct and precise analytical results. We, therefore, recommend to use a good quality ELISA microplate washer maintained at a good level of washing mechanical performance. Generally, 4-5 automatic washing cycles of 0.3 ml/each well are sufficient to avoid false-positive reactions and remove high background. Anyhow, we recommend to calibrate the washing system on the kit itself so to match the declared analytical performances. In case of manual washing, we suggest to perform 5 washing cycles, dispensing and aspirating 0.3 ml/well per cycle and leaving a soak time of 30 sec between each cycle. In any case, the liquid from the plates must be inactivated with a sodium hypochlorite solution at a final concentration of 2.5%, before being thrown away or autoclaved, as it must be considered as potentially infected.

Assay Procedure

1. At least one hour before use, bring all reagents, controls and samples to room temperature (18-30°C). Mixing them carefully on vortex.
2. Do not mix reagents from different lots.
3. For the test, we recommend to distribute the negative control in triplicate, the positive control in single, and samples possibly in duplicate.
4. Distribution and incubation times must be the same for all wells in the same analysis.
5. Avoid long interruptions between each step of the assay procedure.
6. It is suggested to eliminate the excess of washing solution from the microplate after washing by blotting it gently on an absorbent paper pad.
7. The colour developed in the last incubation is stable for a maximum of one hour in the dark.
8. We recommend to read the plate with an ELISA automatic reader able to subtract the background at 620-630 nm and to read the absorbance of samples and controls at 450 nm. The blanking of the instrument is to be carried out in the blank reagent well (well A1).

Assay Scheme

Follow this scheme: Monoclonal antibody coated wells

Reagents	*At Blank*	*Negative control*	*Positive control*	*Sample*
Negative	-	100 µl	-	-
Control positive control	-	-	100 µl	-
Sample	-	-	-	100µl
Cover strips with adhesive film				
Incubate 120 min at + 37°C				
Peel out the adhesive film and aspirate the reaction solution from all wells.				
Wash 4-5 times with 300 µl of diluted washing solution, carefully aspirating off the remaining liquid.				
Diluted conjugate	-	100 µl	100 µl	100 µl
Cover strips with adhesive film				
Incubate 60 min. at + 37°C.				
Contd...				
Wash 4-5 times with 300 µl of diluted washing solution, carefully aspirating off the remaining liquid.				
Chromogen/ substrate Mixed 1:1	100 µl	100 µl	100 µl	100 µl
Incubate 20 min at RT protected from light.				
Stop solution	100 µl	100 µl	100 µl	100 µl
Read the absorbance of each well against A1 blanking-well at 450 nm and 620-630 nm.				

Validity of the Assay

The assay is to be considered valid if:

1. The OD 450 nm of the blanking well is lower than 0.100. Higher values indicate a chromogen/substrate contamination. In such a case, repeat the assay carefully checking the reagent.
2. After subtracting the blank, the mean OD value for the negative control is lower than 0.100. Higher values indicate an uncorrect washing procedure. !n such a case, check the efficiency of the washing device.
3. The OD 450 nm of the positive control is higher than 1000OD 450 nm. Lower values indicate kit or control decay. In such a case, check the expiry date of the kit before repeating the assay.

Calculation of Results

Calculate the mean value of the OD 450 nm negative control (NC), check it is included in the range values of the validity of the assay and calculate the cut-off value through the following formula:

NC + 0.100 = cut off

Samples with 3 mean OD 450 nm lower than cut-off are considered negative.

Samples with a mean OD 450 nm higher than cut-off are considered positive.

Example of Calculation

Negative Control Mean OD 450 nm	0.030
Positive Control OD 450 nm	2.100
Cut-off =	0.130
Sample 1 OD 450 nm 0.045	negative
Sample 2 OD 450 nm 0.876	positive

Characteristics of the Assay

1. **Sensitivity:** The sensitivity of the assay has been calculated by means of the international standard for HBeAg supplied by Paul Erlich Institute.
   The test shows a sensitivity at the cut-off of about 0.5 PEI U/ml.
2. **Specificity:** It has been calculated on panels of negative and positive samples, pre-classified with an FDA-approved kit present on the market. The assay shows a specificity > 99% on plasma and sera.
3. **Reproducibility:** It has been calculated on the negative and positive controls tested in replicates in different days. CVs between 4-15% have been obtained depending on their OD 450 nm value.

HBe Ag/Ab, Courtesy: Lilac Medicare

Enzyme Immunoassay for the Determination of Hepatitis B "e" Antigen and antibody or HBeAg/Ab
— For *"in vitro"* diagnostic use only

Introduction

Hepatitis B "e" Antigen or HBeAg is known to be intimately associated with hepatitis B virus or HBV replication and the presence of infective Dane particles in the blood.

Recently, it has been found that HBeAg is a product of proteolytic degradation of hepatitis B core antigen or HBcAg, occurring in hepatocytes, whose expression is under the control of the precore region of HBV genome.

If HBeAg is considered a specific marker of infectivity, the presence of anti-HBeAg antibodies in blood is recognised to be a clinical sign of recovery from infection to convalescence.

The determination of these too analytes in samples from HBV patients has become important for the classification of the phase of illness and as a prognostic value in the follow-up of infected patients.

Principle of the Assay HBeAg

The solid phase is coated with a specific anti-HBeAg monoclonal antibody that in the 1st incubation captures the antigen if present in the sample.

After washing, a second monoclonal antibody, labelled with peroxidase (HRP) binds the antigen captured on the solid phase by means of a second binding site.

In the 3rd incubation, the enzyme bound generates a colour by acting on the substrate/chromogen mixture that can be detected by a photometer. The intensity of the colour is proportional to the concentration of the antigen in the sample.

HBeAb

Anti-HBeAg antibodies, if present in the sample, compete with a recombinant HBeAg preparation for a fixed amount of an anti-HBeAg antibody, coated on the microplate wells.

The competitive assay is carried out in two incubations, the first with the sample and recHBeAg, and the second with a tracer, composed of two anti-HBeAg monoclonal antibodies, labelled with peroxidase (HRP).

The concentration of the bound enzyme on the solid phase becomes inversely proportional to the amount of anti-HBeAg antibodies in the sample and its activity is detected by adding the chromogen/substrate in the third incubation.

The concentration of HBeAg specific antibodies in the sample is determined by means of a cut-off value that allows for the semiquantitative detection of anti-HBeAg antibodies.

Test Conditions and Notices

1. All the reagents contained in the kit are for *"in vitro"* diagnostic use only.
2. Do not use the kit or reagents after the expiry date stated on labels. Do not mix reagents of different lots.
3. Procedures should be performed carefully in order to obtain reliable results and clinical interpretations.
4. Bring all the reagents to room temperature for at least 60 min, before the test is started.
5. Avoid any contamination of reagents when taking them out of vials. We recommend to use automatic pipettes and disposable tips. When dispensing reagents, do not touch the wall of microplate wells with tips, in order to avoid any cross contamination.
6. In the washing procedure, use only the washing solution provided with the kit and follow carefully the indications reported in the washing instructions section of this insert.

7. Ensure that the substrate/chromogen mixture does not come in contact with oxidising agents or metallic surfaces; avoid any intense light exposure during the incubation step or the reagent preparation.
   When preparing the substrate/chromogen mixture for the analysis, use only plastic, disposable, clean or sterile containers.
8. Samples and materials potentially infective have to be handled with care as they could transmit infection.
   All objects come in direct contact with samples and all residuals of the assay should be treated or wasted as potentially infective. Best procedures for inactivation are treatments with autoclave at 121°C for 30 min or with sodium hypochlorite at a final concentration of 2.5% for 24 hr. This last method can be used for the treatment of the liquid waste after that it has been neutralised with NaOH.
9. Avoid any contact of liquids with skin and mucosas.
   Use always protective talk-free gloves, glasses and laboratory coats, according to the safety regulations.

Content of the Kit

a. **Strips microplate:** 12 × 8 wells strips coated with purified anti-HBeAg antibody. The plate is contained in a sealed bag with dessicant. Bring the plate to room temperature before use, to prevent any moisture formation inside the bag.
b. **Enzyme conjugate:** 1 vial of 1.5 ml proteic buffer solution containing anti HBeAg monoclonal antibodies, labelled with HRP, 20x concentrated. It contains proteic stabilisers, 0.2 mg/ml gentamicin sulphate and 0.1% Kathon GC as preservatives.
c. **Conjugate diluent:** 1 vials of 30 ml proteic buffer solution for the dilution of the concentrated tracer. It contains proteic stabilisers, 0.2 mg/ml gentamicin sulphate and 0.1% Kathon GC as preservatives.
d. **Washing solution:** 1 vial of 50 ml 25x concentrated solution to be diluted up to 1250 ml with EIA grade water. It contains a phosphate buffer, Tween 20 and Kathon GC as preservatives.
   The diluted solution, when stored at room temperature, is stable for at least 1 week.
e. **Chromogen:** 1 vial of 12 ml the solution contains telramethylbenzidine (TMB) with activators and stabilisers, diluted in a phosphate/citrate buffer.
   Warning: Store protected from light.
f. **Substrate:** 1 vial of 12 ml the solution contains stabilised hydrogen peroxide diluted in a phosphate/citrate buffer.
g. **Stop solution:** 1 vial of 12 ml it contains 1NHCI
   Warning: Handle with care.
h. **Negative control:** 1 vial of 2.5 ml human serum base not reactive for HBeAb. It contains 0.2 mg/ml gentamicin sulphate and 0.1% Kathon GC as preservatives.
i. **HBeAb positive control:** 1 vial of 1.5 ml human serum base reactive for HBeAb at about 0.3 PEI U/ml it contains 0.2 mg/ml gentamicin sulphate and 0.3% Kathon GC as preservatives.
l. **HBeAg positive control:** 1 vial of 1.5 ml human serum base reactive for rec-HBeAg. It contains 0.2 mg/ml gentamicin sulphate and 0.1% Kathon GC as preservatives.
m. **Neutraliser:** 1 vial of 0.9 ml 20 x concentrated proteic solution containing noninfective rec-HBeAg. It contains 0.09% sodium azide and 0.1% Kathon GC as preservatives.
n. **Neutraliser diluent:** 1 vial of 18 ml proleic buffered solution containing 0.09% sodium azide and 0.1% Kathon GC as preservatives; used to dilute the neutralises
o. **Cardboard sealers:** 2 plastic transparent sealers to cover plates when incubating at + 37°C.

Note: All the materials of human origin have been tested and found negative for HBsAg, HCV Ab and HIV Ab with FDA-approved kits.

Storage and Stability

1. The kit has to stored at 2 to 8°C and used before the expiration date declared on the external label.
2. Unused strips have to be returned into their bag containing the dessicant and firmly sealed with tape before store them back at 2 to 8°C. After the bag has been opened the first time, strips are stable till the dessicant turns pink.

3. The diluted washing solution is stable at room temperature for 1 week or for 3 weeks at 2 to 8°C.
4. The chromogen/substrate mixture is stable for 4 hr at rt when stored protected from light.
5. The diluted conjugate is stable for 1 week at 2 to 8°C, when stored in a sterile disposable container.
6. All the other liquid reagents are stable at 2 to 8°C when handled carefully to avoid contaminations.

Materials not Provided

1. Micropipettes of 10, 100 and 1000 µl
2. Vortex mixer and adsorbent papers
3. ELISA grade water for dilutions
4. Timer
5. Photometric ELISA reader linear up to at least 2 OD and supplied with filters of 450 nm and 620-630 nm
6. Incubator set at +37°C
7. Automatic microplate washer or manual apparatus capable to deliver 300 µl and aspirate.

Samples

Either fresh sera or plasma can be used for the assay. If not used immediately, they can be stored at 2 to 8°C for 1 week. In case of longer storage freeze them at –30°C. Samples should be dear and not contaminated by micro-organisms.

If necessary, remove contaminating particles by centrifugation at 2000 g x 20 min at rt or by filtration on 0.22 µ filters. Highly lipaemic, icteric or haemolysed samples should not be used as they can give false results in the assay.

Preparation of Reagents

a. **Washing solution:** The concentrated solution has to be diluted 25 x in ELISA grade water before use.
b. **Conjugate:** Dilute the concentrated conjugate 20x with the conjugate diluent and mix gently on vortex. Prepare only the volume necessary to the test.
c. **Chromogen/substrate:** About 5 minutes before use, prepare this reagent in a disposable plastic container by mixing 1 volume of chromogen with 1 volume of substrate. Prepare only the volume necessary to the test.
d. **Neutralisers** Before use, prepare this reagent in a disposable plastic container by diluting the concentrate 20x in its diluent. Prepare only the volume necessary to the test.

Washing Instructions

A good washing procedure is essential to obtain correct and precise analytical data. We, therefore, recommend to use a good quality ELISA microplate washer, maintained at the best level of washing performances.

Generally, 4-5 automatic washing cycles of 300 µl/well are sufficient to avoid false-positive reactions and high background. Anyhow, we recommend to calibrate the washing system on the kit itself so to match the declared analytical performances. In case of manual washing, we suggest to carry out 5 cycles, dispensing 300 µl/well and aspirating the liquid for 5 times. In any case, the liquid aspirated out the strips must be treated with a sodium hypochlorite solution at a final concentration of 2.5% for 24 hr, before liquids are wasted in an appropriate way.

Assay Procedure

Important notes

At least 1 hr before use, bring all the components of the kit to rt and mix the liquid reagents carefully on vortex.

Do not mix reagents of different lots.

We recommend to distribute the controls in duplicate. Distribution and incubation times should be the same for all the wells. Avoid long interruptions among the different steps of the assay.

It is suggested to eliminate the excess of washing solution from wells by blotting them gently on a paper adsorbent pad.

The colour developed in the last incubation is stable for maximum 1 hr in the dark. We recommend to read the microplate at 450 nm (reading filter) and subtract the blank at 620-630 nm (blanking filter). Use well A1 to carry out blanking operations.

HBeAg Test

1. Leave the A1 well empty for blanking operations. Dispense controls and samples in the proper wells necessary for the assay, according to the following scheme:

Position	Calibrator/sample
A1	blanking well
B1+C1	200 µl of HBeAg negative control
D1+E1	200 µl of HBeAg positive control
F1... H12	200 µl of samples

Incubate the microplate sealed for 120 min at + 37°C.

2. Peel out the plate sealer and wash the microplate according to instructions. In the meantime dilute the concentrated conjugate.
3. Add 200 µl of diluted conjugate in all the wells, but A1. Cover the microplate with the plate sealer and incubate strips for 60 min at + 37°C.
4 Peel out the plate sealer and wash the microplate according to instructions. In the meantime, prepare the chromogen/substrate mixture.
5 Add 200 µl of the chromogen/substrate mixture to all the wells, A1 included, incubate the microplate for 20 min at rt, protected from light.
6 Stop the enzymatic reaction by adding 100 µl stop solution to all the wells, A1 included. Read the microplate at 450 nm and 620-630 nm blanking the instrument on A1 well.

HBeAb Test

1. Leave the A1 well empty for blanking operations. Dispense controls and samples in the proper wells necessary for the assay, according to the following scheme:

Position	Calibrator/sample
A1	blanking well
B1+C1	100 µl of HBeAb negative control
D1+E1	100 µl of HBeAb positive control
F1...H12	100 µl of samples

Then add 100 µl of diluted neutralizers in all control and sample wells. Incubate the microplate sealed for 120 min at + 37°C.

2. Peel out the plate sealer, wash the microplate according to instructions and then proceed as described for the antigen test.

Validity of the Assay

The assay is considered valid if:

HBeAg Test

1. The OD 450 nm of the A1 blank well is < 0.100.
2. After blanking on A1, the OD 450 nm mean value of the negative control or NC is < 0.200.
3. The OD 450 nm of the positive control (PC) is > 1.000.

HBeAb Test

1. The OD 450 nm of the A1 blank well is < 0.100.
2. After blanking on A1, the OD 450 nm mean value of the negative control or NC is > 1.000.
3. The OD 450 nm ratio between the negative control (NC) and the positive one (PC) is higher than 2; that is as OD 450 nm NC/OD 450 nm > 2.

In case data above do not match the correct values, before repeating the test check carefully the expiration date of the kit, the performances of the instruments used for the assay and the procedure of distribution of controls and samples.

Calculation of Results

If the test turns out to be valid, calculate the cut-off value through the following formula:

HBeAg Test

NC + 0.100 = cut-off

Samples with an OD 450 nm value lower than the cut-off are classified as negative for HBeAg.

Samples with an OD 450 nm value higher than the cut-off are classified as positive for HBeAg.

Example of calculation

Negative control mean OD 450 nm	0.050
Positive control mean OD 450 nm	1.800
Cut-off = NC + 0.100 =	0.150
Sample # 1 OD 450 nm =	0.060 negative
Sample # 2 OD 450 nm =	1.325 positive

HBeAb Test

PC = cut-off

Samples with an OD 450 nm value higher than the cut-off are classified as negative for HBeAb.

Samples with an OD 450 nm value lower than the cut-off are classified as positive for HbeAb (content of antibodies higher than 0.3 PEI U/ml).

Example of calculation

Negative control mean OD 450 nm	1.800
Positive control mean OD 450 nm	0.400
Cut-off =	0.400
Sample # 1 OD 450 nm =	1.680 negative
Sample # 2 OD 450 nm =	0.158 positive

Assay Performances

HBeAg Test

1. **Sensitivity:** The sensitivity of the assay has been calculated by means of the international standard for HBeAg supplied by Paul Erlich Institute.
   The test shows a sensitivity at the cut-off of about 0.5 4PEI U/ml.
2. **Specificity:** It has been calculated on panels of negative and positive samples, preclassified with an FDA-approved kit present on the market. The assay shows a specificity > 98% on plasma and sera.
3. **Reproducibility:** It has been calculated on the negative and positive controls tested in replicates in different days. CVs between 6-15% have been obtained depending on their OD 450 nm value.

HBeAb Test

1. **Sensitivity:** The sensitivity of the assay has been calculated by means of the international standard for HBeAb supplied by Paul Erlich Institute.
   The test shows a sensitivity at the cut-off of about 0.3 PEI U/ml.
2. **Specificity:** It has been calculated on panels of negative and positive samples, preclassified with an FDA-approved kit present on the market. The assay shows a specificity > 98% on plasma and sera.
3. **Reproducibility:** It has been calculated on the negative and positive controls tested in replicates in different days. CVs between 6-15% have been obtained depending on their OD 450 nm value.

HBs Ab, Courtesy: Lilac Medicare

Enzyme Immunoassay for the Quantitative Determination of Antibodies to Hepatitis B Virus or HBs Ab
—For *"in vitro"* diagnostic use only

Introduction

Hepatitis B surface antigen (HBsAg) is the major structural polypeptide of the envelope of the hepatitis B virus (HBV). This antigen is composed mainly of the type common determinant "a" and the type specific determinants "d" and "y", present only on the specific serotypes.

Upon infection, a strong immunological response develops firstly against the type-specific determinants and in a second time against the "a" determinant.

Anti "a" antibodies are, however, recognised to be most effective in the neutralisation of the virus, protecting the patient from other infections and leading it to convalescence.

The detection of HBsAb has become important for the follow up of patients infected by HBV and the monitoring of recipients upon vaccination with synthetic and natural HBsAg.

Principle of the Assay

Microplates are coated with a preparation of highly purified HBsAg that in the first incubation with sample specifically captures anti-HBsAg antibodies to the solid phase.

After washing, captured antibodies are detected by an HBsAg, labelled with peroxidase (HRP), that specifically binds the second available binding site of these antibodies.

The enzyme specifically bound to wells, by acting on the substrate/chromogen mixture, generates an optical signal that is proportional to the amount of HBsAb in the sample and can be detected by an ELISA reader.

The amount of antibodies may be quantitated by means of a standard curve calibrated against the WHO reference preparation.

Samples are pretreated in the well with an additive able to block interferences present in vaccinated individuals.

Test Conditions and Notices

1. All the reagents contained in the kit are for *"in vitro"* diagnostic use only.
2. Do not use the kit or reagents after the expiry date stated on labels. Do not mix reagents of different lots.
3. Procedures should be performed carefully in order to obtain reliable results and clinical interpretations.
4. Firing all the reagents to room temperature for at least 60 min, before the test is started.
5. Avoid any contamination of reagents when taking them out of vials. We recommend to use automatic pipettes and disposable tips.

When dispensing reagents, do not touch the wall of microplate wells with tips, in order to avoid any cross contamination.

6. In the washing procedure, use only the washing solution provided with the kit and follow carefully the indications reported in the "washing instructions " section of this insert.
7. Ensure that the substrate/chromogen mixture does not come in contact with oxidising agents or metallic surfaces; avoid any intense light exposure during the incubation step or the reagent preparation.
   When preparing the substrate/chromogen mixture for the analysis, use only plastic, disposable, clean or sterile containers.
8. Samples and materials potentially infective have to be handled with care as they could transmit infection.
   All objects come in direct contact with samples and all residuals of the assay should be treated or wasted as potentially infective. Best procedures for inactivation are treatments with autoclave at 121°C for 30 min or with sodium hypochlorite at a final concentration of 2.5% for 24 hr. This last method can be used for the treatment of the liquid waste after that it has been neutralised with NaOH.
9. Avoid any contact of liquids with skin and mucosas. Use always protective talk-free gloves, glasses and laboratory coats, according to the safety regulations.

Content of the Kit

Strips microplate: 1 :12 × 8 wells strips coated with purified not infective HBsAg. The plate is contained in a sealed bag with dessicant. Bring the plate to room temperature before use, to prevent any moisture formation inside the bag.

Enzyme conjugate: 1 vial of 0.8 ml proteic buffer solution containing not infective purified HBsAg, labelled with HRP, 20 x concentrated. It contains proteic stabilisers, 0.2 mg/ml gentamicin sulphate and 0.3% Kathon GC as preservatives.

Conjugate diluent: 1 vial of 16 ml proteic buffer solution for the dilution of the concentrated conjugate. It contains proteic stabilisers, 0.2 mg/ml gentamicin sulphate and 0.3% Kathon GC as preservatives.

Washing solution: 1 vial of 50 ml 25 x concentrated solution to be diluted up to 1250 ml with EIA grade water. It contains a phosphate buffer. Tween 20 and Kathon GC as preservative. The diluted solution, when stored at room temperature, is stable for at least 1 week.

Chromogen: 1 vial of 8 ml the solution contains tetramethylbenzidine (TMB) with activators and stabilisers, diluted in a phosphate/citrate-buffer.

Warning: Store protected from light.

Substrate: 1 vial of 8 ml the solution contains stabilised hydrogen peroxide diluted in a phosphate/citrate buffer.

Stop solution: 1 vial of 12 ml it contains 1N HCl.

Warning: Avoid contact with eyes and skin.

Additive: 1 vial of 10 ml buffer solution for the pretreatment of controls and samples right in the well, blocking interferences present in vaccinated individuals.

Calibration curve: 5 vials of 2 ml each the set contains the following standards: 0-10-50-100-250 WHO mIU/ml

Cardboard sealers: 2 plastic transparent sealers to cover plates when incubating at +37°C.

Note: All the materials of human origin have been tested and found negative for HBsAg. HCV Ab and HIV Ab with FDA-approved kits.

Storage and Stability

1. The kit has to be stored at 2 to 8°C and tried before the expiration date declared on the external label.
2. Unused strips have to be returned into their bag containing the dessicant and firmly sealed with tape before store them back at 2 to 8°C. After the bag has been opened the first time, strips are stable till the dessicant turns pink.
3. The diluted washing solution is stable at room temperature for 1 week or for 3 weeks at 2 to 8°C.
4. The chromogen/substrate mixture is stable for 4 hr at rt. when stored protected from light.
5. The diluted conjugate is stable for 1 week at 2 to 8°C, when stored in a sterile disposable container.

6. All the other liquid reagents are stable at 2 to 8°C when handled carefully to avoid contaminations.

Materials not Provided

1. Micropipettes of 50, 100 and 1000 µl.
2. Vortex mixer and adsorbent papers.
3. ELISA grade water for dilutions.
4. Timer.
5. Photometric ELISA reader linear up to at least 2 OD and supplied with filters of 450 nm and 620-630 nm.
6. Incubator set at +37°C
7. Automatic microplate washer or manual apparatus capable to deliver 300 µl and aspirate.

Samples

Either fresh sera or plasma can be used for the assay.

If not used immediately, they can be stored at 2 to 8°C for 1 week. In case of longer storage freeze them at –30°C. Samples should be clear and not contaminated by micro-organisms.

If necessary, remove contaminating particles by centrifugation at 2000 g × 20 min at rt or by filtration on 0.22 µ filters.

Highly lipaemic, icteric or haemolysed samples should not be used as they can give false results in the assay.

Preparation of Reagents

a. **Washing solution:** The concentrated solution has to be diluted 25x in ELISA grade water before use.

b. **Conjugate:** Dilute the concentrated conjugate 20 x with the conjugate diluent and mix gently on vortex. Prepare only the volume necessary to the test.

c. **Chromogen/Substrate:** About 5 minutes before use, prepare this reagent in a disposable plastic container by mixing 1 volume of chromogen with 1 volume of substrate. Prepare only the volume necessary to the test.

Washing Instructions

A good washing procedure is essential to obtain correct and precise analytical results. We, therefore, recommend to use a good quality ELISA microplate washer maintained at a good level of washing mechanical performance. Generally, 4-5 automatic washing cycles of 0.3 ml/each well are sufficient to avoid false-positive reactions and remove high background. Anyhow, we recommend to calibrate the washing system on the kit itself so to match the declared analytical performances eventually adding a soak time between each washing cycle (see manual washing). In case of manual washing, we suggest to perform 5 washing cycles, dispensing and aspirating 0.3 ml/well per cycle and leaving a soak time of 30 sec. between each cycle. In any case the liquid: from the plates must be inactivated with a sodium hypochlorite solution at a final concentration of 25%, before being thrown away or autoclaved, as it must be considered as potentially infected.

Assay Procedure

Important Notes

At least 1 hr before use, bring all the components of the kit to rt and mix the liquid reagents carefully on vortex. Do not mix reagents of different lots. We recommend to distribute calibrators in duplicate.

Distribution and incubation times should be the same for all the wells. Avoid long interruptions among the different steps of the assay.

It is suggested to eliminate the excess of washing solution from wells by blotting them gently on a paper adsorbent pad.

The colour developed in the last incubation is stable for maximum 1 hr in the dark. We recommend to read the microplate at 450 nm (reading filter) and subtract the blank at 620-630 nm (blanking filter). Use well A1 to carry out blanking operations.

1. Add 50 µl of additive in all the wells, except A1 (blanking well). Then distribute calibrators and samples according to the following scheme:

Quantitative Assay:

Position	*Calibrator/sample*
A1+B1	Blanking wells
C1+D1	100 µl of standard 0 mIU/ml
E1+F1	100 µl of standard 10 mIU/ml
G1+H1	100 µl of standard 50 mIU/ml
A2+B2	100 µl of standard 100 mIU/ml
C2+D2	100 µl of standard 250 mIU/ml
E2...H12	100 µl of samples

Qualitative Assay

Position	*Calibrator/sample*
Al	Blanking wells
B1+C1	100 µl of standard 0 mIU/ml
D1+E1	100 µl of'standard 10 mIU/ml
F1	100 µl of standard 250 mIU/ml
G1...H12	100 µl of samples

Then incubate the microplate for 120 min at + 37°C sealed with the plastic cardboard.

2 Peel out the plate sealer and wash the microplate according to instructions. In the meantime, prepare the diluted conjugate as reported.

3 Add 100 µl of the diluted conjugate to all the wells, except A1 + B1 used for blanking. Incubate the microplate for 60 min at +37°C.

4 Peel out the plate sealer and wash the microplate according to instructions. In the meantime, prepare the chromogen/substrate solution as reported.

5 Add 100 µl of the mixed chromogen/substrate reagent to all the wells, A1-B1 included. Incubate the microplate for 20 min at rt.

6 Stop the enzymatic reaction by adding 100 µl stop solution to all the wells, Al-Bl included. Then read the microplate at 450 nm and 620-630 nm blanking the instrument on A1+B1 wells.

Validity of the Assay

The assay is considered valid if:

1. The OD 450 nm of the Al blank well is < 0.100.
2. After blanking on Al, the OD 450 nm mean value of the 0 WHO mIU/ml standard is < 0.200.
3. After blanking on Al, the OD 450 nm mean value of the 10 WHO mIU/ml standard is higher than the mean OD 450 nm of the 0 WHO mIU/ml standard.
4. The OD 450 nm mean value of the 250 WHO mIU/ml standard is > 1.000.

In case data above do not match the correct values, before repeating the test check carefully the expiration date of the kit. The performances of the instruments used for the assay and the procedure of distribution of controls and samples.

Calculation of Results

If the test turns out to be valid, operate as follows.

Quantitative Assay

Elaborate the standard curve mean OD values with the best fitting system available (suggested: 4-parameter). Then calculate the mIU/ml content of samples on the standard curve.

Example of Standard Curve

0	mIU/ml	0.050	OD 450 nm
10	mIU/ml	0.200	OD 450 nm
50	mIU/ml	0.800	OD 450 nm
100	mIU/ml	1.500	OD 450 nm
250	mIU/ml	3.000	OD 450 nm

Qualitative Assay

Use the following formulation to calculate the cut-off:

Cut-off = mean OD 450 nm Std 10 mIU/ml

Samples with an OD 450 nm value lower than the cut-off are considered negative for HBsAb. Samples with an OD 450 nm higher than the cut-off are considered positive for HBsAb.

Example of calculation:

Std 10 mIU/ml OD 450 nm =	0.200
Cut-off =	0.280
Sample # 1 OD 450 nm =	0.070 negative
Sample # 2 OD 450 nm =	0.800 positive

Note: Do not. use these values for the calculation of data. These figures are provided only as an example.

Assay Performances

1. **Sensitivity:** The sensitivity of the assay has been calculated by means of the international standard for HBsAb supplied by WHO. The test shows an analytical sensitivity better than 5 WHO mIU/ml. The international literature has positioned the cut-off for protection in vaccination at minimum 20 WHO mIU/ml
2. **Specificity:** It has been calculated on panels of negative and positive samples, preclassified with an FDA-approved kit present on the market. The assay shows a specificity > 99 % on plasma and sera.
3. **Reproducibility:** It has been calculated on negative and positive controls tested in replicates in different days. CVs between 4-12 % have been obtained depending on their OD 450 nm value.

HBsAG ONE STEP
Courtesy: Lilac Medicare

The 3rd generation ELISA kit for the "one-step" determination of Hepatitis B Surface Antigen or HBsAg in human serum and plasma.

Introduction

Hepatitis B surface antigen (HBsAg) is the most important protein of the envelope component of hepatitis B virus (HBV), responsible for acute and chronic forms of viral hepatitis. The surface antigen contains the determinant "a", common to all the known viral subtypes, immunologically distinguished in three distinct subgroups (a, y and d). This common determinant is further composed of two immunological distinct epitopes. Among the three major forms of viral hepatitis, HBV is responsible for the most frequent transfusion transmitted disease. It induces a spectrum of clinical manifestations, ranging from mild, inapparent disease to fulminant hepatitis, severe chronic liver disease, and cirrhosis. The HBV is also clearly implicated in the development of primary hepatocellular carcinoma. The ability to detect HbsAg revolutionised the prevention of infection and crossinfection by HBV and has led to an understanding of its distribution and epidemiology. High sensitive enzyme immunoassays have provided the clinician with a powerful and reliable analytical system to detect the presence of HBsAg in samples at the ng/ml level.

Principle of the Assay

The HBsAg One Step kit uses two highly specific monoclonal antibodies, directed to different and sterically distant epitopes of the common "a" antigen, that can be found on the surface antigen of HBV. One of the two monoclonal antibodies is bound to the microplate while the second one is conjugated with peroxidase (HRP). The two antibodies form a "sandwich" complex with the antigen when present in the sample, that is mixed with the enzyme conjugate directly, in a simultaneous or "one-step" reaction. After the washing step, the enzymatic activity is detected by incubation with the mixed specific chromogen/substrate (TMB-urea peroxide). The intensity of the generated colour is proportional to the amount of antigen in the specimen.

Content of the Kit and Reagents Preparation

1. **Microtitre strips:** 1 microtitre plates 3 × 8-wells-strips coated with purified anti-HBsAg monoclonal antibody. The plate is contained in a sealed bag with dessicant. Bring the plate to room temperature before using it, so to prevent any moisture formation inside the bag.
2. **Enzyme conjugate:** 1 vial of 0.125 ml. proteic buffer solution containing an anti-HBsAg monoclonal antibody conjugated with HRP, 20 x concentrated. It contains stabilisers, 0.2 mg/ml gentamicin sulphate and 0.1% Kathon GC as preservatives.
3. **Conjugate diluent:** 1 vial of 2.5 ml proteic buffer solution for the dilution of the concentrated conjugate. It contains 0.2 mg/ml gentamicin sulphate, 0.1% Kathon GC as preservatives.
4. **Washing solution:** 1 vial of 50 ml It contains a concentrated solution of PBS and Tween 20. This solution must be diluted 1 25 with ultra-pure water before use. The diluted solution, when stored at room temperature, is stable for at least 1 week.
5. **Chromogen:** 1 vial of 2.5 ml. The solution contains tetramethyl benzidine (TMB) with activators and stabilisers, diluted in phosphate/citrate buffer.
   Warning: Store protected from light.
6. **Substrate:** 1 vial of 2.5 ml. The solution contains hydrogen peroxide diluted in phosphate/citrate buffer.
7. **Stop solution:** 1 vial of 12 ml. It contains 1 N HCI.
   Warning: Avoid contact with eyes and skin.
8. **Negative control:** 1 vial of 0.5 ml. Human serum base, non-reactive to HBsAg and containing 0.2 mg/ml gentamicin sulphate and 0.1% Kathon GC as preservatives.
9. **Positive control:** 1 vial of 0.5 ml. Human serum base reactive for not infected recHBsAg. It contains 0.2 mg/ml gentamicin sulphate and 0.1% Kathon GC as preservatives.
10. **Cardboard sealer:** 1 cardboard sealer to be used for protecting the plate during the incubations.

Note: All materials of human origin were tested and found negative to anti-HIV and anti-HCV antibodies.

Conditions and Notices

1. All the reagents contained in the kit are for *in vitro* diagnostic use only.
2. Do not use the kit or reagents after the expiry date stated on the labels. Do not mix reagents from different lots.
3. Procedure should be performed carefully in order to obtain reliable results and interpretations.
4. Bring all reagents to room temperature at least 60 minutes before the analysis.
5. Avoid contaminating reagents when taking them from the vials. We recommend to use automatic pipettes with disposable tips. When dispensing reagents, do not touch with tips the wall of wells in order to avoid cross contaminations.
6. For the washing step use only the washing solution provided in the kit and follow carefully the indications reported at point "washing instruction". It is recommended anyway to use a good quality microplate washer.
7. Avoid the substrate/chromogen to come in contact with oxidising agents or metallic surfaces. Avoid intense light exposure during incubation or reagent preparation. When preparing chromogen/substrate we recommend the use of plastic disposable sterile containers.
8. Samples and materials potentially infected have to be handled with care as they could transmit the infection. All objects come in direct contact with samples and all residuals of the assay should be treated or eliminated as potentially infected. Best procedures for inactivation are treatments in autoclave at 121°C for 30 minutes or with sodium hypochlorite at a final concentration of 2.5% for 24 hours. This last method can be used for treating the liquid washes that have to be neutralised before with sodium hydroxide.
9. Avoid contact with skin and mucosas, especially with the blocking reagent.
10. In any case, use protective talc-free gloves.

Storage and Stability of the Kit

1. The HBsAg One Step kit must be stored at 2 to 8°C and used before the expiry date stated on the label.
2. Unused strips have to be placed in the bag containing dessicant and firmly sealed before re-store at 2 to 8°C. After opening, strips are stable until the dessicant turns pink.
3. The diluted washing solution can be stored for one week at room temperature or 3 weeks at +2 to 8°C.
4. The chromogen/substrate solution is stable for 4 hours at room temperature, protected from light.
5. The diluted conjugate is stable for one week at 2 to 8°C when stored in sterile disposable container. We recommend to dilute only the quantity necessary to the test.
6. All other liquid reagents are stable when stored at 2 to 8°C up to the expiry date, provided that they are handled carefully to avoid any environment contamination.

Materials not Provided in the Kit

1. Semiautomatic pipettes of 10, 200 and 1000 µl.
2. Vortex mixer and absorbent paper.
3. Bidistilled water.
4. Chronometer.
5. Photometric reader of microplates or microstrips, linear up to at least 2 OD and provided with filters of 450 nm and 620-630 nm.
6. Incubator set + 37°C.
7. Microplates automatic washing device or manual apparatus capable of aspirating and dispensing volumes of 500 µl.

Samples

Either fresh sera or plasma can be used. If not used immediately they can be stored at 2 to 8°C for 1 week in case of longer storage, freeze at –20°C. Samples should be without microbial contaminations. In case, centrifuge at 2000 g for 20 minutes or filtrate with a 0.2 µ filter. Highly lipaemic or haemolysed samples can give uncorrect analytical results. Samples containing high titres of rheumatoid factor and anti-mouse heterophylous antibodies could give false-positive results.

Reagents Preparation

1. Washing solution: Dilute 1:25 with bidistilled water and mix carefully before use.
2. Conjugate: Dilute the conjugate 1:20 with corresponding diluent. Mix carefully on vortex.

3. Chromogen/substrate: About 5 minutes before use, prepare this reagent in a disposable plastic container, according to needs by mixing the chromogen with the substrate in equal volumes.

Washing Instruction

A good washing procedure is essential to obtain correct and precise analytical results. We, therefore, recommend to use a good quality ELISA microplate washer maintained at a good level of washing mechanical performance. Generally, 4-5 automatic washing cycles of 0.3 ml/each well are sufficient to avoid false-positive reactions and remove high background. Anyhow we recommend to calibrate the washing system on the kit itself so to match the declared analytical performances eventually adding a soak time between each washing cycle (see manual washing). In case of manual washing, we suggest to perform 5 washing cycles, dispensing and aspirating 0.3 ml/well per cycle and leaving a soak time of 30 sec. between each cycle. In any case, the liquid from the plates must be inactivated with a sodium hypochlorite solution at a final concentration of 25%, before being thrown away or autoclaved, as it must be considered as potentially infected.

Assay Procedure

Important Notes

1. The microplate or the strips have to be pre-washed before the test is run with one cycle of 500 µl. This step is very important in order to obtain the expected and declared specificity. Missing this operation can generate false-positive reactions to come up. This step is essential for the assay.
2. At least one hour before use, bring all reagents, controls and samples to room temperature (18-30°C), mixing them carefully on vortex.
3. Do not mix reagents from different lots.
4. We recommend to distribute the negative control in triplicate, the positive control in single, and samples possibly in duplicate.
5. Distribution and incubation times must be the same for all wells in the same analysis.
6. Avoid long interruptions between each step of the assay procedure.
7. It is suggested to eliminate the excess of washing solution from the microplate after washing by blotting it gently on an absorbent paper pad.
8. The colour developed in the last incubation is stable for a maximum of one hour in the dark.
9. We recommend to read the plate with an ELISA automatic reader able to subtract the background at 620-630 nm and to read the absorbance of samples and controls at 450 nm. The "blanking" of the instrument is to be carried out in the blank reagent well (well A1).

Assay Scheme

Pre-washed Monoclonal antibody coated wells

Reagents	A1 *Blank*	Negative *Control*	Positive *Control*	Sample
Negative control	-	150 µl	-	-
Positive control	-	-	150 µl	-
Sample	-	-	-	150 µl
Diluted conjugate	-	50 µl	50 µl	50 µl
Gently mix, then cover strips with adhesive film				
Incubate 120 mm, at + 37°C.				
Peel out the adhesive film and aspirate the reaction solution from all wells				
Wash 4-5 times with 500ul of diluted washing solution, carefully aspirating off the remaining liquid.				
Reagents chromogen/substrate mixed 1:1	150 µl	150 µl	150 µl	150 µl
Cover strips with a new adhesive film				
Incubate 20 mm. at room temperature protected from light				
Stop solution	100 µl	100 µl	100 µl	100 µl
Read the absorbance of each well against Al blanking-well at 450 nm and 620-630 nm				

Validity of the Assay

1. The OD 450 nm of the blanking well is lower than 0.100 higher values indicate a chromogen/substrate contamination. In such a case, repeat the assay carefully checking the reagent.
2. After substracting the blank, the mean OD value for the negative control is lower than 0.060. Higher values indicate an uncorrect

washing procedure. In such a case, check the efficiency the washing device.

3. The OD 450 nm of the positive control is higher than 1.000 OD 450 nm. Lower values indicate kit or control decay. In such a case, check the expiry date of the kit before repeating the assay.

Calculation of Results

Calculate the cut-off value through the following formula.

Mean negative control OD 450 nm + 0.040 = cut-off

Samples with an OD 450 nm value lower than the cut-off are classified as negative for HBsAg.

Samples with an OD 450 nm value within a value of cut-off + 20% are considered in a gray-zone. Patients in the gray-zone should be followed up.

Samples with an OD 450 nm higher than the gray-zone upper limit are classified as positive for HBsAg.

Example of Calculation

Negative control mean OD 450 nm	0.040 (NC)
Positive control mean OD 450 nm	1.800
Cut-off = NC + 0.040 =	0.080
Gray-zone = 0.080 + 20% =	0.096
Sample #1 OD 450 nm =	0.030 negative
Sample # 2 OD 450 nm =	1.158 positive

CHARACTERISTICS OF THE ASSAY

Sensitivity

The sensitivity of the EQUIPAR kit was calculated using the reference HBsAg preparations (1978), "ad" and "ay" subtypes, from Paul Ehrlich Institute. Such preparations were aliquoted in serial dilutions in negative human serum. Sensitivity was calculated as minimum detectable concentration expressed in UPEI/ ml. The following sensitivity was found "ay[1] subtype about 0.03 U PEI/ml, "ad" subtype about 0.06 U PEI/ ml. These data were confirmed with the Boston Biomedica Inc. panel showing a sensitivity for both the subtypes of about 0.2 ng/ ml.

Specificity

A study made on a statistically significative population of negative sera and plasma has shown a specificity higher than 99.5%. Normal values were found between 0.010-0.040 OD 450 nm. Serum and plasma panels, found repeatedly positive with reference analytical systems, and coming from different viral Hepatitis B pathologies, were found positive with a specificity higher than 99.5%.

Reproducibility

Negative and low positive samples were controlled repeatedly to determine precise statistic values for precision CV values between 4 and 15% were found depending on the samples OD 450 nm values.

HBsAg, Courtesy: Lilac Medicare

Two Steps Enzyme Immunoassay for the determination of Hepatitis Bs Antigen or HBsAg For *"in vitro"* diagnostic use only

Introduction

Hepatitis B surface Antigen or HBsAg is the most important protein of the envelope component of Hepatitis B Virus of HBV, responsible of acute and chronic forms of viral hepatitis.

The surface antigen contains the determinant "a", common to all the known viral subtypes, immunologically distinguished in three distinct subgroups (a, y and d). This common determinant is further composed of at least two immunologically distinct epitopes.

Among the major forms of viral hepatitis, HBV is responsible of the most frequent transfusion transmitted disease. It induces a spectrum of clinical manifestations ranging from mild, inapparent disease to fulminant hepatitis, severe chronic liver disease and cirrhosis. HBV is also clearly implicated in the development of primary hepatocellular carcinoma.

The ability to detect HBsAg in the last years revolutionized the prevention of infection and crossinfection by HBV and has led to understanding of its distribution and epidemiology.

High sensitive enzyme immunoassays have provided the clinician with a powerful and reliable analytical system to detect the presence of HBsAg in samples at ng/ml levels.

Principle of the Assay

The kit uses two highly specific monoclonal antibodies, directed to different epitopes of the type common "a" antigen, one adsorbed onto the wells of the microplate and the second labelled with horseradish peroxidase (HRP).

The sample is added on the plate in the 1st incubation and the HBsAg, if present, is captured by the adsorbed antibody.

After washing, in the 2nd incubation the conjugate binds to the captured antigen. The presence of a specific immunocomplex on the solid phase is then detected by the action of the captured conjugate on the chromogen/substrate mixture in the 3rd incubation.

The intensity of the colour generated by the enzyme is proportional to the amount of antigen in the sample.

A cut-off value allows the discrimination between the negative and the positive population.

Notices and Warnings

1. All the reagents contained in the kit are for *"in vitro"* diagnostic use only.
2. Do not use the kit or reagents after the expiry date stated on labels or in case the kit is damaged.
   Do not mix reagents of different lots.
3. Procedures should be performed carefully in order to obtain reliable results and clinical interpretations.
   All the instruments (washer, reader, work-station) have to be submitted to maintenance, regularly, and kept at the highest level of performances.
4. Bring all the reagents to room temperature for at least 60 min, before their use in the assay.
5. Avoid any contamination of reagents when taking them out of vials. We recommend to use automatic pipettes and disposable tips.
   When dispensing reagents and in particular the HRP conjugate, do not touch the wall of microplate wells with tips, in order to avoid any contamination and false results.
6. In the washing procedure, use only the washing solution provided with the kit and follow carefully the indications reported in the "washing instructions" section of this insert.
7. Ensure that the substrate/chromogen mixture does not come in contact with oxidizing agents or metallic surfaces. Avoid any intense light exposure during the incubation step or the reagent preparation.
   When preparing the substrate/chromogen mixture for the analysis use only plastic, disposable, clean or sterile containers.
8. Samples have to be treated as potentially infective and therefore, handled with care as they could transmit infections.
   All objects, machines and instrument parts, accidentally come in direct contact with samples, have to be decontaminated with disinfectants certified capable to inactivate HBV, HCV and HIV.
   Residuals of the assay have to be treated and then wasted as potentially infective.
   Best procedures for inactivation are treatments with autoclave at 121°C for 30 min or with sodium hypochlorite at a final concentration of 2.5% for 24 hr. This last method can be used for the treatment of liquid wastes after they have been neutralised to pH 6-8 with NaOH.
9. Avoid any contact of liquids with skin and mucosas. Use protective talk-free gloves, glasses and laboratory coats when working with samples.
   Always apply the standard laboratory safety procedures for biohazard containment and protection and report any accident according to.

CONTENT OF THE KIT

Strips microplate: 1:12 × 8:6 × 8 wells strips coated with purified anti HBsAg antibody. The plate is contained in a sealed bag with dessicant. Bring the plate to room temperature before use, to prevent any moisture formation inside the bag.

Enzyme conjugate: 1 vial of 1.0 ml 1 × 0.5 ml Proteic buffer solution containing an anti HBsAg monoclonal antibody, labelled with HRP, 20x concentrated. It contains proteic stabilizers, 0.2 mg/ml gentamicine sulphate and 0.1% Kathon GC as preservatives.

Conjugate diluent: 1 vial of 20 ml 1 × 10 m Proteic buffer solution for the dilution of the concentrated conjugate. It contains proteic stabilizers, 0.2 mg/ml gentamicine sulphate and 0.1% Kathon GC as preservatives.

Washing solution: 1 vial of 50 ml It contains a concentrated solution of PBS and Tween 20. This solution must be diluted 1:25 with distilled water before use. The diluted solution, when stored at room temperature, is stable for at least 1 week.

Chromogen: 1 vial of 8 ml 1 × 4 ml The solution contains tetramethylbenzidine (TMB) with activators and stabilizers, diluted in 0.1 M phosphate/citrate buffer.
Warning: store protected from light.

Substrate: 1 vial of 8 ml (code 1900BGTS) 1 × 4 ml The solution contains stabilised hydrogen peroxide diluted in 0.1 M phosphate/citrate buffer.

Stop solution: 1 vial of 12 ml. It contains a ready-to-use solution of 1N HCI. Handle with care.

Negative control: 1 vial of 2 ml 1 × 1 ml. Human serum base not reactive for HBsAg. It contains 0.2 mg/ml gentamicine sulphate and 0.1% Kathon GC as preservatives.

Positive control: 1 vial of 1 ml 1 × 0.5 ml. Human serum base positive for HBsAg. It contains not infective recombinant HBsAg, 0.2 mg/ml gentamicine sulphate and 0.1% Kathon GC as preservatives.

Cardboard sealers: 2 Plastic transparent sealers to cover plates when incubating at +40°C.

Note: All the materials of human origin have been tested and found negative for HBsAg, HCV Ab and HIV Ab with FDA approved kits.

Storage and Stability

1. The kit has to stored at 2 to 8°C and used before the expiration date declared on the external label.
2. Unused strips have to be returned into their bag containing the dessicant and firmly sealed with tape before store them back at 2 to 8°C. After the bag has been opened the first time, strips are stable till the dessicant turns pale pink.
3. The diluted washing solution is stable at room temperature for 1 week or for 3 weeks at 2 to 8°C.
4. The chromogen/substrate mixture is stable for 4 hr at rt when stored protected from light.
5. The diluted conjugate is stable for 1 week at 2 to 8°C, when stored in a sterile disposable container.
6. All the other liquid reagents are stable at 2 to 8°C when handled carefully to avoid contaminations.

Material not Provided

1. Micropipettes of 100 and 1000 ul disposable tips.
2. Vortex mixer and adsorbent papers.
3. ELISA grade water for dilutions.
4. Timer.
5. Photometric ELISA reader linear up to at least 2 OD and supplied with filters of 450 nm and 620-630 nm.
6. Incubator set at + 40°C.
7. Automatic microplate washer or manual apparatus capable to deliver 300 ul and aspirate.

Samples

Either fresh sera or plasma can be used for the assay.

If not used immediately, they can be stored at 2 to 8°C for 1 week without any loss of reactivity.

In case of longer storage freeze samples at -30°C. Samples should be clear and not contaminated by microrganisms and clots.

If necessary, remove contaminating particles by centrifugation at 2000 g × 20 min at r.t. or by filtration on 0.22 μ filters.

Highly lipemic, icteric or hemolised samples should not be used as they can give false results in the assay.

Samples showing high titres of heterophilic antibodies (HAMA) may interfere in the assay system and give false positive results.

Preparation of Reagents

Washing Solution: The concentrated solution has to be diluted 25x in ELISA grade water before use and carefully mixed.

Conjugate: Dilute 20x the necessary amount of the concentrated conjugate with the conjugate Diluent and mix gently on vortex.

Chromogen/substrate: About 5 minutes before use, prepare this reagent in a disposable plastic container, according to needs, by mixing 1 volume of Chromogen with 1 volume of substrate.

Washing Instructions

A good washing procedure is essential to obtain correct and precise analytical data.

We therefore, recommend to use a good quality ELISA microplate washer, maintained at the best level of washing performances.

Generally, 4-6 automatic washing and soaking (30 sec.) cycles of 300 ul/well are sufficient to avoid false positive reactions and high background.

Anyhow, we recommend to calibrate the washing system on the kit itself so to match the declared analytical performances. In case of manual washing, we suggest to carry out 5 cycles, dispensing 300 ul/ well and aspirating the liquid for 5 times leaving a soak time of 30 sec.between each cycle.

In any case, the liquid aspirated out the strips must be treated with a sodium hypochlorite solution at a final concentration of 2.5% for 24 hrs, before liquids are wasted in an appropriate way.

Assay Procedure

Important Notes

At least 1 hr before use, bring all the components of the kit to rt and mix the liquid reagents carefully on vortex.

Do not mix reagents of different lots.

Distribution and incubation times should be the same for all the wells of the microplate. When using automatic work-stations program the instrument to operate according to the assay procedure described in the insert. Avoid long interruptions among the different steps of the assay.

It is suggested to eliminate the excess of washing solution from wells by blotting them gently on a paper adsorbent pad. Omit this operation in automated systems and when no residue is seen on the bottom of the well.

The colour developed in the last incubation is stable for maximum 1 hr in the dark.

We recommend to read the microplate at 450 nm (reading filter) and subtract the blank at 620-630 nm (blanking filter).

Use well A1 to carry out blanking operations.

Operative Instructions

1. Leave the A1 well empty for blanking operations. Dispense 150 ul of controls and samples in the proper wells necessary for the assay, according to the following scheme:

Position	Calibrator/sample
A1	blanking well
B1+C1+D1	150 ul of negative control
E1	150 ul of positive control
F1...H12	150 ul of Samples

Incubate the microplate sealed for

A. Standard procedure: 120 min at + 37°C.
B. Short procedure: 60 min at + 37°C.
C. Long procedure: overnight at room temperature
D. Fast procedure: 60 min at + 37°C

Important note The standard and the long procedure are recommended for blood screening.

2. Peel out the plate sealer and wash the microplate according to instructions. In the meantime dilute the concentrated conjugate.
3. Add 150 ul of diluted conjugate to all the wells, A1 excluded. Incubate the microplate for
   60 min at + 37°C.(procedure A -B -C)
   30 min at + 37°C. (procedure D)
4. Peel out the plate sealer and wash the microplate according to instructions.
5. Add 150 ul of chromogen/substrate mixture to all the wells, A1 included. Incubate the microplate for 20 min at rt (procedure A -B - C) 15 min at rt (procedure D) protected from light.
6 Stop the enzymatic reaction by adding 100 ul stop solution to all the wells, A1 included.
7. Read the microplate at 450 nm and 620-630 nm blanking the instrument on A1 well.

Validity of the Assay

The assay is considered valid if:

1. The OD 450 nm of the A1 blank well is < 0.100. If higher check for contaminations of the solution of chromogen/substrate mixture before repeating the test.
2. After blanking on A1, the OD 450 nm mean value of the negative control or NC is < 0.060. If higher, control the performances of the washing device and in case increase the number of washing cycles, according to point I.
3. The OD 450 nm mean value for the positive control is > 1.000.

If lower, check for the expiration date of the kit and control the performances of the instruments used.

Important Note

It is essential for the user to verify that all the operative conditions are carefully checked before using the kit the very first time. Instruments in part icular have to be adapted to the assay procedures in order to match the validity values reported above.

Calculation of Results

If the test is confirmed valid, calculate the cut-off value through the following formula:

NC + 0.040 = cut-off

Samples with an OD 450 nm value lower than the cut-off are classified as negative for HBsAg.

Samples with an OD 450 nm value within the cut-off + 20% are considered in a gray-zone.

Samples with an OD 450 nm value higher than the upper limit of the gray-zone are classified positive for HBsAg.

Example of Calculation

Negative control mean OD 450 nm	0.020 (NC)
Positive control mean OD 450 nm	1.800
Cut-off = NC +0.040 =	0.060
Gray-zone = 0.060 + 20% =	0.072
Sample #1 OD 450 nm =	0.020 negative
Sample # 2 OD 450 nm =	1.158 positive

ASSAY PERFORMANCES

Sensitivity

The sensitivity of the assay has been calculated by means of the International standard for HBsAg supplied by Paul Erlich Institute.

The test shows a sensitivity of about:

Procedure A 0.03 PEI U/ml

Procedure B 0.04 PEI U/ml

Procedure C 0.02 PEI U/ml

Procedure D 0.06 PEI U/ml

These data were confirmed with the Boston Biomedica Inc. panel for HBsAg. The test shows a sensitivity of about 0.2 ng/ml (procedure C) and 0.5 ng/ml for the procedure D.

Specificity

It has been calculated on panels of negative samples from normal individuals and blood donors, preclassified negative with an FDA approved kit present on the market.

Both plasma, derived with different standard techniques of preparation, and sera have been used to determine the value of specificity. Fresh and frozen specimens have been tested too to check for interferences due to collection and storage.

The assay shows a specificity > 99% on plasma and sera. All the HBsAg known subtypes, "ay" and "ad", and isoforms "w" and "r", supplied by CNTS—France, have been tested in the assay and determined as positive at the concentrations supplied.

Reproducibility

It has been calculated on the Negative and the Positive Controls and on a sample close to the cut-off.

These samples have been tested in replicates, in different days and with different lots of kits.

CV's value have been shown in the following ranges:

NC	mean OD 450 nm	0.030	mean	CV 15%
Cut-off	mean OD 450 nm	0.100	mean	CV 7%
PC	mean OD 450 nm	2.900	mean	CV 4%

Assay Scheme

Method	*A*	*B*	*C*	*D*
Controls and samples	150 µl	150µl	150 µl	150 µl
1st incubation	120 min	60 min	o.n.	60 min
Temperature	+37°C	+37°C	room	+37°C
2nd incubation	60 min	60 min	60 min	30 min
Temperature	+37°C	+37°C	+37°C	+37°C
3rd incubation	20 min	20 min	20 min	15 min
Temperature	r.t.	r.t.	r.t.	r.t.
Stop solution	100 µl	100 µl	100 µl	100 µl
Reading OP	450 nm	450 nm	450 nm	450 nm
SensitivityPEI U/ml		0.03	0.04	0.02 0.06

HBsAg CONFIRMATORY TEST
Courtesy: Lilac Medicare

Enzyme immunoassay for the confirmation of the HBsAg Positivity in human sera and plasma For *in vitro* diagnostic use only.

Introduction

In the screening of blood units for Hepatitis B Surface Antigen, or HBsAg, some false reactivity may happen, leading to a misinterpretation of the assay results and a misclassification of the blood unit and of the donor. To confirm the positivity of a screened sample or to confirm the presence of an ongoing HBV infection in an hospitalised patient, a confirmatory test has to be run. A simple procedure based on an immunoreaction of neutralisation is used in combination with the HBsAg assay.

Principle of the Assay

The same immunoenzymatic method for the determination of HBsAg in serum or plasma is used in combination with a neutralizing polyclonal antibody, able to block any specific reactivity if present in the sample. The positive sample is incubated in the microplate in the presence of a goat anti HBsAg antiserum that prevents any HBsAg present in the sample from binding to the solid phase, in this case no further immunological reaction happens and no signal is generated, in case the positivity is due to some interfering substance present in the sample, the specific neutralisation reaction will not take place and therefore, a non specific signal will be generated by the enzime conjugate.

Content of the Kit and Reagents Preparation

1. **Microtitre Strips:** 1 microtitre plate. 12 × 8-wells-strips coated with anti-HBsAg monoclonal antibody. The plate is contained in a sealed bag with dessicant. Bring the plate to room temperature before using it, so to prevent any moisture formation inside the bag.
2. **Negative Control:** 1 vial of 2 ml. Human serum base non-reactive to HBsAg. It contains 0.2 mg/ml gentamicin sulphate and 0.1% Kathon GC as preservatives.
3. **Positive Control:** 1 vial of 1 ml. Human serum base reactive to HBsAg. synthetic and not infective. It contains 0.2 mg/ml gentamicin sulphate and 0.1% Kathon GC as preservatives.
4. **Enzyme Conjugate:** 1 vial of 0.8 ml. It contains a stabilised 20x concentrated solution of monoclonal antibody conjugated with HRP. It contains 0.2 mg/ml gentamicin sulphate and 0.1% Kathon GC as preservatives.
5. **Conjugate Diluent:** 1 vial of 16 ml. Proleic buffer solution for the dilution of the concentrated enzyme conjugate. It contains 0.2 mg/ml gentamicin sulphate and 0.1% Kathon GC as preservatives.
6. **Stop Solution:** 1 vial of 12 ml. It contains 1N HCl. Warning avoid contact with eyes and skin.
7. **Washing Solution:** 1 vial of 50 ml. It contains a concentrated solution of PBS and Tween 20. The solution has to be diluted 1:25 with ultrapure water before use. The diluted solution, when stored at room temperature, is stable for at least 1 week.
8. **Neutralizing Reagent:** 1 vial of 1 ml. It contains a solution of goat antiserum neutralizing HbsAg. It contains 0.2 mg/rnl gentamicin sulphate and 0.1% Kathon GC as preservatives.
9. **Control Reagent:** 1 vial of 1 ml. It contains a solution of normal goat serum not reactive used as negative control of neutralisation. It contains 0.2 mg/mi gentamicin sulphate and 0.1% Kathon GC as preservatives.
10. **Chromogen:** 1 vial of 8 ml. The solution contains tetramethylbenzidine (TMB) with activators and stabilizers diluted in phosphate/citrate buffer.
    Warning: Store protected from light
11. **Substrate:** 1 vial of 8 ml. The solution contains urea peroxide diluted in phosphate/citrate buffer.
12. **Cardboard Sealers:** n.° 2 plastic transparent sealers to cover plates when incubating at +40°C.

N.B. All materials of human origin were tested and found negative to anti-HIV, anti-HCV and anti-HbsAg antibodies with FDA approved kits.

Conditions and Notices

1. All the reagents contained in the kit are for *in vitro* diagnostic use only.
2. Do not use the kit or reagents after the expiry date stated on the labels. Do not mix reagents from different lots.
3. Procedure should be performed carefully, in order to obtain reliable results and clinical interpretations.
4. Bring all reagents to room temperature at least 60 minutes before the analysis.
5. Avoid contaminating reagents when taking them out of vials. We recommend to use automatic pipettes with disposable tips. When

dispensing reagents do not touch with tips the wall of wells in order to avoid cross-contaminations.

6. For the washing step, use only the Washing Solution provided in the kit and follow carefully the indications reported at point "Washing Instruction". It is recommended anyway to use a good quality microplate washer.
7. Avoid the substrate/chromogen to come in contact with oxidizing agents or metallic surfaces; avoid intense light exposure during incubation.or reagent preparation. When preparing chromogen/substrate we recommend the use of plastic disposable sterile containers.
8. Samples and materials potentially infected have to be handled with care as they could transmit the infection. All objects come in direct contact with samples and all residuals of the assay should be treated or eliminated as potentially infected. Best procedures for inactivation are treatments in autoclave at 121°C for 30 minutes or with sodium hypochlorite at a final concentration of 2.5% for 24 hours. This last method can be used for treating the liquid washes that have to be neutralised before with sodium hidroxyde.
9. Avoid contact with skin and mucosas, specially with the blocking reagent.
10. In any case, use protective talc-free gloves, glasses and laboratory coats, according to the safety regulations.

Storage and Stability of the Kit

1. The HBsAg Confirmatory kit must be stored at 2 to 8°C and used before the expiry date stated on the label.
2. Unused strips have to be placed in the bag containing dessicant and firmly sealed before restore at 2 to 8°C. After opening, strips are stable until the dessicant turns pink.
3. The diluted washing solution can be stored for one week at room temperature or 3 weeks at +2 to 8°C.
4. The diluted conjugate is stable for one week at 2 to 8°C when stored in sterile disposable container. Anyway, we suggest to dilute only the quantity necessary to the assay.
5. The chromogen/substrate mixture is stable for 4 hrs at R.T. when stored protected from light.
6. All other liquid reagents are stable when stored at 2 to 8'C, provided that they are handled carefully to avoid any environment contamination.

Materials not Provided in the Kit

1. Semi-automatic pipettes of 100, 200 and 1000 µl and disposable tips.
2. Vortex mixer and absorbent paper.
3. ELISA grade water for dilutions.
4. Timer.
5. Incubator +40°C.
6. Photometric reader of microplates or microstrips, linear up to at least 2 OD and provided with filters of 450 nm and 620-630 nm.
7. Microplates automatic washing device or manual apparatus capable of aspirating and dispensing volumes of 300 µl.

Samples

Either fresh HBsAg positive sera or plasma can be used. If not used immediately, they can be stored at 2 to 8ºC for 1 week; in case of longer storage, freeze at –30°C. Samples should be without microbial contaminations. In case, centrifuge at 2000 g for 20 minutes or filtrate with a 0.22 filter. Highly lipemic, I icteric or hemolised samples can give uncorrect analytical results.

Reagents Preparation

1. Washing solution: dilute 1:25 with bidistilled water and mix carefully before use.
2. Conjugate: mix carefully the concentrated conjugate on vortex and then dilute 1:20 the volume needed for the assay with its diluent. Mix. again on vortex.
3. Chromogen/substrate: about 5 minutes before use prepare in a disposable plastic container, according to needs, the substrale/chromogen solution by mixing the two reagents in equal volumes.

Washing Instruction

A good washing procedure is essential to obtain correct and precise analytical results. We therefore, recommend to use a good quality ELISA. microplate washer, maintained at the best level of washing mechanical performance. Generally, 4-5 automatic washing cycles of 0.3 ml/each well are sufficient to avoid fates positive reactions and remove high background. Anyhow we recommend to calibrate the washing system on the kit itself so to match the declared analytical performances eventually adding the soak time (see manual washing). In case of manual washing, we suggest to perform 5 washing cycles, dispensing and aspiiating 0.3 ml/well per cycle and leaving a soak time of 30 sec.after each cycle. In any case the liquid from the plates must be inactivated with a sodium hypochlorite solution at a final concentration of 2.5%, before being thrown away or autodaved, as it must be considered as potentially infected. It is suggested to eliminate the excess of washing solution from the microplate after washing by blotting it gently on an absorbent paper pad.

ASSAY PROCEDURE

Important notes

1. At least 1 hr before use bring all the components of the kit to rt and mix the liquid reagents carefully on vortex.
2. Do not mix reagents of different lots.
3. Distribution and incubation times should be the same for all the wells.
4. Avoid long interruptions among the different steps of the assay.
5. It is suggested to eliminate the excess of washing solution from wells by blotting them gently on a paper adsorbent pad.
6. The colour developed in the last incubation is stable for maximum 1 hr in the dark. We recommend to read the microplate at 450 nm (reading filter) and subtract the blank at 620-630 nm (blanking filter).
7. Use well A1 to carry out blanking operations.

Positive Samples with OD 450 nm higher than 2 to 3

1. Dilute the positive sample 1:10, 1:100 and 1:1000 in the negative control in order to have at least 250 ul of each dilution.
2. To the wells A1+B1+C1+D1 add 20 u! of the Neutralising Reagent; to the wells E1+F1+G1-I-H1 add 20 ul of the Control Reagent. Then add 100 ul of the positive sample not diluted in A1 and E1 and the same diluted 1 10. 1:100 and 1:100 in B1, C1, D1 and F1, G1, H1.
   The following scheme is reported as exemplification well Neutralising Control Sample # 1

	Reagent	Reagent	100 ul
A1	20ul		undiluted
B1	20ul		1 10
C1	20ul		1:100
D1	20ul		1:1000
E1		20ul	undiluted
F1		20ul	1 10
G1		20ul	1:100
H1		20ul	1:1000

   Proceed with the other positive samples according to the scheme descnbed above. Cover the strip with the plastic film and incubate for 120 min at + 37°C. Alternatively, incubate the microplate at room temperature overnight.
3. Peel out the plate sealer and wash the microplate according to instructions, in the meantime dilute the concentrated enzyme.
4. Add 100 ul of diluted conjugate to all the wells. Incubate the microplate for 60 min at + 37°C.
5. Peel out the plate sealer and wash the microplate according to instructions.
6. Add 100 ul of chromogen/substrate mixture to all the wells. Incubate the microplate for 20 min at rt., protected from light.
7. Stop the enzymatic reaction by adding 100 ul stop solution to all the wells. Read optical densities of the microplate wells at 450 nm.

Positive samples with OD 450 nm lower than 2 to 3

1. Dispense 20 ul Neutralising Reagent in A1 and 20 ul Control Reagent in B1. Then add 100 ul positive sample in A1 and B1.
2. Cover the strip with the plastic film and incubate for 120 min. at + 37°C. Alternatively, incubate the microplate at room temperature overnight.

Proceed as described above for the other steps.

Calculation of Results

A. Positive samples with OD 450 nm higher than 2 to 3
   Identify which control well among E, F, G or H shows a OD 450 nm value lower than 2.0. Then use the OD 450 nm value of the corresponding neutralisation well, where the sample has been dispensed at the same dilution, for the calculation.

B. Positive samples with OD 450 nm lower than 2 to 3
In this case use the OD 450 nm values of the control and the neutralisation wells for calculation.

The positive sample is considered confirmed for HBsAg if a value of at least 50% neutralisation is observed.

In mathematical terms a positive result is confirmed for HBsAg if the following values are obtained.

The positive sample is confirmed if
OD 450 nm controUOD 450 nm neutralisation > 2

The positive sample is not confirmed (false positive) if
OD 450 nm control/OD 450 nm neutralisation < 2

Example

Sample #1 shows a value higher than 2 OD 450 in the first screening assay. The sample is diluted as reported in the method.

Sample dilution 1:10
well B1 OD 450 nm = 0.100 (neutralisation)
well FI OD 450 nm = 1.000 (control)
Ratio control/neutralisation = 1.000/0.100 = 10
Positivity of the sample confirmed

Sample #2 shows a value lower than 2 OD 450 nm in the first screening assay. The sample is used without dilution as reported in the method.

Undiluted sample
well AI OD 450 nm = 0.100 (neutralisation)
well B1 OD 450 nm = 1.600 (control)
Ratio control/neutralisation = 1.600/0.100 = 16
Positivity of the sample confirmed

Sample #3 shows a value lower than 2 OD 450 nm in the first screening assay. The sample is used without dilution as reported in the method.

Well AI OD 450 nm = 1.600 (neutralisation)
Well B1 OD4SO nm = 2.000 (control)
Ratio control/neutralisation = 2.000/1.600 = 1.25
Positivity of the sample not confirmed.

Test Performances

The assay is capable to confirm positive samples containing up to 0.1 ug/ml HBsAg, subtype "ay" and "ad" as well.

High HBsAg content samples have to be diluted in Negative Control according to the procedure reported for OD values higher than 2.

Samples showing very low positivity in the screening" assays, ranging 1-2 S/Co values, may be difficult to be confirmed due to very low OD signals.

In this case it is suggested to examine the sample by prolonging the 1st incubation overnight at room temperature and then by following the instructions from point n° 3.

In this specific case, if the OD 450 nm signal for the control well is lower than 0.200 it is not recommended to use the results obtained for the diagnosis of confirmation.

MICRO ELISA HCV
Courtesy: Lilac Medicare

3rd generation Enzyme Immunoassay for the determination of Antibodies to Hepatitis C Virus or HCV Ab For *"in vitro"* diagnostic use only

Introduction

Hepatitis C Virus or HCV is an enveloped RNA virus recently classified in the family of Flaviviridae.

The genome encodes for structural components, a nucleocapsid protein and two envelope glycoproteins, and functional constituents involved in the virus replication and protein processing. The nucleocapsid-encoding region seems to be the most conservative among the isolates obtained all over the world.

HCV accounts for about 95% of hepatitis infections in recipients of blood transfusion and 50% of cases of sporadic NANB hepatitis. HCV commonly gives origin to asymptomatic hepatitis and chronicity develops in a high number of cases, sometime evolving in severe forms of illness, as hepatocarcinoma.

Antibodies directed to the major immunodominant determinants of the viral proteins are detected in patients infected with HCV, early in the course of infection.

The determination of antibody to HCV has become mandatory in the screening of blood units to prevent post-transfusion hepatitis. It is also currently used to follow-up risk individuals and patients under treatment with interferon.

Principle of the Assay

Microplates are coated with HCV-specific synthetic antigens derived from "core" and "ns" regions encoding for conservative immunodominant antigenic determinants (Core, NS3, NS4 and NS5).

The solid phase is first treated with the diluted sample and HCV Ab are captured, if present, by the antigens. After washing out all the other components of the sample, in the 2nd incubation bound HCV Ab are detected by the addition of anti lgG and M antibody, labelled with peroxidase (HRP). The enzyme captured on the solid phase, acting on the substrate/chromogen mixture, generates an optical signal that is proportional to the amount of anti HCV antibodies present in the sample.

Test Conditions and Notices

1. All the reagents contained in the kit are for "*in vitro*' diagnostic use only.
2. Do not use the kit or reagents after the expiry date stated on labels. Do not mix reagents of different lots.
3. Procedures should be performed carefully in order to obtain reliable results and clinical interpretations.
4. Bring all the reagents to room temperature for at least 60 min, before the test is started.
5. Avoid any contamination of reagents when taking them out of vials. We recommend to use automatic pipettes and disposable tips. When dispensing reagents, do not touch the wall of microplate wells with tips, in order to avoid any cross-contamination.
6. In the washing procedure, use only the Washing Solution provided with the kit and follow carefully the indications reported in the "Washing Instructions" section of this insert.
7. Ensure that the substrate/chromogen mixture does not come in contact with oxidizing agents or metallic surfaces; avoid any intense light exposure during the incubation step or the reagent preparation.
   When preparing the substrate/chromogen mixture for the analysis use only plastic, disposable, clean or sterile containers.
8. Samples and materials potentially infective have to be handled with care as they could transmit infection.
   All objects come in direct contact with samples and all residuals of the assay should be treated or wasted as potentially infective. Best procedures for inactivation are treatments with autoclave at 121°C for 30 min or with sodium hypochlorite at a final concentration of 2.5% for 24 hr. This last method can be used for the treatment of the liquid waste after that it has been neutralised with NaOH.
9. Avoid any contact of liquids with skin and mucosas. Use always protective talk-free gloves, glasses and laboratory coats, according to the safety regulations.

CONTENT OF THE KIT

a. **Strips microplate:** n°1 12 × 8 wells strips coated with synthetic HCV antigens. The plate is contained in a sealed bag with desiccant. Bring the plate to room temperature before use, to prevent any moisture formation inside the bag.

b. **Enzyme conjugate:** n°1 vial of 15 ml Proteic buffer solution containing a specific anti-h lgG and M antibody, labelled with HRP, ready to use. It contains proteic stabilizers, 0.2 mg/ml gentamicine sulfate and 0-3% Kathon GC.

c. **Washing solution:** n°1 vial of 50 ml 25 x concentrated solution to be diluted up to 1250 ml with EIA grade water It contains an imidazole buffer, Tween 20 and Kathon GC as preservative.
   The diluted solution, when stored room temperature, is stable for at least 1 week.

d. **Chromogen/substrate:** n°1 vial of 15 ml The solution contains tetramethyil benzidine (TMB)and hydrogen peroxide with activators and stabilizers, diluted in phosphate/citrate buffer.
   Warning: Store protected from light.

e. **Stop solution:** n°1 vial of 12 ml It contains 1 N HCI.
   Warning: Avoid contact with eyes and skin.

f. **Negative control:** n°1 vial of 4 ml Human serum base not reactive for anti-HCV antibodies. It contains, 0.09% sodium azide and 0.3% Kathon GC as preservatives.

g. **Positive control:** n°1 vial of 2 ml Human serum base highly reactive for HCV Ab. It contains, 0.09% sodium azide and 0.3% Kathon GC as preservatives. The Control has been chemically inactivated for HCV. Anyway handle this component as potentially infective.

h. **Sample diluent:** n°1 vial of 50 ml Proteic solution for the preparation of samples. It contains a detergent, proteic stabilizers, 0.09% sodium azide and 0.3% Kathon GC as preservatives.

i. **Cardboard sealers:** n°2 Plastic transparent sealers to cover plates when incubating at + 37°C.

Note: All human serum derived materials have been tested as negative for HBsAg, and HIV antibodies with FDA approved kits. The positive control has been inactivated for HCV. Anyway, handle these components as potentially infective.

Storage and Stability

1. The kit has to stored at 2 to 8°C and used before the expiration date declared on the external label.
2. Unused strips have to be returned into their bag containing the desiccant and firmly sealed with tape before store them back at 2 to 8°C. After the bag has been opened the first time, strips are stable till the desiccant turns pink.
3. The diluted washing solution is stable at room temperature for 1 week or for 3 weeks at 2 to 3°C.
4. All the other liquid reagents are stable tl 2 to 8°C when handled carefully to avoid contamination.

Material not Provided

1. Micropipettes of 10, 100 and 1000 ul.
2. Vortex mixer and adsorbent papers.
3. ELISA grade water for dilutions.
4. Timer.
5. Pnotometric ELISA reader linear up to at least 2 OD and supplied with filters of 450 nm and 620-630 nm.
6. Incubator set at + 37°C.
7. Automatic microplate washer or manual apparatus capable to deliver 300 ul and aspirate.

Samples

Either fresh sera or plasma can be used for the assay. If not used immediately, they can be stored at 2 to 8°C for 1 week. In case of longer storage freeze them at –30°C.

Samples should be clear and not contaminated by microorganisms. Do not freeze and thaw samples more than one time, as IgM may get damaged .

If necessary, remove contaminating particles by centrifugatton at 2000 g × 20 min at rt or by filtration on 0.22 u filters.

Highly lipemic, icteric or hemolised samples should not be used as they can give false results in the assay.

Preparation of Reagents

a. Washing Solution: The concentrated solution has to be diluted 25x in ELISA grade water before use.

Washing Instructions

A good washing procedure is essential to obtain correct and precise analytical data. We therefore, recommend to use a good quality ELISA microplate washer, maintained at the best level of washing performances.

Generally, 4-5 automatic washing cycles of 300 ul/well are sufficient to avoid false positive reactions and high background. Anyhow, we recommend to calibrate the washing system on the kit itself so to match'the declared analytical performances.

In case of manual washing, we suggest to carry out 5 cycles, dispensing 300 ul/well and aspirating the liquid for 5 times, leaving a soak time of 30' between each cycle.

In any case, the liquid aspirated out the strips must be treated with a sodium hypochlorite solution at a final concentration of 2.5% for 24 hrs, before liquids are wasted in an appropriate way.

ASSAY PROCEDURE

Important Notes

At least 1 hr before use, bring all the components of the kit to rt and mix the liquid reagents carefully on vortex. Do not mix reagents of different lots. Distribution and incubation times should be the same for all the wells; avoid long interruptions among the different steps of the assay.

It is suggested to eliminate the excess of washing solution from wells by blotting them gently on a paper adsorbent pad. The colour developed in the last incubation is stable for maximum 1 hr in the dark.

We recommend to read the microplate at 450 nm (reading filter) and subtract the blank at 620-630 nm (blanking filter).

Use well A1 to carry out blanking operations.

Automated Assay

The assay procedure may be automated in all the analytical steps on most of the ELISA work stations available.

When the test is run automatically with an ELISA system we suggest to make the work-station aspirate 240 ul of Sample Diluent and then 10 ul of sample (final dilution of 1:25).

All the mixture is then carefully dispensed directly into the appropriate well of the microplate and the dispensation needle extensively washed, before processing the next sample.

Do not dilute Controls as they are ready-to-use.

Dispense 250 ul controls in the appropriate control wells.

For the next operations follow the instructions reported below for the standard manual procedure.

It is strongly recommended to make the work-station operate in order to keep the same incubation time from the first to the last well dispensed, by washing the microplate strips-by-strips and insert ing time-laps (soaking) among them.

Standard Manual Procedure

1. Leave the A1 well empty for blanking operations. Dilute samples 1:25 with the Sample Diluent (240 ul diluent + 10 ul sample) directly in the appropriate sample well. Alternatively dilute the samples in dilution tubes (i.e. 480 ul diluent + 20 ul sample), mix on vortex and then dispense 250 µl per well. Do not dilute controls as they are ready-to-use. Then dispense controls into the appropriate control wells according to the following table:

position	calibrator/sample
A1	blanking well
B1+C1+D1	250 ul of negative control
E1	250 ul of Positive Contra!
F1	H12240 ul Diluent + 10 ul Sample

   Shake gently the microplate in order to mix the sample into the diluent, carefully

   Cover the microplate with the plate sealer and incubate strips for 60 min at + 37°C.
2. Peel out the plate sealer and wash the microplate according to instructions.
3. Add 100 ul of Enzyme to all the wells, but A1. Incubate the microplate sealed for 30 min at + 37°C.
4. Peel out the plate sealer and wash the microplate according to instructions.
5. Add 100 ul of chromogen/substrate to all the wells, A1 included. Incubate the microplate for 15 min at room temperature, protected from light.
6. Stop the enzymatic reaction by adding 100ul stop solution to all the wells, A1 included.

Read the microplate at 450 nm and 620-630 nm blanking the instrument on A1 well.

Validity of the Assay

The assay is considered valid if

1. The OD 450 nm of the A1 blank well is < 0.100.
2. After blanking on A1, the OD 450 nm mean value of the negative control (NC) is < 0.200.
3. The OD 450 nm mean value of the positive control (PC) is > 0.800.

In case data above do not match the correct values, before repeating the test check carefully the expiration date of the kit, the performances of the instruments used for the assay and the procedure of distribution of controls and samples.

Calculation of Results

If the validity of the assay is confirmed, calculate the cut-off value through the following formula

NC + 0.200 = cut-off

Samples with an OD 450 nm value lower than the cut-off are classified as negative for anti-HCV antibodies.

Samples with an OD 450 nm value within the cut-off + 20% are considered in a gray-zone. Patients in this zone should be followed up.

Samples with an OD 450 nm value higher than the upper limit of the gray-zone are consider positive for anti-HCV antibodies. As some false positivity has been reported by Literature for HCV Ab (ranging 2-7% depending on the screened population) any ELISA positive sample has to be confirmed by an alternative method.

Example of Calculation

Negative control mean OD 450 nm	0.060 NC
positive control OD 450 nm	2.800
Cut-off = NC + 0.200 =	0.260
Gray-zone = 0.260 + 20% =	0.312
Sample # 1 OD 450 nm =	0.050 negative
Sample #2 OD 450 nm =	1.250 positive
Sample #3 OD 450 nm =	0.270 irigtayzone

Assay Performances

Sensibility: The sensitivity of the assay has been calculated on a panel of seroconversion and of positive samples by comparing with a FDA approved kit on the market. The test shows a sensitivity > 99%.

Sensibility: It has been calculated on panels of negative samples, preclassified with an FDA approved kit present on the market. The assay shows a specificity > 99.6% on plasma and sera.

Reproducibility: It has been calculated on the negative and positive controls tested in replicates in different days. CV's between 2.5-10% have been obtained depending on their OD 450 nm value.

HCV IgM, Courtesy: Lilac Medicare

Enzyme Immunoassay for the *Determination of IgM antibodies to Hepatitis C Virus or HCV IgM For "in vitro"* diagnostic use only-96 tests.

Introduction

Hepatitis C Virus or HCV is an enveloped RNA virus recently classified in the family of Flaviviridae. The genome encodes for structural components, a nucleocapsid protein and two envelope glycoproteins, and functional constituents involved in the virus replication and protein processing. The nucleocapsid-encoding region seems to be the most conservative among the isolates obtained all over the world. HCV accounts for about 95% of hepatitis infections in recipients of blood transfusion and 50% of cases of sporadic NANB hepatitis. HCV commonly gives origin to asymptomatic hepatitis and chronicity develops in a high number of cases, sometime evolving in severe forms of illness, as hepatocarcinoma. IgM antibodies directed to the major immunodominant determinants of the viral proteins are detected in patients infected with HCV, early in the course of infection and in patients upon reactivation of viral replication in hepatocites. The determination of IgM antibody to HCV has become currently in use to follow-up patients under treatment with interferon.

Principle of the Assay

Microplates are coated with HCV-specific immuno-dominant synthetic antigens. The solid phase is first treated with the diluted sample and HCV IgM are captured, if present, by the antigens. After washing out all the other components of the sample, in the 2nd incubation bound HCV IgM are detected by the addition of anti-h lgM antibody, labelled with peroxidase (HRP). The enzyme captured on the solid phase, acting on the substrate/chromogen mixture, generates an optical signal that is proportional to the amount of anti HCV IgM antibodies present in the sample. Interferences due to IgG and RF in samples are blocked directly into the well by a Neutralizing Reagent.

Test Conditions and Notices

1. All the reagents contained in the kit are for *"in vitro"* diagnostic use only.
2. Do not use the kit or reagents after the expiry date stated on labels. Do not mix reagents of different lots.
3. Procedures should be performed carefully in order to obtain reliable results and clinical interpretations.
4. Bring all the reagents to room temperature for at least 60 min, before the test is started.
5. Avoid any contamination of reagents when taking them out of vials. We recommend to use automatic pipettes and disposable tips. When dispensing reagents, do not touch the wall of microplate wells with tips, in order to avoid any cross-contamination.
6. In the washing procedure, use only the washing solution provided with the kit and follow carefully the indications reported in the "Washing Instructions' section of this insert.
7. Ensure that the substrate/chromogen mixture does not come in contact with oxidizing agents or metallic surfaces; avoid any intense light exposure during the incubation step or the reagent preparation. When preparing the substrate/chromogen mixture for the analysis use only plastic, disposable, clean or sterile containers.
8. Samples and materials potentially infective have to be handled with care as they could transmit infection. All objects come in direct contact with samples and all residuals of the assay should be treated or wasted as potentially infective. Best procedures for inactivation are treatments with autoclave at 121°C for 30 min or with sodium hypochlorite at a final concentration of 2.5% for 24 hr. This last method can be used for the treatment of the liquid waste after that it has been neutralised with NaOH.
9. Avoid any contact of liquids with skin and mucosas. Use always protective talk-free

gloves, glasses and laboratory coats, according to the safety regulations.

Content of the Kit

1. **Strips Microplate:** 12 × 8 wells strips coated with synthetic HCV antigens. The plate is contained in a sealed bag with dessicant. Bring the plate to room temperature before use, to prevent any moisture formation inside the bag.
2. **Enzyme Conjugate:** Proteic buffer solution containing a specific anti-IgM antibody, labelled with HRP, 20x concentrated. It contains proteic stabilizers, 0.2 mg/ml gentamicine sulphate and 0.3% Kathon GC.
3. **Conjugate Diluent:** Proteic buffered solution for the dilution of the concentrated tracer. It contains proteic stabilizers, 0.2 mg/ml gentamicine sulphate and 0.3% Kathon GC as preservatives.
4. **Washing Solution:** 25 × concentrated solution to be diluted up to 1250 ml with EIA grade water. It contains a phosphate buffer, Tween 20 and Kathon GC as preservative. The diluted solution, when stored at room temperature, is stable for at least 1 week.
5. **Chromogen:** The solution contains tetramethylbenzidine (TMB) with activators and stabilizers, diluted in a phosphate/citrate buffer. Warning Store protected from light.
6. **Substrate:** The solution contains stabilised hydrogen peroxide diluted in a phosphate/ citrate buffer.
7. **Stop solution:** It contains 1N HCI. **Warning** avoid contact with eyes and skin.
8. **Negative control:** Human serum base not reactive for anti-HCV antibodies. It contains 0.2 mg/ml gentamicin sulphate and 0.3% Kathon GC as preservatives.
9. **Positive control:** Human serum base reactive for HCV IgM. It contains 0.2 mg/ml gentamicine sulphate and 0.3% Kathon GC as preservatives.
10. **Sample Diluent:** Proteic solution for the preparation of samples. It contains a detergent, proteic stabilizers, 0.09% sodium azide and 0.3% Kathon GC as preservatives.
11. **Neutralizing Reagent**: Proteic solution for the neutralisation of IgG and RF in samples. It contains a detergent, proteic stabilizers, 0.09% sodium azide and 0.3% Kathon GC as preservatives.
12. **Cardboard** Sealers Plastic transparent sealers to cover plates when incubating at + 37°C.

Note: All human serum derived materials have been tested as negative for HBsAg, and HIV antibodies with FDA approved kits. The positive control has been inactivated for HCV. Anyway, handle this component as potentially infective.

Storage and Stability

1. The kit has to stored at 2 to 8°C and used before the expiration date declared on the external label.
2. Unused strips have to be returned into their bag containing the dessicant and firmly sealed with tape before store them back at 2 to 8°C. After the bag has been opened the first ' time, strips are stable till the dessicant turns pink.
3. The diluted washing solution is stable at room temperature; for 1 week or for 3 weeks at 2 to 8°C.
4. The chromogen/substrate mixture is stable for 4 hr at r. t. when stored protected from light.
5. The diluted conjugate is stable for 1 week at 2 to 8°C, when stored in a sterile disposable container.
6. All the other liquid reagents are stable at 2 to 8°C when handled carefully to avoid contaminations.

Materials not Provided

1. Micropipettes of 10, 100 and 1000 ul.
2. Vortex mixer and adsorbent papers.
3. ELISA grade water for dilutions.
4. Timer.
5. Photometric ELISA reader linear up to at least 2 OD and supplied with filters of 450 nm and 620-630 nm.
6. Incubator set at + 37°C.
7. Automatic microplate washer or manual apparatus capable to deliver 300 ul and aspirate.

Samples

Either fresh sera or plasma can be used for the assay. If not used immediately, they can be stored at 2 to 8°C for 1 week. In case of longer storage freeze them at –30°C. Samples should be clear and not contaminated by microrganisms. Do not freeze and thaw samples more than one time, as IgM may get damaged. If necessary, remove contaminating particles by centrifugation at 2000 g x 20 min at rt or by filtration on 0.22u filters. Highly lipemic, icteric or hemolised samples should not be used as they can give false results in the assay.

Preparation of Reagents

a. **Washing Solution:**The concentrated solution has to be diluted 2and in ELISA grade water before use.
b. **Conjugate:** Dilute the concentrated conjugate 1 20 with its Diluent. Mix gently on vortex before use. Prepare only the volume necessary to the test.
c. **Chromogen/Substrate:** About 5 minutes before use, prepare this reagent in a disposable plastic container, according to needs, by mixing 1 volume of Chromogen with 1 volume of Substrate. Prepare only the volume necessary to the test.

Washing Instructions

A good washing procedure is essential to obtain correct and precise analytical data. We therefore, recommend to use a good quality ELISA microplate washer, maintained at the best level of washing performances. Generally, 4-5 automatic washing cycles of 300 ul/well are sufficient to avoid false positive reactions and high background. Anyhow, we recommend to calibrate the washing system on the kit itself so to match the declared analytical performances. In case of manual washing, we suggest to carry out 5 cycles, dispensing 300 ul/well, **leaving a soak time of 30 sec** and aspirating the liquid for 5 times. In any case, the liquid aspirated out the strips must be treated with a sodium hypochlorite solution at a final concentration of 2.5% for 24 hrs, before liquids are wasted in an appropriate way.

Assay Procedure Important Notes

- At least 1 hr before use, bring all the components of the kit to rt and mix the liquid reagents carefully on vortex.
- Do not mix reagents of different lots.
- We recommend to distribute the calibrators in duplicate. Distribution and incubation times should be the same for all the wells. Avoid long interruptions among the different steps of the assay.
- It is suggested to eliminate the excess of washing solution from wells by blotting them gently on a paper adsorbent pad.
- The colour developed in the last incubation is stable for maximum 1 hr in the dark. We recommend to read the microplate at 450 nm (reading filter) and subtract the blank at 620-630 nm (blanking filter). Use well A1 to carry out blanking operations.

1. Leave the A1 well empty for blanking operations. Dilute samples 1: 101 with the Sample Diluent (10 ul sample + 1000 ul diluent). Do not dilute controls as they are prediluted and ready-to-use.
   Dispense 50 ul of Neutralizing Reagent in all the wells of the samoles do not add it to A1, used for blanking, and the wells for the controls. Then dispense controls and samples into wells according to the following table

Position	Calibrator/sample
A1	blanking well
81+C1	100 ul of negative control
D1	100 ul of positive control
E1 H12	100 ul of Samples

   Cover the microplate with the plate sealer and incubate strips for 60 min at + 37°C.
2. Peel out the plate sealer and wash the microplate according to instructions. In the meantime prepare the enzyme conjugate by diluting it 1: 20 as described.
3. Add 100 ul diluted conjugate to all the wells, but A1. Incubate the microplate sealed for 60 min at + 37°C.
4. Peel out the plate sealer and wash the microplate according to instructions. In the meantime prepare the chromogen/substrate mixture as described.
5. Add 100 ul of the chromogen/substrate mixture to all the wells, A1 included. Incubate the microplate for 20 min at rt, protected from light.
6. Stop the enzymatic reaction by adding 100 ul stop solution to all the wells, A1 included.

Read the microplate at 450 nm and 620-630 nm blanking the instrument on A1 wed.

Validity of the Assay

The assay is considere valid if:

1. TheOD 450 nm of the Al blank well is < 0.100.

2. After blanking on A1, the OD 450 rt m mean value of the negative control (NC) is < 0.200.
3. The OD 450 nm mean value of the positive control (PC) is > 0.500.

In case data above do not match the correct values, before repeating the test check carefully the expiration date of the kit, the performances of the instruments used for the assay and the procedure of distribution of controls and samples.

Calculation of Results

If the validity of the assay is confirmed, calculate the cut-off value through the following formula.

NC + 0.250 = cut-off

Samples with an OD 450 nm value lower than the cut-off are classified as negative for HCV IgM.

Samples with an OD 450 nm value higher than the cut-off are classified as positive for HCV IgM.

Note: Some, false positivity has been reported by Literature for "sandwhich" IgM assays due to very high concentrations of interferents.

Example of calculation

Negative control mean OD 450 nm	0.050 NC
Positive control OD 450 nm	1.200
Cut-off = NC + 0.250 =	0.300
Sample # 1 OD 450 nm =	0.080 negative
Sample #2 OD 450 nm =	1.158 positive

Assay Performances

Sensibility: The sensitivity of the assay has been calculated on a panel of positive samples by comparing with a FDA approved kit on the market. The test shows a sensitivity > 98%.

Specificity: It has been calculated on panels of negative and positive samples, preclassified with an FDA approved kit present on the market. The assay shows a specificity > 98% on plasma and sera.

Reproducibility: It has been calculated on the Negative and positive controls tested in replicates in different days. CVs between 4-12% have been obtained depending on their OD 450 nm value.

HCV-Ab CONFIRMATORY TEST
Courtesy: Lilac Medicare

Enzyme Immunoassay of the **Confirmation of Antibody Positivity to Hepatitis C Virus** For *"in vitro"* diagnostic use only.

Introduction

Hepatitis C Virus or HCV is an enveloped RNA virus recently classified in the family of Flaviviridae.

The genome encodes for structural components, a nucleocapsid protein and two envelope glycoproteins, and functional constituents involved in the virus replication and protein processing. The nucleocapsid-encoding region seems to be the most conservative among the isolates obtained all over the world.

HCV accounts for about 95% of hepatitis infections in recipients of blood transfusion and 50% of cases of sporadic NANB hepatitis. HCV commonly gives origin to asymptomatic hepatitis and chronicity develops in a high number of cases, sometime evolving in severe forms of illness, as hepatocarcinoma.

The determination of antibody to HCV has become mandatory in the screening of blood units to prevent post-transfusion hepatitis. It is also currently used to follow-up risk individuals and patients under treatment with interferon.

Conformation of any positive result is strongly recommended in the clinical laboratory practice before considering the patient truly positive for anti HCV antibodies.

Principle of the Assay

Microplates are coated by strips with HCV-specific synthetic antigens derived from "core", "ns" and "env" regions encoding for conservative immuno-dominant antigenic determinants (Core, NS3, NS4, NS5 and Env).

Antigens are adsorbed to the wells composing the strips as follows:

Position	*Antigen*	*Composition*
A	None	Well for blanking operations
B	Casein	Negative internal control
C	Core	Specific synthetic antigen
D	NS3	Specific synthetic antigen
E	NS4	Specific synthetic antigen
F	NS5	Specific synthetic antigen
G	Env	Specific synthetic antigen
H	hlgG	Positive Internal Control

The strip is first treated with the sample turned out to be positive in the screening assay, Anti HCV antibodies are captured, if present, by the specific antigens.

After washing out all the other components of the sample, in the 2nd incubation bound HCV Ab are detected by the addition of anti hlgGandM antibody, labeled with peroxidase (HRP).

The enzyme captured on the solid phase, acting on the substrate/chromogen mixture, generates an optical signal that is proportional to the amount of anti HCV antibodies present in the sample.

Controls are included to provide an internal check of the analytical system.

The sample is confirmed positive if at least two specific reactivities are present.

Test Conditions and Notices

1. AH the reagents contained in the kit are for *"in vitro"* diagnostic use only.
2. Do not use the kit or reagents after the expiry date stated on labels. Do not mix reagents of different lots.
3. Procedures should be performed carefully in order to obtain reliable results and clinical interpretations.
4. Bring all the reagents to room temperature for at least 60 min, before the test is started.
5. Avoid any contamination of reagents when taking them out of vials. We recommend to use automatic pipettes and disposable tips. When dispensing reagents, do not touch the wall of microplate wells with tips, ir order to avoid any cross-contamination.
6. In the washing procedure, use only the Washing Solution provided with the kit and follow carefully the indications reported in the "Washing Instructions" section of this insert.
7. Ensure that the Substrate/Chromogen mixture does not come in contact with oxidizing agents or metallic surfaces; avoid any intense light exposure during the incubation step or the reagent preparation.
   When preparing the Substrate/Chromogen mixture for the analysis use only plastic, disposable, clean or sterile containers.
8. Samples and materials potentially infective have to be handled with care as they could transmit infection.
   All objects come in direct contact with samples and all residuals of the assay should be treated or wasted as potentially infective. Best procedures for inactivation are treatments with autoclave at 121°C or 30 min or with sodium hypochlorite at a final concentration of 2.5% for 24 hr. This last method can be used for the treatment of the liquid waste after that it has been neutralised with NaOH.
9. Avoid any contact of liquids with skin and mucosas. Use always protective talk-free gloves, glasses and laboratory coats, according to the safety regulations.

CONTENT OF THE KIT

a. **Strips Microplate:** n°1 12 × 8 wells strips coated by strip with synthetic HCV antigens. Strips are contained in a sealed bag with a dessicant and a frame. Bring the strips necessary to the test to room temperature before use, and close firmly the bag to prevent any moisture formation inside.

b. **Enzyme conjugate:** n°1 vial of 1 ml Proteic buffer solution containing a specific anti-h IgG and M antibody, labeled with HRP, 20x concentrated. It contains proteic stabilizers, 0.2 mg/ml gentamicine sulphate and 0.3% Kathon GC.

c. **Conjugate Diluent:** n°1 vial of 20 ml Proteic buffered solution for the dilution of the concentrated conjugate. It contains proteic stabilizers, 0.2 mg/ml gentamicine sulphate and 0.3% Kation GC as preservatives.

d. **Washing Solution:** n°1 vial of 5 ml 20 x concentrated solution to be diluted up to 1000 ml with EIA grade water. It contains a phosphate buffer, Tween 20 and Kathon GC as preservative.

   The diluted solution, when stored at room temperature, is stable for at least 1 week.

e. **Chromogen:** n°1 vial of 5 ml The solution contains tetrametrylbenzidine (TMB) with activators and stabilizers, diluted in a phosphate/citrate buffer.

   Warning: Store protected from light.

f. **Substrate:** n°1 vial of 8 ml The solution contains stabilised hydrogen peroxide diluted in a phosphate/citrate buffer.

g. **Stop solution:** n°1 vial of 12 ml It contains a solution of 1N HCI. Warning avoid contact with eyes or skin.

h. **Negative control:** n°1 vial of 3 ml Human serum base not reactive for anti-HCV antibodies. It contains 0.2 mg/ml gentamicine sulphate and 0.3% Kathon GC as preservatives.

i. **Positive control:** n°1 vial of 3 ml Human serum base highly reactive for HCV Ab. It contains 0.2 mg/ml gentamicine sulphate and 0.3% Kathon GC as preservatives.

j. **Sample Diluent:** n°1 vial of 20 ml Proteic solution for the preparation of samples. It contains a detergent, proteic stabilizers, 0.1% sodium azide and 0.3% Kathon GC as preservatives.

Note: All human serum derived materials have been tested as negative for HBsAg, and HIV antibodies with FDA approved kits. The positive control has been inactivated for HCV. Anyway, handle these components as potentially infective.

Storage and Stability

1. The kit has to stored at 2 to 8°C and used before the expiration date declared on the external label.
2. Unused strips have to be returned into their bag containing the dessicani and firmly sealed with tape before store them back at 2 to 8°C.
3. After the bag has been opened the first time, strips are stable till the dessicant turns pink.
4. The diluted washing solution is stable at room temperature for 1 week or for 3 weeks at 2 to 8°C.
5. The chromogen/substrate mixture is stable for 4 hr at rt when stored protected from light.
6. The diluted conjugate is stable for 1 week at 2 to 8°C, when stored in a sterile disposable container.
7. All the other liquid reagents are stable at 2 to 8°C when handled carefully to avoid contaminations.

Material not Provided

1. Micropipettes of 10, 100 and 1000 ul.
2. Vortex mixer and adsorbent papers.
3. ELISA grade water for dilutions.
4. Timer.
5. Photometric ELISA supplied with filters of 450 nm and 620-630 nm.
6. Incubator set at + 37°C.
7. Automatic microplate washer or manual apparatus capable to deliver 300 ul and aspirate.

Samples

Either fresh sera or plasma can be used for the assay. If not used immediately, they can be stored at 2 to 8°C for 1 week. In case of longer storage freeze them at –30°C.

Samples should be clear and not contaminated by microrganisms.

Do not freeze and thaw samples more than one time, as antibodies may get damaged .

If necessary, remove contaminating particles by centrifugation at 2000 g × 20 min at rt or by filtration on 0.22 u filters.

Highly lipemic, icteric or hemolised samples should not be used as they can give false results in the assay.

Preparation of Reagents

a. **Washing Solution:** The concentrated solution has to be diluted 20x in ELISA grade water before use.

b. **Conjugate:** Dilute the concentrated conjugate 1:20 with the Tracer Diluent.
Mix gently on vortex before use. Prepare only the volume necessary to the test.

c. **Chromogen/Substrate:** About 5 minutes before use, prepare this reagent in a disposable plastic container, according to needs, by mixing 1 volume of Chromogen with 1 volume of Substrate. Prepare only the volume necessary to the test.

Washing Instructions

A good washing procedure is essential to obtain correct and precise analytical data. We therefore, recommend to use a good quality ELISA microplate washer, maintained at the best level of washing performances.

Generally, 4-5 automatic washing cycles of 300 ul/well are sufficient to avoid false positive reactions and high background.

Anyhow, we recommend to calibrate the washing system on the kit itself so to match the declared analytical performances. In case of manual washing, we suggest to carry out 5 cycles, dispensing 300 ul/well and aspirating the liquid for 5 times.

In any case, the liquid aspirated out the strips must be treated with a sodium hypochlorite solution at a final concentration of 2.5% for 24 hrs, before liquids are wasted in an appropriate way.

ASSAY PROCEDURE

Important Notes

At least 1 hr before use, bring all the components of the kit to rt and mix the liquid reagents carefully on vortex.

Do not mix reagents of different iots.

We recommend to distribute the calibrators in duplicate. Distribution and incubation times should be the same for all the wells. Avoid long interruptions among the different steps of the assay.

It is suggested to eliminate the excess of washing solution from wells by blotting them gently on a paper adsorbent pad. The colour developed in the last incubation is stable for maximum 1 hr in the dark. We recommend to read the microplate at 450 nm (reading filter) and subtract the blank at 620-630 nm (blanking filter).

Use well A1 to carry out blanking operations.

1. Leave the A1 well empty for blanking operations. Dilute 10 µl sample to confirm with 1 ml diluent (1 :101 dilution).

   Do not dilute controls (if tested) as they are prediluted and ready-to-use.

   Then dispense the diluted sample to confirm into one strip module according to the following table:

Position	Sample
A1	blanking well
B1	100 ul diluted sample to confirm
C1	100 ul diluted sample to confirm
D1	100 ul diluted sample to confirm
E1	100 ul diluted sample to confirm
F1	100 ul diluted sample to confirm
G1	100 ul diluted sample to confirm
H1	100 ul diluted sample to confirm

   Cover the strip with the sealer and incubate the strip module for 60 min at + 37°C.
2. Peel out the plate sealer and wash the strip module according to instructions. In the meantime prepare the conjugate by diluting it 1: 20 as described.
3. Add 100 ul diluted conjugate to all the wells, except A1. Incubate the module sealed for 60 min at 37°C.
4. Peel out the plate sealer and wash the strip according to the instructions. In the meantime prepare the chromogen/substrate mixture as described.
5. Add 100 ul of the chromogen/substrate mixture to all the wells, A1 included. Incubate the strip module for 20 min at rt. temp, protected from light.
6. Stop the enzymatic reaction by adding 100 ul Stop Solution to all the wells, A1 included.

Read the strip module at 450 nm and 620-630 nm blanking the instrument on A1 well.

Validity of the Assay

The assay is considered valid if:

1. The OD 450 nm in A1 blank well is < 0.100.
2. After blanking, the OD 450 nm in HI well is > 0.800.
3. After blanking, the OD 450 nm mean value of the negative control (if tested) is < 0.200.
4. After blanking, the OD 450 nm value of the positive control (if tested) is > 0.800 in at least two positions from B1 to F1.

In case data above do not match the correct values, before repeating the test check carefully the expiration date of the kit, the performances of the instruments used for the assay and the procedure of distribution of controls and samples.

Interpretation of Results

If the validity of the assay is confirmed, examine the following table for the interpretation of results.

Classification	Results
Negative	Wells from C1 to G1 with OD 450 nm < B1 + 0.250
False Positive	B1 well with bD450 nm > 0.250
Indeterminate	One well from C1 to G1 with OD 450 nm > B1 + 0.250. B1 well must have OD 450 nm < 0.250
Positive	At least 2 wells from C1 to G1 with 1 OD 450 nm > 81 +0.250 B 1 well must have OD 450 nm< 0.250

HDV Ab, Courtesy: Lilac Medicare

Enzyme Immunoassay for the **Determination of Antibodies to Hepatitis Delta Virus or HDV Ab-For *"in vitro"* diagnostic use only**

Introduction

The Hepatitis Delta Virus or HDV is a RNA defective virus composed of a core presenting the delta-specific antigen, encapsulated by HBsAg, that requires the helper function of HBV to support its replication. Infection by HDV occurs in the presence of acute or chronic HBV infection. When acute delta and acute HBV simultaneously occur, the illness becomes severe and clinical and biochemical features may be indistinguishable from those of-HBV infection alone. In contrast, a patient with chronic HBV infection can support HDV replication indefinitely, usually with a less severe illness appearing as a clinical exacerbation.

The determination of HDV specific serological markers (HDV Ag, HDV Ab, HDV IgM and HDV IgG represents in these cases an important tool to the clinician for the classification of the etiological agent, for the follow up of infected patients and their treatment. The detection of HDV total antibodies allows the classification -of the illness and the monitoring of the seroconversion event.

Principle of the Assay

Anti-HDV antibodies, if present in the sample, compete with a virus-specific polyclonal IgG, labelled with peroxidase (HRP) for a fixed amount of recHDV, coated on the microplate.

The concentration of the bound enzyme on the solid phase becomes inversely proportional to the amount of anti-HDV antibodies in the sample and its activity is detected by adding the chromogen/ substrate in the last incubation.

The concentration of HDV-specific antibodies in the sample is determined by means of a cut-off value that allows for the semiquantitative detection of anti-HDV antibodies.

Test Conditions and Notices

1. All the reagents contained in the kit are for *"in vitro"* diagnostic use only.
2. Do not use the kit or reagents after the expiry date stated on labels. Do not mix reagents of different lots.
3. Procedures should be performed carefully in order to obtain reliable results and clinical interpretations.
4. Bring all the reagents to room temperature for at least 60 min, before the test is started.
5. Avoid any contamination of reagenis when taking them out of vials. We recommend to use automatic pipettes and disposable tips. When dispensing reagents, do not touch the wall of microplate wells with tips, in order to avoid any cross-contamination.
6. In the washing procedure, use only the washing solution provided with the kit and follow carefully the indications reported in the "washing instructions" section of this insert.
7. Ensure that the substrate/chromogen mixture does not come in contact with oxidizing agents or metallic surfaces; avoid any intense light exposure during the incubation step or the reagent preparation.
   When preparing the substrate/chromogen mixture for the analysis use only plastic, disposable, clean or sterile containers.
8. Samples and materials potentially infective have to be handled with care as they could transmit infection.
   All objects come in direct contact with samples and all residuals of the assay should be treated or wasted as potentially infective. Best procedures for inactivation are treatments with autoclave at 121°C for 30 min or with sodium hypochlorite at a final concentration of 2.5% for 24 hr. This last method can be used for the treatment of the liquid waste after that it has been neutralised with NaOH.
9. Avoid any contact of liquids with skin and mucosas. Use always protective talk-free gloves, glasses and laboratory coats, according to the safety regulations.

CONTENT OF THE KIT

a. **Strips Microplate:** n°1 12 × 8 wells strips coated with not infective recombinant HDV antigen. The plate is contained in a sealed bag with dessicant. Bring the plate to room temperature before use, to prevent any moisture formation inside the bag.
b. **Enzyme conjugate:** n°1 vial of 0.8 ml Proteic buffer solution containing anti-HDV polyclonal antibody, labelled with HRP, 20x concentrated. It contains proteic stabilizers, 0.2 mg/ml gentamicine sulphate and 0.1% Kathon GC as preservatives.
c. **Conjugate diluent:** n°1 vial of 16 ml Proteic buffer solution for the dilution of the

concentrated tracer. It contains proteic stabilizers, 0.2 mg/ml gentamicine sulphate and 0.1% Kathon GC as preservatives.

d. **Washing solution:** n°1 vial of 50 ml 25x concentrated solution to be diluted up to 1250 ml with EIA grade water. It contains a phosphate buffer and a detergent (Tween 20). The diluted solution, when stored at room temperature, is stable for at least 1 week.

e. **Chromogen:** n°1 vial of 8 ml The solution contains tetramethylbenzidine (TMB) with activators and stabilizers, diluted in a phosphate/citrate buffer.
Warning: Store protected from light

f. **Substrate:** n°1 vial of 8 ml The solution contains stabilised hydrogen peroxide diluted in a phosphate/citrate buffer

g. **Stop solution:** n°1 vial of 12 ml It contains a solution of 1N HCI
Warning: Caustic Handle with care

h. **Negative control:** n°1 vial of 2 ml Human serum base not reactive for anti-HDV antibodies. It contains 0.2 mg/ml gentamicin sulphate and 0.1% Kathon GC as preservatives.

i. **Positive control:** n°1 vial of 2 ml Human serum base reactive for anti-HDV antibodies. It contains 0.2 mg/ml geniarnicine sulphate and 0.1% Kathon GC as preservatives.

j. **Cardboard sealers:** n°2 Plastic transparent sealers to cover plates when incubating at + 37°C.

Note: All the materials of human origin, have been, tested and found negative for HBsAg, HCV Ab and HIV Ab with FDA approved kits.

Storage and Stability

1. The kit has to stored at 2 to 8°C and used before the expiration date declared on the external label.
2. Unused strips have to be returned into their bag containing the dessicant and firmly sealed with tape before store them back at 2 to 8°C. After the bag has been opened the first time, strips are stable till the dessicant turns pink.
3. The diluted washing solution is stable at room temperature for 1 week or for 3 weeks at 2 to 8°C.
4. The chromogen/substrate mixture is stable for 4 hr at rt when stored protected from light.
5. The diluted conjugate is stable for 1 week at 2 to 8°C, when stored in a sterile disposable container.
6. All the other liquid reagents are stable at 2 to 8°C when handled carefully to avoid contaminations.

Material not Provided

1. Micropipettes of 50, 100 and 1000 ul.
2. Vortex mixer and adsorbent papers.
3. ELISA grade water for dilutions.
4. Timer.
5. Photometric ELISA reader linear up to at least 2 OD and supplied with filters of 450 nm and 620-630 nm.
6. Incubator set at + 37°C.
7. Automatic microplate washer or manual apparatus capable to deliver 300 ul and aspirate.

Samples

Either fresh sera or plasma can be used for the assay. If not used immediately, they can be stored at 2 to 8°C for 1 week. In case of longer storage freeze them at –30°C.

Samples should be clear and not contaminated by microrganisms.

If necessary, remove contaminating particles by centrifugation at 2000 g × 20 min at rt or by filtration on 0.22 μ filters.

Highly lipaemic, icteric or haemolised samples should not be used as they can give false results in the assay.

Preparation of Reagents

a. **Washing Solution:** The concentrated solution has to be diluted 25x in ELISA grade water before use.

b. **Enzyme Conjugate**: Dilute the concentrated conjugate 20x with the conjugate diluent and mix gently on vortex.

c. **Chromogen/substrate:** About 5 minutes before use, prepare this reagent in a disposable plastic container, according to needs, by mixing 1 volume of Chromogen with 1 volume of substrate.

Washing Instructions

A good washing procedure is essential to obtain correct and precise analytical data.

We therefore, recommend to use a good quality ELISA microplate washer, maintained at the best level of washing performances.

Generally, 4-5 automatic washing cycles of 300 ul/well are sufficient to avoid false positive reactions and high background.

Anyhow, we recommend to calibrate the washing system on the kit itself so to match the declared analytical performances.

In case of manual washing, we suggest to carry out 5 cycles, dispensing 300 ul/well and aspirating the liquid for 5 times and leaving a soak time of 30 sec.between each cycle.

In any case, the liquid aspirated out the strips must be treated with a sodium hypochlorite solution at a final concentration of 2.5% for 24 hrs, before liquids are wasted in an appropriate way.

ASSAY PROCEDURE

Important Notes

- At least 1 hr before use, bring all the components of the kit to rt and mix the liquid reagents carefully on vortex.
- Do not mix reagents of different lots.
- We recommend to distribute the controls in duplicate. Distribution and incubation times should be the same for all the wells. Avoid long interruptions among the different steps of the assay. It is suggested to eliminate the excess of washing solution from wells by blotting them gently on a paper adsorbent pad.
- The colour developed in the last incubation is stable for maximum 1 hr in the dark. We recommend to read the' microplate at 450 nm (reading filter) and subtract the blank at 620-630 nm (blanking filter). Use well A1 to carry out blanking operations.

1. Distribute controls and samples according to the following scheme:

Position	Calibrator/sample
A1	blanking well
B1+C1	100 µl of negative control
D1+E1	100 µl of Positive Control
F1 H12	100 µl of Samples

Incubate the microplate for 60 min at and 37°C.

2. Peel out the plate sealer and wash the microplate according to instructions. In the meantime, dilute the enzyme conjugate as described.
3. **Add 100 µl of diluted enzyme to all the wells. A1 excluded, incubate. Incubate the microplate for 60 min at 37°C.**
4. Peel out the plate sealer and wash the microplate according to instructions. In the meantime, prepare the chromogen/substrate mixture as described.
5. Add 100 µl of the chromogen/substrate mixture to all the wells, A1 included. Incubate the microplate for 20 min at room temperature, protected from light.
6. Stop the enzymatic reaction by adding 100 µl stop solution to all the wells, A1 included. Read the microplate at 450 nm and 620-630 nm blanking the instrument on A1 welt.

Validity of the Assay

The assay is considered valid if

1. The OD 450 mn of the A1 blank well is < 0.100.
2. After blanking on A1, the OD 450 nm mean value of the negative control or NC is > 1.000.
3. After blanking on A1, the OD 450 nm mean value of the positive control or PC is < NIC/10.

In case data above do not match the correct values, before repeating the test check carefully the expiration date of the kit, the performances of the instruments used for the assay and the procedure of distribution of controls and samples.

Calculation of Results

If the test turns out to be valid, calculate the cut-off value through the following formula

Cut-off = (NC + PC)/4

Samples with an OD 450 nm value equal or higher than the cut-off are classified as negative for anti-HDV Ab. Samples with an OD 450 nm value lower than the cut-off are classified as positive for anti-HDV Ab.

Example of Calculation

Negative control mean OD 450 nm 1.900

Positive control mean OD 450 nm	0.100
Cut-off = (NC+PC)/4 =	0.500
Sample # 1 OD 450 nm =	1.680 negative
Sample #2 OD 450 nm =	0.158 positive

Assay Performances

Sensibility: The sensitivity of the assay has been calculated on a panel of positive samples by limiting dilution with reference to a FDA approved kit on the market. The assay shows a sensibility > 98%.

Specificity: It has been calculated on panels of negative and positive samples, preclassified with an FDA approved kit present on the market. The assay shows a specificity > 98% on plasma and sera.

Reproducibility: It has been calculated on the Negative and positive controls run in replicates in different days. CV's between 6-15% have been obtained depending on their OD 450 nm value.

HDV Ag, Courtesy: Lilac Medicare

Enzyme immunoassay for the **determination of Hepatitis Delta Antigen or HDVAg in human serum and plasma** For *in vitro* **diagnostic use only**

Introduction

The hepatitis delta virus (HDV) is an RNA defective virus composed of a delta-specific antigen expressing core, encapsulated by HBsAg, that requires the helper function of HBV to support its replication.

Infection by HDV occurs in the presence of acute or chronic HBV infection. When acute delta and acute HBV simultaneously occur , the illness becomes severe where clinical and biochemical features may be indistinguishable from those of HBV infection alone.

In contrast, a patient with chronic HBV infection can support HDV replication indefinitely, usually with a less severe illness appearing as a clinical exacerbation.

The determination of HDV-specific serological markers (HDVAg, IgM and IgG) represents in these cases an important tool to the clinician for the classification of the etiological agent, for the follow up of infected patients and their treatment.

The detection of HDV-specific antibodies allows the classification of the illness and the monitoring of the seroconversion event.

Principle of the Assay

The HDV Ag, if present in the sample, is captured by a specific monoclonal antibody, in the 1st incubation. In the 2nd incubation, after washing, a tracer, composed of a second anti HDV Ag antibody, labeled with peroxidase (HRP) is added to the microplate and binds to the captured HDV Ag. The concentration of the bound enzyme on the solid phase is proportional to the amount of HDV Ag in the sample and its activity is detected by adding the chromogen/ substrate in the 3rd incubation.

The presence of HDV Ag in the sample is determined by means of a cut-off value that allows for the semiquantitative detection of the antigen.

Content of the Kit and Reagents Preparation

1. **Microtitre strips:** 1 microtitre plate. 12 × 8/6 × 8/3 × 8-wells-strips coated with purified anti-HDVAg monoclonal antibody. The plate is contained in a sealed bag with dessicant. Bring the plate to room temperature before using it, so to prevent any moisture formation inside the bag.
2. **Enzyme Conjugate:** 1 vial of 1.5 ml/ × 0.8 ml/ 1 × 0.35 ml Proteic buffer solution containing an anti-HDV Ag antibody conjugated with HRP, 20 x concentrated. It contains stabilisers, 0.2 mg/ml gentamicin sulphate, 0.1% Kathon GC and as preservatives.
3. **Conjugate diluent**: 1 vial of 30 ml/1 × 15 ml/ 1 × 7 ml Proteic buffer solution for the dilution of the concentrated tracer. It contains 0.2 mg/ ml gentamicin sulphate, 0.1% Kathon GC and as preservatives.
4. **Wash Solution** 1 vial of 50 ml 25x concentrated solution of phosphate buffer containing Tween 20 as detergent. It has to be diluted up to 1250 ml with distilled water before use. The diluted solution, when stored at room temperature is stable for at least 1 week.
5. **Chromogen:** 1 vial of 12 ml/1 × 6 ml/1 × 3 ml The solution contains tetramethyltabq enzidine (TMB) with activators and stabilisers, diluted in phosphate/citrate buffer. Warning store protected from light.
6. **Substrate:** 1 vial of 12 ml/1 × 6 ml/1 × 3 ml The solution contains hydrogen peroxide diluted in phosphate/citrate buffer.

7. **Stop solution:**1 vial of 12 ml It contains 1N HCI. Handle with care. Avoid contact with eyes and skin.
8. **Negative control:** 1 vial of 1.5 ml/1 × 0.8 ml/ 1 × 0.4 ml Human serum base, nonreactive to HDVAg and containing 0.2 mg/ml gentamicin sulphate, 0.1% Kathon GC and as preservatives.
9. **Positive control:**1 vial. Lyophilised non infective recombinant HDV Ag.lt contains 0.2 mg/ml gentamicin sulphate, 0.1% Kathon GC.
10. **Detergent** 1 vial of 15 ml/1 × 7 ml/1 × 3.5 ml 6% NP40 solution containing 0.09% Na-azide
11. **Cardboard sealers:** 2 cardboard sealers to be used for protecting the plate during the incubations.

NB: All materials of human origin were tested and found negative to anti-HIVand anti-HCV antibodies.

Conditions and Notices

1. All the reagents contained in the kit are for *in vitro* diagnostic use only.
2. Do not use the kit or reagents after the expiry date stated on the labels. Do not mix reagents from different lots.
3. Procedure should be performed carefully, in order to obtain reliable results and interpretations.
4. Bring all reagents to room temperature at least 60 minutes before the analysis.
5. Avoid contaminating reagents when taking them from the vials. We recommend to use automatic pipettes with disposable tips. When dispensing reagents, do not touch with tips the wall of wells in order to avoid crosscontaminations.
6. For the washing step, use only the washing solution provided in the kit and follow carefully the indications reported at point "washing instruction". It is recommended anyway to use a good quality microplate washer.
7. Avoid the substrate/chromogen to come in contact with oxidising agents or metallic surfaces; avoid intense light exposure during incubation or reagent preparation. When preparing chromogen/substrate, we recommend the use of plastic disposable sterile containers.
8. Samples and materials potentially infected have to be handled with care as they could transmit the infection. All objects come in direct contact with samples and all residuals of the assay should be treated or eliminated as potentially infected. Best procedures for inactivation are treatments in autoclave at 121°C for 30 minutes or with sodium hypochlorite at a final concentration of 2.5% for 24 hours. This last method can be used for treating the liquid washes that have to be neutralised before with sodium hydroxide.
9. Avoid contact with skin and mucosas especially with the blocking reagent.
10. In any case, use protective talc-free gloves.

Storage and Stability of the Kit

1. The kit must be stored at 2 to 8°C and used before the expiry date stated on the external label.
2. Unused strips have to be placed in the bag containing dessicant and firmly sealed before re-store at 2 to 8°C.
   After opening, strips are stable until the dessicant turns pink.
3. The diluted washing solution can be stored for one week at room temperature or 3 weeks at +2 to 8°C.
4. The chromogen/substrate solution is stable for 4 hours at room temperature, protected from light.
5. The diluted conjugate is stable for one week at 2 to 8°C when stored in sterile disposable container. We recommend to dilute only the quantity necessary to the test.
6. The dissolved positive control is not stable. Store in aliquots at –20°C.
7. All other liquid reagents are stable when stored at 2 to 8°C up to the expiry date, provided that they are handled carefully to avoid any environment contamination.

Materials not Provided in the Kit

1. Semiautomatic pipettes of 50, 100 and 1000 µl.
2. Vortex mixer and absorbent paper
3. Bidistiiled water.
4. Chronometer.
5. Photometric reader of microplates or microstrips, linear up to at least 2 OD and provided with filters of 450 nm and 620-630 nm.

6. Incubator set + 37°C
7. Microplates automatic washing device or manual apparatus capable of aspirating and dispensing volumes of 300 µl.

Samples

Either fresh sera or plasma can be used. If not used immediately, they can be stored at 2 to 8°C for 1 week in case of longer storage, freeze at –20°C. Samples should be without microbial contaminations. In case, centrifuge at 2000 g for 20 minutes or filtrate with a 0.2 µ filter. Highly lipaemic or haemolised samples can give uncorrect analytical results. Samples containing high titres of rheumatoid factor and anti-mouse heterophylous antibodies could give false positive results.

Reagents Preparation

1. **Washing solution:** Dilute 1:25 with bidistilled water and mix carefully before use.
2. **Conjugate:** Dilute 1:20 with corresponding diluent. Mix carefully on vortex.
3. **Chromogen/substrate:** About 5 minutes before use, prepare in disposable plastic container, according to needs, the substrate/chromogen solution by mixing the chromogen and the substrate in equal volumes.
4. **Positive control:** Dissolve the content of the lyphosilised vial with 1.5 ml of EIA grade water and mix on vortex.The dissolved control is not stable. Store in aliquots at –20°C.

Washing Instruction

A good washing procedure is essential to obtain correct and precise analytical results. We, therefore, recommend to use a good quality ELISA microplate washer, maintained at a good level of washing mechanical performance. Generally, 4-5 automatic washing cycles of 0.3 ml/each well are sufficient to avoid false-positive reactions and remove high background. Anyhow, we recommend to calibrate the washing system on the kit itself so to match the declared analytical performances. In case of manual washing, we suggest to perform 5 washing cycles, dispensing and aspirating 0.3 ml/well per cycle and leaving a soak time of 30 sec between each cycle, in any case the liquid from the plates must be inactivated with a sodium hypochlorite solution at a final concentration of 2.5%, before being thrown away or autoclaved, as it must be considered as potentially infected.

Assay Procedure

1. At least one hour before use, bring all reagents, controls and samples to room temperature (18-30°C) mixing them carefully on vortex.
2. Do not mix reagents from different lots.
3. We recommend to distribute the negative control in triplicate, the positive control in single, and samples possibly in duplicate.
4. Distribution and incubation times must be the same for all wells in the same analysis.
5. Avoid long interruptions between each step of the assay procedure.
6. It is suggested to eliminate the excess of washing solution from the microplate after washing by blotting it gently on an absorbent paper pad.
7. The colour developed in the last incubation is stable for a maximum of one hour in the dark.
8. We recommend to read the plate with an ELISA automatic reader able to substract the background at 620-630 nm and to read the absorbance of samples and controls at 450 nm. The "blanking" of the instrument is to be carried out in the blank reagent well (well A1).

Assay Scheme

Leave the A1 well empty for blanking. When controls and samples have been distributed, add the detergent as described below.

Monoclonal antibody-coated wells

Reagents	*A1 Blank*	*Controls*	*Sample*
Controls	-	100 µl	-
Sample	-	-	100 µl
Detergent	-	100 µl	100 µl
Cover strips with adhesive film			
Incubate 120 min. at 37°C			
Peel out the adhesive film and aspirate the reaction solution from all wells			
Wash 4-5 times with 300 µl of diluted washing solution, carefully aspirating off the remaining liquid			

Contd...

Contd...

Diluted conjugate	-	200 µl	200 µl
Cover strips with adhesive film			
Incubate 60 min. at + 37°C			
Peel out the adhesive film and aspirate the reaction solution from all wells			
Wash 4-5 times with 300 µl of diluted washing solution, carefully aspirating off the remaining liquid.			
Reagents chromogen/ substrate mixed 1:1	200 µl	200 µl	200 µl
Cover strips with a new adhesive film			
Incubate 20 min at room temperature, protected from light.			
Stop solution	100 µl	100 µl	100 µl
Read the absorbance of each well against A1 blanking-well at 450 nm and 620-630 nm.			

Validity of the Assay

The assay is to be considered valid if:

1. The OD 450 nm of the blanking well is lower than 0.100. Higher values indicate a chromogen/substrate contamination. In such a case, repeat the assay carefully checking the reagent.
2. After subtracting the blank, the mean OD value for the negative control is lower than 0.100. Higher values indicate an uncorrect washing procedure. In such a case, check the efficiency of the washing device.
3. The OD 450 nm of the positive control is higher than 0.800 OD 450 nm. Lower values indicate kit or control decay, in such a case, check the expiry date of the kit before repeating the assay.

Calculation of Results

Calculate the cut-off value through the following formula:

Mean negative control OD 450 nm + 0.100 = cut-off

Samples with OD values equal to or higher than cut-off are to be considered positive to HDVAg.

Samples with OD values lower than cut-off are to be considered negative.

Example of calculation

Negative control mean OD 450 nm	0.050
Positive control mean OD 450 nm	1.800
Cut-off =	0.150
Sample # 1 OD 450 nm =	0.080 negative
Sample # 2 OD 450 nm =	1.158 positive

Assay Performances

1. **Sensitivity:** The sensitivity of the assay has been calculated by means of a panel of positive samples by limiting dilution, with reference to a kit present on the market and FDA approved.
   The sensitivity of the assay is >99%.
2. **Specificity:** It has been calculated on panels of negative and positive samples, preclassified with an FDA-approved kit present on the market. The assay shows a specificity > 99% on plasma and sera.
3. **Reproducibility:** It has been calculated on the negative and positive controls tested in replicates in different days. CVs between 4-15% have been obtained depending on their OD 450 nm value.

HDV IgG, Courtesy: Lilac Medicare

Enzyme Immunoassay for the Determination of IgG Class Antibodies to Hepatitis Delta Virus

For *in vitro* diagnostic use only

Introduction

The hepatitis delta virus (HDV) is a RNA defective virus composed of a delta-specific antigen expressing core, encapsulated by HBsAg, that requires the helper function of HBV to support its replication. Infection by HDV occurs in the presence of acute or chronic HBV infection. When acute delta and acute HBV simultaneously occur, the illness becomes severe where clinical and biochemical features may be indistinguishable from those of HBV infection alone. In contrast, a patient with chronic HBV infection can support HDV replication indefinitely, usually with a less severe illness appearing as a clinical exacerbation. The determination of HDV-specific serological markers (HDVAg, IgM and IgG) represents in these cases an important tool to the clinician for the classification of the aetiological agent, for the follow-up of infected patients and their treatment. The detection of HDV-specific antibodies allows the classification of the illness and the monitoring of the seroconversion.

Principle of the Assay

Microplates are coated with a purified preparation of HDV-specific synthetic antigens which, in the first incubation, capture specifically the antibody if present in the sample. After washing out the other components of the sample, specific anti-HDV antibodies are detected with a goat anti-human IgG antibody conjugated with peroxidase (HRP). The intensity of the colour, generated by the enzyme on the substrate/chromogen mixture in the last incubation, is proportional to the content of anti-HDV antibodies in the sample. Quantitative results may be calculated by means of 3 standard curve calibrated in arbitrary units, providing a quantitative determination of HDV-specific IgG.

Content of the Kit and Reagents Preparation

1. **Microtitre strips:** 1 microtitre plate. 12 × 8-wells strips coated with HDV-specific synthetic antigens. The plate is contained in a sealed bag with dessicant. Bring the plate to room temperature before use, to prevent any moisture formation inside the bag.
2. **Enzyme conjugate:** 1 vial of 0.8 ml. Proteic buffer solution containing human anti-IgG polyclonal antibodies, conjugated with HRP, 20 x concentrated, it contains proteic stabilisers, 0.2 mg/ml gentamicin sulphate and 0.1% Kathon GC as preservatives.
3. **Conjugate diluent:** 1 vial of 16 ml. Proteic buffer solution for the dilution of the concentrated tracer. It contains 0.2 mg/ml gentamicin sulphate and 0.1% Kathon GC as preservatives.
4. **Wash solution:** 1 vial of 50 ml 25x concentrated solution of phosphate buffer containing Tween 20 as detergent. It has to be diluted up to 1250 ml with distilled water. The diluted solution, when stored at room temperature, is stable for at least 1 week.
5. **Chromogen:** 1 vial of 8 ml. The solution contains tetramethylbenzidine (TMB) with activators and stabilisers, diluted in phosphate/citrate buffer.
   Warning store protected from light.
6. **Substrate:** 1 vial of 8 ml. The solution contains urea peroxide diluted in phosphate/citrate buffer.
7. **Stop solution:** 1 vial of 12 ml. It contains a solution of 1N HCI. Handle with care.
8. **Negative control:** 1 vial of 2 ml.Human serum base not reactive for HDV IgG; it contains 0.09% Na-azide and 0.1% Kathon GC.
   The control is prediluted and ready to use.
9. **Positive control:**1 vial of 2 ml. Human serum base positive for HDV IgG; it contains 0.09% Na-azide and 0.1% Kathon GC. The control is prediluted and ready to use.
10. **Sample diluent:** 1 vial of 50 ml Proteic solution for samples preparation; it contains a detergent, proteic stabilisers, 0.09% sodium azide and 0.1% Kathon GC as preservatives.
11. **Cardboard sealers:** 2 cardboard sealers to be used to cover the plate during the incubations.

Conditions and Notices

1. All the reagents contained in the kit are for *in vitro* diagnostic use only.
2. Do not use the kit or reagents after the expiry date stated on the labels. Do not mix reagents from different lots.
3. Procedures should be performed carefully, in order to obtain reliable results and clinical interpretations.
4. Bring all reagents to room temperature at least 50 minutes before the analysis.
5. Avoid contaminating reagents when taking them from the vials. We recommend to use automatic pipettes with disposable tips. When dispensing reagents, do not touch with tips the wall of wells in order to avoid crosscontaminations.
6. For the washing step, use only the washing solution provided in the kit and follow carefully the indications reported at point "washing instruction". It is recommended anyway to use a good quality microplate washer.
7. Avoid the substrate/chromogen to come in contact with oxidising agents or metallic surfaces, avoid intense light exposure during incubation or reagent preparation. When preparing chromogen/substrate we recommend the use of plastic disposable sterile containers.
8. Samples and materials potentially infected have to be handled with care as they could transmit the infection. All objects come in direct contact with samples and all residuals of the assay should be treated or eliminated as potentially infected. Best procedures for inactivation are treatments with autoclave at

121°C for 30 minutes or with sodium hypochlorite at a final concentration of 2.5% for 24 hours. This last method can be used for treating the liquid washes that have to be neutralised before with sodium hydroxide.
9. Avoid any contact with skin and mucosas, especially with the blocking reagent.
10. In any case, use protective talk-free gloves.

Storage and Stability of the Kit

1. The HDV IgG kit has to be stored at 2 to 8°C and used before the expiry date stated on the label.
2. Unused strips have to be placed in the bag containing the dessicant and firmly sealed before re-store at 2 to 8°C. After opening, strips are stable until the dessicant turns pink.
3. The diluted washing solution can be stored for one week at room temperature or 3 weeks at +2 to 8°C.
4. The chromogen/substrate solution is stable for 4 hours at room temperature, protected from light.
5. The diluted conjugate is stable for 1 week at 2 to 8°C, when stored in disposable sterile container.
6. All other liquid reagents are stable when stored at 2 to 8°C provided that they are handled carefully to avoid any enviro nment contamination.

Materials not Provided in the Kit

1. Semiautomatic pipettes of 10, 200 and 1000 µl.
2. Vortex mixer and absorbent paper
3. Ultrapure water (bidistilled).
4. Chronometer.
5. Photometric reader of microplates or microstrips, linear up to at least 2 OD and supplied with filters of 450 nm and 620-630 nm.
6. Incubator set at + 37°C.
7. Automatic microplates washing device or manual apparatus capable of aspirating and dispensing volumes of 300 µl.

Samples

Either fresh sera or plasma can be used. If not used immediately, they can be stored at 2 to 8°C for 1 week; in case of longer storage, freeze at –20°C. Samples should be without particles or microbial contaminations; in case, centrifuge at 2000 g for 20 minutes or filtrate with a 0.2 µl filter. Highly lipaemic or haemolised samples can give uncorrect analytical results.

Reagents Preparation

1. Wash solution dilute 1:25 with distilled water and mix carefully before use.
2. Conjugate: Dissolve 1:20 the concentrated conjugate with its diluent. Mix carefully on vortex.
3. Chromogen/substrate: Prepare in disposable plastic container according to needs, the substrate, chromogen solution by mixing the chromogen with the substrate in equal volumes.

Washing Instruction

A good washing procedure is essential to obtain correct and precise analytical results. We therefore, recommend to use a good quality ELISA microplate washer, maintained at a good level of washing mechanical performances. Generally, 4-5 automatic washing cycles of 0.3 ml/well are sufficient to avoid false-positive reactions and remove high background. Anyhow, we recommend to calibrate the washing system on the kit itself so to match the declared analytical performances in case adding a soak time between each cycle (see manual washing). In case of manual washing, we suggest to perform 5 washing cycles, dispensing and aspirating 0.3 ml/well per cycle, leaving 3 soak time of 30 sec. between each cycle. In any case the liquid washed out from the plates must be inactivated with a sodium hypochlorite solution at a final concentration of 2.5%, before being thrown away or autoclaved, as it must be considered as potentially infected.

Assay Procedure

1. At least one hour before use, bring all reagents, calibration set and samples to room temperature (18-30°C), mixing them carefully on vortex.
2. Do not mix reagents from different lots.
3. We recommend to distribute the calibration set and the samples in duplicate.
4. Distribution and incubation times must be the same for all wells in the same analysis.

5. Avoid long interruptions between each step of the assay procedure.
6. It is suggested to eliminate the excess of washing solution from the microplate after washing by blotting it gently on an absorbent paper pad.
7. The colour developed in the last incubation is stable for a maximum of one hour in the dark.
8. We recommend to read the plate with an ELISA automatic reader able to subtract the background at 620-630 nm and to read the absorbance of samples and standards at 450 nm. The "blanking" of the instalment is to be carried out in the blank reagent well (well A1).

Assay Scheme

1. Dilute the sample 1:51 with the sample diluent (e.g. 10 µl sample + 0.5 ml diluent). The calibration set is ready-to-use; do not dilute! Mix carefully on vortex before dispensing.
2. Follow this scheme:

HDV antigens-coated wells

Reagents	*A1 Blank*	*Calibrators*	*Sumple*
Calibrators	-	100 µl	
Sample	-	-	100 µl
Cover strips Wifo adhesive film			
Incubate 60 min. at + 37°C			
Peel out the adhesive film arid aspirate the reaction solution from all wells. Wash 4-5 times with 300 pi of diluted washing solution, carefully aspirating off the remaining liquid.			
Diluted conjugate	-	100 µl	100 µl
Cover strips witn adhesive film			
Incubate 30 min, at+37°C			
Peel out the adhesive film and aspirate the reaction solution from all wells.			
Wash 4-5 times with 300 pi of diluted washing solution, carefully aspirating off the remaining liquid.			
Reagents chromogen/ substrate mixed 1:1	100 µl	100 µl	100 µl
Cover strips with a new adhesive film.			
Incubate 15 min at room temperature, protected from light.			
Stop solution	100 µl	100 µl	100 µl
Read the absorbance of each well against A1 blanking-well at 450 nm and 620-630 nm.			

Validity of the Assay

The assay is to be considered valid if:

1. The OD 450 nm of the blanking well is lower than 0.100. Higher values indicate a chromogen/substrate contamination, in such a case, repeat the assay carefully checking the reagent.
2. After substracting the blank, the mean OD value for the negative control and the 0 Uarb/ml standard is lower than 0.200. Higher values indicate an uncorrect washing procedure. In such a case, check the efficiency of the washing device.
3. The value of the positive control is higher than 1.000 OD 450 nm. Lower values indicate kit or calibrator decay, in such a case, check expiry date of the kit before repeating the assay.

Calculation of Results

Check for the validity of the test and then calculate the cut-off value with the following formulation :
Negative control mean OD 450 nm + 0.150
= cut-off

Samples with an OD 450 nm value lower than the cut-off are not reactive for anti-HDV IgG.

Samples with an OD 450 nm value higher than the cut-off are considered positive.

Assay Performances

Specificity: It has been calculated on panels of negative, samples preclassified with an FDA-approved kit present in the market. Results show a value > 98%.

Sensitivity: The sensitivity of the assay has been calculated on a panel of seroconversion and of positive samples by comparing with an FDA-approved kit in the market. The test shows a sensitivity >98%.

Reproducibility: It has been calculated on the negative and positive controls tested in replicates in different days. CVs between 4-12% have been obtained depending on their OD 450 nm value.

Example of calculation

Negative control (NC)	0.050 OD 450 nm Mean Value
Positive control (PC)	1.200 OD 450 nm
Cut-off = NC + 0.150	0.200
Sample n°1	0,072 OD 450 nm negative
Sample n°2	0.678 OD 450 nm positive

HDV IgM, Courtesy: Lilac Medicare

Enzyme "Capture" Immunoassay for the Determination of IgM Class Antibodies to Hepatitis Delta Virus or HDV IgM

For *in vitro* diagnostic use only

Introduction

The hepatitis delta virus (HDV) is an RNA defective virus composed of a delta-specific antigen expressing core, encapsulated by HBsAg, that requires the helper function of HBV to support its replication. Infection by HDV occurs in the presence of acute or chronic HBV infection. When acute delta and acute HBV simultaneously occur, the illness becomes severe where clinical and biochemical features may be indistinguishable from those of HBV infection alone. In contrast, a patient with chronic HBV infection can support HDV replication indefinitely, usually with a less severe illness appearing as a clinical exacerbation. The determination of HDV-specific serological markers (HDVAg, IgM and IgG) represents in these cases an important tool to the clinician for the classification of the aetiological agent, for the follow-up of infected patients and their treatment. The detection of HDV-specific IgM antibodies allows the classification of the illness and the monitoring of the seroconversion.

Principle of the Assay

Microplates are coated with a monoclonal anti-IgM antibody that in the first step captures specifically this class of antibodies. After washing out all the other components of the sample, in the 2nd incubation bound anti-HDV IgM are detected by the addition of recombinant HDV antigen immunocomplexed with a specific antibody, labelled with peroxidase (HRP). After washing, the enzyme captured on the solid phase, acting on the substrate/chromogen mixture, generates an optical signal that is proportional to the amount of IgM antibodies present in the sample.

Content of the Kit and Reagents Preparation

1. **Microtitre strips:** 1 microtitre plate. 12 × 8-wells strips coated with anti human IgM monoclonal antibody. The plate is contained in a sealed bag with dessicant. Bring the plate to room temperature before use, to prevent any moisture formation inside the bag.
2. **Enzyme conjugate:** 1 vial of 0.8 ml 20x. Proteic buffer solution containing a specific anti-HDV antibody, labelled with HRP. It contains proteic stabilisers, 0.2 mg/ml gentamicin sulphate and 0.1% Kathon GC as preservatives.
3. **Antigen conjugate:** Diluent 1 vial of 16 ml. Proteic buffered solution for the preparation of the diluted conjugate. It contains 0.2 mg/ml gentamicin sulphate and 0.1% Kathon GC as preservatives.
4. **HDV Antigen:** 6 vials. Lyophillised recombinant HDVAg. The content of the vial has to be dissolved with 1.9 ml antigen/conjugate diluent before use.
5. **Washing solution:** 1 vial of 50 ml 25x concentrated solution to be diluted up to 1250 ml with bidistilled water. It contains a phosphate buffer, a detergent and preservatives (0.1% Kathon GC).
6. **Chromogen:** 1 vial of 8 ml. The solution contains tetramethyl benzidine (TMB) with activators and stabilisers, diluted in phosphate/citrate buffer.
   Warning: store protected from light.
7. **Substrate:** 1 vial of 8 ml. The solution contains stabilised hydrogen peroxide diluted in phosphate/citrate buffer.
8. **Stop solution:** 1 vial of 12 ml. It contains 1 NHCl.
   Warning avoid contact with eyes and skin.
9. **Negative control:** 1 vial of 2 ml. Human serum base not reactive for anti-HDV IgM antibodies, predicted and ready for use. It contains 0.09% sodium azide and 0.1% Kathon GC as preservatives.
10. **Positive control:** 1 vial of 2 ml. Human serum base reactive for anti-HDV IgM antibodies, prediluted and ready to use. It contains 0.09% sodium azide and 0.1% Kathon GC as preservatives.
11. **Sample diluent:** 2 vials of 50 ml each. Proteic solution for samples preparation; it contains a detergent, proteic stabilisers, 0.09% sodium azide and 0.1% Kathon GC as preservatives.
12. **Cardboard sealers:** 2 cardboard sealers to be used to cover the plate during the incubations.

Note All the materials of human origin have been tested as negative for HBsAg, HIV and HCV with FDA approved kits.

Conditions and Notices

1. All the reagents contained in the kit are for *in vitro* diagnostic use only.
2. Do not use the kit or reagents after the expiry date stated on the labels. Do not mix reagents from different lots.
3. Procedures should be performed carefully, in order to obtain reliable results and clinical interpretations.
4. Bring all reagents to room temperature at least 60 minutes before the analysis.
5. Avoid contaminating reagents when taking them from the vials. We recommend to use automatic pipettes with disposable tips. When dispensing reagents, do not touch with tips the wall of wells in order to avoid cross contaminations.
6. For the washing step, use only the washing solution provided in the kit and follow carefully the indications reported at point "washing instruction". It is recommended anyway to use a good quality microplate washer.
7. Avoid the substrate/chromogen to come in contact with oxidising agents or metallic surfaces; avoid intense light exposure during incubation or reagent preparation. When preparing chromogen/substrate, we recommend the use of plastic disposable sterile containers.
8. Samples and materials potentially infected have to be handled with care as they could transmit the infection. All objects come in direct contact with samples and all residuals of the assay should be treated or eliminated as potentially infected. Best procedures for inactivation are treatments with autoclave at 121°C for 30 minutes or with sodium hypochlorite at a final concentration of 2.5% for 24 hours. This last method can be used for treating the liquid washes that have to be neutralised before with sodium hydroxide.
9. Avoid any contact with skin and mucosas, especially with the blocking reagent.
10. In any case, use protective talk-free gioves, glasses and laboratory coats, according to the safety regulations.

Storage and Stability of the Kit

1. The kit has to be stored at 2 to 8°C and used before the expiry date stated an the label.
2. Unused strips have to be placed in the bag containing the dessicant and firmly sealed before re-store at 2 to 8°C. After opening, strips are stable until the dessicant turns pink.
3. The diluted washing solution can be stored for one week at room temperature or 3 weeks at +2 to 8°C.
4. The chrornogen/substrate solution is stable for 4 hours at room temperature, protected from light.
5. The antigen/conjugate immunocomplex is not stable. Prepare only the volume needed for the test.
6. All the other liquid reagents are stable when stored at 2 to 8°C, provided that they are handled carefully to avoid any environment contamination.

Materials not Provided in the Kit

1. Semiautomatic pipettes of 10, 200 and 1000 (jl.
2. Vortex mixer and absorbent paper.
3. Ultrapure water (bidistilled).
4. Chronometer.
5. Photometric reader of microplates or microstrips, linear up to at least 2 OD and supplied with filters of 450 nm and 620-630 nm.
6. Incubator set at + 37°C.
7. Automatic microplates washing device or manual apparatus capable of aspirating and dispensing volumes of 300 µl.

Samples

Either fresh sera or plasma can be used, if not used immediately, they can be stored at 2 to 8°C for 1 week; in case of longer storage, freeze at 20°C. Samples should be without particles or microbial contaminations; in case, centrifuge at 2000 g for 20 minutes or filtrate with a 0.2 µl filter. Highly lipaemic or haemolysed samples can give uncorrect analytical results.

Reagents Preparation

1. Washing solution: Dilute 1:25 with bidistilted water and mix care fully before use.
2. Antigen/conjugate immunocomplex: Before running the test dissolve the lypholised antigen with 1.9 ml of the proper diluent. Let the content fully dissolve; then add 0.1 ml of concentrated conjugate and mix carefully on

vortex. Prepare only the volume necessary to the test.

3. Chromogen/substrate: 5 min before use, prepare in disposable plastic container, according to needs, the substrate/chromogen solution by mixing the chromogen with the substrate in equal volumes.

Washing Instruction

A good washing procedure is essential to obtain correct and precise analytical results. We, therefore, recommend to use a good quality ELISA microplate washer, maintained at a good level of washing mechanical performances. Generally, 4-5 automatic washing cycles of 0.3 ml/well are sufficient to avoid false-positive reactions and remove high background. Anyhow, we recommend to calibrate the washing system on the kit itself so to match the declared analytical performances. In case of manual washing, we suggest to perform 5 washing cycles dispensing and aspirating 0.3 ml/well per cycle and leaving a soak time of 30 sec.between each cycle; in any case, the liquid washed from the plates must be inactivated with a sodium hypochlorite solution at a final concentration of 2.5%, before being thrown away or autoclaved, as it must be considered as potentially infected.

Assay Procedure

Important Notes

1. At least one hour before use, bring all reagents, calibration set and samples to room temperature (18-30°C), mixing them carefully on vortex.
2. Do not mix reagents from different lots.
3. We recommend to distribute the calibration set and the samples in duplicate. The calibration set is prediluted and ready to use. Samples have to be diluted 1:201 by mixing 5 µl sample with 1 ml sample diluent into a disposable tube on vortex.
4. Distribution and incubation times must be the same for all wells in the same analysis.
5. Avoid long interruptions between each step of the assay procedure.
6. It is suggested to eliminate the excess of washing solution from the microplate after washing by blotting it gently on an absorbent paper pad.
7. The colour developed in the last incubation is stable for a maximum of one hour in the dark.
8. We recommend to read the plate with an ELISA automatic reader able to substract the background at 620-630 nm and to read the absorbance of samples and standards at 450 nm. The "blanking" of the instrument is to be carried out in the blank reagent well (well A1).

Assay Procedure

1. Dilute samples 1:101 by mixing 10 µl sample with 1 ml sample diluent. Do not dilute the controls as they are ready-to-use. Leave empty the A1 well for blanking. Dispense 100 µl of the controls in duplicate and then 100 µl of the samples.
2. Cover the microplate with the plate sealer and incubate at + 37°C for 60 min.
3. Wash the plate according to the washing procedure described.
4. Add 100 µl antigen/conjugate immunocomplex, prepared as described before, to all the wells, except for A1. Incubate the microplate sealed at + 37°C for 60 min
5. Wash the plate according to the washing procedure described. In the meantime mix 1 volume of TMB chromogen with 1 volume of substrate in a sterile disposable tube on vortex.
6. Dispense 100 µl of the mixture in all the wells, A1 included. Incubate the microplate at room temperature for 20 min, in the dark.
7. Add 100 µl of stop solution in all the wells. Read the microplate at 450 nm as reading filter and 620-630 nm as reference filter. Use the A1 well for blanking.

Validity of the Test

The test is considered valid if:

1. The OD 450 nm of the A1 well is lower than 0.100. Higher values are indicative of contamination of the chromogen/substrate mixture or of a bad procedure for washing. Check for them before repeating the test.
2. The OD 450 nm of the negative control is lower than 0.200 after blanking on A1. Higher values are indicative of a bad procedure of washing. Check for it before repeating the test.

3. The OD 450 nm of the positive control is higher than 0.500. Lower values are indicative of an abnormal decay of the kit or the control. Check carefully the date of expiration.

Results

Check first for the validity of the test.

Calculate the mean OD 450 nm value of the negative control (NC) and then use the following formula for the calculation of the cut-off:

NC + 0.250 = cut-off

Samples with an OD 450 nm value lower than the cut-off are considered negative for anti-HDV IgM antibodies. **Samples** with an OD 450 nm value higher than the cut-off are considered positive for the presence of anti-HDV IgM antibodies.

Example of calculation

Negative control	OD 450 nm 0.120
Positive control	OD 450 nm 1.230
Cut-off	0.120 + 0.250 = 0.370
Sample 1	OD 450 nm 0.135 negative
Sample 2	OD450 nm 1.345 positive

Assay Performances

Sensitivity The sensitivity of the assay has been calculated on a panel of seroconversion and of positive samples by comparing with a FDA approved kit on the market. The test shows a sensitivity > 98%.

Specificity: It has been calculated on panels of negative and positive samples,preclassified with an FDA-approved kit present on the market. The assay shows a specificity >98% on plasma and sera.

Reproducibility: It has been calculated on the negative and positive controls tested in replicates in different days. CV's between 4-12% have been obtained depending on their OD 450 nm value.

HEV Ab, Courtesy: Lilac Medicare

Enzyme mmunoassay for the Determination of Antibodies to Hepaittis E Virus

For *in vitro* diagnostic use only

Introduction

Hepatitis E virus (HEV) is a recently discovered agent of the enterically transmitted non-A, non-B, non-C and non-D viral hepatitis. The HEV infection has a worldwide distribution and a predominant waterbone route of transmission. The first reported outbreak of this infection occurred in 1955 in New Delhi; since that time, epidemics of hepatitis E have been documented in many countries (Somalia, Borneo, Pakistan, Mexico). The HEV shows morphological and biophysical properties in common to viruses found in the family Caliciviridae. The viral genome consists in a single-stranded RNA molecule that contains three open reading frames (ORF 1, 2 and 3) that encode for nonstructural and structural proteins. Epitope mapping of the viral genome has lead to the identification of the presence of highly immuno-reactive type-specific epitopes. Synthetic peptides and recombinant proteins have been used to develop immunoenzymatic assays for the detection of HEV antibodies (IgG and IgM). These tests have been recently introduced in many countries to screen blood units for HEV antibodies.

Principle of the Assay

Microtitre plates are coated with HEV specific synthetic antigens derived from "ORF2" and "ORF3". The solid phase is first treated with the diluted sample. After the washing step, the specifically bound antibodies are detected with goat anti-human IgG/IgM antibodies, conjugated to peroxidase (HRP). A substrate/chromogen solution is added and the intensity of the colour developed by the bound enzyme is proportional to the amount of anti-HEV antibodies in the sample. Results are evaluated against a cut-off value able to discriminate HEV negative from positive individuals.

Content of the Kit and Reagents Preparation

1. **Microtitre strips:** 1 microtitre plate 12 × 8-wells strips 6 × 8 microplale coated with HEV/ specific synthetic antigens. The plate is contained in a sealed bag with dessicant. Bring the plate to room temperature before use, to prevent any moisture formation inside the bag.
2. **Enzyme conjugate:** 1 vial of 0.8 ml 1 × 0.4 ml. Proteic buffer solution containing anti-human IgG; IgM antibodies, conjugated with HRP, 20x concentrated. It contains proteic stabi-lisers, 0-2 mg/ml gentamicin sulphate, 0.1% Kathon GC and 0.01% Cialit as preservatives.
3. **Conjugate diluent:** 1 vial of 16 ml 1 × 8 ml. Proteic buffer solution for the dilution of the

concentrated tracer. It contains 0.2 mg/ml gentamicin sulphate, 0.1% Kathon GC and 0.01% Cialit as preservatives.

4. **Washing solution:** 1 vial of 50 ml 25x concentrated solution to be diluted up to 1250 ml with bidistilled water. It contains phosphate buffer, Tween 20 and 0.1% Kathon GC. The diluted solution, when stored at room temperature, is stable for at least 1 week.
5. **Chromogen:** 1 vial of 8 ml 1 × 4 ml. The solution contains tetramethyl, benzidine (TMB) with activators and stabilisers, diluted in phosphate/citrate buffer.
   Warning: Store protected from light.
6. **Substrate:** 1 vial or 8 ml 1 × 4 ml. The solution contains urea peroxide diluted in phosphate/citrate buffer.
7. **Stop solution:** 1 vial of 12 ml. It contains 1 N HCl.
   Warning: Avoid contact with eyes and skin
8. **Negative control:** 1 vial of 2 ml 1 ×1 ml. Ready-to-use prediluted serum base, not-reactive to anti-HEV antibodies. It contains 0.2 mg/ml gentamicin sulphate and 0.1% Kathon GC as preservatives. Do not dilute again.
9. **Positive control:** 1 vial of 1 ml 1 × 0.5 ml. Ready-to-use predicted serum base, reactive to anti-HEV antibodies. It contains 0.2 mg/ml gentamicin sulphate and 0.1% Kathon GC as preservatives. Do not dilute again.
10. **Sample diluent:** 2 vials of 50 ml 1 × 50 ml. Proteic solution for samples preparation; it contains a detergent, proteic stabilisers, 0.09% sodium azide and 0.1% Kathon GC as preservatives.
11. **Cardboard sealers:** 2 cardboard sealers to be used to cover the plate during the incubations.

Conditions and Notices

1. All the reagents contained in the kit are for *in vitro* diagnostic use only.
2. Do not use the kit or reagents after the expiry date stated on the labels. Do not mix reagents from different lots.
3. Procedures should be performed carefully, in order to obtain reliable results and clinical interpretations.
4. Bring all reagents to room temperature at least 60 minutes before the analysis.
5. Avoid contaminating reagents when taking them from the vials. We recommend to use automatic pipettes with disposable tips. When dispensing reagents, do not touch with tips the wall of wells in order to avoid cross contaminations.
6. For the washing step, use only the washing solution provided in the kit and follow carefully the indications reported at point "washing instruction". It is recommended anyway to use a good quality microplate washer.
7. Avoid the substrate/chromogen to come in contact with oxidising agents or metallic surfaces; avoid intense light exposure during incubation or reagent preparation. When preparing chromogen/substrate, we recommend the use of plastic disposable sterile containers.
8. Samples and materials potentially infected have to be handled with care as they could transmit the infection. All objects come in direct contact with samples and all residuals or the assay should be treated or eliminated as potentially infected. Best procedures for inactivation are treatments with autoclave at 121°C for 30 minutes or with sodium hypochlorite at a final concentration of 2.5% for 24 hours. This last method can be used for treating the liquid washes that have to be neutralised before with sodium hydroxide.
9. Avoid any contact with skin and mucosas, especially with the blocking reagent.
10. In any case, use protective talk-free gloves.

Storage and Stability of the Kit

1. The kit has to be stored at 2 to 8°C and used before the expiry date stated on the label.
2. Unused strips have to be placed in the bag containing the dessicant and firmly seated before re-store at 2 to 8°C. After opening, strips are stable until the dessicant turns pink.
3. The diluted washing solution can be stored for one week at room temperature or 3 weeks at +2 to 8°C.
4. The chromogen/substrate solution is stable for 4 hours at room temperature, protected from light.

5. The diluted conjugate is stable for one week at 2 to 8°C when stored in a sterile disposable container.
6. All other liquid reagents are stable when stored at 2 to 8°C provided that they are handled carefully to avoid any environment contamination.

Materials not Provided in the Kit

1. Semiautomatic pipettes of 10, 200 and 1000 µl.
2. Vortex mixer and absorbent paper.
3. Ultrapure water (bidistilled).
4. Chronometer.
5. Photometric reader of rnicroplates or microstrips, linear up to at least 2 OD and supplied with filters of 450 nm and 620-630 nm.
6. Incubator set at + 37°C.
7. Automatic microplates washing device or manual apparatus capable of aspirating and dispensing volumes of 300 µl.

Samples

Either fresh sera or plasma can be used. If not used immediately, they can be stored at 2 to 8°C for 1 week; in case of longer storage, freeze at –20°C. Avoid repeated freeze-thawing cycles. Samples should be without particles or microbial contaminations; in case, centrifuge at 2000 g for 20 minutes. Highly lipaemic or haemolised samples can give uncorrect analytical results.

Reagents Preparation

1. Washing solution: Dilute 1:25 with bidistilled water and mix carefully before use. Dissolve crystals if present.
2. Conjugate: Dilute 1:20 the concentrated conjugate with its diluent and mix carefully on vortex.
3. Chromogen/substrate: Prepare in disposable plastic container, according to needs, the substrate/chromogen solution by mixing the chromogen with the substrate in equal volumes.

Washing Instruction

A good washing procedure is essential to obtain correct and precise analytical results. We, therefore, recommend to use a good quality ELISA microplate washer, maintained at a good level of washing mechanical performances. Generally, 4-6 automatic washing cycles of 0.3 ml/well are sufficient to avoid false-positive reactions and remove high background. Anyhow, we recommend to calibrate the washing system on the kit itself so to match the declared analytical performances. In case of manual washing, we suggest to perform 5 washing cycles, dispensing and aspirating 0.3 ml/well per cycle, leaving a soak time of 30 sec.between each cycle. In any case the liquid washed out from the plates must be inactivated with a sodium hypochlorite solution at a final concentration of 2.5%, before being thrown away or autoclaved, as it must be considered as potentially infected.

Assay Procedure

1. At least one hour before use, bring all reagents, controls and samples to room temperature (18-30°C), mixing them carefully on vortex.
2. Do not mix reagents from different lots.
3. We recommend to distribute the negative and the cut-off controls in duplicate.
4. Distribution and incubation times must be the same for all wells in the same analysis.
5. Avoid long interruptions between each step of the assay procedure.
6. It is suggested to eliminate the excess of washing solution from the microplate after washing by blotting it gently on an absorbent paper pad.
7. The color developed in the last incubation is stable for a maximum of one hour in the dark.
8. We recommend to read the plate with an ELISA automatic reader able to subtract the background at 620-630 nm and to read the absorbance of samples and standards at 450 nm. The "blanking" of the instrument is to be carried out in the blank reagent well (well A1).
9. In case the assay is processed by an automatic EIA system, we recommend to dilute automatically the sample by aspirating 10 µl sample followed by 1 ml diluent and dispensing all into the appropiate dilution tube. Do not dilute the controls present in the kit as they are prediluted ready to use.

Assay Scheme

Dilute the sample 1:101 with the sample diluent (Ex. 10 µl sample + 1000 pi diluent). Controls are ready-to-use. Do not dilute! Mix carefully on vortex before dispensing.

HEV synthetic antigens=coated wells

Reagents	*A1 Blank*	*Controls*	*Sample*
Standards	-	100 µl	-
Sample	-	-	100 µl
Cover strips with adhesive film			
Incubate 60 min. at + 37°C			
Peel out the adhesive film and aspirate the reaction solution from all wells. Wash 4-5 times with 300 µl of diluted washing solution, carefully aspirating off the remaining liquid			
Diluted conjugate	-	100 µl	100 µl
Cover strips with adhesive film			
Incubate 30 min. at + 37°C			
Peel out the adhesive film and aspirate the reaction solution from all wells. Wash 4-5 times with 300 µl of diluted washing solution, carefully aspirating off the remaning liquid			
Reagerrt Chromogen/ Substrate Mixed 1 :1	100 µl	100 µl	100 µl
Cover strips with a new adhesive film			
Incubate 15 min at room temperature, protected from light			
Stop solution	100 µl	100 µl	100 µl
Read the absorbance of each well against A1 blanking-well at 450 nm, 405 nm and 620-630 nm			

Validity of the Assay

1. The OD 450 nm of the blanking well is lower than 0.100. Higher values indicate a chromogen/substrate contamination. In such a case, repeat the assay carefully checking the reagent.
2. After subtracting the blank, the mean OD value for the negative control is lower than 0.200. Higher values indicate an uncorrect washing procedure; check the efficiency of the washing device.
3. The OD 450 nm of the positive control is higher than 0.800; lower signals are due to uncorrect washing procedure or assay decay.

Calculation of Results

Calculate the mean OD 450 nm values of the negative control (NC), the positive control (PC) and samples. Check for the validity of the assay and then calculate the cut-off value through the following formula:

NC + 0.250 = cut-off

Samples with OD 450 nm values lower than cut-off are to be considered not reactive to anti-HEV antibodies. Samples with OD 450 nm values higher than the cut-off are to be considered reactive to anti-HEV antibodies.

Example of Calculation

Controls	OD
NC	0.050
PC	1.200
Cut-off = NC + 0.250 =	0.300
Sample 1 OD 450 nm = 0.080 negative	
Sample 2 OD 450 nm = 1.158 positive	

Assay Performances

Sensitivity: It has been calculated on a panel of seroconversion and of positive samples by comparing with an FDA-approved reference kit and data show a value better than 98%.

Specificity: It has been calculated as above on panels of negative and positive samples, preclassified with an FDA-approved reference kit. Data show a value better than 98% on plasma and sera.

Reproducibility: It has been calculated on the negative and positive controls ran in replicates in different days. Data show values ranging 4-12% depending on OD 450 nm values.

HEV IgG, Courtesy: Lilac Medicare

Enzyme Immunoassay for the Detection of IgG antibody to Hepatitis E Virus

For *in vitro* diagnostic use only.

Introduction

Hepatitis E virus (HEV) is a recently discovered agent of entencally transmitted non-A, non-B hepatitis. The HEV infection has a worldwide distribution and a predominant waterborne route of transmission. The first reported outbreak of this infection occurred in 1955 in New Delhi; since this time, epidemics of hepatitis E have been documented in many countries (Somalia, Borneo, Pakistan, Mexico).

The HEV shows morphological and biophysical properties similar to viruses found in the family Caliciviridae. The HEV genome consists of a single-stranded RNA molecule that contains 3 open reading frames (ORF 1, ORF 2, ORF 3) that encode for non-structural and structural proteins. Epitope mappings of the viral genome have lead to identify the presence of highly immunoreactive type-common epitopes. Synthetic peptides or recombinant expressed proteins, derived from these regions, have been used to develop enzyme immunoassay for the detection of IgG and IgM antibody. Antibody to HEV of IgM class appears associated to acute stage of infection, while antibody to IgG class characterises previous HEV exposure.

Principle of the Assay

The kit HEV IgG for the detection of antibodies to hepatitis E virus, or HEV, is based on the principle of enzyme-linked immunoassay, or ELISA. The assay is used to determine specific IgG both in sera and plasma. The microplate is activated with HEV specific synthetic peptides from ORF 2 and ORF 3 encoding conservative immunodominant epitopes. In the first incubation solid phase specifically captures the antibodies in the sample. In the following step, an anti-human IgG, labelled with HRP, binds to the immunocomplex formed in solid phase. In the last incubation, the enzyme bound on the plate acts on the substrate generating an optical signal, that can be measured by an ELISA reader.

Content of the Kit and Reagents Preparation

1. **Microtitre strips**: 1 microtitre plate. 12 × 8-wells/6 × 8 -wells/3 × 8-wells/strips activated with synthetic HEV specific peptides. The plate is contained in a sealed bag with dessicant. Bring the plate to room temperature before use, to prevent any moisture formation inside the bag.
2. **Enzyme conjugate**: 1 vial of 0.8 ml/1 × 0.4 ml/1 × 0.2 ml/20 x concentrated solution of goat anti-human IgG, labelled with HRP. It contains proteic stabilisers, 0.2 mg/ml gentamicin sulphate and 0.1% Kathon GC as preservatives.
3. **Conjugate diluent** 1 vial of 16 ml/1 × 8 ml/1 × 4 ml. Proteic buffer solution for the dilution of the concentrated tracer. It contains proteic stabilisers 0.2 mg/ml gentamicin sulphate and 0.1% Kathon GC as preservatives.
4. **Washing solution**: 1 vial of 50 ml 25x concentrated solution to be diluted up to 1250 ml with bidistilled water, containing PBS and detergents.
5. **Chromogen:** 1 vial of 8 ml/1 × 4 ml/1 × 2 ml. The solution contains tetramethyl benzidine (TMB) with activators and stabilisers, diluted in phosphate/citrate buffer.
   Warning: Store protected from light.
6. **Substrate**: 1 vial of 8 ml/1 × 4 ml/1 × 2 ml. The solution contains urea peroxide diluted in phosphate/citrate buffer.
7. **Stop solution:** 1 vial of 12 ml. It contains 1N HCl.
   Warning: The reagent is irritant. Handle with care.
8. **Negative control:** 1 vial of 2 ml /1 × 1 ml /1 × 0.5 ml. Human serum base, nonreactive to anti-HEV, ready to use. It contains 0.2 mg/ml gentamicin sulphate and 0.1% Kathon GC as preservative.
9. **Positive control:** 1 vial of 2 ml/1 × 1 ml/1 × 0.5 ml. Human serum base reactive to anti-HEV IgG (heat inactivated), ready to use. It contains 0.2 mg/ml gentamicin sulphate and 0.1% Kathon GC as preservative. **Warning:** Handle as a potentially infective material.
10. **Sample:** Diluandnt 2 vials of 50 ml.1 × 50 ml/1 × 25 ml. Proteic buffer solution for the dilution of the samples. It contains 0.09% sodium azide and 0.1% Kathon GC as preservative.
11. **Cardboard sealers:** 2 cardboard sealers to be used to cover the plate during incubations.

Conditions and Notices

1. All the reagents contained in the kit are for *in vitro* diagnostic use only.
2. Do not use the kit or reagents after the expiry date stated on the labels. Do not mix reagents from different lots.
3. Procedures should be performed carefully, in order to obtain reliable results and clinical interpretations.

4. Bring all reagents to room temperature at least 60 minutes before the analysis.
5. Avoid contaminating reagents when taking them from the vials. We recommend to use automatic pipettes with disposable tips. When dispensing reagents, do not touch with tips the wall of wells in order to avoid crosscontaminations.
6. For the washing step, use only the washing solution provided in the kit and follow carefully the indications reported at point "washing instruction". It is recommended anyway to use a good quality microplate washer.
7. Avoid the substrate/chromogen to come in contact with oxidising agents or metallic surfaces; avoid intense light exposure during incubation or reagent preparation. When preparing chromogen/substrate, we recommend the use of plastic disposable sterile containers.
8. Samples and materials potentially infected have to be handled with care as they could transmit the infection. All objects come in direct contact with samples and all residuals of the assay should be treated or eliminated as potentially infected. Best procedures for inactivation are treatments with autoclave at 121°C for 30 minutes or with sodium hypochlorite at a final concentration of 2.5% for 24 hours. This last method can be used for treating the liquid washes that have to be neutralised before with sodium hydroxide.
9. Avoid any contact with skin and mucosas, especially with the blocking reagent.
10. In any case, use protective talk-free gloves.

Storage and Stability of the Kit

1. The HEV IgG kit is stable for 12 months when stored at +4°C. The expiration date is printed on the kit package.
2. Unused strips have to be placed in the bag containing the dessicant and firmly sealed before re-store at 2 to 8°C. After opening, strips are stable until the dessicant turns pink.
3. The diluted washing solution can be stored for one week at room temperature or 3 weeks at +2 to 8°C.
4. The chromogen/substrate solution is stable for 4 hours at room temperature, protected from light.
5. The dissolved conjugate is not stable. We suggest to dilute only the quantity necessary to the test.
6. All other liquid reagents are stable when stored at 2 to 8°C, provided that they are handled carefully to avoid any microbial contamination.

Materials not Provided in the Kit

1. Semiautomatic pipettes of 100, 200 and 1000 µl.
2. Vortex mixer and absorbent paper.
3. Ultrapure water (bidistilled).
4. Chronometer.
5. Photometric reader of microplates or microstrips, linear up to at least 2 OD and supplied with filters of 450 nm, 405 nm and 620-630 nm.
6. Incubator set at + 40°C.
7. Automatic microplates washing device or manual apparatus capable of aspirating and dispensing volumes of 300 µl.

Samples

Either fresh sera or plasma can be used, indifferently. If not used immediately, they can be stored at 2 to 8°C for 1 week; in case of any longer storage, freeze at –20°C. Samples should be without particles or microbial contaminations; in case, centrifuge at 2000 g for 20 minutes or filtrate with a 0.2 µ filter. Highly lipaemic or haemolysed samples can give uncorrect analytical results.

Reagents Preparation

1. Washing solution: Before use, dilute 1:25 with bidistilled water and mix carefully before use. The diluted solution can be stored at room temperature.
2. Conjugate: Before use, mix the 20 x concentrated, then dilute 1 20 with the conjugate diluent and mix with care. The diluted solution is not stable, dilute only the amount necessary to the test.
3. Chromogen/substrate: Just before use, mix together the two reagents in equal volumes in a sterile disposable tube. The stability of the mixture is limited, prepare only the volume necessary to the test.

Washing Instruction

A good washing procedure is essential to obtain correct and precise analytical results. We therefore, recommend to use a good quality ELISA microplate washer, maintained at a good level of washing mechanical performances. Generally, 4-5 automatic washing cycles of 0.3 ml/well are sufficient to avoid false-positive reactions and remove high background. Anyhow, we recommend to calibrate the washing system on the kit itself so to match the declared analytical performances eventually adding a soak time between each washing cycle (see manual washing). In case of rnanual washing, we suggest to perform 5 washing cycles, dispensing and aspirating 0.3 ml/well per cycle and leaving a soak time of 30 sec between each cycle. In any case the liquid washed out from the plates must be inactivated with a sodium hypochlorite solution at a final concentration of 2.5%, before being thrown away or autoclaved, as it must be considered as potentially infected.

Assay Procedure

1. At least one hour before use, bring all reagents and samples to room temperature (18-30°C), mixing them carefully on vortex.
2. Do not mix reagents from different lots.
3. We recommend to distribute controls and samples in duplicate.
4. Distribution and incubation times must be the same for all wells in the same analysis.
5. Avoid long interruptions between each step of the assay procedure.
6. It is suggested to eliminate the excess of washing solution from the microplate after washing by blotting it gently on an absorbent paper pad.
7. The colour developed in the last incubation is stable for a maximum of one hour in the dark.
8. We recommend to read the plate with an ELISA automatic reader able to substract the background at 620-630 nm and to read the absorbance of samples and standards at 450 nrn and 405 nm. "Blanking" is carried out on the blank well, A1.

Assay Scheme

1. Dilute samples 1:101 with the sample diluent (e.g. 10 µl sample + 100 µl diluent) and mix on vortex. Controls are ready to use.
2. Follow this scheme:

HEV-coated wells

Reagents	*A1 blank*	*Controls*	*Sample*
Controls	100 µl		
Sample	-	-	100 µl
Cover strips with adhesive film			
Incubate 60 min at + 37°C			
Peel out the adhesive film and aspirate the reaction solution from all wells. Wash 4-5 times with 300 µl of diluted washing solution, carefully aspirating off the remaining liquid.			
Diluted conjugate	-	100 µl	100 µl
Cover strips with adhesive film			
Incubate 60 min. at + 37°C			
Peel out the adhesive film and aspirate the reaction solution from all wells.Wash 4-5 times with 300 µl of diluted washing solution, carefully aspirating off the remaining liquid			
Reagent chromogen/substrate mixed 1:1	100 µl	100 µl	100 µl
Cover strips with a new adhesive film			
Incubate 20 min. at RT, protected from light			
Stop solution	100 µl	100 µl	100 µl
Read the absorbance of each well against A1 blanking-well at 450 nm and 620-630 nm			

Validity of the Assay

The assay is to be considered valid if:

1. The OD 450 nm of the blanking well is lower than 0.100. Higher values indicate a chromogen/substrate contamination. In such a case, repeat the assay carefully checking the reagent.
2. After subtracting the blank, the OD 450 nm value of the negative control is lower than 0.200. Higher values indicate an uncorrect washing procedure. In such a case, check the efficiency of the washing device.
3. The OD 450 nm value of the positive control is higher than 0.800. Lower values indicate kit or controls decay. In such a case, check expiry date of the kit before repeating the assay.

Calculation of Results

Cut-off = Negative control (NC) + 0.250

Samples with OD values higher than cut-off are to be considered positive to HEV.

Samples with OD values lower than cut-off are to be considered negative to HEV

Example of calculation

Controls	OD
NC	0.062
PC	1.600
CO = NC + 0.250	0.312
Sample # 1	0.080 negative
Sample # 2	1.158 positive

Assay Performances

Sensibility: The sensitivity of the assay has been calculated on a panel of seroconversion and of positive samples by comparing with an FDA-approved kit on the market. The test shows a sensitivity > 98%.

Specificity: It has been calculated on panels of negative and positive samples, preclassified with an FDA-approved kit present on the market. The assay shows a specificity > 98% on plasma and sera.

Reproducibility: It has been calculated on the negative and positive controls tested in replicates in different days. CVs between 4-12 % have been obtained depending on their OD 450 nm value.

HEV IGM, Courtesy: Lilac Medicare

Enzyme Immunoassay for the Determination of IgM antibodies to Hepatitis E Virus or HEV IgM

For *"in vitro"* diagnostic use only

Introduction

Hepatitis E virus or HEV is a recently discovered agent of enterically transmitted viral hepatitis. The HEV is a serious problem in many developing countries and its first outbreak was reported in 1955 in New Delhi, India. Hepatitis E has never been associated with chronic infection; however, a high case-fatality rate has been found among pregnant women. The cloning and sequencing of HEV genome have lead to the development of serological tests for the detection of anti-HEV IgG and IgM antibodies. These tests are based on synthetic immunodominant antigens derived from conservative regions of the virus.

Principle of the Assay

Microplates are coated with HEV-specific immunodominant synthetic antigens. The solid phase is first treated with the diluted sample and HEV IgM are captured, if present by the antigens.

After washing out all the other components of the sample, in the 2nd incubation bound HEV IgM are detected by the addition of anti-IgM antibody, labelled with peroxidase (HRP). The enzyme captured on the solid phase, acting on the substrate/ chromogen mixture, generates an optical signal that is proportional to the amount of anti-HEV IgM antibodies present in the sample. Interferences due to IgG and RF in samples are blocked directly into the well by a neutralising reagent.

Test Conditions and Notices

1. All the reagents contained in the kit are for *"in vitro"* diagnostic use only.
2. Do not use the kit or reagents after the expiry date stated on labels. Do not mix reagents of different lots.
3. Procedures should be performed carefully in order to obtain reliable results and clinical interpretations.
4. Bring all the reagents to room temperature for at least 60 min, before the test is started.
5. Avoid any contamination of reagents when taking them out of vials. We recommend to use automatic pipettes and disposable tips. When dispensing reagents, do not touch the wall of microplate wells with tips, in order to avoid any crosscontamination.
6. In the washing procedure, use only the washing solution provided with the kit and follow carefully the indications reported in the "washing instructions" section of this insert .
7. Ensure that the substrate/chromogen mixture does not come in contact with oxidising agents or metallic surfaces; avoid any intense light exposure during the incubation step or the reagent preparation. When preparing the substrate/chromogen mixture for the analysis use only plastic, disposable, clean or sterile containers.
8. Samples and materials potentially infective have to be handled with care as they could transmit infection. All objects come in direct contact with samples and all residuals of the assay should be treated or wasted as potentially infective. Best procedures for inactivation are treatments with autoclave at 121°C for 30 min or with sodium hypochlorite

at a final concentration of 2.5% for 24 hr. This last method can be used for the treatment of the liquid waste after that it has been neutralised with NaOH.

9. Avoid any contact of liquids with skin and mucosas. Use always protective talk-free gloves, glasses and laboratory coats, according to the safety regulations.

Content of the Kit

Strips microplate: 12 × 8 wells strips coated with synthetic HEV antigens. The plate is contained in a sealed bag with dessicant. Bring the plate to room temperature before use, to prevent any moisture formation inside the bag.

Enzyme conjugate: 1 vial of 0.8 ml. Proteic buffer solution containing a specific anti-h IgM antibody, labelled with HRP, 20 x concentrated. It contains proteic stabilisers, 0.2 mg/ml gentamicin sulphate and 0.1% Kathon GC.

Conjugate diluent: 1 vial of 16 ml. Proteic buffered solution for the dilution of the concentrated tracer. It contains proteic stabilisers, 0.2 mg/ml gentamicin sulphate and 0.1% Kathon GC as preservatives.

Washing solution: 1 vial of 50 ml. 25 x concentrated solution to be diluted up to 1250 ml with EIA grade water. It contains a phosphate buffer and Tween 20. The diluted solution, when stored at room temperature, is stable for at least 1 week.

Chromogen: 1 vial of 8 ml. The solution contains tetramethyl benzidine (TMB) with activators and stabilizers, diluted in a phosphate/citrate buffer.
Warning: Store protected from light.

Substrate: 1 vial of 8 ml. The solution contains stabilised hydrogen peroxide diluted in a phosphate/citrate buffer.

Stop solution: 1 vial of 12 ml. It contains a solution of 1N HCl
Warning: Avoid contact with eyes or skin.

Negative control: 1 vial of 2 ml. Human serum base not reactive for anti-HEV antibodies. It contains 0.2 mg/ml gentamicin sulphate and 0.1% Kathon GC as preservatives.

Positive control: 1 vial of 2 ml. Human serum base reactive for HEV IgM. It contains 0.2 mg/ml gentamicin sulphate and 0.1% Kathon GC as preservatives.

Sample diluent: 2 vials of 50 ml. Proteic solution for the preparation of samples. It contains a detergent, proteic stabilisers, 0.09% sodium azide and 0.1% Kathon GC as preservatives.

Neutralizing reagent: 1 vials of 8 ml. Proteic solution for the neutralisation of IgG and RF in samples. It contains a detergent, proteic stabilisers, 0.09% sodium azide and 0.1% Kathon GC as preservatives.

Cardboard sealers: 2. Plastic transparent sealers to cover plates when incubating at + 37°C.

Note: All human serum derived materials have been tested as negative for HBsAg, and HIV antibodies with FDA-approved kits. The positive control has been inactivated for HEV. Anyway, handle this component as potentially infective.

Storage and Stability

1. The kit has to be stored at 2 to 8°C and used before the expiration date declared on the external label.
2. Unused strips have to be returned into their bag containing the dessicant and firmly sealed with, tape before store them back at 2 to 8°C. After the bag has been opened the first time, strips are stable till the dessicant turns pink.
3. The diluted washing solution is stable at room temperature for 1 week or for 3 weeks at 2 to 8° C.
4. The chromogen/substrate mixture is stable for 4 hr at rt when stored protected from light.
5. The diluted conjugate is stable for 1 week at 2 to 8°C, when stored in a sterile disposable container.
6. All the other liquid reagents are stable at 2 to 8°C when handled carefully to avoid contaminations.

Materials not Provided

1. Micropipettes of 10, 100 and 1000 µl.
2. Vortex mixer and adsorbent papers
3. ELISA grade water for dilutions
4. Timer
5. Photometric ELISA reader linear up to at least 2 OD and supplied with filters of 450 nm and 620-630 nm.

6. Incubator set at + 37°C.
7. Automatic microplate washer or manual apparatus capable to deliver 300 µl and aspirate.

Samples

Either fresh sera or plasma can be used for the assay. If not used immediately, they can be stored at 2 to 8°C for 1 week. In case of longer storage freeze them at –30°C. Samples should be clear and not contaminated by microorganisms. Do not freeze and thaw samples more than one time, as IgM may get damaged. If necessary, remove contaminating particles by centrifugation at 2000 g x 20 min at rt or by filtration on 0.22 µ filters. Highly lipaemic, icteric or haemolised samples should not be used as they can give false results in the assay.

Preparation of Reagents

a. **Washing solution:** The concentrated solution has to be diluted 25 x in ELISA grade water before use.
b. **Conjugate:** Dilute the concentrated conjugate 1: 20 with the diluent. Mix gently on vortex before use.
c. **Chromogen/Substrate:** About 5 minutes before use, prepare this reagent in a disposable plastic container, according to needs, by mixing 1 volume of chromogen with 1 volume of substrate.

Washing Instructions

A good washing procedure is essential to obtain correct and precise analytical data. We, therefore, recommend to use a good quality ELISA microplate washer, maintained at the best level of washing performances. Generally, 4-5 automatic washing cycles of 300 µl/well are sufficient to avoid false-positive reactions and high background. Anyhow, we recommend to calibrate the washing system on the kit itself so to match the declared analytical performances, adding in case a soak between each cycle (see manual washing). In case of manual washing, we suggest to carry out 5 cycles, dispensing 300 µl/well and aspirating the liquid for 5 times, leaving a soak time of 30 sec between each cycle. In any case, the liquid aspirated out the strips must be treated with a sodium hypochlorite solution at final concentration of 2.5% for 24 hr, before liquids are wasted in an appropriate way.

Assay Procedure

- At least 1 hr before use, bring all the components of the kit to rt and mix the liquid reagents carefully on vortex.
- Do not mix reagents of different lots.
- We recommend to distribute the calibrators in duplicate.
- Distribution and incubation times should be the same for all the wells. Avoid long interruptions among the different steps of the assay.
- It is suggested to eliminate the excess of washing solution from wells by blotting them gently on a paper adsorbent pad.
- The colour developed in the last incubation is stable for maximum 1 hr in the dark. We recommend to read the microplate at 450 nm (reading filter) and subtract the blank at 620-630 nm (blanking filter). Use well A1 to carry out blanking operations.

1. Leave the A1 well empty for blanking operations. Dilute samples 1 :101 with the sample diluent (10 µl sample + 1000 µl diluent). Do not dilute controls as they are prediluted and ready-to-use. Dispense 50 µl of neutralising reagent in all the wells, but A1 used for blanking. Then dispense controls and samples into wells according to the following table position

Calibrator/sample	
A1	Blanking well
B1+C1	100 µl of negative control
D1	100 µl of positive control
E1 H12 100 µl of samples	

   Cover the microplate with the plate sealer and incubate strips for 60 min at + 37°C.
2. Peel out the plate sealer and wash the microplate according to instructions. In the meantime, prepare the conjugate by diluting it 1:20 as described.
3. Add 100 µl diluted conjugate to all the wells, but A1. Incubate the microplate seated for 60 min at + 37°C.
4. Peel out the plate sealer and wash the microplate according to instructions. In the meantime, prepare the chromogen/substrate mixture as described.

5. Add 100 µl of the chromogen/substrate mixture to all the wells, A1 included. Incubate the microplate for 20 min at rt protected from light.
6. Stop the enzymatic reaction by adding 100 µl stop solution to all the wells, A1 included.

Read the microplate at 450 nm and 620-630 nm blanking the instrument on A1 well.

Validity of the Assay

The assay is considered valid if:

1. The OD 450 nm of the A1 blank well is < 0.100.
2. After blanking on A1, the OD 450 nm mean value of the negative control (NC) is < 0.200.
3. The OD 450 nm mean value of the positive control (PC) is > 0.500.

In case data above do not match the correct values, before repeating the test, check carefully the expiration date of the kit. The performances of the instruments used for the assay and the procedure of distribution of controls and samples.

Calculation of Results

If the validity of the assay is confirmed, calculate the cut-off value through the following formula: NC + 0.250 = cut-off

Samples with an OD 450 nm value lower than the cut-off are classified as negative for HEV IgM. Samples with an OD 450 nm value higher than the cut-off are classified as positive for HEV IgM.

Note: Some false positivity has been reported by Literature for "sandwhich" IgM assays due to very high concentrations of interferents.

Example of Calculation

Negative control mean OD 450 nm	0.050 NC
Positive control OD 450 nm	1.200
Cut-Off = NC + 0.250 = 0300	
Sample # 1 OD 450 nm = 0.080	negative
Sample # 2 OD 450 nm = 1.158	positive

Assay Performances

Sensibility: The sensitivity of the assay has been calculated on a panel of positive samples by comparing with an FDA-approved kit in the market. The test shows a sensitivity > 98%.

Specificity: It has been calculated on panels of negative and positive samples, preclassified with an FDA-approved kit present in the market. The assay shows a specificity > 98% on plasma and sera.

Reproducibility: It has been calculated on the negative and positive controls tested in replicates in different days. CVs between 4-12% have been obtained depending on their OD 450 nm value.

TORCH INFECTIONS
Courtesy: Tulip Group of Companies

Slide Test for Antibodies to *Toxoplasma gondii*

Summary

Toxoplasmosis is an infectious disease caused by the parasite *Toxoplasma gondii* and affects both animals and humans. In humans this infection is usually acquired by ingesting inadequately cooked meat or from feces of infected cats. Approximately 25 to 50% of the adult population are asymptomatically affected with Toxoplasmosis.

Acquired Toxoplasmosis is usually asymptomatic and benign. In pregnant women, however, the infection acquires a special significance as the parasite may enter the fetal circulation throug placenta and cause congenital Toxoplasmosis.

The consequences of congenital Toxoplasmosis range from spontaneous abortion and prematurity to generalised and neurological symptoms. Some infants with congenital Toxoplasmosis may also remain asymptomatic at birth and develop the disease durinc childhood or adolescence.

Reagent

1. Toxogen latex reagent: A uniform suspension of polystyrene latex particles coated with *Toxoplasma gondii* soluble antigens.
2. Positive control, reactive with the Toxogen latex reagent.
3. Negative control, non reactive with the Toxogen latex reagent.

TOXOGEN latex reagent is standardised to detect 10-15 IU/ml or more of *Toxoplasma* antibodies. Each batch of reagents undergoes rigorous quality control at various stages of manufacture for its specificity, sensitivity and performance.

Reagent Storage and Stability

1. Store the reagent at 2 to 8°C. Do not freeze.
2. The shelf life of the reagent is as per the expiry date mentioned on the reagent vial label.

Principle

Latex particles coated with *Toxoplasma gondii* antigens will agglutinate when mixed with serum containing antibodies to *Toxoplasrm gondii.* Agglutination is absent when antibodies to *Toxoplasma gondii* are absent.

Note

1. *In vitro* diagnostic reagent for laboratory and professional use only. Not for medicinal use.
2. All the reagents derived from human source have been tested for HBsAg and antibody to HIV and found to be non reactive. However, handle the material as if infectious.
3. Reagent contains 0.1% Sodium Azide as preservative. Avoid contact with skin and mucosa. On disposal flush with large quantities of water.
4. Shake the latex/reagent vial gently before use to disperse the latex particles uniformly and improve the test readability.
5. Recap the reagent vials immediately after performing the test.
6. Use only a clean and dry glass slide. Clean the slide with distilled water and wipe dry before use.
7. Accessories provided with the kit only must be used for optimum results.
8. The positive control is pre-diluted and ready to use.

Specimen Collection and Storage

No special preparation of the patient is required prior to sample collection by approved techniques. Fresh serum should be used for testing. In case of delay in testing, store the sample at 2 to 8°C for upto 48 hours.

MATERIAL PROVIDED WITH THE KIT

Reagent Pack

Toxoplasma gondii latex reagent, Positive control, Negative control.

Accessories Pack

Glass slide with six reaction circles, Mixing sticks, Rubber teats, Sample dispensing pipettes.

Additional Material Required

Test tubes (10 × 75 mm), Pipettes, Isotonic saline, Stop watch, Direct light source, 5% 2-Mercaptoethanol solution.

Test Procedure

Bring reagent and samples to room temperature before use. Dilute sample to be tested 1: 16 with 0.9% saline (0.1 ml of serum+1.5 ml of 0.9% saline).

Qualitative Method

1. Place one drop of diluted serum on the reaction circle of the glass slide using a disposable pipette provided with the kit.
2. Add one drop of well mixed latex reagent to the drop of diluted serum sample.
3. Using a mixing stick, mix the sample and the latex reagent uniformly over the entire circle.
4. Immediately start a stopwatch. Rock the slide gently back and forth. Observe for agglutination macroscopically at five minutes.

Semi Quantitative Method

1. Using isotonic saline, prepare serial dilutions of the serum samples positive in the qualitative method starting frorn 1:32, 1:64, 1:128, 1:256 and so on.
2. Pipette each dilution of the serum sample onto separate reaction circles of the slide.
3. Add one drop of well mixed latex reagent to each dilution of the serum sample.
4. Using a mixing stick, mix the sample and the latex reagent uniformly over the entire circle.
5. Immediately, starta stopwatch. Rock the slide gently back and forth. Observe for agglutination macroscopically at five minutes.

INTERPRETATIONS OF RESULTS

Qualitative Method

Agglutination is a positive test result and indicates presence of diagnostically significant level of antibodies to *Toxoplasma gondii.* No agglutination is a negative test result and indicates absence of diagnostically significant level of antibodies to *Toxoplasma gondii.*

Semi Quantitative Method

The highest dilution of serum showing agglutination corresponds to the titre of antibodies to *Toxoplasma gondii*.

Differentiation IgG - IgM

By previous treatment of the sera with reducing agents, such as 2-mercaptoethanol, it is possible to observe the type of immunoglobulins responsible for the reaction.

Add 50 µl of the 2-mercaptoethanol solution to 1 ml of 1:16 diluted serum under test. Incubate for 60 minutes at 37°C.

At the end of the incubation period, proceed using the semi quantitative test procedure as outlined above.

When antibody titre drops 2 or more dilutions after mercaptoethanol treatment, it can be considered IgM positive.

Significance of Test Results

a. Serum samples that test negative in 1:16 dilution indicate absence of diagnostically significant anti toxoplasma titre.
b. Serum samples positive at 1:16 dilution indicate residual titre due to past exposure.
c. Positive titres from 1:32 -1:128 dilution should be suspect of incipient toxoplasmosis. Evolution of titre 3 weeks later should be determined. Increase of atleast two dilutions should be considered indicative of acute toxoplasmosis.
d. Titre of 1:256 or more suggest possible active infection.
e. Determination of IgM antibodies is also advisable in (c) and (d) cases.

Remarks

1. Markedly lipaemic, haemolysed and contaminated serum samples could give rise to non-specific result.
2. Use of plasma rather than serum can lead to false positive results.
3. Positive and negative controls should be run with each series of tests to validate the results.
4. It is recommended that results of the tests should be correlated with clinical findings to arrive at the final diagnosis.

TORCH INFECTIONS—INTRODUCTION

Toxoplasma Infection

Toxoplasma gondii is an obligate intracellular protozoan parasite that is probably capable of infecting all species of mammals, including man. The detection of IgM antibodies to *T. gondii* is particularly helpful for the diagnosis of acute/primary infections in "risk" individuals in association with AIDS, organ transplantation and pregnancy. As most of Toxoplasma infections are mild or asymptomatic in otherwise healthy individuals, the detection of *T. gondii*-specific IgM, in absence of detectable specific IgG, has become important for the monitoring of primary infections in pregnant women, as the parasite can lead to birth defects. Moreover, as *T. gondii* infections are most severe in immunocompromised patients, where the disease can be fatal, acute infections due to this parasite have to be distinguished from other disorders. Recently developed, IgM capture assays provide the clinician with a helpful and reliable test, not affected by rheumatoid factor.

Rubella Infection

Infection with Rubella virus in children and adults is a self-limited, mild disease characterized by an erythematous rash, mild upper respiratory symptoms and suboccipital lymphadenopathy. After recovery, the individual is immune to subsequent infection with rubella virus. Primary infection of a pregnant woman, however, particularly in the first trimester of pregnancy, may result in a high risk of fetal infection with severe complications. Congenital Rubella is characterized by cataracts, deafness, congenital heart disease and other malformations which may occur singularly or in combination (1). It is extremely important therefore, to identify those women who are not immune to rubella and to immunize them well before they become pregnant. This can be achieved by screening the serum for the presence of antibodies to Rubella and a positive result is indicative of immunity. The ELISA has been shown to be a sensitive and reliable procedure for detection of antibodies to Rubella.

Cytomegalovirus Infection

Cytomegalovirus (CMV) infections are widespread and approximately half of the adult population have antibodies to CMV. The majority of CMV infections are asymptomatic but CMV infections can cause serious disease in the newborn infant and the immunocompromised individual. About 2% of pregnant women have either a primary or a reactivated CMV infection during pregnancy and it is estimated that 10 to 20% of congenitally infected newborns will show evidence of disease. Clinical symptoms may range from severe disease with jaundice, hepatosplenomegaly, and central nervous system inolvement, to asymptomatic infants who will, however, later develop hearing defects. CMV infections are frequent in individuals with deficient cellular immunity such as cancer patients or person with Acquired Immunodeficiency Syndrome, or those receiving immunosuppresive agents. The detection of antibodies against CMV may be of value as an aid in the diagnosis and in determining the immune status of the patient. Various procedures such as complement fixation, indirect hemagglutination, and indirect immunofluorescent assay have been used to detect CMV antibody. More recently, the enzyme-linked immunosorbent assay (ELISA) has been developed and utilised for serological detection of CMV.

Herpes Simplex Virus (1 + 2) Infections

Herpes Simplex Virus types 1 (HSV-1) and 2 (HSV-2) are large complex DNA-containing viruses which have been shown to induce during infection the synthesis of several proteins, possessing an high number of crossreactive determinants and just a few of type-specific sequences. The majority of primary genital herpes infections and recurrent genital herpes infections are caused by HSV-2. Nongenital herpes infections such as common cold sores are caused primarily by HSV-1. The detection of virus-specific IgM antibodies is important In the diagnosis of acute/primary virus infections or reactivation of a latent one, in the absence of evident clinical symptoms, Asymptomatic infections may happen for HSVrin apparently of healthy individuals and during pregnancy. Severe herpes infections may happen in immunosuppressed or immunocompromised patients. Recently developed, IgM enzyme-immunoassays provide the clinician with a helpful and reliable diagnostic test for the monitoring of "risk" population.

TORCH SCREEN EIA KIT
Courtesy: Lilac Medicare

Enzyme Immunoassay (EIA) procedure for the determination of IgM Antibodies to TORCH infections (*Toxoplasma gondii,* Rubella Virus, Cytomegalovirus and Herpes Simplex Virus respectively). *For in Vitro Diagnostic Use Only.*

Introduction

TORCH is an acronym for Toxoplasmosis, Rubella, Cytomegalovirus and Herpes Simplex Virus. *Toxoplasma gondii* is an obligate parasite infecting a wide variety of birds and mammals including man. Infection is passed through contact with contaminated cat feces or eating raw or uncooked meat. Infection can be passed transplacently or via organ and blood products.

Rubella is an acute viral infection of children and adults that characteristically include rash, fever and resembles a mild attack of measles. Infection during pregnancy particularly the first trimester, can result in fetal death or severe anatomical deformity and mental retardation. Therefore, early detection of Rubella infection is extremely important.

Cytomegalovirus (CMV) is a member of the beta herpesvirus group and causes similar disease in various animals. All are associated with the production of enlarged cells—hence, the name Cytomegalovials. Infection can spread through aerosol, sexual intercourse, blood and organ products.

Herpes Simplex Virus (HSV-1 and HSV-2) produce a variety of infections involving mucocutaneous surfaces, the central nervous system (CNS), and on occasion visceral organs. Infection is acquired through close contact with the carrier or through sexual transmission. Both viral subtypes can cause genital and orofacial infections, and the infection caused by the two subtypes are clinically indistinguishable. However, the frequency of reactivation of infection is influenced by the by the anatomic site and the virus subtype.

Principle of the EIA Test

TORCH antigens (*Toxoplasma*, Rubella, Cytomegalovirus and Herpes Simplex Virus) are fixed separately to the interior surface of respective microwells strips (separate strips for *Toxoplasma*, Rubella, Cytomegalovirus and Herpes Simplex Virus). Patient's serum is added and any antibody present to respective

TORCH antigens will bind to these antigens in the specific microwells.

The microwells are washed to remove unbound serum proteins. Antibodies conjugated with Horseradish Peroxidase enzyme and directed against human IgM are added and will in turn bind to any human IgM present.

The microwells are washed to remove unbound conjugate and then chromogen/substrate is added. In the presence of peroxidase enzyme the colourless substrate is hydrolysed to a coloured end-product. The colour intensity is proportional to the amount of antibodies present in the patient's serum.

Components

Each kit contains sufficient reagents to perform 24 tests of individual TORCH analytes.

1. Antigen coated microwell: 12 colour coded microwell strips, 3 strips (8 wells × strips) each of *Toxoplasma* (Blue band), Rubella (Red band), Cytomegalovirus (Green band) and Herpes Simplex Virus (Black band) respectively in a flexible bag with desiccant. (Allow the microwells to reach room temperature before opening; reseal unused microwells in the bag with desiccant and store at 4°C).
2. Negative control: 1 × 2.0 ml/vial. Ready to use. AI Value 0.3. Contains serum proteins and Thimerosal as preservative.
3. Low Positive Standard (Cut-Off): 1 × 1.0 ml/vial each for *Toxoplasma*, Rubella, Cytomegalovirus and Herpes Simplex Virus. Ready to use. AI Value = 1.0. Contains serum proteins and Thimerosal as preservative.
4. High Positive Standard 1 × 1.0 ml/vial each for *Toxoplasma*, Rubella, Cytomegalovirus and Herpes Simplex Virus. Ready to use. AI Value reported on the label of the vial. Contains serum proteins and Thimerosal as preservative.
5. Serum Diluent: 2 × 50 ml/bottles. Ready to use. Contains PBS/Tween and protein stabilizers and absorbent solution for correcting intererence due to RF and IgG.
6. Wash buffer concentrate: 1 × 50 ml/bottle × 20 concentrate. Contains PBS/Tween (Dilute to 1 liter with distilled water before use).Once diluted, the wash solution is stable for 1 month at 4 to 8°C. or 1 week at room temperature.
7. Enzyme conjugate: 1 × 6 ml/vial combi conjugate for *Toxoplasma* IgM and CMV IgM, 1 × 4 ml/vial for Rub IgM, 1 × 4 ml/vial conjugate for HSV IgM. Ready to use. Horseradish peroxidase conjugated goat anti-human IgM (FC μ chain specific).
8. 1 MB Substrate solution: 1 × 12 ml/vial TMB combi for Toxo IgM and Rub IgM, 1 × 12 ml/vial TMB combi for CMV IgM and HSV IgM.
9. Stop solution: 1 × 12 ml/vial. Contains 1N HCl solution.
   Warning: Avoid contact with eyes or skin.
10. Instruction manual.
11. Graph paper to prepare standard curve.

Material Required but not Provided

1. 10 ul and 100 ul micropipettes.
2. Test tubes for sample dilution.
3. Disposable pipettes graduated for dispensing 1 ml.
4. Distilled or deionized water.
5. Wash bottle.
6. Timer with 60 minute range.
7. Absorbent paper.
8. Microwell reader with 450 nm filter.

Precautions

1. Upon receipt, store the kit at 2°-8°C.
2. Do not interchange components between different kits.
3. When using the kit check that the reagent solutions are clear. Any cloudiness or odor is indicative of contamination.
4. Avoid cross-contamination between serum specimens.
5. Avoid cross-contamination between conjugate and substrate.
6. Do not use the kit after the expiration date.
7. Treat all specimens and kit reagents as potentially infectious. Although the human sera utilised in preparing the kit reagents have been tested and found to be negative to Hepatitis B and to HIV, there is no testmethod available that can offer complete assurance that hepatitis B virus, HIV or other infectious agents are absert. Therefore, all human serum specimens and kit reagents should be handled at the Biosafety Level 2 as recommended by the Centers for Disease Control/US. Institutes of Health publication "Biosafety in Microbiological and Biomedical Laboratories", 1984.

8. Never pipette by mouth, and use gloves when handling human blood or serum specimens and other potentially infectious materials.
9. The use of disposable glass or plastic-ware is recommended in order to avoid contamination.
10. The wash solutions and reagents utilised in the assay should be discarded into a disinfectant solution such as sodium hypochlorite (i.e. 50 ml household bleach in 950 ml water) before disposal. Other materials should be treated as biohazard waste and also disposed according to recommended procedures.

Specimen Preparation

Aseptically draw blood by venipuncture and collect the serum using standard techniques. Avoid using haemolysed or hyperlipaemic sera which may give erroneous results. Serum specimens can be stored at 2°C to 8°C for up to five days after collection. For longer periods the specimen should be stored frozen. Avoid preservatives, particularly sodium azide which will inhibit the enzyme reaction.

Assay Procedure

1. Place the required number of respective Microwells in the microwell holder. Mark one end of each strip for orientation.
2. Dilute the samples 1:100 with Serum Diluent (10ul serum to 1ml serum diluent). Do not dilute the calibrators. They are ready for use. Incubate the diluted samples for 30' at room temperature.
3. Pipette 100 ul of specific negative control, low positive standard (cut-off), high positive standard and serum specimens in respective wells.
4. Incubate at room temperature (23-25°C) for 15 minutes (30 minutes for Rubella IgM).
5. Wash microwells by inverting and flicking into a sink. Completely fill with wash buffer and repeat washes × 3. Refill with Wash buffer and soak for 5 minutes. Empty wells and blot with absorbent paper. Repeat wasing 5 times without soak.
6. Pipette 100 ul of respective enzyme conjugate into each well.
7. Incubate at room temperature (23-25°C) for 15 minutes (30 minutes for Rubella IgM).
8. Wash microwells as in step 5.
9. Pipette 100 ul 1 MB substrate in each well.
10. Incubate at room temperature (23-25°C) for 10 minutes.
11. Pipette 100 ul stop solution into each well using the same pipetting sequence as in step 9 and 10.
12. Measure the colour intensity of the solution in each well using a microwell reader with a 450 nm filter (referencing at 630 nm). (Before reading carefully wipe the exterior of the wells and check that there is no residue or scratches that may give erroneous readings).
13. Prepare the standard curve and calculate results.

Quality Control

Each time the assay is run the Positive Standards should be run in duplicate. The mean OD values should fall within the following ranges:

	OD Range
Negative control	< 0.250
Low positive standard	> 0.300
High positive standard	> 0.500

Results

The results are reported as Activity Index Values. The AI compares the binding activity (positivity) of the test sample to the cut-off level of activity that is defined as positive (Activity Index Value=1.0).

Calculation

Graph the absorbance readings of the calibrators against the assigned Activity Index Value listed on the vials using semilog graph paper.

Table 1

Samples	*OD at 450 nm*	*Result*
Neg. Ctrl.	0.100	(To prepare the curve)
Low Pos.Std.	0.500	(To prepare the curve)
High Pos. Std.	1,100	(To prepare the curve)
Patient 1	0.337	< 1.0AI
Patient 2	1,000	3.3AI

Reporting Results

The Activity Index Values (AI) of the controls and the serum samples are read from the standard curve prepared for each run. Check that the values of the negative control and positive calibrator are within limits listed in the QC before reporting out the test results as Activity Index (AI) (Fig. 23.37).

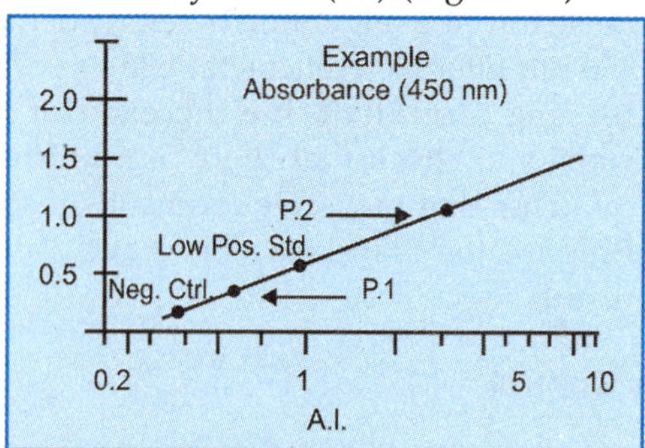

Fig. 23.37: Result reporting

Interpretation of Results

AI	Interpretation
< 0.90	Negative
0.91-1.10	Equivocal
> 1.1	Positive

1. A negative result indicates that there is no recent or current infection with TORCH agent. Samples taken too early in the course of a primary infection with TORCH may not have detectable levels of IgM-specific antibody.
2. A positive result indicates that there is a recent infection with TORCH. Low levels of TORCH-specific IgM antibodies may be detectable for up to one year following primary infection in some patients. In other patients IgM specific antibody titres may revert to negative levels within three weeks after infection.
3. Specimens showing equivocal results must be retested: if they remain equivocal after repeat testing they should be tested by an alternate serologic procedure.

Note: Serological assays alone can only determine past exposure to the TORCH and should not be used as the sole basis for a diagnosis of recent or current infection. All other appropriate clinical findings and laboratory data must be considered in order to establish a diagnosis.

Performance Characteristics

Linearity

Dilution of serum tested

	1:100	1:200	1:400
Serum A	2.4	1.2	
Serum B	1.8	0.9	-
Serum C	4.0	2.1	1.2

Evaluation of Intra-Assay Variation

	Mean (AI) Value	CV
Serum A	3.3	6.8%
Serum B	1.4	10.1%
Serum C	1.9	7.2%

TORCH SCREEN IgG EIA KIT
Courtesy: Lilac Medicare

Intended Use

Enzyme Immunoassay (EIA) procedure for the determination of IgG Antibodies to TORCH infections (*Toxoplasma gondii,* Rubella Virus, Cytomegalovirus and Herpes Simplex Virus respectively). *For in Vitro Diagnostic Use Only.*

Introduction

TORCH is an acronym for Toxoplasmosis, Rubella, Cytomegalovirus and Herpes Simplex Virus. *Toxoplasma gondii* is an obligate parasite infecting a wide variety of birds and mammals including man. Infection is passed through contact with contaminated cat feces or eating raw or uncooked meat. Infection can be passed transplacently or via organ and blood products.

Rubella is an acute viral infection of children and adults that characteristically include rash, fever and resembles a mild attack of measles. Infection during pregnancy particularly the first trimester, can result in fetal death or severe anatomical deformity and mental retardation. Therefore, early detection of Rubella infection is extremely important.

Cytomegalovirus (CMV) is a member of the beta herpesvirus group and causes similar disease in various animals. All are associated with the production of enlarged cells—hence the name Cytomegalovirus. Infection can spread through aerosol, sexual intercourse, blood and organ products.

Herpes Simplex Virus (HSV-1 and HSV-2) produce a variety of infections involving mucocutaneous surfaces, the central nervous system (CMS), and on occasion visceral organs. Infection is acquired through close contact with the carrier or through sexual transmission. Both viral subtypes can cause genital and orofacial infections, and the infection caused by the two subtypes are clinically indistinguishable. However, the frequency of reactivation of infection is influenced by the by the anatomic site and the virus subtype.

Principle of the EIA Test

TORCH antigens (*Toxoplasma*, Rubella, Cytomegalovirus and Herpes Simplex Virus) are fixed separately to the interior surface of respective microwell strips (separate strips for *Toxoplasma*, Rubella, Cytomegatovirus and Herpes Simplex Virus).

Patient's serum is added and any antibody present to respective TORCH antigens will bind to these antigens in the specific microwells.

The microwells are washed to remove unbound serum proteins. Antibodies conjugated with Horseradish Peroxidase enzyme and directed against human IgG are added and will in turn bind to any human IgG present.

The microwells are washed to remove unbound conjugate and then chromogen/substrate is added. In the presence of peroxidase enzyme the colourless substrate is hydrolysed to a coloured end-product. The colour intensity is proportional to the amount of antibodies present in the patient's serum.

Components

Each kit contains sufficient reagents to perform 24 tests of individual TORCH analytes.

1. *Antigen coated microwell:* 12 colour coded microwell strips, 3 each of *Toxoplasma* (Blue band). Rubella (Red band), Cytomegalovirus (Green band) and Herpes Simplex Virus (Black band) respectively in a flexible bag with desiccant. (Allow the microwells to reach room temperature before opening; reseal unused microwells in the bag with desiccant and store at 4°C).
2. *Negative control*: 1 × 2.0 ml/vial. Ready to use. AI Value = 0.3. Contains serum proteins and thimerosal as preservative.
3. *Low positive standard (Cut-Off)* :1 × 1.0 ml/vial each for *Toxoplasma*, Rubella, Cytomegalovirus and Herpes Simplex Virus. Ready to use. AI Value = 1.0. Contains serum proteins and Thimerosal as preservative. (*)
4. *High positive standard:* 1 x 1.0 ml/vial each for *Toxoplasma*, Rubella, Cytomegalovirus and Herpes Simplex Virus. Ready to use. AI Value reported on the label of the vial. Contains serum proteins and Thimerosal as preservative. (*)
5. *Serum diluent:* 2 × 50 ml/bottles. Ready to use. Contains PBS/Tween and protein stabilizers.
6. *Wash buffer concentrate:* 1 × 50 ml/bottle × 20 concentrate. Contains PBS/Tween (Dilute to 1 liter with distilled water before use). Once diluted, the wash solution is stable for 1 month at 4-8° C. or 1 week at room temperature.
7. *Enzyme conjugate:* 1 × 12 ml/vial combi conjugate for *Toxoplasma* IgG and HSV IgG, CMV IgG and Rubella IgG. Ready to use. Horseradish peroxidase conjugated goat anti-human IgG (FC g chain specific).
8. *TMB substrate solution:* 1 × 12 ml/vial. TMB.
9. *Stop solution:* 1 × 12 ml/vial. Contains 1N HCl solution.
   Warning: Avoid contact with eyes or skin.
10. *Instruction manual.*
11. *Graph paper* to prepare standard curve.
    (*) The reference sera for *Toxoplasma* IgG and Rubella IgG are standardized against the WHO 3rd Reference Preparation,1994.

Material Required but not Provided

1. 10 ul and 100 ul micropipettes.
2. Test tubes for sample dilution.
3. Disposable pipettes graduated for dispensing 1 ml.
4. Distilled or deionized water.
5. Wash bottle.
6. Timer with 60 minute range.
7. Absorbent paper.
8. Microwell reader with 450 nm filter.

Precautions

1. Upon receipt, store the kit at 2 to 8° C.
2. Do not interchange components between different kits.
3. When using the kit check that the reagent solutions are clear. Any cloudiness or odor is indicative of contamination.
4. Avoid cross-contamination between serum specimens.
5. Avoid cross-contamination between conjugate and substrate.

6. Do not use the kit after the expiration date.
7. Treat all specimens and kit reagents as potentially infectious. Although the human sera utilised in preparing the kit reagents have been tested and found to be negative to Hepatitis B and negative to HIV, there is no test method available that can offer complete assurance that Hepatitis B virus, HIV or other infectious agents are absent. Therefore, all human serum specimens and kit reagents should be handled at the Biosafety Level 2 as recommended by the Centers for Disease Control/U.S. Institutes of Health publication "Biosafety in Microbiological and Biomedical Laboratories", 1984.
8. Never pipette by mouth and use gloves when handling human blood or serum specimens and other potentially infectious materials.
9. The use of disposable glass or plastic-ware is raccommended in order to avoid contamination.
10. The wash solutions and reagents utilised in the assay should be discarded into a disinfectant solution such as sodium hypochlorite (i.e. 50 ml household bleach in 950 ml water) before disposal. Other materials should be treated as biohazard waste and also disposed according to recommended procedures.

Specimen Preparation

Aseptically draw blood by venipuncture and collect the serum using standard techniques. Avoid using hemolysed or hyperlipemic sera which may give erroneous results. Serum specimens can be stored at 2°C to 8°C for up to five days after collection. For longer periods the specimen should be stored frozen. Avoid preservatives, particularly sodium azide which will inhibit the enzyme reaction.

Assay Procedure

1. Place the required number of respective Microwells in the microwell holder. Mark one end of each strip for orientation.
2. Dilute the samples 1:100 with Serum Diluent (10 ul serum to 1 ml serum diluent). Do not dilute the standards. They are ready for use.
3. Pipette 100 ul of the specific serum standards and serum specimens in respective wells.
4. Incubate at room temperature (23-25°C) for 15 minutes.
5. Wash microwells by inverting and flicking into a sink. Completely fill with wash buffer and repeat washes × 3. Refill with wash buffer and soak for 5 minutes. Empty wells and blot with absorbent paper. Wash 5 times without soak.
6. Pipette 100 ul respective Enzyme Conjugate into each well.
7. Incubate at room temperature (23-25°C) for 15 minutes.
8. Wash microwells as in step 5.
9. Pipette 100 ul TMB Substrate in each well.
10. Incubate at room temperature (23-25°C) for 5 minutes.
11. Pipette 100 ul Stop Solution into each well using the same pipetting sequence as in step 9.
12. Measure the colour intensity of the solution in each well using a microwell reader with a 450 nm filter (referencing at 630 nm). (Before reading carefully wipe the exterior of the wells and check that there is no residue or scratches that may give erroneous readings).
13. Prepare the standard curve and calculate results.

Quality Control

Each time the assay is run the Positive Standards should be run in duplicate. The mean OD values for the Standards should fall within the following ranges.

	OD Range
Negative control	< 0.250
Low positive standard	> 0.300
High positive standard	> 0.500

Results

The results are reported as Activity Index Values. The AI compares the binding activity (positivity) of the test sample to the cut-off level of activity that is defined as positive (Activity Index Value = 1.0). It is possible to convert the Activity Index into International Units multiplying it by a Conversion Factor (*Toxoplasma* = 12.5 and Rubella = 10.0).

Calculation

Graph the absorbance readings of the standards against the assigned Activity Index value listed on the vials using semilog graph paper and trace the curve.

Table 1

Samples	*OD 450 nm*	*at Result*
Neg. Ctrl. (AI 0.3)	0.100	
LowPos. Std. (AI 1.0)	0.500	(To prepare the curve)
High Pos. (AI 6.5)	1.300	(To prepare the curve)
Patient 1	0.337	< 1.0AI
Patient 2	1.000	3.3 A I.

Reporting Results

The Activity Index Values (AI) of the controls and the serum samples are read from the standard curve prepared for each run. Check that the values of the negative control and positive calibrators are within limits listed in the QC (Fig. 23.38).

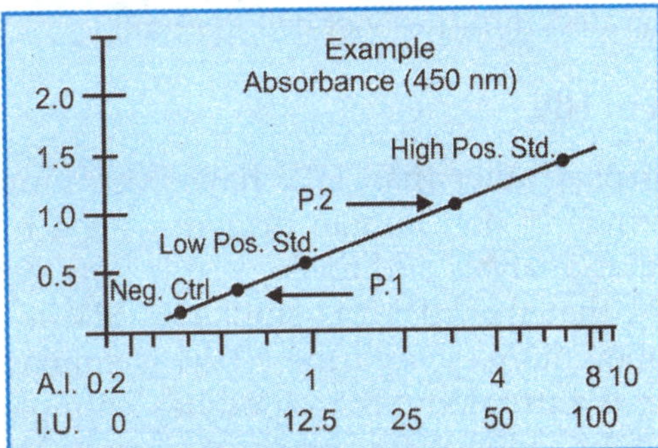

Fig. 23.38: Result reporting

Interpretation of Results

AI	Interpretation
< 0.9	Negative
0.91 -1.10	Equivocal
> 1.1	Positive

1. A negative result indicates that there was no prior exposure to the TORCH agents. These individuals are presumed to be susceptible to a primary infection.
   A negative result, however, does not rule out the possibility of recent infection with the serum being tested before the appearance of IgG antibodies. If recent infection is suspected it is recommended that:
   a. The serum sample be tested for the IgM antibodies.
   b. A second sample taken 1 to 2 weeks later be tested for IgG antibodies to see if seroconversion has occurred.
2. A positive result indicates that there was prior exposure at some undetermined time to the TORCH agent. A highly positive result may indicate acute or recent disease.
3. Specimens showing equivocal results must be retested: if they remain equivocal after repeat testing they should be tested by an alternate serologic procedure.

Note: Serological assays alone can only determine past exposure to the TORCH agent and should not be used as the sole basis for a diagnosis of recent or current infection. All the other appropriate clinical findings and laboratory data must be considered in order to establish a diagnosis.

PERFORMANCE CHARACTERISTICS

Linearity

Serial twofold dilutions of positive sera tested in this assay when plotted against Activity Index Values (serial dilution) on the X-axis (log-scale) gave absorbance values that showed a linear correlation indicating that it was possible to obtain an accurate quantitation of specific antibody present by testing serum at a single dilution. The results obtained when sera tested at different dilutions are shown in Table 2

Dilution of Serum Tested

	1:100	*1:200*	*1:400*	*1:800*
Serum A	4.5	2.2	0.8	
Serum B	2.7	1.0	0.7	-
Serum C	3.8	1.9	1.1	0.8
Serum D	2.8	1.2	0.8	
Serum E	1.8	1.0	10.8	-

Linerity Dilution Test

Table 3 (data listed in OP values)

Dilution	*Expected Values 425*	*Found Values*
1:2	0.712	0.695
1:4	0.356	0.410
1:8	0.178	0.244
1:16	0.089	0.151
1:32	0.044	0.091

Y = 0.8914X + 0.0723 ; r = 0.998; Seriel = Expected Values; Serie 2 = Found Values.

HUMAN IMMUNODEFICIECNY VIRUS

Since its recognition in 1981, the HIV pandemic has spread unabated across continents. The catastrophic potential of the pandemic may still not have been fully realized as it continues to exact enormous toll throughout the world in both human and economic terms.

The demographic characteristics of those affected by the epidemic has changed drastically since the first cases were reported in the year 1981 in the USA comprising overwhelmingly of gay population. Today new cases of HIV infection originate predominantly through heterosexual contacts and injecting drug users. The infection rates amongst women, adolescent girls and children have increased dramatically. It is estimated that in the year 2001 a total of 40 million people worldwide were living with HIV/AIDS and in the year 2001 it is estimated that at least 5 million people were infected with HIV and at least 3 million people perished due to the disease.

The epidemic has negated decades worth of work on controlling diseases, improving nutrition and in many African countries it has become an unprecedented emergency with approximately 25% of the most productive age group between 15 years to 49 years being infected.

It is estimated that in sub-Saharan Africa the life expectancy would reduce from average 64 years to 47 years. If the present warning of epidemiologists go unheeded, South Asia, South East Asia and China may follow the disastrous course of sub-Saharan Africa. The battle against AIDS has to be fought on multiple fronts such as education, counselling, prevention of infection, voluntary testing, treatment and vaccination programmes.

HIV Virus

The HIV-1 and HIV-2 belong to the retrovirus family, sub family lentivirinae. Both retroviruses are so named because one step of their replication cycle is the creation of DNA copy of their RNA genome. The genetic information of a retrovirus therefore flows from RNA to DNA at this step, which is in the opposite direction of the flow in most biological systems. HIV is a lipid enveloped positive stranded RNA virus like all Retroviruses.

RNA viruses are distinguished by the possession of an enzyme viral reverse transcriptase that transcribes the viral RNA into provirus DNA which is integrated into the host cell genome.

People infected with HIV in 2001	Total	5 Million
	Adults	4.3 Million
	Women	1.8 Million
	Children < 15 years	800,000
	Total	40 Million
No. of people living with HIV/AIDS	Adults	37.2 Million
	Women	17.6 Million
	Children < 15 years	2.7 Million
	Total	3 Million
AIDS deaths in 2001	Adults	2.4 Million
	Women	1.1 Million
	Children < 15 years	580,000
	Total	21.8 Million
Total no. of AIDS deaths since the beginning of the epidemic until 2001	Adults	17.5 Million
	Women	9 Million
	Children < 15 years	4.3 Million
Total no. of AIDS orphans since the beginning of the epidemic until 2001	Total	13.2 Million

Fig. 23.39: Summary of the HIV/AIDS epidemic, December 2001

Origin of HIV

Lentiviruses other than HIV have been found in a wide range of non human primates. As a result of molecular analysis and analogy, it is now generally thought that the HIV-2 is similar to SIVsm (Sooty mangabey monkey) and the HIV-1 is similar to the SIVcpz (Pantroglodytes troglodytes chimpanzees), indigenous to the West and West Central Africa.

It is postulated that through Zoonosis these viruses at some point of time crossed over to the humans.

The HIV Virion

The mature HIV-1 virion measures approximately 100 nm in diameter. The HIV-1 genome consists of two identical, noncomplementary sense (+) strands of RNA, each approximately 9.2 kb long, packaged in a cone-shaped protein core, composed of 24kDa capsid (CA) proteins (p24), surrounded by a unique bilayer envelope derived from the host cell membrane. The viral enzymes, Reverse Transcriptase, integrase and protease are packaged with the RNA in the core. The surface (SU) and transmembrane (TM) glycoproteins, gp 120 and gp 41 respectively, form a noncovalent complex. Also incorporated into the envelope are various host proteins including HLA class I and II DR molecules.

Regional HIV/AIDS Statistics, December 2000

Region	Epidemic started	Adults and children living infected with HIV/AIDS (million)	Adults and children newly infected with HIV (million)	Percent Adults prevalence rate	Percent of HIV positive adults who are women	Main mode(s) of transmission for adults living with HIV/AIDS
Sub Saharan Africa	Late 70's Early 80's	28.1	3.4	8.4	55	HTS
North Africa and the Middle East	Late 80's	0.44	0.080	0.2	40	HTS, IDU
South and South East Asia	Late 80's	6.1	0.8	0.6	35	HTS, IDU
East Asia and Pacific	Late 80's	1.0	0.27	0.1	20	IDU, HTS, HMS
Latin America	Late 70's Early 80's	1.4	0.13	0.5	30	IDU, HMS, HTS
Caribbean	Late 70's Early 80's	0.42	0.06	2.2	50	HTS, HMS
Eastern Europe and Central Asia	Early 90's	1.0	0.25	0.5	20	IDU
Western Europe	Late 70's Early 80's	0.56	0.03	0.3	25	HMS, IDU
North America	Late 70's Early 80's	0.94	0.045	0.6	20	IDU, HMS, HTS
Australia and New Zealand	Late 70's Early 80's	15,000	500	0.1	10	HMS
Total		40	5	1.2	48	

HTS = Heterosexual, HMS = Homosexual, IDU = Injecting Drug Users

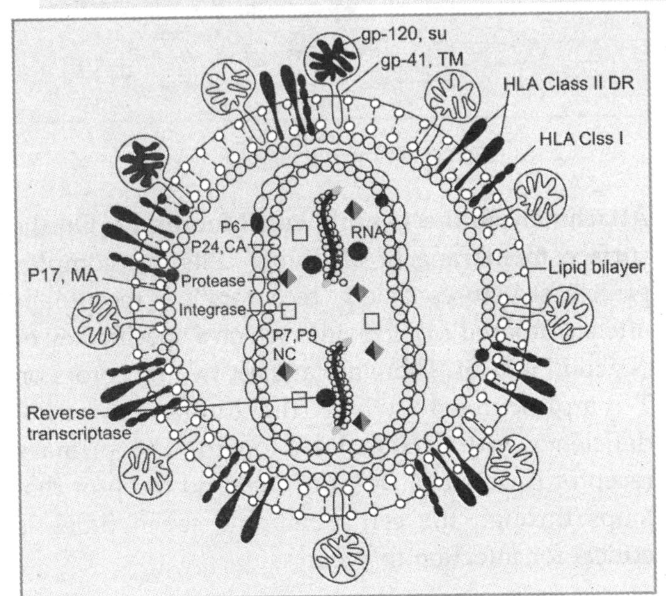

Fig. 23.40: The HIV genome

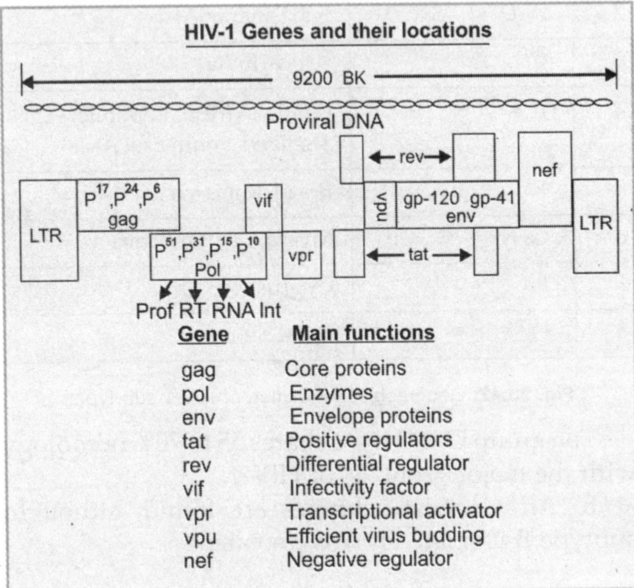

Fig. 23.41: Genetic map of HIV

Biologically HIV-2 is very similar to the HIV-1, with the genome exhibiting about 60% homology in the gag and pol genes and about 30-40% homology in the other viral genes. It is recognized that HIV-2 is less easily transmitted than HIV-1 and the period between infection and illness is relatively longer in the case of HIV-2. While the HIV-1 is widespread globally, the HIV-2 is primarily found in West Africa.

HIV Types and Variants

The HIV virus is a term used to refer collectively to the HIV-1 and HIV-2 retroviruses which are distinct from one another.

The HIV-1 genome is heterogeneous and the envelope gene with its 5 hyper variable region V3 of the surface glycoprotein gp 120, encoding a central loop structure contains the most important site for antibody binding. The phylogenetic analysis of V3 sequences have lead to the identification of three major groups of HIV-1: M (major), O (outlier) and the most recently described group N (New).

Within the major group M, there are nine subtypes A through to K. As the virus continues to mutate and the global epidemic continues, new subtypes are expected to develop and be isolated.

The viruses originally identified as subtype E and I are now considered intersubtype recombinants.

Sr.	HIV-1 Sub Types	Geographical Distribution
1	B	USA, Japan, Australia
2	A, D	Sub Saharan Africa
3	C	Africa, India
4	E	Central African Republic, Thailand, South East Asia
5	F	Brazil, Romania
6	G, H	Russia, Central Africa
7	I	Cyprus
8	O	Cameroon

Fig. 23.42: Geographic distribution of HIV-1 sub types

The group O, of HIV-1 shares 55 to 70% homology with the major group M of HIV-1.

In Africa, most subtypes are found, although, subtype B is relatively less prevalent.

Life Cycle of the HIV

Like all lipid enveloped viruses, the HIV must remain moist to be infectious and it is easily inactivated. For this reason, HIV is primarily transmitted sexually, by exchange of blood, or from mother to child perinatally or by breastfeeding or through sharing infected needles during injecting drug use.

After initial contact and attachment to the hosts immune system (e.g. lymphocytes, monocytes) post infection a cascade of intracellular events within the host are unraveled, the end product being the production of new viral particles, death of the infected cells and the ultimate devastation of the hosts immune system. The main steps in the HIV replication cycle are as follows:

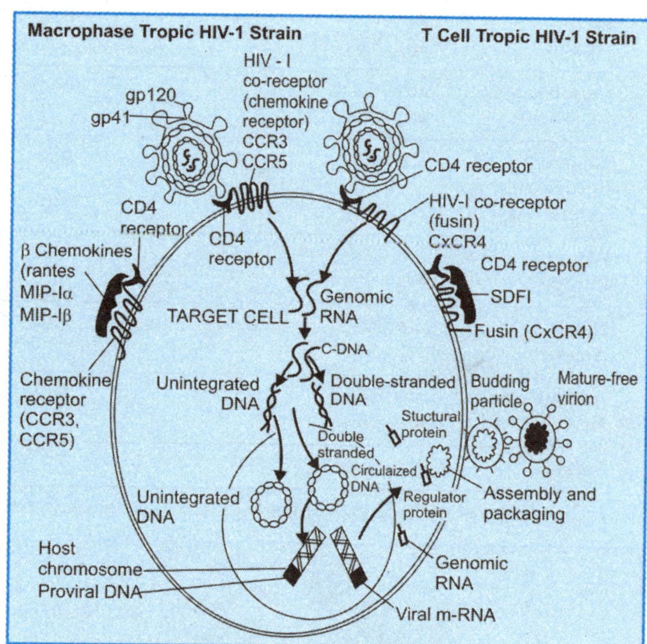

Fig. 23.43: The HIV replication cycle

Attachment to the Lymphocyte Membrane: On the surface membrane of all living cells are complex protein structures called "receptors". A receptor is often compared to a lock into which a specific key or "ligand" will fit. There are at least two receptors on T-lymphocytes to which the human immunodeficiency virus (HIV) locks on to. The primary receptor is called "CD4". But a second receptor that loops through the cell membrane seven times is critical for infection to occur.

HIV Gene	Protein Product	Function in Life Cycle of HIV
gag	Gag/core protein precursor	Viral Core Proteins: p24 : major capsid protein p17 : matrix protein p9 : binds to viral RNA p7 : binds to viral RNA
env	Env./envelope proteins	Viral envelope proteins: gp 120 : major envelope protein, mediates virion binding to cell surface receptor (CD4) gp 41 : mediates fusion of viral envelope and cell membrane
pol	Reverse transcriptase	Converts single-stranded viral RNA into viral DNA duplex.
	Integrase	Integrates viral DNA duplex into host cell genome as provirus DNA
	Protease	Cleaves core precursor polyprotein into functional core proteins
tat	Tat protein	Essential regulatory protein, transactivates expression of all viral genes
rev	Rev protein	Regulatory protein, activates expression of HIV structural and enzymatic genes
vif	Vif protein	Role in viral budding and infectivity of free virions
vpu	Vpu protein	Promotes release of budding virions from host cell
nef	Nef protein	Regulatory protein (essential for pathogenicity of SIV)
vpr	Vpr protein	Regulatory protein, role uncertain

Fig. 23.44: Functions of the HIV gene

HIV infection of a lymphocyte requires attachment of the virus to the cell membrane through both of these "ligand receptor" links. In cells whose "7-transmembrane receptor" is different, the HIV "key" no longer matches the lymphocyte "lock" and attachment is incomplete. Such cells may avoid infection with HIV.

Entry of the Viral RNA: Tight attachment of the viral particle to receptors on the lymphocyte membrane enables fusion with the cell membrane. The viral contents including viral RNA then empty into the cell's cytoplasm, like the other viruses.

Reverse Transcription: Converting viral RNA into DNA.

An enzyme that is part of the human immunodeficiency virus reads the sequence of viral RNA nucleic acids that have entered the host cell and transcribes the sequence into a complementary DNA sequence. This enzyme is called "Reverse transcriptase". Without reverse transcriptase, the viral genome cannot be incorporated into the host cell, and cannot reproduce.

Reverse transcriptase sometimes makes mistakes reading the RNA sequence. The result is that not all viruses produced in a single infected cell are alike. Instead, they end up with a variety of subtle molecular differences in their surface coat and enzymes. Thus through each replication cycle HIV surface molecules are continually changing.

Integration of Viral DNA

Once the viral RNA has been reverse-transcribed into a strand of DNA, the DNA can then be integrated (inserted) into the DNA of the lymphocyte. The virus has its own enzyme called "integrase" that facilitates incorporation of the viral DNA into the host cells DNA. The integrated DNA is called a provirus.

Transcription: Back to RNA

As long as the lymphocyte is not activated or "turned-on", nothing happens to the viral DNA. But if the lymphocyte is activated, transcription of the viral DNA begins, resulting in the production of multiple copies of viral RNA. This RNA codes for the production of the viral proteins and enzymes (translation) and will also be packaged later as new viruses.

Translation: RNA > Proteins

There are nine genes in the HIV RNA. Those genes have the code necessary to produce structural proteins such as the viral envelope, core and the enzymes like reverse transcriptase, integrase, and another crucial enzyme called protease.

Viral Protease: When viral RNA is translated into a polypeptide sequence, that sequence is assembled in a long chain that includes several individual proteins (reverse transcriptase, protease, integrase). Before these enzymes become functional, they must be cut off from the longer polypeptide chain. Viral protease cuts the long chain into its individual enzymes components, which then facilitates the production of new viruses.

Assembly and Budding: Finally, viral RNA and associated proteins are packaged and released from the lymphocyte surface, taking with them a swatch of lymphocyte membrane containing viral surface proteins. These proteins will then bind to the receptors on other immune cells facilitating continued infection and propogation.

Budding viruses are often exactly like the original particle that initially infected the host, however, the resulting viruses also exhibit a range of variations.

During its replication cycle, the HIV is capable of mutating at a rate of approximately one nucleotide substitution per genome per replication cycle; making the virus capable of wide genetic diversity and flexibility to respond to a wide array of selection pressures.

As a consequence drug resistance and immunologic escape mutants are rapidly generated in infected persons through all stages of infection.

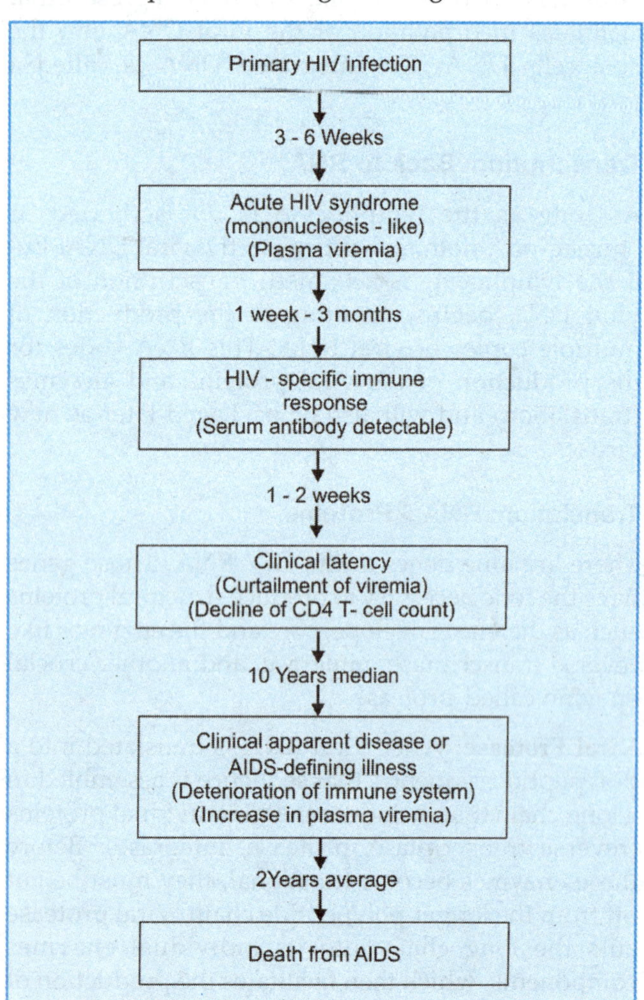

Fig. 23.45: Natural history of HIV infection

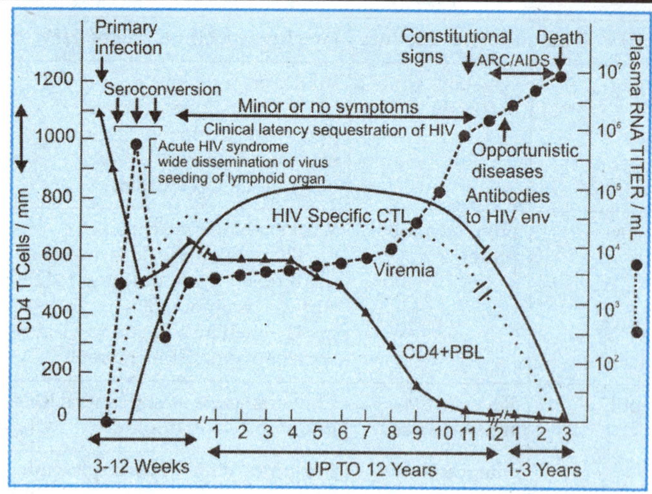

Fig. 23.46: Immuno pathogenesis of HIV infection

The duration of clinical latency following primary HIV infection varies widely among individual persons depending upon many factors; such as exposure categories (blood, sexual contact, mother-to-child), portal of entry, viral pathogenicity and mutation, host resistance, intrinsic and specific immune responsiveness, new treatment strategies with combinations of potent antiretroviral drug therapy etc.

There are also some HIV-seropositive, long-term "non-progressors" who have continued to be healthy without evidence of disease or immune defects for ten or more years after primary HIV infection.

Although reliable clinical data are available for only the past 15 years or so, it is predicted that approximately 95% of HIV-1-infected patients will progressively develop AIDS within 15 years of infection. The first few weeks after primary infection are characterized by an acute mononucleosis or flu-like illness. During this stage seroconversion usually occurs and is associated with a rapid increase in circulating viral titres. This is followed by virus dissemination to lymphoid organs. Adaptive host immunity, including neutralizing antibodies and cytotoxicT lymphocytes (CTL) against virus-infected cell, subsequently develop. While these responses may temporarily control the infection, generally they are unable to eliminate the virus. The patient then enters the stage of clinical latency or the asymptomatic period. A progressive decrease in CD4+ peripheral blood lymphocytes (PBL) continues during the latency stage. When CD4 counts fall below 200/mm^3, the disease usually enters a symptomatic phase, characterized by opportunistic infections and other AIDS-defining conditions in the host.

Clinically Apparent Disease

This clinically apparent, symptomatic stage is a consequence (secondary manifestation) of the progressive and profound deterioration of the immune system that occurs over time in most patients with HIV infection. The CD4 T-cell count continues downward to the range of 200-400/cubic mm. Plasma viremia and p24 antigenemia approach high levels such as seen in the primary infection. Some of the constitutional symptoms, opportunistic infections, and other manifestations of advanced symptomatic HIV disease are given in the following figure.

	(CD4 T – cell count 200-400/cubic mm)
1.	Constitutional symptoms: • Fever • Weight loss • Fatigue • Night Sweats • Diarrhoea • Persistent generalized lymphadenopathy
2.	Infections: • Oral or vaginal candidiasis • Oral hairy leukoplakia • Herpes zoster (shingles) • Herpes simplex • Listeriosis
3.	Other Manifestations: • Cervical dysplasia • Cervical carcinoma in situ • Idiopathic thrombocytopenic purpura (ITP) • Neuropathy • Seborrhea

Fig. 23.47: Manifestations of advanced symptomatic disease

As the CD4 T-cell counts continue to fall, sometimes precipitiously, and reach levels that define AIDS (CD4 T-cell count less than 200/cubic mm), predisposition to AIDS-defining conditions, such as opportunistic infections caused by viruses, bacteria, fungi and protozoa, neoplastic disease, HIV encephalopathy, wasting syndrome, and progressive multifocal leukoencephalopathy that complicate the clinical course and are often the cause of death.

HIV Specific Prognostic Markers

Several HIV specific markers can be used for disease prognosis. Of these declining levels of antibody to p24 (anti-p24) and increasing concentrations of HIV antigen, especially the p24 antigen have been most widely used.

	List of conditions in the 1993 AIDS Surveilliance Case Definition issued by Centers for Disease Control and Prevention
1.	CD4 T-cell count < 200/cubic mm
2.	Opportunistic Infections: • Candidiasis of bronchi, trachea, or lungs • Candidiasis, esophageal • Coccidioidomycosis, disseminated or extrapulmonary • Cryptococcosis, extrapulmonary • Cryptosporidiosis disease (other than liver, spleen, or nodes) • Cytomegalovirus retinitis (with loss of vision) • Herpes simplex: chronic ulcer (s) (>1 month duration); or bronchitis, or esophagitis • Histoplasmosis, disseminated or extrapulmonary • Isopsoriasis, chronic intestinal (>1 month duration) • Mycobacterium avium complex or M. kansasii, disseminated or extrapulmonary • *Pneumocystis carinii* pneumonia • Pneumonia, recurrent • Salmonella septicemia, recurrent • Toxoplasmosis of brain
3.	Neoplastic Disease: • Cervical carcinoma, invasive • Kaposi's sarcoma • Lymphoma, Burkitt's (or equivalent term) • Lymphoma, primary in brain
4.	HIV encephalopathy (AIDS dementia complex)
5.	Wasting syndrome due to HIV
6.	Progressive multifocal leukoencephalopathy (PML)

Fig 23.48: List of CDC conditions

Levels of antibody/antigen however can vary widely between individuals and therefore sequential tests are usually necessary to confirm a trend. Indeed some patients are not measurably antigenaemic until later on in the disease progression, where as others may be antigenaemic for many years. There is still a debate as to the mechanism of these changes. A decline in anti p24 levels could lead to reduced formation of antigen—antibody complexes and hence allow detection of the p24 antigen. Alternatively, the developing p24 antigenaemia may reflect increased virus replication. As the infection progresses, the amount of viral RNA and infectious virus in plasma increases and the proportion of peripheral blood mononuclear cells carrying the provirus also increases.

The prognostic significance of p24 antigenaemia is indicated by a four-fold increase to the progression to AIDS within 3 years, in those who show circulating p24 antigen. However only about 50 percent of patients with ARC and approximately two-thirds of patients with AIDS will be antigenaemic.

A decrease in titre of anti p24 antibody is also associated with disease progression and has been shown to occur before the rise in p24 antigen levels. The decline in titre of anti p24 antibody may therefore be an early indicator of disease progression.

Non Specific Markers of HIV Progression

Markers other than HIV specific antigens and antibodies can be of use in predicting and assessing progression to AIDS.

At present the most commonly used marker is the CD4 cell count, expressed either as an absolute value (normal adult range 600-1700/mm^3) or as a CD4:CD8 ratio (normal adult ratio 1.2 to 3.5).

Similarly, when CD4 cell counts fall to 200/mm^3 or less, prophylaxis against *pneumocystis carnii* is generally initiated.

Measurements of cell counts are, however, subject to potentially large biological and laboratory variation and interpretation should be based on more than one result. A recent prospective study has suggested that combining measurements of the levels of either serum β2-microglobulin or neopterin along with the CD4 cell count improves its prognostic significance. It is likely that a combination of markers rather than a single marker will prove useful for the monitoring of disease progression.

The precise role and practicality of this approach requires for the evaluation.

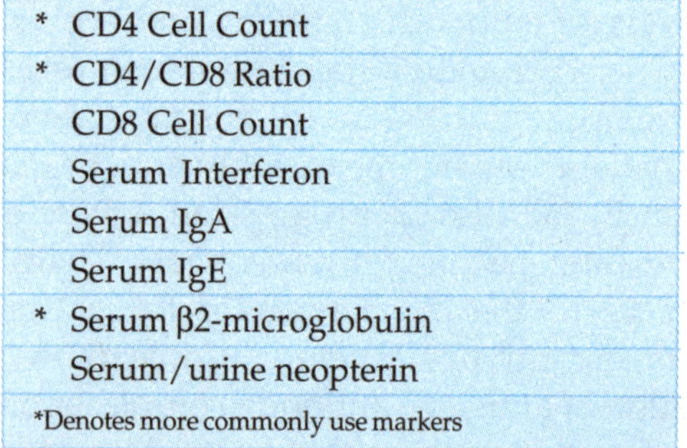

* CD4 Cell Count
* CD4/CD8 Ratio
CD8 Cell Count
Serum Interferon
Serum IgA
Serum IgE
* Serum β2-microglobulin
Serum/urine neopterin
*Denotes more commonly use markers

Fig. 23.49: Non-specific markers of HIV progression

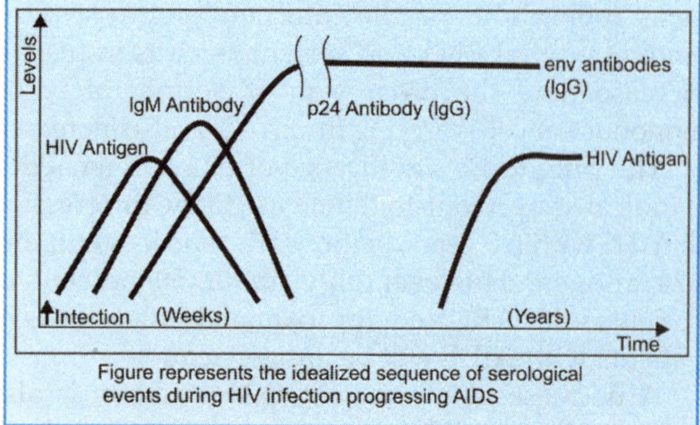

Fig 23.50: Serological profile of HIV infection

Following infection there is evidence of active viral replication as virus can be isolated from cultures of peripheral blood mononuclear cells and p24 antigen can be detected in the serum by immunoassays and viral RNA based assays. This antigenaemia may only last for a week or two and disappears when the antibody response develops following seroconversion. The timing of collection of any blood samples is crucial as prior to or at seroconversion antigen is detected in less than 50% of samples. Seroconversion occurs in most patients by 4-8 weeks after exposure although in some cases antibody may not appear until 6-9 months later. This delay between infection and appearance of antibodies is termed as the "Window Period". At seroconversion, antibody of the IgM class can be detected. Analysis of the reactivity of the IgG response by immunoblotting or enzyme immunoassay based on recombinant proteins shows that antibodies develop rapidly to the principal structural proteins e.g. the envelope glycoproteins gp 160, gp 120 and gp 41 and the core proteins p18, p24. Antibody to the polygene proteins can also be detected. Antibodies to the envelope glycoproteins gp 160, gp 120 and gp 41 incase of HIV-1 and gp 36 in case of HIV-2 infections may appear before antibodies to the core proteins although the time difference is generally only a matter of days or a few weeks.

After seroconversion there is evidence of continued virus replication as virus can be cultured from the plasma as well as detected by PCR based RNA assays. Indirect evidence is provided by the progressive increase in the level of antibodies to all the major virus components during this time.

In neonates the serological profile is complicated by the presence of the maternal anti-HIV antibody.

For some years after seroconversion the patient may remain well or develop persistent generalized lymphadenopathy. Throughout this period viraemia may increase. A reduction in the level of antibody to the p24 core protein and the appearance of p24 Ag are associated with progression to clinically overt disease. In the later stages of AIDS, as the immune system is destroyed, antibody may not be detectable in some patients.

HIV Diagnostic Testing Techniques

As has been discussed that virtually all individuals who become infected with HIV mount an IgG antibody response to the virus which current immunoassays will detect by 4 to 8 weeks after primary infection and in the majority of cases for the remainder of the individuals life. Screening and diagnostic tests thus rely upon the detection of antibodies to HIV. During part of the window period IgM anti-HIV and HIV Ag may be present, but specific screening for them though desirable is not cost effective in low prevalence populations.

During the search for the causative agent of AIDS, tests for anti-HIV detection were developed. Initial testing was by Western Blot analysis. However, the magnitude of the HIV epidemic and the need for extensive screening were not fully understood. By 1983 and 1984, it had become apparent that rapid, simple and inexpensive assays would be required. Research assays were developed and in 1985 several manufacturers introduced enzyme immunoassays for blood donor screening. In the ensuing years these assays have evolved rapidly by utilizing products of modern biotechnology, for screening and confirmation of HIV infection.

Enzyme Immunoassays (EIA)

The diversity of EIA formats make a simple, meaningful definition difficult to formulate, but EIA's can be described as a binding assays that depend upon the antigen-antibody reaction as the basis and the enzyme reaction as a marker for the proof of reaction. Anti-HIV EIA kits in various formats are available. Obtaining high quality results not only depends upon the quality of the kit but also on strict adherence to kit protocols, well-maintained equipments and good performance assurance procedures. Under these conditions many assays currently available will achieve >99% sensitivity and specificity. Typically, a batch of tests takes 1.5-3 hours to complete. Since the EIA's detect Anti-HIV antibodies, the solid phase on the microwell is coated with HIV specific proteins.

Generation of Assays

The terms first, second and third generation have been applied to anti-HIV assays according to the source of the HIV Ag used on the solid phase as opposed to sequential improvements.

First generation assays may lack specificity because of reactions with contaminating cell proteins and lack sensitivity due to the high sample dilution needed to attain acceptable specificity. For second and third generation assays, the identification and sequencing of important antigenic sites, the expression of proteins of precisely targeted portions of HIV cDNA, and the synthesis of oligopeptides containing immunodominant epitopes has provided new antigens for use in the assay systems. When incorporated into EIA's these recombinant proteins and peptides have led to substantial improvements in sensitivity and specificity and have the added advantage of being safer, easier and more reproducible in performance.

Generation of Anti HIV Assays	
First Generation	Native viral antigens from lymphocyte culture
Second Generation	Expression products of recombinant HIV cDNA
Third Generation	Chemically synthesized oligopeptides (approximately 15-40 amino acids) Double antigen sandwich assays

Fig. 23.51: Generations of Anti HIV assays

EIA ASSAY FORMATS

There are four basic assay formats for the detection of antibodies to HIV.

Type 1: Indirect or Antiglobulin

A relatively crude native HIV antigen preparation is immunoabsorbed to the solid phase by pre-coating with HIV antibody. Anti human globulin conjugated to enzymes is used as a tracer, with a compatible substrate as a chromogenic marker.

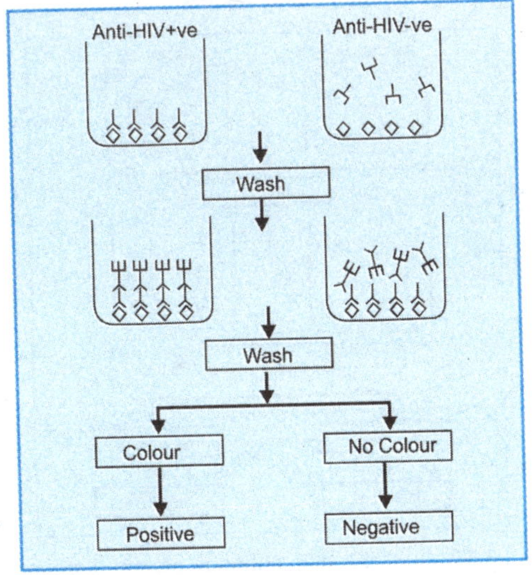

Fig. 23.52: Indirect or antiglobulin assays

Type 2: Competitive Assay

In competitive assays the sample need not be diluted. These assays exhibit high sensitivity. To ensure good specificity and sensitivity the spectrum of anti-HIV detected is predominantly against env. determinants, but because antibodies to env antigens of HIV-1 and HIV-2 show only limited cross reaction the competitive format is unsuitable for combined anti-HIV-1/HIV-2 screening.

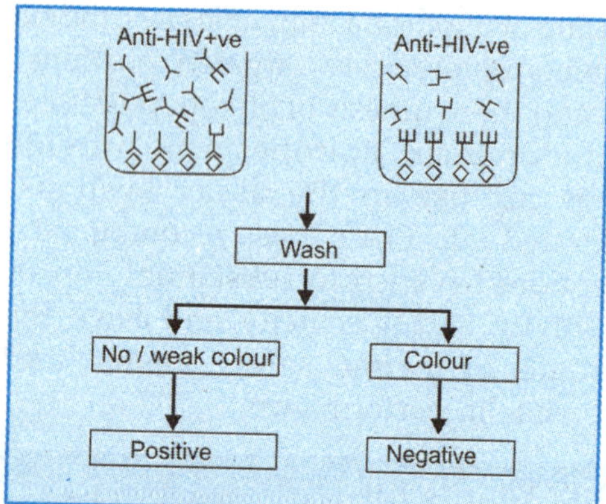

Fig. 23.53: Competitive assays

Type 3: Class Specific Antibody Capture Assay

Class specific antibody capture assays are only available as a research tool. They have proved to be highly accurate for detecting anti-HIV specimen such as saliva and urine and find important applications in epidemiological research and other situations where venipuncture is impractical.

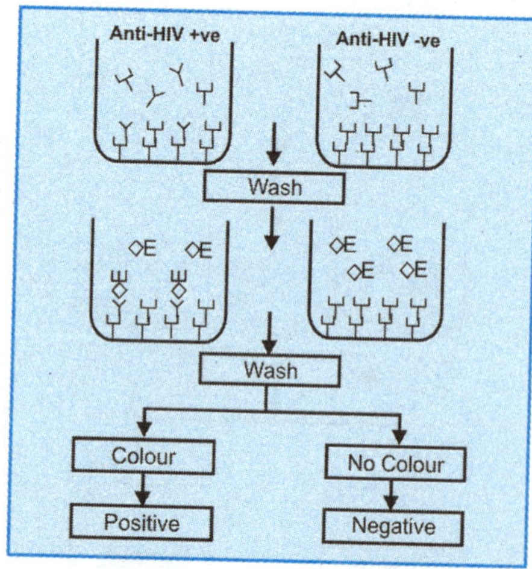

Fig. 23.54: Class specific antibody capture assays

Type 4: Double Antigen Sandwich or Immunometric Assay

A commercially available example of this assay detects anti-HIV-1 and anti-HIV-2 by using recombinant HIV-1 antigens and synthetic oliopeptide antigens from the HIV-2.

These assays are sensitive and specific, an added advantage being that they do react with IgM anti HIV antibodies and they are reported to detect seroconversion earlier.

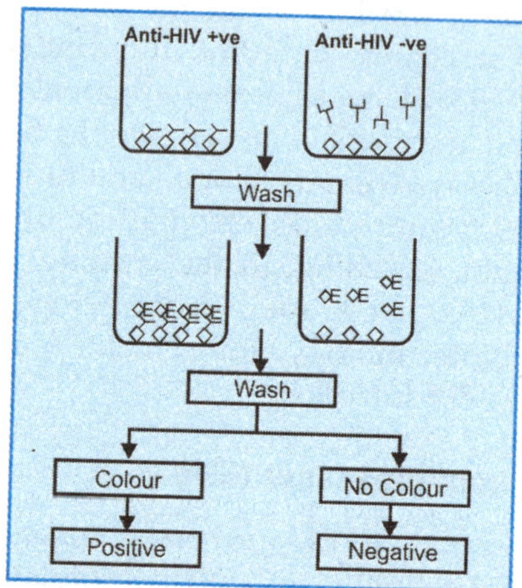

Fig. 23.55: Immunometric Assays

HIV Antigen EIA's

HIV Antigen EIA's have been developed primarily for the purpose of monitoring HIV-infected individuals for antigenaemia, but are also used to monitor growth of HIV in lymphocyte cultures. The methods used are in general modifications of antibody sandwich assays described earlier.

Anti-HIV prepared from the serum of HIV infected individuals, animal antisera raised against purified viral or recombinant antigens and monoclonal antibodies have all been used in various combinations as capture and detector antibody as well as a variety of enzymes and substrates.

The sensitivity of HIV Ag assays can be below 50 pg/ml. It should be noted, however, that standards do vary from one commercial kit to another reflecting the unsuitability of standardizing by weight of a complexed antigen, which will be, measured immunometrically.

Estimations of HIV antigen level can, therefore, be regarded as 'semi quantitative'. Most manufacturers do provide HIV antigen standards, which can be included in assay runs in order to produce a standard curve from which specimen HIV antigen levels can be extrapolated. Despite the 'semi quantitative' nature of the estimation, sequential monitoring of titres may be informative regarding disease progression or efficacy of antiviral therapy.

Confirmation of positive findings is recommended and some manufacturers have reagents available for this purpose, usually a blocking antibody.

Confirmatory/Supplementary Assays

Confirmatory tests are used to confirm whether specimens found reactive with a particular screening test contain antibodies specific to HIV. The most commonly used confirmatory test until recently, was the Western Blot (WB). However, its use has proven to be very expensive and prone to producing large numbers of indeterminate results. The differences in criteria for the interpretation of Western Blot also has lead to classification difficulties of indeterminate samples. Now, studies have shown that combinations of ELISAs or Simple/Rapid assays can provide results as reliable as the WB at a much lower cost.

1. **Western Blot:** The Western Blot was developed to detect antibodies to HIV and to qualitatively determine to which viral proteins the antibody response had been raised. The assay is based on the detection of the reaction of specific antibodies in the sample with viral antigens that have been electrophoretically separated and transferred ("blotted") onto a nitrocellulose sheet on a backing. Antibodies, which react with antigens on the membrane, are visualized with an enzyme labelled anti-human immunoglobulin and an enzyme substrate, which gives an insoluble coloured product at the site of reaction.

   Although WB allows the humoral immune response to HIV to be mapped, there are several problems: Not all sera from infected individuals react with all HIV proteins. Sera from some uninfected individuals may react with one or more HIV proteins or with contaminating residual lymphocyte cell proteins. Large differences between batches and particularly between manufacturers occur in the number of proteins and their relative concentrations and positions on the strips. The assay is read visually. To counter these difficulties, some standardization has been attempted, particularly in terms of interpretation of the reactivity observed. Several sets of criteria have been recommended which differ in details, but commonly require an antibody to at least one env. gene product, and at least one band from gag and/or pol for classifying a positive test result.

Organisation	Criteria	
	Positive (minimum of)	Negative
World Health Organisation	Two env. bands	No HIV specific bands
C.D.C	Any two of p24; gp41; gp 120/160	No bands at all
Consortium for Retrovirus serology standardisation	p24 or p32 and gp 41 or gp 120/160	No bands at all
American Red Cross	At least one from each of gag, pol and env	No bands at all
Food and Drug Administration (USA)	p24, p32 and gp 41 or gp 160	No bands at all

Fig. 23.56: Criteria for interpretation of western blot assay

   Results which neither satisfy 'Positive' nor 'Negative' criteria are termed as 'Indeterminates'. Recently, immunoblots, which resemble WB but utilize a selection of synthetic HIV antigens applied to membrane strips as discrete bands have been developed (LIA/RIBA). These are reportedly comparable to the electrophoterically manufactured traditional blots, with reduction in the proportion of indeterminate results. However these are equally expensive.

2. **Indirect Immunofluorescence:** If has been commonly employed to detect anti-HIV antibodies. Acetone fixed HIV infected lymphocytes are incubated with sample, followed by a fluorescein conjugated anti-human IgG. The cells are then examined using fluorescent microscopy. If anti-HIV is present a typical pattern of fluorescent staining is seen in the cells. If is usually reserved for confirmation as it is time-consuming and requires highly-skilled operators and an expensive, well-maintained fluorescence microscope.

3. **Radioimmunoprecipitation Assay:** RIPA is used by very few laboratories. Initially, HIV Ag is metabolically labelled by substituting one or more S tagged amino acids in HIV culture medium. The labelled cells are then disrupted to release the labelled proteins and the resulting suspension is clarified. The labelled proteins are used for testing the sample. Containment facilities for handling live HIV and radioisotopes are required along with expensive equipment and consumables for immunochemistry, limiting its usage to few reference laboratories.

Virus Detection Methods

Virus isolation has traditionally been achieved by co-cultivation of gradient purified patient's peripheral blood lymphocytes with stimulated lymphocytes from an uninfected individual. To seek evidence of viral replication the cultured cells may be examined by microscopy for cytopathic changes and by HIV immunofluorescence. The culture medium may also be assayed for HIV p24 Ag or reverse transcriptase activity. Isolation of HIV indicates beyond any doubt that the subject is infected with HIV. However, it has a very restricted role to play in confirmatory testing because of its relatively low sensitivity and the cost and complexity of the technique. HIV can sometimes be isolated from fresh or properly stored plasma, but usually a fresh blood sample will be required to provide peripheral blood mononuclear cells for co-cultivation. Very few laboratories claim nearly 100 percent HIV isolation from all anti-HIV positive subject, but most achieve 60-80 percent success. Virus isolation is generally reserved for research purposes due to its expense, low sensitivity, long incubation time and need for high containment facilities.

p24 Antigen and Nucleic Acid Technologies

A number of other assays have been introduced in recent years which assist in the establishment of the diagnosis of HIV infection and may also be used to monitor the progress of the infection and the response to therapy. These include assays that detect virus particles, e.g. the HIV p24 antigen ELISA, or the presence of HIV viral nucleic acid sequences (RNA or DNA) by means of nucleic acid amplification techniques. NAT assays have made it possible to detect minute amounts of viral material - as little as a single viral genome (the detection limit for most assays is around 300 copies/ml). These sensitive procedures are well suited for early diagnosis of mother-to-child transmission and for monitoring the viral load of patients who are on antiretroviral therapy. However, in routine practice this technique can have limited specificity, needs sophisticated equipment, rigorous laboratory conditions and highly trained staff, and is still very expensive.

Rapid Tests for the Detection of Anti-HIV Antibodies

Advances in technology have now made it possible to design rapid HIV antibody assays based on agglutination, immunodot, immunochromatographic and immunoconcentration/filtration techniques, the assays have comparable sensitivity to equivalent generation EIAs.

The assays are easy to perform and ideal for low through put laboratories. Since same day results are offered through the use of these tests, they help in timely detection and treatment intervention of HIV infection.

The overall considerations in rapid test assay development are as follows:

1. The tests should pick up antibody response to HIV-1 and HIV-2.
2. The test when used in areas endemic with variants of HIV 1 such as O and M (Cameroon, Gabon) should be reactive with the antibodies to the variants.
3. The test should increase the sensitivity of detection during the "window period" shortening it as much as possible.
4. The antigenic configuration of the test should preferably use recombinant antigens or peptides from the conserved immunodominant regions of the HIV-1 and HIV-2 genome.
5. The screening test should have sensitivity and specificity in excess of 99 percent.

Well designed rapid tests based on protein A based tracers that pick up IgG class anti-HIV antibodies bound to the solid phase, in general achieve such specifications. However since protein A based assays necessarily map only IgG class anti-HIV antibodies, they tend to be less sensitive than systems having the ability to pick up IgG and IgM class of Anti-HIV antibodies. Third generation rapid tests now utilize the principle of double antigen sandwich immunoassays. In the double antigen sandwich system recombinant proteins from the immunodominant regions of the HIV genome are used on the capture as well as on the tracer reagent. Antibodies to HIV are thus specifically captured and sandwiched during the test specifically between the solid phase and tracer antigens. This third generation system not only improves specificity but also improves sensitivity of the assay since not only IgG but also IgM antibodies react in the system, improving the test sensitivity in the early seroconversion phase of the HIV infection. Such improved third generation rapid tests are being made available now.

Flow Through Technology

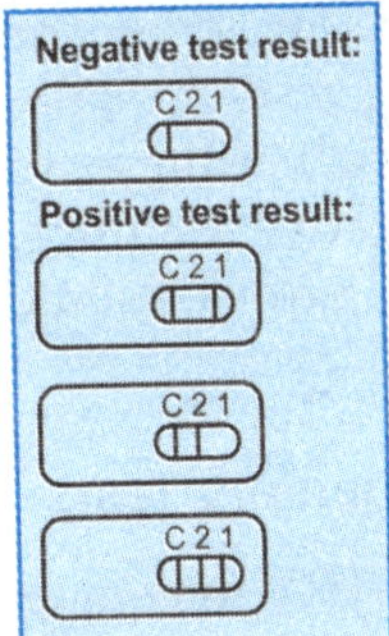

Appearance of only one control band corresponding to control region 'C'

In addition to the control band 'C', appearance of reactive band at test region '1': Specimen positive for Antibodies to HIV 1.

In addition to the control band 'C', appearance of reactive band at test region '2': Specimen positive for Antibodies to HIV 2.

In addition to the control band 'C' appearance of reactive band at test region '1' and test region '2': Specimen positive for Antibodies to HIV 1 and HIV 2.

Invalid test result: The test should be considered invalid if neither the test band nor the control band appears.

Lateral Flow Technology

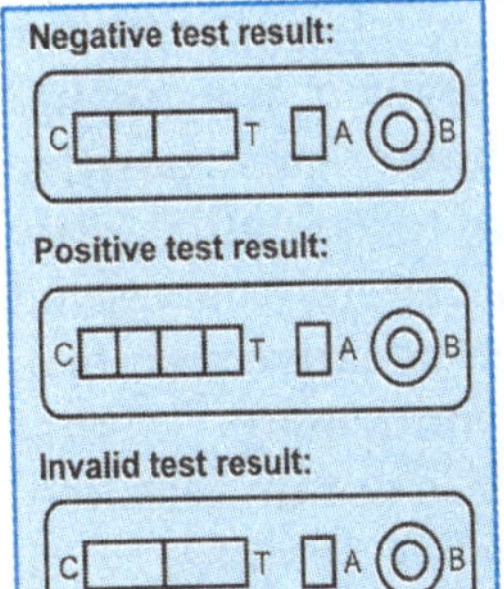

Appearance of only one coloured band at the control region 'C'.

Positive test result:

Appearance of a coloured band at the test region 'T' in addition to the band at control region 'C'.

Invalid test result:

The test should be considered invalid if neither the test band nor the control band appears.

Flow Through v/s Lateral Flow Technology

Rapid tests currently available are based either on the second generation protein A based flow through systems or the third generation lateral flow based double antigen system. The flow through technology based tests are multicomponent, multistep based systems that require cold storage. These tests also require higher degree of laboratarian involvement and can only use serum or plasma as a sample. Since the membrane needs to be rehydrated before use there is a limit on the number of tests that can be run at a time simultaneously. New generation flow through assays, however, have been reported with distinct advantages over second generation flow through assays.

On the other hand lateral flow technology based double antigen sandwich assays are single step/two step and easier to use. Suitability of whole blood as a sample and room temperature storage in addition to higher clinical sensitivity due to anti-HIV IgM detection capability make these tests a method of choice for most settings. These assays have an overall advantage over flow through technology based tests.

Application of HIV Testing

The donor screening tests for anti HIV have been also adopted for clinical diagnosis and for epidemiological prevalence and monitoring studies. Because the consequences of a positive diagnosis of HIV infection are so serious it is generally considered that people who are tested should be asked to give consent to testing only after counselling, which in simple and sensitive terms explains the background to the screening test, the implications of a positive finding and advice on risk avoidance. Follow-up clinical and psychological support for those found to be infected is also essential. Of equal importance is a mechanism for distinguishing which of those samples that react in screening assays are genuine, or true positives.

Screening tests for anti-HIV-1 will not detect all HIV-2 infections and the discovery of HIV-2 infections outside of its recognized endemic regions in West Africa has influenced the decision by many countries to introduce tests which can detect antibody to HIV-2 reliably. There are now many 'combined' HIV-1/HIV-2 EIAs and rapid tests that have become the screening method of choice. Simultaneously test that can in addition detect the antibody to subgroup 'O' are considered "complete" as a screening test.

Screening

Anti-HIV screening assays were primarily developed for blood bank screening with the objective of protecting the recipients of blood or its products from infection with HIV. In addition to screening, vetting of donors and phasing out of inducements to donate are now strongly recommended by WHO.

However, in regions where HIV has spread primarily by heterosexual contacts, vetting of donors is difficult as "high-risk" groups are not easily recognized and more reliance is therefore placed on anti-HIV screening. Nevertheless, anti-HIV screening alone is insufficient to ensure that the blood supply is free from HIV contamination. Even if the assays were 100 percent sensitive, technical and clerical errors can lead to reporting errors. Many considerations affect the choice of screening assay including sensitivity, specificity, ease of performance and cost. Poor sensitivity may jeopardize the safety of recipients of blood or other tissues while, on the other hand, poor specificity is costly in terms of unnecessarily wasted donations, the cost of extra confirmatory testing and the problems of management of donors whose samples are reactive. Limited resources have led some transfusion services to consider the screening test simply as a means to protect recipients. Many however, are also able to assume responsibility for their donors, ensuring that screen-reactive samples are confirmed before counselling the donor and offering referral to an expert HIV clinic.

Worldwide application of anti-HIV screening assays outside the strictly clinical arena are increasing: many life insurance companies require anti-HIV screening before offering cover to applicants, and some authorities require HIV testing before issuing marriage licences, immigration documents or admitting recruits to armed services. Some controversy surrounds these applications of HIV screening with respect to their moral, ethical and legal justification. If carried out, confirmation of a screen reactive finding is an absolute requirement, especially as these tests are applied to populations in which HIV prevalence is generally low and therefore false positive reactions are common relative to genuine positive reactions.

Diagnosis

When screening tests for anti-HIV first made it possible to identify HIV-infected individuals who did not manifest the classical signs and symptoms of AIDS, there was some debate whether testing was worthwhile for them. However, improvements in predicting the progression of disease by use of prognostic markers and continuous improvements in treatment, both with Antiretroviral and prophylactic treatment of opportunistic infections, now favour the policy of early identification of all HIV-infected individuals.

There are three main diagnostic applications of anti HIV testing:

a. To confirm that a patient presenting with symptoms associated with HIV infection is infected with HIV
b. To investigate a person who has been exposed to infection because of exposure to body fluids from a known HIV-infected individual, perhaps by sexual intercourse or by inoculation.
c. And to test those who belong to one of the recognized risk groups, are healthy and have no definite history of exposure, but are anxious and present themselves for testing in the hope of gaining the reassurance of a negative result.

Many diagnostic laboratories now take the precaution of running two screening tests (usually different manufacturers kits) on each sample to decrease the possibility of false negative findings, whether due to a technical or clerical error or some inherent fault in an assay.

Approach to Confirmatory Supplementary Tests

The best of the currently available anti-HIV screening assays will give rise to less than 1 in 1,000 repeatable false positive reactions. Although this represents excellent specificity, when such a test is applied to a low prevalence population only a small proportion of reactive samples will be genuine. To avoid the potentially serious consequences of a false diagnosis, several strategies have been devised for further testing to determine the authenticity of a positive screening reaction. This is referred to as confirmatory or supplementary testing. It is generally accepted that only positive and unexpected negative results in screening assays need to be confirmed. So that unnecessary confirmatory testing is not undertaken, most laboratories first retest reactive samples twice or more in the screening assay. Unrepeatable reactions are reported as negative. Whatever confirmatory strategy is employed, it is good practice to seek a follow-up sample from any individuals found to be reactive. this is to primarily safeguard against a false diagnosis due to technical or clerical errors, but also to check that an uncomfirmable positive reaction on a screening assay is not a result of sampling too early during seroconversion. Cases of dual infectivity with HIV-1 and HIV-2 have been reported and thus in some instances this may require confirmation.

Western Blot (WB)

The most widely accepted 'confirmatory' test is Western Blot. A reaction in a screening assay simply indicates that antibody from the specimen is bound to the solid phase: this can be an HIV-specific or non-specific reaction. WB provides additional information about specificity, in terms of reactivity with particular HIV proteins. The reaction pattern obtained may be interpreted as positive, negative or indeterminate according to the application of one of several sets of accepted criteria. The disadvantages of WB are its cost, subjectivity and high rate of indeterminate reactions. Stringent criteria, while achieving high specificity, lead to low sensitivity. Thus, some sera from infected subjects only give indeterminate results. Conversely, low stringency criteria lead to some false positive diagnosis by WB. A further disadvantage is that criteria have usually been determined using a particular manufacturer's product. When these are applied to a different WB they may not be valid.

Line immunoassays resembling WB and 'dot-immunoblots', each using several synthetic antigens derived from different HIV genes are now being widely used. They are usually more rapid and at least as sensitive as WB. Interpretative criteria vary but are generally similar to WB, with the same three possible outcomes.

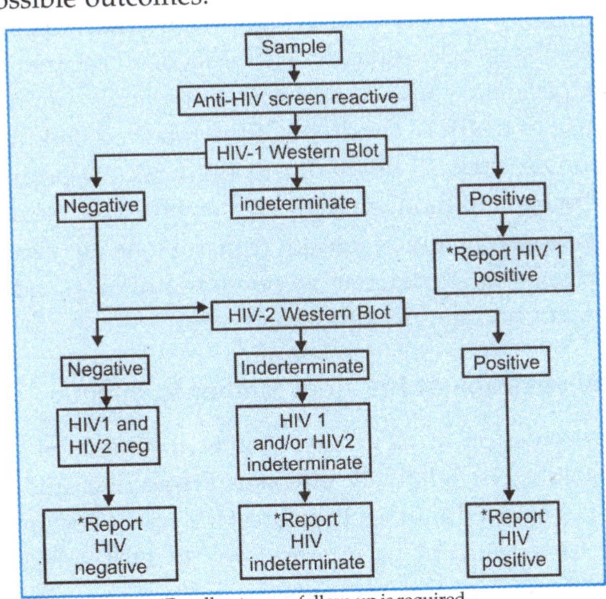

Fig. 23.57: Approach to confirmatory tests

NAT-PCR Based Methods

The NAT-PCR based assays detect the nucleic acid of HIV directly in an infected patient's sample and is employed as a confirmatory method. The expense and technical demands of PCR will, for the foreseeable future restrict its use to carefully selected cases and to providing support to investigations of simpler, less expensive confirmatory strategies.

Alternative Approach to Confirmatory Testing

This approach seeks to determine if a sample reaction in a screening test will also give a positive signal in at least two further 'independent' screening assays. Assays were originally defined as 'independent' if they were each of a different type. But this concept has recently been broadened to incorporate assays using antigens from different sources, e.g. viral, recombinant DNA expression products and synthetic peptides. Just as there have to be trials of WB to develop accurate interpretive criteria, particular combinations of assays must be examined to demonstrate that they are generally independent of each other, i.e. they are not susceptible to the same non-specific effects.

It has recently been shown that a combination of rapid screening assays can also give diagnosis as accurate as WB, and more cheaply. This option should be particularly useful for anti-HIV confirmation especially in the developing world, as a cost effective solution.

WHO/UNAIDS Strategies for HIV Antibody Screening

These three strategies take into account the objective of testing (i.e. whether for transfusion safety, surveillance or diagnosis) and the local seroprevalence rate. Depending on these factors, three different algorithms for repeat and confirmatory testing have been proposed to confirm initial screening results.

They avoid the use of the Western Blot for confirmation of positive screening test result; although Western Blot confirmation is still the rule in the USA, Germany and other countries, it can be replaced by more economical testing algorithms using ELISA-type assays and/or rapid/simple test devices.

Strategy I requires only one test. It is to be used for:

- Transfusion screening (if no results are to be provided)
- Surveillance (if prevalence > 10% and no results are to be provided)
- Diagnosis (only if patient is symptomatic and population HIV prevalence > 30%)
  NB: This is not normally adequate for diagnosis!

Strategy II requires up to two tests and is to be used for:

- Surveillance (if prevalence ≤ 10% and no results are to be provided)
- Diagnosis if patient symptomatic and population prevalence ≤ 30%, or if patient asymptomatic and population prevalence > 10%.

Strategy III requires up to three tests for:

- Diagnosis if patient asymptomatic and population HIV prevalence ≤ 10%.

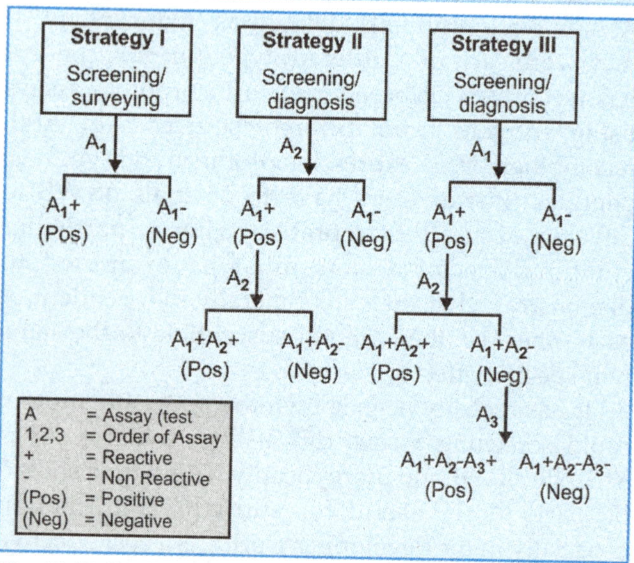

Fig. 23.58: WHO/UNAIDS Strategies for HIV Antibodies Screening

The successful confirmation using these strategies requires the user to distinguish strictly between assay results (non-reactive or reactive) and patient diagnosis ("Positive" or "Negative").

For all strategies, the first (screening) test (Test 1) should be chosen for its very high sensitivity (>99%) (to avoid false-negative results), while the confirmatory tests (Tests 2 and 3) must have a high specificity (> 99%). No test performance characteristic must be <95%. Furthermore, the different tests used for each strategy must employ different formats.

Discrimination Between HIV-1 and HIV-2 Infection

Tests that claim to distinguish HIV-1 from HIV-2 infection cannot necessarily be regarded as confirmatory tests. Some of them rely on a reaction with a single short length oligopeptide and may lack sensitivity for antibody from all individuals infected by the homologous HIV type. However, most of the confirmatory methods already mentioned will discriminate to some degree between HIV-1 and HIV-2. Cross reactions, between env and gag antigens in WB make it less efficient than other approaches such as utilizing a pair of type-specific competitive EIAs or a line immunoassay employing HIV-1 and HIV-2 specific synthetic antigens. Also, the cost of two WB strips or PCR for HIV-1 and HIV-2 is high and it is doubtful whether such expenditure should be committed to making a differential diagnosis for the small proportion of cases in which more simple and inexpensive approaches fail.

Paediatric HIV Infection

Since the first report of an infant with AIDS in November 1982, the incidence of HIV infection in the pediatric population has increased exponentially. By the year 2000, it is estimated that HIV pandemic was responsible for the deaths of 3 million women and more than 2.5 million children worldwide. Additionally about 5.5 million children might have been orphaned because of premature death of their parents.

It has been proposed that when maternal infection rates reach 2-3% globally, HIV infection acquired by the perinatal route could become the most common cause of death in children. Of the reported children, younger than 13 years old in the USA, 90 percent were born to mothers with HIV or HIV risk factors, 5 percent received blood transfusions or tissue transplants, 3 percent were hemophiliacs and 1 percent had no identified risk factor.

Transmission of HIV from Mother to Infants

Transmission of HIV from mother to infants is not absolute but relatively efficient. Propective studies have reported mother to infant HIV transmission in 13 to 39 percent of infants born to HIV infected mothers. Perinatal transmission may occur before, during or after birth. Many characteristics of the

HIV infected mothers may be associated with increased risk of perinatal HIV transmission; women with symptomatic HIV infections or AIDS may have an increased risk of transmitting infection to their infants as compared to asymptomatic pregnant mothers.

Higher transmission rates have been reported for infants delivered vaginally than those by cesarean section. In some studies presence of other STD's during pregnancy, such as syphilis, appear to increase the likelihood of HIV transmission possibly due to placentitis associated with Treponema pallidum coinfection. Other ulcerative genital infections may also increase the transmission rates.

Perinatal feeding practices can also affect vertical HIV transmission as HIV infection does occur via breastfeeding. Type of milk ingested (colostrum versus later milk) duration of breastfeeding, duration of mother's HIV infection, her viral load and the antibody content in her milk influences mother to infant transmission rates.

The working definition of intrauterine infection as suggested by experts is a positive PCR or HIV culture or a p24 antigen test on the infants blood within 48 hours of life. Perinatal infection is defined as negative assays shortly after birth and positive results occurring later. Voluntary testing for HIV to recognize HIV infected mothers can benefit through antiretroviral therapies, early prophylaxis of genital infections, providing passive HIV antibody to pregnant women, fetus and the newborn and providing active or passive enhancement of fetal and neonatal anti HIV specific immunity.

Diagnostic Challenges: Child Born to a HIV Infected Mother

Diagnosis of HIV infection in children born to HIV infected mothers is complicated by the presence, in almost all cases, of the maternal anti HIV antibody which crosses the placenta to the fetus. Over all, less than one third of the children are actually infected. Since HIV antibody assays such as EIA, immunoblots primarily detect IgG class of antibodies and in infants, this class of antibody may persist from upto 9-18 months, conventional antibody tests cannot be used to reliably predict the HIV infection in children under 18 months of age. In the first year of life, HIV infection can be reliably diagnosed by PCR and viral culture, since they can correctly identify upto 50 percent of the infected infants at birth and nearly 100 percent of the infected infants by 6 months of age. It must be however recognized that false positive PCR results occur in the first week of life and the standard p24 antigen assay is less sensitive than culture or PCR as it fails to detect immuno complexed p24 antigen.

The additional potentially useful methods currently under development and evaluation are:

a. Test based on in vitro production of virus specific antibodies by patients lymphocytes.
b. Detection of patient specific IgA antibodies to HIV, since the IgA does not cross the placenta.

Anti Retroviral Therapy

The treatment of HIV infection requires an understanding of viral replication, dynamics, antiviral potency, pharmacokinetics and toxicities of individual drugs, interactions between drugs when used in combination and the limitations imposed by failure of one drug on the future use of same and related drugs. Most of the anti retroviral drugs available today exert their anti retroviral action by disrupting the viral replication cycle of the HIV within the infected host. Broadly these drugs can be classified into:

- Inhibitors of viral reverse transcriptase that block the conversion of the viral RT dependent genomic RNA into double stranded DNA notable amongst those being:
  - Non nucleoside RT inhibitors, and
  - Nucleoside analogue RT inhibitors, and
  - Nucleotide analogue RT inhitors.
- Inhibitors of the viral protease enzyme to prevent the cleavage of poly proteins and conversion of viral particle into an mature infectious virion (protease inhibitors). The inhibitors of viral transcriptase compete with

natural enzyme substrates *in vivo*, leading to perinatal DNA chain termination of the HIV life cycle. On the other hand, action of the protease inhibitors does not let the viral particles mature and remain replication defective.

Since HIV infection is a dynamic process with high rates of replication and great potential for genetic mutation, a major determinant of anti retroviral drug failure is viral genotypic variation conferring drug resistance.

When a patient starts a drug regime, the regime selects for pre existing mutation as well as additional mutants that may appear in different genetic backgrounds. Mutations continue to appear unless rate of replication is curtailed enough to retard genetic variation.

Use of Highly Active Anti Retroviral Therapy (HAART)

Combination regimes that produce more potent inhibition of viral replication may delay or prevent resistance from arising by limiting the new mutations from occurring or accumulating. Because of high cost and limited availability HAART is beyond reach of most infected individuals or individuals at risk for HIV infection.

The recent widespread use of plasma HIV-RNA levels to monitor infection and therapy has transformed clinical management of infected individuals. Therapy for persons with HIV infection is based upon CD4 cell counts and HIV-RNA plasma levels.

CD 4 cells/ml	Plasma HIV-1 RNA levels (copies/ml)		
	< 5000	5000-30000	>30000
< 350	Recommend therapy	Recommend therapy	Recommend therapy
350-500	Consider therapy	Recommend therapy	Recommend therapy
>500	Defer therapy	Recommend therapy	Recommend therapy

Fig. 23.59: Plasma HIV RNA levels

The level of HIV-RNA reflects the magnitude of viral replication. It correlates with the rate of CD4 T cell decline, the relative risk of clinical disease progression and the time to death.

Baseline RNA levels are measured before the anti retroviral therapy is started and during drug therapy to guide subsequent steps. A consistent increase in viral load of more than 0.5 log 10 usually suggests a failing anti retroviral regimen. The RNA viral load test is currently available for HIV 1 infection only.

The CD4 T cell count on the other hand refelcts the extent of immune damage that has already occurred because of HIV infection. CD4 T cell counts correlate with the risk of developing opportunistic infections, neoplasms and with time to death. Base line CD4 T cell counts are measured before anti retroviral therapy is initiated to assess prognosis and guide prophylaxis of opportunistic infections.

Vaccines for HIV Infection

It is clear, that attempts to modify high risk behaviour amongst population has met with variable success. Because of the high cost and limited availability, HAART is beyond the reach of most individuals at risk for HIV infection. Effective vaccination probably offers the best hope for containing the HIV epidemic.

The development of vaccines against HIV poses a formidable, scientific, logistic and social challenge and the most important problems are:

- Lack of understanding of the critical parameters of immunity that would protect against the infection/disease or both.
- Substantial genotypic variations occur among the infective HIV strain along with high level of mutation and recombination in the replication of individual isolates.
- The relationship of these genotypic variations to the expression of antigens that might induce protective immunity remains poorly defined.
- An effective vaccine would have to stimulate broadly directed immune response so as to be able to inhibit diverse strains of HIV.

A large body of information continues to be generated concerning the immune response to HIV infection as various phase I, II, and III efficacy trials are under way in addition to the development of vaccines based on diverse approaches.

It is hoped that an effective vaccines is closer than never before, to contain the pandemic of HIV and AIDS.

RAPID IMMUNOCONCENTRATION TEST FOR HIV I AND HIV 2 ANTIBODIES. FLOW THROUGH METHOD

RETROQUICK-HIV, Courtesy: Tulip Group of Companies

Introduction

Retroquic-HIV is a membrane based flow through immunoassay for the detection of antibodies to HIV 1 and HIV 2 in human serum and plasma. Highly purified synthetic peptides of gp 120 and gp 41 (HIV 1) and gp 36 (HIV 2) corresponding to the immunodominant regions of the HIV 1 and HIV 2 utilised in the test system assist in visual, qualitative, simultaneous detection and differentiation of antibodies to HIV 1 and 2.

Summary

Acquired Immunodeficiency syndrome (AIDS) is caused by at least two retroviruses, the HIV 1 and the HIV 2, collectively referred to as HIV 1/2. Antibodies to HIV 1 envelope protein (gp 120), transmembrane protein (gp 41) and HIV 2 transmembrane protein (gp 36) are prevalent in sera of individuals with AIDS or ARC or who are at high risk of contracting AIDS. Detection of these antibodies indicates exposure to the HIV 1/2 virus.

Principle

Retroquic-HIV test comprises of a test device striped with distinct bands of purified gp 120 and gp 41 synthetic peptide specific to HIV 1 at test region '1' and gp 36 synthetic peptide specific to HIV 2 at test region '2'. The third band striped at region 'C' corresponds to the assay performance control. First the membrane assembly is hydrated with wash buffer and then the specimen is added. Antibodies to HIV 1 and/or 2 if present, are captured by the respective antigens. After washing with wash buffer, Protein A conjugated gold sol reagent is added to reveal the presence/ absence of bound antibodies. Post final wash a positive reaction is visualised by the appearance of purple coloured bands at the test region '1' and/or '2'. The absence of bands at test region '1' and '2' is a negative test result. The appearance of control band serves to validate sample addition, reagent and assay performance.

REAGENTS AND MATERIALS SUPPLIED

Kit components

Retroquic-HIV immunoconcentration test kit for HIV 1 and HIV 2 antibodies comprises of the following components:

1. Ready to use individually pouched, flow through test devices striped with HIV 1 specific purified synthetic peptides at test region '1' and HIV 2 specific purified synthetic peptides at test region '2' and a blue dyed protein A based control band at region 'C' along with a specimen dropper and dessicant.
2. Dropper bottle with ready to use wash buffer solution.
3. Dropper bottle with ready to use protein A conjugated gold sol solution.
4. Package insert.

Storage and Stability

The unopened Retroquic-HIV kit, as well as kit components upon opening, must be stored at 2 to 8°C, till the duration of the shelf life as indicated on the kit/kit component labels.

1. *In vitro* diagnostic test. Not for medicinal use.
2. Read package insert carefully before performing the test.
3. Do not use beyond expiry date.
4. Flow through device, wash buffer and protein A conjugate of the same lot are optimized as a system. It is important that the kit components of the same lot are used for achieving accurate and reproducible results. Do not intermix reagents from different lots.
5. The sequence of addition of reagents should be followed meticulously for achieving accurate results.
6. Handle all specimen as potentially infectious.
7. Follow standard bio safety guidelines for personal protection, handling and disposal of potentially infectious material.
8. After use, the kit components must be returned to the recommended storage temperature immediately.

Specimen Collection and Preparations

1. No prior preparation of the patient is required before sample collection by approved techniques.

2. Fresh serum/plasma is preferable. Serum/ plasma may be stored at 2 to 8° C upto 24 hours in case of delay in testing. For long term storage, freeze the specimen at -20°C.
3. Repeated freezing and thawing of the specimen should be avoided.
4. Do not use haemolysed, clotted, contaminated, viscous/turbid specimen.
5. Specimen containing precipitates or particulate matter must be centrifuged and the clear supernatant only used for testing.
6. Do not heat -inactivate the specimen.
7. Frozen samples for retrospective studies must be centrifuged at 3000 rpm for 15 minutes and the clear supernatant must be used for tests.

Test Procedure

1. Bring all reagents and specimen to room temperature (25 - 30°C) before use. Tighten the Wash Buffer solution and Protein A Gold Conjugate dropper bottle caps in a clockwise direction to pierce the respective dropper bottle nozzles. The addition of specimen/ reagents must be done at the centre of the reaction port, holding the sample dropper/dropper bottles in a vertical position. Ensure the drops are free falling. Use a new sample dropper for each specimen to avoid cross contamination.
2. Tear open the foil pouches and retrieve the required number of Retroquic-HIV membrane test devices and label appropriately.
3. Add two drops of wash buffer into the reaction port of the device and allow to soak through completely.
4. Using the sample dropper provided, add one drop of the serum/plasma specimen into the reaction port. Allow to soak through completely.
5. Add three drops of wash buffer to the reaction port and allow to soak through completely.
6. Add two drops of protein A gold conjugate to the reaction port and allow to soak through completely.
7. Add two drops of wash buffer and allow the wash buffer to soak through completely.
8. Read and record the results immediately.

INTERPRETATION OF RESULTS

Negative Test result

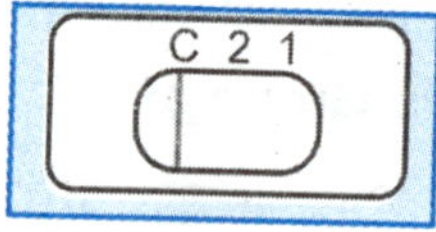

Appearance of only one control band corresponding to control region 'C'.

Positive Test results

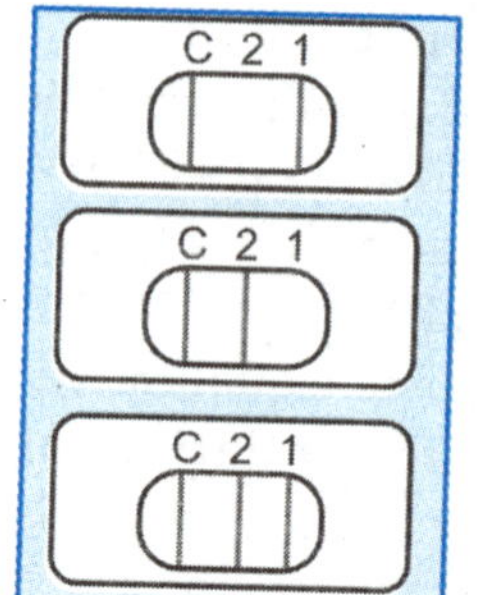

In addition to the control band 'C', appearance of reactive band at test region '1': Specimen positive for Antibodies to HIV 1.

In addition to the control band 'C', appearance of reactive band at test region '2': Specimen positive for Antibodies to HIV 2.

In addition to the control band 'C', appearance of reactive bands at test region '1' and test region '2' Specimen positive for Antibodies to HIV 1 and HIV 2.

Invalid Test result

The test should be considered invalid if neither the test band nor the control band appears. In case of invalid results, the test should be repeated using a fresh device.

Performance Characteristics

In an in-house trial, one thousand and sixty four specimen negative for antibodies to HIV 1 and HIV 2 and hundred and forty five specimen positive for antibodies to HIV 1 and ninteen specimen positive for antibodies to HIV 1 and .HIV 2 were run in parallel with a licensed, commercially available test and Retroquic-HIV. The results obtained are as follows:

Specimen	*No. of samples*	*Licensed Test*	*Retroquic -HIV*
Negative for Ab. to HIV.1/2		1064	1064 1064
Positive for Ab. to HIV 1	145	145	145
Positive for Ab. to HIV 1 and HIV 2	19	19	19

Based on the above study the sensitivity and specificity of Retroquic-HIV is 100% each.

Remarks

1. The addition of reagents must be accomplished without interruptions.
2. After addition of the wash buffer, in step 7 of the procedure, if the background in the reaction port is high, the samples must be recentrifuged appropriately so as to pellet invisible particulate matter. Test should be rerun with the clear supernatant.
3. The presence of antibodies to HIV 1/2 indicates previous exposure to HIV 1 and/or HIV 2 virus but does not constitute a diagnosis of AIDS.
4. Absence of antibodies to HIV 1/2 does not indicate that an individual is absolutely free of HIV 1 or HIV 2 as the collection of sample and its timing vis-a-vis sero-conversion will influence the test outcome.
5. Since HIV 1 and HIV 2 viruses are similar in genomic structure and morphology and antibodies to them have (30-70%) cross reactivity, reactive test bands for HIV 1 and HIV 2 do not necessarily imply mixed infection with HIV 1 and HIV 2.
6. Though Retroquic-HIV is a reliable and sensitive screening test, it should not be used as a sole criterion for diagnosis of HIV infection.
7. All positive specimen should be further tested using appropriate supplemental confirmatory tests.
8. As in all tests the results must be correlated with clinical findings before arriving at the final diagnosis.
9. Since various tests for HIV 1/2 differ in their performance characteristics and antigenic composition, the reactivity patterns may differ.
10. The results of Retroquic-HIV must be read within 30 minutes of test completion.
11. Do not compare the intensity of the test lines and the control lines to judge the concentration of the antibodies in the test sample.
12. Testing of pooled specimen is not recommended.
13. The control band in fresh unused membrane test devices is blue coloured and changes to blackish purple colour after test performance.
14. The control band would not develop if the sample addition has not been done.

RAPID IMMUNOCHROMATOGRAPHIC TEST FOR HIV 1/2 ANTIBODIES LATERAL FLOW METHOD

RETROCHECK HIV, Courtesy: Tulip Group of Companies

Introduction

Retrocheck HIV - WB is a third generation, rapid, self performing, qualitative, two site, sandwich immunoassay for the simultaneous detection of antibodies specific to the HIV 1 and HIV 2 virus in serum, plasma or whole blood. The test employs recombinant proteins representing the highly immunodominant envelope and core regions of HIV 1 (gp 41 and p24-0-subtype fusion polypeptide) and the envelope region of HIV 2 (gp 36). Combination of these proteins in a third generation double antigen sandwich format affords specific and early detection of seroconversion following exposure to HIV 1 and HIV 2.

Summary

Acquired immunodeficiency syndrome (AIDS) is caused by at least two retroviruses, the HIV 1 and the HIV 2, collectively referred to as HIV 1:12. Antibodies to HIV 1 core protein p24, transmembrane protein (gp 41) and/or antibodies to HIV 2 transmembrane protein (gp 36) are prevalent in the sera of individuals with AIDS, ARC or at high risk of contracting AIDS. Detection of these antibodies indicates exposure to the HIV 1/2 virus.

Principle

Retrocheck HIV-WB utilises the principle of lateral flow immunochromatography, a unique two site, double antigen sandwich immunoassay on a membrane. As the test specimen flows through the membrane of the test assembly, the coloured HIV specific recombinant antigen-colloidal gold conjugate complexes with HIV antibodies in the sample. This complex moves further on the membrane to the test region 'T' where it is immobilised by the HIV specific recombinant antigens coated on the membrane leading to formation of a coloured band which confirms a positive test result. Absence of the coloured band in the test region 'T' indicates a negative test result. The unreacted conjugate and unbound complex if any, move further on the membrane and are subsequently immobilised by the anti-rabbit antibodies coated on the membrane at the control region 'C', forming a coloured band. This control band serves to validate the reagent and assay performance.

REAGENTS AND MATERIAL SUPPLIED

Kit Components

1. Retrocheck HIV-WB membrane test assembly comprises of HIV specific recombinant antigen-colloidal gold conjugate co-dispensed with rabbit IgG gold conjugate; pre dispensed with HIV specific recombinant antigen at region 'T' and anti-rabbit antiserum pre dispensed at the region 'C', along with a sample dropper and desiccant.
2. Sample Running Buffer.
3. Package insert.

Storage and Stability

The test kit may be stored between 4 and 30°C for the duration of the shelf life of the kit as indicated on the pouch/kit label.

Note

1. In vitro diagnostic test.
2. Do not use beyond expiry date.
3. Read the package insert carefully before performing the test.
4. Handle all specimen as potentially infectious.
5. Follow standard biosafety guidelines for personal protection, handling and disposal of potentially infectious material.

Specimen Collection and Preparation

1. No prior preparation of the patient is required before sample collection by approved techniques.
2. Fresh serum/plasma is preferable. Anticoagulated whole blood can also be used as specimen. Serum/plasma may be stored at 2 to 8°C upto 24 hours in case of delay in testing. For long term storage, freeze the specimen at -20°C. Whole blood should be used immediately and should not be frozen.
3. Repeated freezing and thawing of the specimen should be avoided.
4. Do not use haemolysed, clotted, contaminated, viscous/turbid specimen.
5. Specimen containing precipitates or paniculate matter must be centrifuged and the clear supernatant only used for testing.
6. Do not heat inactivate the sample.
7. Frozen samples for retrospective studies must be centrifuged at 3000 rpm for 15 minutes and the clear supernatant must be used for tests.

Test Procedure and Interpretation of Results

1. Let the sealed pouches attain room temperature (25-30°C). Tighten the cap of sample running buffer bottle to pierce the dropper bottle nozzle. The addition of the specimen and buffer must be done at the center of the sample/reagent addition ports holding the sample dropper/dropper bottles in a vertical position. Ensure the drops are free falling. Use a new sample dropper for each specimen to avoid cross contamination.
2. Tear open the sealed pouches and retrieve the appropriate number of membrane test assemblies as required. Label the membrane test assembly appropriately. Once opened the assemblies must be used immediately.
3. Dispense one drop of serum/plasma or whole blood using the sample dropper provided into the sample port 'A'.
4. Dispense five drops of sample running buffer into reagent port 'B'.
5. At the end of fifteen minutes, read the results as follows:

   Negative test result

   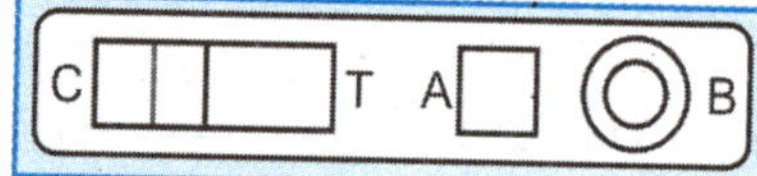

   Appearance of only one coloured band at the control region 'C'. Specimen negative for antibodies to HIV 1/2.

   Positive test result.

   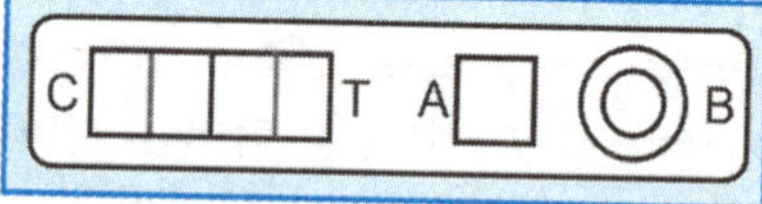

   Appearance of a coloured band at the test region 'T' in addition to the band at control region 'C'. Specimen positive for antibodies to HIV 1/2.
6. The test should be considered invalid if neither the test nor the control band appear. Repeat the test with a new device.
7. Based on the concentration of antibodies to HIV 1 and HIV 2 in the specimen a positive result may start appearing as early as two minutes, negative results must, however, be confirmed only at the end of fifteen minutes.

8. In case of doubtful results at fifteen minutes, the test may be extended up to a maximum of 30 minutes, if required.

Performance Characteristics

In an in-house clinical trial, one thousand and sixty four known negative specimens for antibodies to HIV 1 and HIV 2, one hundred and four known positive specimen for antibodies to HIV 1 and nineteen known positive specimens for antibodies to HIV 1 and HIV 2 were tested with Retrocheck HIV-WB in parallel with a licensed commercially available test. The results obtained are as follows:

Specimen	*No. of samples*	*Licensed Test*	*Retrocheck HIV - WB*
Negative for Ab's. to HIV 1 and HIV 2	1064	1062	1062
Positive for Ab's. to HIV 1	104	104	104
Positive for Ab's. to HIV and HIV 2	19	19	19

Based on the above study the sensitivity of Retrocheck HIV - WB is 100% and specificity is 99.8%.

Remarks

1. Though Retrocheck HIV - WB is a sensitive and reliable screening test, it should not be used as a sole criterion for diagnosis of HIV infection.
2. All positive specimen should be further tested using appropriate supplemental confirmatory tests. Test samples that are positive by third generation double antigen sandwich based assays may be reactive with very early seroconversion samples, which are negative/ indeterminate with blot based assays. Such samples should be reconfirmed with a RNA-PCR based method or must be followed up for seroconversion later.
3. As with all diagnostic tests, results must be correlated with clinical findings to arrive at the final diagnosis.
4. Absence of antibodies to HIV 1/2 does not indicate that an individual is absolutely free of HIV 1/2 infection, as the collection of sample and its timing vis-à-vis seroconversion will influence the test outcome.
5. Do not compare the intensity of test lines and the control lines to judge the concentration of antibodies in the test specimen.
6. Since various tests for HIV differ in their performance characteristics and antigenic composition, their reactivity patterns may differ.
7. Testing of pooled samples is not recommended.
8. The presence of antibodies to HIV indicates previous exposure to HIV 1 and/or HIV 2; but does not constitute a diagnosis of AIDS.
9. The results of Retrocheck HIV-WB must be read within 30 minutes of the test completion.
10. The membrane is laminated with an adhesive tape to prevent surface evaporation. Air pockets or patches may appear, which do not interfere with the test results. Presence of a band at the test region even if low in intensity or formation is a positive result.
11. The deliberate slow reaction kinetics of Retrocheck HIV - WB is designed to maximize and enhance reaction time between sample capture and tracer elements to improve test sensitivity.
12. Retrocheck HIV-WB is also reactive with HIV 1 group 'O' subtype samples.

TUBERCULOSIS

TB IgG, IgA, IgM Ab, Mfd. ANDA
Courtesy: Lilac Medicare

In vitro diagnostic test Enzyme-immuno-assay for the Determination of IgA, IgG or IgM Antibodies against Mycobacteria in Human Serum.

Serodiagnosis of Mycobacterial Infections

The A60 antigen complex is an inter-specific antigen found in the cytosol of typical and atypical mycobacteria. It reacts with antibodies created during mycobacterial intections (tuberculosis, leprae,....), and also reacts with the antibodies produced during Nocardia intections.

Antimycobacterial antibodies are absent in healthy individuals. However, inapparent or abortive infections due to mycobacteria are much more frequent than usually suspected. In particular, IgM antibodies are frequently observed after a contact inherent to professional occupations (e.g. hospital personnel and social workers) or to adverse social conditions.

In the latter case, the positive IgM reaction is observed most readily among babies and infants growing in unhealthy conditions. A positive IgM test observed in the serum and CSF is most useful in establishing the diagnosis of tuberculous meningitis for the serodiagnosis of latent pulmonary or extrapulmonary tuberculous primary infection and for the prognosis of relapses.

The large amount of work that has been carried out to establish the clinical validity of the Anda.Tb IgG test allowed the following conclusions to be drawn:

- Healthy people are negative, even if they have a positive intraderma reaction and even if they live in a country with severe endemy.
- The prevalence of inapparent subclinical infections is largely under-evaluated in the third-world, but also in developed countries among certain social and professional groups: people in regular contact with individuals belonging to the third or fourth-world (e.g. food store employees, hospital personnel an jailed people), non-tuberculous diseased people, positive HIV patients in hospitals and others. All show a percentage of A60 seropositives, sometimes well superior to that seen in the population at large which presents a frequency of positives fluctuating between 1.5 percent and 3 percent.
- In patients suffering from a tuberculous infection, the test shows the presence of IgG antibodies if the patient has undergone an antigenic booster stimulus. The test will be positive mostly in cases of patent active infection. It will also be positive in case of a booster vaccination in healthy people.
- In patients affected by extra-pulmonary tuberculosis, the test will be effective according to the organ infected.
- In 10 to 20 percent of the patients, the humoral immunologic activity is weak. Patients showing such an anergy may appear negative.
- Tuberculous meningitis provokes the formation of antibodies in the cerebro-spinal fluid (CSF), detectable at a 1:10 dilution.

The presence of IgG antibodies indicates a good immunological response of the patient to the infection. An energy affecting some patients before or at the beginning of the treatment concerns as well the cellular immunity (PPD) as the IgG output. The production of IgA antibodies is largely independent from the production of IgG antibodies and may occur while the patient is in an IgG anergic state. IgA antibodies easily form complexes with antigen and are at the origin of inflammatory processes in various organs. IgA antibodies are readily detected in the serum of some apparently healthy individuals at risk, in the sputum of some patients suffering from a pulmonary tuberculous infection and in biological fluids of patients suffering from extra-pulmonary infections. In particular, specific IgA antibodies are detected in about 30 percent of the patients suffering from Crohn's disease. Interestingly, people in contact with these patients only show elevated IgG antibodies. Note that the presence of anfi-A 60 antibodies in those patients is probably due to secondary mycobacterial infections, as other studies do not report their presence and as nucleic acids specific to mycobacteria have never been discovered in that type of patient.

Principle of the Method

Anda Tb is an immuno-enzymatic test with dosage on a solid phase. Samples of diluted human sera, sputum (IgA) or cerebrospinal fluid (CSF) are distributed in the wells of the microtitration plates coated with the A60 mycobacterial complexes. Their incubation allows for the formation of antigen-antibodies complexes. The unbound components of the sera are eliminated by washing. The wells are thereafter incubated with peroxidase-labelled anti-human IgA, IgG or IgM antibodies that bind to the antibody complexes present. The unbound antibodies are eliminated by washing. A solution of tetra-methyl-benzidine (TMB) containing hydrogen peroxide, is thereafter introduced in the wells. A colour develops during the reaction of peroxidase with TMB, whose quantity is proportional to that of specific antibodies present in the sample.

For IgA and IgG tests, a reference curve is constructed by plotting the optical densities of the references. The concentration of the unknown sera analysed at the same time as the references is then determined from the reference curve and transformed into relative sero-units, which allows the user to take into account the inevitable daily variations which occur during the determinations.

For IgM tests, a threshold value is determined from the optical density obtained with a positive reference. The sample whose optical density is equal to or greater than this value is considered positive.

The controls included in the IgG tests are intended to verify if the test was properly carried out. They are not to be used as references.

Reagents

A. For IgA tests

1. 2 bottles (2 × 50 ml) of sample diluent (serum or sputum).
   Preservatives: Sodium azide and sodium mercurothiolate. A black deposit may appear in this reagent. It has no influence on the quality of the reagent.
2. 1 bottle (13 ml) of peroxidase-labelled anti-human IgA (anti-human IgA-POD) in protein-stabilised buffer *(blue cap)*.
   Preservatives: Thymol. A precipitate may form in this solution, which has no incidence on the quality of the reagent.
3. 1 bottle (1.6 ml) of 10-fold concentrated TMB (tetramethylbenzidine) (IRRITANT: R 20/21/22-36/37/38, S 23-26-36).
4. 1 bottle (16 ml) of TMB diluent. Citric acid-phosphate buffer containing 0.02 percent of H_2O_2 *(white cap)*.
5. 1 bottle (1.6 ml) sulfuric acid (H_2SO_4) (0.5 N) *(red cap)*.
6. 1 vial (1, 4 ml) of negative reference *(yellow cap)*.
   Preservatives: Sodium azide and sodium mercurothiolate. Ready for use.
7. 1 vial (1, 4 ml) of reference containing 1 unit/ml *(white cap)*.
   Preservatives: Sodium azide and sodium mercurothiolate. Ready for use.
8. 1 vial (1, 4 ml) of reference containing 2 units/ml *(purple cap)*.
   Preservatives: Sodium azide and sodium mercurothiolate. Ready for use.
9. 1 vial (1, 4 ml) of reference containing 4 units/ml *(pink cap)*.
   Preservatives: Sodium azide and sodium mercurothiolate. Ready for use.
10. 1 vial (1,4 ml) of reference containing 8 units/ml *(red cap)*.
    Preservatives: Sodium azide and sodium mercurothiolate. Ready for use.
11. 1 vial (1, 4 ml) of reference containing 16 units/ml *(blue cap)*.
    Preservatives: Sodium azide and sodium mercurothiolate. Ready for use.
12. 1 bottle (50 ml) of 20-fold concentrated washing buffer solution.
13. 12 strips of 8 wells coated with antigen A60 from *Mycobacterium bovis* (BCG).

B. For IgG tests

1. 2 bottles (2 x 50 ml) of sample diluent (serum, CSF., sputum or other biological fluid).
   PRESERVATIVES: Sodium azide and sodium mercurothiolate. A black deposit may appear in this reagent. It has no influence on the quality of the reagent.
2. 1 bottle (13 ml) of peroxidase-labelled anti-human IgG (anti-human IgG-POD) in protein-stabilised buffer *(blue cap)*.
   Preservative: thymol. A precipitate may form in this solution, which has no incidence on the quality of the reagent.
3. 1 bottle (1.6 ml) of 10-fold concentrated TMB (tetramethyl benzidine) (IRRITANT: R 20/21/22-36/37/38, S 23-26-36).
4. 1 bottle (16 ml) of TMB diluent. Citric acid-phosphate buffer containing 0,02 percent of H_2O_2 *(white cap)*.
5. 1 bottle (16 ml) sulfuric acid (H2SO4) (0.5N) *(red cap)*.
6. 1 vial (0,15 ml) of weak positive control (225-375 U/ ml) *(green cap)*.
   Preservative: sodium azide.
7. 1 vial (0,15 ml) of strong positive control (600-1100 U/ ml) (orange cap).
   Preservatives: Sodium azide.
8. 1 vial (1, 4 ml) of negative reference (yellow cap).
   Preservatives: Sodium azide and sodium mercurothiolate. Ready for use.
9. 1 vial (1, 4 ml) of reference containing 1 unit/ml *(white cap)*.
   Preservatives: Sodium azide and sodium mercurothiolate. Ready for use.
10. 1 vial (1, 4 ml) of reference containing 2 units/ml *(purple cap)*.
    Preservatives: Sodium azide and sodium mercurothiolate. Ready for use.

11. 1 vial (1, 4 ml) of reference containing 4 units/ml *(pink cap).*
    Preservatives: Sodium azide and sodium mercurothiolate. Ready for use.
12. 1 vial (1, 4 ml) of reference containing 8 units/ml *(red cap).*
    Preservatives: Sodium azide and sodium mercurothiolate. Ready for use.
13. 1 vial (1,4 ml) of reference containing 16 units/ml *(blue cap).*
    Preservatives: Sodium azide and .sodium mercurothiolate. Ready for use.
14. 1 bottle (50 ml) of 20-fold concentrated washing buffer solution.
15. 12 strips of 8 wells coated with antigen A60 from *Mycobacterium bovis* (BCG).

C. For IgM tests

1. 2 bottles (2 × 50 ml) of sample diluent (serum or CSF).
   Preservative: sodium mercurothiolate. A black deposit 'may appear in this reagent. It has no influence on the quality of the reagent.
2. 1 vial (13 ml) of peroxidase-labelled anti-human IgM (anti-hu mlgM-POD) in protein-stabilised buffer *(blue cap).*
   Preservative: thymol. A precipitate may form in this solution, which has no incidence on the quality of the reagent.
3. 1 bottle (1.6 ml) of 10-fold concentrated TMB (tetramethyl benzidine) (IRRITANT: R 20/21/22-36/37/38, S 23-26-36).
4. 1 bottle (16 ml) of TMB diluent. Citric acid - phosphate buffer containing 0,02 percent of H_2O_2 *(white cap).*
5. 1 bottle (16 ml) sulfuric acid (H_2SO_4J- (0.5 N) *(red cap).*
6. 1 vial (1, 4 ml) of negative reference (*grey cap*).
   Preservative: sodium mercurothiolate. Ready for use.
7. 1 vial (l, 4 ml) of positive limit reference (*brown cap*).
   Preservative: sodium mercurothioiate. Ready for use.
8. 1 bottle (50 ml) of 20-fold concentrated washing buffer solution.
9. 12 strips of 8 wells coated with antigen A60 from *Mycobacterium bovis* (BCG).

Material Required but not Provided

- Pipettes of l0µl, 100 µl and 1000 µl
- A photometer that can measure absorbances at 450 nm
- Tubes for serum dilutions
- Distilled or demineralised water
- A 37° C incubator.

Specimen Collection and Preparation

1. The samples to be analysed should be either serum, sputum, cerebrospinal fluid (CSF) or other biological fluids. Collect the specimens using normal techniques. Avoid haemolysis. Let the blood clot at room temperature in a sterile vessel and then extract the serum.
2. Sputum can be used in the IgA and IgG tests at a 1:20 dilution. CSF can be used in the IgG and IgM tests at a 1:10 dilution.
3. Use material for single use only.
4. Store the samples in the cold and keep an aliquot frozen.

Precautions of Use

1. Do not pipet by mouth.
2. Do not mix reagents from different batches.
3. Do not use the components beyond their expiration date.
4. Keep reagents at +4°C in the dark. Only the sulphuric acid, the washing buffer solution and the coated wells can be kept at room temperature.
5. Bring reagents to room temperature just before use.
6. Avoid microbial contamination of the reagents when opening and removing aliquots from primary vials.
7. Change the tips of the pipettes after each operation in order to avoid cross-contamination.
8. Be sure that all the wells are submitted to the same operational conditions and the same incubation periods.
9. A determination cannot be interrupted once started and must be brought to its completion.
10. Incubate the wells in the shadow or the dark.
11. Avoid physical contact with the sulphuric acid and the TMB stock solution. In case of contact, wash the contaminated surface abundantly with water.

12. The products of human origin have been found devoid of the following infections: HIV I and II, hepatitis B and C. They have however, to be manipulated as infectious products. Wear gloves, protective clothes and other appropriate material while using them. Clean up spills with appropriate antiviral products.
13. The time limit for use of an open kit is six months or the expiry date of the kit, whichever comes first, provided all constituents have been properly closed, have not been contaminated and have been stored properly (see point 4).

Preparation of the Reagents

a. Washing solution

Add 19 volumes of distilled water to one volume of concentrated (20x) washing buffer.

b. TMB work solution

Add 9 volumes of TMB diluent to one volume of concentrated (10x) TMB solution. This solution is to be prepared just before use. It must be colourless and homogeneous.

Preparation of Diluted TMB solution

Number of wells	*TMB concentrated*	*TMB diluent*
8	0.10 ml	0.9 ml
16	0.20 ml	1.80 ml
32	0.35 ml	3.15 ml
48	0.50 ml	4.50 ml
64	0.70 ml	6.30 ml
80	0.90 ml	8.10 ml
96	1.00 ml	9.00 ml

Test Procedure

A. For the IgA tests

1. Bring the A60 sensitised wells to room temperature.
2. Dilute the sera to be tested 1:100 in the sample medium (10 µl of serum in 1000 µl of medium). Sputum should be diluted 1:20 in the same medium. Mix well. In some regions, the presence of antibodies at a low level is very common in healthy individuals and the dilutions necessary to avoid false positives will need to be higher. This must be determined by an analysis at various dilutions, for example, 1:100, 1:200, 1:500 and 1:1000, of a panel of negative sera originating from that region. A dilution of 1:50 or 1:25 may be better suited for children and new-born babies.
3. The references are already diluted and should be used as such.
   Note : IgA determination is semi-quantitative and based on the use of the furnished references. A rougher determination can be obtained by using only the 2 and 16 U references.
4. Introduce 100 µl of diluted sample into a microtitration well. Use two wells per sample and identify each well. Proceed in the same way for the references.
5. Incubate 1 hour at 37°C.
6. Dilute the concentrated washing buffer solution during this incubation period.
7. Wash the wells under a light stream of diluted washing buffer: fill and empty the wells 5 times (3 times with an automatic plate washer). At the end of the washing process, the wells must be entirely dry.
   Note: turn the plates and hit them on a sheet of absorbing paper. Do not rub inside the wells.
8. Distribute 100 µl of anti-human IgA-POD conjugate in each well. Incubate 30 minutes at 37°C.
9. Dilute the TMB just before the end of the 30 minutes.
10. Wash the wells under a light stream of diluted washing buffer: fill and empty the wells 5 times (3 times with an automatic plate washer). At the end of the washing process, the wells must be entirely dry.
11. Distribute rapidly 100 µl of the diluted TMB solution in each well of the microtitration plate. Incubate at 37°C during exactly 15 minutes.
12. Add rapidly 100 µl of H_2SO_4.
13. Measure the absorbances at 450 nm.
14. The blank of the photometer is adjusted on air (empty, unused wells)

B. For the IgG Tests

1. Bring the A60 sensitised wells to room temperature.

2. Dilute the positive controls and the sera to be tested 1:100 in the sample medium (l0µl of serum in l000 µl of medium). Sputum should be diluted 1:20 and CSF 1:10 in the same medium. Mix well. In some regions, the presence of antibodies at a low level is very common in healthy individuals and the dilutions necessary to avoid false positives will need to be higher. This must be determined by an analysis at various dilutions, for example 1:100, 1:200, 1:500 and 1:1000, of a panel of negative sera originating from that region. A dilution of 1:50 or 1:25 may be better suited for children and new-born babies.
3. The references are already diluted and should be used as such.
   Note : IgG determination is semi-quantitative and based on the use of the furnished references. A rougher determination can be obtained by using only the 2 and 16 U references.
4. Introduce 100 µl of diluted sample into a microtitration well. Use two wells per sample and identify each well. Proceed in the same way for the references and the controls.
5. Incubate 1 hour at 37°C.
6. Dilute the concentrated washing buffer solution during this incubation period.
7. Wash the wells under a light stream of diluted washing buffer: fill and empty the wells 5 times (3 times with an automatic plate washer). At the end of the washing process, the wells must be entirely dry.
   Note: turn the plates and hit them on a sheet of absorbing paper. Do not rub inside the wells.
8. Distribute 100 µl of anti-human IgG-POD conjugate in each well. Incubate 30 minutes at 37°C.
9. Dilute the TMB just before the end of the 30 minutes.
10. Wash the wells under a light stream of diluted washing solution: fill and empty the wells 5 times (3 times with an automatic plate washer). At the end of the washing process, the wells must be entirely dry.
11. Distribute *rapidly* l00 µl of the diluted TMB solution in each well of the microtitration plate. Incubate at 37°C during exactly 15 minutes.
12. Add *rapidly* 100 µl of H_2SO_4.
13. Measure the absorbances at 450 nm.
14. The blank of the photometer is adjusted on air (empty, unused wells).

C. For the IgM tests

1. Bring the A60 sensitised wells to room temperature.
2. Dilute the sera to be tested 1:100 in the sample medium (l0 µl of serum in l00 µl of medium). CSF should be diluted 1:10 in the same medium. Mix well. In some regions, the presence of antibodies at a low level is very common in healthy individuals and the dilutions necessary to avoid false positives will need to be higher. This must be determined by an analysis at various dilutions, for example 1:100, 1:200,1:500 and 1:1000, of a panel of negative sera originating from that region. A dilution of 1:50 or 1:25 may be better suited for children and new-born babies.
3. The references are already diluted and should be used as such.
4. Introduce l00 µl of diluted sample into a microtitration well. Use two wells per sample and identify each well. Proceed in the same way for the references.
5. Incubate 1 hour at 37°C.
6. Dilute the concentrated washing buffer solution during this incubation period.
7. Wash the wells under a light stream of diluted washing buffer: fill and empty the wells 5 times (3 times with an automatic plate washer). At the end of the washing process, the wells must be entirely dry.
   Note: turn the plates and hit them on a sheet of absorbing paper. Do not rub inside the wells.
8. Distribute 100 µl of anti-hu mlg M-POD conjugate in each well. Incubate 30 minutes at 37°C.
9. Dilute the TMB just before the end of the 30 minutes.
10. Wash the wells under a light stream of diluted washing solution: fill and empty the wells 5 times (3 times with an automatic plate washer). At the end of the washing process, the wells must be entirely dry.
11. Distribute rapidly-100 µl of the diluted TMB solution in each well of the microtitration plate. Incubate at 37°C during 15 minutes.

12. During colour development, read the absorbance of the positive reference after 15 minutes (without adding sulphuric acid) in the blue range, i.e. at 620 nm. If the observed absorbance is below 0.13, continue the incubation for a further 10 minutes at 37°C (25 minutes total).
13. Add rapidly 100 µl of H_2SO_4.
14. Measure the absorbances at 450 nm.
15. The blank of the photometer is adjusted on air (empty, unused wells).

Summary of the Procedure

Step	*Calibrators*	*Samples*
References, Ready for use	100 µl	
Diluted samples And controls	-	100 µl

Incubate 1 hour at 37°C

Wash 5 times with washing buffe		
Addition of		
PODase-labelled	100 µl	100 µl
Anti-human Ig		

Incubate 30 Minutes at 37°C

Wash 5 times with washing buffer		
Diluted TMB	100 µl	100 µl
Incubate 15 minutes at 37°C for IgA, IgG		

Incubate 15-25 minutes at 37°C for IgM

H_2SO_4	100 µl	100 µl
Read at 450 NM		

Determination of Results

A. IgA and IgG tests

1. Calculate the mean absorbance (OD at 450 nm) for each sample and reference.
2. On semi-log graph paper, plot the OD result of each reference, except for the negative reference, on the vertical axis (arithmetic ordinate = Y) in relation to the number of corresponding units on the horizontal axis (logarithmic abscissa = X). This reference curve should essentially be a straight line between 2 and 16 units with IgG but is not necessary so with IgA. The extrapolation of the results beyond 16 units is not recommended because of the loss in precision of the measures at high densities. Sera whose OD is superior to that obtained for *16* units should be further diluted and reanalysed on the basis of the new dilution factor.
3. Using the mean absorbance value for each sample, determine the corresponding concentration of antibodies expressed in units/ml as follows. From the reference curve, find the absorbance value on the Y axis and extend a horizontal line down to the reference curve. At the intersection point, extend a vertical line to the X axis and read the corresponding concentration in specific Igs for the unknown. Multiply by the applied dilution factor (normally 100) to obtain the ELISA units.
4. Controls: The weak positive control for IgG should give results between 225 and 375 U, the strong positive control for IgG should give results between 600 and 1100 U.

B. IgM Tests

1. Calculate the mean absorbance (OD at 450 nm) tor each sample and reference.
2. Normalised values: To reduce daily variations and for comparison of data obtained on different days, divide the absorbance of the analysed samples by the absorbance of the positive reference obtained during the analysis.

$$\frac{\text{A 450 nm sample}}{\text{A 450 nm positive reference.}}$$

The normalised value of the positive reference is 1. All samples whose normalised absorbance value is below 0, 8 are considered negative, indicating levels of specific antibodies inferior to those expected to confirm an infection. All samples whose normalised value is comprised between 0, 8 and 1, 0 are considered dubious and all samples whose normalised value is above 1.0 are considered positive for IgM globulins. The test is positive provided interfering pathological conditions are excluded.

C. Limits of the Methods

The results obtained with this test are to be estimated in conjunction with clinical observations and the results of other tests.

1. The concentration of circulating antibodies must be used as a complement to other information available to the physician (symptoms, results of other tests, clinical observations.).
   - As an example, the absence of IgG or IgA antibodies in a patient showing other symptoms characteristic of TB infection should not be considered as a false negative, but rather as a case of anergy indicating that the infection is at an advanced state and/or that the patient needs external help to overcome his illness.
   - Similarly, the presence of IgM antibodies in an otherwise healthy individual indicates the start of an infection. This person should therefore, be watched to determine if the infection is benign and transitory of if it will develop into an illness.
   - Finally, a high level of IgG of IgA antibodies in an otherwise healthy individual indicates that he has regular contacts with an infectious source and that he should be watched.
2. Haemolysed samples or samples showing strong lipemia or turbidity may yield false values.

D. Specificity

1. Mycobacterioses other than those caused by M tuberculosis (typical tubercolosis) and *M bovis* may yield positive results with the Anda elisa test. This is the case for organisms of the *M avium* (atypical tuberculosis), *M paratuberculosis* and *M. leprae* groups. It is also the case for other mycobacteria, such as *M xenopi*, *M chelonei* or *M kansasii*, that rarely cause illnesses. These atypical mycobacteria sometimes cause secondary infections in immunodepressed/patients (cancer, HIV, etc.) or inapparent infections in healthy persons.
2. Cross-reaction by non-tuberculous diseases caused by *Nocardia* is reported, as are frequent and inapparent secondary infections caused by mycobacteria during leishmaniasis.
3. Interference by non-tuberculosis pulmonary diseases is possible. These are caused by secondary infections by a mycobacterial species listed above and are often benign and transient.
4. Immuno-depressive treatments presumably alter the immuneresponse to infection, inducing negative results in IgG, IgA or both in tuberculous patients.
5. All IgM-sero-positive samples should be submitted to a confirmation test after their absorbance on protein G to eliminate the possible interferences due to rheumatoid factor or high levels of IgG. Anda Biologicals provides such a protein G suspension (Anda. Bind Filtration and Anda. Bind Sedimentation).
6. Specificity of Anda ELISA mycobacteria depends on the studied population and on the chosen control groups in each clinical trial. Some examples are presented in the table on the following page.

E. Sensitivity

The sensitivity of the Anda ELISA mycobacteria kits depends on the cut off values used. These cut-off values must be determined separately in each population as it varies with exposure level to the TB bacillus and other environmental mycobacteria. Similarly, positive and negative predictive values vary with the prevalence of TB in the population.

'Interpretation of the Results

A. Cut off

Serological data are a measure of the humoral immune status of a patient or of a population. They are not a substitute to antigen detection but are comparable to tuberculin tests, which evaluate the cellular immune status of a patient or of a population. The difference resides in the long-lasting skin reactivity after exposure, which is not found in humoral immunity. In this case, the antibody production appears to depend on the antigenic load. A second difference is the possibility to analyse three different gamma-globulin classes. As with the skin reactions, the clinician must adapt the cut-off of serological measurements to the level of endemy observed in the region or within the analysed population. In general, the following cut-offs have been found applicable:

IgM

Absorbance	Normalised values	
Neg. <Ref. Pos. - 20%	< 0.8	
Ret. Pos. - 20%<Borderline <Ref.Pos.	-	0.8 - 1.0
Positive>Ref. Pos.	> 1.0	

	IgA Sero - Units	**IgG** Sero - Units	
Neg.	Neg. <200	< 125	
Borderline	neg: 201-300 pos.: 301-350	125 - 225	
Positive	>350	-	> 225

Children and HIV-infected people: the positive cut-off is reduced to 120 U/ ml for IgG and 200 U/ ml for IgA.

The search for IgG antibodies should be completed by a search for IgM antibodies: both classes of antibodies should be analysed together. For diagnostic purposes, analysis of both IgG and IgA antibodies will greatly increase the specificity and sensitivity of the results.

Serological data must always be integrated with clinical, imaging, microbiological and tuberculin skin tests in order to reach the most accurate diagnostic conclusion.

B. Healthy People

In healthy people, an IgM positive result may be observed without consequences in the following situations:

a. A transient IgM answer may be observed 7 to 10 days after a tuberculin skin test.
b. The presence of rheumatoid factor may yield a positive result.
c. A BCG vaccination may readily induce the synthesis of antibodies, specially of the IgM class.
d. Contacts with a mycobacterial focus may be betrayed by a short transient outburst of IgM antibodies.
e. An Inapparent infection, without symptons, of atypicol mycobacteria, will cause production of antibodies.

People with negative X-rays and absence of symptoms may yield the following results: (1)

IgM - IgG - IgA-: skin test positive: previous contact. No infection, no action advised.

IgM + IgG - IgA -: Skin test negative or positive. This pattern denotes a recently jnfected subject. Action may be advised.

IgM - IgG + IgA +/-: Skin test positive: previous contact with a good immunological response . No action advised.

IgM + IgG + IgA +/-: Previous contact and recent re-exposure. Action may be advised.

C. Tuberculous States

It is now established that mycobacterial infections reach a state of active disease when the immune defences of the host are reduced. The disease appears most readily in the presence of cofactors which favour the evolution of the infection (cancer, HIV, malnutrition, unhealthy living conditions, etc.). This prerequisite immunological weakness is further amplified by the immunological energy induced by the invading *Mycobacterium* itself which, under favourable circumstances, is able to inhibit the humoral and cellular immunities of the host. The immunological energy is usually abolished after about 2 weeks of efficacious chemotherapy. Nevertheless, it may last much longer when the treatment is inappropriate or when the treatment has been applied at a later stage of the infection (6).

a. A **R**eactive (**R**) tuberculosis evolves positively because the immunity of the patient is efficient (1). Clinically, the disease is present as a localised form.
b. An **A**nergic (**A**) tuberculosis occurs when a pre-existing immune depression, sometimes amplified by the bacillus, favours the disease. The illness is then characterised by several non-circumscribed localisations. There are cavities, parenchymal destruction and abundant presence of mycobacteria. In the most severe cases, IDR and antibodies are absent.
c. Intermediate situations, Intermediary **R**eactive (**IR**) and Intermediary **A**nergic (**IA**), are of course also observed.

	R	**A**	**IR**	**IA**
Mantoux 51U	+	-	+/-	
Mantouxl 10 IU	+	-	+	+/-
Multitestl MC	+	-	+	+/-
Serology IgM	-	+/-	+/-	+
Serology IgG	+/-	-	+	+/-
Microbiology	-	+	+/-	+
Response to therapy	+	-	+	+/-

R: reactive illness—**A**: inactice illness (anergy)

IR: reactive intermediate stage—IA: inactive intermediate stage

Conclusion (1)

M-, G + and Mantoux + : past infection without clinical signs or ongoing disease of the Reactive type.

M -, G + and Mantoux + : either TB in terminal phase or disease in progress, of the **R** or **IR** type.

M +, G + and Mantoux + : ongoing disease of the **IR** or **IA** type

M +, G - and Mantoux + : ongoing disease of the **IA** type

M +, G - and Mantoux - : ongoing disease of the **A** or **IA** type

M -, G - and Mantoux - : non-tuberculous disease, or anergic tuberculosis of the **A** type

M +, G + and Mantoux - : ongoing disease, of the **IR** or **IA** type.

M -, G + and Mantoux -: ongoing disease, of the **IR** type.

D. HIV Cases

People infected by HIV often suffer from reduced immunological functions. In these cases, the Mantoux intradermal reaction must be considered positive when the diameter of the induration reaches 5 mm. The only anti-mycobacterial antibodies we may expect to detect are of the IgM class. IgG antibodies are produced in little amounts: they must be looked for at a low serum dilution. IgM positivity in a HIV patient is sufficient to start a prophylaxis, even if the tuberculin results are negative.

E. IgA Antibodies

IgA has a potent inflammatory potential: polymeric IgA and immune complexes with IgA activate complement and can trigger inflammatory mechanisms in different organs. Increased synthesis of specific IgA antibodies is experimentally associated with increased susceptibility to infection. During an infection (symptomatic or not), the production of IgA antibodies'occurs normally after the initial surge of IgM antibodies. Production-of IgA antibodies is not strongly affected by the anergy that may reduce the IgG production and hypersensitivity reactivity observed at the onset of infection in some patients. Apparently, IgA antibodies are part of the misdirected immunological TH 2-response affecting some patients: in extreme cases, some anergic patients devoid of cutireactivity and with low IgGs may abundantly produce IgA antibodies. In contrast, people responding adequately to a mycobacterial challenge may show high levels of IgG antibodies and no IgAs.

The presence of IgA antibodies in the serum of healthy people has been correlated with a frequent contact with infectious foci. IgA antibodies are often observed together with low but significant levels of IgG antibodies and these antibodies may betray an inflammatory process in other organs than the lungs in apparently healthy people.

The presence of IgA antibodies in the serum, sputum, or other biological fluids of tuberculous patients indicates that the immunological response of these patients has been partially or totally misdirected. On rare occasions, it is the only specific antibody that can be detected. Its search is thus, warranted when immune anergy has depressed the synthesis of IgM and IgG antibodies.

In patients suffering from extrapulmonary infections, the presence of IgA antibodies detected in bodily fluids (pleural fluid, pericardial fluid, etc.) at a 1:20 dilution is a major sign of mycobacterial infection. Detection of IgAs in these fluids is, in difficult cases, a precious diagnostic clue that complements the detection of IgM and IgG antibodies in serum.

F. Interpretations of Serological Results

1. Serologicaliy positive cases in a healthy population betray recent infection. IgM seropositivity is very frequent but transient. It is found for example among children and babies living in unhealthy conditions, among student nurses learning to handle mycobacterial cultures or among soldiers. This IgM positivity normally disappears after 1 to 2 months provided the subject is no longer in contact with an infectious focus.

   IgA seropositivity is scarce and found for example among the flight crew of airlines regularly flying to Third-World countries. IgG seropositivity is even more scarce among healthy subjects and denotes a frequent exposure to infectious foci (policemen, hospital personnel, mycobacteriologists, supermarket employees, etc.).

2. Positive serology is frequently observed in some well defined diseases (cystic fibrosis, leishmaniasis, cancer pneumopathy, sarcoidosis, AIDS). This seropositivity denotes a mycobacterial colonisation. This infection is most often inapparent, but the patient should be followed just in case it develops into an illness.
3. Positive serology in some patients may indicate an infection or secondary infection, inapparent or not, by mycobacteria other than *M. tuberculosis*.
4. Presence of IgM antibodies points to the beginning of a primary infection. The IgM test is particularly useful for the early diagnosis of tuberculous meningitis. The IgM antibodies are superior to IgG to detect mycobacterial colonisation in AIDS patients.
5. IgG antibodies appear when an infection is well established. They indicate that the patient produces a good immunological response against the infection.
6. IgM plus IgG measurements are analysed together to detect reactivation cases in chronic infections.
7. IgG antibodies are routinely analysed both in chronic infections and to measure the effects of therapy. Immunologically weak patients will develop an anergic condition brought about, at least in part, by the bacillus itself. A successful therapy, observed through improving clinical signs and culture negativisation, is often accompanied by first an increase in IgG titres, followed by a decrease in titres during therapy, provided the therapy was not given too late. If the therapy is failing, or if the patient is relapsing, the IgG titres will again increase.
8. Persistence of low levels of antibodies after therapy is supposed to indicate the presence of non-evacuated antigenic pouches.
9. IgA antibodies are most helpful in difficult cases presenting an anergy, i.e. lack of tuberculin reactivity and no synthesis of IgG antibodies.
10. Detection of IgA antibodies in bodily fluids other than serum or sputum strengthen the diagnosis of mycobacteriai infection in cases of:
    - suspected meningitis
    - pleuresy and pericarditis
    - renal tuberculosis
    - AIDS syndrome

TUMOUR MARKERS

ALPHA-FETOPROTEIN (AFP) ELISA

Courtesy: Lilac medicare

Intended Use: The Quantitative Determination of Alpha-Fetoprotein (AFP) Concentration in Human Serum by a Microplate Immunoenzymometric Assay

Summary and Explanation of the Test

Alpha-Fetoprotein (AFP) is a glycoprotein with a molecular weight of 70 kDA. AFP is normally produced during fetal development by the hepatocytes, yolk sac and to a lesser extent by the gastrointestinal tract. Serum concentrations reach a peak level of up to 10 mg/ml at twelve weeks of gestation. This peak level gradually decreases to less than 25 ng/ml after one year of postpartum. Thereafter, the levels reduce further to less than 10 ng/ml.

Elevated levels of AFP are found in patients with primary heptatoma and yolk sac-derived germ tumors. AFP is the most useful marker for the diagnosis and management of hepatocellular carcinoma.

AFP is also elevated in pregnant women. Presence of abnormally high AFP concentrations in pregnant women provides a risk marker for Down syndrome.

In this method, AFP calibrator, patient specimen or control is first added to a streptavidin coated well. Biotinylated monoclonal and enzyme labeled antibodies (directed against distinct and different epitopes of AFP) are added and the reactants mixed. Reaction between the various AFP antibodies and native AFP forms a sandwich complex that binds with the streptavidin coated to the well.

After the completion of the required incubation period, the enzyme-AFP antibody bound conjugate is separated from the unbound enzyme-AFP conjugate by aspiration or decantation. The activity of the enzyme present on the surface of the well is quantitated by reaction with a suitable substrate to produce colour.

The employment of several serum references of known carcinoembryonic antigen (AFP) levels permits the construction of a dose response curve of activity and concentration. From comparison to the dose response curve, an unknown specimen's activity can be correlated with AFP concentration.

PRINCIPLE

Immunoenzymometric Assay

The essential reagents required for an immunoenzymometric assay include high affinity and specificity antibodies (enzyme and immobilised), with different and distinct epitope recognition, in excess, and native antigen. In this procedure, the immobilisation takes place during the assay at the surface of a microplate well through the interaction of streptavidin coated on the well and exogenously added biotinylated monoclonal anti-AFP antibody.

Upon mixing monoclonal biotinylated antibody, the enzyme-labeled antibody and a serum containing the native antigen, reaction results between the native antigen and the antibodies, without competition or steric hindrance, to form a soluble sandwich complex. The interaction is illustrated by the following equation

$$^{Enz}Ab_{(p)} + Ag_{A}FP + {}^{Btn}Ab_{<(m)} \underset{k\text{-}a}{\overset{k_a}{\rightleftharpoons}} {}^{Enz}Ab_{(p)}\text{-}Ag_{AF}p\text{-}{}^{Btn}Ab_{(m)}$$

$^{Btn}Ab_{(m)}$ = Biotinylated monoclonal antibody (excess quantity)
AgApp = Native antigen (variable quantity)
$^{Enz}Ab_{(p)}$ = Enzyme labeled polyclonal antibody (excess quantity)
$^{Enz}Ab_{(p)}$-AgAFP-$^{Btn}Ab_{(m)}$ = Antigen-antibodies sandwich complex
k_a = Rate constant of association
k_{-a} = Rate constant of dissociation

Simultaneously, the complex is deposited to the well through the high affinity reaction of streptavidin and biotinylated antibody. This interaction is illustrated below.

$$^{Enz}Ab_{(p)}\text{-}Ag_{A}Fp\text{-}{}^{Btn}Ab_{(m)} + \text{Streptavidin cw} \rightarrow \text{Immobilised complex}$$

Streptavidin cw = Streptavidin immobilised on well

Immobilised complex = sandwich complex bound to the solid surface.

After equilibrium is attained, the antibody-bound fraction is separated from unbound antigen by decantation or aspiration. The enzyme activity in the antibody-bound fraction is directly proportional to the native antigen concentration. By utilising several different serum references of known antigen values, a dose response curve can be generated from which the antigen concentration of an unknown can be ascertained.

Reagents for 96-Well Microplate

A. Alpha-Fetoprotein (AFP) -1.0 ml/vial Six vials of references fB-AFP Antigen at levels of 0(A), 5(B), 25(C), 50(D), 250(E) and 500(F) ng/ ml. Store at 2 to 8°C. A preservative has been added.

B. Enzyme Conjugate and Biotinylated Monoclonal antibody—11 ml/vial One (1) vial containing enzyme labeled antibody, biotinylated monoclonal mouse IgG in buffer, dye, and preservative. Store at 2 to 8°C.

C. Streptavidin Coated Microplate-96 wells One 96-well microplate coated with Streptavidin and packaged in an aluminum bag with a drying agent. Store at 2 to 8°C.

D. Wash Solution Concentrate -20 ml One (1) vial containing a surfactant in phosphate buffered saline. A preservative has been added. Store at 2 to 30°C.

E. Substrate A -7.0 ml/vial One (1) bottle containing tetramethylbenzidine (TMB) in buffer. Store at 2 to 8°C .

F. Substrate B - 7.0 ml/vial One (1) bottle containing hydrogen peroxide (H_2O_2) in buffer. Store at 2 to 8°C.

G. Stop Solution - 6.0 ml/vial One (1) bottle containing a strong acid (1N HCI). Store at 2 to 30°C.

Note 1: Do not use reagents beyond the kit expiration date.

Note 2: Opened reagents are stable for sixty (60) days when stored at 2 to 8°C.

FOR IN VITRO DIAGNOSTIC USE NOT FOR INTERNAL OR EXTERNAL USE IN HUMANS OR ANIMALS

Precautions

All products that contain human serum have been found to be non-reactive for Hepatitis B Surface Antigen, HIV 1 and 2 and HCV Antibodies by FDA required tests. Since no known test can offer complete assurance that infectious agents are absent, all human serum products should be handled as potentially hazardous and capable of transmitting disease. Good laboratory procedures for handling blood products can be found in the Center for Disease Control/ National Institute of Health, "Biosafety in Microbiological and Biomedical Laboratories," 2nd Edition, 1988, HHS.

Specimen Collection and Preparation

The specimens shall be blood serum in type and the usual precautions in the collection of venipuncture samples should be observed. For accurate comparison to established normal values, a fasting morning serum sample should be obtained. The blood should be collected in a plain redtop venipuncture tube without additives or gel barrier. Allow the blood to clot. Centrifuge the specimen to separate the serum from the cells.

Samples may be refrigerated at 2 to 8°C for a maximum period of five (5) days. If the specimen(s) can not be assayed within this time, the sample(s) may be stored at temperatures of -20°C for up to 30 days. Avoid repetitive freezing and thawing. When assayed in duplicate, 0.050 ml of the specimen is required.

Materials Provided

1. Six (6) vials of AFP serum calibrators.
2. One (1) vial of combined biotinylated monoclonal antibody and enzyme labeled polyclonal reagent.
3. One 96-well Streptavidin Coated Microplate.
4. One (1) bottle of Wash Buffer Concentrate.
5. One (1) bottle of Substrate A.
6. One (1) bottle of Substrate B.
7. One (1) bottle of Stop solution.
8. Instructions.

Required But Not Provided

1. Pipette(s) capable of delivering 25 µl and 100 µl volumes with a precision of better than 1.5%.
2. Dispenser(s) for repetitive deliveries of 0.100 ml and 0.300 ml volumes with a precision of better than 1.5% (optional).
3. Microplate washer or a squeeze bottle (optional).
4. Microplate Reader with 450 nm wavelength absorbance capability.
5. Container(s) for mixing of reagents (see below).
6. Absorbent Paper for blotting the microplate wells.
7. Plastic wrap or microplate cover for incubation steps.
8. Vacuum aspirator (optional) for wash steps.
9. Timer.
10. Storage container for storage of wash buffer.
11. Distilled or deionized water.

Reagent Preparation

1. Working Reagent 1 - Wash buffer
   Dilute contents of Wash concentrate to 1000 ml with distilled or deionized water in a suitable storage container. Store at room temperature.
2. Working Reagent 2-Substrate Solution - Prepare before use
   Determine the amount of reagent needed and prepare by mixing equal portions of Substrate A and Substrate B in a suitable container. For example, add 1ml of A and 1ml of B per two (2) eight well strips (A slight excess of solution is made). Use within one (1) hour of preparation for maximum performance of the assay.

Test Procedure

Before proceeding with the assay, bring all reagents, serum references and controls to room temperature.

1. Format the microplates' wells for each serum reference, control and patient specimen to be assayed in duplicate. Replace any unused microwell strips back into the aluminum bag, seal and store at 2 to 8°C.
2. Pipette 0.025 ml (25 µl) of the appropriate serum reference, control or specimen into the assigned well.
3. Add 0.100 ml (100 µl) of the biotinylated/enzyme labeled antibodies to each well. It is very important to dispense all reagents close to the bottom of the coated well.
4. Swirl the microplate gently for 20 to 30 seconds to mix and cover.
5. Incubate 60 minutes at room temperature.
6. Discard the contents of the microplate by decantation or aspiration. If decanting, tap and blot the plate dry with absorbent paper.
7. Add 300 µl of wash buffer (see Reagent Preparation Section), decant (tap and blot) or aspirate. Repeat two (2) additional times for a total of three (3) washes. An automatic or manual plate washer can be used. Follow the manufacturer's instruction for proper usage. If a squeeze bottle is employed, fill each well by depressing the container (avoiding air bubbles) to dispense the wash. Decant the wash and repeat two (2) additional times.

8. Add 0.100 ml (100 µl) of working substrate solution to all wells (see Reagent Preparation Section). Always add reagents in the same order to minimize reaction time differences between wells.
9. Incubate at room temperature for fifteen (15) minutes.
10. Add 0.050 ml (50 µl) of stop solution to each well and mix gently for 15-20 seconds. Always add reagents in the same order to minimize reaction time differences between wells.
11. Read the absorbance in each well at 450 nm in a microplate reader. The results should be read within thirty (30) minutes of adding the stop solution.

Quality Control

Each laboratory should assay controls at levels in the low, normal and elevated range for monitoring assay performance. These controls should be treated as unknowns and values determined in every test procedure performed. Quality control charts should be maintained to follow the performance of the supplied reagents. Pertinent statistical methods should be employed to ascertain trends. The individual laboratory should set acceptable assay performance limits. Other parameters that should be monitored include the 80, 50 and 20% intercepts of the dose response curve for run-to-run reproducibility. In addition, maximum absorbance should be consistent with past experience. Significant deviation from established performance can indicate unnoticed change in experimental conditions or degradation of kit reagents. Fresh reagents should be used to determine the reason for the variations.

Results

A dose response curve is used to ascertain the concentration of AFP in unknown specimens.

1. Record the absorbance obtained from the printout of the microplate reader as outlined in Example 1.
2. Plot the absorbance for each duplicate serum reference versus the corresponding AFP concentration in ng/ml on linear graph paper (do not average the duplicates of the serum references before plotting).
3. Draw the best-fit curve through the plotted points.
4. To determine the concentration of AFP for an unknown, locate the average absorbance of the duplicates for each unknown on the vertical axis of the graph, find the intersecting point on the curve, and read the concentration (in ng/ml) from the horizontal axis of the graph (the duplicates of the unknown may be averaged as indicated). In the following example, the average absorbance (0.420) intersects the dose response curve at (33.2 ng/ml) AFP concentration (See Figure 23.60).

Note: Computer data reduction software designed for IEMA assays may also be used for the data reduction.

Example 1

Well	*Serum References*	*Absorbance*
1	0.0 ng/ml	0.012
2	0.0 ng/ml	0.011
3	5.0 ng/ml	0.100
4	5.0 ng/ml	0.097
5	25.0 ng/ml	0.336
6	25.0 ng/ml	0.333
7	50.0 ng/ml	0.612
8	50.0 ng/ml	0.577
9	250.0 ng/ml	2.005
10	250.0 ng/ml	1.975
11	500.0 ng/ml	2.664
12	500.0 ng/ml	2.680

Well	**Unknown ID**	**OD**	**Avg OD**	**Value**
13	Unknown #1	0.427		
14	Unknown #1	0.413	0.420	33.2 ng/ml

*The data presented in Example 1 and Figure 23.60 are for illustration only and should not be used in lieu of a dose response curve prepared with each assay.

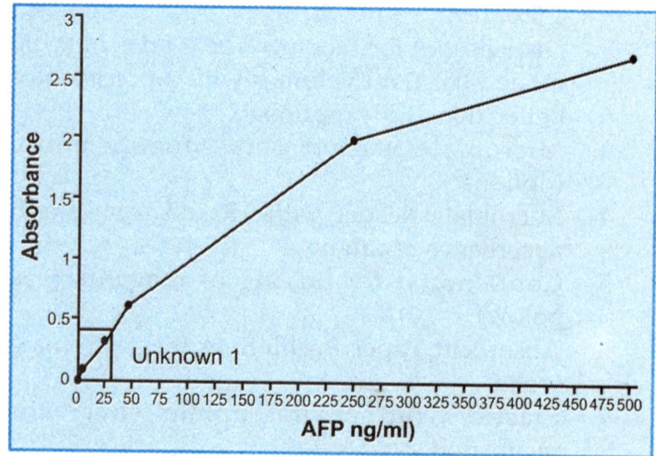

Fig. 23.60

QC Parameters

Maximum Absorbance (500ng/ml) = >1.5

Limitations of Procedure

A. Assay Performance

It is important that the time of reaction in each well is held constant for reproducible results. Pipetting of samples should/not extend beyond ten (10) minutes to avoid assay drift. If more than one (1) plate is used, it is recommended to repeat the dose response curve.

Addition of the substrate solution initiates a kinetic reaction, which is terminated by the addition of the stop solution. Therefore, the addition of the substrate and the stopping solution should be added in the same sequence to eliminate anytime deviation during reaction.

Plate readers measure vertically. Do not touch the bottom of the wells.

Failure to remove adhering solution adequately in the aspiration or decantation wash step(s) may result in poor replication and spurious results.

Sample(s), which are contaminated microbiologically, should not be used in the assay. Highly lipaemic or haemolysed specimen(s) should similarly not be used.

Patient specimens with AFP concentrations above 500 ng/ml may be diluted (for example 1/10 or higher) with normal male serum (AFP < 10 ng/ml) and re-assayed. The sample's concentration is obtained by multiplying the result by the dilution factor (X10).

Each component in one assay should be of the same 1st number and stored under identical conditions.

B. Interpretation

If computer controlled data reduction is used to interpret the results of the test, it is imperative that the predicted values for the calibrators fall within 10% of the assigned concentrations.

AFP has a low clinical sensitivity and specificity as a tumor marker. Clinically an elevated AFP value alone is not of diagnostic value as a test for cancer and should only be used in conjunction with other clinical manifestations (observations) and diagnostic parameters. AFP levels are known to be elevated in a number of benign diseases and conditions including pregnancy and non-malignant liver diseases such as hepatitis and cirrhosis.

Expected Ranges of Values

Approximately 97 to 98% of the normal healthy population has AFP levels less than 8.5 ng/ml (4). In high risk patients, AFP values between 100 and 350 ng/ml suggest hepatocellular carcinoma. Concentrations over 350 ng/ml usually are indication of the disease.

Expected Values for the AFP ELISA Test System Male and Female <8.5ng/ml (97-98%)

It is important to keep in mind that establishment of a range of values which can be expected to be found by a given method for a population of "normal'-persons is dependent upon a multiplicity of factors the specificity of the method, the population tested and the precision of the method in the hands of the analyst. For these reasons each laboratory should depend upon the range of expected values established by the Manufacturer only until an in-house range can be determined by the analysts using the method with a population indigeneous to the area in which the laboratory is located.

Reference Values

		SI Units
Adult females		
Nonpregnant	0-10 ng/ml	0-10 µg/L
Pregnant		
2 months	<75 ng/ml	<75 µg/L
3 months	<130 ng/ml	<130 µg/L
4 months	<210 ng/ml	<210 µg/L
5 months	<300 ng/ml	<300 µg/L
6 months	<400 ng/ml	<400 µg/L
7 months	<450 ng/ml	<450 µg/L
8 months	<450 ng/ml	<450 µg/L
9 months	<400 ng/ml	<400 µg/L
Immediately postpartum	<375 ng/ml	<375 µg/L
Adult males	0-10 ng/ml	0-10 µg/L
Children	0-30 ng/ml	0-30 µg/L

Increased

Ataxia telangiectasia, cirrhosis, gonadal teratoblastoma, cancer (embryonal, hepatocellular, pancreatic with liver metastases, malignant teratoma of ovary of testes, gastric with liver metastases, biliary system, germ cell tumors), hepatitis (acute, chronic, neonatal), pregnancy (with fetal neural tube defects, multiple fetuses, fetal distress, fetal death), intrauterine death, duodenal atresia, oomphalocele, spontaneous abortion, tetralogy of Fallot (or Turner's syndrome), tyrosinemia, and ulcerative colitis.

Decreased

Has been associated with Down syndrome when less than 0.25 times the normal median.

CA 15-3 (CARCINOGENIC ANTIGEN 15-3) Courtesy: Lilac Medicare

Summary and Explanation of the Assay

The MUC-1 antigen is a membrane-anchored mucin-type glycoprotein present in malignant and normal epithelial cells of certain organs, e.g. breast, lung, ovary and pancreas. The apo-protein of the MUC-1 mucin contains a transmembrane domain, a cytoplasmic domain, and an extracellular carbohydrate rich domain. The extracellular domain is characterised by polymorphism with respect to the number of a 20 amino acid tandem repeat (VNTR polymorphism). The MUC-1 breast cancer mucin < (CA15-3 antigen) is secreted from tumor cells and can be used as a serological marker of breast cancer.

The CanAg CA15-3 El A is based on two mouse monoclonal antibodies, Ma695 as catcher antibody recognising a sialylated carbohydrate epitope expressed on the mucin and Ma552 as a tracer antibody directed towards the TRPAPG heptapeptide of the protein core.

Principles of the CA15-3 EIA

The CA15-3 EIA is a solid-phase, non-competitive assay based upon the direct sandwich technique. Standards and patient samples are incubated together with biotinylated anti-CA15-3 monoclonal antibody and HRP labelled tracer in streptaviclin coated microtitre strips. After washing, buffered Substrate/ Chromogen reagent (hydrogen peroxide and 3, 3', 5, 5' tetra-methyl-benzidine) is added to each well and the enzyme reaction is allowed to proceed. During the enzyme reaction a blue colour will develop if antigen is present. The intensity of the colour is proportional to the amount of CA15-3 present in the samples.

The colour intensity is determined in a microtitre plate spectrophotometer at 620 nm (or optionally at 405 nm after addition of Stop Solution).

Standard curves are constructed for each assay by plotting absorbance value versus the concentration for each standard. The CA15-3 concentrations of patients samples are then read from the standard curve.

Kit Contents

Each CanAg CA15-3 EIA kit contains reagents for 96 tests.

The expiry date of the complete kit is stated on the label on the outside of the kit box.

Do not use the kit components beyond the expiry date.

Do not mix reagents from different lots of kits. Store the kit at + 2- + 8°C.

Component	*Quantity*	*Shelf life and storage*
CA15-3 Standards	5 vials	+2 - +8° until expiry date stated on the vials
CA15-3	OU/ml	0.5 mL
CA15-3	15U/ml	0.5 mL
CA15-3	50U/ml	0.5 mL
CA15-3	125U/ml	0.5 mL
CA15-3	250 U/ml	0.5 mL

Ready for use. The standards are in Tris-HCl buffered salt solution with bovine serum albumin, an inert yellow dye, and 0.01% methyl-isothiazolone (MIT) as preservative.

Sample Diluent 2 vials 50 mL each +2 -+8°C until expiry date stated on the vials

Ready to use for diluting samples. Contains Tris-HCl buffered salt solution with bovine serum albumin, an inert yellow dye, and 0.01% methyl-isothiazolone (MIT) as preservative.

Additional Sample Diluent can be obtained by ordering the product: "Sample Diluent CA15-3 EIA" Prod. No. 200-24 containing 50 mL.

Tracer 1 vial 0.75 mL	+2 -+8°C until expiry date stated on the vial
Stock solution of HRP anti CA15-3 monoclonal antibody from mouse,«= 50 μg/mL. Contains 0.01% methyl-isothiazolone (MIT) as preservative.	
BiotinAnti 1 bottle 15 mL CA15-3 stated on the vial	+2 - +8°C until expiry date
Biotin anti CA15-3 monoclonal antibody from mouse, 2 μg/ml.	
Ready for use phosphate buffered saline (pH 7.2) with bovine serum albumin, bovine immunoglobulin, mouse immunoglubuline, Tween 20, a blue inert dye, and 0.01% methyl-isothiazolone as preservative.	
Streptavidin 1 plate Microtitre Plate	+2 - +8°C until expiry date stated on the label
12 × 8 wells coated with Streptavidin	

Contd...

Contd...

TMB HRP Substrate 1 bottle 12 mL +2 - +8°C until expiry date stated on the vial	
Ready for use. Contains buffered hydrogen peroxide and 3,3',5,5' tetra-methylbenzidine (TMB).	
HRP Stop Solution	1 bottle 15 mL +2 -+8°C until expiry date stated on the vial Ready for use 0.12 M hydrochloric acid.
Wash Concentrate	1 bottle 40 mL +2 - +8°C until expiry date stated on the vial
To be diluted with water 25 times before use. A Tris-HCl buffered salt solution with Tween 20. Contains Germall II as preservative.	

Materials Required but not Supplied with the Kit

1. **Microtitre Plate Shaker** Shaking should be medium to vigorous. Longitudinal shaking approximately 200 strokes/min, oscillations 700-900/min.
2. **Microtitre Plate Wash Device** Either an automatic platewash capable of performing 1 and 6 washing cycles, or semi manual microtitre plate washing device connected to vacuum pump or water-jet vacuum and a liquid trap for retaining aspirated liquid.
   The Nunc Immuno-8 manual strip washer is recommended if an automatic microtitre platewash is not used.
3. **Microtitre plate spectrophotometer reader** with a wavelength of 620 nm and/or 405 nm, and an absorbance range of 0 to 3.0.
4. **Precision pipettes** with disposable plastic tips to deliver 25 µl, 50 µl, 100 µl and 1 ml. An 8-channel pipette or respenser pipette with disposable plastic tips for delivery of 100 µl is useful but not essential,
5. Distilled or deionized water for preparation of diluted Wash solution.

Specimen Collection and Handling

CanAg CA15-3 EIA is intended for use with serum or plasma. Collect blood by venipuncture, allow to clot and separate the serum or plasma by centrifugation. Haemolysed, moderately lipaemic or icteric samples do not affect the results of the assay. Samples containing fibrin, gross haemolysis, gross lipemia, or turbidimetry may give misleading results.

Samples can be stored at +2 - + 8°C for 2 days. For longer periods it is recommended to store the samples aliquoted at - 20°C. Avoid repeated freezing and thawing of the samples. Allow frozen samples to thaw slowly, preferably in a refrigerator over night. Bring the samples to room temperature before analysis.

Warnings and Precautions

For *in vitro* diagnostic use

Please refer to the US Department of Health and Human Services (Bethesda, Md., USA) publication No. (CDC) 88-8395 on laboratory safety or any other local or national regulation. Handle all patient specimens as potentially infectious.

The contents of this kit, and their residues, must not be allowed to come into contact with ruminating animals or swine.

Procedural Notes

1. A thorough understanding of this package insert is necessary to ensure proper use of the CanAg 15-3 EIA kit. The reagents supplied with this kit are intended for use as an integral unit. Do not mix identical reagents from kits having different lot numbers. Do not use the kit reagents after the expiry date printed on the outside of the kit box.
2. Reagents should be allowed to reach room temperature (20-25°C) prior to use. The assay should only be performed at temperatures between 20 and 28°C to obtain accurate results. Frozen specimens should be brought to room temperature slowly and gently mixed by hand. Do not vortex or vigorously mix patient samples or control samples.
3. Before starting to pipette standards and patient specimens it is advisable to mark the strips to be able to clearly identify the samples during and after the assay.
4. A careful washing procedure of the strips is essential. Ensure that each well is filled up completely to the top edge, that the aspiration of the wells between and after the washing cycles is complete and the wells are dry. If there is liquid left in the wells, invert the plate and tap it carefully against absorbing paper.
   Automatic strip washer: Follow the manufacturer's instructions for maintenance, and wash the required number of wash cycles prior to and after each incubation step.

The aspiration/wash device should not be left standing with the wash solution for long periods, as the needles may get clogged giving poor liquid delivery and suction.

5. When handling the TMB HRP Substrate solution make sure to use clean disposable plastic pipette tips (or respenser pipette tip). If the TMB HRP Substrate is transferred from the reagent bottle use only a carefully cleaned reservoir or, preferably a disposable plastic tray to avoid contamination of the reagent. The TMB HRP Substrate should be colourless or slightly bluish. A blue colour indicates that the reagent has been contaminated and should be discarded.
6. Be sure to use a proper pipetting technique when handling samples and reagents. Hold the pipette tip slightly above the top of the well and avoid touching the plastic strip or surface of the liquid to avoid carry over from well to well. A proper pipetting technique is of particular importance when handling the TMB HRP Substrate solution.

Assay Procedure

Perform each determination in duplicate for both standards and patient samples. A standard curve should be run with each assay. All reagents and samples must be brought to room temperature (+20 - + 25°C) before use.

1. Preparation of reagents stability of reconstituted reagent

Wash solution 2 weeks at +2-+25°C in sealed container.

Pour the 40 ml Wash Concentrate into a clean container and dilute 25 -fold by adding 960 mL of distilled or deionised water to give a buffered wash solution.

Sample Preparation

1. Dilute the samples 1:41 by mixing 25 µl of sample with 1 ml of Sample Diluent. Note Standard should not be diluted.

Antibody solution. 3 weeks at +2-+8°C

Prepare the needed volume of Antibody solution by mixing 50 µL of the Tracer solution with 1 mL of the Biotin Anti CA15-3 solution per strip

Strips	*Tracer solution (µL)*	*Biotin Anti CA15-3 (mL)*
1	50	1
2	100	2
3	150	3
4	200	4
5	250	5
6	300	6
7	350	7
8	400	8
9	450	9
10	500	10
11	550	11
12	600	12

Be sure to use a clean plastic or glass bottle for preparation of the Antibody solution.

Alternative: Pour the content of the Tracer solution into the bottle of Bi-otin Anti CA15-3 and mix gently. Make sure that all content of the Tracer solution is transferred to the bottle of Biotin Anti CA15-3 .

Note: The diluted tracer is stable for 3 weeks at +2-+8°C. Do not prepare more Antibody solution than will be used within this period and make sure that it is stored properly.

2. Transfer the required number of microtitre strips to a strip frame. (Return the remaining unused strips to the plastic tray pack and reseal). Wash each strip once with the Wash solution. Do not wash more strips than can be handled within 30 min.
3. Pipette 25 µl of the CA15-3 standards (Std) and the diluted patient samples (unknowns-link) into the strip wells according to the following scheme (Fig. 23.61)
4. Add 100 µl of the Antibody solution to each well using a 100 µL precision pipette (or an 8-channel. 100 µL precision pipette). Avoid carry-over by holding the pipette tip slightly above the top of the well and avoid touching the plastic strip or the surface of the liquid.
5. Incubate the frame for 2 hour (± 5 min) at room temperature (+ 20-+28 C) with constant shaking of the plate using a microtiter plate shaker.
6. Wash each strip 6 times, using the wash procedure described in procedural notes point 4.
7. Add 100 µL of TMB HRP Substrate to each well using the same pipetting procedure as in 4. The TMB HRP Substrate solution should be

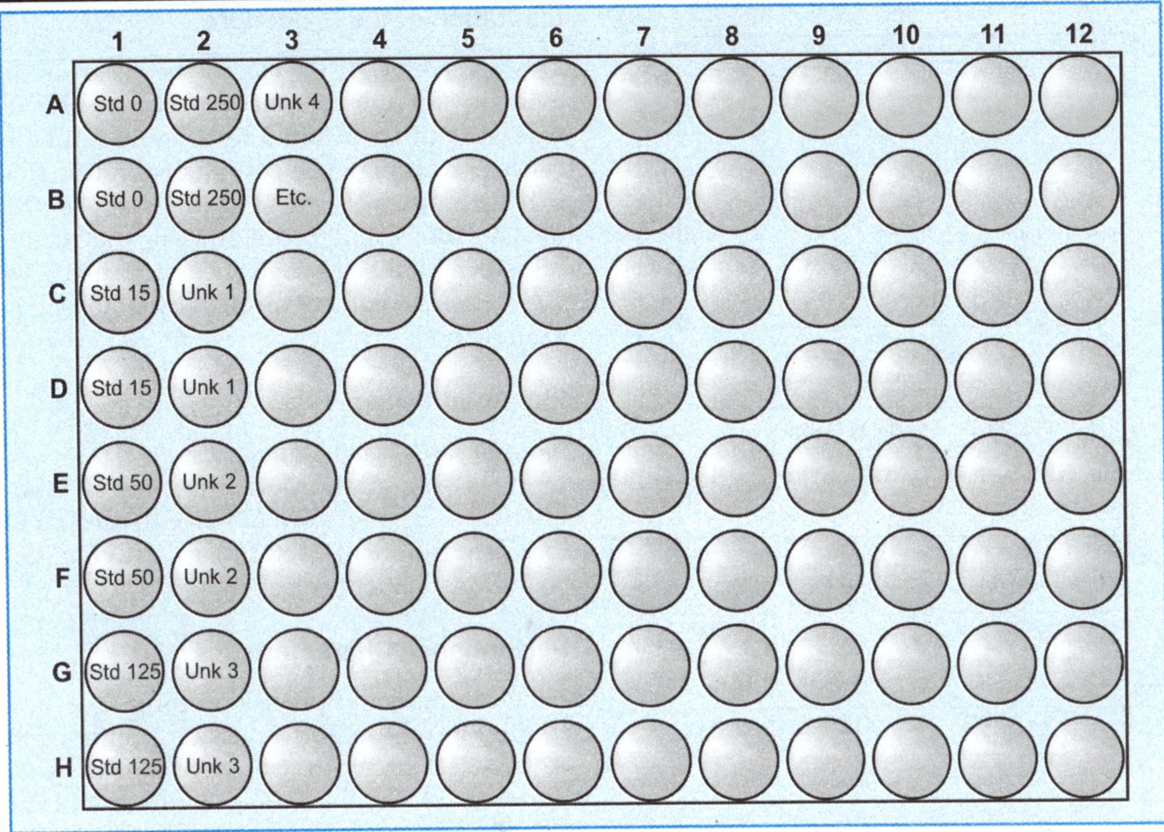

Fig. 23.61: Pipetting scheme

added to the wells as quickly as possible, and the time between the addition to the first and last well should not exceed 10 minutes.

8. Incubate the frame for 30 min (± 5 min) at room temperature with constant shaking.
9. Immediate read the absorbance at 620 nm in a microtiter plate (or micro strip) reader.

Option

If the laboratory does not have access to a microtitre plate reader capable of reading at 620 nm, the absorbance can be determined as in point 10.

10 Add 100 µL of HRP Stop Solution and mix. Thereafter read absorbance at 405 nm in a microtitre plate (or micro strip) reader within 15 min after addition of HRP Stop Solution.

Calculation of Results

If a microtitre plate spectrophotometer reader with built-in data calculation program is used refer to the manual for the plate reader and create a program using the concentration of each of the CA15-3 standards.

For automatic calculation of CA15-3 results it is recommended to use either of the following methods:

- Spline smoothed curve fit method. Standard 0 should be used as plate blank.
- Interpolation with point-to-point evaluation. Standard 0U/ml should be included in the curve with the value 0U/ml.
- Quadratic curve fit method. Standard 0U/ml should be included in the curve with the value 0U/ml

Note: 4-Parametric or Linear regression evaluation methods should not be used

For manual evaluation, a standard curve is constructed by plotting the absorbance (A) values obtained for each CA15-3 standard against the corresponding CA15-3 concentration (in U/ml) (see figure below). The unknown CA15-3 concentrations, in U/ml, can then be read from the standard curve using the mean absorbance value of each patient specimen (Fig. 23.62).

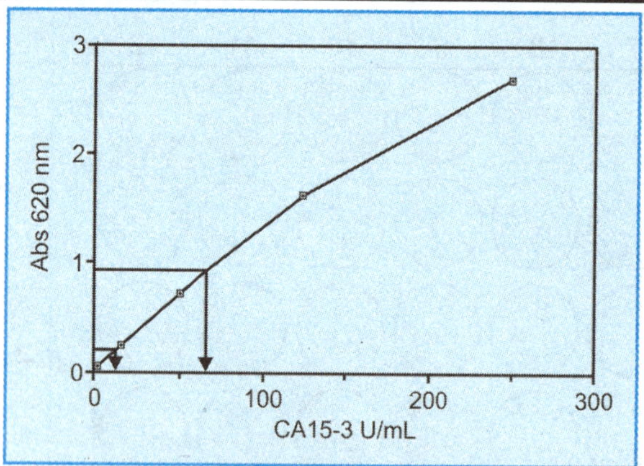

Fig. 23.62: Result calculation

Example (do not use this curve to determine actual assay results)

Specimen	*Standard values*	*Mean abs value (A)*	*CA15-3 U/ml*
Standard	0	0 U/ml	0.044
Standard	15	15 U/ml	0.252
Standard	50	50 U/ml	0.723
Standard	125	125 U/ml	1.612
Standard	250	250 U/ml	2.680
Specimen A		0.241	14.1
Specimen B		0.895	63.1

Calculation of Results with Diluted Samples

If samples in an initial analysis give CA15-3 levels higher than 250 U/n the samples should be diluted 1/10 and 1/100 with CA15-3 U/ml standard to obtain the accurate CA15-3 concentration of the samples.

1:10 dilution = 50 µL of specimen + 450 µL of Sample Diluent

1:100 dilution = 50 µL of 1:10 dilution + 450 µL of Sample Diluent

The CA15-3 concentration of the undiluted sample is then obtained as follows:

Dilution 1/10:10 x Measured value

Dilution 1/100 100 x Measured value

Quality Controls

The use of internal control serum samples is advised to assure the day-to day validity of results. It is recommended that the laboratory prepares its own serum pools at different levels as controls.

Limitation of the Procedure

The level of CA15-3 cannot be used as absolute evidence for the presence or absence of malignant disease, and the CA15-3 test should not be used in cancer screening. The results of the test should be interpreted only in conjunction with other investigations and procedures in the diagnosis of disease and the management of patients, and the CA15-3 test should not replace any established clinical examination.

Expected Values

Normal range < 30 Units.

It is recommended that each laboratory establishes its own normal range to account for such local environment factors as diet, climate, living conditions, patient selection, etc.

Performance Characteristics

Dose-response and precision profile

Dose-response and precision profile of the Can Ag CA15-3 El A kit was determined by random pipetting of standards and controls and analysed according to the assay procedure (Fig. 23.63).

Dose response and precision profile, n = 8

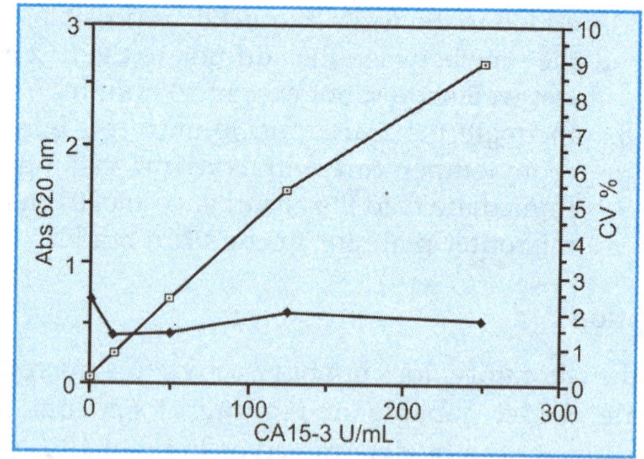

Fig. 23.63: Dose response

Precision

Intra-assay (with-in run) precision of the CanAg CA15-3 EIA kit.

Sample	*Replicates*	*Mean, U/ml*	*SD, U/ml*	*CV%*
1	10	17.5	0.3	1.7
2	10	67.2	1.3	2.0
3	10	86.4	1.5	1.7
4	10	163.5	2.1	1.3

Inter-assay variation of the CanAg CA15-5 EIA kit

Sample	*Replicates*	*Mean, U/ml*	*SD, U/ml*	*CV%*
1	15	16.8	0.8	4.7
2	15	63.9	3.1	4.8
3	15	82.3	4.7	5.7
4	15	155.2	7.5	4.9

Detection Limit

The detection limit of the CanAg CA15-3 EIA is < 1 U/ml defined as the concentration corresponding to the mean of the absorbance values for the 0 standard plus 2 standard deviations of the 0-standard deterrmination (mean value + 2 SD).

Recovery

Spiked serum samples were prepared by adding CA15-3 antigen to normal serum samples. The recovery of the added antigen was in the range 95 - 110%.

Linearity

Patient samples were serially diluted with Sample Diluent and analysed. The obtained values are in the range 91 to 110% of the expected value.

Hook Effect

No hook effect has been noticed with samples up to 7500 U/ml.

Note: In very high samples the colour of the substrate will change from blue to greenish (and eventually yellow in extremely high samples). This will lead to a falsely low absorbance at 620 nm, and in extreme cases the absorbance may fall within the standard curve range and noticed as a hook.

Ca 15-3 (Carcinogenic Antigen 15-3), Serum

Norm <22 U/ ml

Increased

Adenoma of salivary gland; breast cancer; benign breast disease; breast cancer metastasis; lung cancer; ovarian benign disease; recurrence after remission in breast cancer with bone metastasis.

Decreased

Positive response to therapy.

CA 19-9 (CARBOHYDRATE AG 19-9, GICAM GASTROINTESTINAL CANCER ANTIGEN) BLOOD Mfd: Can Ag, Courtesy: Lilac Medicare

Summary and Explanation of the Assay

The CanAg CA19-9 EIA is based on one mouse monoclonal antibody, C192, directed against the sialyl Lewis epitopes of the CA19-9 antigen.

Principles of the CanAg CA19-9 EIA

The CanAg CA19-9 EIA is a solid-phase non-competitive assay based upon the direct sandwich technique. Standards and patient samples are incubated together with biotinylated anti-CA19-9 monoclonal antibody (MAb) C192 (derived from mice) in Streptavidin coated microtitre strips. The CA19-9 in the standards/samples is adsorbed to the Streptavidin coated microtitre strips by the biotinylated anti-CA19-9 MAb during the incubation. The strips are then washed followed by incubation with HRP labelled anti CA19-9 MAb C192. After washing, buffered Substrate/Chromogen reagent (hydrogen peroxide and 3,3',5,5' tetramethyl benzidine) is added to each well and the enzyme reaction is allowed to proceed. During the enzyme reaction a blue colour will develop if antigen is present. The intensity of the colour is proportional to the amount of CA19-9 present in the samples.

The colour intensity is determined in a microtitre plate spectrophotometer at 620 nm (or optionally at 405 nm after addition of Stop Solution).

Standard curves arc constructed for each assay by plotting absorbance value versus the concentration for each standard. The CA19-9 concentrations of patients samples are then read from the standard curve.

Kit Contents

Each CanAg CA19-9 EIA kit contains reagents for 96 tests.

The expiry date of the kit is stated on the label on the outside of the kit box. Do not use the kit components beyond the expiry date. Do not mix reagents from different lots of kits. Store the kit at + 2- + 8°C.

Protocol Sheet

Mix the components directly before use. Use shaking conditions according to the instructions.

Step	Bottle/Plate	Procedure
1. Prepare wash solution	Wash Concentrate	Dilute 40 mL of Wash Concentrate with 960 mL of deionized water.
2. Dilute samples	Sample Diluent Sample(S) Note: Standards should not be diluted.	Dilute the samples 1:41 by mixing 25 µL of sample with 1 mL of sample Diluent.
3. Prepare Antibody solution	Tracer Biotin Anti CA 15-3	Mix Tracer and Biotin Anti CA 15-3 accordingly: no. of strips / Tracer µL / Tracer Diluent mL 1 / 50 / 1 2 / 100 / 2 3 / 150 / 3 4 / 200 / 4 5 / 250 / 5 6 / 300 / 6 7 / 350 / 7 8 / 400 / 8 9 / 450 / 9 10 / 500 / 10 11 / 550 / 11 12 / 600 / 12
4. Wash	Plate	Wash each well once with wash solution.
5. Add standards and sample	0.15, 50, 125, 250	25 µL in each well
6. Add Antibody solution	Antibody solution	100 µL in each well
7. Incubate	Plate	2 hours shaking at room temperature
8. Wash	Plate	Wash each well six times with wash solution.
9. Add TMB HRP substrate	TMB/HRP/SUBSTRATE	100 µL in each well
10. Incubate	Plate	30 min shaking at room temperature
11. Read absorbance	Plate	620 nm
Alt. 11. Add HRP Stop Solution	HRP Stop Solution	100 µL in each well
Alt. 12. Incubate	Plate	1 min shaking at room temperature
Alt. 13. Read absorbance	Plate	Read at 405 nm within 15 min

Component CA19-9 Standards	*Quantity 6 vials*	*Shelf life and storage +2 - +8° until expiry date stated on the vials*
CA19-9	0 U/ml	0.5 mL
CA19-9	15 U/ml	0.5 mL
CA19-9	30 U/ml	0.5 mL
CA19-9	60 U/ml	0.5 mL
CA19-9	120 U/ml	0.5 mL
CA19-9	240 U/ml	0.5 mL

Ready for use. The standards are in Tris-HCl buffered salt solution with bovine serum albumin, an inert yellow dye, and 0.05% sodium azide as preservative. CA19-9 0 U/ml should also be used as Sample Diluent.

Tracer 1 vial 0.75 mL +2 - +8°C until expiry date stated on the vial

Stock solution of HRP anti CA19-9 monoclonal antibody from mouse, 30 µg/mL. Contains 0.1% methyl-isothiazolone (MIT) as preservative. To be diluted with Tracer Diluent prior to use.

Component	*Quantity*	*Shelf life and storage*
Tracer Diluent	1 bottle 15 mL	+2 - +8°C until expiry date stated on the vial
Ready for use phosphate buffered saline (pH 7.5) with bovine serum albumin, bovine immunoglobulin, mouse immunoglubuline, Tween 20, a blue inert dye, and 0.01% methyl-isothiazolone as preservative.		
Biotin Anti CA19-9	1 bottle 15 mL	+2 - +8° until expiry date stated on the vial
Biotin anti CA19-9 monoclonal antibody from mouse, = 2 ug/mL. Ready for use citrate phosphate buffer (pH 7.5) with bovine serum albumin, bovine globulin, mouse immunoglobulin, Tween 40, an inert red dye, and 0.01% methyl-isothiazolone as preservative.		
Streptavidin Microtitre Plate	1 Plate	+2 - +8° until expiry date stated on the plate label

Contd...

Contd...

12 × 8 wells coated with Streptavidin.		
TMB HRP Substrate	1 bottle 12 mL	+2 - +8° until expiry date stated on the vial.
Ready for use. Contains buffered hydrogen peroxide and 3,3',5,5' tetra- methylbenzidine (TMB).		
HRP Stop Solution	1 bottle 15 mL	+2 - +8° until expiry date stated on the vial
Ready for use 0.12 M hydrochloric acid.		
Wash Concentrate	1 bottle 40 mL	+2 - +8° until expiry date stated on the vial
To be diluted with water 25 times before use. A Tris-HCl buffered salt solution with Tween 20. Contains Germall II as preservative.		

Materials Required but not Supplied with the Kit

1. **Microtitre Plate Shaker** Shaking should be medium to vigorous. Longitudinal shaking approximately 200 strokes/min, oscillations 700-900/min.
2. **Microtitre plate wash device** Either an automatic platewash capable of performing 1 and 6 washing cycles, or a semi manual microtitre plate washing device connected to vacuum purnp or water-jet vacuum and a liquid trap for retaining aspirated liquid.
   The Nunc Immuno-8 manual strip washer is recommended if an automatic microtitre platewash is not used.
3. Microtitre plate spectrophotometer reader with a wavelength of 620 nm and/or 405 nm, and an absorbance range of 0 to 3.0.
4. Precision pipettes with disposable plastic tips to deliver 25 µL, 50 µL, 100 µL and 1 mL. An 8-channel pipette or respenser pipette with disposable plastic tips for delivery of 100 µL is useful but not essential.
5. Distilled or deionized water for preparation of diluted Wash solution.

Specimen Collection and Handling

The CanAg CA19-9 EIA is intended for use with serum or plasma. Collect blood by venipuncture, allow to clot and separate the serum or plasma by centrifugation. Haemolysed, moderately lipaemic or icteric samples do not affect the results of the assay. Samples containing fibrin, gross haemolysis, gross lipaemia, or turbidimetry may give misleading results.

Samples can be stored at +2 - + 8°C for 2 days. For longer periods it is recommended to store the samples aliquoted at - 20°C. Avoid repeated freezing and thawing of the samples. Allow frozen samples to thaw slowly, preferably in a refrigerator over night. Then bring the samples to room temperature before analysis.

Warnings and Precautions

For *in vitro* diagnostic use

Please refer to the US Department of Health and Human Services (Bethesda, Md, USA) publication No. (CDC) 88-8395 on laboratory safety or any other local or national regulation. Handle all patient specimens as potentially infectious.

The contents of this kit, and their residues, must not be allowed to come into contact with ruminating animals or swine.

Reagents contain sodium azide (NaN_3) as a preservative. Sodium azide may react with lead and copper plumbing to form highly explosive metal azides. On disposal, flush with a large volume of water to prevent azide build-up.

Procedural Notes

1. A thorough understanding of this package insert is necessary to ensure proper use of the CanAg 19-9 EIA kit. The reagents supplied with this kit are intended for use as an integral unit. Do not mix identical reagents from kits having different lot numbers.
   Do not use the kit reagents after the expiry date printed on the outside of the kit box.
2. Reagents should be allowed to reach room temperature (20-25°C) prior to use. The assay should only be performed at temperatures between 20 and 28°C to obtain accurate results. Frozen specimens should be brought to room temperature slowly and gently mixed by hand. Do not vortex or vigorously mix patient samples or control samples.
3. Before starting to pipette standards and patient specimens it is advisable to mark the strips to be able to clearly identify the samples during and after the assay.
4. A careful washing procedure of the strips is essential. Ensure that each well is filled up completely to the top edge, that the aspiration of the wells between and after the washing cycles is complete and the wells are dry. If

there is liquid left in the wells, invert the plate and tap it carefully against absorbing paper. Automatic strip washer: Follow the manufacturer's instructions for maintenance, and wash the required number of wash cycles prior to and after each incubation step.
The aspiration/wash device should not be left standing with the wash solution for long periods, as the needles may get clogged giving poor liquid delivery and suction.

5. Add 100 µL of Biotin Anti CA19-9 solution to each well using 100 µl precision pipette (or an 8-channel 100 uL precision pipette). Avoid carry-over by holding the pipette tip slightly above the top of the well and avoid touching the plastic strip or the surface of the liquid.
6. Incubate the frame for 2 hours (± 5 min) at room temperature (+ 20 -+28°C) with constant shaking of the plate using a microtitre plate shaker.
7. After the first incubation aspirate and wash each strip 3 times, using a wash procedure as described above in Procedural notes point 4.
8. Add 100 µL of Tracer working solution to each well. Use the same pipetting procedure as in 4.
9. Incubate the frame for 1 hour (± 5 min) at room temperature (+20 + 28°C) with constant shaking.
10. After the second incubation aspirate and wash each strip 6 times, using a wash procedure as described above in Procedural notes point 4.
11. Add 100 µL of TMB HRP Substrate to each well using the same pipetting procedure as in 4. The TMB HRP Substrate solution should be added to the wells as quickly as possible, and the time between addition to the first and last well should not exceed 10 min.
12. Incubate for 30 min (± 5 min) at room temperature with constant shaking.
13. Immediately read the absorbance at 620 nm in a microtitre plate (or micro strip) reader.
Option
If the laboratory does not have access to a microtitre plate reader capable of reading at 620 nm, the absorbance can be determined as in point 14.

CANAG CA19-9 EIA PROD. NO. 120-10

Protocol Sheet September 1998

Mix the components directly before use. Use shaking conditions according to the Instructions.

Step	*Bottle/Plate*	*Procedure*			
1.	Prepare wash solution	Wash Concentrate	Dilute 40 mL of Wash Concentrate with 960 mL of deionized water.		
2.	Wash	Plate	Wash each well once with wash solution. Use manual or automatic washer.		
3.	Add standards	0,15,30,120,240,	25 µL in each well		
4.	Add Biotin Anti CA19-9	Biotin Anti CA19-9	100 µL in each well		
5.	Incubate	Plate	2 hours shaking at room temperature		
6.	Wash	Plate	Wash each well three times with wash solution. Use manual or automatic washer.		
7.	Prepare	Tracer Tracer Diluent	Mix Tracer and accordingly		
	Tracer working solution	Tracer diluent	no. of strips	Tracer µL	Tracer Diluent mL
			1	50	1
			2	100	2
			3	150	3
			4	200	4
			5	250	5
			6	300	6
			7	350	7
			8	400	8
			9	450	9
			10	500	10
			11	550	11
			12	600	12

Contd...

Contd...

8.	Add Tracer working solution	Trace working solution	100 µL in each well
9.	Incubate	Plate	1 hour shaking at room temperature
10.	Wash	Plate	Wash each well six times with wash solution. Use manual or automatic washer
11.	Add TMB HRP substrate	TMB HRP substrate	100 µL in each well
12.	Incubate	Plate	30 min shaking at room temperature
13.	Read absorbance	Plate	620 nm
	Alt.13. Add HRP Stop Solution	HRP stop solution	100 µL in each well
	Alt.14. Incubate	Plate	1 min shaking at room temperature
	Alt. 15. Read absorbance	Plate	Read at 405 nm within 15 min

	1	2	3	4	5	6	7	etc
A	Std 0	Std 120	3rd Unk					
B	Std 0	Std 120	etc					
C	Std 15	Std 240						
D	Std 15	Std 240						
E	Std 30	1st Unk						
F	Std 30	1 s Unk						
G	Std 60	2nd Unk						
H	Std 60	2nd Unk						

14. Add 100 µL of HRP Stop Solution and mix. Thereafter read absorbance at 405 nm in a microtitre plate (or micro strip) reader within 15 min after addition of HRP Stop Solution.

Calculation of Results

If a microtitre plate spectrophotometer reader with built-in data calculation program is used refer to the manual for the plate reader and create a program using the concentration of each of the CA19-9 standards.

For automatic calculation of CA19-9 results it is recommended to use either of the following methods

— Spline smoothed curve fit method. Standard 0 should be used as plate blank.

— Interpolation with point-to-point evaluation. Standard 0 U /mL should be included in the curve with the value 0 U/ml.

— Quadratic curve fit method. Standard 0 U/ml should be included in the curve with the value 0 U/ml.

Note: 4-Parametric or Linear regression evaluation methods should not be used.

For manual evaluation, a standard curve is constructed by plotting the absorbance (A) values obtained for each CA19-9 standard against the corresponding CA19-9 concentration (in U/ml) (see figure below). The unknown CA19-9 concentrations, in U/ml, can then be read from the standard curve using the mean absorbance value of each patient specimen (Fig. 23.64).

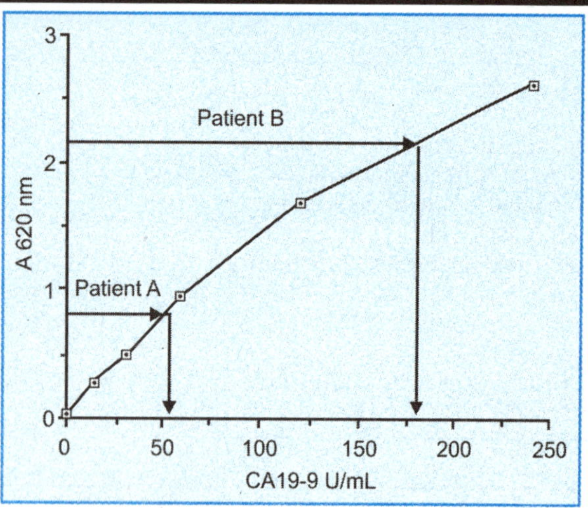

Fig. 23.64: Result calculation

Example (do not use this curve to determine actual assay results)

Specimen	*Standard values*	*Mean abs value (A)*	*CA19-9 U/ml*
Standard 0	0 U/ml	0.036	
Standard 15	15 U/ml	0.276	
Standard 30	30 U/ml	0.508	
Standard 60	60 U/ml	0.928	
Standard 120	120 U/ml	1.665	
Standard 240	240 U/ml	2.583	
Sample A		0.815	52
Sample B		2.130	181

Calculation of Results with Diluted Samples

If samples in an initial analysis give CA19-9 levels higher than 240 U/ mL the samples should be diluted 1/10 and 1/100 with CA19-9 U/ml standard to obtain the accurate CA19-9 concentration of the samples.

1:10 dilution = 50 µL of specimen + 450 µL of Sample Diluent

1:100 dilution = 50 µL of 1:10 dilution + 450 µL of Sample Diluent

The CAt9 9 concentration of the undiluted sample is then obtained as follows:

Dilution 1/10:10 x Measured value

Dilution 1/100:100 x Measured value

Quality Controls

The use of internal control serum samples is advised to assure the day-to-day validity of results. It is recommended that the laboratory prepares its own serum pools at different levels as controls.

Limitation of the Procedure

The level of CA19-9 cannot be used as absolute evidence for the presence or absence of malignant disease, and the CA19-9 test should not be used in cancer screening. The results of the test should be interpreted only in conjunction with other investigations and procedures in the diagnosis of disease and the management of patients, and the CA19-9 test should not replace any established clinical examination.

Expected Values

Normal range < 37 Units.

It is recommended that each laboratory establishes its own normal range.

Performance Characteristics

Dose-response and precision profile

Dose-response and precision profile for CanAg CA19-9 EIA were determined by random pipetting of standards and controls and analysed according to the assay procedure (Fig. 23.65).

Dose-response and precision profile, n= 10

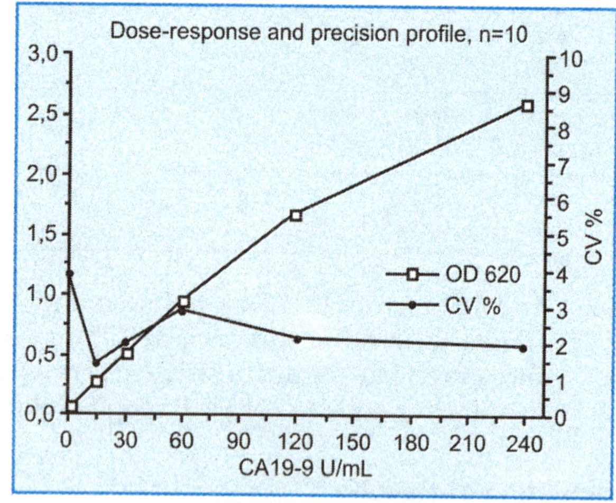

Fig. 23.65: Dose response

Precision

Intra-assay (with-in run) precision of the CanAg C A19-9 EIA kit is shown below

Sample	*Replicates*	*Mean, U/ml*	*SD, U/ml*	*CV%*
1	6	17.4	0.4	2.3
2	6	50.3	0.6	1.3
3	6	166.3	2.7	1.6

Inter-assay (between-run) precision of the CanAg CA19-9 EIA calculated from three separate analyses by three technicians with 6 replicates of each sample during three days is shown below:

Sample	*Replicates*	*Mean, U/ml*	*SD, U/ml*	*CV%*
1	18	17.1	0.5	2.6
2	18	52.3	1.8	3.4
3	18	175.5	7.4	4.2

Detection Limit

The detection limit of the CanAg CA19-9 EIA is < 1 U/ml defined as the concentration corresponding to the mean of the absorbance values for the 0-standard plus 2 standard deviations of the 0-standard determination (mean value + 2 SD).

Recovery

Spiked serum samples were prepared by adding CA19-9 antigen to normal serum samples. The recovery of the added antigen was in the range 90 to 110%.

Linearity

Patient samples were serially diluted with 0-standard and analysed. The obtained values were in the range 96-105% of the expected value.

Hook Effect

No hook effect has been noticed with samples up to 50 000 U/ml.

Note: In very high samples the colour of the substrate will change from blue to greenish (and eventually yellow in extremely high samples). This will lead to a falsely low absorbance at 620 run, and in extreme cases the absorbance may fall within the standard curve range and be noticed as a hook.

		SI Units
Norm	<37 AU/ml	<37 kU/l
Metastasis	>1000 AU/ml	>1000 kU/L

Usage

Tumor marker antigen that is helpful in post-therapeutic monitoring to determine the success of therapy or the presence of cancer recurrence. Useful for monitoring gastrointestinal cancers, head and neck tumors, and gynecologic tumors. Predicts the recurrence of stomach, pancreatic, liver, and colourectal malignancies. Is used in combination with other tumor markers to measure the effectiveness of treatment or earlier detection of recurrence and development of metastases. Most effective for monitoring pancreatic cancer.

Increased

Intra-abdominal carcinoma, pancreatic carcinoma (most frequently elevated marker; elevated levels found in 80 percent of patients with pancreatic cancer), and possibly with other adenocarcinomas such as lung, gastric, biliary, and colonic. Also cholangitis, cirrhosis, and pancreatitis (acute).

Description A carbohydrate antigen, related to the Lewis blood group antigen. CA 19-9 is a carbohydrate antigen that has been shown to be elevated in the sera or some clients with gastro-intestinal tumors. Elevated levels can indicate recurrence of cancer before radiographic or clinical findings by 1 to 7 months.

CA242
Mfd: Can Ag, Courtesy: Lilac Medicare

Summary and Explanation of the Assay

During malignant transformation of cells, substances which are not present or present in very low amounts in normal cells, may be expressed and secreted into body fluids. Tumour-associated substances may be determined with immunological methods using reagents specific for the tumour-associated antigen, and used for detection of malignant cells or presence of tumour in the body, to study the status of the disease and/or follow the effect of therapy.

The CA242 epitope, identified by the C242 monoclonal antibody (MAb), is a sialylated carbohydrate antigen present on mucinous type of glycoprotein (s) (named CanAg) in carcinomas of many organs. The CanAg antigen is shedded from the tumour and the CA242 epitope can be detected in serum from patients with carcinomas using the C242 MAb.

The CA242 levels are low in healthy subjects and subjects with benign diseases, while elevated levels are commonly found in patients with gastrointestinal cance.

The CA242 test may be used as an aid in the diagnosis and management of patients with known or suspected gastrointestinal carcinomas. The test can be used for diagnostic studies of carcinomas in different organs, to monitor the effect of different treatments of cancer, detection of recurrent cancer disease, and for studies of the prognostic significance of pre-and post treatment levels of CA242.

The CA242 test should not be used as a substitute for any established clinical examination of malignancy, but may be used as a complement to existing clinical and laboratory methods.

Principles of the CA242 EIA

The CanAg CA242 EIA is a solid phase non-competitive assay based upon the direct sandwich technique. Standards and patient samples are incubated together with biotinylated anti-CanAg monoclonal antibody (derived from mice) in Streptavidin coated microtitre strips. The CanAg antigert(s) is adsorbed to the Streptavidin coated microtitre strips by the biotinylated anti-CanAg MAb during this incubation. The strips are then washed followed by incubation with HRP labelled. C242-MAb, which reacts with the CA242 antigenic sites on the bound CanAg antigen. After washing, buffered Substrate/Chromogen reagent (hydrogen peroxide and 3,3',5,5' tetra-methylbenzidine) is added to each well and the enzyme reaction is allowed to proceed. During the enzyme reaction a blue colour will develop if antigen is present. The intensity of the colour is proportional to the amount of CA242 antigen present in the samples.

The colour intensity is determined in a microtitre plate spectrophotometer at 620 nm (or optionally at 405 nm after addition of Stop Solution).

Standard curves are constructed for each assay by plotting absorbance value versus the concentration for each standard. The CA242 concentrations of patient samples are then read from the standard curve.

Kit Contents

Each CA242 EIA kit contains reagents for 96 tests.

The expiry date of the complete kit is stated on the label on the outside of the kit box.

Do not use the kit beyond the expiry date.

Do not mix reagents from different lots of kits.

Store the kit at + 2- +8° C.

Component	*Quantity*	*Shelf life and storage*
C242 Standards	5 vials	+2-+8°C until expiry date stated on the vials
CA242 OU/ml	0.5 ml	
CA242 15U/ml	0.5 mL	
CA242 50U/ml	0.5 mL	
CA242 100 U/ml	0.5mL	
CA242 150U/ml	0.5 mL	

Ready for use. The standards are in Tris-HCl buffered salt solution with bovine serum albumin, an inert yellow dye, and 0.05% sodium azide as preservative.

The standards have been calibrated against an internal reference preparation with the arbitrary defined concentration of 500 U/ml.

Tracer	1 vial 0.75 mL	+2 - +8°C until expiry date stated on the vial
Stock solution of HRP anti CA242 monorclonal antibody from mouse, 40-50µg/mL.		
To be diluted with Tracer Diluent prior to use. Contains 0.01% MIT as preservative.		
Tracer Diluent	1 bottle 15 mL	+2 - +8°C until expiry date stated on the vial
Ready for use phosphate buffered saline (pH 7.2) with bovine serum albumin, bovine globulin, mouse immunoglobulin, Tween 20, and 0.01% MIT as preservative.		
ANTICanAg	1 bottle 15 mL	+2 - +8°C until expiry date stated on the vial
Biotin anti CA242 monoclonal antibody from mouse, ≈ 1.5 µg/mL		
Ready for use Tris-HCl buffered saline (pH 7.75) with bovine serum albumin, bovine globulin, Tween 40, an inert red dye, and 0.05% sodium azide as preservative.		
Sample Diluent	1 bottle 8 mL	+2 -+8°C until expiry date stated on the vial
Ready for use solution containing normal human serum and 0.05% sodium azide as preservative.		
Streptavidin Microtitre plate	Plate 1 plate	+2 -+8°C until expiry date stated on the
12 × 8 wells coated with Streptavidin.		

Contd...

Contd...

TMB HRP Substrate	1 bottle 12 mL	+2 - +8°C until expiry date stated on the vial
Ready for use. Contains buffered hydrogen peroxide and 3,3',5,5' tetramethylbenzidine (TMB).		
HRP Stop Solution	1 bottle 15 mL	+2 - +8°C until expiry date stated on the vial
Ready for use 0.12 M hydrochloric acid.		
Wash Concentrate	1 bottle 40 mL	+2 - +8°C until expiry date stated on the vial
To be diluted with water 25 times before use. A Tris-HCl buffered salt solution with Tween 20. Contains Germall II as preservative.		

Materials Required but not Supplied with the Kit

1. **Microtitre Plate Shaker** Shaking should be medium to vigorous. Longitudinal shaking approximately 200 strokes/min, oscillations 700-900/min.
2. **Microtitre Plate Wash Device** Either an automatic platewash capable of performing 1,3 and 6 washing cycles, or a semi manual microtitre plate washing device connected to vacuum pump or water-jet vacuum and a liquid trap for retaining aspirated liquid.
   The Nunc Immuno-8 manual strip washer is recommended if an automatic micro titre platewash is not used.
3. Microtitre plate spectrophotometer reader with a wavelength of 620 nm and/or 405 nm, and an absorbance range of 0 to 2.5 or preferably 3.0.
4. Precision pipettes with disposable plastic tips to deliver 25 µL, 50 µL and 100 µL. An 8-channel pipette or respenser pipette with disposable plastic tips for delivery of 100 µL is useful but not essential.
5. Distilled or deionized water for preparation of diluted Wash solution.

Specimen Collection and Handling

CA242 EIA is intended for use with serum or plasma. Collect blood by venipuncture, allow to clot and separate the serum or plasma by centrifugation. Haemolysed, moderately lipaemic or icteric samples do not influence the results of the assay. Samples containing fibrin, gross haemolysis, gross lipemia, or turbid samples may give misleading results.

Samples can be stored at +2 - +8°C for 2 days. For longer periods it is recommended to store the samples aliquoted at - 20°C. Avoid repeated freezing and thawing of the samples. Allow frozen samples to thaw slowly, preferable in a refrigerator over night. Bring the samples to room temperature before analysis.

Warnings and Precautions

For *in vitro* diagnostic use

Please refer to the US Department of Health and Human Services (Bethesda, Md., US) publication No. (CDC) 88-8395 on laboratory safety or any other local or national regulation.

Handle all patient specimens as potentially infectious.

The contents of this kit, and their residues, must not be allowed to come into contact with ruminating animals or swine.

Reagents contain sodium azide (NaN_3) as a preservative. Sodium azide may react with lead and copper plumbing to form highly explosive metal azides. On disposal, flush with a large volume of water to prevent azide build-up.

Procedural Notes

1. A thorough understanding of this package insert is necessary to ensure proper use of the CanAg CA242 EIA kit. The reagents supplied with this kit are intended for use as an integral unit.
   Do not mix identical reagents from kits having different lot numbers.
   Do not use the kit reagents after the expiry date printed on the outside of the kit box.
2. Reagents should be allowed to reach room temperature (20-25°C) prior to use. The assay should only be performed at temperatures between 20 and 28°C to obtain accurate results.
   Frozen specimens should be brought to room temperature slowly and gently mixed by hand. Do not vortex or vigorously mix patient samples or control samples.
3. Before starting to pipette standards and patient specimens it is advisable to mark the strips to be able to clearly identify the samples during and after the assay.

4. A careful washing procedure of the strips is essential. Ensure that each well is filled up completely to the top edge, and that the aspiration of the wells between and after the washing cycles is complete and the wells are dry. If there is liquid left in the wells, invert the plate and tap it carefully against absorbing paper.
   Automatic strip washer: Follow the manufacturer's instructions for maintenance, and wash the required number of wash cycles prior to and after each incubation step.
   The aspiration/wash device should not be left standing with the wash solution for long periods as the needles may get clogged giving poor liquid delivery and suction.
5. When handling the TMB HRP Substrate solution be sure to use clean disposable plastic pipette tips (or respenser pipette tip). If the TMB HRP Substrate is transferred from the reagent bottle use only a carefully cleaned reservoir or, preferably, disposable plastic tray to avoid contamination of the reagent.
   The TMB HRP Substrate should be colourless or slightly bluish. A blue colour indicates that the reagent has been contaminated and should be discarded.
6. Be sure to use a proper pipetting technique when handling samples and reagents. Hold the pipette tip slightly above the top of the well and avoid touching the plastic strip or surface of the liquid to avoid carry over from well to well. A proper pipetting technique is of particular importance when handling the 1MB HRP Substrate solution.

Assay Procedure

Perform each determination in duplicate for both standards and patient samples. A standard curve should be run with each assay. All reagents and samples must be brought to room temperature (+20-+ 25°C) before use.

1. Preparation of reagents	Stability of reconstituted reagents
Wash solution	2 weeks at +2-+25°C in sealed container

Pour the 40 mL Wash Concentrate into a clean container and dilute 25-fold by adding 960 mL of distilled or deionized water to give a buffered wash solution.

Tracer working solution	3 weeks at +2 -+8°C

Prepare the needed volume of diluted HRP anti CA242 tracer by mixing 50 µL of the Tracer stock solution with 1 mL Tracer Diluent per strip.

Strips	Tracer stock solution (µL)	Tracer Diluent (mL)
1	50	1
2	100	2
3	150	3
4	200	4
5	250	5
6	300	6
7	350	7
8	400	8
9	450	9
10	500	10
11	550	11
12	600	12

Be sure to use a clean plastic or glass bottle for preparation of the HRP Anti-CA242 tracer solution. *Alternative:* Pour the content of the Tracer stock solution into the bottle of Tracer Diluent and mix gently. Make sure that all of the Tracer stock solution is transferred to the bottle of Tracer Diluent.

Note: The diluted tracer is stable for 3 weeks at +2-+8°C. Do not prepare more Tracer working solution than will be used within this period, and make sure that it is stored properly.

2. Transfer the required number of microtitre plate strips to a strip frame. (Return the remaining unused strips to the plastic tray pack and seal). Wash each strip once with the Wash solution. Do not wash more strips than can be handled within 30 min.
3. Pipette-e 25 µL of the CA242 standards (Std) and patient samples (unknowns-Unk) into the strip wells according to the following scheme (Fig. 23.66).
4. Add 100 µL of ANTI CanAg solution to each well using 100 µL precision pipette (or an 8-channel 100 µL precision pipette). Avoid carry-over by holding the pipette tip slightly above the top of the well and avoid touching the plastic strip or the surface of the liquid.
5. Incubate the frame for 2 hours (± 10 min) at room temperature (+ 20 + 28°C) with constant shaking of the plate using a microtitre plate shaker.

Protocol Sheet September 1998

Mix the components directly before use. Use shaking conditions according to the Instructions.

	Step	*Bottle/Plate*	*Procedure*		
1.	Prepare wash solution	Wash concentrate	Dilute 40 mL of Wash Concentrate with 960 mL of deionized water		
2.	Wash	Plate	Wash each well once with wash solution. Use manual or automatic washer		
3.	Add standards and sample	0,15,50,100,150	25 µL each well		
4.	Add Anti CanAg	Anti CanAg	100 µL in each well		
5.	Incubate	Plate	2 hours shaking at room temperature		
6.	Wash	Plate	Wash each well three times with wash solution. Use manual or automatic washer.		
7.	Prepare Tracer working solution	Tracer Tracer Diluent	Mix Tracer and Tracer Diluent accordingly:		
			no. of strips	Tracer µL	Tracer Diluent mL =
			1	50	1
			2	100	2
			3	150	3
			4	200	4
			5	250	5
			6	300	6
			7	350	7
			8	400	8
			9	450	0
			10	500	10
			11	550	11
			12	600	12
8.	Add Tracer working solution	Tracer working solution	100 µL in each well		
9.	Incubate	Plate 1 hour shaking at room temperature			
10.	Wash	Wash each well six times with wash			
	solution		Use manual or automatic washer.		
11.	Add TMB HRP Substrate	TMB HRP substrate	100 µL in each well		
12.	Incubate	PLATE	30 min shaking at room temperature		
13.	Read absorbance	Plate	620 nm		
	Alt.13. Add HRP Stop Solution	HRP stop solution	100 µL in each well		
	Alt.14. Incubate	Plate	1 min shaking at room temperature		
	Alt.15 Read absorbance	Plate	Read at 405 nm within 15 min		

6. After the first incubation aspirate and wash each strip 3 times, using the wash procedure described in Procedural notes point 4.
7. Add 100 µL of Tracer working solution to each well. Use the same pipetting procedure as in 4.
8. Incubate the frame for 1 hour (± 5 min) at room temperature (+ 20 +28°C) with constant shaking.
9. After the second incubation aspirate and wash each strip 6 times, using the wash procedure described in Procedural notes point 4.
10. Add 100 µL of TMB HRP Substrate to each well using the same procedure as in 4. The TMB HRB Substrate solution should be added to the wells as quickly as possible, and the time between the addition to the first and last well should not exceed 5 min.
11. Incubate for 30 min (± 5 min) at room temperature with constant shaking. Avoid exposure to direct sun light.
12. Immediately read the absorbance at 620 nm in a microtitre plate (or microstrip) reader.
    Option
    If the laboratory does not have access to a micro titre plate reader capable of reading at 620 nm, the absorbance can be determined as in point 13.
13. Add 100 µL of HRP Stop Solution and mix. Thereafter, read absorbance at 405 nm in a microtitre plate (or microstrip) reader within 15 min after addition of HRP Stop Solution.

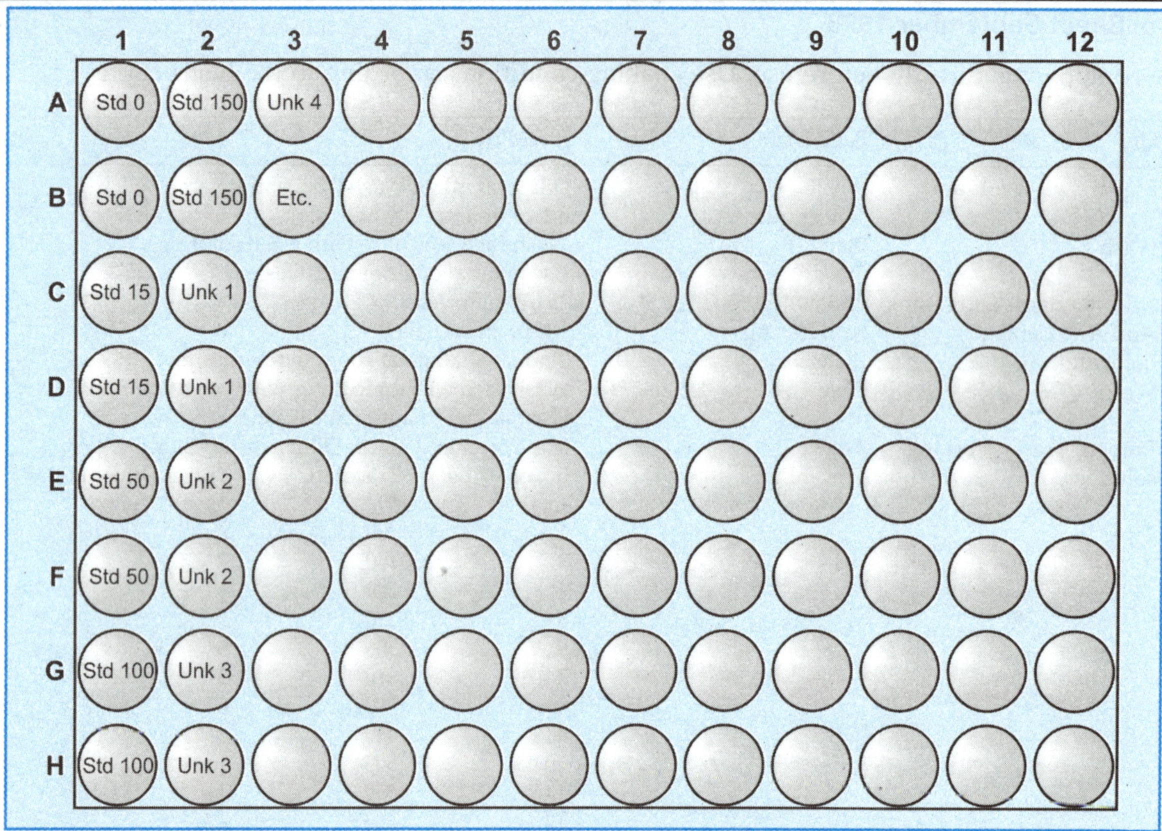

Fig. 23.66: Pipetting scheme

Calculation of Results

If a microtitre plate spectrophotometer reader with built-in data calculation program is used refer to the manual for the plate reader and create a program using the concentration of each of the CA242 standards.

For automatic calculation of CA242 results it is recommended to use either of the following methods

- Spline smoothed curve fit method. Standard 0 should be used as plate blank.
- Interpolation with point-to-point evaluation. Standard 0 U/ml should be included in the curve with the value 0U/ml.
- Quadratic curve fit method. Standard 0 U/ml should be included in the curve with the value 0 U/ml.

Note: 4-Parametric or Linear regression evaluation methods should not be used.

For manual evaluation, a standard curve is constructed by plotting the absorbance (A) values obtained for each CA242 standard against the corresponding CA242 concentration (in U/mL) (see figure below). The unknown CA242 concentrations, in U/ml, can then be read from the standard curve using the mean absorbance value of each patient specimen (Fig. 23.67).

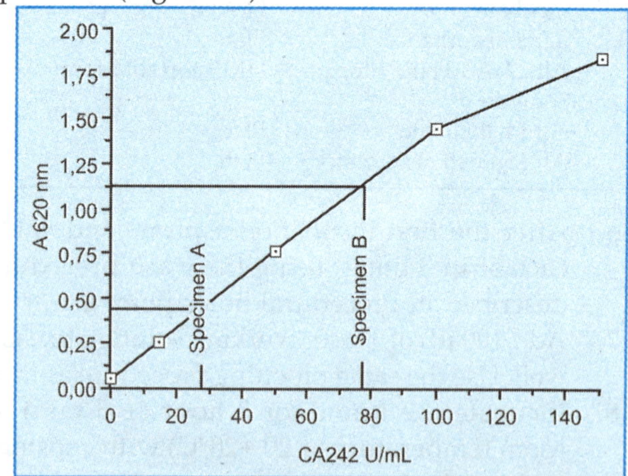

Fig. 23.67: Result calculation

Example (do not use this curve to determine actual assay results)

Specimen	Standard values	Mean abs value (A)	CA242 U/ml
Standard 0	0 U/ml	0.049	
Standard 15	15 U/ml	0.261	

Standard 50	50 U/ml	0.758	
Standard 100	100 U/ml	1.445	
Standard 150	150 U/ml	1.820	
Specimen A		0.445	27.5
Specimen B		1.120	77.2

Calculation of Results with Diluted Samples

If samples in an initial analysis give CA242 levels higher than 150 U/ml the samples should be diluted 1/10 and 1/100 with Sample Diluent to obtain the accurate CA242 concentration of the samples.

1:10 dilution = 50 µL of specimen + 450 µL of Sample Diluent (SD)

1:100 dilution = 50 µL of 1 10 dilution + 450 µL of SD

The CA242 concentration of the undiluted sample is then obtained as follows:

Dilution 1/10:10 x [Measured value-0.9 × CA242 conc., of Sample Diluent]

Dilution 1/100:100 x [Measured value - CA242 conc., of Sample Diluent]

The CA242 concentration of the actual lot of Sample Diluent is stated on the label.

Quality Controls

The use of internal control sera is advised to assure the day-to-day validity of results. It is recommended that the laboratory prepares its-own serum pools at different levels as controls.

Limitations of the Procedure

The level of CA242 cannot be used as absolute evidence for the presence or absence of malignant disease, and the CA242 test should not be used in cancer screening. The results of the test should be interpreted only in conjunction with other investigations and procedures in the diagnosis of disease and the management of patients, and the CA242 test should not replace any established clinical examination.

Reference Value

Normal value: in healthy subjects < 20 Units/mL

CA242 concentration has been determined with the CanAg CA242 EIA kit in 200 serum samples from healthy individuals.

The CA242 level in healthy subjects was 8.0 ± 6.7 U/ml, with a median value of 6.4 U/ml, and the 95th percentile 21.7 U/ml.

It is recommended that each laboratory establishes its own normal range so as to account for such local enviro nmental factors as diet, climate, living conditions, patients selection, etc.

PERFORMANCE OF THE CHARACTERISTICS

Dose-response and Precision Profile

A typical standard curve and precision profile obtained with the CanAg CA242 EIA kit are shown below. The precision profile is based on random pipetting of standards into one microtitre plate, n = 12.

Dose-response and precision profile (Fig. 23.68).

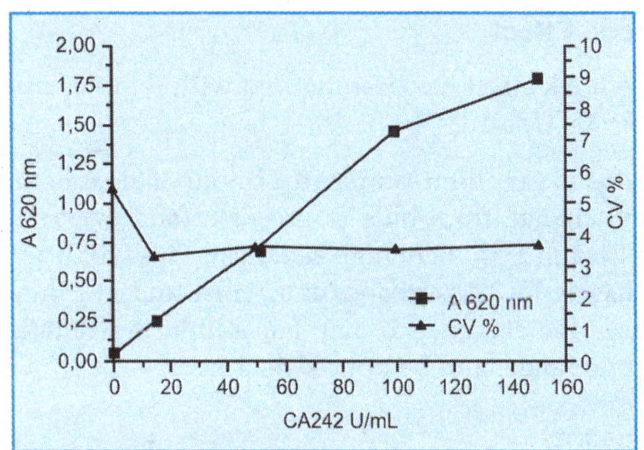

Fig. 23.68: Dose response

CA242 U/ml

Precision

Intra-assay (with-in run) precision of the CanAg CA242 kit is shown below:

Sample	*Number of replicates*	*Mean value U/ml*	*SD U/ml%*	*CV*
1	4	12.7	0.3	2.7
2	4	57.6	1.1	1.9
3	4	78.6	2.9	3.7
4	4	122.3	4.1	3.3

Inter-assay (between run) precision calculated from three separate analyses with 4 replicates of each sample during three days.

Sample	*Number of > replicates*	*Mean value SD U/ml*	*CV U/ml*	*%*
1	12.7	-	0.4	3.5
2	12	59.8	2.7	4.4
3	12	80.2	5.1	6.4
4	12	133.9	8.2	6.1

Detection Limit

The detection limit of the CanAg CA242 EIA assay is < 1 U/ml defined as the concentration corresponding to the mean of the absorbance values for the "0" standard plus 2 standard deviations of the 0 standard determination (mean value + 2 SD).

Recovery

Spiked serum samples were prepared by adding CA242'antigen to normal serum samples. The recovery of the antigen were in the range 92 -102%.

Hook Effect

No hook effect has been noticed with samples up to 150 000 U/ml.

Note: In very high samples the colour of the substrate will change from blue to greenish (and eventually yellow in extremely high samples). This will lead to a falsely low Absorbance at 620 nrn, and in extreme cases the absorbance may fall within the standard curve range, and be noticed as a hook.

Linearity

Patient samples were serially diluted with Sample Diluent and analysed. The obtained values were in the range 93 -109% of the expected values.

CA 50 (CARBOHYDRATE ANTIGEN 50), BLOOD

Norm <17 U/ ml.

Increased

Colourectal adenocarcinomas, digestive tract carcinoma, esophageal squamous cell carcinoma, non-small cell lung carcinoma, pancreatic cancer, transitional cell bladder carcinoma.

Decreased

Positive response to therapy.

Description: A tumor marker that increases with many malignancies, particularly those of the digestive tract. This test is not specific enough for screening and correlates more with tumor progression than with tumor regression.

CA 125 (CANCER ANTIGEN 125)
Mfd: Monobind, Courtesy: Lilac Medicare

Intended Use

The Quantitativ\ Determination of Cancer Antigen 125 (CA-125) Concentration in Human Serum by a Microplate Immunoenzymometric assay

Summary and Explanation of the Test

Cancer Antigen 125 (CA-125) is a glycoprotein that occurs in blood as high molecular weight (M, > 200,000). High concentrations of this antigen are associated with ovarian cancer and a range of benign and malignant diseases. Although the specificity and sensitivity of CA-125 assays are somewhat limited, especially in early diagnosis of ovarian cancer, the assay has found widespread use in the differential diagnosis of adnexal masses, in monitoring disease progression and response to therapy in ovarian cancer, and in the early detection of recurrence after surgery or chemotherapy for ovarian cancer. Published literature has shown that elevated serum CA-125 levels can be observed in patients with serious endometroid, clear cell and undifferentiated ovarian carcinoma. The serum CA-125 is elevated in 1% of normal healthy women, 3% of normal healthy women with benign ovarian diseases, 6% of patients with non-neoplastic conditions (including but not limited to first trimester pregnancy, menstruation, endometriosis uterine fibrosis, acute salphingitis, hepatic diseases and inflammation of peritoneum or pericardium).

In this method, CA-125 calibrator, patient specimen or control is first added to a streptavidin coated well. Biotinylated monoclonal and enzyme labeled antibodies (directed against distinct and different epitopes of CA-125) are added and the reactants mixed. Reaction between the various CA-125 antibodies and native CA-125 forms a sandwich complex that binds with the streptavidin coated to the well.

After the completion of the required incubation period, the enzyme-CA-125 antibody bound conjugate is separated from the unbound enzyme-CA-125 conjugate by aspiration or decantation. The activity of the enzyme present on the surface of the well is quantitated by reaction with a suitable substrate to produce colour.

The employment of several serum references of known Cancer Antigen 125 (CA-125) levels permits the construction of a dose response curve of activity and concentration. From comparison to the dose response curve, an unknown specimen's activity can be correlated with CA-125 concentration.

PRINCIPLE

Immunoenzymometric Assay

The essential reagents required for an immunoenzymometric assay include high affinity and specificity antibodies (enzyme and immobilised), with different and distinct epitope recognition, in excess, and native antigen. In this procedure, the immobilisation takes place during the assay at the surface of a microplate well through the interaction of streptavidin coated on the well and exogenously added biotinylated monoclonal anti-CA-125 antibody.

Upon mixing monoclonal biotinylated antibody, the enzymelabeled antibody and a serum containing the native antigen, reaction results between the native antigen and the antibodies, without competition or steric hindrance, to form a soluble sandwich complex. The interaction is illustrated by the following equation

$$^{Enz}Ab + Ag_{CA\text{-}125} + {}^{Btn}Ab_{(m)} \underset{k_{-a}}{\overset{k_a}{\rightleftharpoons}} {}^{Enz}Ab\text{-}Ag_{CA}\text{-}{}^{Btn}Ab_{(m)}$$

$k_{-a}\ {}^{Btn}Ab_{(m)}$ = Biotinylated monoclonal antibody (excess quantity)

$Ag_{CA\text{-}125}$ = Native antigen (variable quantity)

^{Enz}Ab = Enzyme labeled antibody (excess quantity)

$^{Enz}Ab\text{-}Ag_{CA\text{-}125}\text{-}{}^{Btn}Ab_{(m)}$ = Antigen-antibodies sandwich complex

k_a = Rate constant of association

k_{-a} = Rate constant of dissociation

Simultaneously, the complex is deposited to the well through the high affinity reaction of streptavidin and biotinylated antibody. This interaction is illustrated below

$^{Enz}Ab\ \text{-}Ag_{CA\text{-}125\text{-}}{}^{Btn}Ab_{(m)}$ + $Streptavidin_{cw}$ => Immobilised complex

Streptavidin cw = Streptavidin immobilised on well

Immobilised complex = sandwich complex bound to the well

After equilibrium is attained, the antibody-bound fraction is separated from unbound antigen by decantation or aspiration. The enzyme activity in the antibody-bound fraction is directly proportional to the native antigen concentration. By utilizing several different serum references of known antigen values, a dose response curve can be generated from which the antigen concentration of an unknown can be ascertained.

REAGENTS MATERIALS PROVIDED

A. Cancer Antigen 125 (CA-125) 1 ml/vial

Six (6) vials of references CA-125 Antigen at levels of 0(A), 15(B), 50(C), 100(D), 200(E) and 400(F) U/ml. Store at 2 to 8°C. A preservative has been added.

Note: The standards, human serum based, were made using a >99% pure affinity purified preparation of CA-125. The preparation was calibrated against Centocor CA-125IRMA test.

B. Enzyme-Antibody-Conjugate and Biotinylated Monoclonal antibody—13ml/vial

One (1) vial containing enzyme labeled antibody, biotinylated monoclonal mouse IgG in buffer, dye, and preservative. Store at 2 to 8° C.

C. Streptavidin Coated Microplate—96 wells

One 96-well microplate coated with streptavidin and packaged in an aluminum bag with a drying agent. Store at 2 to 8° C.

D. Wash Solution Concentrate - 20 ml

One (1) vial containing a surfactant in buffered saline. A preservative has been added. Store at 2 to 30°C.

E. Substrate A -7ml/vial

One (1) bottle containing tetramethylbenzidine (TMB) in buffer. Store at 2 to 8°C.

F. Substrate B—7ml/vial

One (1) bottle containing hydrogen peroxide (H_2O_2) in buffer. Store at 2 to 8°C.

G. Stop Solution-8ml/vial

One (1) bottle containing a strong acid (1N HCl). Store at 2 to 30°C.

Product Instructions

Note 1

Do not use reagents beyond the kit expiration date.

Note 2

Opened reagents are stable for sixty (60) days when stored at 2 to 8°C.

Note 3

Above reagents are for a single 96-well microplate

Required But Not Provided

1. Pipette capable of delivering 100 µl volumes with a precision of better than 1.5 %.
2. Dispenser(s) for repetitive deliveries of 0.100 ml and 0.300 ml volumes with a precision of better than 1.5%.
3. Microplate washers or a squeeze bottle (optional).
4. Microplate reader with 450 nm and 620 nm wavelength absorbance capability.
5. Absorbent paper for blotting the microplate wells.
6. Plastic wrap or microplate cover for incubation steps.
7. Vacuum aspirator (optional) for wash steps.
8. Timer.
9. Quality control materials

Precautions

For In Vitro Diagnostic Use

Not for Internal or External Use in Humans or Animals

All products that contain human serum have been found to be non-reactive for Hepatitis B Surface Antigen, HIV 1 and 2 and HCV Antibodies by FDA licensed reagents. Since no known test can offer complete assurance that infectious agents are absent, all human serum products should be handled as potentially hazardous and capable of transmitting disease. Good laboratory procedures for handling blood products can be found in the Center for Disease Control/National Institute of Health, "Biosafety in Microbiological and Biomedical Laboratories," 2nd Edition, 1988, HHS Publication No. (CDC) 88-8395.

Specimen Collection and Preparation

The specimens shall be blood, serum in type and the usual precautions in the collection of venipuncture samples should be observed. For accurate comparison to established normal values, a fasting morning serum sample should be obtained. The blood should be collected in a plain redtop venipuncture tube without additives or anti-coagulants. Allow the blood to clot. Centrifuge the specimen to separate the serum from the cells.

Samples may be refrigerated at 2 to 8°C for a maximum period of five (5) days. If the specimen(s) cannot be assayed within this time, the sample(s) may be stored at temperatures of -20°C for up to 30 days. Avoid repetitive freezing and thawing. When assayed in duplicate, 0.200 ml of the specimen is required.

Reagent Preparation

1. **Wash Buffer** Dilute contents of Wash Concentrate to 1000 ml with distilled or deionized water in a suitable storage container. Store at room temperature 20 to 27°C for up to 60 days.
2. **Working Substrate Solution** Pour the contents of the vial labeled Solution 'A' into the vial labeled Solution 'B'. Mix and store at 2 to 8°C. Use within 60 days. Or for longer periods of usage determine the amount of reagent needed and prepare by mixing equal portions of Substrate A and Substrate B in a suitable container. For example, add 1 ml of A and 1 ml of B per two (2) eight well strips (A slight excess of solution is made. Discard the unused portion).
   Note: Do not use the working substrate if it looks blue.

Test Procedure

Before proceeding with the assay, bring all reagents, serum references and controls to room temperature (20-27°C).

1. Format the microplates wells for each serum reference, control and patient specimen to be assayed in duplicate. Replace any unused microwell strips back into the aluminum bag, seal and store at 2 to 8°C.
2. Pipette 0.025 ml (25 µl) of the appropriate serum reference, control or specimen into the assigned well.
3. Add 0.100 ml (100 µl) of the biotinylated/enzyme labeled antibodies to each well. It is very important to dispense all reagents close to the bottom of the coated-well.
4. Swirl the microplate gently for 20-30 seconds to mix and cover.

5. Incubate 60 minutes at room temperature.
6. Discard the contents of the microplate by decantation or aspiration. If decanting, tap and blot the plate dry with absorbent paper.
7. Add 300 µl of wash buffer (see Reagent Preparation Section), decant (tap and blot) or aspirate. Repeat two (2) additional times for a total of three (3) washes. An automatic or manual plate washer can be used. Follow the manufacturer's instruction for proper usage. If a squeeze bottle is employed, fill each well by depressing the container (avoiding air bubbles) to dispense the wash. Decant the wash and repeat two (2) additional times.
8. Add 0.100 ml (100 µl) of working substrate solution to all wells (see Reagent Preparation Section). Always add reagents in the same order to minimise reaction time differences between wells.
9. Incubate at room temperature for fifteen (15) minutes.
10. Add 0.050 ml (50 µl) of stop solution to each well and mix gently for 15 to 20 seconds. Always add reagents in the same order to minimize reaction time differences between wells.
11. Read the absorbance in each well at 450 nm (using a reference wavelength of 620-630 nm to minimize well imperfections) in a microplate reader. The results should be read within thirty (30) minutes of adding the stop solution.

Quality Control

Each laboratory should assay controls at levels in the low, medium and high ranges of the dose response curve for monitoring assay performance. These controls should be treated as unknowns and values determined in every test procedure performed. Quality control charts should be maintained to follow the performance of the supplied reagents. Pertinent statistical methods should be employed to ascertain trends. Significant deviation from established performance can indicate unnoticed change in experimental conditions or degradation of kit reagents. Fresh reagents should be used to determine the reason for the variations.

Results

A dose response curve is used to ascertain the concentration of follicle stimulating hormone in unknown specimens.

1. Record the absorbance obtained from the printout of the microplate reader as outlined in Example 1.
2. Plot the absorbance for each duplicate serum reference versus the corresponding CA-125 concentration in U/ml on linear graph paper (do not average the duplicates of the serum references before plotting).
3. Draw the best-fit curve through the plotted points.
4. To determine the concentration of CA-125 for an unknown, locate the average absorbance of the duplicates for each unknown on the vertical axis of the graph, find the intersecting point on the curve, and read the concentration (in U/ml) from the horizontal axis of the graph (the duplicates of the unknown may be averaged as indicated). (See Figure 23.69).

Note: Computer data reduction software designed for IEMA assays may also be used for the data reduction.

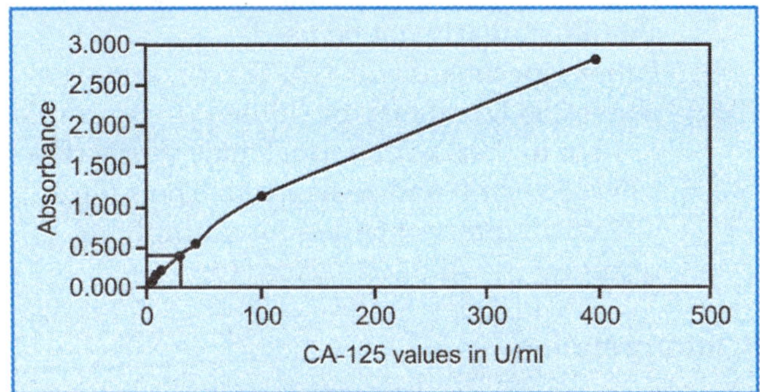

Fig. 23.69: Result calculation

The data presented in Figure 23.69 are for illustration only and should not be used in lieu of a dose response curve prepared with each assay.

QC Parameters

In order for the assay results to be considered valid the following criteria should be met

1. The absorbance (OD) of calibrator F should be ≥ 1.3.
2. Four out of six quality control pools should be within the established ranges.

LIMITATIONS OF PROCEDURE

A. Assay Performance

1. It is important that the time of reaction in each well is held constant for reproducible results.

2. Pipetting of samples should not extend beyond ten (10) minutes to avoid assay drift.
3. If more than one (1) plate is used, it is recommended to repeat the dose response curve.
4. Addition of the substrate solution initiates a kinetic reaction, which is terminated by the addition of the stop solution. Therefore, the addition of the substrate and the stopping solution should be added in the same sequence to eliminate any time-deviation during reaction.
5. Plate readers measure vertically. Do not touch the bottom of the wells.
6. Failure to remove adhering solution adequately in the aspiration or decantation wash step(s) may result in poor replication and spurious results.
7. Use components from the same lot. No intermixing of reagents from different batches.
8. Sample(s), which are contaminated microbiologically, should not be used in the assay. Highly lipemeic or hemolysed specimen(s) should similarly not be used.
9. Patient specimens with CA-125 concentrations above 250 U/ml may be diluted (for example 1/10 or higher) with normal male serum (CA-125 < 5 U/ml) and re-assayed. The sample's concentration is obtained by multiplying the result by the dilution factor (10).

B. Interpretation

1. If computer controlled data reduction is used to interpret the results of the test, it is imperative that the predicted values for the calibrators fall within 10% of the assigned concentrations.
2. CA-125 has a low clinical sensitivity and specificity as a tumor marker. Clinically an elevated CA-125 value alone is not of diagnostic value as a test for cancer and should only be used in conjunction with other clinical manifestations (observations) and diagnostic parameters.

Expected Ranges of Values

The serum CA-125 is elevated in 1% of normal healthy women, 3% of normal healthy women with benign ovarian diseases, 6% of patients with non-neoplastic conditions (including but not limited to first trimester pregnancy, menstruation, endometriosis uterine fibrosis, acute salphingitis, hepatic diseases and inflammation of peritoneum or pericardium).

Expected Values for the CA-125 ELISA Test System

Healthy and non-pregnant subjects ≤ 35 U/ml

It is important to keep in mind that establishment of a range of values which can be expected to be found by a given method for a population of "normal" persons is dependent upon a multiplicity of factors: the specificity of the method, the population tested and the precision of the method in the hands of the analyst. For these reasons each laboratory should depend upon the range of expected values established by the Manufacturer only until an in-house range can be determined by the analysts using the method with a population indigeneous to the area in which the laboratory is located.

CARCINOEMBRYONIC ANTIGEN (CEA)
Mfd: Monobind, Courtesy: Lilac Medicare

Summary and Explanation of the Test

Carcinoembryonic antigen (CEA) is a glycoprotein with a molecular weight of 180 kDA. CEA is the first of the so-called carcinoembryonic proteins that was discovered in 1965 by Gold and Freeman. CEA is the most widely used marker for gastrointestinal cancer.

Although CEA is primarily associated with colorectal cancers, other malignancies that can cause elevated levels of CEA include breast, lung, stomach, pancreas, ovary and other organs. Benign conditions that cause significantly higher than normal levels include inflammation of lung and gastrointestinal (GI) tract and benign liver cancer. Heavy Smokers, as a group, have higher than normal baseline concentration of CEA.

In this method, CEA calibrator, patient specimen or control is first added to a streptavidin coated well. Biotinylated monoclonal and enzyme labeled antibodies (directed against distinct and different epitopes of CEA) are added and the reactants mixed. Reaction between the various CEA antibodies and native CEA forms a sandwich complex that binds with the streptavidin coated to the well.

After the completion of the required incubation period, the enzyme-CEA antibody bound conjugate is separated from the unbound enzyme-CEA conjugate by aspiration or decantation. The activity of the enzyme present on the surface of the well is quantitated by reaction with a suitable substrate to produce colour.

The employment of several serum references of known carcinoembryonic antigen (CEA) levels permits the construction of a dose response curve of activity and concentration. From comparison to the dose response curve, an unknown specimen's activity can be correlated with CEA concentration.

PRINCIPLE

Immunoenzymometric Assay

The essential reagents required for an immunoenzymometric assay include high affinity and specificity antibodies (enzyme and immobilised), with different and distinct epitope recognition, in excess, and native antigen. In this procedure, the immobilisation takes place during the assay at the surface of a microplate well through the interaction of streptavidin coated on the well and exogenously added biotinylated monoclonal anti-CEA antibody.

Upon mixing monoclonal biotinylated antibody, the enzyme-labelled antibody and a serum containing the native antigen, reaction results between the native antigen and the antibodies, without competition or steric hindrance, to form a soluble sandwich complex. The interaction is illustrated by the following equation.

$$^{Enz}Ab_{(p)} + Ag_{CEA} + {}^{Btn}Ab_{(m)} \underset{k\text{-}a}{\overset{k^{a}}{\rightleftharpoons}} EnzAb_{(p)}\text{-}Ag_{CEA}\text{-}{}^{Btn}Ab_{(m)}$$

$^{Btn}Ab_{(m)}$ = Biotinylated monoclonal antibody (excess quantity)
Ag_{CEA} = Native antigen (variable quantity)
$^{Enz}Ab_{(p)}$ = Enzyme labelled polyclonal antibody (excess quantity)
$^{Enz}Ab_{(p)}\text{-}Ag_{CEA}\text{-}{}^{Btn}Ab_{(m)}$ = Antigen-antibodies sandwich complex
ka = Rate constant of association
$k\text{-}_{a}$ = Rate constant of dissociation

Simultaneously, the complex is deposited to the well through the high affinity reaction of streptavidin and biotinylated antibody. This interaction is illustrated below:

$^{Enz}Ab_{(p)}\text{-}Ag_{CEA}\text{-}{}^{Btn}Ab_{(m)}$ + Streptavidin cw => Immobilised complex

Streptavidin cw = Streptavidin immobilised on well Immobilised complex = sandwich complex bound to the solid surface

After equilibrium is attained, the antibody-bound fraction is separated from unbound antigen by decantation or aspiration. The enzyme activity in the antibody-bound fraction is directly proportional to the native antigen concentration. By utilising several different serum references of known antigen values, a dose response curve can be generated from which the antigen concentration of an unknown can be ascertained.

REAGENTS FOR 96-WELL MICROPLATE

A. Carcinoembryonic antigen (CEA) -1.0 ml/vial

Six (6) vials of references S-CEA Antigen at levels of 0(A), 5(B), 10(C), 25(D), 50(E) and 250(F) ng/ ml. Store at 2 to 8°C. A preservative has been added.

B. Enzyme-Polyclonal Conjugate and Biotinylated Monoclonal antibody—11 ml/vial

One (1) vial containing enzyme labelled antibody, biotinylated monoclonal mouse IgG in buffer, dye, and preservative. Store at 2 to 8°C.

C. Streptavidin Coated Microplate - 96 wells

One 96-well microplate coated with Streptavidin and packaged in an aluminum bag with a drying agent. Store at 2 to 8°C.

D. Wash Solution Concentrate - 20 ml

One (1) vial containing a surfactant in phosphate buffered saline. A preservative has been added. Store at 2 to 30°C.

E. Substrate A -7.0 ml/vial

One (1) bottle containing tetramethylbenzidine (TMB) in buffer. Store at 2 to 8°C.

F. Substrate B - 7.0 ml/vial

One (1) bottle containing hydrogen peroxide (HaO_2) in buffer. Store at 2 to 8°C.

G. Stop Solution—6.0 ml/vial

One (1) bottle containing a strong acid (1N HCI). Store at 2 to 30°C.

Note 1: Do not use reagents beyond the kit expiration date.

Note 2: Opened reagents are stable for sixty (60) days when stored at 2 to 8°C.

For In Vitro Diagnostic Use

Not for Internal or External Use in Humans or Animals

Precautions

All products that contain human serum have been found to be non-reactive for Hepatitis B Surface Antigen, HIV 1 and 2 and HCV Antibodies by FDA required tests. Since no known test can offer complete assurance that infectious agents are absent, all human serum products should be handled as potentially hazardous and capable of transmitting disease. Good laboratory procedures for handling blood products can be found in the Centre for Disease Control/ National Institute of Health, "Biosafety in Microbiological and Biomedical Laboratories," 2nd Edition, 1988, HHS

Specimen Collection and Preparation

The specimens shall be blood serum in type and the usual precautions in the collection of venipuncture samples should be observed. For accurate comparison to established normal values, a fasting morning serum sample should be obtained. The blood should be collected in a plain redtop venipuncture tube without additives or gel barrier. Allow the blood to clot. Centrifuge the specimen to separate the serum from the cells.

Samples may be refrigerated at 2 to 8°C for a maximum period of five (5) days. If the specimen(s) can not be assayed within this time, the sample(s) may be stored at temperatures of -20°C for up to 30 days. Avoid repetitive freezing and thawing. When assayed in duplicate, 0.050 ml of the specimen is required.

MATERIALS

Provided

1. Six (6) vials of CEA serum calibrators.
2. One (1) vial of combined biotinylated monoclonal antibody and enzyme labeled polyclonal reagent.
3. One 96-well Streptavidin Coated Microplate.
4. One (1) bottle of Wash Buffer Concentrate.
5. One (1) bottle of Substrate A.
6. One (1) bottle of Substrate B.
7. One (1) bottle of Stop solution.
8. Instructions.

Required But Not Provided

1. Pipette(s) capable of delivering 25 µl and 100 µl volumes with a precision of better than 1.5%.
2. Dispenser(s) for repetitive deliveries of 0.100 ml and 0.300 ml volumes with a precision of better than 1.6% (optional).
3. Microplate washer or a squeeze bottle (optional).
4. Microplate Reader with 450 nm wavelength absorbance capability.
5. Container(s) for mixing of reagents (see below).
6. Absorbent Paper for blotting the microplate wells.
7. Plastic wrap or microplate cover for incubation steps.
8. Vacuum aspirator (optional) for wash steps.
9. Timer.
10. Storage container for storage of wash buffer.
11. Distilled or deionized water.

Reagent Preparation

1. **Working Reagent 1-Wash buffer** Dilute contents of Wash concentrate to 1000 ml with distilled or deionized water in a suitable storage container. Store at room temperature.
2. **Working Reagent 2 - Substrate Solution - Prepare before use** Determine the amount of reagent needed and prepare by mixing equal portions of Substrate A and Substrate B in a suitable container. For example, add 1 ml of A and 1 ml of B per two (2) eight well strips (A slight excess of solution is made). Use within one (1) hour of preparation for maximum performance of the assay.

Test Procedure

Before proceeding with the assay, bring all reagents, serum references and controls to room temperature.

1. Format the microplates' wells for each serum reference, control and patient specimen to be assayed in duplicate. Replace any unused microwell strips back into the aluminum bag, seal and store at 2 to 8°C.
2. Pipette 0.025 ml (25 µl) of the appropriate serum reference, control or specimen into the assigned well.

3. Add 0.100 ml (100 µl) of the biotinylated/enzyme labelled antibodies to each well. It is very important to dispense all reagents close to the bottom of the coated well.
4. Swirl the microplate gently for 20 to 30 seconds to mix and cover.
5. Incubate 60 minutes at room temperature.
6. Discard the contents of the microplate by decantation or aspiration. If decanting, tap and blot the plate dry with absorbent paper.
7. Add 300 µl of wash buffer (see Reagent Preparation Section), decant (tap and blot) or aspirate. Repeat two (2) additional times for a total of three (3) washes. An automatic or manual plate washer can be used. Follow the manufacturer's instruction for proper usage. If a is queeze bottle is employed, fill each well by depressing the container (avoiding air bubbles) to dispense the wash. Decant the wash and repeat two (2) additional times.
8. Add 0.100 ml (100 µl) of working substrate solution to all wells (see Reagent Preparation Section). Always add reagents in the same order to minimize reaction time differences between wells.
9. Incubate at room temperature for fifteen (15) minutes.
10. Add 0.050 ml (50 µl) of stop solution to each well and mix gently for 15 to 20 seconds. Always add reagents in the same order to minimize reaction time differences between wells.
11. Read the absorbance in each well at 450 nm in a microplate reader. The results should be read within thirty (30) minutes of adding the stop solution.

Quality Control

Each laboratory should assay controls at levels in the low, normal and elevated range for monitoring assay performance. These controls should be treated as unknowns and values determined in every test procedure performed. Quality control charts should be maintained to follow the performance of the supplied reagents. Pertinent statistical methods should be employed to ascertain trends. The individual laboratory should set acceptable assay performance limits. Other parameters that should be monitored include the 80, 50 and 20% intercepts of the dose response curve for run-to-run reproducibility. In addition, maximum absorbance should be consistent with past experience. Significant deviation from established performance can indicate unnoticed change in experimental conditions or degradation of kit reagents. Fresh reagents should be used to determine the reason for the variations.

Results

A dose response curve is used to ascertain the concentration of CEA in unknown specimens.

1. Record the absorbance obtained from the printout of the microplate reader as outlined in Example 1.
2. Plot the absorbance for each duplicate serum reference versus the corresponding CEA concentration in ng/ml on linear graph paper (do not average the duplicates of the serum references before plotting).
3. Draw the best-fit curve through the plotted points.
4. To determine the concentration of CEA for an unknown, locate the average absorbance of the duplicates for each unknown on the vertical axis of the graph, find the intersecting point on the curve, and read the concentration (in ng/ml) from the horizontal axis of the graph (the duplicates of the unknown may be averaged as indicated). In the following example, the average absorbance (0.391) intersects the dose response curve at (22.5ng/ml) CEA concentration (See Figure 23.70).

Note: Computer data reduction software designed for IEMA assays may also be used for the data reduction.

Example 1

Well	*Serum References*	*Absorbance*
1	0.0 ng/ml	0.017
2	0.0 ng/ml	0.019
3	5.0 ng/ml	0.160
4	5.0 ng/ml	0.159
5	10.0 ng/ml	0.231
6	10.0 ng/ml	0.224
7	25.0 ng/ml	0.431
8	25.0 ng/ml	0.418
9	50.0 ng/ml	0.776
10	50.0 ng/ml	0.763
11	100.0 ng/ml	2.851
12	100.0 ng/ml	2.885/

Well	**Unknown IU**	**OD**	**Avg OD**	**Value**
13	Unknown #1	0.398		
14	Unknown #1	0.384	0.391	22.5 ng/ml

*The data presented in Example 1 and Figure 23.70 are for illustration only and should not be used in lieu of a dose response curve prepared with each assay.

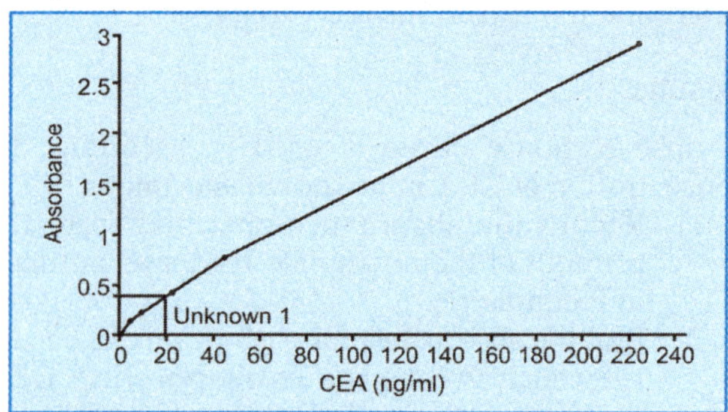

Fig. 23.70: Result calculation

QC Parameters
Maximum Absorbance (250 ng/ml) ⇒ 1.5

LIMITATIONS OF PROCEDURE

A. Assay Performance

It is important that the time of reaction in each well is held constant for reproducible results. Pipetting of samples should not extend beyond ten (10) minutes to avoid assay drift. If more than one (1) plate is used, it is recommended to repeat the dose response curve.

Addition of the substrate solution initiates a kinetic reaction, which is terminated by the addition of the stop solution. Therefore, the addition of the substrate and the stopping solution should be added in the same sequence to eliminate any time deviation during reaction.

Plate readers measure vertically. Do not touch the bottom of the wells.

Failure to remove adhering solution adequately in the aspiration or decantation wash step(s) may result in poor replication and spurious results.

Sample(s), which are contaminated microbiologically, should not be used in the assay. Highly lipaemic or haemolysed specimen(s) should similarly not be used.

Patient specimens with CEA concentrations above 250 ng/ml may be diluted (for example 1/10 or higher) with normal male serum (CEA < 5 ng/ml) and re-assayed. The sample's concentration is obtained by multiplying the result by the dilution factor (10).

Each component in one assay should be of the same lot number and stored under identical conditions.

B. Interpretation

If computer controlled data reduction is used to interpret the results of the test, it is imperative that the predicted values for the calibrators fall within 10% of the assigned concentrations.

CEA has a low clinical sensitivity and specificity as a tumour marker. Clinically an elevated CEA value alone is not of diagnostic value as a test for cancer and should only be used in conjunction with other clinical manifestations (observations) and diagnostic parameters. There are patients with colourectal cancer that do not exhibit elevated CEA values and elevated CEA values do not always change with progression or regression of disease. Smokers demonstrate a higher range of baseline values than non-smokers.

Expected Ranges of Values

Nearly 99% of non-smokers have CEA concentrations less than 5 ng/ml. Similarly 99% of smokers have concentrations less than 10 ng/ml.

Table 1

Expected Values for the CEA ELISA Test System

Non-smokers <5 ng/ml

Smokers <10 ng/ml

It is important to keep in mind that establishment of a range of values which can be expected to be found by a given method for a population of "normal" -persons is dependent upon a multiplicity of factors the specificity of the method, the population tested and the precision of the method in the hands of the analyst. For these reasons each laboratory should depend upon the range of expected values established by the manufacturer only until an in-house range can be determined by the analysts using the method with a population indigeneous to the area in which the laboratory is located.

Normal values

		SI Units
Nonsmoker	<5 ng/ml	<5 mg/L
Smoker	<10 ng/ml	<10 mg/L

Increased

Cancer (breast, oesophageal, gastrointestinal, ovarian, pancreatic, prostate, pulmonary), chronic ischemic heart disease, cirrhosis, hypothyroidism, inflammatory bowel disease, inflammatory processes, leukemia, neuroblastoma, pancreatitis (acute), pneumonia (bacterial), pulmonary emphysema, radiation therapy (recent), renal failure (acute), tobacco smokers (chronic), and trauma. Drugs include antineoplastics and hepatotoxic drugs.

Decreased

Not clinically significant.

Description: CEA is a glycoprotein produced by the fetus from age 2 to 6 months and secreted by gastrointestinal cells. It is an antigen that can be found in trace amounts in healthy adults, but is secreted in greater amounts during rapid multiplication of epithelial cells, especially of the gastrointestinal tract. This test is not diagnostic, but because levels are increased in malignancies, CEA provides a guide to management and helps evaluate the success or surgery and other forms of cancer treatment. This test is most valuable in the early detection of recurrent colourectal cancer because blood levels may rise 3 months before clinical symptoms of the recurrent disease are present. CEA levels many be measured every 1-3 months to monitor response to and direct therapy for colourectal cancer. Normal levels occur within 4 to 6 weeks after effective therapy.

PROSTATE-SPECIFIC ANTIGEN (PSA)

TOTAL PROSTATE SPECIFIC ANTIGEN (TPSA) ELISA, Mfd: Monobind, Courtesy: Lilac Medicare

Summary and Explanation of the Test

Prostate Specific antigen (PSA) is a serine protease with chymotrypsin-like activity. The protein is a single chain glycoprotein with a molecular weight of 28.4 kDA. PSA derives its name from the observation that it is a normal antigen of the prostrate but is not found in any other normal or malignant tissue.

PSA is found in benign, malignant and metastatic prostrate cancer. Since prostate cancer is the second most prevalent form of male malignancy, the detection of elevated PSA levels plays an important role in the early diagnosis. Serum PSA levels have been found to more useful than prostatic acid phosphatase (PAP) in the diagnosis and management of patients due to increased sensitivity. In this method, PSA calibrator, patient specimen or control is first added to a streptavidin-coated tube. Biotinylated monoclonal and enzyme labeled antibodies (directed against distinct and different epitopes of PSA) are added and the reactants mixed. Reaction between the various PSA antibodies and native PSA forms a sandwich complex that binds with the streptavidin coated to the tube.

After the completion of the required incubation period, the enzyme-PSA antibody bound conjugate is separated from the unbound enzyme-PSA conjugate by aspiration or decantation. The activity of the enzyme present on the surface of the tube is quantitated by reaction with a suitable substrate to produce colour.

The employment of several serum references of known prostate specific antigen (PSA) levels permits the construction of a dose response curve of activity and concentration. From comparison to the dose response curve, an unknown specimen's activity can be correlated with PSA concentration.

PRINCIPLE

Immunoenzymometric Assay

The essential reagents required for an immunoenzymometric assay include high affinity and specificity antibodies (enzyme and immobilised), with different and distinct epitope recognition, in excess, and native antigen. In this procedure, the immobilisation takes place during the assay at the surface of a coated tube through the interaction of streptavidin coated on the tube and exogenously added biotinylated monoclonal anti-PSA antibody.

Upon mixing monoclonal biotinylated antibody, the enzyme-labeled antibody and a serum containing the native antigen, reaction results between the native antigen and the antibodies, without competition or steric hindrance, to form a soluble sandwich complex. The interaction is illustrated by the following equation

$$^{Enz}Ab_{(p)} + AgPSA + {}^{Btn}AB_{(m)} \underset{k_{-a}}{\overset{ka}{\rightleftharpoons}} {}^{Enz}Ab_{(p)}\text{-}AgPSA\text{-}{}^{Btn}Ab_{(m)}$$

$^{Btn}Ab_{(m)}$ = Biotinylated antibody (excess quantity)
$Ag_{P}s_{A}$ = Native antigen (variable quantity)
$^{Enz}Ab_{(P)}$ = Enzyme labeled antibody (excess quantity)
$^{Enz}Ab_{(p)}A_{PSA}{}^{Btn}Ab_{(m)}$ = Antigen-antibodies complex
k_a = Rate constant of association
k_{-a} = Rate constant of dissociation

Simultaneously, the complex is deposited to the tube through the high affinity reaction of streptavidin and biotinylated antibody. This interaction is illustrated below:

$^{Enz}Ab_{(p)}$-Ag_{PSA} $^{-Btn}Ab_{(m)}$ + Streptavidin CT immobilised complex

Streptavidin $_{CT}$ = Streptavidin immobilised on tube

Immobilised complex = complex bound to the solid surface

After equilibrium is attained, the antibody-bound fraction is separated from unbound antigen by decantation or aspiration. The enzyme activity in the antibody-bound fraction is directly proportional to the native antigen concentration. By utilising several different serum references of known antigen values, a dose response curve can be generated from which the antigen concentration of an unknown can be ascertained.

MATERIAL PROVIDED

A. Prostrate Specific antigen (PSA) 1.0 ml/vial

Six (6) vials of references PSA Antigen at levels of 0(A), 5(B), 10(C), 25(D). 50(E) and 100(F) ng/ml. Sore at 2 to 8°C. A preservative has been added. (The references are calibrated against WHO International Standard # 96/670).

B. Enzyme-Conjugate/Biotinylated Monoclonal antibody —6.0 ml/vial

One (1) vial containing enzyme labeled antibody, biotinylated monoclonal mouse IgG in buffer, dye, and preservative. Store at 2 to 8°C.

C. Streptavidin Coated Tubes

Fifty (50) 12 × 75 mm plastic tubes coated with streptavidin and packaged in an aluminum bag with a drying agent. Store at 2 to 8ºC.

D. Wash Solution Concentrate - 20 ml

One (1) vial containing a surfactant in Tris/ buffered saline. A preservative has been added. Store at 2 to 30°C.

E. Substrate A -7.0 ml/vial

One (1) bottle containing tetramethyl benzidine (TMB) in buffer. Store at 2 to 8°C.

F. Substrate B - 7.0 ml/vial

One (1) bottle containing hydrogen peroxide (H_2O_2) in buffer. Store at 2 to 30°C.

G. Stop Solution - 8.0 ml/vial

One (1) bottle containing a strong acid (1 N HCI). Store at 2 to 30°C.

H. Product Insert

1. *Note:* Do not use reagents beyond the kit expiration date.
2. *Note:* Opened reagents are stable for sixty (60) days when stored at 2 to 8°C.

For in Vitro Diagnostic Use

Not for Internal or Externai Use in Humans or Animals

Precautions

All products that contain human serum have been found to be nonreactive for hepatitis B surface antigen, HIV 1 and 2 and HCV Antibodies by FDA required tests. Since no known test can offer complete assurance that infectious agents are absent, all human serum products should be handled as potentially hazardous and capable of transmitting disease. Good laboratory procedures for handling blood products can be found in the Center for Disease Control/ National Institute of Health, "Biosafety in Microbiological and Biomedical Laboratories," 2nd Edition, 1988, HHS.

Specimen Collection and Preparation

The specimens shall be blood serum in type and the usual precautions in the collection of venipuncture samples should be observed. For accurate comparison to established normal values, a fasting morning serum sample should be obtained. The blood should be collected in a plain red-top venipuncture tube with or without gel barrier. Allow the blood to clot. Centrifuge the specimen to separate the serum from the cells.

Samples may be refrigerated at 2 to 8°C for a maximum period of five (5) days. If the specimen(s) cannot be assayed within this time, the sample(s) may be stored at temperatures of –20°C for up to 30 days. Avoid repetitive freezing and thawing. When assayed in duplicate, 0.050 ml of the specimen is required.

Materials Required but not Provided

1. Pipette(s) capable of delivering 50 µl and 100 µl volumes with a precision of better than 1.5%.

2. Coated tube washer or a squeeze bottle (optional).
3. Coated tube reader with 450 nm and/or 405 nm wavelength absorbance capability.
4. Container(s) for mixing of reagents (see below).
5. Absorbent paper for blotting the coated tube tubes.
6. Plastic wrap or coated tube cover for incubation steps.
7. Vacuum aspirator (optional) for wash steps.
8. Timer.
9. Storage container for storage of wash buffer.
10. Distilled or deionized water.
11. Quality control materials.
12. Cuvettes or 12 x 75 mm borosilicate glass test tubes.

Reagent Preparation

1. **Wash Buffer** Dilute contents of Wash Concentrate to 1000 ml with distilled or deionised water in a suitable storage container.
2. **Working Substrate Solution-Prepare before use:** Determine the amount of reagent needed and prepare by mixing equal portions of Substrate A and Substrate B in a suitable container. For example, add 1 ml of A and 1 ml of B per two (2) eight tube (A slight excess of solution is made). Use within one hour of preparation for maximum performance of the assay.
3. **Stop Solution Dilution:** The stop solution dilution is dependent on the instrument used for quantitation. After completion of the test procedure, the stop solution is used for two purposes: (i) To stop the kinetic reaction and (ii), to provide sufficient volume for use in a variety of spectrophotometers at different wavelengths (450 nm and 405 nm). The stop solution is diluted to the volume indicated on the following chart. The volume refers to the final volume of the solution. That is, the contents of the stop solution are diluted to 200 ml if a 1 cm cell at 450 nm is used for the measurement or diluted to 100 ml if a 1 cm cell at 405 nm is used for the measurement.

Stop solution dilution

Wavelength	1 cm cell	0.5 cm cell
450 nm	200 ml	100 ml
405 nm	100 ml	50 ml

12 mm × 75 mm disposable borosilicate glass tubes or machine specific cuvettes can be used in manual spectrophotometers. One may also use sipper system based spectrophotometers for reading the absorbances.

Note: The volume of stop solution is not critical to the performance of the assay. The different volumes are used to adapt different configuration for measurement with varied spectrophotometers using diverse cell widths.

*The signal at 405 nm is approximately 30% of the signal at 450 nm.

Test Procedure

Before proceeding with the assay, bring all reagents, serum references and controls to room temperature (20-27°C).

1. Appropriately label coated tubes for each serum reference, control and patient specimen to be assayed in duplicate. Replace any unused tubes back into the ziplock bag, seal and store at 2 to 8°C.
2. Pipette 0.025 ml (25 µl) of the appropriate serum reference, control or specimen into the assigned tube.
3. Add 0.100 ml (100 µl) of the biotinylated/ enzymes labelled antibodies to each tube. It is very important to dispense all reagents close to the bottom of the coated tube.
4. Swirl the tube rack gently for 20-30 seconds to mix and cover.
5. Incubate 60 minutes at room temperature.
6. Discard the contents of the tubes by decantation or aspiration. If decanting, tap and blot the plate dry with absorbent paper.
7. Add 4 ml of wash buffer (see Reagent Preparation Section), decant (tap firmly and blot) or aspirate. An automatic or manual tube washer can be used. A total of three (3) washes should be performed. Follow the manufacturer's instruction for proper usage, if a squeeze bottle is employed, fill each tube to the brim by depressing the container (avoiding air bubbles) to dispense the wash.

Note: It is important that all the droplets of unreacted enzyme reagent are removed in the wash step. The volume of wash solution in an automated tube washer must be sufficient (1 or 2 ml) to completely remove the unreactive enzyme.

8. Add 0.200 ml (200 µl) of working substrate solution to all tubes (see Reagent Preparation Section). Always add reagents to the same order to minimise reaction time differences between tubes.
9. Incubate at room temperature for fifteen (15) minutes.
10. Add the appropriate volume of stop solution (see Reagent Preparation Section) to each tube. Always add reagents in the same order to minimise reaction time differences between tubes.

Stop solution volume

Wavelength	1 cm cell *	0.5 cm cell
450 nm	2 ml /tube	1.0 ml/tube
405 nm	0.8 ml (800 µl tube	0.3 ml (300 µl)/tube
Final total volume in tube		
Wavelength	1 cm cell *	0.5 cm cell
450 nm	2.2 ml	1.2 ml
405 nm	1.0 ml	0.5 ml

11. Transfer to appropriate cell/cuvette or 12 mm × 75 mm borosilicate glass test tubes and read the absorbance in each tube at 450 nm or 405 nm using a spectrophotometer. The results should be read within thirty (30) minutes of adding the stop solution.

Quality Control

Each laboratory should assay controls at levels in the low, normal and elevated range for monitoring assay performance. These controls should be treated as unknowns and values determined in every test procedure performed. Quality control charts should be maintained to follow the performance of the supplied reagents. Pertinent statistical methods should be employed to ascertain trends. The individual laboratory should set acceptable assay performance limits. Other parameters that should be monitored include the 80. 50 and 20% intercepts of the dose response curve for run-to-run reproducibility. In addition, maximum absorbance should be consistent with past experience. Significant deviation from established performance can indicate unnoticed change in experimental conditions or degradation of kit reagents. Fresh reagents should be used to determine the reason for the variations.

Results

A dose response curve is used to ascertain the concentration of PSA in unknown specimens.

1. Record the absorbance obtained from the printout of the tube reader as outlined in Example 1.
2. Plot the absorbance for each duplicate serum reference versus the corresponding PSA concentration in ng/ml on linear graph paper (do not average the duplicates of the serum references before plotting).
3. Draw the best-fit curve through the plotted points.
4. To determine the concentration of PSA for an unknown, locate the average absorbance of the duplicates for each unknown on the vertical axis of the graph, find the intersecting point on the curve, and read the concentration (in ng/ml) from the horizontal axis of the graph (the duplicates of the unknown may be averaged as indicated). In the following example, the average absorbance @ 405 nm (0.370) or @ 450 (0.616) intersects the dose response curve at (16.9 ng/ml) PSA concentration (See Figure 23.71).

Note: Computer data reduction software designed for ELISA assays may also be used for the data reduction.

Example 1

Tube #	*Sample IU*		*1 cm cell 0.8 ml stop OD@405 nm*		*1 cm cell 2.0 ml stop OD@450 nm*
1,2	0 ng/ml		0.002		0.013
3,4	5 ng/ml		0.14		0.217
5,6	10 ng/ml		0.242		0.402
7,8	25 ng/ml		0.53		0.888
9,10	50 ng/ml		0.819		1.331
11,12	100 ng/ml		1.109		1.846
		OD	ng/ml	OD	ng/ml
13,14	Control 1	0.125	4.6	0.208	4.3
15,16	Patient 1	0.37	16.9	0.616	16.9

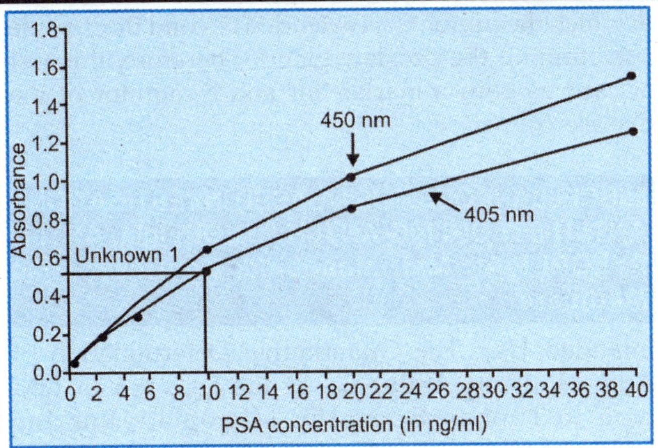

Fig. 23.71: Result calculation

'The data presented in Example 1 and Figure 23.71 are for illustration only and should not be used in lieu of a dose response curve prepared with each assay.

Limitations of Procedure

A. Assay Performance

It is important that the time of reaction in each tube is held constant for reproducible results. Pipetting of samples should not extend beyond ten (10) minutes to avoid assay drift. If more than one (1) plate is used, it is recommended to repeat the dose response curve.

Addition of the substrate solution initiates a kinetic reaction, which is terminated by the addition of the stop solution. Therefore, the addition of the substrate and the stopping solution should be added in the same sequence to eliminate any time deviation during reaction.

Failure to remove adhering solution adequately in the aspiration or decapitation wash step(s) may result in poor replication and spurious results.

Sample(s), which are contaminated microbiologically, should not be used in the assay. Highly lipaemic or haemolysed specimen(s) should similarly not be used.

Each component in one assay should be of the same lot number and stored under identical conditions.

Patient specimens with PSA concentrations above 100 ng/ml may be diluted (for example, 1/10 or higher) with normal female serum (PSA = 0 ng/ml) and re-assayed. The sample's concentration is obtained by multiplying the result by the dilution factor (10).

Each component in one assay should be of the same lot number and stored under identical conditions.

B. Interpretation

If computer-controlled data reduction is used to interpret the results of the test, it is imperative that the predicted values for the calibrators fall within 10% of the assigned concentrations.

PSA is elevated in benign prostrate hypertrophy (BPH). Clinically, an elevated PSA value alone is not of diagnostic value as a specific test for cancer and should only be used in conjunction with other clinical manifestations (observations) and diagnostic procedures (prostate biopsy). Free PSA determinations may be helpful in regard to the discrimination of BPH and prostrate cancer conditions.

Expected Ranges of Values

Healthy males are expected to have values below 4 ng/ ml..

Expected Values for the PSA ELISA Test System Healthy Males <4 ng/ml

It is important to keep in mind that establishment of a range of values which can be expected to be found by a given method for a population of "normal" persons is dependent upon a multiplicity of factors the specificity of the method, the population tested and the precision of the method in the hands of the analyst. For these reasons, each laboratory should depend upon the range of expected values established by the manufacturer only until an in-house range can be determined by the analysed using the method with a population indigeneous to the area in which the laboratory is located.

Usage

Assists in the identification, differentiation, clarification, staging, and localisation of tumour; monitoring preoperatively, postoperatively, and for recurrent tumour; assists in the selection of therapeutic interventions or cytotoxic drug therapy; and assists in assessment of tumour response to treatment protocols.

Increased

Benign prostatic hypertrophy, cirrhosis, impotence,

osteoprosis, prostate cancer or infarct, prostatic needle biopsy, prostatitis, transurethral resection (TUR), urethral instrumentation, and urinary retention.

Description

Prostate-specific antigen (PSA) is a glycoprotein exclusive to the prostate epithelium. It is smaller than the prostatic acid phosphatase molecule, more stable, and does not demonstrate diural variations. Tumour catabolic activity and accelerated metabolic rate in prostate carcinoma elevate the serum value of PSA. PSA is, therefore, a reliable immunocytochemical marker used in the detection to prostate cancer.

PROSTATIC ACID PHOSPHATES (PAP), BLOOD

Norms Values are dependent upon laboratory method

		SI Unit
Fishman-Lerner	0-0.7 U/dl	
Bessey, Lowry, and Brock (BLB)		
Female	0.02-0.55 U at 37°C	0.3-9.2 U/L
Male	0.15-0.65 U at 37°C	2.5-10.8 U/L
Bodansky	0-3 U/dl	0-16.1 U/L
King-Armstrong	0-3 U/dl	0-5.3 U/L
RIA	2.5-3.7 ng/ml	

Increased

Bone cancer (metastatic), hyperparathyroidism, metastatic prostatic carcinoma, multiple myeloma, osteogenesis imperfecta, Paget's disease, prostatic carcinoma (10-25%), and prostatic infarct.

Decreased

Down syndrome. Drugs include oestrogen therapy for prostatic carcinoma, and ethanol.

Description

Prostatic acid phosphatase, an isoenzyme of acid phosphatase, is a lysosomal enzyme that hydrolyses phosphate esters. It is found mainly in the prostate, but is also present in erthrocytes and the kidneys, liver, and spleen. Prostatic tissue has a concentration of acid phosphatase 100 times greater than other tissues. Serum activity of the prostatic isoenzyme is greatly increased in metastatic cancer of the prostate in which the tumour has extended beyond the capsule surrounding the prostate gland. Therefore, this test is used as both a marker for and a monitor of the disease course.

MISCELLANEOUS ELISA-BASED INVESTIGATIONS ANTI-H PYLORI IgG ANTI-H PYLORI IgM, ANTI-H PYLORI IgA, Mfd: Monobind, Courtesy: Lilac Medicare

Intended Use: The Quantitative Determination of Anti- H. pylori Antibodies of the IgG, IgA or IgM type in Human Serum by Microplate Enzyme Immunoassay

Summary and Explanation of the Test

Helicobacter pylori has been shown to be the unidentified curved bacillus that was observed by Warren and Marshall in close contact with gastric epithelium in biopsy studies of patients suffering from chronic gastritis. Although the source of *H. pylori* infection is not known, the evidence is quite convincing that the bacillus can cause acute gastritis and may lead to chronic gasteritis. Sethi et al has reported that *H. pylori* was present in ninety-one (91) percent of patients with chronic superficial gastritis. Marshall determined that *H. pylori* was present in ninety (90) percent of duodenal ulcer and seventy (70) percent of gastric ulcer patients.

The use of serological testing to ascertain the immunologically produced antibody caused by *H. pylori* infection has been suggested as the method of choice to screen large populations. Measurements of the antibodies to *H. pylori* have been done by haemagglutination, serum complement fixation and bacterial agglutination. These tests do not have the sensitivity of enzyme immunoassay and are limited by subjective interpretation. This procedure, with the enhanced sensitivity of EIA, permits easy detectability of antibodies to *H. pylori.* In addition, the results are quantitated by a spectrophotometer, which eliminates subjective interpretation.

Monobind's microplate enzyme immunoassay methodology provides the technician with optimum sensitivity while requiring a few technical manipulations. In this method, serum reference, diluted patient specimen, or control is first added to a microplate well. Biotinylated *H. pylori* is added, then the reactants are mixed. A reaction result between the autoantibodies to *H. pylori* and the biotinylated *H. pylori* to form an immune complex, which is deposited to the surface of streptavidin-coated wells through the high affinity reaction of biotin and streptavidin.

After the completion of the required incubation period, aspiration or decantation separates the reactants that are not attached to the wells. An enzyme anti-human IgG, M or A conjugate is then added to permit quantitation of reaction through interacting with human IgG, M or A of the immune complex. After washing, the enzyme activity is determined by reaction with substrate to produce colour.

The employment of several serum references of known antibody activity permits construction of a graph of enzyme and antibody activities. From comparison to the dose response curve, an unknown specimen's enzyme activity can be correlated with autoimmune antibody level.

PRINCIPLE

A Sequential ELISA Method

The reagents required for the sequential ELISA assay include immobilised antigen, circulating auto-antibody and enzyme-linked specie specific antibody. In this procedure, the immobilisation takes place during the assay at the surface of a microplate well through the interaction c streptavidin coated on the well and exogeneous added biotinylated *H. pylori* antigen.

Upon mixing biotinylated antigen, and a serum containing the antibody reaction results between the antigen and the antibody to form an immune complex. The interaction is illustrated by the followed equation :

$$\text{h-Ab}_{(X\text{-}H.\ pylori)} + {}^{Btn}\text{Ag}_{(H.\ pylori)} \underset{k_{-a}}{\overset{k_a}{\rightleftharpoons}} \text{h-Ab}_{(X\text{-}H.\ pylori)}\text{-}{}^{Btn}\text{Ag}_{(H.\ pylori)}$$

${}^{Btn}\text{Ag}_{(H.\ pylori)}$ = Biotinylated antigen (constant quantity)

$\text{h-Ab}_{(x\text{-}H.\ pylori)}$ = Human auto-antibody (variable quantity)

$\text{Ab}_{(x\text{-}H.\ pylori)}\text{-}{}^{Btn}\text{Ag}_{(H.\ pylori)}$ = Immune complex (variable quantity)

ka = Rate constant of association

k_{-a} = Rate constant of disassociation

Simultaneously, the complex is deposited to the well through the high affinity reaction of streptavidin and biotinylated antigen. This interactions illustrated below:

$\text{h-Ab}_{(x\text{-}H.\ pylori)}\text{-}{}^{Btn}\text{Ag}_{(H.\ pylori)}\text{-Streptavidin}_{cw} \Rightarrow$ immobilised complex (IC)

Streptavidincw = Streptavidin immobolised on well

Immobilised complex = sandwich complex bound to the solid surface

After the incubation time, the well is washed to separate the unboum components by aspiration and/or decantation. The enzyme linked specie specific antibody (anti-h-IgG, M or A) is then added to the microwells. The conjugates binds to the immune complex that formed.

$$\text{IC}_{(h\text{-}IgG,\ M\ or\ A)} + {}^{ENZ}\text{Ab}_{(X\text{-}h\text{-}IgG,\ M\ or\ A)} \Rightarrow {}^{ENZ}\text{Ab}_{(x\text{-}h\text{-}IgG,\ M\ or\ A)}\text{-IC}_{(h\text{-}IgG,\ M\ or\ A)}$$

$\text{IC}_{(h\text{-}IgG,\ M\ or\ A)}$ = Immobilised immune complex (variable quantity)

${}^{ENZ}\text{Ab}_{(X\text{-}h\text{-}IgG,\ M\ or\ A)}$ = Enzyme-antibody conjugate (constant quantity)

${}^{ENZ}\text{Ab}_{(X\text{-}h\text{-}IgG,\ M\ or\ A)}\text{-}\ \text{IC}_{(h\text{-}IgG,\ M\ or\ A)}$ = Antigen-antibody complex (variabli quantity)

The anti-h-IgG, IgM or IgA enzyme conjugate that binds to the immune complex in a second incubation is separated from unreacted material by wash step. The enzyme activity in this fraction is directly proportional to the antibody concentration in the specimen. By utilising several different serum references of known antibody activity, a reference curve can be generated from which the antibody activity of an unknown can be ascertained.

Reagents for 96-Well Microplate

A. Anti-H. pylori Calibrators—1.0 ml/vial

Five (5) vials of references for anti-*H. pylori* at levels of 0(A), 10(B), 25(C), 50(D) and 100 (E) U/ml* of the IgG, IgM or IgA type. Store 2 to 8°C. A preservative has been added.

Manufacturers' Reference Value

B. H.Pylori Biotin Conjugate- 11 ml/vial

One (1) vial of biotinylated inactivated *H. pylori* in a buffering matrix. A preservative has been added. Store at 2 to 8°C.

C. Enzyme-antigen Conjugate - 11 ml/vial

One (1) vial of anti-human IgG, IgM or IgA-horseradish peroxidase (HRP) conjugate in a buffering matrix. A preservative has been added. Store at 2 to 8°C.

D. Streptavidin-Coated Microplate - 96 wells

One 96-well microplate coated with Streptavidin and packaged in an aluminum bag with a drying agent. Store at 2 to 8°C.

E. Serum Diluent Concentrate— 20 ml

One (1) vial of serum diluent containing buffer salts and a dye. Store at 2 to 8°C.

F. Wash Solution Concentrate—20 ml

One (1) vial containing a surfactant in phosphate buffered saline. A preservative has been added. Store at 2 to 30°C.

G. Substrate A ~7.0 ml/vial

One (1) bottle containing tetramethyl benzidine (TMB) in buffer. Store at 2 to 8°C.

H. Substrate B - 7.0 ml/vial

One (1) bottle containing hydrogen peroxide (H_2O_2) in buffer. Store at 2 to 8°C.

I. Stop Solution - 6.0 ml/vial

One (1) bottle containing a strong acid (1N HCl). Store at 2 to 30°C.

Note 1: Do not use reagents beyond the kit expiration date.

Note 2: Opened reagents are stable for sixty (60) days when stored at 2 to 8°C.

Precautions

For In Vitro Diagnostic Use
Not for Internal or External
Use in Humans or Animals

All products that contain human serum have been found to be non-reactive for hepatitis B surface antigen, HIV 1 and 2 and HCV antibodies by FDA required tests. Since no known test can offer complete assurance that infectious agents are absent, all human serum products should be handled as potentially hazardous and capable of transmitting disease. Good laboratory procedures for handling blood products can be found in the Center for Disease Control/ National Institute of Health, "Biosafety in Microbiological and Biomedical Laboratories," 2nd Edition, 1988, HHS Publication No. (CDC) 88-8395.

Specimen Collection and Preparation

Collect sample(s) by venipuncture in ten (10) ml silicone evacuated tube(s). The usual precautions in the collection of venipuncture samples should be observed. Separate the red blood cells by centrifugation and use the serum obtained for the anti-*H. pylori* procedure. Specimen(s) may be refrigerated at 2 to 8°C for a maximum period of 48 hours. If the specimen(s) cannot be assayed within 48 hours, the sample(s) may be stored at temperatures of -20°C for up to 30 days.

Materials

Provided

1. Five (5) vials of serum reference for Anti-*H. pylori* (IgG, M or A type)
2. One (1) vial of *H. pylori* Biotin Conjugate
3. One (1) vial of Enzyme-Anti-h-IgG, M or A Conjugate
4. One 96-well Streptavidin-coated Microplate
5. One (1) vial of Serum Diluent Concentrate
6. One (1) bottle of Wash Buffer Concentrate
7. One (1) bottle of Substrate A
8. One (1) bottle of Substrate B
9. One (1) bottle of Stop solution
10. Instructions

Required but not Provided

1. Pipette(s) capable of delivering 10 µl and 25 µl volumes with a precision <1.5%
2. Dispenser(s) for repetitive deliveries of 0.100 ml, 0.300 ml and 1.0 ml volumes with a precision of better than 1.5%
3. Microplate washer (optional) or squeeze bottle to wash plates
4. Microplate reader with 450 nm wavelength absorbance capability
5. Test tubes for dilution of patient samples and substrate A and B
6. Absorbent paper for blotting the microplate wells
7. Plastic wrap or microplate cover for incubation steps
8. Vacuum aspirator for wash steps (optional)
9. Timer

Reagent Preparation

1. Serum Diluent

Dilute the serum diluent concentrate to 200 ml in a suitable container with distilled or deionized water. Store at 2 to 8°C.

2. Wash Buffer

Dilute contents of wash concentrate to 1000 ml with distilled or deionized water in a suitable storage container. Store at room temperature until expiration date printed on concentrate label.

3. Patient Sample Dilution (1/100)

Dispense 0.010 ml (10 µl) of each patient specimen into 1 ml of serun diluent. Cover and vortex or mix thoroughly by inversion. Store at 2 to 8°C for up to forty-eight (48) hours.

4. Working Substrate Solution -Prepare Immediately Before Use

Determine the amount of reagent needed and prepare by mixini equal portions of substrate A and substrate B in a suitable container. For example, add 1 ml of A and 1 ml of B per two (2) eight well strips (a slight excess of solution is made). Use within one (1) hour of preparation for maximum performance of the assay.

Test Procedure

Before proceeding with the assay, bring all reagents, serum reference and controls to room temperature.

1. Format the microplates' wells for each serum reference, control and patient specimen to be assayed in duplicate.
2. Pipette 0.025 ml (25 µl) of the appropriate serum reference, control or diluted patient specimen into the assigned well for IgG determination. For IgM or IgA, pipette 0.050 ml (50 µl) of the appropriate serum reference, control or diluted patient specimen into the assigned well.
3. Add 0.100 ml (100 µl) of *H. pylori* biotinylated conjugate solution.
4. Swirl the microplate gently for 20-30 seconds to mix and cover.
5. Incubate 60 minutes at room temperature.
6. Discard the contents of the microplate by decantation or aspiration. If decanting, blot the plate dry with absorbent paper.
7. Add 300 µl of wash buffer (see Reagent Preparation Section), decant (blot) or aspirate. Repeat two (2) additional times for a total of three (3) washes. An automatic or manual plate washer can be used. Follow the manufacturer's instruction for proper usage. If a squeeze bottle is employed, fill each well by depressing the container (avoiding air bubbles) to dispense the wash. Decant the wash and repeat two (2) additional times.
8. Add 0.100 ml (100 µl) of Enzyme anti-h-IgG, M or A Conjugate Solution to all wells. Always add reagents in the same order to minimize reaction time differences between wells.
9. Swirl the microplate gently, cover and incubate for thirty (30) minutes at room temperature.
10. Repeat steps (6 and 7) as explained above.
11. Add 0.100 ml (100 µl) of Working Substrate Solution to all wells (see Reagent Preparation Section). Always add reagents in the same order to minimise reaction time differences between wells.
12. Incubate at room temperature for fifteen (15) minutes.
13. Add 0.050 ml (50 µl) of stop solution to each well and swirl the microplate gently for 15-20 seconds to mix. Always add reagents in the same order to minimize reaction time differences between wells.
14. Read the absorbance in each well at 450 nm in a microplate reader. The results should be read within thirty (30) minutes of adding the stop solution.

Note: For re-assaying specimens with concentrations greater than 100 U/ml, dilute the sample an additional 1:10 or 1:100 using the original diluted material. Multiply by the dilution factor to obtain the concentration of the specimen.

Quality Control

Each laboratory should assay and establish reference intervals for clinically relevant controls to monitor assay performance. These controls should be treated as unknowns and values determined in every test procedure performed. Quality control charts should be maintained to follow the performance of the supplied reagents. Pertinent statistical methods should be employed to ascertain trends. Maximum absorbance should be consistent with past experience. Significant deviation from established performance can indicate unnoticed change in experimental conditions or degradation of kit reagents. Fresh reagents should be used to determine the reason for the variations.

Results

A reference curve is used to ascertain the concentration of anti-*H. pylori* in unknown specimens.

1. Record the absorbance obtained from the printout of the microplate reader as outlined in Example 1.
2. Plot the absorbance for each duplicate serum reference versus the corresponding anti *H. pylori* activity in U/ml on linear graph paper (do not average the duplicates of the serum references before plotting).
3. Draw the best-fit curve through the plotted points.
4. To determine the level of anti *H. pylori* activity for an unknown, locate the average absorbance of the duplicates for each unknown on the vertical axis of the graph, find the intersecting point on the curve, and read the concentration (in U/ml) from the horizontal axis of the graph (the duplicates of the unknown may be averaged as indicated). In the following example, the average absorbance 1.56 (intersects the dose response curve) at 44.5 U/ml anti- *H. pylori* concentration (See Figure 23.72).

Example 1 (Typical results for IgG, M or A)

Well	*Calibrator*	*Absorbance*
1	0 U/ml	0.007
2	0 U/ml	0.007
3	10 U/ml	0.453
4	10 U/ml	0.443
5	25 U/ml	1.053
6	25 U/ml	1.037
7	50 U/ml	1.678
8	50 U/ml	1.664
9	100U/ml	2.281
10	100 U/ml	2.181

Well	**Unknown ID**	**OD**	**Avg. OD**	**Value**
11	Unknown #1	1.493		
12	Unknown #1	1.618	1.556	44.5 U/ml

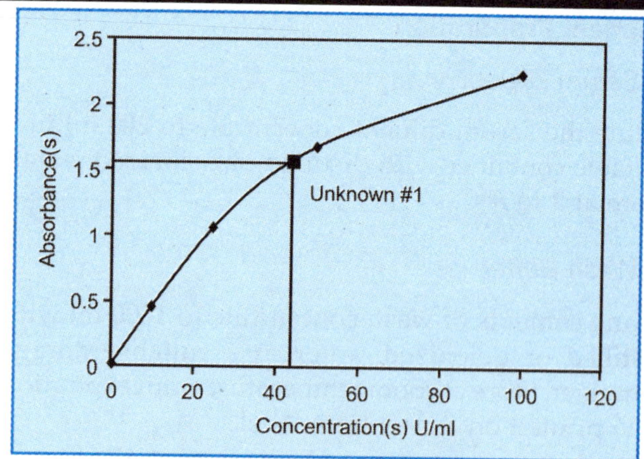

Fig. 23.72: Result calculation

The data presented in Example 1 and Figure 23.72 are for illustration only and should not be used in lieu of a standard curve prepared with each assay.

QC Parameters

Maximum Absorbance (100 U/ml calibrator) = 1.8-2.7

Limitations of Procedure

A. Assay Performance

It is important that the time of reaction in each well is held constant for reproducible results. Pipetting of samples should not extend beyond ten (10) minutes to avoid assay drift. If more than one (1) plate is used, it is recommended to repeat the dose response curve.

Addition of the substrate solution initiates a kinetic reaction, which is terminated by the addition of the stop solution. Therefore, the addition of the substrate and the stopping solution should be added in the same sequence to eliminate any time deviation during reaction.

Plate readers measure vertically. Do not touch the bottom of the wells.

Failure to remove adhering solution adequately in the aspiration or decantation wash step(s) may result in poor replication and spurious results.

Very high concentration of anti-*H. pylori* in patient specimens can contaminate samples immediately following these extreme levels. Bad duplicates are indicative of cross contamination. Repeat any sample which follows any patient specimen with over 3.0 units of absorbance.

Samples, which are contaminated microbiologically, should not be used.

B. Interpretation

If computer-controlled data reduction is used to interpret the results of the test, it is imperative that the predicted values for the calibrators fall within 10% of the assigned concentrations.

The presence of antibodies to *H. pylori* is confirmed when the serum level exceeds 20 U/ml. The clinical significance of the result should be used in evaluating the possible presence of gastrointestinal disease. However, clinical inferences should not be solely based on this test but rather as an adjunct to the clinical manifestations of the patient and other relevant tests such as Histology, Urease and Culture. A positive result does not indicate gastrointestinal disease and does not distinguish between the colourisation or infection of *H. pylori.* Similarly, a negative result does not eliminate the absence of *H. pylori* infection but rather; very low titre of antibody that may be related to the early stages of colonisation.

FERRITIN, Mfd: Monobind, Courtesy: Lilac Medicare

Summary and Explanation of the Test

Ferritin, in circulation, as measured in serum levels is a satisfactory index of body's iron storage. The iron storage is directly measured by quantitative phlebotomy, iron absorption studies, liver biopsies and microscopic examinations of bone marrow aspirates. Iron deficiency *(anaemia)* and iron overload *(Haemochromatosis)* are conditions associated with body's iron storage or lack thereof. Measurements of total iron-binding capacity (TIBC) have widely been used as aids in the determination of these conditions. However, an assay of serum *ferritin* is simply more sensitive and reliable means of demonstration these disorders.

Ferritin is present in blood in very low concentrations. Normally, approximately 1% of plasma iron is contained in *ferritin*. The plasma *terrain*, is in equilibrium with body stores, and variations of iron storage. The plasma concentrations of *ferritin* decline very early in anaemic conditions like development of iron deficiency, long before the changes are observed in the blood haemoglobin concentration, size of the erythrocytes and TIBC. Thus measurements of serum *ferritin* can serve as an early indicator of iron deficiency that is uncomplicated by other concurrent conditions. At the same time, a large number of chronic conditions can result in elevated levels of serum *ferritin*. These include chronic infections, chronic inflammatory diseases such as rheumatoid arthritis, heart disease and some other malignancies, especially lymphomas, leukaemias, breast cancer and neuroblastoma. In patients who have these chronic disorders together with iron deficiency, serum *ferritin* levels are often normal. An increase in circulating *ferritin* is observed in patients with viral hepatitis or after, a toxic liver injury as a release of farritin from the injured liver cells. Elevated serum *ferritin* levels are found in patients with haemochromatosis and haemosiderosis.

Circulating *ferritin* levels have been used by clinicians, as an aid, in the diagnosis of several other disorders. It has proved as a valuable tool in differential diagnosis of anaemia due to iron deficiency and anaemias due to other disorders and, in exposing the depletion of iron reserves long before the onset of anaemia. Serial determinations have been used to monitor, non-invasively, the erosion of iron storage during pregnancy and in patients undergoing dialysis. Serum *ferritin* is routinely used as a screen for iron deficiency for a variety of populations like blood donors and people who are receiving regular blood transfusions or iron replacement therapy.

In this method, *ferritin* calibrator, patient specimen or control is first added to a streptavidin-coated well. Biotinylated monoclonal antibody (specific for *ferritin)* is added and the reactants mixed. Reaction results between the biotinylated *ferritin* antibody and native *ferritin* to form an immune complex that is deposited on the streptavidin-coated well. The excess serum proteins are washed away via a wash step. Another *ferritin* specific antibody, labelled with an enzyme, is added to the wells. The enzyme-labelled antibody binds to the *ferritin* already immobilised on the well. Excess enzyme is washed off via a wash step. A colour is generated by the addition of a substrate. The intensity of the colour generation is directly proportional to the concentration of the *ferritin* in the sample.

The employment of several serum references of known *ferritin* levels permits the construction of a dose response curve of activity and concentration. From comparison to the dose response curve, an unknown specimen's activity can be correlated with *ferritin* concentration.

Principle

Immunoenzymometric Sequential Assay

The essential reagents required for an immunoenzymometric assay include high affinity and specificity antibodies (enzyme and immobilised), with different and distinct epitope recognition, in excess, and native antigen. In this procedure, the immobilisation takes place during the assay at the surface of a microplate well through the interaction of streptavidin coated on the well and exogenously added biotinylated monoclonal anti-*ferritin* antibody.

Upon mixing monoclonal biotinylated antibody, and a serum containing the native antigen, reaction results between the native antigen and the antibody, forming an antibody-antigen complex. Simultaneously the biotin attached to the antibody binds to the streptavidin coated on the microwells resulting in immobilisation of the complex. The interaction is illustrated by the following equation:

$$Ag\ (ferritin) + {}^{Btn}Ab_{(m)} \underset{k_{-a}}{\overset{k_a}{\rightleftharpoons}} Ag_{(ferritin)}\text{-}{}^{Btn}Ab_{(m)}$$

${}^{Btn}Ab_{(m)}$ = Biotinylated monoclonal antibody (excess quantity)
$Ag_{(ferritin)}$ = Native antigen (variable quantity)
$Ag_{(ferritin)}\text{-}{}^{Btn}Ab_{(m)}$ = Antigen-antibody complex (variable quantity)
k_a = Rate constant of association
k_{-a} = Rate constant of dissociation

$Ag_{(ferritin)}\text{-}{}^{Btn}Ab_{(m)}$ + Streptavidin$_{cw}$ ⇒ immobilised complex (1C)
Streptavidin$_{cw}$ = Streptavidin immobolised on well
Immobilised complex (1C) = Ag-Ab bound to the well

After a suitable incubation period, the antibody-antigen bound fraction is separated from unbound antigen by decantation or aspiration. Another antibody (directed at a different epitope) labelled with an enzyme is added. Another interaction occurs to form an enzyme-labelled antibody-antigen-biotinylated-antibody complex on the surface of the wells. Excess enzyme is washed off via a wash step. A suitable substrate is added to produce colour measurable with the use of a microplate spectrophotometer. The enzyme activity on the well is directly proportional to the native free antigen concentration. By utilising several different serum references of known antigen concentration, a dose response curve can be generated from which the antigen concentration of an unknown can be ascertained.

$$1c + {}^{Enz}Ab\ (ferritn) \underset{k\text{-}b}{\overset{kb}{\rightleftharpoons}} {}^{Enz}Ab\ (ferritin)\text{-}1c$$

${}^{Enz}Ab(ferritin)$ = Enzyme-labelled antibody (excess quantity)
${}^{Enz}Ab(ferritin)$ = Antigen-antibodies complex
k_b = Rate constant of association
k_{-b} = Rate constant of dissociation

Incubate at room temperature for fifteen (15) minutes.

Add 0.050 ml (50µl) of stop solution to each well and mix gently for 15-20 seconds.

Read the absorbance in each well at 450 nm (using a reference wavelength of 620-630 nm to minimise well imperfections) in a microplate reader. The results should be read within thirty (30) minutes of adding the stop solution.

Note: Always add reagents in the same order to minimise reaction time differences between wells.

Quality Control

Each laboratory should assay controls at levels in the low, medium and high ranges of the dose response curve for monitoring assay performance. These controls should be treated as unknowns and values determined in every test procedure performed. Quality control charts should be maintained to follow the performance of the supplied reagents. Pertinent statistical methods should be employed to ascertain trends. Significant deviation from established performance can indicate unnoticed change in experimental conditions or degradation of kit reagents. Fresh reagents should be used to determine the reason for the variations.

Results

A dose response curve is used to ascertain the concentration of *ferritin* in unknown specimens.

1. Record the absorbance obtained from the printout of the microplate reader as outlined in Example 1.
2. Plot the absorbance for each duplicate serum reference versus the corresponding *ferritin* concentration in ng/ml on linear graph paper.
3. Draw the best-fit curve through the plotted points.
4. To determine the concentration of *ferritin* for an unknown, locate the average absorbance of the duplicates for each unknown on the

vertical axis of the graph, find the intersecting point on the curve, and read the concentration (in ng/ml) from the horizontal axis of the graph (the duplicates of the unknown may be averaged as indicated). In the following example, the average absorbance (1.287) intersects the dose response curve at (154 ng/ml) *ferritin* concentration (See Figure 23.73).

Note: Computer data reduction software designed for IEMA /ELISA assays may also be used for the data reduction.

Example 1

ID	*Well position*	*Absorbance*	*Mean Absorbance (B)*	*Concentration*
Cal A	A1	0.022	0.003	0
	B1	0.003		
Cal B	C1	0.11	0.112	10
	D1	0.113		
Cal C	E1	0.586	0.617	50
	F1	0.647		
Cal D	G1	1.204	1.262	150
	H1	1.32		
Cal E	A2	1.947	1.917	400
	B2	1.887		
Cal F	C2	2.586	2.561	800
	D2	2.536		
Ctrl 1	E2	0.707	0.721	66.1
	F2	0.734		
Patient 1	G2	1.289	1.287	154
	H2	1.285		
Patient 2	A3	1.647	1.659	301.6
	B3	1.671		

*The data presented in Example 1 and Figure 23.73 are for illustration only and should not be used in lieu of a dose response curve prepared with each assay.

QC Parameters

- Maximum Absorbance (Calibrator 'F') >1.2
- Maximum Absorbance (Calibrator 'A') <0.1

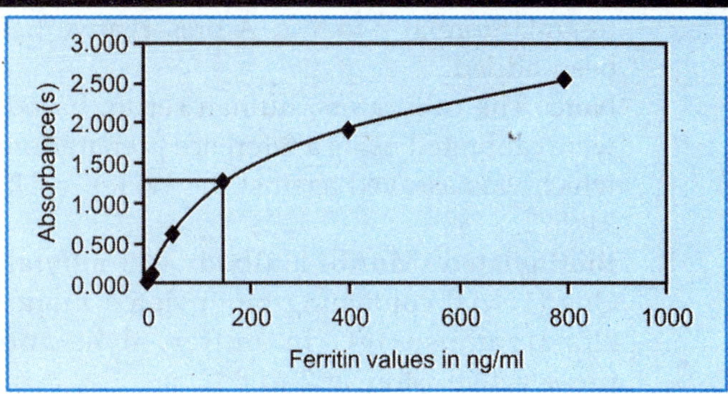

Fig. 23.73: Result calculation

Limitations of Procedure

A. Assay Performance

1. It is important that the time of reaction in each well is held constant for reproducible results. Pipetting of samples should not extend beyond ten (10) minutes to avoid assay drift. If more than one (1) plate is used, it is recommended to repeat the dose response curve.
2. Addition of the substrate solution initiates a kinetic reaction, which is terminated by the addition of the stop solution. Therefore, the addition of the substrate and the stopping solution should be added in the same sequence to eliminate any time deviation during reaction.
3. Plate readers measure vertically. Do not touch the bottom of the wells.
4. Failure to remove adhering solution adequately in the aspiration, or decantation wash step(s) may result in poor replication and spurious results.
5. Sample(s), which are contaminated microbiologically, should not be used in the assay. Highly lipaemic or haemolysed-specimen(s) should similarly not be used.
6. Patient specimens with *ferritin* concentrations above 800 ng/ml may be diluted (for example 1/10) with normal serum stripped of *ferritin* and re-assayed.

Reagents

Provided

A. **Ferritin Calibrators -1 ml/vial**
Six (6) vials of *ferritin* calibrators at levels of 0 (A), 10(B), 50 (C), 150(D), 400(E) and 800(F)

ng/ml. Store at 2 to 8°C. A preservative has been added.

Note: The calibrators, human serum based, were calibrated using a reference preparation, which was assayed against the WHO 3rd IS 94/572

B. **Biotinylated (MoAb) antibody—13 ml/vial**
One (1) vial containing biotinylated monoclonal mouse IgG in buffer, dye, and preservative. Store at 2 to 8°C.

C. **Enzyme-Labelled Anti-Ferritin IgG-13 ml/vial**
One (1) vial containing Horseradish Peroxidase (HRP) labeled Anti-Ferritin IgG in buffer, dye and preservatives. Store at 2 to 8°C.

D. **Streptavidin Coated microplate-96 wells**
One 96-well microplate coated with streptavidin and packaged in an aluminum bag with a drying agent. Store at 2 to 8°C.

E. **Wash Solution Concentrate - 20 ml**
One (1) vial containing a surfactant in buffered saline. A preservative has been added. Store at 2 to 30°C.

F. **Substrate A -7 ml/vlal**
One (1) bottle containing tetramethyl benzidine (TMB) in buffer. Store at 2 to 8°C.

G. **Substrate B - 7 ml/vial**
One (1) bottle containing hydrogen peroxide (H_2O_2) in buffer. Store at 2 to 8°C. One (1) bottle containing a strong acid (1N HCl). Store at 2 to 30°C.

I. **Product Insert**
Note 1: Do not use reagents beyond the kit expiration date.
Note 2: Opened reagents are stable for sixty (60) days when stored at 2 to 8°C.
Note 3: Above reagents are for a single 96-well microplate.

Required but not Provided

1. Pipette capable of delivering 25, 50 µl volumes with a precision of better than 1.5%.
2. Dispenser(s) for repetitive deliveries of 0.100 ml and 0.300 ml volumes with a precision of better than 1.5%.
3. Microplate washers or a squeeze bottle (optional).
4. Microplate reader with 450 nm and 620 nm wavelength absorbance capability.
5. Absorbent paper for blotting the microplate wells.
6. Plastic wrap or microplate cover for incubation steps.
7. Vacuum aspirator (optional) for wash steps.
8. Timer.
9. Quality control materials.

Precautions

For In Vitro Diagnostic Use Not for Internal or External Use in Humans or Animals

All products that contain human serum have been found to be nonreactive for hepatitis B surface antigen, HIV 1 and 2 and HCV antibodies by FDA licensed reagents. Since no known test can offer complete assurance that infectious agents are absent, all human serum products should be handled as potentially hazardous and capable of transmitting disease. Good laboratory procedures for handling blood products can be found in the Center for Disease Control/National Institute of Health, "Biosafety in Microbiological and Biomedical Laboratories,' 2nd Edition, 1988, HHS Publication No. (CDC) 88-8395.

Specimen Collection and Preparation

The specimens shall be blood; serum in type and the usual precautions in the collection of venipuncture samples should be observed. For accurate comparison to established normal values, a fasting morning serum sample should be obtained. The blood should be collected in a plain red-top venipuncture tube without additives or anticoagulants. Allow the blood to clot for samples. Centrifuge the specimen to separate the serum from the cells.

Samples may be refrigerated at 2 to 8°C for a maximum period of five (5) days. If the specimen(s) cannot be assayed within this time, the sample(s) may be stored at temperatures of -20°C for up to 30 days. Avoid repetitive freezing and thawing. When assayed in duplicate, 0.050 ml of the specimen is required.

Reagent Preparation

1. **Wash Buffer** Dilute contents of Wash Concentrate to 1000 ml with distilled or deionized water in a suitable storage

container. Store at room temperature 20-27°C for up to 60 days.

2. **Working Substrate Solution** Pour the contents of the vial labelled Solution 'A' into the vial labelled Solution 'B'. Mix and store at 2 to 8°C. Use within 60 days. Or for longer periods of usage determine the amount of reagent needed and prepare by mixing equal portions of Substrate A and Substrate B in a suitable container. For example, add 1ml of A and 1ml of B per two (2) eight well strips (A slight excess of solution is made. Discard the unused portion).

Note: Do not use the working substrate if it looks blue.

Test Procedure

Before proceeding with the assay, bring all reagents, serum references and controls to room temperature (20-27°C).

1. Format the microplates' wells for each serum reference, control and patient specimen to be assayed in duplicate. Replace any unused microwell strips back into the aluminum bag, seal and store at 2 to 8°C.
2. Pipette 0.025 ml (25 µl) of the appropriate serum reference, control or specimen into the assigned well.
3. Add 0.100 ml (100 µl) of the biotinylated antibody to each well. It is very important to dispense all reagents close to the bottom of the coated well.
4. Swirl the microplate gently for 20-30 seconds to mix and cover.
5. Incubate 30 minutes at room temperature.
6. Discard the contents of the microplate by decantation or aspiration. If decanting, tap and blot the plate dry with absorbent paper.
7. Add 300 µl of wash buffer (see Reagent Preparation Section), decant (tap and blot) or aspirate. Repeat two (2) additional times for a total of three (3) washes. An automatic or manual plate washer can be used. Follow the manufacturer's instruction for proper usage. If a squeeze bottle is employed, fill each well by depressing the container (avoiding air bubbles) to dispense the wash. Decant the wash and repeat two (2) additional times.
8. Add 0.100 ml (100 µl) of the Anti-Ferritin-enzyme-labelled antibody to each well.
9. Swirl the microplate gently for 20-30 seconds to mix and cover.
10. Incubate 30 minutes at room temperature.
11. Discard the contents of the microplate by decantation or aspiration. If decanting, blot the plate dry with absorbent paper.
12. Add 300 µl of wash buffer (see Reagent Preparation Section), decant (tap and blot) or aspirate. Repeat two (2) additional times for a total of three (3) washes.
13. Add 0.100 ml (100 µl) of working substrate solution to all wells (see Reagent Preparation Section) concentration is obtained by multiplying the result by the dilution factor (100).
14. Each component in one assay should be of the same lot number and stored under identical conditions.

B. Interpretation

If computer-controlled data reduction is used to interpret the results of the test, it is imperative that the predicted values for the calibrators fall within 10% of the assigned concentrations.

IMMUNOGLOBULIN E (IgE)
Mfd: Monobind, Courtesy: Lilac Medicare

Intended Use: The Quantitative Determination of Immunoglobulin E (IgE) Concentration in Human Serum by a Microplate Enzyme Immunoassay

Summary and Explanation of the Test

Allergic reactions, which are becoming more widespread, are usually diagnosed on the basis of medical history and clinical symptoms. *In vitro* and *in vivo* testing, however, play a key role in confirming clinical suspicions and tailoring treatment. The measurement of immunoglobulin E (IgE) in serum is widely used in the diagnosis of allergic reactions and parasitic infections. Many allergies are caused by the immunoglobulins of subclass IgE acting as point of contact between the allergen and specialised cells. The IgE molecules (MW 200,000) bind to the surface of the mast cells and basophillic granulocytes. Subsequently, the binding of allergen to cell-bound IgE causes these cells to release histamines and other vasoactive substances. The release of histamines in the body results initiates what is commonly known as an allergic reaction.

Before making any therapeutic determination, it is important, however, to know whether the allergic reaction is IgE mediated or non-IgE mediated. Measurement of total IgE in serum sample, along with other supporting diagnostic information, can help to make that determination. Measurement of total circulating IgE may also be of value in the early detection of allergy in infants and as a means of predicting future atopic manifestations. Before deciding on any therapy it is important to take into consideration all the relevant clinical information as well as information supplied by specific allergy testing.

The IgE levels show a slow increase during childhood, reaching adult levels in the second decade of life. In general, the total IgE levels increase with the allergies a person has and the number of times of exposure to the relevant allergens. Significant elevations may be seen in the sensitised individuals, but also in cases of myeloma, pulmonay aspergillosis, and during the active stages of parasitic infections.

In this method, IgE calibrator, patient specimen or control is first added to a streptavidin coated well. Biotinylated monoclonal antibody (specific for IgE) is added and the reactants mixed. Reaction between the IgE antibodies and native IgE forms complex that binds with the streptavidin coated to the well. The excess serum proteins are washed away via a wash step. Another enzyme-labelled monoclonal antibody specific to IgE is added to the wells. The enzyme-labelled antibody binds to the IgE already immobilised on the well through its binding with the biotinylated monoclonal antibody. Excess enzyme is washed off via a wash step. A colour is generated by the addition of a substrate. The intensity of the colour generation is directly proportional to the concentration of the IgE in the sample.

Principle

Immunoenzymometric Sequential Assay

The essential reagents required for an immunoenzymometric assay include high affinity and specificity antibodies (enzyme and immobilised different and distinct epitnoe recognition, in excess, and native antigen. In this procedure, the immobilisation takes place during the assay at the surface of a microplate well through the interaction of streptavidin coated on the well and exogenously added biotinylated monoclonal anti-IgE antibody.

Upon mixing monoclonal biotinylated antibody, and a serum containing the native antigen, reaction results between the native antigen and the antibody, forming an antibody-antigen complex. The interaction is illustrated by the following equation:

$$Ag_{(IgE)} - {}^{Btn}Ab_{(m)} \underset{k_{-a}}{\overset{k_a}{\rightleftharpoons}} Ag_{(IgE)}\text{-}{}^{Btn}Ab_{(m)}$$

${}^{B}tnAb_{(m)}$ = Biotinylated monoclonal antibody (excess quantity)

$Ag^{(IgE)}$ = Native antigen (variable quantity)

$Ag^{(IgE)\text{-}Btn}Ab_{(m)}$ = Antigen-antibody complex (variable quantity)

k_a = Rate constant of association

k_{-a} = Rate constant of disassotiation

Simultaneously, the complex is deposited to the well through the high affinity reaction of streptavidin and biotinylated antibody. This interaction is illustrated below:

$Ag_{(IgE)}\text{-}{}^{Btn}Ab_{(m)}{}^{+}$ Streptavidin cw $\Rightarrow$ Immobilised complex (1C)

Streptavidin$_{cw}$ = Streptavidin immobilised on well

Immobilised complex (1C) = Ag-Ab bound to the well

After a suitable incubation period, the antibody-antigen bound fraction is separated from unbound antigen by decantation or aspiration. Another antibody (directed at a different epitope) labelled with an enzyme is added. Another interaction occurs to form an enzyme-labelled Antibody-Antigen-Biotinyfated-Antibody complex on the surface of the wells. Excess enzyme is washed off via a wash step. A suitable substrate is added to produce colour measurable with the use of a microplate spectrophotometer. The enzyme activity on the well is directly proportional to the native free antigen concentration. By utilising several different serum references of known antigen concentration, a dose response curve can be generated from which the antigen concentration of an unknown can be ascertained.

$$(IC) + {}^{Enz}Ab_{(x\text{-}IgE)} \underset{k_{-a}}{\overset{k_a}{\rightleftharpoons}} {}^{Enz}Ab_{(x\text{-}IgE)}\text{-}IC$$

${}^{Enz}Ab_{(x\text{-}IgE)}$ = Enzyme-labelled antibody (excess quantity)

${}^{Enz}Ab(x\text{-}IgE)\text{-}IC$ = Antigen-antibodies complex

k_b = Rate constant of association

k_{-b} = Rate constant of dissociation

Reagents Provided

A. Human Serum References-1.0 ml/viat

Six (6) vials of human serum based reference calibrators at concentrations of 0 (A), 5 (B), 25 (C), 50

(D), 150 (E) and 400 (F) IU/ml. Store at 2 to 8°C. A preservative has been added.

(The Calibrators are standardized against WHO'S 2nd IRP 75/502 for IgE).

B. IgE Biotin Conjugate-13 ml/vial

One (1) vial of Anti-Human IgE (MoAb)-Biotin reagent in a protein-stabilised matrix. A preservative has been added. Store at 2 to 8°C.

C. IgE Enzyme Conjugate-13 ml/vial

One (1) vial of Anti-Human IgE-HRP conjugate in a protein- stabilised matrix. A preservative has been added. Store at 2 to 8°C.

D. Streptavidin Microplate - 96 wells

One 96-well microplate coated with streptavidin and packaged in an aluminium bag with a drying agent. Store at 2 to 8°C.

E. Wash Solution Concentrate—20 ml

One (1) vial containing a surfactant in buffered saline. A preservative has been added. Store at 2 to 30°C.

F. Substrate A - 7.0 ml/via

One (1) bottle containing tetramethyl benzidine (1 MB) in acetate buffer. Store at 2 to 8°C.

G. Substrate B - 7.0 ml/vial

One (1) bottle containing hydrogen peroxide (H_2O_2) in acetate buffer. Store at 2 to 8°C.

H. Stop Solution-8.0 ml/vial

One (1) bottle containing a strong acid (1N HCl). Store at 2 to 8°C.

I. Product Insert

Note 1: Do not use reagents beyond the kit expiration date.
Note 2: Opened reagents are stable for sixty (60) days when stored at 2 to 8°C.
Note 3: Above reagents are for a single 96-well microplate.

Required but not Provided

1. Pipette capable of delivering 50 µl volumes with a precision of better than 1.5%.
2. Dispenser(s) for repetitive deliveries of 0.100 ml and 0.300 ml volumes with a precision of better than 1.5%.
3. Microplate washers or a squeeze bottle (optional).
4. Microplate reader with 450 nm and 620 nm wavelength absorbance capability.
5. Absorbent paper for blotting the microplate wells.
6. Plastic wrap or microplate cover for incubation steps.
7. Vacuum aspirator (optional) for wash steps.
8. Timer.
9. Quality control materials.

Precautions

For In Vitro Diagnostic Use Not for Internal or External Use in Humans or Animals

All products that contain human serum have been found to be nonreactive for hepatitis B surface antigen, HIV 1 and 2 and HCV antibodies by FDA licensed reagents. Since no known test can offer complete assurance that infectious agents are absent, all human serum products should be handled as potentially hazardous and capable of transmitting disease. Good laboratory procedures for handling blood products can be found in the Center for Disease Control/National Institute of Health, "Biosafety in Microbiological and Biomedical Laboratories," 2nd Edition, 1988, HHS Publication No. (CDC) 88-8395.

Specimen Collection and Preparation

The specimens shall be blood; serum in type and the usual precautions in the collection of venipuncture samples should be observed. For accurate comparison to established normal values, a fasting morning serum sample should be obtained. The blood should be collected in a plain red-top venipuncture tube without additives or anticoagulants. Allow the blood to clot for samples. Centrifuge the specimen to separate the serum from the cells.

Samples may be refrigerated at 2 to 8°C for a maximum period of five (5) days. If the specimen(s) cannot be assayed within this time, the sample(s) may be stored at temperatures of –20°C for up to 30 days. Avoid repetitive freezing and thawing. When assayed in duplicate, 0.050 ml of the specimen is required.

Reagents Preparation

1. **Wash buffer:** Dilute contents of wash concentrate to 1000 ml with distilled or deionized water in a suitable storage container. Store at room temperature 20-27°C for up to 60 days.
2. **Working substrate solution:** Pour (the contents of the vial labelled Solution 'A' into the vial labelled Solution 'B'. Mix and store at 2 to 8°C. Use within 60 days. Or for longer periods of usage, determine the amount of reagent needed and prepare by mixing equal portions of Substrate A and Substrate B in a suitable container. For example, add 1 ml of A and 1 ml of B per two (2) eight well strips (A slight excess of solution is made. Discard the unused portion).

Note: Do not use the working substrate if it looks blue.

Test Procedure

Before proceeding with the assay, bring all reagents, serum references and controls to room temperature (20-27°C).

1. Format the microplates' wells for each serum reference, control and patient specimen to be assayed in duplicate. Replace any unused microwell strips back into the aluminum bag, seal and store at 2 to 8°C.
2. Pipette 0.025 ml (25 µl) of the appropriate serum reference, control or specimen into the assigned well.
3. Add 0.100 ml (100 µl) of the *IgE Biotin reagent* to each well. It is very important to dispense all reagents close to the bottom of the coated well.
4. Swirl the microplate gently for 20-30 seconds to mix and cover.
5. Incubate 30 minutes at room temperature.
6. Discard the contents of the microplate by decantation or aspiration. If decanting, tap and blot the plate dry with absorbent paper.
7. Add 300 µl of wash buffer (see Reagent Preparation Section), decant (tap and blot) or aspirate. Repeat two (2) additional times for a total of three (3) washes. An automatic or manual plate washer can be used. Follow the manufacturer's instruction for proper usage. If a squeeze bottle is employed, fill each well by depressing the container (avoiding air bubbles) to dispense the wash. Decant the wash and repeat two (2) additional times.
8. Add 0.100 ml (100 ul) of the Anti-IgE-HRP labelled antibody to each well.
9. Swirl the microplate gently for 20-30 seconds to mix and cover.
10. Incubate 30 minutes at room temperature.
11. Discard the contents of the microplate by decantation or aspiration. If decanting, blot the plate dry with absorbent paper
12. Add 300 µl of wash buffer (see Reagent Preparation Section), decant (tap and blot) or aspirate. Repeat two (2) additional times for a total of three (3) washes. An automatic or manual plate washer can be used. Follow the manufacturer's instruction for proper usage. If a squeeze bottle is employed, fill each well by depressing the container (avoiding air bubbles) to dispense the wash. Decant the wash and repeat two (2) additional times.
13. Add 0.100 ml (100 µl) of working substrate solution to all wells-(see Reagent Preparation Section). Always add reagents in the same order to minimise reaction time.
14. Incubate at room temperature for fifteen (15) minutes.
15. Add 0.050 ml (50 µl) of stop solution to each well and gently mix for 15-20 seconds.
16. Read the absorbance in each well at 450 nm (using a reference wavelength of 620-630 nm to minimize well imperfections) in a microplate reader. The results should be read within thirty (30) minutes of adding the stop solution.

Quality Control

Each laboratory should assay controls at levels in the low, mid and high range for monitoring assay performance. These controls should be treated as unknowns and values determined in every test procedure performed. Quality control charts should be maintained to follow the performance of the supplied reagents. Pertinent statistical methods should be employed to ascertain trends. Significant deviation from established performance can indicate unnoticed change in experimental conditions or degradation of kit reagents. Fresh reagents should be used to determine the reason for the variations.

Results

A dose response curve is used to ascertain the concentration of IgE in unknown specimens.

1. Record the absorbance obtained from the printout of the microplate reader as outlined in Example 1.
2. Plot a dose response curve (DRC) using the mean absorbance for each duplicate serum reference versus the corresponding IgE concentration in IU/ml on linear graph paper.
3. Draw the best-fit curve through the plotted points (see Figure 23.74).
4. Interpolate the concentrations of unknown control or patient serum from the dose response curve (see Figure 23.74).

Example 1

ID	*Well Position*	*Absorbance*	*Mean Absorbance (B)*	*Concentration*
Cal A	A1	0.014	0.015	0
	B1	0.016		
Cal B	C1	0.072	0.073	5
	D1	0.074		
Cal C	E1	0.364	0.345	25
	F1	0.326		
Cal D	G1	0.663	0.639	50
	H1	0.614		
Cal E	A2	1.34	1.364	150
	B2	1.388		
Cal F	C2	2.601	2.641	400
	D2	2.682		
Ctrl 1	E2	2.575	2.562	375.3
	F2	2.549		
Ctrl 2	G2	0.818	0.813	71.2
	H2	0.807		
Patient 1	A3	1.322	1.323	142
	B3	1.324		

*The data presented in Example 1 and Figure 23.74 is for illustration only and should not be used in lieu of a standard curve prepared with each assay.

QC Parameters

In order for the assay results to be considered valid, the following criteria should be met.

1. The absorbance (OD) of calibrator 'A' should be < 0.1.
2. The absorbance (OD) of calibrator F should be > 1.2
3. Four out of six quality control pools should be within the established ranges.

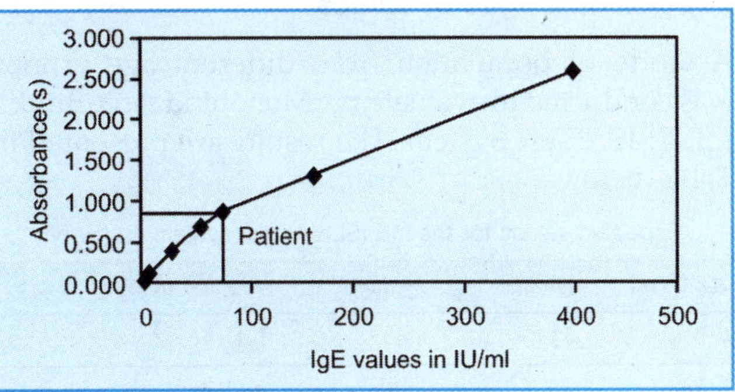

Fig. 23.74: Result calculation

Limitations of Procedure

1. It is important that the time of reaction in each well is held constant for reproducible results.
2. If more than one (1) plate is used, it is recommended to repeat the dose response curve.
3. Addition of the substrate solution initiates a kinetic reaction, which is terminated by the addition of the stop solution. Therefore, the addition of the substrate and the stopping solution should be added in the same sequence to eliminate any time-deviation during reaction.
4. Rate readers measure vertically. Do not touch the bottom of the wells.
5. Failure to remove adhering solution adequately in the aspiration or decantation wash step(s) may result in poor replication and spurious results.
6. Highly lipaemic, haemolysed or grossly contaminated specimen(s) should not be used.
7. Use components from the same lot. No intermixing of reagents from different batches.
8. Serum IgE concentration is dependent upon a multiplicity of factors including if the patient is sensitised, how many times the patient has been exposed to a specific allergen, etc. Total IgE concentration alone is not sufficient to assess the clinical status. All the clinical findings, especially specific allergy testing should be taken into consideration while determining the clinical status of the patient.

9. Since all atopic reactions are not IgE mediated, all relevant clinical information should be taken into consideration before making any determination for patients who may be in the normal range.

Expected Ranges of Values

A study of population from different age groups was conducted to evaluate the Monobind AccuBind™ IgE ELISA Test System. The results are presented in Table below.

Expected values for the IgE (ELISA) test system (in IU/ml)

Age (Yrs)	*Number*	*Median*	*Absolute Range*
0-3	31	6.4	ND-46
3-16	43	25.0	ND-280
Adult	145	43	0-200

Each laboratory is advised to establish its own ranges for normal and abnormal populations. These ranges are always dependent upon locale, population, laboratory, technique and specificity of the method.

Performance Characteristics

A. Precision

The inter- and intra-assay precision of the Accu Bind™ Microplate ELISA Test System were determined by analyses on three different levels of pooled patient sera. The number, mean values, standard deviation (σ) and coefficient of variation for each of these control sera are presented in Tables given below.

Intra-assay precision

In order to validate the within-assay precision of AccuBind™ Microplate ELISA Test System, twenty replicates of each of three pooled sera (low medium and high ranges of the dose response curve) were assayed in the same assay. An intra-assay precision of 1.95 to 5.87% was obtained see table below.

Intra-assay precision (in IU/ml)

	Low	*Medium*	*High*
Number (n)	20	20	20
Mean	48.9	160.5	297.6
1 SD	2.87	6.47	5.810
% CV	5.87	4.03	1.95

Inter-Assay Precision

In order to validate the Inter-assay precision of AccuBind™ Microplate ELISA Test System one duplicate of each of three pooled sera (low medium and high ranges of the dose response curve) was assayed in 10 assays done over a period of six months that involved five different sets of reagents and three different technicians. An inter-assay precision of 3.52 to 8.42% was obtained see table below.

Inter assay precision (in IU/ml)

	Low	*Medium*	*High*
Number (n)	10		10 10
Mean	46.3	157	301
1 SD	3.9	7.3	10.6
% CV	8.42	4.64	3.52

B. Accuracy

The AccuBind™ Microplate ELISA Test System was compared with a coated tube radioimmunoassay (IRMA) method. Biological specimens with IgE levels in the low, medium and high ranges were used (The values ranged from 0.8 to 3100 IU/ml). The total number of such specimens was 219. The least square regression equation and the correlation coefficient were computed for this ELISA Test System in comparison with the predicate method is given in table below.

Linear regression analysis

Method	*Mean(x)*	*Equation*
Monobind EIA "X"	178	x = –12.9 + 1.21 Y
Predicate IRMA "Y"	157	

Only slight amounts of bias between this method and the reference method are indicated by the closeness of the mean values. The least square regression equation and correlation coefficient indicates excellent method agreement.

C. Parallelism

Two patient pools were assayed diluted (in 'O' Calibrator) and undiluted with Monobind AccuBind™ IgE ELISA Microwells Test System. The observed and expected values are listed below.

Sample	Observed	Expected%	Recovery
Pool 1	106.8		
Pool 1/2	50.8	53.4	95.1
Pool 1/4	25.3	26.7	94.8
Pool 1/8	13.4	13.3	100.6
Pool 1/16	6.6	6.7	98.5
Pool 2	395.9		
Pool 2/2	189.5	197.9	95.8
Pool 2/4	106.1	98.9	107.2
Pool 2/8	48.0	49.5	96.9
Pool 2/16	25.8	24.7	104.2

D. Sensitivity

The AccuBind™ Microplate ELISA Test System procedure has a sensitivity of 1.0 (lU/ ml. The sensitivity was ascertained by determining the variability of the 0 IU/ml serum calibrator and using the 2 σ (95% certainty) statistics to calculate the minimum dose.

E. Specificity

The specificity of AccuBind™ IgE Microplate ELISA Test System, to closely related immunoglobulins was evaluated by adding those at twice the physiological concentrations to a serum matrix. No cross reaction between the antibodies used and the related molecules was detected.

F. Linearity

Two patient pools were spiked with known amounts of IgE and assayed with AccuBind™ IgE Microplate ELISA Test System. The observed and expected values are listed below.

Sample	Observed (O) Sample IU/ml	Expected (E) IU/ml	% Recovery (O/E)
Pool 1	25.7	—	—
Pool +25	50.7	50.7	100.0
Pool 1+50	74.8	75.7	101.2
Pool 1+ 100	122.7	125.7	97.6
Pool 1+ 200	232.0	225.7	102.7
Pool 2	12.3	—	—
Pool 2 + 25	41.7	37.3	111.2
Pool 2+50	62.6	62.3	100.6
Pool 2+100	109.4	112.3	97.4
Pool 2+200	197.2	212.3	9

CHAPTER 24

Histopathology

PREPARATION OF TISSUES

Fixation

This is the process of killing and hardening. The first phase of fixation is the rapid killing; the second phase, the hardening of tissue. After removal, the tissue should be put in the fixative immediately. The choice of a fixing agent should be determined by the purpose of which the tissue is to be stained or preserved. If several special stains may be required, small blocks of the tissue should be fixed in each of the following: 10 % neutral formalin, Zenker's fluid, Bouin's fluid and absolute alcohol or Carnoy's fluid.

Blocks should be cut thin enough so that the fixing fluid will penetrate the tissue in a reasonably short time. To this end blocks should not be more than 0.5 cm thick and should be immersed in at least 20 times their volumes of fixative.

Ten per cent formalin is the most widely used fixative because it is compatible with most stains. Length of fixation depends on the size of blocks.

I. *10 % Formalin solution*

37-40% Formaldehyde	100 cc
Tap Water	900 cc

II. *Buffered neutral formalin solution*

37-40% Formaldehyde	100 cc
Distilled water	900 cc
Sodium phosphate monobasic	4 gm
Sodium phosphate dibasic	6.5 gm

III. *Zenker's fluid*

Distilled water	1000 cc
Mercuric chloride	50 gm
Potassium dichromate	25 gm
Sodium sulphate	10 gm

Add 5 cc of glacial acetic acid to 95 cc of Zenker's fluid before use.

IV. *Lugol's solution* (Weigert's Modification)

Potassium iodide	2 gm
Iodine	1 gm
Distilled water	100 cc

V. *Bouin's fluid*

Picric acid, saturated aqueous solution	750 cc
37-40% Formaldehyde	250 cc
Glacial acetic acid	50 cc

VI. *Carnoy's fluid*

Absolute alcohol	60 cc
Chloroform	30 cc
Acetic acid glacial	10 cc

VII. *Absolute alcohol and acetone are also used as fixatives for bacteria, glycogen, and some of the enzymes.*

Decalcification

Bone and calcified tissue should be cut into small pieces with a saw before fixation. After they are thoroughly fixed, they are placed in a gauze bag tied with a string which has been dipped in melted paraffin. The bag is suspended in a large quantity of decalcifying solution, at least a quart for blocks of the average size. Stirring or agitation of the fluid hastens decalcification. Every trace of decalcifying solution must be removed by washing the pieces in running water for several hours before dehydration and embedding.

Nitric Acid Method

1. Decalcify sections in large quantities of 5% aqueous solution of nitric acid for 1 to 4 days. Change the solution daily. Sections of bone may be tested by bending, piercing with a sharp needle or X-ray.
2. Wash in running water for 24 hours.
3. Neutralize in 10% formalin to which an excess of calcium or magnesium carbonate has been added.
4. Wash in running water for 24 to 48 hours.
5. Dehydrate, clear and embed in either paraffin or celloidin.

The method is used only for small pieces of bone which must be processed rapidly. Exposure of nay length to nitric acid impairs or destroys nuclear staining.

Formic Acid Sodium Citrate Method

1. Decalcify for 5-14 days in formic acid-sodium citrate solution. Change solution daily for best results.

Solution A

Sodium citrate	50 gm
Distilled water	250 cc

Solution B

Formic acid (90%)	125 cc
Distilled water	125 cc

Mix solutions A & B for use

2. Wash in running water for 4 to 8 hours
3. Dehydrate, clear and embed.

This technique gives better staining quality than the nitric acid method.

Electrolytic Method

1. Decalcify in the electrolytic apparatus in formic acid-hydrochloric acid for 1 to 4 hours.

Electrolytic decalcifying solution

Formic acid (90%)	100 cc
Hydrochloric acid	80 cc
Distilled water to make	1000 cc

2. Wash in running water for 24 hours.
3. Dehydrate, clear, and embed.

Processing of Tissues

Embedding in paraffin is accomplished most rapidly and gives the best results when thin sections of soft tissues are wanted. Since paraffin is not miscible with water, the tissue must be dehydrated and then cleared in a solution that is miscible with paraffin.

Automatic tissue processing units are usually employed these days. Yorco provides such units (Fig. 24.1). This instrument has several beakers, each filled with a specific fluid in it. The basket containing the tissue sections with identification tags is automatically dipped and revolved in the beakers at preset timings. Usually, paraffin embedding process is started in the afternoon and is complete by mornings on the following day. Various schedules for paraffin processing are given below.

Method I

1. Alcohol 80%	1-2 hours
2. Alcohol 95%- 2 changes	1-2 hours each
3. Alcohol absolute-3 changes	1-2 hours each
4. Xylene-2 changes	1-2 hours each
5. Melted paraffin-3 changes	1-2 hours each
6. Embed in paraffin and cool quickly.	

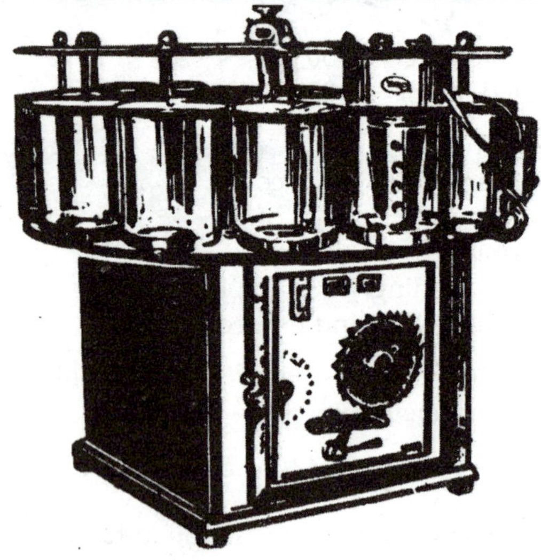

Fig. 24.1: Automatic tissue processing unit (Courtesy: Yorco scientific)

Method II

1. Alcohol 80%-2 changes 1-2 hours each
2. Alcohol 95%-2 changes 1-2 hours each
3. Alcohol, absolute-3 changes 1-3 hours each
4. Chloroform-2 changes 1-2 hours each
5. Paraffin, melted-3 changes 1 hour each
6. Embed and cool quickly

Method III

1. Alcohol 80%-2 changes 1-2 hours each
2. Alcohol 95%-2 changes 1-2 hours each
3. Alcohol, absolute-3 changes 1-2 hours each
4. Benzene-1 change 1-2 hours each
5. Paraffin bath-3 changes 1 hours each
6. Embed and cool immediately
   (In place of alcohol one may use acetone. Xylene and benzene can be used in place of one another).

Preparation of Sections

It is important that the knife used for cutting sections be very sharp and without nicks. A perfect edge for a microtome knife may be defined in simple terms as the junction of two smooth plane surfaces at an angle of about 14 degrees. Knife sharpening may be done by mechanical means on commercial automatic knife sharpeners (Shandon: UK) or done manually called honing and stroping.

Cutting Sections

After the paraffin block has been secured at the appropriate place in the microtome, adjustment of the block and the knife is now required. Keep a piece of cotton in a dish of tap water and an ice cube in a petri dish beside the microtome (Fig. 24.2) at all times.

To facilitate sectioning, apply the wet cotton to the surface of the block after rough cutting. Then place the ice cube directly on the knife to flatten the side of the cube that is to be applied to the surface of the block. Be sure to crank the block back a fraction of a millimeter from the knife edge, so that the first section cut after the block has been soaked and chilled will not be too thick.

Collect the section ribbons in a bowl containing hot water and unfurl or straighten the sections gently with a fine tip camels hair brush.

Attaching Sections to Slides

The glass slides on which tissue sections are to be mounted must be marked beforehand with the identifying case number. A glass marking pencil is used for this purpose.

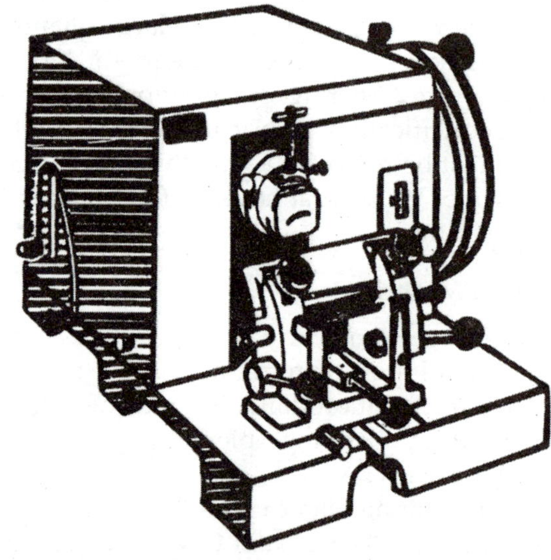

Fig. 24.2: Rotary microtome (Courtesy: Yorco Scientific)

Paraffin sections may be attached to slides in several ways. A small drop of Mayer's egg albumin is smeared over the surface of the slide with the finger and the excess rubbed off with the heel of the hand, or it can be applied with a clean foam rubber sponge. A sponge is usually preferred so that the epithelial cells from the fingers will not adhere to the slide and produce artefacts when stained.

Mayer's egg albumin

Egg white 50 cc
Glycerin 50 cc

Mix well and filter through coarse filter paper, or through several thicknesses of gauze. Add a crystal of thymol to preserve.

Egg adhesive from dried albumin

Albumin, dried	5.0 gm
Sodium chloride	0.5 gm
Distilled water	100.0 cc

Filter on Buchner's funnel with vacuum. To 50 cc of filtrate, and 50 cc glycerin, add a crystal of thymol to preserve.

Slides smeared by one of the above-mentioned egg adhesives are taken below the floating section and the section is placed in the centre of the slide; leave it to dry to be stained subsequently.

Technique for Frozen Sections

1. Fix small blocks of tissue in 10% formalin.
2. Wash blocks in water before freezing.
3. Put a drop of water on the holder and place the block in position parallel to the knife edge.
4. Holding the block with the index finger or a glass slide, turn on the coolant gas/fluid slightly. When block is firmly fixed to holder, release more coolant gas/fluid until the block is frozen.
5. Start sectioning and continue until a complete section is obtained. Usually, the block will have thawed to about right consistency by this time. If it is frozen too hard, the sections may shatter. Allow the block to thaw slightly and try again. If it has become too soft, the sections will also shatter or fracture. The correct temperature can only be judged by experience. Sometimes rubbing the finger across the block will give it the right consistency for good sections to cut. It is best to cut slowly.
6. Lift the sections off the knife edge with the tip of the little or ring finger which has been dipped in distilled water. Place in a Petridish of distilled water. Dry the knife between sections as water will cause the following section to be uneven or perforated.
7. Frozen sections may be stained with polychrome methylene blue, haematoxylin and eosin, or fat stains.

Staining

Staining may be done by the free flotation method or the sections may be picked up on the slide first and stained as usual.

Mounting

Fat stains must be mounted in glycerin jelly. Sections stained by other techniques may also be mounted in glycerin jelly or they may be dehydrated, cleared in xylene and mounted in DPX mountant.

REMOVAL OF PIGMENTS AND PRECIPITATES

Mercury Precipitate

If Zenker-fixed material stored for a long time is to be stained with alum haematoxylin, it will be found that areas where the mercuric chloride is deposited stain deep blue and distort the microscopic picture. Therefore, it is necessary to:

1. Deparaffinise the sections by putting them on a hot plate and then take through 2 changes of xylene, absolute alcohol and 95% alcohol.
2. Place in alcoholic iodine (1 gm iodine in 100 cc of 80% alcohol) for 10 to 15 minutes.
3. Rinse in tap water.
4. Place in 5% aqueous sodium thiosulphfate solution (hypo) for 5 minutes.
5. Wash in running tap water for 10 to 20 minutes and rinse well in distilled water before staining.

Formalin Produced Precipitate

Method I

1. Deparaffinise the sections through 2 changes each of xylene, absolute alcohol, and 95% alcohol.
2. Rinse well in distilled water.
3. Let stand in saturated aqueous picric acid solution for 1 to 3 hours.
4. Wash well in running tap water.

Note

This picric acid solution will not bleach malarial pigment.

Method II

1. Deparaffinise the sections through 2 changes each of xylene, absolute alcohol and 95% alcohol.
2. Rinse well in distilled water.
3. Place in bleaching solution for 5-10 minutes.

   Bleaching solution

Hydrogen peroxide	25.0 cc
Acetone	25.0 cc
Ammonium hydroxide	1 drop.

4. Wash well in running tap water, and stain as desired.

Melanin Pigment

1. Deparaffinise the sections through 2 changes each of xylene, absolute alcohol and 95% alcohol.
2. Rinse well in distilled water.
3. Place in 0.25% aqueous potassium permanganate solution for 1 to 4 hours.
4. Wash well in water.
5. Place in a 5% aqueous oxalic acid solution or a hydrobromic acid solution (HBr 1 part, distilled water 3 parts) until sections are clear (2-5 minutes).
6. Wash in running tap water for 10 minutes, rinse in distilled water, and stain as desired.

Malarial Pigment

Method I

1. Deparaffinise the sections through 2 changes each of xylene, absolute alcohol, and 95% alcohol.
2. Wash well in distilled water.
3. Place in a 5% aqueous solution of ammonium sulphide for 20-24 hours.
4. Wash in running tap water for 15-20 minutes, rinse well in distilled water and stain as desired.

Method II

1. Deparaffinise the sections through 2 changes each of xylene, absolute alcohol, and 95% alcohol.
2. Place in a saturated alcoholic picric acid solution or 1 to 24 hours.
3. Wash well in running tap water and distilled water, and stain as desired.

Method III

1. Deparaffinise the sections through 2 changes each of xylene, absolute alcohol, and 95% alcohol.
2. Rinse well in distilled water.
3. Place in the following bleaching solution for 5 minutes or less.

   Bleaching solution

Acetone	50 cc
Hydrogen peroxide (3%)	50 cc
Ammonia water (28%)	10.cc

4. Wash well in running tap water and distilled water, and stain as desired.

ROUTINE STAINING PROCEDURES

Haematoxylin, a natural dye, is the most important staining reagent used in histologic work. Used alone, it has little affinity for tissue; but in combination with (mordants) aluminium, iron, chromium, copper or tungsten salts, it is a powerful nuclear stain and a chromatin stain. The active colouring agent, haematein, is formed by the oxidation of haematoxylin. This process, known as "ripening", takes several days or weeks unless it is hastened by the addition of an oxidising agent, such as mercuric oxide, hydrogen peroxide, potassium permanganate, sodium perborate or sodium iodate.

Most commonly used haematoxylins are used in combination with aluminium in the form of alum. Various formulations used go by the following names, e.g. Harris, Mayer, Delafield, Ehrlich, Bullard and Bohmer.

Section stained with haematoxylins may be counter-stained with eosin, Congo red, eosinol, safranin or other contrasting media.

There are two methods of staining when haematoxylin is used: progressive and regressive.

Progressive: The haematoxylin contains an excess of aluminium salts or acid, thus increasing the selectivity for nuclei. After staining with haematoxylin, the slides are washed well in water and counterstained.

Regressive: This is accomplished by overstaining in a relatively neutral solution of haematoxylin, then removing the stain from the other constituents with acid alcohol or other differentiating agent.

COMMONLY EMPLOYED HAEMATOXYLINS

Harris's Alum Haematoxylin

Haematoxylin crystals	5.0 gm
Alcohol, absolute	50.0 gm
Ammonium or potassium alum	100.0 gm
Distilled water	1000.0 cc
Mercuric oxide (red)	2.5 gm

Dissolve the haematoxylin in the alcohol, the alum in water by the aid of heat. Remove from heat and mix the two solutions. Bring to a boil as rapidly as possible. Remove from the heat and add the mercuric oxide slowly. Reheat until it becomes dark purple, remove from flame immediately and plunge the vessel into a basin of cold water until cool. The stain is ready for use as soon as it cools. Addition of 2 to 4 cc of glacial acetic acid per 100 cc of solution increases the precision of the nuclear stain. Filter before use.

Mayer's Haematoxylin

Haematoxylin	1 gm
Distilled water	1000 cc
Sodium iodate	0.2 gm
Ammonium or potassium alum	50 gm
Citric acid	1 gm
Chloral hydrate	50 gm

Dissolve the haematoxylin in water, using gentle heat if necessary. Then add the sodium iodate, then the alum. Shake until the alum is dissolved, then add the citric acid, and finally the chloral hydrate. The final colour of the stain is reddish-violet. Stain will keep well.

Counterstains for Haematoxylin Stains

Stock 1% Aqueous Eosin Solution

Eosin Y, water soluble	10 gm
Distilled water	1000 cc
Dissolve and add:	
Glacial acetic acid	2 cc

Stock 1% Alcoholic Eosin Solution

Eosin Y, water soluble	1 gm
Distilled water	20 cc
Dissolve and add:	
Alcohol, 95%	80 cc

Working Eosin Solution

Eosin, 1% stock solution	1 part
Alcohol, 80%	3 parts

If deeper shade of red is desired in staining add 0.5 cc of glacial acetic acid to each 100 cc of stain.

Routine Haematoxylin and Eosin Stain

Fixation: May be used after any fixation

Technique:
Paraffin or frozen.
Cut paraffin sections at 6 microns.

Solution

1. Harris's haematoxylin
2. Acid alcohol
   70% alcohol — 1000 cc
   Hydrochloric acid, concentrated — 10 cc
3. Ammonia water
   Tap water — 1000 cc
   Strong ammonia water — 2 to 3 cc
4. Saturated lithium carbonate solution
   Lithium cabonate
   Distilled water
5. Alcoholic eosin solution
6. Lugol's solution (Weigert's modification)
   Potassium iodide — 2 gm
   Iodine crystals — 1 gm
   Distilled water — 100 gm
7. Alcohol iodine solution
   Iodine crystals — 1 gm
   Alcohol, 95% — 100 cc
8. Sodium thiosulphate solution (Hypo)
   Sodium thiosulphate — 5 gm
   Distilled water — 100 cc

Staining Procedure

1. Xylene, absolute alcohol, 95% alcohol.
2. If sections are Zenker's fixed, treat with either Lugol's solution or 1% alcoholic iodine solution 10-15 minutes. Wash with tap water. Treat with 5% sodium thiosulphate 5 minutes. Wash well with tap water.
3. Harris's haematoxylin for 15 minutes.
4. Rinse in tap water.
5. Differentiate in acid alcohol—3 to 10 quick dips. Check the differentiation with the microscope—nuclei should be distinct and the background very light or colourless.
6. Wash in tap water very briefly.
7. Dip in ammonia water (for 10-20 seconds) saturated lithium carbonate until sections are bright blue.
8. Wash in running tap water for 10-20 minutes.
9. Stain with eosin for 15 seconds to 2 minutes depending on the age of the eosin and the depth of counterstain required.
10. 95% alcohol.
11. Absolute alcohol—at least 2 changes.
12. Xylene—2 changes.
13. Mount in DPX mountant.
    Results Nuclei—blue
    Cytoplasm—pink.

SPECIAL STAINS

Stains for Connective Tissue

a. *Mallory's Phosphotungstic Acid Haematoxylin Stain*
   Discussed in detail later
b. *Mallory's Phosphomolybdic Acid Haematoxylin stain*
   Results:
   Collagen fibres—deep blue.

c. *Heidenhain's Iron Haematoxylin Stain*
Results:
Chromatin, nucleoli, mitochondria, and parts of striated muscle fibres are stained black. Other tissue elements are stained by contrast stain used. Demonstrates amoeba.

d. *Mallory's Aniline Blue Collagen Stain*
Results:
Nuclei—red
Ground substance of cartilage, mucin and amyloid—varying shades of blue
Erythrocytes and myelin—yellow
Elastic fibrils—pale pink, pale yellow or unstained.

e. *Lee-Brown's Modification of Mallory's Aniline Blue Stain*
Results:
Nuclei—orange
Collagen—blue
Glomerular basement membrane of kidney—deep blue.

f. *Van Gieson's Stain for Collagen Fibres*
Discussed in detail later.

h. *Barbeito—Lobez' Trichrome Stain*
Results:
Nuclei—violet red.
Cytoplasm—green to pale blue
Reticulum fibres—deep blue
Collagen—brilliant green
RBCs—brilliant orange
Bacteria—violet red.

i. *Gomori's One-Step Trichrome Stain*
Results:
Muscle fibres—red
Collagen—green
Nuclei—blue to black
Striations of muscle are easily demonstrable.

j. *Heidenhain's Aniline Blue Stain*
Results:
Chromatin, osteocytes and neuroglia —red
Cytoplasm—pink to blue
Collagen and reticulum—blue
Muscle—red to yellow.

k. *Gallego's Iron Fuchsin Stain*
Results:
Nuclei—grey to black
Collagen and reticulum—deep blue
Muscle—greenish to orange yellow
Calcium—reddish to purple brown
Mast cell granules—deep red
Cartilage—purple to violet
Mucus—blue violet
Cytoplasm—olive to brown
Elastic fibres—purple to red.

l. *Weigert's Resorcin Fuchsin Elastic Stain*
Results:
Elastic fibres—blue-black to black
Nuclei—blue to black
Collagen—pink to red
Other tissue elements—yellow.

m. *Gomori's Aldehyde Fuchsin Stain*
Results:
Elastic fibers and mucin—deep blue
Beta cells of pancreas—deep blue
Other—stain of counterstain.

n. *Verhoeff's Elastic Stain*
Discussed in detail later.

o. *Wilder's Reticulum Stain*
Discussed in detail later.

p. *Koneff's Stain for Bone and Cartilage*
Results:
Hyaline cartilage and osteoid—blue
Bone—bright red to reddish brown
Matrix of vesicular zone of epiphyseal disc and remnants of matrix—green
Proliferating cartilage—blue
Hyaline cartilage—blue.

Stains for Cytoplasmic Granules

a. *Gomori's Chromaffin Stain*
Results:
Chromaffin granules—purplish red
Only alpha cells of pancreatic islets, some cells of anterior pituitary and granules of neutrophils and myelocytes stain likewise.

b. *Acid Fushsin Aniline Blue Method for Pituitary Granules*
Results:
Acidophil granules—orange vermillion
Basophil granules—deep cobalt blue
Connective tissue—bright blue
RBCs—intense vermillion

c. *Fontana-Masson Stain for Argentaffin Granules*
Discussed in detail later.

d. *Luna's Mast Cell Stain*
Results:
Mast cells—deep purple-red
Other cellular elements—blue-black.
Background—yellowish orange.

Stains for Fats and Lipoids

a. *Osmium Tetraoxide Stain for Fat*
Results:
Fat—black
Background—yellow to brown

b. *Oil Red O Fat Stain*
Discussed in detail later

c. *Sudan Black B Stain for Fat*
Results:
Fat—black, blue, or blue-black.
Nuclei—red

Stains for Carbohydrates and Mucoproteins

a. *Best's Carmine Stain for Glycogen*
Discussed in detail later.

b. *Periodic Acid-Schiff (PAS) Reaction*
Discussed in detail later

c. Mayer's Mucicarmine Stain
Discussed in detail later.

d. Alcian Blue
Results:
Acid mucopolysaccharides—blue
Nuclei—pink.

e. Alcian Blue-PAS Stain
Results:
Exclusively acid substances (e.g. various connective tissue mucins)-blue.
Neutral polysaccharides (e.g. glycogen and Brunner- gland mucin)-magenta.
Certain substances (e.g. most epithelial mucins and cartilage ground substance) are coloured by both Alcian blue and PAS, yielding varying shades of purple to very deep colour. The cell bodies of fungi are red to purple, while mucoid capsules (e.g., cryptococcus neoformans) are blue.
Other features appear about the same as with the ordinary PAS stain.

f. *Crystal Violet Amyloid Stain*
Discussed in detail later.

g. *Bennhold's Congo Red Amyloid Stain*
Results:
Amyloid—pale pink to red.
Nuclei—blue.

h. *Toluidine Blue Metachromasia Stain*
Results:
Metachromatic tissue–pink.

Stains for Pigments and Minerals

a. *Modification of Mallory's Reaction for Iron*
Results:
Iron pigments—bright blue.
Nuclei—red.
Cytoplasm—pink to rose.

b. *Gomori's Iron Reaction*
Results:
Iron pigments—bright blue.
Nuclei—red.
Cytoplasm—pink to rose.

c. *von Kossa's Method for Demonstrating Calcium*
Discussed in detail later.

d. *Svain's Bile Pigment Stain*
Results:
Bile pigments—emerald green.
(Localisations cannot be considered reliable because of the diffusibility of the reactants and the final colour.)
Nuclei—red.
Cytoplasm—pink to rose.

e. *De Galantha's Method for Demonstration of Urate Crystals*
Results:
Urates—black.
Connective tissue—yellow.

Stains for Bacteria, Fungi and Inclusion Bodies

a. *Kinyoun's Acid-Fast Stain*
Results:
Acid-fast bacteria—bright red.
Background—light blue.

b. *Ziehl-Neelsen Stain for Acid-Fast Bacteria*
Discussed in detail later.

c. *Fite-Faraco Stain for Acid-Fast Bacilli*
Results:
Acid-fast bacilli—red.
Background—light blue.

d. *Brown and Brenn Stain for Bacteria in Tissue*
Results:
Gram-positive bacteria—blue.
Gram-negative bacteria—red.
Nuclei—red.
Other tissue elements—yellow.

e. *Levaditi's Method for Staining Spirochetes in Blocks*
Results:
Spirochetes—intensely black.
Background—yellow to light brown.

f. *Warthin-Starry Method for Staining Spirochetes*
Results:
Spirochetes—black.
Background—pale yellow to light brown.

g. *Silver Method for Spirochetes and Donovan Bodies*
Results:
Spirochetes, Donovan bodies, also fungi and bacteria—black.
Background—yellow to brown.

h. *Gridley's Stain for Fungi*
Results:
Mycelia—deep blue.
Conidia—deep rose to purple.
Background—yellow.
Elastic tissue and mucin also stain deep blue.

i. *Gomori's Methanamine-Silver Nitrate Technique (Grocott's application to Fungi)*
Results:
Fungi—sharply delineated in black.
Mucin—taupe or dark grey.
Inner part of mycelia and hyphae—old rose.
Background—pale green.

j. *Phloxine Toluidine Blue Stain for Malarial Parasites*
Results:
Malarial parasites—pale blue cytoplasmic structures within erythrocytes.
Erythrocytes—orange to red.
Cytoplasm—pale rose with deep red granules.
Nuclei—blue to purple.
Supporting stroma—orange red.

k. *Parson's Stain for Negri Bodies*
Results:
Negri bodies—bright orange-red.
Nuclei—blue.
Erythrocytes—copper.

l. *Haematoxylin-Shorr S 3 Stain for Inclusion bodies*
Results:
Inclusion bodies—brilliant red.
Connective tissue—light red.
Elastic tissue—purplish red.
Muscle—red.
Keratin—orange.
Erythrocytes—orange red.
Nuclei—blue.

m. *Giemsa's Stain for Rickettsiae*
Results:
Rickettsiae—violet.
Nuclei—blue.
Cytoplasm and connective tissue—pink.
Erythrocytes—salmon.

SOME STAINING TECHNIQUES IN DETAIL

Mallory's Phosphotungstic Acid Haematoxylin Stain

PTAH

Fixation: Zenker-fixed best. If formalin-fixed, tissue should be mordanted from 1 to 12 hours in a saturated solution of mercuric chloride or in Zenker's fluid.

Technique: Paraffin, sections cut at 6 microns.

Solutions:	*Phosphotungstic Acid Haematoxylin*
Haematoxylin	1 gm
Phosphotungstic acid	20 gm
Distilled water	1000 cc

Dissolve the solid ingradients in separate portions of the water, the haematoxylin with the aid of gentle heat. When cool, combine. No preservative is necessary. Spontaneous ripening requires several weeks but the addition of 0.177 gm of potassium permanganate will cause the stain to ripen at once.

Staining Procedure

1. Deparaffinise sections through 2 changes of xylene, absolute and 95% alcohol to distilled water as usual.
2. Remove mercury precipitate by placing in alcoholic iodine solution for 5 to 10 minutes.
3. Wash in tap water.
4. Clear off iodine in 5% sodium thiosulphate (hypo) solution for 5 minutes.
5. Wash in running water for 10-20 minutes.
6. Stain for 12 to 24 hours in phosphotungstic acid haematoxylin solution.
7. Differentiate in 95% alcohol—check differentiation under the microscope.
8. Absolute alcohol, 2 changes.
9. Xylene, 2 changes.
10. Mount in D.P.X.

Results

Nuclei—blue
Fibrin—blue
Fibroglia and microglia—blue
Collagen—yellowish to brownish red
Coarse elastic fibrils—purplish tint.

van Gieson's Stain for Collagen Fibres

Fixation: Formalin.

Technique: Paraffin, cut sections at 6 microns.

Solution

Weigert's Iron Haematoxylin

Solution A

Haematoxylin	1 gm
Absolute alcohol	100 cc

Solution B

29% ferric chloride	4 cc
Distilled water	95 cc
Hydrochloric acid, concentrated	1 cc

Working Solution

Equal parts of Solution A and Solution B

van Gieson's Solution

Acid fushsin, 1% aqueous solution 2.5 cc

Picric acid, saturated aqueous solution 97.5 cc

Staining Procedure

1. Xylene.
2. Absolute alcohol.
3. 95% alcohol.
4. Rinse in distilled water.
5. Stain in Weigert's haematoxylin solution for 10 minutes.
6. Wash in distilled water.
7. Counterstain in van Gieson's solution for 1 to 3 minutes.
8. 95% alcohol.
9. Absolute alcohol—2 changes.
10. Xylene—2 changes.
11. Mount in DPX/ Add 3 drops of saturated alcoholic picric acid to each 50 cc of xylene used in clearing. Mount from acidified xylene. This intensifies the background and prevents sections from fading.

Results

Collagen—red

Muscle, cornified epithelium—yellow

Nuclei—blue to black.

Running water will remove van Gieson's solution.

Solution B will remove Weigert's haematoxylin.

Masson's Trichrome Stain

Fixation: Bouin's or formalin. Mordant sections of formalin-fixed material in Bouin's fluid for one hour at 56°C, or overnight at room temperature.

Technique: Paraffin, cut sections at 6 microns.

Solutions

Bouin's solution

Picric acid saturated aqueous solution	75 cc
Formaldehyde, 37-40%	25 cc
Glacial acetic acid	5 cc

Weigert's Iron Haematoxylin

Solution A and B and working solution as in Van Gieson's stain for collagen fibres

Biebrich Scarlet-Acid Fuchsin Solution

Biebrich Scarlet, aqueous 1%	90 cc
Acid fuchsin, aqueous, 1%	10 cc
Glacial acetic acid	1 cc

Phosphomolybdic-Phosphotungstic Acid Solution

Phosphomolybdic acid	5 gm
Phosphotungstic acid	5 gm
Distilled water	200 cc

Aniline Blue Solution

Aniline blue	2.5 mg
Acetic acid	2 cc
Distilled water	100 cc

Light Green Solution

Light green	5 cc
Distilled water	250 cc
Glacial acetic acid	2 cc.

Heat water, dissolve light green, cool, filter and add acid.

1% Acetic Water Solution

Glacial acetic acid	1 cc
Distilled water	100 cc.

Staining Procedure

1. Xylene.
2. Absolute alcohol.
3. 95% alcohol.
4. Rinse in distilled water.
5. Mordant in Bouin's fixative for 1 hour at 56°C, or overnight at room temperature.
6. Cool and wash in running water until yellow colour disappears.

7. Rinse in distilled water.
8. Weigert's iron haematoxylin solution for 10 minutes. Wash in running water 10 minutes.
9. Rinse in distilled water.
10. Biebrich scarlet-acid fuchsin solution for 15 minutes. Save solution.
11. Rinse in distilled water.
12. Phosphomolybdic acid-phosphotungstic acid solution for 10 to 15 minutes before aniline blue solution. Aqueous phosphotungstic acid 5% for 15 minutes before light green counter stain. Discard solution.
13. Aniline blue solution for 5 to 10 minutes or light green solution for 1 minute. Save solution.
14. Rinse in distilled water.
15. Acetic water 1% for 3 to 5 minutes. Discard solution.
16. Alcohol, 95%
17. Absolute alcohol—3 changes.
18. Xylene—2 changes.
19. Mount in DPX.

Results

Nuclei—black
Cytoplasm, keratin, muscle fibres, intercellular fibres—red
Collagen, mucus—blue.

Verhoff's Elastic Stain

Fixation: Formalin.

Technique: Paraffin, sections to be cut at 6 microns.

Solutions

Elastic tissue stain
Dissolve 1 gm of haematoxylin in 22 cc of absolute alcohol in an open dish on a hot plate. Cool, filter and add 8 cc of a 10% aqueous solution of ferric chloride and 8 cc of iodine solution (2 gm iodine, 4 gm potassium iodide dissolved in 100 cc of distilled water). Always use freshly made solutions for better results.

Ferric Chloride Solution

Ferric chloride	2 gm
Distilled water	100 cc

Van Gieson's Stain

Acid fuchsin, aqueous solution 1%	5 cc
Saturated aqueous solution picric acid	100 cc

Sodium Thiosulphate (Hypo) Solution

Sodium thiosulphate	5 gm
Distilled water	100 cc

Staining Procedure

1. As usual deparaffinise and take to water.
2. Verhoff's elastic tissue stain for 15 minutes.
3. Wash in distilled water.
4. Differentiate in 2% ferric chloride–only a few minutes. Check under microscope and if differentiated too far, restain.
5. Place in 5% sodium thiosulphate for 1 minute.
6. Wash in tap water 5 minutes.
7. Counterstain in van Gieson's stain for 1 minute.
8. Absolute alcohol-2 changes.
9. Xylene-2 changes.
10. Mount in DPX.

Results

Elastic fibres—blue-black to black.
Nuclei—blue to black.
Collagen—red.
Other tissue elements—yellow.

Wilder's Reticulin Stain

Fixation: Formalin.

Technique: Paraffin. Sections cut at 6 to 10 microns.

Solutions

Phosphomolybdic Acid Solution

Phosphomolybdic acid	10 mg
Distilled water	100 cc

Uranium Nitrate Solution

Uranium nitrate	1 gm
Distilled water	100 cc

Ammoniacal Silver Solution
To 5 cc of 10.2% aqueous solution of liver nitrate add 28% ammonia water, drop by drop, until the precipitate which forms in almost dissolved. Add 5 cc of 3.1% sodium hydroxide and barely dissolve the resulting precipitate with a few drops of ammonia water. Make the solution up to 50 cc with distilled water. Use at once. Glassware must be clean.

Reducing Solution

Distilled water	50 cc
Neutral formaldehyde, 40%	0.5 cc
Uranium nitrate 1% aqueous solution (Make fresh just before use)	1.5 cc

Gold Chloride Solution

Gold chloride solution, 1%	
[Break glass vial (15 grains) in graduated cylinder with 100 cc distilled water for 10% solution.]	
Distilled water	40 cc

Sodium Thiosulphate (Hypo) Solution

Sodium thiosulphate	5 gm
Distilled water	100 cc

Nuclear Fast Red (Kernechtrot) Stain

Dissolve 0.1 gm nuclear fast red in 100 cc of a 5% solution of aluminium sulphate with aid of heat. Cool, filter, add grain of thymol as a preservative.

Staining Procedure

1. Xylene, absolute alcohol, 95% alcohol, distilled water.
2. Remove mercury precipitates if Zenker-fixed.
3. Wash well in distilled water.
4. Phosphomolybdic acid solution for 1 minute (oxidiser).
5. Rinse well in running water or cells will hold the yellow.
6. Dip in 1% aqueous uranium nitrate for 5 seconds or less (sensitizer).
7. Wash in distilled water for 10 to 20 minutes.
8. Place in ammoniacal silver solution for 1 minute.
9. Dip very quickly in 95% alcohol and go immediately into:
10. Reducing solution for 1 minute.
11. Rinse well in distilled water.
12. Tone in gold chloride solution for 1 minute or until sections lose their yellow colour and turn lavender. Too much toning will make sections red. Check individually under microscope.
13. Rinse in distilled water.
14. Place in 5% sodium thiosulphate for 1 to 5 minutes.
15. Wash well in tap water.
16. Counterstain, if desired, with alum haematoxylin and eosin, or nuclear fast red. Rinse well in distilled water.
17. Alcohol, 95%
18. Absolute alcohol-2 changes.
19. Xylene-2 changes.
20. Mount in DPX.

Results

Reticulin fibres—black
Collagen—Rose colour.
Other tissue elements–depending on counter-stain used.

Fontana-Masson Stain for Argentaffin Granules

Fixation: Formalin.

Technique: Paraffin. Cut sections at 6 microns.

Solutions

Silver Nitrate Solution (Fontana)

Dissolve 10 gm of silver nitrate in 100 cc of distilled water. To 65 cc of this solution, add ammonium hydroxide until a clear solution with no precipitate is obtained. Add, drop by drop, enough of the remaining 5 cc of silver nitrate solution to cause the above solution to become slightly cloudy. Let stand overnight before using. When ready to use, dilute each 25 cc of silver solution with 75 cc of distilled water and filter.

Gold Chloride Solution

Gold chloride solution	10 cc
Distilled water	40 cc

Sodium Thiosulphate Solution

Sodium thiosulphate	5 gm
Distilled water	100 cc

Nuclear Fast Red (Kernechtrot) Solution

Dissolve 0.1 gm of nuclear fast red in a 5% solution of aluminium sulphate with the aid of heat. Cool, filter add a grain of thymol as a preservative.

Staining Procedure

1. Deparaffinise and hydrate to water.
2. Immerse slides in silver nitrate solution for 1 hour at 56°C.
3. Rinse in distilled water.
4. Immerse in gold chloride solution for 10 minutes.
5. Rinse in distilled water.
6. Place in sodium thiosulphate for 5 minutes.
7. Rinse in distilled water.
8. Counterstain with eosin or nuclear fast red, if desired. Rinse in distilled water.
9. Alcohol, 95%.
10. Absolute alcohol.
11. Xylene.
12. Mount in DPX.

Results

Argentaffin granules and melanin—black.
Nuclei—pink.

Oil Red O Fat Stain

Fixation: Formalin.

Technique: Cut frozen sections at 10 to 15 microns. Collect in distilled water.

Solutions

Oil Red O solution

Oil Red O	1 to 2 gm
Alcohol, 70%	50 cc
Acetone	50 cc

Glycerin Jelly

Gelatin	10 gm
Distilled water	60 cc
Heat until gelatin is dissolved. Add:	
Glycerin	70 cc
Phenol	1 cc

Harris's haematoxylin for counterstain

Staining Procedure

1. Carry sections through on an angled glass rod.
2. Dip sections in 70% alcohol for only a second.
3. Place in oil red O in a tightly closed container for 5 minutes.
4. Wash quickly in 70% alcohol-avoid folds in sections.
5. Wash in water.
6. Counterstain in Harris's haematoxylin for a few minutes.
7. Wash in water.
8. Blue in ammonia water. If sections are too dark when removed from the haematoxylin, they may be differentiated in 1% acetic water for a few seconds, then blued in ammonia water.
9. Wash in water.
10. Mount in glycerin jelly.

Results

Fat—orange to bright red.
Nuclei—blue.

Best's Carmine Stain for Glycogen

Fixation: Tissue must be fixed in absolute alcohol or Carnoy's fluid. Since glycogen is soluble in water go directly from fixative to the clearing agent and then to paraffin.

Technique: Paraffin. Cut sections at 6 microns.

Solutions

Carmine Stock Solution

Carmine	2 gm
Potassium carbonate	1 gm
Potassium chloride	5 gm
Distilled water	60 cc

Boil gently and cautiously for several minutes. Cook in open dish (evaporating dish). When cool, add 20 cc of strong ammonia water. Keep in ice box.

Working Solution of Carmine

Stock carmine solution	10 cc
Ammonia water, 28%	15 cc
Methanol	15 cc

Differentiating Solution

Absolute alcohol	20 cc
Methanol	10 cc
Distilled water	25 cc

Staining Procedure

1. Xylene, Absolute alcohol.
2. Dip slides in very thin solution of celloidin—dry for a few seconds.
3. Place in water to harden for a few seconds.
4. Stain in Harris's haematoxylin solution for 15 minutes.
5. Differentiate in acid alcohol. Leave nuclei a little dark because ammonia decolourises them slightly.
6. Place in working solution of carmine for 20 to 30 minutes. Carry a control slide for checking.
7. Place for a few seconds in the differentiating solution.
8. Wash quickly in 80% alcohol.
9. Alcohol 95%.
10. Absolute alcohol-2 changes.
11. Xylene-2 changes.
12. Mount in DPX.

Results

Glycogen—pink to red.
Nuclei—blue.

Periodic Acid-Schiff (PAS) Reaction

Fixation: Formalin.

Technique: Cut paraffin sections at 6 microns.

Solutions

Coleman's Feulgen Reagent

Dissolve 1 gm of basic fuchsin in 200 cc hot distilled water. Bring to boiling point. Cool and add 2 gm potassium metabisulphite, and 10 cc normal hydrochloric acid. Let bleach for 24 hours, then add 0.5 gm activated carbon. Shake 1 minute and filter through coarse filter paper. Repeat filtration until solution is colourless. Store in a refrigerator.

OR

Schiff's Leuco-Fuchsin Solution

Dissolve 1 gm basic fuchsin in 200 cc hot distilled water. Bring to boiling point. Cool to 50°C. Filter and add 20 cc normal hydrochloric acid. Cool further and add 1 gm anhydrous sodium bisulfite, or sodium metabisulphite. Keep in the dark for 48 hours until solution becomes straw coloured. Store in refrigerator.

Test for Schiff's Leuco-Fuchsin Solution

Pour a few drops of Schiff's solution into 10 cc of 37-40% formaldehyde in a watch glass. If the solution turns reddish purple rapidly, it is good. If the reaction is delayed and the resultant colour deep blue-purple, the solution is breaking down.

Normal Hydrochloric Acid Solution

Hydrochloric acid, Conc. Sp. gr. 1.19	83.5 cc
Distilled water	916.5 cc

0.2% Light Green counterstain (Stock)

Light green crystals	0.2 gm
Distilled water	100 cc
Glacial acetic acid	0.2 cc

Working Light Green Solution

Light green, stock solution	10 cc
Distilled water	50 cc

Diastase Solution

Diastase	0.5 gm
Distilled water, sterile	100 cc

Store in refrigerator. Good for 1 week.

(Instead of diastase solution, one can use one's own saliva).

Staining Procedure

1. Xylene
2. Absolute alcohol
3. Alcohol 95%.
4. Rinse in distilled water.
   (If PAS reaction with digestion is needed, place sections in 0.5% diastase for 20 minutes. Saliva can also be used. Rinse in running tap water 10 minutes, and wash in distilled water.)
5. Periodic acid solution for 5 minutes (oxidiser).
6. Rinse in distilled water.
7. Place in Coleman's Feulgen or Schiff's Leuco-Fuchsin for 15 minutes.
8. Place in running tap water for 10 minutes for pink colour to develop.
9. Stain in Harris's haematoxylin for 6 minutes or light green counterstain for a few seconds. Light green is recommended for counterstaining sections in which fungi are to be demonstrated. Omit steps 10 through 14 if light green is used.
10. Rinse in tap water
11. Differentiate in acid alcohol- 3 to 10 quick dips.
12. Wash in tap water.
13. Dip in ammonia water to blue sections.
14. Wash in running tap water for 10 minutes.
15. Alcohol, 95%.
16. Absolute alcohol-2 changes.
17. Xylene-2 changes.
18. Mount in DPX.

Results

Glycogen, mucin, hyaluronic acid, reticulin, fibrin or thrombi, colloid droplets, hyalin of arteriosclerosis, hyalin deposits in glomeruli, cells in renal arterioles where preserved, most basement membranes, colloid of pituitary stalks and thyroid, amyloid infiltration and other elements may show a positive reaction–rose to purplish red.

Nuclei—blue
Fungi—red
Background—pale green (with light green counterstain).

Mayer's Mucicarmine Stain

Fixation: Formalin.

Technique: Cut paraffin section at 6 microns.

Solutions

Weigert's Iron Haematoxylin

Solution A

Haematoxylin	1 gm
Alcohol, 95%	100 cc

Solution B

Ferric chloride 29% aqueous solution	4 cc
Distilled water	95 cc
Hydrochloric acid, concentrated	1 cc

Working Solution

Equal parts of solutions A and B. Prepare fresh.

Metanil Yellow Solution

Metanil yellow	0.25 gm
Distilled water	100 cc
Glacial acetic acid	0.25 gm

Mucicarmine Stain

Carmine	1 gm
Aluminium chloride, anhydrous	0.5 gm
Distilled water	2 cc

Mix stain in small test tube. Heat over small flame for 2 minutes. Liquid becomes almost black and syrupy. Dilute with 100 cc of 50 % alcohol and let stand for 25 hours. Filter. Dilute 1 to 4 with tap water for use.

Staining Procedure

1. Deparaffinise sections through 2 changes of xylene, absolute and 95% alcohol to distilled water as usual. Remove mercury precipitates through iodine and hyposolutions if necessary.
2. Stain for 7 minutes in working solution of Weigert's haematoxylin.
3. Wash in tap water for 5 to 10 minutes.
4. Place in diluted mucicarmine solution for 30 to 60 minutes or longer.

   Check control slide with microscope after 30 minutes.
5. Rinse quickly in distilled water.
6. Stain in metanil yellow solution for 1 minute.
7. Rinse quickly in distilled water.
8. Rinse quickly in 95% alcohol.
9. Dehydrate in 2 changes of absolute alcohol, clear with 2 to 3 changes of Xylene, and mount in DPX.

Results

Mucin—deep rose to red.
Nuclei—black.
Other tissue elements—yellow.

Crystal Violet Amyloid Stain

Fixation: Formalin

Technique: Cut paraffin sections at 6 microns.

Solutions

Stock Crystal Violet Solution

Crystal violet-to saturate-approximately	14 gm
Alcohol, 95%	100 cc

Working Crystal Violet Solution

Crystal violet, stock solution	10 cc
Distilled water	300 cc
Hydrochloric acid, concentrated	1 cc

Abopon Mounting Medium

Abopon	50 gm
Distilled water	25 cc

Dissolve with the aid of heat.

If this medium cannot be obtained, then put a drop of water on the section to be seen and examine under microscope.

Staining Procedure

1. Deparaffinise sections through 2 changes of xylene, absolute and 95% alcohol to distilled water as usual.
2. Stain in working crystal violet solution for 1 to 2 minutes. Use control slide. Check with microscope.
3. Rinse well in tap water.
4. Mount in Abopon.
5. Seal edges of coverslip with nail polish.

Results

Amyloid—purplish violet
Other tissue elements—blue.

von Kossa's Method for Demonstrating Calcium

Fixation: Alcohol or 10% formalin. Alcohols are preferred.

Technique: Cut paraffin sections at 6 microns.

Solutions

5% Silver Nitrate Solution

Silver nitrate	5 gm
Distilled water	100 cc

Solution stable only 2 weeks.

5% Sodium Thiosulphate Solution

Sodium thiosulphate	5 gm
Distilled water	100 cc

Nuclear Fast Red (Kernechtrot) Stain

Dissolve 0.1 gm nuclear fast red powder in 100 cc of a 5% aqueous aluminium sulphate solution with the aid of heat. Cool and filter. Add a crystal of thymol as preservative. Keeps well at room temperature. Can be re-used.

Staining Procedure

1. Deparaffinise sections through 2 changes of xylene, absolute and 95% alcohols to distilled water.
2. Place in 5% silver nitrate solution for 30 to 60 minutes exposed to direct sunlight, ultraviolet lamp, or a 100 watt desk lamp light. Use chemically clean container.
3. Rinse in distilled water.
4. Place in 5% solution thiosulphate for 2 to 3 minutes.
5. Wash well in distilled water.
6. Counterstain in nuclear fast red for 5 minutes.
7. Wash in distilled water.
8. Dehydrate with 2 changes of 95% alcohol, absolute alcohol, clear with 2 changes of xylene and mount in DPX.

Results

Calcium salts—black
Nuclei—red
Cytoplasm—pink to rose.

Ziehl-Neelsen Stain for Acid-Fast Bacteria

Fixation: Formalin

Technique: Paraffin sections at 4 to 6 microns.

Solutions

Carbol Fuchsin solution

Acid carbolic, white fused	
Crystals, melted	2.5 cc
Alcohol, absolute	5 cc
Basic fuchsin	0.5 gm
Distilled water	50 cc

Store at room temperature. Filter before use.

1% Acid Alcohol

Hydrochloric acid, concentrated	1 cc
Alcohol, 70%	99 cc

OR

1% Sulphuric Acid Water

Sulphuric acid concentrated	1 cc
Distilled water	99 cc

Working Methylene Blue Solution

Methylene blue	0.5 gm
Glacial acetic acid, concentrated	0.5 cc
Tap water	100 cc

Staining Procedure

1. Deparaffinise sections through 2 changes of xylene, and run through absolute and 95% alcohols to distilled water as usual. Remove mercury precipitates through iodine and hypo-solutions if necessary.
2. Stain sections with carbol fuchsin solution for 10 minutes. Filter solution before use.
3. Rinse well in tap water.
4. Decolourise with 1% acid alcohol or 1% sulphuric acid water, until sections are pale pink.
5. Wash thoroughly with running water for 8 minutes.
6. Counterstain by dipping one slide at a time in working methylene blue solution. Sections should be pale blue. Overstaining will mask bacilli.
7. Wash with tap water and distilled water.
8. Dehydrate with 2 changes of 95% alcohol and absolute alcohol, clear with 2 changes of xylene, and mount in DPX.

Results

Acid-fast bacilli—bright red.
Erythrocytes—yellowish-orange.
Other tissue elements—pale blue.

AUTOMATION IN HISTOPATHOLOGY

Shandon products outclass all others and are provided in India by Vickers India Ltd. Given below are a few salient features of some of their products.

Hypercentre (Shandon)

Modular enclosed tissue processing system:

- A unique, safe, totally enclosed system that will not release vapours into the laboratory during processing.
- Keyboard programming and memory with video

display and simple tough button controls accept ordinary language.
- Separate command, reaction and storage modules offer flexible choice of layouts
- One command module can control up to 5 reaction and storage modules independently and simultaneously.
- Nine programmes per reaction module—total capacity 45 programmes, each of which can be recalled instantly.
- Programmes can be monitored at every stage.

Histocentre (Shandon)

Integrated tissue embedding centre:
- Provides efficient utilisation of bench space—easy to clean work surfaces all on one level.
- Incorporates processed tissue storage, cassette opening and base.
- Wax temperature can be preset and monitored continually on digital display—can also be switched to monitor hotplate temperature.
- Wax dispenser can be foot operated leaving both hands free.
- Wax flow rate easily adjusted with nozzle heated to prevent wax solidifying.
- Illuminated work area and integral magnifier.

2 LE (Shandon)

2 litre automatic tissue processor
- Simple to use electronic timer and programme controls provide virtually unlimited programming capacity with constant digital read out.
- Capacity of 160 cassettes in double load or up to 336 specimens in divided baskets.
- Antievaporation lids on all beakers reduce fume levels.
- Two independent programme memories can store up to 4 complete processing cycles.
- Vacuum impregnation during processing cycle if optional vacuum pump utilised.

Duplex (Shandon)

1 litre automatic tissue processor
- Economic versatile processing for single or double load operation.
- 12 station cycle—with 9 or 10 one litre beakers and 2 or 3 thermostatically controlled wax baths.
- Automatic agitation ensures efficient impregnation of tissue.
- Wide range of tissue baskets—large capsule and divided types in stainless steel and plastic.
- Standard 24-hour timer plus 24-hour delay.

Hypercut (Shandon)

Rotary Microtome
- Exceptional strength and stability with heavy weight construction which eliminates vibration and chatter.
- Unique linear bearing action provides smooth almost effortless control.
- Sections paraffin wax embedded tissue blocks consistently and accurately from 0.5 to 30.
- Unique easy to adjust knife holder accepts wide range of knives including glass, tungsten carbide tipped, and disposable type.
- Optional lightweight knife holder provides additional access to cutting area.

Autosharp 5 (Shandon)

Automatic microtome knife sharpner
- Rapid high quality consistent sharpening of microtome knives, no special training required.
- Designed to sharpen tungsten carbide tipped as well as conventional steel knives.
- Wide range of knife holders available for C type, D type and knives up to 250 mm long.
- Easy-to-use damper; touch button controls and digital timer control.
- Unique, hard wearing microsharp iron lapping plate with extended life.
- Easy-to-adjust facet angle indicator.

Linistain GLX (Shandon)

Random access stainer for histology
- Special built-in fume extraction system, protects laboratory personnel from xylene fumes.
- Provides consistent uniform staining of specimens on standard microsope slide.
- Random access provides flexibility to use various staining routines and eliminates batching.
- Allows free choice of stain source and type.
- Running water wash selectable at all positions.
- Proven, reliable design with a few moving parts.
- Compact, narrow shape allows wise use of bench space.

Varistain 24 (Shandon)

Automatic 24 position batch stainer

- Simple-to-use electronic timer and programme controls provide virtually unlimited programing capacity with constant digital read out.
- Immersion times can be programmed to the second with all the versatility of hand staining.
- Individual immersion times can be reprogrammed to take account of changing conditions.
- Two independent programme memories can store up to 4 complete staining routines. Three capacities of stainless steel slide carrier available—10 slide, 40 slide and 60 slide.
- Compatible with Autoslip automatic over slipper.

Varistain 12 (Shandon)

Automatic 12 position stainer

- Designed for H and E staining and haematological techniques.
- Equal or unequal times can be selected.
- 224 slides per hour output on continuous loading operation.
- Single load operation for 16 or 32 slides horizontally or 48 slides vertically.
- 60-minute timer with additional option for 30 minutes, or short immersion timers.
- Aeration and agitation provided.

Autoslip (Shandon)

Automatic coverslipper

- Applies mountant and coverslip to standard microscope slides automatically, presenting the finished slide for examination.
- Eliminates hand coverslipping—one of the most unpleasant and hazardous operations in histology and cytology.
- Produces coverslipped slides of consistent high quality at the rate of up to 160 slides per hour.
- Coverslipped slides held in xylene saturated atmosphere to prevent drying out of specimens prior to coverslipping.
- Unique plastic slide clips enable slides to be transferred direct from Varistain 24 series of automatic stainers.

CHAPTER 25

Cytology

Cytology is that branch of diagnostic medicine which deals with the study of individual cells and/or tissue fragments spread on laboratory slide and stained appropriately.

Stains used commonly are Papanicolaou's stain and May-Grünwalds Giemsa (MGG) stain. For the former, alcohol fixation is required; and the latter, fixation should be done by using methanol. For Acid-Fast Bacilli staining, ethanol fixation is used. Wherever ethanol fixation is required, the material obtained and spread on a slide should be immediately immersed into ethanol. For MGG staining, the smears are air dried and methanol fixed.

For fine, needle aspirations and thick cellular discharges/fluids, no centrifugation is required. While relatively watery, thin and hypocellular fluids need centrifugation, the sediment so obtained is smeared on to the slides, stained, and examined.

The advantage of cytological techniques is the rapidity with which the diagnosis can be provided. However, this branch has not, and cannot, replace the ultimate in diagnosis, namely—histopathology.

Cytological study can be done on discharges from the body (vaginal, nipple, sinus, etc.), scrappings obtained (from buccal mucosa, or other mucosal surfaces approachable by employing fibre-optic endoscopes), or by aspirating from palpable lumps (abscesses, growths, etc). In any case, the material obtained is smeared on slides, an easy and convenient way is to put the material between two slides and pull them apart or smearing on the slide by using a coverslip with application of gentle pressure. All liquids (relatively hypocellular, e.g. urine, body cavity fluids, etc.) have to be centrifuged, the sediment is used for smearing. If a bigger chunk of cellular material is obtained, it can be submitted for histopathological examination too. Do not forget to add EDTA to containers in which coagulable fluids are to be collected.

Cytological diagnosis is an important part of cervical (gynaecological) lesions, accessible mucosal lesions and soft tissue tumours palpable superficially or else approached under fluoroscopic guidance. Using vacuum to suck and needle movement in various directions (to dislodge tissue fragments), sufficient amount of material can be obtained.

The commonly used stains are Pap's stain and MGG. Details of Pap's staining are mentioned below. MGG staining is similar to that of blood peripheral smear staining.

Papanicolaou Method of Staining Smears (modified)

Preparation of Smears

1. Exfoliated cells degenerate rapidly; therefore smear should be prepared and fixed immediately. If there is to be any delay, the specimen should be fixed in 95% alcohol and refrigerated until smears can be prepared. Specimens requiring centrifugation (e.g., urine and various fluids) are preserved by adding an equal volume of 50% ethyl alcohol, centrifugation is at 2000 rpm for 30 minutes.
2. Viscid secretions (e.g. vaginal, cervical and prostatic) should be smeared directly onto clean glass slides and fixed immediately.
3. Body fluids and watery exudates (e.g. urine, spinal fluid, pleural fluid, etc.) will not adhere to the glass slides unless the slide is first coated with a layer of Mayer's egg albumin (one drop per slide).
4. The sediment or centrifuged specimen is smeared onto glass slides coated with Mayer's egg albumin. Any remaining sediment should be processed as a biopsy specimen for conventional histology examination.

Fixation

1. Use equal parts of ether and 95% alcohol.
2. Smears should be fixed immediately while still wet, though partial drying along the edges may be permitted to prevent the material from becoming detached from the slide.
3. Fixation time is 30 minutes to 1 week.
4. If unstained slides are to be mailed, they must be placed in the fixative for at least 2 hours, then dried and placed face to face before shipment.

Solutions

1. Harris's haematoxylin (modified)
   - Haematoxylin crystals 5 gm
   - Absolute alcohol 50 cc
   - Ammonium or potassium alum 100 cc
   - Distilled water 1000 cc
   - Mercuric oxide 2.5 gm

   For this purpose, acetic acid should not be added.
2. Orange G6 (OG 6)
   - Orange G6, 0.5% solution in 95% alcohol 100 cc
   - Phosphotungstic acid 0.015 gm
3. Eosin-Azure 50 (EA 50)

   These stains should be purchased readymade. These are ready for use and cannot be equalled by mixture, prepared in laboratory.

Staining Procedure

1. After fixation, transfer slides without drying directly from alcohol—ether solution to 95% alcohol, then through 80% alcohol, 70% alcohol, and water, to distilled water.
2. Stain in Harris's haematoxylin (modified), 8 minutes.
3. Rinse gently in tap water to prevent cells from being washed off.
4. Differentiate carefully the nuclear staining in 1% hydrochloric acid in 70% alcohol; the nuclei should be clear and sharp in detail; the cytoplasm should be light blue and clear.
5. Place in gently running tap water for 5 minutes to wash out the acid thoroughly and to blue the nuclei.
6. Rinse in distilled water and transfer through 70% alcohol, 80% alcohol, to 95% alcohol.
7. Stain in OG 6 for 2 minutes.
8. Rinse 5 times as follows:
   a. Twice in 95% alcohol.
   b. Once in 1% acetic acid in 95% alcohol.
   c. Once in 1% phoshotungstic acid in 95% alcohol.
   d. Once in 95% alcohol.
9. Stain in EA 50 for 3 minutes.
10. Rinse 9 times as follows:
    a. 3 changes of 95% alcohol.
    b. 2 changes of absolute alcohol.
    c. 4 changes of xylene.
11. Mount in DPX.

Results

Nuclei—blue with clear sharp details.

Cytoplasm—varying shades of pink, blue, yellow, green grey. If necessary, slides may be decolourised in acid alcohol, washed thoroughly in tap water to remove all acid and restained.

FNAC

Fine-Needle Aspiration Cytology Transcutaneous Aspiration of Palpable Lesions

Twenty ml plastic disposable syringe with 21 to 23-gauze fine needles of variable length, depending upon the site of tumour, are used for aspiration. The syringe is fitted with a specially designed handle which permits a single hand operation during aspiration. The skin is cleaned with antiseptic solution. No local anaesthesia is required. The tumour mass is fixed with one hand and with the other hand aspiration is carried out. When the needle enters the tumour, the plunger of the syringe is retracted to create a vacuum in the barrel and the needle is moved to and fro 3 to 4 times. For adequate sampling, the needle may be moved in three to four different directions (Fig. 25.1). After completion of aspiration, the plunger is released before taking out the needle in order to equalise the pressure. The needle is disconnected and after filling the syringe with air, it is reconnected. The content of the needle is expressed on clean glass slides. Smears are made by applying a gentle pressure with the flat surface of another glass slide and allowed to air dry. Alternatively, the flat surface of a covership can be used to prepare the smears. Smears are routinely fixed in methanol for MGG staining. Whenever Pap staining is required for better nuclear clarity, wet fixation in absolute alcohol is recommended. Also, smears may be fixed appropriately for various cytochemical stains when fluid aspirated, is discharged into a clean tube and centrifuged at 1500 rpm. Smears are made from the deposits when the aspiration fluid is admixed with blood or frankly haemorrhagic, it may be collected in a heparinised container. Haematocrit method or lymphoprep can be used to separate the tumour cells from RBCs. In case, where cellularity is poor, the deposit is resuspended in 1 ml of supernatant, spun in a cytocentrifuge and processed in a similar manner.

ASPIRATION OF INTRATHORACIC MASSES

Lung

Aspiration cytology of intrathoracic masses is usually performed to diagnose peripheral lung lesions which are not accessible by bronchoscope and which do not desquamate into the bronchial tree. This procedure is usually carried out around the table under television flouroscopy. The skin is cleaned with iodine and spirit and filtration with local anaesthesia is done up to pleura. The needle length can be selected according to the depth of the lesion. The usual internal diameter of the needle is 0.6 to 0.7 mm. When the needle reaches the intrathoracic mass, the aspiration is performed as per palpable lesions. The patient is asked to hold his breath during the aspiration. The entire procedure of inserting the needle and aspirating the lesion should not take more than 20 seconds. The needle may be reinserted in a different direction if no representative material is obtained initially. After the aspiration cytology, the patient needs to be kept under observation for about two hours so as to detect rare complications like bleeding or pneumothorax if any.

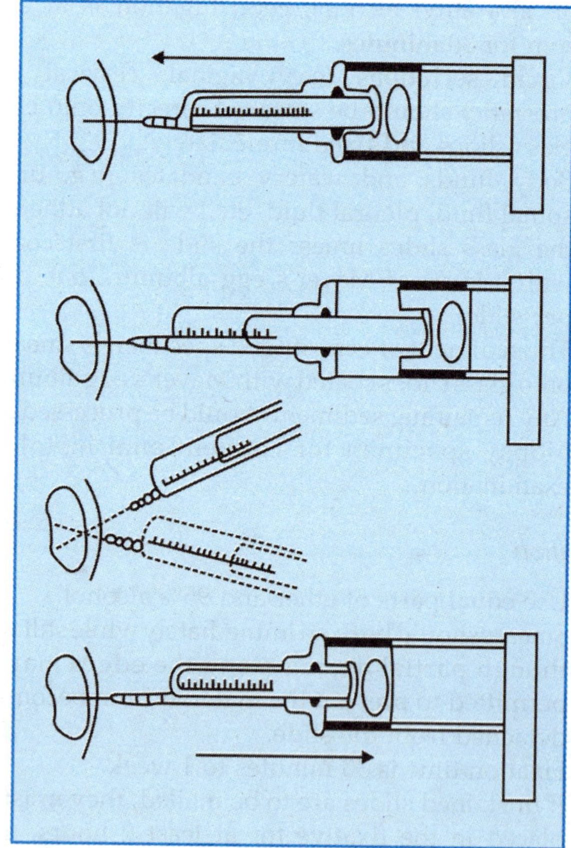

Fig. 25.1: Technique of fine-needle aspiration biopsy

1. Needle within the lymph-node.
2. Retraction of the piston of the syringe in order to create negative pressure in barrel of syringe.
3. Movement of needle in 2 to 3 directions/plains.
4. Release of piston and withdrawal of the needle.

Liver

A 8-16 cm needle with external diameter of 0.6 mm (22 gauze) are used for aspiration of liver. (Usually, a prothrombin time is estimated before liver aspiration. If the value is very low, vitamin K is given to raise it to a satisfactory level).

No local anaesthesia is necessary. Depending upon the site of lesion, the needle is introduced transcostally or subcostally. The ideal transcostal area for entry of needle is 9th intercostal space in midaxillary line. When the liver is enlarged particularly when the tumour mass is palpable, aspiration can be carried out in the subcostal region.

Prostatic: Aspiration is undertaken with the help of a needle guide and long needle (20 cm). The patient is placed in the lithotomy position. The prostate is carefully palpated through rectum before the procedure. Well lubricated gloved index finger of left hand with the needle guide is fixed over the nodule palpable through rectum. Then the needle is introduced through the needle guide and aspiration is performed as described for transcutaneous biopsy.

Ovarian tumour: Large ovarian tumours which are palpable per abdomen can be aspirated transabdominally avoiding the loops of intestine. The lesion can also be approached through the vaginal vault with the help of a needle guide and a long needle as is described under the aspiration of prostate.

Advantages of the Procedure

1. Fine-needle aspiration biopsy is a quick, convenient, economic and almost painless procedure which can be practiced on an outpatient basis.
2. Local anaesthesia is not required.
3. Can be attempted at multiple sites and repeated if necessary.
4. Malignancy can be confirmed or excluded in potentially operable lesions suspicious of malignancy and the extent of surgery can be planned well in advance.
5. Is a good diagnostic aid prior to application of radiation in inoperable cases or where surgery is contraindicated.
6. By way of evacuation of a cyst content, it helps as a therapeutic aid in addition to providing diagnosis.
7. It helps in assessing the stage of the disease prior to surgery or radiotherapy.
8. Local recurrence or metastasis can be detected in postoperative or post-radiation follow up cases, for further management.
9. Aspirated material can be used for immunological, cytochemical, cytogenetical and microbiological studies.

Limitation

False-negative results may be obtained in the following situations:

1. If there is extensive fibrosis and sclerosis in a tumour.
2. If the tumour is highly vascular.
3. If there is tumour necrosis.

To minimise these errors-special precautions can be taken.

ULTRASOUND-GUIDED FINE-NEEDLE ASPIRATION CYTOLOGY

The use of ultrasound as a tool in medical diagnosis is gaining increased acceptance in most medical centres. The chief advantages of ultrasound as a diagnostic modality are three:

1. It is a noninvasive study, causing little or no discomfort to the patient and usually requiring no special preparation.
2. It does not require the use of ionising radiation such as X-rays. Studies to date have shown no proven adverse effects from the ultrasonic beam at the conventional power levels used for diagnosis.
3. Ultrasound is capable of providing some diagnostic information which may not be available using other noninvasive techniques.

The ultrasound beam is in many ways similar to a beam of light. It obeys the laws of optics and can (unlike X-rays) be focussed, reflected, or refracted. The beam consists of high frequency sound waves generated by vibration of a piezoelectric crystal within an ultrasound transducer. The crystal vibrates in response to an electrical signal, the frequency of vibration being a function of the shape and thickness of the crystal itself. This is exactly the same principle that governs the sound of a bell. Bells of differing shapes and sizes have different. For most medical applications, the frequency used is approximately 2.5 million cycles per second (2.5 mega Hertz). The same crystal that transmits the ultrasonic beam also functions as a listening device. For example, a pulse of ultrasound is beamed for a fraction of a second and the crystal then "listens" during a much longer interval for the echo response. Returning sound waves (echoes) strike the transducer, producing vibrations which are transmitted as electrical signals to an oscilloscope or for storage on the screen of a cathode ray tube.

What produces these echoes? The tissues of the body vary from each other in sound-transmission characteristics (acoustic impedance). When two tissues of differing acoustic impedance are apposed, the ultrasonic beam will be partially reflected at the interface between them, returning an echo signal to the transducer. The degree of difference in acoustic impedance will determine the strength of the returning echo. Thus, if soft tissue lies next to bone, which has a very high acoustic impedance, or next to air, which has a very low acoustic impedance, strong interfaces will be formed, and strong echoes will be returned. On the other hand, soft tissues (vessel walls, septa, fat, parenchyma, etc.) differ only slightly from one another in acoustic impedance and the echoes that are returned from their various interfaces are relatively weak. These echoes are recorded as spikes on an oscilloscope or stored as dots on the screen of the cathode ray tube. This latter type of storage display is called a B-scan, B because the brightness (and size) of the dots on the screen varies with the strength of the acoustic interface.

B-Scanning

B-scan displays are used when performing studies of the abdomen, retroperitoneum, and pelvis. The orientation of the dots on the storage screen varies with the orientation of the transducer relative to the patient's body. As the transducer (attached to a rigid hinged arm, which holds it in any plane selected) is moved across a section of the patient's body, it sends a narrow, well-directed ultrasonic beam through the tissues. As this beam traverses the abdomen, it is partially reflected at various interfaces, owing to relative differences in acoustic impedance. These reflected echoes are recorded as dots, which build up an image of the section on a storage screen (Fig. 25.2). When a suitable picture has been made, it may be photographed on either Polaroid or X-ray film, or recorded on heat-sensitive paper.

It is important to remember that relatively inhomogeneous tissues, such as solid organs or masses, will generally have many weak echoes recorded within them, representing small vessels, ducts, and septae traversing the tissue. Relatively homogeneous tissues, such as fluid-filled organs or cystic lesions, show a few internal echoes, even when the sensitivity of the machine is turned up very high ("high gain").

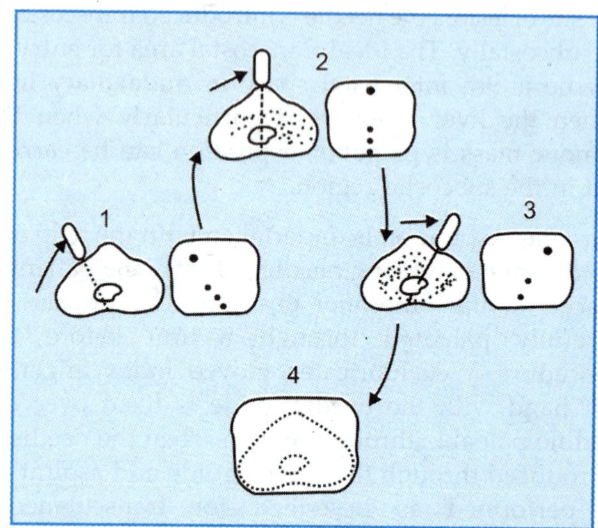

Fig. 25.2: As the transducer is moved across the body, an image of the body section traversed is built up on the storage screen

Ultrasonography-guided fine-needle aspiration cytology is being practised in case of lesions of thyroid, and some selected cases of intrathoracic tumours and also in breast.

Advantages

1. Takes less time than to perform mammography.
2. No radiation hazards.
3. Can be used to guide the aspiration of cyst that could not be drained clinically hence avoids surgery.
4. It can guide placement of wire guide.

Disadvantages

1. Limitations in diagnostic usefulness because benign appearance overlaps, the malignant.
2. Unable to detect lesions less than 1.5 cm in diameter (breast).

Application

Differentiating cyst from solid mass.

Smearing Techniques

One-Step Smearing Technique

The standard overlap and pull-apart method of smear preparation can itself be a source of dilution. Aspirates of poorly vascularised tumours often yield semisolid, undiluted tissue fragments that can be easily expelled from the needle core as a compact drop onto a slide. If standard pull-apart smears are prepared, this material is dispersed onto two slides. A slight modification of the pull-apart technique, called the one-step technique, greatly limits what is in effect a 50% dilution of the material. The two slides are held at right angles. A small drop of aspirate material is placed near the frosted edge of a slide held by one hand at that edge. A second slide is then placed across the first, establishing a fulcrum such that the mobile slide, when carefully rotated away from the observer and downward toward the material, just covers the drop. The smearing slide is then quickly but smoothly brought toward the operator, with a smearing pressure barely greater than that caused by the capillary space dispersion of fluid between the slides. This gentle and smooth stroke yields optimal monolayer smears for semisolid or small-volume specimens. Little material is transferred to smearing slide.

Two-Step Particle Concentration and Smearing Technique

For needle aspirates that are diluted by fluid, a procedure called the two-step smearing technique provides an optimal concentration of cells on the slide.

With the frosted ends away from the observer, each slide is held at the tips of its lateral border by three fingers. The thumb and index finger contact the upper outer frosted corner of each slide, and the fifth finger contacts the underside of the lower outer corner.

First, a drop of the aspirate is placed near the frosted end of a clean, grease-free slide. With the labelled ends still away from the observer, the other hand brings the smearing slide onto the first slide, at a point between the drop of aspiration and the observer. The smearing slide is then passed away from the observer and through the drop so as to collect the drop in the acute angle formed by the two slides.

With the first slide still stationary, the mobile slide begins the concentration procedure by next moving the entrapped material away from the frosted end and toward the observer. This movement disperses much of the fluid over the central portion of the stationary slide, while most of the particles remain with the small amount of residual fluid at the line of slide intersection. At this point, the mobile slide is lifted perpendicularly upward and away from the stationary slide, and the similarities of this technique to preparing peripheral blood smears end. Next, the stationary slide is rotated vertically with its frosted end pointing downward. For 1 to 3 seconds, gravity is allowed to draw any excess fluid further away from the particles, which largely remain at the last line of slide intersection. The particles can frequently be seen by reflected light as small, slightly raised points.

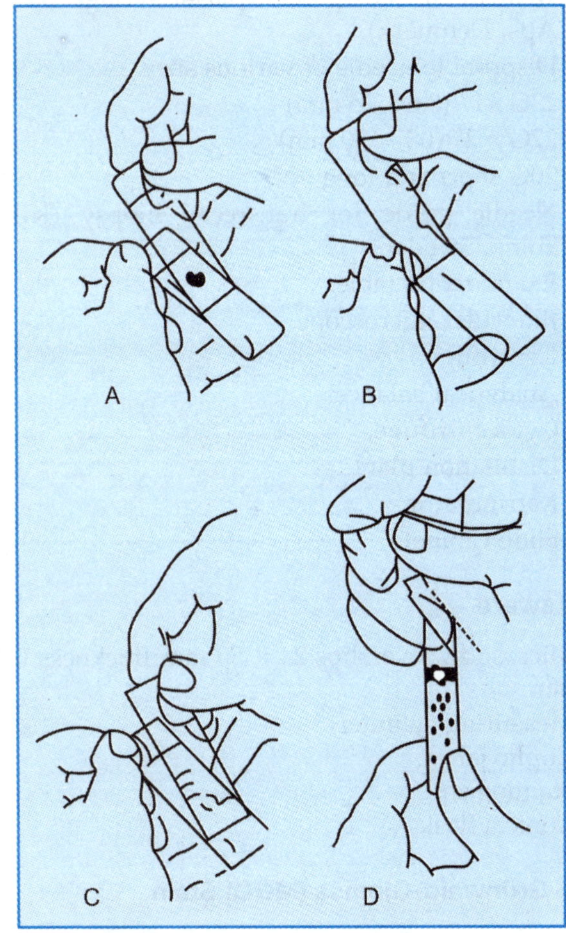

Fig. 25.3: Two-step technique. Line drawing summary. (A) Finger position. (B) Collection of aspirate, (C) Particle concentration smear, and (D) Preparation of a monolayer smear are illustrated for a right-handed operator

At this point the basic concentration manoeuvres (first step of the two-step technique) are complete, and the particles now await monolayer smearing by a slight variation of the standard pull-apart technique (the second step). By fulcrum action, the mobile slide is placed so that when slowly rotated onto the other slide it extends about 1 to 2 mm past the line of concentrated particles. As soon as the two slides come into contact, they are gently pulled apart with minimal additional pressure, yielding a well-formed monolayer (Fig. 25.3).

REQUIREMENTS FOR LABORATORY SET UP

Equipment

1. Handle constructed for disposable 20 ml or 10 ml syringe (Cameco, Enelyberg, Sweden).
2. 10 ml or 20 ml disposable plastic syringe. (ASIK, Aps. Denmark).
3. Disposable needle of various sizes
   23G ×1″ (0.6 × 25 mm)
   22G × 2″ (0.7 × 50 mm)
   20G short and long
4. Needle guide for transrectal biopsy (KIFA, Solna, Sweden).
5. Examination table.
6. Binocular microscope.
7. Centrifuge.
8. Analytical balance.
9. Cytocentrifuge.
10. Distillation plant.
11. Refrigerator.
12. Slide cabinet.

Glassware

1. Microslide coverslips 24 × 50 mm thickness 0.17 mm
2. Measuring cylinder
3. Coplin jar
4. Staining jar
5. Conical flask

May-Grünwald-Giemsa (MGG) Stain

Reagents

1. May-Grünwald stain
2. Giemsa's stain
3. Methanol
4. Glycerol
5. Conical flask
6. Phosphate (pH 6.8)

Preparation of Stains

i. Preparation of May-Grünwald stain: 0.3 gm of powdered dye is weighed out and transferred to a conical flast of 200-250 ml capacity. A volume of 100 ml of methanol is added and the mixture is warmed to 50°C. The flask is then allowed to cool to room temperature and is shaken several times during the day. After standing for 24 hours, the solution is filtered. It is then ready for use, no ripening being required.
ii. Preparation of solution of Giemsa powder is dissolved in 54 ml of glycerol and after cooling, mixed with 84 ml of methanol GR and filtered.

Staining Techniques

Air-dried smears are fixed in a jar of methanol for 5 minutes. Fixed smears are stained as follows:

1. With May-Grünwald stain, freshly diluted with an equal part of phosphate buffer for 5 minutes.
2. With Giemsa's stain, diluted with 9 parts of phosphate buffer for 10 to 15 minutes.
3. Washed with phosphate buffer (pH 6.8).
4. Dried in air.
5. Mounted by a rectangular cover glass using DPX as mountant.

Papanicolaou's Stain

Harris's Haematoxylin

Prepared as follows:

Haematoxylin	1 gm
Absolute alcohol	10 ml
Potassium alum	20 gm
Distilled water	200 ml
Mercuric oxide	0.5 gm

The haematoxylin is dissolved in absolute alcohol and potassium alum in distilled water with the aid of heat. The two solutions are mixed together. The mixture is boiled, removed from the flame and mercuric oxide is added bit by bit. The flask containing the solution is then immersed into cold water bath. After cooling, it is filtered and stored in a coloured bottle.

Orange G-6

Orange G-6 solution is prepared as follows:

Orange G	0.5 gm

95 percent ethyl alcohol	100 ml
Phosphotungstic acid	0.015 gm

Eosin Azure-36 (EA-36)

The stock solutions of light green SF yellowish (A), eosin yellow (B), are prepared as follows:

a. Light green—(SF)

Light green SF yellowish	0.5 gm
95 per cent ethyl alcohol	100 ml

b. Eosin yellow

Eosin yellow	0.5 gm
95 per cent ethyl alcohol	100 ml

From the stock solution, the working solution of EA-36 is prepared as follows:

Light green SF yellowish (A)	45 ml
Eosin yellow (B)	45 ml
Phosphotungstic acid	0.200 gm

All these solutions are kept in the refrigerator when not in use.

Automatic Staining

Automatic stainer can process a large number of smears with excellent results.

Autostainer: Slides held in rack are automatically rotated around baths containing stains and other reagents. Time schedule for staining as mentioned previously in manual process can be obtained by calibrating a timing dial. The reagents are renewed weekly. The instrument has the advantage that it can easily be adapted for staining techniques. It uses laboratory prepared reagents and it allows for complete adaptability in staining, times. After staining the slides are mounted with DPX.

Staining Method

a. *Manual process*

The fixed slides are transferred directly from the fixative into the following solutions:

1. 80 per cent ethyl alcohol	10 dips
2. 70 per cent ethyl alcohol	10 dips
3. 50 per cent ethyl alcohol	10 dips
4. Distilled water	3 minutes
5. Harris's haematoxylin	1 minute
6. Running tap water	1 minute
7. Hydrochloric acid (0.5%)	5 dips
8. Running cap water	1 minute
9. Dilute solution of lithium carbonate	1 minute
10. Running tap water	1 minute
11. 50 per cent ethyl alcohol	10 dips
12. 70 per cent ethyl alcohol	10 dips
13. 80 per cent ethyl alcohol	10 dips
14. 95 per cent ethyl alcohol	10 dips
15. Orange G-6	1 minute
16. 95 per cent ethyl alcohol	10 dips
17. 95 per cent ethyl alcohol	10 dips
18. EA-36	4 minutes
19. 95 per cent ethyl alcohol	10 dips
20. 95 per cent ethyl alcohol	10 dips
21. Absolute alcohol	4 minutes
22. Xylene	5 minutes

Slides are then mounted with DPX.

Results

Nucleus—blue
Cytoplasm of superficial cell— pink
Cytoplasm of intermediate cell—bluish green
Red blood cells—orange

Papanicolaou's Staining Schedule for Automated Stainer (Total Staining Time about 30 min)

Step No.		*Time in minutes*
1.	H_2O	1
2.	Harris's haematoxylin	3
3.	H_2O	1
4.	0.1 % HCl in 70% Ethanol	¼
5.	H_2O	¼
6.	% NH_4OH in 70% Ethanol	1
7.	95% Ethanol	1
8.	95% Ethanol	1
9.	95% Ethanol	1
10.	95% Ethanol	1
11.	OG-Modified	2
12.	95% Ethanol	1
13.	95% Ethanol	1
15.	EA-modified	3
16.	100% Ethanol	1
17.	100% Ethanol	1
18.	100% Ethanol	1
19.	100% Ethanol	1

20. Xylol	1
21. Xylol	1

Papanicolaou's Staining Procedure for Manual Set-up (Total Staining Time Under 7 Min)

	Regressive method	*Progressive method*
1. H_2O	30 dips (seconds)	30
2. Harris's Haematoxylin	60 dips	30
3. H_2O	10 dips	10
4. H_2O	10 dips	10
5. 0.1 % HCl in 70% Ethanol	5 dips	Not Necessary
6. H_2O	10 dips	10
7. 1% NH_4OH in	30 dips	30
8. 95 % Ethanol	10 dips	10
9. 95% Ethanol	10 dips	10
10. 95% Ethanol	10 dips	10
11. OG-Modified	30 dips	30
12. 95% Ethanol	10 dips	10
13. 95% Ethanol	10 dips	10
14. 95% Ethanol	10 dips	10
15. EA-Modified	60 disp	60
16. 100% Ethanol	10 dips	10
17. 100% Ethanol	10 dips	10
18. 100% Ethanol	10 dips	10
19. 100% Ethanol	10 dips	10
20. Xylol	10 dips	30
21. Xylol	10 dips	10
22. Xylol	10 dips	10

Combined Alcian Blue—PAS Technique for Acid and Neutral Mucins

Acid mucin and neutral mucin are clearly separated by this technique. It is also useful as a routine demonstration technique for the presence of any mucin. The acid mucins are first stained with alcian blue and are not available for PAS reaction. Only the neutral mucin is stained by PAS reaction which follows. In this way, a good colour distinction can be made between acid and neutral mucins.

Preparation of Stains

a. Alcian blue : 1 gm
   3% acetic acid : 100 ml
b. Schiff's reagent

Method

1. Wash the fixed smears in distilled water.
2. Stain smear with alcian blue solutions for 5 minutes.
3. Wash in water.
4. Treat with 1% periodic acid for 5 minutes.
5. Rinse in distilled water.
6. Place in Schiff's reagent for 10 minutes.
7. Wash in running water for 10 minutes.
8. Stain nuclei with haematoxylin.
9. Wash in water.
10. Dehydrate, clear and mount.

Results

Acid mucin—Blue
Neutral mucin—Magenta
Nuclei—Pale blue

Naphthol ASBI Phosphate Method for Acid Phosphatase

Acid phosphatase is demonstrated by an Azodye coupling technique which depends upon the hydrolysis of a substrate containing Alpha-napthyol phosphate. As hydrolysis occurs, the liberated napthol couples with a diazotised amine and forms an insoluble coloured precipitate.

Burstone (1958) recommended naphthol ASBI phosphate as substrate—the primary reaction product, produced by the enzyme hydrolysing this substrate is extremely insoluble.

Preparation of Solutions

a. *Substrate solutions*

Naphthol ASBI phosphate	10 mg
Dimethyl formamide	1 ml

b. *Buffer solution*

Sodium acetate	1.17 gm
Sodium barbitone	2.94 gm
Distilled water	100 ml

c. *Sodium nitrite solution*

Sodium nitrite	400 mg
Distilled water	10 ml

d. *Pararosanilin hydrochloride stock solution*

Pararosanilin hydrochloride	1 gm
Distilled water	20 ml
Concentrated HCl	5 ml

Heat gently, cool to room temperature and filter

e. *Distilled water*

Preparation of incubating solution

Solution (A)	0.5 ml
Solution (B)	2.5 ml

Preparation of incubating solution

Solution (A)	0.5 ml
Solution (B)	2.5 ml
Solution (C)	0.8 ml
Solution (D)	0.8 ml
Solution (E)	6 ml

A volume of 0.4 ml of solution C and solution D mixed together and allowed to stand for 2 minutes before adding to incubating solution

The pH should be between 4.7 and 5.0 it is adjusted with 0.1 N NaOH.

Method

1. Incubate smears at 37°C for 60 minutes
2. Wash in water
3. Counterstain in 2% methyl green (chloroform extracted).
4. Wash in running water
5. Dehydrate clear and mount

Results

Acid phosphatase activity : Red
Nuclei : Green

Alkaline Phosphatase: Azo Dye Coupling Method Using Alpha Naphthyl Phosphate

Fixation

Formol calcium at 4°C
Formol vapour

Preparation of incubating medium

Sodium naphthyl phosphate	10 mg
0.2M Tris buffer (Stock solution A) pH	10 ml
Diazonium salt (fast red TR)	10 mg

The final pH of the incubating medium should be between 9.0 and 9.4. The sodium naphthyl phosphate is dissolved in the buffer, the diazonium salt is added and the solution well mixed. The solution is then filtered and used immediately.

Method

a. After fixation, incubate the smears at room temperature for 10-60 minutes.
b. Wash in distilled water.
c. Counterstain in 2 per cent methyl green (chloroform extracted).
d. Wash in running tap water.
e. Mount in glycerin jelly.

Results

Alkaline phosphatase activity : Reddish brown.
Nuclei : Green.

α-Naphthyl Acetate Method for Nonspecific Esterase

This method employs α-naphthyl acetate as the substrate, the enzyme releases α-naphthol during the hydrolysis of the substrate. The α-naphthol is then coupled with a suitable diazonium salt to produce an insoluble azo dye at the site of enzyme activity.

Preparation of Solutions

a. *Substrate solutions*:

α-naphthyl acetate	50 mg
Acetone	5 ml

b. *Buffer solution*:

Sodium dihydrogen orthophosphate	2.75 gm
Distilled water	100 ml

c. *Sodium nitrite solution*:

Sodium nitrite	400 mg
Distilled water	10 ml

d. *Pararosanilin HCl - Stock solution*:

Pararosanilin hydrochloride	2 gm
2 N-hydrochloric acid	50 ml

e. Distilled water.

Preparation of Incubating Medium

Solution	(A)	0.25 ml
Solution	(B)	7.25 ml
Solution	(C)	0.8 ml
Solution	(D)	0.8 ml

A volume of 0.4 ml of solution C and D is mixed together and allowed to stand before adding to incubating medium.

The pH should be 5.8 to 6.1.

Method

a. Incubate smears at 37°C for 20 minutes.
b. Wash in water.

c. Counterstain in 2% methyl green (chloroform extracted)
d. Wash well in water.
e. Dehydrate, clear and mount.

Results

Estarase : Reddish brown
Nuclei : Green.

Diaminobenzidine Method for Peroxidase

Preparation of Incubating Solution

3:3 - diaminobenzibine tetra-hydrochloride	5 mg
Tris buffer (pH 7.6)	10 ml
1 per cent hydrogen peroxidase	0.1 ml

Method

a. Rinse fixed smears in distilled water.
b. Transfer to incubating solution for 5 minutes at room temperature.
c. Rinse in 3 changes of distilled water.
d. Dehydrate clear and mount in DPX.

Result

Peroxidase—fine brownish granules.

Peroxidase Stain

Fixative—95% ethanol : 90 ml
40% HCHO : 10 ml

Preparation of Solutions

To 30 ml of 30% ethanol, add 0.9 gm of Benzidine, mix well and then add 3 ml of zinc sulphate (3.8%). A precipitate is formed then add 3 mg of sodium acetate and 4.5 ml of IN-NaOH (4 gm in 100 ml). The pH should be 6. Filter and store at room temperature.

Method

a. Fix the smear with fixative for one minute.
b. Wash gently with tap water and soak out the excess water.
c. Take 5 mlof staining solution and 3 drops of 3% hydrogen peroxide, mix well and cover the slide for 30 sec at 20ºC.
d. Wash the slide in running tap water for 10 seconds.
e. Counterstain with dituted Giemsa's stain for 2 minutes.
f. Wash with tap water then dried and mounted in DPX.

Results

Peroxidase positive seen as green granules.

Oil Red O Method for Lipids

It is a useful preliminary method to indicate two major lipid classes. For detailed morphology oil red O method is used with Mayer's haemalum.

Preparation of Solution

The working solution is prepared an hour in advance by mixing three parts of a stock solution of oil red O (saturated in 99% isopropanol) with two parts of distilled water and filtering just before use.

Method

Fix the smears in formalin vapour for 5 min and wash in running tap water for 10 minutes.

a. Rinse in 60% isopropanol.
b. Stain for 15 minutes in Oil Red O.
c. Differentiate in 60% isopropanol until a delipidised control section appears colourless.
d. Wash in water and counterstain nuclei with Mayer's haemalum for three minutes.
e. Wash well in water.
f. Rinse in distilled water and mount in glycerine jelly.

Results

Unsaturated hydrophobic lipids and mineral

Oil	red
Phospholipids	pink

Immunoperoxidase Staining

Introduction

This is an immunohistochemical technique, aimed at the specific histological localisation of particular tissue antigens by immunological method. These techniques are being increasingly used for diagnostic histology. The immunoperoxidase test which makes use of specific antibodies conjugated with horse radish peroxidase or alkaline phosphatase enzymes are now a days commonly used for histochemical detection of various antigenic markers.

Direct method: The primary antibody conjugated with enzyme, is used to react with the antigenic sites. The combined antibody-antigen complex with enzyme is developed with specific substrate. Tissues/smears are examined under light microscope to detect the substrate colour at the antigenic site.

Indirect method: It is more sensitive and commonly used. The specific primary antibody is applied directly to the tissues/smears. This is followed by the second antibody (antispecies specific IgG) conjugated with enzyme. The colour of the reaction is developed by using specific substrate and examined under light microscope.

Material

Peroxidase conjugated with antirabbit Igs, PBS (pH 7.2/0.2M), DAB (3.3 Diamino benzidine-4 HCl), normal swine serum, hydrogen peroxidase, antigen specific antibody raised in rabbit.

Indirect Method

1. Dewaxed paraffin sections are hydrated in usual manner. Where prefixed smears are used, these are washed with buffered distilled water.
2. Endogenous peroxidase activity is blocked with a fresh 3% solution of hydrogen peroxide in distilled water for 10-30 minutes or with acid alcohol for 15 minutes. For Cryostat, use acid alcohol or phenylhydrazine (5x10^3 M) for 15-30 minutes.
3. Wash twice with phosphate buffer saline *(pH 7.2, 0.2M).
4. Expose sections/smears to normal swine serum diluted 1:5 with buffer at 22°C, 5-10 minutes. Excess NSS/NGS is removed, without washing prior to stage 4.
5. Sections/smears are treated with optimally diluted primary rabbit antiserum at 22°C, 15-30 minutes or 24-48 hours at 4°C with highly diluted antiserum.
6. Treat sections/smears with horseradish peroxidase labelled swine/antirabbit IgG 1:20-1:100 for 15-30 minutes at 22°C.
7. Wash twice with phosphate buffer saline* (pH 7.2). The end product is revealed with a freshly made solution of 0.05%, 3, 3-diaminobenzidine tetrahydrochloride (DAB) in 0.01% H_2O_2 in wash buffer.

Sections/smears are counterstained with a weak haematoxylin, dehydrated, cleared in xylene and mounted in DPX for the DAB or PDP reactions (brown to dark brown). Aqueous mountants, e.g. glycerine gelatine, are used for the carbazole reaction (red).

* PBS (Phosphate buffer saline) pH 7.2/0.2 M

Solution A:

(Sodium dihydrogen orthophosphate)

$NaH_2PO_4 . 2H_2O$—31.2 gm for 1 litre.

Solution B:

Disodium hydrogen phosphate

$Na_2HPO_4 . 2H_2O$—31.6 gm for 1 litre.

Working solution:

Solution A 70 ml + Solution B 180 ml. Make the volume up to 1 litre and dissolve 5.7 gm NaCl in a litre and filter before use.

Immunofluorescence

Principle: It is a histochemical or cytochemical technique for *in situ* detection and localisation of specific intracellular antigens. Specific antibodies conjugated with fluorescent dyes, such as fluorescein or rhodamine, are used to trace the specific antigenic areas on the tissue smear or section. This can be visualised under the fluorescent microscope, as bright purple green/red colour fluorescence.

A. *Direct Immunofluorescence*: In this method, conjugated antiserum is added directly to the tissue sections or viable cell suspension.

B. *Indirect Immunofluorescence*: It is more sensitive and commonly used. The unlabelled, specific antibody is applied directly to the tissue smears/sections, followed by a second antibody treatment, i.e. antispecies specific Ig conjugated with fluorescein or rhodamine and examined under UV-microscope. Due to the use of second antibody, the sensitivity and specificity of the reaction is highly improved.

Material: FITC/antihuman Igs conjugates, phosphate buffer saline (PBS), specific antibody, glycerol buffer, fluorescent microscope. Smear or section of tissue.

Method

1. Reasonably diluted antibody put on the antigen slide fixed in methanol for half an hour at room temperature in moisture chamber.
2. Wash the slide twice in PBS pH 7.2. All washes are carried out on a magnetic stirrer.
3. Incubate slides for 30 minutes with 1:20 diluted FITC (Fluoroscein isothiocynate) conjugated with Igs in PBS/pH 7.2* containing 0.01%. Evans blue as counterstain at room temperature in a moisture chamber.
4. Wash the slide twice in PBS pH 7.2.
5. Mount the slide with 90% glycerol buffer pH 8.6.
6. Examine the slide under UV-microscope. The antigen positive areas of the cell will show purple green fluorescence, whereas the negative area would appear brick red.

* PBS preparation described earlier.

AUTOMATION IN CYTOLOGY

A programmable cytocentrigue from WESCOR is available which can be used to prepare slide from any body fluid. With the help of cytocentrifuge sample cells, one can safely and quickly deposit a monolayer of cells on to a microscope slide for staining or any other processing.

This can be used on any of the body fluids, such as CSF, urine, synovial fluid, aspirates, washes, etc. and can be programmed as per the requirements.

CHAPTER 26

Microbiology and Bacteriology

In the following pages maximum stress is laid on diagnostic bacteriology.

CLASSIFICATION

Protophyta

Schizomycetes (Bacteria and related forms)

Actinomycetales: These members form elongated cells and have a tendency to branch, produces spores, not all are pathogenic to man

- Actinomycetaceae.
- Mycobacteriaceae.
- Nitrobacteriaceae.

Eubacteriales: This represents the true bacteria forms, classifiable as bacilli, cocci, or vibrios. Their staining reaction can either be gram positive or gram negative. Some are motile and possess peritrichous flagella. They multiply by binary fission. Widely distributed they can be saprophytes, parasites and many are pathogenic to human beings.

- Pseudomonadaceae
- Enterobacteriaceae
- Corynebacteriaceae
- Lactobacillaceae
- Micrococcaceae
- Spirillacea
- Bacteriodaceae
- Bacillaceae
- Neisseriaceae
- Brucellaceae.

Spirochaetales: These are slender, spiral shaped cells, aflagellate but move by flexing or whirling and spinning. Stainable by special stains only, they are free-living and include saprophytic and parasitic forms.

— Treponemataceae.

Microtatobiotes (The smallest living things)

Rickettsiales: Most of these are intracellular pathogens, and filtrable forms and need special methods of culture.

Virales

Thallophyta

These are the Molds and Yeasts.

BACTERIAL CELL CONSTITUENTS

Like other living cells, all bacteria possess the cell membrane, cytoplasm and a nucleus. Special characteristics are seen in certain strains.

Capsule: This is a protective outer covering layer possessed by some bacteria.

Flagella: These assist in locomotion, their arrangement may vary.

Spores: Under unfavourable conditions for growth sporing occurs. Spores are non reproductive. Upon return of favourable environment they are transformed into the reproducible vegetative form. Spores are spherical and have a distinctive placement within the cell. They may be central subterminal or terminal. Knowing their location assists in identification of species.

Inclusion granules: Some of the bacteria show inclusion granules. Volutin granules are metachromatic granules and may appear as aggregates of substances concerned with cell metabolism; when stained with toluidine blue, they stain a red violet colour in contrast to blue staining of the cytoplasm. These are considered to be made of polymerised inorganic phosphate. Lipid granules may be seen in bacteria and stained with sudan black. Polysaccharide granules stainable by iodine (like glycogen or starch) can be seen in cytoplasm of some bacteria.

Shape of Bacteria

1. *Cocci:* Spherical
   (a) Cocci in cluster—Staphylococci
   (b) Cocci in chain—Streptococci
   (c) Cocci in pair—Diplococci
   (d) Cocci in groups of four—Tetrad
   (e) Cocci in groups of eight—Sarcino.
2. *Bacilli:* These are cylindrical or rod shaped organisms. They can be of the following types.
   (a) Length of the cell equalling its breadth, called coccobacilli, e.g., *Brucella*
   (b) Chinese letter arrangement as seen in corynebacteria
   (c) Vibrio are comma shaped, curved, rods and are named so on account of their vibratory movement
   (d) Spirochaetes are relatively longer, thinner, flexible and coil shaped
   (e) Actinomycetes are the branching filamentous bacteria
   (f) Mycoplasma lack cell wall and hence have no definite morphology. They may be round or oval bodies with inter-connecting filaments.

Bacterial reproduction occurs by a simple process of binary fission.

Bacterial physiology: Bacterial physiology and biochemistry are studied by observing cultures grown in the laboratory on artificially prepared nutrient media. Various external factors influencing bacterial growth are—food, moisture, hydrogenion concentration, oxygen, carbondioxide, temperature and light.

1. *Food:* Bacterial growth is to large extent dependent on an adequate supply of suitable food material, the specific nutrient requirements vary from species to species. The important nutrient requirements are carbon, nitrogen, inorganic salts and for certain species, accessory growth factors of bacterial vitamins.
2. *Moisture:* For bacterial growth moisture is essential. Drying in the air damages bacteria.
3. *Hydrogen-ion-concentration or pH:* Most of the microbes growth better at a slightly alkaline pH (pH 7.2-7.6). Some acidophilic bacteria fluorish in acidic pH. Those needing strong alkaline medium are termed basophilic.
4. *Oxygen needs:* Most bacteria can grow in the presence of oxygen and air and also in its absence. Those which grow in the presence of oxygen are called aerobes, while those which grow in its absence are termed anaerobes. Those which can grow under both the conditions are called facultative anaerobes, whereas bacteria that can grow in complete absence of oxygen are named obligatory anaerobes.

5. *Carbon dioxide:* All bacteria need the presence of small amounts of CO_2 for growth, an amount provided by atmosphere or by the metabolic reactions occurring in the bacteria itself. However, some bacteria need a higher concentration of CO_2 (5-10%).
6. *Temperature:* For bacteria there is a range of temperature at which growth can occur. So there is a maximum, a minimum and the intermediate optimum temperature (at which the growth is most rapid). In the laboratory this optimum temperature is maintained in an incubator thermostatically controlled. Majority of bacteria grow between 25°C and 40°C and are termed mesophilic. 30°C is optimal for free living and 37°C is optimal for parasites in man or animals. Bacteria that grow best between 60 and 70°C are called thermophilic, while those growing best between 15 and 20°C are labelled as psychrophilic.
7. *Light:* Darkness is a favourable condition for growth and viability of bacteria. Direct sunlight is injurious to bacterial growth. Some bacteria can produce pigmentation on exposure to light and are called as photochromogens.
8. *Symboisis or mutual beneficial coexistence:* A living organism multiplying in a human body is called as a parasite and the person harboring is the host. When both the parasite and the host derive benefit from each other—it is termed symbiosis. Certain intestinal bacteria provide vitamins to their host without causing any pathogenic effects—a symbiotic relationship.

Products of Bacterial Growth

While thriving in a host or on an artificial culture medium, some bacteria produce substances that exert injurious effects in the host—these are called 'toxins'. In addition certain enzymes may be harmful to the host. Some bacteria produce pigments (harmless, help in bacterial identification).

1. *Bacterial toxins:* These injurious products of bacteria are of two types: (i) exotoxins (extracellular) and (ii) endotoxins (intracellular). Toxins diffuse readily from the living bacteria into the surrounding medium. They can be obtained from the medium after removal of the bacteria. This can be done by centrifugation or by filtering through a Seitz filter. The toxins remain in the supernatant fluid in the case of centrifugation and in the filtrate in the case of filtration. Certain gram positive bacteria secrete *exotoxins*, for example, Corynebacterium diphtheriae. Exotoxins are antigenic and are rapidly destroyed by heat.

   Endotoxins: These are toxins intimately associated with the cell wall of the most gram negative bacteria. They are released after death and disintegration of the bacteria. The majority of pathogenic bacteria produce endotoxins only. As mentioned in the previous paragraph for exotoxins—the endotoxins would be present in the residues and not in the supernatant (centrifugation) or in the filtrate (filtration).
2. *Bacterial enzymes:*
   a. Proteolytic enzymes: An enzyme responsible for decomposition of dead animal and vegetable matter in nature.
   b. Coagulase: This is often demonstrated during the study of biochemical properties of some pathogenic bacteria.
   c. Amylase: This enzyme is capable of splitting starch and is not much used in the study of bacteria.
   d. Lactic acid fermentation.
3. *Bacterial pigments*: Many bacteria have the capacity to produce pigments, e.g. *Staphylococcus aureus*—golden yellow pigment and pseudomonas pyocyaneus-green pigment. Certain pigments are restricted to the bacterial colonies while others can diffuse to surrounding medium.

KOCH'S POSTULATES

The etiologic relationship between pathogen and a disease is established by fulfilling Koch's Postulates, viz.

1. The pathogen must be constantly found in the body of host either alive or dead.
2. It must regularly be isolated and it must be grown in pure culture *in vitro*.
3. When such a pure culture is inoculated into a susceptible animal species, the typical disease must result.
4. From such experimentally induced disease the pathogen must be again isolated.

MORPHOLOGY AND STAINING REACTIONS

Bacterial identification is aided by their staining reactions. Simple stains are used to show the presence of organisms and the nature of the cellular contents in exudates.

1. *Loeffler's Methylene Blue:* Saturated solution of methylene blue in alcohol 30 ml. Potassium hydroxide 0.01% in distilled water—100 ml.

   Method

   Stain for three minutes after making and fixing the smear. This stain does not readily overstain.
2. *Dilute Carbolfuchsin:* This is made by diluting Ziehl-Neelsen's carbolfuchsin stain ten times its volume in water. The smears are stained for 10-25 seconds and are washed well with water. (Overstaining must be avoided here).

The two most frequently used differential stains are the Gram and Ziehl-Neelsen techniques

Gram's Stain

This is the most widely used but not a fully understood technique. Various theories put forward are:

a. It has been shown that gram-positive organisms contain a substance known as magnesium ribonucleate, which gram-negative organisms lack. If this substance is removed from gram-positive bacteria, they will react as gram-negative organisms.
b. When iodine is applied for staining with crystal violet or another stain of that group a compound is formed which is insoluble in water, but soluble in alcohol or acetone. It is said that the more permeable the organism (i.e. the more easily water and other fluids can pass through the cell wall) the more likely it is to be gram-negative, since the acetone or alcohol has easier access to the compound which it will dissolve.
c. It is also thought that the pH of the organism has at least some influence of the reaction. Gram-positive bacteria have a more acid cytoplasm and this is increased by the addition of iodine. According to this school of thought it is the acidity of the cytoplasm which helps the organism to retain the stain.

Method

1. Make a thin smear of the material or culture let dry at room temperature. Heating, should be avoided as this interferes with the staining reaction.
2. Pass the slide through a flame once or twice or until it feels comfortably warm on the back of the hand.
3. Place the slide on the rack and flood with the crystal violet or gentian violet stain—stain for one minute.
4. Wash off the stain with Gram's or Lugol's iodine and leave the slide covered with iodine for one minute.
5. Rinse in water.
6. Pour on acetone or alcohol till no more blue colour comes from the slide (Acetone does this more quickly than alcohol so care should be taken not to use acetone for a longer period). (Serous and mucoid material are more difficult to decolourise than saline suspensions and require a longer exposure to the decolourising agent).
7. Rinse in water again.
8. Stain with one of the following counter-stains: Safranin, Neutral red, or 1:10 Carbolfuchsin.
9. Rinse in water and allow it to dry by standing it vertically, or by blotting it with filter paper.

Results

Because the gram-positive organisms retain the crystal violet after decolourisation, they appear dark blue in colour. The gram-negative organisms are decolourised and take up the counterstain and therefore, appear pink in colour.

Reagents

1. Crystal violet-0.5% solution in distilled water.
2. Iodine-(Lugol's)-10 gm iodine, 20 gm potassium iodide in 1000 ml of distilled water. Dissolve the potassium iodide in 250 ml water and then add 10 gm of iodine. When dissolved make up to 1000 ml with distilled water (This solution is three times stronger than gram's iodine and is preferable).
3. Acetone.

4. Counter stain.
   (a) 1 gm Neutral red
   2 ml 1% Acetic acid
   Distilled water to make 1000 ml
   (b) Safranin
   1.7 gm safranin
   50 ml alcohol
   Distilled water to make 500 ml
   (c) Dilute carbolfuchsin
   1:10 dilution of strong carbolfuchsin.

Ziehl-Neelsen Stain

This stain is another method of categorising certain bacteria, depending on their ability to resist decolourization by acid and alcohol. A very strong stain is used, basic fuchsin in a phenol solution and heat is applied in order that the stain can penetrate the waxy covering certain bacteria.

Method

a. Make a smear of the material and allow to dry at room temperature.
b. Flood the whole slide with strong carbolfuchsin and heat gently underneath the slide until steam is seen rising from the slide. (Do not overheat, avoid boiling of the stain).
c. Rinse in water and flood the slide with 25% sulfuric acid. Leave this until the smear is pale pink in colour.
d. Rinse in water and pour on alcohol for a few minutes.
e. Counterstain with malachite green, methylene blue or picric acid.
f. Dry by standing the slide vertically—do not blot dry as the tubercle organisms may get attached to the paper and later may get transferred to another slide.

Results

The tubercle bacillus resists decolourising by acid and alcohol (i.e it is both acid and alcohol fast) it will remain bright red while all other organisms and material will take on the colour of the counterstain.

Modified Ziehl-Neelsen's Stain

Used for leprosy where the bacteria are less acid fast. The method is as mentioned above except that 5% Sulfuric acid is used instead of 25%.

Reagents

Carbolfuchsin:
Basic fuchsin 10 gm
Alcohol-100 ml
5% aqueous phenol-1000 ml

Decolourising agents:
25% sulfuric acid, or
5% sulfuric acid (for M leprae) or
Acid-alcohol 3% HCI in alcohol

Counterstains:
Loeffler's methylene blue or

Malachite green—0.05% aqueous solution or

Methylene blue—0.1% aqueous solution or
Picric acid-saturated aqueous solution.

RAPID TWO STEP COLD AFB STAIN (Courtesy: Tulip Group of Companies)

Novachrom

Summary

Infection with *Mycobacterium tuberculosis* remains a major public health problem. The epidemic of Tuberculosis and Multi Drug Resistant Tuberculosis reflects the failure of public health and social programs towards prompt treatment of infected cases and screening of high-risk population. While culture, isolation and sensitivity of *Mycobacterium tuberculosis* from patient groups using standard methods remain the gold standard for *Mycobacterium tuberculosis* detection and effective and swift treatment worldwide, Acid Fast Bacilli staining is the first line microscopic procedure performed towards this goal.

Reagent

Microxpress Novachrom is a Reagent for laboratory use only. Novachrom Rapid Two Step Cold AFB Stain comprises of:

a. NOVACHROM AFB stain (A)—carbol fuchsin
b. NOVACHROM AFB stain (B)—counter stain with decolouriser

Rapid Two Step Cold AFB Stain is provided as a ready to use stain set. It is used for screening of *Mycobacterium tuberculosis* from biological specimen such as sputum, CSF and urine. It is also used in the identification of *Mycobacterium tuberculosis* from isolated culture. It is a modification of Kinyoun's cold stain.

Principle

Carbol fuchsin forms acid insoluble complex with Mycolic acid present on the Acid Fast Bacilli and renders red/pinkish red colour to *Mycobacterium tuberculosis.* Other elements present in the smear take up counter stain (Methylene blue) and are stained bluish. NOVACHROM, Rapid Two Step Cold AFB Stain avoids the extra decolourisation step associated with traditional staining techniques as the decolourising component is incorporated within the counter stain. NOVACHROM staining system is simple to perform and very much reproducible. It has a sensitivity comparable to the traditional Ziehl-Neelsen hot staining method and also as compared to Acid Fast Bacilli culture results. It is a clinically proven, easy to use, time, labour and cost saving. This simplicity of staining makes NOVACHROM an ideal screening tool for *Mycobacterium tuberculosis.*

Storage and Stability

1. Store the NOVACHROM Kit at room temperature (25-30°C), away from light
2. Stability of the NOVACHROM Kit is as per the expiry date mentioned on the label.

Additional Material Required

Sterile plating loops (10 µl), biosafety hood with Bunsen burner, activated 2% Glutaraldehyde solution, distilled water, microscope with oil immersion lens, cedar wood oil.

Specimen Collection and Preparation

Collect specimen prior to use of antimicrobial agent. Wherever possible, indicate clearly that patient is on antitubercular drugs.

CSF: Collect as much as possible in a syringe, clean skin with alcohol before aspirating specimen.

Body fluids: Disinfect the site and collect specimen with aseptic precautions.

Sputum: Collect 5 to 10 ml in a sterile container from an early morning specimen of deep productive cough. For induced specimen use sterile saline. Have patients rinse mouth with water to minimize specimen contamination with food particles, mouthwash, or oral drugs.

Urine: As organisms accumulate in the bladder overnight, first morning void provides best yield. Collect midstream clean catch urine, first morning catheterisation/suprapubic taps in sterile containers.

Specimen Preparation

Proper decontamination and concentration of specimen containing normal microbial flora are crucial to detection of *Mycobacterium tuberculosis.* Specimen obtained from sterile sites such as CSF, peritoneal or pleural fluids do not need decontamination. However, since most specimens for Acid Fast Bacilli smear and culture are from respiratory tract and the mucous traps Acid Fast Bacilli and protects other organisms from decontamination and concentration, decontamination and liquefaction is a must Most satisfactory for this purpose is a combination of N-acetyl - L cysteine (mucolytic agent) and 2% NaOH (decontaminant)—(available as LYFECTOL from Microxpress). Petroffs method of decontamination can also be used.

Test Procedure

For direct sputum screening use 10 µl of purulent sputum or use 10 µl of decontaminated and concentrated specimen.

1. Place the specimen under test on a clean, scratchless glass slide using a sterile plating loop.
2. Spread by tracing concentric circles well separated over an area of 200 mm square (200 mm × 1 mm), take care as to not to reach the edge of the slide. Alternatively for dense mucoid specimen press the specimen between two glass slides and pull apart gently to form a thin film of mucous.
3. When the smear is completed, plunge the inoculating loop into liquid disinfectant (2% Glutaraldehyde) and shake to remove any sputum, then flame sterilise loop.
4. Air-dry the smear.
5. Fix the smear by passing the slide approximately three times on the flame.
   (Note: While passing the smear slide on the flame see that the side opposite the smear is facing the flame).
6. Mix well and add NOVACHROM AFB stain (A) over the smear to cover it completely (4-5 drops ≈ 0.2 ml, may be required)
7. Keep for 6 minutes and then rinse with plenty of distilled water slowly to remove excess of NOVACHROM AFB stain (A).

8. Tilt slide to drain, mix well and add NOVACHROM AFB stain (B) over the smear to cover it completely (4-5 drops ≈ 0.2 ml, may be required).
9. Keep for 6 minutes and then rinse the smear once more with distilled water to remove excess of NOVACHROM AFB stain (B).
10. Air-dry and observe under oil immersion (magnification 10. X).

Interpretation of Results

1. Presence of pink to red coloured slender Bacilli - Smear Acid Fast Bacilli positive.
2. Absence of pink to red coloured slender Bacilli - Smear Acid Fast Bacilli negative.
3. Pus cells and other bacteria stain purple to blue colour.

Grading of results

After 5 minutes of examination covering about 10 fields.

Number of Acid Fast Bacilli observed	*Report*
No Acid Fast Bacilli	Negative
1-1 Acid Fast Bacilli	Actual Number
-> 1 Acid Fast Bacilli	+
Masses of Acid Fast Bacilli in several fields	++

Remarks

1. Improper decontamination and concentration procedure will yield erroneous results.
2. Treat the specimens and used slants by immersing in 2% activated Glutaraldehyde for at least two hours before incineration and disposal.
3. Good laboratory practices and hazard precautions must be observed at all times.
4. Observe stain timings which are essential to obtain correct staining results.
5. Under stain or over decolourisafion may give false results.
6. NOVACHROM stains stored between 25°C and 30°C should not show precipitation.
7. Artefacts could be mistaken for Acid Fast Bacilli.

SPECIAL STAINS

Used to stain flagella, capsules, spores and granules.

Stains for Diphtheria Bacillus

Ponder's Stain

Toluidin blue 0.02 gm
Glacial acetic acid 1 ml
Absolute alcohol 2 ml
Distilled water to make 100 ml

Method

Spread the stain on the film for one minute and wash in tap water.

Result

Dark blue granules in pale blue bacillus

Albert's Stain

Solution I	Toluidin blue	0.15 gm
	Malachite green	0.2 gm
	Glacial acetic acid	1 ml
	95% alcohol	2 ml
	Distilled water	100 ml

Dissolve the dyes in alcohol and add to the water and acetic acid. Let stand for one day and filter.

Solution II	Iodine	2 gm
	Potassium iodide	3 gm
	Distilled water	300 ml

Method

Apply solution I for 3 to 5 minutes wash in tap water, blot and dry. Apply solution II for one minute wash, blot and dry.

Result

The granules stain bluish black, the cytoplasm green and other organism light green.

Modified Neisser's Method

Neisser's methylene blue:

Methylene blue	1 gm
Ethyl alcohol (95%)	50 ml
Glacial acetic acid	50 ml
Distilled water	1000 ml

Method

a. Stain with Neisser's methylene blue for 3 minutes.

b. Wash off with iodine solution used in Gram's method and leave some solution on the slide for one minute.
c. Wash in water and counterstain with neutral red solution used in Gram's method for 3 minutes.
d. Wash in water and dry.

Result

The bacilli show deep blue granules, the remainder of the organism assumes a pink colour.

Staining of Capsules

Hiss's Method

a. Saturated alcoholic solution of basic fuchsin or gentian violet 1 part to distilled water 19 parts.
b. 20% aqueous copper sulphate solution.

Method

Place a few drops of solution (a) on slide. Heat to steaming and leave on slide 30 seconds.

Wash off with solution (b).

Result

Capsule appears as faint blue halo around dark purple cell.

India Ink Method

The capsule is seen as a clear halo around the microorganism against the black background. This method may be used for demonstrating cryptococci.

Staining of Spores

Modified Ziehl-Neelsen's Method

1. Ziehl-Neelsen's carbolfuchsin
2. Sulfuric acid 0.5% or methylated spirit.
3. Loeffler's methylene blue.

Method

1. Stain with carbolfuchsin for 5-10 minutes, heating until steam rises.
2. Wash in tap water.
3. Decolourise with 0.5% sulfuric acid or methylated spirit. If the acid is stronger than 1%, spores of many bacilli are decolourised.
4. Wash in tap water. Now the smear is examined and if both bacilli and spores are red, it is decolourized again. If the spores alone are stained, it is counterstained. Let the counterstain to act for 2 minutes. Wash in water, blot and dry.

Result

The spores are stained bright red and the bacilli blue.

Staining of Spirochaetes

Fontana's Method

(a) Fixative	Acetic acid	1 ml
	Formalin	2 ml
	Distilled water	100 ml
(b) Mordant	Phenol	1 gm
	Tannic acid	5 gms
	Distilled water	100 gms

(c) Ammoniated silver nitrate

Add 10% ammonia to 0.5% solution of silver nitrate in distilled water until the precipitate formed just dissolves. Now add more silver nitrate solution drop by drop until the precipitate returns and does not redissolve.

Method

1. Treat the film 3 times, thirty seconds each time, with the fixative.
2. Wash off the fixative with absolute alcohol to act for 3 minutes.
3. Drain off the excess of alcohol and carefully burn off the remainder until the film is dry.
4. Pour on the mordant, heating till steam rises and allow to act for 30 seconds.
5. Wash well in distilled water and again dry the slide.
6. Treat with ammoniated silver nitrate, heating till steam rises, for half minute, when the film becomes brown in colour.
7. Wash well in distilled water and dry.

Result

The spirochaetes are stained brownish black on a brownish yellow background.

Staining of Fungi

Lactophenol Cotton Blue

Phenol crystals	20 gms
Lactic acid	20 ml
Glycerol	40 ml
Cotton blue/methylene blue	0.05 gm
Distilled water	20 ml

Dissolve the phenol crystals in the liquids by gently heating and then add the dye.

Take a portion from the fungal growth and place it on a drop of lactophenol cotton blue on a slide. Then place a cover slip over the drop and press gently. Blot to remove excess stain. Seal with varnish or nail polish.

Staining of Flagella

Loeffler's Method

Loeffler's Flagella Mordant

Tannic acid 20% aqueous	100 ml
Ferrous sulphate crystals	20 gm

Loeffler's Flagella Stain

10% alcoholic solution of	
Basic fuchsin	10 ml
Distilled water	40 ml

Method

Flood the smear with the mordant for 5 minutes. Wash with distilled water. Add heated Loeffler's Flagella Stain and allow to act for 3 minutes. Wash with distilled water and dry. (The slides should be very clean).

Result

Organisms stain red and flagella pink.

Negative Staining

Negating Staining is a technique by which organisms remain unstained against a dark background.

India Ink method

A small quantity of India ink 10% nigrosin is mixed with the material on a slide. A smear is made by means of another slide and the preparation is allowed to dry. The smear is examined and the spirochaetes are seen as clear transparent objects against a dark brown background. Capsules may also be demonstrated by this method.

MOTILITY OF BACTERIA

Hanging Drop Method

This method is used to observe the morphology but also demonstrates the motility of organisms. A special slide with a concave centre is used or else a ring of plasticine can be placed on the slide. A drop of the culture of bacterial suspension is placed on a coverslip. Vaseline is placed near the concave area of the slide approximately the corners of the coverslip. The slide is placed over the coverslip so that the drop of culture is directly under the concave area and the vaseline adheres to the coverslip.

The slide is then quickly inverted and placed under the microscope Motile organisms will be seen darting through the medium in which they are suspended. Motility should be differentiated from Brownian movement which is caused by bombardment of the molecules of the fluid. In motility the organisms move in a definite direction, whereas in Brownian movement they show no direction.

CULTURE

Four factors are to be taken into account

1. Media providing optimum growth.
2. Temperature.
3. Atmosphere.
4. Cultural characteristics, e.g. size, shape and pigmentation of colonies.

Media

Media can be (a) basic (b) enrichment (c) selective and (d) indicater media.

1. *Basic media:* These contain the necessary constituents for growth— meat extract, peptone and salt, and these are nutrient broth (liquid) or nutrient agar (solid). Many organisms would grow on these type of media and need no other factors.
2. *Enrichment media:* Are used for organisms which need an additional source of nutrition. This can be done by adding blood or serum to the nutrient agar or broth. An enrichment medium used for growth of the *Mycobacterium tuberculosis* contains eggs.
3. *Differential and selective media:* These media by virtue of their chemical composition inhibit the growth of some organisms while at the same time support the growth of others. Examples: eosin-methylene blue agar and MacConkey agar contains lactose and dye or an indicator in the decolourised state. Bacteria which ferment lactose with the production of acid will produce red colour or colonies with metallic sheen differen-

tiates the lactose fermenting coliform bacilli from colonies of lactose non-fermenting organisms. Some media which are used are also highly selective in their action on other organisms. Such media as S.S. agar, desoxycholate citrate agar and bismuth sulphite agar will inhibit the growth of the majority of coliform bacilli along with many strains of proteus and will permit the successful isolation of enteric pathogens. Tellurite glycerin agar and mannitol salt agar are selective media for the isolation of coagulase positive *Staphylococcus* from material containing other organisms. Phenyl-ethyl-alcohol agar is a selective medium for the isolation of gram-positive cocci in specimens or cultures contaminated with gram-negative organisms particularly proteus. Infusion agar containing potassium tellurite and blood/serum inhibits the growth of normal throat commensals and encourages the growth of *C. diphtheriae*. Some medias make use of the selective antimicrobial activity of some antibiotics and are useful for isolating certain pathogenic organisms from material containing mixed flora. Sabouraud dextrose agar containing cyclohexamide and chloramphenicol will support the growth of dermatophytes and most fungi, while markedly inhibiting the growth of many saprophytic fungi and bacteria.

4. *Indicator media:* These are largely used for biochemical reactions. The most common example is sugar media containing various carbohydrates such as glucose, lactose, maltose etc. Christensen's urea medium is used mainly in the identification of *Proteus* which has the ability to hydrolyse the urea and consequently because of the presence of phenolphthalein in the medium, a change of colour is produced.

Temperature

Most bacteria, pathogenic in humans, give optimum growth when incubated at body temperature, i.e., 37°C. Some saprophytes, however, grow best at lower temperatures, even as low as 4°C and others at high temperatures. The latter are known as thermophilic bacteria and are used in testing effectiveness of sterilisation techniques.

Atmosphere

Most organisms need oxygen for growth and are incubated in normal atmospheric conditions. Some pathogens, e.g. tetanus bacilli, will grow only in the absence of oxygen. This is achieved by using McIntosh and Fildes' jar, a thick metal or glass jar with a metal lid which can be clamped down tightly by bolts. On this lid are 2 holes-one an air inlet and the other an outlet. There are also 2 electric terminals. On the underside of the lid is a piece of asbestos saturated with palladium and covered by wire gauze. This is connected to the terminals, and acts as a catalyst in combining any oxygen still present after evacuation of the jar with the hydrogen which is passed into the jar.

The method is given below.

1. Keep the plates upside down in the jar.
2. Place in the jar an indicator-equal parts of 10% NaOH, 6% glucose and 0.5% methylene blue, boiled until the solution becomes colourless. It should remain colourless throughout incubation. If it turns to its original blue colour during incubation, complete anaerobiosis (oxygenless state) has not been achieved.
3. Tightly clamp down the lid.
4. Open the air outlet valve and close the air inlet valve.
5. Attach the apparatus to an exhaust pump, and slowly evacuate the jar. (If a glass jar is used, it should be evacuated while enclosed in a padded box to avoid danger of explosion).
6. Allow hydrogen obtained from hydrogen cylinders or Kipp's apparatus in through the inlet valve after closing the outlet valve.
7. Attach the terminals to the main current and leave for 20 minutes. This heats the palladiumized asbestos to assist the combination of hydrogen with any remaining oxygen.
8. Allow a little more hydrogen in via the inlet valve.
9. Put the jar in the incubator overnight. The present day McIntosh-Filde's jars have room temperature catalysts and need no electrical charge. They are left at room temperature for 15-30 minutes before allowing more hydrogen into the jar. *There are other, less complicated methods of achieving anaerobiosis (i.e., an oxygenless state) e.g.*
   1. Boil a tube of nutrient broth and layer over it sterile vaseline. The boiling removes the oxygen and the vaseline prevents more entering as the broth cools. The tube is inoculated using a sterile pasteur pipette.

2. A sterile iron nail placed in glucose broth which has been treated as in method (1), will maintain anaerobic conditions for some time.
3. Robertson's cooked meat medium and Brewer's thioglycollate broth are frequently used in the culture of anaerobic organisms.

Some organisms are not anaerobic, but do grow better when the amount of oxygen has been reduced. One simple technique is to place the plates in a tin or wide mouthed bottle with a tight fitting lid. A candle is lit inside the container and the lid replaced firmly. The candle flame will use off the oxygen and give an atmosphere of 5-10% CO_2. The container is placed in the incubator.

Cultural Characteristics

Bacteria grown artificially (*in vitro*) on agar plates are described as colonies. These colonies vary in size, shape, pigment production, and haemolysis on blood agar depending on the type of media.

Colonies are described as:

1. *Shape:* Circular, regular, radiating or rhizard.
2. *Surface:* Smooth, rough, fine, granular shiny, dull, etc.
3. *Size:* Usually colonies are 2-3 mm in diameter, smaller ones may be less than 1 mm.
4. *Contiguity:* Colonies may be discrete or swarming.
5. *Consistency:* May be mucoid, tenacious dry or adherent to the medium.
6. *Pigmentation:* Some organisms produce pigmented colonies (*Staphylococci, Pseudomonas*).
7. *Opacity:* On nutrient agar they may be transparent, translucent or opaque.
8. *Elevation:* Colonies may be raised, low convex, umblicated or dome shaped.
9. *Media changes:* Colonial growth may bring about colour changes in the media themselves, e.g. hemolysis on blood agar by haemolytic streptococci. With Pseudomonas the green pigment produced may diffuse into the medium.

Biochemical Reactions

Organisms that are alike in microscopic and cultural characteristic are often differentiated by their reactions in various biochemical tests.

1. *Sugar fermentation:* Specific carbohydrate fermentation is a property of some organisms when grown in sugar media. Sugars most frequently employed are glucose, sucrose, lactose, mannite, maltose and dulcite. Usually these are incorporated into peptone water, but for the more delicate organisms, Hiss's serum water must be used. Meningococci and gonococci will only react in solid serum-sugar media. Each sugar medium has a coloured stopper and a set 'colour scheme' may be established for the following sugars.
   Glucose (green), Lactose (red), Sucrose (blue), Mannite (mauve), Maltose (blue and white), Dulcite (pink).
   The organism ferments sugar and produces acid and, in certain groups, gas. Acid production is indicated by a colour change of the medium, due to inclusion of a pH indicator. Gas production is shown by placing a small Durham's tube upside down in the medium during its production. Before inoculating the medium the tube should be completely filled with the medium. If gas is produced, small bubbles of gas will be seen in the inverted tube.
2. *Other biochemical tests:* Organisms may further be identified biochemically by their production of indole, change in pH (as shown by the methyl red test), by their utilisation of citrate and by another test called the Voges-Proskauer reaction. These 4 tests are especially useful in the differentiation of intestinal pathogens.

Serology

Bacteriologic diagnosis can also be confirmed by estimating antibodies to specific antigens of the bacteria. Examples: VDRL and Kahn tests for syphilis. ASO for β-haemolytic streptococci and Widal for typhoid.

PREPARATION OF CULTURE MEDIA

Anything used for preparing culture media should be free from living organisms. All media prepared should be sterilised according to instructions for each type of media. pH adjustment should be correct for all media. Since most organisms grow at a slightly alkaline pH, it should therefore be adjusted between pH 7.2-7.6. Time can be saved by using dehydrated culture media: as per the manufacturer's instructions, weigh the dehydrated medium, add the requisite amount of boiled distilled water, mix the two and sterilise the solution. Given below are methods for preparation of culture media

Peptone Water

This medium is used for the testing of indole production, for the preparation of sugar media, and when made highly alkaline (pH 8.0-8.4) is used for the cultivation of *Vibrio cholerae.*

Peptone	10 gm
Sodium chloride	5 gm
Distilled water	1000 ml

Dissolve by steaming. Adjust the pH to 7.5. Filter through paper. Distribute in tubes or bottles. Sterilise at 15 lb. pressure for 20 minutes. The commercially available peptone water consists of water soluble products obtained from lean meat or other protein materials by digestion mainly with a proteolytic enzyme like pepsin, trypsin or papain. The important constituents are peptones, proteoses, amino acids and inorganic salts.

Nutrient Broth

Peptone	10 gm
Sodium chloride	5 gm
Meat extract	10 gm
Distilled water	1000 ml.

Mix the ingredients and allow to dissolve (can be accomplished by steaming it). Adjust pH to 7.6. Phosphates may precipitate out and should be extricated by filtration. Distribute the medium in large bottles and then sterilize at 15 lb. for 20 minutes. *When 1% glucose is added to this nutrient broth it becomes glucose broth.*

Nutrient Agar

Agar-agar, is a long chain polysaccharide substance from certain seaweeds. It forms a firm gel in watery solution at concentrations of about 2%. Agar alone has no nutritive properties. It melts at about 95°C and solidifies only when cooled.

To the nutrient broth add 2% of agar—it then becomes nutrient agar. After addition of 2% agar, autoclave at 15 lb. for 20 minutes. Clear with white of egg. Autoclave and filter. Distribute into flasks and sterilise at 15 lb. for 20 minutes.

Blood Agar

Melt the nutrient agar and cool to 50°C. Aseptically add 5-10% sterile defibrinated blood. Mix and pour into petridishes or tubes which are sloped. Bank blood or rabbit blood may be used.

Chocolate Agar

Add blood to nutrient agar as for blood agar. Mix well and raise the temperature to 80°C keeping well mixed. Leave at 80°C for 10 minutes. Pour into petridishes or tubes as needed.

Sugar Media

Sugar media are used to study the biochemical reactions of bacteria. To sterilized peptone water add 1% of the required sugar and 1% Andrade's indicator. Distribute into sterile tubes containing inverted Durham's fermentation tubes. Indicator is used to study the acid formation by bacteria. If acid is produced media becomes reddish pink. Instead of Andrades indicator the following indicators can also be used.

Neutral red 0.25% to 1% solution—if acid is produced—pink colour.

Phenol red 0.01%—if acid is produced—yellow colour.

The sugar media are sterilised by fractional sterilisation or tyndallisation. The sugar may be carmolised or charred at a temperature higher than 100°C, so it is steamed on three consecutive days in Arnold's steam steriliser.

Preparation of Andrade's Indicator

Dissolve 0.5 gram of acid fuchsin in 100 ml of distilled water. Add 16 ml of normal Sodium Hydroxide (NaOH) and leave overnight. The colour should change from pink to brownish red and then to yellow.

Hiss's Serum Water Sugars

This is used for biochemical reaction of Neisseriae. Corynebacterium and other organisms requiring serum for growth.

Ox serum	1 part
Distilled water	3 part

Adjust reaction to pH 7.5 and Andrades indicator 1% and sugar 1%. Sterilise as for peptone water/sugar media.

Loeffler's Serum Slopes

(Used for cultivating diphtheria bacilli)

Ox serum	3 parts
Glucose broth 1%	1 part

Blood is collected from ox under sterile conditions and serum separated aseptically. Inspissate the medium at 75°C for 1 hour.

Media for Identification of Fungi

Sabouraud's Glucose Agar

Glucose	40 grams
Peptone	10 grams
Agar	20 grams
Water to	1000 ml

Dissolve peptone in water and adjust the pH to 5.4. Add agar and melt it at 15 lb. for 20 minutes. Then add glucose and sterilise by fractional sterilisation.

READY TO POUR, STERILISED POUCHED MEDIA FOR MICROBIOLOGICAL APPLICATIONS (Courtesy: Tulip Group of Companies

Instaprep

Summary

Cultivation and isolation of bacteria from pathological samples is many a times key to the identification of the underlying infections. With ever increasing strains of resistant microorganisms, susceptibility testing to antimicrobials agents complements selecting appropriate drugs/drug regimens to treat infections.

Availability of microbiology testing and such procedures being available in routine laboratories has been limited due to the availability of dehydrated media which can be put to use only after substantial procedural and preparatory requirements. INSTAPREP media are ready to use/ready to pour and fill this long felt need using a unique proprietary technology for routine microbiological testing.

Reagent

MICROXPRESS INSTAPREP are Reagents for laboratory use only.

INSTAPREP is a ready to pour sterilised pouched media for microbiological applications such as cultivation/isolation/selective growth/susceptibility tests.

Nutrient Agar

Nutrient Agar is used as a general culture medium. It can be used for maintaining microorganisms for prolonged survival of cultures. It can be used for cultivation of nor fastidious organisms. Addition of sheep blood/or serum makes it suitable for cultivation of related fastidious organisms. The poured medium is light straw coloured, slightly opalescent with a pH at 7.4 ± 0.2. Product Code: NA

MacConkey Agar

MacConkey Agar is the standard medium for the cultivation of enterobacteria. It is a selective and differential medium. It contains a bile salt to inhibit non intestinal bacteria with neutral red to distinguish the lactose fermenting conliforms from the lactose non fermenting *Salmonella* and *Shigella* species. The poured medium is a distinct dear reddish brown colour with a pH at 7.4 ± 0.2.

CLED Agar with Andrade's Indicator

CLED Agar with Andrade's Indicator is a medium of choice, recommended for use in urinary bacteriology as it promotes the growth of all urinary pathogens. Additionally since it is an electrolyte deficient medium swarming due to Proteus species is prevented and direct colony count is facilitated. For direct colony count the medium is inoculated by proper dilution of the sample. Additionally CLED Agar helps identify the organism directly from the first isolate based on colony morphology and colour within 24 hours. The poured medium is slightly opalescent greenish/grey with a pH at 7.5 ± 0.2. Product Code: CA

Sabouraud Dextrose Agar

Sabouraud Dextrose Agar is the standard agar for the cultivation and growth of fungi; particularly those associated with skin infections. The poured medium is light straw coloured slightly opalescent with a pH at 5.6 ± 0.2. Product Code: SA

Mueller Hinton Agar

Mueller Hinton Agar is the standard agar recommended for susceptibility tests using antibiotic sensitivity disks. Mueller Hinton agar is recommended by NCCLS and WHO Committee on standardisation of susceptibility testing for determining the susceptibility of microorganisms because of its reproducibility. The poured medium is light amber coloured to slightly opalescent with a pH of 7.3 ± 0.1. Product Code: MH

Principle

INSTAPREP ready to pour media are presterilised media with standard proven formulations. The pouched media only need to be kept in boiling (100ºC) water for ten minutes and they become ready to pour into sterile plates. A result of TULIP'S long research the INSTAPREP pouched media accord flexibility to the laboratories, thereby avoiding laborious preparatory steps and wastage. INSTAPREP media also help laboratories to set up cultures on a random basis and not to be restricted to batching of cultures. As compared to prepoured plates and dehydrated media, variability, contamination and wastage is also avoided.

Storage and Stability

a. Store the pouches at room temperature (25 and 30ºC).
b. Stability of the unopened pouch is as per the expiry date mentioned on the label.

Additional Material Required

Water bath (250 ml beaker) at 100ºC, vertical laminar air flow/biosafety hood with Bunsen burner, forceps/tongs, sterile petridishes (disposable/glass), scissors, disinfectant (70ºC alcohol), absorbent sterile gauze, plastic/glass/wire rod for hanging pouches in water bath.

Procedure

1. Retrieve the required number of pouches from the carton.
2. Gently squeeze the gelled media to the bottom of the (Dip side) pouch, upto 'SQZ' mark.
3. Hang the pouches vertically'using a hanging rod in a boiling water bath (at 100ºC) with the 'DIP side into the water and the water level upto the 'MAX' mark, for 1 minutes. Ensure that the heat source is not directly applied to the pouch. Retrieve the pouches after 10 minutes. (In case rod hanger is not used for the pouches, remove the pouches using forceps/tongs). After retrieving the pouch it should be dried diligently with gauze and then disinfected. Any residual water from the water bath should not be allowed to drip on to the poured plate to avoid contamination.
4. Wipe dry the pouch corner at the 'CUT' mark and disinfect with 70 % iso-propyl alcohol (IPA).
5. Cut the pouch across the 'CUT' mark with disinfected scissors.
6. Prise open the opening at the 'CUT' mark, squeeze and pour out media aseptically into a sterile 9 mm (diameter) petridish, taking care not to splash or form air bubbles while pouring.
7. Cover the petridish and allow the poured media to set.
8. The poured plate is now ready to use.
9. The samples should be collected and processed asceptically before plating.

Interpretation of Results

1. Gramstain, biochemical or serological studies should be performed for the characterisation and identification of the growth.
2. For CLED and MacConkey agar the micro-organisms can be identified as in (Table 26.1):
3. For susceptibility tests on Mueller Hinton (MH) Agar the size of the zone of inhibition corresponds to the sensitivity of the micro-organism to the particular antibiotic.

Remarks

1. The temperature of waterbath must be at 100ºC to liquefy the media. Cooler waterbaths will provide lumpy, uneven media.
2. Since all Agar based media solidify rapidly, it is important that the minimum time be lost between retrieval of the pouch from boiling water bath and pouring asceptically into the sterile plates. This will produce evenly surfaced medium.
3. The poured plates on solidification can be used for plating specimens or for antibiotic susceptibility tests (Mueller Hinton Agar).
4. Good laboratory practices and hazard precautions must be observed at all times.
5. With CLED medium, use 10 μl urine inoculum

MEDIUM	Morpho-logy	E. coli	Proteus	Klebsielia	Candida	Pseudomonas	Salmonella	Shigella	Streptococci	Staphyloccocci
CLED	Colonies	Pink Regular	Green Irregular	Dull large mucous	White Regular	Colourless Convex	-	-	Pink regular	Pink regular
	Medium	Pink /Red	Blue /Green	Green /Grey	Pink	Blue /Green	-	-	Pink/red	Pink/red
MacConkey Agar	Colonies	Red Convex	Transparent Irregular	Pink large Mucous	- -	Transparent Irregular	Transparent Irregular	Transparent Irregular		
	Medium	Red	Colourless	Pink/red	-	Colourless	Original Red/brown	Original Red/brown	-	-

and observe the growth at 24 hours. The colony count multiplied by 100 will correspond to CFU/ ml of organism in the urine sample.

6. 15 ml media is sufficient for the standard 90 mm petridishes. In case smaller petridishes are being used more number of plates can be poured with a single pouch, proportionately.
7. The identity of the medium is imprinted on the sealing band as a product code, where as the lot. number is mentioned on the carton label.

MEDIA FOR GROWTH OF ANAEROBES

Thioglycollate Medium

To nutrient broth add 0.1% sodium thioglycollate.

0.05% powdered agar.

1% glucose.

1/500000 methylene blue. Sterilize at 10 lb. for 15 minutes. The sodium thioglycollate maintains anaerobic conditions present after autoclaving assisted by glucose and the agar which prevents convection currents in the medium; methylene blue acts as an indicator.

Robertson's Cooked Meat Medium

Mince 500 grams of fat free ox heart (fresh) and place in 500 ml of boiling distilled water and allow it to boil for some time. Drain off the liquid through a muslin filter and while still hot, press the minced meat in a cloth and dry partially by spreading it on a cloth or filter paper. In this condition it can be introduced into the bottle. Place about 2.9 gm of dried meat in a bottle and cover with 10 ml of nutrient broth or the infusion broth filtered from the meat to which is added 0.25% Sodium chloride, 0.5% peptone and pH is adjusted to 7.7. Put the caps on the bottles and autoclave at 15 lb. for 20 minutes. The material to be inoculated is introduced towards the bottom of the tube in contact with the meat.

MacConkey's Medium

(For enteric gram-negative bacilli)

Peptone	20 gms
Sodium taurocholate	5 gms
Distilled water	1000 ml
Sodium chloride	5 grams

Dissolve this in a steamer and adjust the reaction to pH 7.5. After this, add 2% agar and melt in the autoclave at 15 lb. for 20 minutes. Clear with white of eggs. Than add lactose 10 gms and 1% solution of neutral red, 7-10 ml to the media. Distribute in 200 ml flasks and sterilize by steaming on 3 consecutive days in the Arnold's steam steriliser. Organisms which produce acid from lactose e.g., *E. coli* form rose pink coloured colonies are called lactose fermenters. Non-lactose fermenters, such as *Salmonella typhi,* produce colourless colonies. Sodium taurocholate is a bile salt which inhibits the growth of gram-positive bacteria and promotes the growth of enteric gram-negative bacteria.

LOWENSTEIN JENSEN MEDIUM

(For cultivation and differentiation of human and bovine types of tubercle bacilli).

Mineral salt solution

Potassium dihydrogen phosphate	0.4%
Magnesium sulphate	0.04%
Magnesium citrate	0.1%
Asparagine	0.6%
Glycerol	2% (in distilled water)

Heat to dissolve. Boil the solution by placing a steamer for 2 hours and allow it to cool overnight. 600 ml is a convenient quantity to prepare. Asparagine gives the source of nitrogen and glycerol the source of carbon. To each 600 ml of mineral salt solution add 30 grams of potato starch.

A luxuriant growth can be obtained even without the addition of potato starch. Eggs are washed with soap water and immersed in 5% carbolic acid for half an hour. After this wash the eggs in distilled water and break them and filter. For 600 ml of mineral salt solution, 1000 ml of egg fluid is required. Add 40 ml of 1% malachite green solution to this solution. Inspissate the media at 80-85°C for 50 minutes on three consecutive days.

METHOD OF INOCULATION

Streak Plate Method

The streak plate if properly prepared offers a most practical way of obtaining discrete colonies and pure culture. But is of no use if plate is not inoculated properly. The plates may be prepared in advance in any desired quantity and stored in the refrigerator until inoculation. The agar surface should be free of water of condensation before the streaking is done.

Method I: This method is designed for culture from broth, agar plates or slopes.

1. Place one loopful of the inoculum near the periphery of the plate.
2. With a loop spread the inoculum over the upper portion of the plate.
3. Stab the loop into the agar several times and continue streaking overlapping the previous streak.
4. Stab the loop as before and continue streaking.
5. Flame the loop allow it to cool and overlap the last streak and complete streaking.
6. Lift the loop and streak the centre of the plate with zigzag motions.
7. Discrete colonies should be found in the central portion of the plate while additional importance on hemolytic activity may be gained from the effect of a reduced oxygen tension on the organism stabbed into the media.

Method II: This method of streaking may be used either for culture from solid media or for heavy broth cultures.

1. Select the wanted colony from a crowded plate or pick up growth from a slant with a needle. Streak this carefully on a restricted area of the plate. Flame the needle and put it away.
2. With the sterile cool loop make one light sweep through the needle inoculated area and streak with close parallel strokes the top one fourth of the plate surface. Flame the loop and allow it to cool.
3. Turn the plate and streak the remainder of the plate with the same loop. Avoiding any areas previously streaked.
4. Discrete colonies should appear in the areas which was last streaked.

Method III: This method constitutes a simple technique and is used for liquid culture largely but it may also be used for culture from solid media.

1. Place a loopful of inoculum near the periphery of the plate and cover approximately 1/4 of the plate with close parallel streaks. Flame the loop and allow it to cool.
2. Make one light sweep through the lower portion of this streaked area. Turn the plate at right angles and streak approximately 1/2 of the remaining portion without overlapping previous streaks.
3. Turn the plate and streak the remainder of the plate avoiding previously streaked area.
4. The appearance of this plate will resemble that obtained in method II.

PRECAUTIONARY MEASURES TO BE UNDERTAKEN IN A MICROBIOLOGY LABORATORY

The infected material obtained from patients is to be treated with utmost care. In fact, all individuals working in such a laboratory should wear laboratory coats, wear gloves, use nose and mouth masks and be immunized regularly for prophylaxis against communicable diseases. Outlined below are the rules which *MUST* be observed.

1. Have an air pressure flow (air curtain) at the entry and exit doors of the laboratory. Being expensives, if this can not be installed, the other precautions mentioned below are to be rigidly followed.
2. Change clothing before entering and leaving the laboratory. If this is not possible use a laboratory apron to be worn over the outdoor clothing.
3. After working with cultures, and always before one leaves the laboratory, hands should be well washed, first in some disinfectant solution and then with soap and water.
4. Do not eat or drink in the laboratory.
5. The pipettes graduated or pasteur, should be

operated with rubber teats, and should always be plugged at the mouth piece with cotton wool.

6. Do not use tongue to moisten gummed labels, envelopes, etc.
7. Discarded cultures and contaminated material should be placed in disinfectant for 24 hours or autoclaved before the containers are washed.
8. Wrapping from contaminated material should also be placed in disinfectant and not in the waste paper basket.
9. A bowl of strong disinfectant should be readily available on the working bench, so that supernatant fluids, etc. may be poured there rather than into the sink.
10. Wire loops should be sterilised before and after use and the mouths of tubes and bottles should be passed through the flame on opening and closing.
11. While working there should not be any current of breeze, hence fans should be off and windows shut.

SPECIMEN COLLECTION

As far as possible obtain specimens before the commencement of therapy. This is important especially for CSF cultures. Often a purulent CSF will reveal no bacterial pathogens on smear or culture when an antibiotic has been given within the previous 24 hours. A patient with enteric fever may show a negative stool culture if the specimen has been collected while the patient was receiving suppressive antibiotics. Another important factor for the successful isolation of organisms is the stage of the disease at which the specimen is collected for culture, enteric pathogens are present in much greater numbers during the acute or diarrheal stage of intestinal infections and they are more likely to be isolated at that time. Specimens should be inoculated as soon as possible. If it is not possible then refrigerate the specimens at 4-6oC. Swabs from wounds, urogenital tract, throat, rectum and samples of feces or sputum can be refrigerated for 2-3 hours after procuring them without appreciable loss of pathogens. Urine specimens may be refrigerated for 12 hours without affecting the bacterial flora. On the other hand, cloudy C.S.F from a patient with purulent meningitis should be examined immediately. Gastric washing, for culture of *Mycobacterium tuberculosis* should be processed soon after delivery as the Mycobacteria die quickly in gastric washing. Specimens submitted for isolation of viruses should be frozen immediately. Specimens of hair scrapings may be submitted for isolation of fungi may be kept at room temperature before inoculation. Sputum, bronchial secretions, bone marrow and purulent material from patients suspected of having a systemic fungal infection should be inoculated to appropriate media as soon as possible.

All receptacles (containers) for collection of specimens must be sterile otherwise contaminants from the container will also be grown.

URINE

Organisms found in a normal urine are staphylococci (coagulase negative), diphtheroid bacilli and coliform bacteria. The important pathogens are *Escherichia coli, Proteus, Citrobacter, Pseudomonas, Klebsiella. Moraxella, Acinetobacter, Staphylococcus, Streptococcus faecalis, Salmonellae, Mycobacterium tuberculosis,* etc. For non-tuberculosis patients a mid stream fresh urine specimen is good enough. Urine samples are streaked on Blood Agar and MacConkey agar plates. At the same time microscopic examination of the urine should also be carried out. Catheterisation is indicated only when a mid stream specimen (MSS) can not be obtained, if done—all aseptic precautions must be undertaken. Before collecting the specimen, the area is washed well with soapy water and dried and then the MSS collected. A Gram's stain should be done on the centrifuged sediment.

If tuberculous nephritis is suspected, a 24 hour specimen, or preferably 5 consecutive early morning specimens are sent to the laboratory. The specimens are centrifuged and the deposits pooled. A Ziehl-Neelsen stain is done and the deposits concentrated before culturing for tubercle bacilli.

EASYBACT Courtesy: Tulip Group of Companies

Chromogenic, Differential, Semi-quantitative bacteriuria collection and screening system

Summary

Urinary tract infection is one of the most common infections encountered in clinical practice. Cultivation and isolation of bacteria from pathological urine samples is many a times the key to identification of underlying pathogens. With ever increasing strains of resistant microorganisms, susceptibility testing to antimicrobial agents for selecting appropriate drugs/ drug regimens is routinely indicated. EASYBACT a ready to use CLED agar slants, fills this long felt need using a unique proprietary technology for routine bacteriuria screening.

Reagent

EASYBACT is a ready to use, pre-calibrated CLED medium with a pH indicator, for easy isolation, identification and enumeration of bacteriuria in urine within 18 to 24 hours. Colonies obtained from this medium can be further processed for antibiotic sensitivity testing directly using the plate method. The standard medium is slightly opalescent greenish / grey in colour. EASYBACT is suitable for urinary bacteriology and supports the isolation and growth of most common urinary tract pathogens such as *E. coli, Klebsiella, Proteus, Candida, Pseudomonas, Streptococci* and *Staphylococci.*

Principle

As the urine sample is voided/placed in the EASYBACT vial and subsequently emptied, bacteria if present get seeded onto the medium and start growing. EASYBACT has been calibrated to yield colony counts similar to the standard plate methods. EASYBACT has a double indicator system that allows differentiation of various urinary pathogens by differential colour formation within the colony as well as the medium. Study of colony morphology allows further identification. Since swarming of *Proteus* species is prevented on this media, this media is convenient for colony count.

Storage and Stability

(a) Store the EASYBACT slants at 2-8ºC, away from light. DO NOT FREEZE, (b) Stability of the unused slants is as per the expiry date mentioned on the vial/ carton labels, (c) Avoid jerks and vibrations while storage, shipping and incubation, (d) Upon opening, the medium must be put into use immediately.

Additional Materials Required

Incubator (37ºC), blotting/filter paper, activated 2% Glutaraldehyde solution.

Specimen Collection and Preparation

As pathogens accumulate in the patient's bladder overnight, first morning voided urine samples provide the best yield. Asceptically collect midstream clean catch urine or first morning catheterisation/ suprapubic taps in sterile containers. Fresh urine specimen is recommend for testing. Samples may be tested upto 3 hours when stored at 2-8ºC. If the patients can be explained clearly, EASYBACT vial may be used to directly collect the midstream clean catch samples.(Refer Notes for collection of midstream clean catch urine).

TEST Procedure

1. Retrieve the required number of EASYBACT vials from the carton.
2. Bring the slants to room temperature (25-30°C) prior to testing.
3. Label the EASYBACT vials appropriately with the patient's I.D.
4. Open the EASYBACT vial observing asceptic conditions.
5. Directly collect clean catch midstream urine into the EASYBACT vial or add urine samples from catheterisation/suprapubic taps into the EASYBACT vial, right up to the brim.
6. Empty the urine sample from the EASYBACT vial immediately, observing asceptic conditions.
7. In case small amount of urine is retained in the vial, drain the excess urine by ***gently tapping*** the mouth of the EASYBACT vial on to a fresh clean blotting/filter paper. This is done to ensure no excess urine remains on the slant/ in the bottle.
8. Recap the vial immediately.
9. Incubate the vial in an incubator, preset at 37°C for 18 to 24 hours, ***in an inverted position*** with the ***cap facing downwards***
10. Read the results at the end of the incubation period.

Interpretation of Results

Density Count: Read the density of the colonies as per the chart given below:

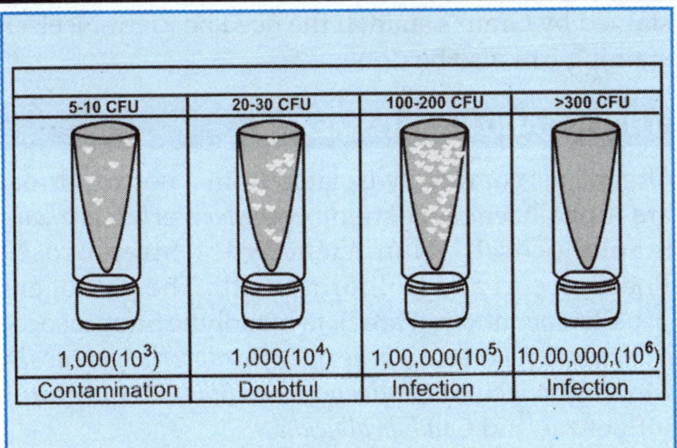

Identification of Bacteria

The pathogenic organisms can be identified as per the colour chart provided with the EASYBACT kit and the table mentioned below:

Remarks

1. Discoloured, dislodged, or contaminated medium should not be used.
2. Ensure that clean catch midstream urine samples are used so that surrounding external microbial flora do not give discrepant results.
3. Observe asceptic conditions while performing the test to avoid contamination with non-pathogenic bacteria.
4. Urine specimens should be collected and cultured immediately. Prolonged storage of urine samples at room temperature (25-3°C) may result in multiplication of contaminating organisms and raise the bacterial count leading to discrepancies.
5. Cultures of three consecutive first morning urine specimens are universally recommended since the reliability of the test increases to approximately 100 %.
6. Whenever possible indicate if the patient is on antibiotic therapy, since urine samples of patients on antibiotic therapy may not show bacterial growth or may have low colony count.
7. Treat the specimens and used slants by immersing in 2% activated Glutaraldehyde for at least two hours before incineration and disposal.
8. For confirmation and identification of the isolated organism, it is recommended to perform gram stain, biochemical or serological studies.
9. Good laboratory practices and hazard precautions must be observed at all times.
10. When performed correctly, EASYBACT results correlate with standard plate method using calibrated loop.
11. Optionally calibrated loops can also be used for inoculating the sample.

Notes

Procedure for collection of clean catch midstream urine samples. The objective is to collect a specimen, which will reflect as much as possible only the urine present in the urinary bladder.

Thus, a clean midstream void is recommended. Instruct the patient as follows:

1. Wash and clean the private parts with a dilute soap. Remove all traces of soap by washing with large quantity of water. Wipe dry.
2. Void out, into the toilet, the first stream of urine. This will flush out dead epithelial cells of the urinary bladder, microparticulates and normal microbial flora, which may have collected in the urine. Then hold the remaining urine in the bladder.
3. Next, void the second stream of urine aseptically into the EASYBACT vial right upto the brim. Again hold the remaining urine in the bladder.
4. Lastly, void out the remaining third stream, into the toilet.
5. This procedure ensures that the urine is voided as three discreet segments. (First stream to flush out contaminants, second stream as the clean midstream for test).
6. Follow instructions as mentioned in the Test Procedure for performance of the test.

	E. coli	*Proteus*	*Klebsiella*	*Candida*	*Pseudomonas*	*Streptococci*	*Staphylococci*
Colonies	Pink Regular	Green Irregular	Dullarge Mucous	White Regular	Colourless Convex	Pink Regular	Pink Regular
Medium	Pink/ Red	Blue/ Green	Green/ Grey	Pink	Blue/ Green	Pink/ Red	Pink/ Red

FECES

Most of the organisms which make up the intestinal flora in man belong to the family Enterobacteriaceae. These may include the intestinal commensals (the coliform bacilli and *Proteus* species) as well as the enteric pathogens of *Salmonella* and *Shigella*, intestinal streptococci, clostridia and various yeasts including *Candida albicans* may be present. The cholera vibrio may also be isolated.

Samples of feces should be sent to the laboratory in disposable containers, e.g. cartons of waxed cardboard which are incinerated after use. Since feces contain inummerable bacteria, and since selective media for enteric (intestinal) pathogens are almost invariably used, aseptic precautions are rather futile and unnecessary. It should be remembered, however, that where blood and mucus are present in the stool, this part should be especially selected for culture, since the pathogens are most likely to be found there.

The feces are inoculated into a solid bile salt medium such as MacConkey agar or desoxycholate-citrate-agar (DCA) and also onto Wilson and Blair's bismuth sulphite medium. Liquid media such as Selenite F which will inhibit the growth of the coliform bacilli or brilliant green broth which will enhance the growth of the pathogens: are also inoculated. These are all incubated at 37°C over-night. A Gram stain of the feces is of little value except in cases of fungi and staphylococci infections.

SPUTUM

The commonly isolated organisms from sputum are Pneumococci, Beta-Hemolytic Streptococci and *Mycobacterium tuberculosis*. If the culture for organisms other than *M. tuberculosis* is needed, all possible care has to be taken while doing so. Rinse the mouth with an antiseptic or clean water to avoid contamination from the oral cavity. The specimen should be collected in a wide mouthed sterile jar with a screw-cap lid. If the sample has to be concentrated when culturing for *M. tuberculosis*, there is less need for a sterile jar, in fact, disposable waxed cartons are preferable since they and their contents can safely be incinerated.

For routine cultures, a loopful of the sputum is inoculated onto one/two blood agar plates. When two are inoculated one is incubated in a 5-10% CO_2 atmosphere. A smear is made from specimen and stained by Gram's stain. If the need be Ziehl-Neelsen staining can also be done.

THROAT AND NASAL SMEARS

Organisms commonly isolated from a normal throat are Alpha-haemolytic streptococci, *Neisseria catarrhalis*, Staphylococci, Non-haemolytic Streptococci, Pneumococci and Coliform bacilli. The pathogens usually encountered are Beta hemolytic Streptococci, *Corynebacterium diphtheriae, Bordetella pertussis*, Meningococci, *Staphylococcus aureus*, Hemophilus influenzae and *Candida albicans*.

The sterile swabs should be first moistened with normal saline (sterile) and then rubbed over the infected area.

A blood agar plate is inoculated. A Gram's stain is rarely necessary except in cases where Diphtheria or Vincents angina are suspected. If Diphtheria is suspected the smears should by stained by Albert's, Ponder's or Neisser's techniques.

PUS SWABS

The infected area is carefully swabbed with spirit before the swab is taken, or the pus aspirated. Carry out a Gram's stain, streak on blood agar, MacConkey agar and then place into nutrient broth or, if anaerobes are suspected, into thioglycollate broth or Robertson's cooked meat medium. In cases of suspected gangrene or tetanus: two blood agar plates should be inoculated, one for aerobic culture and the other for incubation in an anaerobic atmosphere.

BLOOD CULTURES

Bacteremia is an important part of any systemic infection and hence, blood culture acquires similar significance. Blood culture permits the prompt commencement of specific treatment against the offending organism and may prove to be lifesaving.

Bacteremia occurs transiently in pneumococcal pneumonia, bacterial meningitis, urinary tract infections, enteric fever and generalized *Salmonella* infections. A mild transitory bacteremia is a frequent finding in many infectious diseases but a persistent bacteremia points towards a more serious infection. When the classic syndrome of a septicemia is due to pyogenic organism, chills, fever prostration is found, one rarely finds difficulty in isolation of the causative organism. In some diseases the chances of isolating bacteria from blood culture depends on the stage of the disease at which the culture is done. For example, bacteria can be cultured during the early course of the disease, thus the cultivation of the bacteria from the blood is important since it may be the only reliable means of making an early diagnosis available for the physician. A diagnosis of bacteremia can only be made by growing the pathogenic agents on suitable culture media. Perfect aseptic conditions must be observed while collecting blood for blood culture. Enriched aerobic and anaerobic culture media must be utilised in order to provide optimal conditions for bacterial growth. Commonly isolated pathogens from blood cultures are:

- Alpha and Beta hemolytic streptococci.
- Staphylococci, pathogenic and saprophytic.
- Coliform bacilli and related organisms.
- Pneumococci.
- *Hemophilus influenzae.*
- *Enterococci.*
- *Clostridium perfringens.*
- *Pseudomonas species.*
- *Bacteroides species.*
- *Neisseria meningitidis*
- *Salmonella species.*
- *Pasteurella tularensis.*
- *Leptospira species.*
- Pathogenic yeasts and molds.

Keep all the required things—the culture media (nutrient or glucose broth), spirit lamp, pen for labelling, etc.—by the bedside of the patient. Three bottles of broth should be incubated, on for aerobic cultivation, one for anaerobic and other for incubation in 5-10% CO_2. The site selected for venipuncture is well swabbed with cotton moistened in spirit and with tincture of iodine. The needle is fitted onto the syringe without touching the needle or the nozzle of the syringe. Blood is withdrawn—about 15 ml. After withdrawing needle from arm the needle is passed through the flame. Remove protective covering from culture bottle. The top of the screw-capped bottle is flamed and the needle inserted into the bottle through the rubber washer and 5 ml of blood is placed in each bottle. The bottle is again flamed and protective covering replaced on the bottle-top. The same procedure is carried out for each of the three bottles.

Once collected the cultures should be incubated at 37°C immediately and left overnight in the appropriate atmospheres. Subcultures are made every two days, either until growth is found or until 2 weeks have elapsed. Only after two weeks have elapsed can a report of 'No growth' be sent.

If the patient has already been on penicillin or sulphonamide therapy, penicillianse or para-minobenzoic acid may be added respectively. These substances will counteract the effect of any of the drugs present in the serum. Counteracting agents for other antibiotics are not yet known.

CSF, PLEURAL FLUID AND OTHER BODY FLUIDS

The aspirated material should be sent to the laboratory immediately in sterile tubes or bottles.

They are cultured on blood agar, aerobically, anaerobically and in 5-10% CO_2. Gram and Ziehl-Neelsen stains are done on smears prepared from centrifuged sediments.

Broth cultures should also be set up. The plates and subcultures of the broth should be incubated for 48 hours before reporting as negative (i.e. No growth). Organisms isolated from CSF are: *Hemophilus influenzae, Pneumococcus, Neisseria meningitidis, Mycobacterium tuberculosis, Staphylococcus, Streptococcus,* Coliform bacilli, Pseudomonas and Viruses.

EAR DISCHARGE CULTURES

Organisms isolated from the ear are:

Non pathogenic

- Coagulase negative Staphylococci and Diphtheroids.

Pathogenic

- *Pseudomonas, Staphylococcus, Proteus, Pneumococci,* Alpha and Beta hemolytic Streptococci and Coliform bacilli.

Material from ear is taken by swab sticks. Do a Gram stain and culture to a nutrient broth, blood agar and MacConkeys agar.

EYE CULTURES

Organisms isolated from the infections of the eyes are *Staphylococcus aureus, Neisseria gonorrheae,* Pneumococci, Alpha and Beta hemolytic Streptococci and Hemophilus. Purulent material may be obtained from the conjunctiva with the help of a cotton swab stick. This should be inoculated to blood agar and chocolate agar and to thioglycollate media. Chocolate agar should be incubated in a 10% CO_2 jar.

GRAM-POSITIVE COCCI

Staphylococci

Morphology

Gram-positive cocci, mainly arranged in cluster, but also found in pairs or singly.

Culture

Colonies measure 2-4 mm in diameter, and are thick opaque, shiny discs. Each species produces a characteristic pigment, e.g.,

Staph. aureus	golden yellow
Staph. albus	white
Staph. citrous	lemon yellow
Staph. roseus	pink

The organism grows well on basic media, can be grown on nutrient agar, milk agar and also on MacConkey agar, although on MacConkey the colonies are much smaller and appear deep pink in colour.

Coagulase Test

This test is employed to differentiate pathogens from non-pathogens. It depends on the production of an enzyme coagulase, which coagulates blood plasma. This test may be done in 2 ways.

1. *Slide test:* A suspension of staphylococcal colonies is made in a loopful of saline on a slide, and a loopful of undiluted plasma is added.
   Positive reactions are seen as 'clumping' of the suspension in a few seconds. In negative reactions the suspension remains uniform.
2. *Tube test:* The organism should preferably be cultured in nutrient broth overnight, but if urgent results are needed, a suspension made in broth can be used.

About 1 ml of the culture (or broth suspension) is placed in a sterile tube and an equal quantity of plasma (1/10 dilution) is added. The tube is incubated for at least four, but not more than six hours. If the tube is incubated longer, another enzyme fibrinolysin produced by the bacteria will dissolve the clot formed in a positive reaction, thus giving a false-negative reaction.

The tube test is more reliable as it has less false-positives. Negative control organisms should always be set up, which ever method is used.

Staphylococci liquefy gel and hemolyse blood.

Pathogenicity

Staphylococcus aureus is usually the pathogenic variety causing inflammatory lesions with pus formation e.g. boils, furuncles, blepheritis, pemphigus. It may also produce food poisoning due to enterotoxin.

Streptococci

Morphology

Streptococci are gram-positive cocci, arranged mainly in chains of varying length. They may be roughly divided into 3 groups by their effect on blood agar.

Alpha-hemolysis—a green colouration of the medium around the colonies, e.g. *Streptococcus viridans.*

Beta-hemolysis—a clear zone of hemolysis around the colonies, e.g. *Strep. pyogenes.*

Gamma-hemolysis—no obvious alteration of medium around the colonies, e.g., *Strep. fecalis.*

Culture

In culture, they are all small (1 mm diameter), discrete, shiny, regular and semitransparent colonies, *Strept. pyogenes* and *Strep. viridans* require blood or serum for growth, but *Strept. fecalis* will grow easily both on nutrient agar and MacConkey's agar. Another means of differentiating *Strep. fecalis* from the other two is by heating a broth culture or suspension of the organism to 60°C for 30 minutes. Only *Strep. fecalis* will withstand this heating and grow subsequently if cultured. Such means of differentiating are important, as *Strep. fecalis* may appear alpha or beta haemolytic and be mistaken for one of the other streptococci.

However, the most reliable way of differentiating the beta-hemolytic streptococci is by serological testing. Lancefield divided this group (of which there are many types) into several serological types, designated A-Q by precipitation reactions between the antigenic extract of the organism and antisera.

Pathogenicity

Strep. pyogenes: This frequently is a cause of sore throat, tonsillitis and scarlet fever. It may also give rise to cellulitis and also be responsible for infection of burns and septicemia.

Strep. viridans: This is usually a commensal in the upper respiratory tract but is sometimes the cause of subacute bacterial endocarditis, in which the organism is isolated from blood cultures (up to 3 successive cultures may be needed for isolating the organism).

*Strep. fecalis:*This is a commensal of the intestine, but is known to cause urinary tract infections or may be a secondary invader in such causes.

Pneumococci

Morphology

Diplococcus pneumoniae are oval shaped, gram-positive diplococci, the more virulent strains being capsulated. The diplococci are placed end to end, and in culture, may be arranged in short chains (usually).

Culture

After overnight incubation, the colonies appear similar to Strep. viridans, and show the same alpha hemolysis, but on further incubation the centre and edge of the colony become raised, with concentric rings.

The organism is aerobic and needs the enrichment of blood/serum for growth. Pneumococci may be differentiated from *Strep. viridans* by their solubility in bile salts (e.g. sodium taurocholate). When the bile salt is added to a broth culture of the organism, lysis can be observed within 15 minutes. The test may be carried out by adding 0.1 ml of a 10% solution of sodium desoxycholate to 5 ml of broth culture.

Other differences between Pneumococci and Strep. viridans.

Pneumococci	*Strep. viridans*
1. Soluble in bile	Not soluble
2. Sensitive to optochin	Not sensitive
3. Ferments inulin	Does not ferment inulin
4. Draughtman colonies	Small convex colonies.

Pathogenicity

Pneumococci are frequently the cause of pneumonia, empyema, meningitis. They also cause subacute-bacterial endocarditis and sometimes septicemia.

GRAM-NEGATIVE COCCI

Neisseria

Bacteria belonging to this group are gram-negative diplococci, arranged side-by-side and tending to be rather kidney shaped. Clinically three of them are important. viz. *N. catarrhalis*—a commensal in throat and upper respiratory tract: *N. meningitidis* causing meningitis; and *N. gonorrhoea* causing gonorrhoea.

N. catarrhalis

Mistakingly it was thought to cause catarrh but is no longer incriminated as the causative organism.

Morphology

In morphology, it is typical of the group, gram-negative diplococcus (sometimes also in tetrads) with long axes, parallel (i.e., side-by-side).

Culture

In culture, it differs from *N. meningitidis* and *N. gonorrhoea* is that it will grow at room temperature and needs no enrichment medium. Colonies are 1-2 mm in diameter, very dry and difficult to emulsify in saline. They have a wrinkled, shrivelled up appearance.

N. Meningitidis

Morphology

The morphology is typical of *Neisseria* group. They may be present intracellularly within neutrophils of CSF in a case of meningitis.

Culture

It is best to isolate them on chocolate agar in 5-10% CO_2 atmosphere. The colonies are approximately 1 mm in diameter, shiny, smooth and easily emulsified in saline. The organism can not grow at room temperature.

N. meningitidis and *N. gonorrhoea* can be distinguished from others by morphological and cultural characteristics alone by oxidase reaction can also be used for differentiating them. In this test, a weak solution of tetramethyl para phenylenediamine is poured over the culture plate. *Neissseria* colonies turn purple in colour, other colonies retain their normal colours.

(If subcultures are to be made, the colonies must be picked off from the medium, and subcultured onto another plate as soon as possible after the solution has been added).

Biochemical (sugar) reactions are best done on solid sugar media although the reason for this is still obscure. *N. meningitidis* ferments glucose and maltose.

N. Gonorrhoea

Morphology

The morphology is similar to *N. meningitidis*. Intracellular forms may be seen in polymorphs in the exudate from the gonorrhoeal sore.

Culture

Serum, blood or chocolate agar is used for the isolation of the organism. The colonies of which are very smooth, regular, shiny in appearance at first, but later become crenated at the edge, with a raised opaque centre. The colonies give a positive oxidase reaction. The organisms ferment glucose only, with best results obtained using solid sugar media.

Comparison of meningococci and gonococci

	Meningococci	*Gonococci*
1.	Ferments maltose and glucose	Ferments glucose only
2.	pH of the medium should be between 7.0 and 7.4	pH of the medium should be 7.5
3.	Causes meningitis, conjunctivitis, endocarditis	Causes gonorrhoea in the genitalia; conjunctivitis and arthritis.

N. gonorrhoeae is very susceptible to drying and hence, material obtained should be processed immediately. One may even take the plates to be streaked at the patient's bedside or else the swab may be placed in Stuart's transport medium and sent to the laboratory in this. If the samples have to be sent by post then the latter method is most suitable and ideal.

Veilonella

These are minute, gram negative, spherical diplococci found in the digestive tract and vagina. They are generally regarded as non-pathogenic but it is possible that at times they may be associated with disease states. They are anaerobic and produce acid and gas in glucose.

ANAEROBIC SPORE BEARING BACILLI

Clostridia

Clostridia comprise the gram-positive spore bearing anaerobic bacilli. some of them decompose protein and may form exotoxins. Majority of them are saprophytes in oil and a few are pathogenic to man.

Pathogenic clostridia

Tetanus—*Clostridium tetani*

Gas gangrene—*Clostridium welchii/perfringens, Clostridium novyi* and *Clostridium septicum*

Botulism—*Clostridium botulinum.*

Clostridium tetani

Clostridium tetani is causative organism of tetanus in man and animals. Tetanus is usually the result of contamination of a wound with *Cl. tetani* spores. The source of the infection may be soil, dirty clothing or dust spore of *Cl. tetani.*

Morphology

It is a gram-positive bacillus 2.5 x 0.4-0.5 and possesses a spherical terminal spore. The terminal spore gives it a drumstick appearance. *Clostridium tetani* is motile organism.

Culture

Cl. tetani is an obligatory anaerobe. It is readily grown on cooked-meat medium. On blood agar, under anaerobic conditions, *Cl. tetani* grows and produces hemolysis. In cooked meat medium, there is slight digestion and blackening of meat.

Clostridium tetani does not ferment any sugar. These bacilli, however, slowly liquefy gelatin. Coagulated serum is rendered more transparent and softened but is not liquefied. *Cl. tetani* is a proteolytic organism.

Clostridium tetani toxins are extremely harmful to man as well as animals. Man is, however, more susceptible to toxins.

Laboratory Diagnosis

The material is obtained from the wound.

a. *Microscopic diagnosis:* Material obtained from the wound is smeared on to a slide and stained by Gram's method. The presence of drumstick bacilli is suggestive of *Cl. tetani,* but it is not conclusive as other organisms having terminal spores as *Cl. tetani* may be present. Culture, therefore, becomes mandatory.
b. *Cultural techniques:* The most ideal medium for this purpose is the cooked-meat medium. Strict anaerobic conditions are a must. The cooked-meat medium is heated to 75-80ºC for about 20-30 minutes to destroy the vegetative organisms. After inoculation, incubate for 4 to 5 days. Make smears from culture, stain and examine for typical gram-positive bacilli with spherical terminal spores.
c. *Animal inoculation:* Toxin formation may be studied by culturing the organism in a suitable liquid medium and injecting the bacteria-free filtrate into a susceptible animal (white mouse) which will develop the signs and symptoms of tetanus. It is always necessary to use two animals, one with the toxin alone and the other which has been given a prophylactic dose of antitoxin.

Toxin produced

Tetanospasmin—is neurotoxin and tetanolysin — lytic for RBC's.

Gas Gangrene Causing Organisms

Gas gangrene is a massive necrosis of tissues with gas formation and associated with an extreme toxemia. The main factor in gas gangrene is infection by anaerobic bacteria which leads to the death of tissues and gas formation. The gas is produced by organisms by fermenting tissue carbohydrates, *Clostridium welchii/perfringens, septicum* and *novyi;* all belong to this group.

Clostridium welchii (or C. perfringens)

Morphology

It is a long rod-shaped gram positive bacillus forming a large oval and central or sub-terminal spore. It is non-motile.

Culture

Cl. welchii grows on all the usual laboratory media but needs strict anaerobic atmosphere and rather prolonged incubation, may need as long as 15 days. Best growth is obtained by using glucose agar or glucose blood agar. On cooked-meat medium it has a luxuriant growth, produces gas and a sour odour, the meat being turned pink in colour. On blood agar marked hemolysis is produced.

The organism is mainly saccharolytic with little or no proteolytic action. It ferments glucose, maltose, lactose and saccharose with formation of acid and gas. It liquefies gelatin. On coagulated serum medium their is no digestion or liquefaction of proteins. In litmus milk, *Cl. welchii* produces acid, gas and clotting. The formation of gas is so abundant that its action on this medium is referred to as stormy fermentation.

Toxins produced

Alpha, beta, epsilon, iota, theta, gamma, delta, etc.

Clostridium septicum

Morphology

This is a moderately large bacillus, with rounded ends and is motile. In the tissues it develops into large, swollen, gram-positive citron bodies. Spores are readily formed and are oval, central or subterminal and bulging.

Culture

It is an obligatory anaerobe which grows on ordinary media. Glucose promotes the growth of the organism. In litmus milk medium, slight acid is formed, and the milk is slowly clotted, but often the change is minimal. Gelatin is liquefied. In cooked-meat medium the meat is reddened but not digested. *Cl. septicum* may be associated with gas gangrene in man..

Clostridium novyi

Morphology

This resembles *Cl. welchii* morphologically, but is somewhat larger and more pleomorphic. The spores are oval, central or subterminal.

Culture

It is an obligatory anaerobe and grows well on ordinary media.

In litmus milk, late clotting may occur. It liquefies gelatin.

Clostridium novyi is associated with a markedly toxic form of gas gangrene in man.

Diagnosis of Gangrene

The bacteriological diagnosis of gas gangrene is usually combined with a general bacteriological examination of the infected wound with which this condition is associated. Specimens of the exudate should be taken from deeper parts of the wound and where the infection is most pronounced. These may be obtained in capillary tubes, but sterile swabs rubbed over the wound surface and soaked in the exudate, serve well for the purpose. At least 2 swabs should be taken from the wound, one for direct smear and another for culture. If there are necrotic tissue fragments in the wound, small pieces should be placed in a sterile screw capped bottle and used for microscopic examination and culture.

Microscopy

Gram's staining of the films should be done. If gas gangrene is present, gram-positive bacilli predominate and show subterminal spores.

Culture

The material is inoculated into cooked-meat medium. In this all organisms will grow. The mixed growth is heated to 75-80°C for half an hour and then plated on blood or glucose agar and incubated anaerobically. The single colonies are stained and studied by biochemical reactions.

Clostridium botulinum

This is the causative organism of botulism, a kind of food poisoning due to eating tinned meat or improperly cooked meat which had been previously infected with the bacilli. The organism is widely distributed in soil and may sometimes be found in the intestinal tracts of certain domestic animals.

Morphology

It is a fairly large bacillus, 4-6 μ long and about 1 μ thick, arranged either singly or in short chains. It forms an oval terminal spore which is thicker than the bacillus. It has slight motility.

Culture

It is a strict anaerobe. It grows well at low temperature of 20°C, although the optimum temperature is 35°C. The organism grows on ordinary media, abundant growth is produced in cooked-meat medium.

The organism is both proteolytic and saccharolytic, the former property predominating.

In cooked-meat medium, vigorous growth takes place with the blackening of the meat. Gelatin is readily liquefied.

Laboratory Diagnosis

Botulism is a food poisoning, the suspect food should therefore be examined bacteriologically. It may occasionally be possible to demonstrate the presence of toxin in the patient's blood or in the post-mortem material, e.g. blood, liver—by direct animal inoculation. Gram stained film of the food may first be examined for spore forming gram-positive bacilli.

A portion of the suspected food stuff may be given to a susceptible animal, which on feeding on it, may show signs and symptoms of botulism. The food can be injected into the peritoneal cavity of a mouse after suspending it in saline and obtaining supernatant fluid. After death, post-mortem is carried out and the infected lesions are cultured and *Cl. botulinum* is obtained in pure culture in case of botulism.

AEROBIC SPORE FORMING BACILLI

These organisms are gram-positive spore forming bacilli which may be arranged in chains. The majority of them are non-pathogens barring Bacillus anthracis which causes anthrax.

Bacillus anthracis

This is the causative organism of anthrax in cattle, sheep and other animals. It is infective for man, generally by spores entering through injured skin or by inhalation of the spores from infected animals.

Morphology

The organism is an aerobic, large, non-motile bacillus with a cylindrical spore. The bacteria may often be arranged in chains and may often be arranged in chains and may be surrounded by a capsule.

Culture

On agar the colonies are white, granular and circular with wavy margins like "medusa head".

Gelatin stab shows an "inverted fur tree appearance".

Diseases Caused

1. Malignant pustule.
2. Wool sorter's disease.

Laboratory Diagnosis

1. Smear from exudate to demonstrate the bacilli
2. Cultures
3. Guinea pig or mouse inoculation
4. Ascoli's precipitin test.

Bacillus subtilis

This organisms is commonly found in air and soil. This species of often found as a contaminant in the laboratory. Morphologically it is a long slender, motile bacillus which may be found in chains. The colonies are large, flat and dull with a typical ground glass appearance.

Bacillus cereus

This species is a common contaminant in the laboratory. Morphologically it is a large, motile bacillus which usually occurs in tangled chains. The colonies are small and smooth, however, some of the colonies may be spreading.

GRAM-POSITIVE BACILLI

Corynebacteria

Corynebacteria are gram-positive rod-like forms. They are aerobic, non-motile, non-sporing, non acid fast, often staining irregularly and having a beaded appearance. Frequently, irregular swelling at one end gives the organism a club-shaped appearance. *Corynebacterium diphtheriae* is the most important in this species and there are three types, gravis, intermedius and mitis. Gravis is the most virulent and mitis the least.

Morphology

Slender, straight or slightly curved rods, non-motile and non-sporing. They may show a beaded appearance due to uneven staining and arranged in a "chinese letter" formation pattern. Albert's stain is the stain of choice, the bacilli appearing green with blue-black beading due to volutin granules.

Culture

Various media on which they can be grown are:

1. Ordinary nutrient media, e.g. nutrient agar and blood agar.
2. Loeffler serum agar—on this the colonies are small, circular, white and opaque with thick centres and crenated borders.
3. Potassium tellurite—on this three types of colonies are seen:
   a. Gravis—Relatively large, greyish black, flat lusterless colonies appearing like "daisy heads".
   b. Intermedius—Relatively small, black, lusterless colonies with domed centres resembling "poached eggs".
   c. Mitis—Convex, smooth, translucent colonies.

Elek's gel precipitin test is positive and demonstrates the powerful exotoxin produced. Some strains produce hemolysis.

Diseases Caused

1. Diphtheritic inflammations, e.g. pseudomembranous inflammation in the fauces.
2. Acute myocarditis.

Laboratory Diagnosis

1. Elek's test.
2. Intradermal injection (of material to be tested) into guinea pig.
3. Schick test: Intradermal injection of toxin. Positive reaction is an area of redness 1-5 cm in diameter by the fourth day.

Diphtherioid bacilli

These are non toxigenic corynebacteria with little or no pathogenicity.

Corynebacterium hoffmanni

This is a commensal of the throat. Morphology and staining—Compared to the diphtheria bacillus it is shorter and may present an oval shape. It is strongly gram-positive and no volutin granules are detected by Albert's staining. It grows on ordinary media aerobically.

Corynebacterium xerosis

This is a commensal in the conjunctival sac. Closely resembles diphtheria bacillus and many show volutin granules.

Corynebacterium acne

This is an organism associated with acne. It is gram-positive, rod-shaped and shows marked pleomorphism. some show beaded appearance.

MYCOBACTERIUM

Mycobacteria are non-motile, rod-shaped bacteria, usually slender, straight or slightly curved, but occasionally with slender filaments or even branching. Most species do not stain easily, but when stained with strong dyes resist decolourization with acid, and hence the name-Acid fast bacilli (AFB). They are aerobic, non-spore bearing, and most strains grow slowly, but a few stains grow rapidly, not only at 37°C but even at 22°C.

Strains of Mycobacteria

a. Pathogenic species
- *M. tuberculosis:* *hominis*, *bovis*, *avium*
- *M. fortuitum*
- *M. paratuberculosis*
- *M. ulcerans*
- *M. blanei*
- *M. leprae*
- *M. lepraemurium*

b. Non-pathogenic species
- *M. smegmatis*
- *M. phlei*
- *M. butyricum*

c. Anonymous strains
- Photochromogens
- Scotochromogens
- Battey types
- Rapid growing saprophytes.

Morphology

It is a slender or slightly curved bacillus, in direct smears measuring about 2.5 to 3.5 by 0.3µ although both shorter and longer forms may be seen. In cultures, short forms are found especially on solid media, but longer forms may be found in liquid media. The bacillus may occur singly, or in pairs, or in larger or smaller masses.

The tubercle bacillus (T.B. or Koch's Bacillus) does not stain easily by the ordinary dyes, but it stains well with a strong dye with a mordant, such as carbol fuchsin when the stain is hot but it takes a longer time when the stain is cold. When once it has been stained it resists decolourisation with 20% H_2SO_4 or HNO_3 (Nitric acid); it also resists decolourisation with alcohol, and so it is both acid and alcohol fast. The method generally used for staining is Ziehl-Neelsen's method or one of its modifications. The bacilli may stain evenly, or they may show beading or barred staining or sometimes may have terminal granules. The bacilli are gram-positive but by this method they are stained only with great difficulty and Gram's method is of no use for their identification. A more recent method is the use of auramine-phenol florescent stain.

Cultures

The tubercle bacillus will not grow on ordinary media. Primary cultures are usually made on some form of egg medium of which Lowenstein-Jensen (L.J.) medium is probably the most widely used. Dorset's egg medium or Petragnani's media may also be used. After the primary culture has been established it is possible to make subcultures on media without egg, such as Dubos, Proskauer and Beck, Kirschner and Youman's media.

All the varieties, viz. hominis, bovis and avium may be found in man but in India the bovine seems to be rare in man, and the avian is not a common finding.

Cultural charactristics: M. tuberculosis is aerobic, and the optimum temperature for the human and bovine varieties is 37°C, and for the avian 40-44°C. It grows slowly. It does not grow on ordinary media but for the primary isolation requires an enriched medium, a medium including eggs is used most commonly. Glycerol stimulates the growth of the human and avian varieties but not the bovine. On L.J. medium, the general appearance of the growth is dry, irregular, tough and tenacious, a buff to light orange in colour, but if the surface of the medium is moist the appearance of the colony is smoother. The growth is said to be eugonic that is growing well. The bovine variety is dysgonic that is growing with difficulty and the colonies are smaller, discrete, rather smooth, slightly moist, and greyish yellow in colour. The avian grows rapidly, the colonies are moister, more luxuriant and individual colonies have a smooth shiny surface, yellowish to faint pink in colour.

Laboratory Diagnosis

In many specimens the finding of acid-fast bacilli typical in shape and staining, is accepted as sufficient for calling them tubercle bacilli, but it must always be remembered that there are many other acid-fast bacilli which may be found particularly in stomach-wash, urine, feces, and even in sputum. Also when bacilli are few in number, they may not be found in direct smear. Concentration methods such as sodium hydroxide and trisodium phosphate may help but on the whole considerable labour is involved without a great increase in positive findings. Therefore, cultures are being increasingly used even if 3 to 4 weeks elapse before a positive result is given, and most workers report a negative only after 6 to 8 weeks.

The specimens most commonly examined for tubercle bacilli are sputum, stomach wash, laryngeal swabs, urine, CSF, pleural or peritoneal fluid, pus and tissue. The specimens are collected in clean, sterile vessels, and most are treated with 4% NaOH or 6% H_2SO_4 (v/v) before the culture is made. The treatment homogenises the specimen and also destroys organisms other than mycobacteria.

Concentration Methods

Except in very severe cases, the organism is not always present in large numbers and for this reason, techniques have been devised for concentrating the organisms present to facilitate their detection and isolation. Concentration serves two other purposes.

1. The mucoid material is broken down and the sample homogenised.
2. Other unwanted bacteria are killed, thus allowing the tubercle bacillus to grow in pure culture.

Petroff's method

This is considered to be one of the most reliable methods.

1. Half fill a universal container with the sputum (or other material) and add an equal quantity of 4% NaOH. (For lesser samples a proportionately equal quantity should be added).
2. Invert the closed container twice or three times and place in the incubator for 30 minutes, inverting it every 10 minutes.
3. Centrifuge at 3000 rpm for 30 minutes. (The centrifuge must be completely at a standstill before opening it again after centrifuging tubercular samples.
4. Discard the supernatant.
5. Add a few drops of neutral red indicator to the deposit.
6. Neutralise with 8% HCl.
7. Inoculate neutralised deposit on the L.J. or some other egg medium.

Oxalic acid method

This is primarily used for laryngeal swabs, but is rather unreliable in that it does not completely ensure the destruction of untoward organisms.

The swab is simply left in oxalic acid for 30 minutes, and then smeared on the egg medium.

Trisodium phosphate method

This, too, is less preferable than Petroff's method, because it needs much longer incubation periods.

An equal quantity of sample and 10% trisodium phosphate are incubated for 24 hours, after which the container is centrifuged for 30 minutes and the supernatant discarded.

The deposit is neutralised with 8% HCl using bromthymol as indicator.

Other Pathogenic Mycobacteria

M. fortuitum: This bacillus has been isolated from soil and from suppurative infections in men and animals and also in glandular infections. It grows rapidly and is not pathogenic for guinea-pigs.

M. paratuberculosis: This is also known as bacillus of Johne's disease and is the cause of a chronic enteritis in cattle and sheep. The primary isolation is difficult and medium has to contain mycobactin—an extract from other mycobacteria.

M. ulcerans: This produces a chronic or subacute ulceration in both the skin and the adjacent subcutaneous tissue, particularly of legs and arms. Incubation temperature should be between 25°C and 35°C and the best growth is at 33°C. It grows on glycerine agar.

M. balnei: This bacillus has been isolated from swimming pools and produces ulcerative lesions on the extremities. It grows more rapidly than *M. ulcerans,* but will not grow above 35°C.

M. leprae: This is also known as Hansen's bacillus and causes leprosy. Smears are made from a scraping from the skin of suspected lesions and from nasal smears. It has been found in sputum. The usual method is skin clips from the affected areas.

Films are stained by Z-N stain, but it is customary to use 5% sulphuric acid for decolourising as *M. leprae* is not so strongly acidfast as *M. tuberculosis,* but stained M. leprae bacilli may resist decolourisation with 20% sulphuric acid. The bacilli are usually present in large numbers (in lepromatous leprosy) and are generally found in packets like cigar bundles within phagocytic cells called lepra cells. They may stain uniformly but there is often marked beading. The bacilli may also be stained fairly easily by Gram's method.

Until recently no claims of culture were substantiated but it is now believe that the organism may be isolated on the foot pads of mice.

M. lepraemurium

This is an organism found in rats in a disease somewhat resembling leprosy. It can be passed on experimentally to other animals of the same species.

Non-Pathogenic Species

M. smegmatis

The smegma bacillus is an acid-fast bacillus found in the smegma secretion around the genital and anal parts of human beings and in some animals such as dogs. It can also be found in other parts of the body, e.g., in the ear. The bacillus may be found in the urine, but if the urine is carefully collected after cleansing the external parts it can usually be avoided.

It is generally shorter and thicker than the tubercle bacillus, and many strains of the smegma bacillus are decolourised by alcohol which distinguishes them from the tubercle bacillus. They grow rapidly in culture.

M. butyricum

The butter bacillus. These bacilli may be found in grass, water, butter, milk, ,manure etc. They grow rapidly in culture.

Acid-fast bacilli can frequently be found in the mouths of water taps, but some at least seem to be affected by 6% H_2SO_4 when an attempt is made to grow them, but survive treatment with weaker acid.

Anonymous Strains

Many of the so-called anonymous strains are classified by their reaction to light. Photo-chromogens are those which produce orange colonies when they are exposed to light (day-light/artificial light). Scotochromogens are those which produce coloured colonies even in the dark. It is therefore, important in dealing with this classification not to grow them in an incubator that is opened frequently, not to let them stand on the laboratory bench unless the observation is actually being made. The yellow-orange pigment develops after exposure to light in 6-24 hours. The scotochromogens produce a yellow growth but this turns more orange on exposure to light. The Battey type either does not change, or if it does, the change is very slow.

Animal Inoculation

Sometimes for final identification it is necessary to inoculate an animal to see if the organism will produce disease. The human strain of *M. tuberculosis* will produce disease in both guinea pigs and rabbits, but the rabbit will show little sign of tuberculosis. With the bovine strain, however, the rabbit is also highly susceptible. In some specimens the material may be directly inoculated, in other only after a primary culture has been grown.

OVERVIEW OF M. TUBERCULOSIS DIAGNOSTIC APPROACH AFB STAINING, CULTURE AND SENSITIVITY

INTRODUCTION

Humans are very susceptible to the *Tuberculosis* infection but are remarkably resistant to the *Tuberculosis* disease; which is dependent largely on the state of the hosts immune system. Of all the *Mycobacterial* species *Mycobacterium tuberculosis* remains the most common cause of pulmonary tuberculosis and remains the most virulent of all the *Mycobacterial* species.

The disease, as now well known, is highly contagious. Although the disease involves all susceptible individuals, the incidence is higher amongst disadvantaged minorities. Industrialisation, increased crowded housing and nutritional deprivation have influenced the spread. With the emergence of HIV and resultant immunocompromise, TB has emerged as a major killer not only in the third world countries but is also resurging in the western world. According to World Health Organisation (WHO) reports, each year an estimated eight million new cases of *Tuberculosis* occur, leading to three million deaths; and almost a third of the world's population is infected by the causative organism, *Mycobacterium tuberculosis.*

According to a study, in India, the number of *Tuberculosis* patients is increasing at the rate of 1.5 million per year, and a quarter of these are sputum positive. Thus, about 4 per cent of all Indians are infected with *Mycobacterium tuberculosis.*

With the emergence of the multiple drug resistant strains due to poorly administered therapeutic measures and patient non-compliance, *Mycobacterium tuberculosis* is challenging its containment, on the basis of empirical treatment alone.

BRIEF MICROBIOLOGY

The genus *Mycobacterium* is composed of slow growing organisms, which are "acid fast". Currently about 55 species of *Mycobacteria* are recognised. They are non-motile, slightly curved or straight rods (0.2-0.6 × 1-10 mm) and may occasionally demonstrate branching. The organisms are aerobic and have a gram positive cell wall, although they do not gram stain well.

The *Mycobacteria* contain a lipid rich cell surface which includes true waxes and glycolipids 60-90 carbon, long chain Mycolic acids, unique to the *Mycobacterial* cell wall are responsible for their:

- Acid fastness;
- Failure to react with gram stains;
- Resistance to the action of antibodies and complement.

The four species in the *Mycobacterium tuberculosis* complex are *M. tuberculosis, M. microtic, M. africanum* and *M. bovis.* Laboratories can use biochemical tests for differentiation between isolated strains.

DIAGNOSIS OF *MYCOBACTERIUM TUBERCULOSIS* INFECTION

The diagnosis of *Tuberculosis* is often made on the basis of clinical symptoms, chest X-ray and sputum AFB, since available tests based on immunological principles for *Mycobacterium tuberculosis* diagnosis have yet to over come the problem of poor sensitivity and specificity associated with them. For the time being, speedy and appropriate laboratory diagnosis of *Tuberculosis* infection through AFB staining, culture and sensitivity have more and more important role to play in sensitive detection and appropriate treatment of patients with *Tuberculosis.* However, sample collection, preparation, processing techniques and detection methods employed have a profound effect on the sensitivity and specificity of the results for the detection of *Mycobacterium tuberculosis* infection by AFB and culture methods.

SPECIMEN SELECTION

A critical factor in the ability of laboratories to isolate *Mycobacterium tuberculosis* is obtaining appropriate specimen for AFB smear and culture. Approximately 85% of the TB cases are pulmonary. However, many patients cannot produce sputum spontaneously and alternative respiratory tract specimens such as induced sputum, gastric lavage or fiberoptic bronchoscopy may be needed. As the proportion of patients with extrapulmonary form of *Tuberculosis* is increasing, adequate specimen from extrapulmonary sites need to be provided.

SAMPLE CONCENTRATION AND DECONTAMINATION

Specimens obtained from sterile sites such as CSF, peritoneal or pleural fluids do not require decontamination. However, most specimens for AFB smear and culture are from the respiratory tract and do contain mixed microbial flora. Successful recovery of *Mycobacteria* depends upon properly collected specimen and suppression of contaminating bacteria.

Since mucous traps AFB and protects other organisms from effective decontamination a combination of 2% NaOH (decontaminant) and 0.5% N-acetyl-L-cysteine (mucolytic agent) is preferably employed. Neutralisation of strong decontaminating solutions before using the sample for AFB stain and culture is usually accompanied with sequential buffered wash of the concentrated sample because if the pH of the concentrate remains alkaline or acidic it can destroy the culture medium and prevent the growth of *Mycobacteria* and staining efficiency of the AFB smears. The buffered wash also helps in reducing the specific gravity of specimen and sediments the *Mycobacterium* more effectively.

Another important aspect post decontamination is the specimen concentration and relative centrifugal force applied to the specimen. Improvement in correlation between specimen showing a positive smear for AFB and a positive culture has been demonstrated by increasing the centrifugal force applied to pellet the specimen.

MUCOLYTIC, DISINFECTANT, SPECIMEN PRETREATMENT AND BUFFERING SYSTEM FOR AFB STAINING AND CULTURE (Courtesy: Tulip Group of Companies)

Lyfectol

Summary

Infection with *Mycobacterium tuberculosis* remains a major public health problem. The epidemic of

Recommendations for Sample Collection for *Mycobacterial* isolation and Acid Fast Staining

Specimen type	*Specimen requirements*	*Special Instructions*	*Unacceptable Specimen*
Abscess contents aspirated fluid.	As much as possible in syringe with Luer tip cap.	Cleanse skin with alcohol before aspirating sample. Laboratory may provide 7H9 broth/Kirchner medium for transport of small volumes of aspirates.	Dry swab.
Blood.	10 ml SPS (yellow top) blood collection tube or 10 ml Isolator tube.	Disinfect site as for routine blood culture. Mix tube contents immediately after collection. SPS is preferred anticoagulant Heparinized blood is also acceptable.	Blood Collected in EDTA, which greatly inhibits Mycobacterial growth even in trace amounts. Coagulated blood.
Body fluids (pleural, pericardial, peritoneal).	As much as possible (10-15 ml min.) in sterile container or syringe with Luer tip cap. Collect bloody specimens into SPS blood collection tubes.	Disinlect site with alcohol it collecting by needle and syringe.	
Bone	Bone in sterile container without fixative or preservative.	—	Specimen submitted in formalin.
Bone arrow.	As much as possible in SPS blood collection tube or 1.5 ml in pediatric Isolator tube.	Collect aseptically. Mix SPS tube contents immediately following collection.	
Bronchoalveolar lavage or bronchial washings.	≥ 5 ml in sterile containers.	Avoid contaminating bronchoscope with tap water, Saprophytic mycobacteria may produce false-positive culture or smear results.	
Bronchial brushings	Sterile container or Middlebrook 7H9 broth or Kirchner medium	—	—
CSF	≥ 2 ml in sterile container.	Use maximum volume attainable	
Gastric lavage fluid	≥ 5-10 ml in sterile container. Collect in the morning soon after the patient awakens in order to obtain sputum swallowed during sleep.	Collect fasting early morning specimen on three consecutive days. Use sterile saline. Adjust to neutral pH with 10 mg to sodium carbonate immediately following collection. Laboratory should provide collection tube containing sodium carbonate.	Specimen that has not been neutralised.
Lymph node.	Node or portion on sterile container without fixative or preservative.	Collect aseptically, and avoid indigenous microbiota. Select caseous portion if available. Do not immerse in saline or other fluid or wrap in gauze.	Specimen submitted in formalin.

Contd...

Contd...

Skin lesion	Submit biopsy specimen in sterile container without fixative or preservative. Submit aspirate in syringe with Luer tip cap.	Swabs in transport medium (Amies or Stuarts) are acceptable only if biopsy sample or aspirate is not obtainable. For cutaneous ulcer, collect biopsy sample from periphery of lesion, or aspirate material from under margin or lesion.	Dry swab.
Smear on slides.	Smear specimen over 1.5 by 1.5 cm area of clear slide.	Heat fix smears. Transport in slide container taped closed and labeled BIOHAZARD.	
Sputum.	5-10 ml in sterile wax-free disposable container. Collect an early morning specimen from deep, productive cough on at least three consecutive days. Do not pool specimens. For follow-up of patients on therapy, collect at weekly intervals beginning three weeks after initiation of therapy.	For expectorated sputum, instruct patient on how to produce sputum specimen as distinct from saliva or nasopharyngeal discharge. Have patient rinse mouth with water before collecting sputum to avoid contaminating specimen with food particles, mouthwash or oral drugs, which may inhibit the growth of mycobacteria. For induced sputum, use sterile hypertonic saline. Indicate on request if specimen is induced sputum.	24 hour pooled specimens; saliva,
Stool.	≥ 1 g in sterile, wax-free, disposable container.	Collect specimen directly into container or transfer from bedpan or plastic wrap stretched over toilet bowl. Wax from container may produce false positive smear.	Frozen specimen. Utility of culturing stool for acid-fast bacilli remains controversial,

Tuberculosis and Multi Drug Resistant Tuberculosis reflects the failure of public health and social programs towards prompt treatment of infected cases and screening of high-risk population. Culture, isolation and sensitivity of *Mycobacterium tuberculosis* from patient groups using standard methods remain the gold standard for *Mycobacterium tuberculosis* detection and effective and swift treatment worldwide.

Reagent

MICROXPRESS LYFECTOL is a reagent for laboratory use only. LYFECTOL is provided as a three component reagent.

a. Reagent A (2% NaOH solution)
b. Reagent B (N- acetyl L-cysteine)
c. Reagent C (Phosphate buffer pH 6.8)

Accessories: Spatula for approximate weighing (12 mg) and transfer of Reagent B.

LYFECTOL is used for decontamination and concentration of specimen containing normal microbial flora such as sputum as per international recommendation.

Principle

Proper decontamination and concentration of specimen containing normal microbial flora such as sputum are crucial in detecting *Mycobacterium tuberculosis.*

LYFECTOL provides a liquefaction-decontamination and specimen buffering procedure that maintains the viability and pathogenecity of *Mycobacterium tuberculosis,* simultaneously eliminating all unwanted microorganisms. Since mucous is sticky, Acid Fast Bacilli trapped in mucoid portion of sputum are released by mucolytic action of N-acetyl L-cysteine. NaOH decontaminates other microorganisms, and final wash with phosphate buffer ensures that specimen is at optimum pH for staining and culturing. Specimen pretreatment and disinfection with LYFECTOL increases relative Add Fast Bacilli concentration and ensures its more sensitive detection during Add Fast Bacilli staining and culture.

Storage and Stability

1. Store the LYFECTOL kit at 2-8°C, away from light.
2. Stability of the LYFECTOL kit is as per the expiry date mentioned on the label.

Additional Material Required

Sterile plating loops (10 µl), biosafety hood with Bunsen burner, centrifuge at 3000-4000 g, activated 2% Glutaraldehyde solution. 5 ml measuring cylinder, vortex mixer, 1 ml micropipette, 15-25 ml universal container.

Specimen Collection

Collect specimen prior to use of antimicrobial agent. Wherever possible, indicate clearly that patient is on antitubercular drugs. Sputum: Collect 5 to 1 ml in a sterile container from an early morning specimen of deep productive cough. For induced specimen use sterile saline. Have patients rinse mouth with water to minimize specimen contamination with food particles, mouthwash, or oral drugs.

Procedure

The procedure mentioned below is for 2.5 ml of the sputum sample. In case of variation in quantity of specimen used, process using proportionate amounts of reagent, mucolytic and disinfection reagent.

Preparation of Mucolytic Reagent

The mucolytic reagent must be prepared just prior to use.

1. Bring the reagents to room temperature.
2. Add one scoop full (~12 mg) of reagent B to 2.5 ml of Reagent A with the provided spatula.
3. Mix to dissolve.
4. The mucolytic Reagent can be used within 24 hours of preparation, if stored at 2-8°C.

Processing of Specimen

1. Take approximately 2.5 ml of the specimen in a clean sterile 15-25 ml universal container.
2. Add 2.5 ml of the mucolytic Reagent and close the container tightly with a screw cap fitted with an intact liner.
3. Mix well by gently vortexing at every 5 minutes interval for 20 minutes.
4. After 20 minutes, unscrew the cap of the container carefully and add 5 ml of Reagent C.
5. Close again the container tightly as in step 2.
6. Mix well and centrifuge for 25 minutes at 3000-4000 g.
7. After centrifugation unscrew the cap of the container with the content carefully and discard the supernatant gently in an activated 2% Glutaraldehyde solution, taking care as not to disturb the pellet at the bottom.
8. To the pellet at the bottom add 1 ml distilled water and re-suspend the contents.
9. Use this suspended material for microscopy (Acid Fast Bacilli), Acid Fast Bacilli culture or Polymerase Chain Reaction.

Remarks

1. Treat the unused specimen and contaminated containers by immersing in 2% activated Glutaraldehyde for atleast two hours before incineration and disposal.
2. Good laboratory practices and hazard precautions must be observed at all times.
3. Discoloured or contaminated Reagent should not be used.
4. The Reagent containing the phosphate buffer may appear turbid on prolonged storage at 2-8°C. Gently warm at 25-30°C before usage to remove such a appearance.

EFFECT OF CENTRIFUGAL FORCE ON POSITIVE SMEARS/CULTURES FOR *MYCOBACTERIA*

Specimen	Relative Centrifugal Force (g)		
	1260	3000	3800
Positive smear	1.8%	4.5%	9.6%
Positive cultures	7.1%	11.2%	11.6%
Correlation of positive smear/cultures	25%	4 0. %	82%

* Adapted from Clinical Diagnosis and Management by Laboratory Methods, Todd, Sanford and Davidsohn, 17th Edition 1998, Edited by John Bernard Henry.

Thus, proper decontamination and preparation of specimen is crucial to AFB detection by culture and AFB staining.

THE AFB SMEAR

The sensitivity of AFB smear for specimen from extra pulmonary sites is lower than from sputa. The lipid-containing cell walls of *Mycobacteria* have a unique characteristic in binding carbolfuchsin stain so tightly that it resists de-staining with strong decolourising agents such as strong alcohols and strong acids. This "acid-fast" staining reaction of *Mycobacteria,* along with their unique beaded and slightly curved shape, is a valuable aid in the early detection of infection and monitoring of therapy.

It has been estimated that there must be 10,000 acid-fast bacilli per milliliter of sputum to be detected by microscopy. Patients with extensive disease will shed large numbers of *Mycobacteria* and show a good correlation between a positive smear and a positive culture. In patients with minimal or less advanced disease, the correlation of positive smears to positive cultures may range from 30 to 80 per cent.

Acid-fact stains performed on a weekly basis are also useful in following the response of patients to drug therapy. After drugs are started, cultures will became negative before smears, indicating that the bacilli are injured sufficiently to prevent replication but not to the point of preventing binding of the stain. With continued drug treatment, more organisms are killed and fewer shed, hence monitoring the number of stainable organisms in the sputum during treatment can provide an early and objective measure of response.

It should be noted that in patients receiving antimycobacterial therapy not all stainable organisms are viable. Should the number of organism fail to decrease after therapy is started, the possibility of drug resistance must be considered. Additional cultures should be taken and drug susceptibility studies obtained.

Two types of acid-fast stains are frequently used:

1. Carbolfuchsin based stains;
2. Fluorochrome based stains.

1. The carbolfuchsin stains, so called because of the Reagent formed by mixing of the stain Basic Fuchsin with the disinfectant Phenol (carbolic acid). Carbolfuchsin stained *Mycobacteria* appear bright red/ pinkish against a bluish background.

Two procedures using carbolfuchsin based stains are in common use:

(a) Three component Ziehl-Neelsen, or "hot stain", and

(b) Three component Kinyoun or "cold stain".

The Kinyoun stain is a modification of the classical Ziehl-Neelsen "hot stain". The classical Ziehl-Neelsen "hot stain" requires application of heat to the fixed smears flushed with the stains during staining process, where as the Kinyoun stain does not require the application of heat and is less tedious to perform and standardise.

Recent advances in staining techniques have been reported where the cold Kinyoun stain has been further modified to accommodate the decolouriser within the counter stain. The novel two component two step stain is time, labour and cost saving, more user friendly and easy to standardise. It also has good correlation with the classical Ziehl-Neelsen "hot stain" and AFB cultures.

RAPID TWO STEP COLD AFB STAIN (Courtesy: Tulip Group of Companies)

Novachrom

Summary

Infection with *Mycobacterium tuberculosis* remains a major public health problem. The epidemic of tuberculosis and Multi Drug Resistant Tuberculosis reflects the failure of public health and social programs towards prompt treatment of infected cases and screening of high-risk population. While culture, isolation and sensitivity of *Mycobacterium tuberculosis* from patient groups using standard methods remain the gold standard for *Mycobacterium tuberculosis* detection and effective and swift treatment worldwide, Acid Fast Bacilli staining is the first line microscopic procedure performed towards this goal.

Reagent

MICROXPRESS NOVACHROM is a Reagent for laboratory use only. NOVACHROM Rapid Two Step Cold AFB Stain comprises of:

a. NOVACHROM AFB stain (A) - carbol fuchsin
b. NOVACHROM AFB stain (B) - counter stain with decolouriser

Rapid Two Step Cold AFB Stain is provided as a ready to use stain set. It is used for screening of *Mycobacterium tuberculosis* from biological specimen such as sputum, CSF and urine. It is also used in the identification of *Mycobacterium tuberculosis* from isolated culture. It is a modification of Kinyoun's cold stain.

Principle

Carbol fuchsin forms acid insoluble complex with Mycolic add present on the Acid Fast Bacilli and renders red/pinkish red colour to *Mycobacterium tuberculosis.* Other elements present in the smear take up counter stain (Methylene blue) and are stained bluish. NOVACHROM, Rapid Two Step Cold AFB Stain avoids the extra decolourisation step associated with traditional staining techniques as the decolourising component is incorporated within the counter stain. NOVACHROM staining system is simple to perform and very much reproducible. It has a sensitivity comparable to the traditional Ziehl Neelsen hot staining method and also as compared to Acid Fast Bacilli culture results. It is a clinically proven, easy to use, time, labour and cost saving. This simplicity of staining makes NOVACHROM an ideal screening tool for *Mycobacterium tuberculosis.*

Storage and Stability

1. Store the NOVACHROM Kit at room temperature (25-30°C), away from light.
2. Stability of the NOVACHROM Kit is as per the expiry date mentioned on the label.

Additional Material Required

Sterile plating loops (10 µl), biosafety hood with Bunsen burner, activated 2% Glutaraldehyde solution, distilled water, microscope with oil immersion lens, cedar wood oil.

Specimen Collection and Preparation

Collect specimen prior to use of antimicrobial agent. Wherever possible, indicate clearly that patient is on antitubercular drugs.

CSF: Collect as much as possible in a syringe, clean skin with alcohol before aspirating specimen.

Body fluids: Disinfect the site and collect specimen with aseptic precautions.

Sputum: Collect 5 to 10 ml in a sterile container from an early morning specimen of deep productive cough. For induced specimen use sterile saline. Have patients rinse mouth with water to minimise specimen contamination with food particles, mouthwash, or oral drugs.

Urine: As organisms accumulate in the bladder overnight, first morning void provides best yield. Collect midstream clean catch urine, first morning catheterisation/suprapubic taps in sterile containers.

Specimen Preparation

Proper decontamination and concentration of specimen containing normal microbial flora are crucial to detection of *Mycobacterium tuberculosis.* Specimen obtained from sterile sites such as CSF, peritoneal or pleural fluids do not need decontamination. However, since most specimens for Acid Fast Bacilli smear and culture are from respiratory tract and the mucous traps Acid Fast Bacilli and protects other organisms from decontamination and concentration, decontamination and liquefaction is a must. Most satisfactory for this purpose is a combination of N-acetyl—L cysteine (mucolytic agent) and 2% NaOH (decontaminant)—(available as LYFECTOL from Microxpress). Petroffs method of decontamination can also be used.

Test Procedure

For direct sputum screening use 10 µl of purulent sputum or use 10 µl of decontaminated and concentrated specimen.

1. Place the specimen under test on a clean, scratchless glass slide using a sterile plating loop.
2. Spread by tracing concentric circles well separated over an area of 200 mm square (20 mm × 10 mm), take care as to not to reach the edge of the slide. Alternatively for dense mucoid specimen press the specimen between two glass slides and pull apart gently to form a thin film of mucous.
3. When the smear is completed, plunge the inoculating loop into liquid disinfectant (2% Glutaraldehyde) and shake to remove any sputum, then flame sterilise loop.
4. Air-dry the smear.
5. Fix the smear by passing the slide approximately three times on the flame.
   (Note: While passing the smear slide on the flame see that the side opposite the smear is facing the flame).
6. Mix well and add NOVACHROM AFB stain (A) over the smear to cover it completely (4-5 drops ≈ 0.2 ml, may be required).
7. Keep for 6 minutes and then rinse with plenty of distilled water slowly to remove excess of NOVACHROM AFB stain (A).
8. Tilt slide to drain, mix well and add NOVACHROM AFB stain (B) over the smear

to cover it completely (4-5 drops ≈ 0.2 ml, may be required).

9. Keep for 6 minutes and then rinse the smear once more with distilled water to remove excess of NOVACHROM AFB stain (B).
10. Air-dry and observe under oil immersion (magnification 100 X).

Interpretation of Results

1. Presence of pink to red coloured slender Bacilli—Smear Acid Fast Bacilli positive.
2. Absence of pink to red coloured slender Bacilli—Smear Acid Fast Bacilli negative.
3. Pus cells and other bacteria stain purple to blue colour.

Grading of Results

After 5 minutes of examination covering about 100 fields.

Number of Acid Fast Bacilli observed	REPORT
No Acid Fast Bacilli	Negative
1-10 Acid Fast Bacilli	Actual Number
> 10 Acid Fast Bacilli	+
Masses of Acid Fast Bacilli in several fields	++

Remarks

1. Improper decontamination and concentration procedure will yield erroneous results.
2. Treat the specimens and used slants by immersing in 2% activated Glutaraldehyde for at least two hours before incineration and disposal.
3. Good laboratory practices and hazard precautions must be observed at all times.
4. Observe stain timings which are essential to obtain correct staining results.
5. Under stain or over decolourisation may give false results.
6. NOVACHROM stains stored between 25 and 30°C should not show precipitation.
7. Artefacts could be mistaken for Acid Fast Bacilli.

2. The fluorochrome based stains for AFB comprise of Auramine O, sometimes used in combination with a second fluorochrome stain, Rhodamine.

Smears stained with Auramine O can be scanned using a 25 × objective. Fluorochrome-stained *Mycobacteria* appear bright yellow against a dark background obtained by counterstaining with potassium permanganate, thereby permitting the slide to be scanned under the lower magnification without loosing sensitivity. The sharp visual contrast between the bright coloured *Mycobacteria* and the dark background offers a distinct advantage in scanning a much larger area of the slide during the same time necessary for looking at the carbolfuchsin stain.

When using the Auramine stain, a significantly larger area of the smear can be scanned in the same period of time used to scan a carbolfuschin-stained smear.

Enthusiasm for the carbolfuchsin and fluorochrome staining methods varies between laboratories, with different professionals strongly partial to one method or the other. Specificity for *Mycobacteria* seems to be the same for both.

The crucial factors in maximising smear sensitivity and specificity are:

- Centrifugation of digested fluid specimen at a minimum of 3000 g;
- The smear should be prepared on a new clean undamaged glass slide;
- Scanning of at least 3000 fields per slide.

The reporting of the AFB smear should be preferably done according to the CDC, USA method, or as per the National Reference Institution norms.

Quantitation Scale for Acid-Fast Bacillus Smears according to stain used

Carbolfuchsin (X 1000)	Fluorochrome (X 250)	Quantity Reported
No AFB/3 fields	No AFB/30 fields	No AFB seen
1 -2 AFB/300 fields	1 -2 AFB/30 fields	Doubtful; repeat test
1-9AFB/100 fields	1-9 AFB/10 fields	Rare(1+)
1 -9 AFB/10 fields	1-9 AFB/field	Few (2+)
1 -9 AFB/fields	10-90 AFB/field	Moderate (3+)
>9 AFB/fields	>9 AFB/field	Numerous (4+)

However, Indian Reference Institutions recommend reporting after 5 minutes of examination covering about 100 fields. Grading is done as follows:

Number of Acid Fast Bacilli observed	Report
No Acid Fast Bacilli	Negative
1-10 Acid Fast Bacilli	Actual Number
>10 Acid Fast Bacilli	+
Masses of Acid Fast Bacilli in several fields	+ +

* Adapted trom National Tuberculosis Institute Monograph Series: 1, Manual for Establishment and Functioning of a Tuberculosis Culture Laboratory, Govt. Of India National Tuberculosis Institute, No. 8, Bellary Road, Bangalore 560 003, August 1993.

Smears with fewer than 3 AFB per slide account for about 85% of false positive smear reporting and are considered doubtful. A repeat specimen should be registered. However, *Mycobacterium tuberculosis* infection must be considered for any patient with repeat smear AFB positive regardless of the number of AFB observed.

FACTORS INFLUENCING SENSITIVITY AND SPECIFICITY OF AFB SMEARS

FALSE POSITIVE RESULTS

Acid fast particles other than tubercle bacilli

Occasionally, a sputum specimen or smear may contain particles that are acid-fast, i.e. when treated with the Ziehl-Neelsen method, they retain the red stain (carbolfuchsin) and resist decolourisation with acid-alcohol. These red particles may sometimes resemble tubercle bacilli. They include certain food particles (e.g., waxes, oils), precipitates, other micro-organisms, inorganic materials and artifacts.

Food particles: To eliminate these, the patient should rinse their mouth with pure water and clean their teeth (without using tooth-paste or disinfectant) before producing the sputum specimen. It is even better if the patient produced the specimen before breakfast or on an empty stomach.

Precipitated stains: Though these are quite easy to differentiate from acid-fast bacilli, they may hamper reading or occasionally mislead an inexperienced microscopist. Precipitates can be removed by filtration of staining solutions. However, it is safer to use freshly prepared solutions, filled into carefully cleaned bottles, rather than stale staining solutions.

Saprophytic acid-fast bacilli: These occur in soil and water, and may occasionally get into the specimen or smear during processing. This can be avoided by using distilled or boiled water from scrupulously clean containers.

***Mycobacterium kansasii* or *Nocardia* species:** These occasionally occur in specimens. When they cause pulmonary disease, they are usually present in large numbers.

Spores of *Bacillus subtilis*: These are very rare, mostly of ovoid shape, and larger than tubercle bacilli.

Fibres and pollens: Fibres, including those of wood, cotton, filter paper and bamboo, usually occur singly, most often in only one microscopic field. The pollen of certain pine trees is seen as short, coccoid rods occurring very rarely in specimens.

Scratches on the slide: Scratches may sometimes retain the red stain and confuse beginners. They are usually seen in parallel rows, are generally longer than acid-fast bacilli, and are undulated. They can be identified easily, because they are found in a deeper layer on the slide, below the smear disappearing when the cells (e.g., leucocytes) in the smear get focused on.

Contamination through the transfer of bacilli from one smear to another

It may happen that acid-fast bacilli are transferred accidentally from a positive slide to a negative one, when several slides are treated simultaneously in staining or decolourisation tanks. This can be avoided by processing each slide separately, e.g., on a rack. Such racks are usually made of wire and can be decontaminated easily by flaming.

Acid-fast bacilli may also be transferred accidentally when the glass rod or dropper used for placing immersion oil on the slide touches the surface of a positive slide and rubs off some material. The same can happen when blotting paper is used for drying several stained smear consecutively. Therefore, the blotting paper should not be used at all, or for no more than one slide. The oil dropper should not touch the smear, and the oil should be allowed to drip freely on to the slide. For the same reason, the surface of the slide should not be rubbed with the oil immersion objective. Before a new slide is examined, the oil should be wiped off the lens with a piece of cotton tissue or, even better, with special lens-cleaning paper.

When microscopy is used for the detection of acid-fast bacilli, slides should never be used more than once.

FALSE NEGATIVE RESULTS

False negative results are commonly due to deficiencies in the preparation of the smear, in staining, and in scanning. Adequate collection of the specimen and subsequent "selection of sputum particles are essential to the preparation of a smear and should receive special attention.

Deficiencies leading to false negative results include the following:

Inadequate sputum collection

The patient is sometimes not told clearly enough what constitutes a proper sputum specimen and how he should produce one. It must be made clear to him that saliva and nasopharyngeal discharge are unsuitable for examination. Patients should be encouraged and given time to produce bronchial sputum from the "depths of the chest". If repeated attempts have failed, tickling of the inner surface of the epiglottis or trachea with a swab, or intratracheal instillation of 5-10 ml of cool saline or sterile water may provoke a vigorous cough with sputum. Other techniques to stimulate the production of sputum, such as aerosol induction, gastric aspiration, and bronchoscopy, require more complex equipment or special skills.

If a patient discharges acid-fast bacilli in his sputum, these are more likely to be found in a specimen produced in the early morning than in one produced later in the day. If early-morning sputum in required, the patient should be given a container and instructed to place in it the very first sputum he produces in the morning, before breakfast and before taking any medicaments.

Improper storage of sputum specimens and stained smears

Acid-fast bacilli may lose their acid-fastness as a result of exposure of the specimen to direct sunlight, radiation (e.g., ultraviolet light), excessive heat, or storage for more than a week in hot and dry conditions.

If Ziehl-Neelsen stained smears have to be stored for re-examination, the immersion oil must be washed from the smears with xylol because the immersion oil removes the stain from the acid-fast bacilli.

Fluorochrome stained smears will lose their fluorescence with storage.

Failure to select suitable sputum particles for smear preparation

Tubercle bacilli are most likely to be found in little blobs ("lentils") of greenish-grey or yellowish matter of a thick, creamy consistency. (Such blobs usually consist of dead caseous tissue eliminated from a cavity in the lung). If the sputum is not treated by a special concentration procedure involving centrifugation, these blobs have to be carefully separated from the rest of the sputum and transferred to a slide. They can be seen more easily in the sputum against a dark background.

Inadequate preparation of smear or staining of slides

False negative results may be obtained also when:

a. Too little material has been spread on the slide, so that the smear is too thin;
b. The smear is too thick, so that sufficient light cannot pass through it;
c. The slide has been over heated when fixing the smear;
d. The smear has not been sufficiently fixed and parts of the material have been washed off;
e. The staining with carbolfuchsin was too short or was overdone by boiling;
f. The counterstaining was too intensive, so that the acid-fast bacilli have been obscured;
g. Staining and counterstaining times have not been followed precisely.

Inadequate examination of the smear

If the scanning is done erratically or too briefly, too few fields may be examined. (Occasionally the examiner is unable to distinguish the red-stained acid-fast bacilli because of colour blindness or other visual disturbances).

Other reasons for false results

Administrative errors: Such errors may include:

a. Misidentification of patients, misspelling of names, or confusion of names or of codes numbers of specimens and slides;
b. Mistakes in labeling containers;
c. False recording of reporting.

Reading errors: Reader or observer error, which is mainly due to visual or psychological reasons, occurs in practically all diagnostic, clinical and laboratory work. The nature of this phenomenon, sometimes called the "human factor", is to a large extent unknown. Nevertheless, under certain conditions it is measurable. The degree and frequency of error-overreading as well as under-reading varies from one person to another and also within the same individual at different times.

Inter-individual reader variations in smear microscopy has been repeatedly studied and its frequency has been found relatively low compared, for instance, with inter-individual error in say, chest radiography.

It seems likely that many reader errors would be avoided if each microscopist were properly trained and strongly advised to report what he actually saw, and never what he thought he was expected to see. However, discrepancies in the results of smear microscopy are far more often due to deficient sputum collection and smear preparation than due to reader error.

AFB CULTURE AND ISOLATION

The modern bacteriology has many mycobacteriological media available to it. An ideal medium should be able to produce rapid and abundant growth, enhance phenotype characteristics, inhibit the growth of contaminants and should be usable for antimicrobial techniques. However, despite advances, the isolation of *Mycobacterium tuberculosis* is still a slow process ranging from 10 days to 8 weeks.

Solid media: LJ medium produces a slightly higher rate of TB isolation however, it is prone to slant contamination. A good LJ medium is non-selective, light green in colour, smooth slant without bubble formation so as to view *Mycobacterial* growth easily. The concentration of Malachite green is critical for achieving a good colour contrast for visualisation of *Mycobacterial* colonies. Sub optimal concentration of Malachite green in the medium produces higher contamination rates whereas excessive Malachite green can suppress and delay the *Mycobacterium* growth itself.

Agar based medium such as Middlebrook are transparent, allow quicker examination of colony morphology. Middlebrook is more resistant to contamination and produces growth of *Mycobacterium tuberculosis* faster than L.J. medium. Some commercially available 7H11 medium have been modified to increase the amount of Malachite green. Laboratory workers should be careful to determine this, for while the increase content of aniline dye retards growth of contaminating bacteria, it can also inhibit the growth of *Mycobacterium*.

When laboratories rely primarily on solid medium it will take a minimum of 3 weeks to produce colonies of *Mycobacterium tuberculosis*.

READY TO USE LJ SOLID MEDIUM FOR *MYCOBACTERIUM TUBERCULOSIS* ISOLATION (Courtesy: Tulip Group of Companies)

Mycocult

Summary

Infection with *Mycobacterium tuberculosis* remains a major public health problem. The epidemic of Tuberculosis and Multi Drug Resistant Tuberculosis reflects the failure of public health and social programs towards prompt treatment of infected cases and screening of high-risk population. Culture, isolation and sensitivity of *Mycobacterium tuberculosis* from patient groups using standard culture methods remain the gold standard for *Mycobacterium tuberculosis* detection and effective and swift treatment worldwide.

Reagent

MICROEX PRESS MYCOCULT is a Reagent for laboratory use only.

MYCOCULT Lowenstein-Jensen medium is provided as a ready to use slant. It is a standard non-selective inspissated egg based solid medium for the isolation of *Mycobacterium tuberculosis* from biological specimen such as sputum, CSF, urine.

Principle

Lowenstein-Jensen medium supports the growth of *Mycobacterium tuberculosis*.

The glycerol present in the medium enhances the growth of *Mycobacterium tuberculosis*. Accurate amount of malachite green not only has an inhibitory effect on growth of organisms other than *Mycobacterium tuberculosis*, but also provides the desired colour contrast for easy identification of *Mycobacterium tuberculosis* colonies.

Storage and Stability

a. Store the MYCOCULT - LJ kit at 2-8°C away from light.

b. Stability of the unopened medium is as per the expiry date mentioned on the label.
c. Avoid jerks and vibration while storage, shipping and incubation.
d. Upon opening, the medium must be put into use instantly.

Additional Material Required

Sterile plating loops (10 (µl), incubator at 37± 0.5°C, biosafety hood with Bunsen burner, activated 2% Glutaraldehyde solution, 0.2 ml micropipettes.

Specimen Collection and Preparation

Collect specimen prior to use of antimicrobial agent. Wherever possible, indicate clearly that patient is on antitubercular drugs.

CSF: Collect as much as possible in a syringe, clean skin with alcohol before aspirating specimen.

Body fluids: Disinfect the site and collect specimen with aseptic precautions.

Sputum: Collect 5 to 10 ml in a sterile container from an early morning specimen of deep productive cough. For induced specimen use sterile saline. Have patients rinse mouth with water to minimise specimen contamination with food particles, mouthwash, or oral drugs.

Urine: As organisms accumulate in the bladder overnight, first morning void provides best yield. Collect midstream clean catch urine, first morning catheterisation/suprapubic taps in sterile containers.

Specimen Preparation

Proper decontamination and concentration of specimen containing normal microbial flora are crucial to detection of *Mycobacterium tuberculosis*. Specimen obtained from sterile sites such as CSF, peritoneal or pleural fluids do not need decontamination. However, since most specimens for AFB smear and culture are from respiratory tract and mucous traps AFB and protects other organisms from decontamination and concentration, decontamination and liquefaction is a must. Most satisfactory for this purpose is a combination of N-acetyl-cysteine (mucolytic agent) and 2% NaOH (decontaminant)-(available as LYFECTOL from Microxpress). Petroffs method of decontamination can also be used.

Test Procedure

1. Bring the Lowenstein-Jensen medium slant to room temperature.
2. Label the Lowenstein-Jensen medium slant appropriately.
3. Draw 10 µl of the decontaminated and concentrated specimen from the reconstituted pellet with a sterile calibrated loop and plate it on the Lowenstein-Jensen medium slant aseptically.
4. For quantitative evaluation prepare bacterial suspension to match McFari land 0.5 standard, dilute this 1:10000 and Seed 100 µl on the Lowenstein-Jensen medium slant aseptically (seed stock consists of approx.-15000 organisms/ml).
5. Close the Lowenstein-Jensen slant cap tightly and incubate at 37± 0.5°C.
6. Observe for growth weekly till 8 weeks.

Interpretation of Results

1. *Mycobacterium tuberculosis* colonies may be detected from third week onwards up to eight weeks. The colonies are characterised by rough granular buff coloured growth, which has an initial size of 1-3 mm and full-grown size of 5-8 mm.

Remarks

1. Discoloured, dislodged, or contaminated medium should not be used.
2. Improper decontamination and concentration procedure will yield erroneous results.
3. Treat the specimens and used slants by immersing in 2% activated Glutaraldehyde for at least two hours before incineration and disposal.
4. Good laboratory practices and hazard precautions must be observed at all times.
5. In specimens from patients already on antitubercular drugs, the initial growth may be further delayed.
6. Growth on the Lowenstein-Jensen slant within the first week post inoculation usually indicates atypical *Mycobacterium* or contamination due to insufficient decontamination of specimen.
7. All culture growth should be characterized based on morphology, AFB stain and biochemical tests.

Liquid media: Such as Middlebrook 7H9, Dubos Tween albumin broth and Kirchner medium have been developed for the enrichment of growth of small number of *Mycobacteria.* They are valuable in isolating bacteria from uncontaminated specimen such as CSF, pleura and peritoneal fluids. There is an increased growth rate of *Mycobacterium tuberculosis* in liquid medium. Inclusion of Antibiotic cocktails such as PACT (Polymyxin B, Amphotericin B, Carbenicillin, Trimethoprim) or PANTA (Polymyxin B, Amphotericin B, Nalidixic Acid, Trimethoprim, Azlocillin) is required to make the liquid media sufficiently inhibitory to the growth of other bacteria and fungi especially when sputum specimens are used.

It is recommended internationally that specimen for *Mycobacterial* culture should be inoculated in both types of media. According to DIN and DZK guidelines atleast 3 different media should be inoculated, and atleast one of them being a liquid medium.

The different composition of the media and combination of different media have an impact on the yield and positive cultures, thereby increasing sensitivity of culture and *Mycobacterial* isolation.

Recent Indian studies have also indicated that *'Lowenstein-Jensen'* medium and *'Kirchner's* liquid medium are the best combination for the isolation of *Mycobacteria* from specimens other than sputum.

Ideally the cultures are incubated at 36±10ºC; with an atmosphere of 5-10% of CO_2 being stimulating to the growth of *Mycobacteria.*

COMBIPACK OF SOLID AND LIQUID MEDIUM FOR *MYCOBACTERIUM TUBERCULOSIS* ISOLATION (Courtesy: Tulip Group of Companies)

Combicult

Summary

Infection with *Mycobacterium tuberculosis* remains a major public health problem. The epidemic of Tuberculosis and Multi Drug Resistant Tuberculosis reflects the failure of public health and social program's towards prompt treatment of infected cases and screening of high-risk population. Culture, isolation and sensitivity of *Mycobacterium tuberculosis* from patient groups using standard culture methods remain the gold standard for *Mycobacterium tuberculosis* detection and effective and swift treatment worldwide.

Reagent

MICROXPRESS COMBICULT is a Reagent for laboratory use only. Lowenstein-Jensen medium is provided as a ready to use slant Kirchner medium is provided as a three-component medium.

a. Kirchner medium base
b. Kirchner selective enrichment containing antibiotic cocktail Polymyxin B, Amphotericin B, Carbenicillin, Trimethoprim (PACT)
c. Sterile distilled water for reconstitution of Kirchner selective enrichment

Lowenstein-Jensen medium is a standard non-selective inspissated egg based solid medium for the isolation of *Mycobacterium tuberculosis* from biological specimen such as sputum, CSF, urine. Lowenstein-Jensen medium supports the growth of *Mycobacterium tuberculosis.* The glycerol present in the Lowenstein-Jensen medium enhances the growth of *Mycobacterium tuberculosis.* Accurate amount of malachite green not only has an inhibitory effect on growth of organisms other than *Mycobacterium* but also provide the desired colour contrast for easy identification of *Mycobacterium* colonies.

Kirchner medium is a liquid medium enriched with serum. Kirchner medium has Polymyxin B, Amphotericin B, Carbenicillin, Trimethoprim as inhibitory antibiotic cocktail for most of the bacteria and fungus other than *Mycobacterium.* Being a buffered medium, it allows direct inoculation of larger inoculum upto 500 µl, and also keeps up the acid base balance during the growth phase.

Principle

The gold standard for primary isolation of *Mycobacterium tuberculosis* is the use of liquid media in conjunction with solid media. Most *Mycobacterium* species grow more quickly in liquid media than solid media. Liquid media also support higher detection rates especially with specimen material containing smaller number of bacilli. Simultaneous inoculation of solid media and liquid media yields significantly higher recovery rates for *Mycobacterium tuberculosis* growth as compared to when each media is used independently.

Storage and Stability

1. Store the COMBICULT kit at 2-8°C, away from light

2. Stability of the unopened media is as per the expiry date mentioned on the label.
3. Avoid jerks and vibrations while storage, shipping and incubation.
4. Upon opening, the media must be put into use instantly.

Additional Material Required

Sterile plating loops (10 µl), incubator at 37± 0.5° C, biosafety hood with Bunsen burner, activated 2% Glutaraldehyde solution, 0.2 ml micropipettes.

Specimen Collection and Preparation

Collect specimen prior to use of antimicrobial agents. Wherever possible, indicate clearly that patient is on antitubercular drugs.

CSF: Collect as much as possible in a syringe, clean skin with alcohol before aspirating specimen.

Body fluids: Disinfect the site and collect specimen with aseptic precautions.

Sputum: Collect 5 to 10 ml in a sterile container from an early morning specimen of deep productive cough. For induced specimen use sterile saline, have patients rinse mouth with water to minimize specimen contamination with food particles, mouthwash, or oral drugs.

Urine: As organisms accumulate in the bladder overnight, first morning void provides best yield. Collect midstream clean catch urine, first morning catheterisation/suprapubic taps in stetile containers.

Specimen Preparation

Proper decontamination and concentration of specimen containing normal microbial flora are crucial to detection of *Mycobacterium tuberculosis*. Specimen obtained from sterile sites such as CSF, peritoneal or pleural fluids do not need decontamination. However, since most specimens for AFB smear and culture are from respiratory tract and the mucous traps AFB and protects other organisms from decontamination and concentration, decontamination and liquefaction is a must. Most satisfactory for this purpose is a combination of N-acetyl - L cysteine (mucolytic agent) and 2% NaOH (decontaminant)-(available as LYFECTOL from Microxpress). Petroffs method of decontamination can also be used.

Preparation of Kirchner Medium

1. Reconstitute the Kirchner selective enrichment with 1 ml of sterile distilled water provided with the kit.
2. Transfer reconstituted selective enrichment aseptically to the Kirchner medium base, which is now ready to use as 'Kirchner Medium'.

Test Procedure

Kirchner medium

1. Bring the Kirchner medium to room temperature.
2. Label the Kirchner medium appropriately.
3. Draw 10 µl of the decontaminated and concentrated specimen from the reconstituted pellet with a sterile calibrated loop.
4. Inoculate in Kirchner medium aseptically.
5. Close the Kirchner medium cap tightly and incubate at 37 ± 0.5° C.
6. Observe for growth every third day till 8 weeks.

Lowenstein-Jensen slant

1. Bring the Lowenstein-Jensen medium slant to room temperature.
2. Label the Lowenstein-Jensen medium slant appropriately.
3. Draw 10 µl of the decontaminated and concentrated specimen from the reconstituted pellet with a sterile calibrated loop and plate it on the Lowenstein-Jensen medium slant aseptically.
4. For quantitative evaluation prepare bacterial suspension to match McFari land 0.5 standard, dilute this 1:10000 and Seed 100 µl on the Lowenstein-Jensen medium slant aseptically (seed stock consists of approx.-15000 organisms/ml).
5. Close the Lowenstein-Jensen slant cap tightly and incubate at 37± 0.5°C.
6. Observe for growth weekly till 8 weeks.

Interpretation of Results

a. *Mycobacterium tuberculosis* colonies on Lowenstein-Jensen slant may be detected from third week onwards up to eight weeks. The colonies are characterised by rough granular buff coloured growth, which has initial size of 1-3 mm and full-grown size of 5-8 mm.
b. *Mycobacterium tuberculosis* growth in Kirchner medium is characterised by fluffy growth to

small granules. The granules sediment to the bottom.

c. Since both the media differ in their composition, growth of *Mycobacterium tuberculosis* in either medium should be considered as a positive culture result. The growth needs to be identified.

Remarks

1. Discoloured, dislodged, contaminated or turbid medium should not be used.
2. Improper decontamination and concentration procedure will yield erroneous results.
3. Good laboratory practices and hazard precautions must be observed at all times.
4. While observing growth in liquid medium, care needs to be taken to differentiate between *Mycobacterium* growth and specimen material's own turbidity.
5. Treat the specimens and used slants by immersing in 2% activated Glutaraldehyde for at least two hours before incineration and disposal.
6. Preparation of Kirchner medium has to be carried out just prior to inoculation of specimen or culture.
7. In specimens from patient, already on antitubercular drugs the initial growth may be further delayed.
8. Growth on the Lowenstein-Jensen slant/ Kirchner medium within the first week post inoculation usually indicates atypical *Mycobacterium* or contamination due to insufficient decontamination of specimen.
9. All culture growth should be characterised based on morphology, AFB stain and biochemical tests.

Radiometric media: Developed in 1970, represent a significant improvement in the rapid isolation of *Mycobacterium tuberculosis.* Detection time is directly proportional to the number of metabolically active bacteria present and the metabolic rate is influenced by the type of specimen, number of organisms, therapy status of patient, decontamination procedures and the incubation temperature.

The average time for reporting the isolation of *Mycobacterium tuberculosis* using radiometric technique is reportedly 22±9 days as compared to 31 ±9 days for solid media.

However, the radiometric system is more labour intensive, requires disposal of radioactive material and still cannot detect some *Mycobacterium tuberculosis* isolates that can only be detected on agar slants. Some laboratories prefer to use LJ slants as a backup to Radiometric media. Considering the cost aspects and the fact that *Mycobacterium tuberculosis* is largely a problem of the third world, use of radiometric media is still restricted and use of solid and liquid media is widely practiced.

SUSCEPTIBILITY TESTING OF *MYCOBACTERIUM TUBERCULOSIS*

Resistance to antitubercular agents was recognised soon after their introduction in early 1960s, and standardized methods for antimicrobial susceptibility have been developed. Routine laboratory susceptibility testing of primary TB isolates has not been generally suggested unless drug resistance in a particular community exceeds 5%. However with the resurgence of TB drug resistance, C.D.C. USA has recently recommended that susceptibility tests should be performed on all primary isolates.

In a recent Indian study, a total of 3181 samples were processed for isolation of tubercle bacilli; and 707 samples were culture positive. The pattern of drug resistance is shown in the following table:

Pattern of Drug Resistance for *Mycobacterium tuberculosis*

Drug	Percent Resistance
Isoniazid	30.41
Rifampin	58.55
Streptomycin	46.95
Ethambutol	3.67
D Cycloserine	24.32
Kanamycin	14.42
Ethionamide	60.67
Amikacin	15.84
Ciprofloxacin	7.49

* Adapted from Bombay Hospital Journal; Drug Resistance in Tuberculosis; by Lina Deodhar et al. April 1999.

In India, it has been observed that private practitioners use different drug regimens to treat tuberculosis and very few regimens match with the standard (recommended by WHO).

The problem of acquired drug resistance (ADR) is truly man made. Poor administered *Tuberculosis* control programme, inadequate dosages, monotheraphy, insufficient durations of treatment, irregularity in drug intake, frequent defaults are some of the common reasons for emergence of ADR. In addition, HIV is quickening the pace at which *Tuberculosis* is spreading. Therefore, *Tuberculosis* is becoming the leading killer disease of HIV-positive people.

Clinicians should ensure that *Mycobacterium tuberculosis* susceptibility tests are carried out for patients:

- Who fail to respond after 3 months of treatment;
- Who do not convert to having negative smears after 3 months of treatment; with regimens that include INH and Rifampin, and 5 months for treatment without INH and Rifampin.
- Whose smears demonstrate increasing number of AFB after an initial decrease
- Patients whose cultures do not become negative after 4-6 months
- Patients who relapse.

TB susceptibility testing has three main goals:

- It provides data as to what drug should be used for treatment;
- Screens for drug resistance;
- Measures incidence and prevalence of drug resistance within the community.

Susceptibility Testing Methodology

Susceptibility tests can be performed directly, from a smear positive specimen, or indirectly, from the growth of colonies from the specimens. The former has the advantage of measuring the sensitivity prior to cultivation on laboratory media. The direct method also produces results more rapidly but; because of uncertainly of the species of *Mycobacterium*, and due to less control of the viable inoculum size, the results require confirmation with an indirect test, the direct test is not generally utilised.

Three methods make use of critical concentrations to define drug resistance and can be performed directly or indirectly:

- Absolute concentration method
- Resistance ratio method
- Proportion method.

The absolute concentration method determines if 1% or more of an inoculum will grow after being cultured on media containing critical concentrations of a drug on the plate. It requires growth of the patient strain on drug free medium to demonstrate the viability, but does not compare the colony numbers on drug free and drug containing media so that the inoculum must be carefully standardised.

The resistance ratio is similar to the absolute concentration method except that the patient strain is compared with the growth of a standard laboratory strain. Results are reported as the ratio of the MIC of the patient strain to that of the laboratory strain. A patient strain with a ratio of 8:1 is considered resistant, while 4:1 is suggestive of resistance. This method is more tolerant to variation in concentration of drugs within different batches of media.

The proportion method compares the growth of a patient strain in the presence and absence of a drug. If 1% or more of the inoculum produces colonies on media that contains an agent at the critical concentration compared with controls, the isolate is considered to be resistant. This method is the most popular and is relatively simple to perform and interpret.

SUSCEPTIBILITY TESTING OF *MYCOBACTERIA*

Eleven drugs are used in the treatment of *Tuberculosis.* Five are considered "primary" and include Streptomycin, Isoniazid, Rifampicin, Pyrazinamide and Ethambutol, while the remaining six, Ethionamide, Ciprofloxacin, Kanamycin, D cycloserine, para-Aminosalicylic acid and Amikacin are considered "secondary" and used only when resistance develops to the primary drugs.

Although drugs have been incorporated in inspissated egg-based media for conducting susceptibility tests, many laboratories internationally now prefer using Middlebrook 7H11 or 7H10 as a base medium, adding the drugs after cooling the agar to 45°C. Adding the drugs to the agar medium after autoclaving decreases the loss of activity that can occur in egg-based medium such L.J. during inspissation. An additional loss of drug activity may occur in egg-based media with binding of some agents to egg albumin and other proteins.

Drug Concentrations for Proportion Method Susceptibility Testing using various culture media*

Drug Concentration (µg/ml)

Drug	*7H10*	*7H11*	*Lowenstein -Jensen*
Isoniazid	0.2,1.0	0.2,1.0	0.2,1.0
p-Aminosalicylic Acid	2.0	8.0	0.5
Streptomycin	2.0	2.0	4.0
Rifampicin	1.0	1.0	40.0
Ethambutol	2.0	7.5	2.0
Ethionamide	5.0	10.0	20.0
Kanamycin	5.0	6.0	20.0
Capreomycin	10.0	10.0	20.0
D Cycloserine	20.0	30.0	30.0
Pyrazinamide	50.0	—	100.0

A simplified method for preparing drug susceptibility plates has also been developed. This method uses filter paper disks containing the primary antitubercular drugs, and the test for susceptibility is run in a similar fashion as the Kirby Bauer method for routine drug susceptibility tests.

As discussed, the direct *Mycobacterial* susceptibility test is inoculated from digested and concentrated sputum found to be positive for acid-fast bacilli. The indirect susceptibility test is inoculated from colonies isolated from a primary culture. The direct test will usually give good results only if large numbers of *Mycobacteria* are present in the specimen. The advantage of the direct susceptibility test is an earlier report (three to four weeks) in contrast to the indirect test, which may take up to six to eight weeks. The disadvantage of the direct susceptibility test is that it usually requires a large number of *Mycobacteria* for successful growth and is often overgrown by large numbers of contaminating bacteria.

Other novel methods of susceptibility testing have been developed based on the mycobacteriophage technique, using the luminiscent luciferase activity. Other researchers have localized specific *Mycobacterium tuberculosis* mutations responsible for drug resistance. These sites have been used as amplification targets and promise to provide a rapid method for testing the suspecibility of patient isolates to these drugs.

PRIMARY/SECONDARY DRUG CONTAINING LOWENSTEIN-JENSEN MEDIA PANEL MTB SENSITIVITY TESTS

Courtesy: Tulip Group of Companies

Sensicult

Summary

Inadequate chemotherapy, irregularity of treatment and use of improper antitubercular regimen lead to high failure rates of antitubercular treatment. As a result, the prevalence of chronic patients discharging drug-resistant organisms increases. Alarming figures of drug resistance in newly detected patients are being reported, mainly from developing countries. This calls for testing of antibiotic sensitivity in vitro prior to starting therapy.

Reagent

MICROXPRESS SENSICULT - LJ Primary/secondary drug panels are Reagents for laboratory use only. Primary/secondary drug containing Lowenstein-Jensen media panel for MTB sensitivity tests is a set of ready to use Lowenstein-Jensen solid medium slants incorporated with individual antitubercular drugs of recommended specified strength.

Contents

I. Primary drug Lowenstein-Jensen medium panel contains Lowenstein-Jensen medium with the following antibiotics/antitubercular drugs.

Drug	Symbol	pH	Concentration
1. Isoniazid	IN	7.0+ 0.1	1.0 ng/ml
2. Ethambutol	EB	7.0± 0.1	2.0 µg/ml
3. Rifampicin	RP	7.0± 0.1	4.0 µg/ml
4. Streptomycin	ST	7.0 ± 0.1	4.0 µg/ml
5. Pyrazinamide	PY	5.5 ± 0.1	100. µg/ml
6. Control for Pyrazinamide	P.C.	5.5 ± 0.1	
7. L. J. Control	LJ	7.0 ± 0.1	-
8. Sterile distilled water with glass beads for inoculum preparation			

II. Secondary drugs Lowenstein-Jensen media panel contains Lowenstein-Jensen medium with the following antibiotics/antitubercular drugs.

Drug	Symbol	pH	Concentration
1.p-Aminosalicylic acid	PA	7.0 ± 0.1	0.5 µg/ml
2.Ciprofloxacin	CP	7.0± 0.1	2 0. µg/ml
3.Amikacin	AM	7.0 ± 0.1	20.0 µg/ml
4.D cycloserine	DC	7.0 ± 0.1	30.0 µg/ml
5.Kanamycin	KA	7.0 ± 0.1	20.0 µg/ml
6.Ethionamide	ET	7.0 ± 0.1	20.0 µg/ml
7.L. J. Control	LJ	7.0 ± 0.1	—
8.Sterile distilled water with glass beads for inoculum preparation			

Principle

Due to increase in drug resistant strains of *Mycobacterium tuberculosis* and increasing failure rates of antitubercular drug regimens, it is desirable to start antitubercular therapy only after sensitivity assay of the most suitable drug against particular isolate infecting the patient.

Storage and Stability

1. Avoid jerks and vibration while storage, shipping and incubation.
2. Store the SENSICULT - LJ kits at 2-8°C, away from light.
3. Stability of the unopened media is as per the expiry date mentioned on the label.
4. Upon opening, the medium must be put into use instantly.

Additional Material Required

Sterile plating loops (10 µl), incubator at 37± 0.5°C, biosafety hood with Bunsen burner, activated 2% Glutaraldehyde solution, vortex mixer, 0.1 ml - 0.5 ml micropipettes, sterile micropipette tips.

Inoculum Preparation for Sensitivity Testing

a. Take a loopful asceptically from the *Mycobacterium tuberculosis* colony grown on Lowenstein-Jensen slant.
b. Transfer it asceptically to the screw capped bottle containing 0.1 ml of sterile distilled water and glass beads, for inoculum preparation.
c. Close cap tightly and subject the contents of the bottle to mechanical shaking (vortex) for 10 minutes.
d. Keep standing for 10 minutes before opening the bottle.
e. Dilute this in saline to match Me Farland 0.5 Standard. This contains approximately 1.5×10^8 org/ml.
f. Further dilute to 1: 10000 with saline. This is seed culture. (10000 -12000 org/ml)
g. Mix well and use this as inoculum.
h. Discard the container with glass beads in 2% activated Glutaraldehyde solution.

Test Procedure

1. Bring the primary/secondary drug containing Lowenstein-Jensen media panel for MTB sensitivity tests slants to room temperature.
2. Apply 100 µl from the seed stock to each slant of primary/secondary drug containing Lowenstein-Jensen media panel for MTB sensitivity tests also control LJ.
3. A fresh disposable loop should be used for each slant.
4. Close the cap tightly and incubate at 37± 0.5° C.
5. Observe for the growth after 2 weeks till 8 weeks, every week.

Interpretation of Results

As and when there is sufficient growth on control (>100 colonies) compare the growth with the antibiotic containing media.

1. If ratio of the growth in antibiotic containing media as compared to control is less than 0.01 the isolate will be termed as sensitive.
2. If ratio of the growth in antibiotic containing media as compared to control is more than 0.01 the isolate will be termed as resistant.

Example :-

$$\text{Ratio} = \frac{\text{No. of colonies on antibiotic containing media}}{\text{No. of colonies on control media}}$$

Sensitive if ratio is less than 0. 01

Resistant if ratio is more than 0.01

Border line if ratio is equal to 0.01

Remarks

1. Discoloured, dislodged or contaminated medium should not be used.
2. Good laboratory practices and hazard precautions must be observed at all times.
3. Treat the specimen and used slants by immersing in 2% activated Glutaraldehyde for at least two hours before incineration and disposal.

OTHER MARKERS

Adenosine deaminase, a surrogate marker, for the diagnosis of Tuberculosis has also shown promise. It is based on the measurement of activity of Adenosine deaminase, an enzyme produced by lymphocytes. The test has excellent sensitivity for TB meningitis and for examining pleural infections.The sensitivity and specificity is reported well above 90%, the test is easy to perform and relatively inexpensive.

To conclude, the objective of adapting different types of technology and instruments is to shorten the times for isolation, identification and susceptibility testing of bacteria and other microorganisms has been particularly relevant for *Mycobacteria*. Hopefully alternative methods to the standard procedures now used, could be developed soon enough for routine use, to provide cultures and susceptibility information in a shorter time interval. Till such time the AFB staining, culture and sensitivity remain the gold standard for accurate and early diagnosis of *Tuberculosis*, improvements and standardisation of techniques for these classical methods is important for better laboratory diagnosis and clinical information support. Significant cost savings might be effected by a reduction in hospitalisation and return of the patient to a productive career.

IN DETERMINATION OF ADENOSINE DEAMINASE ACTIVITY IN SERUM, PLASMA AND BIOLOGICAL FLUIDS ADA-MTB® (Courtesy: Tulip Group of Companies)

ADA-MTB®

Summary

Tuberculosis occurs worldwide and is rampant in many countries. Though curable, its infection is on the rise. The most specific test is the positive bacterial culture of a patient's sputum sample. This is cumbersome and time consuming. X-rays, smears for AFB and Tuberculin tests though comparatively rapid are not conclusive. Adenosine Deaminase (ADA) is an enzyme widely distributed in mammalian tissues, particularly in T Lymphocytes. Increased levels of ADA are found in various forms of tuberculosis making it a marker for the same. Though ADA is also increased in various infectious diseases like Infectious Mononucleosis, Typhoid, Viral Hepatitis, initial stages of HIV, and in cases of malignant tumours, the same can be ruled out clinically.

Reagent

MICROXPRESS ADA-MTB is a reagent for laboratory use only.

ADA-MTB comprises of:

a. ADA-MTB reagent (L1)—Buffer reagent, ready to use.
b. ADA-MTB reagent (L2)—Adenosine reagent, ready to use.
c. ADA-MTB reagent (L3)—Phenol reagent.
d. ADA-MTB reagent (L4)—Hypochlorite reagent.
e. ADA-MTB standard (S)—ADA standard, ready to use.

Principle

Adenosine Deaminase hydrolyses adenosine to ammonia and inosine. The ammonia formed further reacts with a phenol and hypochlorite in an alkaline medium to form a blue indophenol complex with sodium nitroprusside acting as a catalyst. Intensity of the blue coloured indophenol complex formed is directly proportional to the amount of ADA present in the sample.

$$\text{Adenosine} + H_2O \xrightarrow{\text{ADA}} \text{Ammonia} + \text{Inosine}$$

$$\text{Ammonia} + \text{Phenol} + \text{Hypochlorite} \xrightarrow[\text{Medium}]{\text{Alkaline}} \text{Blue Indophenol Complex}$$

Reference Values

Serum, Plasma, Pleural, Pericardial and Ascitic Fluids	Normal	< 30 U/L
	Suspect	30 U/L to 40 U/L
	Strong Suspect	>40 U/L to 60 U/L
	Positive	> 60 U/L
	Normal	< 10 U/L
CSF	Positive	> 10 U/L

It is recommended that each laboratory establish its own normal range representing its patient population.

Storage and Stability

1. Store the ADA-MTB kit at 2-8°C, away from light.
2. Stability of the ADA-MTB kit is as per the expiry date mentioned on the label.

Note

1. It is important that kit components from the same lot are used for achieving accurate and

reproducible results Do not intermix reagents from different lots.
2. The sequence of addition of Reagents should be followed meticulously for achieving accurate results.

Additional Material Required

Test tubes, test tube stand, waterbath/incubator (37°C), distilled or deionised water, variable volume pipettes, spectrophotometer with filter at 570-630 nm (Hg 578 or 623 nm) at 37°C or colourimeter with yellow or red filter, stopwatch.

Reagent Preparation

Reagents L1, L2 and standard are ready to use. **Adenosine Reagent (L2) may form crystals at 2-8°C. Dissolve the same by gently warming (37°C to 50°C) the Reagent for some time before use.** Both the Phenol Reagent (L3) and Hypochlorite Reagent (L4) need to be diluted 1:5 with distilled water before use (1 part of Reagent + 4 parts of distilled water). The Working Phenol Reagent and Working Hypochlorite Reagent are stable for at least 6 months when stored at 2-8°C in tightly closed bottles.

Specimen Collection and Preparation

Collect specimen prior to use of antimicrobial agent. Wherever possible, indicate clearly that patient is on antitubercular drugs.

CSF: Collect as much as possible in a syringe, clean skin with alcohol before aspirating specimen.

Body fluids: Disinfect the site and collect specimen with aseptic precautions.

Serum, Plasma: No special preparation of the patient is required prior to sample collection by approved techniques. It is recommended to use fresh sample specimen for testing. Do not use haemolyzed, contaminated or turbid sample specimens. Fresh EDTA, citrate, heparinised oroxalate anticoagulated (dry anticoagulant) plasma specimens are suitable for performing the test.

ADA is reported to be stable in serum for 3 days at 2-8°C and in biological fluids for 2 days at 2-8°C, as after this, ammonia may be released in the samples even without any microbial contamination.

Test Procedure

1. Bring all Reagents and samples to room temperature before use.
2. Prepare the Working Phenol Reagent and Working Hypochlorite Reagent.
3. Set the spectrophotometer filter at 570-630 nm (Hg 578 or 623 nm) at 37°C
4. Pipette into clean dry test tubes labeled Blank (B), Standard (S), Sample Blank (SB) and Test (T) as follows:

Additional Sequence	B ml	S ml	SB ml	T ml
Buffer Reagent	0.20	0.20	—	—
Adenosine Reagent	--	--	0.20	0.20
Deionised Water	0.20			
Standard	—	0.20	—	
Sample	—	—	—	0.20
5.Mix well and incubate at 37°C for exactly 60 minutes, and then add the following:				
Working Phenol Reagent	1.00	1.00	1.00	1.00
Sample	—	—	0.02	—
Working Hypochlorite /reagent	1.00	1.00	1.00	1.00
6Mix well and incubate at 37°C for 15 minutes or at R.I for 3 minutes.				
7Measure the absorbance of the Blank (Abs. B), Standard (Abs. S), Sample Blank (Abs. SB) and Test (Abs. T) against distilled water.				

Calculations

$$\text{Total ADA activity in U/L} = \frac{\text{Abs.T-Abs.SB}}{\text{Abs. S-Abs. B}} \times 50$$

Linearity

The procedure is linear upto 150 U/L. If values exceed this limit dilute the sample with deionised water and repeat the assay. Calculate the value using the appropriate dilution factor.

Remarks

1. One unit of ADA activity releases three nanomoles of ammonia in the reaction in 1 hour at 37° C
2. Patients with hyperamoniemia, kidney disorders and hepatitis can present high level of ADA values. Patients with chronic malnutrition or HIV can present low levels of ADA values.

3. Higher levels of ADA are also found in leprosy, brucellosis, HIV infections, viral hepatitis, infectious mononucleosis and liver cirrhosis. Before arriving to a diagnostic decision, these clinical conditions must be ruled out.
4. Using a cut off level of 60 units/L of ADA, values has been reported to show the specificity and the sensitivity of the test as above 90% for the MTB infection.
5. Below 60 U/L of ADA, the serum of ADA specificity and sensitivity is lower and should be interpreted in the light of other tests for confirmation of *Mycobacterium tuberculosis* infection.

GRAM-NEGATIVE BACILLI

The organisms mentioned below can be divided into five families according to the criteria given.

A. The organisms which grow well on any ordinary media containing peptone.
   1. The organisms which ferment few or no carbohydrates.
      a. Achromobacteriaceae.
   2. The organisms which ferment many carbohydrates.
      b. Enterobacteriaceae.
B. The organisms which are obligate parasites requiring body fluids for growth. These are small gram-negative rods.
   a. Brucellaceae.
C. The organisms which tend to elongate and are motile and most species produce water soluble pigments.
   a. Pseudomonadaceae.
D. Miscellaneous rod-shaped organisms (both gram-positive and gram-negative)

ACHROMOBACTERIACEA

This family contains three genera of which only one is encountered in human microbiology.

Alcaligens fecalis

This is a gram-negative rod inhabiting the intestinal tract of man and animals. It is motile and like all members of this family fails to ferment most carbohydrates. It is non-pathogenic in the stool of man because it fails to ferment lactose, it may at first have the appearance of a pathogenic stool organisms. It is readily distinguished, however, because it not only fails to ferment lactose but it also fails to ferment dextrose and other sugar which are commonly used for species identification, and it fails to grow on the selective media designed for the isolation of intestinal pathogens.

ENTEROBACTERIACEAE

(Gram-negative intestinal bacilli) These organisms comprise the following main groups:

1. The coliform bacilli which include the common commensal aerobic bacteria of the colon of man and animals.
2. The Salmonella group which includes the typhoid-paratyphoid bacilli (of enteric fever) and the organisms of bacterial enteritis or food poisoning.
3. The *Shigella* or dysentery group. General characteristics: gram-negative, non-sporing bacillary organisms, about 2-4 microns by 0.5 micron (average), aerobes and facultative anaerobes growing best at about 37ºC fermenting various carbohydrates but not usually liquefying gelatin or serum.

Proteus vulgaris

Straight rods about the same size as *Pseudomonas aeruginosa,* pleomorphic, motile with numerous lateral flagella, non-sporing, gram-negative. Members of this genus grow abundantly at 37ºC on the usual cultural media. They are actively motile and have a tendency to swarm, causing spreading of their colonies over the media, often obscuring other organisms. It is important to remember that these organisms do not ferment lactose despite the fact that they are not intestinal pathogens. They can be readily distinguished from the pathogenic non-lactose fermenters because they do not grow readily on the selective media to be described, but they split urea. That is colonies of organisms produce urease which have the property to break down urea to ammonia. Pathogenic non-lactose fermenters lack this property.

The next three genera, closely related, are *Escherichia, Aerobacter* and *Klebsiella*. These organisms have the following features in common—they are all non-pathogenic in stool, they all ferment lactose actively, and they grow abundantly on ordinary media at 37ºC.

Escherichia coli

These gram-negative rods are found in almost every stool specimen and are of the utmost importance to medical microbiology. They are frequently pathogenic when found in either the urinary tract or in purulent material from other sources. Their growth on blood agar is rather non-specific and they may occasionally show true hemolysis. They are usually motile, they do not produce hydrogen sulphide, and they produce promptly both acid and gas from lactose. On EMB media they are highly pigmented and have a metallic sheen. They are important as an indication of fecal contamination of water, food and milk and is therefore, important that this organism be distinguished from some others which are closely related. They IMVC is a group of tests which are useful as a means of distinguishing *E. coli* from other members of this group.

Indole

This can be tested for by growing the organism in peptone water and after two days, withdrawing with a sterile pipette 2 to 3 ml into a test tube. An equal volume of Ehrlich's reagent is then added. A rose colour develops in the presence of indole, and can be separated out with amyl alcohol. The addition of a saturated solution of potassium persulphate hastens the reaction. If the indole reaction is negative after two days growth, the test should also be repeated after seven days, as some strains are slow in their production of indole.

Methyl Red

This test is dependent upon the degree of acidity produced by the organism in dextrose broth. The indicator methyl red is red on the acid side and yellow on the alkaline side but the shift is at about pH 3. Therefore, an organism which ferments dextrose with small amount of acidity approximately 5, is negative to methyl red, whereas one which ferments, dextrose with the production of a high degree of acidity, approximately pH 2, is positive methyl red.

Voges-Prokaeur Reaction

This is a qualitative test for the presence of acetyl-methyl-carbinol. In the fermentation of glucose some organisms form this chemical, which gives a purple colour when added to peptone in a strongly alkaline medium. The test is performed by growing the organisms in a glucose-peptone broth for about 48 hours. At the end of this time, if the medium is alkalinised by adding 5 cc of 10% KOH, a deep pink colour develops after some standing. The culture must be at least 48 hours old.

Citrate Test

This is a test to determine the ability of an organism to utilise citrate as the sole source of carbon in a synthetic medium. The medium is prepared containing inorganic substances and sodium citrate.

The characteristic IMVC formula for *E. coli* is +, +, –, –.

Aerobacter aerogenes

The organism is ubiquitous in nature found in the soil and upon many grains. It resembles *E. coli* although it usually forms a more gelatinous colony on EMB. The IMVC test is –, –, +, +. Some organisms are intermediate in their IMVC reactions. Bergey separates these two genera according to Methyl Red and Voges-Proskaeur, therefore of the four tests, these two are the most reliable.

Klebsiella pneumoniae

This organism is rather variable in some of its physiologic characteristics. It usually closely resembles *Aerobacter aerogenes* but IMVC often intermediate or variable. *Klebsiella pneumoniae* should be suspected in the following instances:

a. In culture material obtained from lungs.
b. In culture material from a patient with crusting lesions of the nose.

Morphology

A small non-motile, non-sporing gram-negative bacillus with rounded ends and varying greatly in size 1-4 µ by 0.5 µ. The shorter forms simulate cocci. The bacilli occur usually in pairs but also singly, and in short chains. They are typically capsulated, especially when seen in tissues.

Klebsiella rhinoscleromatis

This organism closely resembles the pneumobacillus in morphology and cultural characteristics, but produces no gas from glucose, and does not ferment lactose. It does not grow in media containing bile, and does not give the Indole and Voges-Proskaeur reactions. The organism is associated with a chronic granuloma of the mucus membrane of the nose, mouth or throat.

Klebsiella Ozaene

Closely resembles the pneumobacillus, but is non-gas producing in glucose. It is found associated with ozaenae, but is not to be regarded as the causative agent of this condition.

Paracolon Bacilli

These organisms occupy a borderline position. In all essential features they resemble either *E. coli* or *Aerobacter aerogenes*, with one important exception, they ferment lactose very slowly and weakly. Since one species of the enteric pathogens may also ferment lactose very slowly there is a possibility of confusion. They following features serve to distinguish the paracolon organisms from this one pathogenic species (*Shigella shigae*).

1. Growth on selective media: *Shigella* grows well on SS media, while paracolon organisms do not.
2. Motility: *Shigella* is always non-motile. The paracolon may or may not demonstrate motility.

The paracolon group of organisms represents a variant of the *Escherichia* tribe. They are named according to which the common genera, the unknown most closely resembles for example *Paracolobacterium aerogenodies* or *P. coliforms*.

ENTERIC FEVER BACILLI-TYPHOID AND PARATYPHOID

These include *Salmonella typhi, Salmonella paratyphi* A and *Salmonella paratyphi* B.

Salmonella typhi

This is the pathogen responsible for typhoid fever.

Morphology

A gram-negative non-sporing bacillus about 2-4 μ, actively motile, with numerous long peritrichous flagella as observed in special stained preparations.

Cultures

Aerobe and facultative, grows well on ordinary media at optimum temperature of 37°C. Colonies on agar-like those of coliform bacilli, but smaller, thinner and most transparent. No liquefaction of gelatin. Colonies on MacConkeys are smaller than those of coliform bacilli and pale or colourless, the typhoid bacillus being a non-lactose fermenter. Colonies are pale or colourless on descoxycholate citrate medium. *S. typhi* ferments glucose and mannitol with acid, but no gas formation; does not ferment lactose or sucrose and does not produce indole.

Salmonella paratyphi A and *Salmonella paratyphi* B

The morphology and general characters are identical with those of the typhoid bacillus. Important reactions are no change on lactose, glucose and mannitol—acid and gas production, sucrose—no change. The typhoid bacilli do not produce gas while the paratyphoid bacilli produce gas.

Pathogenicity

The diseases of typhoid fever and paratyphoid fever are characterised by widespread dissemination of the organisms by the blood-stream, with production of a systemic febrile disease. The common symptoms are headache, anorexia, muscular weakness, diarrhea and development of typical 'rose spots' on the abdominal skin. After the general invasion of the body, the bacteria tend to localise in the lymphatic system. The symptoms of the disease are apparently the result of toxemia from the endotoxin of the organisms. The organisms may be found in the blood cultures during the first 10 days. They are found in the urine, especially during the second week, and they are found in the stool from about the second week on, with increasing frequency as the organisms tend to localise in the lymphoid tissue of the intestinal wall. After recovery from the disease, many people harbour a few bacteria in the intestinal tract and especially in the gallbladder. These people are not sick, for they have developed an adequate immunologic protection to the organism. Artificial immunisation is established by the use of typhoid vaccine.

Diagnosis of Enteric Infections

The bacteriological diagnosis depend upon

1. The isolation from the body and the identification of the causative organisms.
2. The demonstration of its presence in the body by the Widal agglutination reaction, which is

based on the occurrence of specific agglutinins to the organism in the serum of the infected person.

Blood Culture

In the early stages of illness, blood culture is the best diagnostic method, and should be used in all cases met with during the first 10 days of fever.

Feces Culture

Typhoid and paratyphoid bacilli can be isolated from the feces and are most frequent at the end of the second week or during the third week, but may be detected at all stages of the disease. Examination of feces however, may yield negative results unless repeated, and the isolation of typhoid-paratyphoid bacilli from this source is often rendered difficult owing to their being relatively scanty as compared with coliform bacilli. MacConkeys bile salt, neutral red, lactose agar is a medium used for the differentiation of typhoid-paratyphoid bacilli, and ordinary coliform bacilli. Desoxycholate-citrate agar is also used. Wilson and Blairs Bismuth sulphite method may also be used. Special media includes selenite F medium and tetrathionate broth which gives very good results when used as an enrichment. In the examination of feces from enteric cases the best results are obtained by employing two or three different methods simultaneously.

Urine Culture

Typhoid-paratyphoid bacilli may also be isolated from urine. The specimen is centrifuged, several loopfuls of the deposit are inoculated on a plate of desoxycholate-citrate medium and successive strokes made in the usual way so that isolated colonies are obtained.

Widal Reaction

Discussed in detail in Serology chapter.

ORGANISMS OF BACTERIAL ENTERITIDIS OF FOOD POISONING

These organisms are found in the intestinal contents during the disease and in some cases, in the food.

Salmonella enteritidis

The organism is generally similar to *S. paratyphi* B in various cultural and biochemical characters but does not ferment inositol.

Salmonella typhimurium

Resembles *S. paratyphi* B in cultural and biochemical reactions. The identification of *S. typhimurium* and other *Salmonella* types is carried out by the method of antigenic analysis. *S. typhimurium* produces enteritidis in a wide variety of animals.

Diagnosis of Salmonella Food Poisoning

The stool is cultured on desoxycholate citrate medium as in the diagnosis of enteric fever, pale colonies are subinoculated and the resulting cultures are tested and identified. Blood culture may in some cases yield positive results and should be carried out as a routine measure.

GROUP OF DYSENTERY BACILLI

The causative organisms of an acute form of dysentry most prevalent in tropical countries. In some instances, particularly those caused by *Shigella shigae*, the disease may be virulent, characterised by high fever and toxemia. The stool is characteristically full of pus cells, without much blood or mucus. In severe cases the stool may resemble purulent material. The degree of toxemia may be extreme so as to cause death. These generalised effects are probably the result of absorption of endotoxins.

Shigella shigae or dysenteriae and Shigella flexneri or paradysenteriae

Morphology

Non-motile, non-sporing, gram-negative bacilli about 2-4 μ x 0.5 μ but often showing a tendency to shorter coccobacillary forms.

Culture

Resembles the *Salmonella* group. Gelatin is not liquefied. Biochemical reactions—the dysentery bacilli ferment glucose without gas production, and in the case of sugar fermentations generally are non-gas producing. H_2S is not produced.

BRUCELLACEAE

These organisms are small gram negative coccoid to rod-shaped cells which may be found either singly or in pairs or short chains. The organisms may either be aerobic or facultative anaerobes. An increased

CO_2 tension is necessary for the growth of some of the species. Most of the species require additional nutritional factors for growth.

Pasturella Pestis

This organism is the causative agent of plague in man and rats.

Morphology

The plague bacilli are short plump, non-motile, gram negative rods which may be very pleomorphic. They may appear singly or in pairs or short chains. A capsule may be demonstrated especially from animal tissues.

Culture

This organism grows best at 30°C. The colonies produced on blood agar are small and round and are transparent and glistening with a wavy margin.

Pasturella Tularensis

This organism causes tularemia which is a disease of rodents that is easily transmitted to man, through handling of infected animals or blood sucking insects.

Morphology

This organism is a minute, pleomorphic, non-motile, gram negative rod with capsules occurring *in vivo.*

Culture

The organism requires a special enrichment medium for growth. The colonies produced are minute transparent drop-like colonies which appear 2-5 days after incubation. The optimal growth temperature is 32°C.

Bordetella pertussis

This is the causative agent of whooping cough.

Morphology

These organisms are minute gram negative, motile or non-motile coccobacilli.

Culture

The organism requires special enrichment media (potato-blood glycerol agar) called Bordet-Gengou agar for growth.

Brucella

This genus consists of three species of small gram negative coccoid bacilli. All 3 are strict parasites and are pathogenic for man and animals. This genus is divided into species by their action on sugar and by their additional requirements of CO_2. The organisms are aerobic and grow best at 37°C.

Brucella abortus, *Br. melitensis* and *Br. suis* cause contagious abortion in cattle and undulent fever in man.

Laboratory Diagnosis

Blood culture should be carried out repeatedly in all cases during the febrile phase and it is essential that at least 10 ml of blood should be withdrawn for this purpose, as the organisms may be relatively scanty. In suspected *Br. abortus* infection, the blood culture must be incubated in an atmosphere of 10% CO_2, in *Br. melitensis* the organism may be isolated from urine.

An agglutination reaction may be done with *Brucella* antigen after 7-10 days from the onset of illness. It has to be noted that normal serum may agglutinate *Brucella* suspensions in low dilutions. In cases of undulant fever, however, the serum often agglutinates both *Br. abortus* and *Br. melitensis* in high dilutions 1:1000. In suspected cases, if the reaction occurs only with low dilutions, e.g. less than 1:80, the result can not be regarded as conclusive. When the test is repeated, a rising titre should be observed.

HAEMOPHILUS

This genus includes the small non-motile, gram-negative bacilli which require the presence of haemoglobin for growth. Some of the species require additional factors for growth. This factor is Factor X which is a heat stable substance associated with haemoglobin and Factor V which is a heat labile substance found in yeasts and vegetable extracts. All of the species of this genus are parasites and will grow only in the presence of growth accessory substances. They may or may not be pathogenic for man.

Haemophilus influenzae

This organism is commonly isolated from the respiratory tract. It plays an important role in acute respiratory infections, conjunctivitis and purulent meningitis. This organism grows well on chocolate agar enriched with a yeast supplement. The colonies grow in 24 hours and resemble droplets of moisture on agar plates. If the colonies are growing near colonies of staphylococci or pneumococci, they will be large. These colonies produce an extra supply of Factor V which stimulates the growth of *Hemophilus influenzae.* This phenomenon is called as satellitism.

Haemophilus aegypticus (Koch-week bacillus)

This organism is the causative agent of conjunctivitis (pink eye). This organism closely resembles *H. influenzae* and needs both factors X and V for growth.

Haemophilus ducreyi

This organism is the cause of chancroid in man, a sexually transmitted disease. The small Gram negative rods may be found in smears from a genital ulcer. *H. ducreyi* is grown on chocolate enriched agar only with considerable difficulty.

Donovania granulomatis

This too causes a venereal disease—Granuloma Venereum. Laboratory diagnosis of this disease is made by demonstrating 'Donovan bodies' which are bacillary bodies surrounded by a dense capsule in the mononuclear cells from the lesion which have been stained with Leishman's stain. The organism will not grow on ordinary media.

Moraxela lacunate (Morax-Axenfeld bacillus)

This is the causative agent of conjunctivitis. In stained smears of pus, the organisms appear as short, thick gram-negative diplobacilli. It grows on Loeffler's serum medium and the colonies appear as small indentations indicating liquefaction of the medium.

PSEUDOMONADACEAE

This group includes a large number of bacilli which tend to elongate and some of these may produce a water soluble pigment. The majority of these species are not pathogenic to man.

Pseudomonas aeruginosa (Bacillus pyocyaneus)

The organism is commonly found in air and water but is frequently encountered in urinary, eye and ear infections.

Morphology

This is a gram-negative motile rod with 1-3 polar flagella occurring singly, in pairs and chains. The colonies give a ground glass blue green appearance. This organism can often be distinguished by the characteristic grape-like odour. It should be remembered, however that a few of the species are non-chromogenic and therefore, the identification on the basis of pigment production may be difficult.

Culture

Pseudomonas grows well on ordinary media. It does not ferment lactose and since on MacConkey agar the pigment may be masked or absent, it may be confused with enteric pathogens. *Pseudomonas* strains isolated from clinical material are hemolytic on blood agar.

BACTERIACEAE

The members of this group include the small gram-negative, non-sporing bacteria with rounded or pointed ends. They vary in size from filtrable forms to long filamentous branching organisms. Majority of them are strict anaerobes and are found in mouth, vagina and intestinal tract of man. These organisms can cause abscesses and occasionally septicemia. Complex culture media are needed for isolating these bacteria.

Fusibacterium Fusiforme

A gram-negative bacilli with pointed ends. It is found in the normal mouth and is especially associated with the fusospirochaetal disease, Vincent's angina. This organism may be seen in smears from Vincent's lesions.

Vibrio cholerae

Vibrio cholerae, or the comma bacillus is the causative agent of cholera. This disease is characterised by an acute gastroenteritis of sudden onset and often running a fatal course.

Morphology

It is a bent or slightly curved bacillus, resembling very closely a comma, from which it derived its name, comma bacillus. It is about 2 μ in length. It is actively motile, and the movement is of a darting or scintillating type. It is a gram-negative bacteria.

Culture

It is aerobic and slight growth also occurs under anaerobic conditions. It grows on ordinary media at a temperature range of 16-40ºC. Abundant growth occurs on highly alkaline media of pH 8.2. Colonies on nutrient agar are white circular discs and transparent. True *V. cholerae* is non-haemolytic. It ferments glucose, sucrose, mannitol, and maltose with only acid production. *V. cholerae* can produce indole and nitrites in peptone water. This is studied by cholera red reaction. Add a few drops of H_2SO_4 to 4 day's peptone water culture. A reddish-pink colour develops due to the formation of nitrose indole.

Laboratory Diagnosis

Collection of materials, from infected patient; 'rice water' stool, vomit and other fomites; from suspected water: About a litre should be collected from the surface in a sterile vessel, and packed in ice until used for examination.

Methods of Examination

Microscopic examination of fresh stool. This gives an idea of the character of the cellular exudate and is very helpful to differentiate the condition from acute bacillary dysentery. There are very few leucocytes or macrophages but only mucus and degenerated epithelial cells. In some cases, red cells may be present. Many bacilli with characteristic morphology and well marked motility may be seen.

A white flake of mucus is taken and smeared over a clear slide which is allowed to dry in the air. The film is then fixed over a flame and stained with dilute carbol fuchsin for a minute or two. After a through wash, when the slide is dry, it is examined under an oil immersion lens. The typical comma shaped, gram-negative vibrios are found in a case of cholera. A hanging drop preparation is useful to observe motility.

Cultural Methods

An alkaline peptone water tube is inoculated with a flake of mucus and incubated for 8-10 hours. A drop from the surface should be examined for the vibrios. Subcultures are made from this to Dieudonne's medium. The resultant growth is identified by smear and biochemical reactions. From the peptone water culture, a cholera red reaction may be done to identify the organism.

SPIROCHAETES

These are spiral, elongated, motile, flexible, organisms. They are not easily stained and are best demonstrated by dark field microscopy or silver impregnation methods. The three important groups are (1) *Treponema*. (2) *Leptospira*, and (3) *Borrelia.*

Treponema

These are slender spirals about 0.2 μ in width and 5-15 μ in length, causing syphilis and related diseases. The spirals are so thin that dark field microscopy is used. They are actively motile.

Treponema pallidum

This is the causative organism of syphilis, a human infection, transmitted sexually. It occurs in three stages, namely primary, secondary and tertiary stages.

Primary Stage

2-10 weeks after infection an ulcer is formed which heals spontaneously. Spirochaetes can usually be demonstrated in the serous exudate from the lesion.

Secondary Stage

2-10 weeks after healing, skin eruption may occur giving rise to a red rash with papules. Spirochaetes can be demonstrated in the serous exudate from these skin lesions.

Tertiary Stage

About 50% of the untreated cases proceed to this stage which is characterised by degenerative changes in the central nervous system, bones and liver. Spirochaetes are very rarely demonstrated, serological reactions such as Kahn, VDRL are usually positive after about 2 weeks from the onset of the primary stage.

Congenital syphilis: is caused by the transference of *T. pallidum* by a syphilitic women to the fetus through the placenta.

Morphology

An exceedingly delicate, spiral filament. 6-14 μ by 0.13 μ with 6-12 coils which are comparatively sharp and regular. In the unstained material it requires dark field illumination for its demonstration. *T. pallidum* can not be demonstrated by the ordinary staining methods. The organism may be demonstrated by Fontana's method or the India Ink method, using the exudate from the chancre.

Laboratory Diagnosis of Syphilis

In primary stage, where there is an ulcerated sore, *T. pallidum* can usually be demonstrated in the serous exudate from the lesion. The dark ground illumination method is the most suitable technique for the purpose, and provides a convenient means of diagnosis. The procedure of dark field illumination has been discussed under special uses of a microscope.

Material Collection

The material consists of scrapings from primary or secondary lesions or from aspirations from glands. In the case of a primary chancre the part above the ulcer is constricted with fingers (make sure to wear gloves) and the scrapings taken from the depth of the ulcer. In the case of the secondary lesions on skin or mucous membrane the tissue may be scraped taking precautions to avoid secondary contamination. In all cases several preparations should be made and the specimens examined immediately. The examiner should protect himself against infection by wearing gloves and by washing his hands in an antiseptic immediately after the examination.

In the dark field microscopy *T. pallidum* appears as bright and corkscrew like, slowly revolving and occasionally flexible. The ends are pointed and tapering. The undulating movement is characteristic.

Treponema pertenue

This is the cause of yaws, a tropical disease, an ulcerating papule occurring on the arms or legs. In morphology it is identical to *T. pallidum.*

Treponema curateum

Causative organism of pinta, a disease giving rise to non-ulcerating papule. It is seen predominantly in negros and has highest incidence in Mexico.

Treponema microdentum

This organism may flourish in caries teeth and may be found in secretions between teeth.

Treponema calligyrum

These organisms may occur in secretions of the genitals.

Leptospira

These are tightly coiled, thin spirochaetes with one end often turned at a sharp angle resembling, when at rest, a button hook. They vary from 5-15 μ in length and are about 0.1 μ in width. They can be stained by Giemsa, but are best demonstrated by silver impregnation.

Leptospira Icterohemorrhagiae

This is the causative organism of infectious jaundice (Weil's disease) and is transmitted to man by ingestion of water or food contaminated from animal sources. Urine and feces excreted by infected rats, mice or dogs contain the leptospira, which may remain viable for many weeks.

Laboratory Diagnosis

Examination of blood by dark field microscopy. During the first week of the disease, Leptospira can be detected in blood by the dark field illumination. Only a very small percentage can be diagnosed this way. After this the urine is examined.

Cultivation

The *Leptospira* medium is inoculated with 2-3 ml of blood. The organisms are searched for dark ground microscopy weekly, at least for 4 weeks. The *Leptospira* are best demonstrated by examining the centrifuged deposit of urine by the dark field method.

Borrelia

These spirochaetes are large, 10 to 30μ in length with irregular wide open coils staining easily with aniline and in Romanowsky stains. They can be cultured in blood or serum and also in tissue culture.

Borrelia vincenti

Occurs in Vincent's angina, a pseudomem-branous condition of the throat. Appearance of the spirochaetes together with large fusiform bacilli are indicative of infection. Sputum and throat swabs are examined for the diagnosis of Vincent's angina.

Borrelia recurrentis

This is the causative organism of European relapsing fever transmitted by body lice either by bite or by scratching with infected fingers by bite or by scratching with infected fingers after crushing the lice. Incubation period is 3-10 days after which chills and fever arise.

Borrelia duttonii

This is the causative organism of West African relapsing fever. The organisms are transmitted by ticks.

Laboratory Diagnosis of Relapsing Fevers

During the pyrexial phases, the spirochaetes may be frequently demonstrated in the blood. Thin and thick films are made, as for malaria, and stained by Leishman's or Giemsa's stain. Better methods, however, are dark ground or phase contrast microscopy.

Spirillum minus

This is the causative organism of rat bite fever. It is a short, spiral organism about 2-5 μ in length and relatively broad, with regular short coils. This organism is actively motile and is included in the group *Spirillum.* It can be demonstrated by dark field illumination.

In rat bite fever the *Spirillum* may be demonstrated in the local lesion, the draining lymph nodes, and even the blood, either by direct microscopic examination or by animal inoculation. The organism is transferred to human beings by the bite of a rat, causing a local lesion which leads to swelling of glands, skin rashes and a relapsing type of fever.

GRAM STAINER

Gram stainer: Aerospray Microbiology can be used for quick and high quality Gram Staining and offers advantages over hand staining or dip type stainer, like speed, economy, consistent performance and no cross contamination. It can stain 12 slides in 5 minutes and the slides are ready for microscopy.

The instrument is available from WESCOR USA.

Chapter 27

Mycology

In evolutionary set up fungi are placed higher in plant kingdom than bacteria. They exist in two distinct morphological forms: 1. the yeast form, and 2. the mycelium—which consists of a mass of long, branching tube-like filamentous structures called hyphae. Hyphae can be divided into segments—septate, or may not have any divisions—aseptate. Some fungi exist only as yeast forms when growing at 37°C but grow as mycelial forms at room temperatures. Other fungi grow only as hyphae at all temperatures. The yeast form of fungi generally multiply by budding; the bud is known as a blastospore. The hyphae have specialised structures known as conidia. They may also develop resting spores, especially when they are exposed to a hostile environment, which have thick walls, called chalmydospores. A colony of yeast-like fungi resembles a bacterial colony in culture. A colony of hyphae with its conidia and spores presents a filamentous growth, or mould.

All fungi are gram-positive and give a positive PAS reaction. Most fungi are aerobic with the exception of *Actinomyces*. Some species of *Nocardia* are acid fast, but most fungi are acid fast.

Barring a few of fungi, most are nonpathogenic to man. They are classified according to their medical importance as follows:

1. Superficial mycoses and dermatophytes.
2. Deep or systemic mycoses.
3. Contaminant (opportunistic) fungi which under special circumstances cause disease.

SUPERFICIAL MYCOSES AND DERMATOPHYTES

The fungi infect the skin, hair and nails. They do not involve deeper structures. They are subdivided into three genera:

a. **Microsporum:** This invades hair and skin, but not nails. This causes 'ringworm' infection. Colonies on Sabouraud's agar are a reddish-brown in colour, and often a reddish-brown pigment is produced in the medium. They produce powdery aerial mycelium.

b. **Trichophyton:** This fungus invades skin, hair and nails. They cause various types of ringworm, athlete's foot, etc. Colonies are powdery or waxy with pigmentation from white, pink, red to brown and yellow.

c. **Epidermophyton:** This fungus invades skin and nails, but not hair. Colonies are slow-growing with a green, slightly granular appearance.

Laboratory Diagnosis

- Scrapings of skin and nails.
- Hair plucked from infected area.
- Culture on Sabouraud's, agar for 2-3 weeks at room temperature.

Hair and scrapings are placed on a slide in a drop of 10% NaOH or KOH, coverslip, and examined after 10-30 minutes. In skin and nails branching hyphae are seen. In hairs, spores are seen. If they are all on the outside of the hair, it is called ectothrix infection. If they have developed and grown inside the hair, it is called endothrix infection. Some species cause the infected hair to fluoresce under ultraviolet light.

INTERMEDIATE SUPERFICIAL DEEP MYCOSES

Candida albicans (Monilia)

This is an oval budding, yeast-like fungus. It may be a commensal or part of the normal flora in small numbers in the GIT, mouth and vagina; but it can also cause disease in the skin, nails, mucous membranes (thrush of the mouth, vagina or anus), rarely it may take the form of systemic disease and involve heart, lungs or other structures in the body. On Sabouraud's agar soft, cream-coloured colonies develop at both 37°C and room temperature.

Examine swabs and scrapings from surface lesions, sputum or pus from deeper tissues. Sputum or exudates may be examined by Gram's stain for presence of budding, gram-positive, yeast-like fungus. Skin or nail scrapings are first placed in a drop of 10% NaOH or KOH and then examined for the yeast-like fungi.

Specimens are cultured on Sabouraud's agar at room temperature and at 37°C. At both temperatures, the colonies consist of yeast-like cells, though at room temperature small 'pseudomycelia' (nonseptate projections from yeast-like cells) are produced.

DEEP OR SYSTEMIC MYCOSES

Actinomyces

These organisms are related to true bacteria, but because of filamentous branching mycelial growth resemble fungi. The filaments sometimes break up into bacteria-like pieces. It causes actinomycosis, which is characterised by chronic sinuses, draining pus, leading from deep abscess cavities, usually in the neck, chest or abdomen. Actinomyces are sometimes normal inhabitants—commensals or saprophytes—in the mouth, throat and tonsils but under impaired host resistance, they become opportunistic pathogens and invade tissues. Direct examination of sputum or pus from a draining abscess will reveal small yellow granules, called 'sulphur granules'. When they are found and examined microscopically after crushing between two glass slides, the granules are seen to be made up of thin interlacing strands or branching filaments (about 1 μ in diameter) with club-shaped expansions at the end of the filaments at the periphery giving a ray-like appearance to the edge of the granule. The filaments are gram-positive and nonacid fast. Culture must be made anaerobically since this organism is an obligate anaerobe, usually in thioglycollate broth or on blood agar, at 37°C.

Laboratory Diagnosis

Examine pus or sputum for 'sulphur granules' and Gram's stain for gram-positive branching filaments.

Nocardia

These are morphologically similar to *Actinomyces*, though they; (i) found in soil and not as commensal in the body, (ii) are aerobic rather than anaerobic, (iii) may have granules in the pus though less frequently and those present not usually as yellow in colour, and (iv) some of the organisms may be weakly acid fast.

Nocardia is one of the organisms causing Madura foot.

Cryptococcus neoformans

It causes cryptococcosis or torulosis. It can cause a pulmonary infection and often spreads to the meninges and brain. It is a yeast-like budding fungus which is characterised by a large capsule both as it grows in tissue and in culture. Even in culture, it does not produce mycelia, but the colonies on Sabouraud's agar are smooth and glistening and cream-coloured. The capsule can be best identified by mixing the specimens of sputum, pus, or CSF with India ink.

Laboratory Diagnosis

Sputum, CSF and tissue are examined for these budding yeast-like organisms (5-20 μ). They are not refractile like red blood cells (RBCs), and neither RBCs nor lymphocytes show budding like these organisms. Toluidine blue 0.1% colours these organisms pink, stains lymphocytes blue and does not give any colour to red cells. India ink will reveal the wide capsules. Culture is done on Sabouraud's agar at 37°C and growth is rapid (1-2 days).

Histoplasma capsulatum

This organism causes histoplasmosis, which can be both a pulmonary infection (similar to tuberculosis) or show widespread dissemination throughout the body. The organism generally lives intracellularly in cells of the reticuloendothelial system; in macrophages, reticulum cells in bone marrow, spleen, etc. They appear as tiny (1 μ) intracellular oval bodies with a recognisable clear halo or capsule surrounding the small central stained organism. They cannot be seen in the unstained material, but can be seen in Giemsa, Leishman, haematoxylin and PAS stained preparations. Culture in broth or blood agar, plates at 37°C growth is yeast-like with smooth, white coloured colonies. On Sabouraud's agar at room temperature, there is mycelial growth of septate hyphae with spores.

Laboratory Diagnosis

Sputum, pus, blood and bone marrow smears, and tissue specimens are examined as stained preparations for the presence of the small, ovoid, capsulated intracellular organism.

Coccidioides

This organism causes coccidioidomycosis, which like *Histoplasma* can cause pulmonary, disseminated disease or occasionally deep skin ulcers. In tissue the organism is typified by the presence of thick-walled spherules (10-80 μ) which are filled with endospores (2-5 μ).

Laboratory Diagnosis

Examination of sputum, gastric washings or pus for the presence of these spherules. Culture at room temperature on Sabouraud's agar gives white cottony growth which soon becomes brown and microscopic examination reveals septate hyphae and spores.

FUNGI USUALLY PRESENT AS CONTAMINANTS BUT WHICH RARELY CAUSE DISEASE—USUALLY IN PATIENTS CHRONICALLY ILL FROM OTHER DISEASES

1. *Geotrichum*: Occasionally causes pulmonary, bronchial or oral disease. Direct examination of sputum reveals rectangular cells (4-8 m) with rounded edges.
2. *Penicillium*
3. *Aspergillus*
4. *Mucor:* The common mould on bread.

MYCOLOGICAL METHODS

Collection and Despatch of Specimens

Skin, Nail and Hair: Scrape the skin, into piece of clean and sterile tissue paper. Fold the paper and send to the laboratory. Debris beneath the nail after clipping off the affected nail and hair from infected parts are also collected in the same way.

Sputum, Pus, Spinal Fluid Exudates and Biopsy Materials: These are collected in sterile bottles.

Microscopic Examination

Skin, Nail and Hair: The specimens are placed into a clean slide and one drop of 10-20% NaOH or KOH is added and is covered with a coverslip. The slide is heated over a flame to soften and clear the material. Examine the slides microscopically.

The slides are stained by adding one drop of lactophenol cotton blue to one edge of the coverslip. Mycelial structure takes the blue stain.

Sputum, Pus and Exudates: Wet mount preparations are made on clean slide and examined microscopically. Gram's stain is also used to stain the fungus materials.

Cultural Examination

The most common medium is Sabouraud's agar. The scrapings from skin and nails and hairs are planted onto medium and are incubated for 2-3 weeks. Sputum, pus and exudates are cultured and incubated at room temperature and at 37°C.

CHAPTER 28

Diagnostic Skin Tests

Skin tests are diagnostic procedures performed by the intradermal administration of diagnostic materials or their application to the surface of the skin. In order to the useful, skin tests have to be properly performed, accurately read, and correctly interpreted.

TECHNIQUE OF SKIN TESTS

Instruments and materials must be sterile. The skin must be carefully cleaned, but irritation is to be avoided. Gentle sponging with 70% alcohol is sufficient. Most skin tests are performed on the forearm but other skin areas are equally satisfactory.

Intracutaneous Injection

A short bevel, fine gauge (No. 26 or 27) needle is introduced below the upper layers of the epithelium but not into the subcutis. A properly placed needle permits the injection of 0.1 ml of fluid, raising a round bleb. This is the most reliable technique, and is commonly used for tuberculin purified protein derivative (PPD) and histoplasmin tests, coccidioidin test in adults and many others.

Transcutaneous Administration

The site is cleaned and dried with a lance or needle, short scratches are made in the epidermis, not deeply enough to draw blood. The scratches should be 1/8 inch long and about 2 inches apart on the flexor aspect of the forearm. One drop of the allergen test fluid is applied to each scratch and left undisturbed for 10 minutes. This technique is used commonly in testing for pollen or food allergens.

Patch Tests

These depend on the ability of the test substance to diffuse into the skin. The test substance is adsorbed onto a small patch of gauze which is affixed to the skin with adhesive tape. Allowing the patch to remain in contact with the skin for 24 hours. Sterile, unimpregnated gauze must surround the patch and separate it from the area where the adhesive tape touches the skin (to distinguish reactions to the test substance from reactions to adhesive). This technique is used sometimes for tuberculin tests in children, but it is less reliable than the intradermal test.

IMMUNOLOGIC BASIC FOR SKIN TESTS

Most skin tests may be placed in one of the following three groups

Toxin—Antitoxin Neutralisation

The action of toxin or antitoxin is responsible for the observed reaction. In the Schick and Dick tests, toxin is injected into the skin. Unless neutralised by circulating antitoxin, the toxin provokes erythema and induration within 12-72 hours. A positive reaction thus indicates the absence of adequate antitoxin levels. In the Schültz-Charlton reaction, antitoxin is injected into an area of suspected scarlet fever rash. If blanching occurs, the erythrogenic toxin has been neutralised by specific antitoxin. This identifies the rash and confirms the diagnosis.

Anaphylatic Type of Hypersensitivity (Immediate Reactions)

This type of reaction is characterised by the following features:

a. The reaction is "immediate." Erythema and wheal formation appear within 5-20 minutes and disappear within 1 hour after injection or application of the allergen.
b. The reaction is associated with specific circulating antibodies and can be passively transferred by means of serum (see Prausnitz-Kustner reaction).
c. The reaction is mainly a vascular one, without much cellular infiltration and induration.

Examples of "immediate reactions" of this type are allergy to pollen and house serum sensitivity.

Tuberculin Type of Hypersensitivity (Delayed Reactions)

This type of reaction is characterised by the following features:

a. The reaction is "delayed". Erythema and induration appear in 24-48 hours and may last for several days.
b. The reaction is not intimately associated with circulating antibodies and cannot be transferred passively by means of serum. Passive transfer is possible by means of leucocytes or leucocyte extracts from a sensitised person.
c. The reaction is largely infiltrative and inflammatory with little acute change in vascular permeability (which is paramount in the anaphylactic type).

Examples of "delayed reactions" and tuberculin, coccidioidin, histoplasmin and Frei's tests.

COMMON SKIN TESTS

Toxin—Antitoxin Neutralisation Tests

Schick Test

For determining susceptibility to diphtheria.

1. *Material:* Diluted diphtheria toxin containing 1/50 MLD (minimal lethal dose for a guinea pig) in 0.1 ml, available commercially.
2. *Technique:* After cleansing the skin of the forearm, 0.1 ml is injected intradermally. A positive test consists of an area of erythema 1-2 cm in diameter reaching its maximum intensity about the fourth day. Pigmentation of the area may persist for weeks.
3. *Interpretation:* A positive test means that the individual does not have sufficient circulating antitoxin to neutralise the injected toxin and therefore that he is susceptible to diphtheria. The converse is true for the negative reaction.
   Present-day purified toxins rarely give false-positive reactions attributable to sensitivity tend to fade much quickly than a positive Schick test. If it is desired to include a check on possible sensitivity, 0.1 ml of heated (and therefore inactivated) toxin is injected into the other arm. If the control site develops the same reactions as the site injected with active toxin, sensitivity is present to the injected protein.
4. *Test for toxoid sensitivity:* Before immunisation of adults, the Mononey test for sensitivity to toxoid should be performed. This is usually done by injecting 0.1 ml diphtheria toxoid diluted 1:20

instead of the heated toxin control. A positive test indicates sensitivity to the toxoid, and immunisation has to start with exceedingly small doses.

Dick Test

For the determination of susceptibility to the erythrogenic toxin of haemolytic streptococci. It consists of observing the reaction to intradermally injected erythrogenic streptococcus toxin. The development of erythema indicates as positive test. A negative Dick test merely indicates probable immunity to the erythrogenic toxin but not to streptococcal infection. A Dick-negative person is unlikely to develop scarlet fever but is as likely as a Dick-positive person to develop other streptococcal diseases or sequelae. Therefore, the test is of little importance and is rarely done.

Schültz-Charlton Reaction

For the diagnosis of scarlet fever rash. The test consists of the injection of antitoxin to streptococcal erythrogenic toxin (or scarlet fever convalescent serum) into an area of rash. Blanching in 12 hours suggests specific neutralisation and confirms the diagnosis of scarlet fever. This test is of little importance and is rarely done.

Immediate Reaction Type of Skin Tests

Test for Sensitivity to Horse Serum

Before injecting horse serum (e.g., tetanus or diphtheria antitoxin) into any patient, ascertain possible sensitivity to horse serum. Similar precautions and tests apply to certain drugs, especially penicillin. Inquire about previous injections of serum or reactions to drugs, history of allergy, hay fever, etc., and perform sensitivity test as follows:

1. *Technique:* Always have a vial of 1:1000 epinephrine and a small syringe and needle ready when doing any test for serum sensitivity or administering serum. Of the two tests skin is more reliable. If no evidence of hypersensitivity is obtained by the tests, serum is administered undiluted by the route indicated.
   a. *Skin test:* Cleanse skin, then inject intradermally 0.1 ml of horse serum diluted 1:30 with saline. Appearance of wheal 1-3 cm in diameter within 15 minutes suggests sensitivity to horse serum.
   b. *Conjunctival test:* Examine conjunctivas for presence of inflammation. Instill 1 drop of horse serum diluted 1:10 into the conjunctival sac, 1 drop of saline into the other as control. The control conjunctiva should appear normal after 3-5 minutes. In persons hypersensitive to horse serum, the test conjunctiva will show reddening, itching and lacrimation within 15-30 minutes.
2. Unfavourable reactions following serum administration.
   a. *Immediate anaphylaxis:* Exceedingly rare if skin tests are negative. Consists of difficulty in breathing, nausea, vascular collapse, and shock within 5-60 minutes after serum administration. Give 1 ml of 1:1000 epinephrine subcutaneously at the first sign of reaction and other supportive measures. Unless the patient responds promptly, give hydrocortisone 100 mg I/V.
   b. *Febrile reaction:* Occurs even when skin test was negative. Chills, fever, nausea within 1-6 hours after serum was given intravenously. Use supportive measures, no epinephrine.
   c. *Serum sickness:* Occurs often, even when skin test was negative. Fever, pruritus, oedema, urticaria, lymphadenopathy, arthralgia, and occasionally arthritis with effusion develop 7-11 days after serum injection. Rarely, an accelerated reaction of the same type develops 1-6 days after injection of serum or drug (penicillin).
   d. *Treatment:* Epinephrine is helpful. Corticotropin adrenocorticitrophin hormone (ACTH) or corticosteroids tend to suppress the symptoms of hypersensitivity reactions.
3. If the skin test is positive:
   a. Obtain antiserum from another animal species (e.g., rabbit or goat) and repeat skin test with it.
      Avoid implicated drug.
   b. Desensitise the patient to horse serum.
4. Desensitisation is done as follows: Inject gradually increasing doses of horse serum diluted 1:10. Begin

with 0.1 ml, then 0.2 ml and 0.5 ml subcutaneously at 30 minute intervals. If no significant reaction is observed, give 0.1 ml undiluted horse serum followed by 0.2 ml and 0.5 ml at 30 minute intervals. If a given dose is followed by a slight reaction, give the same or a smaller dose after 30-60 minutes together with 1 ml of 1:1000 epinephrine. Increase doses steadily until 2 or 3 ml can be given without reaction. Repeat every 30-60 minutes until the full dose of serum has been given. Similar desensitisation is possible with drugs, e.g., streptomycin.

5. *Treatment of severe reactions:* After a severe reaction, it is unwise to continue serum administration and desensitisation. If severe reaction should occur during desensitisation, treat with:
   a. Epinephrine, 1:1000, 1 ml S/C or I/V.
   b. Atropine sulphate, 0.5 mg S/C.
   c. Antihistaminic drugs, e.g., diphenhydramine, I/V.
   d. Artificial respiration and oxygen if necessary; external warmth.
   e. Hydrocortisone, 50-100 mg I/V.

Direct Skin Tests for Allergens (Respiratory, contact, drug, or food)

1. *Technique:* In allergic work-up, the patient is ordinarily tested either with the scratch or the intradermal method for sensitivity to a variety of allergens. Test substances are available commercially or may be specially prepared. The usual positive response consists of a wheal and erythema appearing 5-30 minutes after contact with the allergen.
2. *Interpretation:* In interpreting such reactions, the following must be kept in mind:
   a. A negative skin test does not rule out systemic sensitivity.
   b. A positive skin test does not necessarily mean that allergic symptoms are related to the particular allergen.
   c. Individuals may at times give positive reactions to many substances, at other times to none.

Prausnitz-Kustner Reactions

A method used to demonstrate presence of a substance by passive transfer of serum. Used in dermatology and investigations of allergy.

1. *Technique:* Obtain serum from the patient and inject 0.2-0.3 ml intradermally into a normal person. Twelve to 18 hours later, inject the suspected antigen into the area thus prepared with the serum and into another comparable skin area, as control.
2. *Interpretation:* A positive reaction (erythema, wheal) at the test (but not the control site) indicates successful transfer of specific antibodies and, by inference, demonstrates that the patient possesses anaphylactic hypersensitivity to the allergen.

Penicillin Hypersensitivity

Use skin test of penicilloyl-polylsine, native penicillin, or its degradation products.

Foshay's Test

Rarely used in tularaemia and brucellosis for the detection of circulating specific antigen. Immediate positive reaction to intradermal injection of specific antiserum is considered useful in diagnosis.

Extracts of Parasitic Worms (e.g. *Trichinella*)

It may give immediate and delayed reactions (see below).

Delayed Reaction Type of Skin Tests

Tuberculin test (Mantoux test, Pirquet Reaction)

An individual who has been infected with the tubercle bacillus given a skin reaction of the delayed type when tuberculoprotein is administered. In addition to the local skin reaction, focal and general reactions may occur in very hypersensitive individual, e.g. persons with erythema nodosum or phlyctenular conjunctivitis. In such persons, therefore, only very minute quantities of test substances must be injected.

1. *Test materials*
   a. Old tuberculin (OT), a concentrated filtrate of broth in which tubercle bacilli have been grown.
   b. Purified protein derivative (PPD), obtained by chemical fractionation of OT. Both OT and PPD are available commercially, standardised in terms of biologic reactivity as tuberculin units (TU). Equivalent values are given below.

Approximate tuberculin equivalents

TU	*"Strength"*	*PPD mg/dose*	*OT dilution*
1	First	0.00002	1: 10,000
5	Inter-mediate	0.0001	1:2000
250	Second	0.005	1: 100

2. *Technique:* The initial test dose most commonly used is 5 TU, but this should be reduced to 1 TU, if the individual is expected to be hypersensitive. Higher doses are injected when lower doses have given negative results. Test material of suitable strength, 0.1 ml, is injected into the cleansed skin of forearm. Readings are taken 48 and 72 hours later.
3. *Reading and interpretation:* The tuberculin test is considered positive if induration of 10 mm diameter or more follows injection of 5 TU. Erythema has no specific meaning. In very strongly positive reactions, there may be central necrosis. A positive tuberculin test indicates only that the individual has been infected with tubercle bacilli in the past; it does not indicate present, active disease, resistance, or immunity. The test is most helpful if there is evidence of recent "conversion", i.e. change from tuberculin-negative to tuberculin-positive in a few months. This clearly indicates recent infection and requires study to rule out active disease.

Tuberculin tests may be falsely negative during illnesses which induce "anergy", e.g., milliary tuberculosis, measles and other exanthems, Boeck's sarcoid, and Hodgkin's disease, or in persons receiving immunosuppressants, e.g., corticosteroids.

Candida

Skin test material used to test for reactivity to a universal antigen or the presence of anergy.

Filariasis

Dirofilaria immitus. Skin test (CDC, Atlanta) supports diagnosis.

Ducrey Test (Ito-Reenstierna test, chancroid skin test, dmelcos test; for the diagnosis of chancroid)

Ducrey vaccine (a suspension of *H. ducreyi*) is injected intradermally. A positive reaction (erythema and induration) in 1-3 days denotes past infection with *H. ducreyi*; hypersensitivity may persist for years.

Brucellergen Test (For the diagnosis of brucellosis)

Intradermal injection of a suspension of *Brucella* organisms may give positive results in 12-48 hours. However, the test is not reliable and agglutination reactions are usually preferred if the organism cannot be isolated from the patient: Skin tests may raise agglutination titre.

Tularaemia Skin Test

Highly specific. Remains positive longer than agglutination titre.

Frei Test (For the diagnosis of lymphogranuloma venereum)

The antigen consists of suspension prepared from infected chick embryos and is injected intradermally. A control injection with uninfected chick embryo material must be included in the test. A positive reaction consists of induration and erythema 5-20 mm in diameter in 48 hours. Reading of the control injection must be negative. A positive reaction is suggestive of past infection with one of the agents of the lymphogranuloma—psittacosis group.

Mumps and Herpes Simplex Tests

Skin tests for infections are available, denoting past infections with these viruses. The reaction (after intracutaneous infection of virus material) is often faint and fleeting. It may reach its maximum erythema in 6-48 hours.

Echinococcus Skin Test (Casoni reaction; for the diagnosis of hydatid disease)

Antigen (hydatid fluid) obtained from human or animal sources gives immediate or delayed reactions after intradermal injection.

Trichinella Skin Test (For the diagnosis for trichinosis)

Commercial antigens can be used but an acid-soluble protein fraction (self-prepared) of *Trichina* larvae gives good specificity of delayed reaction

Coccidioidin Test (For diagnosis of past infection with Coccidioides immitus)

This test is essentially similar to the tuberculin test. The fungus is grown in synthetic medium for a long period and the broth is filtered and concentrated. Usual test strength is 1:100, giving a positive reaction with induration and erythema in 24-48 hours. Hypersensitivity is commonly acquired as a result of subclinical infection following transient and minimal exposure to infectious arthrospores. Hypersensitivity persists for life. The test is occasionally negative in disseminated coccidioidomycosis. Cross-reactions with other fungal infections are noted with lower dilutions of coccidioidin.

Histoplasmin Test (For the diagnosis of past infection with Histoplasma capsulatum)

Histoplasmin is prepared similarly to tuberculin and coccidioidin. Usual test strength is 1:100. Positive test indicates past infection. Cross-reactions with other fungal infections are apparently rather high.

Blastomycin Test (For the diagnosis of past infection with Blastomyces)

Test material is a suspension of yeast phase of *Blastomyces*. Test interpretation and reading are similar to those of the coccidioidin test.

Kveim-Siltzbach Test (For the diagnosis of sarcoidosis)

An extract of sarcoid tissue (especially lymph node of spleen) injected into the skin of a person with sarcoidosis results in a small papule which persists for months. Excision of this papule after 4-8 weeks discloses a microscopic pattern resembling other sarcoid lesions. The basis of the reaction is uncertain, and the test not quite reliable.

Toxoplasma Skin Test

Injection of test material prepared from a suspension of killed organisms gives a delayed reaction in some persons with positive serologic tests. No reaction in others. The test is unreliable for diagnosis and is used mainly for epidemiology.

Nonbacterial Regional Lymphadenitis ("Cat Scratch Fever") Test

Pus from active cases is diluted 1:5, heated at 60°C for 10 hours, and stored at 4°C. Intradermal injection of 0.1 ml gives a delayed reaction in persons with this disorder, no reaction in others.

THESE INVESTIGATIONS HAVE NOW LARGELY BEEN REPLACED BY MORE ACCURATE (AND NOT AT ALL DANGEROUS) ENZYME-LINKED IMMUNOSORBENY ASSAY (ELISA) TESTS.

CHAPTER 29

Diagnostic Immunology
(Immunodiffusion, Electrophorsis and Turbidimetry)

QUALITATIVE DETERMINATION OF PLASMA PROTEINS BY IMMUNOPRECIPITATION

The principle of immunoprecipitation was first described by Kraus. Originally, immunoprecipitation reactions carried out in test tubes were detected by the fact that turbidity can be observed following the mixing of antigen (Ag) and antibody (Ab) solutions. Centrifugation of such samples results in an insoluble sediment. Layering the antigen solution on top of the antibody solution in a narrow test tube, without mixing, results in a ring-like turbidity at the contact area within a short time. This so-called "ring test" reveals the presence of Ag-Ab precipitation in the solution studied. A distinction of characteristics between the various antigens and antibodies cannot be made.

Immunodiffusion Method of Oudin

With this method, the Ag-Ab precipitation takes place in a gel medium. Due to the different diffusion rates of heterogeneous antigens (e.g. the proteins of blood serum) the differentiation of the various antigens is rendered possible. The linear (one dimensional) double diffusion technique, i.e. diffusion of antigens and antibodies from opposite directions, results in the formation of multilayered precipitations if heterologous Ag solutions and multivalent antisera are used.

Agar is most frequently employed for the gel because of its transparency and solidification characteristics.

Double Diffusion Method of Ouchterlony

Agar gel is poured uniformly onto glass plates or into Petri dishes and allowed to solidify. Holes (wells) are cut into the agar gel which are filled with Ag and Ab solutions, respectively. Both the antigens and antibodies diffuse radially, and form, upon confluence, immunoprecipitates. These immunoprecipitates often take the form of a curved line. Because of its numerous possible modifications, the versatile arrangement of Ag-Ab containing wells, etc. this technique is widely applied in immunological, biochemical and medical laboratories.

Grabar and Williams's Method of Immunoelectrophoresis

This represents a combination of physicochemical and immunochemical techniques. The material to be examined (e.g. tissue exudates, serum, etc.) is separated electrophoretically on agar gel and, subsequently, subjected to the effect of a precipitating antiserum. This is done by placing antiserum in a trough in the agar parallel to the electrophoretically separated proteins. Both the antibodies and antigens diffuse toward one another, forming, upon confluence, well-defined precipitin lines.

To date, approximately 30 different precipitin lines in human serum can be detected by immunoelectrophoresis (IEP), indicating an equal number of individuals serum proteins. Of late, many of these serum proteins have been characterised.

The immunoelectrophoretic technique is a valuable addition to available methods for characterisation of proteins. This technique is usefully employed in all areas of protein chemistry and in connection with the investigation of a large number of clinical problems connected with protein metabolism. In particular, the microtechnique of IEP has found widespread acceptance.

METHODOLOGY

Double Diffusion of Ouchterlony

Macrotechnique

Reagents

1. Phosphate buffer solution 0.15 mol/L, pH 7.1. This solution is obtained by mixing 67 ml of solution I with 33 ml of solution II.
   Solution I: Distilled water is added to 26.70 gm of $Na_2 HPO_4 . 2H_2O$ to total 1,000 ml.
   Solution II: Distilled water is added to 20.41 gm of KH_2PO_4 to total 1,000 ml.
2. Agar
   Behringwerke agar purum or agar of equal quality which possesses satisfactory transparency.
3. Antisera
   Antisera to plasma proteins.

Preparation of Agar Gel Slides

Four grams of purified agar is mixed with 100 ml of phosphate buffer solution 0.15 mol/L, pH 7.1, and 300 ml of distilled water. Approximately 40 mg of Thimerosal are added as a preservative. This mixture is heated at 100°C until the solution is clear. Undissolved particles can be removed by centrifugation of the hot solution at 3,000 rpm for 2-3 minutes.

Twenty two millilitres of the hot agar solution is then pipetted into level Petri dishes of 8 cm diameter. Upon standing for a short time, the agar solution will solidify, forming a gel. Holes (wells) are cut into the agar gel by means of a glass or metal punch. For routine examinations, it is best to cut holes of 0.6 to 0.7 cm in diameter approximately 2 cm apart (as measured from the centre of the holes). Punch sets of various patterns are available commercially. After cutting the holes, a small amount of agar gel is heated with several drops of water in a test tube. A few drops of this diluted agar solution are added to each hole to seal the gaps between the agar gel and the bottom of the Petri dish.

Gel Diffusion Procedure

Petri dishes prepared in this manner can be used for nay type of immunoprecipitation reaction. Multivalent antisera (e.g. antiserum to human serum), heterogeneous antigen solution (e.g. human serum), purified proteins (human IgG, human IgA, or human albumin), or specific antisera (e.g, antisera to plasma proteins) can be analysed by this method.

The wells in the agar plate are filled completely with approximately 0.1 ml of antigen solution or antiserum. Highly precipitating antisera react optimally with antigen solutions of concentrations between 1 and 10 mg/ml. The Petri dish is covered to prevent drying of the agar, then allowed to stand at room temperature for 2-3 days.

During this period, immunoprecipitates form. Each individual antigen produces a single precipitin line, the location of which depends upon the rate of diffusion and the concentration of the antigen. The diffusion rate of protein depends primarily upon the molecular weight. High molecular globulins (e.g. macroglobulins) are precipitated in the proximity of the point of application, in contrast to antigens of lower molecular weight (e.g. albumin) which are precipitated nearer to antibody well. Immunologically, identical proteins in adjacent wells form precipitin lines which merge completely ("reaction of identity"). Partial immunological identity (partially shared antigenic determinants) is reflected by formation of precipitin arcs, which partially fuse and partially intersect forming so-called "spurs" (e.g. γ G-globulin) and γ A-globulin). Immunological non-identity is reflected by intersection of the precipitin lines without fusion (e.g. albumin and γ G-globulin).

Microtechnique

A microtechnique, using small agar gel plates, with smaller Ag wells and shorter distances between them, is applicable, under certain circumstances. Examples include the need to examine small amounts of test material, or if test results are needed in a short time period. Plates for this microtechnique may be prepared with a 2% agar solution as used for immunoelectrophoresis. Three ml quantities of the hot agar solution are pipetted onto precleaned glass slides (2" × 2") and the agar is then allowed to solidify. The agar wells are cut either individually or by means of a template.

Recording of Results

Photographic recording of results of gel diffusion tests is the most satisfactory method of documentation. Precipitin lines can be copied directly onto photographic paper. For this purpose, the surface of the agar gel is carefully rinsed with tap water to remove dust or other undissolved particles in the antisera or antigen solutions. To obtain an optically uniform surface, the agar is covered by tap water or physiological saline solution. The Petri dish is then placed on photographic paper (extra hard) in a dark room and illuminated from above with a lamp of approximately 200 watts. When optimally exposed and developed, the photographic paper will exhibit even fine precipitin lines with great sharpness.

Staining of the precipitin patterns of gel diffusion preparations can be achieved by the methods described under "immunoelectrophoresis" if this should prove necessary.

Possible Sources of Error

1. Specific antisera to plasma proteins are obtained by immunising rabbits or goats with highly purified plasma proteins. Frequently, traces of contaminating antibodies in such antisera must be removed by absorption. Absorbed antisera may contain minute amounts of antigens (human plasma proteins) used for this purpose. This possibility must be considered when precipitin lines occur between the antisera wells, where two or more types of antisera are used.
2. Occasionally, circular precipitates develop around the antigen wells. These "hallos" occur particularly when markedly lipemic or aged samples of sera or plasma are used. These non-specific precipitations are easily distinguished from specific immunoprecipitates by their circular arrangements. Strongly haemolytic sera may mimic nonspecific precipitates on photographic records.

IMMUNOELECTROPHORESIS

Reagents and Equipment

Agar

Agar used for IEP should have a low calcium concentration and should yield a transparent gel with a low solidifications point. Agar of good quality can be prepared by washing commercially available agar. It is important to wash agar thoroughly with distilled water since electrophoretic separation of serum proteins depends partly upon the purity of agar. For example, in unwashed agar the protein migration to the anode in the electrical field is limited; the majority of proteins migrate to the cathode due to the marked electro-osmotic potential. Agar specifically prepared for IEP is available from Behring diagnostics.

Particularly suitable as a carrier medium for IEP is the low-ion agarose, which is obtained by the removal of the agaropectin moiety of agar.

Buffer

Michaelis diethylbarbiturate acetate buffer solution pH = 8.2, μ = 0.1.

A total of 13.38 gm of sodium 5, 5-diethylbarbiturate and 8.83 gm of sodium acetate trihydrate are dissolved in distilled water to yield 1.5 litres. The pH is adjusted to 8.2 by adding approximately 180 ml 0.1 N hydrochloric acid. This solution possesses an ionic strength of μ = 0.1.

Antisera

Depending upon the specific problem to which the technique is being applied (e.g. IEP analysis of human serum) either the multivalent antisera (i.e. antisera containing numerous antibodies, such as those directed against the various proteins of human serum) or the specific antisera (i.e. antisera directed against specific antigens, such as albumin, Ig G, etc.) can be employed. Such antisera can be prepared in horses, rabbits, goats chickens, or other suitable animals. The higher the immunoprecipitation titre of the antiserum (as shown by the ring test), the stronger are the precipitin lines on IEP.

With rabbit antiserum to human serum, approximately 30 different human serum proteins can be demonstrated by IEP. A somewhat different immunoelectrophoretic pattern is obtained with horse antihuman antiserum. This difference is due to an altered Ag-Ab ratio which is dependent upon the species specific differences of antibody structures. Rabbit antisera form strong precipitin lines in a wide range of Ag-Ab ratios, whereas horse antisera produce finer and sharper precipitin lines in a rather narrow range of Ag-Ab ratios. For this reason, it may be advisable to use various dilutions when using horse antisera.

A list of antisera to plasma protein made by Behringwerke can be had from Behring diagnostics.

Immunoelectrophoresis Equipment

The equipment for IEP with all needed accessories is commercially available. It can be obtained from: Mass Diagnostics, Delhi.

Preparation of Agar Gel Slides

Two grams of pure agar is dissolved in 50 ml of diethylbarbiturate acetate buffer, pH 8.2 (μ = 0.1) (can check by pH meter), and 50 ml of distilled water. This solution is heated for 15 minutes in a water bath of 100°C. Any undissolved particles can be removed from the heated agar by centrifugation at 3,000 rpm for 2-3 minutes. Ten mg of Thimerosal is added as a preservative. The hot agar solution is applied by pipette to alcohol cleansed, level glass slides. 3 ml of agar are placed onto each glass slide. After a few minutes the agar solidifies and the glass slides thus prepared are put into moisture chamber. A simple plastic container with Petri dish of water could serve as a moisture chamber.

It is advisable to prepare just sufficient agar solution to cover the glass slides since repeated heating of the gel leads to alterations which interfere with electrophoretic process. Holes and troughs are punched trough the agar layer with a die or suitable modification. On both sides of the through, a hole is made. Agar remaining in the punch is aspirated by a syringe connected to the barrel of the punch by rubber tubing.

Application of Antigens

The antigen mixture, e.g. serum, to be electrophoresed is introduced into the wells by a 26-gauge needle attached to a tuberculin syringe or by means of an appropriate micropipette. Complete fillings of the wells require about 0.002 ml of serum or protein solution. Each slide provides two Ag wells, permitting antigen analysis in duplicates or comparison of two different antigens. For the analysis of enzymatically cleaved agents or substances which diffuse readily, it is recommended that only one antigen be electrophoresed, since migration to the other side of the Ab trough is a possibility.

Electrophoresis

In principle the apparatus used for IEP is similar to that used for paper electrophoresis. The ends of the antigen-containing agar covered microscope slides are placed on two parallel bars. Filter paper strips establish the contact between the agar on the slides and the buffer in the troughs. The slides must be horizontal in position. The voltage between the ends of the slides is 45 V (6 volts/cm). Adequate electrophoretic separation is achieved within 45 minutes. Under these conditions the agar slides warm to approximately 25-28°C. Therefore, the application of a lid is necessary to prevent dessication.

Application of Antiserum

Subsequent to electrophoretic separation, the agar strip from the precut centre trough is removed with a 19-gauge injection needle attached to tuberculin syringe. The amount of antiserum applied is approximately 0.04 to 0.06 ml. It is advantageous to vary the antigen and antiserum concentrations. A shorter antibody trough can be used to examine only one serum fraction (e.g. IgG) in order to economise on antisera. After application of antiserum, the slides are placed in a moisture chamber for diffusion. The electophoretically separated proteins (i.e. antigens) and the antiserum diffuse toward one another and the homologous agents undergo an Ag-Ab reaction by forming precipitin lines at the points of confluence. Depending upon the concentration of antigens and antisera, optimal immunoprecipitates are formed between 20 hours and longer.

Possible Sources of Errors

1. Slides must be cleaned with chromic sulphuric acid.
2. The electrophoretic separation of the serum protein must be within an optimal range. Too short or too long a separation distance may be caused by faulty buffer composition (pH, μ), by incomplete contact between agar slides and filter paper strips, or by improper voltage. It is important to maintain uniform distribution of voltage (not of current) through the agar.
3. Wells of proper diameters and the correct distance between the Ag well and Ab trough are decisive for satisfactory IEP. Deviation from these specifications may result in marked dislocations and/or distortion of precipitin patterns.
4. The agar gel slides should be used within 2 or 3 days after preparation and must be stored in moisture-containing sealed containers, preferably at 4°C.
5. The sera to be examined should be fairly fresh or stored by freezing at –20°C. Bacterial contamination or autocatalytic processes may result in marked alterations of serum samples, leading to changes in electrophoretic mobility, solubility, etc.
6. Normal control sera should be examined simultaneously with abnormal sera.

Fixation of Precipitin Patterns

Immunoelectrophoretic patterns can be recorded by photographing the unstained or stained precipitin lines. For most purposes, direct photography of the slide is sufficient.

Staining of the precipitin patterns is occasionally of value for chemical characterisation of the precipitin lines. The agar slides are washed with physiological saline for one or two days, in order to remove the nonprecipitated protein from the agar. They are then covered by the filter paper and dried completely either in the incubator at 37°C (or in air at room temperature). After removal of the filter paper, the agar slides are placed in 2% acetic acid solution for approximately 5 minutes. The various staining techniques performed are as follows.

Protein Stains

Amidoschwarz (*Amido black*): 0.5% amidoschwarz 10B in methanol-glacial acetic acid (9:1). Stain for 5-10 minutes, then wash with methanolglacial acetic acid (9:1), for approximately 15 minutes.

Azocarmine: 0.5% azocarmine B in methanol-glacial acetic acid (9:1). Stain for 15 minutes; wash with methanol-glacial acetic acid solution (9:1).

Light green: 0.5% green SF in 5% trichloroacetic acid. Stain for one hour; wash with 5% trichloroacetic acid solution.

Bromophenol blue: 0.1% bromophenol blue in $HgC1_2$-saturated methanol. Wash with methanol. Green stain results from acid solution, blue stain from alkaline solution.

Lipoprotein Stains

Oil red: 0.5% oil red O in 50% ethanol (filtered). Stain for approximately two hours. Wash with 50% ethanol.

Sudanblack: Sudanblack (0.1%) is dissolved in 60% ethanol at 37°C, with occasional stirring, during a 24-hour time period. This solution is then filtered at 25°C and stored in dark containers. Before use, 0.1 ml of a 30% sodium hydroxide solution is added to 160 ml of the sudanblack solution. After staining for 2 hours, the slides are then washed using 50% ethanol.

Peroxidase Reaction (for haptoglobin and haemopexin)

Benzidine: Dissolve 0.2 gm benzidine in 100 ml of distilled water, then add 0.5 ml glacial acetic acid and 0.2 ml hydrogen peroxide 30%. When stained for 10-20 minutes, the specific precipitates become dark greenish-blue in colour.

Fixation of the colour: Wash briefly with distilled water, stain for 10 minutes in a 0.1% solution of $Ni(NH_4)_2$ $(SO_4)_2$, thereafter for 12 hours in 0.2% $Ni(NH_4)_2(SO_4)_2$. The specific colour is bluish black.

Ceruloplasmin Stain

p-Phenylenediamine: Solution must be prepared immediately before use. Dissolve 21.6 mg of p-phenylenediamine in 100 ml of sodium acetate buffer solution (pH 5.7, $\mu = 0.1$); add 10 ml of a solution consisting of 0.65 gm sodium azide in 1,000 ml of distilled water, and warm to 37°C. Stain for 2 hours at 37°C. Wash twice for 2 hours in sodium acetate buffer (pH 5.7). This technique is suitable for fresh samples only.

Cholinesterase Stain

Indoxylacetate: Five mg indoxylacetate is dissolved in 0.5 ml acetone, to which are added immediately thereafter 22 ml of a diethylbarbiturate acetate buffer solution pH 8.2, $\mu = 0.05$ (1 volume of buffer $\mu = 0.1$ and one volume of distilled water) and 2.5 ml of copper acetate solution 0.1 µmol/L (0.018) gm copper acetate in 100 ml distilled water). This solution must be used within 8 hours after preparation. After staining for 2 hours, and subsequent washing in tap water for one hour, cholinesterase is indicated by blue colour.

Lipid-Protein Double Staining

A volume of 0.5% oil red solution in 50% ethanol is suitable as a lipid stain. Place the slide in the dye mixture for approximately 2 hours, then wash 50% ethyl alcohol. A volume of 0.5% light green solution in 5% trichloroacetic acid is then immediately applied to achieve the specific protein stain. The staining time for proteins is approximately one hour. Wash with trichloroacetic acid.

The slides must be photographed after for keeping a permanent record.

Identification and Interpretation of Precipitin Lines

The analysis of immunoelectrophoretic patterns requires a certain degree of experience and training. It is imperative to be able to recognise the various specific precipitin lines. Various techniques are available to achieve identification of given precipitin line by experimental means:

1. Employment of specific antisera
2. Specific stains
3. Selective absorption
4. Employment of purified proteins.

PRACTICAL APPLICATION OF IMMUNOELECTROPHORESIS

Increased immunoglobulin concentrations are indicated by elongated and thickened precipitin lines of IgG, IgA and IgM immunoglobulins and antigen excess result in positions of these precipitin lines closer to the antibody trough in comparison with those obtained with normal sera. Although IEP does not lend itself to precise quantitation of serum proteins, marked deviations from normal concentrations may be recognised.

Increased IgG, IgA and IgM are frequently associated with acute and chronic liver diseases. This is the case in acute hepatitis, in which a particularly impressive increase in IgM occurs. In infectious mononucleosis, chronic hepatitis and Leannec's cirrhosis all three major immunoglobulins are frequently, but not invariably, increased. In lipoid hepatitis the IgG-globulin precipitin line may be markedly accentuated. Collagen diseases, including Sjögren's syndrome and systemic lupus erythematosus (SLE), as well as certain infections, may be associated with hyperimmunoglobulinaemia as indicated by IEP. In trypanosomiasis, the IgM may be excessively increased. Certain virus diseases, such as Coxsackie infections, are often associated with increased immunoglobulins.

In most cases of sarcoidosis IEP has not revealed abnormal serum protein changes, though definite IgA increases have been observed by some. IEP revealed increased immunoglobulin contents in a variety of additional diseases such as dermatitis herpetiformis and dermatitis gestationis and pernicious anaemia in which IgA, and mongolism in which the IgA and IgG were increased. Besides all the causes mentioned above, the disorders mentioned under hypoalbunaemia, monoclonal and polyclonal gammopathies discussed under serum protein in clinical chemistry chapter can also be assessed by using IEP techniques.

QUANTITATIVE DETERMINATION OF PLASMA PROTEINS BY IMMUNOPRECIPITATION

The reagents used for quantitative determination are specific antisera which react stoichiometrically with the proteins to be determined and form precipitates with them. These immune reactions may occur either in solutions or in gels which contain the antiserum in even distribution. In the first case, the quantity of immune precipitate, measurable at appropriate dilutions as turbidity or by other means, gives a quantitative measure of the antigen concentration. By using, as the reaction medium, a gel containing antiserum, the reagent is arranged in the form of a stationary phase into which the antigen can penetrate either by diffusion or under the influence of an electrical field. The resulting precipitates, which assume different configurations depending on the method used, can be quantitatively evaluated.

In the four most widely used methods to be described, reaction conditions have been selected which ensure that the quantity of specific antiserum is constant and exceeds the quantity of antigen, while the concentrations of the antigens to be determined can vary within wide ranges.

FUNDAMENTAL QUANTITATIVE CONSIDERATIONS

Photometric Method

Principle: This method is a modification based on the determination of the nitrogen content of isolated immunoprecipitates as described by Heidelberger. In contrast to the tedious technique, the antigen and antibody are allowed to react together at high dilution. Under these conditions, the reaction product of the immune reaction does not result in the formation of the precipitate which sediments, but merely in the appearance of tubidity. The extinction (e.g. at 450 nm) can be used as a measure of the turbidity. If the quantity of antiserum is kept constant and the antigen concentration is varied, a curve can be obtained. When the antigen is present in excess, soluble reaction products are formed. For this reason, only the ascending limb of the curve can be used for quantitative determinations. By reference to this part of the curve, the concentration of antigen in an unknown solution can be determined.

Single Linear Immunodiffusion of Oudin

Principle: Gel containing the antiserum is allowed to solidify in a test tube, and the antigen solution is poured on top of it. The precipitate formed at the boundary layer migrates into gel zone. The distance of the front of the precipitate from the boundary surface is proportional to the square root of the diffusion time, t.

$$h = k \times \sqrt{t}$$

As the migration velocity of the antigen

$$k \frac{h}{\sqrt{t}}$$

is proportional to the logarithm of its concentration CAg and the distance h through which the precipitate migrates may be expressed by the following equation:

$$\log CAg = a \times k + b = a \times \frac{h}{\sqrt{t}} + b$$

Accordingly, if CAg as a function of $\frac{h}{\sqrt{t}}$, is plotted in a semilogarithmic system, the result is a straight line. Its slope is represented by a and it intersects the ordinate at b. The slopes a and b are thus constants determined by the Ag-Ab system under consideration. The length of the cylinder of precipitate is proportional to the negative logarithm of antibody concentration.

The fundamental difference between the techniques of single linear immunodiffusion and single radial immunodiffusion and electroimmunodiffusion (EID) described below is simply that in the former the antigen concentration is determined from the speed of migration of an immunoprecipitate; while in the latter methods, it is determined by measuring the precipitin area on the length of a precipitate which remains constant after a certain time period.

Since the diffusion velocity of any molecule is dependent on temperature, it is essential in using Oudin's technique that the temperature be kept strictly constant during the reaction period.

The results of EID by Laurell's method and single radial immunodiffusion as described by Mancini, Cabonara and Heremans are not significantly affected by temperature fluctuations. One advantage of Oudin's method is that the solutions require less exact volume measurements, and pipetting errors which may affect other methods are of minor importance.

Single Radial Immunodiffusion

Principle: Dissolved antigen molecules diffuse radially from a cylindrical well into an agar gel layer of uniform thickness containing the corresponding antiserum. The resulting precipitate assumes the form of a cylinder or ring. When diffusion ceases, the surface area of the base of the cylinder is directly proportional to the quantity of antigen, at a predetermined concentration of antiserum in the reaction gel.

If the circular area πr^2 (i.e., area of central well + area of precipitate) is plotted on a graph as a function of the quantity of antigen QAg (i.e., antigen concentration × volume of antigen solution), the result is a straight line relationship expressed by the equation $\pi r^2 = k \times QAg + S$

The point S at which the straight line intercepts the ordinate is a function of the size of the central well. And the slope k is inversely proportional to the antiserum concentration in the gel and the gel thickness. By standardising the technical conditions, it is possible to keep constant the variables contained in k and S so that the measured radius or diameter of the precipitate ring is a function solely of the quantity of antigen introduced. With the aid of standardised protein preparations, it is possible to construct a reference curve which can be used to determine the antigen concentrations of unknown solutions. It is essential, however, to deliver identical volumes of the antigen solutions, standard and test solutions, into central wells.

Differences in temperature do not affect the results of this reaction. The only effect of a rise in temperature is to accelerate diffusion and thereby the appearance of a measurable precipitin ring. However, the temperature should not be allowed to rise above 37°C because the gel may melt and because of the risk of irreversible damage to the thermolabile proteins.

Electroimmunodiffusion

Principle: In the course of the electrophoretic migration of an antigen through agarose gel containing the corresponding antiserum, it produces an extended trail of an immunoprecipitate. The length 'I' of the precipitate is a measure of the antigen concentration provided that the latter is contained in a fixed volume of solvent.

Depending on the electrophoretic migration rate of an antigen, the precipitin peaks may appear more or less rapidly. Fast moving proteins usually produce long narrow precipitin bands ending in a point, while proteins of lower eletrophoretic mobility produce broader precipitates with rounded ends. Because of their slow migration rates, elctrophoresis takes longer; diffusion of the antigen at right angles to the direction of electrophoresis may be responsible for the broadening of the peaks. The migration velocity of the antigens is affected by the field strength and the pH of the buffer solution employed. Careful standardisation of these factors is essential for reproducible results. This makes the method somewhat more elaborate than comparable methods based on diffusion alone. On the other hand, the results are usually available in 2 or 3 hours, while the methods of Oudin and Mancini require at least 20-30 hours.

Single Radial Immunodiffusion

Equipment

Antiserum-agar gel plates of single radial immunodiffusion by the method of Mancini, Carbonara and Heremans as modified by Augener can be prepared in polystyrene Petri dishes (8 cm diameter) having perfectly flat bottoms.

Application of exact amounts of antigen samples is best achieved by the use of a microlitre syringe with which exact amounts of 1 µL can be delivered (provided by Behring diagnostics).

The immunoprecipitin rings can be measured with a measuring microscope or a magnifying lens with 0.1 mm scale. A simple way of measuring is by using a measuring template (with *Tripartigen* plates from Behring Diagnostics, these are given as part of the kit for immunoglobulin, etc., quantitations).

Procedure

A microlitre syringe is used to fill holes in the agar gel layer with 2 µL of antigen solution. At least three different dilutions of each standard solution are required to plot a curve. The remaining holes are used for the solutions being analysed. Each is filled with 2 µL of the test specimen in suitable dilution; the diluent is physiological saline. After introducing the reagents, the plates are left in a moisture chamber at room temperature. The results are preferably read after 2 days, although an approximate reading can be obtained in one day. After 2 days, the circular immunoprecipitates in the gel layer are distinct and can easily be measured. For *Tripartigen* (from Behring Diagnostics) a Tripartigen ruler (scale) is provided to read the ring diameter and the quantitation is done by noting the corresponding value given in appropriate units from the reference chart provided. With every kit, a standard serum/specific protein solution can also be had for comparing results.

TUBIDIMETRY

Introduction

Diagnosis is a decision point. The decision is the intention to treat. It is the point at which sufficient evidence has been accumulated to state, beyond reasonable doubt, that the patient is or is not suffering from a particular disease.

Laboratory tests remain one of the mainstays on which the clinicians rely for diagnosis and management of the patient. Laboratory tests are indicated for:

1. **Detection:** The presence or absence of a particular substance, e.g., testing for infectious diseases like Veneral Diseases Research Laboratory (VDRL), Hepatitis B surface antigen (HBsAg).
2. **Quantification:** Accurately determining the concentration of a particular substance as an aid to diagnosis or differential diagnosis (e.g., Concentration of CRP in differential diagnosis of viral and bacterial infections) and for establishing the extent of the clinical condition (e.g., IgA in measuring disease severity).
3. **Monitoring:** The course of clinical condition or response to therapy.
4. **Prognosis:** For predicting the probability of occurrence of a disease/disorder (e.g., microalbuminuria for predicting diabetic nephropathy) or predicting the outcome of a disease/disorder.

Microscopy, biochemical assays, microbiology procedures, and immunoassays are various techniques that fulfil the requirements of routine laboratory tests to meet the needs of the clinicians.

Certain clinical analytes can be measured by specific techniques only, whereas for the measurement of certain analytes options exist for selecting the techniques of measurement. For example, urinary albumin can be measured by biochemical methods such as pyrogallol red or coumassie blue. But for the diagnosis of microalbuminuria, a condition where urinary excretion of albumin is in the range of 30-300 mg/L, the accuracy of the measurements by biochemical methods is questionable because these methods also react with other proteins in addition to albumin which are frequently found to be present in urine. Immunochemical methods (immunoassays) which are more sensitive and specific have a distinct advantage and, hence, are preferred.

Immunoassays

Immunoassays are assays that detect the presence of an antigen in the human body with the help of an antibody or detect the presence of an antibody with the help of an antigen. In this text for simplicity, all further information provided is based on considering antibody as a reagent to detect antigen in the human body fluids.

The first reported immunoassays were homogeneous. They are attributed to Kraus (1897), who coined the term **'precipitin'** for the precipitate formed upon mixing an antigen and an antibody.

Meyer in 1922 employed sheep erythrocytes to serve as a label and conjugated human immunoglobulin to them. Anti-immunoglobulin antibodies appearing in rheumatoid arthritis patients were shown to cause visible clumping of these erythrocytes. This method was known as **haemagglutination.**

Singer and Plotz replaced the erythrocytes with latex particles, which were easier to standardise, and these assays are popularly known as **latex agglutination tests.** High degree of sensitivity for a wide variety of antigens/antibodies, which can be detected by these latex agglutination assays, has promoted their usage worldwide for screening since 1956 in clinical laboratories. The simplicity of performance and obviating the need for equipments, have made these assays extremely popular.

The need for quantitative estimation, and higher sensitivity led to the development of **radioimmunoassays** (RIA) first in 1959 by Berson and Rosalyn Yalow. The first RIA developed was used to detect and quantify insulin.

Since then immunoassays have been used to detect and quantify a variety of molecules native to humans such as proteins, hormones as well as foreign molecules such as bacteria, viruses and parasites.

Qualitative Immunoassays

Qualitative immunoassay techniques provide test results, which only help to dentify or indicate the presence of analytes. Various techniques for qualitative detection of antigens have been in use, which include latex agglutination, passive gel diffusion, IEP and Western blotting. These techniques at the best can give a semiquantitative or comparative information about analytes under assay.

Single immunodiffusion technique uses the diffusion of an antigen into agar impregnated with antibody. **Double immunodiffusion technique** allows the direct comparison of two or more test materials providing a simple and direct method for determining whether the antigens in the test specimens are identical, cross-reactive, or non-identical. **Immunoelectrophoresis** has been used over the years for detection of several different antigens present in a common solution. The latex agglutination assays though simple to use are subject to variations in results as the interpretation pattern between negative and weakly reactive samples may vary between laboratory to laboratory and person to person.

Lower sensitivity for many analytes and the need for correct quantification of analytes for:

- Effective monitoring of disease
- For differential diagnosis to aid correct therapy, have created the need for more sensitive and precise quantitative immunoassays

Quantitative Immunoassays

Quantitative results of immunoassays are extremely useful in:

- Establishing the extent of severity of a disease
- Assessing the course and stage of clinical condition
- Differential diagnosis of many diseases
- Monitoring response to therapy
- Accurate prognosis of disease

Various techniques have been used to develop quantitative methods that include radial immunodiffusion (RID) and electroimmunoassays, turbidimetric and nephelometric assays and labelled immunochemical assays.

The RID and electroimmunoassay (rocket electrophoresis) though reliable, are slow, relatively involvement intensive, and expensive. This limits their usage in routine laboratories. In many laboratories the gel-based techniques are restricted to qualitative studies or are used as reference methods.

During the last decade, the gel techniques are increasingly being replaced by optical detection methods.

The various techniques by which quantitative immunoassays are performed can be broadly grouped as follows;

Heterogeneous Immunoassays: These assay systems employ an antibody immobilised on a solid phase, which captures the corresponding antigen from the sample. A second labelled antibody specific to a different epitope of the antigen is used as a basis for signal generation. After the immunochemical reaction has taken place, the bound-and unbound-labelled antibodies are separated. The concentration of antigen is then estimated by measuring bound or unbound-labelled antibodies through an appropriate signal generation and measurement system.

Heterogeneous immunoassays can be performed by various techniques such as:

- Radioimmunoassays (RIA)
- Enzymeimmunoassays (EIA)
- Fluorescent enzyme immunoassay
- Chemiluminescent enzyme immunoassay

The difficulties associated with separation of bound-and unbound-labelled antibodies, the need for dedicated instrumentation and labour intensive procedures has prompted the usage of heterogeneous assays in speciality laboratories mainly through use of expensive automation.

The need for simpler, affordable, user-friendly assay techniques for detection of routinely encountered clinical analytes still remained to be explored. With the tremendous progress made in instrumentation technology, ootics, and software, the face of quantitative estimation for routine parameters has changed dramatically in the recent years. Simultaneous development in purification techniques for polyclonal antibodies, emergence of monoclonal antibodies with high specificity and avidity have been instrumental in the development of homogeneous assay techniques which are simple to perform and easily adaptable for routine laboratory analysis.

Homogeneous Immunoassays: These assays require only the mixing of a sample (antigen) and the immunochemical reagents (antibody) followed by detection of signal. These assays do not require separation of free or bound-labelled materials in the test system for the detection or measurement of the antigen. In homogeneous immunoassays the immunochemical binding produces a detectable signal (agglutination, absorbance, fluorescence, etc.). The simplicity and flexibility associated with the performance of homogeneous assays has made their usage popular with laboratarians worldwide.

The homogeneous assays can be performed by different techniques such as:

- Turbidimetry
- Nephelometry
- Homogeneous enzyme immunoassays
- Enzyme-multiplied immunoassay technique (EMIT)
- Enzyme inhibitor immunoassay
- Enzyme complementation immunoassay
- Substrate linked fluorescence immunoassay (SLFIA)
- Scintillation proximity assay (SPA)
- Electrochemiluminiscence (ECL)
- Luminescent oxygen channelling immunoassay (LOCI)

The clinical chemistry analysers (photometers) were originally developed for colourimetric estimation of chemical or enzymatic reactions. Subsequently, it was shown that the visible scattered light in Kraus's precipitin reaction could be measured by turbidimetry and nephelometry on photometers, to quantitate the immune complex formation. These systems utilise the fast reaction between an antigen with their corresponding antibodies in a liquid phase.

The technique of quantitation by turbidimetry and nephelometry is apparently similar to the popular absorption spectrophotometry used in routine clinical laboratories and hence, adaptable by high throughput as well as small and medium laboratories easily.

SPECTROPHOTOMETRY

Spectrophotometers work on the basis of the Beer's and Lambert's law.

Beer's law: When a coloured solution is illuminated with a monochromatic light (light of a single wavelength), its absorbance is proportional to the concentration of the coloured solution when the light path is constant, i.e. $A \alpha C$ where A is the absorbance of light, C is the concentration of solution.

Lambert's law: When a coloured solution is illuminated with a monochromatic light, its absorption is proportional to the length of the light path, when the concentration of the solution is constant, i.e. $A \alpha L$, Where A is the absorbance of light, L is the length of the light path.

Beer-Lambert law: Combining the two laws together, we have the Beer-Lambert's law, which states that when a coloured solution is illuminated by a monochromatic light, its absorbance is proportional to the concentration of the solution and the length of the light path, i.e. $A \alpha C \alpha L$.

$$A = K \times C \times L \text{ .....Equation (1)}$$

where K is a constant

In all photometric estimations a reference standard whose concentration is known is used and its colour intensity is compared with the colour intensity of the test sample, i.e. $A_t = K \times C_t \times L$

$$A_s = K \times C_s \times L$$

where at—Absorbance of test, C_s—Concentration of test, A_s—Absorbance of standard, *C_s—Concentration of the standard.*

Since the pathlength is constant (1 cm) in the spectrophotometer, L is constant, concentration of the standard C_s is known, therefore,

$$C_t = \frac{A_t}{A_s} \times C_s \text{ ......Equation (2)}$$

It has been observed with most biochemistry analytes that as the concentration of analyte increases linearly, the absorbance also increases linearly within the pathophysiological concentration. When a graph of concentration vs absorbance is plotted, a straight-line graph is obtained (Fig. 29.1A). A single standard method using a standard of known concentration or a factor method can be employed for calculating the concentration of the unknown.

Certain reactions, however, may not follow the Beer-Lambert law within the pathophysiological concentration for an analyte and, hence, do not provide a straight-line graph. For such analytes, the unknown cannot be determined using a single standard. A graph using different concentration of standards vs absorbance has to be plotted on a graph paper. The plotted curve is known as the standard curve (Fig. 29.1B).

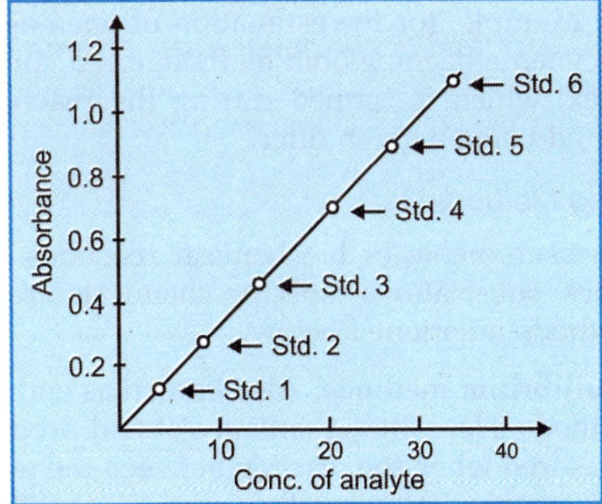

Fig. 29.1A: Illustration of a straight-line graph obtained by plotting absorbance vs concentration of analyte for reactions which obey Beer-Lambert law.

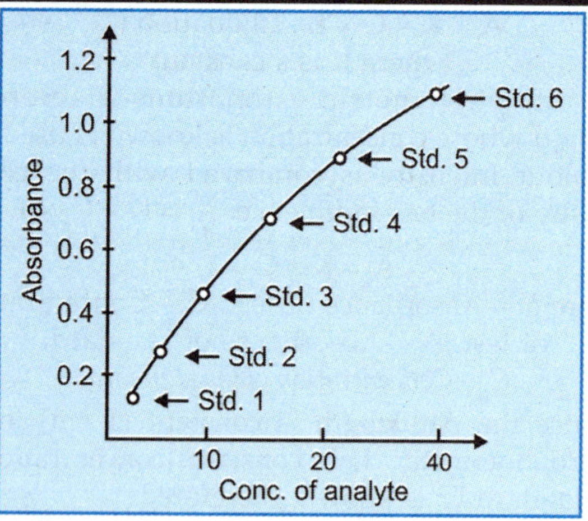

Fig. 29.1B. Illustration of a standard curve obtained by plotting absorbance vs concentration of analyte for reactions which do not obey Beer-Lambert law.

The concentration of the unknown can be interpolated from this standard curve.

Measuring Principles in Biochemistry

Criteria for Wavelength Selection

It has been established that when the wavelength of light used is complementary to the colour of the chemical complex to be measured, peak absorbance is obtained. Thus, selection of the wavelength depends on the colour of the complex to be measured. ***Complementary filters for measuring colour complexes***

Colour of the complex	Wavelength/Colour
Yellow	405/Violet
Red	505/Green
Blue-violet	546/Green
Green	630/Red

For example, for the estimation of haemoglobin using cynamethaemoglobin method, a red coloured complex, which is formed during the reaction, is measured using a green filter.

Reading Methods

The measurements of biochemical reactions using enzymes, substrates or specific chemicals are read by methods mentioned below.

1. **Equilibrium methods:** Also known as end point methods. Here, the absorbance of end product is measured when the reaction between the reagent and sample has virtually come to equilibrium (end) and the substrate has been converted into a stable end product. The reaction ceases when equilibrium is reached. The concentration of the test specimen can be calculated by using the equation 2 as described earlier.
2. **Kinetic methods:** Also known as rate methods where the rate of change of absorbance (ΔA) produced in a fixed time interval is measured. The kinetic measurements are of two types:
   - *Fixed time analysis*—where the ΔA produced by the reaction between the reagent and the substrate is measured by stopping the reaction at a fixed time interval.
   - *Continuous monitoring*—where the ΔA produced is monitored continuously as the reaction proceeds.

   Results of the unknown are derived using a factor (K) in the kinetic methods, which is usually provided by the manufacturer or can be calculated as:

$$K = \frac{V_{total} \times 1000}{V_{sample} \times t \times \epsilon \times d}$$

V_{tolal}= total volume of the reaction mixture, V_{sample}= Volume of sample, t = time, ϵ = molar extinction coefficient of the chromogen, d = length of the light path

Standarisation of Time Interval for Rate Reactions

Determination of the reaction rate involves the measurement of the amount of change in absorbance (ΔA) produced in a defined time interval. Depending on the reaction, kinetics between a specific reagent and the substrate, the time interval for reading the ΔA can be selected to measure the reaction rate. The different types of reaction curves, which can be obtained as the reaction progresses, typically follow the following patterns (Fig. 29.2).

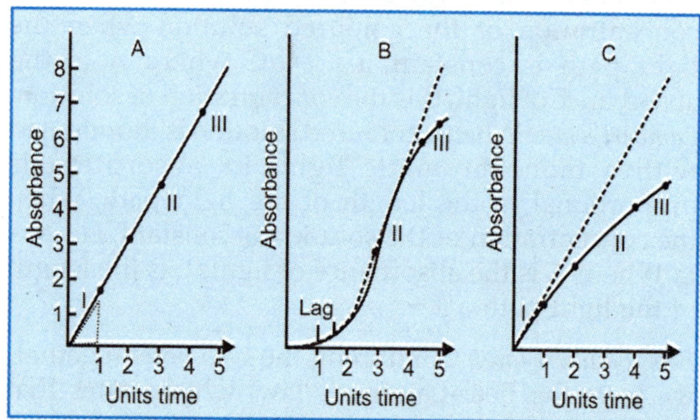

Fig. 29.2: Forms of graphs showing change in reaction rate as a function of time. In A, the rate is constant in all the segments I, II and III. In B, a measurement at segment II will be representative of constant rate, but at segment I (lag phase) and segment III it will be less. In C, the rate falls of continuously

Curve A: If a graph similar to 'curve A' is obtained then any time interval can be selected for reading reactions, as the rate of change is constant during the entire reaction run.

Curve B: Correct results can be obtained only if the rate is measured along segment II. Incorrect results are obtained if the ΔA is measured during the lag phase (I) or during the phase III.

Curve C: Deviates from linearity over its entire course and ΔA fall off with time. At no time does it give rate of constant changes. Such reaction curves are not suitable for measurements and the reagent systems have to be optimised to obtain correct reaction curves.

Measurement of Immune Complexes by Spectrophotometry

Unlike in classical biochemistry, where the reactants are clear and endpoints are expressed as absorbances, the behaviour of light differs for solutions containing suspensions or particulates. Such particles (insoluble immune complexes) are formed as the reaction between antigens and antibodies takes place.

When light of suitable wavelength is allowed to pass through a reaction solution containing antigens (analytes) and the initial absorbance is measured, the absorbance is minimum at this point (Fig. 29.3).

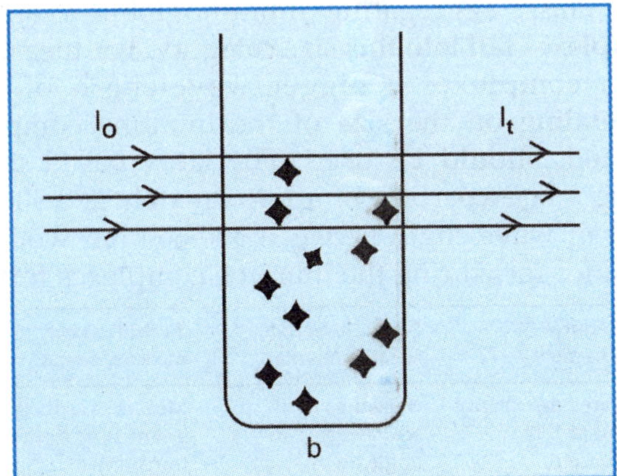

Fig. 29.3: Behaviour of light in solution containing antigens where I_o is the intensity of incident light, I_t is the intensity of transmitted light and 'b' is the cuvette containing antigens in the reaction solution

Subsequently, the reagent containing corresponding antibody solution is then added to the antigen in the cuvette and allowed to react. An agglutination reaction begins when a single molecule of antibody binds to at least two corresponding binding sites on different antigen particles. As the reaction proceeds, the agglutinating particles aggregate and form immune complexes. Immune complexes increase in size, become larger, resulting in an increase in turbidity and the scattering of the incident light. Thus, a decreasing part of the incident light (I_o) is transmitted as the reaction proceeds. Spectrophotometers read this decrease in the intensity of the transmitted light as absorbance (Fig. 29.4).

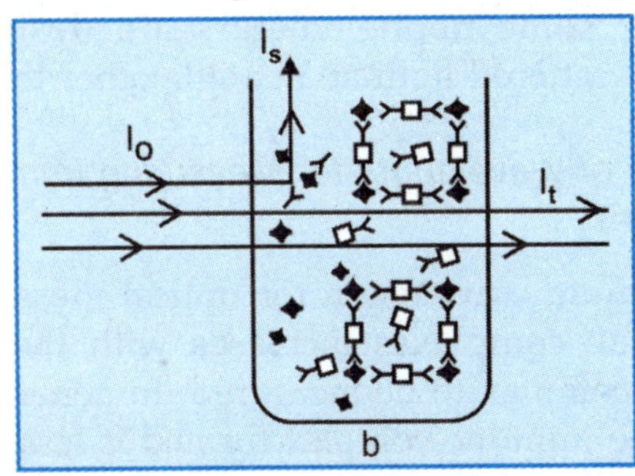

Fig. 29.4: Behaviour of light in solution containing immune - complexes (Ag-Ab), where I_o is the intensity of incident light, I_t is the intensity of transmitted light, I_s is the intensity of scattered light and 'b' is the cuvette containing immune complexes in the reaction solution

This measurement of reduction in the intensity of the transmitted light at 180° is defined as *turbidimetry*. The turbidity is proportional to the analyte concentration, which in turn is proportional to the amount of agglutination. Based on this proportional relationship, the amount of analyte in the sample causing the turbidity can be easily determined. It should be noted that the nature of immunochemical reaction is exactly the same in turbidimetry and nephelometry. However, it is the detection principle applied for measurement, which differentiates turbidimetry from nephelometry (Fig. 29.5):

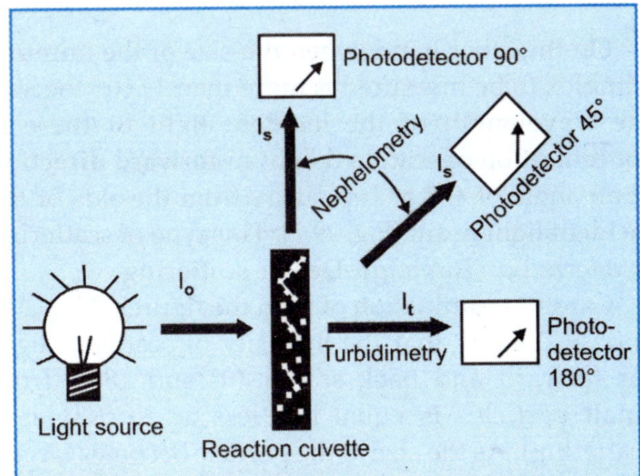

Fig. 29.5: Detection principles in turbidimetry and nephelometry where I_o is the intensity of incident light, 'b' is the reaction cuvette, I_t is the intensity of transmitted light measured by detector at 180°, I_s is the intensity of scattered light measured by detectors placed at 90° and 45°

Nephelometry measures light scattered or reflected towards the detector, which is away from direct path of the transmitted light. Routine spectrophotometers cannot be used for nephelometry and hence, nephelometers are required. Most nephelometers measure light scattering at a 90° angle. However, in order to measure the forward scatter intensity caused by light scattering from large particles, some nephelometers are designed to measure scattered light at an angle other than 90°.

Selection of Wavelength for Measuring Immune Complexes

The optimum wavelength for optical measurement of immune complexes increases with the size of immune complex to be measured. In general, if the size of the immune complex formed is less than 1/10th the size of the wavelength of incident light, then the light scattering is relatively symmetrical (Fig. 29.6). This **uniform scattering** of light is known as **Rayleigh scattering.**

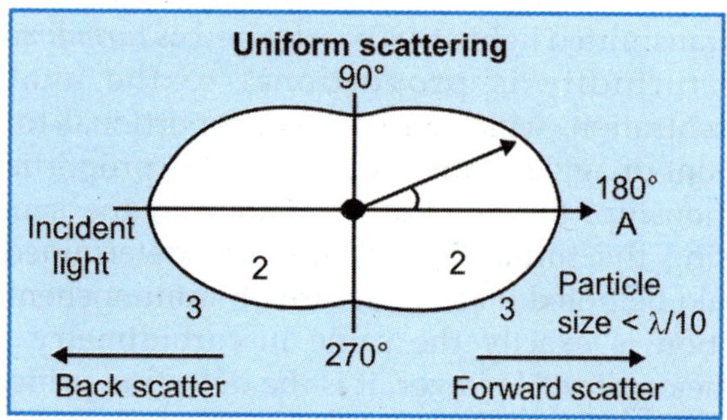

Fig. 29.6: Illustrating Rayleigh scattering for a immune complex with particle size < λ/10 of the wavelength of incident light.

On the other hand, when the size of the immune complex to be measured is more than 1/10th the size the wavelength of the incident light of there is concentration of scattered light in **forward direction** at an angle of 45° or less, away from the axis of the incident light beam (Fig. 29.7). This type of scattering is referred as **Rayleigh-Debye scattering.**

Careful examination of both the figures (Figs 29.6 and 29.7) show that the intensity of scattered light for forward and back scatter (0° and 180°) from small particles is equal but less at 90°(Rayleigh scattering). As the size of the particle becomes larger, the angular dependence of light scattering becomes dissymetrical, increasing in forward scattering and decreasing in backward scattering.

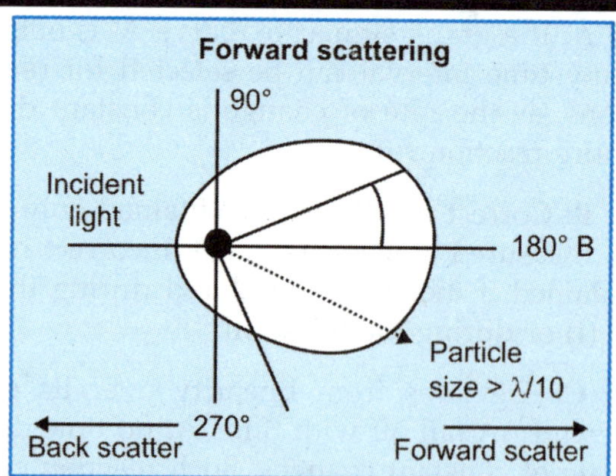

Fig. 29.7: Illustrating Rayleigh-Debye scattering for a immune complex with particle size > λ/70 of the wavelength of incident light

The Rayleigh and Rayleigh-Debye expressions provide useful information about scattering of light by small and intermediate size particles and are important for the optimisation of analytical instrumentation for measuring light using turbidimetric and nephelometric assays.

The upper limit on size of immune complexes exhibiting Rayleigh scattering is about 40 nm when a visible light at 400 nm is used. Many of the plasma proteins such as immunoglobulins, albumin, etc. fall below this limit. As the immune complexes, become larger in size from 40 to 400 nm, the angular dependence of scattered light at 400 nm looses the symmetry around the 90°axis, and shows an increase in forward scattering. Some plasma proteins of the IgM class, aggregating immunoglobulin/antigen complexes fall into this size category. For measuring such complexes a bigger wavelength of light depending on the size of the immune complexes formed, should be used. For latex based assays using a latex particle of approximately 200-300 nm, light of wavelength between 500-600 nm would be ideal for measuring the immune complexes formed.

Biochemical measurements	Nephelometric measurements	Turbidimetric measurements
Measures absorbance of light at 180°, by coloured complexes formed as a result of biochemical reactions	Measures light scattering at an angle away from the incident light due to formation of immune complexes	Measures reduction in intensity of light transmitted (as absorbance) at 180°due to the formation of immune complexes
Selection of wavelength of light is complementary to the colour of the chemical complex to be measured.	Selection of wavelength of light depends on the size of the immune complex formed,	Selection of wavelength of light depends on the size of the immune complex formed.

The choice between turbidimetry and nephelometry will depend on application and the available instrumentation. Until recently, it was assumed that for relatively clear solutions in which the transmission of light in the forward direction is greater than 95 per cent small changes in absorption due to turbidity were difficult to measure with precision. The stability and resolution of modern microprocessor driven spectrophotometers and automated clinical chemistry analysers have greatly improved their ability to measure turbidity with dependable accuracy and precision. Turbidimetric methods have today become competitive in sensitivity with nephelometric methods for immunological quantitation of such solutions.

For some analytes, the signal amplification and assay sensitivity requires the usage of conjugation chemistry to attach antibodies to inert and uniform latex particles. Such reagent systems are referred to as particle enhanced turbidimetry (PET).

PET reagents usually use latex of approximately 200-300 nm for conjugating antibodies to facilitate formation of larger immunecomplexes and thereby generate detectable signals. This leads to decrease in scattering of light at 90° and increase in forward scattering. Turbidimetric assays, therefore, have better precision for measuring larger immune complexes.

In the context of contemporary technology, turbidimetric assays are gaining popularity over nephelometric determination due to their simplicity and overall consistency.

Turbidimetry vs Nephelometry

Turbidimetry	*Nephelometry*
Measures reduction in intensity of transmitted light at 180° due to the formation of immune complexes	Measures scattering of light at an angle (usually 90°) away from the incident light, due to the formation of immune complexes
Can be performed on most spectrophotometers	Requires dedicated nephelometers
Sensitivity competitive with nephelometric for small immune complexes such as serum proteins	Sensitive for measuring small immune measurements complexes such as serum proteins
More precise for measuring large immune complexes	Less precise for measuring large immune complexes due to forward scattering of light
Blanking and reading reaction can be performed in the same measuring cuvette	Blanking has to be performed in separate measuring cuvette
Provides better precision due to slower reaction kinetics as blanking of immunochemical reaction can be monitored in a single cuvette	Because of the fast reaction kinetics it is difficult to obtain a sample and a reagent, sample and reagent blank in case of nephelometry

Contd...

CONSIDERATIONS FOR MEASUREMENTS OF TURBIDIMETRIC IMMUNOASSAYS (TIA)

As far back in the year 1929, Heidelberger and Kendall have quantitatively described the formation of a precipitate when reacting an antigen with an antibody. They demonstrated that when an increasing amount of an antigen is added to a constant amount of corresponding antibody, the resulting degree of precipitate formed follows a bell-shaped curve as shown in Fig. 29.8. To obtain the Heidelberger curve, the antigen concentration is plotted against the absorbances obtained from measuring the Ag-Ab reaction.

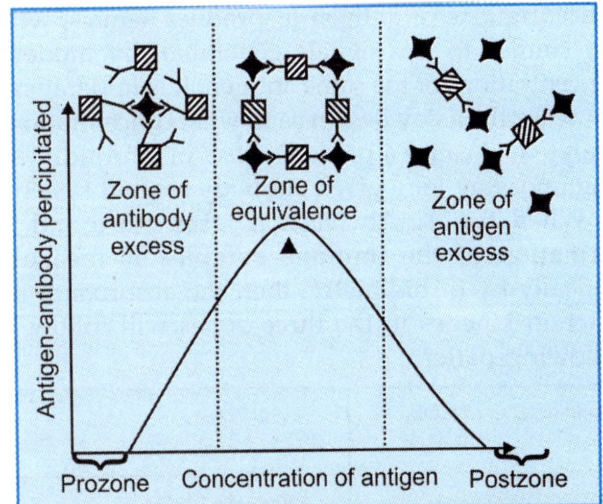

Fig. 29.8: The quantitative immunoprecipitin curve (Heidelberger-Kendall curve)

The Heidelberger-Kendall curve can be divided in three zones as follows:

The Antibody Excess Zone

In the first stage of the reaction, there is a large excess of binding sites in the reaction mixture available for the antigen to bind. First the antigen binding sites are quickly saturated by antibody before cross-linking begins to occur. This results in formation of small Ag-Ab complexes. In this zone the absorbances increase proportionally to the analyte concentration.

Zone of Equivalence

In the second stage of reaction binding sites available for the antigen are proportionate to the antigen concentration. Here, the probability of cross-linking is more likely resulting in formation of large immune complexes. As the saturation point is reached, there is neither free antigen nor free antibody in the reaction mixture. To this zone, the absorbances increase with the increasing analyte concentration, but does not increase proportionally.

The Antigen Excess Zone

In the third stage of the reaction, the relative concentration of the antigen is so high that most of the binding sites are overcrowded, hindering the formation of real precipitate and favouring the formation of small immune complexes. This is called the prozone effect or the hook effect. The term "prozone" is inappropriately used to describe "postzone" or "antigen excess" in day-to-day parlance. The existence of prozone effect causes very high concentrations of antigen to produce signals, which are similar to the signals generated, by moderate concentrations of the same antigen. It is imperative to know for the assay design as to what concentration of analyte will cause a prozone effect in a turbidimetric immunoassay for a given antibody reagent system.

When the Ag-Ab reaction takes place and the formation of the immune complex is measured optically by turbidimetry, then the absorbance and reaction kinetics in the three zones will follow the following pattern:

Heidelberger- Kendall curve	*Absorbance*
Antibody excess zone	Increases towards maximum
Equilibrium	Reaches maximum
Antigen excess zone	Decreases below maximum

The Heidelberger-Kendall immunoprecipitin curve forms the fundamental basis for all homogeneous Ag-Ab assays including turbidimetry and is usually referred to as the **dose response curve.**

For many analytes of diagnostic importance, the Ag-Ab reactions neither follow the Beer-Lambert law nor provide a linear relationship between concentration and turbidity. Estimating the concentrations of analytes using a single standard, as in biochemical analysis therefore, results in inaccurate results near the zone of equivalence. The ΔA is directly proportional to the concentration of analyte only in the initial region of the antibody excess zone. Use of single standard for calculating concentration of analyte may be acceptable only for lower analyte concentrations. As the analyte concentrations increase, the error in measurement will start to magnify. Therefore, for having a larger measuring range, the turbidimetric assays use that part of the dose response curve, which covers the maximum portion of the antibody excess region and demonstrates a linear reaction as the standard curve.

The standard curve is plotted using a number of standards containing different concentrations of analyte being measured (usually 5-6). The highest concentration of the standard is chosen in such a way that the analyte absorbance at that concentration will lie on the linear extreme of the standard curve. The lowest concentration of the analyte is usually selected below the reference values of the analyte of interest.

The linear range between the highest and lowest standards used for the preparation of standard curve is referred to as the **measuring range** of the assay (Fig. 29.9).

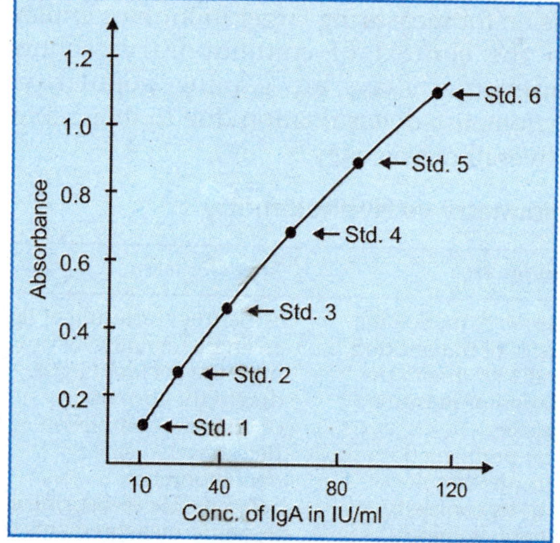

Fig. 29.9: Illustrating standard curve for IgA using lowest standard as 7 IU/ml and highest standard as 120 IU/ml

Optimisation, Standardisation and Quality Control of Turbidimetric Assays

To measure the Ag-Ab reactions, reliably all the factors that affect the reaction rate, other than the concentration of the antibody, must be optimised and controlled. As the reaction velocity is at its maximum under optimal conditions, a larger analytical signal is obtained that can be more accurately and precisely measured as compared to a smaller signal obtained under suboptimal assay conditions.

Investigations, of the factors affecting Ag-Ab reactions were extensively studied by Heidelberger and Kendall. In addition to the relative proportions of immune reactants, other conditions such as temperature, ionic strength of the medium, characteristics of the antibody such as avidity and affinity are important for formation of Ag-Ab immune complex. These principles need to be applied to the reagent system optimisation for immunoturbidimetry.

Ionic Strength: It has been observed that the Ag-Ab reactions are strongly influenced by the nature of ionic medium in which the reaction is carried out. The ionic strength of the reaction environment has a profound effect on the quantum and the rate of the Ag-Ab reaction. As the ionic strength increases, the depth of the electrical double layer that forms around the charged molecules is compressed, reducing the distance over which repulsive forces that keep the molecules apart can act. This in effect leads to the promotion of aggregation. The reduction in charge on the other hand influences the electrostatic attraction between oppositely charged species, thereby reducing the specific binding between antigen and antibody.

pH: The reaction pH also influences the rate of aggregate formation. The rate of reaction is found to be fairly consistent at a pH of 6.0-8.0. Reduction in pH leads to some proteins having net positive charge (those with a pH above the reaction pH) leading to nonspecific agglutination with negatively charged proteins or particles.

Temperature: As is well known, temperature influences the rate of formation of immune complexes and it should be optimised to obtain accurate results. Assays are usually designed with an incubation temperature of 37°C because it is the most common temperature used in the routine of clinical laboratories for clinical assays.

Enhancers: For enhancing the Ag-Ab reactions, polymeric compounds, such as PEG and BSA, may be included in the buffer system. These compounds facilitate the formation of immune complex and help in amplification of signals and improve the assay system sensitivity.

Interference: Many interfering factors, such as bilirubin and lipids, are normally present in the samples apart from the analyte of interest. High concentrations of some of these interfering factors are frequently encountered in clinical samples. They may influence signal generation and, therefore, can interfere in the assay result. Minimising the influence of these factors help provide accurate and precise assay results.

Turbidimetric assays usually employ a suitable buffer in the assay design to optimise assay conditions and the desired ionic strength, pH and enhancement required for the reaction medium. In addition, the buffer is also useful in reducing the influence of interfering factors present in the sample. The buffer used in turbidimetric assays is generally referred to as *activation buffer*.

Characteristics of antibody used as a reagent: Intrinsic characteristics of antibody employed as reagents have a profound effect on the Ag-Ab reactions. The specificity and affinity of the antibody to the antigenic sites affect the sensitivity of the assay and signal generation time. Usually, when high specificity and affinity antibodies are used, a strong agglutination reaction will readily result. In contrast, antibodies with low affinity, even if highly specific, tend to react slowly and form a weak immune complex, thereby lowering the detectable signal. The avidity of antibody is also an important consideration in the formation of immune complexes. This characteristic of the antibody determines the degree of stability of the Ag-Ab complexes at the antigen-binding sites. The tendency of the complexes to dissociate and disperse decreases substantially as the avidity of the antibody increases.

An antibody without cross-reactivity and with a good titre is a prerequisite for a reliable turbidimetric assay utilising antibody as a principal reagent. In addition, the antibody must be formulated as a clear solution to give a low reagent blank and should be free from particulate matter.

Standarisation and Calibration: During the course of treatment, individual patients are likely to have tests carried out for the same analyte by different methods, and to have results checked against reference intervals that were set elsewhere. To achieve agreement between different methods, a single recognised source of reference preparation is needed.

The reference preparation should:

- Have value assignment in meaningful units
- Be stable and identical to the analyte in the test samples
- Be free of interference from the test sample matrix
- Be standardised by a reference method
- Demonstrate inter-method agreements

Most International Reference Preparations (IRPs) and Certified Reference Materials (CRMs) such as CRM 470 for immunoassay analytes, can be obtained from the main custodians of International Biological Standards such as National Institute for Biological Standards and Controls (NIBSC) or WHO and Community Bureau of Reference of the Commission of European Communities (BCR) or the IFCC.

As the availability of International Standards is limited, it is a practice to prepare sets of secondary standards, from which future lots of calibrators can be assigned values. The secondary standards act as an intermediate between IRP primary standard and future lots of calibrators for assay runs. The calibrator sets are made in bulk and values are assigned with reference to the secondary standards.

As discussed, the immunoturbidimetric assays require a set of five or six calibrators to obtain a standard curve. The quantitative values of unknown analyte obtained from the standard curve will be highly dependent on correct assignment of values to the calibrator used for preparing the standard curve.

Quality Control: The tendency of most immunological reagents to produce changes in reactivity over time requires the application of quality control procedures to ensure the satisfactory analytical performance of immunometric assays on a day-to-day basis. Similarly, in the case of turbidimetric immunoassays reagent stability within a defined usable time span is a prime requirement of the reagent systems, so is the need for accurate and stable controls to validate reagent functioning, precision and accuracy.

Reading Principles in Turbidimetry

For turbidimetric measurements, both end point and rate measurements are applicable. However, the factor method for calculating the concentration of the unknown is not preferred in the kinetic methods by turbidimetry due to the nonlinear nature of relationship between absorbance and analyte concentrations.

Once the assay system has been designed, the analysers used for reading must be able to operate according to the principles mentioned below with respect to the addition of reagents and reading of signals (absorbance).

Real Sample Blanking

In this system first the activation buffer (R1) is added to the sample cuvette (S). Then the sample is added, mixed and allowed to stabilise (preincubation period). The first reading (A1) is then taken at the end of preincubation period.

The antibody reagent (R2) is subsequently added, to the above mixture and mixed gently. Turbidity develops due to the reaction between the antigen and the antibody over a short period of time. A second reading is taken at the defined time interval (usually 2-10 minutes).

Table 29.1: Real sample blanking system: using sample cuvette

	Signals		
	First reading (A1)	*Second reading (A2)*	*ΔA_s (A2-A1)*
Sample cuvette (S)	Absorbance due to: • Sample • Buffer	Absorbance due to: • Sample • Buffer • Reagent • Immune complexes	Absorbance due to: • Reagent • Immune complexes

The difference ΔA_S (refer Table 29.1) between the two readings represents the absorbance generated as a result of Ag-Ab reaction.

If required, the absorbance due to the reagent ΔA_B can be measured by running in parallel a reagent blank in a separate cuvette (R) using saline in place of sample (refer Table 29.2)

Table 29.2: Real sample blanking system: using reagent cuvette

	Signals		
	First reading (A1)	*Second reading (A2)*	*ΔA_R (A2-A1)*
Reagent cuvette (R)	Absorbance due to: • Buffer • Blank sample (saline)	Absorbance due to: • Buffer • Blank sample • Reagent	Absorbance due to: • Reagent

ΔA_R thus obtained of the reagent blank can be subtracted from ΔA_S of the sample to calculate the absorbance generated due to the Ag-Ab reaction in the sample.

The reagent blank facility may not be available in many semiautomated analysers. However, the reagent assay system can be optimised to provide a very low reagent blank in order to obviate the need for correcting the reagent blank signals which can contribute to the complete reaction absorbance.

The principle of taking a reading just before the addition of antibody solution (R2) is referred to as *'true sample blanking'* or *'real sample blanking'*.

Immediate Mixed Blanking

In this system initially the activation buffer, sample and the antibody reagent solution are all mixed simultaneously. Then as fast as possible usually 10 to 20 seconds after mixing, the first reading A1 is taken. This 10 to 20 seconds delay time in taking a reading is referred to as **lag phase.** The reaction is allowed to proceed further and the second reading A2 is measured at the preselected time interval. The increase in absorbance ΔA (A2-A1) represents the signal generated due to the Ag-Ab reaction (refer Table 29.3).

Table 29.3: Immediate mixed blanking system

	Signals		
	First reading (A1)	*Second reading (A2)*	*ΔA_s (A2-A1)*
Sample cuvette	Absorbance due to: • Reagent • Buffer • Sample	Absorbance due to: • Reagent • Buffer • Sample • Ag-Ab reaction	Absorbance due to: • Ag-Ab reaction

This method eliminates the need for determination of reagent blank as it measures the increase in absorbance after equilibration of all the reagents and sample. Hence, absorbance generated both due to interfering substances in the sample and the reagent would be blanked during the first reading.

In all Ag-Ab reactions in the initial contact phase the reaction kinetics do not follow a systematic pattern. As this initial chaotic phase settles, the reaction pattern and the absorbances move proportionately. This pattern depends upon the intrinsic nature of the antibody, such as affinity, avidity, etc., and also the concentration of the analyte being measured.

Depending on the assay system requirements, it is desirable that the initial chaotic phase is not included in the measurement of absorbance. Typically, a lag phase would vary from ten to thirty seconds from analyte to analyte. It is, therefore, imperative to follow diligently the recommended time assigned for the lag phase for precise blanking in the *"immediate mixed blanking"* method.

Reaction Kinetics and its Effect on Blanking

The reaction kinetics of an antigen-antibody also guides as to the appropriateness of the blanking system. As the reaction kinetics is not the same for all Ag-Ab systems, for a system with slow reaction kinetics, e.g., IgA, a first reading 10 to 20 seconds after mixing with the antibody is not very critical (Fig. 29.10).

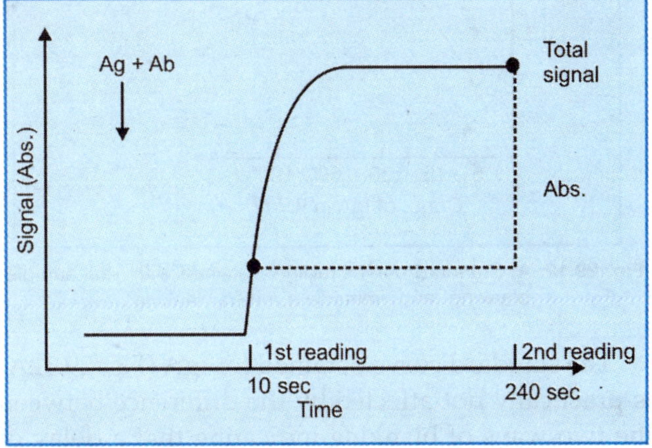

Fig. 29.10: Signal development as a function of time. Fig. illustrating 'immediate mixed blanking' using IgA as an example

However, for a system with fast reaction kinetics, e.g., IgG (Fig. 29.11), half of the reaction would have taken place within 10 to 20 seconds when the first reading is taken. Here, a poorly defined point for the first reading would be obtained.

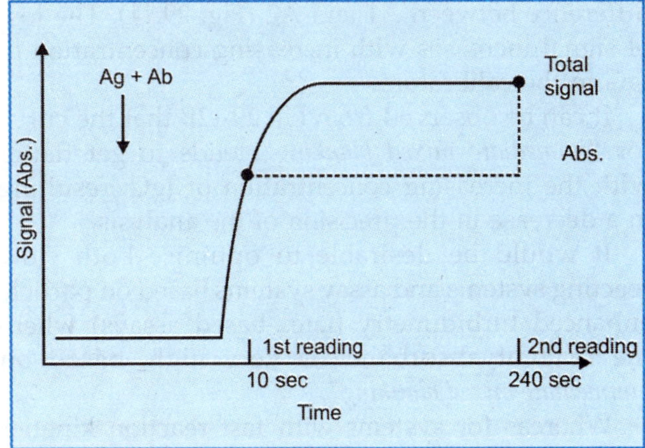

Fig. 29.11: Signal development as a function of time. Fig. illustrating 'immediate mixed blanking' using IgG as an example

The implications of *'immediate mixed blanking'* can be demonstrated by comparing the standard curves obtained for the six calibrators of latex enhanced reagent system for measurement of IgA (Fig. 29.12A) and IgG (Fig. 29.12B) at zero seconds and ten seconds respectively.

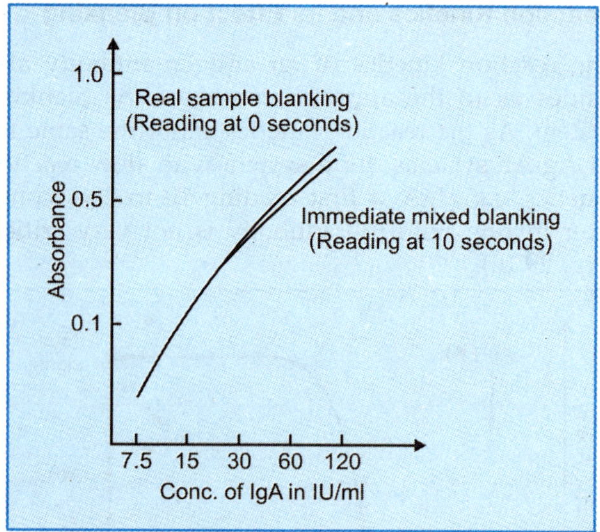

Fig. 29.12: A: Standard curves for IgA obtained with 'real sample blanking' and 'immediate mixed blanking'.

The standard curve obtained for IgA (Fig. 29.12A) is practically not affected by the difference between the two ways of blanking indicating that a delay of ten seconds is not very significant.

Whereas for a non-enhanced system with fast reaction kinetics for measurement of analytes such as IgG (Fig. 29.12B), a delay of ten seconds becomes very critical.

There is considerable signal development during the first ten seconds. This results in decreased difference between A1 and A2 (Fig. 29.11). The loss of signal increases with increasing concentration of IgG in the calibrators.

It can be observed from Fig.29.12B that the curve for *"immediate mixed blanking"* tends to get flatter with the increasing concentration of IgG, resulting in a decrease in the precision of the analysis.

It would be desirable to optimise both slow reacting systems and assay systems based on particle enhanced turbidimetry (latex-based assays) where the reagent absorbance is very high, based on *"immediate mixed blanking"*.

Whereas for systems with fast reaction kinetics such as IgG, the assays should be optimised using the *"real sample blanking"* principle as the sample blanking and the immunochemical reaction can be optimised separately.

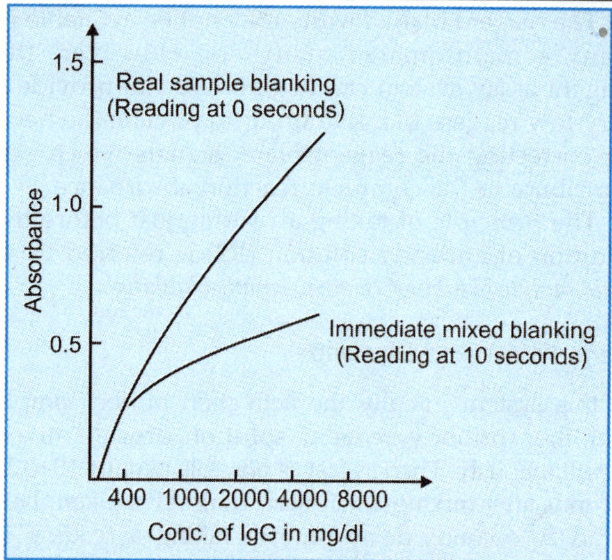

Fig. 29.12B: Standard curves for IgG obtained with 'real sample blanking' and 'immediate mixed blanking'

CONCEPTS OF ASSAY OPTIMISATION

While optimising reagent system for immunoturbidimetric assays, it is important to optimise the dose-response curve by iterating the amount of sample (antigen) and the antibody concentration in the reagent until a dose-response curve as shown in Fig. 29.13 is obtained.

A portion of the antibody excess zone of dose-response curve is then selected as the *"range for the standard curve"*.

Detection Limit

The lowest concentration of an antigen, which gives a detectable signal compared to the background noise, is defined as the detection limit or analytical sensitivity of the analysis. It is defined as the minimum concentration of analyte that is statistically unlikely to form part of the range of signals seen in absence of analyte. Usually, the detection limit is set as the lowest signal where the standard deviation around that signal is less than one third of the signal itself. The lowest concentration selected for the calibration of the assay is usually above the detection limit.

Measuring Range

As long as the analyte signal is higher than the signal of the lowest calibrator and lower than the signal of the highest calibrator, the assay system will operate accurately for the said analyte and a concentration value of the sample can be interpolated.

The interval between the signal generated by the lowest calibrator to the signal generated by the highest calibrator, which gives proportionate and measurable and a linear signal, is referred to as the measuring range of the assay system.

Security Range

The critical point (Cx in Fig. 29.13), in the antigen excess zone of the dose-response curve corresponds to the maximum concentration value of analyte, which gives a signal value higher than the signal value of the calibrator of highest concentration, and just before the value (B_1 in Fig. 29.13) at which erroneous interpolation begins. The interval between the signal of highest standard and the signal of the critical concentration can be referred to as the security range of the assay system for the analyte.

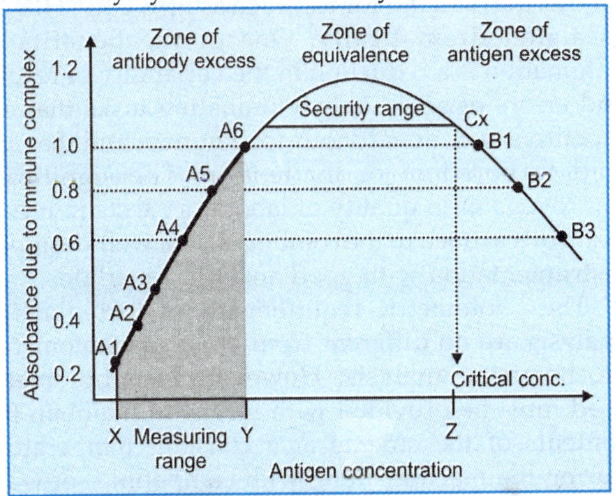

Fig. 29.13: Dose-response curve Fig. illustrating measuring range (X-Y), Critical concentration (Z), standard curve (A1-A6), erroneous interpolation (where Abs. val.1.0 corresponds to A6 and B1, Abs. val. 0.8 corresponds to A5 and B2 and Ab5 val. 0.6 corresponds to A4 and B3), security range (Y-Z)

Reagent Optimisation

The risk of obtaining signals in the antigen excess zone are more relevant in analytes like C-reactive protein or immunoglobulins such as IgG where the concentration between normal and pathological sample can differ by manifolds. It is necessary to make sure that the concentration values lying in the antigen excess zone (critical point) are beyond the concentrations which can be expected to occur in clinical samples during routine analysis.

The relation between the security range and measuring range is very important in optimising assay systems. As mentioned earliers the shape of the dose-response curve depends on the ratio between the antigen and the antibody. At a constant antibody concentration, an increase in the measuring range will result in a narrower security range, leading to antigen excess at a lower antigen concentration (refer Fig. 29.14).

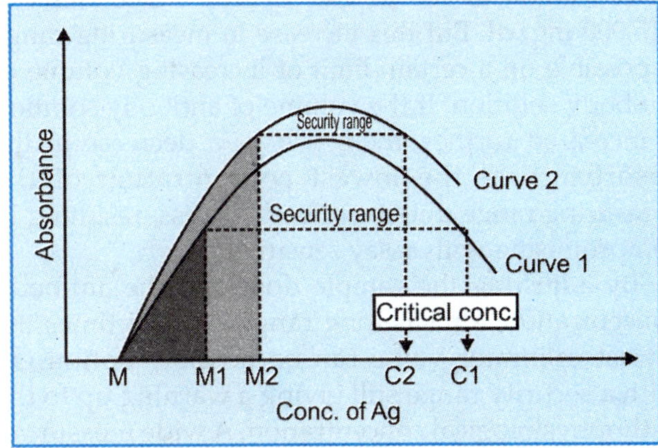

Fig. 29.14: Effect of increasing measuring range on security range. M-M1 = measuring range for curve 1, C1 = critical concentration for curve 1 M-M2 = Measuring range of curve 2, C2 = critical concentration for curve 2

The implications of increasing the antibody reagent concentrations can be practically demonstrated using IgG as an analyte and antihuman IgG as a reagent. The measuring range and the security range can be expanded by increasing the antibody concentration. However, this expansion can only be done to a point where it is still possible to have the desired sensitivity for lower analyte concentration.

Fig. 29.15 shows the effect of increasing the antibody concentration on the security ranges while keeping constant, the measuring range of the dose-response curve.

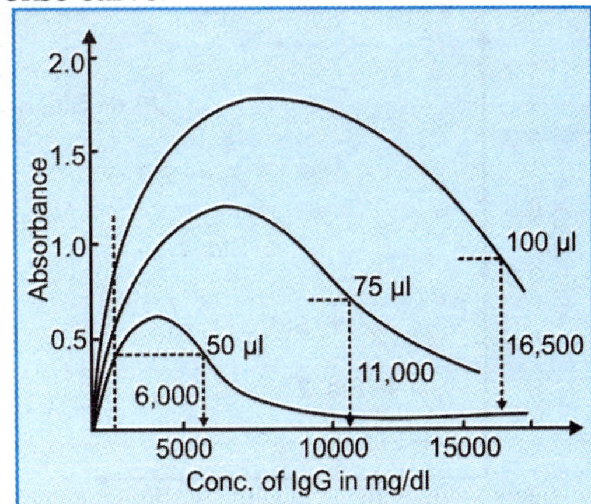

Fig. 29.15: Effect of increasing antibody concentration on security range. Where 50, 75 and 100 (µl are volumes of antibody and 6000, 11000 and 16500 are their respective critical concentrations.

When the volume of an antibody solution of concentration 'X' used is 50 µl, the security range obtained is around 5000 mg/dl. As the volume of the same antibody concentration is increased to 75 µl, the security range increases to > 10,000 mg/dl. With a further increase in volume of the same antibody concentration to 100 µl, the security range shifts to >15,000 mg/dl. But this increase in measuring range is possible till a certain limit of increasing volume of antibody solution. If the volume of antibody solution is increased further, there will be a decrease in the absorbance at the lowest concentration of the measuring range due to antibody excess, resulting in compromising with assay sensitivity.

By adjusting the sample dose and the antibody concentration, a measuring range 20 to 25 times the lowest calibrator value can be possibly optimised, with a security range still giving a warning up to the pathophysiological concentration. A wide measuring range combined with a wide security range offer the advantage of a few reruns and maximum security against antigen excess problems.

Standard Curve

Once the dose-response curve for a reagent has been optimised, a standard curve can be obtained by using a number of dilutions of the calibrator (preferably 5-6) covering the optimal measuring range. The lowest calibrator should be chosen to give a signal significantly higher than the background noise. The highest calibrator should be selected to allow measurements for a reasonably wide range of analyte concentrations, and still leaving space for a fair security range (Fig. 29.16).

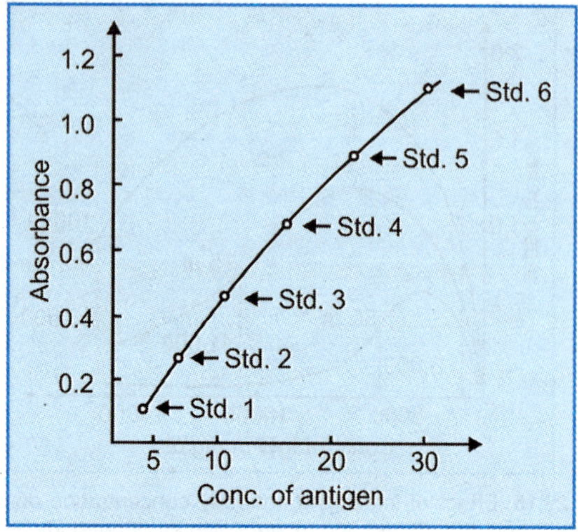

Fig. 29.16: Illustrating Standard Curve

A curve is fitted to the signals obtained for calibrator dilutions and can be stored in the memory of the instrument. Different curve fitting programmes can be made available in instrument software.

Many of the instruments are equipped with a facility to give a 'warning' that indicate reruns of the test with dilution of the sample with high concentration values of analyte. This warning is given as long as the sample signal is higher than the signal of the highest calibrator.

The validity of the stored standard curve should be checked with known controls at regular time intervals.

INSTRUMENTATION FOR TURBIDIMETRY

The development of automated instruments for the clinical laboratory began in the 1950s at the same time as the demand for test such as IgA, CRP, HBsAg escalated dramatically. One of the benefits of automation is a reduction in the variability of results and errors of analysis by eliminating tasks that are repetitive and monotonous for a human and that can lead to boredom or inattention. The significant improvement in quality of laboratory tests in recent years owes much to the combination of well-designed instrumentation with good analytical methods.

The photometric requirements of turbidimetric analysis are no different from those of photometric biochemistry analysis. However, the photometer used must be provided with means to maintain the contents of the cuvette at a constant temperature during the reaction along with compatible software to run the various steps of the reagent and reagent kinetics appropriately.

The chemistry analysers (spectrophotometers) available utilise either or both of the two modes of measuring absorbance.

Aspiration Mode

In this mode the chemical reaction is carried out in a test tube/cuvette. The instrument aspirates the reaction mixture from the test tube/cuvette, which enters into the flow cell (internally built reading chamber), where the absorbance is measured. After the absorbance is measured, the reaction mixture is passed through a different outlet and is collected in a waste collecting bottle. As all the measurements are done in a single flow cell, the flow cell has to be washed after each test. Improper washing may affect the test results of the subsequent tests. Especially, if latex enhanced tests are used, the latex has a tendency to stick and form a permanent coating on the internal walls of the flow cell resulting in variation in the wavelength of the incident light, and hence, lead to erroneous results. Even non-enhanced antibody reagents are proteinacious and cleaning of the flow cell would remain a critical issue.

When Ag-Ab complexes are aspirated, because of the force of aspiration, the formed immune complexes would be structurally disturbed and may break down into smaller complexes, which would result in lower absorbance values. Moreover, the immune precipitates formed may block the aspiration tube or the flow cell itself.

For turbidimetric assays designed with real sample blanking reading principle, it would be inconvenient to run the test in the aspiration mode. Initially, the sample mixed with the activation buffer would have to be aspirated first and absorbance A1 measured. Then again the activation buffer and the sample will have to be taken in another test tube and the principle reagent added and the reaction read after a fixed time interval. Hence, for running one assay twice, the amount of activation buffer and sample will have to be used.

Cuvette Mode

In this mode, the reaction of the reagent and sample takes place in a measuring cuvette, and absorbance is read in the same measuring cuvette itself. Hence, assays using any of the reading principles can be conveniently read in cuvette mode without wastage of reagents.

Instruments applying this mode of measuring have an advantage. As the reactions are run in external cuvettes, the instruments are safe from the effects of reagents. Moreover, availability of standardised optically clean disposable cuvettes eliminates the carryover effects of the previous tests.

Classification of Analysers

There are several types of analysers available in the market. They may be grouped in two categories:

- Semiautomated analysers
- Automated analysers

Semiautomated Analysers

Instruments with an absorbance linearity of 2.0 are suitable for turbidimetric estimations of both particle enhanced and non-particle enhanced reagent systems. Most of the instruments with the above specification can be used for turbidimetric measurements using the absorbance mode. In the absorbance mode as the calibration curve cannot be stored, it has to be drawn manually.

Among the instruments working on cuvette mode for measuring absorbance, very few instruments have software interface programmed with a facility to store the calibration curve utilising both the principles of reading, i.e. 'real sample blanking' and 'immediate mixed blanking' in the multistandard mode. Many instruments with cuvette modes are known to have programmes in multistandard mode to store calibration curve for assay systems using the real sample blanking techniques only.

Automated Analysers

The automated analyzers can be grouped in two categories:

- Centrifugal analysers
- Static instruments (non-centrifugal analysers)

Centrifugal Analysers

In these analysers the cuvettes are arranged in circle (rotor) that can be rotated at a velocity of about 1000 rpm. The shape of each cuvette allows application of sample and reagent (reaction buffer, antibody) in separate compartments. When the rotor starts to spin, the contents of these compartments are mixed simultaneously and held in place in the cuvette by centrifugal force. Readings of all the cuvettes are performed at essentially the same time (i.e when the rotating cuvettes are passing the optical measuring device). Two reading systems are used: either parallel to the length of the cuvette where the volume in the cuvette is proportional to the light path or perpendicular to the length of the cuvette where the width of the cuvette equals the light path.

Static Instruments

In these instruments the cuvettes are mostly arranged in a circle (rotor), and this is slowly rotated in step at a fixed time interval (cycle time). Access to the cuvette is possible only at these intervals for sample or reagent application and reading. Mixing is in most cases performed with a mechanical stirring device. Modern instruments seem more and more to be based on these principles.

All instruments operate under software control. A part of this software is the user interface that makes it possible to programme the instrument to perform analysis and calculation according to an

Table 29.4: Applications, reference values of important clinical analytes

Analyte	*Description*	*Reference values*	*Applications*
RF	Quantitation of rheumatoid factors	< 10 IU/ml	Detection of RA, differential diagnosis of RA from rheumatic fever and other rheumatic disorders
CRP	Quantitation of C-reactive protein	Adults and children < 0.6 mg/dl	Detection of inflammatory conditions, measuring the severity of conditions, differential diagnosis of bacterial and viral infections Monitoring the response to therapy
CRP US	Quantitation of ultrasensitive levels of C-reactive protein	< 0.05 mg/dl	Prognostic cardiac marker
ASO	Quantitation of antistreptolysin 'O'	Children : < 150 IU/ml Adults : < 200 IU/ml	Detection of Group A streptococcal infections such as sore throat, rheumatic fever, rheumatic heart disease
MA	Quantitation of urinary albumin	< 20 mg/L	Detection of microalbuminuria Monitoring the effect of ACE inhibitor or intervention strategies for reducing UAE
IgA	Quantitation of immunoglobulin IgA	70-400 mg/dl	Chronic infections of GI and respiratory tract, anaphylactic transfusion reactions, monitoring progress of IgA myeloma
IgG	Quantitation of immunoglobulin IgG	700-1600 mg/	IgG myeloma, IgG deficiency, assessment of the progression and response to treatment of IgG myeloma
IgM	Quantitation of immunoglobulin IgM	40-230 mg/dl	Monitoring patients with Waldenström's macroglobulinaemia Estimating frequent, chronic and acute infections
IgD	Quantitation of immunoglobulin IgD	3-14 mg/dl	Screening for congenital infection Monitoring IgD myeloma
IgE	Quantitation of IgD immunoglobulin IgE	Adult 3-423 IU/ml	Assessment of atopic diseases, dermatologic and parasitic infections
C3	Quantitation of complement component C3	90-180 mg/dl	C3 deficiency, recurrent infections detection and monitoring of immune complex disorders such as SLE, vasculitis, glomerulonephritis, autoimmune haemolytic anaemia
C4	Quantitation of complement component C4	10-40 mg/dl	Congenital deficiency in lupus erythromatosus Hereditary angioneurotic oedema Recurrent infections
AT III	Quantitation of antithrombin II	17-30 mg/dl	Evaluating patient at risk of developing thrombotic-embolic disease. In surgical patients receiving heparin, assessment of thrombotic risk of contraceptive or oestrogen therapy

Contd...

Contd...

Analyte	*Description*	*Reference values*	*Applications*
Apo A-1	Quantitation of apolipoprotein A-1	Males: 105-175 mg/d Females: 105-205 mg/dl	Independent risk factor for coronary artery disease
Apo B	Quantitation of apolipoprotein B	Males: 60-140 mg/dl Females: 55-130 mg/dl	Elevated Apo B levels are associated with atherosclerosis
Lp(a)	Quantitation of lipoprotein(a)	< 300 mg/L	Risk factor for coronary heart disease that is independent of all other lipid parameters
b2-M	Quantitation of β2-Microglobulin	< 60 yr : 0.8-2.4 mg/L > 60 yr : < 3.0 mg/L	Prognosis of multiple myeloma Early detection of renal transplant rejection, differentiation of glomerular and tubular nephropathies, Monitoring therapeutic response of patients with nonsecretory myeloma or light chain disease
Cp	Quantitation of ceruloplasmin	20-60 mg/dl	Diagnosis of Wilson's disease, Menkes disease, nutritional copper deficiency
Hp	Quantitation of haptoglobin	30-200 mg/dl	Diagnosis and of monitoring of haemolytic diseases

Note: The above reference values are for guidance only. As the reference values are related to age, geographical and methodological differences and vary widely. Each laboratory should define its own reference range for the relevant population.

Table 29.5: Serum proteins in different clinical conditions

Protein	*Increased in*	*Decreased in*
Serum albumin	Rare, usually associated with haemoconcentration	Acute phase response, severe liver disease, nephrotic syndrome, other renal diseases, malnutrition, pregnancy, premature infants
Complement		
Complement C3	APR (infection, inflammation etc.), biliary obstruction, obstructive jaundice, diabetes mellitus, gout, some connective diseases (excluding SLE)	Autoimmune diseases, immune complex diseases, mixed cryoglobulinaemia, serum sickness, chronic renal failure, thrombotic thrombocytopenic purpura, neonatal respiratory distress syndrome, genetic deficiency
Complement C4	APR, RA, SLE, rheumatic fever, ankylosing spondylitis, temporal arteritis, acute viral hepatitis, MI, DM, malignancies, thyroiditis, irritable bowel syndrome, pneumonia, pregnancy	Acquired deficiencies resulting from: ***Hypercatabolism:*** Disease in which circulating immunecomplexes are likely to lead to acquired hypocomplementaemia, subacute bacterial endocarditis, mixed cryoglobulinaemia, hereditary angioneurotic edema, progressive glomerulonephritis ***Hyposynthesis:*** Protein calorie malnutrition, liver disease, Sjögren's syndrome ***Congenital deficiencies:*** Associated with increased frequency of scleroderma, chronic hepatitis, autoimmune hepatitis, Henoch-Schönlein purpura

Contd...

Contd...

Protein	*Increased in*	*Decreased in*
Lipoproteins		
Apolipoprotein A-1	Familial hyper-alphalipoproteinaemia, modest alcohol intake, oestrogen use, exercise, thyroid hormones	Chronic renal failure, tangier disease, diabetes, hypertriglyceridaemia, liver diseases, familial and non-familial hypoalphalipoproteinaemia, certain drugs, androgen use
Apolipoprotein B	Premature atherosclerosis, familial defective Apo B_{100}, hyper-apobetalipoproteinaemia, tendon xanthomata, hepatosplenomegaly, diabetes mellitus, chronic renal disease, tangier disease, hypothyroidism, nephrotic syndrome, familial hypercholesterolaemia	Familial hypobetalipoproteinaemia, abetalipoproteinemia, neuromuscular degeneration, chronic anaemia, exercise, liver disease, acute inflammation, certain drugs, neurologic disease
Lipoprotein (a)	Coronary artery disease, cerebrovascular disease, peripheral vascular disease, nephrotic syndrome, DM (variable), cancer, gout, APR, familial hypercholesterolaemia	Cirrhosis (particularly primary biliary cirrhosis), certain drugs (nicotinic acid, neomycin, oral oestrogen), some steroids such as stanozolol
Immunoglobulins		
IgA class	*Polyclonal*: Chronic liver disease, alcoholic and non-alcoholic cirrhosis, chronic respiratory infections, GI diseases, some immnodeficiency states, RA, ankylosing spondylitis, nephropathy ***Oligoclonal:*** May be observed in electrophoresis of IgA myeloma ***Monoclonal:*** Multiple myeloma (IgA type)	Infancy and early childhood, selective IgA deficiency, protein-losing syndromes, congenital rubella, macroglobulinaemia or non-IgA multiple myeloma
IgG class	***Polyclonal:*** Autoimmune diseases, chronic liver disease, chronic or recurrent infections, sarcoidosis, some parasitic infections, intrauterine contraceptive devices ***Oligoclonal:*** Lymphoid or non-lymphoid malignancies, various autoimmune disorders, infections ***Monoclonal:*** IgG myeloma, lymphoma, Monogammopathies of unknown significance	Agammaglobulinaemia, hypogammaglobulinaemia, omenn's syndrome, X-linked hyper-IgM syndrome, nephrotic syndrome, non-IgG myelomas, infancy, pregnancy
IgM class	***Polyclonal:*** Viral infections (hepatitis A, CMV), parasitic infections (filariasis, malaria), chronic liver disease, hyper-IgM dysgammaglobulinaemia, collagen vascular disease, primary biliary cirrhosis, primary sclerosing cholangitis ***Monoclonal:*** Waldenström's macroglobulinaemia, malignant lymphoma, reticulosis, cold agglutinin/ haemolysin disease	Immunodeficiency states (Wiskott-Aldrich syndrome), non-I_gM IgM myeloma, infancy and early childhood, lymphoma

Contd...

Contd...

Protein	*Increased in*	*Decreased in*
IgD class	IgD myeloma, chronic infections (pyelonephritis), connective tissue disease, Hodgkin's disease, some forms of liver disease	Various hereditary and acquired deficiency syndromes
IgE class	IgE myeloma, allergic rhinitis, atopic dermatitis, bronchial asthma, hay fever, thymic dysplasia, selective IgA immnodeficiency, eosinophilic gastroenteritis, Wiskott-Aldrich syndrome, Loffler's syndrome, hyper-IgE syndrome, active SLE nephritis, certain drugs (particularly gold compounds)	Some progressive neoplastic diseases, ataxia-telangiectasia, hypogammaglobulinaemia, hypersensitivity
CRP	APR, bacterial infections, viral infections, rheumatic fever, active RA, vascular disorders, MI, Crohn's disease, ulcerative colitis, renal transplant failure, early pregnancy, intrauterine devices, malignancies with widespread metastases	None described
Fibrinogen	APR, nephrotic syndrome, haemodialysis patients, pregnancy, oestrogen therapy, contraceptives, acromegaly	Consumption coagulopathies, recurrent pulmonary embolism, recurrent stroke, DIC, incompatible blood transfusion reactions, obstetrical complications, inherited deficiency, prostatic carcinoma, liver disease, certain drugs (e.g., tamoxifen, anabolic steroids, nicotinic acid)
Haptoglobin (Hp)	APR, RA, biliary obstruction, nephritis, ulcerative colitis, aplastic anaemia. Major depression, corticosteroid therapy, androgen use	Ineffective erythropoiesis (sickle cell anaemia, folic acid deficiency), intravascular haemolysis, progressive tumours of liver and marrow, severe liver disease, pregnancy, oestrogen therapy, newborns
Proteinase Inhibitor		
AT III	APR, Vit K deficiency	Inherited deficiency, acute thrombosis, DIG, consumptive coagulopathies, certain chemotherapeutic drugs, severe liver disease, oestrogen therapy, nephrotic syndrome, heparin therapy, some contraceptive medications
Other Markers		
Serum β2 - microglobulin	Decreased glomerular filtration, lymphoproliferative disorders, myeloma, RA, viral infections, anticancer drugs, newborns, ESRD, Crohn's disease, Sjögren's syndrome, dialysis related amyloidosis, certain anti-inflammatory drugs	None reported

optimised protocol. The analytical parameters available for user control vary from instrument to instrument.

Some instruments, however, are "closed instruments" which implies that all parameter settings are read into the instruments by bar coded reagents. In this case the user cannot control the assay and will have to rely entirely on the manufacturer and their instructions.

TURBIDIMETRIC IMMUNOASSAY FOR DETERMINATION OF RHEUMATOID FACTORS

Summary

In rheumatoid arthritis (RA), diagnostically useful autoantibodies termed as rheumatoid factors (RF) can be detected which are immunoglobulins of the class IgG, IgM, IgA and IgE. IgM class IgA with specificity to human IgG Fc is the most useful prognostic marker for RA.

RF play a role in perpetuating the rheumatoid inflammatory process, the severity of joint damage could be predicted according to the strength of RF reactivity. A significant decline of RF with the remission of disease activity has also been demonstrated. Therefore, quantified serial determinations of RF are more meaningful for the diagnosis, prognosis, and assessment of therapeutic efficacy of rheumatoid arthritis. Initial RF positivity has been a sensitive predictor for later joint destruction. Quantified measurement of initial RF level and especially repeated measurements of RF at regular intervals seems to add significantly to the prognostic value of RF in distinguishing between progressive and non-progressive disease in early RA.

QUANTIA-RF is a turbidimetric immunoassay for quantitative detection of rheumatoid factors of the IgM class.

Reagent

1. *QUANTIA-RF activation buffer (R1):* Ready-to-use buffer.
2. *QUANTIA-RF latex reagent (R2):* Ready-to-use uniform suspension of polystyrene latex particles coated with suitably modified Fc fraction of human IgG.
3. *QUANTIA-RF calibrator:* Lyophilised preparation of RF positive serum, which is equivalent to stated amount of RF on IU/ml basis, when hydrated appropriately. The QUANTIA-RF calibrator is traceable to the WHO, International Reference Preparation of Rheumatoid Arthritis Serum.

Each batch of reagents undergoes rigorous quality control at various stages of manufacture for its specificity, sensitivity and performance.

Reagent Storage and Stability

1. Store the reagents at 2 to 8°C. Do not freeze.
2. The shelf-life of the reagent, activation buffer and the calibrator is as per the expiry date mentioned on the respective vial labels.
3. The reconstituted QUANTIA-RF calibrator is stable for 7 days at 2 to 8°C and 48 hours at 25 to 30°C (RT).
4. The working reagent for QUANTIA-RF can be prepared by mixing R2 and R1 in the ratio 1:5.
5. The mixed stability of the working reagent (R1+ R2) is 7 days when stored at 2 to 8°C.

Principle

QUANTIA-RF is a turbidimetric immunoassay for the determination of rheumatoid factors and is based on the principle of agglutination reaction. The test specimen is mixed with QUANTIA RF latex reagent (R2) and activation buffer (R1) and allowed to react. Presence of RF in the test specimen results in formation of an insoluble complex resulting in an increase in turbidity, which is measured at wavelength 505 to 578 nm. The increase in turbidity corresponds to the concentration of RF in the test specimen.

Note

1. *In vitro* diagnostic reagent for laboratory and professional use only. Not for medicinal use.
2. All the reagents derived from human source have been tested for HBsAg and HIV antibodies and are found to be non-reactive. However, handle the material as if infectious.
3. Reagents contain 0.1 per cent sodium azide as preservative. Avoid contact with skin and mucosa. On disposal, flush with large quantities of water.
4. The reagents can be damaged due to microbial contamination or on exposure to extreme temperatures. It is recommended that the performance of the reagents be verified using known controls periodically.

5. Gently mix the QUANTIA-RF latex reagent well before use to disperse the latex particles uniformly to improve test performance.
6. The working reagent should be mixed gently.
7. Do not use vortex mixers for mixing. Gently mix the reagents and samples during test procedures.
8. As the reagents within lots have been matched, reagents from different lots must not be interchanged.
9. Calibrators of different manufacturers must not be used with QUANTIA-RF reagents.
10. The calibration curve must be validated periodically with known controls.
11. The QUANTIA-RF assay is recommended only for analysers with cuvette mode. Though any semiautomated analyser with appropriate programming facility can be used, for best results it is recommended to use; **Quantiamate** analyser. Fully automated analysers may be used, provided the reagent has been standardised on the system.
12. The procedures mentioned in the pack insert are based on a minimum reading volume of 500 µl (0.5 ml). In case of instruments where minimum volume required for reading absorbance is 1.0 ml, use double the quantity of reagents and samples mentioned in the test procedure.

Specimen Collection and Preparation

No special preparation of the patient is required prior to specimen collection by approved techniques.

Only serum should be used for testing. Should a delay in testing occur, store the samples at 2 to 8°C. Samples can be stored for up to three days at 2 to 8°C, provided they are not contaminated. Do not use haemolysed, icteric or highly turbid sera. Turbid or paniculate serum samples must be clarified by centrifugation at 2000 rpm for 15 minutes. Use the clear supernatant for testing.

Additional Material Required

Spectrophotometer with 505 to 578 nm wavelength filters and cuvette mode, stopwatch, well-calibrated micropipettes, disposable tips, isotonic saline, paniculate free distilled water, test tube rack, incubator/waterbath set at 37°C, optically clean disposable cuvettes such as **Quantiamate semimicro-cuvettes/**glass cuvettes.

Note: Though any filter between the wavelengths 505 to 578 can be used, optimum results are obtained with a filter with 546 nm wavelength.

Test Procedure

Bring reagents and specimen to room temperature before use.

Assay Conditions

Wavelength	546 nm
Reaction temperature	37°C
Cuvette	1 cm path length

Method for Preparation of RF Calibration Curve

The QUANTIA-RF calibrator must be reconstituted exactly with 1.0 ml of distilled water, wait for 10 minutes, gently swirl the vial till the solution attains homogeneity. Once reconstituted, it is ready to use for preparation of RF calibration curve. The concentration (S) of RF in the reconstituted calibrator is as mentioned at the end of the package insert.

Dilute the calibrator serially as mentioned below for preparation of calibration curve.

Test tube No.	1	2	3	4	5
Calibrator dilution No.	D1	D2	D3	D4	D5
Isotonic saline	-	100 µl	100 µl	100 µl	100 µl
Calibrator	100 µl	100 µl	100 µl	100 µl	100 µl
Conc. of IgA in IU/ml	120	60	30	15	7.5

The above five dilutions of the calibrator including the highest 120 IU/ml (D1) and lowest 7.5 IU/ml (D5) concentrations of measuring range must be used for the preparation of the calibration curve.

Test Procedure for Preparation of Calibration Curve

1. Zero the instrument with distilled water.
2. Pipette 400 µl of QUANTIA-RF activation buffer (R1) and 100 µl of QUANTIA-RF latex reagent (R2) in the measuring cuvette. Mix well and incubate for five minutes at 37°C.

   or

   Pipette 500 µl of QUANTIA-RF working reagent in the measuring cuvette. Mix well and incubate for five minutes at 37°C.

3. Add 10 µl of calibrator (D1), mix gently and start the stopwatch simultaneously.
4. Read absorbance (A1), *exactly* at ten seconds, and absorbance (A2) again at the end of *exactly* four minutes.
5. Repeat steps No. 2 to 4 for each diluted calibrator (D2 to D5) for preparing calibration curve.
6. Calculate ΔA (A2-A1) for each calibrator (D1 to D5). Plot a graph of ΔA versus concentration of RF on the graph paper provided with the kit.

"The calibration curve" so obtained is valid only for the same lot of QUANTIA-RF reagents.

Test Procedure for Specimen

For determination of RF concentration in the test specimen:

1. Follow steps 2 to 4 as mentioned in the above procedure for calibration curve using the test specimen in place of the calibrator.
2. Calculate ΔA (A2-A1) for the test specimen.

Validation Criteria

If the ΔA of the test specimen is less than ΔA obtained for the standard of highest concentration (D1) then the concentration of IgA in the test specimen can be determined directly by interpolating ΔA of the test specimen from the calibration curve.

If the ΔA of the diluted test specimen is higher than ΔA of standard with highest concentration (D1), then the test has to be rerun by carrying out further dilution of test specimen such as 1:10, 1:20, etc., till the DA of the diluted test specimen is less than ΔA of D1. Then proceed for calculations.

Calculations

1. Interpolate ΔA of the diluted test specimen on the calibration curve and obtain the RF concentration 'C' of the diluted test specimen.
2. Multiply the RF concentration 'C' with the dilution factor (F) of the test specimen for obtaining the concentration of RF in the neat test specimen.

Concentration of RF in the neat test specimen in IU/ml = C × F

(where 'F' is the dilution factor of the test specimen, i.e. 10 for 1:10 dilution of test specimen and so on.)

Specific Performance Characteristics

Measuring Range

The QUANTIA-RF reagent has been designed to measure RF concentrations in the range 7.5-120 IU/ml and is linear between the measuring range.

Detection Limit/Analytical Sensitivity

Detection limit: 7.5 IU/ml

The detection limit represents the lowest measurable RF concentrations that can be distinguished from zero.

Prozone Limit

No prozone effect was observed up to a concentration of 1250 IU/ml of RF.

Precision

Intra-assay precision	*n*	*Mean IU/ml*	*SD*	*CV (%)*
Sample 1	15	14.47	1.06	7.33
Sample 2	15	50.80	4.44	8.74
Sample 3	15	99.20	6.53	6.58
Inter-assay precision	*n*	*Mean IU/ml*	*SD*	*CV (%)*
Sample 1	15	14.88	0.91	6.2
Sample 2	15	51.00	3.39	65.5
Sample 3	15	100.60	4.07	4.04

Interference

No interference was observed with:

Interference factor	**No interference up to**
Glucose	500 mg/dl
Albumin	10 g/dl
Bilirubin	50 mg/dl
Haemoglobin	500 mg/dl
Triglycerides	1000 mg/dl

Reference Values

The reference values of RF in normal population are ≤ 10 IU/ml.

Each laboratory should define its own reference range for relevant population.

Remarks

1. Usage of well-calibrated equipment and accessories and procedures is critical for achieving correct results.

2. When ΔA obtained for the test specimen is greater than the ΔA of the standard with highest concentration then, it indicates that the concentration of IgA in the test specimen is beyond the measuring range of the QUANTIA-RF assay. Such specimens should be rerun with further dilutions.
3. Markedly lipaemic, haemolysed, and contaminated serum samples could produce non-specific values.
4. Use of plasma rather than serum can lead to non-specific values.
5. Do not read results beyond four minutes.
6. Rheumatoid factors are not exclusively found in rheumatoid arthritis but sometimes in syphilis, systemic lupus erythromatosus, hepatitis and hypergammaglobulinaemia also.
7. It is recommended that results of the tests should be correlated with clinical findings to arrive at the final diagnosis.
8. QUANTIA-RF assay is sensitive to the presence of IgM IgA with heterogenous specificity.

TURBIDIMETRIC IMMUNOASSAY FOR DETERMINATION OF C-REACTIVE PROTEIN, QUNATIA CRP®, Courtesy: Tulip Group of Companies

Summary

C-reactive protein (CRP) is an acute phase protein synthesised in the liver. Its rate of synthesis increases within hours of acute injury or the inflammation and may reach as high as 20 times the normal levels. A rapid fall of CRP indicates recovery. The degree of elevation of CRP level directly reflects the mass or activity of inflamed tissue. And its ability to fall to normal levels on resolution of the condition renders quantified CRP values to be a good indicator to allow rapid selection of appropriate anti-inflammatory therapy in several rheumatic diseases, which are, clinically difficult to assess. Apart from indicating inflammatory disorders, CRP levels help in differential diagnosis, in the management of neonatal septicaemia and meningitis where standard microbiological investigations are difficult. CRP levels rise invariably after major surgery, but fall to normal within 7-10 days. Absence of this fall is indicative of septic or inflammatory postoperative complications. Serum CRP concentration provides useful information in patients with myocardial infarction there being an excellent correlation between peak levels of CRP and creatine phosphokinase.

Reagent

1. *QUANTIA-CRP activation buffer (R1)* : Ready-to-use
2. *QUANTIA-CRP reagent (R2)*: Ready-to-use solution of anti-CRP antibody.
3. *QUANTIA-CRP calibrator:* A lyophilised preparation of serum equivalent to the stated amount of CRP on a mg/dl basis, when hydrated appropriately. The QUANTIA-CRP calibrator is traceable to the WHO International Reference Standard (85/506) for Human C-reactive protein.

Each batch of reagents undergoes rigorous quality control at various stages of manufacture for its specificity, sensitivity and performance.

Reagent Storage and Stability

1. Store the reagents at 2 to 8°C. Do not freeze.
2. The shelf-life of the reagent, activation buffer and the calibrator is as per the expiry date mentioned on the respective vial labels.
3. The reconstituted QUANTIA-CRP calibrator is stable for 7 days at 2 to 8°C and 48 hours at 25 to 30°C (RT).

Principle

QUANTIA-CRP is a turbidimetric immunoassay for determination of C-reactive protein in human serum and is based on the principle of agglutination reaction. The test specimen is mixed with activation buffer (R1). QUANTIA-CRP reagent (R2) is then added and allowed to react. Presence of CRP in the test specimen results in the formation of an insoluble complex producing a turbidity, which is measured at 340 nm wavelength. The increase in turbidity corresponds to the concentration of CRP in the test specimen.

Note

1. *In vitro* diagnostic reagent for laboratory and professional use only. Not for medicinal use.
2. All the reagents derived from human source have been tested for HBsAg and HIV antibodies and are found to be non-reactive. However, handle the material as if infectious.
3. Reagents contain 0.1 per cent sodium azide as preservative. Avoid contact with skin and mucosa. On disposal, flush with large quantities of water.
4. The reagents can be damaged due to microbial contamination or on exposure to extreme temperatures. It is recommended that the per-

formance of the reagents be verified using known controls periodically.

5. Gently mix the QUANTIA-CRP reagent well before use to improve test performance.
6. Do not use vortex mixers for mixing. Gently mix the reagents and samples during test procedures.
7. As the reagents within lots have been matched, reagents from different lots must not be interchanged.
8. Calibrators of different manufacturers must not be used with QUANTIA-CRP reagents.
9. The calibration curve must be validated periodically with known controls.
10. The QUANTIA-CRP assay is recommended only for analysers with cuvette mode. Though any semiautomated analyser with appropriate programming facility can be used; for best results it is recommended to use **Quantiamate** analyser. Fully automated analysers may be used, provided the reagent has been standardised on the system.
11. The procedures mentioned in the pack insert are based on a minimum reading volume of 500 µl (0.5 ml). In case of instruments where minimum volume required for reading absorbance is 1.0 ml, use double the quantity of reagents and samples mentioned in the test procedure.

Specimen Collection and Preparation

No special preparation of the patient is required prior to specimen collection by approved techniques. Only serum should be used for testing. Should a delay in testing occur, store the samples at 2 to 8°C. Samples can be stored for up to a week at 2 to 8°C, provided they are not contaminated. Do not use haemolysed, icteric, or highly turbid serum. Turbid or paniculate serum samples must be clarified by centrifugation at 2000 rpm for 15 minutes. Use the clear supernatant for testing.

Additional Material Required

Spectrophotometer with 340 nm wavelength filter and cuvette mode, stopwatch, well-calibrated micropipettes, disposable tips, isotonic saline, particulate free distilled water, test-tube rack, incubator/waterbath set at 37°C, optically clean disposable cuvettes such as **Quantiamate semimicro-cuvettes/**glass cuvettes.

Test Procedure

Bring reagents and sample to room temperature before use.

Assay Conditions

Wavelength	340 nm
Reaction temperature	37°C
Cuvette	1 cm path length

Method for Preparation of CRP Calibration Curve

The QUANTIA-CRP calibrator must be reconstituted exactly with 1.0 ml of distilled water, wait for 10 minutes, gently swirl the vial till the solution attains homogeneity. Once reconstituted, it is ready to use for preparation of the CRP calibration curve.

The concentration (S) of CRP in the reconstituted calibrator is as mentioned at the end of the package insert.

Dilute the calibrator serially as mentioned below for preparation of calibration curve.

Test tube no.	*1*	*2*	*3*	*4*	*5*	*6*
Calibrator dilution No.	D1	D2	D3	D4	D5	D6
Isotonic saline	-	100 µl	100 µl	100 µl	100 µl	100 µl
Calibrator (S)	100 µl	100 µl	100 µl	100 µl	100 µl	100 µl
Conc. of CRP in mg/dl	10	5	2.5	1.2	0.6	0.3

Five dilutions of the calibrator including the highest concentration 10 mg/dl (D1) and the lowest concentration 0.3 mg/dl (D6) of the measuring range must be used for the preparation of the calibration curve. Select any of the three dilutions from D2 to D4 in addition to D1 and D6 to prepare the calibration curve.

Test Procedure for Preparation of Calibration Curve

1. Zero the instrument with distilled water
2. Pipette 500 µl of QUANTIA-CRP activation buffer (R1) and 50 µl of diluted calibrator D1 from tube No. 1 in the measuring cuvette. Mix well and incubate for five minutes at 37°C.
3. Read absorbance (A1).
4. Add 50 µl of QUANTIA-CRP reagent (R2) (preincubated at 37°C), mix gently and start the stopwatch simultaneously.
5. Read absorbance (A2) at the end of *exactly* five minutes.

6. Repeat steps No. 2 to 5 for each diluted calibrator selected for preparing the calibration curve.
7. Calculate ΔA (A2-A1) for each of the diluted calibrator selected for preparing the calibration curve. Plot a graph of ΔA versus concentration of CRP on the graph paper provided with the kit.

"The calibration curve" so obtained is valid only for the same lot of QUANTIA-CRP reagents.

Test procedure for specimen

For determination of CRP concentration in the test specimen;

1. Follow steps 2 to 5 using the test specimen in place of the calibrator.
2. Calculate ΔA (A2-A1) for the test specimen.

Validation Criteria

If the ΔA of the test specimen is less than ΔA obtained for the calibrator of highest concentration (D1), then the concentration of CRP in the test specimen can be determined directly by interpolating ΔA of the test specimen from the calibration curve. If the ΔA of the test specimen is higher than ΔA of the calibrator with highest concentration (D1), then the test has to be rerun by carrying out serial dilutions such as 1:2, 1:4, etc. of test specimen till the ΔA of the diluted test specimen is less than ΔA of D1. The CRP concentration for such samples can be determined as mentioned below in **calculations.**

Calculations

1. Interpolate ΔA of the diluted test specimen on the calibration curve and obtain the CRP concentration 'C' of the diluted test specimen.
2. Multiply the CRP concentration 'C' with the dilution factor (F) of the test specimen for obtaining the concentration of CRP in the neat test specimen.

Concentration of CRP in the neat test specimen in mg/dl = C × F

(where 'F' is the dilution factor of the test specimen, e.g., 2 for 1:2 dilution of test specimen and so on).

Specific Performance Characteristics

Measuring Range

The QUANTIA-CRP reagent has been designed to measure CRP concentrations in the range of 0.3-10 mg/dl.

Detection Limit/Analytical Sensitivity

Detection limit: 0.3 mg/dl

The detection limit represents the lowest measurable CRP concentrations that can be distinguished from zero.

Prozone Limit

No prozone effect was observed with CRP concentration up to 100 mg/dl.

Precision

Intra-assay precision	*n*	*Mean mg/dl*	*SD*	*CV (%)*
Sample 1	15	0.55	0.01	2.08
Sample 2	15	1.64	0.03	1.77
Sample 3	15	9.82	0.12	1.23
Inter-assay precision	*n*	*Mean mg/dl*	*SD*	*CV (%)*
Sample 1	15	0.55	0.01	2.08
Sample 2	15	1.64	0.03	1.77
Sample 3	15	9.82	0.12	1.23

Interference

No interference was observed with:

Interference factor	*No interference up to*
Bilirubin	50 mg/dl
Glucose	400 mg/dl
Haemoglobin	500 mg/dl
Creatinine	6 gm/L
Urea	2 gm/L

Reference Values

The reference values of CRP in normal population are ≤ 0.6 mg/dl.

Remarks

1. Usage of well-calibrated equipment and accessories and procedures is critical for achieving correct results.
2. When ΔA obtained for the test specimen is greater than the ΔA of the standard with highest concentration, then it indicates that the concentration of CRP in the test specimen is beyond the measuring range of the QUANTIA-

CRP assay. Such specimens should be rerun with further dilutions.
3. Markedly lipaemic, haemolysed, and contaminated serum samples could produce non-specific CRP values.
4. Use of plasma rather than serum can lead to erroneous CRP values.
5. Elevated levels of CRP are found to be present after the 1st trimester of pregnancy and persists until delivery.
6. CRP levels are elevated in women who are on oral contraceptives.
7. The commonly used anti-inflammatory drugs or immunosuppressive drugs, including steroids do not affect CRP response, unless the disease activity is affected and it covers an exceptionally broad incremental range up to 3000 times.
8. Do not read results beyond five minutes.
9. Since CRP production is a non-specific response to tissue injury, it is recommended that results of the test should be correlated with clinical findings to arrive at the final diagnosis.

TURBIDIMETRIC IMMUNOASSAY'FOR ULTRASENSITIVE DETERMINATION OF C-REACTIVE PROTEIN

Quantia CRP-US, Courtesy: Tulip Group of Companies

Summary

C-reactive protein (CRP), the classical acute phase protein is an extremely valuable marker for underlying systemic inflammation. The median value for serum CRP in apparently healthy adults is approximately 0.08 mg/dl, the 90th centile of distribution in such subjects is approximately 0.03 mg/dl. The baseline values for CRP in a healthy individual remain stable over a long period of time. The **baseline serum concentration of CRP** predicts the risk of future myocardial infarction and stroke independent of other risk factors, in apparently healthy subjects.

Increased values of CRP below 0.5 mg/dl previously considered to be within the reference interval are strongly associated with increased risk of atherothrombotic events. Several prospective studies suggest that in apparently healthy individuals, as the concentration of CRP increases from greater than 0.055 to 0.211 mg/dl, the probability for developing AMI increases significantly from a factor of 1 to 2.9. Apparently, healthy individuals in the highest quartile (the upper 25 per cent) of the above-mentioned range have 2 to 3 times higher risk of developing subsequent atherosclerotic diseases compared to those in the lowest quartile. Simultaneous ultrasensitive measurements of CRP and total HDL cholesterol predict future vascular risk better than lipid measurements alone.

Such low levels of CRP in apparently healthy adults can be determined by **ultrasensitive immunoassays** such as QUANTIA-CRP US.

Reagent

1. *QUANTIA-CRP US activation buffer (R1)* : Ready-to-use
2. *QUANTIA-CRP US latex reagent (R2)* : Ready-to-use uniform suspension of polystyrene latex particles coated with anti-CRP antibodies.
3. *QUANTIA-CRP US calibrator:* A lyophilised preparation of serum equivalent to the stated amount of CRP on a mg/dl basis, when hydrated appropriately. The QUANTIA-CRP US calibrator is traceable to the WHO International Reference Standard (85/506) for Human C-reactive protein.

Each batch of reagents undergoes rigorous quality control at various stages of manufacture for its specificity, sensitivity and performance.

Reagent Storage and Stability

1. Store the reagents at 2 to 8°C. Do not freeze.
2. The shelf-life of the reagent, activation buffer and the calibrator is as per the expiry date mentioned on the respective vial labels.
3. The reconstituted QUANTIA-CRP US calibrator is stable for 7 days at 2 to 8°C and 48 hours at 25 to 30°C (RT).
4. The working reagent for QUANTIA-CRP US can be prepared by mixing R2 and R1 in the ratio 1:5.
5. The mixed stability of the working reagent (R1 + R2) is 7 days when stored at 2 to 8°C.

Principle

QUANTIA-CRP US is a turbidimetric immunoassay for the ultrasensitive determination of C-reactive protein in human serum and is based on the principle of agglutination reaction. The test specimen is mixed with QUANTIA-CRP US latex reagent and activation buffer and allowed to react. Presence of CRP in the test specimen results in the formation of an insoluble complex producing a turbidity, which is measured at wavelength between 505 and 578 nm. The increase in turbidity corresponds to the concentration of CRP in the test specimen.

Note

1. *In vitro* diagnostic reagent for laboratory and professional use only. Not for medicinal use.
2. All the reagents derived from human source have been tested for HBsAg and HIV antibodies and are found to be non-reactive. However, handle the material as if infectious.
3. Reagents contain 0.1 per cent sodium azide as preservative. Avoid contact with skin and mucosa. On disposal, flush with large quantities of water.
4. The reagents can be damaged due to microbial contamination or on exposure to extreme temperatures. It is recommended that the performance of the reagents be verified using known controls periodically.
5. Gently mix the QUANTIA-CRP US latex reagent well before use to disperse the latex particles uniformly to improve test performance.
6. The working reagent should be mixed gently.
7. Do not use vortex mixers for mixing. Gently mix the reagents and samples during test procedures.
8. The QUANTIA-CRP US assay is recommended only for analyzers with cuvette mode. Though any semiautomated analyser with appropriate programming facility can be used; for best results it is recommended to use **Quantiamate** analyser. Fully automated analysers may be used, provided the reagent has been standardised on the system.
9. Calibrators of different manufacturers must not be used with QUANTIA-CRP US reagents.
10. The calibration curve must be validated periodically with known controls.
11. As the reagents within lots have been matched, reagents from different lots must not be interchanged.
12. The procedures mentioned in the pack insert are based on a minimum reading volume of 500 µl (0.5 ml). In case of instruments where minimum volume required for reading absorbance is 1.0 ml, use double the quantity of reagents and samples mentioned in the test procedure.

Specimen Collection and Preparation

No special preparation of the patient is required prior to specimen collection by approved techniques. Only serum should be used for testing. Should a delay in testing occur, store the samples at 2 to 8°C. Samples can be stored for up to a week at 2 to 8°C, provided they are not contaminated. Do not use haemolysed, icteric, or highly turbid serum. Turbid or particulate serum samples must be clarified by centrifugation at 2000 rpm for 15 minutes. Use the clear supernatant for testing.

Additional Material Required

Spectrophotometer with 505 to 578 nm wavelength filters and cuvette mode, stopwatch, well-calibrated micropipettes, disposable tips, isotonic saline, particulate free distilled water, test-tube rack, incubator/waterbath set at 37°C, optically clean disposable cuvettes such as **Quantiamate semi micro cuvettes**/glass cuvettes.

Note: Though any filter between the wavelengths 505 and 578 can be used, optimum results are obtained with a filter with 546 nm wavelength.

Test Procedure

Bring reagents and sample to room temperature before use.

Assay Conditions

Wavelength	546 nm
Reaction temperature	37°C
Cuvette	1 cm path length

Method for Preparation of CRP US Calibration Curve

The QUANTIA-CRP US calibrator must be reconstituted exactly with 1.0 ml of distilled water, wait for 5 minutes, gently swirl the vial till the solution attains homogeneity. Once reconstituted, it is ready to use for preparation of the CRP calibration curve.

The concentration of CRP (S) in the reconstituted calibrator is as mentioned at the end of this package insert. Dilute the reconstituted calibrator serially as mentioned below for preparation of calibration curve.

Test tube No.	*1*	*2*	*3*	*4*	*5*	*6*	*7*
Calibrator dilution No.	D1	D2	D3	D4	D5	D6	D7
Isotonic saline	-	100 µl	100 µl	100 µl	100 µl	100 µl	100 µl
Calibrator (S)	100 µl	100 µl	100 µl	100 µl	100 µl	100 µl	100 µl
Conc. of CRP in mg/dl	1.0	0.5	0.25	0.125	0.0625	0.031	0.015

Five dilutions of the calibrator including the highest concentration 1.0 mg/dl (D1) and the lowest concentration 0.015 mg/dl (D7) of the measuring range *must* be used for the preparation of the calibration curve. Select any of the three dilutions from D2 to D6 in addition to D1 and D7 to prepare the calibration curve.

Test Procedure for Preparation of Calibration Curve

1. Zero the instrument with distilled water
2. Pipette and 400 µl of QUANTIA-CRP US activation buffer (R1) and 100 µl of QUANTIA-CRP US latex reagent (R2) in the measuring cuvette. Mix well and incubate for five minutes at 37°C.

   or

   Pipette 500 µl of the QUANTIA-CRP US working reagent in the measuring cuvette. Mix well and incubate for five minutes at 37°C.
3. Add 5 µl of calibrator D1, mix gently and start the stopwatch simultaneously.
4. Read absorbance (A1), *exactly* at 10 seconds, and absorbance (A2) again at the end of *exactly* four minutes.
5. Repeat steps No. 2 to 4 for each of the diluted calibrator selected for preparing the calibration curve.
6. Calculate ΔA (A2-A1) for each of the diluted calibrator selected for preparing the calibration curve. Plot a graph of ΔA versus concentration of CRP on the graph paper provided with the kit.

"The calibration curve" so obtained is valid only for the same lot of QUANTIA-CRP US reagents.

Test Procedure for Specimen

For determination of CRP concentration in the test specimen:

1. Follow steps 2-4 as mentioned in the above procedure for calibration curve using the test specimen in place of the calibrator.
2. Calculate ΔA (A2-A1) for the test specimen.

Validation Criteria

If the ΔA of the test specimen is less than ΔA obtained for the calibrator of highest concentration (D1), then the concentration of CRP in the test specimen can be determined directly by interpolating ΔA of the test specimen from the calibration curve. If the ΔA of the test specimen is higher than ΔA of the calibrator with highest concentration (D1), then the test has to be rerun by carrying out serial dilutions such as 1:2, 1:4, etc. of test specimen till the ΔA of the diluted test specimen is less than ΔA of D1. The CRP concentration for such samples can be determined as mentioned below in **calculations.**

Calculations

1. Interpolate ΔA of the diluted test specimen on the calibration curve and obtain the CRP concentration 'C' of the diluted test specimen.
2. Multiply the CRP concentration 'C' with the dilution factor (F) of the test specimen for obtaining the concentration of CRP in the neat test specimen.

Concentration of CRP in the neat test specimen in mg/dl = C × F

(where 'F' is the dilution factor of the test specimen, e.g., 2 for 1:2 dilution of test specimen and so on)

Specific Performance Characteristics

Measuring Range

The QUANTIA-CRP US reagent has been designed to measure CRP concentrations in the range 0.015 - 1.0 mg/dl and is linear within the measuring range.

Detection Limit/Analytical Sensitivity

Detection limit: 0.015 mg/dl

The detection limit represents the lowest measurable CRP concentrations that can be distinguished from zero.

Prozone Limit

No prozone effect was observed up to a CRP concentration of 2.0 mg/dl.

Precision

Intra-assay precision	n	Mean mg/dl	SD	CV (%)
Sample 1	15	0.029	0.002	6.02
Sample 2	15	0.349	0.028	8.17
Sample 3	15	0.797	0.058	7.28
Inter-assay precision	*n*	*Mean mg/dl*	*SD*	*CV (%)*
Sample 1	15	0.029	0.002	5.42
Sample 2	15	0.346	0.017	5.03
Sample 3	15	0.812	0.035	4.27

Interference

No interference was observed with :

Interference factor	No interference up to
Albumin	10 g/dl
Bilirubin	50 mg/dl
Glucose	500 mg/dl
Haemoglobin	500 mg/dl
Triglycerides	1000 mg/dl
IgA	120 IU/ml

Reference Values

Males

CRP in mg/dl	Relative risk factor	
	Future MI	Future Stroke
>0.211 mg/dl	2.9	1.9
0.115-0.210	2.6	1.9
0.056-0.114	1.7	1.7
< 0.055	1.0	1.0

Females

CRP in mg/dl	Relative risk factor Future MI or Future Stroke
>0.73	5.5
0.38-0.73	3.5
0.15-0.37	2.7
<0.15	1.0

The above-mentioned reference values are for guidance only. It is recommended that each laboratory should define its own reference range for relevant population.

Remarks

1. Usage of well-calibrated equipment and accessories and procedures is critical for achieving correct results.
2. When ΔA obtained for the test specimen is greater than the ΔA of the standard with highest concentration, then it indicates that the concentration of CRP in the test specimen is beyond the measuring range of the QUANTIA-CRP assay. Such specimens should be rerun with further dilutions.
3. When using CRP to assess risk of cardiovascular and peripheral vascular disease, measurements should be compared to previous values. Recent medical events resulting in tissue injury, infections and inflammation, which may cause elevated CRP levels, should also be considered when interpreting results.
4. Markedly lipaemic, haemolysed, and contaminated serum samples could produce nonspecific CRP values.
5. Use of plasma rather than serum can lead to erroneous CRP values.
6. Elevated levels of CRP are found to be present after the 1st trimester of pregnancy and persists until delivery.
7. CRP levels are elevated in women who are on oral contraceptives.
8. The commonly used anti-inflammatory drugs or immunosuppressive drugs, including steroids do not affect CRP response, unless the disease activity is affected and it covers an exceptionally broad incremental range up to 3000 times.
9. Do not read results beyond five minutes.
10. Since CRP production is a nonspecific response to tissue injury, it is recommended that results of the test should be correlated with clinical findings to arrive at the final diagnosis.

TURBIDIMETRIC IMMUNOASSAY FOR DETERMINATION OF ANTISTREPTOLYSIN 'O' IN HUMAN SERUM

Quantia CRP-US, Courtesy: Tulip Group of Companies

Summary

The group A, β-haemolytic streptococci produce various exotoxins such as Streptolysin O, Steptolysin

S that can act as antigens. The affected individuals produce specific antibodies against Streptolysin 'O' that has clinical significance namely Antistreptolysin 'O'. Antistreptolysin 'O' can be detected 1-3 weeks after infection, attaining a maximum levels at around 3-6 weeks. Determination of these antibodies is very useful for the diagnosis of streptococcal infections and their relative effects such as rheumatic fever and acute glomerulonephritis.

Reagent

1. *QUANTIA-ASO activation buffer (R1)* : Ready-to-use buffer.
2. *QUANTIA-ASO latex reagent (R2)* : Ready-to-use uniform suspension of polystyrene latex particles coated with stabilised Streptolysin 'O'.
3. *QUANTIA-ASO calibrator:* A lyophilised preparation of ASO positive serum, which is equivalent to stated amount of ASO on IU/ml basis, when hydrated appropriately. The QUANTIA-ASO calibrator is traceable to the International Standard for Antistreptolysin 'O' (97/662).

Each batch of reagents undergoes rigorous quality control at various stages of manufacture for its specificity, sensitivity and performance.

Reagent Storage and Stability

1. Store the reagents at 2 to 8°C. Do not freeze.
2. The shelf-life of the reagent, activation buffer and the calibrator is as per the expiry date mentioned on the respective vial labels.
3. The reconstituted QUANTIA-ASO calibrator is stable for 7 days at 2 to 8°C and 48 hours at 25 to 30°C (RT).
4. The working reagent for QUANTIA-ASO can be prepared by mixing R2 and R1 in the ratio 1:11.
5. The mixed stability of the working reagent (R1 + R2) is 7 days when stored at 2 to 8°C.

Principle

QUANTIA-ASO is a turbidimetric immunoassay for determination of Antistreptolysin 'O' and is based on the principle of agglutination reaction. The test specimen is mixed with QUANTIA-ASO latex reagent (R2) and activation buffer (R1) and allowed to react. Presence of ASO in the test specimen results in the formation of an insoluble complex resulting in an increase in turbidity, which is measured at 505 to 578 nm wavelength. The increase in turbidity corresponds to the concentration of ASO in the test specimen.

Note

1. *In vitro* diagnostic reagent for laboratory and professional use only. Not for medicinal use.
2. All the reagents derived from human source have been tested for HBsAg and HIV antibodies and are found to be non-reactive. However, handle the material as if infectious.
3. Reagents contain 0.1 per cent sodium azide as preservative. Avoid contact with skin and mucosa. On disposal, flush with large quantities of water.
4. The reagents can be damaged due to microbial contamination or on exposure to extreme temperatures. It is recommended that the performance of the reagents be verified using known controls periodically.
5. Gently mix the QUANTIA-ASO latex reagent well before use to improve test performance.
6. The working reagent should be mixed gently.
7. Do not use vortex mixers for mixing reagents. Gently mix the reagents and samples during test procedures.
8. As the reagents within lots have been matched, reagents from different lots must not be interchanged.
9. Calibrators of different manufacturers must not be used with QUANTIA-ASO reagents.
10. The calibration curve must be validated periodically with known controls.
11. The QUANTIA-ASO assay is recommended only for analysers with cuvette mode. Though any semiautomated analyser with appropriate programming facility can be used; for best results it is recommended to use **Quantiamate** analyser. Fully automated analysers may be used, provided the reagent has been standardised on the system.
12. The procedures mentioned in this pack insert are based on a minimum reading volume of 500 µl (0.5 ml). In case of instruments where minimum volume required for reading absorbance is 1.0 ml, use double the quantity of reagents and samples mentioned in the test procedure.

Specimen Collection and Preparation

No special preparation of the patient is required prior to specimen collection by approved techniques. Only serum should be used for testing. Should a delay in testing occur, store the samples at 2 to 8°C. Samples can be stored for up to a week at 2 to 8°C, provided they are not contaminated. Do not use haemolysed, icteric, or highly turbid serum. Turbid or particulate serum samples must be clarified by centrifugation at 2000 rpm for 15 minutes. Use the clear supernatant for testing.

Additional Material Required

Spectrophotometer with 505 to 578 nm wavelength filters and cuvette mode, stopwatch, well calibrated micropipettes, disposable tips, isotonic saline, particulate free distilled water, test-tube rack, incubator/waterbath set at 37°C, optically clean disposable cuvettes such as **Quantiamate semimicro-cuvettes/**glass cuvettes.

Note: Though any filter between the wavelength 505 and 578 nm can be used, optimum results are obtained with a filter with 546 nm wavelength.

Test Procedure

Bring reagents and sample to room temperature before use.

Assay Conditions

Wavelength	546 nm
Reaction temperature	37°C
Cuvette	1 cm path length

Method for Preparation of ASO Calibration Curve

The QUANTIA-ASO calibrator must be reconstituted exactly with 1.0 ml of distilled water, wait for 10 minutes, gently swirl the vial till the solution attains homogeneity. Once reconstituted, it is ready to use for preparation of the ASO calibration curve. The concentration (S) of ASO in the reconstituted calibrator is as mentioned at the end of this package insert. Dilute the calibrator serially as mentioned below for preparation of calibration curve.

Test tube No.	1	2	3	4	5
Calibrator dilution No.	D1	D2	D3	D4	D5
Isotonic Saline	-	100 µl	100 µl	100 µl	100 µl
Calibrator (S)	100 µl	100 µl	100 µl	100 µl	100 µl
Conc. of ASO in IU/ml	800	400	200	100	50

The above five dilutions of the calibrator including the highest concentration 800 IU/ml (D1) and the lowest concentration 50 IU/ml (D5) of the measuring range *must* be used for the preparation of the calibration curve.

Test Procedure for Preparation of Calibration Curve

1. Zero the instrument with distilled water.
2. Pipette 500 µl of activation buffer (R1) and 50 µl of QUANTIA-ASO latex reagent (R2) in the measuring cuvette. Mix well and incubate for five minutes at 37°C.
   Or
   Pipette 550 µl of the QUANTIA-ASO working reagent in the measuring cuvette. Mix well and incubate for 5 minutes at 37°C.
3. Add 10 µl of calibrator D1, mix gently and start the stopwatch simultaneously.
4. Read absorbance (A1), **exactly at ten seconds,** and absorbance (A2) again at the end of **exactly four minutes.**
5. Repeat steps No. 2 to 4 for each diluted calibrator (D2 to D5) for preparing the calibration curve.
6. Calculate ΔA (A2-A1) for each calibrator (D1 to D5). Plot a graph of ΔA versus concentration of ASO on the graph paper provided with the kit.
   "The calibration curve" so obtained is valid only for the same lot of QUANTIA-ASO reagents.

Test Procedure for Specimen

For determination of ASO concentration in the test specimen:

1. Follow steps 2 to 4 as mentioned in the above procedure for calibration curve using the test specimen in place of the calibrator.
2. Calculate ΔA (A2-A1) for the test specimen.

Validation Criteria

If the ΔA of the test specimen is less than ΔA obtained for the calibrator of highest concentration (D1), then the concentration of ASO in the test specimen can be determined directly by interpolating ΔA of the test specimen from the calibration curve. If the ΔA of the test specimen is higher than ΔA of the calibrator with highest concentration (D1), then the test has to be rerun by carrying out serial dilutions of test specimen such as 1:2, 1:4, etc., till the ΔA of the diluted test specimen is less than ΔA of D1. Then proceed for calculations.

Calculations

1. Interpolate ΔA of the diluted test specimen on the calibration curve and obtain the ASO concentration 'C' of the diluted test specimen.
2. Multiply the ASO concentration 'C' with the dilution factor (F) of the test specimen for obtaining the concentration of ASO in the neat test specimen.

Concentration of ASO in the neat test specimen in IU/ml = C × F

(where 'F' is the dilution factor of the test specimen, for example, 2 for 1:2 dilution of test specimen and so on)

Specific Performance Characteristics

Measuring Range

The QUANTIA-ASO reagent has been designed to measure ASO concentrations in the range of 50 to 800 IU/ml and is linear between the measuring range.

Detection Limit/Analytical Sensitivity

Detection limit: 50 IU/ml

The detection limit represents the lowest measurable ASO concentrations that can be distinguished from zero.

Prozone Limit

No prozone effect was observed up to a concentration of 1250 IU/ml of ASO.

Precision

Intra-assay precision	*n*	*Mean IU/ml*	*SD*	*CV (%)*
Sample 1	10	98.6	3.37	3.42
Sample 2	10	298.8	7.82	2.61
Samples	10	699.2	10.12	1.4

Inter-assay precision	*n*	*Mean IU/ml*	*SD*	*CV (%)*
Sample 1	10	98.6	3.73	3.42
Sample 2	10	298.8	7.82	2.61
Sample 3	10	699.2	10.12	1.4

Interference

No interference was observed with :

Interference factor	*No interference up to*
Bilirubin	50 mg/dl
Glucose	500 mg/dl
Haemoglobin	500 mg/dl
Triglycerides	1000 mg/dl
Albumin	10 g/dl

Reference Values

The reference values of ASO in normal population are ≤ 200 IU/ml.

Each laboratory should define its own reference range for relevant age groups and population.

Remarks

1. Usage of well-calibrated equipment and accessories and procedures is critical for achieving correct results.
2. When ΔA obtained for the test specimen is greater than the ΔA of the calibrator with highest concentration, then it indicates that the concentration of ASO in the test specimen is beyond the measuring range of the QUANTIA-ASO assay. Such specimens should be rerun with further dilutions.
3. Markedly lipaemic, haemolysed, and contaminated serum samples could produce erroneous ASO values.
4. Use of plasma rather than serum can lead to erroneous ASO values.
5. Do not read results beyond four minutes.
6. It is recommended that results of the test should be correlated with clinical findings to arrive at final diagnosis.

TURBIDIMETRIC IMMUNOASSAY FOR DETERMINATION OF MICROALBUMINURIA

Quantia MA®, Courtesy: Tulip Group of Companies

Summary

Urinary albumin excretion between 30 and 300 mg/day (microalbuminuria), far below the levels found in clinical proteinuria (> 300 mg/day) is a strong predictor of development of diabetic nephropathy and vascular complications. diabetic nephropathy leads to progressive loss of renal function or end-stage renal disease (ESRD) and may necessitate need for dialysis or transplantation in most cases. The progression of microalbuminuria is closely associated with progressive hypertension and loss of blood glucose control. The early presence of microalbuminuria can be reversed by strict metabolic control and timely intervention of drugs early in the course of disease can arrest the progression of diabetic renal disease. Quantitative values of albumin are useful for differentiating microalbuminuria from clinical proteinuria and the effective monitoring of intervention strategies.

Annual screening of microalbuminuria is recommended by the 'WHO' and 'International Diabetes Foundation' in all patients with IDDM over the age of 12 years and who have had diabetes for five years or more.

Microalbuminuria is also a significant risk marker of cardiovascular diseases. Its presence can be regarded as an index of increased cardiovascular vulnerability and a signal for correction of known risk factors.

Information regarding the concentration of albumin in urine for the detection of microalbuminuria can be obtained by using QUANTIA-MA reagents.

Reagents

QUANTIA-MA assay contains:

1. *QUANTIA-MA activation buffer (R1)* : Ready-to-use.
2. *QUANTIA-MA anti-human albumin reagent (R2)* : A ready-to-use solution of anti-human albumin antibody.
3. *QUANTIA-MA calibrator:* Ready-to-use albumin solution and is equivalent to the stated amount of albumin on mg/L basis. The QUANTIA-MA calibrator is traceable to the IFCC reference material CRM 470.

Each batch of reagents undergoes rigorous quality control at various stages of manufacture for its specificity, sensitivity, and performance.

Storage and Stability

Store the reagents at 2 to 8°C. Do not freeze.

The shelf-life of the reagents is as per the expiry date mentioned on the reagent vial labels.

Principle

QUANTIA-MA is a turbidimetric immunoassay for the detection of albumin in urine and is based on the principle of agglutination reaction. The test specimen is mixed with the activation buffer (R1) and QUANTIA-MA antihuman antibody solution (R2) and allowed to react. Presence of albumin in the test specimen forms an insoluble complex producing a turbidity, which is measured at wavelength 340 nm. The resulting turbidity corresponds to the concentration of albumin in the test specimen.

Note

1. *In vitro* diagnostic reagent for laboratory and professional use only. Not for medicinal use.
2. All the materials derived from human source have been tested for HBsAg and anti-HIV antibodies and found to be nonreactive.
3. The reagents contain 0.1 per cent sodium azide as preservative. Avoid contact with skin or mucosa. On disposal, flush with large quantities of water.
4. The reagents can be damaged due to microbial contamination or on exposure to extreme temperatures. It is recommended that the performance of reagents be verified by testing with known controls periodically.
5. Shake the QUANTIA-MA anti-human albumin reagent well before use to improve test performance.
6. Do not use vortex mixers for mixing. Gently mix the reagents and samples during test procedures.
7. The QUANTIA-MA assay is recommended only for analysers with cuvette mode. Though any semiautomated analyser with appropriate programming facility can be used, for best results it is recommended to use **Quantiamate** analyser. Fully automated analysers may be used, provided the reagent has been standardised on the system.
8. Calibrators of different manufacturers must not be used with QUANTIA-MA reagents.
9. The calibration curve must be validated periodically with known controls.
10. As the reagents within lots have been matched, reagents from different lots must not be interchanged.
11. The procedures mentioned in the pack insert are based on a minimum reading volume of 500 µl (0.5 ml). In case of instruments where minimum volume required for reading absorbance is 1.0 ml, use double the quantity of reagents and samples mentioned in the test procedure.

Sample Collection and Preparation

Though random urine specimen can be used, preferably first morning urine specimen should be collected in clean dry glass or plastic containers free from detergents and even traces of proteins. Specimen should be tested immediately preferably within 12 hours of collection. Specimen can be stored up to 2 days at 2 to 8°C provided they are not contaminated. Specimen should be free from particulate matter. Turbid or particulate urine specimen must be clarified by centrifugation at 2000 rpm for 10 minutes. Use the clear supernatant for testing.

Additional Material Required

Spectrophotometer with 340 nm wavelength and cuvette mode, stopwatch, well calibrated micropipettes, disposable tips, isotonic saline, particulate free distilled water, test-tube rack, incubator/waterbath set at 37°C, optically clean disposable cuvettes such as **Quantiamate semimicro-cuvettes/**glass cuvettes.

Test Procedure

Bring reagents and specimen to room temperature before use.

Assay Conditions

Wavelength	340 nm
Reaction temperature	37°C
Cuvette	1 cm path length

Method for Preparation of MA Calibration Curve

The concentration (S) of QUANTIA-MA calibrator is as mentioned at the end of the package insert.

Dilute the QUANTIA-MA calibrator serially as mentioned below for preparation of calibration curve.

Test tube No.	*1*	*2*	*3*	*4*	*5*
Calibrator dilution No.	01	D2	D3	D4	D5
Isotonic saline	-	100 µl	100 µl	100 µl	100 µl
Calibrator	100 µl	100 µl	100 µl	100 µl	100 µl
Conc. of albumin in mg/L	400	200	100	50	25

The above five dilutions of the calibrator including the highest 400 mg/L (D1) and lowest 25 mg/L (D5) concentrations of measuring range **must** be used for the preparation of the calibration curve.

Test Procedure for Preparation of Calibration Curve

1. Zero the instrument with distilled water
2. Pipette 500 µl of QUANTIA-MA activation buffer (R1) and 10 µl of standard D1 from tube No. 1 in the measuring cuvette. Mix well and incubate for five minutes at 37°C.
3. Read absorbance (A1).
4. Add 100 µl of QUANTIA-MA antihuman albumin reagent (R2), mix gently and start the stopwatch simultaneously.
5. Read absorbance (A2) at the end of *exactly* two minutes
6. Repeat steps No. 2 to 5 for each diluted calibrator (D2 to D5) for preparing calibration curve.
7. Calculate ΔA (A2-A1) for each diluted calibrator for preparing the calibration curve. Plot a graph of ΔA versus concentration of albumin on the graph paper provided with the kit.

"The calibration curve" so obtained is valid only for the same lot of QUANTIA-MA reagents.

Test Procedure for Specimen

1. For determination of albumin concentration in the test specimen please follow steps 2 to 5 using the test specimen in place of the calibrator.
2. Calculate ΔA (A2-A1) for the test specimen.

Validation Criteria

If the ΔA of the test specimen is less than ΔA obtained for the calibrator of highest concentration (D1), then the concentration of albumin in the test specimen can be determined directly by interpolating ΔA of the test specimen on the obtained calibration curve.

If the ΔA of the test specimen is higher than ΔA of standard with highest concentration (D1), then the test has to be rerun by carrying out serial dilutions of test specimen such as 1:2, 1:4, etc. till the ΔA of the diluted test specimen is less than ΔA of D1.

The albumin concentration for such samples can be determined as mentioned in **calculations.**

Calculations

1. Interpolate ΔA of the diluted test specimen on the calibration curve and obtain the albumin concentration 'C' of the diluted test specimen.
2. Multiply the albumin concentration 'C' with the dilution factor (F) of the test specimen for obtaining the concentration of albumin in the neat test specimen.

Concentration of albumin in the neat test specimen in mg/L = C × F

(where 'F is the dilution factor of the test specimen, for example, 2 for 1:2 dilution of test specimen and so on)

Specific Performance Characteristics

Measuring Range

The QUANTIA-MA reagent has been designed to measure albumin concentrations in the range of 25 to 400 mg/L and is linear within the measuring range.

Detection Limit/Analytical Sensitivity

Detection limit: 20 mg/L

The detection limit represents the lowest measurable albumin concentrations that can be distinguished from zero.

Prozone Limit

No prozone effect was observed with albumin concentration up to 1000 mg/L.

Precision

Intra-assay precision	*n*	*Mean mg/L*	*SD*	*CV (%)*
Sample 1	15	30	1.53	5.16
Sample 2	15	150	3.6	2.41
Sample 3	15	325	7.18	2.22
Inter-assay precision	*n*	*Mean mg/L*	*SD*	*CV (%)*
Sample 1	15	30.07	2.31	7.68
Sample 2	15	150.53	5.71	379
Sample 3	15	325.47	12.99	3.99

Interference

No interference was observed with:

Interference factor	*No interference up to*
Glucose	400 mg/dl
Bilirubin	50 mg/dl
Haemoglobin	500 mg/dl
Creatinine	6 g/L
Urea	2 g/L

Reference Values

The reference values of urinary albumin in normal population are ≤ 20 mg/L. The reference values vary with regards to the time of collection of the urine sample.

Remarks

1. Microalbuminuria is classified as:
   - Albumin excretion rate : 20-200 µg/min
   - Albumin/Creatinine ratio : 2.5-25 mg/mmol
   - Albumin/Creatinine ratio : 30-300 mg/g
   - Albumin concentration (early morning urine): 30-300 mg/L
2. For determining albumin excretion rate, ideally a 24-hr urine must be used as a sample.
3. Usage of well-calibrated equipment and accessories and procedures is critical for achieving correct results.
4. When DA obtained for the test specimen is greater than the DA of the standard with highest concentration, then it indicates that the concentration of albumin in the test specimen is beyond the measuring range of the QUANTIA-MA assay. Such specimens should be rerun with further dilutions.
5. Microalbuminuria also occurs in response to acute inflammatory conditions such as ischaemia, trauma and thermal injury, surgery, pancreatitis and inflammatory bowel diseases. In many of these conditions the albumin excretion increases within minutes or hours of the initiating stimulus and only last for 24-72 hours.
6. Albumin excretion has also been associated with urinary tract infection.
7. Use only urine as test specimen. Do not use serum.
8. Contaminated and turbid urine samples could produce erroneous albumin valves.
9. Albumin excretion is subject to physical activity. It is therefore recommended to use urine sample that has been produced at rest whenever random urine specimen is used.
10. As albumin excretion is subject to physiological fluctuations it is necessary to take two measurements in consecutive days, in case of contradictory results three measurements on different days must be done preferably within a week.
11. Liquid intake of the patient must be in the normal range, i.e. 1.5-2 litres/day.
12. To diagnose incipient nephropathy microalbuminuria must be present in at least 2 out of 3 specimens over a 3-6 month period.

13. It is recommended that result of the test should be correlated with clinical findings to arrive at the final diagnosis.
14. Do not read results beyond two mites.

TURBIDIMETRIC IMMUNOASSAY FOR ESTIMATION OF IMMUNOGLOBULIN IgA IN HUMAN SERUM

Quantia IgA, Courtesy: Tulip Group of Companies

Summary

Persistently elevated immunoglobulin levels indicate an ongoing response of the immune system, whereas a decline in immunoglobulin levels hints at a recovery from the infectious process. The absolute levels of immunoglobulin concentration are a measure of the severity of the inflammatory process, especially in virally induced chronic liver disease, chronic bacterial infections, collagen vascular diseases and other autoimmune diseases. In diseases that cause hypergammaglobulinaemia quantitative determination in conjunction with the clinical presentation as well as analysis of serological and clinical chemistry results may not only help in diagnosis, differential diagnosis, but may also prove to be useful for disease monitoring and prognosis.

IgA is the second most abundant immunoglobulin (approximately 10 per cent of the total Ig mass) and is the major immunoglobulin found in mucosal surfaces. Patients with congenital IgA deficiency are prone to autoimmune diseases, and may develop antibodies to IgA and anaphylaxis if transfused. Approximately 10 to 15 per cent of all myeloma are of the IgA type. Polyclonal increase in serum IgA may be observed in chronic inflammatory disease of gastrointestinal and respiratory tracts and liver. IgA may be decreased in patients with chronic sinopulmonary disease, ataxia-telangiectasia or congenital. Information regarding the concentration of IgA can be obtained by using QUANTIA-lgA reagents.

Reagent

1. *QUANTIA-lgA activation buffer (R1):* Ready-to-use.
2. *QUANTIA-lgA antihuman IgA reagent (R2):* Ready-to-use solution of antihuman IgA antibody.
3. *QUANTIA-lgA calibrator:* Lyophilised preparation of serum equivalent to the stated amount of IgA on a mg/dl basis, when hydrated appropriately. The QUANTIA-lgA calibrator is traceable to CRM 470.

Each batch of reagents undergoes rigorous quality control at various stages of manufacture for its specificity, sensitivity, and performance.

Reagent Storage and Stability

1. Store the reagents at 2 to 8°C. Do not freeze.
2. The shelf-life of the reagent, activation buffer and calibrator is as per the expiry date mentioned on the respective vial labels.
3. The reconstituted calibrator is stable for 7 days at 2 to 8°C and 48 hours at 25 to 30°C (RT).

Principle

QUANTIA-lgA is a turbidimetric immunoassay for the detection of immunoglobulin IgA in human serum and is based on the principle of agglutination reaction. The test specimen is mixed with the activation buffer (R1). Antihuman IgA reagent (R2) is then added and allowed to react. Presence of IgA in the test specimen results in the formation of an insoluble complex producing a turbidity, which is measured at wavelength 340 nm. The extent of turbidity corresponds to the concentration of IgA in the test specimen.

Note

1. *In vitro* diagnostic reagent for laboratory and professional use only. Not for medicinal use.
2. All the reagents derived from human source have been tested for HBsAg and HIV antibodies and are found to be nonreactive. However, handle the material as if infectious.
3. Reagents contain 0.1 percent sodium azide as a preservative. Avoid contact with skin and mucosa. On disposal, flush with large quantities of water.
4. The reagents can be damaged due to microbial contamination or on exposure to extreme temperatures. It is recommended that the performance of the reagents be verified using known controls periodically.
5. The QUANTIA-IgA reagents should be mixed well before use to improve test performance.
6. Do not use vortex mixers for mixing reagents. Gently mix the reagents and samples during test procedures.
7. Calibrators of different manufacturers must not be used with QUANTIA-IgA reagents.
8. The calibration curve must be validated periodically with known controls.

9. As the reagents within lots have been matched, reagents from different lots must not be interchanged.
10. The QUANTIA-IgA assay is recommended only for analysers with cuvette mode. Though any semiautomated analyser with appropriate programming facility can be used; for best results it is recommended to use **Quantiamate** analyser. Fully automated analysers may be used, provided the reagent has been standardised on the system.
11. The procedures mentioned in the pack insert are based on a minimum reading volume of 500 µl (0.5 ml). In case of instruments where minimum volume required for reading absorbance is 1.0 ml, use double the quantity of reagents and samples mentioned in the test procedure.

Specimen Collection and Preparation

No special preparation of the patient is required prior to specimen collection by approved techniques.

Only serum should be used for testing. Should a delay in testing occur, store the samples at 2 to 8°C. Samples can be stored for up to a week at 2 to 8°C, provided they are not contaminated. Do not use haemolysed, icteric, or highly turbid sera. Turbid or particulate serum samples must be clarified by centrifugation at 2000 rpm for 15 minutes prior to testing. Use the clear supernatant for testing.

Additional Material Required

Spectrophotometer with 340 nm wavelength and cuvette mode, stopwatch, well-calibrated micropipettes, disposable tips, isotonic saline, particulate free distilled water, test-tube rack, incubator/waterbath set at 37°C, optically clean disposable cuvettes such as **Quantiamate semimicro-cuvettes/**glass cuvettes.

Test Procedure

Bring reagents and samples to room temperature before use.

Assay Conditions

Wavelength	340 nm
Reaction temperature	37°C
Cuvette	1 cm path length

Method for Preparation of IgA Calibration Curve

The QUANTIA-IgA calibrator must be reconstituted exactly with 1.0 ml of distilled water, wait for five minutes, gently swirl the vial till the solution attains homogeneity. Once reconstituted it is ready to use for preparing the IgA calibration curve. The concentration (S) of IgA in the reconstituted calibrator is as mentioned at the end of the package insert.

Prepare 1.0 ml of 144 mg/dl IgA **working standard (Sw)** from the reconstituted calibrator as mentioned at the end of the package insert. The working standard (Sw) is stable for eight hours at 2 to 30°C.

Prepare dilutions of the working standard (Sw) as mentioned below for preparation of calibration curve.

Test tube No.	1	2	3	4	5
Calibrator dilution No.	D1	D2	D3	D4	D5
Isotonic saline	-	100 µl	100 µl	100 µl	200 µl
Working standard (Sw)	100 µl	100 µl	100 µl	100 µl	100 µl
Conc. of IgA in mg/dl	144	72	36	18	6

The above five dilutions of the calibrator including the highest 144 mg/dl (D1) and lowest 6 mg/dl (D5) concentrations of measuring range *must* be used for the preparation of the calibration curve.

Test Procedure for Preparation of Calibration Curve

1. Zero the instrument with distilled water
2. Pipette 500 µl of QUANTIA-IgA activation buffer (R1) and 10 µl of working standard (D1) in the measuring cuvette. Mix well and incubate for five minutes at 37°C.
3. Read absorbance (A1).
4. Add 50 µl of QUANTIA-IgA reagent (R2), mix gently and start the stopwatch simultaneously.
5. Read absorbance (A2) at the end of *exactly* five minutes.
6. Repeat steps No. 2 to 5 for each diluted working standard (D2 to D5) for preparing calibration curve.
7. Calculate ΔA (A2-A1) for each dilution of the working standards (D1 to D5). Plot a graph of ΔA versus concentration of IgA on the graph paper provided with the kit.

"The calibration curve" so obtained is valid only for the same lot of QUANTIA-IgA reagents.

Test Procedure for Specimen

For determination of IgA concentration in the test specimen, dilute the test specimen 1:10 with normal saline.

1. Follow steps 2 to 5 as mentioned in the above procedure for calibration curve using the diluted test specimen in place of the working standard.
2. Calculate ΔA (A2-A1) for the diluted test specimen.

Validation Criteria

If the ΔA of the diluted test specimen is less than ΔA obtained for the standard of highest concentration (D1) then proceed directly for calculations of results.

If the ΔA of the diluted test specimen is higher than ΔA of the standard with highest concentration (D1) then the test has to be rerun by carrying out further dilution of test specimen such as 1:20, 1:40, 1:60, etc., till the DA of the diluted specimen is less than ΔA of D1.

Calculations

For determination of IgA concentration in the test specimen:

1. Interpolate ΔA of the diluted test specimen on the calibration curve and obtain the IgA concentration 'C' of the diluted test specimen.
2. Multiply the IgA concentration 'C' with the dilution factor (F) of the test specimen for obtaining the concentration of IgA in the neat test specimen.

Concentration of IgA in the neat test specimen in mg/dl = C × F

(where 'F' is the dilution factor of the test specimen, i.e. 10 for 1:10 dilution of test specimen and so on).

Specific Performance Characteristics

Measuring Range

The QUANTIA-IgA reagent has been designed to measure serum IgA concentrations in the range 60 to1440 mg/dl, and is linear between the measuring range.

Detection Limit/Analytical Sensitivity

Detection limit: 6 mg/dl

The detection limit represents the lowest measurable IgA concentrations that can be distinguished from zero.

Prozone Limit

No prozone effect was observed up to an IgA concentration of 3500 mg/dl.

Precision

Intra-assay precision	*n*	*Mean mg/dl*	*SP*	*CV (%)*
Sample 1	10	51	4	7.8
Sample 2	10	600	30	5
Sample 3	10	1050	34	3.2
Inter-assay precision	*n*	*Mean mg/dl*	*SD*	*CV (%)*
Sample 1	10	50	4	7
Sample 2	10	610	15	2.4
Samples	10	1410	21	1.48

Interference

No interference was observed with :

Interference factor	*No interference up to*
Glucose	500 mg/dl
Albumin	10 g/dl
Bilirubin	50 mg/dl
Haemoglobin	500 mg/dl
Triglycerides	1000 mg/dl

Reference Values

The interim reference values for immunoglobulin IgA in normal populations are 70-400 mg/dl.

The reference values are related to age, geographical and methodological differences and vary widely in different circumstances. Each laboratory should define its own reference range for the relevant population.

Remarks

1. Usage of well-calibrated equipment and accessories and procedures is critical for achieving correct results.
2. When ΔA obtained for the test specimen is greater than the ΔA of the standard with highest concentration, then it indicates that the concentration of IgA in the test specimen is beyond the measuring range of the QUANTIA-IgA assay. Such specimens should be rerun with further dilutions.

3. Markedly lipaemic, haemolysed, and contaminated serum samples could produce nonspecific values.
4. Use of plasma rather than serum can lead to erroneous values.
5. Do not read results beyond five minutes.
6. It is recommended that results of the tests should be correlated with clinical findings to arrive at the final diagnosis.

TURBIDIMETRIC IMMUNOASSAY FOR ESTIMATION OF IMMUNOGLOBULIN IgG IN HUMAN SERUM

Quantia IgG, Courtesy: Tulip Group of Companies

Summary

Persistently elevated immunoglobulin levels indicate an ongoing response of the immune system, whereas a decline in immunoglobulin levels hints at a recovery from the infectious process. The absolute levels of immunoglobulin concentration are a measure of the severity of the inflammatory process, especially in virally induced chronic liver disease, chronic bacterial infections, collagen vascular diseases and other autoimmune diseases. In diseases that cause hypergammaglobulinaemia quantitative determination in conjunction with the clinical presentation as well as analysis of serological and clinical chemistry results may not only help in diagnosis, differential diagnosis, but may also prove to be useful for disease monitoring and prognosis.

Deficiency of IgG is associated with frequent and occasionally severe pyogenic infections. Increased levels of IgG are associated with chronic or recurrent infections, various autoimmune disorders, lymphoid or nonlymphoid malignancies and IgG myeloma.

IgG is the only immunoglobulin to cross the placenta and provide protection from intrauterine infections to the foetus, and is of importance in defence against infections in newborns.

Decreased levels of IgG are observed in agammaglobulinaemia, hypogammaglobulinaemia, and nephrotic syndrome. Information regarding the concentration of IgG can be obtained by using QUANTIA-IgG reagents.

Reagent

1. *QUANTIA-IgG activation buffer (R1):* Ready-to-use.
2. *QUANTIA-IgG antihuman IgG reagent (R2):* Ready-to-use solution of anti-human IgG antibody.
3. *QUANTIA-IgG calibrator:* Lyophilised preparation of serum equivalent to the stated amount of IgG on a mg/dl basis, when hydrated appropriately. The QUANTIA-IgG calibrator is traceable to CRM 470.

Each batch of reagents undergoes rigorous quality control at various stages of manufacture for its specificity, sensitivity and performance.

Reagent Storage and Stability

1. Store the reagents at 2 to 8°C. Do not freeze.
2. The shelf-life of the reagent, activation buffer and calibrator is as per the expiry date mentioned on the respective vial labels.
3. The reconstituted calibrator is stable for 7 days at 2 to 8°C and 48 hours at 25 to 30°C (RT).

Principle

QUANTIA-IgG is a turbidimetric immunoassay for the detection of Immunoglobulin IgG in human serum and is based on the principle of agglutination reaction. The test specimen is mixed with the Activation buffer (R1) and then with antihuman IgG reagent (R2) and allowed to react. Presence of IgG in the test specimen results in the formation of an insoluble complex producing a turbidity, which is measured at wavelength 340 nm. The extent of turbidity corresponds to the concentration of IgG in the test specimen.

Note

1. *In vitro* diagnostic reagent for laboratory and professional use only. Not for medicinal use.
2. All the reagents derived from human source have been tested for HBsAg and HIV antibodies and are found to be nonreactive. However, handle the material as if infectious.
3. Reagents contain 0.1 percent sodium azide as a preservative. Avoid contact with skin and mucosa. On disposal, flush with large quantities of water.
4. The reagents can be damaged due to microbial contamination or on exposure to extreme temperatures. It is recommended that the performance of the reagents be verified using known controls periodically.

5. The QUANTIA-IgG reagents should be mixed well before use to improve test performance.
6. Do not use vortex mixers for mixing reagents. Gently mix the reagents and samples during test procedures.
7. Calibrators of different manufacturers must not be used with QUANTIA-IgG reagents.
8. The calibration curve must be validated periodically with known controls.
9. As the reagents within lots have been matched, reagents from different lots must not be interchanged.
10. The QUANTIA-IgG assay is recommended only for analysers with cuvette mode. Though any semiautomated analyser with appropriate programming facility can be used; for best results it is recommended to use **Quantiamate** analyser. Fully automated analysers may be used, provided the reagent has been standardised on the system.
11. The procedures mentioned in the pack insert are based on a minimum reading volume of 500 µl (0.5 ml). In case of instruments where minimum volume required for reading absorbance is 1.0 ml, use double the quantity of reagents and samples mentioned in the test procedure.

Specimen Collection and Preparation

No special preparation of the patient is required prior to specimen collection by approved techniques. Only serum should be used for testing. Should a delay in testing occur, store the samples at 2 to 8°C. Samples can be stored for up to a week at 2 to 8°C, provided they are not contaminated. Do not use haemolysed, icteric, or highly turbid sera. Turbid or particulate serum samples must be clarified by centrifugation at 2000 rpm for 15 minutes prior to testing. Use the clear supernatant for testing.

Additional Material Required

Spectrophotometer with 340 nm wavelength and cuvette mode, stopwatch, well-calibrated micropipettes, disposable tips, isotonic saline, particulate free distilled water, test-tube rack, incubator/waterbath set at 37°C, optically clean disposable cuvettes such as **Quantiamate semimicrocuvettes/**glass cuvettes.

Test Procedure

Bring reagents and specimen to room temperature before use.

Assay Conditions

Wavelength	340 nm
Reaction temperature	37°C
Cuvette	1 cm path length

Method for Preparation of IgG Calibration Curve

The QUANTIA-IgG calibrator must be reconstituted exactly with 1.0 ml of distilled water, wait for five minutes, gently swirl the vial till the solution attains homogeneity. Once reconstituted, it is ready to use for preparing the IgG calibration curve. The concentration (S) of IgG in the reconstituted calibrator is as mentioned at the end of the package insert.

Prepare 1.0 ml of 800 mg/dl IgG **working standard (Sw)** from the reconstituted calibrator as mentioned at the end of the package insert. The working standard (Sw) is stable for eight hours at 2 to 30°C.

Prepare dilutions of the working standard (Sw) as mentioned below for preparation of calibration curve.

Test tube No.	*1*	*2*	*3*	*4*	*5*
Calibrator dilution No.	D1	D2	D3	D4	D5
Isotonic Saline	-	100 µl	100 µl	100 µl	95 µl
Working standard (Sw)	100 µl	100 µl	100 µl	100 µl	5 µl
Conc. of IgG in mg/dl	800	400	200	100	40

The above five dilutions of the calibrator including the highest 800 mg/dl (D1) and lowest 40 mg/dl (D5) concentrations of measuring range *must* be used for the preparation of the calibration curve.

Test Procedure for Preparation of Calibration Cvurve

1. Zero the instrument with distilled water.
2. Pipette 500 µl of QUANTIA-IgG activation buffer (R1) and 5 µl of working standard (D1) in the measuring cuvette. Mix well and incubate for five minutes at 37°C.
3. Read absorbance (A1).
4. Add 50 µl of QUANTIA-IgG reagent (R2), mix gently and start the stopwatch simultaneously.

5. Read absorbance (A2) at the end of *exactly* five minutes.
6. Repeat steps No. 2 to 5 for each diluted working standard (D2 to D5) for preparing calibration curve.
7. Calculate ΔA (A2-A1) for each dilution of the working standard (D1 to D5). Plot a graph of ΔA versus concentration of IgG on the graph paper provided with the kit.

"The calibration curve" so obtained is valid only for the same lot of QUANTIA-IgG reagents.

Test Procedure for Specimen

For determination of IgG concentration in the test specimen, dilute the test specimen 1:10 with normal saline.

1. Follow steps 2 to 5 as mentioned in the above procedure for calibration curve using the diluted test specimen in place of the working standard,
2. Calculate ΔA (A2-A1) for the diluted test specimen.

Validation Criteria

If the ΔA of the diluted test specimen is less than ΔA obtained for the standard of highest concentration (D1) then proceed directly for calculations of results.

If the ΔA of the diluted test specimen is higher than ΔA of the standard with highest concentration (D1) then the test has to be rerun by carrying out further dilution of test specimen such as 1:20, 1:40, 1:60 etc., till the DA of the diluted specimen is less than DA of D1.

Calculations

For determination of IgG concentration in the test specimen:

1. Interpolate ΔA of the diluted test specimen on the calibration curve and obtain the IgG concentration 'C' of the diluted test specimen.
2. Multiply the IgG concentration 'C' with the dilution factor (F) of the test specimen for obtaining the concentration of IgG in the neat test specimen.

Concentration of IgG in the neat test specimen in mg/dl = C × F

(where 'F' is the dilution factor of the test specimen, i.e. 10 for 1:10 dilution of test specimen and so on).

Specific Performance Characteristics

Measuring Range

The QUANTIA-IgG reagent has been designed to measure serum IgG concentrations in the range 400-8000 mg/dl, and is linear between the measuring range.

Detection Limit/Analytical Sensitivity

Detection limit: 40 mg/dl

The detection limit represents the lowest measurable IgG concentrations that can be distinguished from zero.

Prozone Limit

No prozone effect was observed up to a IgG concentration of 16,000 mg/dl.

Precision

Intra-assay precision	*n*	*Mean mg/dl*	*SD*	*CV (%)*
Sample 1	10	410	36	8.7
Sample 2	10	2020	100	5
Sample 3	10	7480	240	3.2
Inter-assay precision	*n*	*Mean mg/dl*	*SD*	*CV (%)*
Sample 1	10	510	40	8
Sample 2	10	2000	100	5
Sample 3	10	8120	210	3

Interference

No interference was observed with:

Interference factor	*No interference up to*
Glucose	500 mg/dl
Albumin	10 g/dl
Bilirubin	50 mg/dl
Haemoglobin	500 mg/dl
Triglycerides	1000 mg/dl

Reference Values

The interim reference values for immunoglobulin IgG in normal populations are 700 to 1600 mg/dl.

The reference values are related to age, geographical and methodological differences and vary widely in different circumstances. Each laboratory should define its own reference range for the relevant population.

Remarks

1. Usage of well-calibrated equipment and accessories and procedures is critical for achieving correct results.
2. When ΔA obtained for the test specimen is greater than the ΔA of the standard with highest concentration then, it indicates that the concentration of IgG in the test specimen is beyond the measuring range of the QUANTIA-IgG assay. Such specimens should be rerun with further dilutions.
3. Markedly lipaemic, haemolysed, and contaminated serum samples could produce nonspecific values.
4. Use of plasma rather than serum can lead to erroneous values.
5. Do not read results beyond four minutes.
6. It is recommended that results of the tests should be correlated with clinical findings to arrive at the final diagnosis.

TURBIDIMETRIC IMMUNOASSAY FOR ESTIMATION OF IMMUNOGLOBULIN IgM IN HUMAN SERUM

Quantia IgM, Courtesy: Tulip Group of Companies

Summary

The absolute levels of immunoglobulin concentration are a measure of the severity of the inflammatory process, especially in virally induced chronic liver disease, chronic bacterial infections, collagen vascular diseases and other autoimmune diseases. In diseases that cause hypergammaglobulinaemia quantitative determination in conjunction with the clinical presentation as well as analysis of serological and clinical chemistry parameters or test results may not only help in diagnosis, differential diagnosis, but may also prove to be useful for disease monitoring and prognosis.

Immunoglobulin IgM comprises approximately 7 to 10 per cent of normal serum immunoglobulins and are the prominent antibody class in primary response to most antigenic stimuli. As IgM does not cross the placenta, presence of virus specific IgM in cord blood or neonatal serum is indicative of congenital infection. IgM levels may be increased in chronic liver disease, infections, Waldenström's macroglobulinaemia, and malignant lymphoma. Decreased levels are observed in immune deficiency states, non-IgM myeloma, infancy and early childhood lymphoma.

Quantified IgM measurements are useful for the detection of frequent chronic or acute infections, suspected immunodeficiency, screening for congenital infections and monitoring patients with Waldenström's macroglobulinaemia. Information regarding the concentration of IgM can be obtained by using QUANTIA-IgM reagents.

Reagent

1. *QUANTIA-IgM activation buffer (R1):* Ready-to-use buffer.
2. *QUANTIA-IgM antihuman IgM reagent (R2):* Ready-to-use solution of Antihuman IgM antibody.
3. *QUANTIA-IgM calibrator:* Lyophilised preparation of serum equivalent to the stated amount of IgM on a mg/dl basis, when hydrated appropriately. The QUANTIA-IgM calibrator is traceable to CRM 470.

Each batch of reagents undergoes rigorous quality control at various stages of manufacture for its specificity, sensitivity and performance.

Reagent Storage and Stability

1. Store the reagents at 2 to 8°C. Do not freeze.
2. The shelf-life of the reagent, activation buffer and calibrator is as per the expiry date mentioned on the respective vial labels.
3. The reconstituted calibrator is stable for 7 days at 2 to 8°C and 48 hours at 25 to 30°C (RT).

Principle

QUANTIA-IgM is a turbidimetric immunoassay for the detection of immunoglobulin IgM in human serum and is based on the principle of agglutination reaction. The test specimen is mixed with the activation buffer (R1). Antihuman IgM reagent (R2) is then added and allowed to react. Presence of IgM in the test specimen results in the formation of an insoluble complex producing a turbidity, which is measured at wavelength 340 nm. The extent of turbidity corresponds to the concentration of IgM in the test specimen.

Note

1. *In vitro* diagnostic reagent for laboratory and professional use only. Not for medicinal use.
2. All the reagents derived from human source have been tested for HBsAg and HIV antibodies and are found to be nonreactive. However, handle the material as if infectious.
3. Reagents contain 0.1 percent sodium azide as a preservative. Avoid contact with skin and mucosa. On disposal, flush with large quantities of water.
4. The reagents can be damaged due to microbial contamination or on exposure to extreme temperatures. It is recommended that the performance of the reagents be verified using known controls periodically.
5. The QUANTIA-IgM reagents should be mixed well before use to improve test performance.
6. Do not use vortex mixers for mixing reagents. Gently mix the reagents and samples during test procedures.
7. Calibrators of different manufacturers must not be used with QUANTIA-IgM reagents.
8. The calibration curve must be validated periodically with known controls.
9. As the reagents within lots have been matched, reagents from different lots must not be interchanged.
10. The QUANTIA-IgM assay isrecommended only for analysers with cuvette mode. Though any semiautomated analyser with appropriate programming facility can be used, for best results it is recommended to use **Quantiamate** analyser. Fully automated analysers may be used, provided the reagent has been standardised on the system.
11. The procedures mentioned in the pack insert are based on a minimum reading volume of 500 µl (0.5 ml). In case of instruments where minimum volume required for reading absorbance is 1.0 ml, use double the quantity of reagents and samples mentioned in the test procedure.

Specimen Collection and Preparation

No special preparation of the patient is required prior to specimen collection by approved techniques. Only serum should be used for testing. Should a delay in testing occur, store the samples at 2 to 8°C. Samples can be stored for up to a week at 2 to 8°C, provided they are not contaminated. Do not use haemolysed, icteric or highly turbid sera. Turbid or particulate serum samples must be clarified by centrifugation at 2000 rpm for 15 minutes prior to testing. Use the clear supernatant for testing.

Additional Material Required

Spectrophotometer with 340 nm wavelength and cuvette mode, stopwatch, well-calibrated micropipettes, disposable tips, isotonic saline, particulate free distilled water, test-tube rack, incubator/waterbath set at 37°C, optically clean disposable cuvettes such as **Quantiamate semimicro-cuvettes/**glass cuvettes.

Test Procedure

Bring reagents and specimen to room temperature before use.

Assay Conditions

Wavelength	340 nm
Reaction temperature	37°C
Cuvette	1 cm path length

Method for Preparation of IgM Calibration Curve

The QUANTIA-IgM calibrator must be reconstituted exactly with 1.0 ml of distilled water, wait for five minutes, gently swirl the vial till the solution attains homogeneity. Once reconstituted it is ready to use for preparing the IgM calibration curve. The Concentration (S) of IgM in the reconstituted calibrator is as mentioned at the end of the package insert.

Prepare 1.0 ml of 80 mg/dl IgM **working standard (Sw)** from the reconstituted calibrator as mentioned at the end of the package insert. The working standard (Sw) is stable for eight hours at 2 to 30°C.

Prepare dilutions of the working standard (Sw) as mentioned below for preparation of calibration curve.

Test tube No.	*1*	*2*	*3*	*4*	*5*
Calibrator dilution No.	D1	D2	D3	D4	D5
Isotonic Saline	-	100 µl	100 µl	100 µl	95 µl
Working standard (Sw)	100 µl	100 µl	100 µl	100 µl	5 µl
Conc of IgM in mg/dl	80	40	20	10	4

The above five dilutions of the calibrator including the highest 80 mg/dl (D1) and lowest 4 mg/dl (D5) concentrations of measuring range *must* be used for the preparation of the calibration curve.

Test Procedure for Preparation of Calibration Curve

1. Zero the instrument with distilled water.
2. Pipette 500 µl of QUANTIA-IgM activation buffer (R1) and 25 µl working standard (D1) in the measuring cuvette. Mix well and incubate for five minutes at 37°C.
3. Read absorbance (A1).
4. Add 50 µl of QUANTIA-IgM reagent (R2), mix gently and start the stopwatch simultaneously.
5. Read absorbance (A2) at the end of *exactly* five minutes.
6. Repeat steps No. 2 to 5 for each diluted working standard (D2 to D5) for preparing calibration curve.
7. Calculate ΔA (A2-A1) for each dilution of the working standard (D1 to D5). Plot a graph of ΔA versus concentration of IgM on the graph paper provided with the kit.

"The calibration curve" so obtained is valid only for the same lot of QUANTIA-IgM reagents.

Test Procedure for Specimen

For determination of IgM concentration in the test specimen, dilute the test specimen 1:10 with normal saline.

1. Follow steps 2 to 5 as mentioned in the above procedure for calibration curve using the diluted test specimen in place of the working standard.
2. Calculate ΔA (A2-A1) for the diluted test specimen.

Validation Criteria

If the ΔA of the diluted test specimen is less than ΔA obtained for the standard of highest concentration (D1) then proceed directly for calculations of results.

If the ΔA of the diluted test specimen is higher than ΔA of the standard with highest concentration (D1) then, the test has to be rerun by carrying out dilution of test specimen such as 1:20, 1:40, 1:60, etc., till the ΔA of the diluted test specimen is less than ΔA of D1.

Calculations

For determination of IgM concentration in the test specimen :

1. Interpolate ΔA of the diluted test specimen on the calibration curve and obtain the IgM concentration 'C' of the diluted test specimen.
2. Multiply the IgM concentration 'C' with the appropriate dilution factor (F) of the test specimen for obtaining the concentration of IgM in the neat test specimen.

Concentration of IgM in the neat test specimen in mg/dl = C × F

(where 'F' is the dilution factor of the test specimen, i.e. 10 for 1:10 dilution of test specimen and so on)

Specific Performance Characteristics

Measuring Range

The QUANTIA-IgM reagent has been designed to measure serum IgM concentrations in the range 40 to 800 mg/dl, and is linear between the measuring range.

Detection Limit/Analytical Sensitivity

Detection limit: 4 mg/dl

The detection limit represents the lowest measurable IgM concentrations that can be distinguished from zero.

Prozone Limit

No prozone effect was observed up to a IgM concentration of 3200 mg/dl.

Precision

Intra-assay precision	*n*	*Mean mg/dl*	*SD*	*CV (%)*
Sample 1	10	74	4	5.6
Sample 2	10	200	10	4.9
Sample 3	10	710	30	4.2
Inter-assay precision	*n*	*Mean mg/dl*	*SD*	*CV (%)*
Sample 1	10	45	4	9
Sample 2	10	200	11	5.4
Sample 3	10	810	25	3

Interference

No interference was observed with :

Interference factor	*No interference up to*
Glucose	500 mg/dl
Albumin	10 g/dl
Bilirubin	50 mg/dl
Haemoglobin	500 mg/dl
Triglycerides	1000 mg/dl

Reference Values

The interim reference values for immunoglobulin IgM in normal populations are 40-230 mg/dl.

The reference values are related to age, geographical and methodological differences and vary widely. Each laboratory should define its own reference range for the relevant population.

Remarks

1. Usage of well-calibrated equipment and accessories and procedures is critical for achieving correct results.
2. Markedly lipaemic, haemolysed, and contaminated serum specimen could produce non-specific values.
3. Use of plasma rather than serum can lead to erroneous values.
4. Do not read results beyond four minutes.
5. When ΔA obtained for the test specimen is greater than the ΔA of the standard with highest concentration, then it indicates that the concentration of IgM in the test specimen is beyond the measuring range of the QUANTIA-IgM assay. Such specimens should be rerun with further dilutions.
6. It is recommended that results of the tests should be correlated with clinical findings to arrive at the final diagnosis.

TURBIDIMETRIC IMMUNOASSAY FOR ESTIMATION OF COMPLEMENT C3 IN HUMAN SERUM

Quantia C3, Courtesy: Tulip Group of Companies

Summary

Clinically, complement determination helps to detect whether the complement system has been activated. A decrease in complement components due to the activation of complement system or a hereditary deficiency and/or dysfunction of a complement component is of clinical significance. C3 is a central component of the complement system. C3 is the rate-limiting factor for both the alternate and the classical complement pathways. C3 is often decreased in active forms of SLE and membranoproliferative glomerulonephritis. C3 fixation on red cells and on tissue may result in autoimmune haemolytic disorder or severe tissue damage. Increased levels of C3 are observed in biliary obstruction, nephrotic syndrome and during corticosteroid therapy.

Information regarding the concentration of C3 can be obtained by using QUANTIA-C3 reagents.

Reagent

1. *QUANTIA-C3 activation buffer (R1)*: Ready-to-use.
2. *QUANTIA-C3 anti-human C3 reagent (R2)*: Ready-to-use solution of antihuman C3 antibody.
3. *QUANTIA-C3 calibrator:* Lyophilised preparation of serum equivalent to the stated amount of C3 on a mg/dl basis, when hydrated appropriately. The QUANTIA-C3 calibrator is traceable to CRM 470.

Each batch of reagents undergoes rigorous quality control at various stages of manufacture for its specificity, sensitivity and performance.

Reagent Storage and Stability

1. Store the reagents at 2 to 8°C. Do not freeze.
2. The shelf life of the reagent, activation buffer and calibrator is as per the expiry date mentioned on the respective vial labels.
3. The reconstituted calibrator is stable for 7 days at 2 to 8°C and 48 hours at 25 to 30°C (RT).

Principle

QUANTIA-C3 is a turbidimetric immunoassay for the estimation of C3 in human serum and is based on the principle of agglutination reaction. The test specimen is mixed with the Activation buffer (R1). Antihuman C3 reagent (R2) is then added and allowed to react. Presence of C3 in the test specimen results in the formation of an insoluble complex producing a turbidity, which is measured at wavelength 340 nm. The extent of turbidity corresponds to the concentration of C3 in the test specimen.

Note

1. *In vitro* diagnostic reagent for laboratory and professional use only. Not for medicinal use.

2. All the reagents derived from human source have been tested for HBsAg and HIV antibodies and are found to be nonreactive. However, handle the material as if infectious.
3. Reagents contain 0.1 percent sodium azide as a preservative. Avoid contact with skin and mucosa. On disposal, flush with large quantities of water.
4. The reagents can be damaged due to microbial contamination or on exposure to extreme temperatures. It is recommended that the performance of the reagents be verified using known controls periodically.
5. Do not use vortex mixers for mixing reagents. Gently mix the reagents and samples during test procedures.
6. Calibrators of different manufacturers must not be used with QUANTIA-C3 reagents.
7. The calibration curve must be validated periodically with known controls.
8. As the reagents within lots have been matched, reagents from different lots must not be interchanged.
9. The QUANTIA-C3 assay is recommended only for analysers with cuvette mode. Though any semiautomated analyser with appropriate programming facility can be used; for best results it is recommended to use **Quantiamate** analyser. Fully automated analysers may be used, provided the reagent has been standardised on the system.
10. The procedures mentioned in the pack insert are based on a minimum reading volume of 500 µl (0.5 ml). In case of instruments where minimum volume required for reading absorbance is 1.0 ml, use double the quantity of reagents and samples mentioned in the test procedure.

Specimen Collection and Preparation

No special preparation of the patient is required prior to specimen collection by approved techniques. Only serum should be used for testing. Should a delay in testing occur, store the samples at 2 to 8°C. Samples can be stored for up to a week at 2 to 8°C, provided they are not contaminated. Do not use haemolysed, icteric or highly turbid sera. Turbid or paniculate serum samples must be clarified by centrifugation at 2000 rpm for 15 minutes prior to testing. Use the clear supernatant for testing.

Additional Material Required

Spectrophotometer with 340 nm wavelength and cuvette mode, stopwatch, well-calibrated micropipettes, disposable tips, isotonic saline, particulate free distilled water, test-tube rack, incubator/waterbath set at 37°C, optically clean disposable cuvettes such as **Quantiamate semimicro-cuvettes/**glass cuvettes.

Test Procedure

Bring reagents and specimen to room temperature before use.

Assay Conditions

Wavelength	340 nm
Reaction temperature	37°C
Cuvette	1 cm path length

Method for Preparation of C3 Calibration Curve

The QUANTIA-C3 calibrator must be reconstituted exactly with 1.0 ml of distilled water, wait for five minutes, gently swirl the vial till the solution attains homogeneity. Once reconstituted it is ready to use for preparing the C3 calibration curve. The concentration (S) of C3 in the reconstituted calibrator is as mentioned at the end of the package insert.

Prepare 1.0 ml of 36 mg/dl C3 **working standard (Sw)** from the reconstituted calibrator as mentioned at the end of the package insert. The working standard (Sw) is stable for eight hours at 2 to 30°C.

Prepare dilutions of the working standard (Sw) as mentioned below for preparation of calibration curve.

Test tube No.	1	2	3	4	5
Calibrator dilution No.	D1	D2	D3	D4	D5
Isotonic saline	-	100 µl	100 µl	100 µl	350 µl
Working standard (Sw)	100 µl	100 µl	100 µl	100 µl	10 µl
Conc. of C3 in mg/dl	36	18	9	4.5	1

The above five dilutions of the calibrator including the highest 36 mg/dl (D1) and lowest 1.0 mg/dl (D5) concentrations of measuring range *must* be used for the preparation of the calibration curve.

Test Procedure for Preparation of Calibration Curve

1. Zero the instrument with distilled water
2. Pipette 500 µl of QUANTIA-C3 activation buffer (R1) and 25µl of diluted working standard (D1)

in the measuring cuvette. Mix well and incubate for five minutes at 37°C.

3. Read absorbance (A1).
4. Add 50 µl of QUANTIA-C3 reagent (R2), mix gently and start the stopwatch simultaneously.
5. Read absorbance (A2) at the end of *exactly* five minutes.
6. Repeat steps No. 2 to 5 for each diluted working standard (D2 to D5) for preparing calibration curve.
7. Calculate ΔA (A2-A1) for each dilution of the working standard (D1 to D5). Plot a graph of ΔA versus concentration of C3 on the graph paper provided with the kit.

"The calibration curve" so obtained is valid only for the same lot of QUANTIA-C3 reagents.

Test Procedure for Specimen

For determination of C3 concentration in the test specimen, dilute the test specimen 1:10 with normal saline.

1. Follow steps 2 to 5 as mentioned in the above procedure for calibration curve using the diluted test specimen in place of the working standard.
2. Calculate ΔA (A2-A1) for the diluted test specimen.

Validation Criteria

If the ΔA of the diluted test specimen is less than ΔA obtained for the standard of highest concentration (D1) then proceed directly for calculations of results.

If the ΔA of the diluted test specimen is higher than ΔA of the standard with highest concentration (D1) then the test has to be rerun by carrying out further dilution of test specimen such as 1:20, 1:30, etc., till the ΔA of the diluted specimen is less than ΔA of D1.

Calculations

For determination of C3 concentration in the test specimen :

1. Interpolate ΔA of the diluted test specimen on the calibration curve and obtain the C3 concentration 'C' of the diluted test specimen.
2. Multiply the C3 concentration 'C' with the dilution factor (F) of the test specimen for obtaining the concentration of C3 in the neat test specimen.

Concentration of C3 in the neat test specimen in mg/dl = C × F

(where 'F' is the dilution factor of the test specimen, i.e. 10 for 1:10 dilution of test specimen and so on.)

Specific Performance Characteristics

Measuring Range

The QUANTIA-C3 reagent has been designed to measure serum C3 concentrations in the range 10-360 mg/dl, and is linear between the measuring range.

Detection Limit/Analytical Sensitivity

Detection limit: 1.0 mg/dl

The detection limit represents the lowest measurable C3 concentrations that can be distinguished from zero.

Prozone Limit

No prozone effect was observed up to a C3 concentration of 2500 mg/dl.

Precision

Intra-assay precision	*n*	*Mean mg/dl*	*SD*	*CV (%)*
Sample 1	10	25	2.0	8.6
Sample 2	10	90	2.7	3.0
Sample 3	10	333	3.7	1.1
Inter-assay precision	*n*	*Mean mg/dl*	*SD*	*CV (%)*
Sample 1	1010	0.9	9.3	
Sample 2	1091	1.6	1.8	
Sample 3	10	355	4	1.1

Interference

No interference was observed with:

Interference factor	*No interference up to*
Glucose	500 mg/dl
Albumin	10 g/dl
Bilirubin	50 mg/dl
Haemoglobin	500 mg/dl
Triglycerides	1000 mg/dl

Reference Values

The interim reference values for C3 in normal populations are 90 to 180 mg/dl. When fresh serum samples (less than 8 hours old) are used, lower values than those mentioned above can be expected.

The reference values are related to age, geographical and methodological differences and vary widely. Each laboratory should define its own reference range for the relevant population.

Remarks

1. Usage of well-calibrated equipment and accessories and procedures is critical for achieving correct results.
2. When ΔA obtained for the test specimen is greater than the ΔA of the standard with highest concentration, then it indicates that the concentration of QUANTIA C3 in the test specimen is beyond the measuring range of the assay. Such specimens should be rerun with further dilutions.
3. Markedly lipaemic, haemolysed, and contaminated serum samples could produce nonspecific values.
4. Use of plasma rather than serum can lead to erroneous values.
5. Do not read results beyond four minutes.
6. It is recommended that results of the tests should be correlated with clinical findings to arrive at the final diagnosis.

TURBIDIMETRIC IMMUNOASSAY FOR ESTIMATION OF COMPLEMENT C4 IN HUMAN SERUM

Quantia C4, Courtesy: Tulip Group of Companies

Summary

Clinically, complement determination helps to detect whether the complement system has been activated. A decrease in complement components due to activation of complement system or a hereditary deficiency and/or dysfunction of a complement component is of clinical significance.

C4 is essential for activation of the classical complement pathway. Most of the conditions, which result in decreased levels of C3 also, result in decrease of C4. However, in cases of Auto immune haemolytic anaemia (AIHA) and hereditary angioneurotic edema (HAE), C3 is usually normal while C4 is decreased.

Information regarding the concentration of C4 can be obtained by using QUANTIA-C4 reagents.

Reagent

1. *QUANTIA-C4 activation buffer (R1) :* Ready-to-use.
2. *QUANTIA-C4 antihuman C4 reagent (R2) :* Ready-to-use solution of antihuman C4 antibody.
3. *QUANTIA-C4 calibrator:* Lyophilised preparation of serum equivalent to the stated amount of C4 on a mg/dl basis, when hydrated appropriately. The QUANTIA-C4 calibrator is traceable to CRM 470.

Each batch of reagents undergoes rigorous quality control at various stages of manufacture for its specificity, sensitivity and performance.

Reagent Storage and Stability

1. Store the reagents at 2 to 8°C. Do not freeze.
2. The shelf-life of the reagent, activation buffer and calibrator is as per the expiry date mentioned on the respective vial labels.
3. The reconstituted calibrator is stable for 7 days at 2 to 8°C and 48 hours at 25 to 30°C (RT).

Principle

QUANTIA-C4 is a turbidimetric immunoassay for the estimation of C4 in human serum and is based on the principle of agglutination reaction. The test specimen is mixed with the activation buffer (R1). Antihuman C4 reagent (R2) is then added and allowed to react. Presence of C4 in the test specimen results in the formation of an insoluble complex producing a turbidity, which is measured at wavelength 340 nm. The extent of turbidity corresponds to the concentration of C4 in the test specimen.

Note

1. *In vitro* diagnostic reagent for laboratory and professional use only. Not for medicinal use.
2. All the reagents derived from human source have been tested for HBsAg and HIV antibodies and are found to be nonreactive. However, handle the material as if infectious.
3. Reagents contain 0.1 percent sodium azide as a preservative. Avoid contact with skin and mucosa. On disposal flush with large quantities of water.
4. The reagents can be damaged due to microbial contamination or on exposure to extreme tem-

peratures. It is recommended that the performance of the reagents be verified using known controls periodically.

5. The QUANTIA-C4 reagents should be mixed well before use to improve test performance.
6. Do not use vortex mixers for mixing reagents. Gently mix the reagents and samples during test procedures.
7. Calibrators of different manufacturers must not be used with QUANTIA-C4 reagents.
8. The calibration curve must be validated periodically with known controls.
9. As the reagents within lots have been matched, reagents from different lots must not be interchanged.
10. The QUANTIA-C4 assay is recommended only for analysers with cuvette mode. Though any semiautomated analyser with appropriate programming facility can be used, for best results it is recommended to use **Quantiamate** analyser. Fully automated analysers may be used, provided the reagent has been standardised on the system.
11. The procedures mentioned in the pack insert are based on a minimum reading volume of 500 µl (0.5 ml). In case of instruments where minimum volume required for reading absorbance is 1.0 ml, use double the quantity of reagents and samples mentioned in the test procedure.

Specimen Collection and Preparation

No special preparation of the patient is required prior to specimen collection by approved techniques. Only serum should be used for testing. Should a delay in testing occur, store the samples at 2 to 8°C. Samples can be stored for up to two days at 2 to 8°C, provided they are not contaminated. Do not use haemolysed, icteric, or highly turbid sera. Turbid or particulate serum samples must be clarified by centrifugation at 2000 rpm for 15 minutes prior to testing. Use the clear supernatant for testing.

Additional Material Required

Spectrophotometer with 340 nm wavelength and cuvette mode, stopwatch, well-calibrated micropipettes, disposable tips, isotonic saline, particulate free distilled water, test-tube rack, incubator/waterbath set at 37°C, optically clean disposable cuvettes such as **Quantiamate semi micro cuvettes/** glass cuvettes.

Test Procedure

Bring reagents and specimen to room temperature before use.

Assay Conditions

Wavelength	340 nm
Reaction temperature	37°C
Cuvette	1 cm path length

Method for Preparation of C4 Calibration Curve

The QUANTIA-C4 calibrator must be reconstituted exactly with 1.0 ml of distilled water, wait for five minutes, gently swirl the vial till the solution attains homogeneity. Once reconstituted it is ready to use for preparing the C4 calibration curve. The concentration (S) of C4 in the reconstituted calibrator is as mentioned at the end of the package insert.

Prepare 1.0 ml of 12 mg/dl C4 **working standard (Sw)** from the reconstituted calibrator as mentioned at the end of this package insert. The working standard (Sw) is stable for eight hours at 2 to 30°C.

Prepare dilutions of the working standard (Sw) as mentioned below for preparation of calibration curve.

Test tube No.	1	2	3	4	5
Calibrator dilution No.	D1	D2	D3	D4	D5
Isotonic saline	-	100 µl	100 µl	100 µl	150 µl
Working standard (Sw)	100 µl	100 µl	100 µl	100 µl	10 µl
Conc. of C4 in mg/dl	12	6	3	1.5	0.8

The above five dilutions of the calibrator including the highest 12 mg/dl (D1) and lowest 0.8 mg/dl (D5) concentrations of measuring range *must* be used for the preparation of the calibration curve.

Test Procedure for Preparation of Calibration Curve

1. Zero the instrument with distilled water.
2. Pipette 500 µl of QUANTIA-C4 activation buffer (R1) and 50 µl of working standard (D1) in the measuring cuvette. Mix well and incubate for five minutes at 37°C.
3. Read absorbance (A1).
4. Add 50 µl of QUANTIA-C4 reagent (R2), mix gently and start the stopwatch simultaneously.
5. Read absorbance (A2) at the end of *exactly* five minutes.

6. Repeat steps No. 2 to 5 for each diluted working standard (D2 to D5) for preparing calibration curve.
7. Calculate ΔA (A2-A1) for each dilution of the working standard (D1 to D5). Plot a graph of ΔA versus concentration of C4 on the graph paper provided with the kit.

"The calibration curve" so obtained is valid only for the same lot of QUANTIA-C4 reagents.

Test Procedure for Specimen

For determination of C4 concentration in the test specimen, dilute the test specimen 1:10 with normal saline.

1. Follow steps 2 to 5 as mentioned in above procedure for calibration curve using the diluted test specimen in place of the working standard.
2. Calculate ΔA (A2-A1) for the diluted test specimen.

Validation Criteria

If the ΔA of the diluted test specimen is less than ΔA obtained for the standard of highest concentration (D1) then proceed directly for calculations of results.

If the ΔA of the diluted test specimen is higher than ΔA of the standard with highest concentration (D1) then the test has to be rerun by carrying out further dilution of test specimen such as 1:20, 1:40, 1:60, etc., till the ΔA of the diluted specimen is less than ΔA of D1.

Calculations

For determination of C4 concentration in the test specimen:

1. Interpolate DA of the diluted test specimen on the calibration curve and obtain the C4 concentration 'C' of the diluted test specimen.
2. Multiply the C4 concentration 'C' with the dilution factor (F) of the test specimen for obtaining the concentration of C4 in the neat test specimen.

Concentration of C4 in the neat test specimen in mg/dl = C × F

(where 'F' is the dilution factor of the test specimen, i.e. 10 for 1:10 dilution of test specimen and so on)

Specific Performance Characteristics

Measuring Range

The QUANTIA-C4 reagent has been designed to measure serum C4 concentrations in the range 8-20 mg/dl and is linear between the measuring range.

Detection Limit/Analytical Sensitivity

Detection limit: 0.8 mg/dl.

The detection limit represents the lowest measurable C4 concentrations that can be distinguished from zero.

Prozone Limit

No prozone effect was observed up to a C4 concentration of 350 mg/dl.

Precision

Intra-assay precision	*n*	*Mean mg/dl*	*SD*	*CV (%)*
Sample 1	10	8	0.8	9.6
Sample 2	10	30	1.5	5
Sample 3	10	100	2.7	2.5
Inter-assay precision	*n*	*Mean mg/dl*	*SD*	*CV (%)*
Sample 1	10	8	0.3	4
Sample 2	10	30	1.0	3.3
Sample 3	10	122	2	1.7

Interference

No interference was observed with:

Interference factor	*No interference up to*
Glucose	500 mg/dl
Albumin	10 g/dl
Bilirubin	50 mg/dl
Haemoglobin	500 mg/dl
Triglycerides	1000 mg/dl

Reference Values

The interim reference values for C4 in normal populations are 10 to 40 mg/dl.

The reference values are related to age, geographical and methodological differences and vary widely. Each laboratory should define its own reference range for the relevant population.

Remarks

1. Usage of well-calibrated equipment and accessories and procedures is critical for achieving correct results.
2. When ΔA obtained for the test specimen is greater than the ΔA of the standard with highest

concentration, then it indicates that the concentration of C4 in the test specimen is beyond the measuring range of the QUANTIA-C4 assay. Such specimens should be rerun with further dilutions.
3. Markedly lipaemic, haemolysed, and contaminated serum samples could produce nonspecific values.
4. Use of plasma rather than serum can lead to erroneous values.
5. Do not read results beyond four minutes.
6. It is recommended that results of the tests should be correlated with clinical findings to arrive at the final diagnosis.

TURBIDIMETRIC IMMUNOASSAY FOR ESTIMATION OF ANTITHROMBIN III IN HUMAN SERUM

Quantia AT III, Courtesy: Tulip Group of Companies

Summary

Antithrombin (AT) formerly referred to as antithrombin III, a proteinase inhibitor is the most important inhibitor of the plasma coagulation system. The action of AT III in presence of heparin is directed against thrombin, Xa and IX leading to an effective inhibition of coagulation. Concentration of AT III is useful in differential diagnosis of congenital AT deficiencies. In type I congenital deficiency the AT III concentration is reduced, whereas in type II AT deficiency the AT III concentration is normal. Estimation of AT III is useful in diagnosis of disseminated intravascular coagulation (DIC) and monitoring of the course of treatment of DIC, monitoring of AT III replacement therapy and in cases of heparin resistance. Information regarding the concentration of AT III can be obtained by using QUANTIA-AT III reagents.

Reagent

1. *QUANTIA-AT III activation buffer (R1)* : Ready-to-use.
2. *QUANTIA-AT III antihuman AT III reagent (R2)* : A ready-to-use solution of anti human antithrombin III antibody.
3. *QUANTIA-AT III calibrator:* A lyophilised preparation of serum equivalent to the stated amount of antithrombin III on a mg/dl basis, when hydrated appropriately. The QUANTIA-AT III calibrator is traceable to the 2nd International Standard for Antithrombin', Plasma (93/768).

Each batch of reagents undergoes rigorous quality control at various stages of manufacture for its specificity, sensitivity and performance.

Reagent Storage and Stability

1. Store the reagents at 2 to 8°C. Do not freeze.
2. The shelf-life of the reagent, activation buffer and calibrator is as per the expiry date mentioned on the respective vial labels.
3. The reconstituted calibrator is stable for 7 days at 2 to 8°C and 48 hours at 25 to 30°C (RT).
4. The working reagent can be prepared by mixing R2 and R1 in the ratio 1:11.
5. The mixed stability of the working reagent (R1+R2) is 7 days when stored at 2 to 8°C.

Principle

QUANTIA- AT III is a turbidimetric immunoassay for the estimation of AT III in human serum and is based on the principle of agglutination reaction The test specimen is mixed with the activation buffer (R1) and antihuman AT III reagent (R2) and allowed to react. Presence of AT III in the test specimen results in the formation of an insoluble complex producing a turbidity, which is measured at wavelength 340 nm. The extent of turbidity corresponds to the concentration of antithrombin III in the test specimen.

Note

1. *In vitro* diagnostic reagent for laboratory and professional use only. Not for medicinal use.
2. All the reagents derived from human source have been tested for HBsAg and HIV antibodies and are found to be nonreactive. However, handle the material as if infectious.
3. Reagents contain 0.1 percent sodium azide as a preservative. Avoid contact with skin and mucosa. On disposal, flush with large quantities of water.
4. The reagents can be damaged due to microbial contamination or on exposure to extreme temperatures. It is recommended that the performance of the reagents be verified using known controls periodically.
5. The QUANTIA-AT III reagents should be mixed well before use to improve test performance.

6. Do not use vortex mixers for mixing reagents. Gently mix the reagents and samples during test procedures.
7. Calibrators of different manufacturers must not be used with QUANTIA-AT III reagents.
8. The calibration curve must be validated periodically with known controls.
9. As the reagents within lots have been matched, reagents from different lots must not be interchanged.
10. The QUANTIA-AT III assay is recommended only for analysers with cuvette mode. Though any semiautomated analyser with appropriate programming facility can be used, for best results it is recommended to use **Quantiamate** analyser. Fully automated analysers may be used, provided the reagent has been standardised on the system.
11. The procedures mentioned in the pack insert are based on a minimum reading volume of 500 µl (0.5 ml). In case of instruments where minimum volume required for reading absorbance is 1.0 ml, use double the quantity of reagents and samples mentioned in the test procedure.

Specimen Collection and Preparation

No special preparation of the patient is required prior to specimen collection by approved techniques. Only serum should be used for testing. Should a delay in testing occur, store the samples at 2 to 8°C. Samples can be stored for up to a week at 2 to 8°C, provided they are not contaminated. Do not use haemolysed, icteric, or highly turbid sera. Turbid or particulate serum samples must be clarified by centrifugation at 2000 rpm for 15 minutes prior to testing. Use the clear supernatant for testing.

Additional Material Required

Spectrophotometer with 340 nm wavelength and cuvette mode, stopwatch, well calibrated micropipettes, disposable tips, isotonic saline, particulate free distilled water, test-tube rack, incubator/waterbath set at 37°C, optically clean disposable cuvettes such as **Quantiamate semimicro-cuvettes**/glass cuvettes.

Test Procedure

Bring reagents and specimen to room temperature before use.

Assay Conditions

Wavelength	340 nm
Reaction temperature	37°C
Cuvette	1 cm path length

Method for Preparation of AT III Calibration Curve

The QUANTIA-AT III calibrator must be reconstituted exactly with 1.0 ml of distilled water, wait for 5 minutes, gently swirl the vial till the solution attains homogeneity. Once reconstituted it is ready to use for preparing the AT III calibration curve.

The concentration (S) of AT III in the reconstituted calibrator is as mentioned at the end of the package insert.

Prepare 1.0 ml of 20 mg/dl AT III **working standard (Sw)** from the reconstituted calibrator as mentioned at the end of this package insert. The working standard (Sw) is stable for eight hours at 2 to 30°C.

Prepare serial dilutions of the working standard (Sw) as mentioned below for preparation of calibration curve.

Test tube No.	1	2	3	4	5
Calibrator dilution No.	D1	D2	D3	D4	D5
Saline	-	100 µl	100 µl	100 µl	100 µl
Working standard (SW)	100 µl	100 µl	100 µl	100 µl	100 µl
Conc. of antithrombin III in mg/dl	20	10	5	2.5	1.2

The above five dilutions of the calibrator including the highest 20 mg/dl (D1) and lowest 1.25 mg/dl (D5) concentrations of measuring range *must* be used for the preparation of the calibration curve.

Test Procedure for Preparation of Calibration Curve

1. Zero the instrument with distilled water.
2. Pipette 500 µl of QUANTIA-AT III activation buffer (R1) and 50 µl of Quantia-AT III reagent (R2) in the measuring cuvette. Mix well and incubate for five minutes at 37°C.
   or
   Pipette 550 µl of QUANTIA-AT III working reagent in the measuring cuvette. Mix well and incubate for five minutes at 37°C.
3. Add 50 µl of working standard (D1), mix gently and start the stopwatch simultaneously.
4. Read absorbance (A1), *exactly* at thirty seconds, and absorbance (A2) again at the end of *exactly* five minutes.

5. Repeat steps No.1 to 4 for each diluted working standard (D2 to D5) for preparing calibration curve.
6. Calculate ΔA (A2-A1) for each dilution of the working standard (D1 to D5). Plot a graph of ΔA versus concentration of AT III on the graph paper provided with the kit.

"The calibration curve" so obtained is valid only for the same lot of QUANTIA-AT III reagents.

Test Procedure for Specimen

For determination of AT III concentration in the test specimen, dilute the test specimen 1:5 with normal saline.

1. Follow steps 2 to 5 as mentioned in the above procedure for calibration curve using the diluted test specimen in place of the working standard.
2. Calculate ΔA (A2-A1) for the diluted test specimen.

Validation Criteria

If the ΔA of the diluted test specimen is less than ΔA obtained for the standard of highest concentration (D1) then proceed directly for calculations of results.

If the ΔA of the diluted test specimen is higher than ΔA of the standard with highest concentration (D1), then the test has to be rerun by carrying out further dilution of test specimen such as 1:10, 1:20, etc., till the ΔA of the diluted specimen is less than ΔA of D1.

Calculations

For determination of AT III concentration in the test specimen:

1. Interpolate ΔA of the diluted test specimen on the calibration curve and obtain the AT III concentration 'C' of the diluted test specimen.
2. Multiply the AT III concentration 'C' with the dilution factor (F) of the test specimen for obtaining the concentration of AT III in the neat test specimen.

Concentration of AT III in the neat test specimen in mg/dl = C × F

(where 'F' is the dilution factor of the test specimen, i.e. 5 for 1:5 dilution of test specimen and so on)

Specific Performance Characteristics

Measuring Range

The QUANTIA-AT III reagent has been designed to measure serum AT III concentrations in the range 6.25-100 mg/dl, and is linear between the measuring range.

Detection Limit/Analytical Sensitivity

Detection limit: 1.25 mg/dl

The detection limit represents the lowest measurable AT III concentrations that can be distinguished from zero.

Prozone Limit

No prozone effect was observed up to an AT III concentration of 160 mg/dl.

Precision

Intra-assay precision	*n*	*Mean mg/dl*	*SD*	*CV (%)*
Sample 1	10	7.5	0.1	5.0
Sample 2	10	23	0.25	1.0
Sample 3	10	75	0.4	0.6
Inter-assay precision	*n*	*Mean mg/dl*	*SD*	*CV (%)*
Sample 1	10	13	0.9	8.0
Sample 2	10	25	1.0	5.0
Sample 3	10	100	3.0	3.0

Interference

No interference was observed with

Interference factor	*No interference up to*
Glucose	500 mg/dl
Albumin	10g/dl
Bilirubin	50 mg/dl
Haemoglobin	500 mg/dl
Triglycerides	1000 mg/dl

Reference Values

The interim reference values of AT III in normal populations are 17 - 30 mg/dl.

The reference values are related to age, geographical and methodological differences and vary widely in different circumstances. Each laboratory should define its own reference range for the relevant population.

Remarks

1. Usage of well-calibrated equipment and accessories and procedures is critical for achieving correct results.
2. When ΔA obtained for the test specimen is greater than the ΔA of the standard with highest concentration, then it indicates that the concentration of AT-III in the test specimen is beyond the measuring range of the QUANTIA AT-III assay. Such specimens should be rerun with further dilutions.
3. Markedly lipaemic, haemolysed, and contaminated serum samples could produce nonspecific values.
4. Use of plasma rather than serum can lead to values.
5. Do not read results beyond four minutes.
6. Rheumatoid factors are not exclusively found in rheumatoid arthritis but sometimes in syphilis, systemic lupus erythromatosus, hepatitis and hypergammglobulinaemia also.
7. It isrecommended that results of the tests should be correlated with clinical findings to arrive at the final diagnosis.

AUTOMATION IN TURBIDIMETRY

Quantimate Turbidimetry Analyser

Optimised Measuring System

- Preprogrammed for Quantia reagents
- Adaptable turbidimetric immunoassay reagents
- Backup analyser for routine chemisteries
- Endpoint, kinetic, fixed time, multistandard (MSD) and absorbance modes
- 90 open locations including 40 open locations for MSD
- Six programming modes in MSD
- Automatic flagging of outlying results
- Plug and play system

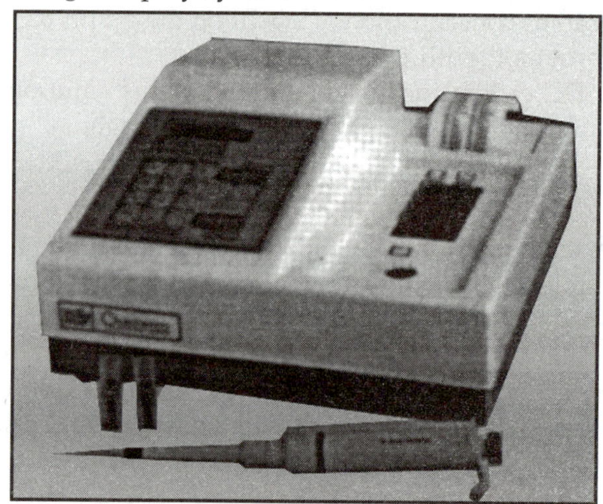

Fig. 29.17

Instrument specifications

- Measuring system : Cuvette mode
- Filter range : 340, 405, 505, 546, 630, 578
- Temperature : 37°C
- Measuring range : –200 to +2000 OD
- Photometric accuracy : 2% from 0 to 2000 OD
- Photometric linearity : ±1%
- Reading volume : Minimum 1.0 ml in macro cuvettes, Minimum 0.3 ml in semimicro cuvettes
- Keyboard : 10 digital keys and 8 functional keys
- Display : Back illuminated LCD with 32 characters
- Thermal printer : 20 columns

IMMUNOGLOBULIN CONCENTRATIONS IN DISEASE

Disease	*IgG*	*IgA*	*IgM*
1. Frequent severe acute infections	N—↑↓	N—↑↓	N—↑↓
2. Chronic infections (e.g., chronic bronchitis, osteromyelitis, tuberculosis, malaria, leprosy)	↑—↑↑	↓—N—↑↑	N—↑
3. Liver diseases:			
*Portal cirrhosis	↑—↑↑	↑↑↑	N—↑
* Viral hepatitis	N—↑	N—↑	↑↑
* Chronic active hepatitis	↑—↑↑	↑	N—↑
* Biliary cirrhosis	N	N	↑↑↑
* Repeated tapping of ascitic fluid	↓	↓	↓
4. Renal diseases:			
* Acute pyelonephritis	N	N	↑↑
* Chronic pyelonephritis	↑↑	↑	↑↑
* Glomerulonephritis	↑	↑↑	N—↓
* Nephrotic syndrome	↓	↓	N
5. Intra-uterine infection (cord blood)	N	N—↑	↑↑
6. Severe burns	↓—↓↓↓	↓—↓↓↓	↓—↓↓↓
7. Protein losing gastroenteropathies	N—↓↓	N—↓	N—↓
8. Multiple myeloma IgG	↓↓↓	↓	↓
IgA	↓	↑↑↑	↓
9. Waldenströem's macroglobulinaemia	↓	↓	↑↑↑
10. Chronic lymphocytic leukaemia	N—↓↓↓	N—↓↓↓	N—↓↓↓
11. Hodgkin's disease	↓—↑↑	↓—↑	↓—↑↑
12. Collagen diseases			
* Rheumatoid arthritis	N—↑↑↑	N—↑↑↑	N—↑↑
* Systemic lupus	↑—↑↑	N—↑	N—↑↑

N = Normal ↑ = Slight increase ↑↑ = Moderate increase ↑↑↑ = Marked increase
↓ = Slight decrease ↓↓ = Moderate decrease ↓↓↓ = Marked decrease

Chapter 30

Cytogenetics

INTRODUCTION

Human cytogenetics is study of chromosomes (*chroma*-colour; *soma*-body) of man. Human beings possess 46 chromosomes (or 23 pairs); of these, 44 are autosomes and 2 are sex chromosomes. Sex chromosomes are XX in females and XY in males. Approximately 1% of newborns are now found to have chromosomal defects which in many cases allow possible prevention of recurrence of the disease with counselling and prenatal diagnosis.

Many clinical entities are found to be associated with specific chromosomal abnormalities. Several chromosomal disorders like trisomy 21 in Down's, XO in Turner's, XXY in Klinefelter's, etc. have been discovered. Some neoplasms are associated with nonrandom chromosomal changes like Philadelphia chromosome (Ph.) in chronic myeloid leukaemia, an interstitial deletion on chromosome 13 in retinoblastoma, etc. Amniocentesis and culturing of chorionic villi are now common techniques for detection of abnormalities in early foetus. Recent advances in banding techniques allow detection of chromosomal abnormalities from a minute defect to complex derangements. Chromosomal study by *in situ* molecular hybridisation has made it possible even to localise gene on the chromosomes and their transpositions. So much so that one thinks in terms of genetic engineering these days, i.e. replacement of defective genes by the correct ones—this will go a long way in eliminating the genetic disorders when it becomes possible.

Cell Division

There are two types of cell division: mitosis and meiosis.

Mitosis occurs in somatic cells (Fig. 30.1 and 30.2), while meiosis is seen in germ cells. Mitosis involves a single division, whereas, meiosis entails two divisions (1. heterotypical or reduction division and 2. homotypical or equational division). The number of chromosomes remains same in mitosis, but is halved in meiosis, leading to formation of two cells in the former and four in the latter. The chromosomal

Somatic cell division (Mitosis) ↓ 46 chromosomes

Gonadal cell division (Meiosis) ↓ 23 bivalents

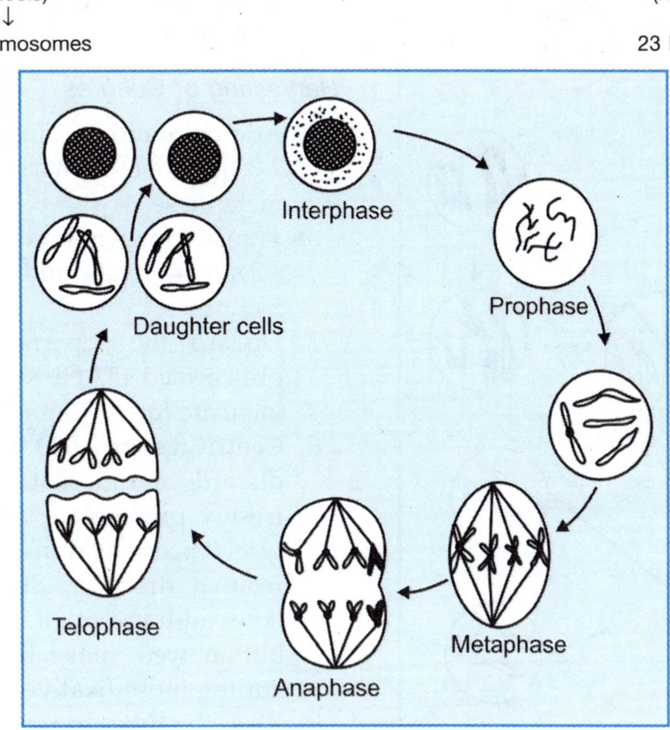

Fig. 30.1: Schematic diagram of miotic cell division

behaviour is independent of each other in mitosis but in meiosis homologous chromosomes get paired together.

BLOOD LYMPHOCYTE CULTURE

The preparative procedure for observation of chromosomes involves four important steps:

a. arresting dividing cells at metaphase.
b. treatment with hypotonic solution.
c. fixation of cells in acetomethanol.
d. spreading of chromosomes on slide surface.

Most commonly, peripheral blood lymphocytes and bone marrow cells are utilised for preparation of mitotic chromosomes and gonadal tissues for meiotic chromosomes.

Chromosome Preparation from Bone Marrow

In a normal healthy adult, bone marrow contains sufficient number of dividing cells for direct observation of chromosomes.

1. Add 5 to 10 drops of bone marrow aspirate in prewarmed 5 ml of TC-199 media containing 40-50 units of heparin per ml and 0.02 µg/ml of colcemid.
2. Mix the material thoroughly by pipetting and incubate at 37°C for 1-2 hours.
3. Centrifuge the suspension for 5 minutes at 1000 rpm.
4. Suspend the cell button with 0.075M (0.56 gm/100 ml) potassium chloride for hypotonic treatment for 10-15 minutes.
5. Centrifuge and discard the supernatant.
6. Add methanol: glacial acetic and (: : 3:1) fixative, fix gradually, mix thoroughly by pipetting and keep for 30 minutes in refrigerator.
7. Change fixative at least 3-4 times.
8. Prepare slides by air-dry method by dropping two or three drops of cell suspension on a clean slide.
9. Stain slides with Giemsa and mount with DPX.

Chromosome Preparation from Whole Blood Culture

Peripheral blood lymphocytes are the most convenient source of mitotic chromosomes.

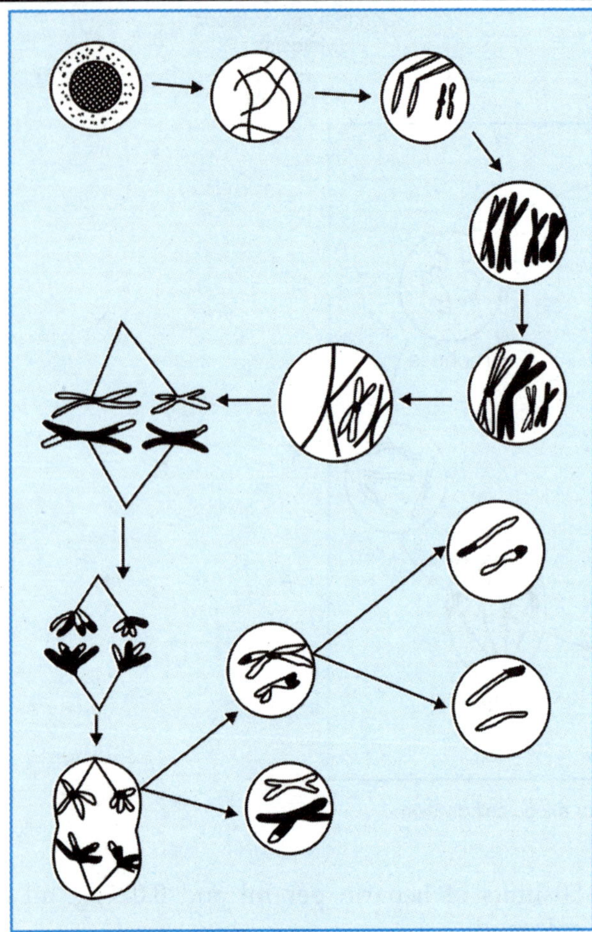

Fig. 30.2: Schematic diagram of mitotic cell division

Chromosomes are prepared after the lymphocytes are stimulated to grow and divide by a suitable mitogen. Phytohaemagglutinin (PHA) is the most commonly employed mitogen. All glassware and reagent including the media to be used for leucocyte culture must be sterilised.

1. Draw about 2 ml of venous blood under aseptic conditions. Transfer the blood into a tube containing heparin (40-50 units/ml) and mix gently to avoid clotting.
2. Add about 0.3 ml of whole blood into a sterile 15 ml screw-capped culture bottle containing 5 ml of TC-199 medium with Hanks base (pH 7.2-7.4) supplemented with 20% foetal calf serum or human serum, 0.1 ml of PHA and 100 µg/ml streptomycin and 200 units/ml of penicillin.
3. Set up at least two parallel cultures for each test sample.
4. Incubate the culture bottles at 37°C for 72 hours with caps tightly closed. Shake the bottles every 12 hours.

Harvesting of Cultures

5. Add colcemid 0.02 µg/ml to each culture bottle 2-3 hours before harvesting to arrest mitosis at metaphase.
6. Transfer the whole content of culture bottle into a centrifuge tube and centrifuge at 1000 rpm for 5 minutes.
7. Discard the supernatant and add 5 ml of prewarmed (37°C) KCl solution (0.075 M) and incubate for 10-15 minutes at 37°C.
8. Centrifuge at 1000 rpm for 5 minutes and discard the supernatant. Fix the cells by adding freshly prepared fixative (methyl alcohol and glacial acetic acid in a ratio of 3:1). Add chilled fixative drop by drop with gentle shaking. After adding 1 ml of fixative and mixing the cell button well, make the volume to 5-10 ml by adding more fixative.
9. Keep the tubes in refrigerator for 30 minutes to fix the cells. Resuspend the cells in fresh fixative and centrifuge as before. Repeat the process until a colourless cell pellet is obtained.

Preparation of Chromosome Slide

10. Discard the supernatant completely without disturbing the cell button. Finally add 0.5 to 1.0 ml of freshly prepared fixative. The final concentration of the cell suspension has to be adjusted depending on the cellular concentration.
11. Keep the precleaned slides in absolute alcohol.
12. Place 2-3 drops of the cell suspension with a pasteur pipette on the slide from a distance to facilitate better spreading.
13. Allow the slides for air drying on heat drying.
14. Stain with buffered Giemsa solution (1:10) at pH 6.8.
15. Dry and pass the slides through xylene and mount in DPX.

Cleaning and Preparation of Slides

1. New slides are kept in concentrated nitric acid for overnight.

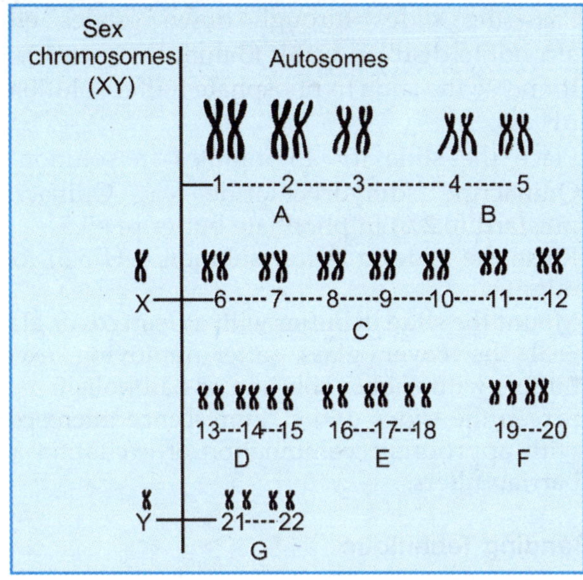

Fig. 30.3: The human male karyotype

2. Keep the slides in horizontal coplin jar under running tap water for 2-3 hours.
3. Rinse in distilled water and store in 90% ethyl alcohol.
4. Wipe off and dry it with a clean cloth or tissue paper.

Procedure of Giemsa Staining

1. Commercial Giemsa solution is diluted 1:10 in phosphate buffer (pH 6.8).
2. Place a few drops of freshly prepared stain on the slide sufficient to cover the entire surface for 5-10 minutes.
3. Rinse in distilled water.
4. Air dry at room temperature.
5. Pass the slide through xylene and mount in DPX.

Preparation of Phosphate Buffer Solution

Solution A: 0.067 M KH_2PO_4 (9.08 gm/litre of distilled water)

Solution B: 0.067 M Na_2HPO_4 (11.88 gm/litre of distilled water)

Mix the solutions as given below:

For pH 6.4—73.2 ml Sol. A + 26.8 ml Sol. B.

For pH 6.8—50.8 ml Sol. A + 49.2 ml Sol. B.

KARYOTYPING

After doing Giemsa staining, the chromosomes are photographed. The individual chromosomes are cut out from the photograph. The chromosomes are then arranged in an orderly fashion, in homologous pairs, to produce a standard arrangement called as karyotype.

The cut out photomicrographs of the 46 chromosomes of a spread are at first arranged in pairs. Thereafter, these pairs are arranged in descending order in relation to their total lengths, placing all their centromeres along the same horizontal line. When arm lengths are unequal, shorter arm is made to point upwards and the longer one downward. The 22 pairs can be arranged in 7 groups. These are as follows:

1. A group: 1 to 3 pairs—metacentric
2. B group: 4 to 5 pairs—submetacentric
3. C group: 6 to 12 pairs—submetacentric
4. D group: 13 to 15 pairs—acrocentric
5. E group: 16 to 18 pairs—submetacentric
6. F group: 19 to 20 pairs—metacentric
7. G group: 21 to 22 pairs—acrocentric.

Group A consists of the longest metacentric chromosomes.

Group G consists of the shortest acrocentric chromosomes.

In males, group G includes Y chromosome. Y chromosome is an acrocentric chromosome like others in the group, but it showns two differences:

a. It is usually the longest in group G.
b. Its long arms are usually parallel to each other, which are divergent in the other members of group G (Fig. 30.3).

The X chromosome is a member of group C and can be distinguished from other members of the group by banding techniques and by using special stains.

Parameters used to characterise a chromosome in the karyotype:

1. Shape of the chromosome.
2. Length of the chromosome.
3. Centromeric index: This index is expressed in the form of the short arm length to the total chromosome length. So,

$$\text{Centromeric index} = \frac{\text{Short arm length}}{\text{Total chromosome length}}$$

For example, this, in a metacentric chromosome is 0.5.

4. Proportion of the arms: It is the ratio between the long and short arms of the chromosome. In a typical metacentric chromosome, this ratio is 1:1.

G AND Q BANDINGS

G and Q bandings are the commonly employed techniques usually asked for chromosomal studies.

G Banding

Trypsin Digestion method (Modified, Seabright, 1971)

1. Slides are allowed to age for 4-5 days before banding technique is employed.
2. Slides are dipped in 15% hydrogen peroxide (H_2O_2) for 5 minutes.
3. Rinse the slides for about 10-15 seconds in normal saline.
4. Immerse the slides in 0.2% trypsin (pH 6.8) solution at 20°C for about 7-10 seconds (if the slides are older, trypsin treatment may be prolonged).
5. Rinse the slides for about 10-15 seconds in normal saline and distilled water and allow to dry.
6. Dry slides for about 10-15 minutes in 5% buffered Giemsa solution at pH 6.8.
7. Wash the slides in running tap water to remove excess stain and dry.
8. Pass the slides through xylene and mount with DPX.

G banding makes identification of each chromosome possible by its characteristic dark and light bands.

Q Banding (Quinacrine Banding Technique)

This reveals bright fluorescent bands throughout the entire length of chromosomes. The long arm of Y chromosomes shows bright fluorescence. Identification of each chromosome and its regions is possible by its characteristic fluorescence bands.

1. Slides are allowed to age 2-3 for days before banding technique is performed.
2. Pass the slides through down grades ethyl alcohol to distilled water (3 minutes in each).
3. Immerse the slide in phosphate buffer solution at pH 5.5.
4. Place the slide for 15 minutes in solution of Quinacrine dihydrochloride, a Quinacrine mustard (0.2%) in phophate buffer pH 5.5.
5. Rinse the slide in buffer solution (pH 5.5) for 5 minutes.
6. Mount the slide in buffer with a clean cover glass.
7. Seal the cover glass (after removing excess buffer) with rubber solution or nail polish.
8. Screen the slides under fluorescence microscope with appropriate combination of excitation and barrier filters.

C Banding Technique

This is used for demonstrating centromeric hetero-chromatin. The chromosomes show dark staining at centromeric heterochromatic regions.

1. Air dried or heat dried chromosomes slides are allowed to age for 7-10 days before banding technique is employed.
2. Put the slides in 0.2 N HCI for 1 hour at room temperature.
3. Rinse the slides thoroughly in distilled water.
4. Rinse the slides in 5% aqueous solution of barium hydroxide at 50°C for 5-7 minutes in water bath (before dipping the slides, keep aqueous solution of barium hydroxide in water bath at 50°C).
5. Wash the slides with several changes of distilled water to remove the precipitate of barium hydroxide.
6. Incubate the slide in 2 x SSC for about 1 hour in coplin jar at 60°C (2 x SSC should be kept at 60°C well in advance). 2 x SSC: 1.754 gram of sodium chloride and 0.882 gram of trisodium citrate in 100 ml of distilled water
7. Rinse the distilled water and pass the slides briefly in 70% and 90% ethanol and allow the slides to dry.
8. Stain with 5% buffered Giemsa solution at pH 6.8, for 10-15 minutes.
9. Rinse the slides in distilled water, dry and pass through xylene and mount in DPX.

Importance of Chromosomal Studies

Chromosomal studies are useful.

(i) In diagnosis of various chromosomal abnormalities like Turner's syndrome, Down's syndrome, Klinefelter's syndrome, etc.

(ii) Clinically, in investigation of patients with abnormalities of sexual developments or infertility.
(iii) In determination of sex of an unborn child.
(iv) In larger scale population surveys, e.g. to detect the effects of occupational hazards on chromosomes in relation to various environmental factors like cold, heat, chemicals, dust, etc.
(v) In new fields involving separation of X or Y bearing sperms.

Variations in the Chromosome Number

Polyploidy

It is used to denote presence of multiples of haploid number of chromosomes. For example, a tetraploid cell has four times the haploid number.

Aneuploidy

It is used to indicate absence of the property of being a normal multiple of haploid number of chromosomes. Thus, a human cell with 45,47 or any other number of chromosomes that is not exact multiple of 23 is an aneuploid cell.

Aneuploidy can be of two types.

1. *Hyperploidy:* It is the condition in which there is addition of one or more chromosomes to the diploid number. It may be called:
   (i) Trisomy (2n + 1) when one chromosome is added to the diploid number. Such a cell would have 47 chromosomes.
   (ii) Tetrasomy (2n + 2) when two chromosomes of a homologous pair are added to the diploid number. Such a cell would have 48 chromosomes.
2. *Hypoploidy:* It involves the loss of one or more chromosomes to the diploid number. It may be called:
   (i) Monosomy (2n-1) when there is loss of one chromosome from the diploid set. A cell exhibiting this condition would contain 45 chromosomes.
   (ii) Nullisomy (2n-2) when both the chromosomes of a homologous pair are lost from the diploid set. Such a cell would have 44 chromosomes.

Barr Body Analysis Buccal Smear for Staining Sex Chromatin Mass

Normal values	*Number of Barr Bodies*
Normal female (XX)	1
Normal male (XO)	0
Turner syndrome (female) (XO)	0
Klinefelter's syndrome (male) (XXY)	1
Klinefelter's syndrome (male) (48 XXXY)	2
Klinefelter's syndrome (male) (49 XXXYY)	2
Klinefelter's syndrome (male) (49 XXXXY)	3

Usage: Screening for sex chromosome abnormalities.

Description: A Barr body, or sex chromatin body, is a tightly coiled, X chromosome lying against the nuclear membrane of female cells or any cell with more than one X chromosome. It shows up as a dark-staining body in the shape of a half-moon and is absent in male cells. Barr bodies are believed to function in early embryonic development and later become inactivated to maintain gene balance of Xs to autosomes. The number of Barr bodies in a client is one less than the number of Xs.

Preparation

a. Rinse the mouth with mouthwash.
b. Obtain a metal spatula saline, two sides, and preservative.

Procedure

a. Gently scrape the buccal mucosa with the metal spatula dipped in saline.
b. Clean the spatula and repeat the procedure gently but firmly.
C. Smear the material on the two slides and place them in the preservative.

Postprocedure Care

a. Label the container of the slides with the client's name, the date, and the contents.

Client and Family Teaching

a. Refer the patient with abnormal results for genetic courseling.

Factors that Affect Results

a. None known.

Other Data

a. Barr bodies do not give any information about Y chromosomes.
b. Human chromosome analysis, rather than buccal smears, should be used for evaluations of newborns with ambiguous genitalia.

Appendices

Appendix I Drug Affecting Laboratory Tests Values

DRUGS AFFECTING RESULTS OF BLOOD STUDIES, ELECTROLYTES, BLOOD GAS ANALYSES, AND ISOTOPE STUDIES

Substances with an asterisk in this table reportedly influence the laboratory test, but further study is needed to determine the exact effect and mechanism of action.

Substance Determined	Drugs Causing Increased Values False Positives	Drugs Causing Decreased Values False Negatives
Acetoacetate decarboxylase riboflavin		Urea
Acid phosphatase	Androgens (in women) Clofibrate	Alcohol Arsenicals Fluorides Heparin Oxalates Phosphates
Albumin	Heparin Phenazopyridine	Ascorbic acid Penicillin Salicylic acid Sulfonamides
Alkaline phosphatase	Acetohexamide Albumin Allopurinol Aluminum nicotinate Amitriptyline Anabolic androgenic agents Azathioprine Bromsulphalein Carbamazepine Cephaloridine Chlorpropamide	Fluorides Oxalates Phosphates Placebo Propranolol Vitamin D

Contd...

Contd...

Substance Determined	Drugs Causing Increased Values False Positives	Drugs Causing Decreased Values False Negatives
	Clindamycin Colchicine Ergosterol Erythromycin (Ilosone) Estrogens Flurazepam Gold Salts N-hydroxyacetamide Imipramine Indomethacin (rare) Isoniazid Lincomycin Methyldopa Methyltestosterone Mithramycin Nicotinic acid (large doses; 3-6 g/day) Nitrofurantoin Novobiocin Oxacillin Oxyphenisatin Papaverine (reversible) PAS Penicillamine Petrofane Phenothiazines Phenylbutazone Procainamide Progestin-estrogen combinations (oral contraceptives) Propranolol Rifampicin Sulfonamides Sulfamethoxazole Sulfisoxazole Tetracycline Thiothixene Tolazamide Tolbutamide	
Alpha amino nitrogen	Sulfamethoxazole Sulfonamides	
Amino acids	ACTH Ampicillin Bismuth 11-oxysteroids Sulfonamides Uric acid	
Ammonia	Acetazolamide (Diamox) Ammonium salts (ammonium chloride in cough preparations) Asparagine Barbiturates	Epinephrine Insulin Acetohydroxamic acid (AHA:urease inhibitor) Arginine Diphenhydramine

Contd...

Contd...

Substance Determined	Drugs Causing Increased Values False Positives	Drugs Causing Decreased Values False Negatives
	Colistimethate sodium (colistin sulfate) Diuretics (*oral*) Chlortalidone (Hygroton) Clopamide Ethacrynic acid (Edecrin) Furosemide (Lasix) Glucose Glutamine Heparin Isoniazid (INH) Lipomul (oil injection) Methicillin (Dimocillin, Staphcillin) Morphine Oral resins Polymyxin B Thiazide diuretics Chlorothiazide (Diuril) Tetracycline (large doses produce hepatic damage with elevated ammonia levels [+]) Urea	(Benadryl) Glutamate sodium Glutamic acid Histidine *Lactobacillus acidophilus* (Lactinex) Methionine Monoamine oxidase inhibitors Iproniazid Neomycin (Mycifradin) Phosphates Potassium salts Sodium salts Tetracycline (reduces ammonia production by gut bacteria [-1]) Tromethamine
Amylase	ACTH Aminosalicylic acid (PAS) Bethanechol Chlorides *Codeine Corticosteroids Cyproheptadine Diatrizoate sodium Diuretics (oral) Chlorthalidone Furosemide Ethanol (gross intake) Histamine Hypaque Indomethacin Isoniazid Lipemia *Meperidine Methylcholine *Morphine Oxyphenbutazone Pancreatic extracts Pentazocine Phenylbutazone	Citrates Diuretics (oral) Ethacrynic acid Fluorides Oxalates

Contd...

Contd...

Substance Determined	Drugs Causing Increased Values False Positives	Drugs Causing Decreased Values False Negatives
	Salicylates	
	Salicylazosulfapyridine	
	Sulfamethizole	
	Tetracycline	
	Thiazide diuretics	
	Chlorothiazide	
	Hydrochlorothiazide	
Bicarbonate	Aldosterone	Metformin
	Viomycin	Phenformin
		Triamterene
Bilirubin (and icteric index)	Acetaminophen (overdose)	Barbiturates
		Caffeine
	Acetazolamide	Chlorine
	Acetohexamide	Citrate
	Allopurinol	Dicophane
	Aluminum nicotinate (rare)	Ethanol (pregnant woman near delivery)
	Aminosalicylic acid (PAS)	
	Amitriptyline	Placebos*
	Amphotericin B	Protein
	Anabolic/androgenic steroids (reversible, conjugated)	Salicylates(large amounts)
		Sodium chloride
	Fluoxymesterone	Sulfisoxazole and penicillin
	Methandriol	
	Methandrostenolone	Urea
	Norethandrolone	
	Norethisterone	
	Norethynodrel	
	Oxymetholone	
	Stanozolol	
	Ascorbic acid	
	Aspidium (unconjugated)	
	Azathioprine	
	Barbiturates	
	Carbamazepine	
	Carotin	
	Chlordiazepoxide	
	Chloroquine	
	Chlorpropamide	
	Clindamycin	
	Desipramine	
	Dextran	
	Diazepam	
	Diphenylhydantoin	
	Epinephrine	
	Erythromycin	
	Ethacrynic acid	
	Ethambutol	
	Ethionamide	
	Ethoxazene	
	Fluorouracil	
	Flurazepam	
	Gentamicin	
	Gold therapy (rare)	
	Halothane (rare)	
	Histidine	
	Idoxuridine	

Contd...

Contd...

Substance Determined	Drugs Causing Increased Values False Positives	Drugs Causing Decreased Values False Negatives
	Imipramine	
	Indandione anitcoagulants	
	Indomethacin	
	Isoniazid	
	Isoproterenol	
	Levodopa	
	Lincomycin	
	Lipochrome	
	Menadiol sodium diphosphate (large doses)	
	Menadione	
	Menadione sodium bisulfite	
	Mercaptopurine	
	Methimazole	
	Methotrexate	
	Methyldopa	
	Mithramycin	
	Monoamine oxidase inhibitors	
	Nicotinic acid (large doses)	
	Nitrofurans	
	Nitrofurantoin	
	Furazolidone	
	Novobiocin	
	Oxacillin	
	Oxyphenisatin	
	Papaverine	
	Penicillin and sulfisoxazole combination	
	Phenacetin (rare)	
	Phenazopyridine	
	Phenelzine	
	Phenothiazines (methotrimeprazine, unconjugated)	
	Phenylbutazone	
	Phytonadione (high dose)	
	Piprobroman	
	Placebos*	
	Primaquine	
	Procainamide	
	Procarbazine	
	Progestin-estrogen combinations (oral contraceptives)	
	Propylthiouracil	
	Protriptyline	
	Pyrazinamide	
	Quinacrine	
	Radiopaque contrast media (sodium, calcium ipodates, competition for excretion)	
	Rifampin (unconjugated)	

Contd...

Contd...

Substance Determined	Drugs Causing Increased Values False Positives	Drugs Causing Decreased Values False Negatives
	Sulfonamides Gantanol Gantrisin Sulfamethizole Tetracyclines Tolbutamide Trifluperidol Troleandomycin Vitamin A Vitamin K,K_1 (large doses in newborn) Xanthophyll	
Blood urea nitrogen (BUN)	Acetohexamide Acetone Alkaline antacids Aminosalicylic acid Ammonium salts Amphotericin B Antimony compound Arginine Arsenicals Ascorbic acid Bacitracin Blood, whole Capreomycin (reversible) Cephaloridine (high doses) Chloral hydrate Chloramphenicol Chlorobutanol Chlorthalidone Colistimethate sodium Creatinine Dextran Doxapram Ethacrvnic acid Fluid therapy Fluorides Furosemide Gentamicin Guanachlor Guanethidine Hydantoins Hydroxyurea Indomethacin Kanamycin Lipomul (oil injection) Lithium carbonate Mercury compounds Methicillin Methyldopa Methysergide Mithramycin Morphine Nalidixic acid Neomycin Nitrofurantoin Pargyline	Chloramphenicol Dextrose infusions Phenothiazines (fluphenazine) Thymol

Contd...

Contd...

Substance Determined	Drugs Causing Increased Values False Positives	Drugs Causing Decreased Values False Negatives
	Polymyxin B Propranolol Radiopaque contrast media Salicylates Spectinomycin Streptokinase-streptodornase Sulfamethoxazole Sulfisoxazole Sulfonamides Tetracyclines (doxycycline does not gives significant increase) Thiazide diuretics Triamterene Vancomycin	
Bromsulphalein (BSP) retention	Acetohexamide Aluminum nicotinate Amidone Anabolic androgenic steroids Fluoxymesterone Methandriol Methandrostenolone Norethandrostenolone Norethisterone Norethynodrel Antifungal agents Aspidium (if absorbed) Barbiturates (stop drug 24 hr. before test) Capreomycin sulfate Carbamazepine (Tegretol) Cardiotonic glycosides Chlorpropamide (cholestatic jaundice) Chlortetracycline Choleretics Clofibrate hepatic damage; cholestatic jaundice) Clomiphene citrate (Clomid) Dehydrocholic acid (interferes with hepatic uptake or biliary excretion of BSP) Diphenylhydantoin (Dilantin) Estrogens (intrahepatic cholestatic jaundice; depress hepatic secretory transport) Ethambutol Ethoxazene Guanoxan Halogen compounds	Albuminuria Kanamycin Phenazopyridine Placebos

Contd...

Contd...

Substance Determined	Drugs Causing Increased Values False Positives	Drugs Causing Decreased Values False Negatives
	Heparin	
	Hydroxyurea (suppresses renal tubular function)	
	Indomethacin	
	Kanamycin*	
	Lipemia	
	Meperidine	
	Mercaptopurine	
	Metaxalone (jaundice)	
	Methadone	
	Methotrexate	
	Methyldopa (Aldomet)	
	Mithramycin	
	Monoamine oxidase inhibitors	
	Isocarboxazid	
	Nialamide	
	Phenelzine sulfate	
	Trancylpromine sulfate	
	Morphine	
	Nicotinic acid (Niacin; large doses)	
	Novobiocin	
	Oxacillin	
	Phenazopyridine (Pyridium)	
	Phenolphthalein	
	Phenolsulfonphthalein (PSP)	
	Placebos*	
	Probenecid	
	Procainamide	
	Progestational agents	
	Progestin-estrogen combinations (oral contraceptives)	
Bromsulphalein (BSP) retention	Pyridium	
	(Radiopaque contrast media	
	Bunamiodyl	
	lopanoic acid (Telepaque)	
	Sodium ipodate	
	Riboflavin	
	Rifamycin	
	Sulfonamides	
Calcium	Alkaline antacids	Acetazolamide
	Ammonium oxalate	Aspirin
	Anabolic/androgenic steroids	BSP (interfers 24 hr.-48 hr.after test)
	Calcium salts	Citrate
	Copper*	Copper*
	Dihydrotachysterol	Corticosteroids
	Estrogens	Edathamil
	Hydralazine	Fluorides
	Iron*	Gentamicin

Contd...

Contd...

Substance Determined	Drugs Causing Increased Values False Positives	Drugs Causing Decreased Values False Negatives
	Magnesium salts	Heparin
	Parathyroid injection	Insulin
	Potassium	Iron*
	Progestins	Laxatives (excessive use)
	Sodium	Lipomul (oil injection)
	Thiazide diuretics (early in therapy)	Magnesium
	Urea	Methicillin
	Vitamin D	Mithramycin
	Zinc*	Oxalate
		Phosphorous (large amounts)
		Sodium polystyrene sulfonate
		Sulfadiazine
		Sulfadimethoxine
		Sulfates
		Sulfisoxazole sulfonamides
		Zinc*
Catecholamines	Ascorbic acid	Cyclopropane
	Levodopa	Ether
	Mehtenamine	
	Methyldopa	
	Niacin	
	Oxytetracycline	
	Protamine	
	Quinidine	
	Riboflavin	
	Sulfadundine	
	Tetracycline	
	Vitamin B	
	Vitamin K	
Cephalin flocculation	Ampicillin*	
	Kanamycin*	
	Oxacillin*	
	Pargyline*	
	Penicillamine*	
	Placebo*	
	Procainamide	
	Thiabendazole	
	Tolbutamide	
	Troleandomycin (TAO; stop drug for 5 wk.)	
	Nicotinic acid (large doses)	
Chloride	Acetazolamide	ACTH/corticosteroids
	Ammonium chloride	Bicarbonate
	Boric acid	Bromides
	Bromides	Ethacrynic acid
	Carbromal	Furosemide
	Chlorides	Mercurial diuretics
	Iodides	Saline infusions
	Ion exchange resins	

Contd...

Contd...

Substance Determined	Drugs Causing Increased Values False Positives	Drugs Causing Decreased Values False Negatives
	Oxyphenbutazone	Thiazide diuretics
	Phenylbutazone	Triamterene
	Protein	Water, glucose
	Steroids	infusions
	Triamterene	(prolonged)
	(prolonged use)	
Cholesterol	ACTH cortico-	ACTH cortico-
	steroids	steroids
	Amino-	Aluminum
	pyrine	nicotinate
	Anabolic	Aminopyrine
	agents	bicamphorate
	Androgens	Para-aminosalicylic
	Aspirin	acid (PAS)
	Bile salts	Androsterone
	Bilirubin	Antidiabetic drugs
	Bromides	Ascorbic acid
	Chlorpromazine	Bile salts
	Clofibrate	Bromides
	Corticosteroids	Chlortetracycline
	Cortisone	Cholestyramine
	Epinephrine	resin
	(indirect effect	Clofibrate
	through ACTH	Colchicine
	stimulation)	Cortisone
	Ether anesthesia	Dextrothyroxine
	Iodides	Diphenyl-
	Lipomul	hydantoin
	Methandro-	EDTA
	stendolone	Estrogens
	Norepinephrine	Glucagon
	Paramethadione	Glucose
	Penicillamine	Haloperidol
	Phenothiazines	Heparin
	Chlorpromazine	Kanamycin
	Trifluoperazine	Neomycin
	Progestin-estrogen	Nicotinic acid
	combination (oral	Nitrates
	contraceptives)	Nitrites
	Protein	Paromomycin
	Salicylates	Pentylenetetrazol
	Thiouracil	Phenformin
	Trimethadione	Phenyramidol
	Tryptophan	Salicylates
	Urea	Sodium chloride
	Viomycin	
	Vitamin A	
	Vitamin D	
Cortisol	Fenfluramine	
	Prednisolone	
	Prednisone	
	Quinacrine	
	Spironolactone	
Creatine	Urea	

Contd...

Contd...

Substance Determined	Drugs Causing Increased Values False Positives	Drugs Causing Decreased Values False Negatives
Creatine phospho-kinase (CPK)	Amphotericin B	Heparin
	Ampicillin(IM administration)	
	Carbenicillin (IM administration)	
	Chlorpromazine (IM administration)	
	Clofibrate	
Creatinine	Albumin	Marijuana
	p-Aminohippurate	Viomycin
	Amphotericin B	
	Arginine	
	Ascorbic acid	
	Barbiturates	
	BSP	
	Clofibrate	
	Colistin	
	Diacetic acid	
	Gentamicin sulfate	
	Glucose	
	Glycerin	
	Hydroxyurea	
	Kanamycin	
	Levodopa	
	Levulose	
	Lipomul (oil injection)	
	Lithium carbonate	
	Mannitol	
	Methicillin	
	Methyldopa	
	Mithramycin	
	Protein	
	PSP	
	Pyruvate	
	Streptokinase streptodornase	
	Triamterene	
Erythrocyte G6PD		Heparin
Folate		Ampicillin
		Chloramp-henicol
		Erythromycin
		Lincomycin
		Penicillin
		Sulfisoxazol
		Tetracycline
Glucose (fasting)	Acetaminophen	Acetaminophen
	Acetazolamide (prediabetics and diabetics)	Acetohexamide (overdose)
	ACTH	Aminosalicylic acid (in diabetics)
	Aluminum nicotinate	Anabolic steroids
	Aminosalicylic acid	Ascorbic acid
		BAL (toxic levels)

Contd...

Contd...

Substance Determined	Drugs Causing Increased Values False Positives	Drugs Causing Decreased Values False Negatives
	Ascorbic acid	Carbutamide
	L-Arginine	Chlorpropamide (overdose)
	BAL (toxic levels)	Clofibrate
	Caffeine	Cyproheptadine
	Chlorthalidone	Dextropropoxyphene
	Clopamide	Ethacrynic acid (large doses)
	Corticosteroids	Ethanol
	Dextran	Fructose
	Dextrothyroxine	Guanethidine
	Diazoxide	Haloperidol
	Diphenylhydantoin	Insulin (overdose)
	Epinephrine	Isocarboxazid
	Estrogens	Isoniazid
	Ethacrynic acid	Levodopa
	Ethionamide	Marihuana
	Ferrous ascorbinate	Metformin (overdose)
	Furosemide	Monoamine oxidase inhibitors
	Hydralazine	Nialamide
	Imipramine	Pargyline
	Indomethacin (rare)	Phenelzine
	Iron dextran	Tranylcypromine
	Iron sorbitex	Nitrazepam
	Isoniazid (excessive doses)	Phenacetin
	Isoproterenol	Phenazopyridine
	Levarterenol	Phenformin
	Levodopa	Phosphorus
	Lithium carbonate	Potassium chloride
	Mercaptopurine	Potassium oxalate
	Methyldopa	Potassium para-amino benzoate (prolonged use)
	Morphine	Propoxyphene
	Nalidixic acid	Propranolol
	Nicotinic acid (large doses)	Reserpine
	Nicotinyl alcohol (large doses)	Salicylates (diabetics; toxic doses)
	Nitrofurantion	Sulfaphenazole
	Paraldehyde (transient)	Tolazamide
	Phenolphthalein	Tolbutamide
	Physostigmine	Tromethamine
	Progestin-estrogen combinations (oral contraceptives)	
	Propylthiouracil	
	Quinethazone	
	Salicylates (toxic doses)	
	Tetracycline	
	Thiabendazole	
	Thiazide diuretics	

Contd...

Contd...

Substance Determined	Drugs Causing Increased Values False Positives	Drugs Causing Decreased Values False Negatives
	Thyroid preparations/synthetic analogues	
	Tolbutamide	
	Triamterene	
	Trioxazine	
Glucose tolerance curve	Corticosteroids* estrogens (decrease tolerance)	Corticosteroids*
	Ferrous ascorbinate	Lithium carbonate
	Nicotinic acid and derivatives (resembles diabetic curve)	Metyrapone
	Phenothiazines	
	Progestin-estrogen combinations (oral contraceptives; increased peripheral resistance to hypoglycemic action of insulin)	
	Salicylates	
	Thiazide diuretics	
17-Hydroxycorticosteroids	Acetazolamide (Diamox)	Aminoglutethimide
	Ascorbic acid	Calcium
(17-OHCS)	(Vitamin C)	gluconate
Chloral	Corticosteroids hydrate	Dexamethasone
	Chloramphenicl (Chloromycetin)	Diphenylhydantion (Dilantin)
	Chlordiazepoxide (Librium)	Mitotane
	Chlormerodrin	Phenothiazines (Chlorpromazine)
	Chlorthalidone (Hygroton;?)	Progestin-estrogen combinations (oral contraceptives)
	Cloxacillin	Reserpine
	Colchicine	
	Cortisone	
	Digitoxin	
	Digoxin	
	Erythromycin (no supporting evidence)	
	Ethinamate	
	Glutethimide (interferes with absorbance)	
	Gonadotropins	
	Hydralazine	
	Hydroxyzine	
	Methenamine Mandelamine	
	Spironolactone	

Contd...

Contd...

Substance Determined	Drugs Causing Increased Values False Positives	Drugs Causing Decreased Values False Negatives
Insulin	Heparin (immuno-assay method)	Heparin
Iron and iron binding assay	Chloramphenicol Fluorides Iron dextran complex Oxalate Progestin-estrogen combinations (oral contraceptives) Tungstate	ACTH Fluorides* Hydroxyurea Oxalate* Steroids Tungstate
^{131}I thyroid uptake (24-hr.)	Barbiturates Estrogens (not persistently) Lithium carbonate (3 mo.-4 mo.) Phenothiazine (1 wk.) Thyroid-stimulating hormone	ACTH Adrenocortical steroids Corticosterone Cortisone Desoxycortico-sterone Prednisolone (1 wk. or less) Prednisone Aminosalicylic acid (prolonged use), 1 wk Amphenone (2-3 days) Antihistamines Chlortrimeton (1 wk. or less) Antithyroid drugs Carbimazole Iothiouracil Mercazole Methimazole Methylthiouracil Muracil Propylthiouracil Chlordiazepoxide Cobalt (1 wk. or less) Coumarin anticoagulants Iodine-containing compounds (general preparations, 1 wk.-3 wk.) Antitussives Diiodohydro-xyquin Enterosept Indocyanine green Iodochlorhydr-oxyquin Iothiouracil Lugol's solution

Contd...

Contd...

Substance Determined	Drugs Causing Increased Values False Positives	Drugs Causing Decreased Values False Negatives
		Neo-penil Isoniazid Meprobamate Mercurials (1 wk.) Nitrate Nitroprusside sodium Orinase Pentothal (1 wk.) Perchlorate (1 wk.) Phenothiazine (1 wk) Phenylbutazone (1 wk.) Progesterone Radiopaque contrast media Cholografin (3 mo.) Diodrast (1-3 mo.) Dionosil (2-4 mo.) Hypaque (1-2 wk.) Mediopaque (1-2 wks.) Neo-iopax (1-2 wk.) Oily solutions (upto 1 yr. or more-Ethiodol, Iodochloral, Lipiodol, Pantopaque, Visciodol) Priodax (1 -3 mo.) Renographin (1-2 wk) Salpix (1 mo.) Skiodan acacia Resorcinol Salicylates Sulfonamides (1 wk) Thiocyanates Thyroid medication (1 wk. - 2 wk.) Desiccated thyroid Thyroglobulin L-Thyroxine Triiodothyronine
Lactic dehy-drogenase (LDH)	Clofibrate Codeine Meperidine Mithramycin Morphine Procainamide Triamterine	Ascorbic acid Oxalate Urea
Lipase	Albumin Cholinergics (Bentanechol, Methacholine) Deoxycholate	Calcium ions

Contd...

Contd...

Substance Determined	Drugs Causing Increased Values False Positives	Drugs Causing Decreased Values False Negatives
	Opiates and analogues Codeine Meperidine Morphine	
Lipids (total)	Heparin	Cholestyramine resin
Lipoproteins	Progestin-estrogen combination (oral contraceptives)	Estrogens Fenfluramine (slight decrease) Phosphates
Magnesium	Lithium carbonate Magnesium products Magnesium antacids Magnesium sulfate Milk of magnesia Salicylates (prolonged use)	Amphotericin B Aldosterone Calcium gluconate Ethacrynic acid Ethanol Insulin Mercurial diuretics (Mercaptomerin) Neomycin
Nonprotein nitrogen (NPN)	Acetophenetidin (azotemia) Amphotericin B Capreomycin (reversible) Edathamil Gentamicin (nephrotoxic) Kanamycin Lipomul (oil injection) Methicillin (azotemia) Neomycin Nitrofurantoin* Sulfonamides Tetracyclines Vitamin D	Nitrofurantoin*
Osmolality	Urea	
Partial pressure of carbon dioxide pCO_2		Heparin
pH	Potassium oxalate Sodium bicarbonate Sodium oxalate	Acetazolamide Ammonium chloride Ammonium oxalate Calcium chloride EDTA Methyl alcohol Paraldehyde Salicylates Sodium citrate

Contd...

Contd...

Substance Determined	Drugs Causing Increased Values False Positives	Drugs Causing Decreased Values False Negatives
Phosphate (inorganic phosphorus) Lipomul	Alkaline antacids Dilatin Heparin Heparin (oil injection) Mannitol* Methicillin Pituitrin Vitamin D Tetracyclines	Aluminium hydroxide Epinephrine Insulin Mannitol* Mithramycin Parathyroid injection Phenothiazine Promethazine
Potassium	Amiloride Aminocaproic acid Boric acid Bromides Calcium Carbacrylamine resin Cephaloridine Copper Epinephrine Heparin Iron Isoniazid Lipomul (oil injection) Mannitol infusions Metformin Methicillin Penicillin G potassium Phenformin Protein Sodium Spironolactone Succinylcholine Triamterene Urea*	Acetazolamide ACTH Aminsalicyclic acid (PAS) Ammonium chloride (rare) Amphotericin Amphotericin B Carbenoxolone Cathartics Chlorthalidone Corticosteroids Dextrose infusions Dichlorphenamide Diuretics (oral) Ethacrynic acid Furosemide Edathamil (EDTA) Epinephrine Glucagon Glucose Insulin Laxatives (excessive use) Licorice Lithium carbonate Methazolamide (prolonged use) Mithramycin Penicillin G sodium (massive IV) Phosphate Polymyxin B Salicylates Sodium glutamate Sodium phytate Sodium polystyrene sulfonate Sulfates Tetracyclines Thiazide diuretics Urea* Viomycin

Contd...

Contd...

Substance Determined	Drugs Causing Increased Values False Positives	Drugs Causing Decreased Values False Negatives
Protein-bound iodine (PBI)	ACTH Barbiturates Barium sulfate Bromide BSP Chlormadinone Clofibrate* Cod liver oil Corticosteroids large doses; lasts 8 days) Dextrothyroxine Dimethisterone Dithiazanine Erythrosine Estrogens Iodides Iodine-containing compounds Isopropamide Levodopa Liothyronine Meprobamate Mercurial diuretics (digestion techniques) Metrecal (iodo-casein in the preparation; lasts 30 days) Penicillin Perphenazine (proloned use) Povidone-iodine (even topically) Progestin-estrogen combinations (oral contraceptives) Pyrazinamide Radiopaque contrast media (lasts from days to mth. to years) Thyroid therapy L-thyroxine Undeceylenium chloride-iodine (even topically) Vitamins A and D	ACTH Aminobenzoate Aminoglutethimide Aminosalicyclic acid Anabolic agents Androgens Antithyroid drugs Methimazole Methylthiouracil Propylthiouracil BSP Chlorate Chlormerodin Clofibrate* Cobalt Cold preparations Corticosteroids (large doses; lasts 8 days) Diphenylhydantoin 1 wk. therapy; lasts 7-10days) Disulfiram Ethionamide Fluorides (massive dose) Glucocorticoids Gold Isoniazid Lithium carbonate Meralluride Mercaptomerin Mercurial diuretics (effect lasts 2 days in vitro) Mephenytoin Nitroprusside, sodium metabolite Phenothiazines (large doses) Phenylbutazone Resorcinol Salicylates (high-dose) Sulfonamides Sulfonylurea (rare) Thiazide diuretics Thiocyanates Thyroid therapy Triiodothyronine
Protein, total	ACTH Anabolic steroids	Ammonium ion Dextran

Contd...

Contd...

Substance Determined	Drugs Causing Increased Values False Positives	Drugs Causing Decreased Values False Negatives
	Androgenic steroids Bilirubin BSP Clofibrate Corticosteroids Dextran Growth hormone Heparin Insulin Lipemia Mercuric chloride Penicillin (massive doses) Phenazopyridine Radiographic contrast media Thyroid preparations Tolbutamide	Progestin-estrogen combinations (oral contraceptives) Pyrazinamide Salicylates
Serum glutamic-oxaloacetic trans-aminase (SGOT)	Acetaminophen Aluminium nicotinate Amantadine Aminosalicyclic acid (PAS) Ampicillin Anabolic agents Androgens Ascorbic acid Aspartate aminotransferase Carbenicillin (high dose) Cardiotonic glycoside Cephalothin Chlorquine Chloroquine Clindamycin Clofibrate Cloxacillin Colchicine Cortisone Cycloserine Desipramine Diphenylhydantoin Epinephrine Erythromycin Ethambutol Ethionamide Flurazepam Gentamicin Guanethidine analogs Hydralazine N-hydroxyacetamide Ibufenac Indomethacin Isoniazid Isoproterenol Levodopa	Salicylates*

Contd...

Contd...

Substance Determined	Drugs Causing Increased Values False Positives	Drugs Causing Decreased Values False Negatives
	Lincomycin	
	Lipemia (alcoholic patient)	
	Methotrexate	
	Methyldopa	
	Mithramycin	
	Nafcillin	
	Nalidixic acid	
	Nicotinic acid	
	Nitrofurantoin	
	Opiates	
	Codeine	
	Meperidine	
	Morphine	
	Oxacillin	
	Phenelzine	
	Phenothaizines	
	Placebo	
	Polycillin	
	Procainamide	
	Progestin-estrogen combinations (oral contraceptives)	
	Propranolol	
	Prostaphlin	
	Pyrantel pamoate	
	Rifampicin	
	Salicylates*	
	Stibocaptate	
	Sulfamethazole	
	Sulfathiazole	
	Tetracycline	
	Theophylline	
	Thiabendazole	
	Thiothixine	
	Tolbutamide	
	Troleandomycin (1-wk, dose)	
	Vitamin A	
Serum glutamic pyruvic transaminase (SGPT)	Aluminium nicotinate	Salicylates*
	Anabolic agents	
	Androgens	
	Carbenicillin (high doses)	
	Cardiotonic glycosides	
	Clindamycin	
	Clofibrate	
	Codeine	
	Cycloserine	
	Desipramine	

Contd...

Contd...

Substance Determined	Drugs Causing Increased Values False Positives	Drugs Causing Decreased Values False Negatives
	Erythromycin (lauryl salt)	
	Ethionamide	
	Flurazepam	
	Gentamicin	
	Guanethidine analogs	
	N-hydroxyacetamide	
	Ibufenac	
	Indomethacin	
	Isoniazid	
	Lincomycin	
	Lipemia	
	Meperidine	
	Methyldopa	
	Mithramycin	
	Morphine	
	Phenothiazines	
	Procainamide	
	Progestin-estrogen combinations (oral contraceptives)	
	Propranolol	
	Pyrazinamide	
	Rifampin	
	Salicylates*	
	Spectinomycin	
	Stibocaptate	
	Tetracycline	
	Thiothixene	
	Troleandomycin (effect lasts 1 wk.)	
Sodium	Anabolic agents	Ammonium chloride
	Boric acid	Carbacrylamine resin
	Calcium	Dichlorphenamide
	Copper	Diuretics (oral)
	Corticosteroids	Carbonic anhydrase inhibitors
	Glucose*	
	Iron	Ethacrynic acid
	Marihuana	Furosemide
	Methyldopa	Glucose*
	Oxyphenbutazone	Heparin
	Phenylbutazone	Laxatives (excessive use)
	Potassium	Mannitol
	Progestin-estrogen combinations (oral contraceptives)	Mercurial diuretics
		Phosphates
		Quinethazone
	Protein	Spironolactone

Contd...

Contd...

Substance Determined	Drugs Causing Increased Values False Positives	Drugs Causing Decreased Values False Negatives
	Rauwolfia alkaloids Saline infusions Sulfate Urea*	Thiazide diuretics Triamterene Urea*
Thymol turbidity (cephalin flocculation)	Adrenocortico-tropic hormones Albumin Aluminium nicotinate (large doses; rare) Anabolic/androgenic steroids Bilirubin Cephalothin Chlorpropamide Clofibrate Erythromycin Florantyrone Growth Hormone Heparin* Indomethacin Insulin Lincomycin Lipemia Nalidixic acid Penicillamine Thyroid preparation Tolbutamide Troleandomycin	Albumin (high) Heparin* Oxalated plasma
Thyroxine-binding globulin	Chlormadinone Progestin-estrogen combinations (oral contraceptives)	Anabolic agents Androgens
Thyroxine T_4	Chloramidone Cliofibrate Diethylstilbestrol Diphenyl-hydantoin Estradiol Estrogens (Oral contraceptives) Perphenazine Progestine Sulfamethoxazole	Aminosalicyclic acid Chlorpromazine Cortisone Diphenyldantoin Heparin Lithium Methylthiouracil Oxyphenbutazone Prednisone Reserpine Sulfonamides Testosterone Tolbutamide

Contd...

Contd...

Substance Determined	Drugs Causing Increased Values False Positives	Drugs Causing Decreased Values False Negatives
Triiodothy-ronine (T_3) uptake	ACTH (conflic-ting reports) Anabolic agents Androgens Anticoagulants,oral Corticosteroids	ACTH (conflicting reports) Antihyroid drugs Methimazole Methylthiouracil Prophylthiouracil
Triiodothy-ronine (T_3) uptake	(conflicting reports) Dextrothyroxine Diphenylhydantoin Estrogens Heparin Iodate Phenylbutazone Salicylates (high doses) Thyroid therapy L-thyroxine Triiodothyronine	BAL Chlordiazepoxide Corticosteroids (conflicting reports) Estrogens Ipodate Perphenazine Progestine-estrogen combinations (oral contraceptives) Thiazide diuretics Sulfonylureas
Uric acid	Acetazolamide Acetaminophen Adrenocortical steroids Aluminium nicotinate Aminophylline Ampicillin Angiotensin Ascorbic acid Aspirin Azathioprine Bishydroxycoumarin Blood, whole Busulfan Carbenicillin Chloral hydrate Coffee Corticosteroids Dextran Diazoxide Diuretics, oral Epinephrine Ethacrynic acid Ethambutol Ethanol Fructose Furosemide	Acetohexamide ACTH Adrenocortical steroids Allopurinol Anticoagulants Benziodarone Chlorine Chlorprothixene Chlorthalidone Cincophan Corticosteroids Coumarin Ethacrynic acid (IV administration) Furosemide Glucose Lithium carbonate (in manic depressives) Mannitol Marihuana Oxyphenbutazone Phenothiazines Phenylbutazone Phenylmercuric acetate Piperazine Potassium oxalate

Contd...

Contd...

Substance Determined	Drugs Causing Increased Values False Positives	Drugs Causing Decreased Values False Negatives
	Gentamicin	Salicylates (large doses)
	Glucose	Saline infusions
	Griseofulvin	Sodium oxalate
	Hydralazine	Sulfinpyrazone
	Hydroxyurea	Thiazide diuretics (Chlorothiazide, 500 mg. IV)
	Ibufenac	
	Lead intoxication	
	Levodopa	Triamterne*
	Lipomul (oil injection)	
	Mecamylamine	
	Mercaptopurine	
	Methicillin	
	Methotrexate	
	Methyldopa	
	Norepinephrine	
	Nicotinic acid	
	Nitrogen mustards	
	Penicillin	
	Phenacetin	
	Phenelzine	
	Phenothiazines	
	Potassium salts	
	Probenecid	
	Propylthiouracil antimetabolites	
	Azathioprine	
	6-Mercaptopurine	
	6-Thioguanine	
	Pyrazinamide	
	Quinethazone	
	Reducing substances	
	Rifampin	
	Salicylates (low doses)	
	Salicyclic acid	
	Spironolactone	
	Thiazide diuretics (Chlorothiazide, 1.5 gm in divided doses)	
	Triamterene*	
	Vincristine	

DRUGS AFFECTING RESULTS OF URINE STUDIES

Substances with an asterisk in this table reportedly influence the laboratory test, but further study is needed to determine the exact effect and mechanism of action.

Substance Determined	Drugs Causing Increased Values False Positives	Drugs Causing Decreased Values False Negatives
Acetone (ketones)	Aspirin	
	BSP (colour interference on nitroprusside test, Ketosix, Labstix, Acetest, Bili-Labstix)	
	Ether anesthesia	
	Inositol or methionine	
	Insulin (excessive doses)	
	Isoniazid intoxication (produces acetonuria)	
	Isopropyl alcohol	
	Levodopa (L-Dopa, brown on Ketostix or Labstix)	
	Metformin	
	Methyldopa	
	Paraldehyde	
	Increased acetaldehyde; nitroprusside reaction, Acetest	
	Phenazopyridine (Pyridium)	
	Interfering colours on Ketostix	
	Phenacetin	
	Phenformin	
	Phenothiazines	
	PSP (possible colour interference on nitroprusside test, Ketostix, Labstix, Acetest, Bili-Labstix)	
Aldosterone	Progesterone	
Alkaline phosphatase		Ethionamide
		Nitrofurantoin
Alpha amino nitrogen	Sulfonamides	
Amino acids	ACTH	Epinephrine
	Amphetamine	Insulin
	Ampicillin (false-positive spots on paper chromatograms)	
Amino acids continued	Cephalexin	
	Colistin	
	Cortisone	
	Dopamine	
	Ephedrine	
	Epinephrine	
	Gentamicin	
	Kanamycin	
	Levarterenol	
	Levodopa	
	Mafenide	
	Methamphetamine	
	Methyldopa	
	Neomycin	
	Penicillamine	

Contd...

Contd...

Substance Determined	Drugs Causing Increased Values False Positives	Drugs Causing Decreased Values False Negatives
	Phenacetin Phenylephrine Phenylpropanol Polymyxin Sulfonamide Tetracycline	
Amino levulinic acid	Penicillin	
Bacteria		Phenazopyridine
Benzidine	Bromides Copper Ferricyanide Formalin Iodides Permanganate	
Bile	Aminosalicylic acid Aspirin Chlorpromazine Chlorprothixene Chloroxazone Flufenamic acid Mefenamic acid Phenazopyridine Phenothiazines Thymol	
Bilirubin	Acetophenazine Aspirin Chlorprothixine Ethoxazene reddish colour (Bili-Labstix) Flufenazine Mefenamic acid (Ponstel) Perphenazine Phenazopyridine (Pyridium; false positive)– "foam test." atypical colour reaction on talc-disk-Fouchet-spot test and Franklin's tablet-Fouchet test; red colour–Ictotest, Bili-Labstix) Phenothiazines Chlorpromazine (Bili-Labstix; Ictotest is unaffected)	
Calcium	Cholestyramine Dihydrotachysterol Nandrolone (in some cancer patients) Parathyroid injection Vitamin D	Alkaline urine Phosphates Sodium phytate Thiazide diuretics Viomycin

Contd...

Contd...

Substance Determined	Drugs Causing Increased Values False Positives	Drugs Causing Decreased Values False Negatives
Catechol-amines	Aminophylline Aspirin Caffeine Carbon tetrachloride Chloral hydrate Demeclocycline Dopamine Epinephrine inhalation (Dylephrin, Mehaler-Epinephrine, Micronephrine, Vaponephrine) Erythromycin Ethanol Formaldehyde Gaunethidine (Ismelin; elevated epinephrine, decreased norepinephrine) Hydralazine (Aspresoline) Hydroquinone Hypertensive agents Imipramine (Tofranil) Isoproterenol Levodopa (L-dopa) Methenamine Methyldopa (Aldomet) Niacin Nitroglycerin Phenothiazines Quinidine Quinine Tetracyclines Chlortetracycline Oxytetracycline B complex vitamins (nicotinic acid, riboflavin) Reserpine (large dose)	Bethanedine Chlorpromazine Guanethidine (Ismelin), elevated epinephrine decreased norepinephrine Guanoxan Reserpine
Chloride	Bromides	
Cortisol	Quinacrine Spironolactone	Dextran Ethacrynic acid Hydrochloro-thiazide
Creatine and creatinine	Androgens Corticosteroids Histidine Levodopa Methyldopa Nitrofuran derivatives Nitrofurazone Urea	Thiazide diuretics
Crystals	Acetazolamide Aminosalicylic acid	

Contd...

Contd...

Substance Determined	Drugs Causing Increased Values False Positives	Drugs Causing Decreased Values False Negatives
	Ampicillin Methenamine mandelate Sulfonamides Thiabendazole	
Diacetic acid	Acetate* Antipyrine* Sodium bicarbonate* Cyanate* Coaltar drugs* Levodopa (L-dopa) Phenazopyridine (Pyridium) Phenothiazines Salicylates	Acetate* Antipyrine* Sodium bicarbonate Cyanate*
Diagnex blue	Aluminium salts Antacids Cremomycin Donnagel Kaolin Kaopectate Atabrine Barium B complex vitamins Nicotinic acid Riboflavin Calcium Iron Magnesium Methylene blue Phenazopyridine Potassium salts (larger amounts) Quinacrine (Mepacrine) Quinidine Quinine Sodium salts (large amounts) Triamterene	Caffeine sodium benzoate Phenazopyridine
Estradiol	Levodopa Crystals (probable for drug)	Cascara Methotrexate
Estriol		Aspirin Glucose Hydrochlorothiazide Methenamine
Estrogens	Anthraquinone Cascara Chlortetracycline Levodopa Methenamine	Acetazolamide Cascara Danthron Glucose Hydrochlorothiazide

Contd...

Contd...

Substance Determined	Drugs Causing Increased Values False Positives	Drugs Causing Decreased Values False Negatives
	Phenothiazines* (prochlorperazine, Kober method) Tetracyclines* Vitamins	Methenamine Phenothiazines (prochlorperazine) Tetracyclines Vitamins*
Estrone		Senna
Ferric chloride test	Aminosalicylic acid Antipyretics Aspirin Levodopa Methotrimeprazine Methyldopa Perphenazine Phenothiazines Salicylates	
Fouchet test	Aspirin	
FPN	Aminosalicylic acid Chlorpromazine Fluphenazine Methdilazine Perphenazine Prochlorperazine Promazine Promethazine Thiopropazate Thioridazine Trifluoperazine Triflupromazine	
Glucose	Acetanilid (Benedict's) Amino acids Aminopyrine Aminosalicylic acid (PAS), reducing agent (Benedict's; glucose oxidase not affected) Antipyrine Ascorbic acid (large doses produce false positive with Benedict's or Clinitest) Aspedium oleoresin Aspirin Bismuth Carbamazepine (Tegretol) Carinamide Cephalexin Cephaloglycin	Ampicillin Ascorbic acid Aspirin Bisacodyl Cephaloridine Cephalothin Chloral hydrate Dipyrone Epinephrine Flurazepam Furosemide Glucose Hydroquinone Levodopa (L-dopa) Meralluride sodium (Mercuhydrine; glucose oxidase) Mercurial diuretics

Contd...

Contd...

Substance Determined	Drugs Causing Increased Values False Positives	Drugs Causing Decreased Values False Negatives
	Cephaloridine	Oxytetracycline
	Cephalothin Clinitest-black brown, interpreted as positive glucose or as false negative)	Phenazopyridine (Pyridium; glucose oxidase negative, Tes-Tape positive; copper reduction test not affected)
	Chloral betaine	Phenobarbital
	Chloral hydrate (Noctec; Benedict's large doses, positive Clinitest; glucose oxidase not affected)	Prednisone
		Propoxyphene
		Salicylates (glucose oxidase negative)
	Chloramphenicol (Chloromycetin; Benedict's, Clinitest)	Tetracycline
	Chloroform	
	Chlortetracycline	
	Cinchophen	
	Corticosteroids (increased production of glucose, lower renal threshold)	
	Corticotropin	
	Creatinine	
	Dextrothyroxine	
	Edathamil (EDTA)	
	Ephedrine (large doses)	
	Ethacrynic acid	
	Formaldehyde	
	Gluconates	
	Glucuronic acid	
	Hippuric acid	
	Histidine	
	Homogentisic acid	
	Hydrogen peroxide (Benedict's glucose oxidase)	
	Hypochlorites (Benedict's glucose oxidase)	
	Indomethacin	
	Isoniazid (INH; Benedict's,Clinitest, or glucose oxidase not affected; hyperglycemic, may produce true glucosuria)	
	Levodopa (L-dopa; Clinitest positive, glucose oxidase negative)	
	Lithium carbonate	
	Methaproterenol	
	Metaxalone (Skelarin; reducing substance interferes-(Benedict's Clinitest-glucose oxidase not affected)	
	Methenamine products	
	Methyldopa (Aldomet)	
	Methyprylon	
	Morphine (Benedict's)	
	Nalidixic acid	
	Neocinchophen	
	Niacin	
	Nicotinic acid (large doses)	
	Nitrofurans	
	Nitrofurantoin (Furadantin)	
	Furazolidine (Furoxone) metabolite (Benedict's)	
	Furazolidone histidine	
	Nitrofurazone	
	Nucleoproteins	
	Oxalic acid	
	Oxazepam	
	Oxytetracycline	
	Penicillin (Benedict's) Clinitest)	
	Phenacetin	
	Phenazopyridine (Pyridium; glucose oxidase negative, Tes-Tape positive; copper reduction test not affected)	
	Phenols	
	Phenothiazines	
	Probenecid (reducing substance in the urine; Benedict's, Clinitest; glucose oxidase not affected)	
	Protein	
	Pyrazolones	
	Quinethazone (glucosuria)	
	Salicylates (Clinitest positive, large doses)	
	Streptomycin (Benedict's, Clinitest; glucose oxidase not affected)	
	Sulfamethoxazole	
	Sulfathiazole	
	Sulfonamides (Sulfanilamide; Benedict's, Clinitest; large doses interfere with copper reduction test)	
	Tetracycline (large amounts of ascorbic	

Contd...

Contd...

Substance Determined	Drugs Causing Increased Values False Positives	Drugs Causing Decreased Values False Negatives
	acid in preparations of tetracycline; Benedict's, Clinitest positive; Clinistix, Tes-Tape negative) Thiazide diuretics Trimethozine (Trioxazine; Combistix, glucose oxidase) Uric acid Vaginal powders (contain glucose)	
Guaiac (blood) Iodides	Bromides Copper Oxidizing agents (excreted in urine)	Ascorbic acid (high doses)
Guaicols spot test	Aspirin Chlorpromazine Glyceryl guaiacolate Methyldopa Monoamine oxidase inhibitor Morphine Phenacetin Reserpine Thiopental	Dopamine Epinephrine Levarterenol Levodopa
Haemoglobin	Imipramine	Ascorbic acid Tetracycline
Hippuric acid	Aspirin	
Homogentisic acid	Ascorbic acid Aspirin Hydroquinone Levodopa	
Homovanillic acid	Aspirin Ascorbic acid	Aspirin Aspirin
17-Hydroxycorticosteroids (17-OHCS)	Chloral hydrate Chloramphenicol Chlordiazepoxide Chlormerodrin Colchicine Dextroamphetamine* Digitoxin Digoxin Erythromycin Ethinamate Glutethimide Hydralazine Iodides Menadione Meprobamate Methyprylon Metyrapone Phenothiazines (Chlorpromazine)	Estrogens Promethazine Reserpine

Contd...

Contd...

Substance Determined	Drugs Causing Increased Values False Positives	Drugs Causing Decreased Values False Negatives
	Potassium iodide Spironolactone Sulfamerazine Thiazide diuretics (Chlorothiazide) Troleandomycin (TAO) Quindine Quinine Paraldehyde Phenazopyridine (Pyridium)	
5-Hydroxy-indoleacetic acid (HIAA; serotonin) Serotonin 5 HIAA continued	Acetaminophen Acetanilid Acetazolamide Caffeine Ephedrine Fluorouracil (5-FU) Glyceryl guaiacolate Lugol's solution Melphalan Mephenesin Methamphetamine Methocarbamol Methysergide maleate Phenacetin Phenmetrazine (Preludin) Reserpine Serotonin in food amounts of serotonin present in avocados, bananas, plums, walnuts, pineapples, and eggplants)	Aspirin p-Chlorophenyl-alanine Chlorpromazine Corticotropin (ACTH; pharmacologic effect) Ethanol Heparin Imipramine (Tofranil) Isoniazid (INH) Levodopa Methenamine mandelate (Mandelamine) Methyldopa Monoamine oxidase inhibitors Phenothiazines (Chlorpromazine Thorazine) Prochlor-perazine Promazine Promethazine
17-Keto-steorids (17-KS)	Acetazolamide Androgenic steroids Ascorbic acid Cephaloridine Cephalothin Chlordiazepoxide Chlorothiazide* Chlorpromazine (Thorazine) Cloxacillin (Tegapen) Corticotropin (ACTH) Cortisone Dextroamphet-amine* Digitoxin	Aminaglute-thimide Betamethasone Chlordiazepo-xide (Librium) Chlorpromazine Chlormerodrin Chlorothiazide* Corticosteroids Cortisone derivatives of high potency) Dexamethasone Digoxin Diphenylhy-dantoin Estrogens

Contd...

Contd...

Substance Determined	Drugs Causing Increased Values False Positives	Drugs Causing Decreased Values False Negatives
	Erythromycin Ethinamate (Valmid) Gonadotropin Hydralazine Hydroxyzine Meprobamate Methicillin Methyprylon Metyrapone Morphine Nalidixic acid Oleandomycin Oxacillin Paraldehyde* Penicillin G (large dose)	Glucose Meprobamate (Equanil, Miltown) Metyrapone Paraldehyde* Piperidine Probenecid Progestin-estrogen combinations (oral contraceptives) Promazine Propoxyphene Pyrazinamide Quinine* Quinidine Reserpine
Phenaglycodol	Salicylates Phenazopyridine (Pyridium) Phenothiazines Piperidine Quinine* Salicylates Secobarbital* Spironolactone Testolactone Testosterone Troleandomycin (TAO)	Secobarbital* Spironolactone
Lactic acid dehydrogenase (LDH)		Ehionamide Nitrofurantoin
Melanogen	Methyldopa	
Mucopolysaccharides	Heparin	
Occult urine cast	Antimony compounds Arsenicals Bacitracin (renal tubular damage) Capreomycin (reversible renal toxicity) Chloroguanide Colistimethate Edathamil Isoniazid Kanamycin (nephrotoxic) Melarsopral Methicillin Neomycin Paramethadione Polymyxin B* Rifampin Trimethadione	
Osmolality	Glucose	

Contd...

Contd...

Substance Determined	Drugs Causing Increased Values False Positives	Drugs Causing Decreased Values False Negatives
PAH clearance	Aminosalicylic acid Sulfonamides	
Phenolsulfonphthalein (PSP)	Anthraquinone derivatives BSP Cascara (urine discoloration) Danthron Ethoxazene (Serenium; urine discoloration) Formaldehyde-forming drugs Methenamine Novobiocin Phenazopyridine (Pyridium) Phenolphthalein Radiographic contrast media Rhubarb extracts Sulfonamides Sulfinpyrazone	Alkali (excess) Carinamide Diodrast Diuretics Iodopyracet Penicillin Probenecid Salicylates Sulfonamides Thiazide diuretics
Phenyl ketone	Aminosalicylic acid Antipyrine Aspirin Chlorpromazine* Epinephrine Histidine metabolites Methotrimeprazine Nialamide Phenacetin Phenothiazines Prochlorperazine Salicylates*	Aminosalicylic acid Aspirin Bilirubin (high concentration) Chlorpromazine* Phenothiazines Salicylates*
Porphyrins	Acriflavine Alcohol Antipyretics Barbiturates Chloroquine Chlorpromazine Chlorpropamide Estrogens Ethoxazene Griseofulvin Oxytetracycline Phenazopyridine Phenothiazines Phenylhydrazine Penicillin Procaine Progestin–estrogen combinations (oral contraceptives) Sedatives and hypnotics	

Contd...

Contd...

Substance Determined	Drugs Causing Increased Values False Positives	Drugs Causing Decreased Values False Negatives
	Sulfamethoxazole Sulfonamides Sulphonal Tetracycline Tolbutamide	
Pregnancy test	Aspirin Chlordiazepoxide Chlorpromazine Fluphenazine Pentylenetetrazole Phenothiazines Promethazine (Gravindex) Thioridazine	Promethazine
Porphobilinogen	Aminosalicylic acid Cascara Chlorpromazine Phenothiazines Procaine	Ascorbic acid Urea
Protein (as albumin)	Acetazolamide (Diamox) Aminophylline Aminosalicylic acid (PAS) Amphotericin B Antimony compounds Arsenicals Aspirin Bacitracin Bicarbonates Bismuth triglycollamate Capreomycin Carbarsone Carbon tetrachloride Carbutamide Carinamide Cephaloridine Chlorpromazine Chlorpropamide Colistimethate Colymicin (Colistin) Corticosteroids Dihydrotachysterol Doxapram Edathamil Ethosuximide Gentamicin Gold salts nephrotoxic Griseofulvin Iron sorbitex (Jectofer) Isoniazid Kanamycin Lipomul (oil injection) Lithium carbonate Mefenamic acid Mercuric chloride Metahexamide Metaxalone Methenamine (large doses) Methsuximide Mithramycin	

Contd...

Contd...

Substance Determined	Drugs Causing Increased Values False Positives	Drugs Causing Decreased Values False Negatives
	Mitotane Neomycin Paraldehyde Paramethadione (Paradione) Penicillamine Penicillin (large doses) Methicillin Oxacillin Phenacemide Phenazopyridine Phenindione Phenylbutazone Phosphorus Polymyxin B Promazine (quarterly ammonium compounds) Pyrazolone derivatives Radiopaque contrast media Sodium diatrizoate (Hypaque) Iopanoic acid (Telepaque) Salicylates (overdosage) Salyrgan-theophylline Sodium bicarbonate Streptomycin Sulfamethoxazole Sulfisoxazole Sulfonamides Sulfameter Sulfones Suramin Tetracyclines (degraded) Theophylline sodium glycinate (high doses) Thiabendazole Thiosemicarbazones Thymol Tolbutamide Trimethadione Turpentine Viomycin Vitamin D Zoxazolamine	
RBC or haemoglobin	Aminosalicylic acid (large doses) Amphotericin B Bacitracin Chloroguanide Colchicine Colistimethate (Colistin) Corticosteroids Coumarin derivatives Cyclophosphamide Gold salts Indomethacin	Ascorbic acid

Contd...

Contd...

Substance Determined	Drugs Causing Increased Values False Positives	Drugs Causing Decreased Values False Negatives
	Kanamycin (renal injury) Lipomul Mandelic acid derivatives Mefenamic acid Mephenesin Mersalyl theophylline Methenamine Methicillin Mitotane Oxyphenbutazone Phenindione derivatives Phenylbutazone PhisoHex Phosphorus Phytonadione Polymyxin B Primaquine (high dosage) Probenecid Proguanil Pyrazoline derivatives Rifampin Sulfonamides Sulfones Suramin Thiabendazole Thiazide diuretics Viomycin	
Specific gravity	Albumin Dextran Glucose Radiopaque contrast media Sucrose	
Tyrosine	Aspirin	
Uric acid	Ascorbic acid Aspirin Bishydroxycoumarin Corticosteroids Dopamine Mercaptopurine Methyldopa* Probenecid Salicylates Sulfinpyrazone Thiazide diuretics Thiothixene	Acetazolamide Alcohol (chronic consumption can interfere with test results) Allopurinol Ethacrynic acid Methyldopa* Triamterene
Urobilin	Fluorescein Merbromin Riboflavin	
Urobilinogen	Acetazolamide (Diamox) Amidopyrine Aminosalicylic acid (PAS) Antipyrine Bile salts	Ammonium chloride Antibiotics Ascorbic acid Chloramphenicol (large doses)

Contd...

Contd...

Substance Determined	Drugs Causing Increased Values False Positives	Drugs Causing Decreased Values False Negatives
	BSP Cascara Chlorophyl Chlorpromazine Diatrizoate Drugs that cause hemolysis of RBC's Epinephrine Formalin* Hypaque Methenamine compounds Novocaine Phenazopyridine Phenothiazines Procaine Pyradone Pyramidon Sodium bicarbonate Sulfadiazine Sulfamethizole Sulfamethoxazole Sulfapyridine Sulfathiazole Sulfisoxzole Sulfonamides Tetracycline Thoradex	Formalin* Tetracycline (possible)
Vanillylmandelic acid (VMA)	Aminosalicylic acid (PAS) Anileridine Aspirin BSP Cough medicines (some) Disulfiram (Antabuse) Epinephrine (Adrenaline) Foods and beverages (bananas, chocolate, coffee, tea vanilla extract) Glyceryl guaiacolate Insulin (large doses) Levodopa (L-dopa) Lithium carbonate Mandelamine Mephenesin Methocarbamol Methyldopa Morphine Nalidixic acid Nitroglycerin Norepinephrine Oxytetracycline Phenazopyridine	Aspirin Chlorpromazine Guanethidine Imipramine Levodopa Monoamine oxidase inhibitors Morphine Pentobarbital Reserpine

Contd...

Contd...

Substance Determined	Drugs Causing Increased Values False Positives	Drugs Causing Decreased Values False Negatives
	PSP Reserpine Salicylates Stibophen	
Xylose excretion	Glucose Phenazopyridine	

DRUGS THAT MAY AFFECT COLOUR OF URINE

Colour of Urine	Drug
Reddish brown	Aminopyrine Cascara and senna laxatives in acid urine
Orange	Aminopyrine Phenazopyridine
Orange to orange red	Ethoxazine Phenindione Pyridium Rifampin Senna
Orange to purple red	Chlorzoxazone
Orange yellow	Anisindione Fluorescein (after IV administration) Phenindione Salicylazosulfapyridine (in alkaline urine)
Rust yellow to brownish	Primaquine Nitrofurantions Salicylazosulfapyridine Sulfonamides
Pink to red or red brown	Danthron Dilantin Doxidan Phenolphthalein Phenothiazine Phensuximide
Magenta Red	Phenolphthalein Amidopyrine Aniline dyes Desferal Neotropin Phenolphthalein and pyridium in acid urine Prontosil PSP and BSP dyes in alkaline urine Pyridium
Purple red	Chlordiazepoxide Ibuprofen (also pink, red) Phenolphthalein in alkaline urine

Contd...

Contd...

Colour of Urine	Drug
Dark brown	Phenolic drugs Phenylhydrazine
Brown black	Amitriptyline Cascara Jecotofir Methylene blue Pyridium (in alkaline urine) Ribloflavin
Pink to brown	Phenothiazine tranquillizers
Pale blue	Dyrenium (Triamterene)
Reddish iron chelate	Deferoxamine
Dark coloured	Iron salts
Urine that darkens on standing	Antiparkinson drugs Levodopa Sinemet
Blue or green	Methylene blue Amitriptyline Triamterene
Bright yellow	Riboflavin Pyridium in alkaline urine
Yellow/pink-alkaline Brown	Cascara Chloroquine Iron salts Metronidazole Sulfamethoxazole Sulfonamides (some)
Red brown	Cinchophen
Brown, green, blue	Nitrofurans
Pink red	Diphenylhydantoin Phenacetin
Dark green	Phenylsalicylate

DRUGS AFFECTING RESULTS OF FECAL STUDIES

Drugs Affecting Fecal Studies

Substance Determined	Drugs Causing Increased Values False Positives	Drugs Causing Decreased Values False Negatives
Occult blood -benzidine or guaiac test	Boric acid (toxicity) Bromides	Ascorbic acid (high doses) Colchicine (toxicity)
	Iodides Iodine Iron (inorganic) Oxidizing agents (excreted in urine) Pyridium	

Drugs Affecting Colour or Feces

Color of Stool	Drug
Whitish discolouration or speckling	Aluminum hydroxide, antacids
Pink or red to black	Anticoagulants (excess dose) Salicylates (causing internal bleeding)
Black	Bismuth salts, iron salts, charcoal
Brownish staining	Dihydroxyanthraquinones
Green to blue	Dithiazanine
Green	Mercurous chloride, indomethacin, calomel
Orange red	Phenazopyridine
Red	Phenolphthalein, pyruvium pamoate, tetracyclines in syrup, Bromsulphalein
Yellow	Rhubarb,santonin
Yellow to brown	Senna
Pink to red to black (resulting from internal bleeding)	Salicylates
Light	Sitosterols

DRUGS AFFECTING RESULTS OF HAEMATOLOGIC AND SEROLOGIC STUDIES

Substance Determined	Drugs Causing Increased Values False Positives	Drugs Causing Decreased Values False Negatives
Bleeding	Acetysalicylic acid Dextran Mithramycin Pantothenyl alcohol and derivatives Streptokinase-streptodornase	
Coagulation time	All cause positive Coombs' test Anticoagulants Azathioprine Carbenicillin (high doses in impaired renal function) Cephalexin Cephaloglycin Cephaloridine Cephalothin Chlorpromazine Diphenylhydantoin Dipyrone Ethosuximide Hydralazine Isoniazid Levodopa Mefenamic acid	Corticosteroids Epinephrine

Contd...

Contd...

Substance Determined	Drugs Causing Increased Values False Positives	Drugs Causing Decreased Values False Negatives
	Mephalan Methyldopa (effect lasts 6mo.) Mithramycin Oxyphenisatin Penicillin Procainamide Quinidine Rifampin Streptomycin Sulfonamides Tetracyclines	
Erythrocyte count or haemoglobin	Gentamicin Methyldopa (Aldomet)	Acetaminophen Acetophenazine maleate Acetophenetidin Aminosalicylic acid
Erythrocyte count or haemoglobin		Amphotericin B Antimony compounds Antineoplastic agents Azathioprine Fluorouracil Floxuridine Hydroxyurea Mechlorethamine Mithramycin Triethylene-melamine Urethan Arsenicals Carbamazepine Chloramphenicol Chloroquine Diiodohydroxyquin Doxapram Ethosuximide Furazolidone Glucosulfone Haloperidol Hydantoin derivatives Hydralazine Hydroxychloroquine sulfate Indomethacin Isoniazid (rare) MAO inhibitors Mefenamic acid Mepacrine (quinacrine) Mephenoxalone Mercurial diuretics (prolonged use)

Contd...

Contd...

Substance Determined	Drugs Causing Increased Values False Positives	Drugs Causing Decreased Values False Negatives
		Metaxalone
		Methaqualone
		Methsuximide
		Methyldopa (Aldomet)
		Nitrites
		Nitrofurantoin (rare)
		Novobiocin
		Oleandomycin
Erythrocyte count or haemoglobin		Oxyphenbutazone
		Paramethadione, trimethadione
		Penicillamine
		Penicillin
		Phenacemide
		Phenobarbital (rare)
		Phenylbutazone
		Phytonadione (large doses in infants)
		Primaquine
		Primidone
		Pyrazolone derivatives
		Pyrimethamine
		Radioactive agents (large doses)
		Rifampin
		Spectinomycin
		Sulfameter
		Sulfonamides (rarely with sulfathiazole)
		Sulfones
		Sulfonylureas (oral hypoglycemic agents)
		Tetracycline
		Thiazide diuretics (rare)
		Thiocyanates
		Thiosemicarbazones
		Trimethadione
		Tripelennamine
		Troleandomycin
		Vitamin A (excess dose and use)
Leukocytes	Aollpurinol (hypersensitivity)	Acetaminophen
		Acetohexamide
	Aminosalicylic acid	Acetophenetidin
	Ampicillin	Allopurinol

Contd...

Contd...

Substance Determined	Drugs Causing Increased Values False Positives	Drugs Causing Decreased Values False Negatives
	Atropine (in children)	(hypersensitivity)
	Barbiturates	Aminoglutethimide
	Capreomycin	
	Cardiotonic glycosides	Aminopyrine
		Aminosalicylic acid
	Cephalothin	
	Chlorpropamide	Amodiaquine
	Clindamycin	Antineoplastic agents
	Cloxacillin	Chlorambucil
	Desipramine, imiprazine	Cyclophosphamide
		Cytoxan
	Diethylcarbamacine	Fluorouracil
		Floxuridine
	Digitalis (rare)	Hydroxyurea
	Diphenhydramine	Mechlorethamine
	Dipyrone	Mithramycin
	Epinephrine	Triethylenemelamine
	Erythromycin	
	Florantyrone (in patients with pre-existing liver disease)	Antipyrine
		Azathioprine
		Bismuth
		Carbamazepine
	Gold compounds	Carbimazole
	Hydantoin derivatives	Cephalothin
		Chloramphenicol
	Iodides	
	Iron dextran injection (Imferon)	Chlordiazepoxide
		Chloroquine
	Isoniazid	Chlorpropamide
	Kanamycin	Chlorprothixene
	Lincomycin (one case reported)	Chlorthalidone
		Clindamycin
	Methicillin	Clofibrate
	Methyldopa	Cloxacillin
	Methysergide	Colistin
	Nalidixic acid	Corticosteroids reported for prednisolone; Prednisone)
	Novobiocin	
	Phenothiazines (large doses)	Desipramine, imipramine
	Potassium iodide	Diazepam
	Primaquine	Dichlorphenamide
	Procainamide	Diethazine
	Streptodornase streptokinase	Diiodohydroxyquin
	Ristocetin	Diphenhydramine
	Streptomycin	Doxapram
	Stibocapate (antimony)	Ethacrynic acid
		Ethoxzolamide

Contd...

Contd...

Substance Determined	Drugs Causing Increased Values False Positives	Drugs Causing Decreased Values False Negatives
	Sulfonamides (long-acting) Tetracyclines (prolonged use) Triamterene Trifluperidol Vancomycin Viomycin	Furosemide Glaucarubin Glucosulfone Gold compounds Griseofulvin Haloperidol Hydantoin derivatives Hydralazine Hydroxychloroquine Idoxuridine (in high concentration) Indandione derivatives (oral anticoagulants) Indomethacin Iothiouracil Mefenamic acid Mepacrine (Quinacrine) Mepazine Mephenesin Meprobamate Mercurial diuretics (rare) Metaxalone Methampyrone Methazolamide Methimazole Methocarbamol Methsuximide Methyldopa Methylthiouracil Methyprylon (metabolite: methicillin sodium, oxacillin) Methysergide Metronidazole Monoamine oxidase inhibitors Nitrofurantoin (rare) Novobiocin Oleandomycin Oxandrolone Oxazepam Oxyphenbutazone Paraldehyde Penicillamine Penicillins Phenothiazines (large doses) Phenylbutazone

Contd...

Contd...

Substance Determined	Drugs Causing Increased Values False Positives	Drugs Causing Decreased Values False Negatives
		Potassium perchlorate Primaquine Primidone (rare) Procainamide (both reported) Procarbazine Propylthiouracil Protriptyline Pyrathiazine (prolonged use) Pyrazolone derivatives Pyrimethamine (Daraprim) Quinine Radioactive agents Rifampin Ristocetin Sulfonamides* Sulfonylureas (oral hypoglycemic agents) Sulthiame Thiabendazole Thiazide diuretics (rare) Thiosemicarbanzones Thiothixene Tripelennamine Vitamin A (prolonged use)
Lupus erythematosus or antinuclear antibodies	Acetazolamide Aminosalicylic acid Birth control pills Chlorothiazide Chlorprothixene Griseofulvin Hydralazine Isoniazid Methyldopa	Penicillin Phenylbutazone Phenytoin sodium Procainamide Streptomycin Sulfonamides Tetracyclines Thiouracil Trimethadione
Prothrombin time	ACTH Alcohol (large quantities) Aluminum nicotinate 50% decreased Amidopyrine Aminosalicylic acid (PAS) Anabolic steroids Antibiotics Anticoagulants (oral)	Antihistamines Diphenhydramine (Benadryl) Barbiturates (enzyme induction) Chloral hydrate Corticosteroids Digitalis (in cardiac failure) Glutethimide

Contd...

Contd...

Substance Determined	Drugs Causing Increased Values False Positives	Drugs Causing Decreased Values False Negatives
	Benziodarones Carbenicillin (high doses with renal failure) Cathartics Clordiazepoxide (Librium)* Cloramphenicol (Chloromycetin) Chlorpromazine* Cholestyramine Clofibrate Diphenidol Diphenylhydantoin (Dilantin) Edathamil Heparin Hydroxyzine Indomethacin (Indocin) Iothiouracil Kanamycin Lipomul (oil injection)* Mefenamic acid (Ponstel) Metandienone Metaproterenol* Methimazole Methyldopa (Aldomet) effect on liver Methylthiouracil Mineral oil Mithramycin Monoamine oxidase inhibitors Morphine Naloxone Neomycin Oxyphenbutazone Penicillin Phenylbutazone Phenyramidol Phosphorus Propylthiouracil Proteolytic enzymes* (e.g., papase, ananase) Pyrazinamide Quinidine Quinine Reserpine Salicylates Streptomycin	Griseolfulvin Lipomul (oil injection)* Metaproterenol* Progestin-estrogen combinations (oral contraceptives) Proteolytic enzymes*(e.g. papase, ananase) Rifampin Theophylline (xanthines may increase plasma prothrombin and factor V,but therapeutic doses have small effect on the response to oral anticoagulants) Thiothixene Vitamin K

Contd...

Contd...

Substance Determined	Drugs Causing Increased Values False Positives	Drugs Causing Decreased Values False Negatives
	Sulfonamides (sulfameter) Tetracyclines Thyroid hormones D-thyroxine (Choloxin) Vitamin A	
Sedimentation rate;erythrocyte sedimentation rate (ESR)	Dextran Methyldopa Methysergide Penicillamine Procainamide Progestin-estrogen combination (oral contraceptives) Theophylline Trifluperidol Vitamin A	Drugs that cause a high blood glucose level (cortisone and ACTH) Ethambutol Quinine Salicylates
Thrombocytes (platelets)	Aspirin	Acetazolamide Acetohexamide Aminosalicylic acid Amphotericin B Antazoline Antimony compounds Antineoplastic agents Azathioprine Busulfan (Myleran; large doses) Chlorambucil Cyclophosphamide (Cytoxan) Flurouracil Floxuridine Mechlorethamine Mithramycin Hydroxyurea Arsenicals Benzene Bismuth Busulfan Carbamazepine Cardiotonic glycosides Chloramphenicol Chloroquine Chlorothiazide Chlorpropamide Chlorthalidone

Contd...

Contd...

Substance Determined	Drugs Causing Increased Values False Positives	Drugs Causing Decreased Values False Negatives
		Colchicine
		DDT
		Diazoxide
		Dipyrone
		Ethacrynic acid
		Ethoxzolamide
		Diethylstilbestrol
		Diphenylhydantoin
		Gentamicin
		Gold salts
		Heparin
		Iothiouracil sodium
		Lincomycin
		Lipomul (oil injection)
		Mefenamic acid
		Mepazine
		Mephenytoin
		Meprobamate
		Methazolamide
		Methimazole
		Methotrexate
		Methyldopa (Aldomet)
		Novobiocin
		Oxyphenbutazone
		Penicillamine
		Penicillins
		Phenindione (indane derivative)
		Phenothiazines
		Phenylbutazone
		Potassium perchlorate
		Prednisone
		Procainamide
		Propranolol
		Propynol-cyclohexanol carbamate
		Pyrazinamide
		Pyrimethamine
		Quinidine sulfate
		Quinine
		Rifampin
		Ristocetin A & B
		Salicylates
		Smallpox vaccine

Contd...

Contd...

Substance Determined	Drugs Causing Increased Values False Positives	Drugs Causing Decreased Values False Negatives
		Sulfonamides
		Sulfadimethoxine
		Sulfameter
Thrombocytes, Platelets continued		Sulphamethoxypyridazine
		Sulphisoxazole
		Sulfonyl ureas (oral hypoglycemic agents)
		Sulphamethoxazole
		Thiazide diuretics (rare)
		Thiourea
		Tolbutamide
		Toluene diisocyanate

DRUGS AFFECTING CEREBROSPINAL FLUID STUDIES

Substance Determined	Drugs Causing Increased Values False Positives	Drugs Causing Decreased Values False Negatives
Proteins	Aminosalicylates	Albumin
	Aminosalicylic acid	Acetophenetidin
	Anesthetics (local), contaminant	Cytarabine
	Aspirin	
	Chloramphenicol	
	Chlorpromazine	
	Epinephrine	
	Lidocaine	
	Methotrexate	
	Penicillin	
	Phenacetin	
	Phenothiazines	
	Procaine	
	Salicylates	
	Streptomycin	
	Sulfadiazine	
	Sulfanilamide	
	Sulfisoxazole	
	Tetracycline	
	Tolbutamide	
	Tryptophan	

Appendices

Appendix II

Maximum permissible transport and storage times for analytes in blood (serum, plasma) and cerebrospinal fluid.

Clinical chemistry, serum, plasma and blood

Analyte	*Stability In blood at room temperature and tendency of change thereafter*	*Stability In serum/plasma -20°C 4-8°C 20-25°C*	*Stabilizer*	*Comments*
Acid phosphatase, prostatic. immunol	1 h, unstable ↓	Without stabilizer 1 d 8 h 2h Stabilized to pH 4-5 4m 8d 8 d	5 mg $NaHSO_4$/ ml serum or 20 µl 10 % acetic acid/ ml serum	Serum > plasma Add stabilizer after-separation of serum
Adrenocorticotropic hormone (ACTH)	Unstable↓, stabilize in aprotinin/EDTA plus mercaptoethanol	6w ? ?	Aprotinin 400 kU/ml mercap-toethanol 2 µl/ml	
Alanine aminotrans-ferase (ALAT. ALT)	4 d ↓	2d 7d 3d		
Albumin	6d	3m 3m 3m		
Aldosterone	1 d ↓	4d 4d 4d	EDTA	Not applicable to outpatients
Alkaline phosphatase total bone	4 d ↓ 4d	2m 7d 7d 2m 7d 7d		
Alubminium	Days	1 yr 2 w 1 w		
Ammonia	15 min in EDTA, Heparin ↑	3 w 2 h 15 min Stabilized by serine and borate	Serine 5 mmol/1 and borate 2 mmol/1	Easily contaminated by sweat ammonia
α-Amylase (AMYL). total pancreatic	 4d↓ 7d ↓	 1 yr 7d 7d 1 yr 7d 7d		

Contd...

Contd...

Analyte	*Stability In blood at room temperature and tendency of change thereafter*	*Stability In serum/plasma -20°C*	*4-8°C*	*20-25°C*	*Stabilizer*	*Comments*
Androstendione	1d ↓	1yr	4d	1 d		
Antislreptolysin	?	?	2d	2d		
α_1-Antitrypsin	?	3 m	3 m	7d	Heparin plasma recommended	EDTA and citrate↓
Apolipoprotein A-l	?		3 d	1d		Do not freeze
Apolipoprotein B	?		3d	1d		Do not freeze
Aspartate Aminotransferase (ASAT, AST)	7d↓	2w	7d	4d		
Bicarbonate	Unstable (+ 4°C, 30 min)	6m	7d	1d	Keep closed	1 h after opening the tube
Bilirubin, conjugated total	 7d in dark ↓ 7d in dark ↓	 6m 6m	 7d 7d	 2d 1 d	 Darkness required when stored > 8 h	
C-peptide	?	4 w	d	h		
C-reactive protein (CRP)	?	3yr	8d	3d		
C3 complement	1h	8d	8d	4d		Dependent on antibody. during storage C3 increases –C3 decreases
C4 complement	1h	?	2d	2d		
CA 125	?	3m	5d	3d		
CA 15-3	?	3m	5d	?		
CA 19-9	?	3m	5d	?		
CA 72-4	?	3m	7d	?		
Cadmium	1 d in trace element tube	?	?	?	Special tube	Released from red stopper
Calcitonin	1h, stabilized with aprotinin (400 kU/ml)	?	?	?	Aprotinin 400 kU/ml	
Calcium, total	2d ↓	8m	3 w	7d		
Calcium. ionized (actual)	15 min ↑	2h			Use Ca-litrated heparin; keep light	pH-dependent Whole blood recommended only. Stable in gel tubes as primary tubes for 8h after centrifugation.
Carbohydrate-deficient transferin (CDT)	? /	yrs	7d	?		
Carcinoembryonic antigen (CEA)	?	6 m	7d	1 d		
Catecholamines Noradrenaline Adrenaline Dopamine	1 h if not stabilized	4 w 6 m if stabilized	2d	1 d	Glutathione + EGTA, 1.2 mg/ml	Special tube necessary EGTA plasma separated within 15 min and frozen at –20°C.

Contd...

Contd...

Analyte	*Stability In blood at room temperature and tendency of change thereafter*	*Stability In serum/plasma* -20°C	4-8°C	20-25°C	*Stabilizer*	*Comments*
Chloride	1 d ↓	yrs	7d	7d		
Cholesterol, total HDL- LDL-	7d↑ 2d↑ 1d↑	3m 3m 3m	7d 7d 7d	7d 2d 1d		
Cholinesterase (CHE)	7d ↓	3m	17d	17d		
Coeruloplasmin	?	3m	2w	8d		
Copper	7d	yrs	2w	2w	Special tube	Contamination
Corticotropin						See ACTH
Cortisol	7d	3m	7d	7d		
Creatine kinase (CK) total	7d ↓	4w in dark	7d	2d	Darkness	CK-BB not stable without stabilizer
MB (CK-MB)	7d ↓	4 w in dark	7d	2d	SH reagent	Including immunoassays
Creatinine	3d↑	3m	7d	7d		Also enzymatic procedure
CYFRA 21-1	?	6m	4w	2d		
Dehydroepiandrosterone sulfate (DHEA-S)	2 d ↓	yrs	2w	1d		
Electrophoresis. Protein-	?	3 w	3 d	1d		
Erythropoietin	?	?	?	2w		Shipped frozen
Estradiol	1 d	1 yr	3d	1 d		
Estriol	?	1 yr	2d	1 d		
Ethanol	2 w	?	6 m	2 w	EDTA/Heparin	Evaporation, closed tubes
Fatty acids, free	30 min ↑	2d	12	30 min		Freeze serum immediately
Ferritin	?	1yr	7d	7d		
α-Fetoprotein (AFP)	?	3m	3d	3d		
Folic acid	30 min ↓ add ascorbate	8w	6h	30 min	Ascorbate 20 rng/ml	Light ↓
Follitropin (FSH)	7d↓	1yr	2w	2w		
Free thyroxine (FT_4)	?	3 m	8 d	2d		
Free triiodothyronine (FT_3)	?	3 m	2w	1d		
Fructosamine	12 h↑	2m	2w	3d		
Gastrin	2 h	?	?	1 w		Serum frozen as soon as possible
Glucose, blood (capillary)	10 min↓	Hemolysate stabilized ?	2 d	2 d		Hemolysate

Contd...

Contd...

Analyte	*Stability In blood at room temperature and tendency of change thereafter*	*Stability In serum/plasma -20°C 4-8°C 20-25°C*	*Stabilizer*	*Comments*
Glucose, plasma (venous)	10 min ↓ appropriate 7d with glycolysis inhibitor	Stabilized 1d↓ 7d 1d	Fluoride, monoiodo-acetate, mannose	Loss by non-enzymatic glycation (protein matrix)
Glutamate dehydrogenase	?	2 w 7d 7d		
Glutamate oxaloacetic transaminase (GOT)				See ASAT (AST)
Glutamate pyruvate transaminase (GPT)				See ALAT (ALT)
γ-Glutamyl) transferase (γ-GT. GGT)	1d ↓	yrs 7d 7d		
Glycated albumin	?	? ? ?		See fructosamine
Growth hormone (STH, somatotropin)	1 d	3m 8 d 1 d		Separate serum immediately
Haptoglobin	Unstable	3m 3d 4d		Method-dependent; 3 types
HbA_{1c}	3d (EDTA blood)	6m 7d 3d		
Human chorionic gonadotropin (hCG)	?	1 yr 3 d 1 d		
Immunoglobulins IgA IgD IgE IgG IgM	 ? ? ? ? ?	 6 m 3 m 3 m 6m 7d 7d 6m 7d 7d 6 m 3 m 3 m 6m 3m 7d		
Insulin	63 min	6m 1 d 4 h	Plasma preferable	
Iron	2h↑	yrs 3w 7d		EDTA, oxalate, citrate interfere
Lactate	< 5 min, unstable ↑↑ deproteinization recommended, glycolysis inhibitors	? 3d 3d ? 6 d 3d	Mannose-fluoride, oxalate iodoacetate, deproteinization	
Lactate dehydro-genase (LDH)	1 h ↑	4 w 4 d		All isoenzymes serum > plasma
Lead	?	? ? 7 d		Special tubes
Lipase	? h	1 yr 7 d 7 d		
Lipoprotein (a) (Lpa)	?	3 m 2 w ?		
Lutropine (LH)	7d	1 yr 3d 1 d		
Magnesium	1d↑	1 yr 7d 7d		
Myoglobin	1 h ↓	3m 1 d 2h		
Neuron-specific enolase	2 h ↑ (heparin)	3m 3d ?	Heparin plasma	Serum > plasma (platelets, hemolysis)
Osmolality	?	3m 1 d 3 h		

Contd...

Contd...

Analyte	*Stability In blood at room temperature and tendency of change thereafter*	*Stability In serum/plasma -20°C*	*4-8°C*	*20-25°C*	*Stabilizer*	*Comments*
Osteocalcin	15 min	Stabilized 14 d	?	Unstable	EDTA (5 mmol/1) and aprotinin (2500 kU/ml)	
Parathyrin (PTH) intact	6 h (24 h in EDTA blood)	?	1 d	6 h	EDTA	Method-dependent
Phosphate, inorganic	1 h ↑↑	1 yr	4 d	1 d		
Potassium	1 h ↑↑	1 yr	1 w	1 w		Serum > plasma
Progesterone	7d	1 yr	3 d	1 d		
Prolactin	2 d	1 yr	3 d	1 d		No EDTA. citrate
Prostatic-specific antigen (PSA)	1d	3m	2 d	1 d		
Protein electrophoresis	?	3w	3d	1d		
Protein total	1 d	yrs	4 w	6 d		Plasma > serum (fibrinogen)
Rheumatoid factor (RF)	?	4 w	3 d	1d		
Selenium	2 d	1 yr	2 w	1 w		Contamination
Sodium-	4 d ↓	1yr	2 w	2 w		
Testosterone	7d 1 day in women ↑	1yr	3d	1d		
Thyroglobulin	2d	4 w	3d	1d		
Thyrotropine (TSH)	7d	3m	3d	1d		
Thyroxine (T_4)	7d	4 w	7d	2d		
Thyroxine-binding globulin (TBG)	7d	4 w	5d	5d		
Transferrin	?	6 m	8 d	8 d		
Triglycerides	7d ↑	yrs	7d	2d		Decrease ol triglycerides, increase of free glycerol, but only minor increase of total glycerol
Triiodothyronine (T_3)	?	3m	8d	2 d		
Troponin T	?	3 m	1 d	?		
Troponin I	?	?	?	?		
Urea	1 d ↑	1 yr	7d	7d		
Uric acid	7d↑	6m	7d	3d		
Vitamin A	?	2 yrs	4 w	?		Light ↓.
Vitamin B1 (thiamin)	?	1 yr	?	?		
Vitamin B2 (riboflavin)	?	4 w	?	?		Light ↓

Contd...

Contd...

Analyte	*Stability In blood at room temperature and tendency of change thereafter*	*Stability In serum/plasma -20°C 4-8°C 20-25°C*			*Stabilizer*	*Comments*
Vitamin B6 (pyridoxal phosphate)	Unstable, use EDTA plasma	Days	hs	30 min	EDTA plasma darkness	Light ↓
Vitamin B12	Unstable, use EDTA	8w	4h	15 min	EDTA, darkness	Light ↓
Vitamin C	3 h (4°C)	3 w only with stabilizers	3 h	?	Metaphosphate 63 mg/ml; deproteinized	
Vitamin D, 1.25-Dihydroxy-cholecalciferol	3d	?	?	2d		
25-Hydroxy-cholecalciferol	3d	?	?	2d		
Vitamin E (tocopherol)	8h↓	1 yr	4 w	?		
Vitamin K (transphyllochinone)	Unstable	3m	Unstable	?		UV light ↓, use extraction
Zinc	30 min ↑	1 yr	2 w	1 w	Special tubes	Contamination from stoppers

Hematology, EDTA blood

Analyte	*Stability in blood at 20-25°C*					*Stability in blood at 4-8°C*	*Stabilizer*	*Comments*
	M	*C*	*B*	*S*	*O*			
Differential leukocyte count						Do not store at refrigerator temperature	Dry blood smear stable	Lower filling (higher EDTA concentration) decreases stability.
Band neutrophils	3h	8h	12h	2h	4h			
Segmented neutrophils	3h	9h	12h	8h				
Eosinophils		9h	12h	7d	2d			
Basophils			12h	2d	1 d↑			
Monocytes	3h	7h	12h	2h	↑↑			
Lymphocytes	3h	9h	12h	7d	4d			
Erythrocytes	7d					7d		Analyzer-dependent
Haematocrit (Hct, PCV)	1 d					7d	K_2-EDTA superior to K_3-EDTA with centrifuge	
Haemoglobin (Hb)	7d					7d		
Leukocytes	7d					7d		
MCV	1d					7d		
Reticulocytes	1 d					1 d		
Thrombocytes	7d					7d		

M = Microscopic
C = Coulter (STKS®)
B = Bayer/Technicon (H2®))
S = Sysmex (NE 8000)
O = Others (COBAS® Argos)

Coagulation and ESR, citrated blood/plasma

Analyte	*Stability In blood at room temperature and tendency of change thereafter)*	*Stability In plasma −20°C*	*4-8°C*	*20-25°C*	*Stabilizer*	*Comments*
Antithrombin 111	8h	4w	2w	7d		
D-Dimer	8 h	6 m	4d	8 h		
Erythrocyte sedimentation rate (ESR)	2 h	-	-	-		Temperature-dependent
Factor II	?	4w	?	6h		
Factor V	?	4 w	4 h	4 h		Centrifuge at 4°C
Factor VII	?	?	Unstable	8h		
Factor VIII	?	2 w	4 h	4 h		Freeze to store > 4h
Factor IX	4w	?	?	4h		
Factor IX: Ag	?	?	?	?		
Factor X		4w	?	6 h		
Factor XI	?	?	?	?		
Factor XII	?	4w	?	2h		
Factor XIII	?	4w	?	4h		
Fibrin monomers	Unstable ↑↑	?	?	3h	See FDP	
Fibrinogen	8 h	4 w	7d	7d		
Fibrin(ogen) degradation products (FDP)	Unstable ↑↑	4w	1d	?	10 U thrombin and 150 IU Kallikrein/ml blood	Heparin inhibits thrombin effect
Fibrinopeptide A	?	?	2h	?		
Capillary Ouick	?	4 w	2d	6 h		
Hepato Quick						
Partial thromboplastin time (APTT)	4h	4w	8h	4 h		
Protein C	?	4w	7d	8h		
Protein S	?	4 m	4 h	4 h		
Quick, prothrombin time (PT)	8 h	4 w	1d	1d		Reagent-dependent
Reptilase time	?	4w	4 h	8 h		
Thrombin coagulase	?	?	?	8h		
Thrombin time	2h	4 w	8 h	4h		Reagent-dependent
von Willebrand factor (vWF)	?	6m	7 d	2d		

***) Do not cool whole blood samples, global tests are accelerated (activation of factor VII, XI, XII).*

Blood gases and whole blood electrolytes

Analyte	*Stability In blood at room temperature and tendency of change thereafter*	*Stability In blood at refrigerator temperature*	*Stabilizer*	*Comments*	
pH	15 min* ↓	2h**		Decrease due to formation of lactate. Increase due to loss of CO_2.	
pCO_2	15 min* ↑	2 h**	Close, cooling to 6°C	4-Decrease due to loss into surrounding air.	Do not cool plastic containers, and do not store them for more than 15 min.
Bicarbonate, base excess	15 min* ↓	4- 2h**		pH-dependent change.	If the storage interval is longer, use
pO_2	15 min* ↓	2h**		Increase, if not tightly closed.	glass containers and cool them.
Calcium ion, actual	15 min* ↑	2 h**	Heparinate, Ca-titrated and		
Sodium	1h*	1h**	elecIrolyte-balanced.		
Potassium	1 h* ↑↑	1 h**			
Chloride	1 h*	1h**			

*) Stored in closed plastic tubes
**) Stored in ice-water cooled glass

Therapeutic drug monitoring, toxicology (blood)

Analyte	*Stability in blood at room temperature and tendency of change thereafter*	*Stability In serum/plasma* -20°C	4-8°C	20-25°C	*Stabilizer*	*Comments*
Acetylsalicylic acid	?	?	?	?		
Carbamazepine	2d	4w	7d	2d		
Cocaine		4 d	4 w	<30 min	Fluoride, pH 5	
Cyclosporine	?	?	3d	?	EDTA	Monoclonal
Diazepam			5 m	5 m		
Digitoxin	?	6m	3 m	2 w		
Digoxin	?	6 m	3 m	2 w		
Disopyramide	?	5 m	2 w	?		
Ethosuximide	?	5 m	4 w	?		

Contd...

Contd...

Analyte	*Stability In blood at room temperature and tendency of change thereafter*	*Stability In serum/plasma* -20°C	4-8°C	20-25°C	*Stabilizer*	*Comments*
Gentamicin	4h	4w	4w	4h		
Lidocaine	?	?	6 h	?		
Lithium	1h↓	6m	7d	24 h		Accumulates in red cells
Methotrexate	?	6m	3d	?		Protect from light
Nitrazepam		1 w	1 w		Light	
Phenobarbital	2d	6m	6m	6m		
Phenytoin	2d	5m	4 w	2 d		Not stable in SST-tubes
Primidone	?	5m	4 w	?		
Procainamide	?	6m	2 w	?		
Quinidine	?	?	1 d	?		
Tetrahydrocannabinol (THC)		6m	6m	2m	Sodium azide	
Tetrahydrocannabinol)-9-carboxylic acid (THCA)		6 m				
Theophylline		3m	12 w	12 w		
Tobramycin	?	4w	3 d	Unstable		
Valporic acid	2 d	3 m	7 d	2 d		
Vancomycin	?	?	?	?		

Urine

Analyte	*Stability In urine at* -20°C	4-8°C	20-25°C	*Stabilizer*	*Comments*
Albumin	6 m	4 w	7d		Do not freeze (nephelometry)
Aluminium	1 yr	7d	3 d		
δ-Aminolaevulic acid	4w	4d	1d	pH 6-7, stabilized with 0.3 % $NaHCO_3$	Drugs Light↓
α Amlylase	3w	10d	2d		
Amphetamine	1 yr	?	?		
Bence Jones-Protein (light chains κ, γ)	6m	4w	7d		
Benzoylecgonine	4 m	?	?	pH 5, ascorbic acid	Unsilanized glass containers
Calcium	3 w	4 d	2 d	Acidified, pH < 2	Crystallization at cool temperature

Contd...

Contd...

Analyte	*Stability In urine at* -20°C	4-8°C	20-25°C	*Stabilizer*	*Comments*
Catecholamines (noradrenaline, adrenaline, dopamine)	Unstabilized 20 d Stabilized 1 yr	 4 d 1 yr	Acidified, pH < 2 4 d 3 w		
Citrate	4 w')	?	1 d**)	5 ml 1 % thymol	Storage acidified
Cocaine	4 m	3 w	?	pH 5, ascorbic acid	Unsilanized glass containers
Codeine	1 yr	?	?		
Copper	1 yr	7d	3d		
Cortisol	Stable	?	Unstable		
Creatinine	6m	6d	2d		
Cystine	1 yr	3m	7d	HCI	
Glucose	2 d	2d	2h	Pregnancy, diet	Bacteria decrease stability
5-Hydroxyindole acetic acid	2 d	2 d	2 h	Acidified	

**) Stored with HCI (pH< 1.7)*
***) Thymol added*

Analyte	*Stability in urine at* -20°C	4-8°C	20-25°C	*Stabilizer*	- *Comments*
Hydroxyproline	5 d	5 d	5 d	Acidified	
Iron	yrs	7d	3d		
Immunoglobulin G (IgG)	Unstable	4w	7d		Do not freeze (nephelometry)
Lysergic acid diethylamide (LSD)	2m	4 w	4 w		
α2-Macroglobulin	?	7d	7d		
Magnesium	1 yr	3d	3d	Acidified, pH < 2	
α1-Microglobulin	6m	4w	7d		
Morphine	1 yr	?	?		
N-Acetyl-β-D-glucosaminidase (β-NAG)	4 w	7d	1 d		
Osmolality	3m	7d	3h		
Oxalate	4 m (at pH 1.5)		Unstable 1 h	pH < 2 (HCI)	Vitamin C ↑
pH	Unstable↑			Thymol	Increase by NH_4 formation
Phosphate, inorganic	?	?	2 d at pH <5.0	Add thymol	Precipitates at alkaline pH

Contd...

Contd...

Analyte	*Stability In urine at* -20°C	4-8°C	20-25°C	*Stabilizer*	*Comments*
Porphobilinogen	4 w at pH 6-7	7d	4d at pH 6-7	pH 6 - by adding 0.3 % $NaHCO_3$	Acid pH↓
Porphyrins	4w	7d	4d at	pH 6- by adding 0.3 %	Light↓
Total porphyrin Uroporphyrin Heptacarboxyporphyrin Hexacarboxyporphyrin Pentacarboxyporphyrin Coproporphyrin Tricarboxyporphyrin Dicarboxyporphyrin	Stabilized		pH 6-7	$NaHCO_3$	
Potassium	1 yr	2m	45d		
Protein	4 w	7d	1d		
Pyridinium crosslinks (collagen crosslinks)	?	?	7d	5 mmol/l Na-formate	UV-sensitive, stable at day light
Sediment Bacteria Casts (hyaline and others) Epithelial cells Erythrocytes Leukocytes	 24 h days hours 1-4 h 1-4h	 24 h at osm >300 24 h at pH< 6.5 < 1 h at pH > 7.5		50% glycerol in 7% gelatine with 0.5 % thymol (storage in closed glass slides)	Do not feeze
Sodium	1 yr	45 d	45 d		
Test-strip fields Bacteria Erythrocytes Ketone bodies (acetoacetate) Leukocytes Protein Specific gravity		 24 h 1-4 h 1-4 h	 hours ? 1 d hours at pH < 7.5 Unstable (pH effect)		
Tetrahydrocannabinol-9 carboxylic acid (THCA)	1 yr	1 yr	10 w	Albumin	
Urea	4w	7d	2d	pH< 7	Stability less if ammonia is not included
Uric acid	Unstable, unless alkalized 4d			pH > 8	precipitation at pH < 7
Vanilmandelic acid (VMA)	yrs	7d at pH 3-5	7d at pH 3-5	pH 3-5	

CSF

Analyte	*Stability In CSF* -20°C	4-8°C	20-25°C	*Stabilizer*	*Comments*
Albumin	1 yr	2m	1 d	EDTA tubes Up to 1 h: Do not cool. Up to 3 h: Transport on ice. No additives. No partial fixation. Long-term storage: -70°C in glass or polypropylene vessels that can be tightly closed	Glucose, lactate: Stability depends on cell content. IgG: Freezing is not recommended. Leukocytes, tumor cells: Store cells as dry smears.
Glucose	Months	3d	5h↓		
IgG	Unstable	7d	1d		
Lactate	Months	24 h	3h↑		
Leukocytes tumours cells	—	3.5 h	1-2h		
Protein, total	1 yr	6 d	1 d		

Appendix III

TOTAL MEDICAL DIAGNOSTIC LABORATORY SOLUTIONS FROM THE TULIP GROUP OF COMPANIES

IMMUNOHAEMATOLOGY

Reagents for Forward/Subgrouping

Product	*Description*	*Pack*
Eryclone Anti-A	Murine monoclonal IgM blood grouping reagent for slide and tube tests	5 ml, 10 ml 10 × 5 ml 6 × 10 ml
Eryclone Anti-B	Murine monoclonal IgM blood grouping reagent for slide and tube tests	5 ml, 10 ml 10 × 5 ml 6 × 10 ml
Eryclone Anti-A + B	Murine monoclonal IgM blood grouping reagent for slide and tube tests	5 ml, 10 ml 10 × 5 ml 6 × 10 ml
Eryclone Anti-D	Albumin reacting monoclonal IgG Rho(D) typing reagent for slide and modified tube tests	5 ml, 10 ml 10 × 5 ml, 6 × 10 ml
Eryclone Anti-D	Saline reacting monoclonal IgM Rho(D) typing reagent for slide and tube tests	5 ml, 10 ml 10 × 5 ml, 6 × 10 ml
Rhofinal	Monoclonal IgM + IgG reagent blend for routine typing and confirmation of Rho(D) phenotypes by slide and tube tests	5 ml, 10 ml 10 × 5 ml 6 × 10 ml
Eryscreen	Reagent combipack for ABO grouping and Rho (D)(IgM) typing by slide and tube tests	3 × 5 ml 3 × 10 ml 3 × 12 ml
Eryscreen Plus	Reagent combipack for ABO grouping and Rho (D)(IgM + IgG) typing by slide and tube tests	3 × 10 ml 3 × 12 ml

Contd...

Contd...

Product	*Description*	*Pack*
Erybank Rh-hr control	Negative control for Rho(D) typing and serological applications	5 ml
Erybank Anti-A	Conventional polyclonal IgM reagent for slide and tube tests	5 ml 10 ml
Erybank Anti-B	Conventional polyclonal IgM reagent for slide and tube tests	5 ml 10 ml
Erybank Anti-A, B	Conventional polyclonal IgM reagent for slide and tube tests	5 ml 10 ml
Erybank Anti-D	Conventional polyclonal IgG Rho(D) typing reagent for slide and modified tube tests	5 ml 10 ml
Erybank bovine serum albumin	22% bovine serum albumin for serological applications	5 ml, 10 ml, 10 × 5 ml 6 × 10 ml
Erybank Anti-A_1 lectin	Purified *Dolichos biflorus* seed extract reagent for differentiating A_1 and A_2 subgroups	5 ml
Erybank Anti-H lectin	Purified *Ulex europaeus* seed extract reagent for H antigen determination and subgroup differentiation	5 ml

Reagents for Rh Typing Cross Matching

Product	*Description*	*Pack*
Anti-C + D + E	Monoclonal Rh typing reagent for slide and tube tests	2 ml
Eryclone Anti-C, Anti-c, Anti-E, Anti-e	Murine monoclonal IgM reagents for Rh genotyping	2 ml each
Eryclone Antihuman globulin	Polyspecific reagent (anti-IgG + anti-C3d) for direct and indirect AHG (Coombs') tests	2 ml 5 ml, 10 × 5 ml
Eryclone Monospecific Coombs' sera	Murine monoclonal Anti-C3d antibodies for direct and indirect Coombs' tests	2 ml
Erybank Monospecific Coombs' sera	Polyclonal Anti-IgG antibodies for direct and indirect Coombs' tests	2 ml
Liquipap	Liquid stable papain enzyme for serological applications	5 ml

Reagents for Special Applications

Product	*Description*	*Pack*
Osmosol	Concentrated 20x phosphate buffered saline for immunohaematological applications	25 ml
Agtrol	Appropriately diluted monoclonal Anti-D IgG and red cell preserving solution starter pack for preparation of Coombs' control cells *in situ*	5 ml

Contd...

Contd...

Product	*Description*	*Pack*
Tuliss	Low ionic strength solution for serological applications	5 ml
Erywell	Red cell preserving solution for preparation of cell panels *in situ* for serological applications	20 ml

HAEMATOLOGY

Haematology Reagents

Product	*Description*	*Pack*
Sicklevue	Hb S solubility tests for screening sickle cell anaemia	10 tests

IMMUNOLOGY

Infectious Diseases Reagents

Product	*Description*	*Pack*
Virutex	Latex agglutination slide tests for detection of HBsAg in serum and plasma (sensitivity~10 15 ng/ml)	35/70/ 140 tests
Trepolipin	Modified VDRL reagent for the detection of antilipoidal antibodies in serum and plasma during syphilis	25/50/ 100 tests
Syphfinal	Latex agglutination slide tests for detection of antilipoidal antibodies in serum and plasma during syphilis	25/50/ 100 tests
Carbogen	RPR card tests for detection of antilipoidal antibodies in serum and plasma during syphilis	5 ml 50/100/250 tests
Redgen	TRUST antigen card tests for detection of antilipoidal antibodies in serum and plasma during syphilis	75 tests
Tydal	Ready-to-use, colour coded killed suspension of *S.typhi* 'O', *S.typhi* 'H', *S.paratyphi* 'AH' and *S.paratyphi* 'BH' antigens for slide and tube tests	Set-4 × 5 ml O and H-2 × 5 ml O-5 ml, H-5 ml
Typhochek	Ready-to-use, colour coded killed suspension of *S.typhi* 'O', *S.typhi* 'H', *S.paratyphi* 'AH' and *S.paratyphi* 'BH' antigens for tube tests	4 × 50 ml
Vital widal	Vitally stained smooth suspension of *S.typhi* 'O' *S.typhi* 'H', *S.paratyphi* 'AH' and *S.paratyphi* 'BH' antigens for tube tests	Set-4 × 10 ml O and H-2 × 10 ml
Brucel-A	Smooth killed suspension of *Brucella abortus* antigen for slide and tube tests	5 ml
Brucel-M	Smooth killed suspension of *Brucella melitensis* antigen for slide and tube tests	5 ml

Contd...

Contd...

Product	*Description*	*Pack*
Brucel-RB	Smooth killed suspension for *Brucella abortus* antigen stained with rose bengal dye for slide tests	5 ml
Toxogen	Latex agglutination slide tests for screening and semiquantitation of antibodies to *T. gondii* in serum	10/25 tests
Immutex	Haemagglutination slide tests for detecting heterophile antibodies in serum during infectious mononuclosis	20 tests
Salmonella Positive control	Polyspecific serum control reactive with *S.typhi* and *S.paratyphi* antigens	1 ml
Brucella Positive control	Polyspecific serum control reactive with *Brucella* antigens	1 ml

Fertility Reagents

Product	*Description*	*Pack*
Foretel	Latex agglutination inhibition slide tests for detection of hCG in urine during pregnancy (sensitivity~0.3 IU/ml of hCG)	35/70/ 140 tests
Foresight	Direct latex agglutination slide tests for detection of hCG in urine during pregnancy (sensitivity~ 0.2 IU/ml of hCG)	25/50/ 100 tests

Rheumatology Reagents

Product	*Description*	*Pack*
Rhelax-RF	Latex agglutination slide tests for detection and semiquantitation of IgM rheumatoid factors in serum (sensitivity~10 IU/ml)	10/25/50/100 tests
Rhelax-CRP	Latex agglutination slide tests for detection and semiquantitation of C-reactive protein in serum (sensitivity~0.6 mg/dl)	10/25/50/100 tests
Rhelax-ASO	Latex agglutination slide tests for detection and semiquantitation of Anti-streptolysin 'O' in serum (sensitivity~200 IU/ml)	10/25/50/100 tests
Rhelax-SLE	Latex agglutination slide tests for detection of anti-DNP in serum during SLE	10/25 tests

Other Markers

Product	*Description*	*Pack*
Microtex	Latex agglutination inhibition slide tests for detection of microalbuminuria in urine (sensitivity~25 mg/L)	25 tests

IMMUNOTURBIDIMETRY

Quantia Range

Product	*Description*	*Pack*
Quantia-RF	Quantitative immunoturbidimetric assay for detection of IgM rheumatoid factors in serum	25/50 tests
Quantia-CRP	Quantitative immunoturbidimetric assay for detection of C-reactive protein in serum	25/50 tests
Quantia-CRP-US	Quantitative immunoturbidimetric assay for the ultrasensitive detection of C-reactive protein in serum	25/50 tests
Quantia-ASO	Quantitative immunoturbidimetric assay for detection of Anti-streptolysin 'O' in serum	25/50 tests
Quantia-MA	Quantitative immunoturbidimetric assay for detection of microalbuminuria in urine	25/50 tests
Quantia-IgM	Quantitative immunoturbidimetric assay for detection of IgM antibodies in serum	25/50 tests
Quantia-IgA	Quantitative immunoturbidimetric assay for detection of IgA antibodies in serum	25/50 tests
Quantia-IgG	Quantitative immunoturbidimetric assay for detection of IgG antibodies in serum	25/50 tests
Quantia-IgE	Quantitative immunoturbidimetric assay for detection of IgE antibodies in serum	25/50 tests
Qunatia-AT III	Quantitative immunoturbidimetric assay for detection of antithrombin III in human serum/plasma	25/50 tests
Quantia-C3	Quantitative immunoturbidimetric assay for detection of C3 complement component in human serum	25/50 tests
Quantia-C4	Quantitative immunoturbidimetric assay for detection of C4 complement component in human serum	25/50 tests
Quantia-Lpa	Quantitative immunoturbidimetric assay for quantitation of lipoprotein a (Lpa) in serum	50 tests

HAEMOSTASIS

Reagents for Routine Screening

Product	*Description*	*Pack*
Uniplastin	Ready-to-use, calcified, sensitive rabbit brain thromboplastin reagent for PT determination in plasma, (ISI~1.0)	5 ml, 12 × 5 ml
Liquiplastin	Ready-to-use, calcified rabbit brain thromboplastin reagent for PT determination plasma, (ISI~1.5)	5 ml 12 × 5 ml

Contd...

Contd...

Product	*Description*	*Pack*
Liquicelin-E	Ready-to-use, cephaloplastin reagent with ellagic acid as an activator for APTT determination in plasma	3 ml, 12 × 3 ml
Liquiplastin Precision Combipack	Combipack of ready-to-use liquid stable liquiplastin (PT) reagent and 3.2% (0.109 M) buffered trisodium citrate blood collection anticoagulant	25 tests
Uniplastin Precision Combipack	Combipack of ready-to-use liquid stable uniplastin (PT) reagent and 3.2% (0.109 M) buffered trisodium citrate blood collection anticoagulant	25 tests
Liquicelin-E Precision Combipack	Combipack of ready-to-use liquid stable Liquicicelin-E (APTT) reagent and 3.2% (0.109 M) buffered trisodium citrate blood collection anticoagulant	25 tests
Calcium chloride	Recalcification solution for use with APTT reagent (0.02 M)	10 ml, 10 × 10 ml
Profact	3.2% (0.109 M) buffered trisodium citrate anticoagulant for blood collection in routine coagulation assays and ESR by Westergren method	20 ml

Reagents for Special Applications

Product	*Description*	*Pack*
Refractin	0.02 M calcium choloride recalcification solution containing heparin neutralising substance for use with two stage thromboplastin reagent	10 ml
Fibroscreen	Lyophilised bovine thrombin reagent for qualitative estimation and evaluation of use with two stage thromboplastin reagent	6 × 1 ml
Fibroscreen	Lyophilised bovine thrombin reagent for qualitative estimation and evaluation of fibrinogen in plasma	6 × 1 ml
Fibroquant	Reagent for quantitative estimation of fibrinogen in plasma	20 tests
Tulip-XL FDP	Latex agglutination slide tests for detection and semiquantitation of cross-linked fibrin degradation products in plasma (sensitivity~200 ng/ml)	15 tests
LADS	DRVVT tests for screening and confirmation of lupus anticoagulants	10 tests
LA reference plasma	Control plasma for calibration and quality control of DRVVT based LA detection tests	0.5 ml
Plasmatrol-H I/II	Normal and abnormal control plasma for calibration and quality control for with use with PT, APTT, TT and fibrinogen assays	Level 1-6 × 1 ml Level II- 6 × 1 ml

MICROBIOLOGY

Pouched Media for Essential Microbiology

Product	Description	Pack
Instaprep nutrient agar	General culture medium for bacteriology	20 × 15 ml pouches
Instaprep MacConkey agar	Selective and differential medium for *Enterobacteria*	20 × 15 ml pouches
Instaprep Sabourauds dextrose agar	Agar for the cultivation and growth of fungi	20 × 15 ml pouches
Instaprep CLED agar	Preferred medium for urinary bacteriology, differentiation and colony court of isolated organism	20 × 15 ml pouches
Instaprep Muller-hinton agar	Preferred antibiotic suspecting medium	20 × 15 ml pouches
Instaprep SS agar	Differential agar for *Salmonella* and *Shigella*	20 × 15 ml pouches

Culture Systems

Product	Description	Pack
Easy bact	Ready-to-use sterile CLED agar slopes for quantitation of urinary bacteria and identification and differentiation of organisms	12 slants
Blood culture bottle	Trypticase soy broth with SPS	6 × 50 ml

Mycobacteriology Reagents

Product	Description	Pack
Lyfectol	Mucolytic, disinfectant, specimen pretreatment and buffering system for AFB staining and culture	12 tests
Novachrom	Rapid two step cold AFB stain	125 tests
Combicult	Ready-to-use combipack of LJ solid and Kirchner's liquid medium for *Mycobacterium tuberculosis* isolation	One set
Mycocult	Ready-to-use LJ solid medium for *Mycobacterium tuberculosis* isolation	6 slants
Sensicult primary	LJ solid media based, five primary drug panel for MTB sensitivity tests with 2 controls and sample preparation facility	One set
Sensicult secondary	LJ solid media based, six secondary drug panel for MTB sensitivity tests with control and sample preparation facility	One set

Contd...

Contd...

Product	*Description*	*Pack*
ADA-MTB	Colorimetric tests for the determination of adenosine deaminase activity in serum, plasma and biological fluids	15 tests

RAPID TESTS

Fertility

Product	*Description*	*Pack*
Clue (Device)	Rapid one-step device for detection of hCG in urine during pregnancy (sensitivity~10 mIU/ml of hCG)	25 tests, 100 tests
Clue (Dipstick)	Rapid one-step dipstick for detection of hCG in urine during pregnancy (sensitivity~10 mIU/ml of hCG)	25 tests, 100 tests
Insight	Immunoconcentration flow through device for detection of hCG and simultaneous semiquantitation (sensitivity~25 mIU/ml of hCG)	25 tests
Gravicheck (Device)	Rapid one-step device for detection of hCG in serum, urine during pregnancy (sensitivity~10 mIU/ml of hCG)	25 tests
Graviscreen (Dipstick)	One-step tests for detection of hCG in urine (sensitivity~20 mIU/ml of hCG)	25 tests
Ferticheck-LH	Rapid tests for hLH in urine, serum (sensitivity~40 mIU/ml of hLH)	10 tests, 25 tests

Infectious Disease

Product	*Description*	*Pack*
Virucheck (Device)	Rapid one-step device for the detection of HBsAg in serum, plasma (sensitivity~0.5 ng/ml of HBsAg ad/ay subtypes)	25 tests
Virucheck (Dipstick)	Rapid one-step dipstick for the detection of HBsAg in serum, plasma (sensitivity~0.5 ng/ml of HBsAg ad/ay subtypes)	25 tests
Paracheck Pf (Device)	Rapid one-step device for the detection of *P. falciparum* specific HRP 2 antigen in whole blood	10 tests, 25 tests

Infectious Disease

Product	*Description*	*Pack*
Paracheck Pf (Dipstick)	Rapid one-step dipstick for the detection of *P. falciparum* specific HRP 2 antigen in whole blood	10 tests, 25 tests

Contd...

Contd...

Product	*Description*	*Pack*
Parascreen (Device)	Rapid immunochromatographic tests for the detection of *P.falciparum* specific pLDH antigen and pan specific pLDH antigen in whole blood	10 tests
Paramax-3 (Device)	Rapid immunochromatographic tests for the detection of *P.falciparum* specific HRP-2 antigen and *P.vivax* specific pLDH antigen and pan specific pLDH antigen in whole blood	10 tests
Virdict 3	Rapid tests for the simultaneous and differential detection of HIV 1/2, HCV and HBsAg in serum, plasma and whole blood	10 tests, 50 tests
Retroquic	Rapid immunoconcentration flow through tests for HIV 1 and HIV 2 antibodies	10 tests, 50 tests 100 tests
Retrocheck-WB	Third generation, rapid immunochromatographic for HIV 1/2 antibodies	10 tests, 50 tests 100 tests
Syphicheck-WB (Device)	Third generation rapid tests for detection of *T. pallidum* specific antibodies in serum plasma and whole blood	10 tests, 25 tests
Syphicheck-WB (Dipstick)	Third generation rapid tests for detection of *T. pallidum* specific antibodies in serum plasma and whole blood	10 tests,
Dengucheck-WB	Rapid tests for detection of IgM and IgG antibodies to dengue virus in serum, plasma and whole blood	10 tests, 25 tests
Leptocheck-WB	Rapid for detection of IgM antibodies to leptospira in serum, plasma and whole blood	10 tests, 25 tests

Cancer Markers

Product	*Description*	*Pack*
Cancheck-CEA	Rapid tests for CEA in serum, plasma, whole blood. Sensitivity $\geq$ 5 ng/ml CEA	10 tests, 25 tests
Cancheck	Rapid test for AFP in serum, plasma whole blood. Sensitivity $\geq$ 25 ng/ml AFP	10 tests, 25 tests
Cancheck-FOBT	Rapid test for faecal occult blood in faeces. Sensitivity ~ 200 ng/gm of faeces	10 tests, 25 tests
Cancheck-PSA	Rapid tests for PSA in serum, plasma, whole blood. Sensitivity $\geq$ 4 ng/ml PSA	10 tests, 25 tests

Cardiac Marker

Product	*Description*	*Pack*
Cardiacheck -Trop 1	Rapid tests for the detection of cardiac trophnin in serum, plasma, whole blood. Sensitivity 0.1 ng/ml	3 tests 10 tests, 25 tests
Cardiacheck -Myo	Rapid tests for the detection of myoglobin in serum, plasma, whole blood. Sensitivity 100 IU/ml	10 tests, 25 tests

Contd...

Contd...

Product	*Description*	*Pack*
Cardiacheck -M + T	Rapid tests for the simultaneous detection of troponin 1 and myoglobin in serum, plasma, whole blood	3 tests 10 tests, 25 tests

BIOCHEMISTRY

Enzymes

Product	*Description*	*Pack*
Acid phosphatase	Liquid stable, modified King's colorimetric end point method	10 tests
Acid phosphatase	Kinetic method using α naphthyl phosphate for the determination of acid phosphatase acitivity in serum	10 × 2 ml, 30 × 2 ml
Alkaline phosphatase	Liquid stable, modified Kind and King's colorimetric end point method for the determination of alkaline phosphatase activity in serum	15 tests
Alkaline phosphatase (DEA buffer)	Liquid stable, kinetic method using p-nitro phenyl phosphate for the determination of alkaline phosphatase activity in serum	25 ml, 75 ml
Alkaline phosphatase (AMP buffer)	Liquid stable, kinetic method using p-nitro phenyl phosphate for the determination of alkaline phosphatase activity in serum	25 ml, 75 ml
α-Amylase	Liquid stable, direct substrate method using Gal-G2-CNP for the determination of α-amylase activity in serum, plasma and urine	2 × 10 ml, 2 × 30 ml
Creatinine kinase (CK) (NAC act)	Liquid stable, modified IFCC method for the determination of CK activity in serum	2 × 10 ml, 2 × 25 ml
Creatinine kinase -(MB) (CK-MB)	Liquid stable, modified IFCC (immunoinhibition) method for the determination of CK-MB activity in serum	2 × 10 ml, 2 × 25 ml
γ-Glutamyl transferase	Liquid stable, kinetic method using carboxy substrate for the determination of γ-glutamyl transferase activity in serum	1 × 25 ml 1 × 75 ml
Lactate dehydrogenase (P-L)	Liquid stable, modified IFCC, pyruvate to lactate method for the determination of lactate dehydrogenase activity in serum	25 ml
SGOT (ASAT)	Liquid stable, Reitmen and Frankel's (colorimetric) method for the determination of SGOT (ASAT) activity in serum	40 assay
SGOT (ASAT)	Liquid stable, modified IFCC (UV kinetic) method for the determination of SGOT (ASAT) activity in serum	25 ml, 75 ml
SGPT (ALAT)	Liquid stable, Reitmen and Frankel's (colorimetric) method for the determination of SGPT (ALAT) activity in serum	40 assay

Contd...

Contd...

Product	*Description*	*Pack*
SGPT (ASAT)	Liquid stable, modified IFCC (UV kinetic) method for the determination of SGPT (ALAT) activity in serum	25 ml, 75 ml

Substrates

Product	*Description*	*Pack*
Cholesterol	Liquid stable, CHOD/PAP method for the determination of cholesterol in serum, plasma	75 ml 2 × 75 ml, 2 × 150 ml
HDL-cholesterol	Liquid stable, PEG precipitation method for the determination of HDL cholesterol in serum, plasma	10 ml, 75 ml
Glucose	Liquid stable, glucose oxidase/peroxidase method for the determination of glucose in serum, plasma and CSF	2 × 150 ml 3 × 150 ml 1000 ml
Triglycerides	Liquid stable, GPO/PAP method for the determination of triglycerides in serum, plasma	25 ml 75 ml, 2 × 75 ml
Urea	Liquid stable, end point method using diacetyl monoxime for the determination of urea in serum, plasma	25 ml, 50 ml
Urea	Liquid stable, modified Berthelot method for the determination of triglycerides in serum, plasma and urine	75 ml, 3 × 75 ml
Urea	Liquid stable, GLDH (UV kinetic) method for the determination of urea in serum, plasma	75 ml 2 × 75 ml
Uric acid	Liquid stable, phosphotungstate method for the determination of uric acid in serum, plasma	10 ml, 25 ml 25 ml
Uric acid	Liquid stable, uricase/PAP method for the determination of uric acid in serum, plasma	75 ml 2 × 75 ml

Other Metabolities

Product	*Description*	*Pack*
Albumin	Liquid stable, BCG method for the determination of albumin in serum, plasma	1 × 150, 2 × 150
Bilirubin direct and total	Liquid stable, modified Jendrassik and Grof's method for the determination of direct and total bilirubin in serum	30 ml, 75 ml
Calcium	Liquid stable, Arsenazo III method for the determination of calcium in serum, plasma	75 ml
Calcium	Liquid stable, O-cresolphthalein complexone method for the determination of calcium in serum, plasma	2 × 35 ml 2 × 75 ml
Creatinine	Liquid stable, alkaline picrate end point method for the determination of creatinine in serum, plasma	15 tests, 2 × 75 ml
Creatinine	Liquid stable, modified Jaffe's kinetic method using alkaline picrate for the determination of creatinine in serum, urine	2 × 75 ml

Contd...

Contd...

Product	*Description*	*Pack*
Microproteins	Liquid stable, colorimetric method using pyrogallol red for the determination of proteins in urine and CSF	25 ml
Total protein	Liquid stable, Biuret method for the determination of total protein in serum, plasma	1 × 150 ml, 2 × 150 ml

Metals and Ions

Product	*Description*	*Pack*
Chloride	Liquid stable, colorimetric thiocyanate method for the determination of chloride in serum	75 ml 3 × 75 ml
Copper	Liquid stable, colorimetric method using Di-Br-PAESA for the determination of copper in serum	2 × 12.5 ml
Elyte 2	Liquid stable, combo kit for the determination of sodium and potassium in serum	15 ml
Elyte 3	Liquid stable, combo kit for the determination of sodium, potassium and chloride in serum	15 ml
Iron and TIBC	Colorimetric method of using ferrozine for the determination of iron and total iron-binding capacity in serum	35 ml
Magnesium	Liquid stable, colorimetric method using calmagite for the determination of magnesium in serum	2 × 12.5 ml
Phosphorus (inorganic)	Liquid stable, molybdate UV method for the determination of inorganic phosphorus in serum, plasma and urine	75 ml
Phosphorus (inorganic)	Liquid stable, modified Gomorri's (colorimetric) method for the determination of inorganic phosphorus in serum, plasma and urine	10 tests
Potassium	Liquid stable, colorimetric (turbidimetric) method using tetra phenyl boron for the determination of potassium in serum	15 tests
Sodium	Liquid stable, colorimetric method for the determination of sodium in serum	15 tests
Zinc	Liquid stable, colorimetric method using nitro-PAPS for the determination of zinc in serum	25 ml

ELISA

Infectious Disease

Product	*Description*	*Pack*
Qualisa HIV 1/2	Elisa tests for the simultaneous detection of HIV 1/2 antibodies in human serum/plasma	96 tests 192 tests, 496 tests
Qualisa HCV 3.0	Third generation Elisa for the detection of antibodies of HCV antibodies in human serum/plasma	96 tests, 192 tests 496 tests

Contd...

Contd...

Product	*Description*	*Pack*
Qualisa HBsAg	Elisa tests for the detection of HBsAg in human serum/plasma. Sensitivity 0.05 ng/ml of HBsAg	96 tests 192 tests, 496 tests
Heptra HBsAg	Visual rapid HBsAg elisa for human serum or plasma. Sensitivity 0.25 ng/ml of HBsAg	48 tests

Fertility

Product	*Description*	*Pack*
Vectra hCG	Visual rapid Elisa for the detection of hCG in urine. Sensitivity 25 mlU/ml of hCG	48 tests

INSTRUMENTATION

Haemostasis

Product	*Description*	*Pack*
Hemostar	Single channel coagulometer with turbophotometric detection	1 No
Hemostar XF	Single channel coagulometer with turbophotometric detection and direct result display through on-board printer	1 No
Coalab 6000	Fully automated turbodensitometric, opto-mechanical coagulation analyser with automatic adjustment and magnetic stir bar to homogenise the sample	1 No

Clinical Chemistry

Product	*Description*	*Pack*
Screen Master 3000	Auto analyser for clinical chemistry biochemical tests, enzymes and drug assay with on-board printer	1 No
Map Lab plus	Auto analyser for clinical chemistry, biochemical tests, enzymes and drug assay with built in microwell strip reader port, with printer	1 No
Clin check plus	Mini analyser for clinical chemistry is an interferential filter photometer with powered handling, managed by microprocessor.	1 No

Immunoturbidimetry

Product	*Description*	*Pack*
Quantiamate	Optimised analyser preprogrammed for Quantia reagents adaptable for turbidimetric immunoassay reagents. Back up analyser for routine chemistries	1 No

BIOCHEMISTRY

Haemoglobin Estimation

Product	*Description*	*Pack*
Hemocor-C	Liquid stable 25x concentrated cyanmethaemoglobin reagent for the determination of Hb in whole blood	5 × 12.2 ml
Hemocor-D	Liquid stable, ready-to-use cyanmethaemoglobin reagents for the determination of Hb in whole blood	1000 ml
Hemocor standard	Liquid stable, haemoglobin standard for quantitative estimation of Hb in whole blood	10 ml
Hemosafe-SLS	Liquid stable cyanide free, SLS reagent for the determination of Hb in whole blood	1000 ml

Controls and Calibrators

Product	*Description*	*Pack*
Flamecal	Trilevel calibrating solution for flame photometer for Na + , K, LI +	3 × 250 ml
Bili CAL	Trilevel lyophilised bilirubin calibrator for photometric validation	3 × 1 ml
Hb CAL	Trilevel liquid stable haemoglobin calibrator for photometric validation	3 × 10 ml
Patholyte	Lyophilised assayed abnormal serum control for validation of clinical biochemistry reagents	1 ml 3 ml 6 × 1 ml
Normalyte	Lyophilised assayed normal serum control for validation of clinical biochemistry reagents	1 ml 3 ml, 6 × 1 ml
Multidet	Concentrated 10x neutral lab detergent for cleaning glassware, labware and instruments	1000 ml

OTHERS

Microkrom Microscopy Stains

Product	*Description*	*Pack*
Giemsa stain	Ready-to-use Romanowsky stain for thick and thin blood smears	250 ml

Contd...

Contd...

Product	*Description*	*Pack*
Leishman stain	Ready-to-use Romanowsky stain for thick and thin blood smears	250 ml
Field stain	Ready-to-use Romanowsky stain for thick and thin blood smears	250 ml
Field stain	Ready-to-use Romanowsky stain for thick and thin blood smears	250 ml
Weiss buffer	Concentrated 200x buffer solution for use with Romanowsky stains	10 ml

Special Tests

Product	*Description*	*Pack*
Haemospot	Two field standard guaiac method for detecting occult blood in stool	50 tests
G-SIX	Methaemoglobin reduction based method for screening and quantitation of G-6PD deficiency	Monopack, 10 × 1 tests

RAPID TESTS

In Pipeline

Description
Rapid tests for the detection of malaria Pv/Pf
Rapid tests for the detection of antibodies to *M. tuberculosis*
Rapid tests for the detection of IgM antibodies to *S.typhi*
Rapid tests for the detection of IgM antibodies of *Brucella SPP*
Rapid tests for the simultaneous detection of troponin, myoglobin and CK MB
Rapid tests for the detection of antibodies to cysticercosis
Rapid tests for the detection of XL FDP.

IMMUNOTURBIDIMETRY

In Pipeline

Description
Turbidimetric immunoassay for the quantitation of XL FDP in human plasma
Turbidimetric immunoassay for the quantitation of protein C in human plasma
Turbidimetric immunoassay for the quantitation of protein S in human plasma

BIOCHEMISTRY

In Pipeline

Description
Enzymatic assay for the quantitation of G-6PD activity
Ion exchange resin-based tests for the quantitation of glycated haemoglobin

MANUFACTURING LOCATIONS

Tulip Diagnostics (P) Ltd
Plot Nos. 92/96; Phase II C, Verna Industrial Estate,
Verna, Goa-403722, India Tel: (0832) 2783508-10 Fax: (0832) 2783511
E-mail: tulip@sancharnet. in

Microxpress
A Division of Tulip Diagnostics (P) Ltd, Plot Nos. S-126, Phase III B,
Verna Industrial Estate Verna, Goa-403722, India, Tel: (0832) 2782847 Fax: (0832) 2782836
E-mail:Tulip@sancharnet. in

Orchid Biomedical Systems
Plot Nos. 88/89, Phase II C, Verna Industrial Estate, Verna, Goa-403722, India
Tel: (0832) 2783140, 2782140 Fax: (0832) 2783139
E-mail: orchid@sancharnet.in

Qualpro Diagnostics
Plot Nos. 88/89 Phase II C, Verna Industrial Estate,
Verna, Goa, 403722, India Tel: (0832) 2783140, Fax: (0832) 2783139
E-mail: qualpro@sancharnet.in

Zephyr Biochemical
Plot Nos. M 46-67, Phase IIIB, Verna Industrial Estate,
Verna, Goa, 403722, India, Tel: (0832) 2783140 Fax: (0832) 2783139
Email: zephyr@sacharnet.in

Coral Clinical Systems
Plot Nos. 92/96, phase IIC, Verna Industrial estate,
Verna, Goa, 403722, India, Tel: (0832) 2782124, 2782125 Fax: (0832) 2782123
Email: coral@sacharnet.in

Lilac Medicare (P) Ltd. Provides Complete ELISA/CLIA Based Solutions for the Medical Diagnostic Laboratories
Lilac Medicare (P) Ltd. B Sungold, 303 Sher E Punjab, Mahakali Caves Road,
Andheri (E), Mumbai-400093

THYROID IMMUNOASSAYS

- 3rd Generation ultrasensitive assays
- Microwell and coated tube assays
- Breakable wells/individual tube
- Manual and automated kit format
- Simple methodology
- Ready-to-use reagents
- Long shelf-life
- Read at 450 nm/read tubes at 405 nm
- Different pack sizes
- US-FDA approved products

Thyroid Microwell ELISA

Product	*Pack size*	*Description*	*Calibrators*	*Assay time*
Tri-iodothyronine	96 Tests 192 Tests 480 Tests 960 Tests	3rd Generation Ultrasensitive Microwell Elisa	Six human serum based ready-to-use calibrators	75 Minutes
Free Tri-iodothyronine (FT3)	96 Tests 192 Tests 480 Tests	3rd Generation Ultrasensitive Microwell Eiisa	Six human serum based ready-to-use calibrators	75 Minutes
Thyroxine (T4)	96 Tests 192 Tests 480 Tests 960 Tests	3rd Generation Ultrasensitive Microwell Elisa	Six human serum based ready-to-use calibrators	75 Minutes
Free Thyroxine (FT4)	96 Tests 192 Tests 480 Tests	3rd Generation Ultrasensitive Microwell Elisa	Six human serum based ready-to-use calibrators	75 Minutes
Thyrotropin (TSH / US-TSH)	48 Tests 96 Tests 192 Tests 480 Tests 960 Tests	3rd Generation Streptavidin-Biotin Based ultrasensitive Microwell Elisa	Seven human serum based ready-to-use calibrators	75 Minutes
Thyroset (T3 + T4 + TSH)	192 Tests 480 Tests 960 Tests	3rd Generation Ultrasensitive Microwell Elisa	Six human serum based ready-to-use calibrators	75 Minutes
Anti-Thyroglobulin (Tg)	48 Tests 96 Tests	3rd Generation Streptavidin-Biotin Based ultrasensitive Microwell Elisa	Six human serum based ready-to-use calibrators	105 Minutes
Anti-Thyroglobulin (Tg)	48 Tests 96 Tests	Indirect Solid Phase Microwell Elisa	Six ready-to-use calibrators and two controls	65 Minutes
Anti-Thyroperoxidase (TPO)	48 Tests 96 Tests	3rd Generation Streptavidin-Biotin Based ultrasensitive Microwell Elisa	Six human serum based ready-to-use calibrators	105 Minutes

Contd...

Contd...

Product	Pack size	Description	Calibrators	Assay time
Anti-Thyroperoxidase (TPO)	48 Tests 96 Tests	Indirect Solid Phase Microwell Elisa	Six ready-to-use calibrators and two controls	65 Minutes

Thyroid Microwell Elisa

Product	Pack Size	Description	Calibrators	Assay time
T-Uptake	96 Tests	3rd Generation Ultrasensitive Microwell Elisa	Six human serum based ready-to-use calibrators	75 Minutes
T3 + T4 MAPS*	48 + 48 Tests	3rd Generation Ultrasensitive Microwell Elisa	Six human serum based ready-to-use calibrators	75 Minutes
T4 + TSHMAPS*	48 + 48 Tests	3rd Generation Ultrasensitive Microwell Elisa	Six human serum based ready-to-use calibrators	75 Minutes

* MAPS: Multiple Analyte Plate System

Thyroid Coated Tube Assay

Product	Pack size	Description	Calibrators	Assay time
TRUECOAT Tri-iodothyronine (T3)	50 Tests 100 Tests 200 Tests 500 Tests 1000 Tests 2000 Tests	3rd Generation Coated tube Solid Phase EIA*	Six human serum based ready to use calibrators	80 Minutes
TRUECOAT Thyroxine (T4)	50 Tests 100 Tests 200 Tests 500 Tests 1000 Tests 2000 Tests	3rd Generation Coated tube Solid Phase EIA*	Six human serum based ready to use calibrators	80 Minutes
TRUECOAT Thyrotropin (TSH)	50 Tests 100 Tests 200 Tests 500 Tests 1000 Tests 3000 Tests	3rd Generation Streptavidin-Biotin Based Coated Tube EIA*	Seven human serum based ready to use calibrators	80 Minutes

* Read Colorimetrically at 405 nm

FERTILITY IMMUNOASSAYS

- 3rd Generation ultrasensitive assays
- Microwell and coated tube assays
- Breakable wells/individual tube
- Manual and automated kit format
- Simple methodology
- Ready-to-use reagents
- Long shelf-life
- Read at 450 nm/read tubes at 405 nm
- Different pack sizes
- US-FDA approved products

Pituitary Hormone Microwell Elisa

Product	*Pack size*	*Description*	*Calibrators*	*Assay time*
Lutropin (LH)	96 Tests 192 Tests	3rd Generation Streptavidin-Biotin Based ultrasensitive Microwell Elisa	Six human serum based ready-to-use calibrators	75 Minutes
Follitropin (FSH)	96 Tests 192 Tests	3rd Generation Streptavidin-Biotin Based ultrasensitive Microwell Elisa	Six human serum based ready-to-use calibrators	75 Minutes
Prolactin (PRL)	48 Tests 96 Tests 192 Tests	3rd Generation Streptavidin-Biotin Based ultrasensitive Microwell Elisa	Six human serum based ready-to-use calibrators	75 Minutes
LH + FSH MAPS	96 Tests	3rd Generation Streptavidin-Biotin Based ultrasensitive Microwell Elisa	Six human serum based ready-to-use combi calibrators	75 Minutes
Human Chorionic Gonadotrophin (β-hCG)	48 Tests 96 Tests 192 Tests	3rd Generation Streptavidin-Biotin Based ultrasensitive Microwell Elisa	Six human serum based ready-to-use calibrators	75 Minutes

PITUITARY HORMONE COATED TUBE ASSAY

LH + FSH	50 Tests	3rd Generation Streptavidin-Biotin Based ultrasensitive Coated tube EIA*	Six human serum based ready-to-use combi calibrators	80 Minutes
Prolactin (PRL)	50 Tests	3rd Generation Streptavidin-Biotin Based ultrasensitive Coated tube EIA*	Six human serum based ready-to-use calibrators	80 Minutes

* Read colorimetrically at 405 nm

STEROID HORMONE MICROWELL ELISA

Product	*Pack size*	*Description*	*Calibrators*	*Assay time*
Testsosterone	48 Tests 96 Tests	Competitive Assay Microwell Elisa	Five ready to use calibrators	75 Minutes
Androstenedione	48 Tests 96 Tests	Competitive Assay Microwell Elisa	Six ready to use calibrators	75 Minutes
DHEA-S	48 Tests 96 Tests	Competitive Assay Microwell Elisa	Five ready to use calibrators	30 Minutes
1-*β Estradiol(E2)	48 Tests 96 Tests	Competitive Assay Microwell Elisa	Five ready to use calibrators	2 Hours 30 Minutes
Estriol (E3)	48 Tests 96 Tests	Competitive Assay Microwell Elisa	Five calibrators lyophilized	75 Minutes
Progesterone	48 Tests 96 Tests	Competitive Assay Microwell Elisa	Six ready to use calibrators	75 Minutes
17-OH Progesterone	48 Tests 96 Tests	Competitive Assay Microwell Elisa	Five calibrators lyophilized	75 Minutes
Cortisol	48 Tests 96 Tests	Competitive Assay Microwell Elisa	Five ready to use calibrators	75 Minutes

ONCO IMMUNOASSAYS

- 3rd Generation ultrasensitive assays
- Microwell and coated tube assays
- Breakable wells/individual tube
- Manual and automated kit format
- Simple methodology
- Ready-to-use reagents
- Long shelf-life
- Read at 450 nm/read tubes at 405 nm
- Different pack sizes
- US-FDA approved products

Tumour Marker Microwell Elisa

Product	*Pack size*	*Description*	*Calibrators*	*Assay time*
Prostate specific antigen (PSA)	48 Tests 96 Tests 192 Tests	3rd Generation Streptavidin-Biotin Based Elisa	Six human serum based ready to use calibrators	475 Minutes
Alpha Fetoprotein (AFP)	48 Tests 96 Tests	3rd Generation Streptavidin-Biotin Based Elisa	Six human serum based ready to use calibrators	75 Minutes
Carcino Embryonic Antigen (CEA)	48 Tests 96 Tests	3rd Generation Streptavidin-Biotin Based Elisa	Six human serum Based ready to use calibrators	75 Minutes
Human Chorionic Gonadotrophin (*β-hCG)	48 Tests 96 Tests 192 Tests	3rd Generation Streptavidin-Biotin Based Elisa	Six human serum Based ready to use calibrators	75 Minutes

Contd...

Contd...

Product	*Pack size*	*Description*	*Calibrators*	*Assay time*
Ferritin	48 Tests 96 Tests	Indirect Solid Phase Enzyme Immunometric assay	Six ready to use calibrators	65 Minutes
CA 125	48 Tests 96 Tests	3rd Generation Streptavidin-Biotin Based Elisa	Five ready to use calibrators	3 Hours 30 Minutes
CA 15-3	48 Tests 96 Tests	3rd Generation Streptavidin-Biotin Based Elisa	Five ready to use calibrators	2 Hours 30 Minutes
CA 19-9	48 Tests 96 Tests	3rd Generation Streptavidin-Biotin Based Elisa	Six ready to use calibrators	3 Hours 30 Minutes
CA 242	48 Tests 96 Tests	3rd Generation Streptavidin-Biotin Based Elisa	Five ready to use calibrators	3 Hours 30 Minutes
NSE	48 Tests 96 Tests	3rt Generation Streptavidin-Biotin Based Elisa	Five ready to use calibrators	3 Hours 30 Minutes
Free PSA	48 Tests 96 Tests	3rd Generation Streptavidin-Biotin Based Microwell Elisa	Five ready to use calibrators	2 Hrs 30 Minutes

Tumour Markers Coated Tube Assay

Prostate Specific Antigen (PSA)	50 Tests	3rd Generation Streptavidin-Biotin Based Coated Tube EIA	Six human serum based ready to use calibrators	75 Minutes
Alpha Fetoprotein (AFP)**	50 Tests	3rd Generation Streptavidin-Biotin Based Coated Tube EIA	Six human serum based ready to use calibrators	80 Minutes
Carcino Embryonic Antigen (CEA)**	50 Tests	3rd Generation Streptavidin-Biotin Based coated Tube EIA	Six human serum based ready to use calibrators	80 Minutes

TORCH IMMUNOASSAYS

- Two different assay principles:
  1. Interference corrected elisa
  2. Immunocapture elisa
- Accurate and reproducible results
- Breakable wells
- Quantitative and qualitative assays
- Internationally accepted reporting units
- Long shelf-life
- Different pack sizes
- TORCH screen: Single kit for estimation of ToRCH panel IgG to ToRCH panel IgM

TORCH Panel Microwell ELISA

Product	*Pack size*	*Description*	*Calibrators*	*Assay time*
Toxoplasma IgG	24 Tests 48 Tests 96 Tests 192 Tests 480 Tests	Interference Corrected Microwell Elisa	Six human serum based ready-to-use calibrators	375 Minutes
Toxoplasma IgM	24 Tests 48 Tests 96 Tests 192 Tests 480 Tests	Interference Corrected Microwell Elisa	Three human serum based ready-to-use controls	70 Minutes
Rubella IgG	24 Tests 48 Tests 96 Tests 192 Tests 480 Tests	Interference Corrected Microwell Elisa	Six human serum based ready-to-use calibrators	375 Minutes
Rubella IgM	24 Tests 48 Tests 96 Tests 192 Tests 480 Tests	Interference Corrected Microwell Elisa	Three human serum based ready-to-use controls	100 Minutes
Cytomegalovirus IgG	24 Tests 48 Tests 96 Tests 192 Tests 480 Tests	Interference Corrected Microwell Elisa	Three human serum based ready-to-use controls	35 Minutes
Cytomegalovirus IgM	24 Tests 48 Tests 96 Tests 192 Tests 480 Tests	Interference Corrected Microwell Elisa	Three human serum based ready-to-use controls	70 Minutes
Herpes simplex virus (HSV-1 IgG)	24 Tests 48 Tests 96 Tests 192 Tests 480 Tests	Interference Corrected Microwell Elisa	Three human serum based ready-to-use use controls	35 Minutes

Contd...

Contd...

Product	*Pack size*	*Description*	*Calibrators*	*Assay time*
Herpes simplex virus (HSV-1 IgM)	24 Tests 48 Tests 96 Tests 192 Tests 480 Tests	Interference Corrected Microwell Elisa	Three human serum based ready-to-use controls	70 Minutes
Herpes simplex virus (HSV- 2 IgG)	24 Tests 48 Tests 96 Tests 192 Tests 480 Tests	Interference Corrected Microwell Elisa	Three human serum based ready-to-use controls	35 Minutes
Herpes simplex virus (HSV-2 IgM)	24 Tests 48 Tests 96 Tests 192 Tests 480 Tests	Interference Corrected Microwell Elisa	Three human serum based ready-to-use controls	70 Minutes
TORCH Screen (24 tests each)				
Product	*Pack size*	*Description*	*Calibrators*	*Assay time*
TORCH IgG Screen	24 Tests Each	Interference Corrected Microwell Elisa	Human serum based ready-to-use calibrators and controls	35 Minutes
TORCH IgM Screen	24 Tests Each	Interference Corrected Microwell Elisa	Human serum based ready-to-use controls	70 Minutes

TORCH Combination ELISA

Product	*Pack size*	*Description*	*Calibrators*	*Assay time*
Herpes simplex virus HSV (1 + 2) IgG	24 Tests 48 Tests 96 Tests 192 Tests 480 Tests	Interference Corrected Microwell Elisa	Three human serum based ready-to-use controls	35 Minutes
Herpes simplex virus HSV (1 + 2) IgM	24 Tests 48 Tests 96 Tests 192 Tests 480 Tests	Interference Corrected Microwell Elisa	Three human serum based ready-to-use controls	70 Minutes
Herpes simplex virus HSV (1 + 2) IgG + IgM	48 Tests 96 Tests 192 Tests 480 Tests	Interference Corrected Microwell Elisa	Three human serum based ready-to-use controls	35 Minutes

HEPATITIS MARKER IMMUNOASSAYS

- Complete range of viral hepatitis markers-A, B, C, D, E
- 3rd Generation ELISA
- Immunocapture IgM assays
- Available in 24, 48, 96 tests pack sizes
- Ready-to-use calibrators and controls
- Qualitative and quantitative assays
- Breakable wells
- ISO 9001 certification
- EC approved

Hepatitis Marker Microwell ELISA

Product	*Pack size*	*Description*	*Controls*	*Assay time*
HAV Ab	24 Tests 48 Tests 96 Tests	Competitive Microwell Elisa	Human serum based ready-to-use controls	140 Minutes
HAV IgM	24 Tests 48 Tests 96 Tests	Immunocapture Microwell Elisa	Human serum based ready-to-use controls	140 Minutes
HBcAb	24 Tests 48 Tests 96 Tests	Competitive Microwell Elisa	Human serum based ready-to-use controls	105 Minutes
HBc IgM Qualitative	24 Tests 48 Tests 96 Tests	Immunocapture Microwell Elisa	Human serum based ready-to-use controls	140 Minutes
HBc IgM Quantitative	96 Tests	Immunocapture Microwell Elisa	Six ready-to-use calibrators	140 Minutes
HBeAb	24 Tests 48 Tests 96 Tests	Neutralisation Based Microwell Elisa	Human serum based ready-to-use controls	200 Minutes
HBeAg	24 Tests 48 Tests 96 Tests	Antigen Sandwich Based Microwell Elisa	Human serum based ready-to-use controls	140 Minutes
HBe Ag/Ab	48 Tests 96 Tests	Antigen Sandwich/ Competitive Microwell Elisa	Human serum based ready-to-use controls	200 Minutes
HBsAb	24 Tests 48 Tests 96 Tests	Antigen Sandwich Based Microwell Elisa	Five ready-to-use calibrators	140 Minutes
HBsAg one-step	96 Tests	Antigen Sandwich	Human serum based	140 Minutes
Simultaneous	192 Tests	Based Microwell Elisa	ready-to-use controls	75 Minutes
HBsAg Sequential	96 Tests 192 Tests	Antigen Sandwich Based Microwell Elisa	Human serum based ready-to-use controls	140 Minutes 80 Minutes

Contd...

Contd...

Product	*Pack size*	*Description*	*Controls*	*Assay time*
HBsAg Confirmatory	48 Tests	Antigen Sandwich Based Microwell Elisa	Human serum based ready-to-use controls	300 Minutes
HCVAb	96 Tests 192 Tests	Second Antibody Sandwich Microwell Elisa	Human serum based ready-to-use controls	105 Minutes
HCV IgM	96 Tests 192 Tests	Second Antibody Sandwich Microwell Elisa	Human serum based ready-to-use controls	140 Minutes
HCV Profile Elisa Confirmatory	8 × 12 Tests	Second Antibody Sandwich Microwell Elisa	Human serum based ready-to-use controls	140 Minutes
HDV Ab	24 Tests 48 Tests 96 Tests	Competitive Microwell Elisa	Human serum based ready-to-use controls	140 Minutes 96 Tests
HDV Ag	24 Tests 48 Tests 96 Tests	Antigen Sandwich Microwell Elisa	Human serum based ready-to-use controls	200 Minutes
HDV IgG	24 Tests 48 Tests 96 Tests	Second Antibody Sandwich Microwell Elisa	Human serum based ready-to-use controls	140 Minutes
HDV IgM	24 Tests 48 Tests 96 Tests	Immunocapture Microwell Elisa	Human serum based ready-to-use controls	140 Minutes
HEV Ab	24 Tests 48 Tests 96 Tests	Second Antibody Sandwich Microwell Elisa	Human serum based ready-to-use controls	105 Minutes
HEV IgG	24 Tests 48 Tests 96 Tests	Second Antibody Sandwich Microwell Elisa	Human serum based ready-to-use controls	140 Minutes
HEV IgM	24 Tests 48 Tests 96 Tests	Second Antibody Sandwich Microwell Elisa	Human serum based ready-to-use controls	140 Minutes

AUTOIMMUNE IMMUNOASSAYS

- Latests differentiated antigen assay technology
- Breakable wells
- Long shelf-life
- Simple methodology
- Reproducible results
- High sensitivity and reproducible results
- US-FDA approved
- DIN EN 46001 certification
- Quality control assessment schemes from:
  - UK NEQAS (Great Britain)
  - RCPA (Australia)
  - CAP survey (USA)
  - Instand (Germany)

Autoimmune ELISA Kits

Product	*Pack size*	*Description*	*Calibrators*	*Assay time*
Total ANA Screen	48 Tests 96 Tests	Indirect Solid Phase EIA	Ready-to-use controls	65 Minutes
ANA Combi (8 Antigen)	6 Profile	Indirect Solid Phase EIA	Ready-to-use controls	65 Minutes
Anti-dsDNA	48 Tests 96 Tests	Indirect Solid Phase EIA	Ready-to-use calibrators and controls	65 Minutes
Anti-Cardiolipin IgG/IgM	48 Tests 96 Tests	Indirect Solid Phase EIA	Ready-to-use calibrators and controls	65 Minutes
Anti-Cardiolipin IgA	48 Tests 96 Tests	Indirect Solid Phase EIA	Ready-to-use calibrators and controls	65 Minutes
Anti-SS-A	48 Tests 96 Tests	Indirect Solid Phase EIA	Ready-to-use calibrators and controls	65 Minutes
EIA Anti-SS-B	48 Tests 96 Tests	Indirect Solid Phase EIA	Ready-to-use calibrators and controls	65 Minutes
ElAAnti-Sm	48 Tests 96 Tests	Indirect Solid Phase EIA	Ready-to-use calibrators and controls	65 Minutes
EIA Anti-Sm/RNP	48 Tests 96 Tests	Indirect Solid Phase EIA	Ready-to-use calibrators and controls	65 Minutes
EIA Anti-Scl-70	48 Tests 96 Tests	Indirect Solid Phase EIA	Ready-to-use calibrators and controls	65 Minutes
EIA Anti-Jo-1	48 Tests 96 Tests	Indirect Solid Phase EIA	Ready-to-use calibrators and controls	65 Minutes
EIA Anti-ssDNA	48 Tests 96 Tests	Indirect Solid Phase EIA	Ready-to-use calibrators and controls	65 Minutes
Anti-Phospholipid Screen	48 Tests 96 Tests	Indirect Solid Phase EIA	Ready-to-use calibrators and controls	65 Minutes
Anti-Insulin	48 Tests 96 Tests	Indirect Solid Phase EIA	Ready-to-use calibrators and controls	65 Minutes

Contd...

Contd...

Product	*Pack size*	*Description*	*Calibrators*	*Assay time*
Anti-β2-Microglobulin	48 Tests 96 Tests	Indirect Solid Phase EIA	Ready-to-use calibrators and controls	65 Minutes
P-ANCA (MPO)	48 Tests 96 Tests	Indirect Solid Phase EIA	Ready-to-use calibrators and controls	65 Minutes
C-ANCA (PR 3)	48 Tests 96 Tests	Indirect Solid Phase EIA	Ready-to-use calibrators and controls	65 Minutes
ANCA COMBI (P + C)	48 Tests 96 Tests	Indirect Solid Phase EIA	Ready-to-use controls	65 Minutes
Micro-Albumin	48 Tests 96 Tests	Indirect Solid Phase EIA	Ready-to-use calibrators and controls	45 Minutes

OTHER IMMUNOASSAYS

- Breakable wells
- Simple methodology
- Ready-to-use reagents
- Long shelf-life
- Read at 450 nm
- Different pack sizes
- US-FDA approved products
- ISO 9001 certification

Other ELISA

Product	*Pack size*	*Description*	*Calibrators*	*Assay time*
Insulin	48 Tests 96 Tests	3rd Generation Streptavidin-Biotin Based Microwell Elisa	Six human serum based lyophilized calibrators	2 Hrs 15 Minutes
Human Growth Hormone (GH) Moe-GH-096	48 Tests 96 Tests	3rd Generation Streptavidin-Biotin Based Microwell Elisa	Six human serum based ready-to-use calibrators	75 Minutes
Digoxin	48 Tests 96 Tests	3rd Generation Streptavidin-Biotin Based Microwell Elisa	Six human serum based ready-to-use calibrators	60 Minutes
Anti-*H.pylori* IgG	48 Tests 96 Tests	3rd Generation Streptavidin-Biotin Based Microwell Elisa	Six human serum based ready-to-use calibrators	105 Minutes
Anti-*H.pylori*/IgM	48 Tests 96 Tests	3rd Generation Streptavidin-Biotin Based Microwell Elisa	Six human serum based ready-to-use calibrators	105 Minutes

Contd...

Contd...

Product	*Pack size*	*Description*	*Calibrators*	*Assay time*
Anti-*H.pylori* IgA	48 Tests 96 Tests	3rd Generation Streptavidin-Biotin Based Microwell Elisa	Six human serum based ready-to-use calibrators	105 Minutes
Syphilis IgG + IgM	96 Tests	Direct antigen Selection EIA	Three ready-to-use controls	70 Minutes
Syphilis IgG	96 Tests	Direct Antigen Selection EIA	Three ready-to-use controls	70 Minutes
Syphilis IgM	96 Tests	Direct Antigen Selection EIA	Three ready-to-use controls	70 Minutes

LIQUITECH QUALITY CONTROL PACKAGES

- Referral/accuracy quality control sera (Ex. QC)
- Precision quality control sera (in QC)
- Liquid and lyophilised format
- Human and animal matrix formats
- Assayed and unassayed formats
- Different pack sizes
- Long shelf-life with high batch-to-batch consistency

Referral/Accuracy Control

Product	*Pack size*	*Level*	*Format*	*Matrix*
Seronorm™ Immunoassay	12 × 3 ml	Level 1	Lyophilised	Human
Seronorm™ Immunoassay	12 × 3 ml	Level 2	Lyophilised	Human
Seronorm™ Immunoassay	12 × 3 ml	Level 3	Lyophilised	Human
Seronorm™ Human	10 × 5 ml	Level 1	Lyophilised	Human
Seronorm™ Human	10 × 5 ml	Level 2	Lyophilised	Human
Seronorm™	10 × 5 ml	Normal	Lyophilised	Animal
Pathonorm™ H	10 × 5 ml	High	Lyophilised	Animal
Pathonorm™ L	10 × 5 ml	Low	Lyophilised	Animal
Seronorm™ Lipid	12 × 3 ml	Normal	Lyophilised	Animal
Seronorm™ Hb/GI	50 × 1 ml	Level 1	Liquid	Animal
Seronorm™ Hb/GI	50 × 1 ml	Level 2	Liquid	Animal
Seronorm™ Hb/GI	2 × 3 × 1 ml	Level 1/2	Liquid	Animal
Seronorm™ Bilirubin Paediatric	6 × 3 ml	Normal	Lyophilised	Human
Seronorm™ Protein	6 × 1 ml	Normal	Lyophilised	Human
Seronorm™ Protein High	6 × 1 ml	High	Lyophilised	Human

Contd...

Contd...

Product	*Pack size*	*Level*	*Format*	*Matrix*
Seronorm™ Protein Low	6 × 1 ml	Low	Lyophilised	Human
Seronorm™ Lipoprotein	4 × 3 ml	Normal	Liquid	Human
Seronorm™ CRP	12 × 1 ml	Level 1	Liquid	Human
Seronorm™ CRP	12 × 1 ml	Level 2	Liquid	Human
Seronorm™ CRP	6 × 2 × 1 ml	Combi	Liquid	Human
Seronorm™ Urine	10 × 5 ml	Level 1	Lyophilised	Human
Seronorm™ Urine	10 × 5 ml	Level 2	Lyophilised	Human
Seronorm™ TE Urine	10 × 5 ml		Lyophilised	Human
Seronorm™ TE Urine Blank	10 × 5 ml	Blank	Lyophilised	Human
Seronorm™ TE Serum	6 × 3 ml	Level 1	Lyophilised	Human
Seronorm™ TE Serum	6 × 3 ml	Level 2	Lyophilised	Human
Seronorm™ TE WB	10 × 5 ml	Level 1	Lyophilised	Human
Seronorm™ TE WB	10 × 5 ml	Level 2	Lyophilised	Human
Seronorm™ TE WB	10 × 5 ml	Levels	Lyophilised	Human
Seronorm™ Pharmaca Blank	10 × 5 ml	Blank	Lyophilised	Animal
Seronorm™ Pharmaca	10 × 5 ml	Level 1	Lyophilised	Animal
Seronorm™ Pharmaca	10 × 5 ml	Level 2	Lyophilised	Animal

Referral/Accuracy Control (Ex. QC)

Seronorm™ PSA	6 × 1 ml	Level 1	Lyophilised	Human
Seronorm™ PSA	6 × 1 ml	Level 2	Lyophilised	Human
Seronorm™ Cardiac Marker	10 × 3 ml	Level!	Lyophilised	Human
Seronorm™ Cardiac Marker	10 × 3 ml	Level 2	Lyophilised	Human
Seronorm™ Prenatal	6 × 2 ml	Level 1	Lyophilised	Human
Seronorm™ Prenatal	6 × 2 ml	Level 2	Lyophilised	Human
Seronorm™ Prenatal	6 × 2 ml	Level	Lyophilised	Human

Precision Control (In. QC)

Autonorm™ Human	10 × 8 ml	Level 1	Liquid	Human
Autonorm™ Human	10 × 8 ml	Level 2	Liquid	Human
Autonorm™ Human	6 × 10 ml	Normal	Lyophilised	Human
Autonorm™ Human H	6 × 10 ml	High	Lyophilised	Human
Autonorm™	6 × 10 ml	Level 1	Lyophilised	Animal

Contd...

Contd...

Autonorm™	6 × 10 ml	Level 2	Lyophilised	Animal
Autonorm™	6x10 ml	Level 3	Lyophilised	Animal
Autonorm™ Hormone M	10 × 3 ml	Level 1	Lyophilised	Human
Autonorm™ Hormone M	10 × 3 ml	Level 2	Lyophilised	Human
Autonorm™ Hormone F	10 × 3 ml	Level 1	Lyophilised	Human
Autonorm™ Hormone F	10 × 3 ml	Level 2	Lyophilised	Human
Autonorm™ Tumour Marker	12 × 1 ml		Lyophilised	Human

Reconstituted stability/Open Vial stability at –20°C : 30 Days
Reconstituted stability/Open Vial stability at 2 to 8°C: 14 Days Shelf-life: 2 Years

LIQUITECH VARIFIX

- New generation micropipettes
- Durable, nonplastic components
- Fully autoclavable
- Both variable and fixed volume in one pipette
- Digital variable volume setting controller
- No gear jamming
- Separate fixed volume controllers
- 1/3rd plunger activation force
- Air-vent technology
- Easy calibration
- Very few components
- Easy to maintain

CAPP Varifix Single Channel Standard Micropipette

Product	*Description*	*Range*	*Controller*	*Colour Code*
Single Channel Standard 0.2-2 µl	New Generation Fixed and Variable Micropipette	0.2-2 µl	V1F1	
Single Channel Standard 1-10 µl	New Generation Fixed and Variable Micropipette	1-10 µl 1-10 µl	V1F1 V1F3	
Single Channel Standard 5-50 µl	New Generation Fixed and Variable Micropipette	5-50 µl 5-50 µl 5-50 µl	V1F1 V1F3 V1F5	
Single Channel Standard 10-100 µl	New Generation Fixed and Variable Micropipette	10-100 µl 10-100 µl 10-100 µl	V1F1 V1F3 V1F5	
Single Channel Standard 25-200 µl	New Generation Fixed and Variable Micropipette	25-200 µl 25-200 µl 25-200 µl	V1F1 V1F3 V1F5	
Single Channel Standard 100-1000 µl	New Generation Fixed and Variable Micropipette	100-1000 µl 100-1000 µl 100-1000 µl	V1F1 V1F3 V1F5	

Contd...

Contd...

Single Channel Standard 1-5 ml	New Generation Fixed Micropipette	1-5 ml	VOF5	

CAPP Varifix Single Channel Short Micropipette

Product	*Description*	*Range*	*Controller*	*Colour code*
Single Channel Short 1-10 µl	New Generation Fixed and Variable Micropipette	1-10 µl 1-10 µl	V1F1 V1F3	
Single Channel Short 5-50 µl	New Generation Fixed and Variable Micropipette	5-50 µl 5-50 µl 5-50 µl	V1F1 V1F3 V1F5	
Single Channel Short 10-100 µl	New Generation Fixed and Variable Micropipette	10-100 µl 10-100 µl 10-100 µl	V1F1 V1F3 V1F5	
Single Channel Short 25-200 µl	New Generation Fixed and Variable Micropipette	25-200 µl 25-200 µl 25-200 µl	V1F1 V1F3 V1F5	
Single Channel Short 100-1000 µl	New Generation Fixed and Variable Micropipette	100-1000 µl 100-1000 µl 100-1000 µl	V1F1 V1F3 V1F5	

CAPP Varifix Single Channel Colourline Micropipette

Product	*Description*	*Range*	*Controller*	*Colour code*
Single Channel Colourline 0.2-2 µl	New Generation Fixed and Variable Micropipette	0.2-2 µl	V1F1	
Single Channel Colourline 1-10 µl	New Generation Fixed and Variable Micropipette	1-10 µl 1-10 µl	V1F1 V1F3	
Single Channel Colourline 5-50 µl	New Generation Fixed and Variable Micropipette	5-50 µl 5-50 µl 5-50 µl	V1F1 V1F3 V1F5	
Single Channel Colourline 10-100 µl	New Generation Fixed and Variable Micropipette	5-50 µl 5-50 µl 5-50 µl	V1F1 V1F3 V1F5	
Single Channel Colourline 25-200 µl	New Generation Fixed and Variable Micropipette	25-200 µl 25-200 µl 25-200 µl	VIF1 V1F3 V1F5	
Single Channel Colourline 100-1000 µl	New Generation Fixed and Variable Micropipette	100-1000 µl 100-1000 µl 100-1000 µl	V1F1 V1F3 V1F5	

Contd...

Contd...

Product	*Description*	*Range*	*Controller*	*Colour code*
Single Channel Colourline 1-5 ml	New Generation Fixed Micropipette	1-5 ml	V0F5	

In addition to CAPP Colourline Micropipettes, also available under similar specifications CAPP Softline Micropipettes under the same category of Varifix new generation micropipettes.

CAPP Varifix Multichannel Micropipette

Product	*Description*	*Range*	*Controller*	*Colour code*
8 Channel 1 -10 µl	New Generation Fixed and Variable Micropipette	1-10 µl 1-10 µl	V1F1 V1F3	
8 Channel 5-50 µl	New Generation Fixed and Variable Micropipette	5-50 µl 5-50 µl 5-50 µl	V1F1 V1F3 V1F5	
8 Channel 25-200 µl	New Generation Fixed and Variable Micropipette	25-200 µl 25-200 µl 25-200 µl	V1F1 V1F3 V1F5	
8 Channel 50-300 µl	New Generation Fixed and Variable Micropipette	50-300 µl 50-300 µl	V1F1 V1F3	
12 Channel 1-10 µl	New Generation Fixed and Variable Micropipette	1-10 µl 1-10 µl	V1F1 V1F3	
12 Channel 5-50 µl	New Generation Fixed and Variable Micropipette	5-50 µl 5-50 µl 5-50 µl	V1F1 V1F3 V1F5	
12 Channel 25-200 µl	New Generation Fixed and Variable Micropipette	25-200 µl 25-200 µl 25-200 µl	V1F1 V1F3 V1F5	
12 Channel 50-300 µl	New Generation Fixed and Variable Micropipette	50-300 µl 50-300 µl	V1F1 V1F3	
16 Channel 1-10	New Generation Fixed and Variable Micropipette	1-10 µl 1-10 µl	V1F1 V1F3	
16 Channel 5-50 µl	New Generation Fixed and Variable Micropipette	5-50 µl 5-50 µl 5-50 µl	V1F1 V1F3 V1F5	

CAPP VARIFIX-HLA TERASAKI PIPETTE

Product	*Description*	*Range*	*Controller*	*Colour code*
Terasaki 6 Channel 1-10 µl	New Generation Fixed and variable Micropiptte	1-10 µl 1-10 µl	V1F1 VIG3	

TRANSPLANTATION DIAGNOSTICS

- Microplates with pre-loaded Anti-HLA sera
- Complete reagents and accessories for HLA typing
- Lymphocyte isolation and other accessories
- SSP-typing systems
- SSO-typing systems
- Free software

Pre-Dropped HLA Typing Sera

Product	*Pack*	*Description*
Lymphotype ABC 60 (60 Specificities)	6 plates	Microtests plate with pre-dropped HLA-ABC antisera for typing of one specimen
Lymphotype ABC 72 (72 Specificities)	6 plates	Microtests plate with pre-dropped HLA-ABC antisera for typing of one specimen
Lymphotype AB 72 AN (72 Specificities)	6 plates	Microplate with pre-dropped HLA-AB antisera for typing of one specimen
Lymphotype ABC 72 (72 Specificities)	6 plates	Microtests plate with pre-dropped HLA-ABC antisera for orienta typing of one specimen
Lymphotype ABC 120 (120 Specificities)	3 × 2 plates	Microtests plate with pre-dropped HLA-ABC antisera for typing of one specimen
Lymphotype ABC 120 (120 Specificities)	3 × 2 plates	Microplates with 120 pre-loaded HLA-AB antisera for typing of one specimen
Lymphotype ABC 144 (144 Specificities)	3 × 2 plates	Microplate with pre-dropped HLA-ABC antisera for typing of one specimen
Lymphotype AB 144 (144 Specificities)	3 × 2 plates	Microplate with pre-dropped HLA-ABA antisera for typing of one specimen
Lymphotype ABC 180 (180 Specificities)	2 × 3 plates	Microtests plate with pre-dropped HLA-ABC antisera for typing of one specimen
Lymphotype B 27 single	6 plates	Microtests plate with pre-dropped antisera for determination of HLA B 27 for one specimen each
Lymphotype B 27	6 plates	Microtests plate with pre-dropped antisera for determination of HLA B 27 for five specimen each
Lymphotype B 27 special	6 plates	Microtests plate with pre-dropped antisera for determination of HLA B 27 for three specimen each
Lymphotype DR 60 (60 Specificities)	6 plates	Microtests plate with absorbed HLA-DR-DQ antisera for typing of one specimen

Contd...

Contd...

Lymphotype DR 72 (72 Specificities)	6 plates	Micratests plate with absorbed HLA-DR.-DQ antisera for typing of one specimen
Lymphoscreen ABC 60	6 plates	Microtests plate for detection of HLA-ABC antibodies in one specimen (1 package = 6 plates)
Lymphoscreen DR 30 × 2	6 plates	Microtests plate for detection of HLA-Class II antibodies in two specimen each

HLA-SSO/SSP TYPING SYSTEMS

Product	*Pack*	*Description*
Biotests ELPHA Reagent Set	1 set	Washing buffers and staining reagents for HLA - DNA typing of 12 specimen with the ELPHA system
Biotests ELPHA Bulk Reagent Set	1 set	Washing buffers and staining reagents for HLA - DNA typing with the ELPHA system
Biotests ELPHA DQB	1 kit	Microtests plates for HLA - DNA - DQ typing of 12 specime with the ELPHA system
Biotests ELPHA DQB Bulk	1 kit	Microtests plates for HLA - DNA - DQ typing of 120 specimen with the ELPHA system
Biotests ELPHA DRB Low Resolution	1 kit	Microtests plates for HLA- DNA - DR Low resolution typing of 12 specimen with the ELPHA system
Biotests ELPHA DRB Low Resolution Bulk	1 kit	Microtests plates for HLA- DNA - DR Low resolution typing of 120 specimen with the ELPHA system
Biotests ELPHA DRB High Resolution	1 kit	Microtests plates for HLA- DNA - DRB High resolution typing of 6 specimen with the ELPHA system
Biotests ELPHA DR2 Subtyping	1 kit	Microtests plates for HLA- DNA - DR2 subtyping of 12 specimen with the ELPHA system
Biotests ELPHA DR3/11/6 Subtyping	1 kit	Microtests plates for HLA-DNA-DR3/11/6 subtyping of 12 specimen with the ELPHA system
Biotests ELPHA DR4 Subtyping	1 kit	Microtests plates for HLA-DNA - DR4 subtyping of 12 specimen with the ELPHA system
Biotests ELPHA DR 8 + 12 Subtyping	1 kit	Microtests plates for HLA- DNA - DR8 + 12 subtyping of 12 specimen with the ELPHA system
Biotests ELPHA DRB 3 Subtyping	1 kit	Microtests plates for HLA-DNA - DRB3 subtyping of 12 specimen with the ELPHA system
Biotests ELPHA HLA-AB	1 kit	Microtests plates for HLA-A and HLA- B typing of 30 specimen with the ELPHA system
Biotests ELPHA HLA - C	1 kit	Microtests plates for HLA-C typing of 30 specimen with the ELPHA system
Biotests DRB SSP Kit	1 kit	23 amplifications for the determination of DR1-18 DR51, DR52, DR53, incl. negative control, 24 tests
Biotests DQB SSP Kit	1 kit	21 amplifications for the determination of DQ1-9 incl. negative control, 24 tests

Contd...

Contd...

Biotests HLA-A SSP Kit	1 kit	24 amplifications for the determination of HLA- A*01 -A*80, incl. negative control, 24 tests
Biotests HLA-B SSP Kit	1 kit	24 amplifications for the determination of HLA- B*07 - B*82, Bw4, Bw6, incl. negative control, 24 tests
Biotests HLA-C SSP Kit	1 kit	16 amplifications for the determination of HLA- Cw* 01-Cw*18, incl .negative control, 24 tests
Biotests HLA-A2, 28 Sero Add	1 kit	4 amplifications for the differentiation of HLA-A2 A68, A69, incl. negative control, 24 tests
Biotests HLA-ABC SSP Kit	1 kit	96 amplifications for the determination of HLA-A, B and C, incl. negative control, 24 tests
Biotests HLA-AB DR SSP Kit	1 kit	96 amplifications for the determination of HLA-A, B and DR, incl. negative control, 24 tests

Lyophilised Sera for HLA Typing, HLS Control Sera and Accessories

Product	*Pack*	*Description*
Anti-HLA-Sera Category A	0.5 ml	Lyophilized sera for HLA-Typing
Anti-HLA-Sera Category Z	0.5 ml	Lyophilized sera for HLA-Typing
Control-HLA (Positive)	0.5 ml	Lyophilized positive control for HLA-Typing
Control-HLA (Negative)	0.5 ml	Lyophilized negative control for HLA-Typing
Control-HLA-DR (Positive)	0.5 ml	Lyophilized positive control for HLA-DR typing
Complement (Rabbit)	5 ml 10 × 1 ml	Lyophilized rabbit Complement for HLA-Typing
Lymphobeads HLA Class I (CD 8)	5 ml	Immunomagnetic beads for isolation of T-cells for HLA-ABC Typing
Lymphobeads HLA Class II (CD 19)	5 ml	Immunomagnetic beads for isolation of B-cells for HLA - DQ/-DR Typing
Biotests MSD	1 piece	Magnet for immunomagnetic separation (for 6 tubes)
Lymphoflot	100 ml 300 ml	Density gradient medium
Nylon Wool	25 g	For separation of lymphocytes in T and B cells
Lymphostabil	100 ml	Preservation of lymphocytes
Hanks solution	100 ml 500 ml	Free of Ca and Mg
Microtests Plates, 60 Wells	480 Plates	Empty plates for HLA-Typing
Microtests Plates, 2 Wells	20 Plates	Empty plates for HLA-Typing
Cover Oil	1000 ml	Paraffin oil of low viscosity
Cover Glasses	2 ×50 Units	

IMMUNOASSAY AUTOMATION

- Fully automated walkaway systems
- Highly accurate and reproducible results
- True open system
- Single tests as well as multi-tests capability
- Zero consumables
- User friendly/software
- Easy start up and shut down procedure
- Application support
- Complete engineering back up

Triturus: Fully Automated Walkaway Enzyme Immunoassay Automation

Triturus is a true open, fully automated walkaway immunoassay system, designed exclusively for handling multiple parameters in a clinical laboratory. Introduced in the world market after years of meticulous research by diagnostic Grifols, Triturus is absolutely unique in its capabilities as a true open immunoassay system. With increasing complexities in clinical laboratories of today, Triturus stands apart from all other immunoassay systems in handling complex laboratory situation in an easy and simple way with very high degree of operator flexibility. With multi tests and continuous loading of sample and reagent facilities, guided by an extremely simple and effective software, Triturus becomes an indispensable part of any laboratory involved in immunoassays.

Triturus is an engineering marvel and a class of its own.

Triturus

- Fully automated system
- Continuous loading facility
- True open system
- Multitests capability
- Fixed needle/disposable tip option
- Primary tube sampling
- Unique run verification check
- Automatic scheduling and management of different batches
- Online waste disposal
- User- friendly software
- Data storage facility

ALPHA PRIME: MULTIPARAMETRIC IMMUNOASSAY SYSTEM

Alpha Prime, the first multiparametric immunoassay walkaway system, has the ability to consolidate the entire laboratory immunoassay workload in a true open format. With its unique well-by-well management technique, Alpha Prime delivers accurate and reproducible results similar to the high end closed systems.

Designed and launched by SFRI laboratories of France after years of extensive research, Alpha Prime is the first true protocol system in the open immunoassay automation category. Alpha Prime is the only system of its kind with capability of automating all immunoassays in a single system.

The CLIA upgradation option makes Alpha Prime absolutely versatile true open system, even from the technology point of view and gives the user real value for money.

Alpha Prime

- Fully automated system
- 18 Different assays per run
- On-board refrigeration
- True open architecture
- Well-by-well assay management
- True protocol system
- CLIA upgradability option
- Sever probes
- Internal/external teflon coating
- Complete walkaway
- One protocol per strip
- High quality of results

Index

A

Abnormal urine composition in disease 83
ABO grouping 336
ABO testing procedures 324
Achromobacteriaceae 1110
Acid-fast particles 1098
Actinomyces 1119
Actinomycetaceae 1061
Actinomycetales 1061
Activated partial thromboplastin time 310
Acute leukaemias 260
Acute myelomonocytic leukaemias 257
Addison's disease 602
Adenohypophysis 453
ADH 461
Adrenal (suprarenal) gland 463
Adrenal medulla 506
Adrenal steroids 504
Adrenocortical inhibition test 526
Adverse donor reactions 382
Aedes aegypti 780
Aedes albopticus 780
Aerobacter aerogenes 1141
Aerobic spore forming bacilli 1086
AFB culture and isolation 1100
AFB smear 1094
Agglutination tests 1137
Alcaligens fecalis 1110
Aldosterone 505
Alkaline phosphatase isoenzymes 679
Alpha prime 1273
Altered laboratory results in normal pregnancy 440
Amenorrhea 477
Amniocentesis and amniotic fluid analysis 404
Amoebiasis 104
ANA profile 826
  ANA profile positivities 826
ANA profile testing 822
ANA testing 812
Anaemia 202, 1019
Analytical balance 23
Andrade's indicator 1072
Androgens 480
Androstenedione 517
Aneuploidy 1197
  hyperploidy 1197
    tetrasomy 1197
    trisomy 1197
  hypoploidy 1197
    monosomy 1197
    nullisomy 1197
Angina pectoris 711
Anovulation 479
Anterior pituitary 453
Anti-cardiolipin IgM/IgG 841
Anti-human globulin reagents 353
Anti-insulin antibodies 469
Anti-phospholipid syndrome 308
Anti-retroviral therapy 961
Antibody excess zone 1143
Antibody titration studies 362
Anticardiolipin IgA 846
Anticoagulant agents 283
Anticoagulants 197
Antihuman globulin test 348
Antineutrophil cytoplasmic antibodies 827
Antinuclear antibodies 809
Antiphospholipid antibodies 834
Antiphospholipid antibodies and pregnancy 835
Antiphospholipid screen 852
Antiphospholipid syndrome 832
Aortic stenosis 711
Application of HIV testing 957
Ascaris lumbricoides 137
Aspergillus 1121
Aspiration of intrathoracic masses 1050
Assay optimisation 1148
Atomic mass 49
Atomic number 49
Atomic weight 49
Australia antigen HBSAG 856
Autoimmune disorders and ANA 800
Autoimmune ELISA kits 1262
Autoimmune haemylotic anaemia 242
Automation cytology 1060
Automation in blood gas analysis 724
Automation in clinical chemistry 666
Automation in histopathology 1045
  2LE (shandon) 1046
  autosharp 5 (shandon) 1046
  autoslip (shandon) 1047
  duplex (shandon) 1046
  histocentre (shandon) 1046
  hypercentre (shandon) 1045
  hypercut (shandon) 1046

linistain GLX (shandon) 1046
varistain 12 (shandon) 1047
varistain 24 (shandon) 1047
Automation in turbidimetry 1190

B

Bacillaceae 1061
Bacillus anthracis 1086
Bacillus cereus 1087
Bacillus pyocyaneus 1115
Bacillus subtilis 1087
Bacteriaceae 1115
Bacterial cell constituents 1062
Bacterial growth 1063
Bacterial toxins 1063
Bacteriodaceae 1061
Balantidiasis 108
Balantidium coli 108
Barr bodies 1197
Beer's law 617,618
Bence Jones protein tests 55
Best's carmine stain 1042
Bile pigment 63, 609
Bile salts 63
Bilirubin 609
Binding proteins 491
Blackwater fever 121
Bleeding time 265
Blood 181, 223
Blood and its products 388
Blood cell counts 204
Blood collection system 199
Blood cultures 1080
Blood donors 380
Blood film examination 213
Blood flagellate diseases of man 123
American leishmaniasis 123
Chagas' disease 124
kala-azar 123
oriental sore 123
sleeping sickness 123
Blood formation 216
Blood gases 717
blood gas symbols 718
Blood glucose 647
Blood group antibodies 322
Blood group testing in microplates 348
Blood lymphocyte culture 1193
Blood pH 722
Blood transfusion 380
Blood transfusion complications 389
Body fluid and tissue flagellates 161
Bone marrow examination 219
Bone marrow examination and reporting 220
Bordetella pertussis 1114
Borrelia 1117
Borrelia duttonii 1118
Borrelia recurrentis 1118
Borrelia vincenti 1117
Bouin's fluid 1030
Broken bands 735
Bromsulphalein (sulphobromophthalein)
excretion test 611
Brucella 1114
Brucella abortus 779
Brucella melitensis 775
Brucellaceae 1061, 1113
Brucellosis 779
Brucellosis positive control 779
Buffer solution 44

C

C-reactive protein 1159
Calcium in urine 67
Cancer markers 1245
Capillary fragility test of Hess 264
CAPP varifix multichannel micropipette 1268
CAPP varifix single channel colourline micropipette 1267
CAPP varifix single channel short micropipette 1267
Carcinoembryonic antigen 1004
Cardiac marker 1245
Cardiac troponin-1 710
Carnoy's fluid 1030
Case histories 485
Causes of abnormal glucose levels 649
Causes of jaundice 609
Causes of neutropenia 255
Cedar wood oil 1066
Cell division 1192
meiosis 1192
mitosis 1192
Cell sensitization 367
Celloidin 1031
Centrifuge 23
types of 24
Cerebrospinal fluid 391
Ceruloplasmin stain 1134
Cestoda 147
Chaga's disease 130
Chemical examination of semen 409
Chemiluminescence 749
advantages of chemiluminescence technology 751
components of chemiluminescent system 749
enhanced pulse chemiluminescence 751
Chloride 74, 657
Cholesterol 613
Cholesterol: LDL and VLDL 644
Cholinesterase stain 1134
Chorionic gonadotrophin 580
Chronic lymphocytic leukaemia 261
Chronic myeloid leukaemia 261
CK and CK-MB reagent system design 708
CK isoenzymes 707
Classical complement pathway 351
Clearance tests 88
CLED agar 1073
Clinical disorders of mineralocorticoids 506
isolated hypoaldosteronism 506
primary hyperaldosteronism 506
secondary hyperaldosteronism 506
Clostridia 1084
Clostridium botulinum 1086
Clostridium novyi 1085
Clostridium septicum 1085
Clostridium welchii 1085
Clot retraction 268
Clot-based assays 310
Clotting mechanism 275
Clotting process 835
Coagulation time 266
Common respiratory disorders 413
bronchial asthma 415
bronchiectasis 415
chronic bronchitis 416
heart disease 417
lung abscess 416
mycobacteria 413
mycotic (fungal) disease 413
pathological fungi 413
pneumoconiosis 416
pneumonia 416
pulmonary alveolar proteinosis 417
pulmonary embolism 416
viral infections 417
Common skin tests 1124
Complete blood count 208
Complications in malaria 186
Composition on bile 449
Concentration test 86
Conjugated bilirubin 611
Consumer Protection Act 17
Control sera 624
Copper 662
Copper urine 664
Corticotrophin 460, 525
Cortisol 522
Corynebacteriaceae 1061
Corynebacterium acne 1088
Corynebacterium hoffmanni 1087
Corynebacterium xerosis 1088
Creatine kinase 698
Cryptorchidism 474
Crystal violet amyloid stain 1044
Crystals 81
CSF rhinorrhoea and otorrhoea 392
Culture systems 1243
Cushing's syndrome 474
Cyclophyllidean tapeworms of man 147
Cystine 69
Cytology 1048
Cytomegalovirus 939
Cytomegalovirus infection 938

D

Deep or systemic mycoses 1120
Actinomyces 1120
Coccidioides 1121
Cryptococcus neoformans 1121
Histoplasma capsulatum 1121
Nocardia 1120
Delirium tremens 711
Density 49

Dermatomyositis 809
Dermatophytes 1119
Determination of microalbuminuria 1168
Device ICT urine/serum pregnancy test 438
Dexamethasone 526
Diabetes mellitus 598
 classification and causes 599
 diagnosis 600
 diagnostic tests 600
 screening tests 599
Diabetic control index 603
Diagnosis for APLS 838
Diagnosis of infectious mononucleosis 256
Diagnosis of sickle cell anaemia 246
Diagnosis of sickle cells trait 246
Diagnosis of unstable Hb haemoglobinopathy 248
Diaphoresis 711
Differential cell count 221
Dilute blood clot lysis time 301
Diphtherioid bacilli 1087
Direct anti-human globulin test 354
Disinfection 29
Disorders of the pituitary system 463
 gonadotrophin disorders 463
 growth hormone disorders 463
 prolactin disorders 463
 TSH disorders 463
Disseminated intravascular coagulation 305
Distribution of malaria infection 183
Distribution of malarial disease 185
DNA 946
Donovania granulomatis 1115
Drabkin's reagent 200
Dracunculus medinensis 144
Drug affecting laboratory tests values 1199
Drug induced immune thrombocytopenia 305
Drugs affect colour of urine 1219
Drugs affecting cerebrospinal fluid studies 1224
Drugs affecting results of blood studies 1199
Drugs affecting results of fecal studies 1219
Drugs affecting results of haematologic and serologic studies 1220
Drugs affecting results of urine studies 1211
dRVVT test 313
Dubin-Johnson syndrome 611
Dysentery bacilli 1113
Dyspnoea 711

E

Ear discharge cultures 1081
Early pregnancy loss 432
Echinococcus granulosus 150
Ectopic pregnancy 431
EIA assay formats 953
Electron configuration 49
Electron microscope 23
Electrophoresis 1132
ELISA 454, 736, 1248, 1263
 classification of 736
  capture 737
  competitive 737
  direct 736
  heterogeneous 740
  homogeneous 739
  immunocapture 739
  indirect 736
  interference corrected 739
  qualitative 741
  semi-quantitative 740
  streptavidin-biotin 737
 ELISA:
  practical aspects 741
 steps in 742
ELISA-based investigations 1014
ELISA-based tests 862
Elution techniques 365
Endocarditis 711
Endocardium 711
Endocrine system 452
Endotoxins 1063
Enhancement techniques 350
Entamoeba hartmanni 100
Entamoeba histolytica 102
Enterobacteriaceae 1061, 1110
Enterobius vermicularis 135
Enzyme deficiency related anaemias 242
Enzyme immunoassay (EIA) 735
Enzymes 1246
Eosin stain 1035
Epicardium 711
Epigastrium 711
Epinephrine 507
Erythrocyte indices 208
Erythrocyte sedimentation rate (ESR) 210
Erythropoiesis 217
Esbach's albuminometer 56
Escherichia coli 1141
Estimated urobilinogen 64
Estriol 511
Euglobulin lysis time 300
Examination of a blood film 219
Examination of duodenal contents 447
Examination of foetal haemoglobin 233
Excretion test 611
Extrinsic pituitary disorders 454
Eye cultures 1081

F

Faecal fat 96
Faecal occult blood 94
Faecal urobilinogen 611
Faint ghost bands 735
Fasciola hepatica 157
Fat in urine 70
Female fertility 475
Female hormone system 475, 477
Ferric chloride testing 70
Ferritin 1018, 1019
Fertility 1244
Fertility factor 2 474
Fertility reagents 1240
Fibronogn estimation 298
Fibroscreen thrombin time test for qualitative estimation of fibrinogen 296
Filarial worms 141
Flame photometer 129, 726
Flotation concentration methods 98
Flukes of man 155
Fluorescence microscopy 22
FNAC 1050
Follicle stimulating hormone 75, 570
Fontana-Masson stain 1041
Formalin produced precipitate 1033
Formed urinary sediment 82
Free thyroxine (FT4) 545
Fresh blood 388
FSH and LH pituitary hormones 479
Functional platelet disorders 305
Functions of the kidney 85
Fusibacterium fusiforme 1115

G

G and Q bandings 1196
G6PD deficiency 230
Gamma-glutamyl transpeptidase (GGTP) 690
Gas gangrene causing organisms 1085
Gastric constituents 442
 abnormal gastric constituents 443
Gastric juice examination 443
Gastric test meals 444
Genetic map of HIV 947
Genetics of ABO system 323
Geotrichum 1121
Germ cell aplasia 474
Giemsa's stain 214
Gilbert's disease 611
Globulin test 394
Glucagon 607
Glucocorticoids 464
Glutamyl transferase 690
Glycogenosis type V 711
Glycohaemoglobin 603
Glycosylated hemoglobin kit 604
Gomori's trichrome stain 179
Gonadotrophin-releasing hormone (GnRH) 488
Gram's stain 1064
Gram-negative bacilli 1110
Gram-positive bacilli 1087
Gram-positive cocci 1082
 pneumococci 1083
 staphylococci 1082
 streptococci 1082
Growth hormone 454

H

Haemagglutination 1137
Haematocrit 203
Haematology reagents 1239
Haematoxylin stain 180
Haematoxylin stains 1035
Haematuria 66
 causes 66

Haemochromatosis 1019
Haemoglobin 200
Haemoglobin estimation 1250
Haemoglobin structure and synthesis disorders 243
Haemolytic anaemias 241
Haemophilus 1114
  Haemophilus aegypticus 1115
  Haemophilus ducreyi 1115
  Haemophilus influenzae 1114
Hazardous reagents/chemicals 9
HBc Ab 888
HBc IgM 872
HBeAb 876
HBsAg 894
HBsAg confirmatory test 896
HCV IgM 906
HCV-Ab confirmatory test 909
HDL cholesterol 641
HDV Ag 916
HDV IgG 919
Heidelberger-Kendall curve 1143
Helicobacter pylori 1014
Hemolytic disease of the newborn 390
Hemorrhagic disease of newborn 307
Hemostar 318
Hemostar XF 319
Heparin therapy 269
Hepatitis A virus 862
Hepatitis B core antigen 872
Hepatitis markers 856
Hereditary elliptocytosis 242
Hereditary metabolic disorders 70
Hereditary spherocytosis 242
Herpes simplex virus (1+2) infection 939
HEV IgG 929
Hippuric acid test 614
Hiss's serum water supars 1072
HIV gene 949
HIV genome 947
HIV replication cycle 948
HIV types and variants 948
HIV virion 946
HIV virus 946
HIV-1 946
HIV-2 946
HLA-SSO/SSP typing systems 1270
Hook effect 747
  reduction of 747
Hookworms 134
Hormones and fertility 471
Hormones secreted by the pituitary gland 453
  growth hormone 453
    ACTH 453
    ADH 453
    FSH 453
    LH 453
    MSH 453
    oxytocin 453
    prolactin 453
HSV-1 939
HSV-2 939
Human chorionic gonadotrophin (hCG) 430
Human heart 701
Human intestinal pathogenic protozoans 101
Human male karyotype 1195
Hydatid disease 150
Hymenolepis diminuta 151
Hymenolepsis nana 151
Hyperbilirubinemia 633
  conjugated (direct) hyperbilirubinemia 634
  unconjugated (indirect), hyperbilirubinemia 633
Hyperbilirubinuria 63
Hypernatraemia 729
Hyperparathyroidism 468
Hyperthyroidism 495
Hypoglycaemia 608
  causes of 608
Hyponatraemia 462
Hypoparathyroidism 468
Hypopituitarism 454
Hypothalamus 463

I

ICT techniques for urine/serum sample 436
Icterus index 634
Idiopathic thrombocytopenic purpura 305
Immunoassay automation 1272
Immunochromatographic techniques 731
Immunoelectrophoresis 1131
Immunoenzymometric assay 455
Immunofluorescence 1059
  direct 1059
  indirect 1059
Immunoglobulin E 1023
Immunologic basic for skin tests 1124
Immunopathogenesis of HIV infection 950
Immunoperoxidase staining 1058
Infectious disease 1244
Infectious diseases reagents 1239
Instrumentation for turbidimetry 1150
Insulin 469, 585, 605
  functions of 469
Intermediate superficial deep mycoses 1120
  Candida albicans (Monilia) 1120
International unit 36
Intestinal flagellates 107
Intestinal protozoa of man 100
Intestinal roundworms of man 132
Intrinsic pituitary disease 454
Iron deficiency anaemia 237
Isotope 49

K

17-ketogenic steroids 72
17-ketosteroids 72
Kaolin clotting time 311
Ketone bodies in urine 62
  tests for 62
Ketonuria 62
Klebsiella ozaene 1112
Klebsiella pneumoniae 1141
Klebsiella rhinoscleromatis 1141
Klinefelter's syndrome 474, 1197
Koch's postulates 1063

L

LA reference plasma 317
Laboratory 1
  accidents in the laboratory 11
  code of conduct for medical laboratory personnel 6
  first aid in laboratory accidents 11
  hazards in the clinical laboratory 7
    biological 7
    chemical 7
    physical 7
  laboratory instruments 18
  laboratory set-up 4
    basic laboratory safety 6
    chemicals and radioactive substances 5
    electrical installations 5
    fire prevention 5
    laboratory building and space 4
    liquefied and compressed gases 5
    physical aspects of a laboratory 4
    provisions and precautions 5
    staff safety and facilities 5
    stores 5
  primary laboratory 3
  safety measures in the laboratory 7
  safety with chemicals/reagents 8
  secondary laboratory 3
  tertiary laboratory 3
Laboratory diagnosis of aplastic anaemia 249
Laboratory diagnosis of coagulation disorders 306
Laboratory diagnosis of disorders related to RBCs 237
Laboratory diagnosis of hemophilia 306
Laboratory diagnosis of leukaemias 257
Laboratory diagnosis of platelet disorders 305
Laboratory diagnosis of vascular bleeding disorders 304
Laboratory examination for parasites 179
Lactic dehydrogenase 692
Lactobacillaceae 1061
Lambert's law 618
Lange's colloidal gold test 395
Latex slide test for VDRL 762
LDH isoenzymes 694
LDL-cholesterol 644
Lead poisoning 243
Leishman's stain 214
Leishmania donavani 126
Leishmaniasis 125
  cutaneous leishmaniasis 127
Leptospira 1117
  Leptospira icterohemorrhagiae 1117
Leucopoiesis 217
Leukaemoid reactions 254
Leukoencephalopathy 951
Lipase 675

Lipid-protein double staining 1134
Liquitech quality control packages 1264
LISS phase indirect anti-human globulin test 360
Liver battery (profile) serum 615
Liver disease 713
Liver function tests 609, 614
Low ionic salt solution 375
Lowenstein Jensen medium 1075
Lupus anticoagulants 307
Lupus anticoagulants and bleeding complications 309
Lupus erythematosus cell/phenomenon 256
Luteinising hormone (LH) 75, 566
LYFECTOL 1093
Lyophilised sera for HLA typing 1271

M

MacConkey agar 1073
MacConkey's medium 1075
Magnesium 664
Malaria and its diagnosis 183
Malarial parasites of man 110
  life cycle 116
  P. falciparum 110
  P. malariae 110
  P. ovale 110
  P. vivax 110
Male fertility 471
Male hormone system 472
Malignant hyperthermia 712
Marantic endocarditis 712
MARS 714
Master gland 452
Matrix effects 746
Mayer's haematoxylin 1035
Mayer's mucicarmine stain 1043
Media for growth of anaerobes 1075
Medical diagnostic laboratory solutions 1237
Medico-legal aspects of clinical practice 17
Medium for *Mycobacterium tuberculosis* isolation 1102
Megaloblastic macrocytic anaemias 238
Menstrual cycle 478
Menstrual history 476
Mercury precipitate 1033
Metabolities 1247
Metals and lons 1248
Methods for detecting antinuclear antibodies 811
Metyrapone 526
Microalbuminuria 57, 58
  diagnostic relevance 58
  test for detection 58
Micrococcaceae 1061
Microkrom microscopy stains 1250
Microscope 20
Microtatobiotes 1062
Microxpress INSTAPREP 1073
Mixed connective tissue disease 808
Moraxela lacunate 1115
Motility of bacteria 1069
Mucin clot test 398
Mucor 1121
Mucoviscidosis 451
Mueller Hinton agar 1074
Multiple myeloma 261
Muscular dystrophy 712
Myasthenia gravis 712
Mycobacteria 1088
Mycobacteriaceae 1061
Mycobacteriology reagents 1243
Mycobacterium tuberculosis 1065
Myelosclerosis 262
Myocardial infarction 700
  clinical presentation 701
  diagnosis 701
Myocardial infarction 700
  clinical presentation 701
  diagnosis of MI 701
Myocarditis 712
Myocardium 712
Myocytes 712
Myoglobin 710
Myositis 712
Myotonia congenita 712

N

Naturally occurring antibodies 322
Neisseria 1083
Neisseriaceae 1061
Neubauer's chamber 204
Neurohypophysis 461
Nitrobacteriaceae 1061
Nocardia 1119
Nonpathogenic intestinal amoebae 109
Normal and abnormal control plasmas for coagulation assays 295
Normal saliva 442
Normal values of hCG 419
Novachrom 1065, 1095
Nutrient agar 1072, 1073

O

Ocular myositis 712
Oestrogen 470, 479
Oestrogen fractions 76
Oil red O fat stain 1042
Oral anticoagulant therapy 283
Origin of HIV 946
Ovarian failure 479
Ovary 470
Ovulation 474

P

Pancreas 468
Pancreatic function tests 449
Pancytopenia 250
Papain 361
Papanicolaou's staining 1055
Paracolon bacilli 1112
Paraproteinaemias 261
Parasitism 100
Parathyroid 468, 501
Parkinson's disease 712
Paroxysmal nocturnal hemoglobinuria 243
Partial pressure of carbon dioxide 719
PAS reaction 1056
PAS technique 1056
Pasturella pestis 1114
Pasturella tularensis 1114
Pathogenesis of malaria 117
Pathology of malaria 118
PEG-enhanced indirect anti-human globulin test 360
Penicillium 1121
Pericardial fluid (PF) 402
Pericardial fluid aspiration 402
Pericarditis 712
Periodic acid-Schiff (PAS) reaction 1042
Periodic table elements 47
Peritoneal fluid 403
Peroxidase stain 1058
Phenol red test 87
Phenolsulphonphthalein (PSP) 87
Phlebotomy 269
Phosphatases 675
Phosphorus 654
Photometry 620
Picric acid 1033
Pilocarpine 451
Pineal gland 471
Pipetting scheme 998
Pituitary gland 452
Pituitary hormone coated tube assay 1255
Pituitary hormone microwell ELISA 1255
Plasmid nematodes 134
Platelets 206
Platelets, coagulation and bleeding disorders 264
Pleural fluid 399
Polycythemia 202
Polycythaemia vera 262
Polymerase chain reaction 752
  types of PCR 754
    differential 754
    multiplex 754
    nested 754
Polymyositis 712, 809
    real-time 754
    RT 754
Polyploidy 1197
Porphyrins 65
  causes 65
  clinical relevance 66
  normal values 65
Posterior pituitary 461
Potassium 74
Pouched media 1243
Practical application of immunoelectrophoresis 1134
Pre-dropped HLA typing sera 1269
Precipitin 1137
Pregnancy test 418, 430, 477
  bioassays 418
  device ICT pregnancy test 435
  dipstick ICT pregnancy test 433

ELISA pregnancy test 424
immunologic methods 419
slide test for pregnancy 420
Pregnanediol 75
Pregnanetriol 76
Preparation of culture media 1071
Preparation of tissues 1030
Principle of the EIA test 939
Problems associated with male infertility 471
Processing of tissues 1031
Progesterone 478, 518
17αOH progesterone 520
Prolactin hormone (PRL) 575
Prostate-specific antigen 1009
Prostatic acid phosphates (PAP), blood 1014
Proteinuria 57
glomerular 57
postglomerular 57
tubular 57
Proteus vulgaris 1110
Prothrombin 613
Prothrombin determination 290
Prothrombin time 276
Protophyta 1061
Protozoal diseases of man 101
Pseudomonadaceae 1061
Pseudomonas aeruginosa 1115
PTAH 1038

Q

Quantia range 1241
Quantiamate analyser 1163
Quantitative determintion of plasma proteins 1134

R

Radioimmunoassay (RIA) 754
Rapid diagnostics in electrolyte analysis 729
Rapid plasma reagin (RPR) card test 764
RBC morphology 223
RBC pipette 206
RBCs 205
Reagent for 96-well microplate 455, 537, 562
Reagents for routine screening 1241
Reagents for special applications 1242
Red cell fragility test 227
Red cell preserving solution 335
Refractometer 53
Regurgitation 712
Relative centrifugal force 23
Renal function tests 89
Renal physiology 85
Reporting laboratory tests 27
Requirements for laboratory set up 1054
Reticulocyte count 223
Retrocheck HIV 965
Rh 322
Rh antibodies 339
Rh blood group system 338
Rh(D) grouping procedures 339
Rhabdomyolysis 713
Rheumatology reagents 1240
Rickettsiales 1062
Ring test 1129
RNA 946
Robertson's cooked meat medium 1075
Ropes' test 398
Rotary microtome 1032
Rubella infection 938

S

Sabouraud dextrose agar 1073
Sahli's haemoglobinometer 200
Salmonella typhi 1112
Schiff (PAS) reaction 259
Schistosoma haematobium 84
Schizomycetes 1061
Schlesinger's test 64
Scleroderma 805
causes 805
diagnosis 806
symptoms 806
treatment 806
Screening tests for diagnosis of procoagulant deficiency 303
Sedimentation concentration methods 98
Semen analysis 408
Sensitive thromboplastin reagent 278
Sequential ELISA method 556
Serotonin (5-hydroxytryptamine) 68
Serum albumin 636
Serum cholesterol 638
Serum creatinine 629
Serum iron and TIBC 659
Serum parathyroid hormone 503
Serum proteins 612, 1153
Serum triglycerides 646
Serum-bilirubin 632
SGOT 684
SGOT (AST) 685
SGPT (ALT) 686, 688
Shape of bacteria 1062
bacilli 1062
cocci 1062
Shigella flexneri 1113
Shigella shigae 1113
SI units 35
SIADH 462
Sicklevue solubility test 246
Single channel standard micropipette 1266
Sjögren's syndrome 807
symptoms 807
treatment 808
Skeletal muscle disease 703
Smearing techniques 1053
Sodium 74
Solution strength 45
molar solutions 45
normal solutions 45
part dilutions 45
per cent solutions 45
saturated solution 46
standard solution 46
Special stains 1035
stains for bacteria, fungi and inclusion bodies 1037
stains for carbohydrates and mucoproteins 1037
stains for connective tissue 1035
stains for cytoplasmic granules 1036
Special urine tests 67
Specific hormonal problems 472
congenital adrenal hyperplasia 472
delayed puberty 473
fertile eunuch 474
hyperprolactinaemia 472
hypogonadotrophic hypopituitarism 473
hypothyroidism 472
Kallmann's syndrome 473
panhypopituitarism 473
Spectrophotometer 555, 617, 1185
Spectrophotometry 1139
Sperm counts 409
Sperm morphology 409
Spermatozoa 410
Spinal muscular atrophy 713
Spirillaceae 1061
Spirillum minus 1118
Spirochaetales 1061
Spontaneous abortions 432
Sputum examination 412
Staining reactions 1064
Staining techniques 1038
Status asthmaticus 713
Sterilisation 29
methods commonly used for 29
chemical sterilisation 32
cold 31
dry heat 29
filtration 31
Ionising radiations 31
moist heat 30
sterilisation by heat 29
ultraviolet radiation 31
Steroid hormone microwell ELISA 1256
Stool analysis 91
Stool concentration methods 98
Stool examination 90, 179
inspection of faeces 91
microscopic examination 97
odour and pH 92
specimen collection 90
tests for occult blood 93
Streptococcus 794
Sugars in urine 61
Sulfate 515
Sulkowitch test 67
Susceptibility testing of Mycobacterium tuberculosis 1104
Sweat testing 451
Synovial fluid (SF) 398
Systemic lupus erythematosus 804

T

Tachycardia 713
Taenia saginata 147
Taenia solium 147
Tapeworm diseases of man 146
Tapeworms of man 145
Technique of skin tests 1123
 intracutaneous injection 1123
 patch tests 1123
 transcutaneous administration 1123
Terrain 1019
Test for anti-deoxyribonucleoprotein 799
Test for anti-streptolysin O 794
Test for C-reactive protein 792
Test for HBsAG virucheck® 858
Test for IgM and IgG antibodies 780
Test for IgM antibodies to *Leptospira* 784
Test for infectious mononucleosis 782
Test for malaria 787
Test for malaria PAN/PV/PF 790
Test for *P. falciparum* malaria 786
Test for rheumatoid factors 796
Test for syphilis 756, 766
Testes 469
Testicular enzyme defects 474
Testicular failure 474
Testosterone 469, 510
Tests for chronic pancreatitis 451
Tests for glucose 60
Tests for sickling 234
Tests for thyroid function 491
Tetany 713
Thalassaemias 248
 α thalassaemia 248
 β thalassaemia 248
Thallophyta 1062
Therapeutic drug monitoring 1232
Thioglycollate medium 1075
Thoracentesis 400
Thrombocytopenia 207
Thrombocytosis 207
Thrombogenesis 713
Thromboplastin reagent for prothrombin time determination 280
Thrombopoiesis 218
Thyroglobulin antibodies 555
Thyroid coated tube assay 1254
Thyroid function 467
Thyroid function tests 490
Thyroid gland 465
Thyroid hormone 479
Thyroid microwell ELISA 1253
Thyroid peroxidase antibodies 561
Thyrotropin (TSH) 550
Thyroxine-binding globulin (TBG) test 465
Tissue thromboplastin inhibition test 311
Toluidine red unheated serum test 760
Torch combination ELISA 1259
Torch infections 936
Torch panel microwell ELISA 1258
Torch screen IgG EIA kit 942
Torsion 474
Total carbon dioxide 722
Total protein 635
Total thyroxine (T4) 540
Total triiodothyronine (T3) 526
Toxic/poisoning symptoms and treatment 77
Toxogen latex reagent 936
Toxoplasma gondii 936
Toxoplasma infection 938
Toxoplasmosis 936
Trace elements 661
Transaminases 683
Transcription 949
Transfusion reaction 389
Translation 949
Transplantation diagnostics 1269
Treponema 1116
 calligyrum 1117
 curateum 1117
 microdentum 1117
 pallidum 1116
 pertenue 1117
Treponemataceae 1061
Triage 713
Trichinella spiralis 182
Trichomonas 410
Trichomonas vaginalis 84
Trituras 1272
Trypanosomiasis 128
 African trypanosomiasis 129
 South American type 130
Tuberculosis 967
Tubidimetry 1137
Tumour marker microwell ELISA 1256
Tumour markers 977
Tumour markers coated tube assay 1257
Turbidimetric immunoassays 1143
Turbidimetry vs nephelometry 1143
Turner syndrome 1197
Types of red blood cells 223

U

Ultrasound-guided fine-needle aspiration cytology 1051
Unconjugated bilirubin 609
Urea 625
Uric acid 70, 649
Urinary microscopy constituents 79
 bacteria, fungus and parasites 83
 casts in urine 84
 epithelial cells and epithelial cell casts 80
 granular casts 81
 hyaline casts 80
 oval fat bodies and fatty casts 81
 parasites and parasitic ova 84
 red cells and red cell casts 79
 waxy cysts 81
 white cells and white cell casts 80
Urinary sediment 78
Urine 50
 cells and casts 51
 chemical examination of urine 55
  tests for protein 55
 collection of urine 51
 examination of urine 51
  colour and appearance 51
  odour 53
  reaction 52
  specific gravity 53
  turbidity 54
  urinary volume 54
 physicochemical characteristics of urine 50
 preservation of specimen 51
 urine composition 50
Urinometer 53
Urobilin 64
Urobilinogen (quantitative) 64

V

Vaccines for HIV infection 962
van Gieson's stain 1039
Vanillylmandelic acid (VMA) 71
Varicocoele 474
VDRL reagent 758
VDRL test 756
 conventional test 756
Veilonella 1084
Venereal Disease Research Laboratory 838
Verhoff's elastic stain 1040
Vibrio cholerae 1115
Viral myositis 713
Viral protease 949
Virales 1062
von Kossa's method for demonstrating calcium 1044

W

Water excretion test 524
Ways of obtaining blood 196
 capillary or peripheral blood 196
 venous blood (venipuncture) 196
WBC pipette 204
Weighing scales 23
Weil's disease 1117
Western blot (WB) 959
White blood cells 255
White cell values 251
Whole blood 388
Wilder's reticulin stain 1040
Wright's stain 214
Wuchereria bancrofti 142

Z

Zenker's fluid 1030
Ziehl-Neelsen stain 1045
Zinc (colorimetric method) 661
Zinc sulphate concentration method 98